*Amar* **W9-AXS-788**

**Interactions are written out**

### Drug classifications
Barbiturates, CNS depressants, CYP3A4 inhibitors, selective serotonin reuptake inhibitors: increased toxicity

CNS depressants: increased CNS depression

CYP3A4 inducers (barbiturates): decreased diazepam effect

Oral contraceptives: decreased metabolism of diazepam

### Drug/herb
Cowslip, goldenseal, kava, melatonin, mistletoe, pokeweed, poppy, Queen Anne's lace, valerian: increased diazepam effect

Cola tree, St. John's wort: decreased diazepam effect

### Drug/lab test
Increased: AST/ALT, serum bilirubin

Decreased: radioactive iodine uptake

False increase: 17-OHCS

## NURSING CONSIDERATIONS
### Assessment
• Assess degree of anxiety; what precipitates anxiety and whether product controls symptoms; other signs of anxiety: dilated pupils, inability to sleep, restlessness, inability to focus

• Assess for alcohol withdrawal symptoms, including hallucinations (visual, auditory), delirium, irritability, agitation, fine to coarse tremors

• Monitor B/P (with patient lying, standing), pulse, respiratory rate; if systolic B/P drops 20 mm Hg, hold product, notify prescriber; monitor respirations q5-15 min if given **IV**

• Monitor blood studies: CBC during long-term therapy; blood dyscrasias have occurred (rarely); hepatic studies: ALT, AST

• Monitor for seizure control; type, duration, and intensity of seizures; what precipitates seizures

• Monitor hepatic studies: AST, ALT, bilirubin, creatinine, LDH, alkaline phosphatase

• Assess mental status: mood, sensorium, affect, sleeping pattern, drowsiness, dizziness, suicidal tendencies, and ability of product to control these symptoms; check for tolerance, withdrawal symptoms: headache, nausea, vomiting, muscle pain, weakness after long-term use

• Assess for muscle spasms, pain relief

### Nursing diagnoses
• Anxiety (uses)
• Coping, ineffective (uses)
• Injury, risk for (uses, adverse reactions)
• Knowledge, deficient (teaching)
• Noncompliance (teaching)

**Appropriate nursing diagnoses presented for every drug**

### Implementation

...or GI symptoms
...able to swallow

...candy, frequent sips

• Reduce opioid dosage by one third if given concomitantly with diazepam

• Check to see PO medication has b...lowed

**Detailed IV information**

• Concentrate: use calibrated dropp... with water, juice, pudding, applesauc... immediately

**Rectal route**
• Do not use more than 5×/mo or for an episode q5 days

**IV route**
• Administer **IV** into large vein; do not dilute or mix with any other product; give **IV** 5 mg or less/1 min or total dose over 3 min... (children, infants); CONT INF is n... recommended; inject closest vein... possible; do not dilute or mix wit...

• Check **IV** site for thrombosis o... which may occur rapidly

**Sterile emulsion for injection rout...**
• Use **IV** only, within 6 hr, flush line after use and after 6 hr

**Syringe and IV compatibility entries included**

*Syringe compatibilities:* Cimetidine...

*Syringe incompatibilities:* Benzquina-mide, doxapram, glycopyrrolate, heparin, nalbu-phine

*Y-site compatibilities:* Cefmetazole, DOBUTamine, nafcillin, quinidine, sufentanil

*Y-site incompatibilities:* Hydromor-phone, fluconazole, foscarnet, heparin, pancuro-nium, potassium chloride, vecuronium, vit B with C

*Additive compatibilities:* Netilmicin, verapamil

### Patient/family education
• Advise patient that product may be taken with food; that product is not to be used for everyday stress or used longer than 4 mo unless directed by prescriber; take no more than prescribed amount; may be habit forming

• Caution patient to avoid OTC preparations unless approved by a prescriber; to avoid alcohol, other psychotropic medications unless prescribed; that smoking may decrease diazepam effect by increasing diazepam metabolism; not to discontinue medication abruptly after long-term use, gradually taper

• Inform patient to avoid driving, activities that require alertness; drowsiness may occur; slowly or fainting may occur, especially in ...ric

• Advise patient not to become pregnant using this product

• Inform patient that drowsiness may worsen at beginning of treatment

**Positive results of medication use**

### Evaluation
**Positive therapeutic outcome**
• Decreased anxiety, restlessness, insomnia

**Treatment of overdose:** Lavage, VS, supportive care, flumazenil

❶ Alert    ✦ Canada Only    ⊙ Drug on CD

\* "Tall Man" lettering (See Preface)

# Mosby's Drug Guide for Nurses, Eighth Edition, Companion CD-ROM

Use *Mosby's Drug Guide for Nurses, Eighth Edition, Companion CD-ROM* to find drug information fast! This five-in-one CD-ROM provides you with NCLEX® examination review questions for 63 key drugs, patient teaching guides, a calculation tutorial, a drug card creator, and calculators.

This Companion CD-ROM includes:

- **NCLEX® Examination Review Questions for 63 Key Drugs**
  Includes complete, printable information for the 63 key drugs in the book, matched with 315 NCLEX® examination review questions.

- **Patient Teaching Guides**
  Contains English and Spanish patient teaching guides for the 63 key drugs.

- **Calculation Tutorial**
  Provides calculations and conversions paired with practice problems and answers.

- **Drug Card Creator**
  Features a blank drug card template that is fully customizable and printable.

- **Calculators**
  Contains 30 handy clinical calculators, including several IV and PO dosage calculators, and an IV dose rate calculator.

**Contact Us**
For further information, visit us at http://us.elsevierhealth.com or call us at (800) 545-2522.

**Mini CD-ROM**
This mini CD-ROM will work in your CD-ROM drive. Place it on the inner ring of the tray, as shown, and follow the on-screen installation instructions.

> This mini-CD does not work in:
>     Floppy Drives
>     Slot Drives
>     Zip Drives
>     Stereos
> Insert this mini-CD into your CD-ROM drive as shown at left.

**Important**
No credit or refund will be issued on this book if the CD envelope has been opened, torn, or otherwise tampered with.

**Companion CD-ROM** for *Mosby's Drug Guide for Nurses,* Eighth Edition

## MINIMUM SYSTEM REQUIREMENTS AND SOFTWARE REQUIREMENTS FOR THIS COMPANION CD-ROM:

To use this electronic resource, your computer should meet the following minimum requirements:

This CD will run on both PC and Mac.

**Windows® XP or higher**
Pentium® II 400 MHz or faster processor
At least 64 MB RAM recommended
10 MB free hard disk space
48× or faster CD-ROM drive
800 × 600 monitor with True Color

**Macintosh®**
OS X or greater
Power Macintosh
At least 64 MB RAM recommended
1 GHz+ PowerPC G4
10 MB free hard disk space
48× or faster CD-ROM drive
800 × 600 monitor with millions of colors

## HOW TO RUN THE PROGRAM

**Windows®**
1. Start Microsoft Windows and insert the CD-ROM. The program should run automatically.
2. To manually run the program, double click on your CD-ROM drive. Double click on "Skidmore.exe" to start with the CD-ROM still in the drive.

**Macintosh®**
1. Insert the CD-ROM into the drive.
2. Double click on the CD-ROM icon on your desktop and double click on the file called "Skidmore.osx" (Flash file) to start the program.

## TECHNICAL SUPPORT

Technical support for this product is available between 7:30 AM and 7 PM CST, Monday through Friday. Before calling, be sure that your computer meets the minimum system requirements to run this software. Inside the United States and Canada, call 1-800-692-9010. Outside North America, call 314-872-8370. You may also fax your questions to 314-523-4932, or contact Technical Support through e-mail: technical.support@elsevier.com.

Copyright © 2009 Mosby, Inc., an affiliate of Elsevier Inc.

Pentium, Macintosh, and Windows are registered trademarks.

9996060837

# Mosby's
# Drug Guide
## for Nurses

# Mosby's Drug Guide for Nurses

## EIGHTH EDITION

**Linda Skidmore-Roth, RN, MSN, NP**
**Consultant**
Littleton, Colorado

**Formerly, Nursing Faculty**
New Mexico State University
Las Cruces, New Mexico
El Paso Community College
El Paso, Texas

MOSBY

ELSEVIER

# MOSBY
## ELSEVIER

11830 Westline Industrial Drive
St. Louis, Missouri 63146

MOSBY'S DRUG GUIDE FOR NURSES, EIGHTH EDITION                    ISBN: 978-0-323-06939-7

---

## NOTICE

---

ISBN: 978-0-323-06939-7
Library of Congress Control Number 2008921867

*Executive Publisher:* Darlene Como
*Editor:* Tamara Myers
*Senior Developmental Editor:* Laura M. Selkirk
*Publishing Services Manager:* Melissa Lastarria
*Project Manager:* Mary Pohlman
*Designer:* Maggie Reid

Printed in the United States of America

Last digit is the print number:   9   8   7   6   5   4   3   2   1

# Consultants

**Dana Bartlett, RN, BSN, MSN, MA**
Poison Information Specialist
Children's Hospital of Philadelphia
Philadelphia, Pennsylvania

**Timothy L. Brenner, PharmD**
Hematology/Oncology Clinical Pharmacy
  Specialist
UPMC Cancer Centers
Pittsburgh, Pennsylvania

**Amanda Gross, RPh**
Pharmacist
University of Colorado Hospital
Denver, Colorado

**Dana H. Hamamura, PharmD**
Clinical Pharmacist
University of Colorado Hospital
Denver, Colorado

**Dottie Mathers, RN, MSN**
Associate Professor, Nursing
Pennsylvania College of Technology
Williamsport, Pennsylvania

**Sandra S. Meeker, RN, MSN**
Nursing Professor
Central Texas College
Killeen, Texas

**Amy E. Miller, PharmD, BCPS**
Assistant Professor of Clinical Pharmacy
Philadelphia College of Pharmacy
University of the Sciences in Philadelphia
Philadelphia, Pennsylvania

**Joshua J. Neumiller, PharmD**
Geriatrics Fellow/Clinical Research Associate
Washington State University
Spokane, Washington

**Brenda Pavill, RN, FNP, PhD**
Professor, Nursing
Misericordia University
Dallas, Pennsylvania

**Sarah Reidunn Pool, RN, MS**
Nursing Education Specialist
Mayo Clinic
Rochester, Minnesota

**Randolph E. Regal, BS, PharmD, RPh**
Clinical Assistant Professor
College of Pharmacy
University of Michigan Hospital
Ann Arbor, Michigan

**Stephen M. Setter, PharmD, CDE, CGP, DVM**
Associate Professor
Elder Services/Visiting Nurses Association
Washington State University
Spokane, Washington

**Travis E. Sonnett, PharmD**
Geriatric Fellow
College of Pharmacy
Washington State University
Spokane, Washington

**Sharon Souter, RN, PhD**
Director of the BSN Program
Patty Hanks Shelton School of Nursing
A Consortium of Abilene Christian University,
  Hardin Simmons University, and McMurry
  University
Abilene, Texas

**Patricia R. Teasley, MSN, RN, APRN, BC**
Professor, Nursing Department
Central Texas College
Killeen, Texas

**Cheryle I. Whitney, RN, MSN**
President
ciwhitney & associates, LLC
The Woodlands, Texas

# Preface

*Mosby's Drug Guide for Nurses,* eighth edition, is the most in-depth handbook available for nursing students! Since its first publication in 1996, more than 100 U.S. and Canadian pharmacists and consultants have reviewed the book's content closely. Today, *Mosby's Drug Guide for Nurses* is more up-to-date than ever—with features that make it easy to find critical information fast!

## NEW FEATURES
- There are 19 recent FDA-approved drugs located throughout the book and in Appendix A (see Contents for a complete list). Included are monographs for:
  - lapatinib (Tykerb), a new antineoplastic
  - lisdexamfetamine (Vyvanse), for treatment of ADHD
  - maraviroc (Selzentry), a new class of antivirals (fusion inhibitor)
  - raltegravir (Isentress), a new antiretroviral
  - rotigotine (Neupro), a new agent for Parkinson's disease
- There are 23 clinical drugs, including lubiprostone and varenicline, that have been added to the book.
- There are 50 drug categories, including 11 new entries.
- The latest NANDA nursing diagnoses are included.
- A mini CD-ROM is included that features over 300 NCLEX® examination review questions, patient teaching guides, and drug information for the 63 key drugs that students will encounter most in clinicals. A comprehensive calculation tutorial, a drug card creator, and dosage calculators are also on the CD.

## NEW FACTS
This edition features thousands of new drug facts, including:
- New drugs and new dosage information
- Newly researched adverse effects
- The latest precautions, interactions, and contraindications
- IV therapy updates
- Revised nursing considerations
- Updated patient/family education guidelines
- Updates on key new drug research

## ORGANIZATION
This handbook is organized into four main sections:
- A four-color insert of drug mechanisms and drug administration
- Individual drug monographs (in alphabetical order by generic name)
- Drug Categories
- Appendixes

The guiding principle behind this book is to provide fast, easy access to drug information and nursing considerations. Every detail—from the cover, binding, and paper to the typeface, two-color design, and appendixes—has been carefully chosen with the user in mind.

Here's what you'll find in each section of the handbook:

**Color Insert**

**Mechanisms-of-Action and Sites-of-Action Illustrations**

These 16 detailed, full-color illustrations are added to help enhance the understanding of the mechanism or site of action for the following drugs and drug classes:

- ACE inhibitors
- Adrenocortical steroids
- Anticholinergic bronchodilators
- Antidepressants
- Antidiabetic agents
- Antifungal agents
- Antiinfective agents
- Antiretroviral agents
- Benzodiazepines
- Diuretics
- Drugs used to treat GERD
- Laxatives
- Narcotic agonist-antagonist analgesics
- Narcotic analgesics
- Phenytoin
- Sympatholytics

**Photo Atlas of Drug Administration**

This practical resource for students and practitioners lists standard precautions and provides 30 full-color illustrations depicting the physical landmarks and administration techniques used for **IV**, IM, SUBCUT, and ID drug delivery.

Also included in the color insert are standard precautions and the 2008 Recommended Childhood and Adolescent Immunization Schedule for the United States.

**Individual Drug Monographs**

This book includes monographs for more than 4000 generic and trade medications—those most commonly administered by students. Common trade names are given for all drugs regularly used in the United States and Canada, with drugs available only in Canada identified by a maple leaf icon (✤).

Each monograph provides the following information, whenever possible, for safe, effective administration of each drug:

**High-alert status:** Identifies drugs with the most potential to cause harm to patients if administered incorrectly.

**"Tall Man" lettering:** Uses the capitalization of distinguishing letters to avoid medication errors and is required by the FDA for drug manufacturers.

**Key drug status:** Identifies drugs of special prominence within their functional class that are often encountered by students during clinicals. These drugs are denoted with a special CD icon (🔹) to direct the user to additional materials on the CD.

**Pronunciation:** Helps the nurse master complex generic names.

**Rx, OTC:** Identifies prescription or over-the-counter drugs.

**Functional and chemical classifications:** Helps the nurse recognize similarities and differences among drugs in the same functional but different chemical classes.

**Pregnancy category:** FDA pregnancy categories **A, B, C, D,** or **X** are noted at the beginning of each monograph, as well as under Precautions or Contraindications depending on FDA category. Appendix I provides a detailed explanation of each category.

**Controlled substance schedule:** Includes schedules for the United States and Canada.

**Do not confuse:** Presents drug names that might easily be confused within each appropriate monograph.

**Action:** Describes pharmacologic properties concisely.

**Therapeutic outcome:** Details all possible results of medication use.

**Uses:** Lists the conditions the drug is used to treat.

**Unlabeled uses:** Describes drug uses that may be encountered in practice but are not yet FDA approved.

**Dosages and routes:** Lists all available and approved dosages and routes for adult, pediatric, and geriatric patients.

**Available forms:** Includes tablets, capsules, extended release, injectables (**IV**, IM, SUBCUT), solutions, creams, ointments, lotions, gels, shampoos, elixirs, suspensions, suppositories, sprays, aerosols, and lozenges.

**Adverse effects:** Groups these reactions by alphabetical body system, with common side effects *italicized* and life-threatening reactions in **bold type** for emphasis.

**Contraindications:** Lists conditions under which the drug absolutely should not be given, including FDA pregnancy safety categories **D** or **X.**

**Precautions:** Lists conditions that require special consideration when the drug is prescribed, including FDA pregnancy safety categories **A, B,** and **C.**

**Pharmacokinetics/pharmacodynamics:** Features a quick-reference chart of concise facts of pharmacokinetics (absorption, distribution, metabolism, excretion, half-life) and pharmacodynamics (onset, peak, duration).

**Interactions:** Lists confirmed drug, food, herb, and lab test interactions.

**Nursing considerations:** Identifies key nursing considerations for each step of the nursing process: Assessment, Nursing Diagnoses, Implementation, Patient/Family Education, and Evaluation, including positive therapeutic outcomes. Instructions for giving drugs by various routes (e.g., **IV**, PO, IM, SUBCUT, topically, rectally) appear under Implementation, with route subheadings in bold.

**Compatibilities:** Lists syringe, Y-site, and additive compatibilities and incompatibilities. If no compatibilities are listed for a drug, the necessary compatibility testing has not been done and that compatibility information is unknown. To ensure safety, assume that the drug may not be mixed with other drugs unless specifically stated.

**Nursing Alert icon ◆:** Highlights situations in which the patient could potentially be at risk.

**Treatment of overdose:** Lists drugs and treatments for overdoses where appropriate.

### Drug Categories

The Drug Categories section, following the individual drug monographs, provides general information about the various functional classes to promote learning about the similarities and differences among drugs in the same functional class. It summarizes action, uses, adverse effects, contraindications, precautions, pharmacokinetics, interactions, and nursing considerations for each functional class.

### Appendixes

**Selected new drugs:** Includes comprehensive information on 19 key drugs approved by the FDA during the last 12 months.

**Controlled substance chart:** Covers the drug schedules for the United States, with examples.

**Rarely used drugs:** Provides concise monographs for 78 infrequently used drugs, including dosage and routes, uses, and contraindications.

**Ophthalmic, nasal, topical, and otic products:** Provides essential information for 140 ophthalmic, nasal, topical, and otic products commonly used today, grouped by chemical drug class.

**Vaccines and toxoids:** Features an easy-to-use table with generic and trade names, uses, dosages and routes, and contraindications for 39 key vaccines and toxoids.

**Herbal products:** Features basic usage information for more than 47 common herbs and natural supplements.

**Combination products:** Provides details on the forms and uses of more than 600 combination products.

**High-alert drugs:** Lists the 97 drugs in *Mosby's Drug Guide for Nurses* that are considered high alert because of their potential to cause significant harm to patients.

**Abbreviations and pregnancy categories:** Lists abbreviations alphabetically with their meanings and explains the five FDA pregnancy categories.

The following sources were consulted in the preparation of this edition:

Blumenthal M: *The Complete German Commission E Monographs: Therapeutic Guide to Herbal Medicines,* Austin, 1998, American Botanical Council.

Brunton L, Lazo J, Parker K: *Goodman and Gilman's The Pharmacological Basis of Therapeutics,* ed 11, New York, 2005, McGraw-Hill.

*Clinical Pharmacology* [database online], Tampa, 2007, Gold Standard, Inc. http://www.clinicalpharmacology.com. Updated December 2007.

Gahart BL: *Intravenous Medications,* ed 24, St. Louis, 2008, Mosby.

McKenry LM, Tessier E, Hogan MA: *Mosby's Pharmacology in Nursing,* ed 22, St. Louis, 2006, Mosby.

## Acknowledgments

I am indebted to the nursing and pharmacology consultants who reviewed the manuscript and pages and thank them for their criticism and encouragement. I would also like to thank Darlene Como, Tamara Myers, and Laura Selkirk, my editors, whose active encouragement and enthusiasm have made this book better than it might otherwise have been. I am likewise grateful to Mary Pohlman and Graphic World Inc. for the coordination of the production process and assistance with the development of the new edition.

**Linda Skidmore-Roth**

# Contents

## COLOR INSERT

# Recommended Childhood and Adolescent Immunization Schedule—United States, 2008

## Immunization Schedule for Persons Aged 0-6 Years

| Vaccine ▼    Age ▶ | Birth | 1 month | 2 months | 4 months | 6 months | 12 months | 15 months | 18 months | 19-23 months | 2-3 years | 4-6 years |
|---|---|---|---|---|---|---|---|---|---|---|---|
| Hepatitis B* | HepB | HepB | | | HepB | | | | | | |
| Rotavirus* | | | Rota | Rota | Rota | | | | | | |
| Diphtheria, Tetanus, Pertussis* | | | DTaP | DTaP | DTaP | | DTaP | | | | DTaP |
| Haemophilus Influenzae Type b* | | | Hib | Hib | Hib* | Hib | | | | | |
| Pneumococcal* | | | PCV | PCV | PCV | PCV | | | | PPV | |
| Inactivated Poliovirus | | | IPV | IPV | IPV | | | | | | IPV |
| Influenza* | | | | | Influenza (Yearly) | | | | | | |
| Measles, Mumps, Rubella* | | | | | | MMR | | | | | MMR |
| Varicella* | | | | | | Varicella | | | | | Varicella |
| Hepatitis A* | | | | | | HepA (2 doses) | | | | HepA Series | |
| Meningococcal* | | | | | | | | | | MCV4 | |

**Legend:**
Range of recommended ages
Certain high-risk groups

This schedule indicates the recommended ages for routine administration of currently licensed childhood vaccines, as of December 1, 2007, for children aged 0-6 years. Any dose not administered at the recommended age should be administered at any subsequent visit, when indicated and feasible. Additional vaccines may be licensed and recommended during the year. Licensed combination vaccines may be used whenever any components of the combination are indicated and other components of the vaccine are not contraindicated and if approved by the Food and Drug Administration for that dose of the series. **Providers should consult the respective Advisory Committee on Immunization Practices statement for detailed recommendations, including for high-risk conditions: http://www.cdc.gov/vaccines/pubs/ACIP-list.htm.** Clinically significant adverse events that follow immunization should be reported to the Vaccine Adverse Event Reporting System (VAERS). Guidance about how to obtain and complete a VAERS form is available at http://www.vaers.hhs.gov or by telephone, 800-822-7967.

*For complete information go to http://www.cdc.gov/nip/recs/child-schedule.htm#printable.

# Immunization Schedule for Persons Aged 7-18 Years

| Vaccine ▼                          Age ▶ | 7-10 years | 11-12 years | 13-18 years |
|-------------------------------------------|------------|-------------|-------------|
| Diphtheria, Tetanus, Pertussis*           | *          | Tdap        | Tdap        |
| Human Papillomavirus*                     | *          | HPV (3 doses) | HPV Series |
| Meningococcal*                            | MCV4       | MCV4        | MCV4        |
| Pneumococcal*                             |            | PPV         |             |
| Influenza*                                |            | Influenza (Yearly) |      |
| Hepatitis A*                              |            | HepA Series |             |
| Hepatitis B*                              |            | HepB Series |             |
| Inactivated Poliovirus*                   |            | IPV Series  |             |
| Measles, Mumps, Rubella*                  |            | MMR Series  |             |
| Varicella*                                |            | Varicella Series |        |

Range of recommended ages

Catch-up immunization

Certain high-risk groups

This schedule indicates the recommended ages for routine administration of currently licensed childhood vaccines, as of December 1, 2007, for children aged 7-18 years. Any dose not administered at the recommended age should be administered at any subsequent visit, when indicated and feasible. Additional vaccines may be licensed and recommended during the year. Licensed combination vaccines may be used whenever any components of the combination are indicated and other components of the vaccine are not contraindicated and if approved by the Food and Drug Administration for that dose of the series. **Providers should consult the respective Advisory Committee on Immunization Practices statement for detailed recommendations, including for high-risk conditions: http://www.cdc.gov/vaccines/pubs/ACIP-list.htm.** Clinically significant adverse events that follow immunization should be reported to the Vaccine Adverse Event Reporting System (VAERS). Guidance about how to obtain and complete a VAERS form is available at http://www.vaers.hhs.gov or by telephone, 800-822-7967.

*For complete information go to http://www.cdc.gov/nip/recs/child-schedule.htm#printable.

**STANDARD PRECAUTIONS**

The following precautions are used in the care of all patients regardless of their diagnosis or disease. They are also applied when handling or cleaning equipment or supplies that are potentially contaminated.

1. Wear gloves any time that you may contact blood, any moist body fluid (except sweat), secretions, excretions, nonintact skin, or mucous membranes.

2. Remove your gloves, wash your hands, and reapply clean gloves if your gloves become soiled with infective material.

3. Even if you are wearing gloves, remove them, wash your hands, and apply clean gloves *immediately before* contact with mucous membranes or nonintact skin.

4. Wear a protective cover gown of waterproof material if your clothing is likely to have substantial contact with infective material or if splashing of body fluids is likely.

5. Wear a face shield or goggles to protect your eyes if splashing of secretions is likely.

6. Any time a face shield or goggles is worn, wear a surgical mask to protect the mucous membranes of your nose and mouth. A surgical mask may be worn during certain sterile procedures without protective eyewear. However, protective eyewear is *never* worn without a surgical mask.

7. Handle needles, razors, broken glass, and other sharp objects with care. Needles should never be recapped. All sharps should be disposed of in a puncture-resistant sharps container.

8. Wash your hands before and after each patient contact.

9. Wash your hands before you apply and after you remove gloves. Do not assume that hand washing is unnecessary because gloves were worn. Do not wash your hands with gloves on them.

10. Gloves are used for the care of one patient only, then discarded.

11. Follow your facility policy for disposal of gloves and other contaminated items. These items are generally not disposed of in open trash containers. Facilities have designated disposal sites for these biohazardous waste materials.

12. Use resuscitation barrier devices as an alternative to mouth-to-mouth resuscitation.

13. Linen should be handled in a manner that prevents contamination of the outside of the container. Linen from isolation rooms was previously double bagged. Double bagging is no longer recommended since all linen is handled as potentially infectious. Double bag linen only if the outside of the bag becomes contaminated during the bagging process.

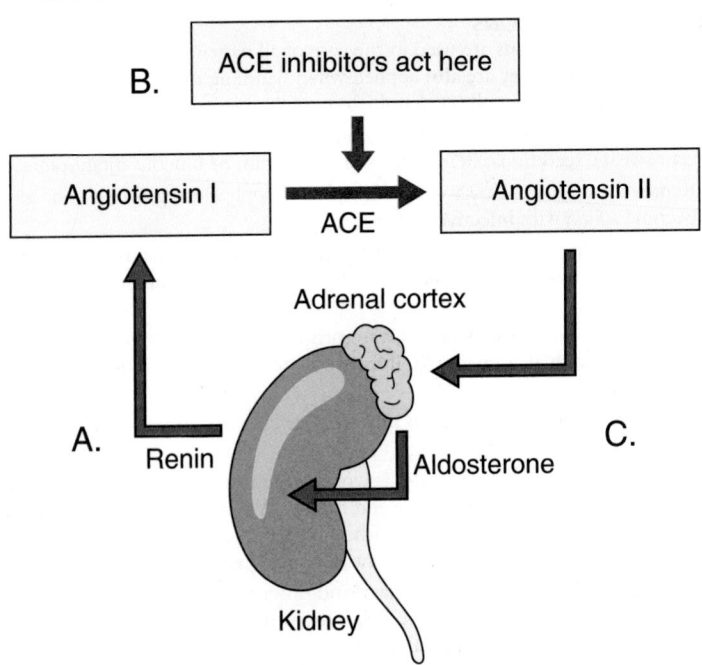

**Plate 1** The renin-angiotensin-aldosterone system plays a major role in regulating B/P. Any condition that decreases renal blood flow, reduces B/P, or stimulates beta$_1$-adrenergic receptors prompts the kidneys to release renin **(A).** Renin acts on angiotensinogen, which is converted to angiotensin I, a weak vasoconstrictor. Angiotensin-converting enzyme (ACE) converts angiotensin I to angiotensin II, which causes systemic and renal blood vessels to constrict **(B).** Systemic vasoconstriction increases peripheral vascular resistance, raising the B/P. Renal vasoconstriction decreases glomerular filtration, resulting in sodium and water retention and increasing blood volume and B/P. In addition, angiotensin II acts on the adrenal cortex, causing it to release aldosterone **(C).** This makes the kidneys retain additional sodium and water, which further increases the B/P. ACE inhibitors, such as captopril, enalapril, and lisinopril, block the action of ACE. As a result, angiotensin II cannot form, which prevents systemic and renal vasoconstriction and the release of aldosterone. (From Prosser S, Worster B, Dewar K: *Applied Pharmacology for Nurses and Other Health Care Professionals*, St. Louis, 2000, Mosby.)

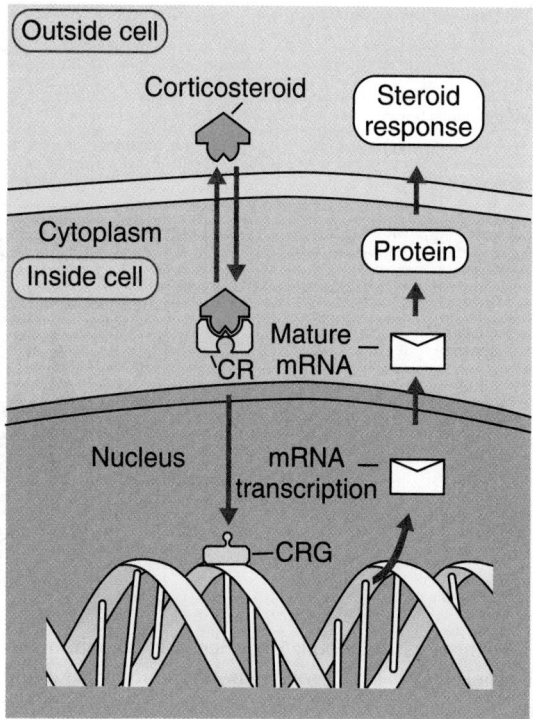

**Plate 2** Adrenocortical steroids (also called corticosteroids) are available in many forms, such as predniSONE, and produce a wide range of effects, such as immunosupression and antiinflammation. Here is how these drugs work at the cellular level.

Corticosteroids are hormones that are naturally produced by the body (endogenous hormones). Synthetic corticosteroids work much the same as the endogenous hormones. When a corticosteroid enters a cell, it binds to corticosteroid receptors (CRs) in the cell's cytoplasm, forming a complex. The complex moves to the nucleus where it causes the transcription of corticosteroid responsive genes (CRGs) to messenger ribonucleic acid (mRNA), eventually translating to a protein that produces a steroid response in target tissues. (From Taylor: *Mosby's Crash Course Pharmacology,* St. Louis, 1998, Mosby.)

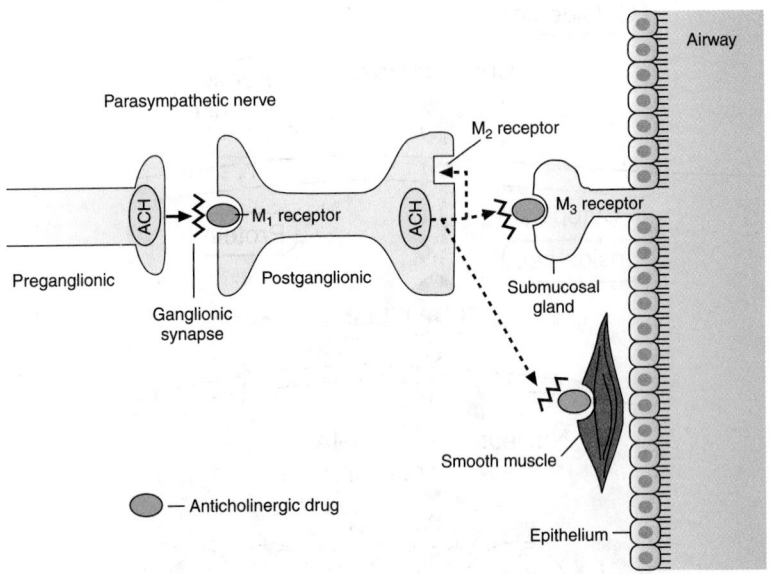

**Plate 3** Anticholinergic bronchodilators, such as ipratropium, work by blocking muscarinic-1 ($M_1$) receptors on postganglionic parasympathetic nerve endings and muscarinic-3 ($M_3$) receptors on the cell membranes of bronchial smooth muscles and submucosal glands. Normally, stimulation of the $M_1$ and $M_3$ receptors by acetylcholine (ACH) causes bronchoconstriction and mucus secretion from submucosal glands. Anticholinergic bronchodilators block these specific muscarinic receptors from the effects of acetylcholine, causing bronchial smooth muscle relaxation, bronchodilation, and decreased mucus production. (From Gardenhire OS: *Rau's Respiratory Care Pharmacology*, ed 7, St. Louis, 2008, Mosby.)

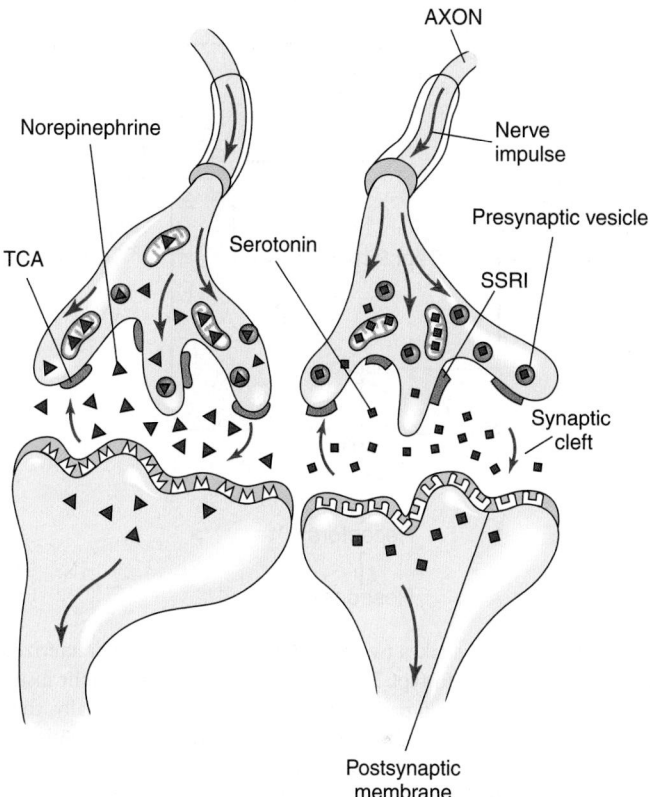

**Plate 4** Depression is thought to occur when levels of neurotransmitters, such as norepinephrine and serotonin, are reduced at postsynaptic receptor sites. These neurotransmitters affect a wide array of functions, including mood, obsessions, appetite, and anxiety. Antidepressants work by increasing the availability of these neurotransmitters at postsynaptic membranes and by enhancing and prolonging their effects. As a result, these agents improve mood, reduce anxiety, and minimize obsessions.

Antidepressants typically are classified as tricyclic antidepressants (TCAs), monoamine oxidase inhibitors (not shown), selective serotonin reuptake inhibitors (SSRIs), and atypical antidepressants (not shown). TCAs, such as amitriptyline and desipramine, primarily block norepinephrine reuptake at presynaptic membranes, thereby increasing the norepinephrine concentration at synapses and making more available at postsynaptic receptors.

SSRIs, such as fluoxetine and paroxetine, selectively inhibit serotonin uptake at presynaptic membranes. This action leads to increased serotonin availability at postsynaptic receptors. (From Gutierrez K: *Pharmacotherapeutics: Clinical Decision Making in Nursing,* ed 2, Philadelphia, 2008, Saunders.)

**Plate 5** Diabetes mellitus takes two forms: type 1 diabetes characterized by a complete lack of insulin and type 2 diabetes marked by insufficient insulin secretion, insulin resistance in peripheral tissues, or both. Normally, the beta cells in the pancreatic islets of Langerhans are responsible for secreting insulin. The rise of glucose levels in the beta cell triggers adenosine triphosphate (ATP)-dependent potassium ($K^+$) channels in the membranes of beta cells to close. Then the beta cells depolarize and calcium ($Ca^{++}$) enters the cell through $Ca^{++}$ channel, and insulin is released from the cell. When circulating insulin engages with insulin receptors on cell membranes, it facilitates the movement of glucose into the cell, among other actions.

Type 1 diabetes is treated with the use of exogenous insulin, which mimics natural insulin in the body. Insulin takes many forms with varying degrees of onset, peak, and duration, including rapid, regular, intermediate, and long acting.

Type 2 diabetes is usually treated with oral agents. Sulfonylureas, such as glyburide, block ATP-dependent $K^+$ channels in the cell membranes of beta cells, ultimately resulting in the release of insulin. (From Taylor: *Mosby's Crash Course Pharmacology*, St. Louis, 1998, Mosby.)

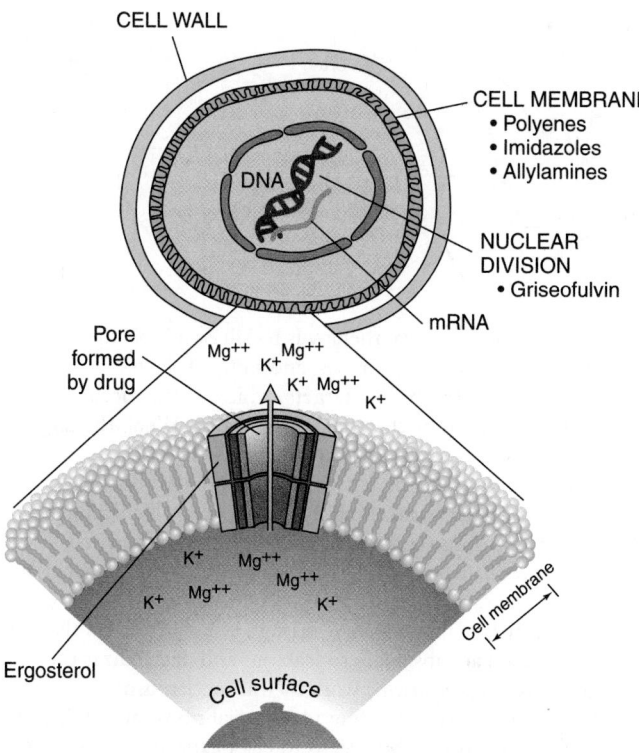

CELL WALL

CELL MEMBRANE
• Polyenes
• Imidazoles
• Allylamines

DNA

NUCLEAR
DIVISION
• Griseofulvin

mRNA

Pore
formed
by drug

$Mg^{++}$   $Mg^{++}$
$K^+$
$K^+$ $Mg^{++}$
$K^+$

$K^+$   $Mg^{++}$
$K^+$   $Mg^{++}$   $Mg^{++}$
$K^+$

Cell membrane

Ergosterol

Cell surface

**Plate 6** Antifungal agents primarily affect fungi at one of two sites: the cell membrane or the cell nucleus. Most of these agents, such as polyene, imidazole, and allylamine antifungals, act on the fungal cell membrane. Polyene antifungals, such amphotericin B, bind to ergosterol and increase cell membrane permeability. Imidazole antifungals, such as fluconazole and ketoconazole, interfere with ergosterol synthesis by inhibiting the cytochrome $P_{450}$ enzyme system, altering the cell membrane, and inhibiting fungal growth. Allylamine antifungals, such as terbinafine, inhibit the enzyme squaline epoxidase, which disrupts ergosterol production—and cell membrane integrity. When cell membrane permeability increases, cellular components, including potassium ($K^+$) and magnesium ($Mg^{++}$), leak out. Loss of these cellular components leads to cell death.

Another antifungal agent, griseofulvin, directly affects the fungal nucleus, interfering with mitosis. By binding to structures in the mitotic spindle, it prevents cells from dividing, which eventually leads to their death. (From Gutierrez K: *Pharmacotherapeutics: Clinical Decision Making in Nursing,* ed 2, Philadelphia, 2008, Saunders.)

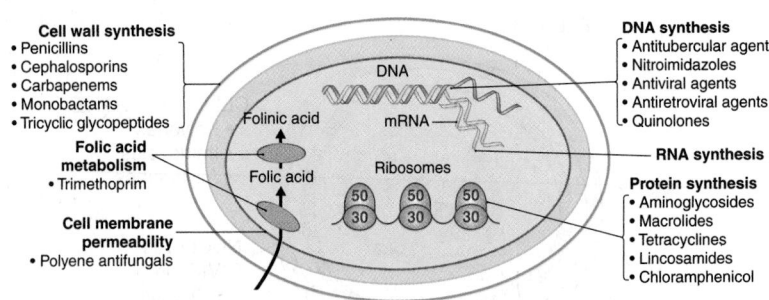

**Cell wall synthesis**
• Penicillins
• Cephalosporins
• Carbapenems
• Monobactams
• Tricyclic glycopeptides

**Folic acid metabolism**
• Trimethoprim

**Cell membrane permeability**
• Polyene antifungals

DNA

Folinic acid    mRNA

Folic acid    Ribosomes

50  50  50
30  30  30

**DNA synthesis**
• Antitubercular agent
• Nitroimidazoles
• Antiviral agents
• Antiretroviral agents
• Quinolones

**RNA synthesis**

**Protein synthesis**
• Aminoglycosides
• Macrolides
• Tetracyclines
• Lincosamides
• Chloramphenicol

**Plate 7** The goal of antiinfective therapy is to kill or inhibit the growth of microorganisms such as bacteria, viruses, and fungi. To achieve this goal, antiinfective agents must reach their targets, which usually occurs through absorption and distribution by the circulatory system. When the target is reached, a drug can kill or suppress microorganisms by:

• Inhibiting cell wall synthesis or activating enzymes that disrupt the cell wall, which leads to cellular weakening, lysis, and death. Penicillins (ampicillin), cephalosporins (cefazolin), carbapenems (imipenem), monobactams (aztreonam), and tricyclic glycopeptides (vancomycin) act in this way.

• Altering cell membrane permeability through direct action on the cell wall, which allows intracellular substances to leak out and destabilizes the cell. Polyene antifungals (amphotericin) work by this mechanism.

• Altering protein synthesis by binding to bacterial ribosomes (50/30) or affecting ribosomal function, which leads to cell death or slowed growth respectively. Aminoglycosides (gentamicin), macrolides (erythromycin), tetracyclines (doxycycline), lincosamides (clindamycin), and the miscellaneous antiinfective chloramphenicol use the action.

• Inhibiting DNA or RNA, including messenger RNA (mRNA), by synthesis by binding to nucleic acids or interacting with enzymes required for their synthesis. Antitubercular agents (rifampin), nitroimidazoles (metronidazole), antiviral agents (acyclovir), antiretroviral agents (stavudine), and quinolones (ciprofloxacin) act like this.

• Inhibiting the metabolism of folic acid and folinic acid or other cellular components that are essential for bacterial cell growth. The miscellaneous antiinfective trimethoprim employs this mechanism of action. (From Page C et al: *Integrated Pharmacology*, ed 3, St. Louis, 2006, Mosby.)

**Plate 8** When viruses reproduce, the infectious viral particle or virion (**A**) enters the host cell. The virion attaches to the cell's surface and then inserts itself into the host cell (**B**). Once inside, the virion uncoats, and the enzyme reverse transcriptase makes two copies of the viral RNA: one copy is identical; the other is a mirror image. These two copies form double-stranded viral DNA that enters the host cell's nucleus, where it inserts itself into the host cell's DNA with the help of the enzyme integrase. Then viral DNA reprograms the host cell to produce additional viral RNA, which begins the process of forming new viruses. Specifically, messenger RNA (mRNA) instructs ribosomal RNA (rRNA) to produce a new chain of proteins and enzymes that are used to form new viruses. Protease cuts the chains, creating individual proteins. These combine with new RNA to create new virions, which bud and are released from the host cell (**C**).

Antiretroviral agents target specific enzymes during viral reproduction. Nucleoside reverse transcriptase inhibitors, such as stavudine, interfere with the action of reverse transcriptase by mimicking naturally occurring nucleosides. Nucleotide reverse transcriptase inhibitors, such as tenofovir, block reverse transcriptase by competing with the natural substrate deoxyadenosine triphosphate and by causing DNA chain termination. Nonnucleoside reverse transcriptase inhibitors, such as delavirdine, work by directly binding to reverse transcriptase. As a result, no viral DNA is available to insert itself into the host cell's DNA. Protease inhibitors, such as indinavir, bind to and interefere with the action of protease; thus, the new chain of proteins formed by rRNA cannot be cut into individual proteins to make new viruses. (From Gutierrez K: *Pharmacotherapeutics: Clinical Decision Making in Nursing,* ed 2, Philadelphia, 2008, Saunders.)

**Plate 9** Benzodiazepines reduce anxiety by stimulating the action of the inhibitory neurotransmitter, gamma-aminobutyric acid (GABA), in the limbic system. The limbic system plays an important role in the regulation of human behavior. Dysfunction of GABA neurotransmission in the limbic system may be linked to the development of certain anxiety disorders.

The limbic system contains a highly dense area of benzodiazepine receptors that may be linked to the antianxiety effects of benzodiazepines. These benzodiazepine receptors are located on the surface of neuronal cell membranes and are adjacent to GABA receptors. The binding of a benzodiazepine to its receptor enhances the affinity of a GABA receptor for GABA. In the absence of a benzodiazepine, the binding of GABA to its receptor causes the chloride channel in the cell membrane to open, which increases the influx of chloride into the cell. This influx of chloride results in hyperpolarization of the neuronal cell membrane and reduces the neuron's ability to fire, which is why GABA is considered an inhibitory neurotransmitter.

A benzodiazepine acts only in the presence of GABA. When it binds to a benzodiazepine receptor, it prolongs the time that the chloride channel remains open. This results in greater depression of neuronal function and a reduction in anxiety. (From Gutierrez K: *Pharmacotherapeutics: Clinical Decision Making in Nursing,* ed 2, Philadelphia, 2008, Saunders.)

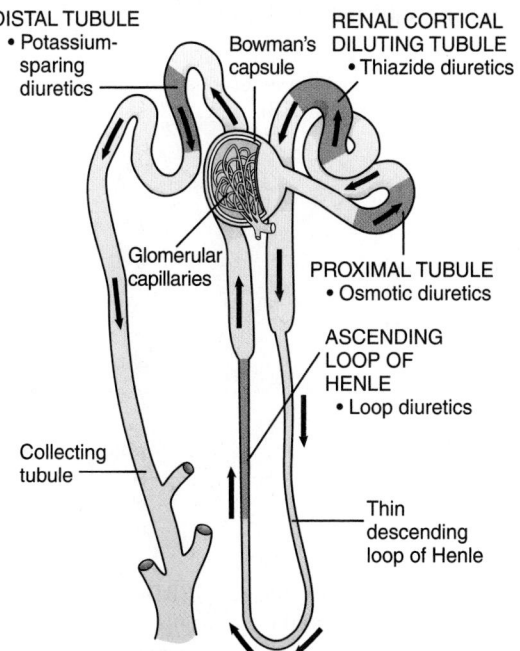

**DISTAL TUBULE**
- Potassium-sparing diuretics

Bowman's capsule

**RENAL CORTICAL DILUTING TUBULE**
- Thiazide diuretics

Glomerular capillaries

**PROXIMAL TUBULE**
- Osmotic diuretics

**ASCENDING LOOP OF HENLE**
- Loop diuretics

Collecting tubule

Thin descending loop of Henle

**Plate 10** Diuretics act primarily to increase water and sodium excretion by the kidneys, thereby increasing urine output. In the process, chloride, potassium, and other electrolytes may also be excreted. Most diuretics act by blocking sodium, water, and chloride reabsorption by peritubular capillaries in the nephrons. As a result, water and electrolytes remain in the convoluted tubules to be excreted as urine. The increased water and electrolyte excretion reduces blood volume—and ultimately blood pressure.

Diuretics belong to four major subclasses:

1. Thiazide diuretics, such as hydrochlorothiazide, act in the early portion of the distal convoluted tubule, called the cortical diluting segment. These drugs block sodium, chloride, and water reabsorption and promote their excretion along with potassium.

2. Loop diuretics, such as furosemide, act primarily in the thick ascending limb of the loop of Henle, blocking sodium, water, and chloride reabsorption. Then these substances are excreted along with potassium.

3. Potassium-sparing diuretics, such as spironolactone, act in the late portion of the distal convoluted tubule and collecting tubule. Here, they inhibit the action of aldosterone, leading to sodium excretion and potassium retention. Although triamterene and amiloride, two other potassium-sparing diuretics, act at the same site, they do not affect aldosterone. Instead, these drugs directly block the exchange of sodium and potassium, leading to decreased sodium reabsorption and decreased potassium excretion.

4. Osmotic diuretics, such as mannitol, work in the proximal convoluted tubule. As their name implies, these diuretics increase the osmotic pressure of the glomerular filtrate, inhibiting the passive reabsorption of water, sodium, and chloride. (From Gutierrez K: *Pharmacotherapeutics: Clinical Decision Making in Nursing,* ed 2, Philadelphia, 2008, Saunders.)

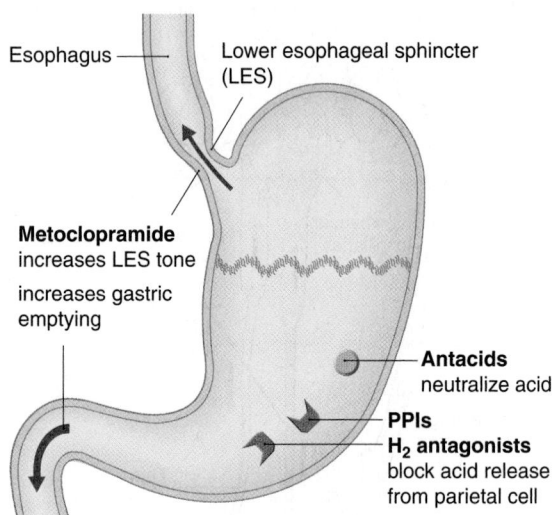

Esophagus — Lower esophageal sphincter (LES)

**Metoclopramide**
increases LES tone

increases gastric emptying

**Antacids** neutralize acid

**PPIs**
**H$_2$ antagonists**
block acid release from parietal cell

**Plate 11** Gastroesophageal reflux disease (GERD) occurs when acidic stomach contents regurgitate into the esophagus, causing heartburn. The disorder may result from a weakness or incompetence of the lower esophageal sphincter (LES). Because the malfunctioning LES makes the reflux leave the stomach and reenter the esophagus slowly, the esophageal mucosa is exposed to the acid for a long time. Because the enzymatic action of parietal cells in the stomach makes the reflux highly acidic, GERD causes irritation and possible erosion of the esophageal mucosa.

Treatment of GERD can employ drugs from several classes: histamine (H$_2$) antagonists, proton pump inhibitors (PPIs), the miscellaneous GI agent metoclopramide, and antacids. H$_2$ antagonists, such as cimetidine, act in parietal cells of the stomach. Normally, H$_2$-receptor stimulation results in gastric acid secretion. By blocking these receptors, H$_2$ antagonists decrease the amount and acidity of gastric secretion, including secretion that occurs with fasting, food consumption at night, and stomach distension.

PPIs, such as esomeprazole, also suppress gastric acid secretion. However, they do it by inhibiting the hydrogen-potassium-adenosine triphsophatase enzyme system, which is located on the surface of parietal cells and controls their gastric acid secretion. PPIs block acid secretion that results from fasting or abdominal distension caused by food ingestion.

Metoclopramide increases the tone and motility of the upper GI tract. It works by stimulating the release of acetylcholine from GI nerve endings, which improves LES tone and leads to decreased reflux. The drug also stimulates gastric emptying, which reduces gastric contents.

Antacids, such as aluminum hydroxide, act primarily in the stomach by chemically combining with the hydrogen ions (H$^+$) in gastric acid and raising the pH of gastric contents. They do not prevent reflux. However, they make the reflux less acidic, so it causes less damage to the esophageal mucosa. (From Page C et al: *Integrated Pharmacology,* ed 3, St. Louis, 2006, Mosby.)

**Plate 12** Laxatives ease or stimulate defecation. Typically, they are classified by their mechanism of action as bulk-forming, osmotic, stimulant, or surfactant laxatives.

Bulk-forming laxatives, such as psyllium, act in the small and large bowel. Because ingredients in these laxatives are undigestible, they remain within the stool and increase the fecal mass by drawing in water. These agents also enhance bacterial growth in the colon, further adding to the fecal mass.

Osmotic laxatives, such as lactulose, draw water into the intestinal lumen, causing the fecal mass to soften and swell. This osmotic action may be enhanced by the metabolism of colonic bacteria to lactate and other organic acids. These acids decrease colonic pH and increase colonic motility.

Stimulant (or irritant) laxatives, such as senna, act on the intestinal wall to increase water and electrolytes in the intestinal lumen. In addition, they directly irritate the colon, increasing motility.

Surfactant laxatives (or fecal softeners), such as docusate, reduce the surface tension of the stool, allowing water to enter it. These laxatives may also help to increase water and electrolyte excretion into the intestinal lumen, softening and increasing the fecal mass. (From Page C et al: *Integrated Pharmacology*, ed 3, St. Louis, 2006, Mosby.)

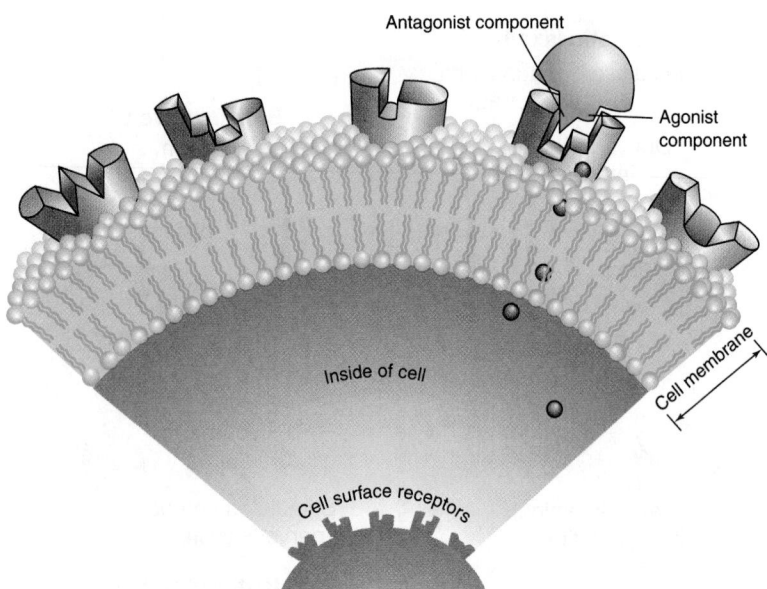

**Plate 13** Cell membranes have different types of opioid receptors, such as mu, kappa, and delta receptors. Opioid agonist-antagonists work by stimulating one type of receptor, while simultaneously blocking another type. As agonists, they work primarily by activating kappa receptors to produce analgesia and such other effects as CNS and respiratory depression, decreased GI motility, and euphoria. As antagonists, they compete with opioids at mu receptors, helping to reverse or block some of the other effects of agonists. (From Gutierrez K: *Pharmacotherapeutics: Clinical Decision Making in Nursing,* ed 2, Philadelphia, 2008, Saunders.)

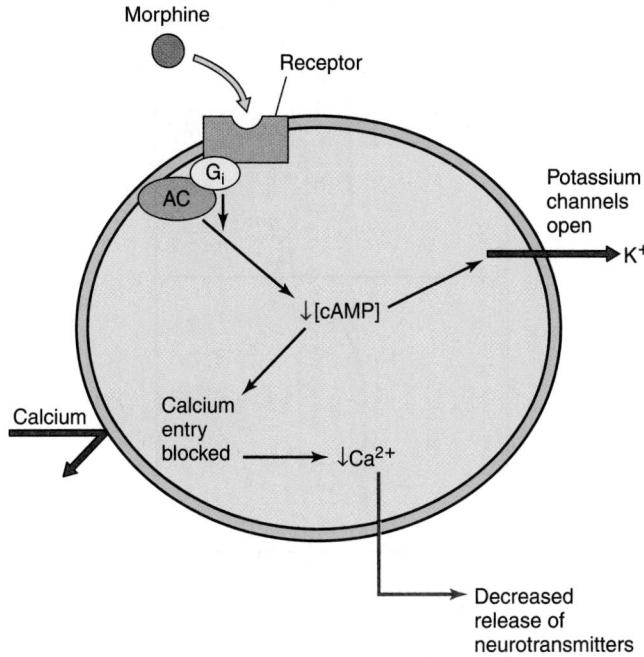

**Plate 14** Narcotic analgesics bind to three types of opioid receptors: mu, kappa, and delta receptors. They produce analgesia primarily by activating mu receptors. However, they also engage with and activate kappa and delta receptors, producing other effects, such as sedation and vasomotor stimulation.

When morphine or another narcotic analgesic binds to opioid receptors, activation occurs. The receptors send signals to the enzyme adenyl cyclase (AC) to slow activity by way of G proteins ($G_i$). Decreased adenyl cyclase activity causes reduced production of cyclic adenosine monophosphate (cAMP). A secondary messenger substance, cAMP is important for regulating cell membrane channels. A reduced cAMP level allows fewer potassium ions to leave the cell and blocks calcium ions from entering the cell. This ion imbalance—especially the reduced intracellular calcium level—ultimately decreases the release of neurotransmitters from the cell, thereby blocking or reducing pain impulse transmission. (From Minneman KP, Wecker L: *Brody's Human Pharmacology: Molecular to Clinical*, ed 4, St. Louis, 2005, Mosby.)

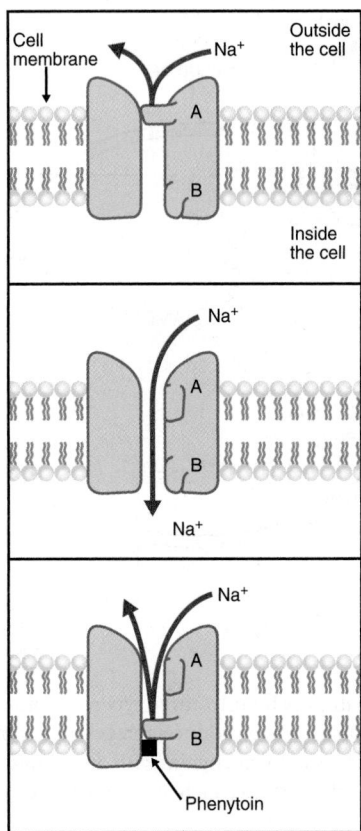

**Plate 15** Phenytoin, which is used to treat tonic-clonic seizures, acts in the motor cortex and brain stem where the tonic phase of tonic-clonic seizures originates. By altering sodium transport across neuronal cell membranes, phenytoin stabilizes the cell membrane, reduces repetitive firing of the neurons, and halts or limits the spread of seizures. The first illustration shows a neuronal cell membrane in its resting state. The activation gate (**A**) of the sodium channel in the cell membrane is closed and blocks sodium ($Na^+$) from entering the cell. In the second illustration, a nerve impulse has caused depolarization and opening of the activation gate, allowing $Na^+$ to move into the cell. In the third illustration, depolarization continues and an inactivation gate (**B**) moves into the channel. This prevents $Na^+$ from moving into the cell. Phenytoin prolongs the inactivated state of the sodium channel by preventing reopening of the inactivation gate. By further preventing $Na^+$ from entering the cell, phenytoin slows impulse transmission, and thus slows the rate at which neurons fire. (From Minneman KP, Wecker L: *Brody's Human Pharmacology: Molecular to Clinical*, ed 4, St. Louis, 2005, Mosby.)

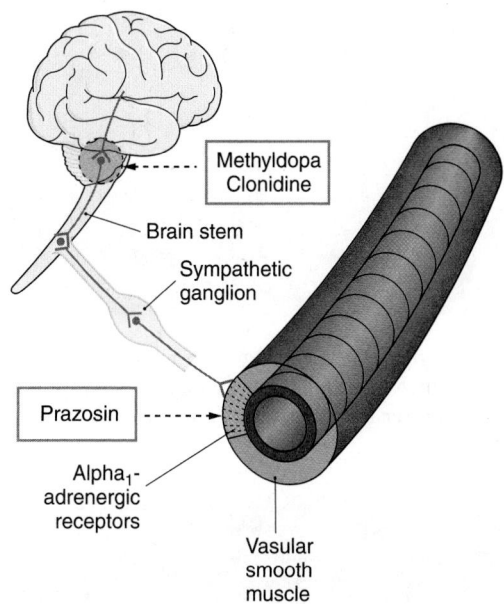

**Plate 16** Sympatholytics inhibit sympathetic nervous system (SNS) activity, which plays a major role in regulating B/P. Normally when the SNS is stimulated, nerve impulses travel from the cardiovascular center of the CNS to the sympathetic ganglia. From there, the impulses travel along postganglionic fibers to specific effector organs, such as the heart and blood vessels. SNS stimulation also triggers the release of norepinephrine, which acts primarily at alpha-adrenergic receptors.

Sympatholytics fall into two subclasses: central-acting alpha$_2$ agonists and peripheral-acting alpha$_1$-adrenergic antagonists. Central-acting alpha$_2$ agonists, such as methyldopa and clonidine, stimulate alpha$_2$-adrenergic receptors in the cardiovascular center of the CNS and reduce activity in the vasomotor center of the brain, interfering with sympathetic stimulation of the heart and blood vessels. This causes blood vessel dilation and decreased cardiac output, which leads to reduced B/P.

Peripheral-acting alpha$_1$-adrenergic antagonists, such as prazosin, inhibit the stimulation of alpha$_1$-adrenergic receptors by norepinephrine in vascular smooth muscle, interfering with SNS-induced vasoconstriction. As a result, the blood vessels dilate, reducing peripheral vascular resistance and venous return to the heart. These effects, in turn, lead to decreased B/P. (From Prosser S, Worster B, Dewar K: *Applied Pharmacology for Nurses and Other Health Care Professionals,* St. Louis, 2000, Mosby.)

**Plate 17** Needles. *Left to right:* 19 gauge, 1½-inch length; 20 gauge, 1-inch length; 21 gauge, 1-inch length; 23 gauge, 1-inch length; and 25 gauge, ⅝-inch length. (From Potter PA, Perry AG: *Fundamentals of Nursing,* ed 7, St. Louis, 2009, Mosby.)

**Plate 18** Needle with plastic guard to prevent needle sticks. **A,** Position of guard before injection. **B,** After injection, the guard locks in place, covering the needle. (From Potter PA, Perry AG: *Fundamentals of Nursing,* ed 7, St. Louis, 2009, Mosby.)

**Plate 19** Preparing an injection from a vial. Remove needle cap from syringe. Pull back on the plunger to draw amount of air into syringe equivalent to volume of medication to be aspirated from vial. **A,** Insert tip of needle, with bevel pointing up, through center of rubber seal. Apply pressure to tip of needle during insertion. **B,** Allow air pressure to fill syringe gradually with medication. Pull back slightly on plunger if necessary. **C,** Remove remaining air from syringe by holding it and needle upright. Tap barrel to dislodge air bubbles. Draw back slightly on plunger and then push plunger upward to eject air. Do not eject fluid. (From Potter PA, Perry AG: *Fundamentals of Nursing,* ed 6, St. Louis, 2005, Mosby.)

**Plate 20** Administering an injection. Cleanse site with antiseptic swab. Apply swab at center of site and rotate outward in circular direction for about 5 cm (2 in). (From Potter PA, Perry AG: *Fundamentals of Nursing,* ed 7, St. Louis, 2009, Mosby.)

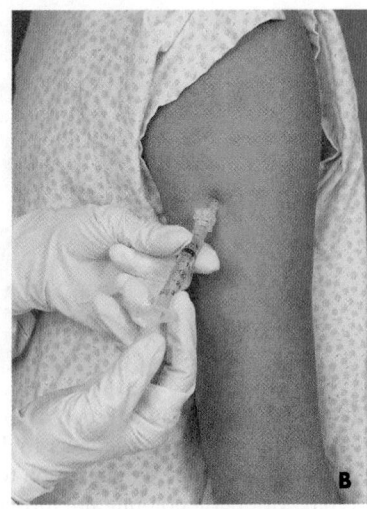

**Plate 21 A,** For a subcutaneous injection, hold the syringe between the thumb and forefinger of the dominant hand as a dart, with the palm down. **B,** After injecting the needle at a 45- to 90-degree angle, grasp lower end of syringe barrel with nondominant hand to end of plunger. Avoid moving syringe while slowly pulling back on plunger to aspirate drug. If blood appears in syringe, remove needle, discard medication and syringe, and repeat procedure. *Exception:* Do not aspirate when giving heparin. (From Potter PA, Perry AG: *Fundamentals of Nursing,* ed 7, St. Louis, 2009, Mosby.)

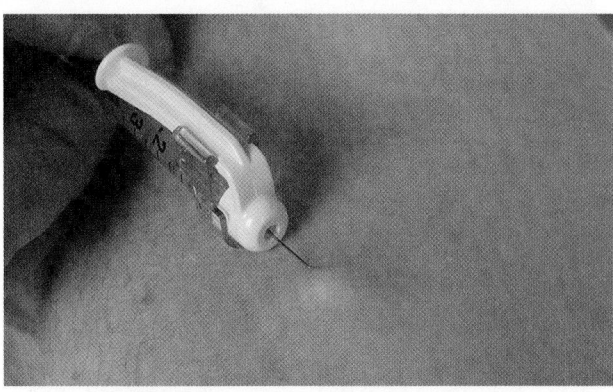

**Plate 22**  For an intradermal injection, note formation of small bleb approximately 6 mm (¼ in) in diameter at injection site. (From Potter PA, Perry AG: *Fundamentals of Nursing,* ed 7, St. Louis, 2009, Mosby.)

**Plate 23 A,** Sites recommended for subcutaneous injections.
**B,** Giving subcutaneous injection in the abdomen. (From
Potter PA, Perry AG: *Fundamentals of Nursing,* ed 6,
St. Louis, 2005, Mosby.)

**Plate 24 A,** Landmarks for IM injection into the deltoid muscle. **B,** Giving IM injection in deltoid muscle. (From Potter PA, Perry AG: *Fundamentals of Nursing,* ed 7, St. Louis, 2009, Mosby.)

**Plate 25** **A,** Landmarks for IM injection in vastus lateralis. **B,** Giving IM injection in vastus lateralis site. (From Potter PA, Perry AG: *Fundamentals of Nursing,* ed 7, St. Louis, 2009, Mosby.)

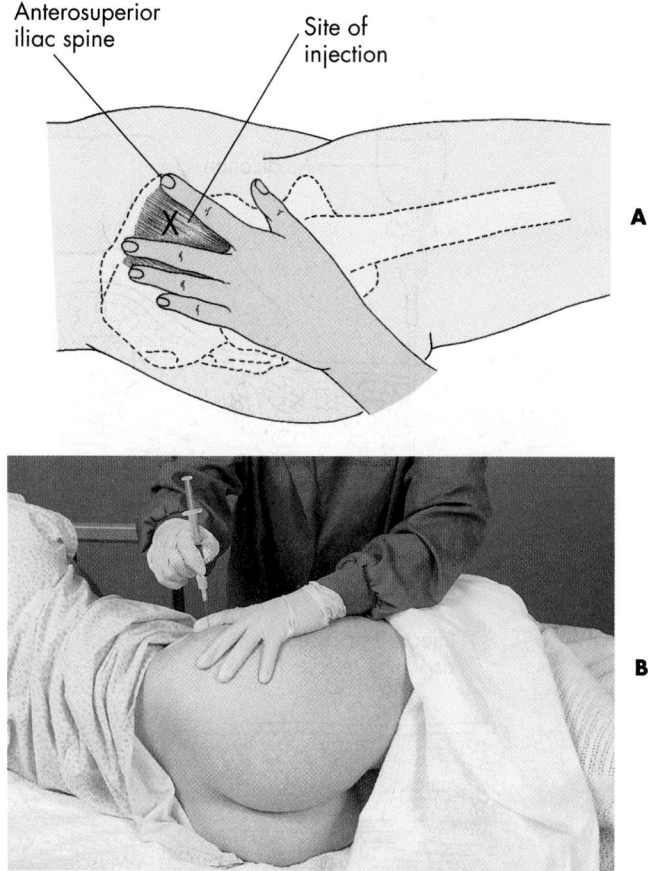

Anterosuperior
iliac spine

Site of
injection

A

B

**Plate 26  A,** Anatomical view of ventrogluteal site. **B,** Giving IM injection into ventrogluteal muscle to avoid major nerves and blood vessels. (From Potter PA, Perry AG: *Fundamentals of Nursing,* ed 7, St. Louis, 2009, Mosby.)

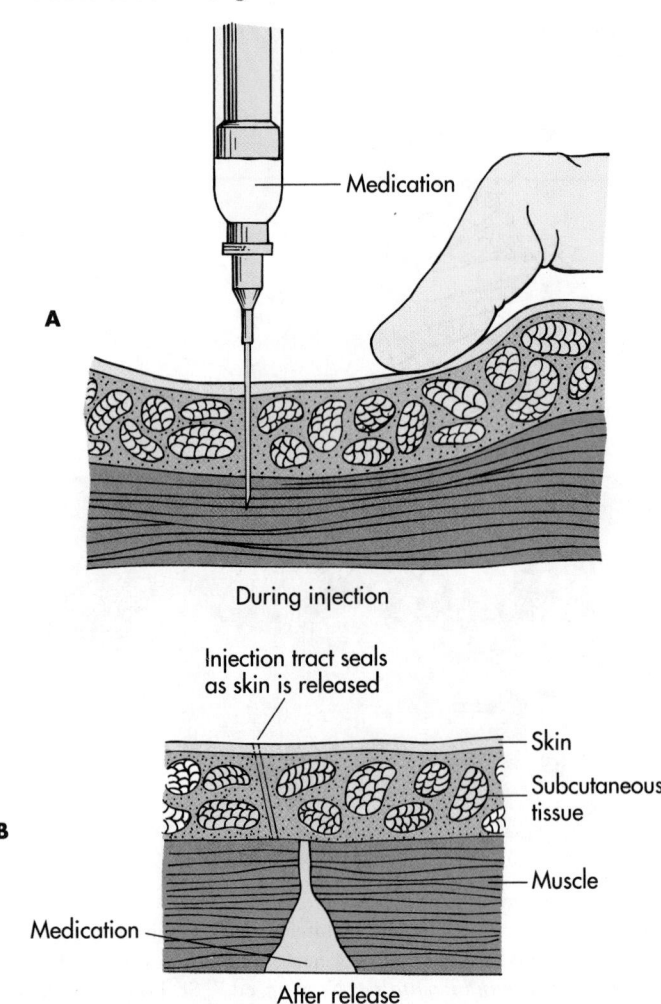

**Plate 27** Z-track method of injection. **A,** Pulling on overlying skin during IM injection moves tissues to prevent later tracking. **B,** The Z-track left after injection prevents the deposit of medication through sensitive tissue. (From Potter PA, Perry AG: *Fundamentals of Nursing,* ed 7, St. Louis, 2009, Mosby.)

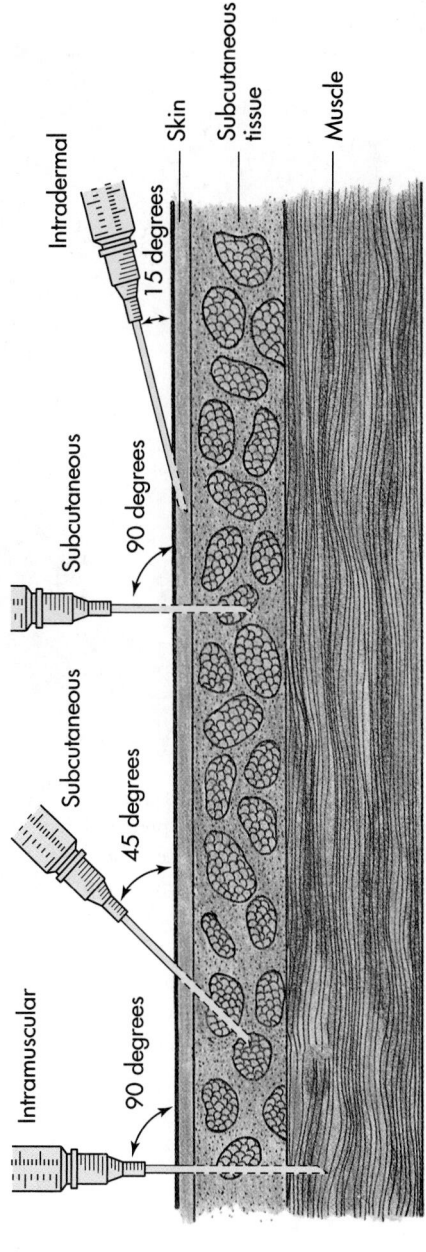

**Plate 28** Comparison of angles of insertion for IM (90 degrees), SUBCUT (45 degrees and 90 degrees), and ID (15 degrees) injections. (From Potter PA, Perry AG: *Fundamentals of Nursing*, ed 7, St. Louis, 2009, Mosby.)

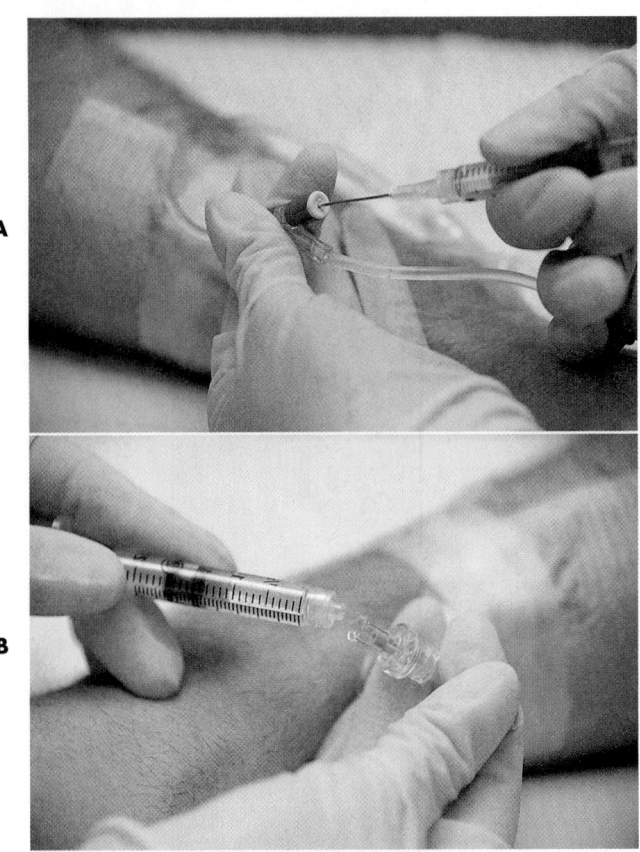

**Plate 29** Administering medication by IV bolus (push). **A,** Needle system: Insert small-gauge needle of syringe containing prepared drug through center of injection port. **B,** Needleless system: Remove cap of needleless injection port. Connect tip of syringe directly. (From Potter PA, Perry AG: *Fundamentals of Nursing,* ed 5, St. Louis, 2001, Mosby.)

*Continued*

**Plate 29  C,** Occlude IV line by pinching tubing just above injection port. Pull back gently on syringe's plunger to aspirate blood return. **D,** After noting blood return, continue to occlude tubing and inject medication slowly over several minutes (read directions on drug package). Use watch to time administration. **E,** IV lock: Insert needle of syringe containing prepared drug through center of diaphragm. (From Potter PA, Perry AG: *Fundamentals of Nursing,* ed 6, St. Louis, 2005, Mosby.)

**Plate 30** Administering IV medication by piggyback, volume administration sets of miniinfusors (syringe pump). Use needle-lock device to secure needle of secondary piggyback line through injection port of main line. (From Potter PA, Perry AG: *Fundamentals of Nursing,* ed 6, St. Louis, 2005, Mosby.)

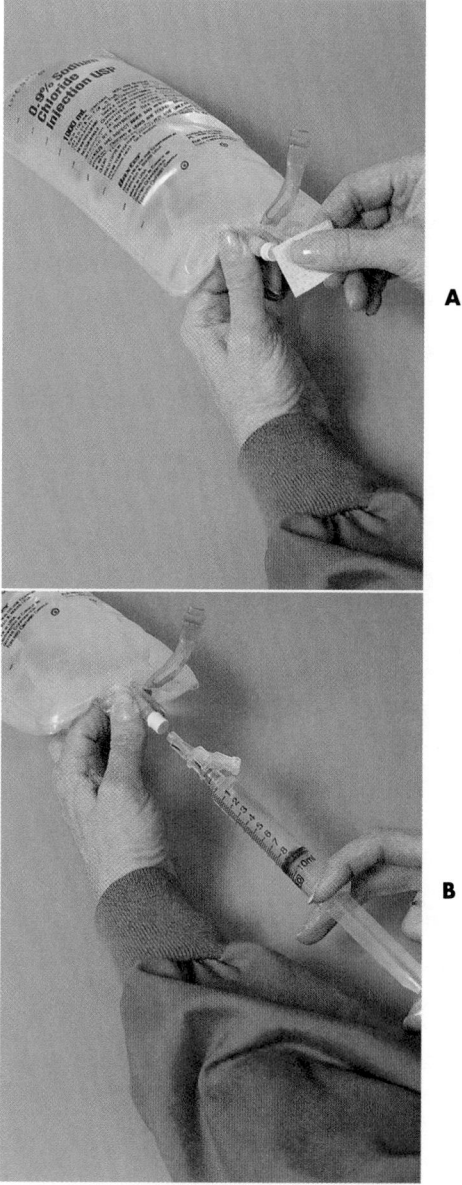

Plate 31 Adding medications to IV fluid containers. **A,** Wipe off port or injection site with alcohol or antiseptic swab. **B,** Remove needle cap from syringe, insert needle of syringe through center of injection port or site, and inject medication. (From Potter PA, Perry AG: *Fundamentals of Nursing,* ed 7, St. Louis, 2009, Mosby.)

## abacavir (Rx)

(aba-ka'veer)

Ziagen

*Func. class.:* Antiretroviral

*Chem. class.:* Nucleoside reverse transcriptase inhibitor (NRTI)

### Pregnancy category C

**Action:** A synthetic, nucleoside analog with inhibitory action against HIV; inhibits replication of HIV by incorporating into cellular DNA by viral reverse transcriptase, thereby terminating the cellular DNA chain

**Therapeutic outcome:** Decreased symptoms of HIV

**Uses:** In combination with other antiretroviral agents for HIV-1 infection (not to be used with lamivudine or tenofovir)

### Dosage and routes

*Adult:* PO 300 mg bid or 600 mg daily with other antiretrovirals

*Adolescents and children ≥3 mo:* PO 8 mg/kg bid, max 300 mg bid with other antiretrovirals

*Hepatic dose*

*Adult:* (Child-Pugh 5-6) PO oral/sol 200 mg bid

**Available forms:** Tabs 300 mg; oral sol 20 mg/ml

### Adverse effects

*CNS: Fever, headache, malaise, insomnia,* paresthesia

*GI: Nausea, vomiting, diarrhea, anorexia, cramps, abdominal pain, increased AST, ALT,* **hepatotoxicity**

*HEMA:* **Granulocytopenia, anemia,** lymphopenia

*INTEG:* Rash, urticaria, hypersensitivity reactions

*META:* **Lactic acidosis**

*MISC:* Increased CPK, **fatal hypersensitivity reactions**

*RESP:* Dyspnea

**Contraindications:** Hypersensitivity, lactic acidosis

**Precautions;** Pregnancy **C,** breastfeeding, child <3 mo, granulocyte count <1000/mm$^3$ or Hgb <9.5 g/dl, severe renal disease, impaired hepatic function

### Pharmacokinetics

| | |
|---|---|
| **Absorption** | Well absorbed (PO) |
| **Distribution** | 50% plasma protein binding |
| **Metabolism** | To inactive metabolite |
| **Excretion** | Kidneys, feces |
| **Half-life** | 1½-2 hr |

### Pharmacodynamics

Unknown

### Interactions

*Individual drugs*

Alcohol: increased abacavir levels; do not use with alcohol

Ribavirin: possible lactic acidosis

Methadone: decreased levels of methadone

### NURSING CONSIDERATIONS
### Assessment

• Assess for symptoms of HIV and possible infection, increased temp

• Assess for lactic acidosis (elevated lactate levels, increased liver function tests) and severe hepatomegaly with steatosis; discontinue treatment and do not restart

⬧ Assess for fatal hypersensitivity reactions: fever, rash, nausea, vomiting, fatigue, cough, dyspnea, diarrhea, abdominal discomfort; treatment should be discontinued and not restarted

⬧ Assess for pancreatitis: abdominal pain, nausea, vomiting, elevated liver enzymes; product should be discontinued because condition can be fatal

• Monitor CBC, differential, platelet count qmo; withhold product if WBC is <4000/mm$^3$ or platelet count is <75,000/mm$^3$; notify prescriber of results; monitor viral load and CD4 counts during treatment

• Monitor renal function studies; BUN, serum uric acid, urine CCr before, during therapy; these may be elevated throughout treatment

• Monitor temp q4hr, may indicate beginning of infection

• Monitor liver function tests before, during therapy (bilirubin, AST, ALT, amylase, alkaline phosphatase, creatine phosphokinase, creatinine prn or qmo)

### Nursing diagnoses

• Infection, risk for (uses)

• Injury, risk for (adverse reactions)

• Knowledge, deficient (teaching)

### Implementation
### PO route

• Give on empty stomach, q12hr around the clock

- Give in combination with other antiretrovirals with or without food
- Store in cool environment; protect from light, do not freeze

## Patient/family education

- Advise patient to report signs of infection: increased temp, sore throat, flulike symptoms; to avoid crowds and those with known infections
- Instruct patient to report signs of anemia: fatigue, headache, faintness, shortness of breath, irritability
- Advise patient to report bleeding; avoid use of razors or commercial mouthwash
- Inform patient that product is not a cure but will control symptoms
- Inform patient that major toxicities may necessitate discontinuing product
- Instruct patient to use contraception during treatment
- Caution patient to avoid OTC products or other medications without approval of prescriber
- Caution patient not to have any sexual contact without use of a condom, needles should not be shared, blood from infected individual should not come in contact with another's mucous membranes
- Give Medication Guide and Warning Card; discuss points on guide
- Advise patient to stop product if skin rash, fever, cough, shortness of breath, GI symptoms occur and notify prescriber immediately; advise all health care providers that allergic reactions have occurred with this product

## Evaluation

**Positive therapeutic outcome**

- Increased CD4 count, decreased viral load

---

## abatacept (Rx)
(ab-a-ta'sept)
Orencia
*Func. class.:* Antirheumatic agent (disease modifying); biologic response modifier

**Pregnancy category** C

**Action:** A selective costimulation modulator, inhibits T-lymphocytes, inhibits tumor necrosis factor (TNF-α), interferon-γ, interleukin-2, that is involved in immune and inflammatory reactions

**Therapeutic outcome:** Decreased pain, inflammation in joints

**Uses:** Acute, chronic rheumatoid arthritis that has not responded to other disease-modifying

agents, may use in combination with DMARDs; do not use with TNF antagonists (adalimumab, etanercept, infliximab) or anakinra

## Dosage and routes

*Adult >100 kg:* **IV** INF 1 g
*Adult 60-100 kg:* **IV** INF 750 mg
*Adult <60 kg:* **IV** INF 500 mg over 30 min; give 2-4 wk after 1st INF, then q4 wk

**Available forms:** Lyophilized powder, single-use vials 250 mg

## Adverse effects

*CNS:* Headache, asthenia, dizziness
*CV: Hypertension, hypotension*
*GI:* Abdominal pain, dyspepsia, nausea
*INTEG:* Rash, *inj site reaction,* flushing, urticaria, pruritus
*RESP: Pharyngitis, cough, URI,* non-URI, *rhinitis,* wheezing
*SYST:* **Anaphylaxis, malignancies, angioedema**

**Contraindications:** Hypersensitivity, TB

**Precautions:** Pregnancy C, breastfeeding, children, geriatric, recurrent infections, COPD

### Pharmacokinetics

| | |
|---|---|
| **Absorption** | Unknown |
| **Distribution** | Unknown |
| **Metabolism** | Unknown |
| **Excretion** | Unknown |
| **Half-life** | Terminal 13-16 days, steady state 60 days |

### Pharmacodynamics

Unknown

## Interactions

*Individual drugs*
Anakinra: do not use
*Drug classifications*
Corticosteroids, immunosuppressives: do not use concurrently
TNF antagonists (adalimumab, etanercept, infliximab): do not use
Vaccines: do not give concurrently; immunizations should be brought up to date before treatment

## NURSING CONSIDERATIONS

**Assessment**

- Assess for latent/active TB before beginning treatment
- Assess for pain, stiffness, ROM, swelling of joints during treatment
- Assess for inj site pain, swelling
- Monitor patient's overall health on each

---

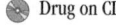

visit; product should not be given with active infections

## Nursing diagnoses
• Knowledge, deficient (teaching)
• Pain, chronic (uses)

## Implementation
• To reconstitute, remove plastic flip top from vial and wipe the top with alcohol wipe; insert syringe needle into vial and direct stream of sterile water for inj on the wall of vial; rotate vial until mixed; vent with needle to rid foam after reconstitution 25 mg/ml; further dilute in 100 ml from a 100 ml infusion bag/bottle; withdraw the needed volume (2 vials remove 20 mg; 3 vials remove 30 ml, 4 vials remove 40 ml); slowly add the reconstituted Orencia sol from each vial into the infusion bag/bottle using the same disposable syringe supplied; mix gently, discard unused portions of vials; do not use if particulate is present or discolored; give over 30 min; use non–protein binding filter (0.2-1.2 mcg)
• Do not admix with other sol or medications
• Store in refrigerator; do not use expired vials

## Patient/family education
• Teach patient that product must be continued for prescribed time to be effective
• Advise patient to use caution when driving; dizziness may occur
• Advise patient not to have vaccinations while taking this product
• Discuss with patient information included in packaging

## Evaluation
**Positive therapeutic outcome**
• Decreased inflammation, pain in joints; decreased erythrocyte sedimentation rate (ESR)

---

## acarbose (Rx)
(a-kar′bose)
Precose
*Func. class.:* Oral antidiabetic
*Chem. class.:* α-Glucosidase inhibitor
**Pregnancy category B**

## Do not confuse:
Precose/PreCare

**Action:** Delays the digestion/absorption of ingested carbohydrates by inhibiting α-glucosidase, results in a smaller rise in blood glucose after meals; does not increase insulin production

**Therapeutic outcome:** Decreased blood glucose levels in diabetes mellitus

**Uses:** Type 2 diabetes mellitus, alone or in combination with a sulfonylurea, metformin

## Dosage and routes
*Initial dose*
*Adult:* PO 25 mg tid with first bite of meal

*Maintenance dose*
*Adult:* PO May be increased to 50-100 mg tid; dosage adjustment at 4-8 wk intervals
*Adult <60 kg:* PO Max 50 mg tid

**Available forms:** Tabs 25, 50, 100 mg

## Adverse effects
*GI: Abdominal pain, diarrhea, flatulence, increased serum transaminase level*

**Contraindications:** Hypersensitivity, diabetic ketoacidosis, cirrhosis, inflammatory bowel disease, ileus, colonic ulceration, partial intestinal obstruction, chronic intestinal disease, serum creatinine >2 mg/dl

**Precautions:** Pregnancy **B**, breastfeeding, children, renal/hepatic disease

### Pharmacokinetics
| | |
|---|---|
| **Absorption** | Unknown |
| **Distribution** | Unknown |
| **Metabolism** | GI tract |
| **Excretion** | Kidneys as intact drug |
| **Half-life** | Elimination 2 hr |

### Pharmacodynamics
| | |
|---|---|
| **Onset** | Unknown |
| **Peak** | 1 hr |
| **Duration** | Unknown |

## Interactions
*Individual drugs*
Digoxin: decreased acarbose effect
Insulin, phenytoin: increased hypoglycemia
Isoniazid, nicotinic acid, thyroid: increased hyperglycemia
*Drug classifications*
Calcium channel blockers, corticosteroids, diuretics, estrogens, oral contraceptives, phenothiazines, progestins, sympathomimetics: increased hyperglycemia
Digestive enzymes, intestinal absorbents, thiazide diuretics, loop diuretics, corticosteroids: decreased effect of acarbose
Sulfonylureas, insulin: increased hypoglycemia
*Drug/herb*
Alfalfa, aloe, basil, bay, bilberry, bitter melon, black cohosh, buchu, burdock, chromium, coenzyme Q10, coriander, eyebright (po), fenugreek, garlic, ginseng, glucomannan,

glucosamine, goat's rue, gymnema, hore-hound, horse chestnut, jambul, myrrh, myrtle, raspberry, Siberian ginseng: increased hypoglycemia

Bee pollen, blue cohosh, broom, chromium, elecampane, eucalyptus, gotu kola, senega: decreased hypoglycemia

**Drug/lab test**
Increased: AST, bilirubin
Decreased: calcium, vit B$_6$

## NURSING CONSIDERATIONS
### Assessment
• Assess for hypoglycemia (weakness, hunger, dizziness, tremors, anxiety, tachycardia, sweating), hyperglycemia; even though this product does not cause hypoglycemia, if on a sulfonylurea or insulin, hypoglycemia may be additive; if hypoglycemia occurs, treat with glucose or if severe, **IV** dextrose or IM glucagon
• Monitor 1 hr postprandial glucose for establishing effectiveness, then glycosylated Hgb q3 mo
• Monitor AST, ALT q3 mo × 1 yr, and periodically thereafter, if elevated dose, may need to be reduced or discontinued; obtain glycosylated Hgb periodically

### Nursing diagnoses
• Knowledge, deficient (teaching)
• Noncompliance (teaching)
• Nutrition: less than body requirements, imbalanced (adverse reactions)
• Nutrition: more than body requirements, imbalanced (uses)

### Implementation
• Give tid with first bite of each meal
• Provide storage in tight container in cool environment

### Patient/family education
• Teach patient the symptoms of hypoglycemia, hyperglycemia and what to do about each
• Instruct that medication must be taken as prescribed; explain consequences of discontinuing the medication abruptly; that insulin may need to be used during stress such as trauma, surgery, fever
• Tell patient to avoid OTC medications, herbal products unless approved by prescriber
• Teach patient that diabetes is a lifelong illness; product will not cure condition; that diet and exercise regimen must be followed
• Instruct patient to carry/wear emergency ID as diabetic

### Evaluation
**Positive therapeutic outcome**
• Improved signs, symptoms of diabetes

mellitus (decreased polyuria, polydipsia, polyphagia; clear sensorium, absence of dizziness, stable gait)

---

**acebutolol (Rx)**
(a-se-byoo' toe-lole)
Monitan ✤, Sectral
*Func. class.:* Antihypertensive
*Chem. class.:* Selective β$_1$-blocker; group II antidysrhythmic (II)

**Pregnancy category  B**

---

**Action:** Competitively blocks stimulation of β-adrenergic receptors within vascular smooth muscle (decreases rate of SA node discharge, increases recovery time), slows conduction of AV node resulting in decreased heart rate (negative chronotropic effect), which decreases O$_2$ consumption in myocardium because of β$_1$-receptor antagonism, also decreases renin-aldosterone-angiotensin system at high doses, inhibits β$_2$-receptors in bronchial system (high doses)

**Therapeutic outcome:** Decreased B/P, heart rate, AV conduction, control of dysrhythmias

**Uses:** Mild to moderate hypertension, management of PVCs

### Dosage and routes
**Hypertension**
*Adult:* PO 400 mg daily or in 2 divided doses; may be increased to desired response; maintenance 200-1200 mg daily in 2 divided doses
*Geriatric:* Max 800 mg daily

**Ventricular dysrhythmia**
*Adult:* PO 200 mg bid, may increase gradually; usual range 600-1200 mg daily; should be tapered over 2 wk before discontinuing
*Geriatric:* PO max 800 mg daily

**PVC management**
*Adult:* PO 200 mg bid, may increase gradually; usual range 600-1200 mg daily in divided doses

**Renal dose**
*Adult:* PO CCr 25-50 ml/min, reduce dose by 50%; if <25 ml/min reduce dose by 75%

**Available forms:** Caps 200, 400 mg; tabs 100, 200, 400 mg ✤

### Adverse effects
*CNS: Insomnia, fatigue, dizziness, mental changes,* memory loss, hallucinations, depres-

sion, lethargy, drowsiness, strange dreams, catatonia, headache
*CV:* **Profound hypotension, bradycardia, CHF,** cold extremities, postural hypotension, **2nd- or 3rd-degree heart block,** edema
*EENT:* Sore throat; dry, burning eyes
*ENDO:* Increased hypoglycemic response to insulin
*GI: Nausea, diarrhea,* vomiting, **mesenteric arterial thrombosis, ischemic colitis,** flatulence
*GU: Impotence,* decreased libido, dysuria, nocturia, polyuria
*HEMA:* **Agranulocytosis, thrombocytopenia, purpura**
*INTEG:* Rash, flushing, pruritus, sweating, alopecia, dry skin
*MISC:* Facial swelling, weight gain, decreased exercise tolerance
*MS:* Joint pain, cramping
*RESP:* **Bronchospasm,** dyspnea, wheezing, cough

**Contraindications:** Hypersensitivity to this agent or β-blockers; cardiogenic shock, heart block (2nd or 3rd degree), sinus bradycardia, CHF, cardiac failure

**Precautions:** Pregnancy **B**, breastfeeding, children, major surgery, diabetes mellitus, renal/hepatic/thyroid disease, COPD, asthma, well-compensated heart failure, peripheral vascular disease

### Pharmacokinetics

| | |
|---|---|
| **Absorption** | Well absorbed |
| **Distribution** | Crosses placenta, minimal CNS; protein binding 26% |
| **Metabolism** | Liver to diacetolol |
| **Excretion** | Urine |
| **Half-life** | 8-13 hr diacetolol, 3-4 hr acebutolol |

### Pharmacodynamics

| | PO (ANTIHYPER-TENSIVE) | PO (ANTIDYS-RHYTHMIAS) |
|---|---|---|
| **Onset** | 1-1½ hr | 1 hr |
| **Peak** | 2-4 hr | 4-6 hr |
| **Duration** | 12-24 hr | 10-12 hr |

### Interactions
#### Individual drugs
Calcium, cholestyramine, colestipol: decreased antihypertensive effect
Cimetidine, diltiazem, hydrALAZINE, methyldopa, prazosin, respirine, verapamil: bradycardia, increased hypotension

Ergots: increased peripheral ischemia
Insulin: increased hypoglycemia
#### Drug classifications
Anticholinergics, cardiac glycosides, diuretics, other antihypertensives, calcium channel blockers: increased hypotension, bradycardia
Antidiabetics, oral: increased hypoglycemic effect
Antihypertensives: increased hypertension
Calcium channel blockers, diuretics, nitrates: increased hypotension
Calcium channel blockers, cardiac glycosides, diuretics: bradycardia
NSAIDs: decreased antihypertensive effect
Oral sulfonylureas: attenuated effects
Theophyllines, β₂-agonists: decreased bronchodilatation
#### Drug/herb
Aconite: increased toxicity, death
Aloe, betel palm, buckthorn bark/berry, butterbur, cascara sagrada bark, cola tree, figwort, guarana, hawthorn, lily of the valley, motherwort, plantain, rhubarb root, senna leaf/fruits: increased acebutolol effect
Astragalus, cola tree: increased or decreased antihypertensive effect
Coenzyme Q10, yohimbe: decreased antihypertensive effect
St. John's wort: decreased acebutolol effect
#### Drug/lab test
Positive: antinuclear antibodies titer
Increased: serum lipoprotein levels, BUN, potassium, triglyceride, uric acid, LDH, AST, ALT, blood glucose, alkaline phosphatase

### NURSING CONSIDERATIONS
#### Assessment
• Monitor B/P during beginning treatment, periodically thereafter; pulse q4hr; note rate, rhythm, quality; apical/radial pulse before administration; notify prescriber of any significant changes (pulse <50 bpm)
• Check for baselines in renal, liver function tests before therapy begins
• Assess for edema in feet, legs daily, monitor I&O, daily weight; check for jugular vein distention, crackles bilaterally, dyspnea (CHF)
• Monitor skin turgor, dryness of mucous membranes for hydration status, especially geriatric

#### Nursing diagnoses
• Cardiac output, decreased (side effects)
• Injury, risk for (side effects)
• Knowledge, deficient (teaching)
• Noncompliance (teaching)

Adverse effects: *italic* = common, **bold** = life-threatening

## Implementation
### PO route
- Given before meals, at bedtime; tablet may be crushed or swallowed whole; give with food to prevent GI upset; reduced dosage in renal dysfunction; check pulse before giving, hold dose and notify prescriber if pulse is <60 bpm
- Store protected from light, moisture; place in cool environment

## Patient/family education
⚠ Teach patient not to discontinue product abruptly, severe cardiac reactions may occur, taper over 2 wk; may cause precipitate angina if stopped abruptly
- Advise patient that product may mask signs of hypoglycemia or alter blood glucose levels
- Teach patient not to use OTC products containing α-adrenergic stimulants (such as nasal decongestants, cold preparations); to avoid alcohol, smoking; to limit sodium intake as prescribed
- Teach patient how to take pulse and B/P at home, advise when to notify prescriber
- Instruct patient to comply with weight control, dietary adjustments, modified exercise program
- Tell patient to carry/wear emergency ID to identify product(s) that patient is taking, allergies; tell patient that product controls symptoms but does not cure
- Caution patient to avoid hazardous activities if dizziness or drowsiness is present; that product may cause sensitivity to cold
- Teach patient to report symptoms of CHF: difficult breathing, especially on exertion or when lying down, night cough, swelling of extremities or bradycardia, dizziness, confusion, depression, fever
- Teach patient to take product as prescribed, not to double or skip doses; take any missed doses as soon as remembered if several hours until next dose
- Advise patient to continue with required lifestyle changes (exercise, diet, weight loss, stress reduction)

## Evaluation
### Positive therapeutic outcome
- Decreased B/P in hypertension (after 1-2 wk)
- Absence of dysrhythmias

**Treatment of overdose:** Lavage, **IV** atropine for bradycardia, **IV** theophylline for bronchospasm, digoxin, $O_2$, diuretic for cardiac failure, hemodialysis, **IV** glucose for hypoglycemia, **IV** diazepam (or phenytoin) for seizures

**acetaminophen**  **(OTC)**
(a-seat-a-mee'noe-fen)
Abenol ♦, Acephen, Aceta, Actimol, Aminofen, Apacet, APAP, Apo-Acetaminophen ♦, Arthritis Foundation Pain Reliever Aspirin-Free, Aspirin-Free Anacin, Aspirin-Free Pain Relief, Atasol ♦, Banesin, Children's Feverall, Dapa, Dapacin, Datril, Exdol ♦, FemEtts, Genapap, Genebs, Halenol, Liquiprin, Mapap, Maranox, Meda, Neopap, Oraphen-PD, Panadol, Redutemp, Robigesic ♦, Rounax ♦, Silapap, Tapanol, Tempra, Tylenol
*Func. class.:* Nonopioid analgesic
*Chem. class.:* Nonsalicylate, paraaminophenol derivative

**Pregnancy category B**

**Action:** May block pain impulses peripherally that occur in response to inhibition of prostaglandin synthesis; does not possess antiinflammatory properties; antipyretic action results from inhibition of prostaglandins in the CNS (hypothalamic heat-regulating center)

**Therapeutic outcome:** Decreased pain, fever

**Uses:** Mild to moderate pain or fever; arthralgia, dental pain, dysmenorrhea, headache, myalgia, osteoarthritis

## Dosage and routes
*Adult and child >12 yr:* PO/RECT 325-650 mg q4-6hr prn, max 4 g/day
*Child 1-12 yr:* PO 10-15 mg/kg q4-6hr, max 5 doses/24 hr; RECT 10-20 mg/kg/dose q4-6hr
*Neonates:* RECT 10-15 mg/kg/dose q6-8hr

**Available forms:** Rectal supp 80, 120, 125, 325, 600, 650 mg; chewable tabs 80, 160 mg; caps 500 mg; elix 120, 160, 325 mg/5 ml; liquid 160 mg/5 ml, 500 mg/15 ml; sol 100 mg/1 ml, 120 mg/2.5 ml; tabs 160, 325, 500, 650 mg

## Adverse effects
*CNS:* Stimulation, drowsiness
*GI:* Nausea, vomiting, abdominal pain; **hepatotoxicity, hepatic seizure (overdose)**
*GU:* **Renal failure** (high, prolonged doses)
*HEMA:* **Leukopenia, neutropenia, hemolytic anemia** (long-term use), **thrombocytopenia, pancytopenia**
*INTEG:* Rash, urticaria
*SYST:* **Hypersensitivity**
*TOXICITY:* **Cyanosis, anemia, neutropenia, jaundice, pancytopenia, CNS stimula-**

tion, delirium followed by vascular collapse, seizures, coma, death

**Contraindications:** Hypersensitivity; intolerance to tartrazine (yellow dye #5), alcohol, table sugar, saccharin, depending on product

**Precautions:** Pregnancy **B**, breastfeeding, geriatric, anemia, renal/hepatic disease, chronic alcoholism

### Pharmacokinetics

| | |
|---|---|
| **Absorption** | Well absorbed (PO), variable (RECT) |
| **Distribution** | Widely distributed; crosses placenta in low concentrations |
| **Metabolism** | Liver 85%-95%; metabolites are toxic at high levels |
| **Excretion** | Kidneys—metabolites, breast milk |
| **Half-life** | 3-4 hr |

### Pharmacodynamics

| | PO | RECT |
|---|---|---|
| **Onset** | ½-1 hr | ½-1 hr |
| **Peak** | 1-3 hr | 1-3 hr |
| **Duration** | 3-4 hr | 3-4 hr |

### Interactions
#### Individual drugs
Alcohol, carbamazepine, diflunisal, isoniazid, rifabutin, rifampin, sulfinpyrazone: increased hepatotoxicity; decreased effect
Colestipol, cholestyramine: decreased absorption of acetaminophen
Warfarin: hypoprothrombinemia; long-term use, high doses of acetaminophen
Zidovudine: increased bone marrow suppression
#### Drug classifications
Barbiturates, hydantoins: decreased effect; increased hepatotoxicity
NSAIDs, salicylates: increased renal adverse reactions
#### Drug/herb
St. John's wort: decreased acetaminophen effect
#### Drug/lab test
Interference: chemstrip G, Dextrostix, Visidex II, 5-HIAA

### NURSING CONSIDERATIONS
#### Assessment
• Monitor liver function studies: AST, ALT, bilirubin, creatinine before therapy if long-term therapy is anticipated; may cause hepatic toxicity at doses >4 g/day with chronic use
• Monitor renal function studies: BUN, urine creatinine, occult blood; albumin indicates nephritis
• Monitor blood studies: CBC, pro-time if patient is on long-term therapy
• Check I&O ratio; decreasing output may indicate renal failure (long-term therapy)
• Assess for fever and pain: type of pain, location, intensity, duration, temp, diaphoresis
• Assess for chronic poisoning: rapid, weak pulse; dyspnea; cold, clammy extremities; report immediately to prescriber
• Assess hepatotoxicity: dark urine, clay-colored stools, yellowing of skin and sclera; itching, abdominal pain, fever, diarrhea if patient is on long-term therapy
• Assess allergic reactions: rash, urticaria; if these occur, product may have to be discontinued

#### Nursing diagnoses
• Injury, risk for (side effects)
• Knowledge, deficient (teaching)
• Mobility, impaired physical (uses)
• Pain, acute (uses)
• Pain, chronic (uses)

#### Implementation
**PO route**
• Administer to patient crushed or whole; chewable tabs may be chewed
• Give with food or milk to decrease gastric symptoms; give 30 min before or 2 hr after meals; absorption may be slowed
• Shake suspension well

#### Patient/family education
⭑ Teach patient not to exceed recommended dosage; acute poisoning with liver damage may result; acute toxicity includes symptoms of nausea, vomiting, and abdominal pain; prescriber should be notified immediately
• Inform patient that toxicity may occur when used with other combination products
• Advise patient not to use with alcohol or herbals without prescriber approval
• Teach patient to recognize signs of chronic overdose: bleeding, bruising, malaise, fever, sore throat
• Inform patient that urine may become dark brown as a result of phenacetin (metabolite of acetaminophen)
• Tell patient to notify prescriber for pain or fever lasting more than 3 days

#### Evaluation
**Positive therapeutic outcome**
• Decreased pain, use pain scoring
• Decreased fever

**Treatment of overdose:** Product level q4hr, gastric lavage, activated charcoal; administer oral acetylcysteine to prevent hepatic damage (*see acetylcysteine monograph,* p. 42)

---

**\*acetaZOLAMIDE** (Rx)
(a-set-a-zole'-a-mide)
Apo-Acetazolamide ✦, acetaZOLAMIDE, Damazide, Diamox, Diamox Sequels
*Func. class.:* Diuretic carbonic anhydrase inhibitor; antiglaucoma agent, antiepileptic
*Chem. class.:* Sulfonamide derivative
**Pregnancy category** C

**Do not confuse:**
acetaZOLAMIDE/acetoHEXAMIDE, Diamox/Dobutrex/Trimox

**Action:** Decreases the aqueous humor in the eye, which lowers intraocular pressure by the inhibition of carbonic anhydrase; also inhibits carbonic anhydrase activity in proximal renal tubules to decrease reabsorption of water, sodium, potassium, bicarbonate; decreases carbonic anhydrase in CNS, increasing seizure threshold; prevents uric acid or cysteine buildup in the renal system by the decrease in pH causing alkaline urine

**Therapeutic outcome:** Decreased intraocular pressure; control of seizures; prevention and treatment of acute mountain sickness; prevention of uric acid/cysteine renal stones; decreased edema in lung tissue and peripherally; decreased B/P

**Uses:** Open-angle glaucoma, angle-closure glaucoma (preoperatively if surgery delayed), epilepsy (petit mal, grand mal, mixed), edema in CHF, product-induced edema, acute altitude sickness

**Unlabeled uses:** Urine alkalinization, metabolic alkalosis in mechanical ventilation, decrease CSF production in infants with hydrocephalus, familial periodic paralysis, nystagmus

**Dosage and routes**
*Angle-closure glaucoma*
**Adult:** PO/**IV** 250 mg q4hr or 250 mg bid, to be used for short-term therapy

*Open-angle glaucoma*
**Adult:** PO/**IV** 250 mg-1 g/day in divided doses for amounts over 250 mg or 500 mg SR bid

*Edema in CHF*
**Adult: IV** 250-375 mg/day in AM
**Child: IV** 5 mg/kg/day in AM

*Seizures*
**Adult:** PO/**IV** 8-30 mg/kg/day in 1-4 divided doses, usual range 375-1000 mg/day; ER not recommended in seizures
**Child:** PO/**IV** 8-30 mg/kg/day in divided doses tid or qid, or 300-900 mg/m²/day, not to exceed 1 g/day

*Altitude sickness*
**Adult:** PO 250 mg q8-12hr; EXT REL 500 mg q12-24hr, start therapy 24-48 hr prior to ascent and ≥48 hr after arrival at high altitude

*Renal dose*
**Adult:** PO/**IV** CCr 10-50 ml/min, give dose q12hr; CCr <10 ml/min, avoid use
**Geriatric:** PO 250 mg bid; use lowest effective dose

*Urine alkalinization (unlabeled)*
**Adult:** PO 5 mg/kg/dose, repeat 2-3× over 24 hr

**Available forms:** Tabs 125, 250 mg; ext rel caps 500 mg; inj 500 mg

**Adverse effects**
*CNS:* Drowsiness, paresthesia, anxiety, depression, headache, dizziness, confusion, stimulation, fatigue, **seizures**
*EENT:* Myopia, tinnitus
*ENDO:* Hyperglycemia
*GI:* Nausea, vomiting, anorexia, diarrhea, melena, weight loss, **hepatic insufficiency, cholestatic jaundice, fulminant hepatic necrosis,** taste alterations
*GU:* Frequency, polyuria, **uremia,** glucosuria, hematuria, dysuria, crystalluria, renal calculi
*HEMA:* **Aplastic anemia, hemolytic anemia, leukopenia, agranulocytosis, thrombocytopenia, purpura, pancytopenia**
*INTEG:* Rash, pruritus, urticaria, fever, **Stevens-Johnson syndrome,** photosensitivity, flushing
*META: Hypokalemia, hyperchloremic acidosis,* hyponatremia

**Contraindications:** Hypersensitivity to sulfonamides, severe renal/hepatic disease, electrolyte imbalances (hyponatremia, hypokalemia), hyperchloremic acidosis, Addison's disease, long-term use in angle-closure glaucoma, adrenalcortical insufficiency

**Precautions:** Pregnancy **C**, breastfeeding, hypercalciuria, respiratory acidosis, COPD

## Pharmacokinetics

| | |
|---|---|
| **Absorption** | GI tract—65% if fasting, 75% with food; **IV**—complete |
| **Distribution** | Crosses placenta; widely distributed |
| **Metabolism** | None |
| **Excretion** | Kidneys, unchanged (80% within 24 hr); breast milk |
| **Half-life** | 2½-5½ hr |

## Pharmacodynamics

| | PO | PO–EXT REL | IV |
|---|---|---|---|
| **Onset** | 1½ hr | 2 hr | 2 min |
| **Peak** | 2-4 hr | 3-6 hr | 15 min |
| **Duration** | 8-12 hr | 18-24 hr | 4-5 hr |

## Interactions
### Individual drugs

CycloSPORINE: increased toxicity
Diflunisal: increased side effects
Flecainide: increased action of flecainide
Lithium: increased excretion of lithium
Memantine: increased action of memantine
Methenamine: decreased acetaZOLAMIDE effect
Phenytoin: increased action of phenytoin
Primidone: decreased primidone level
Quinidine: increased action of quinidine

### Drug classifications

Amphetamines: increased action
Anticholinergics: increased anticholinergic action
Salicylates: increased toxicity
Procainamide: increased action of procainamide
Quinidine: increased action of quinidine

### Drug/lab test

Decreased: thyroid iodine uptake
False positive: urinary protein, 17-hydroxysteroids

## NURSING CONSIDERATIONS
### Assessment

• Assess patient for tinnitus, hearing loss, ear pain; periodic testing of hearing is needed when high doses of this product are given by **IV** route
• Monitor manifestations of hypokalemia: *RENAL:* acidic urine, reduced urine osmolality, nocturia, polyuria, polydipsia; *CARDIAC:* hypotension, broad T wave, U wave, ectopy, tachycardia, weak pulse; *NEURO:* muscle weakness, altered LOC, drowsiness, apathy, lethargy, confusion, depression; *GI:* anorexia, nausea, cramps, constipation, distention, paralytic ileus; *RESP:* hypoventilation, respiratory muscle weakness
• Monitor for CNS, GI, cardiovascular, integumentary, neurologic manifestations of hypocalcemia: *CNS:* personality changes, anxiety, disturbances, depression, psychosis, nausea, vomiting; *GI:* constipation, abdominal pain from muscle spasm; *CV:* decreased contractility, decreased cardiac output, hypotension, lengthened ST segment, prolonged QT interval; *INTEG:* scaling eczema, alopecia, hyperpigmentation; *NEURO:* tetany, muscle twitching, cramping, grimacing, seizure, altered deep tendon reflexes, spasm
• Monitor for manifestations of hypomagnesemia: *CNS:* agitation; *NEURO:* muscle twitching, paresthesias, hyperactive reflexes, positive Babinski's reflex, dysphagia, nystagmus, seizures, tetany; *GI:* nausea, vomiting, diarrhea, anorexia, abdominal distention; *CARDIAC:* ectopy, tachycardia, broad, flat, or inverted T waves, depressed ST segment, prolonged QT, decreased cardiac output, hypotension
• Monitor for manifestations of hyponatremia: *CV:* increased B/P, cold, clammy skin, hypovolemia or hypervolemia, vomiting, diarrhea, abdominal cramps; *NEURO:* lethargy, increased intracranial pressure, confusion, headache, seizures, coma, fatigue, tremors, hyperreflexia
• Monitor for manifestations of hyperchloremia: *NEURO:* weakness, lethargy, coma; *RESP:* deep, rapid breathing
• Assess fluid volume status: I&O ratio and record, count or weigh diapers as appropriate, distended neck veins, crackles in lung, color, quality and specific gravity of urine, skin turgor, adequacy of pulses, moist mucous membranes, bilateral lung sounds, peripheral pitting edema; dehydration symptoms of decreasing output, thirst, hypotension, dry mouth, and mucous membranes should be reported
• Monitor electrolytes: potassium, sodium, calcium, magnesium; also include BUN, blood pH, ABGs, uric acid, CBC, blood glucose
• Assess B/P before and during therapy with patient lying, standing, and sitting as appropriate; orthostatic hypotension can occur rapidly
• Monitor blood, urine glucose in diabetic patients; glucose levels may be increased
• Assess for eye pain, change in vision when using product for intraocular pressure
• Assess neurologic status when using product for seizures
• Assess for decreased symptoms of acute mountain sickness: headache, nausea, vomiting, dizziness, fatigue, drowsiness, shortness of breath, insomnia

Adverse effects: *italic* = common, **bold** = life-threatening

- Assess for cross-sensitivity between other sulfonamides and this product

**Nursing diagnoses**
- Fluid volume, deficient (side effects)
- Fluid volume, excess (uses)
- Knowledge, deficient (teaching)
- Sensory perception, disturbed (uses)

**Implementation**
- Give in AM to avoid interference with sleep
- Administer fluids 2-3 L/day to prevent renal calculi, unless contraindicated
- Potassium replacement if potassium level is <3.0 ml/dl

**PO route**
- Do not crush or chew ext rel caps; caps may be opened and sprinkled on food
- Give with food, if nausea occurs, crush tabs and mix with sweet substance to counteract bitter taste

**IV route**
- Do not use solution that is yellow or has a precipitate or crystals
- Dilute 500 mg of product/5 ml or more sterile water for inj: use within 24 hr

**IV, direct route**
- Give over 1 min or more

**Intermittent IV infusion route**
- May be added to NS, $D_5W$, $D_{10}W$, 0.45% NaCl; give over 4-8 hr

*Additive compatibilities:* Cimetidine, ranitidine

*Additive incompatibilities:* Multivitamins

**Patient/family education**
- Teach patient to take the medication early in the day to prevent nocturia
- Instruct patient to take with food or milk if GI symptoms of nausea and anorexia occur
- Teach patient to maintain a record of weight on a weekly basis and notify prescriber of weight loss of >5 lb
- Caution patient that this product causes a loss of potassium, so food rich in potassium should be added to the diet; refer to a dietitian for assistance in planning
- Advise patient to wear protective clothing and sunscreen in the sun to prevent photosensitivity
- Teach patient not to use alcohol or any OTC medications without prescriber's approval; serious product reactions may occur
- Emphasize the need to contact prescriber immediately if muscle cramps, weakness, nausea, dizziness, or numbness occurs
- Teach patient to take own B/P and pulse and record

- Teach patient to continue taking medication even if feeling better; this product controls symptoms but does not cure the condition
- Teach patient to see ophthalmologist periodically; glaucoma is a slow process
- Advise patient to increase fluids to 2-3 L/day if not contraindicated
- Instruct patient to report nausea, vertigo, rapid weight gain, change in stools

**Evaluation**
**Positive therapeutic outcome**
- Decreased intraocular pressure
- Decreased edema
- Decreased seizures
- Prevention of mountain sickness
- Prevention of uric acid/cysteine stones

**Treatment of overdose:** Lavage if taken orally, monitor electrolytes, administer dextrose in saline, monitor hydration, CV, renal status

## acetylcholine ophthalmic
*See Appendix D*

## acetylcysteine (Rx)
(a-se-teel-sis'tay-een)
Acetadote, Mucomyst ♣, Mucosil, Parvolex ♣
*Func. class.:* Mucolytic; antidote—acetaminophen
*Chem. class.:* Amino acid L-cysteine
**Pregnancy category** B

**Action:** Decreases viscosity of secretions in respiratory tract by breaking disulfide links of mucoproteins; serves as a substrate of glutathione, which is necessary to inactivate toxic metabolites in acetaminophen overdose

**Therapeutic outcome:** Decreased hepatotoxicity from acetaminophen overdose (PO); decreased viscosity of mucus in respiratory disorders (inh)

**Uses:** Acetaminophen toxicity, bronchitis, cystic fibrosis, COPD, atelectasis

**Unlabeled uses:** Prevention of contrast media nephrotoxicity

**Dosage and routes**
*Mucolytic*
*Adult and child:* INSTILL 1-20 ml (10%-20% sol) q2-6hr prn, or 3-5 ml (20% sol) or 6-10 ml (10% sol ) tid or qid; nebulization (face, mask, mouthpiece, tracheostomy) 1-10 ml of a 20% sol or 2-20 ml of a 10% sol

q2-6hr; nebulization (tent, croupette) may require large dose, up to 300 ml/treatment

### Acetaminophen toxicity

**Adult and child:** PO 140 mg/kg, then 70 mg/kg q4hr × 17 doses to total 1330 mg/kg; **IV** loading dose 150 mg/kg over 60 min (dilution 150 mg/kg in 200 ml of $D_5$); maintenance dose 1:50 mg/kg over 4 hr (dilution 50 mg/kg in 500 ml $D_5$); maintenance dose 2:100 mg/kg over 16 hr (dilution 100 mg/kg in 1000 ml $D_5$)

**Available forms:** Oral sol 10%, 20%; inj 20% (200 mg/ml)

### Adverse effects

*CNS: Dizziness, drowsiness,* headache, fever, chills

*CV:* Hypotension

*EENT: Rhinorrhea,* tooth damage

*GI: Nausea,* stomatitis, constipation, vomiting, anorexia, **hepatotoxicity**

*INTEG:* Urticaria, rash, fever, clamminess, pruritus

*RESP:* **Bronchospasm,** burning, **hemoptysis,** chest tightness

**Contraindications:** Hypersensitivity, increased intracranial pressure, status asthmaticus

**Precautions:** Pregnancy **B,** breastfeeding, hypothyroidism, Addison's disease, CNS depression, brain tumor, asthma, renal/hepatic disease, COPD, psychosis, alcoholism, seizure disorders

#### Pharmacokinetics

| | |
|---|---|
| **Absorption** | Extensive (PO), locally (inh) |
| **Distribution** | Unknown |
| **Metabolism** | Liver |
| **Excretion** | Kidneys |
| **Half-life** | 5.6 hr (adult), 11 hr (newborn) |

#### Pharmacodynamics

| | PO | INH |
|---|---|---|
| **Onset** | Unknown | 1 min |
| **Peak** | Unknown | Unknown |
| **Duration** | Up to 4 hr | 100 min |

### Interactions
*Individual drugs*

Iron, copper, rubber: do not use with acetylcysteine

Amphotericin B, chlortetracycline, chymotrypsin, erythromycin lactobionate, hydrogen peroxide, iodized oil, oxytetracycline, sodium ampicillin, tetracycline, trypsin: do not mix with antibiotics

*Drug classifications*

Nitrates: increased effect

### NURSING CONSIDERATIONS
#### Assessment
**Mucolytic use**

• Assess cough: type, frequency, character, including sputum

• Assess characteristics, rate, rhythm of respirations, increased dyspnea, sputum; discontinue if bronchospasm occurs; ABGs for increased $CO_2$ retention in asthma patients

• Monitor VS, cardiac status including checking for dysrhythmias, increased rate, palpitations

**Antidotal use**

• Assess liver function tests, acetaminophen levels, pro-time, glucose, electrolytes; inform prescriber if dose is vomited or vomiting is persistent; provide adequate hydration; decrease dosage in hepatic encephalopathy

• Assess for nausea, vomiting, rash; notify prescriber if these occur

#### Nursing diagnoses

• Airway clearance, ineffective (uses) (mucolytic)

• Gas exchange, impaired (uses) (mucolytic)

• Injury, risk for (uses) (antidote)

• Knowledge, deficient (teaching)

• Poisoning, risk for (uses) (antidote)

#### Implementation

• Give decreased dosage to geriatric patients; their metabolism may be slowed; give gum, hard candy, frequent rinsing of mouth for dryness of oral cavity

• Use only if suction machine is available

**PO route (Antidotal use)**

• Lavage, then give within 24 hr; give with cola or soft drink to disguise taste; can be given with $H_2O$ through tubes; use within 1 hr

**Inhalation route (Mucolytic use)**

• Use before meals ½-1 hr for better absorption, to decrease nausea; only after patient clears airway by deep breathing, coughing

• Give by syringe 2-3 doses of 1-2 ml of 20% or 2-4 ml of 10% sol; 20% sol diluted with NS or water for injection; may give 10% sol undiluted

• Store in refrigerator: use within 96 hr of opening

• Provide assistance with inhaled dose: bronchodilator if bronchospasm occurs; wash face and rinse mouth after use to remove sticky feeling

• Use mechanical suction if cough insufficient to remove excess bronchial secretions

Adverse effects: *italic* = common, **bold** = life-threatening

## IV route

- Dilute with D$_5$, 0.45% NaCl

*Incompatibilities:* Rubber, metals, stability with other products unknown

## Patient/family education

**Mucolytic use**

- Tell patient to avoid driving or other hazardous activities until patient is stabilized on this medication; avoid alcohol, other CNS depressants; will enhance sedating properties of this product
- Teach patient that unpleasant odor will decrease after repeated use; that discoloration of solution after bottle is opened does not impair its effectiveness; avoid smoking, smoke-filled rooms, perfume, dust, environmental pollutants, cleaners
- Teach patient to report vomiting, as dose may need to be repeated

## Evaluation

**Positive therapeutic outcome**

- Absence of purulent secretions when coughing (mucolytic use)
- Clear lung sounds bilaterally (mucolytic use)
- Absence of hepatic damage (acetaminophen toxicity)
- Decreasing blood toxicology (acetaminophen toxicity)

---

## acyclovir (Rx)

(ay-sye′kloe-veer)

Avirax ✤, Zovirax

*Func. class.:* Antiviral

*Chem. class.:* Acylic purine nucleoside analog

### Pregnancy category B

**Action:** Interferes with DNA synthesis by conversion to acyclovir triphosphate, causing decreased viral replication, time of lesional healing

**Therapeutic outcome:** Decreased amount and time of healing of lesions

**Uses:** Mucocutaneous herpes simplex virus, herpes genitalis (HSV-1, HSV-2), varicella infections, herpes zoster, herpes simplex encephalitis

## Dosage and routes

### Renal dose

**Adult and child:** PO/**IV** CCr >50 ml/min 100% dose q8hr; CCr 25-50 ml/min 100% dose q12hr; CCr 10-25 ml/min 100% dose q24hr; CCr 0-10 ml/min 50% of dose q24hr

### *Herpes simplex*

*Adult:* PO 200 mg q4hr

*Adult and child >12 yr:* **IV** INF 10 mg/kg over 1 hr q8hr × 5 days

*Child <12 yr:* **IV** INF 250 mg/m$^2$ or 30 mg/kg/day divided q8hr over 1 hr × 5 days

### *Genital herpes*

*Adult:* PO 200 mg q4hr 5 times a day while awake × 5 days to 6 mo depending on whether initial, recurrent, or chronic; **IV** 5 mg/kg q8hr × 5 days

### *Herpes simplex encephalitis*

*Adult:* **IV** 10 mg/kg over 1 hr q8hr × 10 days

*Child 3 mo-12 yr:* **IV** 20 mg/kg q8hr × 10 days

*Child birth-3 mo:* **IV** 10 mg/kg q8hr × 10 days

### *Herpes zoster*

*Adult:* PO 800 mg q4hr while awake × 7-10 days; **IV** 10 mg/kg q8hr

### *Varicella-zoster*

*Adult:* PO 1000 mg q6hr × 5 days or 600-800 mg q4hr (5×/day while awake); **IV** 20 mg/kg q8hr × 5 days

*Child:* PO 10-20 mg/kg (max 800 mg) qid × 5 days; **IV** 500 mg/m$^2$ q8hr or 10 mg/kg q8hr × 7 days

### *Mucosal/cutaneous herpes simplex infections in immunosuppressed patients*

*Adult and child >12 yr:* **IV** 5 mg/kg q8hr × 7 days

*Child <12 yr:* **IV** 10 mg/kg q8hr × 7 days

### *Chickenpox*

*Adult and child >40 kg:* PO 800 mg qid × 5 days

*Child 2 yr or older <40 kg:* PO 20 mg/kg qid × 5 days

**Available forms:** Caps 200 mg; tabs 400, 800 mg; inj **IV** 500 mg; oral susp

## Adverse effects

***CNS:*** Tremors, confusion, lethargy, hallucinations, **seizures**, *dizziness, headache,* encephalopathic changes

***EENT:*** Gingival hyperplasia

***GI:*** Nausea, vomiting, diarrhea, increased ALT, AST, abdominal pain, glossitis, colitis

***GU:*** **Oliguria, proteinuria, hematuria,** vaginitis, moniliasis, **glomerulonephritis, acute renal failure,** changes in menses, polydipsia

***HEMA:*** **Thrombotic thrombocytopenia purpura, hemolytic uremic syndrome** (immunocompromised patient)

---

***INTEG:*** Rash, urticaria, pruritus, pain or phlebitis at **IV** site, unusual sweating, alopecia
***MS:*** Joint pain, leg pain, muscle cramps

**Contraindications:** Hypersensitivity to this product or ganciclovir, famciclovir, penciclovir, valacyclovir, or valganciclovir

**Precautions:** Pregnancy **B**, breastfeeding, renal/hepatic disease, electrolyte imbalance, dehydration, neurologic disease

### Pharmacokinetics

| | |
|---|---|
| **Absorption** | Minimal (PO) |
| **Distribution** | Widely distributed, crosses placenta; CSF concentration 50% plasma; protein binding 9%-33% |
| **Metabolism** | Liver, minimal |
| **Excretion** | Kidneys, 95% unchanged |
| **Half-life** | 2.0-3.5 hr, increased in renal disease |

### Pharmacodynamics

| | PO | IV |
|---|---|---|
| **Onset** | Unknown | Rapid |
| **Peak** | 1½-2½ | Infusion's end |
| **Duration** | Unknown | Unknown |

### Interactions
*Individual drugs*
Interferon: increased synergistic effect
Probenecid: increased neurotoxicity, nephrotoxicity
Zidovudine: increased CNS side effects

### NURSING CONSIDERATIONS
**Assessment**
• Monitor for signs of infection, type of lesions, area of body covered, purulent drainage
• Check I&O ratio; report hematuria, oliguria, fatigue, weakness; may indicate nephrotoxicity; check for protein in urine during treatment
• Monitor any patient with compromised renal system, since product is excreted slowly in poor renal system function; toxicity may occur rapidly
• Monitor liver studies: AST, ALT
• Monitor blood studies: WBC, RBC, Hct, Hgb, bleeding time; blood dyscrasias may occur; product should be discontinued
• Monitor renal studies: urinalysis, protein, BUN, creatinine, CCr; increased BUN, creatinine indicates renal failure and nephrotoxicity
• Obtain C&S before product therapy; product may be taken as soon as culture is taken; repeat C&S after treatment; determine the presence of other sexually transmitted diseases

• Monitor bowel pattern before, during treatment; if severe abdominal pain with bleeding occurs, product should be discontinued
• Assess allergies before treatment, reaction of each medication; place allergies on chart in bright red letters; allergic reaction: burning, stinging, swelling, redness, rash, vulvitis, pruritus
• Assess neurologic status in herpes encephalitis

### Nursing diagnoses
• Infection, risk for (uses)
• Knowledge, deficient (teaching)

### Implementation
**PO route**
• Do not break, crush, or chew caps
• Give with food to lessen GI symptoms; may give without regard to meals with 8 oz of water
• Store at room temperature in dry place
• May be taken orally before infection occurs or when itching or pain occurs, usually before eruptions
• Must be taken at equal intervals around the clock
• Shake suspension before use
**IV route**
• Provide increased fluids to 3 L/day to decrease crystalluria
• Give by int inf after reconstituting with 10 ml sterile water for injection/500 mg of product (50 mg/ml); shake; dilute in 0.9% NaCl, LR, D₅W, D₅/0.25% NaCl, D₅/0.45% NaCl, D₅/0.9% NaCl (7 mg/ml); give over at least 1 hr (constant rate) by infusion pump to prevent nephrotoxicity; do not reconstitute with sol containing benzyl alcohol or parabens; check infusion site for redness, pain, induration; rotate sites
• Lower dosage in acute or chronic renal failure
• Store at room temperature for up to 12 hr after reconstitution; if refrigerated, sol may show a precipitate that clears at room temperature, yellow discoloration does not affect potency
***Y-site compatibilities:*** Allopurinol, amikacin, ampicillin, amphotericin B cholesteryl sulfate complex, cefamandole, cefazolin, cefonicid, cefoperazone, ceforanide, cefotaxime, cefoxitin, ceftazidime, ceftizoxime, ceftriaxone, cefuroxime, cephapirin, chloramphenicol, cimetidine, clindamycin, cotrimoxazole, dexamethasone sodium phosphate, dimenhyDRINATE, diphenhydrAMINE, doxycycline, DOXOrubicin, erythromycin, famotidine, filgrastim, fluconazole, gallium,

Adverse effects: *italic* = common, **bold** = life-threatening

gentamicin, granisetron, heparin, hydrocortisone sodium succinate, hydromorphone, imipenem/cilastatin, lorazepam, magnesium sulfate, melphalan, methylPREDNISolone sodium succinate, metoclopramide, metronidazole, multivitamin infusion, nafcillin, oxacillin, paclitaxel, penicillin G potassium, pentobarbital, perphenazine, piperacillin, potassium chloride, propofol, ranitidine, remifentanil, sodium bicarbonate, tacrolimus, teniposide, tetracycline, theophylline, thiotepa, ticarcillin, tobramycin, trimethoprim-sulfamethoxazole, vancomycin, zidovudine
*Y-site incompatibilities:* DOBUTamine, DOPamine, ondansetron, verapamil
*Additive compatibilities:* Fluconazole
*Additive incompatibilities:* Blood products, protein-containing solutions, DOBUTamine, DOPamine

**Patient/family education**
**PO route**
• Teach patient that product may be taken orally before infection occurs or when itching or pain occur, usually before eruptions; that partners need to be told that patient has herpes; they can become infected, so condoms must be worn to prevent reinfections; that product does not cure infection, just controls symptoms and does not prevent infection to others
◆ Tell patient to report sore throat, fever, fatigue; may indicate superinfection; that product must be taken at equal intervals around the clock to maintain blood levels for duration of therapy
• Tell patient to notify prescriber of side effects: bruising, bleeding, fatigue, malaise; may indicate blood dyscrasias
• Tell patient to seek dental care during treatment to prevent gingival hyperplasia
• Teach female patients with genital herpes to have regular Pap smears to prevent undetected cervical cancer

**Evaluation**
**Positive therapeutic outcome**
• Absence of itching, painful lesions
• Crusting and healed lesions

**Treatment of overdose:** Discontinue product, hemodialysis, resuscitate if needed

**acyclovir topical**
*See Appendix D*

## adalimumab (Rx)
(add-a-lim'yu-mab)
Humira
*Func. class.:* Antirheumatic agent (disease modifying), immunomodulator

**Pregnancy category B**

**Do not confuse:**
Humira/Humalin

**Action:** A form of human IgG1 monoclonal antibody specific for human tumor necrosis factor (TNF). Elevated levels of TNF are found in patients with rheumatoid arthritis

**Therapeutic outcome:** Decreased pain, inflammation in joints, better ROM

**Uses:** Reduction in signs and symptoms and inhibiting progression of structural damage in patients with moderate to severe active rheumatoid arthritis in patients ≥18 years of age who have not responded to other disease-modifying agents, psoriatic arthritis, Crohn's disease

**Unlabeled uses:** Plaque psoriasis

**Dosage and routes**
*Ankylosing spondylitis/psoriatic arthritis*
*Adult:* SUBCUT 40 mg every other wk

*Crohn's disease*
*Adult:* SUBCUT 160 mg given as 4 inj on day 1, or 2 inj on days 1 and 2, then 80 mg at wk 2 and 40 mg every other wk, starting at wk 4

**Available forms:** Inj 40 mg/0.8 ml

**Adverse effects**
*CNS:* Headache
*EENT:* Sinusitis
*GI:* Abdominal pain, nausea, hepatic damage
*INTEG:* Rash, *inj site reaction*
*MISC:* Flulike symptoms, UTI, hypertension, back pain, lupuslike syndrome, risk of cancer, **risk of infection (TB, invasive fungal infections, other opportunistic infections); may be fatal**
*RESP: URI*

**Contraindications:** Hypersensitivity, active infections

**Precautions:** Pregnancy **B**, breastfeeding, children, geriatric, CNS demyelinating disease, lymphoma, latent TB

## Pharmacokinetics

| | |
|---|---|
| **Absorption** | Unknown |
| **Distribution** | Unknown |
| **Metabolism** | Unknown |
| **Excretion** | Unknown |
| **Half-life** | Terminal 2 wk |

## Pharmacodynamics

Unknown

## Interactions
### Drug classification

Vaccines: do not give concurrently; immunization should be brought up to date before treatment

## NURSING CONSIDERATIONS
### Assessment

- Assess for pain, stiffness, ROM, swelling of joints during treatment
- Check for inj site pain, swelling; usually occur after 2 inj (4-5 days)
- Check for infections, stop treatment if present, some serious infections, including sepsis, may occur; patients with active infections should not be started on this product

### Nursing diagnoses

- Activity intolerance (uses)
- Knowledge, deficient (teaching)
- Mobility, impaired physical (uses)
- Pain, chronic (uses)

### Implementation

- Do not admix with other sol or medications, do not use filter, protect from light

### Patient/family education

- Teach patient about self-administration if appropriate: inj should be made in thigh, abdomen, upper arm; rotate sites at least 1 inch from old site; do not inject in areas that are bruised, red, hard
- Advise patient that if medication is not taken when due, inject next dose as soon as remembered and inject next dose as scheduled

### Evaluation
**Positive therapeutic outcome**

- Decreased inflammation, pain in joints

---

# adefovir (Rx)
(add-ee-foh'veer)
Hepsera
*Func. class.:* Antiviral
## Pregnancy category C

**Action:** Inhibits hepatitis B virus DNA polymerase by competing with natural substrates and by causing DNA termination after its incorporation into viral DNA; causes viral DNA death

**Therapeutic outcome:** Improving liver function tests, lessening symptoms of chronic hepatitis B

**Uses:** Chronic hepatitis B

## Dosage and routes
*Adult:* PO 10 mg daily, optimal duration unknown

### Renal dose
*Adult:* PO CCr ≥50 ml/min 10 mg q24hr; CCr 20-49 ml/min 10 mg q48hr; CCr 10-19 ml/min 10 mg q72hr; hemodialysis 10 mg q7 days following dialysis

**Available forms:** Tabs 10 mg

## Adverse effects
*CNS: Headache*
*GI: Dyspepsia*, abdominal pain, nausea, vomiting, diarrhea, hepatomegaly
*GU:* Hematuria, glycosuria, **nephrotoxicity**
*MISC:* Fever, rash, weight loss

**Contraindications:** Hypersensitivity

**Precautions:** Pregnancy **C**, breastfeeding, children, geriatric, severe renal disease, impaired hepatic disease

## Pharmacokinetics

| | |
|---|---|
| **Absorption** | Rapidly from GI tract |
| **Distribution** | Unknown |
| **Metabolism** | Unknown |
| **Excretion** | Kidneys 45% |
| **Half-life** | 7.48 hr |

## Pharmacodynamics

| | |
|---|---|
| **Onset** | Unknown |
| **Peak** | 1¾ |
| **Duration** | Unknown |

## Interactions
### Individual drugs

Acetaminophen, aspirin, indomethacin: increased granulocytopenia

Acetaminophen, acyclovir, adriamycin, amphotericin B, cimetidine, dapsone, DOXOrubicin, fluconazole, flucytosine, ganciclovir,

---

Adverse effects: *italic* = common, **bold** = life-threatening

indomethacin, interferon, morphine, pent-amidine, phenytoin, probenecid, trimetho-prim, vinBLAStine, vinCRIStine: increased serum concentrations, toxicity

*Drug classifications*

Benzodiazepines, nucleoside analogs (experimental), sulfonamides: increased serum concentrations, toxicity

*Drug/lab test*

Increased: ALT, AST, amylase, creatine kinase

## NURSING CONSIDERATIONS
### Assessment

• Assess for nephrotoxicity: increasing CCr, BUN
• Assess for HIV before beginning treatment because HIV resistance may occur in chronic hepatitis B patients
• Assess for lactic acidosis, severe hepatomegaly with stenosis
• Assess geriatric patients more carefully; may develop renal, cardiac symptoms more rapidly
• Assess for exacerbations of hepatitis after discontinuing treatment, monitor liver function tests

### Nursing diagnoses

• Infection, risk for (uses)
• Knowledge, deficient (teaching)

### Implementation

• Give by mouth without regard to food
• Store in cool environment; protect from light

### Patient/family education

• Advise patient that optimal duration of treatment is unknown
• Advise patient to avoid use with other medications unless approved by prescriber
• Advise patient to notify prescriber of decreased urinary output
• Avoid breastfeeding

### Evaluation

**Positive therapeutic outcome**

• Decreased symptoms of chronic hepatitis B, improving liver function tests

---

**! HIGH ALERT**

## adenosine (Rx)
(ah-den'oh-seen)
Adenocard, Adeno-jec, Adenoscan
*Func. class.:* Antidysrhythmic—miscellaneous
*Chem. class.:* Endogenous nucleoside

**Pregnancy category C**

**Do not confuse:**
Adenocard/adenosine phosphate

**Action:** Slows conduction through AV node, can interrupt reentry pathways through AV node, and can restore normal sinus rhythm in patients with paroxysmal supraventricular tachycardia (PSVT)

**Therapeutic outcome:** Normal sinus rhythm in patients diagnosed with SVT

**Uses:** SVT, as a diagnostic aid to assess myocardial perfusion defects in CAD; Wolff-Parkinson-White (WPW) syndrome

### Dosage and routes
*Antidysrhythmic*
*Adult and child >50 kg:* **IV** BOL 6 mg; if conversion to normal sinus rhythm does not occur within 1-2 min, give 12 mg by rapid **IV** BOL; may repeat 12 mg dose again in 1-2 min
*Infant and child <50 kg:* **IV** BOL 0.05 mg/kg; if not effective, increase dose by 0.05 mg/kg q2 min to a max of 0.25 mg/kg or 12 mg

*Diagnostic use*
*Adult:* **IV** 140 mcg/kg/min × 6 min

*Wolff-Parkinson-White (WPW)*
*Adult/adolescent/child ≥50 kg:* **IV** BOL 6 mg by rapid inf, follow with saline flush; then **IV** BOL 12 mg if needed

**Available forms:** Inj 3 mg/ml (vial); 6 mg/2 ml (vial)

### Adverse effects

*CNS:* Light-headedness, dizziness, arm tingling, numbness, apprehension, blurred vision, headache
*CV:* Chest pain/pressure, **atrial tachydys-rhythmias,** sweating, palpitations, hypotension, *facial flushing*
*GI:* Nausea, metallic taste, throat tightness, groin pressure
*RESP:* Dyspnea, chest pressure, hyperventilation

**Contraindications:** Hypersensitivity, 2nd- or 3rd-degree heart block, AV block, sick sinus syndrome, atrial flutter, atrial fibrillation

---

**Precautions:** Pregnancy **C**, breastfeeding, children, geriatric, asthma

| Pharmacokinetics | |
|---|---|
| Absorption | Complete bioavailability |
| Distribution | Erythrocytes, cardiovascular endothelium |
| Metabolism | Liver, converted to inosine and adenosine monophosphate |
| Excretion | Kidneys |
| Half-life | 10 sec |

| Pharmacodynamics | |
|---|---|
| Onset | Rapid |
| Peak | Unknown |
| Duration | 1-2 min |

### Interactions
*Individual drugs*

Caffeine, theophylline: decreased effects of adenosine
Carbamazepine: increased heart block
Digoxin: increased ventricular fibrillation
Dipyridamole: increased effects of adenosine
Smoking: increased tachycardia
*Drug/herb*

Aconite: increased toxicity, death
Aloe, broom, chronic buckthorn use, cascara sagrada (chronic use), figwort, fumitory, goldenseal, kudzu, licorice, rhubarb, senna: increased effect
Coltsfoot, guarana: decreased effect
Horehound: increased serotonin effect

### NURSING CONSIDERATIONS
Assessment

• Monitor I&O ratio, electrolytes (potassium, sodium, chloride)
• Assess cardiopulmonary status: pulse, respiration, ECG intervals (PR, QRS, QT); check for transient dysrhythmias (PVCs, PACs, sinus tachycardia, AV block)
• Assess respiratory status: rate, rhythm, lung fields for crackles, watch for respiratory depression; bilateral crackles may occur in CHF patient; if increased respiration, increased pulse occurs, product should be discontinued
• Assess CNS effects: dizziness, confusion, paresthesias; product should be discontinued

### Nursing diagnoses
• Cardiac output, decreased (uses)
• Gas exchange, impaired (adverse reactions)
• Knowledge, deficient (teaching)

### Implementation
**IV, direct (bolus) route**
• Give **IV** BOL undiluted; give 6 mg or less by rapid inj; if using an **IV** line, use port near insertion site, flush with 0.9% NaCl (50 ml); warm to room temperature before giving
**Continuous infusion route**
• Give 30-ml vial undiluted via peripheral vein
*Solution compatibilities:* D₅LR, D₅W, LR, 0.9% NaCl
• Store at room temperature; sol should be clear; discard unused product

### Patient/family education
• Tell patient to report facial flushing, dizziness, sweating, palpitations, chest pain
• Instruct patient to rise from sitting or standing slowly to prevent orthostatic hypotension

### Evaluation
**Positive therapeutic outcome**
• Normal sinus rhythm
• Diagnosis of perfusion defect

---

### albumin, normal serum 5%/25% (Rx)
(al-byoo′min)
Albuminar 5%, Albutein 5%, Buminate 5%, Plasbumin 5%, Albuminar 25%, Albutein 25%, Buminate 25%, Plasbumin 25%
*Func. class.:* Blood derivative—volume expander
*Chem. class.:* Placental human plasma

**Pregnancy category C**

**Action:** Exerts colloidal oncotic pressure, which expands volume of circulating blood by pulling fluid from extravascular to intravascular spaces, and maintains cardiac output

**Therapeutic outcome:** Restoration of plasma volume by extravascular to intravascular fluid shift

**Uses:** Restores plasma volume in burns, hyperbilirubinemia, shock, hypoproteinemia, prevention of cerebral edema, cardiopulmonary bypass procedures, ARDS, hemorrhage; also replacement in nephrotic syndrome, hepatic failure

### Dosage and routes
*Burns*
*Adult:* **IV** dose to maintain plasma albumin at 30-50 g/L, use 5% sol initially, then 25% sol after 24 hr

Adverse effects: *italic* = common, **bold** = life-threatening

*Shock*
*Adult:* **IV** 500 ml of 5% sol q30 min, as needed
*Child:* 0.5-1 g/kg/dose

*Hypoproteinemia*
*Adult:* **IV** 1000-2000 ml of 5% sol daily, not to exceed 5-10 ml/min or 25-100 g of 25% sol daily, not to exceed 3 ml/min, titrated to patient response

*Hyperbilirubinemia/ erythroblastosis fetalis*
*Infant:* **IV** 1 g of 25% sol/kg 1-2 hr before transfusion

**Available forms:** Inj 50, 250 mg/ml (5%, 25%)

### Adverse effects
*CNS:* Fever, chills, flushing, headache
*CV:* **Fluid overload,** hypotension, erratic pulse, tachycardia
*GI:* Nausea, vomiting, increased salivation
*INTEG:* Rash, urticaria
*RESP:* Altered respirations, **pulmonary edema**

**Contraindications:** Hypersensitivity, CHF, severe anemia, renal insufficiency, pulmonary edema

**Precautions:** Pregnancy **C,** decreased salt intake, decreased cardiac reserve, lack of albumin deficiency, renal/hepatic disease, chronic anemia

| Pharmacokinetics | |
|---|---|
| **Absorption** | Complete bioavailability |
| **Distribution** | Intravascular spaces |
| **Metabolism** | Liver |
| **Excretion** | Unknown |
| **Half-life** | Unknown |

| Pharmacodynamics | |
|---|---|
| **Onset** | 15-30 min |
| **Peak** | Unknown |
| **Duration** | Unknown |

### Interactions
*Drug/lab test*
Increased: alkaline phosphatase

### NURSING CONSIDERATIONS
#### Assessment
• Monitor blood studies: Hct, Hgb; if serum protein declines, dyspnea, hypoxemia can result; check for decreasing B/P, erratic pulse, respiration
◆ Monitor CVP: pulmonary wedge pressure will increase if overload occurs; I&O ratio:

urinary output may decrease; CVP reading: distended neck veins indicate circulatory overload; shortness of breath, anxiety, insomnia, expiratory crackles, frothy blood-tinged sputum, cough, cyanosis indicate pulmonary overload
• Assess for allergy: fever, rash, itching, chills, flushing, urticaria, nausea, vomiting, hypotension; requires discontinuation of infusion, use of new lot if therapy reinstituted; premedicate with diphenhydrAMINE

#### Nursing diagnoses
• Fluid volume, deficit (uses)
• Fluid volume, excess (adverse reactions)
• Injury, risk for (uses)
• Knowledge, deficient (teaching)

#### Implementation
**IV route**
• Check type of albumin; some are stored at room temperature, some need to be refrigerated; use only amber-colored sol without precipitate; solution should be clear
• Give **IV** slowly to prevent fluid overload; 5% may be given undiluted; 25% may be given diluted ($D_5W$, 0.9% NaCl) or undiluted; give over 4 hr, use infusion pump
• Provide adequate hydration before, during administration; whole blood may need to be given to prevent anemia; monitor hydration during treatment
*Y-site compatibilities:* Diltiazem
*Solution compatibilities:* LR, NaCl, Ringer's, $D_5W$, $D_{10}W$, $D_{2\frac{1}{2}}W$, dextrose/saline, dextran$_6$ $D_5$, dextran$_6$ NaCl 0.9%, dextrose/ Ringer's, dextrose/LR

#### Patient/family education
• Explain use, reason for albumin; provide information on what to report to prescriber (hypersensitivity, fluid overload)

#### Evaluation
**Positive therapeutic outcome**
• Increased B/P, decreased edema (shock, burns)
• Increased serum albumin levels
• Increased plasma protein (hypoproteinemia)

## albuterol ⊕ (Rx)
(al-byoo'ter-ole)
AccuNeb, Airet, albuterol, Gen-
Salbutamol ✦, Novo-Salmol ✦, Proair
HFA, Proventil, Proventil HFA, Salbutamol,
Ventodisk, Ventolin, Ventolin HFA, Vospire
ER
*Func. class.:* Bronchodilator
*Chem. class.:* Adrenergic $\beta_2$-agonist,
sympathomimetic, bronchodilator

**Pregnancy category** C

### Do not confuse:
albuterol/atenolol, Proventil/ Prinivil,
salbutamol/salmeterol, Ventolin/Vantin

**Action:** Causes bronchodilatation by action
on $\beta_2$ (pulmonary) receptors by increasing
levels of cyclic adenosine monophosphate
(cAMP), which relaxes smooth muscle;
produces bronchodilatation; CNS, cardiac
stimulation, increased diuresis, and increased
gastric acid secretion; longer acting than
isoproterenol

**Therapeutic outcome:** Increased ability
to breathe because of bronchodilatation

**Uses:** Prevention of exercise-induced asthma,
acute bronchospasm, bronchitis, emphysema,
bronchiectasis, reversible airway obstruction

**Unlabeled uses:** Hyperkalemia in dialysis
patients

### Dosage and routes
*To prevent exercise-induced*
*bronchospasm*
*Adult:* INH (metered dose inhaler) 2 puffs
15 min before exercising

*Other respiratory conditions*
*Adult and child ≥12 yr:* INH (metered
dose inhaler) 2 puffs q4hr; PO 2-4 mg tid-qid,
not to exceed 8 mg; NEB/IPPB PO 2.5 mg
tid-qid
*Geriatric:* PO 2 mg tid-qid, may increase
gradually to 8 mg tid-qid
*Child 2-12 yr:* INH (metered dose inhaler)
0.1 mg/kg tid (max 2.5 mg tid-qid); NEB/IPPB
0.1-0.15 mg/kg/dose tid-qid or 1.25 mg
tid-qid for child 10-15 kg or 2.5 mg tid-qid
>15 kg

**Available forms:** Aerosol 90 mcg/
actuation; tabs 2, 4 mg; oral sol 2 mg/5 ml; ext
rel 4, 8 mg; inh sol 0.5, 0.83, 1, 2, 5 mg/ml;
powder for inh (Ventodisk) 200, 400 mcg; inh
caps 200 mcg; 100 mcg/spray, 80 inh/canister,
200 inh/canister

### Adverse effects
*CNS: Tremors, anxiety,* insomnia, headache,
dizziness, stimulation, *restlessness,* hallucina-
tions, flushing, irritability
*CV: Palpitations, tachycardia, hypertension,*
angina, hypotension, dysrhythmias
*EENT:* Dry nose, irritation of nose and throat
*GI: Heartburn, nausea, vomiting*
*MISC:* Flushing, sweating, anorexia, bad
taste/smell changes, hypokalemia
*MS:* Muscle cramps
*RESP:* Cough, wheezing, dyspnea, **broncho-
spasm,** dry throat

**Contraindications:** Hypersensitivity to
sympathomimetics, tachydysrhythmias, severe
cardiac disease, heart block

**Precautions:** Pregnancy **C**, breastfeeding,
exercise-induced bronchospasm (aerosol) in
children <12 yr, cardiac disorders, hyperthyroidism, diabetes mellitus, hypertension,
prostatic hypertrophy, angle-closure glaucoma,
seizures, hypoglycemia, seizure disorder

### Pharmacokinetics
| | |
|---|---|
| **Absorption** | Well absorbed (PO) |
| **Distribution** | Unknown |
| **Metabolism** | Liver extensively, tissues |
| **Excretion** | Unknown, breast milk |
| **Half-life** | 3-4 hr |

### Pharmacodynamics
| | PO | PO–EXT REL | INH |
|---|---|---|---|
| **Onset** | ½ hr | ½ hr | 5-15 min |
| **Peak** | 2½ hr | 2-3 hr | 1-1½ hr |
| **Dura-**<br>**tion** | 4-6 hr | 12 hr | 4-6 hr |

### Interactions
*Individual drugs*
Atomoxetine, selegiline: increased CV effects
*Drug classifications*
Adrenergics: increased action of albuterol; do
  not use together
β-Adrenergic blockers: block therapeutic
  effect
Antidepressants (tricyclic): increased chance
  of hypertension, do not use together
Bronchodilators (aerosol): increased action of
  bronchodilator
Diuretics (potassium-losing): increased ECG
  changes/hypokalemia
MAOIs: increased chance of hypertensive
  crisis, do not use together
Oxytocics: severe hypotension, do not use
  together
Theophylline: toxicity

Adverse effects: *italic* = common, **bold** = life-threatening

*Drug/herb*

Black tea, green tea, cola nut, guarana, yerba maté: increased stimulation

*Drug/food*

Caffeine products, chocolate: increased stimulation

## NURSING CONSIDERATIONS
### Assessment

• Assess respiratory function: vital capacity, forced expiratory volume, ABGs, lung sounds; heart rate, rhythm; B/P, sputum (baseline and during therapy)

• Determine that patient has not received theophylline therapy before giving dose, to prevent additive effect; client's ability to self-medicate

• Monitor for evidence of allergic reactions; paradoxic bronchospasm; withhold dose; notify prescriber if bronchospasm occurs

### Nursing diagnoses

• Airway clearance, ineffective (uses)
• Gas exchange, impaired (uses)
• Knowledge, deficient (teaching)

### Implementation
**PO route**

• Do not break, crush, or chew ext rel tabs
• Give PO with meals to decrease gastric irritation; oral sol for children (no alcohol, sugar)
• In geriatric patients, a spacing device is advised

**Aerosol route**

• Give after shaking metered dose inhaler; have patient exhale and place mouthpiece in mouth, inhale slowly while depressing inhaler, hold breath, remove inhaler, exhale slowly; allow at least 1 min between inhalations
• Store in light-resistant container; do not expose to temperatures > 86° F (30° C)

**Nebulizer/IPPB route**

• Dilute 5 mg/ml sol/2.5 ml 0.9% NaCl for inhalation; other solutions do not require dilution for nebulizer $O_2$ flow or compressed air 6-10 L/min

### Patient/family education

• Tell patient not to use OTC medications before consulting prescriber; excess stimulation may occur; instruct patient to use this medication before other medications and allow at least 5 min between each to prevent overstimulation; to limit caffeine products such as chocolate, coffee, tea, and cola
• Teach patient to use inhaler; review package insert with patient; to avoid getting aerosol in eyes or blurring may result; to wash inhaler in warm water and dry daily; to rinse mouth after using; to avoid smoking, smoke-filled rooms, persons with respiratory infections

◆ Teach patient that if paradoxic bronchospasm occurs to stop product immediately and notify prescriber

• Instruct patient on administration of dose, not to use more than prescribed; serious side effects may occur; if taking PO regularly and dose is missed, take when remembered; space other doses on new time schedule; do not double doses

• In geriatric patients, a spacing device is advised

### Evaluation
**Positive therapeutic outcome**

• Absence of dyspnea and wheezing after 1 hr
• Improved airway exchange
• Improved ABGs

**Treatment of overdose:** Administer a $\beta_1$-adrenergic blocker

---

### ⚠ HIGH ALERT

## aldesleukin, IL-2 (Rx)
(al-dess-loo'kin)

Proleukin

*Func. class.:* Antineoplastics—miscellaneous

*Chem. class.:* Interleukin-2, human recombinant, cytokine

**Pregnancy category C**

**Do not confuse:**
aldesleukin/oprelvekin, Proleukin/Oprelvekin/Prokine

**Action:** Enhancement of lymphocyte mitogenesis and stimulation of IL-2–dependent cell lines; enhancement of lymphocyte cytotoxicity; induction of killer cell activity; induction of interferon-γ production; results in activation of cellular immunity and cytokines and inhibition of tumor growth

**Therapeutic outcome:** Prevention of rapid growth of malignant cells

**Uses:** Metastatic renal cell carcinoma in adults, phase II for HIV in combination with zidovudine, melanoma (metastatic)

**Unlabeled uses:** Acute myelogenous leukemia (AML), cutaneous T-cell lymphoma (CTCL), HIV, Hansen's disease (leprosy), mycosis fungoides, non-Hodgkin's lymphoma

---

**A**

## Dosage and routes
### Renal cell cancer/malignant melanoma
*Adult:* **IV** INF 600,000 international units/kg (0.037 mg/kg) over 15 min q8hr × 14 doses; off 9 days; repeat schedule for another 14 doses, for a maximum of 28 doses/course

**Available forms:** Powder for inj 22 million international units/vial

### Adverse effects
*CNS:* Mental status changes, dizziness, sensory dysfunction, syncope, motor dysfunction, fever, chills, headache, impaired memory, depression, sleep disturbances, hallucinations, rigors, neuropathy
*CV:* Hypotension, sinus tachycardia, dysrhythmias, bradycardia, PVCs, PACs, myocardial ischemia, **myocardial infarction, cardiac arrest,** capillary leak syndrome, **CVA**
*EENT:* Reversible visual changes
*GI:* Nausea, vomiting, *diarrhea,* stomatitis, anorexia, GI bleeding, dyspepsia, constipation, **intestinal perforation/ileus,** jaundice, ascites
*GU:* **Oliguria/anuria, proteinuria, hematuria,** dysuria, **renal failure**
*HEMA: Anemia,* **thrombocytopenia, leukopenia, coagulation disorders, leukocytosis, eosinophilia**
*INTEG:* Pruritus, *erythema, rash,* dry skin, **exfoliative dermatitis,** purpura, petechiae, urticaria
*MS:* Arthralgia, myalgia
*RESP:* Pulmonary congestion, dyspnea, **pulmonary edema, respiratory failure,** tachypnea, pleural effusion, wheezing, **apnea**
*SYST:* Infection

**Contraindications:** Hypersensitivity, abnormal thallium stress test or pulmonary function tests, organ allografts

**Precautions:** Pregnancy **C**, breastfeeding, children, CNS metastases, bacterial infections, renal/hepatic/cardiac/pulmonary disease, anemia, thrombocytopenia

### Pharmacokinetics

| | |
|---|---|
| **Absorption** | Complete bioavailability |
| **Distribution** | Rapid extracellular, intravascular |
| **Metabolism** | Kidneys (convoluted tubules) |
| **Excretion** | Kidneys |
| **Half-life** | 85 min |

### Pharmacodynamics

| | |
|---|---|
| **Onset** | 4 wk |
| **Peak** | Unknown |
| **Duration** | ≤12 mo |

### Interactions
#### Individual drugs
Indomethacin, methotrexate, asparaginase, DOXOrubicin: increased toxicity
#### Drug classifications
Aminoglycosides, antineoplastics: increased toxicity
Antihypertensives: increased hypotension
Cytotoxic chemotherapy: increased toxicity
Glucocorticosteroids: decreased tumor effectiveness
Psychotropics: unpredictable reactions
#### Drug/lab test
Increased: bilirubin, BUN, serum creatinine, transaminase, alkaline phosphatase, hypomagnesemia, acidosis hypocalcemia, hypophosphatemia, hypokalemia, hyperuricemia, hypoalbuminemia, hypoproteinemia, hyponatremia, hyperkalemia, alkalosis (toxic effect of product)

### NURSING CONSIDERATIONS
#### Assessment
• Monitor CBC, differential, platelet count weekly; withhold product if WBC is <2000/mm³ or platelet count is <75,000/mm³; notify prescriber of these results; transfusion of RBCs, platelets may be required
◆ Identify capillary leak syndrome (CLS), including a drop in mean arterial pressure (2-12 hr after initiating therapy); hypotension and hypoperfusion will occur; if B/P <90 mm Hg, monitor ECG, CVP in cardiac patients
• Monitor renal function studies: BUN, serum uric acid, urine CCr, electrolytes before, during therapy; I&O ratio; report fall in urine output to <30 ml/hr
• Monitor temp q4hr; fever may indicate beginning infection
• Check liver function tests before, during therapy: bilirubin, AST, ALT, alkaline phosphatase, LDH as needed or monthly
• Monitor ECG; watch for ST-T wave changes, low QRS and T, possible dysrhythmias (sinus tachycardia, PVCs)
• Monitor baselines in pulmonary function; document FEV >2 L or ≥75% before therapy; check daily VS, pulse oximetry, dyspnea, crackles, ABGs, watch for respiratory failure, intubate if necessary
• Obtain stress thallium study before therapy; document normal ejection fraction, unimpaired wall motion

*Adverse effects: italic = common, **bold** = life-threatening*

- Assess for bleeding: hematuria, guaiac, bruising or petechiae, mucosa, or orifices q8hr
- Assess for GI symptoms: frequency of stools, cramping
- Assess for acidosis, signs of dehydration: rapid respirations, poor skin turgor, decreased urine output, dry skin, restlessness, weakness
- Assess for cardiac status: B/P, pulse, character, rhythm, rate, ABGs, ECG
- Assess for infection: sore throat; antibiotics may be prescribed prophylactically

### Nursing diagnoses
- Body image, disturbed (adverse reactions)
- Infection, risk for (adverse reactions)
- Injury, risk for (adverse reactions)
- Knowledge, deficient (teaching)

### Implementation
**Intermittent IV infusion route**
- Give by intermittent IV INF after diluting 22 million international units (1.3 mg)/1.2 ml sterile (1.1 mg/ml) H$_2$O for inj at side of vial and swirl, do not shake; dilute dose with 50 ml D$_5$W and give over 15 min; use plastic bag; do not use an in-line filter; give through Y-tube or 3-way stopcock
- Give DOPamine 1-5 kg/min before onset of hypotension; decreased dose preserves kidney output
- Give hydrocortisone, dexamethasone, or sodium bicarbonate (1 mEq/1 ml) for extravasation, apply ice compresses
- Store any diluted product in refrigerator; do not freeze; administer within 48 hr; bring to room temperature before infusing; discard unused portion

*Y-site compatibilities:* Amikacin, **IV** fat emulsion, gentamicin, morphine, piperacillin, potassium chloride, ticarcillin, tobramycin, TPN #145, amphotericin B, calcium gluconate, diphenhydrAMINE, DOPamine, fluconazole, foscarnet, heparin, magnesium sulfate, metoclopramide, ondansetron, ranitidine, trimethoprim/sulfamethoxazole

### Patient/family education
- Teach patient to avoid use of products containing aspirin or ibuprofen, razors, commercial mouthwash because bleeding may occur; to report symptoms of bleeding, hematuria, tarry stools
- Tell patient to report signs of anemia: fatigue, headache, irritability, faintness, shortness of breath
- Tell patient to report any changes in breathing or coughing even several months after treatment
- Advise patient that contraception will be

necessary during treatment; teratogenesis may occur
- Teach patient to report signs/symptoms of infection: fever, chills, sore throat; patient should avoid crowds or persons with known infections
- Advise patient to avoid alcohol, NSAIDs, salicylates; GI bleeding may occur
- Advise patient that visual problems may occur but are reversible

### Evaluation
**Positive therapeutic outcome**
- Decreased spread of malignancy

## alemtuzumab (Rx)
(al-em-tuz'uh-mab)
Campath
*Func. class.:* Antineoplastic—miscellaneous
*Chem. class.:* Monoclonal antibody
**Pregnancy category** C

**Action:** Composed of recombinant DNA-derived humanized monoclonal antibody (campath-1H), binds to CD52 antigen that is present on surface of B and T lymphocytes, causes lysis of leukemic cells

**Therapeutic outcome:** Decreased in number of white blood cells

**Uses:** B-cell chronic lymphocytic leukemia that has been treated with alkylating agents and that has failed fludarabine therapy, graft-versus-host disease (GVHD)

**Unlabeled uses:** Multiple sclerosis

### Dosage and routes
*Adult:* **IV** 3 mg over 2 hr daily; when tolerated, increase to 10 mg; when 10 mg tolerated, increase to 30 mg daily; maintenance is 30 mg/day 3×/wk on alternate days for 12 wk, titration usually takes 3-7 days, max single dose 30 mg; max weekly dose 90 mg

**Available forms:** Sol for inj 30 mg/ml

### Adverse effects
*CNS: Dizziness,* insomnia, depression, headache, tremor, somnolence, fatigue, drowsiness, weakness
*CV: Hypo/hypertension, tachycardia, edema, chest pain, supraventricular tachycardia*
*GI: Anorexia, diarrhea,* constipation, *nausea, stomatitis, vomiting, abdominal pain, dyspepsia*
*HEMA:* **Anemia, neutropenia, thrombocytopenia, pancytopenia,** purpura, epistaxis
*INTEG: Rash,* local reaction, pruritus
*MISC:* Rigors, fever, *infusion reactions*

*RESP:* Cough, pneumonia, rhinitis, **broncho-spasm,** dyspnea, pharyngitis

**Contraindications:** Hypersensitivity, active systemic infection, immunodeficiency

**Precautions:** Pregnancy **C,** breastfeeding, children

### Pharmacokinetics

| | |
|---|---|
| **Absorption** | Unknown |
| **Distribution** | Unknown; steady state 6 wk |
| **Metabolism** | Unknown |
| **Excretion** | Unknown |
| **Half-life** | 12 days |

### Pharmacodynamics

Unknown

### Interactions
*Individual drugs*
Radiation: increased bone marrow depression
*Drug classifications*
Live virus vaccines: decreased antibody reaction
Other neoplastics: increased bone marrow depression
*Drug/lab test*
Diagnostic tests using antibodies

### NURSING CONSIDERATIONS
### Assessment
• Assess CBC, platelets qwk or more often if myelosuppression occurs; assess CD4+ after therapy until recovery of >200 cells/mcL
• Assess for symptoms of infection; chills, fever, headache, may be masked by product fever; do not administer product if infection is present
• Assess CNS reaction: LOC, mental status, dizziness, confusion
• Assess cardiac status: lung sounds; ECG before and during treatment, especially in those with cardiac disease
• Assess for bone marrow depression: bruising, bleeding, blood in stools, urine, sputum, emesis

### Nursing diagnoses
• Body image, disturbed (adverse reactions)
• Infection, risk for (adverse reactions)
• Injury, risk for (adverse reactions)
• Knowledge, deficient (teaching)
• Nutrition: less than body requirements, imbalanced (side effects)

### Implementation
**IV route**
• Do not give **IV** push or bolus
• Withdraw amount needed; do not shake ampule; use 5 µm filter prior to dilution, check for particulate matter and discoloration; inject into 100 ml sterile 0.9% NaCl or D₅W, invert to mix, do not add other products or infuse in same **IV** tubing
• Store reconstituted sol for ≤8 hr at room temperature, do not freeze; protect from light

### Patient/family education
• Instruct patient to take acetaminophen for fever
• Advise patient to avoid hazardous tasks, since confusion, dizziness may occur
• Instruct patient to report signs of infection: sore throat, fever, diarrhea, vomiting

### Evaluation
**Positive therapeutic outcome**
• Decreased in production of malignant lymphocytes

### alendronate (Rx)
(al-en′droe-nate)
Fosamax
*Func. class.:* Bone-resorption inhibitor
*Chem. class.:* Bisphosphonate
**Pregnancy category C**

**Do not confuse:**
Fosamax/Flomax

**Action:** Decreases rate of bone resorption and may directly block dissolution of hydroxyapatite crystals of bone; inhibits normal and abnormal bone resorption, mineralization

**Therapeutic outcome:** Decreased symptoms of osteoporosis, Paget's disease

**Uses:** Treatment and prevention of osteoporosis in postmenopausal women, treatment of osteoporosis in men, Paget's disease, treatment of corticosteroid-induced osteoporosis in postmenopausal women not receiving estrogen, or in men who are continuing corticosteroid treatment with low bone mass

**Dosage and routes**
*Osteoporosis in postmenopausal women*
*Adult and geriatric:* PO 10 mg daily or 70 mg qwk

*Paget's disease*
*Adult and geriatric:* PO 40 mg daily × 6 mo, consider retreatment for relapse

Adverse effects: *italic* = common, **bold** = life-threatening

*Prevention of osteoporosis*
**Adult:** PO 5 mg daily or 35 mg qwk

*Corticosteroid-induced osteoporosis in postmenopausal women (not receiving estrogen)*
**Adult:** PO 10 mg daily

*Corticosteroid-induced osteoporosis in men or premenopausal women (not receiving estrogen)*
**Adult:** PO 5 mg daily

**Available forms:** Tabs 5, 10, 35, 40, 70 mg; oral sol 70 mg

### Adverse effects

**CNS:** Headache
**GI:** Abdominal pain, anorexia, constipation, nausea, vomiting, esophageal ulceration, acid reflux, dyspepsia, **perforation**, diarrhea
**META:** Anemia, hypokalemia, hypomagnesemia, hypophosphatemia, hypocalcemia
**MS:** Bone pain, osteonecrosis of the jaw
**SYST: Angioedema, Stevens-Johnson syndrome, toxic epidermal necrolysis**

**Contraindications:** Hypersensitivity to bisphosphonates, delayed esophageal emptying, inability to sit or stand for 30 min, hypocalcemia

**Precautions:** Pregnancy **C**, breastfeeding, children, CCr <35 ml/min, esophageal disease, ulcers, gastritis, poor dental health

### Pharmacokinetics

| | |
|---|---|
| **Absorption** | Unknown |
| **Distribution** | Mainly to bones |
| **Metabolism** | Unknown |
| **Excretion** | Via kidneys |
| **Half-life** | Unknown |

### Pharmacodynamics

Unknown

### Interactions
*Individual drugs*
Ranitidine (**IV**): increased alendronate effect
*Drug classifications*
Aminoglycosides, antacids, calcium supplements: decreased absorption
NSAIDs, salicylates: increased GI reactions
*Drug/food*
Caffeine, food, orange juice: decreased product absorption

### NURSING CONSIDERATIONS
**Assessment**
◆ Assess for serious reactions: angioedema, Stevens-Johnson syndrome, toxic epidermal necrolysis
• Assess dental status, regular dental exams should be done
• Hormonal status if a woman, prior to treatment
• For osteoporosis: bone density testing
• For Paget's disease: increased skull size, bone pain, headache
• Monitor renal studies and Ca, P, Mg, K
• Assess for hypercalcemia: paresthesia, twitching, laryngospasm, Chvostek's, Trousseau's signs
• Monitor alkaline phosphatase; level of 2× upper limit of normal is indicated for Paget's disease

**Nursing diagnoses**
• Injury, risk for (uses)
• Knowledge, deficient (teaching)

**Implementation**
• Give PO for 6 mo to be effective in Paget's disease; take with 8 oz of water 30 min before 1st food, beverage, or medication of the day
• Patient to remain upright for 30 min after dose to prevent esophageal irritation
• Store in cool environment out of direct sunlight

**Patient/family education**
• Teach patient to remain upright for 30 min after dose to prevent esophageal irritation; if dose is missed, skip dose, do not double doses or take later in day
• Teach patient to take in AM, only before food, other meds, to take with 6-8 oz of water (not mineral water)
• To take calcium, vit D if instructed by provider
• To use weight-bearing exercise to increase bone density
• Teach patient to let provider know if pregnancy is planned or suspected or if nursing

**Evaluation**
**Positive therapeutic outcome**
• Increased bone mass, absence of fractures

---

### alfuzosin (Rx)
(al-fyoo′zoe-sin)
Uroxatral
*Func. class.:* Antiadrenergic
*Chem. class.:* Quinazolone
**Pregnancy category** B

**Action:** Binds preferentially to $\alpha_{1A}$-adrenoceptor subtype located mainly in the prostate

---

 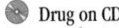

**Therapeutic outcome:** Resolution of symptoms of benign prostatic hyperplasia

**Uses:** Symptoms of benign prostatic hyperplasia; has not been studied for and is not indicated for the treatment of high blood pressure

**Dosage and routes**
*Adult:* PO ext rel 10 mg daily, taken after same meal each day

**Available forms:** Ext rel tabs 10 mg

**Adverse effects**
*CNS: Dizziness, headache,* fatigue
*CV:* Postural hypotension (dizziness, light-headedness, fainting) within a few hours of administration, chest pain, tachycardia
*GI:* Nausea, abdominal pain, dyspepsia, constipation
*GU:* Impotence, priapism
*INTEG:* Rash
*MISC:* Body pain in general
*RESP:* Upper respiratory tract infection, pharyngitis, bronchitis, sinusitis

**Contraindications:** Hypersensitivity, moderate to severe hepatic impairment, not indicated for use in women or children, breastfeeding (but not used in women)

**Precautions:** Pregnancy **B,** geriatric, coronary artery disease, coronary insufficiency, mild hepatic disease, mild/moderate/severe renal disease, history of QT prolongation or coadministration with medications known to prolong QT interval, torsade de pointes, syncope, surgery, prostate cancer, orthostatic hypotension, ocular surgery, CAD, dysrhythmias, angina

**Pharmacokinetics**

| | |
|---|---|
| Absorption | Unknown |
| Distribution | Moderately protein bound (82%-90%) |
| Metabolism | Liver (by CYP3A4 enzyme) |
| Excretion | Urine |
| Half-life | 10 hr |

**Pharmacodynamics**
Unknown

**Interactions**
*Individual drugs*
Alcohol: possible increased effects of alfuzosin
Doxazosin, itraconazole, ketoconazole, prazosin, ritonavir, terazosin: do not take concurrently
*Drug classifications*
CYP3A4 inhibitors (ketoconazole, itraconazole, ritonavir): do not take concurrently

**NURSING CONSIDERATIONS**
**Assessment**
• Assess for prostatic hyperplasia: change in urinary patterns, baseline and throughout treatment
• Monitor CBC with differential and liver function tests; B/P and heart rate; QT prolongation
• Monitor BUN, uric acid, urodynamic studies (urinary flow rates, residual volume)
• Monitor I&O ratios, weight daily, edema; report weight gain or edema

**Nursing diagnoses**
• Urinary elimination, impaired (uses)
• Knowledge, deficient (teaching)

**Implementation**
• Swallow tabs whole; do not break, crush, or chew tabs
• Store in tight container in cool environment

**Patient/family education**
• Advise not to drive or operate machinery for 4 hr after first dose or after dosage increase

**Evaluation**
**Positive therapeutic outcome**
• Decreased symptoms of benign prostatic hyperplasia

**aliskiren**
Tekturna
*See Appendix A, Selected New Drugs*

**alitretinoin (Rx)**
(al-ee-tret'i-noyn)
Panretin
*Func. class.:* Retinoid, 2nd generation, topical antineoplastic
**Pregnancy category D**

**Action:** Controls cellular differentiation and proliferation of neoplastic and healthy cells by binding to retinoid receptors

**Therapeutic outcome:** Decreased size and number of lesions

**Uses:** Kaposi's sarcoma cutaneous lesions

**Dosage and routes**
*Adult:* TOP Apply enough gel to cover lesions with a generous coating, allow to dry for 3-5 min before covering with clothing, do not apply near mucosal areas, apply as long as benefit occurs, do not rub gel into lesion

**Available forms:** Topical gel 0.1%

Adverse effects: *italic* = common, **bold** = life-threatening

**Adverse effects**
***INTEG:*** Rash, stinging, pain, warmth, redness, erythema, blistering, crusting, peeling, dermatitis, pain

**Contraindications:** Pregnancy **D**, hypersensitivity to retinoids

**Precautions:** Breastfeeding, eczema, sunburn, geriatric, cutaneous T-cell lymphoma

| Pharmacokinetics | |
|---|---|
| **Absorption** | Small amounts |
| **Distribution** | Unknown |
| **Metabolism** | Unknown |
| **Excretion** | Kidneys |
| **Half-life** | Unknown |

| Pharmacodynamics |
|---|
| Unknown |

**Interactions**
*Individual drugs*
DEET: do not use around DEET (an insect repellant)

**NURSING CONSIDERATIONS**
**Assessment**
• Assess part of body involved, including time involved, what helps or aggravates condition, cysts, dryness, itching
• Assess for dermal toxicity that may start as erythema, then edema; product may need to be discontinued and restarted

**Nursing diagnoses**
• Body image, disturbed (uses)
• Knowledge, deficient (teaching)
• Skin integrity, impaired (uses)

**Implementation**
• Apply bid initially to lesions, can be increased to tid-qid according to tolerance, discontinue for a few days if severe reactions occur
• Store at room temperature
• Wash hands after application

**Patient/family education**
• Instruct patient to avoid application on normal skin, and to avoid getting cream in eyes, nose, other mucous membranes
• Advise patient to avoid sunlight, sunlamps or to use protective clothing or sunscreen to prevent burns
• Advise patient that treatment may cause warmth, stinging; dryness; peeling will occur
• Caution patient that product does not cure condition; only relieves symptoms; that therapeutic results may be seen in 2-3 wk but may not be optimal until after 6 wk

**Evaluation**
**Positive therapeutic outcome**
• Decrease in size and number of lesions

---

**allopurinol** (Rx)
(al-oh-pure′i-nole)
alloprim, allopurinol, Apo-Allopurinol ✤,
Lopurin, Purinol ✤, Zyloprim
*Func. class.:* Antigout drug, antihyperuricemic
*Chem. class.:* Xanthine enzyme inhibitor
**Pregnancy category** C

**Do not confuse:**
allopurinol/apresoline, Lopurin/Lupron

**Action:** Inhibits the enzyme xanthine oxidase, reducing uric acid synthesis

**Therapeutic outcome:** Decreasing serum uric acid levels, decreasing joint pain

**Uses:** Chronic gout, hyperuricemia associated with malignancies, recurrent calcium oxalate calculi, Chagas disease, cutaneous/visceral leishmaniasis, uric acid calculi

**Dosage and routes**
*Increased uric acid levels in malignancies*
*Adult:* PO 600-800 mg/day in divided doses, start up to 3 days prior to chemotherapy; **IV** INF 200-400 mg/m$^2$/day, max 600 mg/day 24-48 hr prior to chemotherapy
*Child 6-10 yr:* PO 300 mg/day
*Child <6 yr:* PO 150 mg/day
*Child:* **IV** INF 200 mg/m$^2$/day, initially as a single dose or divided q6-12hr

*Gout (mild)*
*Adult:* PO 100-300 mg/day, increase qwk based on uric acid levels, max 800 mg/day, maintenance dose 100-200 mg bid-tid

*Gout (moderate-severe)*
*Adult:* PO 400-600 mg/day in a single dose or divided bid-tid, max 800 mg/day

*Recurrent calculi*
*Adult:* PO 200-300 mg/day in a single dose or divided bid-tid, max 300 mg/dose, 800 mg/day

*Uric acid nephropathy prevention*
*Adult and child >10 yr:* PO 600-800 mg daily × 2-3 days

*Renal dose*
*Adult:* PO CCr ml/min 200 mg/day; CCr 40 ml/min 150 mg/day; CCr 20 ml/min 100 mg/day; CCr 10 ml/min 100 mg every other day; CCr <10 ml/min 100 mg 3×/wk; **IV** CCr

10-20 ml/min 200 mg/day; CCr 3-10 ml/min 100 mg/day; CCr <3 ml/min 100 mg/day at intervals

**Available forms:** Tabs, scored, 100, 300 mg; inj 500 mg/vial

**Adverse effects**
*CNS: Headache,* drowsiness, neuritis, paresthesia
*EENT:* Retinopathy, cataracts, epistaxis
*GI: Nausea, vomiting, anorexia, malaise,* metallic taste, cramps, peptic ulcer, diarrhea, stomatitis
*HEMA:* **Agranulocytosis, thrombocytopenia, aplastic anemia, pancytopenia, leukopenia, bone marrow suppression,** eosinophilia
*INTEG:* Fever, chills, dermatitis, pruritus, purpura, erythema, ecchymosis, alopecia, rash, **Stevens-Johnson syndrome**
*MISC:* Myopathy, arthralgia, hepatomegaly, **cholestatic jaundice, renal failure, exfoliative dermatitis**

**Contraindications:** Hypersensitivity

**Precautions:** Pregnancy **C**, breastfeeding, children, renal/hepatic disease

| Pharmacokinetics | |
| --- | --- |
| **Absorption** | 80% |
| **Distribution** | Widely distributed |
| **Metabolism** | Liver to oxypurinol |
| **Excretion** | Kidneys |
| **Half-life** | 2-3 hr, terminal 18-30 hr |

| Pharmacodynamics | | |
| --- | --- | --- |
| | PO | IV |
| **Onset** | Unknown | Unknown |
| **Peak** | 2-4 hr | Unknown |
| **Duration** | Unknown | Unknown |

**Interactions**
*Individual drugs*
Ammonium chloride potassium/sodium phosphate, vit C: increased kidney stone formation
Ampicillin, amoxicillin: increased risk of rash
Azathioprine: increased bone marrow depression
Mercaptopurine: increased bone marrow depression
Rasburicase: increased xanthine nephropathy, calculi
Theophylline: increased action of theophylline
*Drug classifications*
ACE inhibitors: increased hypersensitivity
Aluminum salts: decreased effects of allopurinol

Anticoagulants (oral): increased action of oral anticoagulants
Antidiabetics (oral): increased action of antidiabetics
Antineoplastics: increased bone marrow suppression
Diuretics (thiazide): increased hypersensitivity

**NURSING CONSIDERATIONS**
**Assessment**
• Assess for pain including location, characteristics, onset/duration, frequency, quality, intensity or severity of pain, precipitating factors
• Monitor uric acid levels q2 wk; normal uric acid levels are 6 mg/dl or less; check I&O ratio; increase fluids to 2 L/day to prevent stone formation, toxicity
• Monitor CBC, AST, BUN, creatinine before starting treatment, monthly; check blood glucose in diabetic patients receiving oral antidiabetic agents
• Monitor nutritional status: discourage organ meat, sardines, salmon, legumes, gravies (high-purine foods), alcohol

**Nursing diagnoses**
• Knowledge, deficient (teaching)
• Nutrition: more than body requirements, imbalanced (uses)

**Implementation**
**PO route**
• Give with meals to prevent GI symptoms; crush and mix with food or fluids for patients with swallowing difficulties
• Increased fluid intake to 2 L/day
• Give a few days before antineoplastic therapy if using for hyperuricemia associated with malignancy
**IV infusion route**
• Reconstitute 30-ml vial with 25 ml of sterile water for inj; dilute to desired conc with 0.9% NaCl for inj or $D_5$ for inj, begin inf within 10 hr
*Solution incompatibilities:* Amikacin, amphotericin B, carmustine, cefotaxime, chlorproMAZINE, cilastatin, cimetidine, clindamycin, cytarabine, dacarbazine, DAUNOrubicin, diphenhydrAMINE, DOXOrubicin, doxycycline, droperidol, floxuridine, gentamicin, haloperidol, hydrOXYzine, idarubicin, imipenem, mechlorethamine, meperidine, metoclopramide, methylPREDNISolone, minocycline, nalbuphine, netilmicin, ondansetron, prochlorperazine, promethazine, sodium bicarbonate, streptozocin, tobramycin, vinorelbine

#### Patient/family education
- Tell patient to increase fluid intake to 2 L/day; to avoid taking large doses of vit C; kidney stone formation may occur; to maintain a diet enhancing urine alkalinity (e.g., milk, other dairy products); if taking for calcium oxalate stones, reduce dairy products, refined sugar, sodium, meat
- Tell patient to report skin rash, stomatitis, malaise, fever, aching; product should be discontinued
- Advise patient to avoid hazardous activities if drowsiness or dizziness occurs; response may take several days to determine
- Tell patient to avoid alcohol, caffeine; these substances increase uric acid levels and decrease allopurinol levels
- Teach patient to report side effects and adverse reactions to prescriber, including rash, itching, nausea, vomiting

#### Evaluation
**Positive therapeutic outcome**
- Decreased pain in joints
- Decreased stone formation in kidney
- Decreased uric acid level to 6 mg/dl

---

### almotriptan (Rx)
(al-moh-trip'tan)
Axert
*Func. class.:* Antimigraine agent
*Chem. class.:* 5-HT$_1$ receptor agonist, triptan

**Pregnancy category** C

**Action:** Binds selectively to the vascular 5-HT$_1$ receptor subtype, exerts antimigraine effect; causes vasoconstriction in cranial arteries

**Therapeutic outcome:** Absence of migraines

**Uses:** Acute treatment of migraine with or without aura

#### Dosage and routes
*Adult:* PO may use 6.25 mg dose initially, but 12.5 mg is more effective; may repeat dose after 2 hr; do not give more than 2 doses/24 hr, 25 mg/day or 4 treatment cycles within any 30-day period

#### Renal/hepatic dose
*Adult:* PO 6.25 mg initially, max 12.5 mg

**Available forms:** Tabs 6.25, 12.5 mg

#### Adverse effects
*CV:* *Flushing,* palpitations, tachycardia, **coronary artery vasospasm, MI, ventricular fibrillation, ventricular tachycardia**

*EENT:* Throat, mouth, nasal discomfort; vision changes
*GI:* Nausea, xerostomia
*INTEG:* Sweating
*MS:* *Weakness, neck stiffness,* myalgia
*NEURO:* *Tingling, hot sensation, burning, feeling of pressure, tightness, numbness, dizziness, sedation,* headache, anxiety, fatigue, cold sensation
*RESP:* Chest tightness, pressure

**Contraindications:** Hypersensitivity, cluster headache, hemiplegia, vascular migraine, ischemic heart disease or risk for, peripheral vascular syndrome; concurrent use of ergotamine-containing preparations, uncontrolled hypertension, basilar or hemiplegic migraine; concurrent MAOI therapy or within 2 wk

**Precautions:** Pregnancy **C,** breastfeeding, children <18 yr, geriatric, postmenopausal women, men >40 yr, risk factors for coronary artery disease, hypercholesterolemia, obesity, diabetes, impaired renal/hepatic function

| Pharmacokinetics | |
|---|---|
| Absorption | Well absorbed (~70%) |
| Distribution | 35% protein bound |
| Metabolism | Liver (metabolite); metabolized by MAO-A, CYP2D6, CYP3A4 |
| Excretion | Urine, feces |
| Half-life | 3-4 hr |

| Pharmacodynamics | |
|---|---|
| Onset | Unknown |
| Peak | 1-3 hr |
| Duration | 3-4 hr |

#### Interactions
*Individual drugs*
Ergot: increased vasospastic effects
Ketoconazole: increased plasma concentration of almotriptan
*Drug classifications*
5-HT$_1$ agonists, ergot derivatives: increased vasospastic effects
CYP2D6 inhibitors: increased almotriptan effect; do not use together
MAOIs: increased almotriptan effect; do not use together
*Drug/herb*
Butterbur, feverfew: increased almotriptan effect

---

## NURSING CONSIDERATIONS
### Assessment

- Assess B/P, signs/symptoms of coronary vasospasms
- Assess for tingling, hot sensation, burning, feeling of pressure, numbness, flushing
- Assess for stress level, activity, recreation, coping mechanisms
- Assess neurologic status: LOC, blurring vision, nausea, vomiting, tingling in extremities preceding headache
- Assess for ingestion of tyramine-containing foods (pickled products, beer, wine, aged cheese), food additives, preservatives, colorings, artificial sweeteners, chocolate, caffeine, which may precipitate these types of headaches

### Nursing diagnoses
- Knowledge, deficient (teaching)
- Pain, acute (uses)

### Implementation
- Swallow tabs whole; do not break, crush, or chew tabs
- Provide quiet, calm environment with decreased stimulation from noise, bright light, excessive talking

### Patient/family education
- Instruct patient to use contraception while taking product, notify prescriber if pregnancy is planned or suspected, avoid breastfeeding
- Advise patient to have dark, quiet environment available
- Inform patient that product does not prevent or reduce number of migraine attacks
- Advise patient to report chest pain, drowsiness, dizziness, tingling, flushing, pressure

### Evaluation
**Positive therapeutic outcome**
- Decreased in severity of migraine

**Treatment of overdose:** Gastric lavage followed by activated charcoal; clinical and ECG monitoring for ≥20 hr after overdose

---

### alprazolam (Rx)
(al-pray'zoe-lam)
Apo-Alpraz ✦, Niravam, Novo-Alprazol ✦, Nu-Alpraz ✦, Xanax, Xanax XR
*Func. class.:* Antianxiety/sedative/hypnotic
*Chem. class.:* Benzodiazepine, short/intermediate acting

**Pregnancy category D**

**Controlled substance schedule IV**

**Do not confuse:**
alprazolam/lorazepam, Xanax/Lanoxin/Tylox/Zantac

**Action:** Depresses subcortical levels of CNS, including limbic system, reticular formation; potentiates GABA (γ-aminobutyric acid)

**Therapeutic outcome:** Decreased anxiety

**Uses:** Anxiety, panic disorders with or without agoraphobia, anxiety with depressive symptoms

**Unlabeled uses:** Premenstrual syndrome, dysphoric disorders, insomnia

### Dosage and routes
*Anxiety disorder*
*Adult:* PO 0.25-0.5 mg tid, may increase q3-4 days if needed, max 4 mg/day in divided doses
*Geriatric:* PO 0.125-0.25 mg bid; increase by 0.125 mg as needed

*Panic disorder*
*Adult:* PO 0.5 mg tid, may increase up to 1 mg/day q3-4 days, max 10 mg/day; EXT REL TABS (Xanax XR) give daily in AM 0.5-1 mg initially, maintenance 1-10 mg daily

*Premenstrual dysphoric disorders (unlabeled)*
*Adult:* PO 0.25 mg bid-qid, starting on day 16-18 of menses, taper over 2-3 days when menses occurs

*Hepatic dose*
Reduce dose by 50%

**Available forms:** Tabs 0.25, 0.5, 1, 2 mg; ext rel tabs (Xanax XR) 0.5, 1, 2, 3 mg; orally disintegrating tabs 0.25, 0.5, 1, 2 mg; oral solution 0.5 mg/5 ml, 1 mg/ml

### Adverse effects
*CNS: Dizziness, drowsiness,* confusion, headache, anxiety, tremors, stimulation, fatigue, depression, insomnia, hallucinations, memory impairment, poor coordination

---

Adverse effects: *italic* = common, **bold** = life-threatening

*CV: Orthostatic hypotension,* **ECG changes, tachycardia,** hypotension
*EENT: Blurred vision,* tinnitus, mydriasis
*GI:* Constipation, dry mouth, nausea, vomiting, anorexia, diarrhea, weight gain/loss, increased appetite
*GU:* Decreased libido
*INTEG:* Rash, dermatitis, itching

**Contraindications:** Pregnancy **D,** breast-feeding, hypersensitivity to benzodiazepines, angle-closure glaucoma, psychosis, addiction

**Precautions:** Geriatric, debilitated, hepatic disease, obesity, severe pulmonary disease

## Pharmacokinetics

| | |
|---|---|
| **Absorption** | Slow, complete |
| **Distribution** | Widely distributed; crosses placenta; crosses blood-brain barrier |
| **Metabolism** | Liver, to active metabolites |
| **Excretion** | Kidneys, breast milk |
| **Half-life** | 12-15 hr |

## Pharmacodynamics

| | |
|---|---|
| **Onset** | 1 hr |
| **Peak** | 1-2 hr |
| **Duration** | 4-6 hr, therapeutic response 2-3 days |

## Interactions
### Individual drugs
Alcohol: increased CNS depression
Cigarette smoking: decreased drug level
CYP3A4 inhibitors (cimetidine, disulfiram, erythromycin, fluoxetine, isoniazid, itraconazole, ketoconazole, metoprolol, propoxyphene, propranolol, valproic acid): increased action of alprazolam
Levodopa: decreased action of levodopa
Rifampin: decreased action of alprazolam
### Drug classifications
Anticonvulsants, antihistamines: increased CNS depression
CYP3A4 inducers (barbiturates): decreased action of alprazolam
Sedative/hypnotics, opioids: increased CNS depression
Xanthines: decreased sedation
### Drug/herb
Cat's claw, chamomile, cowslip, echinacea, goldenseal, hops, kava, licorice, Queen Anne's lace, skullcap, St. John's wort, valerian, wild cherry: increased CNS depression
### Drug/food
Grapefruit juice: increased product level
### Drug/lab test
Increased: ALT, AST, alkaline phosphatase

## NURSING CONSIDERATIONS
### Assessment
🔷 Assess mental status: mood, sensorium, anxiety, affect, sleeping pattern, drowsiness, dizziness, especially geriatric; physical dependency, withdrawal symptoms: anxiety, panic attacks, agitation, seizures, headache, nausea, vomiting, muscle pain, weakness; suicidal tendencies; indications of increasing tolerance and abuse; withdrawal seizures may occur after rapid decrease in dose or abrupt discontinuation; short duration of action makes it the product of choice in the geriatric
• Monitor B/P (with patient lying, standing), pulse; if systolic B/P drops 20 mm Hg, hold product, notify prescriber
• Monitor blood studies: CBC during long-term therapy; blood dyscrasias have occurred rarely; decreased hematocrit, neutropenia may occur
• Monitor hepatic studies: AST, ALT, bilirubin, creatinine LDH, alkaline phosphatase, if on long-term treatment
• Monitor I&O; indicate renal dysfunction if on long-term treatment

### Nursing diagnoses
• Anxiety (uses)
• Injury, risk for (adverse reactions)
• Knowledge, deficient (teaching)

### Implementation
• Give with food or milk for GI symptoms; tab may be crushed, if patient is unable to swallow medication whole, and mixed with foods or fluids; may divide total daily dose into more times/day, if anxiety occurs between doses
• Give sugarless gum, hard candy, frequent sips of water for dry mouth
• Discontinue, decrease by 0.5 mg q3 days
• Place orally disintegrating tabs on tongue to dissolve
• Give ext rel tab in AM

### Patient/family education
• Tell patient that product may be taken with food or fluids, and tabs may be crushed or swallowed whole
• Tell patient not to use for everyday stress or longer than 4 mo unless directed by prescriber; not to take more than prescribed amount; may be habit forming; not to double doses or skip doses; memory impairment is a sign of long-term use
• Tell patient to avoid OTC preparations unless approved by prescriber; alcohol and CNS depressants will increase CNS depression
• Tell patient to avoid driving, activities that require alertness, since drowsiness may occur; to avoid alcohol ingestion or other psychotro-

pic medications; to rise slowly or fainting may occur, especially geriatric; that drowsiness may worsen at beginning of treatment
• Tell patient not to discontinue medication abruptly after long-term use; withdrawal symptoms include vomiting, cramping, tremors, seizures

### Evaluation
**Positive therapeutic outcome**
• Decreased anxiety, restlessness, sleeplessness (short-term treatment only)

**Treatment of overdose:** Lavage, VS, supportive care, flumazenil

---

### ! HIGH ALERT

**alteplase** (Rx)
(al-ti-plaze')
Activase, Activase rt-PA ✤, Lysatec rt-PA ✤, Cathflo, tissue plasminogen activator, t-PA
*Func. class.:* Thrombolytic enzyme
*Chem. class.:* Tissue plasminogen activator (TPA)

**Pregnancy category** C

**Do not confuse:**
alteplace/Altace

**Action:** Produces fibrin conversion of plasminogen to plasmin; able to bind to fibrin, convert plasminogen in thrombus to plasmin, which leads to local fibrinolysis, limited systemic proteolysis

**Therapeutic outcome:** Lysis of thrombi in MI, pulmonary emboli (life threatening)

**Uses:** Lysis of obstructing thrombi associated with acute MI; conditions requiring thrombolysis (e.g., PE, DVT, unclotting arteriovenous shunts, acute ischemic CVA)

**Unlabeled uses:** Arterial thromboembolism, deep vein thrombosis (DVT), occlusion prophylaxis, percutaneous coronary intervention (PCI)

### Dosage and routes
*Pulmonary embolism*
*Adult:* **IV** 100 mg over 2 hr, then heparin

*Acute ischemic stroke*
*Adult:* **IV** 0.9 mg/kg, max 90 mg; give as inf over 1 hr, give 10% of dose **IV** BOL over 1st min

*Myocardial infarction (standard infusion)*
*Adult >65 kg:* **IV** a total of 100 mg; 6-10 mg given **IV** BOL over 1-2 min, 60 mg given over first hr, 20 mg given over second hr, 20 mg given over third hr
*Adult <65 kg:* **IV** 1.25 mg/kg over 3 hr; 60% in first hr (10% as a bolus); remaining 40% over next 2 hr

*Myocardial infarction (accelerated infusion)*
*Adult >67 kg:* 100 mg total dose: give 15 mg **IV** BOL, then 50 mg over 30 min, then 35 mg over 60 min
*Adult <67 kg:* 15 mg **IV** BOL: 0.75 mg/kg over 30 min; 0.5 mg/kg over 60 min

*Occlusion prophylaxis (unlabeled)*
*Adult >30 kg:* Use 110% of internal lumen volume of catheter, max 2 mg in 2 ml; may use up to 2 doses (120 min apart)

**Available forms:** Powder for inj 50 mg (29 million international units/vial), 100 mg (58 million international units/vial), lyophilized powder for injection 2 mg

### Adverse effects
*CV:* **Sinus bradycardia, ventricular tachycardia, accelerated idioventricular rhythm, bradycardia, recurrent ischemic stroke**
*INTEG:* Urticaria, rash
*SYST:* **GI, GU, intracranial, retroperitoneal bleeding, surface bleeding, anaphylaxis**

**Contraindications:** Hypersensitivity, active internal bleeding, recent CVA, severe uncontrolled hypertension, intracranial/intraspinal surgery/trauma (within 3 mo), aneurysm, brain tumor, platelets <100,000 mm$^3$

**Precautions:** Pregnancy **C**, breastfeeding, children, geriatric, neurologic deficits, mitral stenosis, recent GI/GU bleeding, diabetic retinopathy

| Pharmacokinetics | |
|---|---|
| **Absorption** | Complete |
| **Distribution** | Unknown |
| **Metabolism** | >80% liver |
| **Excretion** | Kidneys |
| **Half-life** | 35 min |

| Pharmacodynamics | |
|---|---|
| **Onset** | Immediate |
| **Peak** | 30-45 min |
| **Duration** | 4 hr |

## Interactions
### Individual drugs
Abciximab, aspirin, clopidogrel, dipyridamole, eptifibatide, heparin, plicamycin, ticlopidine, tirofiban, valproic acid: increased bleeding

### Drug classifications
Anticoagulants (oral), cephalosporins (some), NSAIDs, salicylates: increased bleeding

### Drug/herb
Agrimony, alfalfa, angelica, anise, basil, bay, bilberry, black haw, bogbean, bromelain, buchu, chondroitin, cinchona bark, dong quai, fenugreek, feverfew, garlic, ginger, ginkgo, ginseng, horse chestnut, Irish moss, kelp, kelpware, khella, lovage, lungwort, meadowsweet, motherwort, mugwort, nettle, papaya, parsley (large amounts), pau d'arco, pineapple, poplar, prickly ash, safflower, saw palmetto, tonka bean, turmeric, wintergreen, yarrow: increased risk of bleeding

Chamomile, coenzyme Q10, flax, glucomannan, goldenseal, guar gum: decreased anticoagulant effect

### Drug/lab test
Increased: pro-time, APTT, TT

## NURSING CONSIDERATIONS
### Assessment
- Monitor VS q15 min, B/P, pulse, respirations (including peripheral), neurologic signs, temp at least q4hr; temp >104° F (40° C) indicates internal bleeding; monitor rhythm closely; ventricular dysrhythmias may occur with hyperfusion; monitor heart, breath sounds, neurologic status, and peripheral pulses
-  Assess for bleeding during first hr of treatment and 24 hr after procedure: hematuria, hematemesis, bleeding from mucous membranes, epistaxis, ecchymosis, puncture sites; guaiac all body fluids and stools; obtain blood studies (Hct, platelets, PTT, pro-time, TT, APTT) before starting therapy; pro-time or APTT must be less than 2 times control before starting therapy; TT or pro-time q3-4hr during treatment; obtain CPK-MB to identify product effectiveness
- Assess hypersensitivity: fever, rash, facial swelling, dyspnea, itching, chills; mild reaction may be treated with antihistamines; report to prescriber
- Monitor ECG; on monitor, watch for segment changes, changes in rhythm: sinus bradycardia, ventricular tachycardia, accelerated idioventricular rhythm may occur due to reperfusion, cardiac enzymes, radionuclide myocardial scanning/coronary angiography

## Nursing diagnoses
- Injury, risk for (adverse reactions)
- Pain, chronic (uses)
- Tissue perfusion, ineffective (uses)

## Implementation
### Intermittent IV infusion route
- Give after reconstituting with provided diluent; add appropriate amount of sterile water for inj (no preservatives); 20-mg vial/20 ml or 50-mg vial/50 ml (1 mg/ml); mix by slow inversion or dilute with 0.9% NaCl, $D_5W$ to a concentration of 0.5 mg/ml further dilution; 1.5 to <0.5 mg/ml may result in precipitation of product; use 18-G needle; flush line with NaCl after administration; use reconstituted IV sol within 8 hr or discard, within 6 hr of coronary occlusion for best results
-  Do not use 150 mg or more total dose; intracranial bleeding may occur
- Give heparin therapy after thrombolytic therapy is discontinued and when thrombi time, ACT, and APTT less than 2 times control (about 3-4 hr)
- Avoid invasive procedures, inj, rec temp; apply pressure for 30 sec to minor bleeding sites; 30 min to sites of atrial puncture, followed by pressure dressing; inform prescriber if this does not attain hemostasis; apply pressure dressing
- Store powder at room temperature or refrigerate; protect from excessive light

### Y-site compatibilities: Lidocaine, metoprolol, propranolol
### Y-site incompatibilities: DOBUTamine, DOPamine, heparin, nitroglycerin
### Additive compatibilities: Lidocaine, morphine, nitroglycerin

## Patient/family education
- Teach patient reason for alteplase, signs and symptoms of bleeding, allergic reactions, when to notify prescriber

## Evaluation
### Positive therapeutic outcome
- Lysis of pulmonary thrombi
- Adequate hemodynamic state
- Absence of congestive heart failure

## aluminum hydroxide (OTC)

AlternaGEL, Alu-Cap, Alugel ♣, Aluminet, Aluminett, aluminum hydroxide, Alu-Tab, Amphojel, Basal gel, Dialume

*Func. class.:* Antacid, hypophosphatemic, antiulcer

*Chem. class.:* Aluminum product, phosphate binder

### Pregnancy category C

**Action:** Neutralizes gastric acidity, binds phosphates in GI tract; these phosphates are excreted

**Therapeutic outcome:** Decreased acidity, healing of ulcers; decreased phosphate levels in chronic renal failure

**Uses:** Adjunct in peptic, gastric, duodenal ulcers; antacid, hyperphosphatemia in chronic renal failure; reflux esophagitis, hyperacidity, heartburn, stress ulcer prevention in critically ill, GERD

**Unlabeled uses:** GI bleeding

### Dosage and routes

*Adult:* SUSP 5-10 ml 1 hr after meals with a full glass of water, at bedtime; PO 600 mg 1 hr after meals, at bedtime; chewed, max 6 times per day

### Hyperphosphatemia in renal failure

*Adult:* SUSP 500 mg-2 g bid-qid

### GI bleeding (unlabeled)

*Infant:* PO 2-5 ml/dose q1-2hr
*Child:* PO 5-15 ml/dose q1-2hr

**Available forms:** Caps 475, 500 mg; tabs 300, 500, 600 mg; susp 320 mg/5 ml, 450 mg/5 ml, 600 mg/5 ml; 675 mg/5 ml

### Adverse effects

*GI: Constipation,* anorexia, **obstruction,** fecal impaction
*META: Hypophosphatemia,* hypercalciuria

**Contraindications:** Hypersensitivity to this product or aluminum products

**Precautions:** Pregnancy **C,** breastfeeding, geriatric, fluid restriction, decreased GI motility, GI obstruction, dehydration, renal disease, sodium-restricted diets

### Pharmacokinetics

| | |
|---|---|
| **Absorption** | Not usually absorbed |
| **Distribution** | Widely distributed if absorbed; crosses placenta |
| **Metabolism** | Unknown |
| **Excretion** | Feces, kidneys (small amounts), breast milk |
| **Half-life** | Unknown |

### Pharmacodynamics

| | |
|---|---|
| **Onset** | 20-40 min |
| **Peak** | ½ hr |
| **Duration** | 1-3 hr |

### Interactions
#### Individual drugs

Allopurinol: decreased allopurinol effect
Amprenavir: decreased amprenavir effect
Ciprofloxacin: decreased ciprofloxacin effect
Delavirdine: decreased delavirdine effect
Diflunisal: decreased diflunisal effect
Digoxin: decreased digoxin effect
Gabapentin: decreased gabapentin effect
Gatifloxacin: decreased gatifloxacin effect
Isoniazid: decreased isoniazid effect
Ketoconazole: decreased ketoconazole effect
Penicillamine: decreased penicillamine effect
Phenytoin: decreased phenytoin effect
Quinidine: decreased quinidine effect
Ticlopidine: decreased ticlopidine effect
Warfarin: decreased warfarin effect

#### Drug classifications

Cephalosporins: decreased cephalosporin effect
Corticosteroids: decreased corticosteroid effect
$H_2$ antagonists: decreased $H_2$ antagonist effect
Iron salts: decreased iron salt effect
Phenothiazines: decreased phenothiazine effect
Tetracyclines: decreased tetracycline effect
Thyroid hormones: decreased thyroid effect

#### Drug/herb

Buckthorn, cascara sagrada, castor, Chinese rhubarb: decreased action of these herbs

#### Drug/food

High-protein meal: decreased product effect

### NURSING CONSIDERATIONS
#### Assessment

• Assess pain symptoms: location, duration, intensity, alleviating precipitating factors
• Monitor phosphate levels, since product is bound in GI system; urinary pH, calcium, electrolytes; hypophosphatemia: anorexia, weakness, fatigue, bone pain, hyperreflexia
• Monitor constipation; increase bulk in diet if needed

Adverse effects: *italic* = common, **bold** = life-threatening

## Nursing diagnoses
- Constipation (adverse reactions)
- Knowledge, deficient (teaching)
- Pain, chronic (uses)

## Implementation
- 2 tsp (10 ml) will neutralize 20 mEq of acid; 2 tabs will neutralize 16 mEq of acid

**PO route**
- Give laxatives or stool softeners if constipation occurs, especially geriatric
- Give after shaking suspension; follow with water to facilitate passage
- Tab may be chewed if patient is unable to swallow; drink 8 oz of water after chewing; or by nasogastric tube if patient unable to swallow
- Give with 8 oz of water for hyperphosphatemia unless contraindicated
- Give 1 hr before or after other medications to prevent poor absorption
- Give 15 ml 30 min after meals and at bedtime (esophagitis)

**NG tube route**
- May be given as prescribed q1-2hr and given by gastric tube after diluting with water (peptic ulcer)

## Patient/family education
- Instruct patient to increase fluids to 2000 ml/day unless contraindicated
- Instruct patient to avoid phosphate-containing foods (most dairy products, eggs, fruits, carbonated beverages) during product therapy; to add cheese, corn, pasta, plums, prunes, lentils after product (hypophosphatemia)
- Instruct patient not to use for prolonged periods if serum phosphate is low or if on a low-sodium diet; CHF patients should check for sodium content and use sodium-reduced products
- Instruct patient that stools may appear white or speckled; constipation may result; to report black tarry stools, which indicate gastric bleeding
- Instruct patient to check with prescriber after 2 wk of self-prescribed antacid use; may be used for 4-6 wk after symptoms subside or as prescribed
- Instruct patient to separate other medications by 2 hr

## Evaluation
**Positive therapeutic outcome**
- Absence of pain, decreased acidity
- Increased pH of gastric secretions
- Decreased phosphate levels

---

### amantadine (Rx)
(a-man'ta-deen)
amantadine HCl, Symmetrel
*Func. class.:* Antiviral, antiparkinsonian agent
*Chem. class.:* Tricyclic amine

**Pregnancy category** C

**Do not confuse:**
amantadine/ranitidine/rimantidine, Symmetrel/Synthroid

**Action:** Prevents uncoating of nucleic acid in viral cell, preventing penetration of virus to host; causes release of dopamine from neurons

**Therapeutic outcome:** Resolution of infection, lessening of parkinsonism symptoms

**Uses:** Prophylaxis or treatment of influenza type A, extrapyramidal reactions, parkinsonism, Parkinson's disease

**Unlabeled uses:** Neuroleptic malignant syndrome, MS-associated fatigue

### Dosage and routes
*Influenza type A*
**Adult and child >12 yr:** PO 200 mg/day in single dose or divided bid; max 400 mg/day

**Geriatric:** PO No more than 100 mg/day
**Child 9-12 yr:** PO 100 mg bid
**Child 1-9 yr:** PO 5 mg/kg/day divided bid-tid, not to exceed 150 mg/day

*Extrapyramidal reaction/ parkinsonism*
**Adult:** PO 100 mg bid, up to 400 mg/day in EPS; give for 1 wk, then 100 mg as needed up to 400 mg in parkinsonism

*Renal dose*
**Adult:** PO CCr 40-50 ml/min 100 mg/day; CCr 30 ml/min 200 mg 2 times/wk; CCr 20 ml/min 100 mg 3 times/wk; CCr 10 ml/min 100 mg alternating with 200 mg q7 days

*MS-associated fatigue (unlabeled)*
**Adult:** PO 200 mg daily or 100 mg bid

*Neuroleptic malignant syndrome (unlabeled)*
**Adult:** PO 100 mg bid × 3 wk

**Available forms:** Caps 100 mg; syr 50 mg/5 ml

### Adverse effects
*CNS:* Headache, dizziness, drowsiness, fatigue, *anxiety*, psychosis, *depression, hallucinations*, tremors, **seizures,** confusion, *insomnia*
*CV:* Orthostatic hypotension, **CHF**

---

***EENT:*** Blurred vision
***GI:*** *Nausea, vomiting,* constipation, dry mouth, anorexia
***GU:*** *Frequency, retention*
***HEMA:*** **Leukopenia, agranulocytosis**
***INTEG:*** Photosensitivity, dermatitis, livedo reticularis

**Contraindications:** Breastfeeding, child <1 yr, hypersensitivity, eczematic rash

**Precautions:** Pregnancy **C,** geriatric, epilepsy, CHF, orthostatic hypotension, psychiatric disorders, renal/hepatic disease, peripheral edema

| Pharmacokinetics | |
|---|---|
| **Absorption** | Unknown |
| **Distribution** | Crosses placenta |
| **Metabolism** | Not metabolized |
| **Excretion** | Urine unchanged (90%), breast milk |
| **Half-life** | 11-15 hr |

| Pharmacodynamics | |
|---|---|
| **Onset** | 48 hr |
| **Peak** | 2-4 hr |
| **Duration** | Unknown |

### Interactions
#### Individual drugs
Atropine: increased anticholinergic response
Metoclopramide: decreased amantadine effect
Triamterene, hydrochlorothiazide: decreased excretion of amantadine
#### Drug classifications
Anticholinergics (other): increased anticholinergic response
CNS stimulants: increased CNS stimulation
Phenothiazines: decreased amantadine effect
#### Drug/herb
Belladonna, henbane: increased anticholinergic response
Pheasant's eye, quinine, scopolia root: increased action/side effects
Kava: decreased action

### NURSING CONSIDERATIONS
#### Assessment
• Monitor I&O ratio; report frequency, hesitancy; serum BUN, creatinine baseline
• Assess CHF, confusion, mottling of skin
• Assess bowel pattern before, during treatment
• Assess skin eruptions, photosensitivity after administration of product

• Assess respiratory status: rate, character, wheezing, tightness in chest
• Assess allergies before initiation of treatment, reaction of each medication
• Assess signs of infection
• Assess hematologic status for leukopenia, agranulocytosis

#### Nursing diagnoses
• Infection, risk for (uses)
• Knowledge, deficient (teaching)

#### Implementation
• Give before exposure to influenza; continue for 10 days after contact
• Give at least 4 hr before bedtime to prevent insomnia
• Give after meals for better absorption, to decrease GI symptoms
• Give in divided doses to prevent CNS disturbances: headache, dizziness, fatigue, drowsiness
• Store in tight, dry container
• Caps may be opened and mixed with food

#### Patient/family education
• Advise patient to change body position slowly to prevent orthostatic hypotension
• Teach about aspects of product therapy: need to report dyspnea, weight gain, dizziness, poor concentration, dysuria, behavioral changes
• Advise patient to avoid hazardous activities if dizziness, blurred vision occurs
• Advise patient to take product exactly as prescribed; parkinsonian crisis may occur if product is discontinued abruptly; do not double dose; if a dose is missed, do not take within 4 hr of next dose
• Teach to avoid alcohol; do not breastfeed

#### Evaluation
**Positive therapeutic outcome**
• Absence of fever, malaise, cough, dyspnea in infection; tremors, shuffling gait in Parkinson's disease

**Treatment of overdose:** Withdraw product, maintain airway, administer epiNEPHrine, aminophylline, $O_2$, IV corticosteroids, physostigmine

### ambrisentan
Letairis
*See Appendix A, Selected New Drugs*

## amifostine (Rx)
(a-mi-foss'teen)
Ethyol
*Func. class.:* Cytoprotective agent for cis-platin
### Pregnancy category C

**Action:** Binds and detoxifies damaging metabolites of cisplatin by converting this product by alkaline phosphatase in tissue to an active free thiol compound

**Therapeutic outcome:** Decreased toxic reaction from cisplatin

**Uses:** Used to reduce renal toxicity when cisplatin is given in ovarian cancer, reduces xerostomia (dry mouth) in radiation therapy for head, neck cancer

**Unlabeled uses:** To prevent or reduce cisplatin-induced neurotoxicity, cyclophosphamide-induced granulocytopenia; prevent or reduce toxicity of radiation therapy; reduce toxicity of paclitaxel, myelodysplastic syndrome (MDS)

## Dosage and routes
### Reduction of renal damage with cisplatin
*Adult:* **IV** 910 mg/m² daily, within ½ hr before chemotherapy; give over 15 min; may reduce dose to 740 mg/m² if higher dose is poorly tolerated

### Xerostomia
*Adult:* **IV** 200 mg/m² daily over 3 min as inf 15-30 min before radiation therapy

**Available forms:** Powder for inj lyophilized 500 mg/vial

## Adverse effects
*CNS:* Dizziness, somnolence
*CV:* Hypotension
*EENT:* Sneezing
*GI:* Nausea, vomiting, hiccups
*INTEG:* Flushing, feeling of warmth
*MISC:* Hypocalcemia, rash, chills, **anaphylaxis, toxic epidermal necrolysis, Stevens-Johnson syndrome,** *exfoliative dermatitis, erythema multiforme*

**Contraindications:** Breastfeeding, hypersensitivity to mannitol, aminothiol; hypotension, dehydration

**Precautions:** Pregnancy **C,** children, geriatric, CV disease

### Pharmacokinetics
| | |
|---|---|
| **Absorption** | Complete |
| **Distribution** | Unknown |
| **Metabolism** | To free thiol compound |
| **Excretion** | Unknown |
| **Half-life** | 5-8 min |

### Pharmacodynamics
Unknown

## Interactions
### Drug classfications
Antihypertensives: increased hypotension

## NURSING CONSIDERATIONS
### Assessment
• Assess for xerostomia: mouth lesion, dry mouth during therapy
• Assess fluid status before administration; administer antiemetic before administration to prevent severe nausea and vomiting; also, dexamethasone 20 mg **IV** and a serotonin antagonist such as ondansetron, dolasetron, or granisetron
• Monitor calcium levels before and during treatment, may cause hypocalcemia; calcium supplements may be given for hypocalcemia
• Monitor blood pressure before and q5 min during infusion; antihypertensive should be discontinued 24 hr prior to infusion if severe hypotension occurs, give **IV** 0.9% NaCl to expand fluid volume, place in modified Trendelenburg position

### Nursing diagnoses
• Injury, risk for (uses)
• Knowledge, deficient (teaching)

### Implementation
**Intermittent IV infusion route**
• Give by **IV** intermittent inf after reconstituting with 9.5 ml of sterile 0.9% NaCl, further dilute with 0.9% NaCl to a concentration of 5-40 mg/ml, give at a rate over 15 min within ½ hr of chemotherapy
• Patient to be in supine position during infusion

*Y-site compatibilities:* Amikacin, aminophylline, ampicillin, ampicillin/sulbactam, aztreonam, bleomycin, bumetanide, buprenorphine, butorphanol, calcium gluconate, carboplatin, carmustine, cefazolin, cefonicid, cefotaxime, cefotetan, cefoxitin, ceftazidime, ceftizoxime, ceftriaxone, cefuroxime, cimetidine, ciprofloxacin, clindamycin, cyclophosphamide, cytarabine, dacarbazine, dactinomycin, DAUNOrubicin, dexamethasone, diphenhydrAMINE, dobutamine, DOPamine, DOXOrubicin, doxycycline, droperidol, enalaprilat, etoposide, famotidine, floxuridine, fluconazole, fludarabine, fluoro-uracil, furosemide, gallium, gentamicin, granisetron, haloperidol, heparin, hydrocortisone, hydromorphone, idarubicin, ifosfamide, imipenem-cilastatin, leucovorin, lorazepam, magnesium sulfate, mannitol, mechlorethamine, meperidine, mesna, methotrexate, methylPREDNISolone, metoclopramide, metronidazole, mezlocillin, mitomycin, mitoxantrone, morphine, nalbuphine, netilmicin, ondansetron, piperacillin, plicamycin, potassium chloride, promethazine, ranitidine, sodium bicarbonate, streptozocin, teniposide, thiotepa, ticarcillin, ticarcillin/clavulanate, tobramycin, trimethoprim/sulfamethoxazole, trimetrexate, vancomycin, vinBLAStine, vinCRIStine, zidovudine

***Additive incompatibilities:*** Do not mix with other products or solutions

### Patient/family education
• Teach reason for medication and expected results
• Teach that side effects may cause severe nausea, vomiting, decreased B/P, chills, dizziness, somnolence, hiccups, sneezing

### Evaluation
**Positive therapeutic outcome**
• Absence of renal damage

---

### amikacin (Rx)
(am-i-kay'sin)
amikacin sulfate, Amikin
*Func. class.:* Antibiotic
*Chem. class.:* Aminoglycoside
**Pregnancy category D**

### Do not confuse:
Amikin/Amicar

**Action:** Interferes with protein synthesis in bacterial cell by binding to ribosomal subunit, which causes misreading of genetic code; inaccurate peptide sequence forms in protein chain, causing bacterial death

**Therapeutic outcome:** Bactericidal effects for the following organisms: *Pseudomonas aeruginosa, Escherichia coli, Enterobacter, Acinetobacter, Providencia, Citrobacter, Staphylococcus, Serratia, Proteus*

**Uses:** Severe systemic infections of CNS, respiratory, GI, urinary tract, bone, skin, soft tissues caused by *Staphylococcus, Pseudomonas aeruginosa, Escherichia coli, Enterobacter, Acinetobacter, Providencia Citrobacter, Serratia, Proteus, Klebsiella pneumoniae*

**Unlabeled uses:** *Mycobacterium avium* complex (intrathecal or intraventricular) in combination; aerosolization, actinomycotic mycetoma

### Dosage and routes
*Severe systemic infections*
***Adult and child:*** IV INF 15 mg/kg/day in 2-3 divided doses q8-12hr in 100-200 ml D₅W over 30-60 min, not to exceed 1.5 g; use for 7-10 days; decreased dosages are needed in poor renal function as determined by blood levels, renal function studies; IM 15 mg/kg/day in divided doses q8-12hr; daily or extended internal dosing as an alternative dosing regimen
***Infant:*** IV/IM 10 mg/kg initially, then 7.5 mg/kg q12hr
***Neonate:*** IM/IV INF 10 mg/kg initially, then 7.5 mg/kg q12hr
***Premature neonate:*** IV 10 mg/kg initially, then 7.5 mg/kg q8-12hr

*Severe urinary tract infections*
***Adult:*** IM 15 mg/kg/day divided q8-12hr

*Hemodialysis*
***Adult:*** IM/IV 7.5 mg/kg followed by 5 mg/kg 3×/wk after each dialysis session

*TB or other mycobacterial infection*
***Adult and adolescent:*** IV 7.5-15 mg/kg divided q12-24hr as part of a multiple-drug regimen
***Child:*** IV 15-30 mg/kg/day divided q12-24hr as part of a multiple-drug regimen, max 1.5 g/day

*Renal dose*
***Adult:*** IV/IM 7.5 mg/kg initially, then increased as determined by blood levels, renal function studies

**Available forms:** Inj IM, **IV** 50, 250 mg/ml

### Adverse effects
***CNS:*** Confusion, depression, numbness, tremors, **seizures,** muscle twitching, **neurotoxicity,** dizziness, vertigo, tinnitus, **neuromuscular blockade with respiratory paralysis**
***CV:*** Hypotension or hypertension, palpitations
***EENT:*** Ototoxicity, deafness, visual disturbances
***GI:*** *Nausea, vomiting, anorexia,* increased ALT, AST, bilirubin, hepatomegaly, **hepatic necrosis,** splenomegaly
***GU:*** Oliguria, hematuria, **renal damage, azotemia, renal failure, nephrotoxicity**

*HEMA:* **Agranulocytosis, thrombocytopenia, leukopenia, eosinophilia, anemia**
*INTEG:* *Rash,* burning, urticaria, dermatitis, alopecia

**Contraindications:** Pregnancy **D,** mild to moderate infections, hypersensitivity to aminoglycosides, sulfites

**Precautions:** Neonates, breastfeeding, geriatric, mild renal disease, myasthenia gravis, hearing deficits, Parkinson's disease

### Pharmacokinetics

| | |
|---|---|
| **Absorption** | Well absorbed (IM), completely absorbed (**IV**) |
| **Distribution** | Widely distributed in extracellular fluids, poor in CSF; crosses placenta |
| **Metabolism** | Minimal; liver |
| **Excretion** | Mostly unchanged (79%) in kidneys, removed by hemodialysis |
| **Half-life** | 2-3 hr, prolonged up to 7 hr in infants; increased in renal disease |

### Pharmacodynamics

| | IM | IV |
|---|---|---|
| **Onset** | Rapid | Rapid |
| **Peak** | 15-30 min | 1-2 hr |
| **Duration** | Unknown | Unknown |

### Interactions
#### Individual drugs
DimenhyDRINATE, ethacrynic acid: increased masking of ototoxicity
Indomethacin: increased serum trough and peak

#### Drug classifications
Acyclovir, amphotericin B, cycloSPORINE, vancomycin: nephrotoxicity
Cidofovir: do not use together
Aminoglycosides, diuretics (loop): increased ototoxicity
Aminoglycosides: increased neurotoxicity, nephrotoxicity
Anesthetics, nondepolarizing neuromuscular blockers: increased neuromuscular blockade, respiratory depression
Cephalosporins: inactivation of amikacin, nephrotoxicity
Penicillins (parenteral): inactivation of amikacin

#### Drug/herb
Lysine (large amounts): increased toxicity
Acidophilus: do not use with antiinfectives
#### Drug/lab test
Increased: BUN, ALT, AST, bilirubin, LDH, alkaline phosphatase, creatinine

Decreased: calcium, sodium, potassium, magnesium

## NURSING CONSIDERATIONS
### Assessment
• Assess patient for previous sensitivity reaction
• Assess patient for signs and symptoms of infection, including characteristics of wounds, sputum, urine, stool, WBC >10,000/mm$^3$, earache, temp; obtain baseline information before and during treatment
• Obtain C&S tests before beginning product therapy to identify if correct treatment has been initiated
• Assess for allergic reactions: rash, urticaria, pruritus
• Identify urine output; if decreasing, notify prescriber (may indicate nephrotoxicity); also notify prescriber of increased BUN and creatinine, urine CCr <80 ml/min; lower dosage should be given in renal impairment; urinalysis daily for protein, cells, casts, nephrotoxicity may be reversible if product stopped at first sign
• Monitor blood studies: AST, ALT, CBC, Hct, bilirubin, LDH, alkaline phosphatase; Coombs' test monthly if patient is on long-term therapy
• Monitor electrolytes: potassium, sodium, chloride, magnesium monthly if patient is on long-term therapy
• Assess bowel pattern daily; if severe diarrhea occurs, product should be discontinued
• Monitor for bleeding: ecchymosis, bleeding gums, hematuria, stool guaiac daily if on long-term therapy
• Assess for overgrowth of infection: perineal itching, fever, malaise, redness, pain, swelling, drainage, rash, diarrhea, change in cough, sputum
• Obtain weight before treatment; calculation of dosage is usually based on ideal body weight, but may be calculated on actual body weight
• Monitor VS during infusion, watch for hypotension, change in pulse
• Assess **IV** site for thrombophlebitis including pain, redness, swelling q30 min; change site if needed; apply warm compresses to discontinued site
• Obtain serum peak, drawn 30-60 min after **IV** infusion or 60 min after IM injection; trough level drawn just before next dose; 20-30 mcg/ml, trough 4-8 mcg/ml, blood level should be 2-4 times bacteriostatic level
• Urine pH if product is used for UTI; urine should be kept alkaline

⚫ Deafness by audiometric testing, ringing, roaring in ears, vertigo; assess hearing before, during, after treatment
• Dehydration: high specific gravity, decrease in skin turgor, dry mucous membranes, dark urine
• Vestibular dysfunction: nausea, vomiting, dizziness, headache; product should be discontinued if severe

## Nursing diagnoses
• Diarrhea (side effects)
• Infection, risk for (uses)
• Injury, risk for (side effects)
• Knowledge, deficient (teaching)

## Implementation
**IM route**
• Give deeply in large muscle mass, rotate inj sites
**Intermittent IV infusion route**
• Dilute 500 mg of product in 100-200 ml of **IV** D$_5$W, D$_5$NaCl, or 0.9% NaCl and give over ½-1 hr; flush after administration with D$_5$W or 0.9% NaCl
*Syringe compatibilities:* Clindamycin, doxapram
*Y-site compatibilities:* Acyclovir, amifostine, amiodarone, amsacrine, aztreonam, cisatracurium, cyclophosphamide, dexamethasone, diltiazem, enalamprilat, esmolol, filgrastim, fluconazole, fludarabine, foscarnet, furosemide, granisetron, idarubicin, IL-2, labetalol, lorazepam, magnesium sulfate, melphalan, midazolam, morphine, ondansetron, paclitaxel, perphenazine, remifentanil, sargramostim, teniposide, thiotepa, TPN #54, #61, #91, #203, #204, #212, vinorelbine, warfarin, zidovudine

## Patient/family education
• Teach patient to report sore throat, bruising, bleeding, joint pain; may indicate blood dyscrasias (rare)
• Advise patient to contact prescriber if vaginal itching, loose foul-smelling stools, furry tongue occur; may indicate superinfection
• Advise patient to report hypersensitivity: rash, itching, trouble breathing, facial edema and notify prescriber

## Evaluation
**Positive therapeutic outcome**
• Absence of signs/symptoms of infection: WBC <10,000/mm$^3$, temp WNL; absence of red draining wounds; absence of earache
• Reported improvement in symptoms of infection

**Treatment of overdose:** Withdraw product; administer epINEPHrine, O$_2$, hemodialysis, exchange transfusion in the newborn; monitor serum levels of product; may give ticarcillin or carbenicillin

## amiloride (Rx)
(a-mill'oh-ride)
Amiloride HCl, Midamor
*Func. class.:* Potassium-sparing diuretic
*Chem. class.:* Pyrazine
**Pregnancy category B**

**Do not confuse:**
amiloride/amlodipine

**Action:** Inhibits sodium, potassium ATPase in the distal tubule, cortical collecting duct resulting in inhibition of sodium reabsorption and decreasing potassium secretion

**Therapeutic outcome:** Diuretic and antihypertensive effect while retaining potassium

**Uses:** Edema in CHF in combination with other diuretics, for hypertension, adjunct with other diuretics to maintain potassium

**Unlabeled uses:** Ascites

**Dosage and routes**
*Adult:* PO 5-10 mg daily in 1-2 divided doses; may be increased to 10-20 mg daily if needed

**Available forms:** Tabs 5 mg

**Adverse effects**
*CNS: Headache,* dizziness, fatigue, weakness, paresthesias, tremor, depression, anxiety
*CV:* Orthostatic hypotension, dysrhythmias, angina
*EENT:* Blurred vision, increased intraocular pressure
*ELECT:* **Hyperkalemia**
*GI: Nausea, diarrhea,* dry mouth, *vomiting, anorexia,* cramps, constipation, abdominal pain, jaundice
*GU: Polyuria,* dysuria, frequency, impotence
*HEMA:* **Aplastic anemia, neutropenia**
*INTEG: Rash, pruritus,* alopecia, urticaria
*MS: Cramps*
*RESP:* Cough, dyspnea, shortness of breath

**Contraindications:** Anuria, hypersensitivity, hyperkalemia, impaired renal function

**Precautions:** Pregnancy **B**, breastfeeding, geriatric, dehydration, diabetes, acidosis

Adverse effects: *italic* = common, **bold** = life-threatening

| Pharmacokinetics | |
|---|---|
| **Absorption** | Variable (10%-15%) |
| **Distribution** | Widely distributed |
| **Metabolism** | Unchanged in urine (50%), in feces (40%) |
| **Excretion** | Renal; breast milk |
| **Half-life** | 6-9 hr |

| Pharmacodynamics | |
|---|---|
| **Onset** | 2 hr |
| **Peak** | 6-10 hr |
| **Duration** | 24 hr |

## Interactions
### Individual drugs
CycloSPORINE, tacrolimus: increased hyperkalemia

Lithium: increased lithium toxicity
### Drug classifications
ACE inhibitors, diuretics (potassium-sparing), potassium products, salt substitutes: increased hyperkalemia

Antihypertensives: increased action

NSAIDs: decreased effectiveness of amiloride
### Drug/herb
Arginine: fatal hypokalemia

Bearberry, gossypol: increased hypokalemia

Cucumber, dandelion, horsetail, licorice, nettle, pumpkin, Queen Anne's lace: increased amiloride effect

Khella: increased hypotension

St. John's wort: increased severe photosensitivity
### Drug/food
Potassium foods: increased hyperkalemia
### Drug/lab test
Interference: GTT

## NURSING CONSIDERATIONS
### Assessment
• Monitor manifestations of hyperkalemia: *MS:* fatigue, muscle weakness; *CARDIAC:* dysrhythmias, hypotension; *NEURO:* paresthesias, confusion; *RESP:* dyspnea

• Monitor for manifestations of hyponatremia: *CV:* increased B/P, cold, clammy skin, hypovolemia or hypervolemia; *GI:* anorexia, nausea, vomiting, diarrhea, abdominal cramps; *NEURO:* lethargy, increased ICP, confusion, headache, seizures, coma, fatigue, tremors, hyperreflexia

• Monitor for manifestations of hyperchloremia: *NEURO:* weakness, lethargy, coma; *RESP:* deep rapid breathing

• Assess fluid volume status: I&O ratios and record, weight, distended red veins, crackles in lung, color, quality, and specific gravity of urine, skin turgor, adequacy of pulses, moist mucous membranes, bilateral lung sounds, peripheral pitting edema; dehydration symptoms of decreasing output, thirst, hypotension, dry mouth and mucous membranes should be reported

• Monitor electrolytes: potassium, sodium, calcium, magnesium; also include BUN, ABGs, uric acid, CBC, blood glucose

• Assess B/P before and during therapy with patient lying, standing, and sitting as appropriate; orthostatic hypotension can occur rapidly

### Nursing diagnoses
• Fluid volume, deficient (side effects)
• Fluid volume, excess (uses)
• Knowledge, deficient (teaching)

### Implementation
• Give in AM to avoid interference with sleep
• With food; if nausea occurs, absorption may be increased

### Patient/family education
• Teach patient to take medication early in the day to prevent nocturia

• Instruct patient to take with food or milk if GI symptoms of nausea and anorexia occur

• Teach patient to maintain a weekly record of weight and notify prescriber of weight loss >5 lb

• Caution patient that this product causes an increase in potassium levels, so foods high in potassium should be avoided; refer to dietitian for assistance, planning

• Caution patient not to exercise in hot weather or stand for prolonged periods since orthostatic hypotension will be enhanced

• Teach patient not to use alcohol or any OTC medications without prescriber's approval; serious product reactions may occur

• Emphasize the need to contact prescriber immediately if muscle cramps, weakness, nausea, dizziness, or numbness occurs

• Teach patient to take own B/P and pulse and record

• Advise patient that dizziness and confusion may occur; avoid driving or other hazardous activities if alertness is decreased

• Teach patient to continue taking medication even if feeling better; this product controls symptoms but does not cure the condition

• Advise patient with hypertension to continue other medical treatment (exercise, weight loss, relaxation techniques, cessation of smoking)

## Evaluation
**Positive therapeutic outcome**
- Prevention of hypokalemia (diuretic use)
- Decreased edema
- Decreased B/P
- Increased diuresis

**Treatment of overdose:** Lavage if taken orally; monitor electrolytes; administer **IV** fluids; monitor hydration, CV, renal status

## amino acid (Rx)
(a-mee′noe)
Injection: FreAmine, HepatAmine
Solution: Aminess, Aminosyn, BranchAmin, FreAmine III, NephrAmine, Novamine, ProcalAmine, RenAmin, Travasol, Trophamine
*Func. class.:* Caloric agent
*Chem. class.:* Nitrogen product
**Pregnancy category** C

**Action:** Needed for anabolism to maintain structure; decreases catabolism, promotes healing

**Therapeutic outcome:** Positive nitrogen balance, decreased catabolism

**Uses:** Hepatic encephalopathy, cirrhosis, hepatitis, nutritional support in cancer trauma; to prevent nitrogen loss when adequate nutrition by mouth, gastric, or duodenal tube cannot be used; intestinal obstruction, short bowel syndrome, severe malabsorption

## Dosage and routes
*Amino acid injection*
**Adult: IV** 80-120 g/day; 500 ml of amino acids/500 ml D$_{50}$ given over 24 hr

*Amino acid solution*
**Adult: IV** 1-1.5 g/kg/day titrated to patient's needs
**Child: IV** 2-3 g/kg/day titrated to patient's needs

**Available forms:** Inj; many strengths, types

## Adverse effects
*CNS: Dizziness, headache,* confusion, **loss of consciousness**
*CV:* Hypertension, **CHF, pulmonary edema**
*ENDO: Hyperglycemia, rebound hypoglycemia, electrolyte imbalances, hyperosmolar syndrome, hyperosmolar hyperglycemic nonketotic syndrome,* alkalosis, acidosis, hypophosphatemia, hyperammonemia, dehydration, hypocalcemia

*GI:* Nausea, vomiting, liver fat deposits, abdominal pain
*GU:* Glycosuria, osmotic diuresis
*INTEG:* Chills, flushing, warm feeling, rash, urticaria, extravasation necrosis, phlebitis at inj site

**Contraindications:** Hypersensitivity, severe electrolyte imbalances, anuria, severe liver damage, maple syrup urine disease, PKU

**Precautions:** Pregnancy **C,** children, renal disease, diabetes mellitus, CHF

### Pharmacokinetics
| | |
|---|---|
| **Absorption** | Complete bioavailability |
| **Distribution** | Widely distributed |
| **Metabolism** | Anabolism |
| **Excretion** | Kidney to urea nitrogen |
| **Half-life** | Unknown |

### Pharmacodynamics
Unknown

## Interactions
*Drug classifications*
Tetracycline: decreased protein-sparing effects

## NURSING CONSIDERATIONS
**Assessment**
- Monitor electrolytes (potassium, sodium, calcium, chloride, magnesium), blood glucose, ammonia, phosphate, ketones; renal, liver function studies: BUN, creatinine, ALT, AST, bilirubin; urine glucose q6hr using Chemstrips, which are not affected by infusion substances; if BUN increases over 15%, therapy may need to be discontinued
- Check inj site for extravasation: redness along vein, edema at site, necrosis, pain; for a hard, tender area
- Monitor respiratory function q4hr: auscultate lung fields bilaterally for crackles; monitor respirations for quality, rate, rhythm that indicates fluid overload
- Monitor temp q4hr for increased fever, indicating infection; if infection is suspected, infusion is discontinued and tubing, bottle, catheter tip cultured; blood catheter may be obtained
- ◆ Monitor for impending hepatic coma: asterixis, confusion, fetor, lethargy
- Hyperammonemia: nausea, vomiting, malaise, tremors, anorexia, seizures; increased ammonia, ketone levels may occur

**Nursing diagnoses**
- Infection, risk for (adverse reactions)
- Injury, risk for (uses, adverse reactions)

Adverse effects: *italic* = common, **bold** = life-threatening

- Knowledge, deficient (teaching)
- Nutrition: less than body requirements, imbalanced (uses)

## Implementation
**Continuous IV route**
- Give up to 40% protein and dextrose (up to 12.5%) via peripheral vein; stronger solutions require central **IV** administration; TPN only mixed with dextrose to promote protein synthesis
- Use immediately after mixing in pharmacy under strict aseptic technique using laminar flowhood; use infusion pump, in-line filter (0.22 μm) unless mixed with fat emulsion and dextrose (3 in 1)
- ◆ Use careful monitoring technique; do not speed up infusion; pulmonary edema, glucose overload will result
- Storage depends on type of solution; consult manufacturer
- Change dressing and **IV** tubing to prevent infection q24-48hr or q5-7 days if transparent dressing is used

*Y-site compatibilities:* Amikacin, aminophylline, amoxicillin, ampicillin, ascorbic acid inj, atracurium, azlocillin, aztreonam, bumetanide, buprenorphine, calcium gluconate, carboplatin, cefamandole, cefazolin, cefonicid, cefoperazone, cefotaxime, cefotetan, cefoxtin, ceftazidime, ceftizoxime, ceftriaxone, cefuroxime, cephalothin, cephapirin, chloramphenicol, chlorproMAZINE, cimetidine, clindamycin, clonazepam, dexamethasone, diazepam, digoxin, diphenhydrAMINE, DOBUTamine, DOPamine, doxycycline, droperidol, enalaprilat, epINEPHrine, erythromycin lactobionate, famotidine, fentanyl, flucloxacillin, fluconazole, folic acid, foscarnet, gentamicin, granisetron, haloperidol, heparin, hydrocortisone, hydromorphone, hydrOXYzine, idarubicin, ifosfamide, IL-2, imipenem/cilastatin, insulin (regular), isoproterenol, kanamycin, leucovorin, levorphanol, lidocaine, lorazepam, magnesium sulfate, mannitol, meperidine, mesna, methicillin, metronidazole, mezlocillin, miconazole, morphine, moxalactam, multivitamins, nafcillin, netilmicin, nitroglycerin, norepINEPHrine, octreotide, ofloxacin, ondansetron, oxacillin, paclitaxel, penicillin G, penicillin G potassium, pentobarbital, phenobarbital, piperacillin, potassium chloride, prochlorperazine, ranitidine, salbutamol, sargramostim, tacrolimus, thiotepa, ticarcillin, ticarcillin/clavulanate, tobramycin, trimethoprim/sulfamethoxazole, urokinase, vancomycin, vecuronium, zidovudine

*Y-site incompatibilities:* Cephradine
*Additive compatibilities:* Amikacin, aminophylline, aztreonam, calcium gluconate, cefamandole, cefazolin, cefepime, cefotaxime, cefoxitin, cefsulodin, ceftazidime, ceftriaxone, cefuroxime, cimetidine, clindamycin, cyanocobalamin, cyclophosphamide, cycloSPORINE, cytarabine, DOPamine, epoetin, erythromycin, famotidine, folic acid, fosphenytoin, furosemide, heparin, insulin (regular), isoproterenol, lidocaine, meperidine, metaraminol, methicillin, methotrexate, methyldopate, methylPREDNISolone, metoclopramide, morphine, nafcillin, netilmicin, nizatidine, norepinephrine, ondansetron, oxacillin, penicillin G potassium, penicillin G sodium, phytonadione, polymyxin B, sodium bicarbonate, tacrolimus, tobramycin, vancomycin

## Patient/family education
- Teach reason for use of amino acids as part of nutrition (TPN)
- Instruct patient to report at once to prescriber if chills, sweating are experienced

## Evaluation
**Positive therapeutic outcome**
- Weight gain
- Decreased jaundice in liver disorders
- Increased LOC

## aminophylline (theophylline ethylenediamine) (Rx)
(am-in-off'i-lin)
Phyllocontin, Truphylline
*Func. class.:* Bronchodilator, spasmolytic
*Chem. class.:* Xanthine, ethylenediamine
**Pregnancy category C**

**Action:** Exact mechanism unknown; relaxes smooth muscle of respiratory system by blocking phosphodiesterase, which increases cyclic AMP; increased cyclic AMP alters intracellular calcium ion movements; produces bronchodilatation, increased pulmonary blood flow, relaxation of respiratory tract

**Therapeutic outcome:** Increased ability to breathe

**Uses:** Apnea in infancy for respiratory/myocardial stimulation, bronchial asthma, bronchospasm associated with chronic bronchitis, emphysema, bradycardia

**Unlabeled uses:** Methotrexate toxicity, sleep apnea, status asthmaticus

**A**

## Dosage and routes

*Adult:* PO 6 mg/kg, then 3 mg/kg q6hr × 2 doses, then 3 mg/kg q8hr maintenance, max 900 mg/day or 13 mg/kg; PO in CHF 6 mg/kg, then 2 mg/kg q8hr × 2 doses, then 1-2 mg/kg q12hr maintenance; **IV** 4.7 mg/kg, then 0.55 mg/kg/hr × 12 hr, then 0.36 mg/kg/hr maintenance; **IV** in CHF 4.7 mg/kg, then 0.39 mg/kg/hr × 12 hr; then 0.08-0.16 mg/kg/hr maintenance

*Geriatric and in cor pulmonale:* PO 6 mg/kg, then 2 mg/kg q6hr × 2 doses, then 2 mg/kg q8hr maintenance; **IV** 4.7 mg/kg, then 0.47 mg/kg/hr × 12 hr, then 0.24 mg/kg/hr maintenance

*Child 9-16 yr:* PO 6 mg/kg, then 3 mg/kg q4hr × 3 doses, then 3 mg/kg q6hr maintenance, max 18 mg/kg/day 12-16 yr, or 20 mg/kg/day 9-12 yr; **IV** 4.7 mg/kg, then 0.79 mg/kg/hr × 12 hr, then 0.63 mg/kg/hr maintenance

*Child 6 mo-9 yr:* PO 4 mg/kg q4hr × 3 doses, then 4 mg/kg q6hr maintenance, max 24 mg/kg/day; **IV** 4.7 mg/kg, then 0.95 mg/kg/hr × 12 hr, then 0.79 mg/kg/hr maintenance

*Infants 6-52 wk:* Dose (0.2 × age in wk) ÷ 5 × kg = 24 hr dose in mg

*Neonates up to 40 wk premature postconception age:* PO/**IV** 1 mg/kg q12hr

*Neonates at birth or 40 wk postconception age:* PO/**IV** >8 wk postnatal 1-3 mg/kg q6hr; 4-8 wk postnatal 1-2 mg/kg q8hr; up to 4 wk postnatal 1-2 mg/kg q12hr

*Hepatic disease*
*Adult:* PO 6 mg/kg, then 2 mg/kg q8hr × 2 doses, then 1-2 mg/kg q12hr maintenance; **IV** 4.7 mg/kg, then 0.39 mg/kg/hr × 12 hr, then 0.08-0.16 mg/kg/hr maintenance

**Available forms:** Inj 250 mg/10 ml, 500 mg/20 ml, 100 mg/100 ml in 0.45% NaCl; 200 mg/100 ml in 0.45% NaCl; rectal supp 250 mg, 500 mg; oral liq 105 mg/5 ml; tabs 100, 200 mg; cont rel tabs 225, 350 mg

## Adverse effects

*CNS:* Anxiety, restlessness, insomnia, *dizziness,* **seizures,** headache, light-headedness, muscle twitching, tremors
*CV:* *Palpitations, sinus tachycardia,* hypotension, flushing, dysrhythmias, edema
*GI:* *Nausea, vomiting,* diarrhea, dyspepsia, anal irritation (suppositories), epigastric pain, anorexia
*GU:* Urinary frequency, SIADH

*INTEG:* Flushing, urticaria
*RESP:* Tachypnea, increased respiratory rate

**Contraindications:** Hypersensitivity to xanthines, tachydysrhythmias

**Precautions:** Pregnancy **C,** breastfeeding, children, geriatric, CHF, cor pulmonale, hepatic disease, diabetes mellitus, hyperthyroidism, hypertension, seizure disorder, irritation of the rectum or lower colon, alcoholism, active peptic ulcer disease

### Pharmacokinetics

| | |
|---|---|
| **Absorption** | Well absorbed (PO), slow (PO–ext rel), erratic (RECT) |
| **Distribution** | Widely distributed; crosses placenta |
| **Metabolism** | Liver to caffeine |
| **Excretion** | Kidneys |
| **Half-life** | 3-12 hr, increased in renal disease, CHF, geriatric patients, smokers |

### Pharmacodynamics

| | PO | PO–EXT REL | IV |
|---|---|---|---|
| **Onset** | 15-60 min | Unknown | Immediate |
| **Peak** | 1-2 hr | 4-7 hr | Infusion's end |
| **Duration** | 6-8 hr | 8-12 hr | 6-8 hr |

## Interactions
### Individual drugs
Allopurinol (high doses), cimetidine, clarithromycin, disulfiram, erythromycin, fluvoxamine, interferon, mexiletine: decreased metabolism, increased toxicity of aminophylline
Carbamazepine, isoniazid: increased or decreased aminophylline levels
Halothane: increased risk of dysrhythmias
Ketoconazole, phenytoin, rifampin: decreased aminophylline effect
Lithium: decreased effect of lithium
Smoking: increased metabolism, decreased effect

### Drug classifications
Barbiturates, β-adrenergic blockers: decreased effect of aminophylline
Benzodiazepines, corticosteroids, diuretics (loop), fluoroquinolones, influenza vaccines, oral contraceptives: increased aminophylline levels
Corticosteroids, influenza vaccines: increased aminophylline toxicity
Diuretics (loop): may increase or decrease aminophylline levels
Dose-dependent reversal of neuromuscular blockade
Fluoroquinolones: decreased metabolism, increased toxicity

Adverse effects: *italic* = common, **bold** = life-threatening

Sympathomimetics: increased CNS, CV adverse reactions

Tetracyclines: increased adverse reactions

**Drug/herb**

Cola tree, ginseng, guarana, horsetail, Siberian ginseng, tea (black, green), yerba maté: increased effects

St. John's wort: decreased effects

**Drug/food**

High-carbohydrate, low protein diet: decreased elimination

Low-carbohydrate, high-protein diet, charcoal-broiled beef: increased elimination

Xanthines: increased effect

**Drug/lab test**

Increased: plasma free fatty acids

## NURSING CONSIDERATIONS
### Assessment

• Monitor theophylline blood levels (therapeutic level is 10-20 mcg/ml); toxicity may occur with small increase above 20 mcg/ml, especially geriatric; determine whether theophylline was given recently (24 hr); check for toxicity: nausea, vomiting, anxiety, restlessness, insomnia, tachycardia, dysrhythmias, seizures; notify prescriber immediately

• Monitor I&O; diuresis will occur; dehydration may result in geriatric or children in whom diuresis is great

• Monitor respiratory rate, rhythm, depth; auscultate lung fields bilaterally; notify prescriber of abnormalities; check ECG for tachycardia, PVCs, PACs in patients with cardiac problems

• Monitor allergic reactions: rash, urticaria; if these occur, product should be discontinued, prescriber notified

### Nursing diagnoses

• Activity intolerance (uses)
• Airway clearance, ineffective (uses)
• Injury, risk for (uses, adverse reactions)
• Knowledge, deficient (teaching)

### Implementation

• Give around the clock to maintain blood (theophylline) levels

• If switching from **IV** to PO, give controlled-release dose at time of **IV** infusion discontinuation; if giving tab (immediate release), discontinue **IV** and wait >4 hr

• If GI upset occurs, take with 8 oz of water or food

• Increase fluids to 2 L/day

**PO route**

• Do not break, crush, or chew enteric-coated or cont rel tabs

• Avoid giving with food

**Rectal route**

• Rectal dose if patient is unable to take PO; retain rectal dose for ½ hour

**IV route**

• May be diluted for **IV** inf in 100-200 ml in $D_5W$, $D_{10}W$, $D_{20}W$, 0.9% NaCl, 0.45% NaCl, LR

• Give loading dose over ½ hr, max rate of inf 25 mg/min, use infusion pump; after loading dose, give by cont inf

• Avoid IM inj; pain and tissue damage may occur

• Only clear sol; flush **IV** line before dose; store diluted sol for 24 hr if refrigerated

**Syringe compatibilities:** Heparin, metoclopramide, pentobarbital, thiopental

**Y-site compatibilities:** Allopurinol, amifostine, amphotericin B sulfate complex, inamrinone, aztreonam, ceftazidime, cimetidine, cladribine, DOXOrubicin liposome, enalaprilat, esmolol, famotidine, filgrastim, fluconazole, fludarabine, foscarnet, gallium, granisetron, heparin sodium with hydrocortisone sodium succinate, labetalol, melphalan, meropenem, netilmicin, paclitaxel, pancuronium, piperacillin/tazobactam, potassium chloride, propofol, ranitidine, remifentanil, sargramostim, tacrolimus, teniposide, thiotepa, tolazoline, vecuronium

**Y-site incompatibilities:** DOBUTamine, hydrALAZINE, ondansetron

**Additive compatibilities:** Amobarbital, bretylium, calcium gluconate, chloramphenicol, cibenzoline, cimetidine, dexamethasone, diphenhydrAMINE, DOPamine, erythromycin lactobionate, esmolol, floxacillin, flumazenil, furosemide, heparin, hydrocortisone, lidocaine, mephentermine, meropenem, methyldopate, metronidazole/sodium bicarbonate, nitroglycerin, pentobarbital, phenobarbital, potassium chloride, ranitidine, secobarbital, sodium bicarbonate, terbutaline

**Additive incompatibilities:** Ascorbic acid, bleomycin, cephalothin, cefotaxime, chlorproMAZINE, cimetidine, clindamycin, codeine, dimenhyDRINATE, DOBUTamine, DOXOrubicin, doxycycline, epINEPHrine, erythromycin gluceptate, hydrALAZINE, hydrOXYzine, insulin, isoproterenol, meperidine, methicillin, morphine, nafcillin, nitroprusside, norepinephrine, oxytetracycline, papaverine, penicillin G, pentazocine, phenobarbital, phenytoin, prochlorperazine, promazine, promethazine, sulfiSOXAZOLE, tetracycline, vancomycin

### Patient/family education

• Teach patient to take doses as prescribed, not to skip dose; to check OTC medications,

current prescription medications for epHEDrine, which will increase CNS stimulation; advise patient not to drink alcohol or caffeine products (tea, coffee, chocolate, colas), which will increase action
- Teach patient to avoid hazardous activities; dizziness may occur
- Teach patient if GI upset occurs, to take product with 8 oz of water or food; absorption may be decreased
- Teach patient to remain in bed 15-20 min after rect supp is inserted to prevent removal
- Instruct patient to avoid smoking because it increases metabolism; decreases blood levels and terminal half-life; dosage may need to be increased
- Teach patient to obtain blood levels of product every few months to prevent toxicity; not to change brands, since effect may not be the same
- Teach patient to increase fluids to 2 L/day to decrease viscosity of secretions
- Advise patient to report toxicity: nausea, vomiting, anxiety, insomnia, rapid pulse, seizures, flushing, headache, diarrhea

### Evaluation
**Positive therapeutic outcome**
- Decreased dyspnea
- Respiratory stimulation in infants
- Clear lung fields bilaterally

---

### ⚠ HIGH ALERT

## amiodarone (Rx)
(a-mee-oh′da-rone)
Cordarone, Pacerone
*Func. class.:* Antidysrhythmic (Class III)
*Chem. class.:* Iodinated benzofuran derivative

**Pregnancy category D**

### Do not confuse:
amiodarone/inamrinone, Cordarone/Inocor

**Action:** Prolongs action potential duration and effective refractory period, noncompetitive α and β-adrenergic inhibition; increases PR and QT intervals, decreases sinus rate, decreases peripheral vascular resistance

**Therapeutic outcome:** Decreased amount and severity of ventricular dysrhythmias

**Uses:** Severe ventricular tachycardia, supraventricular tachycardia, ventricular fibrillation not controlled by 1st-line agents

### Dosage and routes
*Ventricular dysrhythmias*
*Adult:* PO Loading dose 800-1600 mg/day for 1-3 wk; then 600-800 mg/day × 1 mo; maintenance 400 mg/day; **IV** loading dose (first rapid) 150 mg over the first 10 min then slow 360 mg over the next 6 hr; maintenance 540 mg given over the remaining 18 hr, decrease rate of the slow infusion to 0.5 mg/min
*Child:* PO Loading dose 10-15 mg/kg/day in 1-2 divided doses for 4-14 days then 5 mg/kg/day (not recommended in children)
*Child and infant:* **IV**/INTRAOSSEOUS 5 mg/kg as a bolus (PALS guidelines)

*Perfusion tachycardia:* **IV** 5 mg/kg loading dose given over 20-60 min

*Supraventricular tachycardia*
*Adult:* PO 600-800 mg/day × 7 days or until desired response, then 400 mg/day × 21 days, then 200-400 mg/day maintenance
*Child:* PO 10 mg/kg/day (800 mg/1.72 m²/day) × 10 days or until desired response, then 5 mg/kg/day (400 mg/1.72 m²/day) × 21-28 days, then 2.5 mg/kg/day (200 mg/1.72 m²/day) (not recommended in children)

**Available forms:** Tabs 100, 200, 400 mg; inj 50 mg/ml

### Adverse effects
*CNS: Headache, dizziness,* involuntary movement, tremors, peripheral neuropathy, malaise, fatigue, ataxia, paresthesias, insomnia
*CV: Hypotension,* **bradycardia, sinus arrest, CHF, dysrhythmias, SA node dysfunction**
*EENT:* Blurred vision, halos, photophobia, **corneal microdeposits,** dry eyes
*ENDO:* Hyper/hypothyroidism
*GI:* Nausea, vomiting, diarrhea, abdominal pain, anorexia, constipation, **hepatotoxicity**
*INTEG:* Rash, photosensitivity, blue-gray skin discoloration, alopecia, spontaneous ecchymosis, **toxic epidermal necrolysis**
*MISC:* Flushing, abnormal taste or smell, edema, abnormal salivation, coagulation abnormalities
*MS:* Weakness, pain in extremities
*RESP:* **Pulmonary fibrosis,** pulmonary inflammation, **ARDS, gasping syndrome in neonates**

**Contraindications:** Pregnancy **D,** breastfeeding, neonates, infants, severe sinus node dysfunction, 2nd- or 3rd-degree AV block; bradycardia

---

Adverse effects: *italic* = common, **bold** = life-threatening

**Precautions:** Goiter, Hashimoto's thyroiditis, electrolyte imbalances, CHF, severe hepatic/respiratory disease, children

| Pharmacokinetics | |
|---|---|
| Absorption | Slow, variable (PO) up to 65% |
| Distribution | Body tissues; crosses placenta |
| Metabolism | Liver |
| Excretion | Bile, kidney (minimal) |
| Half-life | 15-100 days |

| Pharmacodynamics | |
|---|---|
| | PO |
| Onset | 1-3 wk |
| Peak | Unknown |
| Duration | Up to months |

## Interactions
### Individual drugs
CycloSPORINE, dextromethorphan, digoxin, disopyramide, flecainide, methotrexate, phenytoin, procainamide, quinidine, theophylline: increased blood levels, increased toxicity

Warfarin: increased bleeding
### Drug classifications
β-Adrenergic blockers, calcium channel blockers: increased bradycardia
### Drug/herb
Aconite: increased toxicity, death

Aloe, broom, buckthorn (chronic use), cascara sagrada (chronic use), Chinese rhubarb, figwort, fumitory, goldenseal, kudzu, licorice, senna: increased effect

Coltsfoot: decreased effect

Horehound: increased serotonin effect
### Drug/food
Grapefruit juice: toxicity
### Drug/lab test
Increased: $T_4$

## NURSING CONSIDERATIONS
### Assessment
• Monitor I&O ratio; monitor electrolytes: potassium, sodium, chloride

• Monitor chest x-ray, thyroid function tests

• Monitor liver function studies: AST, ALT, bilirubin, alkaline phosphatase

• Monitor ECG continuously to determine product effectiveness; measure PR, QRS, QT intervals; check for PVCs, other dysrhythmias; monitor B/P continuously for hypo/hypertension; check for rebound hypertension after 1-2 hr

• Monitor for dehydration or hypovolemia

• Assess for CNS symptoms: confusion, psychosis, numbness, depression, involuntary movements; if these occur, product should be discontinued

• Assess for hypothyroidism: lethargy, dizziness, constipation, enlarged thyroid gland, edema of extremities, cool, pale skin

• Monitor hyperthyroidism: restlessness, tachycardia, eyelid puffiness, weight loss, frequent urination, menstrual irregularities, dyspnea, warm, moist skin

◆ Assess for pulmonary toxicity including ARDS, pulmonary fibrosis: dyspnea, fatigue, cough, fever, chest pain; product should be discontinued if these occur

• Monitor cardiac rate, respiration: rate, rhythm, character, chest pain, ventricular tachycardia, supraventricular tachycardia or fibrillation

• Assess sight and vision before treatment and throughout therapy; microdeposits on the cornea may cause blurred vision, halos, and photophobia

### Nursing diagnoses
• Cardiac output, decreased (uses)
• Gas exchange, impaired (adverse reactions)
• Knowledge, deficient (teaching)

### Implementation
Start with patient hospitalized and monitored
**PO route**
• Give reduced dosage slowly with ECG monitoring only
• Loading dose with food to decrease nausea
**Intermittent IV infusion route**
• 1000 mg/24 hr during loading/maintenance
• Initial loading: add 3 ml (150 mg) 100 ml $D_5W$ (1.5 mg/ml) give over 10 min
• Loading inf: add 18 ml (900 mg) 500 ml $D_5W$ (1.8 mg/ml) give over next 6 hr
• Maintenance inf: Give remainder of loading inf 540 mg over 18 hr (0.5 mg/min)
**Continuous infusion route**
• After 24 hr, give 1-6 mg/ml at 0.5 mg/ml, max 30 mg/min

*Y-site compatibilities:* Amikacin, bretylium, clindamycin, DOBUTamine, DOPamine, doxycycline, erythromycin, esmolol, gentamicin, insulin (regular), isoproterenol, labetalol, lidocaine, metaraminol, metronidazole, midazolam, morphine, nitroglycerin, norepinephrine, penicillin G potassium, phentolamine, phenylephrine, potassium chloride, procainamide, tobramycin, vancomycin

*Additive compatibilities:* DOBUTamine, lidocaine, potassium chloride, procainamide, verapamil

*Solution compatibilities:* $D_5W$, 0.9% NaCl

## Patient/family education

- Instruct patient to report side effects immediately to prescriber
- Instruct patient that skin discoloration is usually reversible, but skin may turn bluish on neck, face, arms when used for long periods
- Advise patient that dark glasses may be needed for photophobia
- Instruct patient to use sunscreen and protective clothing to prevent burning associated with photosensitivity
- Instruct patient to take medication as prescribed, not to double doses
- Instruct patient to complete follow-up appointment with health care provider including pulmonary function studies, chest x-ray, ophthalmic examinations

## Evaluation

**Positive therapeutic outcome**

- Decreased ventricular tachycardia
- Decreased supraventricular tachycardia or fibrillation

**Treatment of overdose:** Administer O₂, artificial ventilation, ECG, DOPamine for circulatory depression, diazepam or thiopental for seizures, isoproterenol

---

## amitriptyline (Rx)

(a-mee-trip′ti-leen)
amitriptyline HCl, Apo-Amitriptyline ✦
*Func. class.:* Antidepressant—tricyclic
*Chem. class.:* Tertiary amine

**Pregnancy category** C

## Do not confuse:

amitriptyline/nortriptyline

**Action:** Blocks reuptake of norepinephrine, serotonin into nerve endings that increase action of norepinephrine, serotonin in nerve cells

**Uses:** Major depression

**Unlabeled uses:** Neuropathic pain, prevention of cluster/migraine headaches, fibromyalgia

**Therapeutic outcome:** Decreased symptoms of depression after 2-3 wk

## Dosage and routes

*Depression*

*Adult:* PO 75 mg/day in divided doses; may increase to 150 mg daily, not to exceed 300 mg/day

*Geriatric and adolescent:* PO 30 mg/day in divided doses; may be increased to 100 mg/day

*Cluster/migraine headaches (unlabeled)*
*Adult:* PO 50-300 mg/day

*Pain (unlabeled)*
*Adult:* PO 75-300 mg/day

*Fibromyalgia/insomnia (unlabeled)*
*Adult:* PO 10-50 mg nightly

**Available forms:** Tabs 10, 25, 50, 75, 100, 150 mg; syr 10 mg/5 ml

## Adverse effects

***CNS:*** *Dizziness, drowsiness,* confusion, headache, anxiety, tremors, stimulation, weakness, insomnia, nightmares, EPS (geriatric), increased psychiatric symptoms, **seizures**

***CV:*** *Orthostatic hypotension,* **ECG changes, tachycardia, hypertension,** palpitations, dysrhythmias

***EENT:*** *Blurred vision,* tinnitus, mydriasis, ophthalmoplegia

***GI:*** *Constipation, dry mouth,* weight gain, nausea, vomiting, **paralytic ileus,** increased appetite, cramps, epigastric distress, jaundice, **hepatitis,** stomatitis

***GU:*** *Urinary retention*

***HEMA:*** **Agranulocytosis, thrombocytopenia, eosinophilia, leukopenia, aplastic anemia**

***INTEG:*** Rash, urticaria, sweating, pruritus, photosensitivity

**Contraindications:** Hypersensitivity to tricyclics, recovery phase of MI

**Precautions:** Pregnancy **C,** breastfeeding, child <12 yr, geriatric, suicidal patients, seizure disorders, prostatic hypertrophy, schizophrenia, psychosis, severe depression, increased intraocular pressure, angle-closure glaucoma, urinary retention, cardiac disease, renal/hepatic disease, hyperthyroidism, electroshock therapy, elective surgery

| Pharmacokinetics | |
|---|---|
| **Absorption** | Well absorbed |
| **Distribution** | Widely distributed; crosses placenta |
| **Metabolism** | Liver, extensively |
| **Excretion** | Kidneys, breast milk |
| **Half-life** | 10-46 hr |

| Pharmacodynamics | |
|---|---|
| | PO |
| **Onset** | 45 min |
| **Peak** | 2-12 hr |
| **Duration** | Unknown |

Adverse effects: *italic* = common, **bold** = life-threatening

### Interactions
#### Individual drugs
Alcohol: increased CNS depression

Carbamazepine: increased amitriptyline levels, increased toxicity

Cimetidine, fluoxetine: increased levels, increased toxicity

Clonidine: decreased effects

Guanethidine: decreased effects

#### Drug classifications
Antidepressants, antidysrhythmics (class IC), phenothiazines: increased amitriptyline levels, toxicity

Antihypertensives: blocked response to antihypertensives

Antithyroid agents: increased risk of agranulocytosis

Barbiturates, benzodiazepines, CNS depressants, opioids, sedative/hypnotics, sympathomimetics (direct acting): increased CNS effects

MAOIs: hypertensive crisis, seizures, hyperpyretic crisis

Oral contraceptives: increased effects, toxicity

Sympathomimetics (indirect acting): decreased effects

#### Drug/herb
Belladonna, henbane, jimsonweed, scopolia: increased anticholinergic effect

Chamomile, hops, kava, lavender, skullcap, valerian: increased CNS depression

SAM-e, St. John's wort: serotonin syndrome

Scopolia: increased amitriptyline action

Yohimbe: increased hypertension

#### Drug/lab test
Increased: serum bilirubin, blood glucose, alkaline phosphatase

### NURSING CONSIDERATIONS
#### Assessment
• Monitor B/P (with patient lying, standing), pulse q4hr; if systolic B/P drops 20 mm Hg, hold product, notify prescriber; take VS q4hr in patients with cardiovascular disease

• Monitor blood studies: CBC, leukocytes, differential, cardiac enzymes if patient is receiving long-term therapy

• Monitor hepatic studies: AST, ALT, bilirubin

• Check weight weekly; appetite may increase with product

• Assess ECG for flattening of T wave, bundle branch block, AV block, prolongation of QTc interval, dysrhythmias in cardiac patients

• Assess for EPS primarily in geriatric: rigidity, dystonia, akathisia

• Assess mental status: mood, sensorium, affect, suicidal tendencies; increase in psychiatric symptoms: depression, panic

• Monitor urinary retention, constipation; constipation is more likely to occur in children or geriatric

• Assess for withdrawal symptoms: headache, nausea, vomiting, muscle pain, weakness; do not usually occur unless product was discontinued abruptly

• Identify alcohol consumption; if alcohol is consumed, hold dose until morning

#### Nursing diagnoses
• Coping, ineffective (uses)
• Injury, risk for (side effects)
• Knowledge, deficient (teaching)
• Noncompliance (teaching)

#### Implementation
• Give with food or milk for GI symptoms
• Crush if patient is unable to swallow medication whole
• Give dosage at bedtime if oversedation occurs during day; may take entire dose at bedtime; geriatric may not tolerate once/day dosing
• Store at room temperature; do not freeze

#### Patient/family education
• Teach patient that therapeutic effects may take 2-3 wk
• Instruct patient to use caution in driving or other activities requiring alertness because of drowsiness, dizziness, blurred vision; to avoid rising quickly from sitting to standing, especially geriatric
• Advise patient to avoid alcohol ingestion, other CNS depressants; overheating
• Teach patient not to discontinue medication quickly after long-term use; may cause nausea, headache, malaise
• Advise patient to wear sunscreen or large hat, since photosensitivity occurs; hyperthermia can occur
• Teach patient to increase fluids, bulk in diet if constipation, urinary retention occur, especially geriatric
• Teach patient to use gum, hard sugarless candy, or frequent sips of water for dry mouth
• Instruct patient to use contraception during treatment

#### Evaluation
**Positive therapeutic outcome**
• Decreased depression
• Absence of suicidal thoughts

#### Treatment of overdose: ECG monitoring, lavage, administer anticonvulsant, sodium bicarbonate

## amlodipine (Rx)
(am-loe′di-peen)

Norvasc

*Func. class.:* Antianginal, calcium channel blocker, antihypertensive

*Chem. class.:* Dihydropyridine

**Pregnancy category** C

### Do not confuse:
amlodipine/amiloride, Norvasc/Navane

**Action:** Inhibits calcium ion influx across cell membrane during cardiac depolarization; produces relaxation of coronary vascular smooth muscle and peripheral vascular smooth muscle; dilates coronary vascular arteries; increases myocardial oxygen delivery in patients with vasospastic angina

**Therapeutic outcome:** Decreased angina pectoris, dysrhythmias, B/P

**Uses:** Chronic stable angina pectoris, hypertension, variant angina (Prinzmetal's angina); may coadminister with other antihypertensives, antianginals

### Dosage and routes
**Angina**
*Adult:* PO 5-10 mg daily

**Hypertension**
*Adult:* PO 5 mg daily initially, max 10 mg/day

**Hepatic dose/geriatric**
*Adult:* PO 2.5 mg/day, may increase to 10 mg/day (antihypertensive); 5 mg/day, may increase to 10 mg/day (antianginal)

**Available forms:** Tabs 2.5, 5, 10 mg

### Adverse effects
*CNS:* Headache, fatigue, dizziness, asthenia, anxiety, depression, insomnia, paresthesia, somnolence

*CV:* Dysrhythmia, peripheral edema, bradycardia, hypotension, palpitations, syncope, chest pain

*GI:* Nausea, vomiting, diarrhea, gastric upset, constipation, flatulence, anorexia, gingival hyperplasia, dyspepsia, dysphagia

*GU:* Nocturia, polyuria, sexual difficulties

*INTEG:* Rash, pruritus, urticaria, hair loss

*MISC:* Flushing, sexual difficulties, muscle cramps, cough, weight gain, tinnitus, epistaxis

**Contraindications:** Sick sinus syndrome, 2nd- or 3rd-degree heart block, hypersensitivity, severe aortic stenosis, severe obstructive coronary artery disease

**Precautions:** Pregnancy **C**, breastfeeding, children, geriatric, CHF, hypotension, hepatic injury

### Pharmacokinetics

| | |
|---|---|
| **Absorption** | Well absorbed up to 90% |
| **Distribution** | Crosses placenta, protein binding 95% |
| **Metabolism** | Liver, extensively |
| **Excretion** | Kidneys to metabolites (90%) |
| **Half-life** | 30-50 hr; increased in geriatric, hepatic disease |

### Pharmacodynamics

| | |
|---|---|
| **Onset** | Unknown |
| **Peak** | 6-10 hr |
| **Duration** | 24 hr |

### Interactions
*Individual drugs*
Alcohol: increased hypotension
Diltiazem: increased amlodipine level
Lithium: increased neurotoxicity
*Drug classifications*
Antihypertensives, nitrates: increased hypotension
NSAIDs: decreased antihypertensive effect
*Drug/herb*
Barberry, betel palm, burdock, goldenseal, khat, khella, lily of the valley, plantain: increased effect
Yohimbe: decreased effect
*Drug/food*
Grapefruit juice: increased hypotension

### NURSING CONSIDERATIONS
**Assessment**
• Assess fluid volume status: I&O ratio and record, weight, distended red veins, crackles in lung, color, quality and specific gravity of urine, skin turgor, adequacy of pulses, moist mucous membranes, bilateral lung sounds, peripheral pitting edema; dehydration symptoms of decreasing output, thirst, hypotension, dry mouth and mucous membranes should be reported
• Monitor B/P and pulse; if B/P drops, call prescriber
• Monitor ALT, AST, bilirubin daily; if these are elevated, hepatotoxicity is suspected
• Monitor if platelet count is <150,000/mm$^3$; product is usually discontinued and another product started
• Monitor cardiac status: B/P, pulse, respiration, ECG

Adverse effects: *italic* = common, **bold** = life-threatening

### Nursing diagnoses
- Cardiac output, decreased (uses)
- Knowledge, deficient (teaching)

### Implementation
- Give once a day, without regard to meals

### Patient/family education
- Advise patient to avoid hazardous activities until stabilized on product, dizziness is no longer a problem
- Instruct patient to avoid alcohol and OTC products unless directed by prescriber
- Advise patient to comply in all areas of medical regimen: diet, exercise, stress reduction, smoking cessation, product therapy; to notify prescriber of irregular heartbeat, shortness of breath, swelling of feet and hands, severe dizziness, constipation, nausea, hypotension
- Teach patient to use as directed even if feeling better; may be taken with other cardiovascular products (nitrates, β-blockers)

### Evaluation
**Positive therapeutic outcome**
- Decreased anginal pain
- Decreased B/P
- Increased exercise tolerance

**Treatment of overdose:** Defibrillation, β-agonists, **IV** calcium inotropic agents, diuretics, atropine for AV block, vasopressor for hypotension

---

## amoxapine (Rx)
(a-mox′a-peen)
amoxapine, Asendin
*Func. class.:* Antidepressant
*Chem. class.:* Dibenzoxazepine derivative, secondary amine

**Pregnancy category C**

### Do not confuse:
amoxapine/amoxicillin/Amoxil

**Action:** Blocks reuptake of norepinephrine, serotonin into nerve endings, thereby increasing action of norepinephrine, serotonin in nerve cells

**Therapeutic outcome:** Decreased symptoms of depression after 2-3 wk

**Uses:** Depression with anxiety or agitation

### Dosage and routes
*Adult:* PO 50 mg bid-tid; may increase to 100 mg tid on third day of therapy; not to exceed 300 mg/day unless lower doses have been given for at least 2 wk; may be given daily dose at bedtime; not to exceed 600 mg/day in hospitalized patients
*Geriatric:* PO 25 mg bid-tid, may increase by 25 mg/wk, up to 400 mg/day in divided doses

**Available forms:** Tabs 25, 50, 100, 150 mg

### Adverse effects
*CNS: Dizziness, drowsiness,* confusion, headache, anxiety, tremors, stimulation, weakness, insomnia, nightmares, EPS (geriatric), increased psychiatric symptoms, paresthesia, impairment of sexual functioning, **neuroleptic malignant syndrome, seizures**
*CV: Orthostatic hypotension, ECG changes, tachycardia,* hypertension, palpitations, **dysrhythmias**
*EENT: Blurred vision,* tinnitus, mydriasis, ophthalmoplegia
*GI: Dry mouth, constipation,* nausea, vomiting, **paralytic ileus,** increased appetite, cramps, epigastric distress, jaundice, **hepatitis,** stomatitis, weight gain
*GU:* Urinary retention, **acute renal failure**
*HEMA:* **Agranulocytosis, thrombocytopenia, eosinophilia, leukopenia**
*INTEG:* Rash, urticaria, sweating, pruritus, photosensitivity
*META:* Increased prolactin levels

**Contraindications:** Hypersensitivity to tricyclics, recovery phase of MI, seizure disorders, prostatic hypertrophy, angle-closure glaucoma

**Precautions:** Pregnancy **C**, geriatric, suicidal patients, severe depression, increased intraocular pressure, urinary retention, cardiac/hepatic disease, hyperthyroidism, electroshock therapy, elective surgery, schizophrenia, urinary retention

| Pharmacokinetics | |
|---|---|
| Absorption | Well absorbed |
| Distribution | Widely distributed, crosses placenta, steady state 2-7 days |
| Metabolism | Liver, extensively |
| Excretion | Kidneys, breast milk |
| Half-life | 8 hr; metabolite 30 hr |

| Pharmacodynamics | |
|---|---|
| Onset | 1-2 wk |
| Peak | 90 min |
| Duration | 6-12 wk |

A

## Interactions
### Individual drugs
Alcohol: increased CNS depression

Cimetidine, fluoxetine, fluvoxamine, paroxetine, sertraline: increased amoxapine levels, increased toxicity of amoxapine

Clonidine, epINEPHrine, norepinephrine: increased hypertensive effect

Guanethidine: decreased effects of amoxapine

### Drug classifications
Barbiturates: decreased amoxapine effect

CNS depressants: increased CNS depression

⬥MAOIs: hypertensive crisis, seizures, hyperpyretic crisis

### Drug/herb
Chamomile, hops, kava, lavender, skullcap, St. John's wort, valerian: increased CNS depression

Belladonna, corkwood, henbane, jimsonweed: increased anticholinergic effect

Scopolia: increased amoxapine action

### Drug/lab test
Increased: blood glucose, liver function tests

Decreased: blood glucose, WBC

## NURSING CONSIDERATIONS
### Assessment
• Monitor B/P (with patient lying, standing), pulse q4hr; if systolic B/P drops 20 mm Hg, hold product, notify prescriber; take vital signs q4hr in patients with cardiovascular disease

• Monitor blood studies: CBC, leukocytes, differential, cardiac enzymes if patient is receiving long-term therapy

• Monitor blood level: therapeutic 20-100 ng/ml

• Monitor hepatic studies: AST, ALT, bilirubin

• Check weight weekly; appetite may increase with product

• Assess ECG for flattening of T wave, bundle branch block, AV block, dysrhythmias in cardiac patients

• Assess for EPS primarily in geriatric: rigidity, dystonia, akathisia

• Assess mental status: mood, sensorium, affect, suicidal tendencies; increase in psychiatric symptoms: depression, panic; confusion (geriatric)

• Monitor urinary retention, constipation; constipation is more likely to occur in children and geriatric

• Assess for withdrawal symptoms: headache, nausea, vomiting, muscle pain, weakness; do not usually occur unless product was discontinued abruptly

• Identify alcohol consumption; if alcohol is consumed, hold dose until morning

## Nursing diagnoses
• Coping, ineffective (uses)
• Injury, risk for (side effects)
• Knowledge, deficient (teaching)
• Noncompliance (teaching)

## Implementation
• Give with food or milk for GI symptoms
• Crush if patient is unable to swallow medication whole
• Store at room temperature; do not freeze

## Patient/family education
• Teach patient that therapeutic effects may take 2-3 wk

• Instruct patient to use caution in driving or other activities requiring alertness because of drowsiness, dizziness, blurred vision; to avoid rising quickly from sitting to standing, especially geriatric

• Teach patient to avoid alcohol ingestion, other CNS depressants, may potentiate effects

• Teach patient not to discontinue medication quickly after long-term use: may cause nausea, headache, malaise

• Teach patient to wear sunscreen or large hat, since photosensitivity occurs

• Teach patient to increase fluids, bulk in diet if constipation, urinary retention occur, especially geriatric

• Advise patient to take gum, hard sugarless candy, or frequent sips of water for dry mouth

## Evaluation
### Positive therapeutic outcome
• Decreased depression
• Absence of suicidal thoughts

**Treatment of overdose:** ECG monitoring, induce emesis, lavage, activated charcoal, administer anticonvulsant

---

## amoxicillin (Rx)
(a-mox-i-sill'in)
amoxicillin, Amoxil, Apo-Amoxi ✦,
DisperMox, Novamoxin ✦, Nu-Amoxi ✦,
Trimox, Wymox
*Func. class.:* Antiinfective, antiulcer
*Chem. class.:* Aminopenicillin
**Pregnancy category B**

**Do not confuse:**
amoxicillin/amoxapine, Amoxil/amoxapine/amoxicillin, Trimox/Diamox/Tylox, Wymox/Tylox

**Action:** Interferes with cell wall replication of susceptible organisms by binding to the bacterial cell wall; the cell wall, rendered

---

Adverse effects: *italic* = common, **bold** = life-threatening

osmotically unstable, swells and bursts from osmotic pressure

**Therapeutic outcome:** Bactericidal effects for the following organisms: effective for gram-positive cocci *(Streptococcus pyogenes, Streptococcus faecalis, Streptococcus pneumoniae)*, gram-negative cocci *(Neisseria gonorrhoeae, Neisseria meningitidis, Escherichia coli)*, gram-negative bacilli *(Haemophilus influenzae, Proteus mirabilis, Salmonella)*, in combination for *Helicobacter pylori*

**Uses:** Infections of respiratory tract, skin, skin structures, genitourinary tract, otitis media, meningitis, septicemia, sinusitis, and bacterial endocarditis prophylaxis

**Unlabeled uses:** Lyme disease, anthrax treatment and prophylaxis

### Dosage and routes
*Renal disease*
*Adult:* PO CCr 10-30 ml/min 250-500 mg q12hr; CCr <10 ml/min 250-500 mg q24hr; do not use 875 mg strength if CCr <50 ml/min

*Systemic infections*
*Adult:* PO 750 mg-1.5 g daily in divided doses q8hr
*Child:* PO 20-50 mg/kg/day in divided doses q8hr

*Gonorrhea/urinary tract infections*
*Adult:* PO 3 g given with 1 g probenecid as a single dose; followed by tetracycline or erythromycin

*Chlamydia trachomatis*
*Adult:* PO 500 mg/day × 1 wk

*Bacterial endocarditis prophylaxis*
*Adult:* PO 2 g 1 hr prior to procedure
*Child:* PO 50 mg/kg/hr 1 hr prior to procedure, max 2 g

*Helicobacter pylori*
*Adult:* PO 1000 mg bid given with lansoprazole 30 mg bid, clarithromycin 500 mg bid × 2 wk; or 1000 mg bid given with omeprazole 20 mg bid, clarithromycin 500 mg bid × 2 wk; or 1000 mg tid given with lansoprazole 30 mg tid × 2 wk

**Available forms:** Caps 250, 500 mg; chewable tabs 125, 200, 250, 400 mg; tabs 500, 875 mg; susp pedidrops 50 mg/ml; susp 125, 200, 250, 400 mg/5 ml

### Adverse effects
*CNS:* Headache, fever, **seizures**
*GI:* *Nausea, vomiting, diarrhea*, increased AST, ALT, abdominal pain, glossitis, colitis, **pseudomembranous colitis**

*HEMA:* Anemia, increased bleeding time, **bone marrow depression, granulocytopenia**
*INTEG:* *Urticaria, rash*
*SYST:* **Anaphylaxis, respiratory distress, serum sickness, Stevens-Johnson syndrome**

**Contraindications:** Hypersensitivity to penicillins

**Precautions:** Pregnancy **B**, breastfeeding, neonates, hypersensitivity to cephalosporins, severe renal disease, acute lymphocytic leukemia

| Pharmacokinetics | |
|---|---|
| **Absorption** | Well absorbed (90%) |
| **Distribution** | Readily in body tissues, fluids, CSF; crosses placenta |
| **Metabolism** | Liver (30%) |
| **Excretion** | Breast milk, kidney, unchanged (70%) |
| **Half-life** | 1-1.3 hr |

| Pharmacodynamics | |
|---|---|
| **Onset** | ½ hr |
| **Peak** | 2 hr |
| **Duration** | Unknown |

### Interactions
*Individual drugs*
Methotrexate: increased methotrexate levels
Probenecid: increased amoxicillin levels, decreased renal excretion
Warfarin: increased anticoagulant effects
*Drug classifications*
Anticoagulants (oral): increased anticoagulant effects
Contraceptives (oral): decreased contraceptive effectiveness
*Drug/herb*
Acidophilus: do not use with antiinfectives, separate by several hours
Khat: decreased absorption, separate by 2 hr
*Drug/lab test*
False positive: urine glucose, urine protein, direct Coombs' test

### NURSING CONSIDERATIONS
### Assessment
• Assess patient for previous sensitivity reaction to penicillins or other cephalosporins; cross-sensitivity between penicillins and cephalosporins is common
• Assess patient for signs and symptoms of infection, including characteristics of wounds, sputum, urine, stool, WBC >10,000/mm³,

 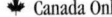

earache, fever; obtain baseline information and monitor symptoms during treatment
- Obtain C&S before beginning product therapy to identify if correct treatment has been initiated
- Assess for allergic reactions during treatment: rash, urticaria, pruritus, chills, fever, joint pain; angioedema may occur a few days after therapy begins; epINEPHrine and resuscitation equipment should be available for anaphylactic reactions
- Identify urine output; if decreasing, notify prescriber (may indicate nephrotoxicity); also, increased BUN, creatinine, urinalysis, protein, blood
- Monitor blood studies: AST, ALT, CBC, Hct, bilirubin, LDH, alkaline phosphatase, Coombs' test monthly if patient is on long-term therapy
- Monitor electrolytes: potassium, sodium, chloride monthly if patient is on long-term therapy
- Assess bowel pattern daily; diarrhea, cramping, blood in stools; if severe diarrhea occurs, notify prescriber; product should be discontinued; pseudomembranous colitis may occur
- Monitor for bleeding: ecchymosis, bleeding gums, hematuria, stool guaiac daily if on long-term therapy
- Assess for overgrowth of infection: perineal itching, fever, malaise, redness, pain, swelling, drainage, rash, diarrhea, change in cough, sputum

### Nursing diagnoses
- Diarrhea (side effects)
- Infection, risk for (uses)
- Injury, risk for (side effects)
- Knowledge, deficient (teaching)
- Noncompliance (teaching)

### Implementation
**PO route**
- Give in even doses around the clock; if GI upset occurs, give with food; product must be given for 10-14 days to ensure organism death and prevent superinfection; store in tight container
- The caps may be opened and contents taken with fluids
- Shake susp well before each dose, may be used alone or mixed in drinks, use immediately; susp may be stored in refrigerator for 14 days

### Patient/family education
- ⬥ Teach patient to report sore throat, bruising, bleeding, joint pain; may indicate blood dyscrasias (rare)
- Advise patient to contact prescriber if vaginal itching, loose foul-smelling stools,

diarrhea, sore throat, fever, fatigue, furry tongue occur; may indicate superinfection or agranulocytopenia
- Instruct patient to take all medication prescribed for the length of time ordered; not to double dose; chew form is available
- Advise patient to notify prescriber of diarrhea with blood or pus, which may indicate pseudomembranous colitis

### Evaluation
**Positive therapeutic outcome**
- Absence of signs/symptoms of infection (WBC <10,000/mm$^3$, temp WNL, absence of red draining wounds or earache)
- Prevention of endocarditis
- Resolution of ulcer symptoms

### Treatment of anaphylaxis: Withdraw
product, maintain airway, administer epINEPHrine, aminophylline, O$_2$, **IV** corticosteroids

---

### amoxicillin/clavulanate (Rx)
(a-mox-i-sill'in)
Augmentin, Augmentin ES-600, Augmentin XR, Clavulin ⬥
*Func. class.:* Broad-spectrum antiinfective (extended spectrum)
*Chem. class.:* Aminopenicillin-β-lactamase inhibitor
**Pregnancy category B**

**Action:** Interferes with cell wall replication of susceptible organisms; the cell wall, rendered osmotically unstable, swells and bursts from osmotic pressure; combination increases spectrum of activity, β-lactamase resistance

**Therapeutic outcome:** Bactericidal effects for the following organisms: *Escherichia coli, Proteus mirabilis, Haemophilus influenzae, Streptococcus faecalis, Streptococcus pneumoniae;* and β-lactamase–producing organisms: *Neisseria gonorrhoeae, Neisseria meningitidis, Shigella, Salmonella, Enterococcus, Streptococcus*

**Uses:** Infections of respiratory tract, skin, skin structures, genitourinary tract; otitis media, meningitis, septicemia, sinusitis, and endocarditis prophylaxis

### Dosage and routes
*Adult:* PO 250-500 mg q8hr or 500-875 mg q12hr depending on severity of infection
*Child ≤40 kg:* PO 20-40 mg/kg/day in divided doses q8hr or 25-45 mg/kg/day in divided doses q12hr

### Renal dose
**Adult:** PO CCr 10-30 ml/min dose q12hr; CCr <10 ml/min dose q24hr; do not use 875 mg strength if CCr <30 ml/min; Augmentin XR is contraindicated in renal disease

**Available forms:** Tabs 250, 500, 875 mg/125 mg clavulanate; chewable tabs 125, 200, 250, 400 mg; powder for oral susp 125, 200, 250, 400 mg/5 ml; (XR) ext rel tabs 1000 mg amoxicillin/62.5 mg clavulanate; (ES) powder for oral susp 600 mg amoxicillin; 42.9 mg clavulanate 5 ml

### Adverse effects
*CNS:* Headache, fever, **seizures**
*GI: Nausea, diarrhea, vomiting,* increased AST, ALT, abdominal pain, glossitis, colitis, black tongue, **pseudomembranous colitis**
*GU:* Oliguria, proteinuria, **hematuria**, *vaginitis, moniliasis,* **glomerulonephritis**
*HEMA:* Anemia, **bone marrow depression, granulocytopenia, leukopenia, eosinophilia, thrombocytopenic purpura**
*INTEG:* Rash, urticaria, dermatitis, **toxic epidermal necrolysis**
*META:* Hyperkalemia, hypokalemia, alkalosis, hypernatremia
*SYST:* **Anaphylaxis, respiratory distress, serum sickness, superinfection, Stevens-Johnson syndrome**

**Contraindications:** Hypersensitivity to penicillins; neonates

**Precautions:** Pregnancy **B**, breastfeeding, neonates, hypersensitivity to cephalosporins, GI/renal disease

| Pharmacokinetics | |
|---|---|
| **Absorption** | Well absorbed (90%) |
| **Distribution** | Readily in body tissues, fluids, CSF; crosses placenta |
| **Metabolism** | Liver (30%) |
| **Excretion** | Breast milk; kidney, unchanged (70%), removed by hemodialysis |
| **Half-life** | 1-1.3 hr |

| Pharmacodynamics | |
|---|---|
| **Onset** | ½ hr |
| **Peak** | 2 hr |
| **Duration** | Unknown |

### Interactions
*Individual drugs*
Allopurinol: increased skin rash
Probenecid: increased amoxicillin levels
Warfarin: increased anticoagulant effect

### Drug classifications
Anticoagulants (oral): increased anticoagulant effects
Contraceptives (oral): decreased contraceptive effectiveness
### Drug/herb
Acidophilus: do not use with antiinfectives; separate by several hours
Khat: decreased absorption, separate by 2 hr
### Drug/lab test
False positive: urine glucose, urine protein, direct Coombs' test

### NURSING CONSIDERATIONS
#### Assessment
• Assess patient for previous sensitivity reaction to penicillins or other cephalosporins; cross-sensitivity between penicillins and cephalosporins is common
• Assess patient for signs and symptoms of infection, including characteristics of wounds, sputum, urine, stool, WBC >10,000/mm³, earache, fever; obtain baseline information and during treatment
• Complete C&S before beginning product therapy to identify if correct treatment has been initiated
• Assess for anaphylaxis: rash, urticaria, pruritus, chills, dyspnea, laryngeal edema, fever, joint pain; angioedema may occur a few days after therapy begins; epINEPHrine and resuscitation equipment should be available for anaphylactic reaction
• Identify urine output; if decreasing, notify prescriber (may indicate nephrotoxicity)
• Monitor renal studies: urinalysis, protein, blood, BUN, creatinine
• Monitor blood studies: AST, ALT, CBC, Hct, bilirubin, LDH, alkaline phosphatase, Coombs' test monthly if patient is on long-term therapy
• Monitor electrolytes: potassium, sodium, chloride monthly if patient is on long-term therapy
• Assess bowel pattern daily; diarrhea, cramping, blood in stools, report to prescriber; if severe diarrhea occurs, product should be discontinued; may indicate pseudomembranous colitis
• Monitor for bleeding: ecchymosis, bleeding gums, hematuria, stool guaiac daily if on long-term therapy
• Assess for overgrowth of infection: perineal itching, fever, malaise, redness, pain, swelling, drainage, rash, diarrhea, change in cough, sputum

#### Nursing diagnoses
• Diarrhea (side effects)
• Infection, risk for (uses)

- Injury, risk for (side effects)
- Knowledge, deficient (teaching)
- Noncompliance (teaching)

## Implementation
### PO route

- Give in even doses around the clock; if GI upset occurs, give with food; product must be taken for 10-14 days to ensure organism death and prevent superinfection; store in tight container; cap can be opened and mixed with food or liquid; chewable tabs should be chewed
- Administer only as directed; two 250-mg tabs not equivalent to one 500-mg tab due to strength of clavulanate
- Shake susp well before each dose; may be used alone or mixed in drinks, use immediately; susp may be stored in refrigerator for 10 days

## Patient/family education

◆ Teach patient to report sore throat, bruising, bleeding, joint pain; may indicate blood dyscrasias (rare)
- Advise patient to contact prescriber if vaginal itching, loose foul-smelling stools occur; may indicate superinfection
- Instruct patient to take all medication prescribed for the length of time prescribed
- Advise patient to notify prescriber of diarrhea with blood or pus, which may indicate pseudomembranous colitis
- Advise patient to use alternative contraceptive measures if using oral contraceptives

## Evaluation
### Positive therapeutic outcome

- Absence of signs/symptoms of infection (WBC <10,000/mm$^3$, temp WNL)
- Reported improvement in symptoms of infection

**Treatment of anaphylaxis:** Withdraw product, maintain airway, administer epINEPHrine, aminophylline, $O_2$, **IV** corticosteroids

## AMPHOTERICIN B

### amphotericin B deoxycholate (Rx)
(am-foh-tehr'ih-sin de-ox-ee-kohl'ate)
Fungizone
### amphotericin B cholesteryl (Rx)
Amphotec
### amphotericin B lipid based (Rx)
Abelcet
### amphotericin B liposome (Rx)
AmBisome
*Func. class.:* Antifungal
*Chem. class.:* Amphoteric polyene

**Pregnancy category** B

**Action:** increased cell membrane permeability in susceptible organisms by binding sterols in fungal cell membrane; decreases potassium, sodium, and nutrients in cell

**Therapeutic outcome:** Fungistatic against histoplasmosis, blastomycosis, coccidioidomycosis, cryptococcosis, aspergillosis, zygomycosis, candidiasis, sporotrichosis, cryptococcal meningitis, mucormycosis caused by mucormycosis, *Rhizopus, Absidia, Entomorphthera, Basidobolus*

**Uses:** Treatment of severe, possibly fatal fungal infections (**IV**); treatment of topical fungal infections

**Unlabeled uses:** Candiduria (bladder irrigation), funguria

**Dosage and routes**
*Fungizone*
*Adult:* **IV** Give test dose of 1 mg (not required); then 0.25 mg/kg, increase daily slowly to 0.5 mg/kg, may give 1 mg/kg/day or 1.5 mg/kg/day, alternate day dosing may be used
*Child:* **IV** 0.25 mg/kg infused initially, increase by 0.25 mg/kg every other day to max of 1 mg/kg/day
*Adult and child:* TOP Apply 2-4 × daily
*Adult and child:* PO 1 ml qid

*Amphotec*
*Adult and child:* **IV** 3-4 mg/kg/day, max 7.5 mg/kg/day

Adverse effects: *italic* = common, **bold** = life-threatening

*Abelcet*
*Adult and child:* **IV** 5 mg/kg/day as a 1 mg/ml inf given 2.5 mg/kg/hr

*AmBisome*
*Fungal infections*
*Adult and child:* **IV** 3-5 mg/kg q24hr

*Visceral leishmaniasis:* 3 mg/kg q24hr days 1-5

**Available forms:** Amphotericin deoxycholate: inj 50-mg vial, oral susp 100 mg/ml; cream, ointment, lotion 3%; amphotericin B cholesteryl: powder for inj 50 mg/20 ml, 100 mg/50 ml; amphotericin B lipid based: susp for inj 100 mg/20-ml vial; amphotericin B lipid complex: susp for inj 100 mg/20 ml vial; amphotericin B liposome: powder for inj 50 mg vial

**Adverse effects**
*CNS: Headache, fever, chills,* peripheral nerve pain, paresthesias, peripheral neuropathy, **seizures,** dizziness
*EENT:* Tinnitus, deafness, diplopia, blurred vision
*GI: Nausea, vomiting, anorexia,* diarrhea, cramps, **hemorrhagic gastroenteritis, acute liver failure**
*GU: Hypokalemia,* axotemia, hyposthenuria, **renal tubular acidosis,** nephrocalcinosis, **permanent renal impairment, anuria, oliguria**
*HEMA:* Normochromic and normocytic anemia, **thrombocytopenia, agranulocytosis, leukopenia, eosinophilia,** hypokalemia, hyponatremia, hypomagnesemia
*INTEG: Burning, irritation,* pain, necrosis at inj site with extravasation, flushing, dermatitis, skin rash (topical route)
*MS: Arthralgia, myalgia,* generalized pain, weakness, weight loss
*SYST:* **Stevens-Johnson syndrome, toxic epidermal necrolysis, exfoliative dermatitis**

**Contraindications:** Hypersensitivity, severe bone marrow depression

**Precautions:** Pregnancy **B,** breastfeeding, children, renal disease, anemia, fungal infection, hypokalemia, hypomagnesium, infections

## Pharmacokinetics

| | |
|---|---|
| **Absorption** | Complete bioavailability (**IV**), rapidly absorbed (TOP) |
| **Distribution** | Body tissues |
| **Metabolism** | Liver |
| **Excretion** | Kidneys, detectable for several weeks |
| **Half-life** | Initial 24-48 hr, terminal 15 days |

## Pharmacodynamics

| | IV | TOP |
|---|---|---|
| **Onset** | Immediate | Unknown |
| **Peak** | 1-2 hr | Unknown |
| **Duration** | Unknown | Unknown |

**Interactions**
*Individual drugs*
Cisplatin, cycloSPORINE, polymyxin B, vancomycin: increased nephrotoxicity
Digoxin: increased hypokalemia
*Drug classifications*
Diuretics, nephrotoxic antibiotics: increased nephrotoxicity
Glucocorticoids, thiazides, skeletal muscle relaxants: increased hypokalemia
*Drug/herb*
Acidophilus: do not use with antiinfectives; separate by several hours
Gossypol: increased risk of nephrotoxicity

**NURSING CONSIDERATIONS**
**Assessment**
• Monitor VS q15-30 min during first inf; note changes in pulse, B/P
• Monitor blood studies: Hgb, Hct, potassium, sodium, calcium, magnesium q2 wk; BUN, creatinine weekly; decreased Hgb, Hct, and magnesium are common with increased potassium
• Monitor weight weekly; if weight increases over 2 lb/wk, edema is present; renal damage should be considered
• Monitor for renal toxicity: increasing BUN, serum creatinine; if BUN is >40 mg/dl or if serum creatinine >3 mg/dl, product may be discontinued or dosage reduced; I&O ratio: watch for decreasing urinary output, change in specific gravity; discontinue product to prevent permanent damage to renal tubules; provide hydration of 2-3 L/day
• Monitor for hepatotoxicity: increasing AST, ALT, alkaline phosphatase, bilirubin
• Monitor for allergic reaction: dermatitis, rash; product should be discontinued, antihistamines (mild reaction) or epINEPHrine (severe reaction) administered; check inj site for thrombophlebitis

• Monitor for hypokalemia: anorexia, drowsiness, weakness, decreased reflexes, dizziness, increased urinary output, increased thirst, paresthesias; if these occur, product should be decreased or discontinued and potassium administered

**Topical route**
• Monitor for allergic reaction: burning, stinging, swelling, redness

## Nursing diagnoses
• Infection, risk for (uses)
• Injury, risk for (adverse reaction)
• Knowledge, deficient (teaching)

## Implementation
**Topical route**
• Provide enough medication to cover lesions completely; do not cover with occlusive dressing; apply liberally and rub thoroughly into affected area; administer after cleansing with soap, water before each application, dry well (as ordered), wear gloves during application
• Store at room temperature in dry place

*Deoxycholate*
**Intermittent IV infusion route**
• Give after diluting 50 mg in 10 ml sterile water (no preservatives) (5 mg-1 ml); shake well, further dilute with 500 ml of $D_5W$ to concentration of 0.1 mg/ml; do not use other diluents or sol; use large needle (20G); change needle for each step; wear gloves
• Use test dosage of 1 mg/20 ml $D_5W$; give over 10-30 min; if no reaction, product is administered as ordered
• Administer **IV** using in-line filter (mean pore diameter >1 μm) using distal veins; check for extravasation, necrosis q8hr; use an infusion pump; administer over 6 hr; rapid inf may result in circulation collapse; may also be given through central line
• Give acetaminophen and diphenhydrAMINE 30 min before inf to reduce fever, chills, headache
• Give product only after C&S confirm organism, product needed to treat condition; make sure product is used in life-threatening infections
• Store protected from moisture and light; diluted sol is stable for 24 hr at room temperature, 1 wk refrigerated

*Syringe compatibilities:* Heparin
*Y-site compatibilities:* Aldesleukin, diltiazem, DOXOrubicin liposome, famotidine, remifentanil, tacrolimus, teniposide, thiotepa, zidovudine
*Y-site incompatibilities:* Enalaprilat, fludarabine, foscarnet, ondansetron

*Additive compatibilities:* Fluconazole, heparin, hydrocortisone, methylPREDNISolone, sodium bicarbonate
*Solution compatibilities:* $D_5W$

*Cholesteryl*
*Liposomal complex*
**IV route**
• Reconstitute with 12 ml sterile water/50 ml vial (4 mg/ml), shake, use 5-micron filter, dilute in $D_5W$ (1-2 mg/ml), give over 2 hr

*Lipid complex*
**IV route**
• Shake vial until dissolved, withdraw dose using 18-G needle, replace needle from syringe with product using 5-micron filter needle (use needle for 4 vials or less), empty contents in **IV** of $D_5W$ (1 mg/ml), give at 2.5 mg/kg/hr, use infusion pump

## Patient/family education
**Topical route**
• Teach patient that skin and clothing may become discolored; to use asepsis (hand washing) before, after each application to prevent further infection
• Instruct patient to apply with glove to prevent further infection; not to cover with occlusive dressing; to continue even if condition improves
• Teach patient to avoid use of OTC creams, ointments, lotions, unless directed by prescriber
• Instruct patient to report increased itching, burning, rash, redness; ointment may irritate most hairy areas; to report if condition worsens
**IV route**
• Advise patient that long-term therapy may be needed to clear infection (2 wk-3 mo depending on type of infection)
• Teach patient side effects and when to notify prescriber

## Evaluation
**Positive therapeutic outcome**
• Decreased in size, number of lesions (TOP)
• Decreased fever, malaise, rash
• Negative C&S for infecting organism

Adverse effects: *italic* = common, **bold** = life-threatening

**ampicillin** (Rx)
(am-pi-sill'in)
Ampicin ✤, Apo-Ampi ✤, Nu-Ampi ✤,
NovoAmpicillin ✤, Omnipen,
Penbriten ✤, Principen
*Func. class.:* Broad-spectrum antiinfective
*Chem. class.:* Aminopenicillin

**Pregnancy category** B

**Do not confuse:**
Omnipen/imipenem

**Action:** Interferes with cell wall replication of susceptible organisms; the cell wall, rendered osmotically unstable, swells, and bursts from osmotic pressure

**Therapeutic outcome:** Bactericidal effects for the following organisms: effective for gram-positive cocci *(Streptococcus pyogenes, Streptococcus faecalis, Streptococcus pneumoniae),* gram-negative cocci *(Neisseria gonorrhoeae, Neisseria meningitidis),* gram-negative bacilli *(Haemophilus influenzae, Proteus mirabilis, Salmonella, Shigella, Listeria monocytogenes),* gram-positive bacilli

**Uses:** Infections of respiratory tract, skin, skin structures, genitourinary tract; otitis media, meningitis, septicemia, sinusitis, and endocarditis prophylaxis

**Dosage and routes**
*Renal dose*
*Adult and child:* CCr 30-50 ml/min q6-8hr; CCr 10-30 ml/min dose q8-12hr; CCr <10 ml/min dose q12hr

*Systemic infections*
*Adult and child ≥40 kg (88 lb):* PO 250-500 mg q6hr; **IV**/IM 2-8 g daily in divided doses q4-6hr
*Child <40 kg:* PO 50-100 mg/kg/day in divided doses q6-8hr; **IV**/IM 100-200 mg/kg/day in divided doses q6-8hr

*Bacterial meningitis*
*Adult:* IM/**IV** 500 mg-3 g q6hr, max 14 g/day
*Child:* IM/**IV** 200-400 mg/kg/day in divided doses q6hr, max 12 g/day

*Gonorrhea*
*Adult and child ≥ 45 kg (99 lb):* PO 3 g given with 1 g probenecid as a single dose or IM/**IV** 500 mg q6hr (≥40 kg); IM/**IV** 50 mg/kg/day in divided doses q6-8hr (<40 kg)

*Prevention of bacterial endocarditis*
*Adult:* IM/**IV** 2 g 30 min before procedure
*Child:* IM/**IV** 50 mg/kg 30 min before procedure, max 2 g

*GI/GU infections other than caused by N. gonorrhoeae*
*Adult and child >20 kg:* PO 250-500 mg q6hr, may use larger dose for more serious infections
*Child ≤20 kg:* PO 50-100 mg/kg/day in divided doses q6hr

**Available forms:** Powder for inj 125, 250, 500 mg, 1, 2, 10 g; **IV** inf 500 mg, 1, 2 g; caps 250, 500 mg; powder for oral susp, 125, 250, 500 mg/5 ml

**Adverse effects**
*CNS:* Lethargy, hallucinations, anxiety, depression, twitching, **coma, seizures**
*GI:* Nausea, vomiting, diarrhea, **pseudomembranous colitis**
*GU:* Oliguria, proteinuria, hematuria, *vaginitis, moniliasis,* **glomerulonephritis**
*HEMA:* Anemia, increased bleeding time, **bone marrow depression, granulocytopenia,** leukopenia, eosinophilia
*INTEG: Rash,* urticaria, **toxic epidermal necrolysis**
*SYST:* Anaphylaxis, **serum sickness, Stevens-Johnson syndrome**

**Contraindications:** Hypersensitivity to penicillins

**Precautions:** Pregnancy **B**, breastfeeding, neonates, hypersensitivity to cephalosporins, renal disease

| Pharmacokinetics | |
|---|---|
| Absorption | Moderate, duodenum (35%-50%) |
| Distribution | Readily in body tissues, fluids, CSF; crosses placenta |
| Metabolism | Liver (30%) |
| Excretion | Breast milk; kidney unchanged (70%), removed by dialysis |
| Half-life | 50-110 min |

| Pharmacodynamics | | | |
|---|---|---|---|
| | PO | IM | IV |
| Onset | Rapid | Rapid | Rapid |
| Peak | 2 hr | 1 hr | Infusion's end |
| Duration | Unknown | Unknown | Unknown |

## Interactions
### Individual drugs
Allopurinol: increased ampicillin-induced skin rash

Probenecid: increased ampicillin levels, decreased renal excretion

### Drug classifications
Contraceptives (oral): decreased contraceptive effectiveness

### Drug/herb
Acidophilus: do not use with antiinfectives; separate by several hours

Khat: decreased absorption, separate by 2 hr

### Drug/lab test
Increased: AST, ALT

Decreased: conjugated estrone in pregnancy, conjugated estriol

False positive: urine glucose, urine protein, direct Coombs' test

## NURSING CONSIDERATIONS
### Assessment
- Assess patient for previous sensitivity reaction to penicillins or other cephalosporins; cross-sensitivity between penicillins and cephalosporins is common
- Assess patient for signs and symptoms of infection, including characteristics of wounds, sputum, urine, stool, WBC >10,000/mm$^3$, earache, fever; obtain baseline information and during treatment
- Obtain C&S before beginning product therapy to identify if correct treatment has been initiated
- Assess for allergic reactions: rash, urticaria, pruritus, chills, fever, joint pain; angioedema may occur a few days after therapy begins; epINEPHrine and resuscitation equipment should be on unit for anaphylactic reaction; also, check for ampicillin rash: pruritic, red, raised
- ❶ Identify urine output; if decreasing, notify prescriber (may indicate nephrotoxicity)
- Monitor renal studies: urinalysis, protein, blood, BUN, creatinine
- Monitor blood studies: AST, ALT, CBC, Hct, bilirubin, LDH, alkaline phosphatase, Coombs' test monthly if patient is on long-term therapy
- Monitor electrolytes: potassium, sodium, chloride monthly if patient is on long-term therapy
- Assess bowel pattern daily; if severe diarrhea occurs, product should be discontinued; may indicate pseudomembranous colitis
- Monitor for bleeding: ecchymosis, bleeding gums, hematuria, stool guaiac daily if on long-term therapy
- Assess for overgrowth of infection: perineal itching, fever, malaise, redness, pain, swelling, drainage, rash, diarrhea, change in cough, sputum

### Nursing diagnoses
- Diarrhea (side effects)
- Infection, risk for (uses)
- Injury, risk for (side effects)
- Knowledge, deficient (teaching)
- Noncompliance (teaching)

### Implementation
**PO route**
- Give in even doses around the clock; product must be taken for 10-14 days to ensure organism death and prevent superinfection; store caps in tight container
- Tabs may be crushed or caps opened and mixed with water
- Shake susp well before each dose; store in refrigerator for 2 wk or 1 wk at room temperature

**IM route**
- Reconstitute with 125 mg/0.9-1.2 ml; 250 mg/0.9-1.9 ml; 500 mg/1.2-1.8 ml; 1 g/2.4-7.4 ml; 2 g/6.8 ml
- Give deep in large muscle mass

**IV route**
- Reconstitute with 125 mg/0.9-1.2 ml; 250 mg/0.9-1.9 ml; 500 mg/1.2-1.8 ml; 1 g/2.4-7.4 ml; 2 g/6.8 ml
- Give by direct **IV** over 3-5 min in lower dosages (125-500 mg) or over 15 min in higher dosages (1-2 g)
- Give by intermittent inf after diluting with 0.9% NaCl, LR, D$_5$W, D$_5$/0.45% NaCl; use 50 ml of sol and dilute to concentration of <30 mg/ml

**Syringe compatibilities:** Chloramphenicol

**Syringe incompatibilities:** Erythromycin, gentamicin, kanamycin, lincomycin, metoclopramide, oxytetracycline, streptomycin, tetracycline

**Y-site compatibilities:** Acyclovir, amifostine, allopurinol, aztreonam, cyclophosphamide, DOXOrubicin liposome, enalaprilat, esmolol, famotidine, filgrastim, fludarabine, foscarnet, granisetron, heparin, regular insulin, labetalol, magnesium sulfate, melphalan, meperidine, morphine, multivitamins, oflaxacin, perphenazine, phytonadione, potassium chloride, propofol, remifentanil, thiotepa, tolazoline, vit B with C

**Y-site incompatibilities:** Calcium gluconate, epINEPHrine, fluconazole, hetastarch, hydromorphone, hydrALAZINE, ondansetron, sargramostim, verapamil, vinorelbine

*Additive compatibilities:* Clindamycin, erythromycin, floxacillin, furosemide, tacrolimus, teniposide, theophylline, verapamil
*Additive incompatibilities:* Amikacin, aztreonam, chlorproMAZINE, DOPamine, gentamicin, hydrALAZINE, hydrocortisone, prochlorperazine

### Patient/family education
◆ Teach patient to report sore throat, bruising, bleeding, joint pain; may indicate blood dyscrasias (rare)
• Advise patient to contact prescriber if vaginal itching, loose foul-smelling stools, furry tongue occur; may indicate superinfection
• Instruct patient to take all medication prescribed for the length of time ordered
• Advise patient to notify prescriber of diarrhea with blood or pus, which may indicate pseudomembranous colitis
• Tab may be crushed; cap may be opened and mixed with water

### Evaluation
**Positive therapeutic outcome**
• Absence of signs/symptoms of infection (WBC <10,000, temp WNL)
• Reported improvement in symptoms of infection

**Treatment of anaphylaxis:** Withdraw product, maintain airway, administer epINEPHrine, aminophylline, O₂, **IV** corticosteroids

---

### ampicillin/sulbactam (Rx)
(am-pi-sill'in/sul-bak'tam)
Unasyn
*Func. class.:* Broad-spectrum antiinfective
*Chem. class.:* Aminopenicillin

**Pregnancy category B**
**(ampicillin)**

**Action:** Interferes with cell wall replication of susceptible organisms; the cell wall, rendered osmotically unstable, swells and bursts from osmotic pressure; this combination extends the spectrum of activity and inhibits β-lactamase that may inactivate ampicillin

**Therapeutic outcome:** Bactericidal against *Pneumococcus, Enterococcus, Streptococcus, Escherichia coli, Proteus mirabilis, Neisseria meningitidis, Neisseria gonorrhoeae, Shigella, Salmonella,* and *Haemophilus influenzae* organisms; use only with β-lactamase–producing strain of infection

**Uses:** Skin and structure infections, intraabdominal infections, pneumonia, gynecologic infections, soft tissue infections, otitis media, sinusitis, meningitis, septicemia

### Dosage and routes
*Adult and child >40 kg:* IM/**IV** 1 g ampicillin and 0.5 g sulbactam to 2 g ampicillin, and 1 g sulbactam q6hr, not to exceed 4 g/day sulbactam
*Child <40 kg:* **IV** 100-200 mg/kg/day (ampicillin component) divided q6hr, max 8 g/day

*Renal dose*
*Adult ≥40 kg:* IM/**IV** CCr 15-29 ml/min dose q12hr; CCr 5-14 ml/min dose q24hr

**Available forms:** Powder for inj 1.5 g (1 g ampicillin, 0.5 g sulbactam), 3 g (2 g ampicillin, 1 g sulbactam), 10 g (10 g ampicillin, 5 g sulbactam)

### Adverse effects
*CNS:* Lethargy, hallucinations, anxiety, depression, twitching, **coma, seizures**
*GI: Nausea, vomiting, diarrhea,* increased AST, ALT, abdominal pain, glossitis, colitis, **pseudomembranous colitis**
*GU:* Oliguria, proteinuria, hematuria, *vaginitis, moniliasis,* **glomerulonephritis,** dysuria
*HEMA:* Anemia, increased bleeding time, **bone marrow depression, granulocytopenia, leukopenia, eosinophilia**
*SYST:* Anaphylaxis, **serum sickness, toxic epidermal necrolysis, Stevens-Johnson syndrome**

**Contraindications:** Hypersensitivity to penicillins, ampicillin, or sulbactam

**Precautions:** Pregnancy **B,** breastfeeding, neonates, hypersensitivity to cephalosporins, renal disease

### Pharmacokinetics
| | |
|---|---|
| Absorption | Well absorbed (IM) |
| Distribution | Readily in body tissues, fluids, CSF; crosses placenta |
| Metabolism | Liver (10%-50%) |
| Excretion | Breast milk; kidney unchanged (75%) |
| Half-life | 50-110 min (ampicillin) |

### Pharmacodynamics
| | IM | IV |
|---|---|---|
| Onset | Rapid | Immediate |
| Peak | 1 hr | Infusion's end |
| Duration | Unknown | Unknown |

---

 Alert     Canada Only    🔘 Drug on CD    * "Tall Man" lettering (See Preface)

### Interactions
*Individual drugs*
Allopurinol: ampicillin-induced skin rash
Methotrexate: increased methotrexate level
Probenecid: increased ampicillin levels, decreased renal excretion
*Drug classifications*
Contraceptives (oral): decreased contraceptive effectiveness
*Drug/herb*
Acidophilus: do not use with antiinfectives; separate by several hours
Khat: decreased absorption, separate by 2 hr
*Drug/lab test*
False positive: urine glucose, urine protein

### NURSING CONSIDERATIONS
**Assessment**
• Assess patient for previous sensitivity reaction to penicillins or cephalosporins; cross-sensitivity between penicillins and cephalosporins is common
• Assess patient for signs and symptoms of infection; including characteristics of wounds, sputum, urine, stool, WBC >10,000/mm³, earache, fever; obtain baseline information and during treatment
• Complete C&S before beginning product therapy to identify if correct treatment has been initiated
• Assess for allergic reactions: rash, urticaria, pruritus, chills, fever, joint pain; angioedema may occur a few days after therapy begins; epINEPHrine and resuscitation equipment should be on unit for anaphylactic reaction
◆ Identify urine output; if decreasing, notify prescriber (may indicate nephrotoxicity)
• Assess renal studies: urinalysis, protein, BUN, creatinine
• Monitor blood studies: AST, ALT, CBC, Hct, bilirubin, LDH, alkaline phosphatase, Coombs' test monthly if patient is on long-term therapy
• Monitor electrolytes: potassium, sodium, chloride monthly if patient is on long-term therapy
• Assess bowel pattern daily; if severe diarrhea occurs, product should be discontinued; may indicate pseudomembranous colitis
• Monitor for bleeding: ecchymosis, bleeding gums, hematuria, stool guaiac daily if on long-term therapy
• Assess for superinfection: perineal itching, fever, malaise, redness, pain, swelling, drainage, rash, diarrhea, change in cough, sputum

**Nursing diagnoses**
• Diarrhea (adverse reactions)
• Infection, risk for (uses)
• Injury, risk for (adverse reactions)
• Knowledge, deficient (teaching)
• Noncompliance (teaching)

**Implementation**
**IM route**
• Reconstitute by adding 3.2 ml/1.5 g or 6.4 ml/3 g; use sterile water, 0.5% or 2% lidocaine; give within 1 hr of preparation; give deep in large muscle mass
• Give after C&S completed; on empty stomach
**IV route**
• Give **IV** after diluting 1.5 g/3.2 ml sterile $H_2O$ for inj; or 3 g/6.4 ml (250 mg ampicillin/125 mg sulbactam); allow to stand until foaming stops; give directly over 15-30 min; dilute further in 50 ml or more of $D_5W$, $D_5$/10.45% NaCl, 10% invert sugar in water, LR, 6% sodium lactate, isotonic NaCl; administer within 1 hr after reconstitution; give as an intermittent inf over 15-30 min
*Y-site compatibilities:* Amifostine, aztreonam, cefepime, enalaprilat, famotidine, filgrastim, fluconazole, fludarabine, granisetron, heparin, regular insulin, meperidine, morphine, paclitaxel, remifentanil, tacrolimus, teniposide, theophylline, thiotepa
*Y-site incompatibilities:* Idarubicin, ondansetron, sargramostim
*Additive compatibilities:* Aztreonam
*Additive incompatibilities:* Aminoglycosides

**Patient/family education**
• Teach patient to report sore throat, bruising, bleeding, joint pain, persistent diarrhea; may indicate blood dyscrasias (rare) or superinfection
• Advise patient to contact prescriber if vaginal itching, loose foul-smelling stools, furry tongue occur; may indicate superinfection
• Instruct patient to use another form of contraception other than oral contraceptives
◆ To report immediately pseudomembranous colitis: fever, diarrhea with pus, blood, or mucus; may occur up to 4 wk after treatment
• To wear or carry emergency ID if allergic to penicillin products

**Evaluation**
**Positive therapeutic outcome**
• Absence of signs/symptoms of infection (WBC <10,000/mm³, temp WNL, absence of red draining wounds, earache)
• Reported improvement in symptoms of infection

Adverse effects: *italic* = common, **bold** = life-threatening

**Treatment of overdose:** Withdraw product, maintain airway, administer epINEPHrine, aminophylline, $O_2$, **IV** corticosteroids for anaphylaxis

---

**amprenavir** (Rx)
(am-pren′-a-ver)
Agenerase
*Func. class.:* Antiretroviral
*Chem. class.:* Protease inhibitor

**Pregnancy category** C

**Action:** Inhibits HIV-1 protease

**Therapeutic outcome:** Prevents maturation of the infectious virus

**Uses:** HIV-1 in combination with other antiretroviral agents

**Dosage and routes**
Caps and solution are not interchangeable
*Adult:* PO (cap) 1200 mg bid; sol 1400 mg bid
*Child >50 kg:* PO (cap) 1200 mg bid; SOL 1400 mg bid
*Child <50 kg:* PO (cap) 20 mg/kg bid or 15 mg/kg tid, max 2400 mg/day; PO (oral sol) 22.5 mg/kg bid or 17 mg/kg tid daily, max 2800 mg/day

*Amprenavir/ritonavir regimen*
*Adult:* PO 600 mg amprenavir, 100 mg ritonavir bid or 1200 mg amprenavir, 200 mg ritonavir bid

*Hepatic dose*
*Child:* PO (Child-Pugh score 5-8) 450 mg bid (caps), 513 mg bid (sol) in combination; (Child-Pugh score 9-12) 300 mg bid (caps) 342 mg bid (sol) in combination

**Available forms:** Cap 50 mg; oral sol 15 mg/ml

**Adverse effects**
*CNS: Paresthesia*
*ENDO:* New-onset diabetes, hyperglycemia, exacerbation of preexisting diabetes mellitus, hypertriglyceridemia
*GI: Diarrhea, abdominal pain, nausea,* **hepatotoxicity**
*HEMA:* **Acute hemolytic anemia**
*INTEG: Rash,* **Stevens-Johnson syndrome**

**Contraindications:** Hypersensitivity; oral sol (infants, child <4 yr, renal/hepatic failure, pregnancy)

**Precautions:** Pregnancy **C**, breastfeeding, children, geriatric, liver/renal disease, hemophilia, sulfonamide sensitivity

**Pharmacokinetics**
| | |
|---|---|
| **Absorption** | Rapidly |
| **Distribution** | 90% protein binding |
| **Metabolism** | Unknown |
| **Excretion** | Unknown |
| **Half-life** | 7-10½ hr |

**Pharmacodynamics**
Unknown

**Interactions**
*Individual drugs*
◆Alprazolam, atorvastatin, bepridil, carbamazepine, clonazepam, clozapine, dapsone, diazepam, diltiazem, ergots, erythromycin, fentanyl, flurazepam, itraconazole, loratadine, lovastatin, midazolam, niCARdipine, NIFEdipine, pimozide, triazolam, verapamil: do not use together; toxicity may occur
Amiodarone, lidocaine, quinidine: serious life-threatening reactions
Cimetidine, clarithromycin, erythromycin, indinavir, itraconazole, ketoconazole, ritonavir: increased amprenavir levels; toxicity may occur
Carbamazepine, didanosine, efavirenz, nevirapine, phenobarbital, phenytoin, methadone, rifamycin: decreased amprenavir levels
Methadone: decreased methadone effect
Warfarin: increased serious life-threatening interactions
*Drug classifications*
Antacids, estrogens: decreased amprenavir levels
Contraceptives (oral): decreased effects of oral contraceptives
Ergots: do not use together; toxicity may occur
Statins: increased myopathy
*Drug/herb*
St. John's wort: decreased amprenavir level
*Drug/food*
Decreased: bioavailability after high-fat meal
*Drug/lab test*
Increased: glucose, cholesterol, triglycerides

**NURSING CONSIDERATIONS**
**Assessment**
• Assess for renal/hepatic failure, pregnancy, or those receiving disulfiram, metronidazole; oral sol contains propylene glycol in greater quantities
• Assess signs of infection, anemia
• Monitor liver studies: ALT, AST; viral load, CD4 count throughout treatment
• Monitor C&S before product therapy; product may be taken as soon as culture is taken; repeat C&S after treatment; determine

---

 Alert    Canada Only   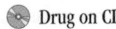 Drug on CD   * "Tall Man" lettering (See Preface)

the presence of other sexually transmitted diseases

• Assess bowel pattern before, during treatment; if severe abdominal pain with bleeding occurs, product should be discontinued; monitor hydration

• Assess skin eruptions, rash, urticaria, itching

• Assess allergies before treatment, reaction of each medication; place allergies on chart

## Nursing diagnoses
• Infection, risk for (uses)
• Knowledge, deficient (teaching)

## Implementation
• Caps and oral sol are not interchangeable on a mg/mg basis

## Patient/family education
• Advise patient to take as prescribed with or without food, avoid high-fat foods; if dose is missed, take as soon as remembered up to 1 hr before next dose; do not double dose, do not share with others

• Advise patient that product must be taken in equal intervals around the clock to maintain blood levels for duration of therapy

• Advise patient to use nonhormonal method of contraception during treatment, use condoms

• Advise patient to notify prescriber of diarrhea, nausea, vomiting, rash

• Teach patient that product does not cure AIDS or prevent transmission to others, only controls symptoms

## Evaluation
**Positive therapeutic outcome**
• Increasing CD4 counts
• Decreased viral load
• Resolution of HIV

## anagrelide (Rx)
(a-na'gre-lide)
Agrylin
*Func. class.:* Antiplatelet
*Chem. class.:* Imidazoquinazolinone
**Pregnancy category** C

**Action:** Reduces platelet count (mechanism not clear) and prevents early platelet shape changes in response to aggregating agents thus inhibiting platelet aggregation

**Therapeutic outcome:** Inhibition of platelet aggregation

**Uses:** Chronic myelogenous leukemia (CML), thrombocytosis, polycythemia vera

## Dosage and routes
*Adult:* PO 0.5 mg qid or 1 mg bid, may be adjusted after 1 wk, max 10 mg/day or 2.5 mg single dose; maintenance: titrate to lowest dose to maintain platelets <600,000

**Available forms:** Caps 0.5, 1.0 mg

## Adverse effects
*CNS: Headache, dizziness,* **seizures,** paresthesia, **CVA,** fever
*CV: Postural hypotension,* tachycardia, palpitations, **CHF, MI,** cardiomyopathy, cardiomegaly, **complete heart block, atrial fibrillation, arrhythmia,** chest pain
*GI:* Diarrhea, abdominal pain, nausea, flatulence, vomiting, anorexia, constipation, pancreatitis
*GU:* Dysuria
*HEMA:* Anemia, **thrombocytopenia,** ecchymosis, lymphadenoma
*INTEG: Rash,* photosensitivity
*MISC:* Edema, pain
*MS:* Asthenia, back pain
*RESP:* Dyspnea

**Contraindications:** Hypersensitivity, hypotension

**Precautions:** Pregnancy C, breastfeeding, child <16 yr, cardiac/renal/hepatic disease

| Pharmacokinetics | |
|---|---|
| Absorption | Unknown |
| Distribution | Unknown |
| Metabolism | Liver, extensively |
| Excretion | Feces/urine |
| Half-life | Terminal half-life 3-4 days |

| Pharmacodynamics | |
|---|---|
| Onset | Unknown |
| Peak | 1 hr |
| Duration | >24 hr |

## Interactions
*Individual drugs*
Abciximab, aspirin, cimetidine, ciprofloxacin, eptifibatide, tirofiban, ticlopidine: increased bleeding risk
Sucralfate: decreased absorption, decreased plasma concentrations
*Drug classifications*
Anticoagulants, NSAIDs, thrombolytics: increased bleeding risk
*Drug/herb*
Arginine: gastric irritation
Bogbean, dong quai, feverfew, ginger, ginkgo: increased effect
Bilberry, saw palmetto: decreased effect
Green tea: increased bleeding risk

Adverse effects: *italic* = common, **bold** = life-threatening

*Drug/food*
Grapefruit juice: avoid use
Decreased: absorption

## NURSING CONSIDERATIONS
### Assessment
• Monitor B/P, pulse baseline and during treatment until stable; take B/P with patient lying, standing; orthostatic hypotension is common
• Assess cardiac status: chest pain, what aggravates or ameliorates condition
• Monitor platelet counts q2 days × 1 wk, and qwk thereafter, response should begin after 1-2 wk; Hgb, WBC

### Nursing diagnoses
• Cardiac output, decreased (uses)
• Knowledge, deficient (teaching)

### Implementation
• May give with food, monitor closely for dosage adjustment, there is better absorption on empty stomach
• Store at room temperature

### Patient/family education
• Teach patient that this medication is not a cure.
• Advise patient that product may have to be taken continuously in evenly spaced doses only as directed; if a dose is missed, take one when remembered up to 4 hr; do not double doses
• Inform patient that it is necessary to quit smoking to prevent excessive vasoconstriction
• Advise patient to rise slowly from sitting or lying down to prevent orthostatic hypotension
• Caution patient not to use alcohol or OTC medication unless approved by prescriber; avoid grapefruit or juice
• Caution patient to avoid hazardous activities until stabilized on medication; dizziness may occur
• Teach patient to report cardiac reactions, increased bruising/bleeding
• Advise patient to use contraception (female, child-bearing age)
• Teach patient to inform health care provider before surgery of medication use
• Advise patient not to double dose; if dose is missed, take as soon as remembered; if close to next dose, omit dose

### Evaluation
**Positive therapeutic outcome**
• Absence of thrombocythemia

---

## anakinra (Rx)
(an-ah-kin'rah)
Kineret
*Func. class.:* Antirheumatic agent (disease modifying), immunomodulator
*Chem. class.:* Recombinant form of human interleukin-1 receptor antagonist (IL-1Ra)

### Pregnancy category B

**Action:** A form of human interleukin-1 receptor antagonist (IL-1Ra) produced by DNA technology; blocks activity of IL-1, resulting in decreased cartilage degradation and decreased bone resorption

**Therapeutic outcome:** Decreased pain, inflammation

**Uses:** Reduction in signs and symptoms of moderate to severe active rheumatoid arthritis in patients 18 years of age or older who have not responded to other disease-modifying agents

### Dosage and routes
*Adult:* SUBCUT 100 mg daily

**Available forms:** Sol for inj, 100 mg/ml

### Adverse effects
*CNS:* Headache
*EENT:* Sinusitis
*GI:* Abdominal pain, nausea, diarrhea
*HEMA:* **Neutropenia**
*INTEG:* Rash, *inj site reaction*, allergic reaction
*MISC:* Flulike symptoms
*MS:* Worsening of RA, arthralgia
*RESP:* URI

**Contraindications:** Hypersensitivity to *Escherichia coli*–derived proteins or this product, sepsis

**Precautions:** Pregnancy **B**, breastfeeding, children, geriatric, renal impairment

| Pharmacokinetics | |
|---|---|
| Absorption | Well absorbed (SUBCUT) |
| Distribution | Unknown |
| Metabolism | Unknown |
| Excretion | Unknown |
| Half-life | 4-6 hr |

| Pharmacodynamics | |
|---|---|
| Onset | Unknown |
| Peak | 3-7 hr |
| Duration | Unknown |

## Interactions
### Drug classifications
Etanercept, TNF blocking agents: increased risk of severe infection

Vaccines: do not coadminister; immunizations should be brought up to date before treatment

## NURSING CONSIDERATIONS
### Assessment
• Assess pain, stiffness, ROM, swelling of joints during treatment
• Assess for inj site pain, swelling; usually occur after 2 inj (4-5 days)
• Assess for infections, stop treatment if present

### Nursing diagnoses
• Injury, risk for (side effects)
• Knowledge, deficient (teaching)
• Mobility, impaired physical (uses)
• Pain, chronic (uses)

### Implementation
• Do not use if cloudy or discolored or if particulate is present, protect from light
• Do not admix with other sol or medications, do not use filter

### Patient/family education
• Teach patient about self-administration if appropriate: inj should be made in thigh, abdomen, upper arm; rotate sites at least 1 in from old site
• Advise patient to notify prescriber if pregnancy is planned or suspected, avoid breastfeeding

### Evaluation
**Positive therapeutic outcome**
• Decreased inflammation, pain in joints

---

### anastrozole (Rx)
(an-ass-stroh'zole)
Arimidex
*Func. class.:* Antineoplastic
*Chem. class.:* Aromatase inhibitor

**Pregnancy category** D

**Action:** Lowers serum estradiol concentrations; many breast cancers have strong estrogen receptors

**Therapeutic outcome:** Prevention of rapidly growing malignant cells

**Uses:** Advanced breast carcinoma that has not responded to other therapy in estrogen-receptor-positive patients (usually postmenopausal); patients with advanced disease on tamoxifen, adjunct therapy in early breast cancer

### Dosage and routes
*Adult:* PO 1 mg daily

**Available forms:** Tabs 1 mg

### Adverse effects
*CNS:* Hot flashes, headache, light-headedness, depression, dizziness, confusion, insomnia, anxiety
*CV:* Chest pain, hypertension, thrombophlebitis, edema
*GI:* Nausea, vomiting, altered taste leading to anorexia, diarrhea, constipation, abdominal pain, dry mouth
*GU:* Vaginal bleeding, pruritus vulvae, vaginal dryness, pelvic pain, UTI
**HEMA:** Leukopenia
*INTEG:* Rash
*MS:* Bone pain, myalgia, asthenia
*RESP:* Cough, sinusitis, dyspnea

**Contraindications:** Pregnancy **D**, hypersensitivity

**Precautions:** Breastfeeding, children, geriatric, renal/hepatic disease

| Pharmacokinetics | |
|---|---|
| Absorption | Adequately absorbed |
| Distribution | Unknown |
| Metabolism | Liver |
| Excretion | Feces, urine |
| Half-life | 50 hr |

| Pharmacodynamics | |
|---|---|
| Onset | Unknown |
| Peak | 4-7 hr |
| Duration | Unknown |

### Interactions
#### Drug/lab test
Increased: GGT, AST, ALT, alkaline phosphatase, cholesterol, LDL

### NURSING CONSIDERATIONS
#### Assessment
• Monitor CBC, differential, platelet count weekly; withhold product if WBC is <4000/mm$^3$ or platelet count is <75,000/mm$^3$; notify prescriber of results; monitor calcium levels (hypercalcemia is common)
• Assess for tumor flare: increase in bone, tumor pain during beginning treatment; give analgesics as ordered to decrease pain
• Assess for bleeding: hematuria, guaiac, bruising or petechiae, mucosa or orifices, q8hr; no rectal temp

Adverse effects: *italic* = common, **bold** = life-threatening

## Nursing diagnoses
- Injury, risk for (adverse reactions)
- Knowledge, deficient (teaching)

## Implementation
- Do not break, crush, or chew enteric products
- Give with food or fluids for GI upset; repeat dose may be needed if vomiting occurs
- Store in light-resistant container at room temperature

## Patient/family education
- Instruct patient to report any complaints, side effects to health care prescriber; if dose is missed, do not double next dose
- Advise patient that vaginal bleeding, pruritus, hot flashes, can occur, and are reversible after discontinuing treatment
- Inform patient about who should be told about tamoxifen therapy
- Advise patient to report vaginal bleeding immediately; that tumor flare—increase in size of tumor, increased bone pain—may occur and will subside rapidly; may take analgesics for pain
- Caution patient to use sunscreen and protective clothing to prevent burns because photosensitivity is common
- Teach patient that hair loss may occur during treatment; a wig or hairpiece may make patient feel better; new hair may be different in color, texture
- Inform patient that rash or lesions are temporary and may become large during beginning therapy

## Evaluation
**Positive therapeutic outcome**
- Decreased spread of malignant cells in breast cancer

---

## anidulafungin (Rx)
(a-nid-yoo-luh-fun'jin)
Eraxis
*Func. class.:* Antifungal, systemic
*Chem. class.:* Echinocandin

**Pregnancy category** C

**Action:** Inhibits fungal enzyme synthesis; causes direct damage to fungal cell wall

**Therapeutic outcome:** Decreased symptoms of candida infection, negative culture

**Uses:** *Candida albicans, C. glabrata, C. parapsilosis, C. tropicalis*

## Dosage and routes
### Candidemia and other candida infections
**Adult: IV** Loading dose 200 mg on day 1, then 100 mg/day until 14 days or more since last positive culture

### Esophageal candidiasis
**Adult: IV** Loading dose 100 mg on day 1, then 50 mg/day for at least 14 days and for at least 7 days after symptoms are resolved

**Available forms:** Powder for injection, lyophilized 50 mg

## Adverse effects
### Candiemia/other candida infections
***CNS:*** **Seizures,** dizziness, *headache*
***CV:*** Deep vein thrombosis, **atrial fibrillation, right bundle branch block,** hypotension, **sinus arrhythmia, thrombophlebitis superficial, ventricular extrasystoles (rare)**
***GI:*** *Nausea; anorexia; vomiting; diarrhea; increased AST, ALT*
***META:*** Hypokalemia
### Esophageal candidiasis
***CNS:*** *Headache*
***GI:*** *Nausea, anorexia, vomiting, diarrhea,* **hepatic necrosis**
***HEMA:*** **Neutropenia, thrombocytopenia, leukopenia, coagulopathy**
***INTEG:*** *Rash*
***META:*** Hypocalcemia, hyperglycemia, hyperkalemia, hypernatremia, hypomagnesium (rare)
***MS:*** *Back pain, rigors*

**Contraindications:** Hypersensitivity to this product or other echinocandins

**Precautions:** Pregnancy C, breastfeeding, children, severe hepatic disease

### Pharmacokinetics
| | |
|---|---|
| Absorption | Unknown |
| Distribution | Steady state after loading dose, protein binding 84% |
| Metabolism | Unknown |
| Excretion | Unknown |
| Half-life | Distribution 0.5-1 hr, terminal 40-50 hr |

### Pharmacodynamics
Unknown

## Interactions
### Individual drugs
CycloSPORINE: increased plasma concentrations

---

*Drug/lab test*
Increased: amylase, bilirubin, CPK, creatinine, ECG, QT prolongation, lipase
Decreased: platelets, magnesium, potassium, transferase, urea

## NURSING CONSIDERATIONS
### Assessment
• Assess for infection, clearing of cultures during treatment; obtain culture baseline and throughout; product may be started as soon as culture is taken
• Monitor CBC (RBC, Hct, Hgb), differential, platelet count periodically; notify prescriber of results
• Monitor renal studies: BUN, serum uric acid, urine CCr, electrolytes before and during therapy
• Monitor hepatic studies before and during treatment: bilirubin, AST, ALT, alk phosphatase, as needed
• Assess for bleeding: hematuria, heme-positive stools, bruising or petechiae, mucosa or orifices; blood dyscrasias can occur
• Assess for GI symptoms: frequency of stools, cramping, if severe diarrhea occurs, electrolytes may need to be given

### Nursing diagnoses
• Infection, risk for (uses)
• Injury, risk for (adverse reactions)
• Knowledge, deficient (teaching)

### Implementation
**IV route**
• Reconstitute with provided dilutent 50 mg vial/5 ml (3.33 mg/ml), dilute with $D_5$ of 0.9% NaCl, only to a concentration of 0.5 mg/ml, run at no more than 1.1 mg/ml
• Do not use if cloudy or precipitated; do not admix
• Store at room temperature, away from light, do not freeze; diluted sol must be used within 24 hr

### Patient/family education
• Advise patient to notify prescriber if pregnancy is suspected or planned; use nonhormonal form of contraception while taking this product
• Instruct patient to avoid breastfeeding while taking this product
• Advise patient to inform prescriber of kidney or liver disease
• Advise patient to report bleeding
• Teach patient to report signs of infection: increased temp, sore throat, flulike symptoms
• Teach patient to notify prescriber of nausea, vomiting, diarrhea, jaundice, anorexia, clay-colored stools, dark urine; heptatotoxicity may occur

### Evaluation
**Positive therapeutic outcome**
• Decreased symptoms of candida infection, negative culture

---

**! HIGH ALERT**

## anistreplase (Rx)
(an-is-tre-plaze')
anisoylated plasminogen, APSAC, Eminase
*Func. class.:* Thrombolytic enzyme
*Chem. class.:* Plasminogen activator

**Pregnancy category C**

**Action:** Promotes thrombolysis by promoting conversion of plasminogen to plasmin; complex is a combination of plasminogen and streptokinase

**Therapeutic outcome:** Thrombolysis in coronary arteries

**Uses:** Management of acute MI; for lysis of coronary artery thrombi

### Dosage and routes
*Adult:* **IV** INJ 30 units over 4-5 min as soon as possible after onset of symptoms

**Available forms:** Powder, lyophilized 30 units/vial

### Adverse effects
*CNS:* Headache, fever, sweating, agitation, dizziness, paresthesia, tremor, vertigo, **intracranial hemorrhage**
*CV:* Hypotension, **dysrhythmias,** conduction disorders
*GI:* Nausea, vomiting
*HEMA:* Decreased Hct, **GI, GU, intracranial, retroperitoneal,** surface bleeding; **thrombocytopenia**
*INTEG:* Rash, urticaria, phlebitis at site, itching, flushing
*MS:* Low back pain, arthralgia
*RESP:* Altered respirations, dyspnea, **bronchospasm, lung edema**
*SYST:* Anaphylaxis (rare)

**Contraindications:** Hypersensitivity, active internal bleeding, intraspinal or intracranial surgery, neoplasms of CNS, severe, uncontrolled hypertension, cerebral embolism, thrombosis, hemorrhage, hypersensitivity to this product or streptokinase, recent trauma/history of CVA

**Precautions:** Pregnancy **C**, breastfeeding, geriatric, arterial emboli from left side of

---

Adverse effects: *italic* = common, **bold** = life-threatening

heart, ulcerative colitis/enteritis, renal/hepatic disease, hypocoagulation, COPD, subacute bacterial endocarditis, rheumatic valvular disease, intraarterial diagnostic procedure or surgery (10 days), recent major surgery

| Pharmacokinetics | |
| --- | --- |
| **Absorption** | Complete bioavailability |
| **Distribution** | Unknown |
| **Metabolism** | Binds to plasmin |
| **Excretion** | Kidneys |
| **Half-life** | 105 min |

| Pharmacodynamics | |
| --- | --- |
| **Onset** | Unknown |
| **Peak** | 45 min |
| **Duration** | Unknown |

## Interactions
### Individual drugs
Abciximab, aspirin, clopidogrel, dipyridamole, eptifibatide, heparin, plicamycin, ticlopidine, tirofiban, valproic acid: increased bleeding risk

Aminocaproic acid, aprotinin, tranexamic acid: decreased action of anistreplase
### Drug classifications
Anticoagulants, antiplatelets, cephalosporins (some), NSAIDs: increased bleeding risk
### Drug/herb
Agrimony, alfalfa, angelica, anise, basil, bay, bilberry, black haw, bogbean, bromelain, buchu, chondroitin, cinchona bark, dong quai, fenugreek, feverfew, garlic, ginger, ginkgo, ginseng, horse chestnut, Irish moss, kelp, kelpware, khella, lovage, lungwort, meadowsweet, motherwort, mugwort, nettle, papaya, parsley (large amounts), pau d'arco, pineapple, poplar, prickly ash, safflower, saw palmetto, tonka bean, turmeric, wintergreen, yarrow: increased risk of bleeding

Chamomile, coenzyme Q10, flax, glucomannan, goldenseal, guar gum: decreased anticoagulant effect
### Drug/lab test
Increased: Pro-time, APTT, TT
Decreased: fibrinogen, plasminogen

## NURSING CONSIDERATIONS
### Assessment
- Monitor VS, B/P, pulse, respirations, neurologic signs, temp at least q4hr, temp >104° F (40° C) or indicators of internal bleeding
- Assess for hypersensitivity: fever, rash, itching, chills; mild reaction may be treated with antihistamines; hypersensitivity reactions/

dyspnea, wheezing, facial swelling should be treated with epINEPHrine
- ⬥ Monitor bleeding during first hr of treatment (hematuria, hematemesis, bleeding from mucous membranes, epistaxis, ecchymosis), continue to monitor for 24 hr after treatment; blood studies (Hct, platelets, PTT, pro-time, TT, APTT) before starting therapy; pro-time or APTT must be <2 × control before starting therapy; TT or pro-time q3-4hr during treatment
- Monitor ECG, treat bradycardia, ventricular changes; assess neurologic status, neurologic change may indicate intracranial bleeding; cardiac enzymes, radionuclide, myocardial scanning/coronary angiography

### Nursing diagnoses
- Injury, risk for (uses, adverse reactions)
- Knowledge, deficient (teaching)
- Tissue perfusion, ineffective (uses)

### Implementation
- Give heparin therapy after thrombolytic therapy is discontinued, TT or APTT <2 × control (about 3-4 hr)
- Avoid invasive procedures: inj, rect temp; about 10% of patients have high streptococcal antibody titers, requiring increased loading doses
- Treat fever with acetaminophen
- Provide pressure for 30 sec to minor bleeding sites, 30 min to sites of arterial puncture followed by dressing; inform prescriber if hemostasis not attained; apply pressure dressing
**IV, direct route**
- Give after reconstituting single-dose vial/5 ml sterile water for inj (not bacteriostatic water), and roll (not shake) to enhance reconstitution, try to minimize foaming; give over 2-5 min by direct **IV**, give within ½ hr of reconstitution or discard, do not add other meds to vial or syringe; give within 6 hr of thrombi identification for best results; cryoprecipitate or fresh frozen plasma if bleeding occurs; store powder in refrigerator; use within 30 min after reconstitution
*Incompatibilities:* Do not mix with other products in sol or syringe

### Patient/family education
- Teach patient action of product and expected outcome; alert patient to possible hypersensitivity reactions and symptoms to report
- Advise patient bed rest is needed during entire course of treatment; handle patient as little as possible during therapy

## Evaluation
**Positive therapeutic outcome**
- Absence of thrombolysis in MI
- Improved ventricular function

---

! HIGH ALERT

## antihemophilic factor VIII (AHF) (Rx)
(an-tee-hee-moe-fill'ik)

Alphanate, antihemophilic factor, Bioclate, Helixate FS, Hemofil M, Humate-P, Hyate:C, Koate-DVI, Kogenate, Kogenate FS, Monoclate-P, Recombinate, ReFacto
*Func. class.:* Hemostatic, blood factor
*Chem. class.:* Factor VIII

**Pregnancy category C**

**Do not confuse:**
Kogenate/Kogenate-2

**Action:** Necessary for clotting. Activates factor X in conjunction with activated factor IX; transforms prothrombin to thrombin

**Therapeutic outcome:** Control of hemorrhage or excessive bleeding in factor VIII deficiency

**Uses:** Hemophilia A, patients with acquired circulating factor VIII inhibitors, factor VIII deficiency; prevention of surgical bleeding, risk of thrombosis (von Willebrand disease)

## Dosage and routes
Depends on severity of deficiency and level of antihemophilic factor

*Massive hemorrhage*
*Adult and child:* **IV** 40-50 units/kg, then 20-25 units/kg q8-12hr

*Bleeding (overt)*
*Adult and child:* **IV** 15-25 units/kg, then 8-15 units/kg q8-12hr × 4 days

*Hemorrhage near vital organs*
*Adult and child:* **IV** 15 units/kg, then 8 units/kg q8hr × 2 days, then 4 units/kg q8hr × 2 days

*Minor hemorrhage*
*Adult and child:* **IV** 8-10 units/kg q24hr × 2-3 days or 8 units/kg q12hr × 2 days, then q24hr × 2 days

*Joint bleeding*
*Adult and child:* **IV** 15 units/kg q8-12hr × 1-2 days

**Available forms:** Inj 250, 500, 1000, 1500 units/vial (number of units noted on label)

## Adverse effects
*CNS:* Headache, *lethargy, chills, fever, flushing,* loss of consciousness
*CV: Hypotension,* tachycardia
*GI:* Nausea, vomiting, abdominal cramps, jaundice, constipation, diarrhea, anorexia, **viral hepatitis**
*HEMA:* **Thrombosis, hemolysis, risk of hepatitis B, risk of HIV**
*INTEG:* Rash, flushing, *urticaria,* stinging at inj site
*MISC:* **Anaphylaxis,** blurred vision, back pain
*RESP:* **Bronchospasm,** rhinitis, dyspnea, nosebleeds, wheezing

**Contraindications:** Hypersensitivity to mouse, hamster, bovine, porcine protein, breastfeeding, HIV, viral infection

**Precautions:** Pregnancy C, neonates/infants, hepatic disease, blood types A, B, AB, factor VIII inhibitor

### Pharmacokinetics
| | |
|---|---|
| Absorption | Complete availability |
| Distribution | Plasma |
| Metabolism | Not metabolized |
| Excretion | No excretion |
| Half-life | Biphasic 4 hr, 15 hr |

### Pharmacodynamics
| | |
|---|---|
| Onset | Immediate |
| Peak | Unknown |
| Duration | 12 hr |

## Interactions
*Drug classifications*
Anticoagulants, NSAIDs, salicylates: increased bleeding

## NURSING CONSIDERATIONS
**Assessment**
- Monitor blood studies (coagulation factors assay by % normal): 5% prevents spontaneous hemorrhage, 30%-50% for surgery, 80%-100% for severe hemorrhage; blood group of patient, donors (if applicable; most factor VIII not from specific blood group donors)
- Monitor I&O, urine color; notify prescriber if urine becomes orange, red; change in urine color signifying hemolytic reaction; patients other than blood type O are more at risk
- Monitor pulse: discontinue infusion if significant increase
- Obtain test for factor VIII inhibitors before starting treatment, may require concomitant antiinhibitor coagulant complex therapy; Hct, Coombs' test with blood types A, B, AB

Adverse effects: *italic* = common, **bold** = life-threatening

- Assess for allergy: fever, rash, itching, jaundice, wheezing, tachycardia, nausea, vomiting; give diphenhydrAMINE (Benadryl); continue therapy if reaction is mild, discontinue if severe; notify prescriber

◆ Monitor bleeding at ankles, knees, elbows, other joints; check for rebleeding after 15-30 min

## Nursing diagnoses
- Injury, risk for (uses, adverse reactions)
- Knowledge, deficient (teaching)
- Tissue perfusion, ineffective (uses)

## Implementation
### IV route
- Administer **IV** slowly; use plastic syringe to reconstitute and administer; do not use glass, product adheres to glass; use another needle as a vent when reconstituting; rotate gently to mix
- Administer after dilution with warm NS, D₅W, LR; give within 3 hr

### IV infusion route
- Administer by **IV** inf: give at ≤2 ml/min if concentration >34 units/ml; or over 3 min if concentration is <34 units/ml; filter before using
- Store in refrigerator; do not freeze; after reconstitution, do not refrigerate; give within 3 hr

*Additive compatibilities:* Do not mix with other products in sol or syringe

## Patient/family education
- Advise patient to report any signs of bleeding: gums, under skin, urine, stools, emesis; review methods to prevent bleeding; to be checked q2-3 mo for HIV screen
- Instruct patient to avoid salicylates/NSAIDs; increases bleeding tendencies, decreases clotting
- Instruct patient to prepare, administer factor VIII concentrates at first sign of danger
- Instruct patient to advise health professionals of treatment for hemophilia
- Advise patient that immunization for hepatitis B may be given first
- Instruct patient to report hives, urticaria, chest tightness, hypotension; may be monoclonal antibody–derived factor VII; signs of viral hepatitis, AIDS
- Advise patient to carry/wear emergency ID describing disease process, products used

## Evaluation
### Positive therapeutic outcome
- Absence of bleeding
- Prevention of rebleeding

## apraclonidine ophthalmic
*See Appendix D*

## aprepitant (Rx)
(ap-re′pi-tant)
Emend
*Func. class.:* Antiemetic—miscellaneous
### Pregnancy category B

**Action:** Selective antagonist of human substance P/neurokinin 1 (NK₁) receptors decreasing emetic reflex

**Therapeutic outcome:** Decreased nausea, vomiting during chemotherapy

**Uses:** Prevention of nausea, vomiting associated with cancer chemotherapy including high-dose cisplatin; used in combination with other antiemetics; postop nausea, vomiting

## Dosage and routes
### Highly emetogenic
*Adult:* PO Day 1 (1 hr prior to chemotherapy) aprepitant 125 mg with 12 mg dexamethasone PO, with 32 mg ondansetron **IV**; day 2 aprepitant 80 mg with 8 mg dexamethasone PO; day 3 aprepitant 80 mg with 8 mg dexamethasone PO; day 4 only dexamethasone 8 mg PO

### Moderately emetogenic
*Adult:* PO Day 1 125 mg aprepitant with dexamethasone 12 mg PO, with ondansetron 8 mg PO × 2; days 2 and 3 80 mg aprepitant only

### Prevention of postop nausea/vomiting
*Adult:* PO 40 mg within 3 hr of induction of anesthesia

**Available forms:** Caps 40, 80, 125 mg

## Adverse effects
*CNS: Headache, dizziness,* insomnia, anxiety, depression, confusion, peripheral neuropathy
*CV:* Bradycardia, tachycardia, DVT, hypertension
*GI: Diarrhea; constipation;* abdominal pain; anorexia; gastritis; increased AST, ALT; *nausea;* vomiting; heartburn
*GU:* Increased BUN, serum creatine, proteinuria, dysuria
*HEMA:* Anemia, **thrombocytopenia, neutropenia**
*MISC:* Asthenia, fatigue, dehydration, fever, hiccups, tinnitus

**Contraindications:** Hypersensitivity

**Precautions:** Pregnancy **B,** breastfeeding, children, geriatric, hepatic disease

### Pharmacokinetics
| | |
|---|---|
| **Absorption** | Unknown |
| **Distribution** | 95% protein bound |
| **Metabolism** | Liver (CYP3A4 enzymes to an active metabolite) |
| **Excretion** | Not in kidneys |
| **Half-life** | 10-12 hr |

### Pharmacodynamics
Unknown

### Interactions
#### Individual drugs
Paroxetine: decreased action of both products
#### Drug classifications
CYP2C9 substrates (phenytoin, TOLBUTamide, warfarin) oral contraceptives: decreased action

CYP3A4 inhibitors (clarithromycin, diltiazem, itraconazole, ketoconazole, nefazodone, nelfinavir, ritonavir, troleandomycin): increased aprepitant action

CYP3A4 inducers (carbamazepine, phenytoin, rifampin): decreased aprepitant action

CYP3A4 substrates (alprazolam, cisapride, dexamethasone, docetaxel, etoposide, ifosfamide, irinotecan, methylPREDNISolone, midazolam, paclitaxel, pimozide, triazolam, vinBLAStine, vinCRIStine, vinorelbine): increased action

#### Drug/food
Grapefruit juice: decreased effect

### NURSING CONSIDERATIONS
#### Assessment
- Assess for absence of nausea, vomiting during chemotherapy
- Advise those on warfarin to have clotting monitored closely during 2-wk period following administration of aprepitant

#### Nursing diagnoses
- Knowledge, deficient (teaching)

#### Implementation
- Give PO on 3-day schedule
- Take first dose 1 hr prior to chemotherapy
- Store at room temperature

#### Patient/family education
- Teach to report diarrhea, constipation
- Advise to take only as prescribed
- Advise to report all medication to prescriber prior to taking this medication
- Instruct to use nonhormonal form of contraception while taking this agent

### Evaluation
#### Positive therapeutic outcome
- Absence of nausea, vomiting during cancer chemotherapy

## arformoterol (Rx)
(ar-for-moe′ter-ole)
Brovana
*Func. class.:* Long-acting adrenergic $\beta_2$-agonist, sympathomimetic, bronchodilator
**Pregnancy category C**

**Action:** Causes bronchodilation by action on $\beta_2$ (pulmonary) receptors by increasing levels of cAMP, which relaxes smooth muscle; produces bronchodilation, CNS, cardiac stimulation, as well as increased diuresis and gastric acid secretion; longer acting than isoproterenol

**Therapeutic outcome:** Absence of dyspnea, wheezing after 1 hr, improved airway exchange, improved ABGs

**Uses:** COPD, including chronic bronchitis, emphysema

### Dosage and routes
#### COPD
*Adult:* NEB 15 mcg, bid, AM, PM

**Available forms:** Inh sol 15 mcg/2 ml

### Adverse effects
*CNS:* Tremors, *anxiety,* insomnia, headache, dizziness, stimulation, *restlessness,* hallucinations, flushing, irritability
*CV:* Palpitations, **tachycardia,** hypo/hypertension, angina, **dysrhythmias**
*EENT:* Dry nose, irritation of nose and throat
*GI:* Heartburn, nausea, vomiting
*MISC:* Flushing, sweating, anorexia, bad taste/smell changes, hypokalemia, **anaphylaxis**
*MS:* Muscle cramps
*RESP:* Cough, wheezing, dyspnea, **bronchospasm,** dry throat

**Contraindications:** Hypersensitivity to sympathomimetics, this product, or racemic formoterol; tachydysrhythmias, severe cardiac disease, heart block, children, actively deteriorating COPD

**Precautions:** Pregnancy **C,** breastfeeding, cardiac disorders, hyperthyroidism, diabetes mellitus, hypertension, prostatic hypertrophy, angle-closure glaucoma, seizures, hypoglycemia

| Pharmacokinetics | |
|---|---|
| **Absorption** | Unknown |
| **Distribution** | Crosses placenta, protein binding 52%-65% |
| **Metabolism** | Direct conjugation by CYP2D6, CYP2C19, extensively |
| **Excretion** | Urine 63%, feces 11% |
| **Half-life** | Terminal (COPD) 26 hr |

| Pharmacodynamics | |
|---|---|
| **Onset** | 5 min |
| **Peak** | 1-1½ hr |
| **Duration** | 4-6 hr |

## Interactions
### Individual drugs
Oxytoxics: increased severe hypotension
Theophylline: increased toxicity
### Drug classifications
Adrenergics, MAOIs, tricyclics: increased action of arformoterol; do not use together
Nebulized bronchodilators: increased action of nebulized bronchodilators
Other β-blockers: decreased arformoterol action
Potassium-losing diuretics: increased ECG changes/hypokalemia
### Drug/herb
Caffeine (cola nut, green/black tea, guarana, yerba maté, coffee, chocolate): increased stimulation

## NURSING CONSIDERATIONS
### Assessment
• Assess respiratory function: vital capacity, forced expiratory volume, ABGs; lung sounds, heart rate and rhythm, B/P, sputum (baseline and peak)
• Determine that patient has not received theophylline therapy or other bronchodilators before giving dose
• Assess patient's ability to self-medicate
• Assess for allergic reactions; anaphylaxis may occur
• Assess paradoxical bronchospasm; hold medication, notify prescriber if bronchospasm occurs

### Nursing diagnoses
• Airway clearance, ineffective (uses)
• Knowledge, deficient (teaching)

### Implementation
• Must be used by nebulization
• Store in refrigerator

### Patient/family education
• Teach patient to use exactly as prescribed; that death has resulted from asthma with products similar to this one
• Advise patient not to use OTC medications; excess stimulation may occur

### Evaluation
**Positive therapeutic outcome**
• Absence of dyspnea, wheezing after 1 hr, improved airway exchange, improved ABGs

---

## ! HIGH ALERT

### argatroban (Rx)
(are-ga-troe′ban)
Argatroban
*Func. class.:* Anticoagulant
*Chem. class.:* Thrombin inhibitor

**Pregnancy category  B**

**Do not confuse:**
argatroban/Aggrastat

**Action:** Direct inhibitor of thrombin that is derived from L-arginine; it reversibly binds to the thrombin active site

**Therapeutic outcome:** Absence or decrease of thrombosis

**Uses:** Thrombosis, prophylaxis or treatment; anticoagulation prevention/treatment of thrombosis in heparin-induced thrombocytopenia; percutaneous coronary intervention (PCI)

### Dosage and routes
#### Heparin-induced thrombocytopenia or heparin-induced thrombocytopenia and thrombosis syndrome
*Adult:* **IV** 2 mcg/kg/min (1 mg/ml) give at 6 ml/hr for 50 kg of weight, at 8 ml/hr for 70 kg of weight, at 11 ml/hr for 90 kg of weight, at 13 ml/hr for 110 kg of weight, at 16 ml/hr for 130 kg of weight

#### Percutaneous coronary intervention (PCI) in HIT
*Adult:* **IV** INF 25 mcg/kg/min and a BOL of 350 mcg/kg given over 3-5 min, check ACT 5-10 min after BOL is completed, proceed if ACT >300 sec

#### Hepatic dose
*Adult:* CONT INF 0.5 mcg/kg/min, adjust rate based on APTT

**Available forms:** Inj 100 mg/ml (must dilute 100-fold)

---

## Adverse effects

*CNS:* Fever

*CV:* **Atrial fibrillation, ventricular tachycardia, coronary thrombosis, MI, myocardial ischemia, coronary occlusion, bradycardia,** chest pain, hypotension

*GI:* Nausea, vomiting, abdominal pain, diarrhea, **GI bleeding**

*GU: Hematuria,* abnormal kidney function, UTI

*HEMA:* **Hemorrhage, thrombocytopenia**

*RESP:* Pneumonia, dyspnea, coughing

*SYST:* **Sepsis**

**Contraindications:** Hypersensitivity, overt major bleeding

**Precautions:** Pregnancy **B,** breastfeeding, children, intracranial bleeding, renal function impairment, hepatic disease

### Pharmacokinetics

| | |
|---|---|
| **Absorption** | Unknown |
| **Distribution** | To extracellular fluid, 54% plasma protein binding |
| **Metabolism** | Liver |
| **Excretion** | Feces |
| **Half-life** | 39-51 min |

### Pharmacodynamics

Unknown

## Interactions

### Individual drugs

Clopidogrel, dipyridamole, heparin, ticlodipine, warfarin: increased bleeding risk

### Drug classifications

Antiplatelets, anticoagulants, thrombolytics: increased risk of bleeding

Glycoprotein IIb/IIIa antagonists (abciximab, eptifibatide, tirofiban), NSAIDs, other anticoagulants, salicylates, thrombolytics (alteplase, reteplase, streptokinase, tenecteplase, urokinase): increased risk of bleeding

### Drug/herb

Agrimony, alfalfa, angelica, anise, basil, bay, bilberry, black haw, bogbean, bromelain, buchu, chondroitin, cinchona bark, dong quai, fenugreek, feverfew, garlic, ginger, ginkgo, ginseng, horse chestnut, Irish moss, kelp, kelpware, khella, lovage, lungwort, meadowsweet, motherwort, mugwort, nettle, papaya, parsley, pau d'arco, pineapple, poplar, prickly ash, safflower, saw palmetto, tonka bean, turmeric, wintergreen, yarrow: increased risk of bleeding

Chamomile, coenzyme Q10, flax, glucomannan, goldenseal, guar gum: decreased anticoagulant effect

## NURSING CONSIDERATIONS

### Assessment

• Obtain baseline APTT before treatment; do not start treatment if APTT ratio ≥2.5, then APTT 4 hr after initiation of treatment and at least daily thereafter; if APTT above target, stop inf for 2 hr, then restart at 50%, take APTT in 4 hr; if below target, increase inf rate by 20%, take APTT in 4 hr, do not exceed inf rate of 0.21 mg/kg/hr without checking for coagulation abnormalities

• Monitor APTT, which should be 1.5-3 × control

⚠ Assess for bleeding gums, petechiae, ecchymosis, black tarry stools, hematuria/epistaxis, B/P, vaginal bleeding and possible hemorrhage

• Fever, skin rash, urticaria

### Nursing diagnoses

• Cardiac output, decreased (uses)
• Diarrhea (adverse reactions)
• Knowledge, deficient (teaching)

### Implementation

• Avoid all IM inj that may cause bleeding

**IV infusion route**

• Dilute in 0.9% NaCl, D₅, LR to a final conc 1 mg/ml; dilute each 2.5-ml vial 100-fold by mixing with 250 ml of diluents, mix by repeated inversion of the diluent bag for 1 min; may be slightly hazy

• Dosage adjustment may be made after review of APTT, not to exceed 10 mcg/kg/min

### Patient/family education

• Advise patient to use soft-bristle toothbrush to avoid bleeding gums, avoid contact sports, use electric razor, avoid IM inj

• Instruct patient to report any signs of bleeding: gums, under skin, urine, stools

### Evaluation

**Positive therapeutic outcome**

• Absence or decrease of thrombosis

---

## aripiprazole (Rx)

(a-rip-ip-pra'zol)

Abilify, Abilify Dismelt

*Func. class.:* Antipsychotic/neuroleptic

**Pregnancy category C**

**Action:** Exact mechanism unknown; may be mediated through both dopamine type 2 (D₂) and serotonin type 2 (5-HT₂) antagonism

---

Adverse effects: *italic* = common, **bold** = life-threatening

**Therapeutic outcome:** Decreased excitement, hallucinations, delusions, paranoia, reorganization of patterns of thought, speech

**Uses:** Schizophrenia, agitation, bipolar disorder, mania

## Dosage and routes
### Schizophrenia
*Adult:* **PO** 10-15 mg/day; if needed, dosage may be increased to 30 mg daily after 2 wk; maintenance 15 mg/day, periodically reassess

### Agitation in bipolar disorder/ schizophrenia
*Adult:* IM 9.75 mg as a single dose, may start with a lower dose

### Bipolar disorder
*Adult:* PO 30 mg/day, may reduce to 15 mg if needed

**Available forms:** Tabs 2, 5, 10, 15, 20, 30 mg; inj 9.75 mg/1.3 ml; orally disintegrating tab 10,15 mg; oral sol 1 mg/ml

## Adverse effects
*CNS:* Drowsiness, insomnia, agitation, anxiety, headache, **seizures, neuroleptic malignant syndrome,** *light-headedness, akathisia, asthenia, tremor,* **stroke, suicidal ideation**
*CV:* Orthostatic hypotension, **tachycardia**
*EENT:* Blurred vision, rhinitis
*GI:* Constipation, *nausea,* vomiting, jaundice, weight gain
*INTEG:* Rash
*RESP:* Cough

**Contraindications:** Hypersensitivity, breastfeeding, seizure disorders

**Precautions:** Pregnancy **C,** children, geriatric, renal/cardiac/hepatic disease

### Pharmacokinetics

| | |
|---|---|
| **Absorption** | Unknown |
| **Distribution** | Protein binding, 90% |
| **Metabolism** | Liver, extensively to major active metabolism |
| **Excretion** | Unknown |
| **Half-life** | Unknown |

### Pharmacodynamics
Unknown

## Interactions
### Individual drugs
Alcohol: increased sedation
Carbamazepine: decreased effects of aripiprazole

Erythromycin, fluoxetine, ketoconazole, quinidine, paroxetine: increased effects of aripiprazole, reduce dose
Famotidine, valproate: decreased aripiprazole level
Lithium: increased EPS
### Drug classifications
Antipsychotics: increased EPS
CNS depressants: increased sedation
CYP3A4/CYP2D6 inhibitors: increased effects of aripiprazole, reduce dose
CYPA34 inducers: decreased effects of aripiprazole; increase dose
### Drug/herb
Betel palm, kava: increased EPS
Cola tree, hops, nettle, nutmeg: increased neuroleptic effect

## NURSING CONSIDERATIONS
### Assessment
• Assess mental status before initial administration
• Check for swallowing of PO medication; check for hoarding or giving of medication to other patients
• Monitor I&O ratio; palpate bladder if urinary output is low
• Monitor bilirubin, CBC, liver function tests qmo
• Assess affect, orientation, LOC, reflexes, gait, coordination, sleep pattern disturbances
• Monitor B/P standing and lying; also pulse, respirations; take q4hr during initial treatment; establish baseline before starting treatment; report drops of 30 mm Hg; watch for ECG changes
• Assess for dizziness, faintness, palpitations, tachycardia on rising
• Assess for EPS, including akathisia (inability to sit still, no pattern to movements), tardive dyskinesia (bizarre movements of the jaw, mouth, tongue, extremities), pseudoparkinsonism (rigidity, tremors, pill rolling, shuffling gait)
◆ Assess for neuroleptic malignant syndrome: hyperthermia, increased CPK, altered mental status, muscle rigidity
• Assess skin turgor daily
• Assess for constipation, urinary retention daily; if these occur, increase bulk and water in diet

### Nursing diagnoses
• Knowledge, deficient (teaching)
• Noncompliance (teaching)
• Sensory perception, disturbed (uses)
• Thought processes, disturbed (uses)

## Implementation

- Administer reduced dose in geriatric
- Decreased stimulus by dimming lights, avoiding loud noises
- Supervise ambulation until patient is stabilized on medication; do not involve in strenuous exercise program because fainting is possible; patient should not stand still for a long time
- Store in tight, light-resistant container

## Patient/family education

- Advise patient that orthostatic hypotension may occur and to rise from sitting or lying position gradually
- Advise patient to avoid hot tubs, hot showers, tub baths; hypotension may occur
- Instruct patient to avoid abrupt withdrawal of this product; EPS may result; product should be withdrawn slowly
- Teach patient to avoid OTC preparations (cough, hayfever, cold) unless approved by prescriber, because serious product interactions may occur; avoid use with alcohol, CNS depressants; increased drowsiness may occur
- Advise patient to avoid hazardous activities if drowsy or dizzy
- Explain importance of compliance with product regimen
- Advise patient, family to report impaired vision, tremors, muscle twitching, urinary retention
- Instruct patient to take extra precautions to stay cool in hot weather, that heat stroke may occur

## Evaluation

**Positive therapeutic outcome**
- Decreased in emotional excitement, hallucinations, delusions, paranoia; reorganization of patterns of thought, speech

**Treatment of overdose:** Lavage if orally ingested; provide airway; *do not induce vomiting*

---

## armodafinil

Nuvigil
*See Appendix A, Selected New Drugs*

---

## ascorbic acid (vitamin C) (OTC, Rx)

(as-kor'bic)

Apo-C ✤, ascorbic acid, Ascorbicap, C-Span, Cebid, Cecon, Cecore 500, Cemill, Cenolate, Cetane, Cevalin, Cevi-Bid, Ce-Vi-Sol, Flavorcee, Mega-C/A Plus, Ortho/CS, Sunkist

*Func. class.:* Vitamin C, water-soluble vitamin

### Pregnancy category C

**Action:** Needed for wound healing, collagen synthesis, antioxidant, carbohydrate metabolism, protein, lipid synthesis, prevention of infection

**Therapeutic outcome:** Replacement and supplementation of vit C

**Uses:** Vit C deficiency, scurvy, delayed wound and bone healing, chronic disease, urine acidification, before gastrectomy; increased need: breastfeeding, pregnancy, hyperthyroidism, emotional stress, trauma, burns, acidification of urine, dietary supplement

**Unlabeled uses:** Common cold prevention

### Dosage and routes
*RDA*
**Neonates and up to 6 mo:** PO 30 mg/day
**Infants 6 mo-1 yr:** PO 35 mg/day
**Child 1-3 yr:** PO 40 mg/day
**Child 4-10 yr:** PO 45 mg/day
**Child 11-14 yr:** PO 50 mg/day
**Adult and child ≥14 yr:** PO 50-500 mg/day
**Pregnancy:** 70 mg/day
**Breastfeeding:** 90 mg/day

*Scurvy*
**Adult:** PO/SUBCUT/IM/**IV** 100 mg-500 mg daily × 2 wk, then 50 mg or more daily
**Child:** PO/SUBCUT/IM/**IV** 100-300 mg daily × 2 wk, then 35 mg or more daily

*Wound healing/chronic disease/fracture*
May be given with zinc
**Adult:** SUBCUT/IM/**IV**/PO 200-500 mg daily for 1-2 mo
**Child:** SUBCUT/IM/**IV**/PO 100-200 mg added doses for 1-2 mo

*Urine acidification*
**Adult:** 4-12 g daily in divided doses
**Child:** 500 mg q6-8hr

---

Adverse effects: *italic* = common, **bold** = life-threatening

**Available forms:** Tabs 25, 50, 100, 250, 500, 1000, 1500 mg; effervescent tabs 1000 mg; chewable tabs 100, 250, 500 mg; time-release tabs 500, 750, 1000, 1500 mg; time-release caps 500 mg; crystals 4 g/tsp; powder 4 g/tsp; liquid 35 mg/0.6 ml; sol 100 mg/ml; syr 20 mg/ml, 500 mg/5 ml; inj SUBCUT, IM, **IV** 100, 250, 500 mg/ml

**Adverse effects**

*CNS:* Headache, insomnia, dizziness, fatigue, flushing
*GI:* Nausea, vomiting, diarrhea, anorexia, heartburn, cramps
*GU:* Polyuria, urine acidification, oxalate or urate renal stones, dysuria
**HEMA: Hemolytic anemia in patients with G6PD**
*INTEG:* Inflammation at inj site

**Contraindications:** Tartrazine, sulfite sensitivity; G6PD deficiency

**Precautions:** Pregnancy **C**, gout, diabetes, renal calculi (large doses)

### Pharmacokinetics

| | |
|---|---|
| **Absorption** | Readily absorbed (PO) |
| **Distribution** | Widely distributed; crosses placenta |
| **Metabolism** | Oxidation |
| **Excretion** | Kidneys, inactive; breast milk |
| **Half-life** | Unknown |

### Pharmacodynamics
Unknown

**Interactions**
*Drug/lab test*
False positive: negatives in glucose tests (Clinitest, Tes-Tape)
False negative: occult blood (large dose), urine bilirubin, leukocyte determination

### NURSING CONSIDERATIONS
**Assessment**
• Assess nutritional status for inclusion of foods high in vit C: citrus fruits, cantaloupe, tomatoes
• Assess for vit C deficiency before, during, and after treatment; scurvy (gingivitis, bleeding gums, loose teeth); poor bone development
• Monitor I&O ratio, polyuria; in patients receiving large doses, renal stones may occur; urine pH (acidification)
• Monitor ascorbic acid levels throughout treatment if continued deficiency is suspected
• Assess inj sites for inflammation, pain, redness, thrombophlebitis if in large doses

**Nursing diagnoses**
• Knowledge, deficient (teaching)
• Nutrition: less than body requirements, imbalanced (uses)

**Implementation**
**PO route**
• Swallow time rel tabs or caps whole; do not break, crush, or chew
• Mix oral sol with foods or fluids
**IM route**
• Not to be diluted; give deep in large muscle mass
**IV, direct route**
• Give undiluted by *direct* **IV** 100 mg over at least 1 min, rapid inf may cause fainting
**Intermittent IV infusion route**
• Give by intermittent inf after diluting with $D_5W$, $D_{10}W$, 0.9% NaCl, 0.45% NaCl, LR, Ringer's sol, dextrose/saline, dextrose/Ringer's combinations; temp will increase pressure in ampules; wrap with gauze before breaking
*Syringe compatibilities:* Metoclopramide, aminophylline, theophylline
*Syringe incompatibilities:* Cefazolin, doxapram
*Additive compatibilities:* Amikacin, calcium chloride, calcium gluceptate, calcium gluconate, cephalothin, chloramphenicol, chlorproMAZINE, colistimethate, cyanocobalamin, diphenhydrAMINE, heparin, kanamycin, methicillin, methyldopate, penicillin G potassium, polymyxin B, prednisoLONE, procaine, prochlorperazine, promethazine, verapamil
*Additive incompatibilities:* Bleomycin, cephapirin, nafcillin, sodium bicarbonate, warfarin
*Y-site compatibilities:* Warfarin

**Patient/family education**
• Teach patient necessary foods to be included in diet that are rich in vit C: citrus fruits, cantaloupe, tomatoes, chili peppers (red)
• Teach patient that smoking decreases vit C levels; not to exceed prescribed dose; increases will be excreted in urine, except time release
• Teach patient not to exceed RDA recommended dose, urinary stones may occur
• Teach patient using ascorbic acid for acidification of urine to test urine pH periodically

**Evaluation**
**Positive therapeutic outcome**
• Absence of anorexia, irritability, pallor, joint pain, hyperkeratosis, petechiae, poor wound healing

A

- Reversal of scurvy: bleeding gums, gingivitis, loose teeth

## aspirin 🔄 (OTC)
(as'pir-in)

acetylsalicylic acid, Acuprin, Apo-ASA ❄, Apo-Asen ❄, Arthrinol ❄, Arthrisin ❄, Artria S.R., A.S.A., Aspergum, Aspirin ❄, Aspir-Low, Aspirtab, Astrin ❄, Bayer Aspirin, Coryphen ❄, Easprin, Ecotrin, 8-Hour Bayer Timed Release, Empirin, Entrophen ❄, Halfprin, Norwich Extra-Strength, Novasen ❄, PMS-ASA ❄, Sloprin, St. Joseph Children's Supasa ❄, Therapy Bayer, ZORprin

*Func. class.:* Nonopioid analgesic
*Chem. class.:* Salicylate

**Pregnancy category** D (3rd trimester)

**Action:** Blocks pain impulses in CNS, reduces inflammation by inhibition of prostaglandin synthesis; antipyretic action results from vasodilatation of peripheral vessels; decreases platelet aggregation

**Therapeutic outcome:** Decreased pain, inflammation, fever; absence of MI, transient ischemic attacks, thrombosis

**Uses:** Mild to moderate pain or fever including rheumatoid arthritis, osteoarthritis, thromboembolic disorders, transient ischemic attacks in men, rheumatic fever, post-MI, prophylaxis of MI, ischemic stroke, angina

**Unlabeled uses:** Prevention of cataracts (long-term use), prevention of pregnancy loss in women with clotting disorders

### Dosage and routes
*Arthritis*
*Adult:* PO 2.6-5.2 g/day in divided doses q4-6hr
*Child >25 kg (55 lb):* PO 2.4-3.6 g/day in divided doses

*Kawasaki disease (unlabeled)*
*Child:* PO 80-100 mg/kg/day in 4 divided doses, maintenance 3-8 mg/kg/day as a single dose × 8 wk, given with gamma globulin

*MI, stroke prophylaxis*
*Adult:* PO 160-325 mg/day

*Pain/fever*
*Adult:* PO/RECT 325-650 mg q4hr prn, not to exceed 4 g/day
*Child 2-11 yr:* PO 10-15 mg/kg/dose q4hr, max 80 mg/kg/day

*Acute rheumatic fever*
*Adult:* PO 5-6 g/day initially
*Child:* PO 100 mg/kg/day × 2 wk, then 75 mg/kg/day × 4-6 wk

*Thromboembolic disorders*
*Adult:* PO 325-650 mg/day or bid

*Transient ischemic attacks (risk)*
*Adult:* PO 160-325 mg/day

*Prevention of recurrent MI*
*Adult:* PO 75-325 mg/day

*CABG*
*Adult:* PO 325 mg/day starting 6 hr postprocedure, continue for 1 yr

*PTCA*
*Adult:* PO 325 mg 2 hr presurgery

**Available forms:** Tabs 81, 162.5, 325, 500, 650, 975 mg; chewable tabs 80, 81 mg; supp 60, 120, 125, 130, 150, 160, 195, 200, 300, 320, 325, 600, 640, 650 mg, 1.2 g; cream; gum 227 mg; dispersible tabs 325, 500 mg; del rel, enteric coated tabs 80, 165, 300, 325, 500, 600, 650, 975 mg; ext rel 325, 650, 800 mg; del rel caps 325, 500 mg

**Adverse effects**
*CNS:* Stimulation, drowsiness, dizziness, confusion, **seizures,** headache, flushing, hallucinations, **coma**
*CV:* Rapid pulse, pulmonary edema
*EENT:* Tinnitus, hearing loss
*ENDO:* Hypoglycemia, hyponatremia, hypokalemia
*GI: Nausea, vomiting,* **GI bleeding,** diarrhea, heartburn, anorexia, **hepatitis**
*HEMA:* **Thrombocytopenia, agranulocytosis, leukopenia, neutropenia, hemolytic anemia,** increased pro-time, PTT, bleeding time
*INTEG: Rash,* urticaria, bruising
*RESP:* Wheezing, hyperpnea
*SYST:* **Reye's syndrome (children), anaphylaxis, laryngeal edema**

**Contraindications:** Pregnancy **D** (3rd trimester), breastfeeding, children <12 yr, children with flulike symptoms, hypersensitivity to salicylates, tartrazine (FDC yellow dye #5), GI bleeding, bleeding disorders, vit K deficiency, peptic ulcer

**Precautions:** Anemia, renal/hepatic disease, Hodgkin's disease, pre/postoperatively, gastritis, asthmatic patients with nasal polyps or aspirin sensitivity

## Pharmacokinetics

| | |
|---|---|
| **Absorption** | Well absorbed, small intestine (PO); erratic (enteric); slow (RECT) |
| **Distribution** | Rapidly, widely distributed; crosses placenta |
| **Metabolism** | Liver, extensively |
| **Excretion** | Inactive metabolites, kidney; breast milk |
| **Half-life** | 15-20 min (low doses); 9 hr (high doses) |

## Pharmacodynamics

| | PO | RECT |
|---|---|---|
| **Onset** | 15-30 min | Slow |
| **Peak** | 1-2 hr | 4-5 hr |
| **Duration** | 4-6 hr | 6-7 hr |

## Interactions
### Individual drugs

Alcohol, cefamandole, clopidogrel, eptifibatide, heparin, plicamycin, ticlopidine, tirofiban: increased risk of bleeding

Ammonium chloride, nizatidine: increased salicylate level

Insulin, methotrexate, phenytoin, valproic acid, warfarin: increased effects of each specific product

Nitroglycerin: increased hypotension

Probenecid: decreased effects of probenecid

Spironolactone, sulfinpyrazone: decreased effects

### Drug classifications

ACE inhibitors: decreased antihypertensive effect

Antacids, corticosteroids, steroids, urinary alkalizers: decreased effects of aspirin

Anticoagulants, thrombolytics: increased risk of bleeding

Diuretics (loop), sulfonylamides, NSAIDs, β-blockers: decreased effect of each specific product

NSAIDs, antiinflammatories, steroids: increased gastric ulcers

Penicillins, oral hypoglycemics, sulfonamides, thrombolytic agents: increased effects of each specific product

Salicylates: decreased blood glucose levels

Urinary acidifiers: increased salicylate levels

### Drug/herb

Anise, arnica, basil, bilberry, bogbean, chamomile, chondroitin, clove, dong quai, fenugreek, feverfew, garlic, ginger, ginkgo, ginseng *(Panax),* horse chestnut, Irish moss, licorice, pansy, red clover: increased risk of bleeding

Arginine, gossypol: gastric irritation

### Drug/food
Foods acidifying urine may increase aspirin levels

### Drug/lab test
Increased: coagulation studies, liver function studies, serum uric acid, amylase, $CO_2$, urinary protein

Decreased: serum potassium, cholesterol

Interference: VMA, 5-HIAA, xylose tolerance test, TSH

## NURSING CONSIDERATIONS
### Assessment
- Assess for pain: character, location, intensity, ROM before and 1 hr after administration
- Monitor liver function studies: AST, ALT, bilirubin, creatinine if patient is on long-term therapy
- Monitor renal function studies: BUN, urine creatinine if patient is on long-term therapy
- Monitor blood studies: CBC, Hct, Hgb, pro-time if patient is on long-term therapy
- Check I&O ratio; decreasing output may indicate renal failure (long-term therapy)
- ◆ Assess hepatotoxicity: dark urine, clay-colored stools, yellowing of the skin and sclera, itching, abdominal pain, fever, diarrhea if patient is on long-term therapy
- Assess for allergic reactions: rash, urticaria; if these occur, product may have to be discontinued; patients with asthma, nasal polyps, allergies; severe allergic reactions may occur
- Assess for ototoxicity: tinnitus, ringing, roaring in ears; audiometric testing needed before, after long-term therapy
- Monitor salicylate level: therapeutic level 150-300 mcg/ml for chronic inflammation
- Check edema in feet, ankles, legs
- Identify prior product history; there are many product interactions

### Nursing diagnoses
- Injury, risk for (side effects)
- Knowledge, deficient (teaching)
- Mobility, impaired physical (uses)
- Pain, acute (uses)
- Pain, chronic (uses)

### Implementation
#### PO route
- Do not break, crush, or chew enteric product
- Administer to patient crushed or whole; chewable tab should be chewed
- Give with food or milk to decrease gastric symptoms; separate by 2 hr of enteric product; absorption may be slowed
- Give antacids 1-2 hr after enteric products

- Give with 8 oz of water and have patient sit upright for 30 min after dose; discard tabs if vinegar-like smell is present; avoid if allergic to tartrazine
- Give ½ hr before planned exercise

**Patient/family education**

- Teach patient to report any symptoms of renal/hepatic toxicity, visual changes, ototoxicity, allergic reactions, bleeding (long-term therapy)
- Instruct patient to take with 8 oz of water and sit upright for 30 min after dose to facilitate product passing into the stomach; to discard tabs if vinegar-like smell is present; to avoid if allergic to tartrazine
- Instruct patient not to exceed recommended dosage; acute poisoning may result
- Advise patient to read label on other OTC products; many contain aspirin
- Inform patient that the therapeutic response takes 2 wk (arthritis)
- Teach patient to report tinnitus, confusion, diarrhea, sweating, hyperventilation
- Advise patient to avoid alcohol ingestion; GI bleeding may occur
- Advise patient with allergies, nasal polyps, asthma, that allergic reactions may develop
- Instruct patient to read labels on other OTC products; may contain salicylates
- Teach patient not to give to children or teens with flulike symptoms or chicken pox; Reye's syndrome may develop

**Evaluation**

**Positive therapeutic outcome**

- Decreased pain
- Decreased inflammation
- Decreased fever
- Absence of MI
- Absence of transient ischemic attacks, thrombosis

**Treatment of overdose:** Lavage, activated charcoal, monitor electrolytes, VS

---

## atazanavir (Rx)
(at-a-za-na'veer)
Reyataz
*Func. class.:* Antiretroviral
*Chem. class.:* Protease inhibitor

**Pregnancy category B**

**Action:** Inhibits human immunodeficiency virus (HIV-1) protease, which prevents maturation of the infectious virus

**Therapeutic outcome:** Decreasing symptoms of HIV

**Uses:** HIV-1 infection in combination with other antiretroviral agents

**Dosage and routes**
*Antiretroviral-naive patients*
*Adult:* PO 400 mg daily
*Antiretroviral-experienced patients*
*Adult:* PO 300 mg daily and ritonavir 100 mg daily
*Hepatic dose*
*Adult:* PO (Child-Pugh B) 300 mg daily; (Child-Pugh C) do not use

**Available forms:** Caps 100, 150, 200, 300 mg

**Adverse effects**
*CNS:* Headache, depression, dizziness, insomnia, peripheral neuropathy
*GI: Diarrhea, abdominal pain, nausea,* vomiting, **hepatotoxicity**
*INTEG: Rash,* **Stevens-Johnson syndrome**, *photosensitivity*
*MISC:* Fatigue, fever, arthralgia, back pain, cough, lipodystrophy, pain, gynecomastia, nephrolithiasis

**Contraindications:** Hypersensitivity

**Precautions:** Pregnancy **B,** breastfeeding, children, geriatric, liver disease

| Pharmacokinetics | |
|---|---|
| Absorption | Rapid, increased with food |
| Distribution | 86% protein bound |
| Metabolism | Liver extensively |
| Excretion | 27% excreted unchanged in urine/feces (minimal) |
| Half-life | 7 hr |

| Pharmacodynamics | |
|---|---|
| Onset | Unknown |
| Peak | 2 hr |
| Duration | Unknown |

**Interactions**
*Individual drugs*
Chlorazepate, clarithromycin, cycloSPORINE, diazepam, irinotecan, midazolam, pimozide, sildenafil, sirolimus, tacrolimus, triazolam, warfarin: increased levels resulting in increased toxicity
Didanosine, efavirenz, rifampin: decreased atazanavir levels
Indinavir: increased hyperbilirubinemia
*Drug classifications*
Antacids, $H_2$-receptor antagonists, proton pump inhibitors: decreased atazanavir levels
Antidepressants (tricyclics), antidysrhythmics,

Adverse effects: *italic* = common, **bold** = life-threatening

ergots, calcium channel blockers, HMG-CoA reductase inhibitors, immunosuppressants: increased levels resulting in increased toxicity

Contraceptives (oral), estrogens: increased effects

***Drug/herb***

St. John's wort: decreased atazanavir levels

***Drug/lab test***

Increased: AST, ALT, total bilirubin, amylase, lipase

## NURSING CONSIDERATIONS
### Assessment
◆ Assess for hepatic failure
• Assess for signs of infection, anemia
• Monitor liver function studies: ALT, AST, bilirubin
• Monitor bowel pattern before, during treatment; if severe abdominal pain with bleeding occurs, product should be discontinued; monitor hydration
• Monitor viral load, CD4 count throughout treatment
• Assess skin eruptions, rash, urticaria, itching
• Identify allergies before treatment, reaction of each medication; place allergies on chart

### Nursing diagnoses
• Injury, risk for (uses, adverse reactions)
• Knowledge, deficient (teaching)

### Implementation
• Administer with food; take 2 hr before or 1 hr after antacid or didanosine

### Patient/family education
• Advise to take as prescribed with other antiretrovirals as prescribed; if dose is missed, take as soon as remembered up to 1 hr before next dose; do not double dose; do not share with others
• Teach that product must be taken daily to maintain blood levels for duration of therapy
• Teach that photosensitivity may occur; use protective clothing or stay out of the sun
• Instruct to notify prescriber if diarrhea, nausea, vomiting, rash occur; dizziness, light-headedness, ECG may be altered
• Inform that product interacts with many products and St. John's wort; advise prescriber of all products, herbal products used
• Advise that redistribution of body fat may occur; the effect is not known
• Teach that product does not cure HIV-1 infection or prevent transmission to others, only controls symptoms
• Advise that if taking sildenafil with atazanavir, there may be an increased risk of sildenafil-associated adverse events, including hypotension and prolonged penile erection; notify physician promptly of these symptoms

### Evaluation
**Positive therapeutic outcome**
• Increasing CD4 counts; decreased viral load, resolution of symptoms of HIV-1 infection

---

### atenolol (Rx)
(a-ten'oh-lole)
Apo-Atenolol ✿, atenolol ✿, Novo-Atenol ✿, Tenormin
*Func. class.:* Antihypertensive
*Chem. class.:* β-Blocker; β₁-, β₂-blocker (high doses)

**Pregnancy category D**

---

**Do not confuse:**
atenolol/albuterol/Altenol, Tenormin/thiamine/Imuran/Trovan

**Action:** Competitively blocks stimulation of β-adrenergic receptor within vascular smooth muscle; produces negative chronotropic activity (decreases rate of SA node discharge, increases recovery time), slows conduction of AV node, decreases heart rate, negative inotropic activity, decreases $O_2$ consumption in myocardium; also decreases renin-aldosterone-angiotensin system at high doses, inhibits β₂-receptors in bronchial system at higher doses

**Therapeutic outcome:** Decreased B/P, heart rate, prevention of angina pectoris, MI

**Uses:** Mild to moderate hypertension; prophylaxis of angina pectoris; suspected or known MI (**IV** use)

### Dosage and routes
*Adult:* PO 50 mg daily, increasing q1-2 wk to 100 mg daily; may increase to 200 mg daily for angina or up to 100 mg for hypertension
*Child:* PO 0.8-1 mg/kg/dose initially
*Geriatric:* PO 25 mg/day initially

***Renal dose***
*Adult:* PO CCr 15-35 ml/min, max 50 mg/day; CCr <15 ml/min max 25 mg/day; hemodialysis 25-50 mg after dialysis

***MI***
*Adult:* **IV** 5 mg over 5 min, then 5 mg over 10 min, then after 10 min give PO dose

**Available forms:** Tabs 25, 50, 100 mg; 500 inj mcg/ml

---

## Adverse effects

*CNS: Insomnia, fatigue, dizziness, mental changes,* memory loss, hallucinations, depression, lethargy, drowsiness, strange dreams, catatonia
*CV:* **Profound hypotension, bradycardia, CHF,** *cold extremities, postural hypotension, 2nd- or 3rd-degree heart block*
*EENT:* Sore throat, dry burning eyes, blurred vision, stuffy nose
*ENDO:* Increased hypoglycemic response to insulin
*GI: Nausea, diarrhea,* vomiting, **mesenteric arterial thrombosis, ischemic colitis**
*GU:* Impotence, decreased libido
*HEMA:* **Agranulocytosis, thrombocytopenia, purpura**
*INTEG:* Rash, fever, alopecia
*RESP:* **Bronchospasm,** dyspnea, wheezing, pulmonary edema

**Contraindications:** Pregnancy **D,** hypersensitivity to β-blockers, cardiogenic shock, 2nd- or 3rd-degree heart block, sinus bradycardia, CHF, cardiac failure, Raynaud's disease, pulmonary edema

**Precautions:** Major surgery, breastfeeding, diabetes mellitus, renal disease, thyroid disease, CHF, COPD, asthma, well-compensated heart failure, dialysis, myasthenia gravis

### Pharmacokinetics

| | |
|---|---|
| Absorption | 50%-60% (PO) |
| Distribution | Crosses placenta; protein binding (5%-15%) |
| Metabolism | Not metabolized |
| Excretion | Breast milk, kidneys (50%), feces (50%—unabsorbed product) |
| Half-life | 6-9 hr |

### Pharmacodynamics

| | PO | IV |
|---|---|---|
| Onset | 1 hr | Rapid |
| Peak | 2-4 hr | 5 min |
| Duration | 24 hr | Unknown |

### Interactions
#### Individual drugs

Atropine: increased atenolol absorption
Digoxin, diltiazem, hydralazine, methyldopa, prazosin, reserpine, verapamil: increased hypotension, bradycardia
#### Drug classifications

Anticholinergics, cardiac glycosides, antihypertensives: increased hypotension, bradycardia

Sympathomimetics (cough, cold preparations): mutual inhibition
#### Drug/herb

Aconite: increased toxicity, death
Betel palm, butterbur, cola tree, figwort, fumitory, guarana, hawthorn, jaborandi tree, lily of the valley, motherwort, plantain: increased atenolol effect
Coenzyme Q10, yohimbe: decreased atenolol effect
#### Drug/lab test

Increased: uric acid, potassium, triglyceride, blood glucose, BUN, ANA titer

### NURSING CONSIDERATIONS
#### Assessment

- Monitor B/P during beginning treatment, periodically thereafter; pulse q4hr; note rate, rhythm, quality: apical/radial pulse before administration; notify prescriber of any significant changes (pulse <50 bpm)
- Check for baselines in renal, liver function tests before therapy begins
- Assess for edema in feet, legs daily; monitor I&O, daily weight; check for jugular vein distention, crackles bilaterally, dyspnea (CHF)

#### Nursing diagnoses

- Cardiac output, decreased (uses)
- Injury, risk for (side effects)
- Knowledge, deficient (teaching)
- Noncompliance (teaching)

#### Implementation
##### PO route

- Given before meals, at bedtime; tablet may be crushed or swallowed whole; give with food to prevent GI upset; reduced dosage in renal dysfunction; take at same time each day
- Store protected from light, moisture; place in cool environment
##### IV route

- Give **IV** direct over 5 min or diluted in 10-50 ml D₅W, 0.9% NaCl, and give at prescribed rate
##### Y-site compatibilities: Meperidine, meropenem, morphine

#### Patient/family education

⚠ Teach patient not to discontinue product abruptly; taper over 2 wk; may cause precipitate angina if stopped abruptly, take at same time each day
- Teach patient not to use OTC products containing α-adrenergic stimulants (such as nasal decongestants, OTC cold preparations); to limit alcohol, smoking; to limit sodium intake as prescribed
- Teach patient how to take pulse and B/P at home; advise when to notify prescriber

Adverse effects: *italic* = common, **bold** = life-threatening

- Instruct patient to comply with weight control, dietary adjustments, modified exercise program
- Advise patient to carry/wear emergency ID for products, allergies, conditions being treated; tell patient product controls symptoms but does not cure
- Caution patient to avoid hazardous activities if dizziness, drowsiness is present
- Teach patient to report symptoms of CHF: difficult breathing, especially on exertion or when lying down, night cough, swelling of extremities or bradycardia, dizziness, confusion, depression, fever
- Teach patient to take product as prescribed, not to double doses, skip doses; take any missed doses as remembered if at least 6 hr until next dose
- Advise patient that product may mask symptoms of hypoglycemia in diabetic patients
- Advise patient to use contraception while taking this product

### Evaluation

**Positive therapeutic outcome**
- Decreased B/P in hypertension (after 1-2 wk)
- Absence of dysrhythmias
- Absence of MI
- Decreased angina

**Treatment of overdose:** Lavage, **IV** atropine for bradycardia, **IV** theophylline for bronchospasm, digoxin, O₂, diuretic for cardiac failure, hemodialysis, **IV** glucose for hyperglycemia, **IV** diazepam (or phenytoin) for seizures

## atomoxetine (Rx)

(at-o-mox'eh-teen)
Strattera
*Func. class.:* Psychotherapeutic—miscellaneous

**Pregnancy category C**

**Action:** A selective norepinephrine reuptake inhibitor; may inhibit the presynaptic norepinephrine transporter; exact mechanism of action is unknown

**Therapeutic outcome:** Decreased hyperactivity, impulsivity, increased attention, organization, ability to complete tasks

**Uses:** Attention deficit hyperactivity disorder

### Dosage and routes

*Child ≤70 kg:* PO 0.5 mg/kg, increase after 3 days to a target daily dose of 1.2 mg/kg in AM or evenly divided doses AM, late afternoon; max 1.4 mg/kg/day or 100 mg daily, whichever is less

*Adult and child >70 kg:* PO 40 mg daily, increase after 3 days to a target daily dose of 80 mg in AM or evenly divided doses AM, late afternoon; max 100 mg daily

**Hepatic dose**

(Child-Pugh B) reduce dose by 50%
(Child-Pugh C) reduce dose by 75%

**Available forms:** Caps 10, 18, 25, 40, 60, 80, 100 mg

### Adverse effects

*CNS: Insomnia,* dizziness, headache, irritability, crying, mood swings, fatigue
*CV: Palpitations,* hot flushes, tachycardia
*ENDO:* Growth retardation
*GI:* Dyspepsia, nausea, anorexia, dry mouth, weight loss, vomiting, diarrhea, constipation, hepatic injury
*GU:* Urinary hesitancy, retention, dysmenorrhea, erectile disturbance, ejaculation failure, impotence, prostatitis, abnormal orgasm
*INTEG: Exfoliative dermatitis,* sweating, rash
*MISC:* Cough, rhinorrhea, dermatitis, ear infection

**Contraindications:** Hypersensitivity, angle-closure glaucoma, arteriosclerosis, cardiac disease, cardiomyopathy, heart failure, jaundice

**Precautions:** Pregnancy C, breastfeeding, children >6 yr, hypertension, hepatic/cardiac/cerebrovascular disease, angioedema, bipolar disorder, dysrhythmias, CAD, hypo/hypertension, suicidal ideation

### Pharmacokinetics

| | |
|---|---|
| Absorption | Unknown |
| Distribution | Protein binding, 98% |
| Metabolism | Liver |
| Excretion | Kidneys |
| Half-life | Unknown |

### Pharmacodynamics

Unknown

### Interactions
*Individual drug*

Albuterol: increased cardiovascular effects
*Drug classifications*

CYP2D6 inhibitors (amiodarone, cimetidine [weak], citalopram, clomiPRAMINE, delavirdine, escitalopram, fluoxetine, gefitinib, imatinib, paroxetine, propafenone, quinidine [potent], ritonavir, sertraline, thioridazine, venlafaxine): increased effects of atomoxetine

◆MAOIs or within 14 days of MAOIs, vasopressors: hypertensive crisis

Pressor agents: increased cardiovascular effects

## NURSING CONSIDERATIONS
### Assessment

• Monitor VS, B/P; check patients with cardiac disease more often for increased B/P
• Monitor height, growth rate q3 mo in children; growth rate may be decreased
• Assess mental status: mood, sensorium, affect, stimulation, insomnia, aggressiveness, suicidal ideation
• Assess appetite, sleep, speech patterns
• Assess for attention span, decreased hyperactivity in ADHD persons

### Nursing diagnoses
• Coping, ineffective (uses)
• Coping, compromised family (uses)
• Knowledge, deficient (teaching)
• Thought processes, disturbed (uses)

### Implementation
• Swallow whole; do not break, crush, or chew
• Give without regard to food
• Provide gum, hard candy, frequent sips of water for dry mouth

### Patient/family education
• Advise patient to avoid OTC preparations unless approved by prescriber
• Advise patient to avoid alcohol ingestion
• Advise patient to avoid hazardous activities until stabilized on medication
• Advise patient to get needed rest; patients will feel more tired at end of day; do not take dose late in day, insomnia may occur

### Evaluation
**Positive therapeutic outcome**
• Decreased hyperactivity (ADHD)

## atorvastatin (Rx)
(a-tore'va-stat-in)
Lipitor
*Func. class.:* Antilipidemic
*Chem. class.:* HMG-CoA reductase inhibitor
**Pregnancy category** X

**Action:** Inhibits HMG-CoA reductase enzyme, which reduces cholesterol synthesis

**Therapeutic outcome:**
Decreased cholesterol levels and LDLs, increased HDLs

**Uses:** As an adjunct in primary hypercholesterolemia (types Ia, Ib), dysbetalipoproteinemia, elevated triglyceride levels; prevention of cardiovascular disease by reduction of heart risk in those with mildly elevated cholesterol

## Dosage and routes
*Adult:* PO 10-20 mg daily, usual range 10-80, dosage adjustments may be made in 2-4 wk intervals, max 80 mg/day; patients requiring >45% reduction in LDL may be started at 40 mg daily

**Available forms:** Tabs 10, 20, 40, 80 mg

### Adverse effects
*CNS:* Headache, asthenia
*EENT:* Lens opacities
*GI: Abdominal cramps, constipation, diarrhea, heartburn,* nausea, dyspepsia, *flatus,* **liver dysfunction,** pancreatitis, increased serum transaminase
*GU:* Impotence
*INTEG:* Rash, pruritus, alopecia
*MISC:* Hypersensitivity
*MS:* Myalgia, **rhabdomyolysis,** arthralgia
*RESP:* Pharyngitis, sinusitis

**Contraindications:** Pregnancy **X**, breastfeeding, hypersensitivity, active liver disease

**Precautions:** Past liver disease, alcoholism, severe acute infections, trauma, severe metabolic disorders, electrolyte imbalance

### Pharmacokinetics
| | |
|---|---|
| **Absorption** | Unknown |
| **Distribution** | Unknown |
| **Metabolism** | Liver |
| **Excretion** | Bile, feces, kidneys |
| **Half-life** | 14 hr |

### Pharmacodynamics
Unknown

### Interactions
*Individual drugs*
Clofibrate, cycloSPORINE, erythromycin, gemfibrozil, niacin: increased risk of rhabdomyolysis
Colestipol: decreased action of atorvastatin
Digoxin: increased action of digoxin
Erythromycin: increased levels of atorvastatin
Warfarin: increased action of warfarin
*Drug classifications*
Antifungals (azole): possible rhabdomyolysis
Contraceptives (oral): increased levels
*Drug/herb*
Glucomannan: increased effect
Gotu kola, St. John's wort: decreased effect

Adverse effects: *italic* = common, **bold** = life-threatening

*Drug/food*
Possible toxicity when used with grapefruit
juice
Oatbran may reduce effectiveness
*Drug/lab test*
Increased: bilirubin, alkaline phosphatase
Interference: thyroid function tests

## NURSING CONSIDERATIONS
### Assessment
• Assess nutrition: fat, protein, carbohydrates;
nutritional analysis should be completed by
dietitian before treatment
• Assess for muscle pain, tenderness, obtain
CPK if these occur, product may need to be
discontinued
• Monitor bowel pattern daily; diarrhea may
be a problem
• Monitor triglycerides, cholesterol at baseline and throughout treatment; LDL and VLDL
should be watched closely; if increased,
product should be discontinued
• Monitor liver function studies q1-2 mo
during the first 1½ yr of treatment; AST, ALT,
liver function tests may be increased
• Monitor renal studies in patients with
compromised renal system: BUN, I&O ratio,
creatinine
• Assess eyes via ophthalmic exam 1 mo after
treatment begins, annually

### Nursing diagnoses
• Diarrhea (adverse reactions)
• Knowledge, deficient (teaching)
• Noncompliance (teaching)

### Implementation
• Administer total daily dose at any time of day
• Store in cool environment in airtight,
light-resistant container

### Patient/family education
• Inform patient that compliance is needed
for positive results to occur, not to double
doses
• Teach patient that risk factors should be
decreased: high-fat diet, smoking, alcohol
consumption, absence of exercise
• Advise patient to notify prescriber if the GI
symptoms of diarrhea, abdominal or epigastric
pain, nausea, vomiting; chills, fever, sore
throat; muscle pain, weakness occur
• Advise patient that treatment will take
several years
• Advise patient that blood work and eye exam
will be necessary during treatment
• Advise not to take if pregnant
• Advise patient to stay out of the sun, use
protective clothing, or use sunscreen to
prevent photosensitivity (rare)

### Evaluation
**Positive therapeutic outcome**
• Decreased cholesterol levels, serum triglyc-
eride
• Improved ratio of HDLs

---

**atovaquone** (Rx)
(a-toe'va-kwon)
Mepron
*Func. class.:* Antiprotozoal
*Chem. class.:* Aromatic diamide derivative;
analog of ubiquinone
**Pregnancy category** C

**Action:** Interferes with DNA/RNA synthesis in
protozoa, specifically ATP and nucleic acid
synthesis

**Therapeutic outcome:** Antiprotozoal
for *Pneumocystis jiroveci* only

**Uses:** *P. jiroveci* infections in patients
intolerant of trimethoprim/sulfamethoxazole
(co-trimoxazole)

**Dosage and routes**
*Acute, mild, moderate*
**Pneumocystis jiroveci *pneumonia*
(PCP)**
*Adult and adolescent 13-16 yr:* PO
750 mg bid with food tid for 21 days

**Pneumocystis jiroveci *pneumonia*
prophylaxis**
*Adult and adolescent:* PO 1500 mg
daily with meal

**Available forms:** Susp 750 mg/5 ml

**Adverse effects**
*CNS: Dizziness, headache, anxiety,* insom-
nia, asthenia, fever
*CV:* Hypotension
*GI: Nausea, vomiting, diarrhea,* anorexia,
increased AST and ALT, acute pancreatitis,
constipation, abdominal pain
*HEMA:* Anemia, **leukopenia, neutropenia**
*INTEG:* Pruritus, urticaria, *rash,* oral monilia,
sweating
*META:* Hyperkalemia, hypoglycemia, hypona-
tremia
*OTHER:* Cough

**Contraindications:** Hypersensitivity or
history of developing life-threatening allergic
reactions to any component of the formulation,
benzyl alcohol sensitivity

**Precautions:** Pregnancy C, breastfeeding,
children, geriatric, blood dyscrasias, GI/

hepatic disease, diabetes mellitus, respiratory insufficiency

### Pharmacokinetics

| | |
|---|---|
| **Absorption** | Poor; increased when taken with fatty foods |
| **Distribution** | Unknown |
| **Metabolism** | Hepatic recycling |
| **Excretion** | Feces, unchanged (94%) |
| **Half-life** | 2-3 days |

### Pharmacodynamics

| | |
|---|---|
| **Onset** | Unknown |
| **Peak** | 1-8 hr |
| **Duration** | Unknown |

### Interactions
*Individual drugs*
Rifampin, rifabutin, tetracycline: decreased effectiveness of atovaquone
*Drug classifications*
Use cautiously with highly protein-bound products with narrow therapeutic indices

### NURSING CONSIDERATIONS
Assessment
• Assess for *Pneumocystis jiroveci:* monitor WBC, bilateral lung sounds, sputum for C&S; these should be checked before, periodically during, and after treatment; after collection of 1st sputum, therapy may begin
• Monitor for symptoms of hyponatremia: *CV:* increased B/P, cold, clammy skin, hypovolemia or hypervolemia; *GI:* anorexia, nausea, vomiting, diarrhea, abdominal cramps; *NEURO:* lethargy, increased ICP, confusion, headache, seizures, coma, fatigue, tremors, hyperreflexia
• Monitor for symptoms of hypoglycemia/hyperglycemia in diabetic patients
• Monitor blood studies: blood glucose, CBC, platelets; I&O ratio; ECG for cardiac dysrhythmias, check B/P; liver function tests: AST, ALT
• Monitor for signs of infection; anemia; monitor bowel pattern before, during treatment
• Monitor respiratory status: rate, character, wheezing, dyspnea; ABGs, chest films
• Assess for dizziness, confusion, hallucination
• Assess for allergies before treatment, reaction of each medication; place allergies on chart; notify all people giving products
Nursing diagnoses
• Diarrhea (adverse reactions)
• Infection, risk for (uses)
• Knowledge, deficient (teaching)

### Implementation
• Give with food (preferably fatty); increased absorption of the product and higher plasma concentrations will occur; give tid × 3 wk
• Give oral suspension after shaken
• Take all contents of foil pouch
### Patient/family education
• Instruct patient to take with food, preferably fatty foods, to increase plasma concentrations
• Advise patient to take product exactly as prescribed
### Evaluation
**Positive therapeutic outcome**
• Decreased temperature
• Ability to breathe
• Three negative sputum cultures

### ! HIGH ALERT

### atropine (Rx)
(a'troe-peen)
atropine sulfate, Atro-Pen, Sal-Tropine
*Func. class.:* Antidsrhythmic, anticholinergic parasympatholytic, mydriatic
*Chem. class.:* Belladonna alkaloid
**Pregnancy category** C

**Do not confuse:**
atropine/Akarpine

**Action:** Blocks acetylcholine at parasympathetic neuroeffector sites; increases cardiac output, heart rate by blocking vagal stimulation in heart; dries secretions, decreases sweating, salivation in low doses; mydriasis, increased heart rate and cycloplegia occur at moderate doses; motility of GI, GU systems at high dose

**Therapeutic outcome:** Drying of secretions, increased heart rate, cycloplegia, mydriasis

**Uses:** Bradycardia <40-50 bpm, bradydysrhythmia, reversal of anticholinesterase agents, insecticide poisoning, blocking cardiac vagal reflexes, decreasing secretions before surgery, antispasmodic with GU and biliary surgery, bronchodilator; ophthalmically for cycloplegia, mydriasis

### Dosage and routes
*Bradycardia/ bradydysrhythmias*
*Adult:* IV BOL 0.5-1 mg given q3-5 min, not to exceed 2 mg
*Child:* IV BOL 0.01-0.03 mg/kg up to 0.4 mg or 0.3 mg/m$^2$; may repeat q4-6hr, min dose 0.1 mg to avoid paradoxical reaction

### Organophosphate poisoning
**Adult and child:** IM/**IV** 2 mg qhr until muscarinic symptoms disappear; may need 6 mg qhr

### Atro-Pen
**Adult and child 90 lb, usually >10 yr:** 2 mg
**Child 40-90 lb, usually 4-10 yr:** 1 mg
**Child 15-40 lb, 6 mo-4 yr:** 0.05 mg

### Presurgery
**Adult and child >20 kg:** SUBCUT/IM/**IV** 0.4-0.6 mg before anesthesia
**Child <20 kg:** IM/SUBCUT 0.01 mg/kg up to 0.4 mg ½-1 hr preop

**Available forms:** Inj 0.05, 0.1, 0.3, 0.4, 0.5, 0.8, 1 mg/ml; tabs 0.4 mg; inj prefilled autoinjectors (Atro-Pen) 0.5, 1, 2 mg

### Adverse effects
***CNS:*** Headache, dizziness, involuntary movement, confusion, psychosis, anxiety, **coma,** flushing, drowsiness, insomnia, weakness, delirium (geriatric)
***CV:*** Hypo/hypertension, paradoxic bradycardia, angina, PVCs, tachycardia, ectopic ventricular beats
***EENT:*** Blurred vision, photophobia, glaucoma, eye pain, pupil dilatation, nasal congestion
***GI:*** Dry mouth, nausea, vomiting, abdominal pain, anorexia, constipation, **paralytic ileus,** abdominal distention, altered taste
***GU:*** Retention, hesitancy, impotence, dysuria
***INTEG:*** Rash, urticaria, contact dermatitis, dry skin, flushing
***MISC:*** Suppression of breastfeeding, decreased sweating

**Contraindications:** Hypersensitivity to belladonna alkaloids, angle-closure glaucoma, GI obstructions, myasthenia gravis, thyrotoxicosis, ulcerative colitis, prostatic hypertrophy, tachycardia/tachydysrhythmias, asthma, acute hemorrhage, severe hepatic disease, myocardial ischemia

**Precautions:** Pregnancy **C,** breastfeeding, child <6 yr, geriatric, renal disease, CHF, tachydysrhythmias, hyperthyroidism, COPD, hypertension, intraabdominal infections, Down syndrome, spastic paralysis, gastric ulcer

## Pharmacokinetics

| | |
|---|---|
| **Absorption** | Well absorbed (PO, SUBCUT, IM) |
| **Distribution** | Crosses blood-brain barrier, placenta |
| **Metabolism** | Liver |
| **Excretion** | Kidneys, unchanged (70%-90%); breast milk |
| **Half-life** | 13-40 hr |

## Pharmacodynamics

| | PO | IM/ SUBCUT | IV | OPHTH |
|---|---|---|---|---|
| **Onset** | ½ hr | 15 min | 2-4 min | ½ hr |
| **Peak** | ½-1 hr | 30 min | 2-4 min | 30-60 min |
| **Duration** | 4-6 hr | 4-6 hr | 4-6 hr | 1-2 wk |

### Interactions
#### Individual drugs
Ketoconazole, levodopa: decreased absorption
Potassium chloride (oral): mucosal lesions
#### Drug classifications
Antacids: decreased absorption of atropine
Antidepressants (tricyclic), antiparkinson agents: increased anticholinergic effect
#### Drug/herb
Aconite: increased toxicity, death
Aloe, buckthorn (chronic use), cascara sagrada (chronic use), figwort, fumitory, goldenseal, jimsonweed, kudzu, licorice, rhubarb, scopolia, senna: increased effect
Black root: forms insoluble complex
Coltsfoot: decreased effect
Horehound: increased serotonin effect

## NURSING CONSIDERATIONS
### Assessment
- Monitor I&O ratio; check for urinary retention and daily output in geriatric or postoperative patients
- Monitor ECG for ectopic ventricular beats, PVC, tachycardia in cardiac patients
- Monitor for bowel sounds; check for constipation; abdominal distention and constipation may occur
- Monitor respiratory status: rate, rhythm, cyanosis, wheezing, dyspnea, engorged neck veins
- Monitor cardiac rate: rhythm, character, B/P continuously
- Monitor allergic reaction: rash, urticaria

### Nursing diagnoses
- Cardiac output, decreased (uses)
- Constipation (adverse reactions)
- Knowledge, deficient (teaching)

---

## Implementation
**PO route**
- PO 30 min before meals
- Give increased bulk, water in diet if constipation occurs (anticholinergic effect)

**IM route**
- Expect atropine flush 15-20 min after inj; it may occur in children and is not harmful

**IV route**
- Give **IV** undiluted or diluted with 10 ml sterile H₂O; give at a rate of 0.6 mg/min; give through Y-tube or 3-way stopcock; do not add to **IV** sol; may cause paradoxic bradycardia lasting 2 min

*Syringe compatibilities:* Benzquinamide, butorphanol, chlorproMAZINE, cimetidine, dimenhyDRINATE, diphenhydrAMINE, droperidol, fentanyl, glycopyrrolate, heparin, hydromorphone, hydrOXYzine, meperidine, metoclopramide, midazolam, milrinone, morphine, nalbuphine, pentazocine, perphenazine, prochlorperazine, promazine, promethazine, propiomazine, ranitidine, scopolamine, sufentanil, vit B with C

*Y-site compatibilities:* Amrinone, etomidate, famotidine, heparin, hydrocortisone sodium succinate, meropenem, nafcillin, potassium chloride, sufentanil, vit B/C

*Additive compatibilities:* DOBUTamine, furosemide, meropenem, netilmicin, sodium bicarbonate, verapamil

## Patient/family education
- Advise patient not to perform strenuous activity in high temperatures; heat stroke may result
- Instruct patient to take as prescribed; not to skip doses
- Instruct patient to report change in vision; blurring or loss of sight; trouble breathing; sweating; flushing, chest pain, allergic reactions, constipation, urinary retention
- Caution patient not to operate machinery if drowsiness occurs
- Advise patient not to take OTC products without approval of physician

## Evaluation
**Positive therapeutic outcome**
- Decreased dysrhythmias
- Increased heart rate
- Decreased secretions, GI, GU spasms
- Bronchodilatation

**Treatment of overdose:** O₂, artificial ventilation, ECG; administer DOPamine for circulatory depression; administer diazepam or thiopental for seizure; assess need for antidysrhythmics

## atropine ophthalmic
*See Appendix D*

### ! HIGH ALERT
### azacitidine (Rx)
(a-za-sie-ti′deen)
Vidaza
*Func. class.:* Antineoplastic hormone
*Chem. class.:* DNA demethylation agent

**Pregnancy category D**

**Action:** Cytotoxic by producing damage to double-strand DNA during DNA synthesis

**Therapeutic outcome:** Improved blood counts in refractor anemia

**Uses:** Myelodysplastic syndrome (MDS)

**Dosage and routes**
*Adult:* SUBCUT 75 mg/m² daily × 7 days, q4 wk, premedicate with antiemetic, dose may be increased to 100 mg/m² if no response is seen after 2 treatment cycles, minimum treatment 4 cycles

**Available forms:** Powdered for inj, lyophilized 100 mg

**Adverse effects**
*CNS:* Anxiety, depression, dizziness, fatigue, headache
*CV:* Cardiac murmur, hypotension, tachycardia
*GI:* Diarrhea, nausea, vomiting, anorexia, constipation, abdominal pain, distention, tenderness, hemorrhoids, mouth hemorrhage, tongue ulceration, stomatitis, dyspepsia, **hepatotoxicity, hepatic coma**
*GU:* **Real failure, renal tubular acidosis**, dysuria, UTI
*HEMA:* **Leukopenia, anemia, thrombocytopenia, neutropenia**, ecchymosis
*INTEG:* Irritation at site, rash, sweating, pyrexia
*META:* Hypokalemia

**Contraindications:** Pregnancy **D**, hypersensitivity to this product or mannitol, advanced malignant hepatic tumors

**Precautions:** Breastfeeding, children, geriatric, renal/hepatic disease; a man should not father a child while taking this product

| Pharmacokinetics | |
|---|---|
| **Absorption** | Rapid |
| **Distribution** | Unknown |
| **Metabolism** | Liver |
| **Excretion** | Urine |
| **Half-life** | 35-49 min |

| Pharmacodynamics | |
|---|---|
| **Onset** | Unknown |
| **Peak** | ½ hr |
| **Duration** | Unknown |

## NURSING CONSIDERATIONS
### Assessment
• Assess for CNS symptoms: fever, headache, chills, dizziness
• Monitor hematologic response with patients with baseline WBC = to $3 \times 10^9$/L, absolute neutrophil count (ANC) = $1.5 \times 10^9$/L, and platelets = $75 \times 10^9$/L, adjust dose; ANC < 0.5 $\times 10^9$/L, platelets < $25 \times 10^9$/L, give 50% dose next course; ANC $0.5 - 1.5 \times 10^9$/L, platelets $25 - 50 \times 10^9$/L, give 67% next course
• Assess buccal cavity q8hr for dryness, sores, or ulceration, white patches, oral pain, bleeding, dysphagia
• Assess for signs of bone marrow depression: bruising, bleeding, blood in stools, urine, sputum, emesis

### Nursing diagnoses
• Body image, disturbed (adverse reactions)
• Infection, risk for (adverse reactions)
• Injury, risk for (adverse reactions)
• Knowledge, deficient (teaching)

### Implementation
• Administer antiemetics and dexamethasone 10 mg at least ½ hr before antineoplastics
**IV route**
• Reconstitute with 4 ml sterile water for inj (25 mg/ml), inject dilutent slowly into vial, invert vial 2-3 times and gently rotate, sol will be cloudy, use immediately, divide doses greater than 4 ml into 2 syringes, resuspend the contents 2-3 times and gently roll syringe between the palms for 30 sec immediately prior to administration
• Rotate injection site
• Increase patient's fluid intake to 2-3 L/day to prevent dehydration, unless contraindicated
• Assist patient with rinsing of mouth tid-qid with water, club soda; brushing of teeth bid-tid with soft brush or cotton-tipped applicator for stomatitis; use unwaxed dental floss
• Provide a nutritious diet with iron, vitamin supplement, low fiber, few dairy products

### Patient/family education
• Instruct patient to avoid foods with citric acid or hot or rough texture if stomatitis is present; to drink adequate fluids
• Instruct patient to report stomatitis; any bleeding, white spots, ulcerations in mouth; tell patient to examine mouth daily, report symptoms
• Advise patient to use contraception during therapy
• Advise patient not to father a child while receiving this product

### Evaluation
**Positive therapeutic outcome**
• Improvement in blood counts in refractory anemia, or refractory anemia with excess blasts

---

## azathioprine (Rx)
(ay-za-thye′oh-preen)
Azusan, Imuran
*Func. class.:* Immunosuppressant
*Chem. class.:* Purine antagonist
**Pregnancy category** D

**Do not confuse:**
Imuran/Imferon/Elmiron/IMDUR/ Enduron/Tenormin

**Action:** Produces immunosuppression by inhibiting purine synthesis, DNA, RNA in cells

**Therapeutic outcome:** Absence of graft rejection, slowing of rheumatoid arthritis

**Uses:** Renal transplants to prevent graft rejection, often used with corticosteroids, cytotoxics; refractory rheumatoid arthritis, refractory ITP, glomerulonephritis, nephrotic syndrome, bone marrow transplant

**Unlabeled uses:** Myasthenia gravis, chronic ulcerative colitis, Crohn's disease, Behçet's syndrome

**Dosage and routes**
*Renal dose*
CCr 10-50 ml/min 75% of dose; CCr <10 ml/min 50% of dose

*Prevention of rejection*
*Adult and child:* **IV** 3-5 mg/kg/day, then maintenance (PO) of at least 1-2 mg/kg/day

*Refractory rheumatoid arthritis*
*Adult:* PO 1/mg/kg/day; may increase dosage after 2 mo by 0.5 mg/kg/day; not to exceed 2.5 mg/kg/day

**Available forms:** Tabs 50, 75, 100 mg; inj **IV** 100 mg

---

### Adverse effects
*GI:* Nausea, vomiting, stomatitis, esophagitis, **pancreatitis, hepatotoxicity, jaundice**
*HEMA:* **Leukopenia, thrombocytopenia, anemia, pancytopenia**
*INTEG:* Rash, alopeia
*MISC:* Raynaud's symptoms, **serum sickness**
*MS:* Arthralgia, muscle wasting

**Contraindications:** Pregnancy **D**, breast-feeding, hypersensitivity

**Precautions:** Severe renal/hepatic disease, geriatric

#### Pharmacokinetics

| | |
|---|---|
| **Absorption** | Readily (PO) |
| **Distribution** | Crosses placenta |
| **Metabolism** | Liver to mercaptopurine |
| **Excretion** | Kidney, minimal |
| **Half-life** | 3 hr |

#### Pharmacodynamics

| | PO | IV |
|---|---|---|
| **Onset** | Unknown | Unknown |
| **Peak** | 4 hr | Unknown |
| **Duration** | Unknown | Unknown |

### Interactions
*Individual drugs*
Do not admix with other products
Allopurinol: increased action of azathioprine
Cotrimoxazole: increased leukopenia
CycloSPORINE: increased myelosuppression
Warfarin: decreased action of warfarin
*Drug classifications*
ACE inhibitors: increased leukopenia
Antineoplastics: increased myelosuppression
Vaccines: decreased immune response
*Drug/herb*
Astragalus, echinacea, melatonin, safflower: increased immunosuppression
Ginseng, maitake, mistletoe, schisandra, St. John's wort, turmeric: decreased effect
*Drug/lab test*
Increased: liver function tests
Decreased: uric acid
Interference: CBC, diff count

### NURSING CONSIDERATIONS
#### Assessment
• Assess symptoms of rheumatoid arthritis: pain in joints, stiffness, poor range of motion, inflammation before and during treatment
• Monitor blood studies: Hgb, WBC, platelets during treatment monthly; if leukocytes are <3000/mm$^3$ or platelets <100,000/mm$^3$,

product should be discontinued or reduced; decreased Hgb level may indicate bone marrow suppression
• Monitor liver function studies: alkaline phosphatase, AST, ALT, amylase, bilirubin; and for hepatotoxicity: dark urine, jaundice, itching, light-colored stools; product should be discontinued
• Monitor I&O, weight daily, report decreasing urine output, toxicity may occur
• Assess for infection: increased temp, WBC; sputum, urine

#### Nursing diagnoses
• Infection, risk for (uses)
• Knowledge, deficient (teaching)
• Mobility, impaired physical (uses)

#### Implementation
**PO route**
• Give all medications PO if possible, avoiding IM inj, since bleeding may occur
• Give with meals to reduce GI upset; nausea is common
• For several days before transplant surgery, patients should be placed in protective isolation
**IV route**
• Prepare in biologic cabinet using gown, gloves, mask; give after diluting 100 mg/10 ml of sterile water for inj; rotate to dissolve; may further dilute with 50 ml or more saline or glucose in saline given over >30 min (intermittent inf)

**Solution compatibilities:** D$_5$W, NaCl 0.9%, NaCl 0.45%

#### Patient/family education
• Teach patient to take as prescribed, do not miss doses; if dose is missed on daily regimen, skip dose; if on multiple dosing/day, take as soon as remembered
• Teach patient that therapeutic response may take 3-4 mo in rheumatoid arthritis, to continue with prescribed exercise, rest, other medications; that product is needed for life in renal transplant
• Instruct patient to report fever, rash, severe diarrhea, chills, sore throat, fatigue, since serious infections may occur; or clay-colored stools and cramping (hepatotoxicity)
• Advise patient to use contraceptive measures during treatment for 12 wk after ending therapy; product is teratogenic
• Advise patient to avoid vaccinations
• Tell patient to avoid crowds and persons with known infections to reduce risk of infection
• Instruct patient not to use OTC medications without approval of prescriber

Adverse effects: *italic* = common, **bold** = life-threatening

• Advise patient to use soft-bristled toothbrush to prevent bleeding

## Evaluation
**Positive therapeutic outcome**
• Absence of graft rejection
• Immunosuppression in autoimmune disorders
• Increased joint mobility without pain in rheumatoid arthritis

---

## azelaic acid topical
*See Appendix D*

---

## azelastine (Rx)
(ay′ze-lass-teen)
Optivar
*Func. class.:* Leukotriene synthesis inhibitor
*Chem. class.:* Phthalazinone derivative

**Pregnancy category** C

**Action:** Inhibits the synthesis and release of leukotrienes; antagonizes action of acetylcholine, histamine, serotonin

**Therapeutic outcome:** Decreased nasal stuffiness, itching, swollen eyes

**Uses:** Seasonal allergic rhinitis

**Dosage and routes**
*Adult and child ≥12 yr:* NASAL 2 sprays/nostril bid

**Available forms:** Spray 137 mcg/actuation

**Adverse effects**
*CNS:* Sedation (more common with increased dosages), drowsiness
*MISC:* Weight increase, myalgia

**Contraindications:** Hypersensitivity

**Precautions:** Pregnancy C

| Pharmacokinetics | |
|---|---|
| Absorption | Unknown |
| Distribution | Unknown |
| Metabolism | Liver, extensively |
| Excretion | Feces |
| Half-life | 25-42 hr |

| Pharmacodynamics | |
|---|---|
| Onset | Unknown |
| Peak | 4-5 hr |
| Duration | Unknown |

## Interactions
*Individual drugs*
Alcohol: increased CNS depression
*Drug classifications*
CNS depressants, opioids, sedative/hypnotics: increased CNS depression

## NURSING CONSIDERATIONS
**Assessment**
• Assess respiratory status: rate, rhythm, increase in bronchial secretions, wheezing, chest tightness; provide fluids to 2 L/day to decrease secretion thickness

**Nursing diagnoses**
• Airway clearance, ineffective (uses)
• Knowledge, deficient (teaching)
• Noncompliance (teaching, overuse)

**Implementation**
• Remove cap/safety clip from spray pump
• Prime pump if using for first time, push 4 times quickly, away from face, blow your nose, then place tip of pump into one nostril, while holding other nostril closed, tilt head forward, and spray into nostril
• Put cover/safety clip back on

**Patient/family education**
• Teach patient all aspects of product uses; to notify prescriber if confusion, sedation occur; to avoid driving and other hazardous activity if drowsiness occurs; to avoid alcohol and other CNS depressants that may potentiate effect
• Caution patient not to exceed recommended dosage; dysrhythmias may occur

**Evaluation**
**Positive therapeutic outcome**
• Absence of runny or congested nose

---

## azelastine nasal agent
*See Appendix D*

---

## azelastine ophthalmic
*See Appendix D*

---

## azithromycin (Rx)
(ay-zi-thro-my'sin)
Zithromax, Zmax
*Func. class.:* Antiinfective
*Chem. class.:* Macrolide (azalide)

**Pregnancy category** B

**Do not confuse:**
azithromycin/erythromycin, Zithromax/Zinacef

**Action:** Binds to 50S ribosomal subunits of susceptible bacteria and suppresses protein synthesis; much greater spectrum of activity than erythromycin; more effective against gram-negative organisms

**Therapeutic outcome:** Bacteriostatic against the following susceptible organisms: *Moraxella catarrhalis, Streptococcus pneumoniae, Streptococcus pyogenes, Staphylococcus aureus, Haemophilus influenzae, Clostridium, Legionella pneumophila, Chlamydia trachomatis, Mycoplasma;* no effect on methicillin-resistant *S. aureus;* in children: acute otitis media *(H. influenzae, M. catarrhalis, S. pneumoniae)* PO, acute pharyngitis/tonsillitis (group A streptococcal) PO; acute skin/soft tissue infections (PO); community-acquired pneumonia *(C. pneumoniae, H. influenzae, M. pneumoniae, S. pneumoniae)* PO; pharyngitis/tonsillitis *(S. pyogenes)*

**Uses:** Mild to moderate infections of the upper respiratory tract, lower respiratory tract; uncomplicated skin and skin structure infections, nongonococcal urethritis, or cervicitis; prophylaxis of disseminated *Mycobacterium avium* complex (MAC)

### Dosage and routes
*Most infections*
*Adult:* PO 500 mg on day 1, then 250 mg daily on days 2-5 for a total dose of 1.5 g
*Child 2-15 yr:* PO 10 mg/kg on day 1, then 5 mg/kg × 4 days

*Pelvic inflammatory disease*
*Adult:* PO/**IV** 500 mg **IV** q24hr × 2 doses, then 500 mg PO q24hr × 7-10 days

*Cervicitis/chlamydia/chancroid/nongonococcal urethritis/syphilis*
*Adult:* PO 1 g single dose

*Gonorrhea*
*Adult:* PO 2 g single dose

*Endocarditis, prophylaxis*
*Adult:* PO 500 mg 1 hr prior to procedure
*Child:* PO 15 mg/kg 1 hr prior to procedure

*Community-acquired pneumonia*
*Adult:* PO/**IV** 500 mg **IV** q24hr × 2 doses, then 500 mg PO q24hr × 7-10 days

*Disseminated MAC infections*
*Adult:* PO 600 mg/day in combination with ethambutol

*Lower respiratory tract infections, acute skin/soft tissue infections, acute pharyngitis/tonsillitis*
*Child:* PO 3-day regimen, 10 mg/kg daily × 3 days

*Acute otitis media*
*Child:* PO 30 mg/kg as a single dose or 10 mg/kg daily × 3 days or 10 mg/kg as a single dose on day 1, max 500 mg/day, then 5 mg/kg on days 2-5, max 250 mg/day

*Prevention of acute otitis media*
*Child:* PO 10 mg/kg qwk × 6 mo

**Available forms:** Tabs 250, 500, 600 mg; powder for inj 500 mg; powder for oral susp 1 g/packet; susp 100, 200 mg/5 ml

### Adverse effects
*CNS:* Dizziness, headache, vertigo, somnolence
*CV:* Palpitations, chest pain
*EENT:* Hearing loss, tinnitus
*GI: Nausea, vomiting, diarrhea,* **hepatotoxicity,** abdominal pain, stomatitis, heartburn, dyspepsia, flatulence, melena, **cholestatic jaundice, pseudomembranous colitis,** tongue discoloration
*GU:* Vaginitis, moniliasis, nephritis
*HEMA:* Anemia
*INTEG:* Rash, urticaria, pruritus, photosensitivity
*SYST:* **Angioedema**

**Contraindications:** Hypersensitivity to azithromycin, erythromycin, or any macrolide

**Precautions:** Pregnancy **B,** breastfeeding, child <6 mo for otitis media, child <2 yr for pharyngitis, geriatric, renal/hepatic/cardiac disease, tonsillitis

| Pharmacokinetics | |
|---|---|
| Absorption | Rapid, (PO) up to 50% |
| Distribution | Widely distributed |
| Metabolism | Unknown, minimal metabolism |
| Excretion | Unchanged (bile); kidneys, minimal |
| Half-life | 11-70 hr |

| Pharmacodynamics | | |
|---|---|---|
| | PO | IV |
| **Onset** | Unknown | Unknown |
| **Peak** | 2-4 hr | End of infusion |
| **Duration** | 24 hr | 24 hr |

## Interactions
### Individual drugs
Bromocriptine, carbamazepine, cycloSPOR-INE, digoxin, disopyramide, methylPRED-NISolone, phenytoin, theophylline, triazolam: increased effects of specific products
Ergotamine: toxicity
◆Pimozide: dysrhythmias; fatal reaction
Triazolam: decreased clearance of triazolam
### Drug classifications
Aluminum, magnesium antacids: decreased levels of azithromycin
Anticoagulants (orals): increased effect of oral anticoagulants
### Drug/herb
Acidophilus: do not use with antiinfectives; separate by several hours
### Drug/lab test
Increased: bilirubin, alkaline phosphatase, CPK, BUN, creatinine, AST, ALT

## NURSING CONSIDERATIONS
### Assessment
• Assess for signs and symptoms of infection: drainage, fever, increased WBC >10,000/mm³, urine culture positive, sore throat, sputum culture positive
• Monitor respiratory status: rate, character, wheezing, tightness in chest; discontinue product if these occur
• Monitor allergies before treatment, reaction of each medication; place allergies on chart, notify all people giving products; skin eruptions, itching
• Monitor I&O ratio, renal studies; report hematuria, oliguria in renal disease; check urinalysis, protein, blood
• Monitor liver studies: AST, ALT, bilirubin, LDH, alkaline phosphatase; CBC with differential
• Monitor C&S before product therapy; product may be taken as soon as culture is taken; C&S may be repeated after treatment
• Monitor bowel pattern before, during treatment
• Assess for superinfection: sore throat, mouth, tongue; fever, fatigue, diarrhea, anogenital pruritus

## Nursing diagnoses
• Diarrhea (adverse reactions)
• Infection, risk for (uses)
• Knowledge, deficient (teaching)

## Implementation
### PO route
• Provide adequate intake of fluids (2 L) during diarrhea episodes
• Give with a full glass of water; give susp 1 hr before or 2 hr after meals; tabs may be taken without regard to food; do not give with fruit juices
• Store at room temperature
• Reconstitute 1 g packet for susp with 60 ml water, mix, rinse glass with more water and have patient drink to consume all medication; packets not for pediatric use
• Do not take aluminum/magnesium-containing antacids or food simultaneously with this product
### IV route
• Reconstitute 500 mg product/4.8 ml sterile water for inj (100 mg/ml), shake, dilute with ≥250 ml 0.9% NaCl, 0.45% NaCl, or LR to 1-2 mg/ml; diluted solution is stable for 24 hr or 7 days if refrigerated
• Give 500 mg or more/1 hr, never give IM or as a bol

## Patient/family education
• Instruct patient to report sore throat, black furry tongue, fever, loose foul-smelling stool, vaginal itching, discharge, fatigue; may indicate superinfection
• Caution patient not to take aluminum/magnesium-containing antacids or food simultaneously with this product; blood levels of azithromycin will be decreased
• Instruct patient to notify prescriber of diarrhea stools, dark urine, pale stools, yellow discoloration of eyes or skin, severe abdominal pain; cholestatic jaundice is a severe adverse reaction
• Teach patient complete dosage regimen; to notify prescriber if symptoms continue
• Teach patient to notify prescriber if pregnancy is suspected
• Inform patient that sunburns may occur; wear protective clothing and sunscreen

## Evaluation
### Positive therapeutic outcome
• C&S negative for infection
• WBC within 5000-10,000/mm³

## azithromycin ophthalmic
*See Appendix D*

 Alert      Canada Only      Drug on CD     * "Tall Man" lettering (See Preface)

## bacitracin topical
*See Appendix D*

---

## baclofen (Rx)
(bak'loe-fen)
Lioresal, Lioresal Intrathecal
*Func. class.:* Skeletal muscle relaxant, central acting
*Chem. class.:* GABA, chlorophenyl derivative
**Pregnancy category C**

**Do not confuse:**
Lioresal/Lotensin

**Action:** Inhibits synaptic responses in CNS by stimulating GABAb receptor subtype, which decreases neurotransmitter function; decreasing frequency, severity of muscle spasms

**Therapeutic outcome:** Decreased spasticity of muscles

**Uses:** Spasticity in spinal cord injury, multiple sclerosis

**Dosage and routes**
*Adult:* PO 5 mg tid × 3 days, then 10 mg tid × 3 days, then 15 mg tid × 3 days, then 20 mg tid × 3 days, then titrated to response, not to exceed 80 mg/day; IT use implantable intrathecal INF pump; use screening trial of 3 separate BOL doses if needed 24 hr apart (50 mcg/ml, 75 mcg/1.5 ml, 100 mcg/2 ml); patients who do not respond to 100 mcg should not be considered for chronic IT therapy; initial double screening dose that produced result and give over 24 hr, increase by 10%-30% q24hr only; maintenance 1200-1500 mcg/day
*Child >2 yr:* PO 10-15 mg/day divided q8hr; titrate every 3 days by 5-15 mg/day to max 40 mg/day
*Child ≥8 yr:* As above, max 60 mg/day
*Child:* IT Initial test dose same as adult; for small children, initial dose of 25 mcg/dose may be used; 25-1200 mcg/day infusion, titrated to response in screening phase
*Geriatric:* PO 5 mg bid-tid

**Available forms:** Tabs 10, 20 mg; intrathecal inj 10 mg/20 ml (500 mcg/ml), 10 mg/5 ml (2000 mcg/ml); pharmacy can prepare extemporaneous liquid preparations

**Adverse effects**
*CNS: Dizziness, weakness, fatigue, drowsiness,* headache, disorientation, insomnia, paresthesias, tremors, **seizures, coma; life-threatening CNS depression, CNS infection (IT)**
*CV:* Hypotension, chest pain, palpitations, edema; **cardiovascular collapse (IT)**
*EENT:* Nasal congestion, blurred vision, mydriasis, tinnitus
*GI: Nausea,* constipation, vomiting, increased AST, alkaline phosphatase, abdominal pain, dry mouth, anorexia
*GU:* Urinary frequency, hematuria
*INTEG:* Rash, pruritus
*RESP:* Dyspnea, respiratory failure (IT)

**Contraindications:** Hypersensitivity

**Precautions:** Pregnancy C, breastfeeding, geriatric, peptic ulcer, renal/hepatic disease, stroke, seizure disorder, diabetes mellitus

| Pharmacokinetics | |
|---|---|
| Absorption | Well (PO) |
| Distribution | Widely, crosses placenta |
| Metabolism | Liver, partially |
| Excretion | Kidney, unchanged 70%-80% |
| Half-life | 2½-4 hr |

| Pharmacodynamics | |
|---|---|
| | PO/IT |
| Onset | 0.5-1 hr |
| Peak | 4 hr |
| Duration | 4-8 hr |

**Interactions**
*Individual drugs*
Alcohol: CNS depression
*Drug classifications*
Antidepressants (tricyclics), antihistamines, barbiturates, MAOIs, opioids, sedative/hypnotics: increased CNS depression
Antihypertensives: increased hypotension
*Drug/herb*
Chamomile, hops, kava, skullcap, valerian: increased CNS depression
*Drug/lab test*
Increased: AST, ALT, alkaline phosphatase, blood glucose

**NURSING CONSIDERATIONS**
**Assessment**
• Monitor B/P, weight, blood glucose, and hepatic function periodically
• Check for increased seizure activity in patients with epilepsy; this product decreases seizure threshold, monitor ECG
• Check I&O ratio; check for urinary retention, frequency, hesitancy

Adverse effects: *italic* = common, **bold** = life-threatening

• Allergic reactions: rash, fever, respiratory distress; severe weakness, numbness in extremities
• Assess CNS depression: dizziness, drowsiness, psychiatric symptoms
• Check dosage, as individual titration is required

## Nursing diagnoses
• Injury, risk for (adverse reactions)
• Knowledge, deficient (teaching)
• Mobility, impaired physical (uses)

## Implementation
**PO route**
• Give with meals for GI symptoms; gum, frequent sips of water for dry mouth
• Store in airtight container at room temperature
**IT route**
• Titration is based on response
• Test dose: Dilute to a concentration of 50 mcg/ml, give over 1 min or more
• Observe for decrease in muscle spasticity
• If response is not adequate, give 2 additional test doses (75 mcg/1.5 ml and 100 mcg/2 ml), maintenance infusion via implantable pump 500-2000 mcg/ml

## Patient/family education
• Give test doses 24 hr apart
• Advise patient not to discontinue medication quickly; hallucinations, spasticity, tachycardia will occur; product should be tapered off over 1-2 wk
**IT route**
• Advise patient not to take with alcohol, other CNS depressants
• Caution patient to avoid altering activities while taking this product; to avoid hazardous activities if drowsiness or dizziness occur
• Advise patient to avoid using OTC medication (cough preparations, antihistamines) unless directed by prescriber

## Evaluation
**Positive therapeutic outcome**
• Decreased pain, spasticity

**Treatment of overdose:** Induce emesis of conscious patient, activated charcoal, dialysis, physostigmine to reduce life-threatening CNS side effects

# balsalazide (Rx)
(ball-sal′a-zide)
Colazal
*Func. class.:* GI antiinflammatory
*Chem. class.:* Salicylate derivative

**Pregnancy category B**

**Do not confuse:**
Colazal/Clozaril

**Action:** Delivered intact to the colon, bioconverted to 5-ASA

**Therapeutic outcome:** Decreased inflammation in colon

**Uses:** Active, mild to moderate ulcerative colitis (adult and child)

**Dosage and routes**
*Adult:* PO 2250 mg, (three 750 mg cap) tid × 8-12 wk
*Adolescent and child 5-12 yr:* PO 2250 mg, (three 750 mg cap) tid × 8 wk

**Available forms:** Tabs 750 mg

**Adverse effects**
*CNS:* Headache, insomnia, fatigue, fever, dizziness
*EENT:* Dry mouth, dry eyes, rhinitis, sinusitis, watery eyes, blurred vision
*GI:* Nausea, vomiting, abdominal pain, diarrhea, rectal bleeding, flatulence, dyspepsia, dry mouth, constipation
*MS:* Arthralgia, back pain, myalgia
*SYST:* Anaphylaxis

**Contraindications:** Hypersensitivity to salicylates

**Precautions:** Pregnancy **B,** breastfeeding, child <14 yr, pyloric stenosis

### Pharmacokinetics
| | |
|---|---|
| **Absorption** | Low, variable |
| **Distribution** | Plasma protein binding 99% |
| **Metabolism** | Unknown |
| **Excretion** | Kidneys, as metabolites |
| **Half-life** | Unknown |

### Pharmacodynamics
Unknown

## Interactions
*Individual drugs*
Mercaptopurine, thioguanine: increased myelosuppression
Azathioprine, warfarin: increased effect

*Drug/lab test*
Increased: AST, ALT, GGT, LDH, bilirubin, alkaline phosphatase
False positive: urinary glucose test

## NURSING CONSIDERATIONS
### Assessment
• Monitor kidney function studies: BUN, creatinine, urinalysis (long-term therapy)
• Assess for allergic reaction: rash, dermatitis, urticaria, pruritus, dyspnea, bronchospasm

### Nursing diagnoses
• Injury, risk for (uses)
• Knowledge, deficient (teaching)

### Implementation
• Give with food in evenly divided doses; swallow tab whole or open cap, sprinkle on applesauce
• Use with resuscitative equipment available; severe allergic reactions may occur
• Give total daily dose evenly spaced to minimize GI intolerance
• Store in tight, light-resistant container at room temperature

### Patient/family education
• Advise patient to notify prescriber if symptoms do not improve, if rash, hives, or respiratory problems occur

### Evaluation
**Positive therapeutic outcome**
• Absence of fever, mucus in stools; resolution of symptoms of ulcerative colitis

---

! HIGH ALERT

## basiliximab (Rx)
(bas-ih-liks′ih-mab)
Simulect
*Func. class.:* Immunosuppressant
*Chem. class.:* Murine/human monoclonal antibody (interleukin-2) receptor antagonist
**Pregnancy category B**

**Action:** Binds to and blocks the IL-2 receptor, which is selectively expressed on the surface of activated T-lymphocytes; impairs the immune system to antigenic challenges

**Therapeutic outcome:** Prevention of graft rejection

**Uses:** Acute allograft rejection in renal transplant patients when used with cycloSPORINE and corticosteroids

### Dosage and routes
*Adult:* **IV** 20 mg × 2 doses; first dose within 2 hr before transplant surgery; second dose given 4 days after transplantation
*Child 2-15 yr:* **IV** 12 mg/m$^2$ × 2 doses; first dose within 2 hr before transplant surgery; second dose given 4 days after transplantation

**Available forms:** Powder for inj 10, 20 mg

### Adverse effects
*CNS: Pyrexia, chills, tremors, headache, insomnia, weakness*
*CV: Chest pain,* angina, **cardiac failure,** hypo/hypertension, edema
*GI: Vomiting, nausea, diarrhea,* constipation, abdominal pain, GI bleeding, gingival hyperplasia, stomatitis
*INTEG: Acne,* pruritus
*META:* Acidosis, hypercholesterolemia, hyperuricemia, hypo/hyperkalemia, hypocalcemia, hypophosphatemia
*MISC:* Infection, moniliasis, **anaphylaxis**
*MS:* Arthralgia, myalgia
*RESP: Dyspnea, wheezing, cough,* **pulmonary edema**

**Contraindications:** Hypersensitivity, exposure to viral infections, breastfeeding

**Precautions:** Pregnancy **B,** children, geriatric, infections

| Pharmacokinetics | |
| --- | --- |
| **Absorption** | Unknown |
| **Distribution** | Unknown |
| **Metabolism** | Unknown |
| **Excretion** | Unknown |
| **Half-life** | 7 days (adult) |
| | 9½ days (child) |

| Pharmacodynamics | |
| --- | --- |
| **Onset** | Unknown |
| **Peak** | ½ hr (adults) |
| **Duration** | Unknown |

### Interactions
*Drug classifications*
Immunosuppressants: increased immunosuppression
*Drug/herb*
Astragalus, echinacea, melatonin, safflower: increased immunosuppression
Ginseng, maitake, mistletoe, schisandra, St. John's wort, turmeric: decreased effect

---

Adverse effects: *italic* = common, **bold** = life-threatening

*Drug/lab test*
Increased: BUN, cholesterol, uric acid, creatinine, potassium, calcium, blood glucose, Hgb, Hct
Decreased: Hgb, Hct, platelets, magnesium, phosphate

## NURSING CONSIDERATIONS
### Assessment
• Assess for infection, increased temp, WBC, sputum, urine
• Monitor blood studies: Hgb, WBC, platelets during treatment qmo; if leukocytes are <3000/mm³, product should be discontinued
• Monitor liver function studies: alkaline phosphatase, AST, ALT, bilirubin
• Assess hepatotoxicity: dark urine, jaundice, itching, light-colored stools; product should be discontinued
◆ Assess for anaphylaxis, hypersensitivity: dyspnea, wheezing, rash, pruritus, hypotension, tachycardia; if severe hypersensitivity reactions occur, product should not be used again

### Nursing diagnoses
• Infection, risk for (adverse reactions)
• Knowledge, deficient (teaching)

### Implementation
• Administer all medications PO if possible; avoid IM inj, since infection may occur
**IV route**
• After adding 5 ml sterile water for inj, shake gently to dissolve, reconstitute to a vol of 50 ml with 0.9% NaCl or D₅, gently invert bag, do not shake, do not admix

### Patient/family education
• Instruct patient to report fever, chills, sore throat, fatigue, since serious infection may occur; avoid crowds, persons with known upper respiratory infections; use contraception during treatment

### Evaluation
**Positive therapeutic outcome**
• Absence of graft rejection

---

## beclomethasone (Rx)
(be-kloe-meth′a-sone)
Beclodisk ✤, Beclovent, QVAR
*Func. class.:* Synthetic glucocorticoid (long acting)
*Chem. class.:* Beclomethasone diester
**Pregnancy category C**

**Action:** Antiinflammatory; vasoconstrictive properties; also immunosuppressive

**Therapeutic outcome:** Decreased inflammation and normal immunity

**Uses:** Seasonal, perennial allergic rhinitis, nasal polyps, chronic steroid-dependent asthma

### Dosage and routes
*Adult and child >12 yr:* INH 48-80 mcg bid (alone) or 40-160 mcg bid (with inhaled corticosteroids), max 320 bid
*Child 5-12 yr:* INH 40 mcg bid, max 80 mcg bid

**Available forms:** Oral inh 40, 80, 250✤ mcg/metered spray; inh cap 100✤, 200✤ mcg

### Adverse effects
*CNS: Headache,*
*EENT: Candidal infection of oral cavity, hoarseness,* sore throat
*GI:* Dry mouth, dyspepsia
*MISC:* **Angioedema adrenal insufficiency,** facial edema, Churg-Strauss syndrome
*RESP:* **Bronchospasm,** wheezing, cough

**Contraindications:** Hypersensitivity, status asthmaticus (primary treatment), nonasthmatic bronchial disease, bacterial, fungal, viral infections of mouth, throat, lungs

**Precautions:** Pregnancy **C**, breastfeeding, child <12, nasal disease/surgery

| Pharmacokinetics | |
|---|---|
| **Absorption** | Locally only |
| **Distribution** | Not distributed |
| **Metabolism** | Lungs, liver (by CYP3A) |
| **Excretion** | Feces, urine |
| **Half-life** | 2.8 hr |

| Pharmacodynamics | | |
|---|---|---|
| | INH | NASAL |
| **Onset** | 1-4 wk | 10 min |
| **Peak** | Unknown | Unknown |
| **Duration** | Unknown | Unknown |

## NURSING CONSIDERATIONS
### Assessment
• Assess adrenal suppression: 17-KS, plasma cortisol for decreased levels, adrenal function periodically for HPA axis suppression during prolonged therapy; monitor growth and development
• Assess blood studies, neutrophils, decreased platelets; WBC with diff baseline and q3 mo; if neutrophils <1000/mm³, discontinue treatment
• Check nasal passages during long-term treatment for changes in mucus; check for

---

burning, stinging; assess for glucocorticoid withdrawal: dizziness, hypotension, fatigue, muscle/joint pain; notify prescriber immediately
• Assess respiratory status: rest, rhythm, characteristics; auscultate lung bilaterally before and throughout treatment
• Assess for fungal infections in mucous membranes

## Nursing diagnoses
• Airway clearance, ineffective (uses)
• Knowledge, deficient (teaching)
• Noncompliance (teaching)
• Oral mucous membrane, impaired (adverse reactions)

## Implementation
• Give PO, using a spacer device for proper dose
• Use after cleaning aerosol top daily with warm water; dry thoroughly
• Store in cool environment; do not puncture or incinerate container
**Inhalation route**
• Shake inhaler, invert, tilt head backward, insert nozzle into nostril, away from septum; hold other nostril closed and depress activator, inhale through nose, exhale through mouth
• Shake oral aerosol well, use spacer

## Patient/family education
• Teach patient to gargle/rinse mouth after each use to prevent oral fungal infections
• Teach patient that in times of stress, systemic corticosteroids may be needed to prevent adrenal insufficiency; do not discontinue oral product abruptly, taper slowly
• Teach patient to continue using product even if mild nasal bleeding occurs; is usually transient
• Teach patient method of administration after providing written instructions from manufacturer
• Clean inhaler by wiping with dry cloth

## Evaluate
**Positive therapeutic outcome**
• Decrease in runny nose, improved symptoms of bronchial asthma

## beclomethasone nasal agent
*See Appendix D*

## benazepril (Rx)
(ben-a′za-pril)
*Func. class.:* Antihypertensive
*Chem. class.:* ACE inhibitor
**Pregnancy category D**

**Action:** Selectively suppresses renin-angiotensin-aldosterone system; inhibits ACE, preventing conversion of angiotensin I to angiotensin II

**Therapeutic outcome:** Decreased B/P in hypertension

**Uses:** Hypertension, alone or in combination with thiazide diuretics

**Unlabeled uses:** CHF

**Dosage and routes**
*Adult:* PO 10 mg daily initially, then 20-40 mg/day divided bid or daily (without a diuretic); 5 mg PO daily (with a diuretic); max 80 mg daily

*Renal dose*
*Adult:* PO 5 mg daily with CCr <30 ml/min; increase as needed to maximum of 40 mg/day
*Geriatric:* PO 5-10 mg/day initially

**Available forms:** Tabs 5, 10, 20, 40 mg

**Adverse effects**
*CNS:* Anxiety, hypertonia, insomnia, paresthesia, headache, dizziness, fatigue
*CV:* Hypotension, postural hypotension, syncope, palpitations, angina
*GI:* Nausea, constipation, vomiting, gastritis, diarrhea
*GU:* Increased BUN, creatinine, decreased libido, impotence, urinary tract infection
*INTEG:* Rash, flushing, sweating
*META:* Hyperkalemia, hyponatremia
*MISC:* **Angioedema**
*MS:* Arthralgia, arthritis, myalgia
*RESP:* Cough, asthma, bronchitis, dyspnea, sinusitis

**Contraindications:** Pregnancy **D,** breastfeeding, children, hypersensitivity to ACE inhibitors

**Precautions:** Impaired renal/liver function, dialysis patients, hypovolemia, blood dyscrasias, CHF, COPD, asthma, geriatric, bilateral renal artery stenosis

## Pharmacokinetics

| | |
|---|---|
| **Absorption** | <40% |
| **Distribution** | Unknown; crosses placenta |
| **Metabolism** | Liver metabolites; protein binding 97% |
| **Excretion** | Kidney, breast milk (minimal) |
| **Half-life** | 10-11 hr (metabolite); increased in renal disease |

## Pharmacodynamics

| | |
|---|---|
| **Onset** | Unknown |
| **Peak** | ½-1 hr |
| **Duration** | Unknown |

## Interactions
### Individual drugs
Alcohol: increased hypotension (large amounts)
Azathioprine: increased myelosuppression
Digoxin, lithium: increased serum levels
### Drug classifications
Antihypertensives, diuretics, nitrates, phenothiazines: increased hypotension
Diuretics (potassium-sparing), potassium supplements: increased hyperkalemia
NSAIDs: decreased hypotensive effects
### Drug/herb
Aconite: increased toxicity, death
Astragalus, cola tree: increased or decreased antihypertensive effect
Barberry, betony, black catechu, black cohosh, bloodroot, broom, burdock, cat's claw, dandelion, goldenseal, Irish moss, Jamaican dogwood, kelp, khella, mistletoe, parsley: increased antihypertensive effect
Coltsfoot, guarana, khat, licorice, pineapple, yohimbe: decreased antihypertensive effect
### Drug/lab test
Increased: AST, ALT, alkaline phosphatase, bilirubin, uric acid, blood glucose
False positive: ANA titer
Positive: ANA titer

## NURSING CONSIDERATIONS
### Assessment
• Monitor blood studies: neutrophils, decreased platelets
• Monitor B/P at peak/trough level of product, check for orthostatic hypotension, syncope; if changes occur, dosage change may be required
• Monitor renal studies: protein, BUN, creatinine; watch for increased levels that may indicate nephrotic syndrome and renal failure; monitor urine for protein; monitor renal symptoms: polyuria, oliguria, frequency, dysuria

• Establish baselines in renal, liver function tests before therapy begins
• Check potassium levels throughout treatment, although hyperkalemia rarely occurs
• Assess for allergic reactions: rash, fever, pruritus, urticaria; product should be discontinued if antihistamines fail to help

### Nursing diagnoses
• Cardiac output, decreased (uses)
• Injury, risk for (side effects)
• Knowledge, deficient (teaching)
• Noncompliance (teaching)

### Implementation
• Store in air-tight container at 86° F (30° C) or less
• Severe hypotension may occur after 1st dose of this medication; decreased hypotension may be prevented by reducing or discontinuing diuretic therapy 3 days before beginning benazepril therapy

### Patient/family education
• Instruct patient not to discontinue product abruptly; advise patient to tell all persons associated with care
• Teach patient not to use OTC products (cough, cold, allergy) unless directed by prescriber; serious side effects can occur; xanthines such as coffee, tea, chocolate, cola can prevent action of product
• Emphasize the importance of complying with dosage schedule, even if feeling better; to continue with medical regimen to decrease B/P: exercise, cessation of smoking, decreasing stress, diet modifications
• Emphasize the need to rise slowly to sitting or standing position to minimize orthostatic hypotension; not to exercise in hot weather because increased hypotension can occur
• Teach patient to notify prescriber of mouth sores, sore throat, fever, swelling of hands or feet, irregular heartbeat, chest pain, coughing, shortness of breath
• Caution patient to report excessive perspiration, dehydration, vomiting, diarrhea; may lead to fall in B/P
• Caution patient that product may cause dizziness, fainting, light-headedness; may occur during first few days of therapy; to avoid activities that may be hazardous
• Teach patient how to take B/P; teach normal readings for age-group; ensure patient takes own B/P
• Advise patient to notify prescriber of pregnancy, product will need to be discontinued

### Evaluation
**Positive therapeutic outcome**
• Decreased B/P in hypertension
Treatment of overdose: 0.9% NaCl
**IV** inf, hemodialysis

---

## benzocaine topical
*See Appendix D*

---

## benztropine  (Rx)
(benz'troe-peen)
Apo-Benztropin ✦, benztropine mesylate
*Func. class.:* Cholinergic blocker, antiparkinson agent
*Chem. class.:* Tertiary amine

**Pregnancy category** C

Action: Blockade of central acetylcholine receptors in the CNS, neurotransmitters are balanced

Therapeutic outcome: Decreased involuntary movements

Uses: Parkinsonian symptoms, EPS associated with neuroleptic products, acute dystonia, hypersalivation

### Dosage and routes
*Drug-induced extrapyramidal symptoms*
*Adult:* IM/**IV** 1-4 mg daily/bid; give PO dose as soon as possible; PO 1-2 mg bid/tid; increase by 0.5 mg q5-6 days
*Child:* IM/**IV** 0.02-0.05 mg/kg/dose 1-2 × 1 day
*Geriatric:* PO 0.5 mg daily/bid, increase by 0.5 mg q5-6 days

*Parkinsonian symptoms*
*Adult:* PO 1-2 mg daily, in 1-2 divided doses; increased 0.5 mg q5-6 days titrated to patient response; max 6 mg daily

*Acute dystonic reactions*
*Adult:* IM/**IV** 1-2 mg, may increase to 1-2 mg bid (PO)

Available forms: Tabs 0.5, 1, 2 mg; inj IM, **IV** 1 mg/ml

### Adverse effects
*CNS:* Confusion, anxiety, restlessness, irritability, delusions, hallucinations, headache, sedation, depression, incoherence, dizziness, memory loss; delirium (geriatric)
*CV:* Palpitations, tachycardia, hypotension, bradycardia
*EENT:* Blurred vision, photophobia, dilated pupils, difficulty swallowing, dry eyes, mydriasis, increased intraocular tension, angle-closure glaucoma
*GI:* *Dryness of mouth, constipation,* nausea, vomiting, abdominal distress, **paralytic ileus,** epigastric distress
*GU:* Hesitancy, retention, dysuria
*INTEG:* Rash, urticaria, dermatoses
*MISC:* Increased temperature, flushing, decreased sweating, **hyperthermia, heat stroke,** numbness of fingers
*MS:* Muscular weakness, cramping

Contraindications: Hypersensitivity, angle-closure glaucoma, myasthenia gravis, GI/GU obstruction, child <3 yr, peptic ulcer, megacolon, prostate hypertrophy

Precautions: Pregnancy **C**, breastfeeding, children, geriatric, tachycardia, renal/hepatic disease, product abuse history, dysrhythmias, hypo/hypertension, psychiatric patients

### Pharmacokinetics
| | |
|---|---|
| **Absorption** | Well (PO, IM), completely (**IV**) absorbed |
| **Distribution** | Unknown |
| **Metabolism** | Unknown |
| **Excretion** | Unknown |
| **Half-life** | Unknown |

### Pharmacodynamics
| | IM/IV | PO |
|---|---|---|
| **Onset** | 15 min | 1 hr |
| **Peak** | Unknown | Unknown |
| **Duration** | 6-10 hr | 6-10 hr |

### Interactions
*Individual drugs*
Disopyramide, quinidine: increased anticholinergic effects
*Drug classifications*
Antidepressants (tricyclic), antihistamines, phenothiazines: increased anticholinergic effects
Antidiarrheals: decreased absorption
*Drug/herb*
Butterbur, jimsonweed: increased benztropine effect
Black catechu: increased constipation
Kava, jaborandi, pill-bearing spurge: decreased benztropine effect

### NURSING CONSIDERATIONS
Assessment
• Monitor I&O ratio; retention commonly causes decreased urinary output, distention, frequency, incontinence

Adverse effects: *italic* = common, **bold** = life-threatening

- Assess for parkinsonism, EPS: shuffling gait, muscle rigidity, involuntary movements, loss of balance, pill rolling, muscle spasms, drooling before and during treatment
- Monitor for urinary hesitancy, retention; palpate bladder if retention occurs
- Monitor for constipation, cramping, pain in abdomen, abdominal distention; increase fluids, bulk, exercise if this occurs
- Assess for tolerance over long-term therapy; dosage may have to be increased or changed
- Assess for mental status: affect, mood, CNS depression, worsening of mental symptoms during early therapy
- Assess for benztropine "buzz" or "high," patients may imitate EPS

## Nursing diagnoses

- Knowledge, deficient (teaching)
- Mobility, impaired physical (uses)
- Noncompliance (teaching)

## Implementation

**PO route**

- Give with or after meals to prevent GI upset; may give with fluids other than water; hard candy, frequent drinks, gum to relieve dry mouth
- Give at bedtime to avoid daytime drowsiness in patient with parkinsonism
- May be crushed and mixed with food
- Store at room temperature

**IM route**

- Give in large muscle mass for dystonic symptoms

**IV route**

- Give parenteral dose with patient recumbent to prevent postural hypotension; give undiluted 1 mg/1 min

*Syringe compatibilities:* Chlorpro-MAZINE, fluphenazine, metoclopramide, perphenazine, thiothixene

*Y-site compatibilities:* Fluconazole, tacrolimus

## Patient/family education

- Teach patient to use caution in hot weather; product may increase susceptibility to stroke since perspiration is decreased; patient should remain indoors
- Advise patient not to discontinue this product abruptly; to taper off over 1 wk to prevent withdrawal symptoms (insomnia, involuntary movements, anxiety, tachycardias)
- Caution patient to avoid driving or other hazardous activities; drowsiness, dizziness may occur
- Teach patient to avoid OTC medication: cough, cold preparations with alcohol, antihis-tamines unless directed by prescriber; increased CNS depression may occur
- Advise patient to rise from sitting or recumbent position slowly to minimize orthostatic hypotension
- Teach patient to use good oral hygiene; to use sugarless gum, hard candy, frequent sips of water to decrease dry mouth; if dry mouth continues, saliva substitutes may be prescribed
- Instruct patient that doses should not be doubled, but missed dose may be taken up to 2 hr before next dose

## Evaluation

**Positive therapeutic outcome**

- Absence of involuntary movements (pill rolling, tremors, muscle spasms)

## betamethasone (Rx)

(bay-tah-meth'ah-sone)
Betnelan ♣, Betnesol ♣, Celestone, Cel-U-Jec, Selestoject ♣
*Func. class.:* Corticosteroid, synthetic; glucocorticoid, long acting

**Pregnancy category** C

**Action:** Decreases inflammation by suppression of migration of polymorphonuclear leukocytes, fibroblasts, reversal of increased capillary permeability and lysosomal stabilization

**Therapeutic outcome:** Decreased inflammation and normal immunity

**Uses:** Immunosuppression, severe inflammation, prevention of neonatal respiratory distress syndrome (by administration to mother), chronic asthma, rhinitis (inh); psoriasis, eczema, contact dermatitis, pruritus (topical)

## Dosage and routes

*Adult:* PO 0.6-7.2 mg daily; IM/**IV** 0.6-7.2 mg daily in joint or soft tissue (sodium phosphate)
*Child:* PO 17.5 mcg/kg/day in 3 divided doses; IM 17.5 mcg/kg/day in 3 divided doses every 3rd day or 5.8-8.75 mcg/kg/day as a single dose (adrenal insufficiency)

*Other uses*
*Child:* PO 62.5-250 mcg/kg/day in 3 divided doses; IM 20.8-125 mcg/kg/day of the base q12-24hr

**Available forms:** Tabs 500, 600 mcg; effervescent tabs 500 mcg ♣; syr 600 mcg/5 ml; ext rel tab 1 mg; sol for inj (phosphate) 3 mg/ml; susp for inj (phosphate/acetate) 6 mg/ml

## Adverse effects

*CNS: Depression, flushing, sweating,* headache, bruising, mood changes
*CV: Hypertension,* **circulatory collapse, thrombophlebitis, embolism,** tachycardia, **necrotizing angiitis, CHF**
*EENT:* Fungal infections, increased intraocular pressure, blurred vision
*GI: Diarrhea, nausea, abdominal distention,* **GI hemorrhage,** increased appetite, **pancreatitis**
*HEMA:* **Thrombocytopenia**
*INTEG: Acne, poor wound healing, bruising,* petechiae
*MS:* Fractures, osteoporosis, weakness

**Contraindications:** Psychosis, hypersensitivity, idiopathic thrombocytopenia, acute glomerulonephritis, amebiasis, fungal infections, nonasthmatic bronchial disease, child <2 yr, AIDS, TB, threadworm

**Precautions:** Pregnancy **C**, diabetes mellitus, glaucoma, osteoporosis, seizure disorders, ulcerative colitis, CHF, myasthenia gravis, renal disease, esophagitis, peptic ulcer

### Pharmacokinetics

| | |
|---|---|
| **Absorption** | Well absorbed (PO); systemic (TOP) |
| **Distribution** | Crosses placenta |
| **Metabolism** | Liver, extensively |
| **Excretion** | Kidney, breast milk |
| **Half-life** | 3-5 hr, adrenal suppression 3-4 days |

### Pharmacodynamics

| | PO | IM | IV | TOP |
|---|---|---|---|---|
| **Onset** | 1-2 hr | Unknown | Rapid | Unknown |
| **Peak** | 2 hr | 4-8 hr | 4-8 hr | Unknown |
| **Duration** | 3 days | 1-1½ days | 1-1½ days | Unknown |

## Interactions
### Individual drugs
Alcohol, indomethacin: increased GI bleeding
Amphotericin B, piperacillin, ticarcillin: increased hypokalemia
CYP3A4 inhibitors (erythromycin, ketoconazole, itraconazole, ritonavir, saquinavir, indinavir): increased effects of betamethasone
Insulin: increased need for insulin
Isoniazid: decreased effect
Phenytoin, rifampin: decreased action; increased metabolism
Somatrem, somatropin: decreased effects
### Drug classifications
Anticoagulants: decreased effect
Barbiturates: decreased action; increased metabolism
Fluoroquinolones: increased tendon rupture
Hypoglycemic agents: increased need for hypoglycemic agents
NSAIDs, salicylates: increased GI bleeding
Salicylates, oral contraceptives: decreased effects
Thiazides, loop diuretics: increased hypokalemia
Toxoids/vaccines: decreased immune response
### Drug/herb
Aloe, buckthorn, cascara sagrada, Chinese rhubarb, senna: increased hypokalemia
Goldenseal, hawthorn, hops, lemon balm, licorice, lily of the valley, mistletoe, perilla, pheasant's eye, squill: increased corticosteroid effect
### Drug/food
Grapefruit juice should be avoided
### Drug/lab test
Increased: cholesterol, sodium, blood glucose, uric acid, calcium, urine glucose
Decreased: calcium, potassium, $T_4$, $T_3$, thyroid $^{131}I$ uptake test, urine 17-OHCS, 17-KS, PBI
False negative: skin allergy tests

## NURSING CONSIDERATIONS
### Assessment
**Systemic route**
• Monitor potassium, blood glucose, urine glucose while on long-term therapy; hypokalemia and hyperglycemia; check weight daily; notify prescriber of weekly gain >5 lb
• Monitor B/P q4hr, pulse; notify prescriber if chest pain occurs
• Monitor I&O ratio; be alert for decreasing urinary output and increasing edema
• Check plasma cortisol levels during long-term therapy (normal level: 138-635 nmol/L [SI units] when drawn at 8 AM); adrenal function periodically for HPA axis suppression
• Assess for symptoms of infection: increased temp, WBC even after withdrawal of medication; product masks infection symptoms
• Assess for symptoms of potassium depletion: paresthesias, fatigue, nausea, vomiting, depression, polyuria, dysrhythmias, weakness
• Monitor for edema, hypo/hypertension, cardiac symptoms
• Assess for mental status: affect, mood, behavioral changes, aggression
**Topical route**
• Check temp; if fever develops, product should be discontinued
• Assess for systemic absorption: increased temp, inflammation, irritation

## Nursing diagnoses
- Infection, risk for (adverse reactions)
- Knowledge, deficient (teaching)
- Noncompliance (teaching)

## Implementation
**PO route**
- Give with food or milk to decrease GI symptoms

**IM route**
- Give IM inj deep in large mass, rotate sites, avoid deltoid, use 21-G needle; in one dose in AM to prevent adrenal suppression; avoid SUBCUT administration; may damage tissue

**Inhalation route**
- Give inh with water to decrease possibility of fungal infections; titrated dose; use lowest effective dose
- Use after cleaning aerosol TOP daily with warm water; dry thoroughly
- Store in cool environment; do not puncture or incinerate container

**Topical route**
- Apply only to affected areas; do not get in eyes; apply medication, then cover with occlusive dressing (only if prescribed), seal to normal skin, change q12hr; systemic absorption may occur
- Apply only to dermatoses; do not use on weeping, denuded, or infected area
- Cleanse before applying product; use treatment for a few days after area has cleared
- Store at room temperature

**IV route**
- Give **IV** (only sodium phosphate product); give over >1 min; may be given by **IV** inf in compatible sol after shaking susp (parenteral)
- Give titrated dose; use lowest effective dose

**Y-site compatibilities:** Heparin, hydrocortisone, potassium chloride, vit B/C

## Patient/family education
**Systemic route**
- Advise patient that long-term therapy may be needed to clear infection (1-2 mo depending on type of infection); that emergency ID as steroid user should be carried or worn; dosage adjustment may be needed
-  Instruct patient to notify prescriber if therapeutic response decreases; caution patient not to discontinue abruptly; adrenal crisis can result
- Instruct patient to avoid OTC products unless directed by prescriber
- Teach patient all aspects of product usage, including cushingoid symptoms
- Teach patient symptoms of adrenal insufficiency: nausea, anorexia, fatigue, dizziness, dyspnea, weakness, joint pain

**Topical route**
- Caution patient to avoid sunlight on affected area; burns may occur

## Evaluation
**Positive therapeutic outcome**
- Ease of respirations, decreased inflammation (systemic)
- Absence of severe itching, patches on skin, flaking (topical)

---

### betamethasone topical
*See Appendix D*

---

### betamethasone (augmented) topical
*See Appendix D*

---

### betaxolol ophthalmic
*See Appendix D*

---

### bethanechol  (Rx)
(be-than'e-kol)
bethanechol chloride, Duvoid, Urebeth, Urecholine
*Func. class.:* Urinary tract stimulant, cholinergic
*Chem. class.:* Synthetic choline ester

**Pregnancy category** C

---

**Action:** Stimulates muscarinic acetylcholine receptors directly; mimics effects of parasympathetic nervous system stimulation; stimulates gastric motility, micturition; increases lower esophageal sphincter pressure

**Therapeutic outcome:** Absence of continued urinary retention

**Uses:** Urinary retention (postoperative, postpartum), neurogenic atony of bladder with retention

**Unlabeled uses:** Ileus

**Dosage and routes**
*Adult:* PO 10-50 mg bid-qid; SUBCUT 5 mg tid-qid prn
*Child:* PO 0.6 mg/kg/day divided in 3-4 doses/day

*Test dose*
*Adult:* SUBCUT 2.5 mg repeated 15-30 min intervals × 4 doses to determine effective dose

---

**Available forms:** Tabs 5, 10, 25, 50 mg; inj SUBCUT 5 mg/ml

**Adverse effects**

*CNS:* Dizziness, headache, malaise
*CV:* Hypotension, bradycardia, reflex tachycardia, **cardiac arrest, circulatory collapse**
*EENT:* Miosis, increased salivation, lacrimation, blurred vision
*GI: Nausea, bloody diarrhea, belching, vomiting, cramps, fecal incontinence*
*GU:* Urgency
*INTEG:* Rash, urticaria, flushing, increased sweating
*RESP:* **Acute asthma, dyspnea, bronchoconstriction**

**Contraindications:** Hypersensitivity, severe bradycardia, asthma, severe hypotension, hyperthyroidism, peptic ulcer, parkinsonism, seizure disorders, CAD, COPD, coronary occlusion, mechanical obstruction, peritonitis, recent urinary or GI surgery, GI/GU obstruction

**Precautions:** Pregnancy **C**, breastfeeding, child <8 yr, hypertension

**Pharmacokinetics**

| | |
|---|---|
| Absorption | Poorly absorbed (PO); well absorbed (SUBCUT) |
| Distribution | Does not cross blood-brain barrier |
| Metabolism | Unknown |
| Excretion | Kidneys |
| Half-life | Unknown |

**Pharmacodynamics**

| | PO | SUBCUT |
|---|---|---|
| Onset | 30-90 min | 5-15 min |
| Peak | 1 hr | 15-30 min |
| Duration | 1-6 hr | 2 hr |

**Interactions**
*Individual drugs*
Procainamide, quinidine: decreased action of procainamide and quinidine
*Drug classifications*
Anticholinergics: decreased action
Cholinergic agonists, anticholinesterase agents: increased action, increased toxicity
Ganglionic blockers: increased severe hypotension
*Drug/herb*
Jaborandi: increased cholinergic effect
Jimsonweed, scopolia: decreased effects
*Drug/lab test*
Increased: AST, lipase/amylase, bilirubin

**NURSING CONSIDERATIONS**
**Assessment**
• Monitor B/P, pulse, respirations; observe after parenteral dose for 1 hr
• Check I&O ratio; check for urinary retention or incontinence; if bladder emptying does not occur, notify prescriber; catheterization may be needed
• Assess for bradycardia, hypotension, bronchospasm, headache, dizziness, seizures, sweating, cramping, respiratory depression; product should be discontinued if toxicity occurs; atropine administration

**Nursing diagnoses**
• Injury, risk for (adverse reactions)
• Knowledge, deficient (teaching)
• Urinary elimination, impaired (uses)

**Implementation**
**PO route**
• Give increased doses if tolerance occurs as prescribed
• To avoid nausea and vomiting, take on an empty stomach; 1 hr before or 2 hr after meals
• Store at room temperature
**SUBCUT route**
⬥ Give parenteral dose by SUBCUT route; use of IM, **IV** may result in cardiac arrest or cholinergic crisis (diarrhea with blood, cramping, hypotension, circulatory collapse)
⬥ Administer only with atropine sulfate available for cholinergic crisis; give only after all other cholinergics have been discontinued
• Do not use sol with a precipitate or if discolored

**Patient/family education**
• Instruct patient to take product exactly as prescribed; 1 hr before meals or 2 hr after meals; do not double doses; if dose is missed, take within 1 hr of scheduled dose
• Caution patient to make position changes slowly; orthostatic hypotension may occur
• Instruct patient to report cramping, diarrhea with blood, flushing to prescriber

**Evaluation**
**Positive therapeutic outcome**
• Absence of urinary retention
• Absence of abdominal distention

**Treatment of overdose:** Administer atropine 0.6-1.2 mg **IV** or IM (adult)

## ⚠ HIGH ALERT

### bevacizumab (Rx)
(beh-va-kiz'you-mab)
Avastin
*Func. class.:* Antineoplastic—miscellaneous
*Chem. class.:* Monoclonal antibody

**Pregnancy category** C

**Action:** DNA-derived monoclonal antibody selectively binds to and inhibits activity of human vascular endothelial growth factor to reduce microvascular growth and inhibition of metastatic disease progression

**Therapeutic outcome:** Decreased tumor size

**Uses:** Metastatic carcinoma of the colon or rectum in combination with 5-FU **IV**

**Unlabeled uses:** Adjunctive in breast, renal cancer

**Dosage and routes**
*Adult:* **IV** INF 5 mg/kg q14 days given over 90 min; if well tolerated, the next infusion may be given over 60 min; if 60 min infusions are well tolerated, subsequent infusions may be given over 30 min

**Available forms:** Inj 25 mg/ml

**Adverse effects**
*CNS: Asthenia, dizziness*
*CV:* **Deep vein thrombosis**, hypo/hypertension, **hypertensive crisis**
*GI:* Nausea, vomiting, anorexia, diarrhea, constipation, abdominal pain, colitis, stomatitis, **GI hemorrhage**
*GU:* Proteinuria, urinary frequency/urgency, **nephrotic syndrome**
*HEMA:* **Leukopenia, neutropenia, thrombocytopenia**
*META:* Bilirubinemia, hypokalemia
*MISC:* **Exfoliative dermatitis, hemorrhage**
*RESP:* Dyspnea, upper respiratory infection

**Contraindications:** Hypersensitivity

**Precautions:** Pregnancy C, breastfeeding, children, geriatric, CHF, blood dyscrasias, CV disease, hypertension

### Pharmacokinetics

| Absorption | Unknown |
|---|---|
| Distribution | Unknown |
| Metabolism | Unknown |
| Excretion | Unknown |
| Half-life | 20 days |

### Pharmacodynamics

| Onset | Unknown |
|---|---|
| Peak | Unknown |
| Duration | Steady state 100 days |

### NURSING CONSIDERATIONS
**Assessment**
• Monitor B/P q 3-4 wk
• Assess for symptoms of infection; may be masked by product
• Monitor CNS reaction: dizziness, confusion
⚠ Assess for GI perforation, serious bleeding, nephrotic syndrome, hypertensive crisis, product should be discontinued permanently; proteinuria, or surgery, product should be discontinued temporarily

**Nursing diagnoses**
• Body image, disturbed (adverse reactions)
• Infection, risk for (adverse reactions)
• Injury, risk for (adverse reactions)
• Knowledge, deficient (teaching)

**Implementation**
**IV route**
• Do not give by **IV** bolus, or **IV** push
• Give as **IV** inf over 90 min for first dose and 60 min thereafter, if well tolerated

**Patient/family education**
• Instruct patient to avoid hazardous tasks, since confusion, dizziness may occur
• Instruct patient to report signs of infection: sore throat, fever, diarrhea, vomiting
• Advise patient not to become pregnant while taking this product, or for several months after discontinuing treatment
• Advise patient to notify prescriber if pregnant or planning a pregnancy

**Evaluation**
**Positive therapeutic outcome**
• Decrease in size of tumors

### bicalutamide (Rx)
(bi-kal-yut'ah-mide)
Casodex
*Func. class.:* Antineoplastic hormone
*Chem. class.:* Nonsteroidal antiandrogen

**Pregnancy category** X

**Action:** Competitively inhibits the action to androgens by binding to cytosol androgen receptors in target tissue

**Therapeutic outcome:** Prevention of growth of malignant cells

B

**Uses:** Prostate cancer in combination with luteinizing hormone-releasing hormone (LHRH) analog

**Dosage and routes**
*Adult:* PO 50 mg daily with LHRH

**Available forms:** Tabs 50 mg

**Adverse effects**
*CV:* Hot flashes, hypertension, chest pain, **CHF,** edema
*CNS:* Dizziness, paresthesia, insomnia, anxiety, neuropathy, headache
*GI: Diarrhea, constipation, nausea,* vomiting, increased liver enzyme test, anorexia, dry mouth, melena, abdominal pain
*GU:* Nocturia, **hematuria,** UTI, impotence, gynecomastia, urinary incontinence, frequency, dysuria, retention, urgency, breast tenderness, decreased libido
*INTEG:* Rash, sweating, dry skin, pruritus, alopecia
*MISC:* Infection, anemia, dyspnea, bone pain, headache, asthenia, *back pain,* flulike symptoms

**Contraindications:** Pregnancy **X,** hypersensitivity

**Precautions:** Breastfeeding, geriatric, renal/hepatic disease

| Pharmacokinetics | |
|---|---|
| **Absorption** | Well absorbed |
| **Distribution** | Unknown |
| **Metabolism** | Liver |
| **Excretion** | Urine, feces |
| **Half-life** | 5.2 days |

| Pharmacodynamics | |
|---|---|
| **Onset** | Unknown |
| **Peak** | 31½ hr |
| **Duration** | Unknown |

**Interactions**
*Drug classifications*
Anticoagulants: increased anticoagulation
*Drug/lab test*
Increased: AST, ALT, bilirubin, BUN, creatinine
Decreased: Hgb, WBC

**NURSING CONSIDERATIONS**
**Assessment**
• Assess for diarrhea, constipation, nausea, vomiting
• Assess for hot flashes, gynecomastia; assure patient that these are common side effects
• Monitor prostate specific antigen (PSA) liver function tests

**Nursing diagnoses**
• Injury, risk for (uses, adverse reactions)
• Knowledge, deficient (teaching)

**Implementation**
• Give at same time each day (for both products) either AM or PM with or without food
• Give only with LHRH treatment

**Patient/family education**
• Teach patient to recognize and report signs of anemia, renal/hepatic toxicity
• Advise patient that hair may be lost, but is reversible after therapy is discontinued
• Advise patient not to use other products unless approved by prescriber
• Advise patient to use contraception

**Evaluation**
**Positive therapeutic outcome**
• Decreased tumor size, spread of malignancy

---

### bimatoprost ophthalmic
*See Appendix D*

---

### bisacodyl (OTC)
(bis-a-koe'dill)
Bisc-Evac, Bisaco-Lax, Bisacolax ♣, Carter's Little Pills, Dacodyl, Deficol, Dulcagen, Dulcolax, Feen-a-Mint, Fleet Laxative, Laxit ♣, Modane, Reliable Gentle Laxative, Therelax
*Func. class.:* Laxative, stimulant
*Chem. class.:* Diphenylmethane
**Pregnancy category C**

**Action:** Acts directly on intestine by increasing motor activity; thought to irritate colonic intramural plexus; increases water in the colon

**Therapeutic outcome:** Decreased constipation

**Uses:** Short-term treatment of constipation, bowel or rectal preparation for surgery, examination

**Dosage and routes**
*Adult ≥12 yr:* PO 5-15 mg in PM or AM; may use up to 30 mg for bowel or rectal preparation; RECT 10 mg (single dose), 30 ml enema
*Child 6-11 yr:* PO 5 mg as a single dose; RECT 5 mg as a single dose

**Available forms:** Tabs 5 mg; enteric coated tabs 5 mg; del rel tabs 10 mg; supp 5, 10 mg; enema 10 mg/30 ml

---

### Adverse effects
*CNS:* Muscle weakness
*GI:* *Nausea, vomiting, anorexia, cramps,* diarrhea, rectal burning (supp)
*META:* Protein-losing enteropathy, alkalosis, hypokalemia, **tetany**, electrolyte and fluid imbalances

**Contraindications:** Hypersensitivity, rectal fissures, abdominal pain, nausea, vomiting, appendicitis, acute surgical abdomen, ulcerated hemorrhoids, acute hepatitis, fecal impaction, intestinal/biliary tract obstruction

**Precautions:** Pregnancy **C**, breastfeeding

| Pharmacokinetics | |
|---|---|
| **Absorption** | Poor |
| **Distribution** | Unknown |
| **Metabolism** | Liver, minimally |
| **Excretion** | Kidneys |
| **Half-life** | Unknown |

| Pharmacodynamics | | |
|---|---|---|
| | PO | RECT |
| **Onset** | 6-10 hr | 15-60 min |
| **Peak** | Unknown | Unknown |
| **Duration** | Unknown | Unknown |

### Interactions
*Drug classifications*
Antacids, gastric acid pump inhibitors, $H_2$-blockers: increased gastric irritation
*Drug/herb*
Flax, lily of the valley, pheasant's eye, senna, squill: increased laxative action
*Drug/food*
Milk: increased gastric irritation

### NURSING CONSIDERATIONS
**Assessment**
• Monitor blood, urine electrolytes if used often by patient; check I&O ratio to identify fluid loss
• Assess cramping, rectal bleeding, nausea, vomiting; if these symptoms occur, product should be discontinued; identify cause of constipation; identify whether fluids, bulk, or exercise missing from lifestyle

**Nursing diagnoses**
• Constipation (uses)
• Diarrhea (side effects)
• Knowledge, deficient (teaching)
• Noncompliance (teaching)

### Implementation
**PO route**
• Swallow tabs whole; do not break, crush, or chew
• Give alone with water only for better absorption; do not take within 1 hr of antacids, milk
• Administer in AM or PM (oral dose)
**Rectal route**
• Lubricate before insertion, patient should retain for ½ hr

### Patient/family education
• Discuss with the patient that adequate fluid and bulk consumption is necessary
• Advise patient that normal bowel movements do not always occur daily
• Teach patient not to use in presence of abdominal pain, nausea, vomiting; tell patient to notify prescriber if constipation unrelieved or if symptoms of electrolyte imbalance occur: muscle cramps, pain, weakness, dizziness, excessive thirst

### Evaluation
**Positive therapeutic outcome**
• Decreased constipation within 3 days

---

## bismuth subsalicylate (OTC)
(bis'meth sub-sa-li'si-late)
Bismatrol, Bismatrol Extra Strength, Bismed, Diotane, Kaopectate, Kao-Tin, Kapectolin, K-pec Peptic Relief, Kola-Pectin, Leader K-pec, Pepto-Bismol, Pepto-Bismol Maximum Strength, Pink Bismuth, PMS-Bismuth Subsalicylate
*Func. class.:* Antidiarrheal/weak antacid
*Chem. class.:* Salicylate

**Pregnancy category C**

**Action:** Inhibits prostaglandin synthesis responsible for GI hypermotility, intestinal inflammation; stimulates absorption of fluid and electrolytes; antimicrobial, antisecretory effects; binds toxins produced by *Escherichia coli*

**Therapeutic outcome:** Absence of loose, watery stools

**Uses:** Diarrhea (cause undetermined); prevention of diarrhea when traveling; may be included to treat *Helicobacter pylori*, heartburn, indigestion, nausea

### Dosage and routes
*Antidiarrheal*
*Adult:* PO 524 mg q30-60min or 1048 mg q1hr, max 4.2 g/24 hr

---

*Child 9-12 yr:* PO 262 mg q½-1hr, max 2.1 g/24 hr
*Child 6-9 yr:* PO 174.6 mg q½-1hr, max 1.4 g/24 hr
*Child 3-6 yr:* PO 88 mg q½-1hr, max 704 mg/24 hr

**Available forms:** Tabs 262 mg; chewable tabs 262, 300 mg; susp 262, 300, 524 mg/15 ml

**Adverse effects**
*CNS:* Confusion, twitching, neurotoxicity (high dose)
*EENT:* Hearing loss, tinnitus, metallic taste, blue gums, black tongue (chew tabs)
*GI:* Increased fecal impaction (high doses), dark stools, constipation, diarrhea, nausea
*HEMA:* Increased bleeding time

**Contraindications:** Child <3 yr; impaction, children, teens with chickenpox, flulike symptoms; hypersensitivity (aspirin), history of GI bleeding; renal disease, varicella, hypersensitivity to this product or salicylates

**Precautions:** Pregnancy **C**, breastfeeding, geriatric, anticoagulant therapy, gout, diabetes mellitus, immobility

| Pharmacokinetics | |
|---|---|
| **Absorption** | Salicylate >90% |
| **Distribution** | None |
| **Metabolism** | None |
| **Excretion** | Feces (unchanged) |
| **Half-life** | Unknown |

| Pharmacodynamics | |
|---|---|
| **Onset** | 1 hr |
| **Peak** | 2 hr |
| **Duration** | 4 hr |

**Interactions**
*Individual drugs*
Tetracycline: decreased absorption
*Drug classifications*
Anticoagulants (oral): increased effect of anticoagulants
Antidiabetics (oral): increased effect of antidiabetics
Salicylates: increased risk of salicylate toxicity
*Drug/herb*
Nutmeg: increased antidiarrheal effect
Sarsaparilla: increased bismuth absorption
*Drug/lab test*
Interference: radiographic studies of GI system

**NURSING CONSIDERATIONS**
**Assessment**
• Monitor skin turgor; dehydration may occur in severe diarrhea; monitor electrolytes (potassium, sodium, chloride) if diarrhea is severe or continues long term
• Assess bowel pattern (frequency, consistency, shape, volume, color) before product therapy, after treatment; check weight, bowel sounds; identify factors contributing to diarrhea (bacteria, diet, medications, tube feedings)

**Nursing diagnoses**
• Constipation (adverse reactions)
• Diarrhea (uses)
• Knowledge, deficient (teaching)

**Implementation**
• Shake susp before use; chewable tabs should not be swallowed whole

**Patient/family education**
• Teach patient to stop use if symptoms do not improve within 2 days or become worse, or if diarrhea is accompanied by high fever
• Teach patient to increase fluids for rehydration
• Tell patient to chew or dissolve chewable tabs in mouth; do not swallow whole; shake susp before using
• Tell patient to avoid other salicylates unless directed by prescriber; not to give to children because of possibility of Reye's syndrome
• Tell patient that stools may turn gray; tongue may darken; impaction may occur in debilitated patients

**Evaluation**
**Positive therapeutic outcome**
• Decreased diarrhea

**bisoprolol** (Rx)
(bis-oh'pro-lole)
Zebeta
*Func. class.:* Antihypertensive
*Chem. class.:* $\beta_1$-Blocker (selective)
**Pregnancy category C**

**Do not confuse:**
Zebeta/Diabeta/Zetia

**Action:** Preferentially and competitively blocks stimulation of $\beta_1$-adrenergic receptor within cardiac muscle (decreases rate of SA node discharge, increases recovery time), slows conduction of AV node, decreases heart rate, which decreases $O_2$ consumption in myocardium; decreases renin-aldosterone-

Adverse effects: *italic* = common, **bold** = life-threatening

angiotensin system; inhibits $\beta_2$-receptors in bronchial and vascular smooth muscle at high doses

**Therapeutic outcome:** Decreased B/P, heart rate

**Uses:** Mild to moderate hypertension

**Unlabeled uses:** Stable angina, stable CHF

## Dosage and routes
### Renal/hepatic dose
*Adult:* PO 2.5 mg, titrate upward

### Hypertension
*Adult:* PO 5 mg/day, may increase if necessary to 20 mg once daily, max 40 mg/day; may need to reduce dose in presence of renal or hepatic impairment

**Available forms:** Tabs 5, 10 mg

## Adverse effects
*CNS:* Vertigo, headache, insomnia, fatigue, dizziness, mental changes, memory loss, hallucinations, depression, lethargy, drowsiness, strange dreams, catatonia, peripheral neuropathy
*CV:* **Ventricular dysrhythmias, profound hypotension, bradycardia, CHF,** cold extremities, postural hypotension, 2nd- or 3rd-degree heart block
*EENT:* Sore throat, dry burning eyes
*ENDO:* Increased hypoglycemic response to insulin
*GI:* Nausea, diarrhea, vomiting, **mesenteric arterial thrombosis,** ischemic colitis, flatulence, gastritis, gastric pain
*GU:* Impotence, decreased libido
*HEMA:* **Agranulocytosis, thrombocytopenia,** purpura, **eosinophilia**
*INTEG:* Rash, flushing, alopecia, pruritus, sweating
*MISC:* Facial swelling, weight gain, decreased exercise tolerance
*MS:* Joint pain, arthralgia
*RESP:* **Bronchospasm,** dyspnea, wheezing, cough, nasal stuffiness

**Contraindications:** Hypersensitivity to β-blockers, cardiogenic shock, heart block (2nd or 3rd degree), sinus bradycardia, CHF, cardiac failure

**Precautions:** Pregnancy **C**, breastfeeding, children, major surgery, diabetes mellitus, renal/hepatic/thyroid/peripheral vascular/aortic or mitral valve disease, COPD, asthma, well-compensated heart failure, myasthenia gravis

### Pharmacokinetics
| | |
|---|---|
| **Absorption** | Well absorbed |
| **Distribution** | Unknown; protein binding (30%) |
| **Metabolism** | Liver, inactive metabolites |
| **Excretion** | Urine, unchanged (50%) |
| **Half-life** | 9-12 hr |

### Pharmacodynamics
| | |
|---|---|
| **Onset** | Unknown |
| **Peak** | 2-4 hr |
| **Duration** | 24 hr |

## Interactions
### Individual drugs
Amiodarone, digoxin: increased bradycardia
Guanethidine, reserpine: increased hypotension
### Drug classifications
ACE inhibitors, α-blockers, calcium channel blockers, diuretics: increased antihypertensive effect
Antidiabetics: increased antidiabetic effect
Calcium channel blockers: increased myocardial depression
Ergots: increased peripheral ischemia
NSAIDs, salicylates: decreased antihypertensive effects
### Drug/herb
Aconite: increased toxicity, death
Betel palm, butterbur, cola tree, figwort, fumitory, guarana, hawthorn, lily of the valley, motherwort, plantain: increased β-blocking effect
Coenzyme Q10, St. John's wort, yohimbe: decreased β-blocking effect
### Drug/lab test
Increased: AST, ALT, blood glucose, BUN, uric acid, potassium, lipoprotein, ANA titer
Interference: glucose/insulin tolerance tests

## NURSING CONSIDERATIONS
### Assessment
• Monitor B/P during beginning treatment, periodically thereafter; pulse q4hr: note rate, rhythm, quality; apical/radial pulse before administration; notify prescriber of any significant changes (pulse <50 bpm)
• Check for baselines in renal, liver function tests before therapy begins
• Assess for edema in feet, legs daily, monitor I&O, daily weight; check for jugular vein distention, crackles, bilaterally, dyspnea (CHF)
• Monitor skin turgor, dryness of mucous membranes for hydration status, especially geriatric

### Nursing diagnoses
• Cardiac output, decreased (uses)
• Injury, risk for (side effects)
• Knowledge, deficient (teaching)
• Noncompliance (teaching)

### Implementation
• Give daily; give with food to prevent GI upset; may be crushed
• Store protected from light, moisture; place in cool environment

### Patient/family education
• Teach patient not to discontinue product abruptly; may cause precipitate angina if stopped abruptly, evaluate noncompliance
• Teach patient not to use OTC products containing α-adrenergic stimulants (such as nasal decongestants, cold preparations); to avoid alcohol, smoking and to limit sodium intake as prescribed
• Teach patient how to take pulse and B/P at home; advise when to notify prescriber
• Instruct patient to comply with weight control, dietary adjustments, modified exercise program
• Tell patient to carry/wear emergency ID to identify product being taken, allergies; tell patient product controls symptoms but does not cure
• Caution patient to avoid hazardous activities if dizziness, drowsiness present
• Teach patient to take product as prescribed, not to double doses, skip doses; take any missed doses as soon as remembered if at least 8 hr until next dose
• Advise patient to report bradycardia, dizziness, confusion, depression, fever, cold extremities
• Teach patient if diabetic, may mask signs of hypoglycemia, or alter blood glucose levels

### Evaluation
**Positive therapeutic outcome**
• Decreased B/P in hypertension (after 1-2 wk)

### Treatment of overdose: Lavage, **IV** atropine for bradycardia, **IV** theophylline for bronchospasm, digoxin, $O_2$, diuretic for cardiac failure, hemodialysis, **IV** glucose for hypoglycemia, **IV** diazepam (or phenytoin) for seizures

---

**! HIGH ALERT**

### bivalirudin (Rx)
(bye-val-i-rue′din)
Angiomax
*Func. class.:* Anticoagulant
*Chem. class.:* Thrombin inhibitor

**Pregnancy category B**

B

**Action:** Direct inhibitor of thrombin that is highly specific; able to inhibit free and clot-bound thrombin

**Therapeutic outcome:** Anticoagulation in percutaneous transluminal coronary angioplasty (PTCA), used with aspirin, heparin-induced thrombocytopenia with thrombosis syndrome

**Uses:** Unstable angina in patients undergoing PTCA

### Dosage and routes
*Adult:* **IV** BOL 0.75 mg/kg, then **IV** INF 1.75 mg/kg/hr for 4 hr; another **IV** INF may be used at 0.2 mg/kg/hr for ≤20 hr; this product is intended to be used with aspirin (325 mg daily) adjusted to body weight

*HIT/HITTS*
*Adult:* **IV** BOL 0.75 mg/kg, then cont inf 1.75 mg/kg/hr for duration of procedure

*Renal dose*
*Adult:* **IV** GFR 30-59 ml/min give 1.75 mg/kg/hr; GFR 10-29 ml/min give 1 mg/kg/hr; dialysis-dependent patients give 0.25 mg/kg/hr

**Available forms:** Inj, lyophilized 250 mg vial

### Adverse effects
*CNS: Headache, insomnia, anxiety, nervousness*
*CV: Hypo/hypertension, bradycardia*
*GI: Nausea, vomiting, abdominal pain, dyspepsia*
**HEMA: Hemorrhage**
*MISC:* Pain at inj site, pelvic pain, urinary retention, fever
*MS: Back pain*

**Contraindications:** Hypersensitivity, active bleeding, cerebral aneurysm, intracranial hemorrhage, recent surgery, CVA, GI bleeding, retroperitoneal bleeding

**Precautions:** Pregnancy **B,** breastfeeding, children, geriatric, renal function impairment, hepatic disease, asthma, blood dyscrasias, thrombocytopenia, GI ulcers, hypertension

---

Adverse effects: *italic* = common, **bold** = life-threatening

## Pharmacokinetics

| | |
|---|---|
| **Absorption** | Unknown |
| **Distribution** | No protein binding |
| **Metabolism** | Unknown |
| **Excretion** | Kidneys |
| **Half-life** | 25 min |

## Pharmacodynamics

| | |
|---|---|
| **Onset** | Unknown |
| **Peak** | Unknown |
| **Duration** | 1 hr |

## Interactions
### Drug classifications
Anticoagulants, thrombolytics: increased risk of bleeding
### Drug/herb
Agrimony, alfalfa, angelica, anise, bilberry, black haw, bogbean, buchu, cat's claw, chamomile, chondroitin, devil's claw, dong quai, evening primrose, fenugreek, feverfew, fish oils, garlic, ginger, ginkgo, ginseng, horse chestnut, Irish moss, kava, kelp, kelpware, khella, licorice, lovage, lungwort, meadowsweet, motherwort, mugwort, nettle, papaya, parsley (large amounts), pau d'arco, pineapple, poplar, prickly ash, red clover, safflower, saw palmetto, senega, skullcap, tonka bean, turmeric, wintergreen, yarrow: increased risk of bleeding
Chamomile, coenzyme Q10, flax, glucomannan, goldenseal, guar gum: decreased anticoagulant effect

## NURSING CONSIDERATIONS
### Assessment
◆ Assess for fall in B/P or Hct that may indicate hemorrhage
• Assess for fever, skin rash, urticaria
• Assess bleeding: check arterial and venous sites, IM inj sites, catheters; all punctures should be minimized

### Nursing diagnoses
• Cardiac output, decreased (uses)
• Knowledge, deficient (teaching)

### Implementation
• Prior to PTCA, give with aspirin, 325 mg **IV** direct 1 mg/kg as a bolus; then intermittent infusion
**Intermittent IV infusion route**
• To each 250-mg vial add 5 ml of sterile water for inj, swirl until dissolved, further dilute reconstituted vial with 50 ml of D$_5$W or 0.9% NaCl (5 mg/ml); the dose is adjusted to body weight, run at 2.5 mg/kg/hr, do not admix before or during administration
• Give reduced dose in renal impairment

## Patient/family education
• Explain reason for product and expected results
## Evaluation
**Positive therapeutic outcome**
• Anticoagulation in PTCA

---

### ❗ HIGH ALERT

**bleomycin** 🔘 (Rx)
(blee-oh-mye'sin)
Blenoxane
*Func. class.:* Antineoplastic, antibiotic
*Chem. class.:* Glycopeptide
**Pregnancy category  D**

**Action:** Inhibits synthesis of DNA, RNA, protein; derived from *Streptomyces verticillus;* replication is decreased by binding to DNA, which causes strand splitting; phase specific in the G$_2$ and M phases; a nonvesicant

**Therapeutic outcome:** Prevention of rapidly growing malignant cells

**Uses:** Cancer of head, neck, penis, cervix, vulva of squamous cell origin, Hodgkin's disease, lymphosarcoma, reticulum cell sarcoma, testicular carcinoma, malignant pleural effusion

**Dosage and routes**
*Adult and child:* IM/SUBCUT/**IV** 0.25-0.5 units/kg q1-2 wk or 10-20 units/m$^2$; then 1 unit/day or 5 units/wk; may also be given by CONT INF; do not exceed total dose, 400 units in lifetime

*Malignant pleural effusion*
*Adult:* 60 units diluted in 100 ml of 0.9% NaCl intrapleural inj given through a thoracotomy tube following drainage of excess pleural fluid and complete lung expansion, remove after 4 hr

**Available forms:** Powder for inj 15, 30 units/vial

**Adverse effects**
*CNS:* Pain at tumor site, headache, confusion
*GI: Nausea, vomiting, anorexia, stomatitis, weight loss,* ulceration of mouth, lips
*IDIOSYNCRATIC REACTION:* Hypotension, confusion, fever, chills, wheezing
*INTEG: Rash, hyperkeratosis, nail changes, alopecia,* pruritus, acne, striae, peeling, hyperpigmentation
*RESP: Fibrosis,* pneumonitis, wheezing, **pulmonary toxicity**

---

◆ Alert    ♣ Canada Only    🔘 Drug on CD    * "Tall Man" lettering (See Preface)

*SYST:* **Anaphylaxis,** radiation recall, Raynaud's phenomenon

**Contraindications:** Pregnancy **D,** hypersensitivity, prior idiosyncratic reaction

**Precautions:** Renal/hepatic/respiratory disease, patients >70 yr old

### Pharmacokinetics

| | |
|---|---|
| **Absorption** | Well absorbed (IM, SUBCUT, intrapleural, intraperitoneal) |
| **Distribution** | Widely distributed |
| **Metabolism** | Liver, 30% |
| **Excretion** | Kidneys, unchanged (50%) |
| **Half-life** | 2 hr; increased in renal disease |

### Pharmacodynamics
Unknown

### Interactions
*Individual drugs*
Fosphenytoin, phenytoin: decreased phenytoin levels
Radiation: increased toxicity, bone marrow suppression
*Drug classifications*
Anesthetics (general), antineoplastics: increased toxicity
*Drug/lab test*
Increased: uric acid

### NURSING CONSIDERATIONS
**Assessment**
• Assess buccal cavity q8hr for dryness, sores or ulceration, white patches, oral pain, bleeding, dysphagia; obtain prescription for viscous lidocaine (Xylocaine)
⬩ Assess symptoms indicating anaphylaxis: rash, pruritus, urticaria, purpuric skin lesions, itching, flushing, wheezing, hypotension; have emergency equipment available
• Monitor CBC, differential, platelet count weekly; withhold product if WBC <4000/mm$^3$ or platelet count <100,000/mm$^3$; notify prescriber of results if WBC <20,000/mm$^3$, platelets <150,000/mm$^3$
• Monitor temp q4hr (may indicate beginning of infection)
• Monitor liver function tests before and during therapy (bilirubin, AST, ALT, LDH) as needed or monthly
• Assess for bleeding: hematuria, stool guaiac, bruising or petechiae, mucosa or orifices q8hr; inflammation of mucosa, breaks in skin
• Identify dyspnea, crackles, unproductive cough, chest pain, tachypnea
• Identify effects of alopecia on body image; discuss feelings about body changes; if edema

in feet, joint pain, stomach pain, shaking present, prescriber should be notified; identify inflammation of mucosa, breaks in skin

**Nursing diagnoses**
• Body image, disturbed (adverse reactions)
• Infection, risk for (adverse reactions)
• Injury, risk for (adverse reactions)
• Knowledge, deficient (teaching)

**Implementation**
• Avoid contact with skin, very irritating; wash completely to remove
• Give fluids **IV** or PO before chemotherapy to hydrate patient
• Give antacid before oral agent; give antiemetic 30-60 min before giving product and prn to prevent vomiting; give antibiotics for prophylaxis of infection
• Provide liquid diet: carbonated beverages, gelatin may be added if patient is not nauseated or vomiting
• Rinsing of mouth tid-qid with water, club soda; brushing of teeth bid-qid with soft brush or cotton-tipped applicators for stomatitis; use unwaxed dental floss
**IM/SUBCUT route**
• IM test dose in lymphoma
• Reconstitute with 1-5 ml sterile water for inj; D$_5$W, 0.9% NaCl, rotate inj sites
**IV route**
• Product should be prepared by experienced personnel using proper precautions
• Two test doses 2-5 units before initial dose in lymphoma; monitor for anaphylaxis
• Give by direct **IV** after reconstituting 15 units or less/5 ml or more of D$_5$W or 0.9% NaCl; give 15 units or less/10 min through Y-tube or 3-way stopcock initial dose; monitor for anaphylaxis
**Intermittent IV infusion route**
• Administer after diluting 50-100 ml 0.9% NaCl, D$_5$W and giving at prescribed rate
**Intrapleural route**
• Give 60 units/50-100 ml of 0.9% NaCl, administered by physician through thoracotomy tube
*Syringe compatibilities:* Cisplatin, cyclophosphamide, DOXOrubicin, droperidol, fluorouracil, furosemide, heparin, leucovorin, methotrexate, metoclopramide, mitomycin, vinBLAStine, vinCRIStine
*Y-site compatibilities:* Allopurinol, amisostine, aztreonam, cisplatin, cyclophosphamide, DOXOrubicin, DOXOrubicin liposome, droperidol, filgrastim, fludarabine, fluorouracil, granisetron, heparin, leucovorin, melphalan, methotrexate, metoclopramide, mitomycin, ondansetron, paclitaxel,

Adverse effects: *italic* = common, **bold** = life-threatening

piperacillin/tazobactam, sargramostim, teniposide, thiotepa, vinBLAStine, vinCRIStine, vinorelbine

*Additive compatibilities:* Amikacin, cephapirin, dexamethasone, diphenhydrAMINE, fluorouracil, gentamicin, heparin, hydrocortisone, phenytoin, streptomycin, tobramycin, vinBLAStine, vinCRIStine

*Additive incompatibilities:* Aminophylline, ascorbic acid inj, carbenicillin, cefazolin, cephalothin, diazepam, hydrocortisone, methotrexate, mitomycin, nafcillin, penicillin G sodium, terbutaline

*Solution compatibilities:* 0.9% NaCl

### Patient/family education

• Teach patient to avoid use of products containing aspirin or ibuprofen, razors, commercial mouthwash; bleeding may occur; to report symptoms of bleeding (hematuria, tarry stools)

• Instruct patient to report signs of anemia (fatigue, headache, irritability, faintness, shortness of breath)

• Instruct patient to report any changes in breathing or coughing even several months after treatment; to avoid crowds and persons with respiratory tract or other infections

• Inform patient that hair may be lost during treatment; a wig or hairpiece may make patient feel better; new hair may be different in color, texture

• Caution patient not to have any vaccinations without the advice of the prescriber; serious reactions can occur

• Advise patient contraception is needed during treatment and for several months after completion of therapy

### Evaluation
**Positive therapeutic outcome**
• Prevention of rapid division of malignant cells

---

### boric acid otic
*See Appendix D*

---

### bortezomib (Rx)
(bor-tez'oh-mib)
Velcade
*Func. class.:* Antineoplastic—miscellaneous
*Chem. class.:* Proteasome inhibitor

**Pregnancy category D**

**Action:** Reversible inhibitor of chymotrypsin-like activity in mammalian cells; causes a delay in tumor growth by disrupting normal homeostatic mechanisms

**Therapeutic outcome:** Decreased growth and spread of malignant cells

**Uses:** Multiple myeloma when at least two other treatments have failed; mantle cell lymphoma

### Dosage and routes
*Mantle cell lymphoma*
**Adult: IV** BOL 1.3 mg/m²/dose (days 1, 4, 8, 11) followed by 10-day rest period (days 12 to 21); max 8 cycles

*Neuropathic pain*
Grade 1 with pain or grade 2, reduce to 1 mg/m²; Grade 2 with pain or grade 3, hold product until toxicity resolves, then start at 0.7 mg/m² qwk; Grade 4 hematologic toxicities, withhold use

**Available forms:** Lyophilized powder for inj 3.5 mg

### Adverse effects
*CNS:* Anxiety, insomnia, dizziness, headache, peripheral neuropathy, rigors, paresthesia
*CV:* Hypotension, edema
*GI:* Abdominal pain, constipation, diarrhea, dyspepsia, nausea, vomiting, anorexia
*HEMA:* Anemia, **neutropenia, thrombocytopenia,**
*MISC:* Dehydration, weight loss, herpes zoster, rash, pruritus, blurred vision
*MS:* Fatigue, malaise, weakness, arthralgia, bone pain, muscle cramps, myalgia, back pain
*RESP:* Cough, pneumonia, dyspnea, URI

**Contraindications:** Pregnancy **D**, hypersensitivity to this product, boron, or mannitol

**Precautions:** Peripheral neuropathy, breastfeeding, children, geriatric, renal/hepatic disease, hypotension

### Pharmacokinetics
| | |
|---|---|
| **Absorption** | Unknown |
| **Distribution** | Protein binding 83% |
| **Metabolism** | P450 enzymes (3A4, 2D6, 2C19, 2C9, 1A2) |
| **Excretion** | Unknown |
| **Half-life** | 9-15 hr |

### Pharmacodynamics
Unknown

### Interactions
*Individual drugs*
Amiodarone, isoniazid, nitrofurantoin: increased peripheral neuropathy

## Drug classifications
Antihypertensives: increased hypotension
Antivirals, statins: increased peripheral neuropathy
Oral hypoglycemics: increased hypo/hyperglycemia
Products that induce or inhibit CYP450 3A4: increased toxicity or decreased efficacy

## NURSING CONSIDERATIONS
### Assessment
• Assess hematologic status: platelets, CBC throughout treatment
• Monitor for extravasation at inj site

### Nursing diagnoses
• Injury, risk for (uses, adverse reactions)
• Knowledge, deficient (teaching)

### Implementation
• Reconstitute each vial with 3.5 ml 0.9% NaCl
• Use protective clothing during handling, preparation; avoid contact with skin

### Patient/family education
• Teach to use contraception while on this product, avoid breastfeeding
• Advise to monitor blood glucose levels if diabetic
• Instruct to contact prescriber if new or worsening peripheral neuropathy, severe vomiting, diarrhea
• Advise to avoid driving, operating machinery until effect is known
• Advise to avoid using other medications unless approved by prescriber

### Evaluation
**Positive therapeutic outcome**
• Improvement of multiple myeloma symptoms

## bosentan (Rx)
(boh-sen-tan)
Tracleer
*Func. class.:* Vasodilator
*Chem. class.:* Endothelin receptor antagonist

**Pregnancy category X**

**Action:** Peripheral vasodilation occurs via antagonism of the effect of endothelin on endothelium and vascular smooth muscle

**Therapeutic outcome:** Decreased pulmonary arterial hypertension

**Uses:** Pulmonary arterial hypertension with class III, IV symptoms

**Unlabeled uses:** Septic shock to improve microcirculatory blood flow

## Dosage and routes
*Adult >40 kg and child >12 yr:* PO 62.5 mg bid × 4 wk, then 125 mg bid
*Adult <40 kg and child >12 yr:* PO 62.5 mg bid

**Available forms:** Tabs 62.5, 125 mg

### Adverse effects
*CNS:* Headache, flushing, fatigue
*CV: Hypotension,* palpitations, edema of lower limbs
*GI:* Abnormal liver function, dyspepsia, **hepatotoxicity**
*INTEG:* Pruritus
*MISC:* Anemia

**Contraindications:** Pregnancy **X**, hypersensitivity, CVA, CAD

**Precautions:** Breastfeeding, children, geriatric, mitral stenosis, impaired hepatic function

### Pharmacokinetics
| | |
|---|---|
| Absorption | 50% absorbed |
| Distribution | Protein binding >98% |
| Metabolism | Liver (metabolites); metabolized CYP2C9, CYP3A4, and possibly CYP2C19; steady state 3-5 days |
| Excretion | Biliary |
| Half-life | 5 hr |

### Pharmacodynamics
Unknown

### Interactions
*Individual drugs*
CycloSPORINE A, glyBURIDE: do not coadminister
CycloSPORINE A, ketoconazole: increased bosentan level
CycloSPORINE: decreased cycloSPORINE level
GlyBURIDE: glyBURIDE level decreased significantly, bosentan also decreased, increased liver function tests
Ketoconazole: increased bosentan level
Simvastatin: decreased effects
Warfarin: decreased anticoagulation
*Drug classifications*
Contraceptives (hormonal), statins: decreased effects
*Drug/lab test*
Increased: ALT, AST
Decreased: Hgb, Hct

## NURSING CONSIDERATIONS
### Assessment
• Assess B/P, pulse during treatment until stable

- Assess hepatic tests: AST, ALT, bilirubin; liver enzymes may increase; if ALT/AST >3 and ≤5 × ULN, confirm lab value, decrease dose or interrupt treatment and monitor AST/ALT q2 wk; if >8 × ULN, stop treatment
- Assess blood studies: Hct, Hgb may be decreased
- Assess hepatic involvement: vomiting, jaundice; product should be discontinued

### Nursing diagnoses
- Knowledge, deficient (teaching)
- Tissue perfusion, ineffective (uses)

### Implementation
- Store at room temperature

### Patient/family education
- Instruct patient to report jaundice, dark urine, joint pain, fatigue, malaise, bruising, easy bleeding; may indicate blood dyscrasias
- Caution patient to avoid pregnancy; to use nonhormonal form of contraception

### Evaluation
**Positive therapeutic outcome**
- Decrease in pulmonary hypertension

## brimonidine ophthalmic
*See Appendix D*

## brinzolamide ophthalmic
*See Appendix D*

## bromfenac ophthalmic
*See Appendix D*

## bromocriptine (Rx)
(broe-moe-krip′teen)
Apo-Bromocriptine ✤, Parlodel, Parlodel Snap Tabs, PMS-Bromocriptine
*Func. class.:* Antiparkinsonian agent; DOPamine receptor agonist
*Chem. class.:* Ergot alkaloid derivative

**Pregnancy category** B

### Do not confuse:
Parlodel/pindolol/Provera

**Action:** Inhibits prolactin release by activating postsynaptic dopamine receptors; activation of striatal dopamine receptors may be reason for improvement in Parkinson's disease

**Therapeutic outcome:** Decreased involuntary movements in Parkinson's disease;

decreased breastfeeding; decreased hormone levels in acromegaly; absence of amenorrhea in hyperprolactinemia

**Uses:** Adjunct with levodopa in Parkinson's disease, amenorrhea/galactorrhea caused by hyperprolactinemia, infertility, acromegaly, pituitary adenomas

**Unlabeled uses:** Neuroleptic malignant syndrome, alcoholism, premenstrual syndrome, mastalgia, cocaine withdrawal, premenstrual breast syndromes

### Dosage and routes
*Hyperprolactinemia*
*Adult:* PO 1.25-2.5 mg with meals; may increase by 2.5 mg q3-7 days; usual dosage 5-7.5 mg

*Acromegaly*
*Adult:* PO 1.25-2.5 mg/day × 3 days at bedtime may increase by 1.25-2.5 mg q3-7 days; usual range 20-30 mg/day; max 100 mg/day

*Parkinson's disease*
*Adult:* PO 1.25 mg bid with meals; may increase q2-4 wk by 2.5 mg/day; not to exceed 100 mg/day

*Pituitary adenoma*
*Adult:* PO 1.25 mg bid-tid, may increase over several weeks to 10-20 mg/day

*Neuroleptic malignant syndrome (unlabeled)*
*Adult:* PO 2.5-5 mg 2-6 ×/day

*Cocaine withdrawal (unlabeled)*
*Adult:* PO 0.625 mg qid × 42 days

*Alcoholism (unlabeled)*
*Adult:* PO 7.5 mg/day

*Mastalgia (unlabeled)*
*Adult:* PO 2.5-7.5 bid, starting 10-14 days prior to menses, discontinue when menses begins

**Available forms:** Caps 5 mg; tabs 2.5 mg

### Adverse effects
*CNS: Headache,* depression, restlessness, anxiety, nervousness, confusion, **seizures,** hallucinations, *dizziness,* fatigue, drowsiness, abnormal involuntary movements, psychosis
*CV: Orthostatic hypotension,* decreased B/P, palpitations, extrasystole, **shock,** dysrhythmias, bradycardia, **MI**
*EENT:* Blurred vision, diplopia, burning eyes, nasal congestion
*GI: Nausea, vomiting, anorexia,* cramps, constipation, diarrhea, dry mouth, GI hemorrhage

*GU:* Frequency, retention, incontinence, diuresis
*INTEG: Rash on face, arms,* alopecia, coolness, pallor of fingers, toes

**Contraindications:** Hypersensitivity to ergot, bromocriptine; severe ischemic disease, severe peripheral vascular disease, hypertension, preeclampsia

**Precautions:** Pregnancy **B,** breastfeeding, children, hepatic/renal disease, pituitary tumors, peptic ulcer disease

Pharmacokinetics

| | |
|---|---|
| **Absorption** | Poorly absorbed |
| **Distribution** | Unknown |
| **Metabolism** | Liver, completely |
| **Excretion** | 85%-98% feces |
| **Half-life** | 4 hr (initial); 50 hr (terminal) |

Pharmacodynamics

| | |
|---|---|
| **Onset** | ½-1½ hr |
| **Peak** | 1-3 hr |
| **Duration** | 8-12 hr |

**Interactions**
*Individual drugs*
Alcohol: increased disulfiram-like reaction
Haloperidol, loxapine, methyldopa, metoclopramide, reserpine: decreased levels of bromocriptine
Levodopa: increased neurologic effects
*Drug classifications*
Antihypertensives: increased hypotension
Contraceptives (oral), estrogens, MAOIs, phenothiazines, progestins: decreased levels of bromocriptine
*Drug/herb*
Chaste tree fruit, kava: decreased bromocriptine effect
Horehound: increased serotonin effect
*Drug/lab test*
Increased: growth hormone, AST, ALT, BUN, CK, uric acid, alkaline phosphatase

**NURSING CONSIDERATIONS**
**Assessment**
• Assess symptoms of Parkinson's disease (EPS): shuffling gait, muscle rigidity, involuntary movements, pill rolling, muscle spasms, drooling before and during treatment
• Assess for resolution of symptoms of neuroleptic malignant syndrome: decreased temp, seizures, sweating, pulse
• Monitor for change in size of soft tissue volume in acromegaly

• Monitor B/P; establish baseline, compare with other readings; this product decreases B/P; patient should remain recumbent for 2-4 hr after first dose; supervise ambulation

**Nursing diagnoses**
• Knowledge, deficient (teaching)
• Mobility, impaired physical (uses)

**Implementation**
• Give with meals or milk to prevent GI symptoms; crush tab if patient has swallowing difficulty
• Give at bedtime so dizziness, orthostatic hypotension do not occur
• Store at room temperature in air-tight container

**Patient/family education**
• Advise patient to change position slowly to prevent orthostatic hypotension
• Tabs may be crushed and mixed with food
• Caution patient to use contraceptives during treatment with this product; pregnancy may occur; to use methods other than oral contraceptives
• Teach patient that therapeutic effect for Parkinson's disease may take 2 mo: galactorrhea, amenorrhea
• Caution patient to avoid hazardous activity if dizziness, drowsiness occurs during treatment start-up
• Advise patient to avoid alcohol and OTC medication unless approved by prescriber
• Teach patients with acromegaly to notify prescriber immediately if severe headache, nausea, vomiting, blurred vision occur; indicates change in enlargement of tumor
• Advise patient to report symptoms of MI immediately

**Evaluation**
**Positive therapeutic outcome**
• Parkinson's disease: decreased slow movements, decreased drooling
• Decreased breast engorgement with accompanied pain, tenderness
• Acromegly: decreased growth hormone levels

Adverse effects: *italic* = common, **bold** = life-threatening

## brompheniramine (OTC, Rx)
(brome-fen-eer′a-meen)
Bidhist, Bromfenac, brompheniramine, Brove X, Brove X CT, Chlorphed, Dehist, Dimetane, Dimetane Extentabs, Dimetapp Allergy Liqui-Gels, Lo Hist 12 Hour, Lodrane 24, Lodrane XR, Nasahist-B, VaZol
*Func. class.:* Antihistamine
*Chem. class.:* Alkylamine, H$_1$-receptor antagonist

**Pregnancy category** C

**Action:** Acts on blood vessels, GI, respiratory system by competing with histamine for H$_1$-receptor site; decreases allergic response by blocking histamine

**Therapeutic outcome:** Absence of allergy symptoms and rhinitis

**Uses:** Allergy symptoms, rhinitis

### Dosage and routes
*Adult and child >12 yr:* PO 4-8 mg bid-qid, not to exceed 36 mg/day; TIME REL 6-12 mg bid-tid, not to exceed 36 mg/day
*Child 6-12 yr:* PO 2 mg bid-qid, max 12 mg/day; EXT REL 6-12 mg/day
*Child 2-6 yr:* 1 mg tid-qid (not to exceed 6 mg/day)
*Child <2 yr:* PO 0.5 mg/kg/day in divided doses (qid)

**Available forms:** Tabs 4 mg; elix 2 mg/5 ml; caps 4 mg; chew tab 12 mg; ext rel tab 6 mg; ext rel cap 12 mg; liquid 8 mg, 12 mg/5 ml

### Adverse effects
***CNS:*** *Dizziness, drowsiness,* poor coordination, fatigue, anxiety, euphoria, confusion, paresthesia, neuritis
***CV:*** Hypotension, palpitations, tachycardia
***EENT:*** Blurred vision, dilated pupils, tinnitus, nasal stuffiness, dry nose, throat, mouth
***GI:*** Nausea, vomiting, anorexia, constipation, diarrhea
***GU:*** Retention, dysuria, frequency, impotence
***HEMA:*** **Thrombocytopenia, agranulocytosis, hemolytic anemia** (rare)
***INTEG:*** Photosensitivity
***RESP:*** Increased thick secretions, wheezing, chest tightness

**Contraindications:** Hypersensitivity to H$_1$-receptor antagonists, acute asthma attack, lower respiratory tract disease, child <2 yr

**Precautions:** Pregnancy C, breastfeeding, increased intraocular pressure, renal/cardiac disease, hypertension, bronchial asthma, seizure disorder, stenosed peptic ulcers, hyperthyroidism, prostatic hypertrophy, bladder neck obstruction, angle-closure glaucoma

### Pharmacokinetics
| | |
|---|---|
| **Absorption** | Well absorbed (PO, IM) |
| **Distribution** | Widely distributed; crosses blood-brain barrier |
| **Metabolism** | Liver, extensively |
| **Excretion** | Kidneys, metabolite; breast milk (minimal) |
| **Half-life** | 12-34 hr |

### Pharmacodynamics
| | PO | SUBCUT/IM | IV |
|---|---|---|---|
| **Onset** | 15-30 min | 30 min | Immediate |
| **Peak** | 2-5 hr | Unknown | Unknown |
| **Duration** | 6-12 hr | 8-12 hr | 8-12 hr |

### Interactions
*Individual drugs*
Alcohol: increased CNS depression
Aminophylline, insulin, pentobarbital: products are incompatible
*Drug classifications*
Barbiturates, opiates, sedative/hypnotics, tricyclics: increased CNS depression
MAOIs: increased anticholinergic effect
*Drug/herb*
Corkwood, henbane leaf: increased anticholinergic effect
Hops, Jamaican dogwood, kava, khat, senega: increased antihistamine effect
*Drug/lab test*
Interference: skin allergy tests (discontinue antihistamines before testing)

### NURSING CONSIDERATIONS
**Assessment**
- Assess respiratory status: rate, rhythm, increase in bronchial secretions, wheezing, chest tightness; provide fluids to 2 L/day to decrease secretion thickness
- Monitor I&O ratio: be alert for urinary retention, frequency, dysuria, especially geriatric; product should be discontinued if these occur
- Monitor CBC during long-term therapy; blood dyscrasias may occur but are rare

### Nursing diagnoses
- Airway clearance, ineffective (uses)
- Injury, risk for (side effects)
- Knowledge, deficient (teaching)
- Noncompliance (teaching, overuse)

## Implementation
- May give with food to prevent GI upset; absorption is not altered by food
- Store in tight, light-resistant container

## Patient/family education
- Teach patient all aspects of product use; to notify prescriber if confusion, sedation, hypotension occur; to avoid driving or other hazardous activity if drowsiness occurs; to avoid alcohol or other CNS depressants that may potentiate effect
- Instruct patient not to exceed recommended dosage; dysrhythmias may occur
- Teach patient hard candy, gum, frequent rinsing of mouth may be used for dryness

## Evaluation
**Positive therapeutic outcome**
- Absence of runny or congested nose, rashes

**Treatment of overdose:** Administer lavage, vasopressors, barbiturates (short acting)

---

## budesonide (Rx)
(byoo-des'oh-nide)
Entocort EC, Pulmicort, Pulmicort Flexhaler, Pulmicort Respules, Rhinocort, Rhinocort Aqua
*Func. class.:* Glucocorticoid

**Pregnancy category** C

**Action:** Prevents inflammation by depression of migration of polymorphonuclear leukocytes, fibroblasts, reversal of increased capillary permeability and lysosomal stabilization; does not suppress hypothalamus and pituitary function

**Uses:** Rhinitis; prophylaxis for asthma; Crohn's disease

## Dosage and routes
*Rhinitis (Rhinocort, Rhinocort Aqua)*
*Adult and child >6 yr:* SPRAY/INH 2 sprays in each nostril AM, PM or 4 sprays in each nostril AM; max 256 mcg/day

*Asthma*
*Adult and child ≥6 yr:* INH 400-600 mcg/day

*Crohn's disease*
*Adult:* PO 9 mg daily AM × 8 wk

**Available forms:** Dry powder for INH 90, 180 mg/actuation, (Pulmicort Flexhaler); inh susp 0.25 mg/2 ml, 0.5 mg/2 ml (Pulmicort Respules); 32 mcg/actuation (Rhinocort Aqua)

## Adverse effects
*CNS: Headache,* insomnia, hypertonia, syncope, dizziness, drowsiness
*CV:* Chest pain, hypertension, sinus tachycardia, palpitation
*EENT: Sinusitis, pharyngitis,* rhinitis, oral candidiasis
*ENDO:* Adrenal insufficiency, growth suppression in children
*GI:* Dry mouth, dyspepsia, nausea, vomiting, abdominal pain
*MISC:* Ecchymosis, fever, *hypersensitivity,* flulike symptoms, epistaxis, dysuria
*MS:* Back pain, myalgias, fractures
*RESP:* Nasal irritation, cough, nasal bleeding, *respiratory infections,* **bronchospasm**

**Contraindications:** Hypersensitivity, status asthmaticus

**Precautions:** Pregnancy C, inhaled form (B); breastfeeding, children, TB, fungal, bacterial, systemic viral infections, ocular herpes simplex, nasal septal ulcers; hepatic disease (caps)

### Pharmacokinetics
| | |
|---|---|
| **Absorption** | 39% |
| **Distribution** | In airways, protein binding 85-90% |
| **Metabolism** | Liver |
| **Excretion** | In urine (60%), small amounts in feces |
| **Half-life** | 2-3.6 hr |

### Pharmacodynamics
| | |
|---|---|
| **Onset** | Respules 2-8 days, Rhinocort Aqua 10 hr |
| **Peak** | Respules 4-6 wk, Rhinocort Aqua 2 wk |
| **Duration** | Unknown |

## Interactions
Avoid using with products metabolized by CYP3A4 inhibition
*Individual drugs*
Cimetidine, ketoconazole: decreased budesonide metabolism
*Drug/herb*
Aloe, buckthorn, Chinese rhubarb, senna: increased hypokalemia

## NURSING CONSIDERATIONS
### Assessment
- Assess respiratory status: rate, rhythm, increase in bronchial secretions, wheezing, chest tightness; provide fluids to 2 L/day to

---

Adverse effects: *italic* = common, **bold** = life-threatening

decrease thickness of secretions; check for oral candidiasis
• For bronchospasm, stop treatment and give bronchodilator
• With viral infections, corticosteroid use can mask infections
• For increased intraocular pressure, discontinue use if increase occurs

### Nursing diagnoses
• Airway clearance, ineffective (uses)
• Injury, risk for (uses)
• Knowledge, deficient (teaching)

### Implementation
**PO route (Crohn's disease)**
• Swallow caps whole; do not break, crush, or chew
• May repeat 8-wk course if needed; may taper to 6 mg/day for 2 wk before cessation
**INH route (asthma)**
• Use scissors to open pouch
• Store at 59°-86° F (15°-30° C); keep away from heat, open flame

### Patient/family education
• Teach patient to notify prescriber of pharyngitis, nasal bleeding, oral candidiasis
• Instruct patient not to exceed recommended dose; adrenal suppression may occur
• Teach patient to carry/wear emergency ID identifying steroid use
• Instruct patient to read and follow package directions
• Instruct patient to prevent exposure to infections, especially viral
• Advise to use good oral hygiene if using by nebulizer or inhaler
• Teach patient to avoid breastfeeding

### Evaluation
**Positive therapeutic outcome**
• Absence of asthma, rhinitis

### budesonide nasal agent
*See Appendix D*

---

### bumetanide (Rx)
(byoo-met'a-nide)
Bumex
*Func. class:* Loop diuretic, antihypertensive
*Chem. class.:* Sulfonamide derivative
**Pregnancy category  C**

**Do not confuse:**
Bumex/Buprenex/Permax

**Action:** Acts on the ascending loop of Henle in the kidney to inhibit the reabsorption of the electrolytes sodium and chloride, causing excretion of sodium, calcium, magnesium, chloride, water, and some potassium; also decreases reabsorption of sodium and chloride and increases the excretion of potassium in the distal tubule of the kidney; responsible for antihypertensive effect and peripheral vasodilatation

**Therapeutic outcome:** Decreased edema in lung tissue and peripherally; decreased B/P

**Uses:** Edema in congestive heart failure, renal/hepatic disease, ascites

### Dosage and routes
*Adult:* PO 0.5-2 mg daily may give 2nd or 3rd dose at 4-5 hr intervals; not to exceed 10 mg/day; may be given on alternate days or intermittently; IM/**IV** 0.5-1 mg; may give 2nd or 3rd dose at 2-3 hr intervals; not to exceed 10 mg/day
*Child:* PO/IM/**IV** 0.02-0.1 mg/kg q12hr, max 10 mg/day

**Available forms:** Tabs 0.5, 1, 2 mg; inj 0.25 mg/ml

### Adverse effects
*CNS:* Headache, fatigue, weakness, vertigo
*CV: Hypotension,* chest pain, ECG changes, **circulatory collapse,** dehydration
*EENT:* Loss of hearing
*ELECT: Hypokalemia, hypochloremic alkalosis, hypomagnesia, hyperuricemia, hypocalcemia, hyponatremia*
*ENDO: Hyperglycemia*
*GI: Nausea,* diarrhea, dry mouth, vomiting, anorexia, cramps, **acute pancreatitis,** upset stomach, abdominal pain, **jaundice**
*GU: Polyuria,* **renal failure,** *glycosuria,* premature ejaculation
*HEMA:* **Thrombocytopenia, leukopenia, granulocytopenia**
*INTEG: Rash, pruritus, purpura,* **Stevens-Johnson syndrome,** sweating, photosensitivity
*MS:* Muscular cramps, stiffness, arthritis

**Contraindications:** Hypersensitivity to sulfonamides, anuria, severe electrolyte deficiency, hepatic coma

**Precautions:** Pregnancy **C**, breastfeeding, neonates, dehydration, severe renal disease, ascites, hepatic cirrhosis, blood dyscrasias, ototoxicity, hyperuricemia, hypokalemia

### Pharmacokinetics

| | PO/IM | | |
|---|---|---|---|
| **Absorption** | Rapidly, completely absorbed | | |
| | PO/IM/IV | | |
| **Distribution** | Crosses placenta, protein binding >91% | | |
| **Metabolism** | Liver (30%-40%) | | |
| **Excretion** | Breast milk, urine (50% unchanged), feces (20%) | | |
| **Half-life** | 1-1½ hr; 6-15 hr neonates | | |

### Pharmacodynamics

| | PO | IM | IV |
|---|---|---|---|
| **Onset** | ½-1 hr | 40 min | 5 min |
| **Peak** | 1-2 hr | 1-2 hr | ½ hr |
| **Duration** | 3-6 hr | 4-6 hr | 3-6 hr |

### Interactions
#### Individual drugs
Digoxin: increased toxicity

Indomethacin: decreased diuretic and antihypertensive effects of bumetanide

Lithium: decreased renal clearance causing increased toxicity

Metolazone: increased diuresis, electrolyte loss

Probenecid: decreased diuretic effect
#### Drug classifications
Aminoglycosides: increased ototoxicity

NSAIDs: decreased diuretic effect

Potassium-wasting products: increased hypokalemia
#### Drug/herb
Aloe, cucumber, dandelion, horsetail, pumpkin, Queen Anne's lace: increased diuretic effect

Khella: increased hypotension

St. John's wort: severe photosensitivity
#### Drug/lab test
Increased: urinary phosphate

### NURSING CONSIDERATIONS
#### Assessment
• Assess patient for tinnitus, hearing loss, ear pain; periodic testing of hearing is needed when high doses of this product are given by **IV** route

• Monitor for manifestations of hypokalemia: *RENAL:* acidic urine, reduced urine osmolality, nocturia, polyuria, polydipsia; *CV:* hypotension, broad T wave, U wave, ectopy, tachycardia, weak pulse; *NEURO:* muscle weakness, altered LOC, drowsiness, apathy, lethargy, confusion, depression; *GI:* anorexia, nausea, cramps, constipation, distention, paralytic ileus; *RESP:* hypoventilation, respiratory muscle weakness

• Monitor for manifestations of hypocalcemia: *CNS:* personality changes, anxiety, disturbances, depression, psychosis; *GI:* nausea, vomiting, constipation, abdominal pain from muscle spasm; *CV:* decreased contractility, decreased cardiac output, hypotension, lengthened ST segment, prolonged QT interval; *INTEG:* scaling eczema, alopecia, hyperpigmentation; *NEURO:* tetany, muscle twitching, cramping, grimacing, seizure, altered deep tendon reflexes, spasm

• Monitor for manifestations of hypomagnesemia: *CNS:* agitation; *NEURO:* muscle twitching, paresthesias, hyperactive reflexes, positive Babinski's reflex, dysphagia, nystagmus, seizures, tetany; *GI:* nausea, vomiting, diarrhea, anorexia, abdominal distention; *CV:* ectopy, tachycardia, broad, flat, or inverted T waves, depressed ST segment, prolonged QT, decreased cardiac output, hypotension

• Monitor for manifestations of hyponatremia: *CV:* increased B/P, cold, clammy skin, hypo/hypervolemia; *GI:* anorexia, nausea, vomiting, diarrhea, abdominal cramps; *NEURO:* lethargy, increased ICP, confusion, headache, seizures, coma, fatigue, tremors, hyperreflexia

• Monitor for manifestations of hyperchloremia: *NEURO:* weakness, lethargy, coma; *RESP:* deep rapid breathing

• Assess fluid volume status: I&O ratio and record, distended red veins, crackles in lung, color, quality and specific gravity of urine, skin turgor, adequacy of pulses, moist mucous membranes, bilateral lung sounds, peripheral pitting edema; dehydration symptoms of decreasing output, thirst, hypotension, dry mouth and mucous membranes should be reported; if urinary output decreases or azotemia occurs, product should be discontinued

• Monitor electrolytes: potassium, sodium, calcium, magnesium; also include BUN, blood pH, ABGs, uric acid, CBC, blood glucose

• Assess B/P before and during therapy with patient lying, standing, and sitting as appropriate; orthostatic hypotension can occur rapidly

• Monitor for digoxin toxicity (anorexia, nausea, vomiting, confusion, paresthesia, muscle cramps) in patients taking digoxin; lithium toxicity in those taking lithium

### Nursing diagnoses
- Fluid volume, deficient (side effects)
- Fluid volume, excess (uses)
- Knowledge, deficient (teaching)
- Urinary elimination, impaired (side effects)

### Implementation
- Give in AM to avoid interference with sleep
- Potassium replacement if potassium level is <3.0 mg/dl whole, or use oral solutions; product may be crushed if patient is unable to swallow

**PO route**
- With food, if nausea occurs; absorption may be reduced; the safest dosage schedule is on alternate days

**IV route**
- Do not use solution that is yellow or has a precipitate or crystals

**IV, direct route**
- Give undiluted through Y-tube or 3-way stopcock; give 20 mg or less/min

**Intermittent IV infusion route**
- May be added to 0.9% NaCl, $D_5W$, $D_{10}W$, $D_{20}W$, invert sugar 10% in electrolyte #1, LR, sodium lactate ⅙ mol/L; use within 24 hr to ensure compatibility; give through Y-tube or 3-way stopcock; give at 4 mg/min or less; use infusion pump

*Syringe compatibility:* Doxapram
*Y-site compatibilities:* Allopurinol, amifostine, aztreonam, cefepime, cisatracurium, cladribine, diltiazem, filgrastim, granisetron, lorazepam, morphine, piperacillin/tazobactam, propofol, remifantanil, teniposide, thiotepa, vinorelbine
*Additive compatibilities:* Floxacillin, furosemide

### Patient/family education
- Teach patient to take the medication early in the day to prevent nocturia
- Instruct the patient to take with food or milk if GI symptoms of nausea and anorexia occur
- Teach patient to maintain weekly record of weight and notify prescriber of weight loss of >5 lb
- Caution the patient that this product causes a loss of potassium, so food rich in potassium should be added to the diet; refer to a dietitian for assistance in planning
- Caution the patient not to exercise in hot weather or stand for prolonged periods since orthostatic hypotension will be enhanced
- Teach patient not to use alcohol or any OTC medications without prescriber's approval; serious product reactions may occur
- Emphasize the need to contact prescriber immediately if muscle cramps, weakness, nausea, dizziness, or numbness occurs
- Teach patient to take own B/P and pulse and record
- Caution the patient that orthostatic hypotension may occur; patient should rise slowly from sitting or reclining positions and lie down if dizziness occurs
- Teach patient to continue taking medication even if feeling better; this product controls symptoms but does not cure the condition
- Advise the patient with hypertension to continue other medical treatment (exercise, weight loss, relaxation techniques, cessation of smoking)

### Evaluation
**Positive therapeutic outcome**
- Decreased edema
- Decreased B/P
- Increased diuresis

---

## buprenorphine (Rx)
(byoo-pre-nor′feen)
Buprenex, Subutex
*Func. class.:* Opioid analgesic, partial agonist
*Chem. class.:* Thebaine derivative

**Pregnancy category** C

**Controlled substance schedule V (parenteral); schedule III (tablet)**

**Do not confuse:**
Buprenex/Bumex

**Action:** Inhibits ascending pain pathways in limbic system, thalamus, midbrain, hypothalamus by binding to opiate receptor sites; this alters pain perception and response; generalized CNS depression

**Therapeutic outcome:** Relief of pain

**Uses:** Moderate to severe pain

### Dosage and routes
*Adult:* IM/IV 0.3 mg q6hr prn; may repeat dose after ½ hr; reduce dosage in geriatric, may repeat after ½ hr; EPIDURAL 60-180 mcg over 48 hr
*Child 2-12 yr:* IM/IV 2-6 mcg/kg q4-6hr
*Geriatric:* PO 0.15 mg q6hr prn

**Available forms:** Inj 0.3 mg/ml (1-ml vials); SL tab 2, 8 mg as base

## Adverse effects
*CNS: Drowsiness, dizziness, confusion, headache, sedation, euphoria,* **increased intracranial pressure,** amnesia
*CV:* Palpitations, bradycardia, change in B/P, tachycardia
*EENT:* Tinnitus, blurred vision, *miosis,* diplopia
*GI: Nausea,* vomiting, anorexia, constipation, cramps, dry mouth
*GU:* Increased urinary output, dysuria, urinary retention
*INTEG: Rash,* urticaria, bruising, flushing, diaphoresis, pruritus
*RESP:* **Respiratory depression,** dyspnea, hypo/hyperventilation

**Contraindications:** Hypersensitivity

**Precautions:** Pregnancy **C**, breastfeeding, addictive personality, increased intracranial pressure, MI (acute), severe heart disease, respiratory depression, renal/hepatic disease, hypothyroidism, Addison's disease, addiction (opioid)

### Pharmacokinetics
| | |
|---|---|
| Absorption | Well absorbed (IM) |
| Distribution | Crosses placenta |
| Metabolism | Liver, extensively |
| Excretion | Kidneys, feces, breast milk |
| Half-life | 2½-3½ hr |

### Pharmacodynamics
| | IM | IV |
|---|---|---|
| Onset | 10-15 min | Immediate |
| Peak | 1 hr | 5 min |
| Duration | 6 hr | 6 hr |

### Interactions
*Individual drugs*
Alcohol: increased respiratory depression, hypotension, sedation
*Drug classifications*
Antihistamines, antipsychotics, CNS depressants, MAOIs, sedatives/hypnotics, skeletal muscle relaxants: increased respiratory depression, hypotension
CYP3A4 inducers (carbamazepine, phenobarbital, phenytoin, rifampin): decreased buprenorphine effect
CYP3A4 inhibitors (erythromycin, indinavir, ketoconazole, ritonavir, saquinavir): increased buprenorphine effect
Opioids: increased CNS depression
*Drug/herb*
Corkwood: increased anticholinergic effect
Gotu kola, Jamaican dogwood, kava, lavender, mistletoe, nettle, pokeweed, poppy, senega, St. John's wort, valerian: increased CNS depression

### NURSING CONSIDERATIONS
#### Assessment
• Assess pain characteristics: location, intensity, type, severity before medication administration and after treatment
• Monitor VS after parenteral route; note muscle rigidity, product history, liver, kidney function tests, respiratory dysfunction: respiratory depression, character, rate, rhythm; notify prescriber if respirations are <10/min
• Monitor CNS changes: dizziness, drowsiness, hallucinations, euphoria, LOC, pupil reaction; withdrawal in opioid-dependent persons; if dependence occurs within 2 wk of discontinuing product, withdrawal symptoms will occur
• Monitor allergic reactions: rash, urticaria

#### Nursing diagnoses
• Breathing pattern, ineffective (adverse reactions)
• Knowledge, deficient (teaching)
• Pain, acute (uses)
• Pain, chronic
• Sensory perception, disturbed (adverse reactions)

#### Implementation
• Give by inj (IM, **IV**), only with resuscitative equipment available; give slowly to prevent rigidity
• Long-term use is not recommended
**IM route**
• Give deep in large muscle mass; rotate sites of inj
**IV route**
• Give **IV** direct undiluted over 3-5 min (0.3 mg/2 min); give slowly
*Syringe compatibility:* Midazolam
*Y-site compatibilities:* Allopurinol, amifostine, aztreonam, cefepime, cisatracurium, cladribine, filgrastim, granisetron, melphalan, piperacillin/tazobactam, propofol, remifentanil, teniposide, thiotepa, vinorelbine
*Additive compatibilities:* Atropine, bupivacaine, diphenhydrAMINE, droperidol, glycopyrrolate, haloperidol, hydrOXYzine, promethazine, scopolamine
*Additive incompatibilities:* Diazepam, floxacillin, furosemide, lorazepam

#### Patient/family education
• Instruct patient to report any symptoms of CNS changes, allergic reactions
• Caution patients to avoid CNS depressants: alcohol, sedative/hypnotics for at least 24 hr after taking this product

Adverse effects: *italic* = common, **bold** = life-threatening

- Discuss with patient that dizziness, drowsiness, and confusion are common; to avoid getting up without assistance, to avoid hazardous activities
- Discuss in detail all aspects of the product

### Evaluation
**Positive therapeutic outcome**
- Relief of pain

**Treatment of overdose:** Naloxone 0.4 mg ampule diluted in 10 ml 0.9% NaCl, give by direct **IV** push 0.02 mg q2min (adult)

---

## *buPROPion (Rx)
(byoo-proe′pee-on)
Budeprion SR, buPROPion, Wellbutrin, Wellbutrin SR, Wellbutrin XL, Zyban
*Func. class.:* Antidepressant—miscellaneous, smoking deterrent
*Chem. class.:* Aminoketone

### Pregnancy category B

**Do not confuse:**
buPROPion/busPIRone, Zyban/Diovan/Zagam

**Action:** Inhibits reuptake of dopamine, serotonin, norepinephrine

**Therapeutic outcome:** Decreased symptoms of depression after 2-3 wk

**Uses:** Depression (Wellbutrin), smoking cessation (Zyban)

**Unlabeled uses:** Neuropathic pain, enhancement of weight loss, attention deficit hyperactivity disorder (ADHD)

### Dosage and routes
*Depression*
*Adult:* PO 100 mg bid initially, then increase after 3 days to 100 mg tid if needed; may increase after 1 mo to 150 mg tid; SR, initially 150 mg AM, increase to 300 mg/day if initial dose is tolerated
*Geriatric:* PO 50-100 mg/day, may increase by 50-100 mg q3-4 days

*Smoking cessation*
*Adult:* PO 150 mg bid, begin with 150 mg daily × 3 days then 300 mg/day continue for 7-12 wk, not to exceed 300 mg/day

**Available forms:** Tabs 75, 100 mg; sus rel tabs (Zyban) 100, 150, 200 mg; ext rel tab (XL) 150, 300 mg (SR-12 hr, XL-24 hr)

### Adverse effects
*CNS: Headache, agitation, confusion,* **seizures,** delusions, *insomnia, sedation, tremors,* dizziness, akinesia, bradykinesia, **suicidal ideation**

*CV:* **Dysrhythmias,** *hypertension,* palpitations, *tachycardia,* hypotension, **complete AV block**
*EENT: Blurred vision, auditory disturbance*
*GI: Nausea, vomiting, dry mouth,* anorexia, diarrhea, increased appetite, *constipation*
*GU:* Impotence, frequency, retention, *menstrual irregularities*
*INTEG: Rash,* pruritus, *sweating,* **Stevens-Johnson syndrome**
*MISC: Weight loss or gain*

**Contraindications:** Hypersensitivity, eating disorders, seizure disorder

**Precautions:** Pregnancy **B,** breastfeeding, children <18 yr, geriatric, renal/hepatic disease, recent MI, cranial trauma, seizure disorders, suicidal thinking/behavior (young adults)

### Pharmacokinetics
| | |
|---|---|
| **Absorption** | Well absorbed; bioavailability poor |
| **Distribution** | Unknown |
| **Metabolism** | Liver extensively |
| **Excretion** | Kidneys |
| **Half-life** | 14 hr, steady state 1½-5 wk |

### Pharmacodynamics
| | |
|---|---|
| **Onset** | Up to 4 wk |
| **Peak** | Unknown |
| **Duration** | Unknown |

### Interactions
*Individual drugs*
Alcohol, levodopa, theophylline: increased risk of seizures
Carbamazepine, cimetidine, phenobarbital, phenytoin: decreased buPROPion effect
Cimetidine: increased buPROPion levels
Ritonavir: increased buPROPion toxicity
*Drug classifications*
Antidepressants, benzodiazepines, MAOIs, phenothiazines, steroids (systemic): increased risk of seizures
CYP450, CYP2D6 products: decreased buPROPion effects
MAOIs: acute toxicity
*Drug/herb*
Belladonna, corkwood, jimsonweed: increased anticholinergic effect
Hops, kava, lavender: increased CNS depression

### NURSING CONSIDERATIONS
**Assessment**
- Monitor B/P (with patient lying, standing), pulse q4hr; if systolic B/P drops 20 mm Hg

---

hold product, notify prescriber; take vital signs q4hr in patients with CV disease
• Assess smoking cessation progress after 7-12 wk, if progress has not been made, product should be discontinued
• Assess for increased risk of seizures; if patient has used CNS depressant or CNS stimulants, dosage of buPROPion should not be exceeded
• Monitor blood studies: CBC, leukocytes, differential, cardiac enzymes if patient is receiving long-term therapy
• Monitor hepatic studies: AST, ALT, bilirubin if on long-term treatment
• Check weight weekly; appetite may increase with product
• Assess ECG for flattening of T wave, bundle branch block, AV block, dysrhythmias in cardiac patients
• Assess for EPS primarily in geriatric: rigidity, dystonia, akathisia
• Assess mental status: mood, sensorium, affect, suicidal tendencies; increase in psychiatric symptoms: depression, panic
• Monitor urinary retention, constipation; constipation is more likely to occur in children or geriatric
• Identify alcohol consumption; if alcohol was consumed, hold dose

### Nursing diagnoses
• Coping, ineffective (uses)
• Injury, risk for (side effects)
• Knowledge, deficient (teaching)
• Noncompliance (teaching)

### Implementation
• Give with food or milk for GI symptoms
• Give sugarless gum, hard candy, or frequent sips of water for dry mouth
• Store at room temperature; do not freeze

### Patient/family education
• Teach patient that therapeutic effects may take 2-3 wk; not to increase dose without prescriber's approval; that treatment for smoking cessation lasts 7-12 wk
• Teach patient to use caution in driving or other activities requiring alertness because of drowsiness, dizziness, blurred vision; to avoid rising quickly from sitting to standing, especially geriatric
• Teach patient to avoid alcohol ingestion; alcohol may increase risk of seizures, obtain approval for other products
• Teach patient to increase fluids, bulk in diet if constipation, urinary retention occur, especially geriatric; notify prescriber immediately if retention occurs

• Teach patient to take gum, hard sugarless candy, or frequent sips of water for dry mouth
• Advise patient not to use with nicotine patches unless directed by prescriber, may increase B/P
• Teach patient that risk of seizures increases when dose is exceeded, or if patient has seizure disorder; suicidal ideas, behavior may occur in children or young adults
• Teach patient to notify prescriber if pregnancy is suspected or planned

### Evaluation
**Positive therapeutic outcome**
• Decrease in depression
• Absence of suicidal thoughts
• Smoking cessation

**Treatment of overdose:** ECG monitoring, induce emesis, lavage, activated charcoal, administer anticonvulsant

---

## *busPIRone (Rx)
(byoo-spye'rone)
BuSpar, BuSpar Dividose, VanSpor
*Func. class.:* Antianxiety, sedative
*Chem. class.:* Azaspirodecanedione
**Pregnancy category B**

**Do not confuse:**
busPIRone/buPROPion

**Action:** Acts by inhibiting the action of serotonin (5-HT) by binding to serotonin and dopamine receptors; also increases norepinephrine metabolism; has shown little potential for abuse

**Therapeutic outcome:** Decreased anxiety

**Uses:** Management and short-term relief of generalized anxiety disorders

**Dosage and routes**
*Adult:* PO 5 mg tid; may increase by 5 mg/day q2-3 days; max 60 mg/day

**Available forms:** Tabs 5, 10, 15, 30 mg

**Adverse effects**
*CNS: Dizziness, headache, depression, stimulation, insomnia, nervousness, lightheadedness, numbness, paresthesia, incoordination, tremors,* excitement, involuntary movements, confusion, akathisia, nightmares, hostility
*CV: Tachycardia, palpitations,* hypo/hypertension, **CVA, CHF, MI**

***EENT:*** *Sore throat, tinnitus, blurred vision, nasal congestion,* red, itching eyes, change in taste, smell

***GI:*** *Nausea, dry mouth, diarrhea, constipation,* flatulence, increased appetite, rectal bleeding

***GU:*** Frequency, hesitancy, menstrual irregularity, change in libido

***INTEG:*** *Rash,* edema, pruritus, alopecia, dry skin

***MISC:*** *Sweating,* fatigue, weight gain, fever

***MS:*** *Pain, weakness,* muscle cramps, spasms

***RESP:*** Hyperventilation, chest congestion, shortness of breath

**Contraindications:** Hypersensitivity, child <18 yr

**Precautions:** Pregnancy **B**, breastfeeding, geriatric, impaired renal/hepatic function

| Pharmacokinetics | |
|---|---|
| **Absorption** | Rapidly absorbed |
| **Distribution** | Unknown |
| **Metabolism** | Liver, extensively |
| **Excretion** | Feces |
| **Half-life** | 2-3 hr |

| Pharmacodynamics | |
|---|---|
| **Onset** | Unknown |
| **Peak** | 40-90 min |
| **Duration** | Unknown |

### Interactions
#### Individual drugs
Alcohol: increased CNS depression

Carbamazepine, dexamethasone, phenobarbitol, phenytoin, rifampin: decreased busPIRone effect

Erythromycin, itraconazole, ketoconazole, nefazodone, ritonavir: increased busPIRone levels

#### Drug classifications
CYP450 products: increased busPIRone levels

MAOIs, procarbazine: increased B/P, do not use together

Products induced by CYP3A4: decreased busPIRone action

Psychotropics: increased CNS depression

Selective serotonin reuptake inhibitors: increase serotonin syndrome

#### Drug/herb
Cowslip, kava, Queen Anne's lace, valerian: increased CNS depression

#### Drug/food
Grapefruit juice: increased peak concentration of busPIRone

## NURSING CONSIDERATIONS
### Assessment
• Assess anxiety reaction: inability to sleep, apprehension, dread, foreboding, or uneasiness related to unidentified source of danger

• Assess for previous product dependence or tolerance; if patient is product dependent or tolerant, amount of medication should be restricted

• Monitor B/P (lying, standing), pulse; if systolic B/P drops 20 mm Hg, hold product, notify prescriber; check I&O; may indicate renal dysfunction

• Monitor mental status: mood, sensorium, affect, sleeping patterns, drowsiness, dizziness, suicidal tendencies; withdrawal symptoms when dose is reduced or product discontinued

• Assess for CNS reaction, some reactions may be unpredictable

### Nursing diagnoses
• Anxiety (uses)
• Knowledge, deficient (teaching)
• Noncompliance (teaching)

### Implementation
• Give with food or milk for GI symptoms; sugarless gum, hard candy, frequent sips of water for dry mouth

• May be crushed

### Patient/family education
• Teach patient that product may be taken with food; if dose is missed take as soon as remembered; do not double doses

• Caution patient to avoid OTC preparations unless approved by the prescriber; to avoid alcohol ingestion and other psychotropic medications unless prescribed; that 1-2 wk of therapy may be required before therapeutic effects occur; to avoid large amounts of grapefruit juice

• Caution patient to avoid driving and activities requiring alertness since drowsiness may occur; until medication response is known, tell patient that drowsiness may worsen at beginning of treatment

• Instruct patient not to discontinue medication abruptly after long-term use; if dose is missed, do not double

• Advise patient to rise slowly or fainting may occur, especially in geriatric

### Evaluation
**Positive therapeutic outcome**
• Increased well-being
• Decreased anxiety, restlessness, sleeplessness, dread

**Treatment of overdose:** Gastric lavage, VS, supportive care

## ⚠ HIGH ALERT

## busulfan (Rx)
(byoo-sul'fan)
Busulfex, Myleran
*Func. class.:* Antineoplastic alkylating agent
*Chem. class.:* Nitrosourea

### Pregnancy category D

### Do not confuse:
Myleran/Leukeran

**Action:** Changes essential cellular ions to covalent bonding with resultant alkylation; this interferes with normal biologic function of DNA; activity is not phase specific; action is due to myelosuppression

**Therapeutic outcome:** Prevention of rapid growth of malignant cells in chronic myelocytic leukemia

**Uses:** Chronic myelocytic leukemia, bone marrow ablation, stem cell transplant preparation in CML

### Dosage and routes
*Chronic myelocytic (granulocytic) leukemia*
*Adult:* PO 4-8 mg/day initially until WBC levels fall to 15,000/mm³; then product is stopped until WBC levels rise over 50,000/mm³; then 1-3 mg/day
*Child:* PO 0.06-0.12 mg/kg or 1.8-4.6 mg/m²/day; dosage is titrated to maintain WBC levels at 20,000/mm³, but never <10,000 mm³

*Allogenic hemopoietic stem cell transplantation in chronic myelogenous leukemia*
*Adult:* **IV** 0.8 mg/kg q6hr × 4 days (total 16 doses); give cyclophosphamide **IV** 60 mg/kg over 1 hr/day for 2 days, starting after 16th dose of busulfan

**Available forms:** Tabs 2 mg; sol for inj 6 mg/ml

### Adverse effects
**PO route**
*CV: Hypotension,* **thrombosis,** *chest pain,* **tachycardia, atrial fibrillation, heart block,** pericardial effusion, **cardiac tamponade** (high dose with cyclophosphamide)
*GI:* Anorexia, constipation, dry mouth, nausea, vomiting, *diarrhea*
*RESP:* **Alveolar hemorrhage,** atelectasis, cough, hemoptysis, hypoxia, pleural effusion, pneumonia, sinusitis, **pulmonary fibrosis**
**IV route**
*CNS:* **Cerebral hemorrhage, coma, seizures,** *anxiety, depression, dizziness, headache,* encephalopathy, weakness, mental changes
*EENT: Pharyngitis, epistaxis, cataracts*
*GI: Diarrhea, nausea, vomiting, weight loss*
*GU:* Impotence, sterility, amenorrhea, gynecomastia, **renal toxicity,** hyperuremia, adrenal insufficiency–like syndrome
*HEMA:* **Thrombocytopenia, leukopenia, pancytopenia, severe bone marrow depression**
*INTEG:* Dermatitis, hyperpigmentation, alopecia
*MISC:* **Chromosomal aberrations**
*RESP:* Irreversible pulmonary fibrosis: pneumonitis

**Contraindications:** Pregnancy **D** (3rd trimester), breastfeeding, radiation, chemotherapy, blastic phase of chronic myelocytic leukemia, hypersensitivity

**Precautions:** Child-bearing-age men and women, leukopenia, thrombocytopenia, anemia, hepatotoxicity, renal toxicity

### Pharmacokinetics

| | |
|---|---|
| **Absorption** | Rapidly absorbed |
| **Distribution** | Unknown; crosses placenta |
| **Metabolism** | Liver, extensively |
| **Excretion** | Kidneys, breast milk |
| **Half-life** | 2.5 hr |

### Pharmacodynamics
Unknown

### Interactions
*Individual drugs*
Acetaminophen, itraconazole: decreased busulfan clearance
Cyclophosphamide: cardiac tamponade
Phenytoin: decreased busulfan level
Radiation: increased toxicity, bone marrow suppression
Thioguanine: hepatotoxicity
*Drug classifications*
Anticoagulants, salicylates: increased risk of bleeding
Antineoplastics: increased toxicity, bone marrow suppression
Live virus vaccines: decreased antibody reaction
*Drug/lab test*
False positive: breast, bladder, cervix, lung cytology tests

### NURSING CONSIDERATIONS
**Assessment**
• Monitor CBC, differential, platelet count weekly; withhold product if WBC <4000/mm³

Adverse effects: *italic* = common, **bold** = life-threatening

or platelets <75,000/mm³; notify prescriber of results if WBC <15,000/mm³, platelets <150,000/mm³; institute thrombocytopenia precautions
• Monitor pulmonary function tests, chest x-ray films before, during therapy; chest film should be obtained q2 wk during treatment; check for dyspnea, crackles, nonproductive cough, chest pain, tachypnea; pulmonary fibrosis may occur up to 10 yr after treatment with busulfan
• Assess for increased uric acid levels, swelling, joint pain primarily in extremities; patient should be well hydrated to prevent urate deposits
• Monitor renal function studies: BUN, serum uric acid, urine CCr before, during therapy; I&O ratio; report fall in urine output of 30 ml/hr; check for decreased hyperuricemia
• Monitor for cold, fever, sore throat (may indicate beginning infection); identify edema in feet, joint or stomach pain, shaking; prescriber should be notified
• Assess for bleeding: hematuria, guaiac, bruising or petechiae, mucosa or orifices q8hr; no rectal temps

### Nursing diagnoses
• Body image, disturbed (adverse reactions)
• Infection, risk for (adverse reactions)
• Injury, risk for (adverse reactions)
• Knowledge, deficient (teaching)

### Implementation
• Give 1 hr before or 2 hr after meals to lessen nausea and vomiting; give at same time daily
• Increased fluid intake to 2-3 L/day to prevent urate deposits, calculus formation
• Administer antibiotics for prophylaxis of infection; may be prescribed since infection potential is high
• Store in tight container
**IV route**
• Prepare in biologic cabinet using gloves, gown, mask; dilute with 10 times volume of product using D₅W or 0.9% NaCl (0.5 mg/ml); when withdrawing product, use needle with 5-micron filter provided, remove amount needed, remove filter, and inject product into diluent; always add product to diluent, not vice versa; stable for 8 hr at room temperature using D₅W or 0.9% NaCl; give by central venous catheter over 2 hr q6hr × 4 days, use infusion pump, do not admix
• Give antiemetic before **IV** route
• Give phenytoin before **IV** to prevent seizures in those with seizure disorders

### Patient/family education
• Teach patient to avoid use of products containing aspirin or ibuprofen, razors, commercial mouthwash since bleeding may occur; to report symptoms of bleeding (hematuria, tarry stools)
• Instruct patient to report signs of anemia (fatigue, headache, irritability, faintness, shortness of breath)
• Instruct patient to report any changes in breathing or coughing even several months after treatment; to avoid crowds and persons with respiratory tract or other infections
• Teach patient that hair loss may occur; discuss the use of wigs or hair pieces
• Caution patient not to have any vaccinations without the advice of the prescriber; serious reactions can occur
• Advise patient that contraception is needed during treatment and for several months after the completion of therapy

### Evaluation
**Positive therapeutic outcome**
• Decreased leukocytes to normal limits
• Absence of sweating at night
• Increased appetite, increased weight

---

## butoconazole vaginal antifungal
*See Appendix D*

---

## butorphanol (Rx)
(byoo-tor′fa-nole)
Stadol
*Func. class.:* Mixed opiate analgesic
*Chem class:* Opioid antagonist, partial agonist
**Pregnancy category** C
**Controlled substance schedule** IV

**Do not confuse:**
Stadol/Haldol/Sotalol

**Action:** Inhibits ascending pain pathways in limbic system, thalamus, midbrain, hypothalamus by binding to opiate receptor sites; this alters pain perception and response

**Therapeutic outcome:** Relief of pain

**Uses:** Moderate to severe pain

**Unlabeled uses:** Migraine headache, pain

**Dosage and routes**
*Adult:* IM 1-4 mg q3-4hr prn; **IV** 0.5-2 mg q3-4hr prn; nasal spray in 1 nostril q3-4hr;

---

may give another dose 1-1½ hr later; may repeat q3-4hr

*Geriatric:* **IV** ½ adult dose at 2× the interval; INTRANASAL may repeat q1-2hr

### Severe pain
*Adult:* INTRANASAL 1 spray in each nostril q3-4hr

### Renal dose
*Adult:* **IV**/IM CCr 10-50 ml/min 75% dose; CCr <10 ml/min 50% dose

**Available forms:** Inj 1, 2 mg/ml; intranasal 10 mg/ml

### Adverse effects
*CNS: Drowsiness, dizziness, confusion, headache, sedation, euphoria, weakness, hallucinations*
*CV:* Palpitations, bradycardia, hypotension
*EENT:* Tinnitus, blurred vision, miosis, diplopia, nasal congestion, unpleasant taste
*GI: Nausea, vomiting, anorexia, constipation, cramps*
*GU:* Increased urinary output, dysuria, urinary retention
*INTEG:* Rash, urticaria, bruising, flushing, diaphoresis, pruritus
*RESP:* **Respiratory depression,** pulmonary hypertension, upper respiratory infection, sinusitis

**Contraindications:** Hypersensitivity to this product or preservative, addiction (opioid), CHF, MI

**Precautions:** Pregnancy **C**, breastfeeding, child <18 yr, addictive personality, increased ICP, respiratory depression, renal/hepatic disease, bowel impaction

| Pharmacokinetics | |
|---|---|
| Absorption | Well absorbed (IM, nasal); complete (**IV**) |
| Distribution | Crosses placenta, protein binding 80% |
| Metabolism | Liver, extensively |
| Excretion | Feces (10%-15%); kidneys, unchanged (small amounts) |
| Half-life | 3-4 hr |

| Pharmacodynamics | | | |
|---|---|---|---|
| | IM | IV | NASAL |
| Onset | 5-10 min | 1 min | 15 min |
| Peak | ½ hr | 5 min | 1-2 hr |
| Duration | 3-4 hr | 2-4 hr | 4-5 hr |

### Interactions
#### Individual drugs
Alcohol: increased respiratory depression, hypotension, sedation
#### Drug classifications
Antipsychotics, CNS depressants, opioids, sedative/hypnotics, skeletal muscle relaxants: increased respiratory depression, hypotension
MAOIs: do not use 2 wk before butorphanol, fatal reaction
#### Drug/herb
Chamomile, kava, Jamaican dogwood, lavender, mistletoe, nettle, pokeweed, poppy, senega, skullcap, St. John's wort, valerian: increased CNS depression
Corkwood: increased anticholinergic effect

### NURSING CONSIDERATIONS
#### Assessment
• Monitor VS after parenteral route; note muscle rigidity, product history, liver, kidney function tests, respiratory dysfunction: respiratory depression, character, rate, rhythm; notify prescriber if respirations are <10/min
• Monitor CNS changes: dizziness, drowsiness, hallucinations, euphoria, LOC, pupil reaction
• Monitor allergic reactions: rash, urticaria

#### Nursing diagnoses
• Injury, risk for (adverse reactions)
• Knowledge, deficient (teaching)
• Pain, acute (uses)
• Pain, chronic (uses)
• Sensory perception, disturbed (adverse reactions)

#### Implementation
• Store in light-resistant container at room temperature
**IM route**
• Give deeply in large muscle mass; rotate inj sites
**Intranasal route**
• Give 1 spray in nostril
• Remove clip and cover, prime before using until spray appears; pump must be reprimed q48hr; close nostril with finger and spray once quickly; have patient sniff
**IV route**
• Give **IV** undiluted at a rate of ≤2 mg/>3-5 min; titrate to patient response
*Syringe compatibilities:* Atropine, chlorproMAZINE, cimetidine, diphenhydrAMINE, droperidol, fentanyl, hydrOXYzine, meperidine, methotrimeprazine, metoclopramide, midazolam, morphine, pentazocine, perphenazine, prochlorperazine, promethazine, scopolamine, thiethylperazine

Adverse effects: *italic* = common, **bold** = life-threatening

*Syringe incompatibilities:* Dimenhy-DRINATE, pentobarbital

*Y-site compatibilities:* Allopurinol, amifostine, azetreonam, cefepime, cisatracurium, cladribine, DOXOrubicin liposome, enalaprilat, esmolol, filgrastim, fludarabine, granisetron, labetalol, melphalan, paclitaxel, piperacillin/tazobactam, propofol, remifentanil, sargramostim, teniposide, thiotepa, vinorelbine

## Patient/family education

- Instruct patient to report any symptoms of CNS changes, allergic reactions; to avoid CNS depressants: alcohol, sedative/hypnotics for at least 24 hr after taking this product
- Discuss with patient that dizziness, drowsiness, and confusion are common; to avoid getting up without assistance, hazardous activities
- Discuss in detail all aspects of the product

**Nasal route**

- Teach patient to blow nose to clear both nostrils before using
- Patient should replace clip and cover after use; caution patient not to shake medication

## Evaluation

**Positive therapeutic outcome**

- Pain relief

**Treatment of overdose:** Narcan 0.2-0.8 **IV**, $O_2$, **IV** fluids, vasopressors

---

## calcitonin (rDNA) (Rx)
(kal-sih-toh'nin)
Fortical

## calcitonin (salmon) (Rx)
Calcimir, Miacalcin, Miacalin Nasal Spray, Osteocalcin, Salmonine

*Func. class.:* Parathyroid agents (calcium regulator)

*Chem. class.:* Polypeptide hormone

**Pregnancy category** C

---

**Action:** Decreases bone resorption, blood calcium levels by direct action on bone, GI system, and kidney; increases deposits of calcium in bones; renal excretion of calcium occurs; opposes parathyroid hormone

**Therapeutic outcome:** Lowered calcium level, decreasing symptoms of Paget's disease

**Uses:** Paget's disease, postmenopausal osteoporosis, hypercalcemia

## Dosage and routes

*rDNA*

*Paget's disease*

*Adult:* SUBCUT 0.5 mg/day initially; may require 0.5 mg bid × 6 mo, then decrease until symptoms reappear

*Salmon*

*Postmenopausal osteoporosis*

*Adult:* SUBCUT/IM 100 international units/day; NASAL 200 international units (1 spray) alternating nostrils daily, activate pump before 1st dose

*Paget's disease*

*Adult:* SUBCUT/IM 100 international units daily, maintenance 50-100 international units daily or every other day

*Hypercalcemia*

*Adult:* SUBCUT/IM 4 international units/kg q12hr, increase to 8 international units/kg q12hr if response is unsatisfactory

**Available forms:** Inj 200 international units/ml; nasal spray 200 international units/actuation

## Adverse effects

*CNS:* Headache, **tetany**, chills, weakness, dizziness, fever

*CV:* Chest pressure

*EENT:* Nasal congestion, eye pain

*GI:* Nausea, diarrhea, vomiting, anorexia, abdominal pain, salty taste, epigastric pain

*GU:* Diuresis, nocturia, urine sediment, frequency

*INTEG:* Rash, flushing, pruritus of earlobes, edema of feet, inj site reaction

*MS:* Swelling, tingling of hands, backache

*RESP:* Dyspnea

*SYST:* **Anaphylaxis**

**Contraindications:** Hypersensitivity

**Precautions:** Pregnancy C, breastfeeding, children, renal disease, osteogenic sarcoma, pernicious anemia

| Pharmacokinetics | |
|---|---|
| **Absorption** | Completely absorbed |
| **Distribution** | Unknown |
| **Metabolism** | Rapid; kidneys, tissue, blood |
| **Excretion** | Kidneys, inactive metabolite |
| **Half-life** | 1 hr |

| Pharmacodynamics | |
|---|---|
| | SUBCUT |
| **Onset** | 15 min |
| **Peak** | 4 hr |
| **Duration** | 8-24 hr |

### Interactions
*Individual drugs*
Lithium: decreased lithium effect

### NURSING CONSIDERATIONS
### Assessment
• Assess for GI symptoms, polyuria, flushing, head swelling, tingling, headache; may indicate hypercalcemia; nervousness, irritability, twitching, seizures, spasm, paresthesia indicate hypocalcemia during beginning of treatment
• Identify nutritional status; check diet for sources of vit D (milk, some seafood), calcium (dairy products, dark green vegetables), phosphates
• Monitor BUN, creatinine, uric acid, chloride, electrolytes, urine pH, urinary calcium, magnesium, phosphate, urinalysis (calcium should be kept at 9-10 mg/dl; vit D 50-135 international units/dl), alkaline phosphatase baseline and q3-6 mo; check urine sediment for casts throughout treatment; monitor urine hydroxyproline in Paget's disease, biochemical markers of bone formation/absorption, radiologic evidence of fracture; bone density (osteoporosis)
• Assess for increased product level, since toxic reactions occur rapidly; have parenteral calcium or gluconate on hand if calcium level drops too low; check for tetany (irritability, paresthesia, nervousness, muscle twitching, seizure, tetanic spasm)

### Nursing diagnoses
• Injury, risk for (adverse reactions)
• Knowledge, deficient (teaching)
• Pain, chronic (uses)

### Implementation
• Store at <77° F (25° C); protect from light
**SUBCUT route (human)**
• Give by SUBCUT route only; rotate inj sites; use within 6 hr of reconstitution; give at bedtime to minimize nausea, vomiting
**IM route (salmon)**
• After test dose of 10 international units/ml, 0.1 ml intradermally; watch 15 min; give only with epINEPHrine and emergency meds available
• IM inj in deep muscle mass slowly; rotate sites; preferred route if volume is >2 ml
**Nasal route**
• Use alternating nostrils for nasal spray; allow to warm to room temperature, prime to get full spray

### Patient/family education
• Teach method of inj if patient will be responsible for self-medication

• Instruct patient to notify prescriber for hypercalcemic relapse: renal calculi, nausea, vomiting, thirst, lethargy, deep bone or flank pain
• Teach patient that warmth and flushing occur and last 1 hr
• Provide a low-calcium diet as prescribed (Paget's disease, hypercalcemia)
• Advise patients with osteoporosis to increase calcium and vit D in diet and to continue with moderate exercise to prevent continued bone loss
• Advise patients to report difficulty swallowing or change in side effects to prescriber immediately

### Evaluation
**Positive therapeutic outcome**
• Calcium levels 9-10 mg/dl
• Decreasing symptoms of Paget's disease, including pain
• Decreased bone loss in osteoporosis

### calcitriol (Rx)
(kal-si-tree'ole)
Rocaltrol, Vitamin D₃
*Func. class.:* Parathyroid agent (calcium regulator)
*Chem. class.:* Vitamin D hormone
**Pregnancy category C**

**Do not confuse:**
calcitriol/Calciferol

**Action:** Increases intestinal absorption of calcium, provides calcium for bones, increases renal tubular resorption of phosphate

**Therapeutic outcome:** Calcium at normal level

**Uses:** Hypocalcemia in chronic renal disease, hyperparathyroidism, pseudohypoparathyroidism

### Dosage and routes
*Hypocalcemia*
*Adult:* **IV** 0.5 mcg tid, initially; may increase by 0.25-0.5 mcg/dose q2-4 wk; 0.5-3 mcg tid maintenance

*Predialysis*
*Adult:* PO 0.25 mcg/day, max 0.5 mcg/day
*Child:* PO 0.25 mcg/day, max 0.5 mcg/day
*Child <3 yr:* PO 10-15 mcg/kg/day

*Hypocalcemia during chronic dialysis*
*Adult:* PO 0.5-3 mcg/day
*Child:* PO 0.25-2 mcg/day

*Renal osteodystrophy*
**Adult:** PO 0.25 mcg every other day-3 mcg/day
**Child:** PO 0.014-0.041 mcg/kg/day

*Hypoparathyroidism*
**Adult:** PO 0.25-2.7 mcg/day
**Child:** PO 0.04-0.08 mcg/kg/day

**Available forms:** Caps 0.25, 0.5 mcg; inj 1 mcg, 2 mcg/ml; oral sol 1 mcg/ml

**Adverse effects**
*CNS:* Drowsiness, headache, vertigo, fever, lethargy, hallucinations
*CV:* Palpitations, hypertension
*EENT:* Blurred vision, photophobia
*GI:* Nausea, diarrhea, vomiting, jaundice, anorexia, dry mouth, constipation, cramps, metallic taste
*GU:* Polyuria, hypercalciuria, hyperphosphatemia, hematuria, thirst
*MS:* Myalgia, arthralgia, decreased bone development, weakness
*SYST:* Anaphylaxis

**Contraindications:** Hypersensitivity, hyperphosphatemia, hypercalcemia, vit D toxicity

**Precautions:** Pregnancy **C**, breastfeeding, renal calculi, CV disease

| Pharmacokinetics | |
| --- | --- |
| **Absorption** | Well absorbed |
| **Distribution** | To liver, crosses placenta |
| **Metabolism** | Liver |
| **Excretion** | Bile |
| **Half-life** | 3-6 hr, undergoes hepatic recycling, excreted in bile |

| Pharmacodynamics | |
| --- | --- |
| **Onset** | 2-6 hr |
| **Peak** | 10-12 hr |
| **Duration** | Up to 5 days |

**Interactions**
*Individual drugs*
Cholestyramine, mineral oil: decreased absorption of calcitriol
Phenytoin: increased vit D metabolism
Verapamil: increased dysrhythmias
*Drug classifications*
Antacids (magnesium): increased hypermagnesemia
Diuretics (thiazide), calcium supplements: increased hypercalcemia
Cardiac glycosides: increased dysrhythmias
Vitamin D products: increased toxicity
Vitamins (fat-soluble): decreased calcitriol absorption

*Drug/food*
Large amounts of high-calcium foods may cause hypercalcemia
*Drug/lab test*
False: increased cholesterol
Interference: alkaline phosphatase, electrolytes

**NURSING CONSIDERATIONS**
**Assessment**
• Assess GI symptoms, polyuria, flushing, head swelling, tingling, headache; may indicate hypercalcemia
• Identify nutritional status; check diet for sources of vit D (milk, some seafood), calcium (dairy products, dark green vegetables), phosphates
• Monitor BUN, creatinine, uric acid, chloride, electrolytes, urine pH, urinary calcium, magnesium, phosphate, urinalysis (calcium should be kept at 9-10 mg/dl; vit D 50-135 international units/dl), alkaline phosphatase baseline and q3-6 mo
◆ Assess for increased product level, since toxic reactions occur rapidly; have calcium chloride on hand if calcium level drops too low; check for tetany

**Nursing diagnoses**
• Injury, risk for (adverse reactions)
• Knowledge, deficient (teaching)
• Pain, chronic (uses)

**Implementation**
**PO route**
• Do not break, crush, or chew caps
• Give with meals for GI symptoms
**IV route**
• Give by direct **IV** over 1 min

**Patient/family education**
• Teach patient the symptoms of hypercalcemia (renal stones, nausea, vomiting, anorexia, lethargy, thirst, bone or flank pain) and about foods rich in calcium
• Advise patient to avoid products with sodium: cured meats, dairy products, cold cuts, olives, beets, pickles, soups, meat tenderizers in chronic renal failure
• Advise patient to avoid products with potassium: oranges, bananas, dried fruit, peas, dark green leafy vegetables, milk, melons, beans in chronic renal failure
• Advise patient to avoid OTC products containing calcium, potassium, or sodium in chronic renal failure
• Instruct patient to avoid all preparations containing vit D
• Instruct patient to monitor weight weekly; maintain fluid intake

## Evaluation
**Positive therapeutic outcome**
- Calcium levels 9-10 mg/dl

---

## calcium carbonate (Rx)
## (PO-OTC, **IV**-Rx)

Alka-Mints, Amitone, Apo-Cal ✤, BioCal, Calcarb, Calci-Chew, Calcilac, Calci-Mix, Calcite ✤, Calglycine ✤, Cal-Plus, Calsan ✤, Caltrate 600, Caltrate Jr., Chooz, Dicarbosil, Equilet, Gencalc, Liquid-Cal, Liquid-Cal-600, Maalox Antacid Caplets, Mallamint, Mylanta Lozenges ✤, Nephro-Calci, Nu-Cal ✤, Os-Cal 500, Oysco 500, Oystercal 500, Oyst-Cal 500, Rolaids Calcium Rich, Titralac, Tums, Tums E-X Extra Strength
*Func. class.:* Antacid, calcium supplement
*Chem. class.:* Calcium product

## calcium acetate (OTC)
(kal'see-um ass'e-tate)
calphron, phoslo

**Pregnancy category  C**

---

**Action:** Neutralizes gastric acidity

**Therapeutic outcome:** Neutralized gastric acidity; calcium at normal levels

**Uses:** Antacid, calcium supplement; not suitable for chronic therapy, hyperphosphatemia, hypertension in pregnancy, osteoporosis, prevention/treatment of hypocalcemia, hyperparathyroidism

## Dosage and routes
*Antacid*
**Adult:** PO 0.5-1.5 g or 2 pieces of gum 1 hr before meals and at bedtime

*Hyperphosphatemia*
**Adult:** PO 1 g or more in divided doses

*Hypertension in pregnancy*
**Adult:** PO 500 mg tid during 3rd trimester

*Prevention of hypocalcemia, depletion, osteoporosis*
**Adult:** PO 1-2 g daily

**Available forms:** Calcium carbonate: chewable tabs 350, 420, 450, 500, 750, 1000, 1250 mg; tabs 500, 600, 650, 1000, 1250 mg; gum 300, 450, 500 mg; susp 1250 mg/5 ml; lozenges 600 mg; caps 1250 mg; powder 6.5 g/packet; calcium acetate: tabs 250 mg (65 mg Ca), 667 mg (169 mg Ca), 668 mg (169 mg Ca), 1 g (250 mg Ca); caps 500 mg (125 mg Ca)

## Adverse effects
*GI: Constipation,* anorexia, nausea, vomiting, flatulence, diarrhea, rebound hyperacidity, eructation

**Contraindications:** Hypersensitivity, hypercalcemia, hyperparathyroidism, bone tumors

**Precautions:** Pregnancy **C,** breastfeeding, geriatric, fluid restriction, decreased GI motility, GI obstruction, dehydration, renal disease

| Pharmacokinetics | |
|---|---|
| **Absorption** | ⅓ absorbed by small intestine |
| **Distribution** | Unknown |
| **Metabolism** | Unknown |
| **Excretion** | Feces, urine, crosses placenta |
| **Half-life** | Unknown |

| Pharmacodynamics | |
|---|---|
| **Onset** | 20 min |
| **Peak** | Unknown |
| **Duration** | 20-180 min |

## Interactions
*Individual drugs*
Ketoconazole: decreased ketoconazole levels
Quinidine: increased quinidine levels
*Drug classifications*
Amphetamines: increased levels of amphetamines
Calcium channel blockers, iron products, salicylates, tetracyclines: decreased levels of each specific product
Quinolone antiinfectives: decreased levels of antiinfectives
*Drug/herb*
Lily of the valley, pheasant's eye, shark cartilage, squill: increased side effect, action
*Drug/lab test*
False increase: increased chloride
False decrease: decreased magnesium, oxylate, lipase
False positive: benzodiazepines

## NURSING CONSIDERATIONS
**Assessment**
- Monitor Ca$^+$ (serum, urine), Ca$^+$ should be 8.5-10.5 mg/dl, urine Ca$^+$ should be 150 mg/day, monitor weekly
◆ Assess for milk-alkali syndrome: nausea, vomiting, disorientation, headache
- Assess for constipation; increase bulk in the diet if needed
- Assess for hypercalcemia: headache, nausea, vomiting, confusion

---

Adverse effects: *italic* = common, **bold** = life-threatening

## Nursing diagnoses
• Knowledge, deficient (teaching)
• Nutrition, less than body requirements, imbalanced (uses)

## Implementation
**PO route**
• Administer as antacid 1 hr after meals and at bedtime
• Administer as supplement 1½ hr after meals and at bedtime
• Administer only with regular tablets or capsules; do not give with enteric-coated tablets
• Administer laxatives or stool softeners if constipation occurs

## Patient/family education
• Advise patient to increase fluids to 2 L unless contraindicated, to add bulk to diet for constipation; notify prescriber of constipation
• Advise patient not to switch antacids unless directed by prescriber, not to use as antacid for >2 wk without approval by prescriber
• Teach patient that therapeutic dose recommendations are figured as elemental calcium

## Evaluation
**Positive therapeutic outcome**
• Absence of pain, decreased acidity

---

## CALCIUM SALTS

**calcium chloride** (Rx)
**calcium gluceptate** (Rx)
**calcium gluconate** (Rx)
Kalcinate
**calcium lactate**
(PO-OTC, **IV**-Rx)
Cal-Lac
*Func. class.:* Electrolyte replacement—calcium product

**Pregnancy category  C**

**Action:** Cation needed for maintenance of nervous, muscular, skeletal systems, enzyme reactions, normal cardiac contractility, coagulation of blood; affects secretory activity of endocrine, exocrine glands

**Therapeutic outcome:** Calcium at normal level, absence of increased magnesium, potassium

**Uses:** Prevention and treatment of hypocalcemia, hypermagnesemia, hypoparathyroidism, neonatal tetany, cardiac toxicity caused by hyperkalemia, lead colic, hyperphosphatemia, vit D deficiency, osteoporosis prophylaxis,
calcium antagonist toxicity (calcium channel blocker toxicity)

## Dosage and routes
*Calcium chloride*
*Adult:* **IV** 500 mg-1 g q1-3 days as indicated by serum calcium levels; give at <1 ml/min; **IV** 200-800 mg injected in ventricle of heart
*Child:* **IV** 25 mg/kg over several min

*Calcium gluceptate*
*Adult:* **IV** 5-20 ml; IM 2-5 ml

*Calcium gluconate*
*Adult:* PO 0.5-2 g bid-qid; **IV** 0.5-2 g at 0.5 ml/min (10% sol); max **IV** dose 3 g
*Child:* PO/**IV** 500 mg/kg/day in divided doses

*Calcium lactate*
*Adult:* PO 325 mg-1.3 g tid with meals
*Child:* PO 500 mg/kg/day in divided doses

**Available forms:** Many; check product listings

## Adverse effects
*CV:* Shortened QT interval, heart block, hypotension, bradycardia, dysrhythmias; **cardiac arrest (IV)**
*GI:* Vomiting, nausea, constipation
*HYPERCALCEMIA:* Drowsiness, lethargy, muscle weakness, headache, constipation, **coma,** anorexia, nausea, vomiting, polyuria, thirst
*INTEG:* Pain, burning at **IV** site, severe venous thrombosis, necrosis, extravasation

**Contraindications:** Hypercalcemia, digoxin toxicity, ventricular fibrillation, renal calculi

**Precautions:** Pregnancy **C,** breastfeeding, children, renal disease, respiratory disease, cor pulmonale, digitalized patient, respiratory failure

### Pharmacokinetics
| | |
|---|---|
| Absorption | Complete bioavailability (**IV**) |
| Distribution | Readily extracellular; crosses placenta |
| Metabolism | Liver |
| Excretion | Feces (80%), kidney (20%), breast milk |
| Half-life | Unknown |

### Pharmacodynamics
| | PO | IV |
|---|---|---|
| Onset | Unknown | Immediate |
| Peak | Unknown | Rapid |
| Duration | Unknown | ½-1½ hr |

---

## Interactions
### Individual drugs
Atenolol: decreased effects of atenolol
Digoxin glycosides: increased dysrhythmias
Phenytoin: decreased absorption of phenytoin when calcium is taken PO
Tetracycline: decreased absorption of tetracycline (PO)
Verapamil: decreased effects of verapamil; increased toxicity
### Drug classifications
Antacids: milk-alkali syndrome (renal disease)
Diuretics (thiazide): increased hypercalcemia
Fluoroquinolones: decreased absorption of fluoroquinolones when calcium is taken PO
Iron salts: decreased absorption of iron when calcium is taken PO
### Drug/herb
Lily of the valley, pheasant's eye, shark cartilage, squill: increased side effects, action
### Drug/lab test
False: decreased magnesium, decreased 17-OHCS, increased 11-OHCS

## NURSING CONSIDERATIONS
### Assessment
• Monitor ECG for decreased QT interval and T-wave inversion: in hypercalcemia, product should be reduced or discontinued
• Monitor calcium levels during treatment (9-10 mg/dl is normal level), urine calcium if hypercaluria occurs
• Assess cardiac status: rate, rhythm, CVP (PWP, PAWP if being monitored directly)
• Assess digitalized patients closely, an increase in calcium increases digoxin toxicity risk

### Nursing diagnoses
• Injury, risk for (uses, adverse reactions)
• Knowledge, deficient (teaching)

### Implementation
**PO route**
• Give PO with or following meals to enhance absorption
• Store at room temperature
**IV route**
• Administer **IV** undiluted or diluted with equal amounts of 0.9% NaCl for inj to a 5% sol; give 0.5-1 ml/min
• Give through small-bore needle into large vein; if extravasation occurs, necrosis will result (**IV**); IM inj may cause severe burning, necrosis, and tissue sloughing; warm sol to body temp before administering (only gluconate/gluceptate)
• Provide seizure precautions: padded side rails, decreased stimuli (noise, light); place

airway suction equipment, padded mouth gag if calcium levels are low
• Patient should remain recumbent 30 min after IV dose
### Calcium chloride
**Syringe compatibilities:** Milrinone
**Y-site compatibilities:** DOBUTamine, epINEPHrine, esmolol, inamrinone, morphine, paclitaxel
**Additive compatibilities:** Amikacin, amphotericin B, ampicillin, ascorbic acid, bretylium, ceftriaxone, cephapirin, chloramphenicol, DOPamine, hydrocortisone, isoproterenol, lidocaine, methicillin, norepinephrine, penicillin G potassium, penicillin G sodium, pentobarbital, phenobarbital, verapamil, vit B/C
### Calcium gluceptate
**Additive compatibilities:** Ascorbic acid inj, isoproterenol, lidocaine, norepinephrine, phytonadione, sodium bicarbonate
### Calcium gluconate
**Syringe compatibilities:** Aldesleukin, allopurinol, amifostine, aztreonam, cefazolin, cefepime, ciprofloxacin, cladribine, DOBUTamine, enalaprilat, epINEPHrine, famotidine, filgrastim, granisetron, heparin/hydrocortisone, labetalol, melphalan, midazolam, netilmicin, piperacillin/tazobactam, potassium chloride, prochlorperazine, propofol, sargramostim, tacrolimus, teniposide, thiotepa, tolazoline, vinorelbine, vit B/C
**Additive compatibilities:** Amikacin, aminophylline, ascorbic acid inj, bretylium, cephapirin, chloramphenicol, corticotropin, dimenhyDRINATE, erythromycin, furosemide, heparin, hydrocortisone, lidocaine, magnesium sulfate, methicillin, norepinephrine, penicillin G potassium, penicillin G sodium, phenobarbital, potassium chloride, tobramycin, vancomycin, verapamil, vit B/C

### Patient/family education
• Caution patient to add food high in vit D content; to add calcium-rich foods to diet: dairy products, shellfish, dark green leafy vegetables; decrease oxalate-rich and zinc-rich foods: nuts, legumes, chocolate, spinach, soy
• Advise patient to prevent injuries, avoid immobilization

### Evaluation
**Positive therapeutic outcome**
• Decreased twitching, paresthesias, muscle spasms
• Absence of tremors, seizures, dysrhythmias, dyspnea, laryngospasm, negative Chvostek's sign, negative Trousseau's sign

Adverse effects: *italic* = common, **bold** = life-threatening

## candesartan (Rx)
(can-deh-sar'tan)

Atacand

*Func. class.:* Antihypertensive

*Chem. class.:* Angiotensin II receptor (Type $AT_1$)

**Pregnancy category**
C (1st trimester),
D (2nd/3rd trimesters)

**Action:** Blocks the vasoconstrictor and aldosterone-secreting effects of angiotensin II; selectively blocks the binding of angiotensin II to the $AT_1$ receptor found in tissues

**Therapeutic outcome:** Decreased B/P

**Uses:** Hypertension, alone or in combination; CHF NYHA Class II-IV and ejection fraction ≤40%

### Dosage and routes

*Adult:* PO (single agent) 16 mg daily initially in patients who are not volume depleted, range 8-32 mg/day; with diuretic or volume depletion 2-32 mg/day as a single dose or divided bid

*Renal dose*
*Adult:* PO Give lowest possible dose

**Available forms:** Tabs 4, 8, 16, 32 mg

### Adverse effects

*CNS: Dizziness,* fatigue, headache
*CV:* Chest pain, peripheral edema, hypotension
*EENT:* Sinusitis, rhinitis, pharyngitis
*GI: Diarrhea,* nausea, abdominal pain, vomiting
*GU:* **Renal failure**
*MS:* Arthralgia, pain
*RESP: Cough, upper respiratory infection*
*SYST:* **Angioedema**

**Contraindications:** Pregnancy **D** (2nd/3rd trimesters), hypersensitivity

**Precautions:** Pregnancy **C** (1st trimester), breastfeeding, children, geriatric, hypersensitivity to ACE inhibitors, volume-depletion, renal/hepatic impairment

### Pharmacokinetics

| | |
|---|---|
| **Absorption** | Well absorbed |
| **Distribution** | Bound to plasma proteins |
| **Metabolism** | Extensive |
| **Excretion** | Feces, urine, breast milk |
| **Half-life** | 9 hr |

### Pharmacodynamics

| | |
|---|---|
| **Onset** | Unknown |
| **Peak** | 2 hr |
| **Duration** | 24 hr |

### Interactions
*Individual drugs*
Lithium: increased lithium level
Potassium: increased hypokalemia
*Drug classifications*
α-blockers, ACE inhibitors, β-blockers, calcium channel blockers: increased hypotension
Diuretics (potassium sparing): increased hypokalemia
NSAIDs, salicylates: decreased effect
*Drug/herb*
Aconite: increased toxicity, death
Astragalus, cola tree: increased or decreased antihypertensive effect
Barberry, betony, black catechu, black cohosh, bloodroot, broom, burdock, cat's claw, dandelion, goldenseal, Irish moss, Jamaican dogwood, kelp, khella, mistletoe, parsley, Queen Anne's lace, rue: increased antihypertensive effect
Coltsfoot, guarana, khat, licorice, yohimbe: decreased antihypertensive effect

### NURSING CONSIDERATIONS
**Assessment**
• Assess B/P, pulse q4hr; note rate, rhythm, quality
• Monitor electrolytes: potassium, sodium, chloride; total $CO_2$
• Obtain baselines in renal, liver function tests before therapy begins
• Assess blood studies: BUN, creatinine, liver function tests before treatment
• Monitor for edema in feet, legs daily
• Assess for skin turgor, dryness of mucous membranes for hydration status; for angioedema: facial swelling, dyspnea
• Assess for pregnancy, this product can cause fetal death when given in pregnancy
• Assess for adverse reactions, especially in renal disease

**Nursing diagnoses**
• Fluid volume, deficient (side effects)
• Knowledge, deficient (teaching)
• Noncompliance (teaching)

**Implementation**
• Administer without regard to meals

**Patient/family education**
• Teach patient not to take the product if breastfeeding or pregnant, or have had an allergic reaction to this product

- If a dose is missed, instruct patient to take as soon as possible, unless it is within an hour before next dose
- Advise patient to comply with dosage schedule, even if feeling better
- Teach patient to notify prescriber of fever, swelling of hands or feet, irregular heartbeat, chest pain
- Advise patient excessive perspiration, dehydration, diarrhea may lead to fall in blood pressure—consult prescriber if these occur
- Inform patient that product may cause dizziness, fainting; light-headedness may occur
- Caution patient to rise slowly to sitting or standing position to minimize orthostatic hypotension
- Advise patient to avoid all OTC medications unless approved by prescriber; to inform all health care providers of medication use
- Teach proper technique for obtaining B/P and acceptable parameters

## Evaluation
**Positive therapeutic outcome**
- Decreased B/P

---

## capecitabine (Rx)
(cap-eh-sit'ah-bean)
Xeloda
*Func. class.:* Antineoplastic, antimetabolite
*Chem. class.:* Fluoropyrimidine carbamate

**Pregnancy category D**

## Do not confuse:
Xeloda/Xenical

**Action:** Competes with physiologic substrate of DNA synthesis, thus interfering with cell replication in the S phase of cell cycle (before mitosis); also interferes with RNA and protein synthesis; product is converted to 5-fluorouracil (5-FU)

**Therapeutic outcome:** Decreasing symptoms of breast cancer

**Uses:** Monotherapy for paclitaxel-anthracycline-resistant metastatic breast, colorectal cancer when 5-FU monotherapy is preferred; treatment of patients with colorectal cancer who have undergone complete resection of their primary tumor

**Unlabeled uses:** Pancreatic cancer

## Dosage and routes:
*Adult:* PO 2500 mg/m$^2$/day in 2 divided doses q12hr at end of meal × 2 wk, then 1 wk rest period; given in 3-wk cycles; may be combined with docetaxel, when capecitalane

dose is lowered; follow the NCIC (National Cancer Institute of Canada) common toxicity criteria

### Renal dose
*Adult:* PO CCr 30-50 ml/min; decrease initial dose to 75% of usual dose

**Available forms:** Tabs 150, 500 mg

## Adverse effects
*CNS:* Dizziness, headache, *paresthesia, fatigue,* insomnia
*GI: Nausea, vomiting, anorexia, diarrhea, stomatitis, abdominal pain, constipation, dyspepsia,* **intestinal obstruction, necrotizing enterocolitis**
*HEMA:* **Neutropenia, lymphopenia, thrombocytopenia,** anemia
*INTEG: Hand and foot syndrome,* dermatitis, nail disorder
*MISC:* Hyperbilirubinemia, eye irritation, edema, myalgia, limb pain, *pyrexia,* dehydration
*RESP: Cough, dyspnea*

**Contraindications:** Pregnancy **D**, infants, hypersensitivity to 5-FU, severe renal impairment (CCr <30 ml/min)

**Precautions:** Renal/hepatic disease, breastfeeding, children, geriatric

| Pharmacokinetics | |
|---|---|
| **Absorption** | Readily, food decreased |
| **Distribution** | Unknown |
| **Metabolism** | Liver, extensively |
| **Excretion** | Kidneys |
| **Half-life** | 45 min |

| Pharmacodynamics | |
|---|---|
| **Onset** | Unknown |
| **Peak** | 1½ hr |
| **Duration** | Unknown |

## Interactions
### Individual drugs
Leucovorin: increased toxicity
Phenytoin: increased phenytoin level
Warfarin: increased risk of bleeding
### Drug classifications
Antacids (aluminum, magnesium): increased capecitabine
### Food/drug
Increased absorption, give within 30 min of a meal

## NURSING CONSIDERATIONS
### Assessment
- Assess buccal cavity q8hr for dryness, sores or ulceration, white patches, pain, bleeding,

---

Adverse effects: *italic* = common, **bold** = life-threatening

dysphagia; obtain prescription for viscous lidocaine (Xylocaine)
• Assess symptoms indicating severe allergic reaction: rash, pruritus, urticaria, purpuric skin lesions, itching, flushing; product should be discontinued
• Monitor CBC, differential, platelet count weekly; withhold product if WBC <4000/mm$^3$ or platelet count is <100,000/mm$^3$; notify prescriber of results if WBC <20,000/mm$^3$, platelet count <150,000/mm$^3$
• Monitor temp q4hr (may indicate beginning of infection)
• Assess for hand/foot syndrome: paresthesia, tingling, painful/painless swelling, blistering, erythema with severe pain of hands/feet
• Assess for toxicity: severe diarrhea, nausea, vomiting, stomatitis
• Assess GI symptoms: frequency of stools, cramping; if severe diarrhea occurs, fluids/electrolytes may need to be given
• Monitor liver function tests before and during therapy (bilirubin, AST, ALT, LDH) as needed or monthly; note jaundice of skin or sclera, dark urine, clay-colored stools, itchy skin, abdominal pain, fever, diarrhea
• Assess for bleeding: hematuria, stool guaiac, bruising or petechiae, mucosa or orifices q8hr; inflammation of mucosa, breaks in skin

### Nursing diagnoses
• Body image, disturbed (adverse reactions)
• Infection, risk for (adverse reactions)
• Injury, risk for (adverse reactions)
• Knowledge, deficient (teaching)

### Implementation
• Give antiemetic 30-60 min before giving product to prevent vomiting and prn; give antibiotics for prophylaxis of infection
• Provide liquid diet: carbonated beverages; gelatin may be added if patient is not nauseated or vomiting
• Help patient to rinse mouth tid-qid with water or club soda, brush teeth bid-qid with soft brush or cotton-tipped applicators for stomatitis, use unwaxed dental floss

### Patient/family education
• Contraceptive measures are recommended during therapy; product is teratogenic to fetus
• Advise patient to avoid use of products containing aspirin or ibuprofen, razors, commercial mouthwash, since bleeding may occur; to report symptoms of bleeding (hematuria, tarry stools)
• Instruct patient to report signs of anemia (fatigue, headache, irritability, faintness, shortness of breath)
• Advise patient not to become pregnant while

taking this product; to avoid using while breastfeeding
• Advise patient not to double dose, if dose is missed
• Advise patient to report immediately severe diarrhea, vomiting, stomatitis, fever ≥100° F, hand/foot syndrome, anorexia

### Evaluation
**Positive therapeutic outcome**
• Prevention of rapid division of malignant cells

---

## captopril  (Rx)
(kap′toe-pril)
Capoten, Novo-Captopril ♣
*Func. class.:* Antihypertensive
*Chem. class.:* Angiotensin-converting enzyme (ACE) inhibitor
**Pregnancy category D**

### Do not confuse:
captopril/Capitrol/carvedilol

**Action:** Selectively suppresses renin-angiotensin-aldosterone system; inhibits ACE; prevents conversion of angiotensin I to angiotensin II

**Therapeutic outcome:** Decreased B/P in hypertension; decreased preload, afterload in CHF

**Uses:** Hypertension, CHF, left ventricular dysfunction (LVD) after MI, diabetic nephropathy

### Dosage and routes
*Malignant hypertension*
*Adult:* PO 25 mg increasing q2hr until desired response; not to exceed 450 mg/day

*Hypertension*
*Adult:* Initial dose: PO 12.5-25 mg bid-tid; may increase to 50 mg bid-tid at 1-2 wk intervals; usual range 25-150 mg bid-tid; max 450 mg
*Child:* PO 0.3-0.5 mg/kg/dose, titrate up to 6 mg/kg/day in 2-4 divided doses
*Neonate:* PO 0.05-0.1 mg/kg bid-tid, may increase as needed

*CHF*
*Adult:* PO 25 mg bid-tid; may increase to 50 mg bid-tid; after 14 days may increase to 150 mg tid if needed

*LVD after MI*
*Adult:* PO 50 mg tid, may begin treatment 3 days after MI; give 6.25 mg as a single dose, then 12.5 mg tid, increase to 25 mg tid for several days, then 50 mg tid

---

 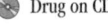

*Diabetic nephropathy*
*Adult:* PO 25 mg tid

*Renal dose*
*Adult:* PO CCr >50 ml/min, no change; CCr 10-50 ml/min, decrease dose by 25%; CCr <10 ml/min, decrease dose by 50%

**Available forms:** Tabs 12.5, 25, 50, 100 mg

### Adverse effects
*CNS:* Fever, chills
*CV: Hypotension,* postural hypotension, *tachycardia,* angina
*GI:* Loss of taste, liver function tests
*GU:* Impotence, dysuria, nocturia, **proteinuria, nephrotic syndrome, acute reversible renal failure,** polyuria, oliguria, frequency
*HEMA:* **Neutropenia, agranulocytosis, pancytopenia, thrombocytopenia,** anemia
*INTEG:* Rash, pruritus
*MISC:* **Angioedema,** hyperkalemia
*RESP:* **Bronchospasm,** *dyspnea, cough*

**Contraindications:** Pregnancy **D,** breastfeeding, children, hypersensitivity, heart block, potassium-sparing diuretics, bilateral renal artery stenosis, angioedema

**Precautions:** Dialysis patients, hypovolemia, leukemia, scleroderma, LE, blood dyscrasias, CHF, diabetes mellitus, renal/hepatic disease, thyroid disease, COPD, asthma

| Pharmacokinetics | |
| --- | --- |
| **Absorption** | Well absorbed |
| **Distribution** | Widely distributed; crosses placenta, excreted in breast milk, small amounts |
| **Metabolism** | Liver (50%) |
| **Excretion** | Kidneys, unchanged (50%) |
| **Half-life** | 2 hr increase in renal disease |

| Pharmacodynamics | |
| --- | --- |
| **Onset** | ¼-1 hr |
| **Peak** | 1 hr |
| **Duration** | 6-12 hr |

### Interactions
*Individual drugs*
Alcohol (acute ingestion): increased hypotension (large amounts)
Digoxin, lithium: increased serum levels, toxicity
Insulin: increased hypoglycemia
*Drug classifications*
Antacids, NSAIDs, salicylates: decreased captopril effect
Antidiabetics (oral): increased hypoglycemia

Antihypertensives, diuretics, nitrates, phenothiazines: increased hypotension
Diuretics (potassium-sparing), potassium supplements: increased toxicity, do not use
Sympathomimetics: do not use
*Drug/herb*
Aconite: increased toxicity, death
Astragalus, cola tree: increased or decreased antihypertensive effect
Barberry, betony, black catechu, black cohosh, bloodroot, broom, burdock, cat's claw, dandelion, goldenseal, Irish moss, Jamaican dogwood, kelp, khella, mistletoe, parsley: increased antihypertensive effect
Coltsfoot, guarana, khat, licorice: decreased antihypertensive effect
*Drug/lab test*
Increased: AST, ALT, alkaline phosphatase, bilirubin, uric acid, glucose
False positive: urine acetone, ANA titer

### NURSING CONSIDERATIONS
**Assessment**
• May be crushed and mixed with food
• Monitor blood studies: decreased platelets; WBC with diff baseline and periodically q3 mo, if neutrophils <1000/mm$^3$, discontinue treatment
• Monitor B/P, check for orthostatic hypotension, syncope; if changes occur, dosage change may be required
• Monitor renal studies: protein, BUN, creatinine; watch for increased levels that may indicate nephrotic syndrome and renal failure; monitor renal symptoms: polyuria, oliguria, frequency, dysuria
• Establish baselines in renal, liver function tests before therapy begins and check periodically; monitor for increased liver function studies; watch for increased uric acid, glucose
• Check potassium levels throughout treatment, although hyperkalemia rarely occurs
• Check for edema in feet, legs daily; monitor weight daily in CHF
• Assess for allergic reactions: rash, fever, pruritus, urticaria; product should be discontinued if antihistamines fail to help

**Nursing diagnoses**
• Cardiac output, decreased (uses)
• Injury, risk for (side effects)
• Knowledge, deficient (teaching)
• Noncompliance (teaching)

**Implementation**
• Store in air-tight container at 86° F (30° C) or less

- Severe hypotension may occur after first dose of this medication; decreasing hypotension may be prevented by reducing or discontinuing diuretic therapy 3 days before beginning captopril therapy
- Administer 1 hr before or 2 hr after meals
- May crush tab and dissolve in water, give within ½ hr, make sure tab is completely dissolved

### Patient/family education

- Caution patient not to discontinue product abruptly; advise patient to tell all persons associated with care
- Teach patient not to use OTC products (cough, cold, allergy) unless directed by prescriber; serious side effects can occur; xanthines such as coffee, tea, chocolate, cola can prevent action of product
- Teach patient importance of complying with dosage schedule, even if feeling better; to continue with medical regimen to decrease B/P: exercise, cessation of smoking, decreasing stress, diet modifications
- Emphasize the need to rise slowly to sitting or standing position to minimize orthostatic hypotension; not to exercise in hot weather or increased hypotension can occur
- Teach patient to notify prescriber of mouth sores, sore throat, fever, swelling of hands or feet, irregular heartbeat, chest pain, coughing, shortness of breath
- Caution patient to report excessive perspiration, dehydration, vomiting, diarrhea; may lead to fall in B/P
- Caution patient that product may cause dizziness, fainting, light-headedness; may occur during first few days of therapy; to avoid activities that may be hazardous
- Teach patient how to take B/P, and teach normal readings for age-group; ensure patient takes regularly
- Advise patient to tell prescriber if pregnancy is suspected or planned

### Evaluation

**Positive therapeutic outcome**

- Decreased B/P in hypertension

**Treatment of overdose:** 0.9% NaCl **IV** infusion, hemodialysis

### carbachol ophthalmic
*See Appendix D*

---

### carbamazepine (Rx)
(kar-ba-maz′e-peen)

Apo-Carbamazepine ✤, Atretol, Carbatrol, Epitol, Equetro ✤, Novo-Carbamaz ✤, Tegretol, Tegretol CR ✤, Tegretol-XR, Teril

*Func. class.:* Anticonvulsant
*Chem. class.:* Iminostilbene derivative

**Pregnancy category D**

**Do not confuse:**
Tegretol/Toradol

**Action:** Exact mechanism unknown; appears to decrease polysynaptic responses and block posttetanic potentiation

**Therapeutic outcome:** Absence of seizures; decreased trigeminal neuralgia pain

**Uses:** Tonic-clonic, complex-partial, mixed seizures; trigeminal neuralgia, bipolar disorder

**Unlabeled uses:** Neurogenic pain, psychotic behavior with dementia, diabetic neuropathy, agitation, hiccups

### Dosage and routes
*Seizures*
*Adult and child >12 yr:* PO 200 mg bid; may be increased by 200 mg/day in divided doses q6-8hr; maintenance 800-1200 mg/day; max 1600 mg/day (adult); max child 12-15 yr 1000 mg/day; max child >15 yr 1200 mg/day; adjustment is needed to minimum dose to control seizures; EXT REL give bid; RECT administration of oral susp 200 mg/10 ml or 6 mg/kg as a single dose
*Child 6-12 yr:* PO tabs 100 mg bid or susp 50 mg qid; may increase by <100 mg qwk, max 1000 mg/day; EXT REL tabs daily-bid
*Child <6 yr:* PO 10-20 mg/kg/day in 2-3 divided doses, may increase qwk

*Trigeminal neuralgia*
*Adult:* PO 100 mg/bid; may increase 100 mg q12hr until pain subsides; not to exceed 1200 mg/day; maintenance is 200-400 mg bid

*Bipolar disorder*
*Adult:* PO (Equetro only) 200 mg bid, may adjust dose by 200 mg daily to desired response; max 1600 mg/day

**Available forms:** Chewable tabs 100, 200 mg; tabs 200 mg; oral susp 100 mg/5 ml; ext rel tabs 100, 200, 400 mg; ext rel caps (Carbatrol) 200, 300 mg

### Adverse effects
*CNS: Drowsiness,* dizziness, confusion, fatigue, **paralysis,** headache, hallucinations,

**worsening of seizures,** unsteadiness, speech disturbances
*CV:* **Hypertension, CHF,** hypotension, aggravation of CAD, dysrhythmias, **AV block**
*EENT:* Tinnitus, dry mouth, blurred vision, diplopia, nystagmus, conjunctivitis
*ENDO:* Syndrome of inappropriate antidiuretic hormone (SIADH) (geriatric)
*GI: Nausea, constipation, diarrhea,* anorexia, vomiting, abdominal pain, stomatitis, glossitis, increased liver enzymes, **hepatitis, hepatic porphyria**
*GU:* Frequency, retention, albuminuria, glycosuria, impotence, increased BUN, **renal failure**
*HEMA:* **Thrombocytopenia,** leukopenia, **agranulocytosis, leukocytosis, aplastic anemia, eosinophilia,** increased pro-time
*INTEG: Rash,* **Stevens-Johnson syndrome,** urticaria, photosensitivity, **toxic epidermal necrolysis**
*RESP:* Pulmonary hypersensitivity (fever, dyspnea, pneumonitis)

**Contraindications:** Pregnancy **D,** hypersensitivity to carbamazepine or tricyclics, bone marrow depression, concomitant use of MAOIs

**Precautions:** Glaucoma, renal/hepatic/cardiac disease, psychosis, breastfeeding, child <6 yr, alcoholism, hematologic disease, hepatic porphyria

### Pharmacokinetics

| | |
|---|---|
| **Absorption** | Slow; completely absorbed |
| **Distribution** | Widely distributed; protein binding 76% |
| **Metabolism** | Extensively, liver, metabolized by CYP3A4 |
| **Excretion** | Urine, feces, breast milk |
| **Half-life** | 12-17 hr or more |

### Pharmacodynamics

| | |
|---|---|
| **Onset** | Slow |
| **Peak** | 4-5 hr |
| **Duration** | Unknown |

### Interactions
*Individual drugs*
Benzodiazepines, darunavir, delavirdine, nefazodone, oxcarbazepine: decreased effect of these products
Cimetidine, clarithromycin, danzol, diltiazem, erythromycin, isoniazid, propoxyphene, valproic acid, verapamil, voriconazole: increased carbamazepine levels
Cisplatin, DOXOrubicin, felbamate, phenobarbitol, phenytoin, primidone, rifampin,

theophylline: increased carbamazepine levels
Contraceptives (oral): decreased effect of oral contraceptives
Desmopressin, lithium, hypressin, vasopressin: increased effects of each specific product
Doxycycline: decreased effect of doxycycline
Fluoxetine, fluroxamine: increased carbamazepine effect
Lithium: increased CNS toxicity
Phenobarbital: increased effect
Phenytoin: increased and decreased plasma levels; decreased carbamazepine plasma levels
Thyroid hormones: decreased effect of thyroid hormones
Valproic acid: decreased plasma levels; increased half-life of carbamazepine
Warfarin: decreased effect of warfarin
*Drug classifications*
CYP3A4 inducers: decreased carbamazepine levels
CYP3A4 inhibitors: increased carbamazepine levels
◆ MAOIs: fatal reaction; do not use together
*Drug/herb*
Ginkgo, quinine: increased anticonvulsant action
Ginseng, santonica: decreased anticonvulsant action
*Drug/food*
Grapefruit juice: increased peak concentration of carbamazepine

### NURSING CONSIDERATIONS
**Assessment**
• Assess for seizures: character, location, duration, intensity, frequency, presence of aura
• Assess for trigeminal neuralgia: facial pain including location, duration, intensity, character, activity that stimulates pain
• Monitor liver function tests (AST, ALT) and urine function tests, BUN, urine protein periodically during treatments
• Assess blood studies: RBC, Hct, Hgb, reticulocyte counts qwk for 4 wk then q3-6 mo if on long-term therapy; if myelosuppression occurs, product should be discontinued
• Check blood levels during treatment or when changing dose; therapeutic level 4-12 mcg/ml
• Assess for blood dyscrasias: fever, sore throat, bruising, rash, jaundice, epistaxis (long-term treatment only)
• Assess seizure activity including type, aura, location, duration, and character; provide seizure precaution

Adverse effects: *italic* = common, **bold** = life-threatening

## Nursing diagnoses
- Injury, risk for (side effects)
- Knowledge, deficient (teaching)

## Implementation
- Do not break, crush, or chew ext rel tabs and caps
- Ext rel caps may be opened and beads mixed with food
- Chewable tabs should be chewed, not swallowed whole
- Give with food for GI symptoms
- Shake oral susp before use
- Mix an equal amount of water, $D_5W$, 0.9% NaCl when giving by NG tube, flush tube with 100 ml of above sol

## Patient/family education
- Teach patient to carry/wear emergency ID stating patient's name, products taken, condition, prescriber's name, phone number
- Caution patient to avoid driving, other activities that require alertness until stabilized on medication
- Teach patient not to discontinue medication quickly after long-term use
- Teach patient to use a nonhormonal type of contraception to prevent harm to the fetus
- Advise patient to use sunscreen to prevent burns
- Teach patient to take exactly as prescribed; do not double or omit doses
- Teach patient to report immediately chills, rash, light-colored stools, dark urine, yellowing of skin/eyes, abdominal pain, sore throat, mouth, ulcers, bruising, blurred vision, dizziness

## Evaluation
**Positive therapeutic outcome**
- Decreased seizure activity

**Treatment of overdose:** Lavage, VS

---

## carbidopa-levodopa (Rx)
(kar-bi-doe'pa lee-voe-doe'pa)
Atamet, carbidopa/levodopa, Sinemet, Sinemet CR
*Func. class.:* Antiparkinsonism agent
*Chem. class.:* Catecholamine

**Pregnancy category** C

**Action:** Decarboxylation of levodopa to periphery is inhibited by carbidopa; more levodopa is made available for transport to brain and conversion to dopamine in the brain

**Therapeutic outcome:** Absence of involuntary movements

**Uses:** Parkinson's disease, parkinsonism resulting from carbon monoxide, chronic manganese intoxication, cerebral arteriosclerosis

**Unlabeled uses:** Restless legs syndrome

## Dosage and routes
### Beginning therapy for those not taking levodopa
*Adult:* PO 25 mg carbidopa/100 mg levodopa tid, may increase daily or every other day by 1 tab to desired response (8 tabs/day); EXT REL tabs carbidopa 5 mg/levodopa 200 mg bid or carbidopa 10 mg/levodopa 100 mg 1 tab tid-qid; may increase by 1 tab daily or every other day until 8 tabs reached

### For those not taking levodopa ER
*Adult:* PO 50 mg carbidopa/200 mg levodopa bid

### For those taking levodopa ER
*Adult:* Begin treatment with 10% more levodopa/day given PO q4-8hr, may increase or decrease dose q3 days

### For those taking levodopa <1.5 g/day
*Adult:* PO 25 mg carbidopa/100 mg levodopa tid-qid, may increase daily to desired response

### For those taking levodopa >1.5 g/day
*Adult:* PO 25 mg carbidopa/250 mg levodopa tid-qid, may increase daily to desired response

### Restless legs syndrome (RLS) (unlabeled)
*Adult:* PO carbidopa 25 mg/levodopa 100 mg, 1 tab at bedtime, may repeat if awakening within 2 hr or 50 mg carbidopa/200 mg levodopa sus rel tab 1-2 tabs 1 hr before bedtime

**Available forms:** Tabs 10 mg carbidopa/100 mg levodopa, 25 mg carbidopa/100 mg levodopa, 25 mg carbidopa/250 mg levodopa; ext rel tab 25 mg/100 mg, 50 mg/200 mg carbidopa/levodopa (Sinemet CR); oral disintegrating tab (Parcopa) 10 mg carbidopa/100 mg levodopa, 25 mg carbidopa/100 mg levodopa; 25 mg carbidopa/250 mg levodopa

## Adverse effects
*CNS: Involuntary choreiform movements, hand tremors, fatigue, headache, anxiety, twitching, numbness, weakness, confusion, agitation, insomnia, nightmares,* psychosis, hallucination, hypomania, severe depression, dizziness

---

**CV:** *Orthostatic hypotension,* tachycardia, hypertension, palpitation
**EENT:** Blurred vision, diplopia, dilated pupils
**GI:** *Nausea, vomiting, anorexia, abdominal distress, dry mouth, flatulence, dysphagia, bitter taste, diarrhea, constipation*
**HEMA: Hemolytic anemia, leukopenia, agranulocytosis**
**INTEG:** Rash, sweating, alopecia
**MISC:** Urinary retention, incontinence, weight change, dark urine

**Contraindications:** Hypersensitivity, angle-closure glaucoma, malignant melanoma, history of malignant melanoma, or undiagnosed skin lesions resembling melanoma

**Precautions:** Pregnancy **C,** breastfeeding, diabetes, renal/cardiac/hepatic/respiratory disease, MI with dysrhythmias, open-angle glaucoma, seizures, peptic ulcer, depression

### Pharmacokinetics

| | |
|---|---|
| **Absorption** | Well absorbed (PO); ER dose slow |
| **Distribution** | Widely distributed |
| **Metabolism** | Liver, extensively |
| **Excretion** | Kidneys, metabolites |
| **Half-life** | Levodopa (1 hr); carbidopa (1-2 hr) |

### Pharmacodynamics

| | PO | PO-ER |
|---|---|---|
| **Onset** | Unknown | Unknown |
| **Peak** | 1 hr | 2½ hr |
| **Duration** | 6-24 hr | Unknown |

### Interactions
*Individual drugs*
Metoclopramide: increased effects of levodopa
Papaverine, pyridoxine: decreased effects of levodopa
*Drug classifications*
Antacids: increased effects of levodopa
Anticholinergics, benzodiazepines, hydantoins: decreased effects of levodopa
MAOIs: hypertensive crisis
*Drug/herb*
Kava, octacosanol: increased Parkinson's symptoms
Indian snakeroot: decreased action; increased EPS
*Drug/food*
Protein: decreased absorption of levodopa
Pyridoxine: decreased levodopa effect
*Drug/lab test*
Increased: AST, ALT, bilirubin, LDH, alkaline phosphatase, BUN
Decreased: VMA, BUN, creatinine
False increase: uric acid, urine protein

False positive: urine ketones (dipstick), Coombs' test
False negative: urine glucose

## NURSING CONSIDERATIONS
### Assessment
- Assess B/P, respiration, orthostatic B/P
- Monitor I&O ratio; retention commonly causes decreased urinary output, distention, frequency, incontinence; palpate bladder if retention occurs
- Assess for muscle twitching, blepharospasm that may indicate toxicity
- Monitor renal, liver, hematopoietic studies, also for diabetes, acromegaly during long-term therapy
- Assess for parkinsonism: shuffling gait, muscle rigidity, involuntary movements, pill rolling, muscle spasms, drooling before and during treatment
- Monitor for constipation, cramping, pain in abdomen, abdominal distention; increase fluids, bulk, exercise if this occurs
- Assess for tolerance over long-term therapy; dose may have to be increased or changed
- Assess for mental status: affect, mood, CNS depression, worsening of mental symptoms during early therapy

### Nursing diagnoses
- Knowledge, deficient (teaching)
- Mobility, impaired physical (uses)

### Implementation
**PO route**
- Swallow ext rel tabs whole; do not break, crush, or chew
- Give product until NPO before surgery; check with prescriber for continuing product
- Adjust dosage depending on patient response
- Give with meals or after meals to prevent GI symptoms; limit protein taken with product
- Give only after MAOIs have been discontinued for 2 wk; if previously on levodopa, discontinue for at least 8 hr before change to levodopa-carbidopa

### Patient/family education
- Teach patient to change positions slowly to prevent orthostatic hypotension
- Teach patient to report side effects: twitching, eye spasms, grimacing, protrusion of tongue, personality changes that indicate overdose
- Instruct patient to use product exactly as prescribed; if product is discontinued abruptly, parkinsonian crisis may occur; do not double doses; take missed dose as soon as remembered up to 2 hr before next dose

Adverse effects: *italic* = common, **bold** = life-threatening

- Teach patient that urine, sweat may darken and is harmless
- Advise patient to use physical activities to maintain mobility and lessen spasms
- Instruct patient that OTC medications should not be used unless approved by prescriber
- Advise patient that drowsiness, dizziness are common; to avoid hazardous activities until response is known
- Explain that sips of water, hard candy, or gum may lessen dry mouth
- Teach patient to take with meals to prevent GI symptoms; to limit protein intake, which impairs product's absorption

### Evaluation
**Positive therapeutic outcome**
- Decrease in akathisia
- Improved mood
- Decreased involuntary movements

---

### ⚠ HIGH ALERT

## carboplatin (Rx)
(kar′boe′pla-tin)
Paraplatin, Paraplatin-AQ ✦
*Func. class.:* Antineoplastic alkylating agent
*Chem. class.:* Platinum coordination compound

**Pregnancy category D**

**Do not confuse:**
carboplatin/cisplatin, Paraplatin/platinol

**Action:** Produces interstrand DNA cross-links and to a lesser extent DNA-protein cross-links; activity is not cell cycle phase specific

**Therapeutic outcome:** Prevention of rapidly growing malignant cells

**Uses:** Initial treatment of ovarian cancer in combination with other agents; palliative treatment of recurrent ovarian carcinoma after treatment with other antineoplastic agents, including cisplatin

### Dosage and routes
(single agent)
*Adult:* **IV** INF initially 300 mg/m² given with cyclophosphamide, q4-6 wk; refractory tumors 360 mg/m² single dose, may repeat q4 wk, as needed; do not repeat until neutrophils >2000 mm³ and platelets >100,000/mm³

### Renal dose
*Adult:* **IV** CCr 41-59 ml/min 250 mg/m², CCr 16-40 ml/min 200 mg/m²; do not use in Ccr <15 ml/min

**Available forms:** Lyophilized powder for inj 50, 150, 450 mg vials; aqueous sol for inj 50 mg/5 ml vial, 150 mg/15 ml vial, 450 mg/45 ml vial, 600 mg/60 ml vial

### Adverse effects
***CNS:*** **Seizures, central neurotoxicity,** peripheral neuropathy, dizziness, confusion
***CV:*** Cardiac abnormalities
***EENT:*** Tinnitus, hearing loss, *vestibular toxicity,* visual changes
***GI:*** Severe nausea, vomiting, diarrhea, weight loss, mucositis, anorexia, constipation, taste change
***HEMA:*** **Thrombocytopenia, leukopenia, pancytopenia, neutropenia, anemia,** bleeding
***INTEG:*** Alopecia, dermatitis, rash, erythema, pruritus, urticaria
***META:*** Hypomagnesemia, hypocalcemia, hypokalemia, hyponatremia, hyperuremia
***SYST:*** Anaphylaxis

**Contraindications:** Pregnancy **D**, hypersensitivity to this product, platinum products, mannitol; severe bone marrow depression, significant bleeding, aluminum products used to prepare or adminster carboplatin

**Precautions:** Radiation therapy within 1 mo, chemotherapy within 1 mo, breastfeeding, liver disease

| Pharmacokinetics | |
|---|---|
| **Absorption** | Complete |
| **Distribution** | Unknown |
| **Metabolism** | Liver |
| **Excretion** | Kidneys |
| **Half-life** | Initial 1-2 hr; postdistribution 2½-6 hr; increased in renal disease |

| Pharmacodynamics | |
|---|---|
| **Onset** | ½ hr |
| **Peak** | Unknown |
| **Duration** | 4-6 hr |

### Interactions
*Individual drugs*
Amphotericin B: increased nephrotoxicity or ototoxicity
Aspirin: increased risk of bleeding
Phenytoin: decreased levels
Radiation: increased toxicity, bone marrow suppression
*Drug classifications*
Aminoglycosides: ototoxicity, increased nephrotoxicity

---

Antineoplastics, bone marrow–suppressing products: increased bone marrow suppression

Myelosuppressives: increased myelosuppression

NSAIDs: increased risk of bleeding

**Drug/lab test**

Increased: AST, BUN, alkaline phosphatase, bilirubin, creatinine

## NURSING CONSIDERATIONS
### Assessment

• Monitor CBC, differential, platelet count weekly; withhold product if neutrophil count is <2000/mm$^3$ or platelet count is <100,000/mm$^3$; notify prescriber of results if WBC <20,000/mm$^3$, platelets <150,000/mm$^3$

• Assess for anaphylaxis: pruritus, wheezing, tachycardia; notify physician after discontinuing products; resuscitation equipment should be available

• Monitor renal function studies: BUN, creatinine, serum uric acid, urine CCr before and during therapy; I&O ratio; report fall in urine output to <30 ml/hr

• Monitor temp q4hr (may indicate beginning of infection)

• Monitor liver function tests before and during therapy (bilirubin, AST, ALT, LDH) as needed or monthly; note jaundice of skin or sclera, dark urine, clay-colored stools, itchy skin, abdominal pain, fever, diarrhea

• Assess for bleeding: hematuria, stool guaiac, bruising or petechiae, mucosa or orifices q8hr; inflammation of mucosa, breaks in skin

• Identify dyspnea, crackles, unproductive cough, chest pain, tachypnea

• Identify effects of alopecia on body image; discuss feelings about body changes

### Nursing diagnoses

• Body image, disturbed (adverse reactions)
• Infection, risk for (adverse reactions)
• Injury, risk for (adverse reactions)
• Knowledge, deficient (teaching)

### Implementation

• Antiemetic 30-60 min before giving product to prevent vomiting, and prn

**IV route**

• Give **IV** after diluting 10 mg/ml of sterile water for inj, D$_5$W, 0.9% NaCl (10 mg/ml); then further dilute with the same sol 1-4 mg/ml; give over 15 min or more (intermittent inf)

• Give **IV** inf over 5-6 hr; do not use needles or **IV** administration sets containing aluminum; may cause precipitate or loss of potency; diuretic (furosemide 40 mg **IV**) after inf

• Store protected from light at room temperature; reconstituted sol is stable for 8 hr at room temperature

**Y-site compatibilities:** Allopurinol, amifostine, aztreonam, cefepime, cladribine, DOXOrubicin liposome, filgrastim, fludarabine, granisetron, melphalan, ondansetron, paclitaxel, piperacillin/tazobactam, propofol, sargramostim, teniposide, thiotepa, vinorelbine

**Additive compatibilities:** Cisplatin, etoposide, floxuridine, ifosfamide, ifosfamide/etoposide, paclitaxel

**Additive incompatibilities:** Fluorouracil, mesna

**Solution compatibilities:** D$_5$/0.2% NaCl, D$_5$/0.45% NaCl, D$_5$/0.9% NaCl, 0.9% NaCl, D$_5$W, sterile water for inj

**Solution incompatibilities:** Sodium bicarbonate

### Patient/family education

• Advise patient to report ringing/roaring in the ears, numbness, tingling in face, extremities, weight gain

• Teach patient to avoid use of products containing aspirin or ibuprofen, NSAIDs, alcohol, razors, commercial mouthwash, since bleeding may occur; to report symptoms of bleeding (hematuria, tarry stools)

• Instruct patient to report signs of anemia (fatigue, headache, irritability, faintness, shortness of breath); sore throat, bleeding, bruising, chills, back pain, blood in stools, dyspnea

• Instruct patient to report any changes in breathing or coughing even several months after treatment; to avoid crowds and persons with respiratory tract or other infections

• Advise patient that hair may be lost during treatment; a wig or hairpiece may make patient feel better; new hair may be different in color, texture

• Caution patient not to have any vaccinations without the advice of the prescriber; serious reactions can occur

• Teach patient that contraception is needed during treatment and for several months after the completion of therapy; not to breastfeed during treatment; to notify prescriber if pregnancy is planned or suspected

### Evaluation
**Positive therapeutic outcome**
• Prevention of rapid division of malignant cells

Adverse effects: *italic* = common, **bold** = life-threatening

## carboprost (Rx)
(kar'boe-prost)
Hemabate, Prostin/15M ♣
*Func. class.:* Oxytocic, abortifacient
*Chem. class.:* Prostaglandin

**Pregnancy category** C

**Action:** Stimulates uterine contractions, causing complete abortion in approximately 16 hr

**Therapeutic outcome:** Loss of fetus; decreased postpartum bleeding

**Uses:** Abortion between 13-20 wk gestation; postpartum hemorrhage caused by uterine atony not controlled by other methods

### Dosage and routes
*To induce abortion*
*Adult:* IM 250 mcg, then 250 mcg q1½-3½ hr, may increase to 500 mcg if no response, not to exceed 12 mg total dose

*Postpartum hemorrhage*
*Adult:* IM 250 mcg, repeat at 15-90 min intervals, max total dosage 2 mg

**Available forms:** Inj 250 mcg/ml

### Adverse effects
*CNS: Fever, chills,* headache
*GI: Nausea, vomiting, diarrhea*

**Contraindications:** Hypersensitivity, severe renal/hepatic/cardiac/respiratory disease, PID

**Precautions:** Pregnancy C, asthma, anemia, jaundice, diabetes mellitus, seizure disorders, past uterine surgery

| Pharmacokinetics | |
|---|---|
| **Absorption** | Well absorbed (nasal) |
| **Distribution** | Widely distributed (extracellular fluid) |
| **Metabolism** | Liver—rapidly |
| **Excretion** | Kidneys |
| **Half-life** | 3-9 min |

| Pharmacodynamics | |
|---|---|
| **Onset** | Unknown |
| **Peak** | 16 hr |
| **Duration** | Unknown |

### Interactions
*Drug classifications*
Oxytocics: increased effects

## NURSING CONSIDERATIONS
### Assessment
- Monitor B/P, pulse; watch for change that may indicate hemorrhage
- Monitor respiratory rate, rhythm, depth; notify physician of abnormalities
- For length, duration of contraction; notify physician of contractions lasting over 1 min or absence of contractions
- Assess for incomplete abortion, pregnancy must be terminated by another method; product is teratogenic

### Nursing diagnoses
- Knowledge, deficient (teaching)

### Implementation
- Give IM inj in deep muscle mass; rotate inj sites if additional doses are given
- Have crash cart available on unit

### Patient/family education
- Advise patient to report increased blood loss, abdominal cramps, increased temp or foul-smelling lochia

### Evaluation
**Positive therapeutic outcome**
- Loss of fetus
- Control of bleeding

## carisoprodol (Rx)
(kar-i-soe-proe'dole)
carisoprodol, Soma, Soprodol 350, Vanadom
*Func. class.:* Skeletal muscle relaxant, central acting
*Chem. class.:* Meprobamate congener

**Pregnancy category** C

**Do not confuse:**
Soma/Soma compound

**Action:** Depresses CNS by blocking interneuronal activity in descending reticular formation of spinal cord, producing sedation

**Therapeutic outcome:** Relaxation of skeletal muscles

**Uses:** Relieving pain, stiffness in musculoskeletal disorders

### Dosage and routes
*Adult and child >12 yr:* PO 350 mg tid and at bedtime
*Child 6-12 yr:* PO 6.25 mg/kg qid

**Available forms:** Tabs 350 mg

### Adverse effects
*CNS: Dizziness, weakness, drowsiness,* headache, tremor, depression, insomnia, ataxia, irritability, **seizures**
*CV:* Postural hypotension, tachycardia
*EENT:* Diplopia, temporary loss of vision
*GI:* Nausea, vomiting, hiccups, epigastric discomfort
*HEMA:* Eosinophilia
*INTEG:* Rash, pruritus, fever, facial flushing, **erythema multiforme**
*RESP:* Asthmatic attack
*SYST:* **Angioedema, anaphylaxis**

**Contraindications:** Hypersensitivity, child <12 yr, intermittent porphyria

**Precautions:** Pregnancy **C**, breastfeeding, geriatric, renal/hepatic disease, addictive personality

#### Pharmacokinetics
| | |
|---|---|
| Absorption | Well absorbed |
| Distribution | Crosses placenta |
| Metabolism | Liver, extensively, substrate of CYP2C19 |
| Excretion | Kidney, unchanged; breast milk |
| Half-life | 8 hr |

#### Pharmacodynamics
| | |
|---|---|
| Onset | ½ hr |
| Peak | 4 hr |
| Duration | 4-6 hr |

### Interactions
*Individual drugs*
Alcohol: increased CNS depression
*Drug classifications*
Antidepressants (tricyclic), barbiturates, opioids, sedative/hypnotics: increased CNS depression
*Drug/herb*
Chamomile, kava, skullcap, valerian: increased CNS depression
*Drug/lab test*
Increased: AST, alkaline phosphatase, blood glucose

### NURSING CONSIDERATIONS
**Assessment**
• Monitor ROM, atrophy, stiffness, and pain in muscles; assess throughout treatment
• Monitor ECG in seizure patients; poor seizure control has occurred with patients taking this product
• Assess for idiosyncratic reaction within a few min or hr of administration (disorientation, restlessness, weakness, euphoria, blurred vision); patient should be reassured that reaction is temporary
• Check for allergic reactions: rash, fever

**Nursing diagnoses**
• Injury, risk for (adverse reactions)
• Knowledge, deficient (teaching)
• Mobility, impaired physical (uses)

**Implementation**
• Give with meals for GI symptoms
• Have patient use gum, frequent sips of water for dry mouth
• Store in tight container at room temperature
• Use for short term (2-3 wk), potential for habituation

**Patient/family education**
• Caution patient not to take with alcohol, other CNS depressants
• Advise patient to avoid altering activities while taking this product
• Caution patient to avoid hazardous activities if drowsiness or dizziness occurs
• Caution patient to avoid using OTC medication such as cough preparations, antihistamines, unless directed by prescriber

**Evaluation**
**Positive therapeutic outcome**
• Decreased pain, spasticity

**Treatment of overdose:** Activated charcoal, lavage, dialysis

### ! HIGH ALERT

### carmustine (Rx)
(kar-mus'teen)
BiCNU, Gliadel
*Func. class.:* Antineoplastic alkylating agent
*Chem. class.:* Nitrosourea
**Pregnancy category D**

**Action:** Alkylates DNA, RNA; inhibits enzymes that allow synthesis of amino acids in proteins; also responsible for cross-linking DNA strands; activity is not cell cycle phase specific

**Therapeutic outcome:** Prevention of rapidly growing malignant cells

**Uses:** Brain tumors such as glioblastoma, medulloblastoma, astrocytoma, ependymoma, metastic brain tumors; multiple myeloma (with prednisone), Hodgkin's disease, other lymphomas; GI, breast, bronchogenic, and renal carcinomas, other lymphomas; wafer, as adjunct to surgery/radiation in newly diagnosed high-grade malignant glioma patients; in recurrent glioblastoma multiforme patients as adjunct to surgery

**Unlabeled uses:** Malignant melanoma

### Dosage and routes

*Adult:* **IV** 75-100 mg/m$^2$ over 1-2 hr × 2 days or 150-200 mg/m$^2$ × 1 dose q6-8 wk or 40 mg/m$^2$/day × 5 days q6 wk; if WBC 3000-3999/mm$^3$ give 50% of dose; if WBC is 2000-2999/mm$^3$ and platelet count is 25,000-75,000/mm$^3$ give 25% of dose; withhold dose if WBC <2000/mm$^3$ and platelets <25,000/mm$^3$

*Adult:* INTRACAVITARY 8 wafers inserted into resection cavity

**Available forms:** Powder for inj 100 mg; wafer 7.7 mg intracavitary

### Adverse effects

*GI: Nausea, vomiting, anorexia, stomatitis,* **hepatotoxicity**
*GU: Azotemia,* **renal failure**
*HEMA:* **Thrombocytopenia, leukopenia, myelosuppression, anemia**
*INTEG:* Pain, burning, hyperpigmentation at inj site
*RESP:* **Fibrosis, pulmonary infiltrate**

**Contraindications:** Pregnancy **D**, breastfeeding, hypersensitivity, leukopenia, thrombocytopenia

#### Pharmacokinetics

| | |
|---|---|
| **Absorption** | Completely absorbed |
| **Distribution** | Readily penetrates CSF |
| **Metabolism** | Liver, rapid |
| **Excretion** | Kidneys, breast milk |
| **Half-life** | Unknown |

#### Pharmacodynamics

Unknown

### Interactions
*Individual drugs*

Aspirin: increased risk of bleeding
Cimetidine, radiation: increased toxicity
Digoxin: decreased effects of digoxin
Phenytoin: decreased effects of phenytoin
*Drug classifications*

Anticoagulants: increased risk of bleeding
Antineoplastics: increased toxicity
Live vaccines: increased adverse reactions; decreased antibody reaction
Myelosuppressive agents: increased myelosuppression

## NURSING CONSIDERATIONS
### Assessment

• Assess buccal cavity q8hr for dryness, sores or ulceration, white patches, pain, bleeding, dysphagia; obtain prescription for viscous lidocaine (Xylocaine)

• Assess symptoms indicating severe allergic reaction: rash, pruritus, urticaria, purpuric skin lesions, itching, flushing; product should be discontinued

• Monitor CBC, differential, platelet count weekly; withhold product if WBC <4000/mm$^3$ or platelet count is <100,000/mm$^3$; notify prescriber of results if WBC <20,000/mm$^3$, platelets <150,000/mm$^3$

• Monitor renal function studies: BUN, creatinine, urine CCr before and during therapy; I&O ratio; report fall in urine output to <30 ml/hr

• Monitor temp q4hr (may indicate beginning of infection)

• Monitor liver function tests before and during therapy (bilirubin, AST, ALT, LDH) as needed or monthly; note yellowing of skin or sclera, dark urine, clay-colored stools, itchy skin, abdominal pain, fever, diarrhea; hepatotoxicity can be serious and fatal

• Assess for bleeding: hematuria, stool guaiac, bruising or petechiae, mucosa or orifices q8hr; inflammation of mucosa, breaks in skin

• Monitor pulmonary function tests, chest x-ray films before, during therapy; chest film should be obtained q2 wk during treatment; monitor for dyspnea, cough, pulmonary fibrosis; infiltrate occurs after high doses or several low-dose courses

• Identify effects of alopecia on body image; discuss feelings about body changes

### Nursing diagnoses

• Body image, disturbed (adverse reactions)
• Infection, risk for (adverse reactions)
• Injury, risk for (adverse reactions)
• Knowledge, deficient (teaching)

### Implementation

• Blood transfusion or RBC colony-stimulating factors to counter anemia may be required

• Give fluids **IV** or PO before chemotherapy to hydrate patient

• Provide antiemetic 30-60 min before giving product to prevent vomiting, and prn; antibiotics for prophylaxis of infection

• Provide liquid diet (carbonated beverages); gelatin may be added if patient is not nauseated or vomiting

• Give all medications PO, if possible, avoid IM inj if platelets <100,000/mm$^3$

### Wafer route
• Foil pouches may be kept at room temperature for 6 hr, if unopened
• If wafers are broken in several pieces, do not use

### IV route
• Prepare in biologic cabinet wearing gown, gloves, mask; avoid contact with skin
• Administer after diluting 100 mg/3 ml ethyl alcohol (provided); then further dilute 27 ml sterile water for inj; then dilute with 100-500 ml 0.9% NaCl or D₅W; give over 1 hr or more; use only glass containers; reduce rate if discomfort is felt
• Flush **IV** line after carmustine with 10 ml 0.9% NaCl to prevent irritation at site
• Store reconstituted sol in refrigerator for 24 hr or room temperature for 8 hr

*Y-site compatibilities:* Amifostine, aztreonam, cefepime, filgrastim, fludarabine, granisetron, melphalan, ondansetron, piperacillin/tazobactam, sargramostim, teniposide, thiotepa, vinorelbine

*Additive incompatibilities:* Sodium bicarbonate

### Patient/family education
• Teach patient to avoid use of products containing aspirin or ibuprofen, razors, commercial mouthwash, since bleeding may occur; to report symptoms of bleeding (hematuria, tarry stools)
• Advise patient to avoid foods with citric acid, hot or rough texture if stomatitis is present
• Instruct patient to report signs of anemia (fatigue, headache, irritability, faintness, shortness of breath); avoid smoking
• Advise patient that hair may be lost during treatment; a wig or hairpiece may make patient feel better; new hair may be different in color, texture
• Caution patient not to have any vaccinations without the advice of the prescriber; serious reactions can occur
• Advise patient that contraception is needed during treatment and for several months after completion of therapy; product has teratogenic properties

### Evaluation
**Positive therapeutic outcome**
• Prevention of rapid division of malignant cells

### carteolol ophthalmic
*See Appendix D*

---

## carvedilol (Rx)
(kar-veh'dee-lol)
Coreg, Coreg CR
*Func. class.:* Antihypertensive α/β-blocker

**Pregnancy category C**

**Do not confuse:**
carvedilol/Captopril/Carteolol

**Action:** A mixture of nonselective β-blocking and α-blocking activity; decreases cardiac output, exercise-induced tachycardia, reflex orthostatic tachycardia; causes reduction in peripheral vascular resistance and vasodilatation

**Therapeutic outcome:** Decreased B/P in hypertension

**Uses:** Essential hypertension alone or in combination with other antihypertensives, CHF, LV dysfunction following MI, cardiomyopathy

### Dosage and routes
*Essential hypertension*
*Adult:* PO 6.25 mg bid × 7-14 days if tolerated well, then increase to 12.5 mg bid × 7-14 days if tolerated well, may be increased if needed to 25 mg bid, max 50 mg daily; EXT REL cap 20 mg/day, may increase after 7-14 days to 40 mg/day

*Congestive heart failure*
*Adult:* PO 3.125 mg bid × 2 wk; if well tolerated, give 6.25 mg bid × 2 wk, then double q2 wk to max dose 25 mg bid <85 kg or 80 mg bid >85 kg; EXT REL cap (Coreg CR) 10 mg/day × 2 wk

*Cardiomyopathy*
*Adult:* PO 6.25-25 mg bid

**Available forms:** Tabs 3.125, 6.25, 12.5, 25 mg; ext rel cap 10, 20, 40, 80 mg

### Adverse effects
*CNS: Dizziness,* somnolence, insomnia, ataxia, hyperesthesia, paresthesia, vertigo, depression, fatigue, weakness, headache
*CV: Bradycardia, postural hypotension,* dependent edema, peripheral edema, **AV block, extrasystoles,** hypo/hypertension, palpitations, peripheral ischemia, **CHF,** pulmonary edema
*GI: Diarrhea,* abdominal pain, increased alkaline phosphatase, increased ALT/AST
*GU:* Decreased libido, *impotence,* UTI
*MISC:* Injury, back pain, viral infection, hypertriglyceridemia, **thrombocytopenia,** *hyperglycemia*
*RESP:* Rhinitis, pharyngitis, dyspnea, **bronchospasm**

Adverse effects: *italic* = common, **bold** = life-threatening

**Contraindications:** Hypersensitivity, bronchial asthma, class IV decompensated cardiac failure, 2nd- or 3rd-degree heart block, cardiogenic shock, severe bradycardia, pulmonary edema

**Precautions:** Pregnancy **C**, breastfeeding, children, geriatric, cardiac failure, hepatic injury, peripheral vascular disease, anesthesia, major surgery, diabetes mellitus, thyrotoxicosis, emphysema, chronic bronchitis, renal disease

### Pharmacokinetics

| | |
|---|---|
| **Absorption** | Readily and extensively absorbed |
| **Distribution** | >98% protein binding |
| **Metabolism** | Extensively liver |
| **Excretion** | Via bile into feces |
| **Half-life** | Terminal half-life 7-10 hr, increased in the geriatric, hepatic disease |

### Pharmacodynamics

Unknown

### Interactions
#### Individual drugs
Alcohol (acute ingestion), cimetidine: increased toxicity

Clonidine: decreased heart rate, B/P

Digoxin: increased concentrations of digoxin

Reserpine, levodopa: increased hypotension, bradycardia

Rifampin: decreased levels of carvedilol
#### Drug classifications
Antihypertensives, nitrates: increased toxicity

Antidiabetic agents: increased hypoglycemia

Calcium channel blockers: increased conduction disturbance

MAOIs: increased bradycardia, hypotension

NSAIDs, thyroid hormones: decreased levels of carvedilol
#### Drug/herb
Aconite: increased toxicity, death

Astragalus, cola tree: increased or decreased antihypertensive effect

Barberry, betony, black catechu, black cohosh, bloodroot, broom, burdock, cat's claw, dandelion, goldenseal, hawthorn, Irish moss, Jamaican dogwood, kelp, khella, mistletoe, parsley: increased antihypertensive effect

Coltsfoot, guarana, khat, licorice: decreased antihypertensive effect

### NURSING CONSIDERATIONS
#### Assessment
• Monitor renal studies including protein, BUN, creatinine; watch for increased levels that may indicate nephrotic syndrome; obtain baselines in renal and liver function tests before beginning treatment; if liver function tests are elevated, product should be discontinued

• Monitor I&O, weight daily

• Monitor B/P during beginning treatment and periodically thereafter; pulse q4hr, note rate, rhythm, quality

• Monitor apical/radial pulse before administration; notify prescriber of significant changes, pulse <50 bpm hold product, notify prescriber

• Assess for edema in feet and legs daily, fluid overload: dyspnea, weight gain, jugular vein distention, fatigue, crackles

#### Nursing diagnoses
• Cardiac output, decreased (uses)
• Injury, risk for (adverse reactions)
• Knowledge, deficient (teaching)
• Noncompliance (teaching)

#### Implementation
• Give PO before meals, at bedtime; tablets may be crushed or swallowed whole, give with food to decrease orthostatic hypotension; do not break, crush, or chew ext rel cap

• Administer reduced dosage in renal dysfunction

#### Patient/family education
• Teach patient not to break, crush, or chew ext rel cap

• Instruct patient to comply with dosage schedule even if feeling better, that improvement may take several weeks

• Teach patient to rise slowly to sitting or standing position to minimize orthostatic hypotension

• Encourage patient to report bradycardia, dizziness, confusion, depression, fever, weight gain, shortness of breath, cold extremities, rash, sore throat, bleeding, bruising

• Teach patient to take pulse at home; advise when to notify prescriber

 Encourage patient not to discontinue product abruptly, taper over 1-2 wk

• Advise patient to avoid hazardous activities until stabilized on medication; dizziness may occur

• Advise patient to avoid all OTC medications unless approved by prescriber

• Advise patient to carry/wear emergency ID with product name, prescriber at all times

• Advise patient to inform all health care providers of products, supplements taken

 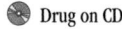

## Evaluation
**Positive therapeutic outcome**
- Decreased B/P
- Decreased symptoms of CHF or angina

---

## cefaclor
*See cephalosporins—2nd generation*

---

## cefadroxil
## cefazolin
*See cephalosporins—1st generation*

---

## cefdinir
## cefditoren pivoxil
## cefepime
## cefotaxime
*See cephalosporins—3rd generation*

---

## cefotetan
## cefoxitin
*See cephalosporins—2nd generation*

---

## cefpodoxime
*See cephalosporins—3rd generation*

---

## cefprozil
*See cephalosporins—2nd generation*

---

## ceftazidime
## ceftibuten
## ceftizoxime
## ceftriaxone
*See cephalosporins—3rd generation*

---

## cefuroxime
*See cephalosporins—2nd generation*

---

### ! HIGH ALERT

## celecoxib (Rx)
(cel-eh-cox'ib)
Celebrex
*Func. class.:* Nonsteroidal antiinflammatory, antirheumatic
*Chem. class.:* COX-2 inhibitor

**Pregnancy category**
**C** (1st/2nd trimesters),
**D** (3rd trimester)

**Do not confuse:**
Celebrex/Celexa/Cerebra/Cerebyx

**Action:** Inhibits prostaglandin synthesis by selectively inhibiting cyclooxygenase 2 (COX-2), an enzyme needed for biosynthesis

**Therapeutic outcome:** Decreased pain, inflammation

**Uses:** Acute, chronic rheumatoid arthritis, osteoarthritis, familial adenomatous polyposis (FAP), acute pain, primary dysmenorrhea, ankylosing spondylitis, juvenile rheumatoid arthritis (JRA)

**Unlabeled uses:** Colorectal adenoma prophylaxis

**Dosage and routes**
**Do not exceed recommended dose, deaths have occurred**

*Acute pain/primary dysmenorrhea*
*Adult:* PO 400 mg initially, then 200 mg if needed on first day, then 200 mg bid prn on subsequent days, if needed

*Osteoarthritis*
*Adult:* PO 200 mg/day as a single dose or 100 mg bid

*Rheumatoid arthritis*
*Adult:* PO 100-200 mg bid

*Ankylosing spondylitis*
*Adult:* PO 200 mg daily or in divided dose (bid)

*FAP*
*Adult:* PO 400 mg bid

*Juvenile rheumatoid arthritis (JRA)*
*Adolescent and child ≥2 yr (>25 kg):* PO 100 mg bid
*Child ≥2 yr (10-25 kg):* PO 50 mg bid

*Colorectal adenoma prophylaxis (unlabeled)*
*Adult:* PO 400 mg bid × 6 mo

---

Adverse effects: *italic* = common, **bold** = life-threatening

**Hepatic dose**
**(Child-Pugh class II)**
*Adult:* PO reduce dose by 50%

**Available forms:** Caps 50, 100, 200, 400 mg

## Adverse effects

*CNS: Fatigue, anxiety, depression, nervousness, paresthesia,* dizziness, insomnia
*CV:* **Stroke, MI, tachycardia, CHF,** angina, palpitations, dysrhythmias, hypertension, fluid retention
*EENT:* Tinnitus, hearing loss, blurred vision, glaucoma, cataract, conjunctivitis, eye pain
*GI: Nausea, anorexia, vomiting, constipation, dry mouth,* diverticulitis, gastritis, gastroenteritis, hemorrhoids, hiatal hernia, stomatitis, **GI bleeding/ulceration**
*GU:* **Nephrotoxicity: dysuria, hematuria, oliguria, azotemia, cystitis, UTI**
*HEMA:* **Blood dyscrasias,** epistaxis, bruising, anemia, **platelet aggregation**
*INTEG:* Purpura, rash, pruritus, sweating, erythema, petechiae, photosensitivity, alopecia, **serious sometimes fatal Stevens-Johnson syndrome, toxic epidermal necrolysis**
*RESP:* Pharyngitis, shortness of breath, pneumonia, coughing

**Contraindications:** Pregnancy **D** (3rd trimester), hypersensitivity to aspirin, iodides, other NSAIDs, sulfonamides, asthma, asthma triad, severe CV disease, CABG

**Precautions:** Pregnancy **C** (1st/2nd trimester), breastfeeding, children <18 yr, geriatric, renal/hepatic disease, hypertension, severe dehydration, bleeding, GI, cardiac disorders, hypersensitivity to other antiinflammatories, glucocorticoids, anticoagulants

| Pharmacokinetics | |
|---|---|
| **Absorption** | Well absorbed (PO) |
| **Distribution** | Crosses placenta, bound to plasma proteins |
| **Metabolism** | Liver |
| **Excretion** | Kidneys |
| **Half-life** | 11 hr |

| Pharmacodynamics | |
|---|---|
| **Onset** | Unknown |
| **Peak** | 3 hr |
| **Duration** | Unknown |

## Interactions
### Individual drugs
Aspirin: decreased effectiveness; increased adverse reactions
Fluconazole: increased celecoxib level
Furosemide: decreased effect of furosemide
Lithium: increased toxicity
Warfarin: increased anticoagulant effects

### Drug classifications
ACE inhibitors: may decrease effects of ACE inhibitors
Anticoagulants: increased risk of bleeding
Antineoplastics: increased risk of hematologic toxicity
Glucocorticoids, NSAIDs: increased adverse reactions
Thiazide diuretics: decreased effectiveness of diuretics

### Drug/herb
Arginine, gossypol: increased gastric irritation
Bearberry, bilberry: increased celecoxib effect
Bogbean, saw palmetto, turmeric: increased bleeding risk
St. John's wort: severe photosensitivity

### Drug/lab test
Increased: ALT, AST, BUN

## NURSING CONSIDERATIONS
### Assessment
• Assess for pain of rheumatoid arthritis, osteoarthritis; check ROM, inflammation of joints, characteristics of pain
◆ Monitor blood counts during therapy; watch for decreasing platelets; if low, therapy may need to be discontinued, restarted after hematologic recovery; and for blood dyscrasias (thrombocytopenia): bruising, fatigue, bleeding, poor healing
• Assess FAP patient for decreasing number of polyps

### Nursing diagnoses
• Injury, risk for (side effects)
• Knowledge, deficient (teaching)
• Mobility, impaired physical (uses)
• Pain, acute (uses)
• Pain, chronic (uses)

### Implementation
• Do not break, crush, chew, or dissolve caps
• Administer with food or milk to decrease gastric symptoms
• Do not increase dose

### Patient/family education
◆ Do not exceed recommended dose; notify prescriber immediately of chest pain, skin eruptions, stop product
• Teach patient that product must be continued for prescribed time to be effective; to avoid other NSAIDs, sulfonamides
• Caution patient to report bleeding, bruising, fatigue, malaise, since blood abnormalities do occur; to report GI symptoms: black tarry stools, cramping

- Teach patient to take with a full glass of water to enhance absorption
- Teach patient to check with prescriber to determine when product should be discontinued before surgery; advise patient to notify prescriber if pregnancy is planned or suspected

**Evaluation**
**Positive therapeutic outcome**
- Decreased pain in arthritic conditions
- Decreased inflammation in arthritic conditions
- Decreased number of polyps (FAP)

## cephalexin
*See cephalosporins—1st generation*

## CEPHALOSPORINS—1ST GENERATION

**cefadroxil** (Rx)
(sef-a-drox'ill)
cefadroxil, Duricef
**cefazolin** (Rx)
(sef-a'zoe-lin)
Ancef, cefazolin
**cephalexin** (Rx)
(sef-a-lex'in)
Apo-Cephalex ✦, cephalexin, Keflex, Keftab, Novo-Lexin ✦, Nu-Cephalex ✦, Panixine
**cephradine** (Rx)
(sef'ra-deen)
cephradine, Velosef
*Func. class.:* Antiinfective
*Chem. class.:* Cephalosporin (1st generation)

**Pregnancy category** B

**Do not confuse:**
cephalexin/cefaclor

**Action:** Inhibits bacterial cell wall synthesis, rendering cell wall osmotically unstable, leading to cell death by binding to cell wall membrane, lysis mediated by cell wall autolytic enzymes

*cefadroxil*
**Therapeutic outcome:** Bactericidal effects for the following: gram-negative bacilli *Escherichia coli, Proteus mirabilis, Klebsiella* (UTI only); gram-positive organisms *Streptococcus pneumoniae, Streptococcus pyogenes, Staphylococcus aureus*

**Uses:** Upper, lower respiratory tract, urinary tract, skin infections; otitis media; tonsillitis, pharyngitis; particularly for UTI

*cefazolin*
**Therapeutic outcome:** Bactericidal effects for the following: gram-negative organisms, *Haemophilus influenzae, Escherichia coli, Proteus mirabilis, Klebsiella;* gram-positive organisms, *Staphylococcus aureus*

**Uses:** Upper, lower respiratory tract, urinary tract, skin infections; bone, joint, biliary, genital infections; endocarditis, surgical prophylaxis, septicemia

*cephalexin*
**Therapeutic outcome:** Bactericidal effects for the following: gram-negative organisms *Haemophilus influenzae, Escherichia coli, Proteus mirabilis, Klebsiella;* gram-positive organisms *Streptococcus pneumoniae, Streptococcus pyogenes, Staphylococcus aureus*

**Uses:** Upper, lower respiratory tract, urinary tract, skin, bone infections; otitis media

*cephradine*
**Therapeutic outcome:** Bactericidal effects for the following: gram-negative bacilli *Haemophilus influenzae, Escherichia coli, Proteus mirabilis, Klebsiella;* gram-positive organisms *Streptococcus pneumoniae, Streptococcus pyogenes, Staphylococcus aureus*

**Uses:** Serious respiratory tract, urinary tract, skin infections; otitis media

**Dosage and routes**
*cefadroxil*
*Adult:* PO 1-2 g daily or q12hr in divided doses, give a loading dose of 1 g initially
*Child:* PO 30 mg/kg/day in divided doses bid

*Renal dose*
*Adult:* PO CCr 25-50 ml/min, 500 mg q12hr; CCr 10-24 ml/min 500 mg q24hr, CCr <10 ml/min 500 mg q36hr

**Available forms:** Caps 500 mg; tabs 1 g; oral susp 125, 250, 500 mg/5 ml
*cefazolin*
*Life-threatening infections*
*Adult:* IM/**IV** 1-2 g q6hr, max 12 g/day
*Child >1 mo:* IM/ 100 mg/kg in 3-4 divided doses, max 6 g/day

*Mild/moderate infections*
*Adult:* IM/**IV** 250 mg-1 g q8hr

*Child >1 mo:* IM/ 25-50 mg/kg in 3-4 equal doses

**Renal dose**
*Adult:* IM/**IV** Following loading dose CCr 35-54 ml/min dose q8hr; CCr 10-34 ml/min 50% of dose q12hr; CCr <10 ml/min 50% of dose q18-24hr
*Child:* IM/**IV** CCr >70 ml/min, no dosage adjustment; CCr 40-70 ml/min following loading dose, reduce dose to 7.5-30 mg/kg q12hr; CCr 20-39 ml/min, give 3.125-12.5 mg/kg after loading dose q12hr; CCr 5-19 ml/min, 2.5-10 mg/kg after loading dose q24 hr

**Available forms:** Inj 250, 500 mg, 1, 5, 10, 20 g; infusion 500 mg, 1 g/50 ml vial

*cephalexin*
**Renal dose**
*Adult:* PO CCr <40 ml/min q8-12hr; CCr 5-10 ml/min q12hr; CCr <5 ml/min q24hr

**Moderate infections**
*Adult:* PO 250-500 mg q6hr
*Child:* PO 25-50 mg/kg/day in 4 equal doses, max 4 g/day

**Moderate skin infections**
*Adult:* PO 500 mg q12hr

**Endocarditis prophylaxis**
2 g 1 hr before procedure

**Severe infections**
*Adult:* PO 500 mg-1 g q6hr
*Child:* PO 50-100 mg/kg/day in 4 equal doses, max 4 g/day

**Available forms:** Caps 250, 500 mg; tabs 250, 500 mg, 1 g; oral susp 125, 250 mg/5 ml

*cephradine*
*Adult:* PO 250 mg-1 g q6-12hr
*Child >1 yr:* PO 6-12 mg/kg q6hr

**Renal dose**
*Adult:* PO CCr >20 ml/min 500 mg q6hr; CCr 5-20 ml/min 250 mg q6hr

**Available forms:** Caps 250, 500 mg; oral susp 125, 250 mg/5 ml

**Side effects/adverse reactions**
*CNS:* Headache, dizziness, weakness, paresthesia, fever, chills, **seizures** (high doses)
*GI:* Nausea, vomiting, *diarrhea, anorexia,* pain, glossitis, bleeding; increased AST, ALT, bilirubin, LDH, alkaline phosphatase; abdominal pain, **pseudomembranous colitis**
*GU:* Proteinuria, vaginitis, pruritus, candidiasis, increased BUN, **nephrotoxicity, renal failure**

*HEMA:* **Leukopenia, thrombocytopenia, agranulocytosis,** anemia, **neutropenia, lymphocytosis, eosinophilia, pancytopenia, hemolytic anemia**
*INTEG:* Rash, urticaria, dermatitis
*RESP:* Dyspnea
*SYST:* **Anaphylaxis, serum sickness,** superinfection, **Stevens-Johnson syndrome**

**Contraindications:** Hypersensitivity to cephalosporins, infants <1 mo

**Precautions:** Pregnancy **B**, breastfeeding, hypersensitivity to penicillins, renal disease

*cefadroxil*

| Pharmacokinetics | |
|---|---|
| **Absorption** | Well absorbed |
| **Distribution** | Widely distributed; crosses placenta |
| **Metabolism** | Not metabolized |
| **Excretion** | Unchanged by kidneys; enters breast milk |
| **Half-life** | 1½-2 hr |

| Pharmacodynamics | |
|---|---|
| | PO |
| **Onset** | Rapid |
| **Peak** | 1½-2 hr |
| **Duration** | 12-24 hr |

*cefazolin*

| Pharmacokinetics | |
|---|---|
| **Absorption** | Well absorbed |
| **Distribution** | Widely distributed; crosses placenta |
| **Metabolism** | Not metabolized |
| **Excretion** | Unchanged by kidneys; enters breast milk |
| **Half-life** | 1½-2½ hr |

| Pharmacodynamics | | |
|---|---|---|
| | IM | IV |
| **Onset** | Rapid | 10 min |
| **Peak** | 1-2 hr | Infusion's end |
| **Duration** | 6-12 hr | Unknown |

*cephalexin*

| Pharmacokinetics | |
|---|---|
| **Absorption** | Well absorbed |
| **Distribution** | Widely distributed; crosses placenta |
| **Metabolism** | Not metabolized |
| **Excretion** | Kidneys, unchanged; enters breast milk |
| **Half-life** | ½-1 hr; increased in renal disease |

| Pharmacodynamics | |
|---|---|
| Onset | 15-30 min |
| Peak | 1 hr |
| Duration | 6-12 hr |

## cephradine

| Pharmacokinetics | |
|---|---|
| Absorption | Well absorbed |
| Distribution | Widely distributed; crosses placenta |
| Metabolism | Not metabolized |
| Excretion | Kidneys, unchanged; enters breast milk |
| Half-life | 1-2 hr |

| Pharmacodynamics | | |
|---|---|---|
| | PO/IM | IV |
| Onset | Rapid | Immediate |
| Peak | 1-2 hr | Infusion's end |
| Duration | 6-12 hr | |

## Interactions
### Individual drugs
Probenecid: increased toxicity
### Drug classifications
Aminoglycosides, diuretics (loop): increased toxicity
### Drug/herb
Acidophilus: do not use with antiinfectives; separate by several hours
### Drug/lab test
Increased: AST, ALT, alkaline phosphatase, LDH, BUN, creatinine, bilirubin
False positive: urinary protein, direct Coombs' test, urine glucose
Interference: cross-matching

## NURSING CONSIDERATIONS
### Assessment
• Assess patient for previous sensitivity reaction to penicillins or other cephalosporins; cross-sensitivity between penicillins and cephalosporins is common
• Assess patient for signs and symptoms of infection including characteristics of wounds, sputum, urine, stool, WBC >10,000/mm$^3$, earache, fever; obtain baseline information and during treatment
• Obtain C&S before beginning product therapy to identify if correct treatment has been initiated
• Assess for anaphylaxis: rash, urticaria, pruritus, chills, fever, joint pain; angioedema may occur a few days after therapy begins; epINEPHrine and resuscitation equipment should be available for anaphylactic reaction

• Identify urine output; if decreasing, notify prescriber (may indicate nephrotoxicity); also check for increased BUN, creatinine
• Monitor blood studies: AST, ALT, CBC, Hct, bilirubin, LDH, alkaline phosphatase, Coombs' test monthly if patient is on long-term therapy
• Monitor electrolytes: potassium, sodium, chloride monthly if patient is on long-term therapy
• Assess bowel pattern daily; if severe diarrhea occurs, product should be discontinued; may indicate pseudomembranous colitis
• Monitor for bleeding: ecchymosis, bleeding gums, hematuria, stool guaiac daily if on long-term therapy
• Assess for superinfection: perineal itching, fever, malaise, redness, pain, swelling, drainage, rash, diarrhea, change in cough, sputum

### Nursing diagnoses
• Diarrhea (side effects)
• Fluid volume, risk for, deficient (side effects)
• Infection, risk for (uses)
• Injury, risk for (side effects)
• Knowledge, deficient (teaching)
• Noncompliance (teaching)

### cefadroxil
### Implementation
• Give in even doses around the clock; if GI upset occurs, give with food; product must be given for 10-14 days to ensure organism death and prevent superinfection
• Shake susp, refrigerate, discard after 2 wk

### cefazolin
### Implementation
**IM route**
• Reconstitute 250-500 mg of product with 2 ml sterile or bacteriostatic water for inj, or 0.9% NaCl; reconstitute 1 g of product with 2.5 ml; give deep in large muscle mass, massage
**IV route**
• Check for irritation, extravasation, phlebitis daily, change site q72hr
• For direct **IV** dilute in 10 ml of sterile water for inj; give over 5 min
• For intermittent inf dilute reconstituted sol (500 mg or 1 mg) in 50-100 ml D$_5$W, D$_{10}$W, D$_5$/0.25% NaCl, D$_5$/0.45% NaCl, D$_5$/0.9% NaCl, D$_5$/LR, or LR, 0.9% NaCl; give over 30-60 min; may be refrigerated up to 96 hr or stored 24 hr at room temperature
**Syringe compatibilities:** Heparin, vit B complex
**Syringe incompatibilities:** Ascorbic acid inj, cimetidine, lidocaine, vit B/C
**Y-site compatibilities:** Acyclovir, allopurinol, amifostine, atracurium, aztre-

onam, calcium gluconate, cyclophosphamide, diltiazem, enalaprilat, esmolol, famotidine, filgrastim, fluconazole, fludarabine, foscarnet, heparin, labetalol, lidocaine, magnesium sulfate, melphalan, meperidine, midazolam, morphine, multivitamins, ondansetron, perphenazine, pancuronium, regular insulin, sargramostim, tacrolimus, teniposide, theophylline, thiotepa, vecuronium, vit B/C

*Y-site incompatibilities:* Amiodarone, hetastarch, hydromorphone, idarubicin, vinorelbine tartrate

*Additive compatibilities:* Aztreonam, clindamycin, famotidine, fluconazole, metronidazole, verapamil

*Additive incompatibilities:* Amikacin, amobarbital, bleomycin, calcium gluceptate, calcium gluconate, colistimethate, erythromycin, kanamycin, oxytetracycline, pentobarbital, polymyxin B, tetracycline

*cephalexin*
## Implementation
• Do not break, crush, or chew caps
• Give in even doses around the clock; if GI upset occurs, give with food; product must be taken for 10-14 days to ensure organism death and prevent superinfection
• Shake susp, refrigerate, discard after 2 wk

*cephradine*
## Implementation
**PO route**
• May be given with food for GI symptoms
• When giving susp, shake well; refrigerate unused portion
**IM route**
• Reconstitute 250 mg/1.2 ml, 500 mg/ml, 1 g/4 ml sterile or bacteriostatic water for inj; give deep in large muscle mass, massage
**IV route**
• Check for irritation, extravasation, phlebitis daily; change site q72hr
• For direct **IV** route, reconstitute 250-500 mg/5 ml sterile water, 0.9% NaCl, $D_5W$, or 1 g/10 ml, 2 g/20 ml; give over 3-5 min
• For intermittent inf, dilute 1 g/10 ml or more sterile water for inj, $D_5W$, $D_{10}W$, or $D_5/0.9\%$ NaCl; give over 30-60 min
• Store refrigerated 96 hr, room temperature 24 hr

*Additive incompatibilities:* Other antibiotics, calcium salts, $D_5W$, epINEPHrine, lidocaine, Ringer's or LR sol, NormosolR, 0.9% NaCl, TPN #61, tetracycline

## Patient/family education
• Teach patient to report sore throat, bruising, bleeding, joint pain; may indicate blood dyscrasias (rare)

• Advise patient to contact prescriber if vaginal itching, loose foul-smelling stools, furry tongue occur; may indicate superinfection
• Instruct patient to take all medication prescribed for the length of time ordered
• Advise patient to notify prescriber of diarrhea with blood, pus, mucus, which may indicate pseudomembranous colitis

## Evaluation
**Positive therapeutic outcome**
• Absence of signs/symptoms of infection (WBC <10,000/mm³, temp WNL, absence of red draining wounds, earache)
• Reported improvement in symptoms of infection
• Negative C&S

**Treatment of anaphylaxis:** EpINEPHrine, antihistamines, resuscitate if needed

---

# CEPHALOSPORINS— 2ND GENERATION

**cefaclor** (Rx)
(sef'a-klor)
Ceclor, Raniclor
**cefotetan** (Rx)
(sef'oh-tee-tan)
Cefotan
**cefoxitin** (Rx)
(se-fox'i-tin)
Mefoxin
**cefprozil** (Rx)
(sef-proe'zill)
Cefzil
**cefuroxime** (Rx)
(sef-yoor-ox'eem)
Ceftin, Cefuroxime, Zinacef
**loracarbef** (Rx)
(lor-a-kar'beff)
Lorabid
*Func. class.:* Antiinfective
*Chem. class.:* Cephalosporin (2nd generation)

**Pregnancy category** B

**Do not confuse:**
cefaclor/cephalexin, Cefotan/Ceftin, cefprozil/cefazolin/cefuroxime, Cefzil/Ceftin/Kefzol

**Action:** Inhibits bacterial cell wall synthesis, rendering cell wall osmotically unstable, leading to cell death by binding to cell wall membrane

---

## cefaclor
**Therapeutic outcome:** Bactericidal effects for the following: gram-negative bacilli *Haemophilus influenzae, Escherichia coli, Proteus mirabilis, Klebsiella;* gram-positive organisms *Streptococcus pneumoniae, Staphylococcus* β-hemolytic; streptococci, anaerobes, *Bacteroides* sp.

**Uses:** Upper and lower respiratory tract, urinary tract, skin infections; otitis media; increased bone, joint, gynecologic infections; septicemia

## cefotetan
**Therapeutic outcome:** Bactericidal effects for the following: gram-negative organisms *Citrobacter, Haemophilus influenzae, Escherichia coli, Enterobacter aerogenes, Proteus mirabilis, Klebsiella, Morganella morganii, Proteus vulgaris, Providencia, Enterobacter, Salmonella, Shigella, Acinetobacter, Bacteroides fragilis, Neisseria, Serratia;* gram-positive organisms *Streptococcus pneumoniae, Streptococcus pyogenes, Staphylococcus aureus;* anaerobes *Bacteroides, Clostridium, Fusobacterium, Peptococcus, Peptostreptococcus*

**Uses:** Serious upper or lower respiratory tract, urinary tract, gynecologic, skin, bone, joint, gonococcal, intraabdominal infections

## cefoxitin
**Therapeutic outcome:** Bactericidal effects for the following: gram-negative bacilli *Bacteroides fragilis, Haemophilus influenzae, Escherichia coli, Proteus, Klebsiella, Providencia, Neisseria gonorrhoeae;* gram-positive organisms *Streptococcus pneumoniae, Streptococcus pyogenes, Staphylococcus aureus;* anaerobes including *Clostridium, Bacteroides, Peptococcus, Peptostreptococcus*

**Uses:** Lower respiratory tract, urinary tract, skin, bone, gynecologic, gonococcal infections; septicemia, peritonitis

## cefprozil
**Therapeutic outcome:** Bactericidal effects for the following: gram-negative bacilli *Haemophilus influenzae, Escherichia coli;* gram-positive organisms *Streptococcus pneumoniae, Streptococcus pyogenes, Staphylococcus aureus*

**Uses:** Pharyngitis/tonsillitis, otitis media, secondary bacterial infection of acute bronchitis, and acute bacterial exacerbation of chronic bronchitis and uncomplicated skin and skin structure infections; acute sinusitis

## cefuroxime
**Therapeutic outcome:** Bactericidal effects for the following: gram-negative bacilli *Haemophilus influenzae, Escherichia coli, Neisseria, Proteus mirabilis, Klebsiella;* gram-positive organisms: *Streptococcus pneumoniae, Streptococcus pyogenes, Staphylococcus aureus*

**Uses:** Serious lower respiratory tract, urinary tract, skin, bone, joint, gonococcal infections, septicemia, meningitis

## loracarbef
**Therapeutic outcome:** Bactericidal effects for the following: gram-negative organisms *Haemophilus influenzae, Escherichia coli, Proteus mirabilis, Klebsiella;* gram-positive organisms *Streptococcus pneumoniae, Streptococcus pyogenes, Staphyloccus aureus*

**Uses:** Upper and lower respiratory tract, urinary tract, skin infections; otitis media, pharyngitis, tonsillitis

## Dosage and routes
### cefaclor
***Adult:*** PO 250-500 mg q8hr, not to exceed 4 g/day or 375-500 mg (ext rel) q12hr × 7-10 days

***Child >1 mo:*** PO 20-40 mg/kg daily in divided doses q8hr, or total daily dose may be divided and given q12hr, not to exceed 1 g/day

**Available forms:** Caps 250, 500 mg; oral susp 125, 187, 250, 375 mg/5 ml; chew tabs (Raniclor) 125, 187, 250, 375 mg

### cefotetan
***Adult:*** IV/IM 1-2 g q12hr × 5-10 days

***Renal dose***
***Adult:*** IM/**IV** CCr 10-30 ml/min q24hr or ½ dose q12hr; CCr <10 ml/min q48hr or ½ dose q24hr

***Perioperative proplylaxis***
***Adult:*** **IV** 1-2 g ½-1 hr before surgery

**Available forms:** Inj 1, 2, 10 g

### cefoxitin
***Adult:*** IM/**IV** 1-2 g q6-8hr

***Uncomplicated gonorrhea***
IM 2 g as single dose with 1 g PO probenecid at same time

***Renal dose***
After loading dose CCr 30-50 ml/min 1-2 g q8-12hr; CCr 10-29 ml/min 1-2 g q12-24hr; CCr <10 ml/min 0.5-1 g q12-24hr

*Severe infections*
*Adult:* IM/**IV** 2 g q4hr
*Child ≥3 mo:* IM/**IV** 80-160 mg/kg/day
divided q4-6hr; max 12 g/day

**Available forms:** Powder for inj 1, 2,
10 g

*cefprozil*
**Renal dose**
CCr <30 ml/min 50% of dose

*Upper respiratory infections*
*Adult:* PO 500 mg q24hr × 10 days

*Otitis media*
*Child 6 mo-12 yr:* PO 15 mg/kg
q12hr × 10 days

*Lower respiratory infections*
*Adult:* PO 500 mg q12hr × 10 days

*Skin/skin structure infections*
*Adult:* PO 250-500 mg q12hr × 10 days

**Available forms:** Tabs 250, 500 mg; susp
125, 250 mg/5 ml

*cefuroxime*
*Adult and child:* PO 250 mg q12hr; may
increase to 500 mg of q12hr in serious infections
*Adult:* IM/**IV** 750 mg-1.5 g q8hr for 5-10
days

*Urinary tract infections*
*Adult:* PO 125 mg q12hr; may increase to
250 mg q12hr if needed

*Otitis media*
*Child <2 yr:* PO 125 mg bid
*Child >2 yr:* PO 250 mg bid

*Surgical prophylaxis*
*Adult:* **IV** 1.5 g ½-1 hr preop

*Severe infections*
*Adult:* IM/**IV** 1.5 g q6hr; may give up to 3 g
q8hr for bacterial meningitis
*Child >3 mo:* IM/**IV** 50-100 mg/kg/day;
may give up to 200-240 mg/kg/day **IV** in
divided doses for bacterial meningitis (not
recommended)
• Dosage reduction indicated in severe renal
impairment (CCr <20 ml/min)

*Uncomplicated gonorrhea*
*Adult:* 1.5 g IM as single dose with oral
probenecid in 2 separate sites

**Available forms:** Tabs 125, 250, 500 mg:
inj 150, 750 mg, 1.5, 7.5 g; inj 750 mg; 1.5 g
powder, susp 125, 250 mg/5 ml

*loracarbef*
*Adult and child >13 yr:* PO 200-400
mg q12hr

*Child to 12 yr:* PO 15-30 mg/kg/day in 2
divided doses q12hr

*Renal dose*
CCr 10-49 ml/min 50% of dose; CCr <10
ml/min q3-5 days

**Available forms:** Caps 200, 400 mg; Oral
susp 100, 200 mg/5 ml

**Side effects/adverse reactions**
*CNS:* Dizziness, headache, fatigue, paresthesia,
fever, chills, confusion
*GI:* *Diarrhea,* nausea, vomiting, anorexia,
dysgeusia, glossitis, bleeding; increased AST,
ALT, bilirubin, LDH, alkaline phosphatase;
abdominal pain, loose stools, flatulence,
heartburn, stomach cramps, colitis, jaundice,
**pseudomembranous colitis**
*GU:* Vaginitis, pruritus, candidiasis, increased
BUN, **nephrotoxicity, renal failure,** pyuria,
dysuria, reversible interstitial nephritis
*HEMA:* **Leukopenia, thrombocytopenia,
agranulocytosis,** anemia, **neutropenia,
lymphocytosis, eosinophilia, pancytopenia, hemolytic anemia, leukocytosis,
granulocytopenia**
*INTEG:* Rash, urticaria, dermatitis, **Stevens-
Johnson syndrome**
*RESP:* Dyspnea
*SYST:* **Anaphylaxis, serum sickness,**
superinfection

**Contraindications:** Hypersensitivity to
cephalosporins or related antibiotics, seizures

**Precautions:** Pregnancy **B,** breastfeeding,
children, renal/GI disease

*cefaclor*

| Pharmacokinetics | |
|---|---|
| **Absorption** | Well absorbed |
| **Distribution** | Widely distributed; crosses pla-
centa |
| **Metabolism** | Not metabolized |
| **Excretion** | Unchanged by kidneys (60%-
80%); enters breast milk |
| **Half-life** | 36-54 min; increased in renal
disease |

| Pharmacodynamics | |
|---|---|
| **Onset** | 15 min |
| **Peak** | ½-1 hr |
| **Duration** | Unknown |

## cefotetan

### Pharmacokinetics

| | |
|---|---|
| **Absorption** | Well absorbed (IM) |
| **Distribution** | Widely distributed; crosses placenta |
| **Metabolism** | Not metabolized |
| **Excretion** | Kidneys, unchanged; enters breast milk |
| **Half-life** | 5 hr; increased in renal disease |

### Pharmacodynamics

| | IM | IV |
|---|---|---|
| **Onset** | Rapid | Immediate |
| **Peak** | 1-3 hr | Infusion's end |
| **Duration** | Unknown | Unknown |

## cefoxitin

### Pharmacokinetics

| | |
|---|---|
| **Absorption** | Well absorbed (IM) |
| **Distribution** | Widely distributed; crosses placenta |
| **Metabolism** | Not metabolized |
| **Excretion** | Kidneys, unchanged; enters breast milk |
| **Half-life** | ½-1 hr; increased in renal disease |

### Pharmacodynamics

| | IM | IV |
|---|---|---|
| **Onset** | Rapid | Immediate |
| **Peak** | ½ hr | Infusion's end |
| **Duration** | Unknown | Unknown |

## cefprozil

### Pharmacokinetics

| | |
|---|---|
| **Absorption** | Well absorbed |
| **Distribution** | Widely distributed; crosses placenta |
| **Metabolism** | Not metabolized |
| **Excretion** | Kidneys, unchanged; enters breast milk |
| **Half-life** | 1-1½ hr; increased in renal disease |

### Pharmacodynamics

Unknown

## loracarbef

### Pharmacokinetics

| | |
|---|---|
| **Absorption** | Well absorbed |
| **Distribution** | Widely distributed; crosses placenta |
| **Metabolism** | Not metabolized |
| **Excretion** | Kidneys, unchanged; enters breast milk |
| **Half-life** | 1 hr; increased in renal disease |

### Pharmacodynamics

| | |
|---|---|
| **Onset** | Rapid |
| **Peak** | 1 hr |
| **Duration** | Unknown |

### Interactions
#### Individual drugs
Alcohol: disulfiram reaction if ingested within 48-72 hr of cephalosporin

Antacids: decreased absorption of cephalosporins

Furosemide: increased toxicity

Plicamycin, valproic acid: increased bleeding

Probenecid: decreased excretion of product and increased blood levels/toxicity

#### Drug classifications
Aminoglycosides: increased toxicity

Anticoagulants, antiplatelets, NSAIDs, thrombolytics: increased bleeding (cefotetan)

$H_2$-blockers: decreased effects of cephalosporins

#### Drug/herb
Angelica, anise, arnica, bogbean, boldo, celery, chamomile, clove, fenugreek, feverfew, garlic, ginger, ginkgo, ginseng *(Panax),* horse chestnut, horseradish, licorice, meadowsweet, onion, papain, passion flower, poplar, prickly ash, red clover, turmeric, willow: increased bleeding risk (cefotetan)

Acidophilus: do not use with antiinfectives; separate by several hours

#### Drug/lab test
False: increased creatinine (serum urine), urinary 17-KS

False positive: urinary protein, direct Coombs' test, urine glucose (Clinitest)

Interference: cross-matching

### NURSING CONSIDERATIONS
#### Assessment
• Assess patient for previous sensitivity reaction to penicillins or other cephalosporins; cross-sensitivity between penicillins and cephalosporins is common

---

Adverse effects: *italic* = common, **bold** = life-threatening

- Assess patient for signs and symptoms of infection including characteristics of wounds, sputum, urine, stool, WBC >10,000/mm$^3$, earache, fever; obtain baseline information and during treatment
- Obtain C&S before beginning product therapy to identify if correct treatment has been initiated
- Assess for anaphylaxis: rash, urticaria, pruritus, dyspnea, chills, fever, joint pain; angioedema may occur a few days after therapy begins; epINEPHrine and resuscitation equipment should be available for anaphylactic reaction
- Identify urine output; if decreasing, notify prescriber (may indicate nephrotoxicity); also check for increased BUN, creatinine
- Monitor blood studies: AST, ALT, CBC, Hct, bilirubin, LDH, alkaline phosphatase, Coombs' test monthly if patient is on long-term therapy
- Monitor electrolytes: potassium, sodium, chloride monthly if patient is on long-term therapy
- Assess bowel pattern daily; if severe diarrhea occurs, product should be discontinued; may indicate pseudomembranous colitis
- Monitor for bleeding: ecchymosis, bleeding gums, hematuria, stool guaiac daily if on long-term therapy
- Assess for overgrowth of infection: perineal itching, fever, malaise, redness, pain, swelling, drainage, rash, diarrhea, change in cough, sputum

### Nursing diagnoses
- Diarrhea (side effects)
- Fluid volume, risk for, deficient (side effects)
- Infection, risk for (uses)
- Injury, risk for (side effects)
- Knowledge, deficient (teaching)
- Noncompliance (teaching)

### Implementation
#### cefaclor
- Do not break, crush, chew, or cut ext rel tabs
- Give in even doses around the clock; if GI upset occurs, give with food; product must be given for 10-14 days to ensure organism death and prevent superinfection
- Shake susp, refrigerate, discard after 2 wk

#### cefotetan
**IM route**
- Reconstitute 1 g/2 ml or 2 g/3 ml of sterile or bacteriostatic water for inj; may be diluted with 0.5% of 1% lidocaine to prevent pain; give deep in large muscle mass, massage

**IV route**
- May be stored 96 hr refrigerated or 24 hr room temperature
- Check for irritation, extravasation, phlebitis daily; change site q72hr
- For direct **IV** dilute in 1 g/10 ml or more and give over 5 min
- For intermittent inf further dilute in 50-100 ml of 0.9% NaCl or D$_5$W; give over 3-5 min; discontinue primary line while running intermittent inf

*Syringe incompatibilities:* Doxapram
*Y-site compatibilities:* Allopurinol, amifostine, aztreonam, diltiazem, famotidine, filgrastim, fluconazole, fludarabine, heparin, regular insulin, melphalan, meperidine, morphine, paclitaxel, sargramostim, tacrolimus, teniposide, theophylline, thiotepa
*Additive incompatibilities:* Aminoglycosides, tetracyclines, heparin

#### cefoxitin
**IM route**
- Reconstitute 1 g/2 ml of sterile water for inj; may be diluted with 0.5% or 1% lidocaine to prevent pain; give deep in large muscle mass, massage

**IV route**
- Check for irritation, extravasation, phlebitis daily; change site q72hr
- For direct **IV**, dilute 1 g/10 ml or 2 g/20 ml of sterile water for inj; shake, let stand until clear; give over 3-5 min
- For intermittent inf further dilute with 50-100 ml of D$_5$W, D$_{10}$W, D$_5$/0.25% NaCl, D$_5$/0.45% NaCl, D$_5$/0.9% NaCl, 0.9% NaCl D$_5$/LR, D$_5$/0.02%, sodium bicarbonate, Ringer's, or LR; give over 15-30 min; may store 96 hr refrigerated or 24 hr room temperature
- For cont inf dilute in 500-1000 ml; give over prescribed rate

*Syringe compatibilities:* Heparin, insulin
*Y-site compatibilities:* Acyclovir, amifostine, aztreonam, cyclophosphamide, diltiazem, famotidine, fluconazole, foscarnet, hydromorphone, magnesium sulfate, meperidine, morphine, ondansetron, perphenazine, temiposide, thiotepa
*Y-site incompatibilities:* Hetastarch
*Additive compatibilities:* Amikacin, cimetidine, clindamycin, gentamicin, kanamycin, multivitamins, sodium bicarbonate, tobramycin, verapamil, vit B/C
*Additive incompatibilities:* Aztreonam

*cefprozil*
**IM route**
• Reconstitute with 1 g/2 ml or 2 g/3 ml of sterile or bacteriostatic water for inj; may be diluted with 0.5% or 1% lidocaine to prevent pain; give deep in large muscle mass, massage
**IV route**
• Check for irritation, extravasation, phlebitis daily; change site q72hr
• For direct **IV**, dilute 1 g/10 ml or more and give over 5 min
• For intermittent inf further dilute with 50-100 ml of 0.9% NaCl or D₅W; give over 3-5 min; discontinue primary line while running intermittent infusion
*Syringe incompatibilities:* Doxapram
*Y-site compatibilities:* Famotidine, fluconazole, fludarabine, regular insulin, meperidine, morphine, sargramostim
*Additive incompatibilities:* Aminoglycosides, tetracyclines, heparin

*loracarbef*
◆ Do not break, crush, or chew caps
• Give on an empty stomach, 1 hr before or 2 hr after a meal
• Oral susp should be shaken before administration; store for 2 wk at room temperature, discard after 2 wk

**Patient/family education**
• Teach patient to report sore throat, bruising, bleeding, joint pain; may indicate blood dyscrasias (rare)
• Advise patient to contact prescriber if vaginal itching, loose foul-smelling stools, furry tongue occur; may indicate superinfection
• Instruct patient to take all medication prescribed for the length of time ordered; to use yogurt or buttermilk to maintain intestinal flora, decrease diarrhea
• Advise patient to notify prescriber of diarrhea with blood or pus, which may indicate pseudomembranous colitis

**Evaluation**
**Positive therapeutic outcome**
• Absence of signs/symptoms of infection (WBC <10,000/mm³, temp WNL, absence of red draining wounds, earache)
• Reported improvement in symptoms of infection
• Negative C&S

**Treatment of anaphylaxis:** EpINEPHrine, antihistamines, resuscitate if needed

## CEPHALOSPORINS— 3RD GENERATION

**cefdinir** (Rx)
(sef'dih-ner)
Omnicef
**cefditoren pivoxil** (Rx)
(sef-dit'oh-ren pih-vox'il)
Spectracef
**cefepime** (Rx)
(sef'e-peem)
Maxipime
**cefixime** (Rx)
(sef-iks'ime)
Cefixime
**cefotaxime** (Rx)
(sef-oh-taks'eem)
Claforan
**cefpodoxime** (Rx)
(sef-poe-docks'eem)
Vantin
**ceftazidime** (Rx)
(sef'tay-zi-deem)
Ceptaz, Fortaz, Tazicef, Tazidime
**ceftibuten** (Rx)
(sef-ti-byoo'tin)
Cedax
**ceftizoxime** (Rx)
(sef-ti-zox'eem)
Cefizox
**ceftriaxone** (Rx)
(sef-try-ax'one)
Rocephin
*Func. class.:* Broad-spectrum antibiotic
*Chem. class.:* Cephalosporin (3rd generation)

**Pregnancy category** B

**Do not confuse:**
ceftazidime/ceftizoxime, Vantin/Ventolin

**Action:** Inhibits bacterial cell wall synthesis, rendering cell wall osmotically unstable, leading to cell death

*cefdinir*
**Therapeutic outcome:** Bactericidal effects for the following: gram-negative organisms *Haemophilus influenzae, Serratia, Salmonella, Klebsiella, Citrobacter, Shigella, Pseudomonas, Haemophilus parainfluenzae, Enterococcus faecalis, Moraxella catarrhalis;* gram-positive organisms *Streptococcus pneumoniae, Streptococcus pyogenes, Staphylococcus aureus*

Adverse effects: *italic* = common, **bold** = life-threatening

**Uses:** Uncomplicated skin and skin structure infections, community-acquired pneumonia, acute exacerbations of chronic bronchitis, acute maxillary sinusitis, pharyngitis, tonsillitis, CNS infections, perioperative prophylaxis

### cefditoren pivoxil
**Therapeutic outcome:** Bactericidal effects for the following organisms: *Haemophilus influenzae, Haemophilus parainfluenzae, Streptococcus pneumoniae, Moraxella catarrhalis, Streptococcus pyogenes, Staphylococcus aureus*

**Uses:** Acute bacterial exacerbation of chronic bronchitis, pharyngitis/tonsillitis; uncomplicated skin, skin structure infections

### cefepime
**Therapeutic outcome:** Bactericidal effects for the following: gram-negative bacilli, *Escherichia coli, Proteus, Klebsiella*; gram-positive organisms *Streptococcus pneumoniae, Streptococcus pyogenes, Staphylococcus aureus*

**Uses:** Lower respiratory tract, urinary tract, skin, bone, gonococcal infections; septicemia, peritonitis

### cefixime
**Therapeutic outcome:** Bactericidal effects for the following organisms: *Escherichia coli, Proteus mirabilis, Streptococcus pyogenes, Haemophilus influenzae, Moraxella catarrhalis, Streptococcus pneumoniae*

**Uses:** Uncomplicated UTI, pharyngitis/tonsillitis, otitis media, acute bronchitis, and exacerbations of chronic bronchitis

### cefotaxime
**Therapeutic outcome:** Bactericidal effects for the following: gram-negative organisms *Haemophilus influenzae, Escherichia coli, Neisseria gonorrhoeae, Neisseria meningitidis, Proteus mirabilis, Klebsiella, Citrobacter, Serratia, Salmonella, Shigella Pseudomonas*; gram-positive organisms *Streptococcus pneumoniae, Streptococcus pyogenes, Staphylococcus aureus*

**Uses:** Lower serious respiratory tract, urinary tract, skin, bone, gonococcal infections; bacteremia, septicemia, meningitis, skin, skin structure infections, CNS infections, perioperative prophylaxis

### cefpodoxime
**Therapeutic outcome:** Bactericidal effects for the following: gram-negative organisms *Neisseria gonorrhoeae, Haemophilus influenzae, Escherichia coli, Proteus mirabilis, Klebsiella*; gram-positive organisms *Streptococcus pneumoniae, Streptococcus pyogenes, Staphylococcus aureus*

**Uses:** Upper and lower respiratory tract, urinary tract, skin infections; otitis media, STDs

### ceftazidime
**Therapeutic outcome:** Bactericidal effects for the following: gram-negative organisms *Haemophilus influenzae, Escherichia coli, Enterobacter aerogenes, Proteus mirabilis, Klebsiella, Citrobacter, Enterobacter, Pseudomonas aeruginosa, Shigella, Acinetobacter, Bacteroides fragilis, Neisseria*; gram-positive organisms *Streptococcus pneumoniae, Streptococcus pyogenes, Staphylococcus aureus*

**Uses:** Serious upper or lower respiratory tract, urinary tract, skin, gynecologic, bone, joint, intraabdominal infections; septicemia, meningitis

### ceftibuten
**Therapeutic outcome:** Bactericidal effects for the following: gram-negative bacilli *Haemophilus influenzae, Escherichia coli*; gram-positive organisms *Streptococcus pneumoniae, Streptococcus pyogenes, Staphylococcus aureus*

**Uses:** Pharyngitis, tonsilitis, secondary bacterial infection of acute bronchitis

### ceftizoxime
**Therapeutic outcome:** Bactericidal effects for the following: gram-negative organisms *Haemophilus influenzae, Escherichia coli, Enterobacter aerogenes, Proteus mirabilis, Klebsiella, Acinetobacter, Neisseria gonorrhoeae, Providencia rettgeri, Pseudomonas aeruginosa, Serratia, Enterobacter*; gram-positive organisms *Streptococcus pneumoniae, Streptococcus pyogenes, Staphylococcus aureus*; anaerobes *Bacteroides, Peptococcus, Peptostreptococcus*

**Uses:** Serious lower respiratory tract, urinary tract, skin, intraabdominal infections; septicemia, meningitis; bone, joint infections; PID caused by *Neisseria gonorrhoeae*

### ceftriaxone
**Therapeutic outcome:** Bactericidal effects on the following: gram-negative organisms *Haemophilus influenzae, Escherichia coli, Enterobacter aerogenes, Proteus mirabilis, Klebsiella, Citrobacter, Enterobacter, Pseudomonas aeruginosa, Neisseria, Serratia*; gram-positive organisms *Strepto-*

*coccus pneumoniae, Streptococcus pyogenes, Staphylococcus aureus;* anaerobes *Bacteroides*

**Uses:** Serious lower respiratory tract, urinary tract, skin, gonococcal, intraabdominal infections; septicemia, meningitis; bone, joint infections

## Dosage and routes
### cefdinir
*Uncomplicated skin and skin structure infections/community-acquired pneumonia*
***Adult and child ≥13 yr:*** PO 300 mg q12hr × 10 days
***Child 6 mo-12 yr:*** PO 7 mg/kg q12hr or 14 mg/kg q24hr × 10 days

*Acute exacerbations of chronic bronchitis/acute maxillary sinusitis*
***Adult and child ≥13 yr:*** PO 300 mg q12hr or 600 mg q24hr × 10 days or 300 mg bid × 5 days in some infections

*Pharyngitis/tonsillitis*
***Adult and child ≥13 yr:*** PO 300 mg q12hr or 600 mg q24hr × 10 days
***Child 6 mo-12 yr:*** PO 7 mg/kg q12hr × 5-10 days or 14 mg/kg q24hr × 10 days

*Renal dose*
CCr <30 ml/min 300 mg daily (adult); 7 mg/kg daily (child)

**Available forms:** Caps 300 mg, oral susp 125 mg/5 ml

### cefditoren pivoxil
***Adult:*** PO 200-400 mg bid

*Renal dose*
***Adult:*** PO CCr 30-50 ml/min, max 200 mg bid; CCr <30 ml/min, max 200 mg daily

**Available forms:** Tabs 200 mg

### cefepime
*Urinary tract infections (mild to moderate)*
***Adult:*** IV/IM 0.5-1 g q12hr × 7-10 days

*Urinary tract infections (severe)*
***Adult:*** IV 2 g q12hr × 10 days

*Pneumonia (moderate to severe)*
***Adult:*** IV 1-2 g q12hr × 10 days
Dosage reduction indicated in renal impairment (CCr <50 ml/min)

*Uncomplicated gonorrhea*
IM 2 g as a single dose with 1 g PO probenecid at the same time

**Available forms:** Powder for inj 500 mg, 1, 2 g

### cefixime
***Adult:*** PO 400 mg/day as a single dose or 200 mg q12hr
***Child >50 kg or >12 yr:*** PO Use adult dosage
***Child <50 kg or <12 yr:*** PO 8 mg/kg/day as a single dose or 4 mg/kg q12hr

*Renal dose*
CCr 21-60 ml/min give 75% of dose; CCr <20 ml/min give 50% of dose

**Available forms:** Tabs 200, 400 mg; powder for oral susp 100 mg/5 ml

### cefotaxime
***Adult:*** IM/IV 1-2 g q12hr
***Child 1 mo-12 yr:*** IM/IV 50-180 mg/kg/day divided q6hr

*Severe infections*
***Adult:*** IM/IV 2 g q4hr, not to exceed 12 g/day
***Child 1 mo-12 yr:*** IM/IV 50-180 mg/kg in 4-6 divided doses

*Uncomplicated gonorrhea*
***Adult:*** IM 1 g; dosage reduction indicated for severe renal impairment (CCr <30 ml/min)

**Available forms:** Powder for inj 500 mg, 1, 2, 10 g; 1, 2 g premixed frozen

### cefpodoxime
*Pneumonia*
***Adult >13 yr:*** PO 200 mg q12hr for 14 days

*Uncomplicated gonorrhea*
***Adult >13 yr:*** PO 200 mg single dose

*Skin and skin structure*
***Adult >13 yr:*** PO 400 mg q12hr for 7-14 days

*Pharyngitis and tonsillitis*
***Adult >13 yr:*** PO 100 mg q12hr for 10 days
***Child 5 mo-12 yr:*** PO 5 mg/kg q12hr (max 100 mg/dose or 200 mg/day) × 5-10 days

*Uncomplicated UTI*
***Adult >13 yr:*** PO 100 mg q12hr for 7 days; dosing interval increased in presence of severe renal impairment

*Acute otitis media*
***Child 5 mo-12 yr:*** PO 5 mg/kg q12hr for 10 days
***Renal dose:*** Reduce dose in renal disease

**Available forms:** Tabs 100, 200 mg/ granules for susp 50, 100 mg/5 ml

### ceftazidime
***Adult:*** IV/IM 1-2 g q8-12hr × 5-10 days

Adverse effects: *italic* = common, **bold** = life-threatening

*Child:* **IV** 30-50 mg/kg q8hr not to exceed 6 g/day

*Neonate:* **IV** 30-50 mg/kg q12hr

*Renal dose*
*Adult:* **IV** CCr <50 ml/min q12hr; CCr 10-30 ml/min q24hr; CCr <10 ml/min q48hr

**Available forms:** Inj 250, 500 mg, 1, 2, 6 g

### ceftibuten
*Adult:* PO 400 mg daily × 10 days
*Child 6 mo-12 yr:* PO 9 mg/kg daily × 10 days

*Renal dose*
*Adult:* PO CCr <50 ml/min 200 mg q24hr; CCr 5-20 ml/min 100 mg q24hr

**Available forms:** Caps 400 mg; susp 90, 180 mg/5 ml

### ceftizoxime
*Adult:* IM/**IV** 1-2 g q8-12hr, may give up to 4 g q8hr in life-threatening infections
*Child >6 mo:* IM/**IV** 50 mg/kg q6-8hr

*Renal dose*
*Adult:* IM/**IV** CCr <80 ml/min 500-1500 mg q8hr; CCr 10-49 ml/min 250-1000 mg q12hr

*PID*
*Adult:* **IV** 2 g q8hr, may increase to 4 g q8hr in severe infections

**Available forms:** Powder for inj 500 mg, 1, 2, 10 g; premixed 1 g, 2 g/50 ml

### ceftriaxone
Reduce dosage in severe renal impairment (CCr <10 ml/min)
*Adult:* IM/**IV** 1-2 g daily, max 2 g q12hr
*Child:* IM/**IV** 50-75 mg/kg/day in equal doses q12hr

*Uncomplicated gonorrhea*
*Adult:* 250 mg IM as single dose

*Meningitis*
*Adult and child:* IM/**IV** 100 mg/kg/day in equal doses q12hr, max 4 g/day

*Surgical prophylaxis*
*Adult:* **IV** 1 g ½-2 hr preop

**Available forms:** Inj 250, 500 mg, 1, 2, 10 g

### Adverse effects
*CNS:* Headache, dizziness, weakness, paresthesia, fever, chills, **seizures,** dyskinesia (cefdinir)
*CV:* **Heart failure,** syncope (cefdinir)
*GI:* *Nausea, vomiting, diarrhea, anorexia,* pain, glossitis, **bleeding;** increased AST, ALT, bilirubin, LDH, alkaline phosphatase; abdomi-

nal pain, **pseudomembranous colitis,** cholestasis (cefotaxime)
*GU:* **Proteinuria,** vaginitis, pruritus, candidiasis, increased BUN, **nephrotoxicity, renal failure**
*HEMA:* **Leukopenia, thrombocytopenia, agranulocytosis,** anemia, **neutropenia,** lymphocytosis, eosinophilia, **pancytopenia, hemolytic anemia**
*INTEG:* Rash, urticaria, dermatitis
*RESP:* Dyspnea
*SYST:* **Anaphylaxis, serum sickness, Stevens-Johnson syndrome**

**Contraindications:** Hypersensitivity to cephalosporins, infants <1 mo

**Precautions:** Pregnancy **B,** breastfeeding, children, hypersensitivity to penicillins, renal/GI disease

### cefdinir

| Pharmacokinetics | |
| --- | --- |
| Absorption | Well absorbed |
| Distribution | Widely distributed; crosses placenta |
| Metabolism | Not metabolized |
| Excretion | Kidneys, unchanged; enters breast milk |
| Half-life | Unknown |

| Pharmacodynamics |
| --- |
| Unknown |

### cefditoren pivoxil

| Pharmacokinetics | |
| --- | --- |
| Absorption | Well absorbed after it is broken down (prodrug) |
| Distribution | Widely |
| Metabolism | Unknown |
| Excretion | Unknown |
| Half-life | 100 mins |

| Pharmacodynamics | |
| --- | --- |
| Onset | Rapid |
| Peak | 0.5-3 hr |
| Duration | 12 hrs |

### cefepime

| Pharmacokinetics | |
| --- | --- |
| Absorption | Well absorbed (IM) |
| Distribution | Widely distributed; crosses placenta |
| Metabolism | Not metabolized |
| Excretion | Kidneys, unchanged; enters breast milk |
| Half-life | 2 hr; increased in renal disease |

### Pharmacodynamics

|  | IM | IV |
|---|---|---|
| Onset | Rapid | Immediate |
| Peak | 79 min | Infusion's end |
| Duration | Unknown | Unknown |

## cefixime

### Pharmacokinetics

| Absorption | Unknown |
|---|---|
| Distribution | Protein binding 65%-70% |
| Metabolism | Unknown |
| Excretion | Urine, bile |
| Half-life | 3-4 hr |

### Pharmacodynamics

| Onset | Unknown |
|---|---|
| Peak | 2-6 hr |
| Duration | Unknown |

## cefotaxime

### Pharmacokinetics

| Absorption | Widely distributed |
|---|---|
| Distribution | Breast milk, small amounts |
| Metabolism | Liver, active metabolites |
| Excretion | 40%-65% unchanged, kidney |
| Half-life | 1 hr |

### Pharmacodynamics

|  | IV | IM |
|---|---|---|
| Onset | 5 min | 30 min |
| Peak | Unknown | Unknown |
| Duration | Unknown | Unknown |

## cefpodoxime

### Pharmacokinetics

| Absorption | Well absorbed |
|---|---|
| Distribution | Widely distributed; crosses placenta |
| Metabolism | Not metabolized |
| Excretion | Kidneys, unchanged; enters breast milk |
| Half-life | 2-3 hr, increased in renal disease |

### Pharmacodynamics

Unknown

## ceftazidime

### Pharmacokinetics

| Absorption | Well absorbed (IM) |
|---|---|
| Distribution | Widely distributed; crosses placenta |
| Metabolism | Not metabolized |
| Excretion | Kidneys, unchanged; enters breast milk |
| Half-life | ½-1 hr; increased in renal disease |

### Pharmacodynamics

|  | IM | IV |
|---|---|---|
| Onset | Rapid | Immediate |
| Peak | 1 hr | Infusion's end |

## ceftibuten

### Pharmacokinetics

| Absorption | Well absorbed |
|---|---|
| Distribution | Widely distributed; crosses placenta |
| Metabolism | Not metabolized |
| Excretion | Kidneys, unchanged; enters breast milk |
| Half-life | 1-1½ hr; increased in renal disease |

### Pharmacodynamics

Unknown

## ceftizoxime

### Pharmacokinetics

| Absorption | Well absorbed (IM) |
|---|---|
| Distribution | Widely distributed; crosses placenta |
| Metabolism | Not metabolized |
| Excretion | Kidneys, unchanged; enters breast milk |
| Half-life | 1½-2 hr; increased in renal disease |

### Pharmacodynamics

|  | IM | IV |
|---|---|---|
| Onset | Rapid | Immediate |
| Peak | 1 hr | Infusion's end |

## ceftriaxone

### Pharmacokinetics

| Absorption | Well absorbed |
|---|---|
| Distribution | Widely distributed; crosses placenta; enters CSF |
| Metabolism | Liver |
| Excretion | Kidneys, partly |
| Half-life | 5-8 hr |

Adverse effects: *italic* = common, **bold** = life-threatening

### Pharmacodynamics

|  | IM | IV |
|---|---|---|
| Onset | Rapid | Immediate |
| Peak | 1 hr | Infusion's end |

### Interactions
#### Individual drugs
Furosemide, probenecid: increased toxicity
Iron: decreased absorption of cefdinir
Plicamycin, valproic acid: increased bleeding
#### Drug classifications
Aminoglycosides: increased toxicity
Anticoagulants, NSAIDs, thrombolytics: increased bleeding
#### Drug/herb
Acidophilus: do not use with antiinfectives; separate by several hours
Angelica, anise, arnica, bogbean, boldo, celery, chamomile, clove, fenugreek, feverfew, garlic, ginger, ginkgo, ginseng *(Panax)*, horse chestnut, horseradish, licorice, meadowsweet, onion, papain, passion flower, poplar, prickly ash, red clover, turmeric, willow: increased risk of bleeding when used with cefoperazone
#### Drug/lab test
Increased: ALT, AST, alkaline phosphatase, LDH, bilirubin, BUN, creatinine
False increase: creatinine (serum urine), urinary 17-KS
False positive: urinary protein, direct Coombs' test, urine glucose
Interference: cross-matching

### NURSING CONSIDERATIONS
#### Assessment
• Assess patient for previous sensitivity reaction to penicillins or other cephalosporins; cross-sensitivity between penicillins and cephalosporins is common
• Assess patient for signs and symptoms of infection including characteristics of wounds, sputum, urine, stool, WBC >10,000/mm$^3$, fever; obtain baseline information and during treatment
• Obtain C&S before beginning product therapy to identify if correct treatment has been initiated
• Assess for anaphylaxis: rash, urticaria, pruritus, chills, fever, joint pain; angioedema may occur a few days after therapy begins; epINEPHrine and resuscitation equipment should be available for anaphylactic reaction
• Identify urine output; if decreasing, notify prescriber (may indicate nephrotoxicity); also check for increased BUN, creatinine
• Monitor blood studies: AST, ALT, CBC, Hct, bilirubin, LDH, alkaline phosphatase, Coombs' test monthly if patient is on long-term therapy
• Monitor electrolytes: potassium, sodium, chloride monthly if patient is on long-term therapy
• Assess bowel pattern daily; if severe diarrhea occurs, product should be discontinued; may indicate pseudomembranous colitis
• Monitor for bleeding: ecchymosis, bleeding gums, hematuria, stool guaiac daily if on long-term therapy
• Assess for overgrowth of infection: perineal itching, fever, malaise, redness, pain, swelling, drainage, rash, diarrhea, change in cough, sputum

#### Nursing diagnoses
• Diarrhea (side effects)
• Infection, risk for (uses)
• Injury, risk for (side effects)
• Knowledge, deficient (teaching)

#### Implementation
##### cefdinir
###### PO route
• Give oral suspension after adding 39 ml water to the 60 ml bottle; 65 ml water to the 12.0 ml bottle; discard unused portion after 10 days

##### cefditoren pivoxil
• Give for 10 days to ensure organism death, prevent superinfection
• Give with food if needed for GI symptoms
• Give after C&S is completed

##### cefepime
###### IM route
• Reconstitute 1 g/2 ml of sterile water for inj; may be diluted with 0.5% or 1% lidocaine to prevent pain; give deep in large muscle mass, massage
###### IV route
• Check for irritation, extravasation, phlebitis daily; change site q72hr
• For intermittent inf dilute with 50-100 ml of D$_5$W, give over 30 min
**Solution compatibilities:** 0.9% NaCl, D$_5$, 0.5, 1.0% lidocaine, bacteriostatic water for inj with parabens/benzyl alcohol

##### cefixime
• Do not break, crush, or chew tab
• Give for 10-14 days to ensure organism death, prevent superinfection

##### cefotaxime
###### IV route
• Dilute 1 g/10 ml D$_5$W, NS, sterile H$_2$O for inj and give over 3-5 min by Y-tube or 3-way stopcock; may be diluted further with 50-100 ml of 0.9% NaCl or D$_5$W; run over ½-1 hr;

discontinue primary inf during administration; or may be diluted in larger volume of sol and given as a cont inf over 6-24 hr
- Give for 10-14 days to ensure organism death, prevent superinfection
- Thaw frozen container at room temperature or refrigeration, do not force thaw by immersion or microwave; visually inspect container for leaks

*Syringe compatibilities:* Heparin, oflaxacin

*Y-site compatibilities:* Acyclovir, amifostine, aztreonam, cyclophosphamide, diltiazem, famotidine, fludarabine, hydromorphone, lorazepam, magnesium sulfate, melphalan, meperidine, midazolam, morphine, ondansetron, perphenazine, sargramostim, teniposide, thiotepa, tolazoline, vinorelbine

*Additive compatibilities:* Clindamycin, metronidazole, verapamil

### cefpodoxime
**IM route**
- Reconstitute 1 g/2 ml or 2 g/3 ml of sterile or bacteriostatic water for inj; may be diluted with 0.5% of 1% lidocaine to prevent pain; give deep in large muscle mass, massage

**IV route**
- Check for irritation, extravasation, phlebitis daily; change site q72hr
- For direct **IV** dilute in 1 g/10 ml or more and give over 5 min
- For intermittent inf further dilute in 50-100 ml of 0.9% NaCl or $D_5W$; give over 3-5 min; discontinue primary line while running intermittent inf

*Syringe incompatibilities:* Doxapram
*Y-site compatibilities:* Famotidine, fluconazole, fludarabine, regular insulin, meperidine, morphine, sargramostim
*Additive incompatibilities:* Aminoglycosides, heparin, tetracyclines

### ceftazidime
**IM route**
- Reconstitute 500 mg/1.5 ml or 1 g/3 ml of sterile or bacteriostatic water for inj; may be diluted with 0.5% or 1% lidocaine to prevent pain; give deep in large muscle mass, massage

**IV route**
- Check for irritation, extravasation, phlebitis daily; change site q72hr
- For direct **IV** dilute 500 mg/5 ml or 1 g/10 ml sterile water for inj; give over 3-5 min; do not use sol with benzyl alcohol for neonates
- For intermittent inf further dilute 1 g/10 ml or more 0.9% NaCl, $D_5W$, $D_{10}W$, $D_5/0.25\%$ NaCl, $D_5/0.45\%$ NaCl, $D_5/0.9\%$ NaCl, or LR; give over 30-60 min

- Store for 96 hr refrigerated, 24 hr room temperature

*Y-site compatibilities:* Acyclovir, allopurinol, amifostine, aztreonam, ciprofloxacin, diltiazem, enalaprilat, esmolol, famotidine, filgrastim, fludarabine, foscarnet, granisetron, heparin, hydromorphone, labetalol, meperidine, melphalan, morphine, ondansetron, paclitaxel, rantidine, tacrolimus, teniposide, theophylline, thiotepa, vinorelbine tartrate, zidovudine

*Y-site incompatibilities:* Amsacrine, fluconazole, idarubicin, sargramostim

*Additive compatibilities:* Ciprofloxacin, clindamycin, fluconazole, metronidazole, ofloxacin

*Additive incompatibilities:* Aminoglycosides, sodium bicarbonate

### ceftibuten
- Administer for 10 days to ensure organism death, prevent superimposed infection
- Administer after C&S

### ceftizoxime
**IM route**
- Reconstitute 250 mg/0.9 ml, 500 mg/1.8 ml, 1 g/3.6 ml, 2 g/7.2 ml; may be diluted with 0.5% or 1% lidocaine to prevent pain; give deep in large muscle mass, massage

**IV route**
- Check for irritation, extravasation, phlebitis daily; change site q72hr
- For intermittent inf reconstitute 250 mg/2.4 ml, 500 mg/4.8 ml, 1 g/9.6 mg/2 g/19.2 ml sterile water for inj, $D_5W$, or 0.9% NaCl; do not use sol with benzyl alcohol for neonates; may be further diluted in 50-100 ml of $D_5W$, $D_{10}W$, 0.9% NaCl, or LR; give over 30-60 min
- May store 96 hr refrigerated, 24 hr room temperature

*Y-site compatibilities:* Acyclovir, allopurinol, amifostine, aztreonam, enalaprilat, esmolol, famotidine, fludarabine, foscarnet, hydromorphone, labetalol, melphalan, meperidine, morphine, ondansetron, sargramostim, teniposide, thiotepa, vinorelbine

*Additive compatibilities:* Clindamycin, metronidazole

*Additive incompatibilities:* Aminoglycosides

### ceftriaxone
- Give IM inj deep in large muscle mass
- Give for 10-14 days to ensure organism death, prevent superinfection

**IV route**
- Give **IV** after diluting 250 mg/2.4 ml of $D_5W$, $H_2O$ for inj, 0.9% NaCl; may be further

diluted with 50-100 ml of 0.9% NaCl, $D_5W$, $D_{10}W$, shake; run over ½-1 hr
• Do not mix with calcium salts

*Y-site compatibilities:* Acyclovir, allopurinol, aztreonam, cisatracurium, diltiazem, DOXOrubicin liposome, fludarabine, foscarnet, heparin, melphalan, meperidine, methotrexate, morphine, paclitaxel, remifentanil, sargramostim, tacrolimus, teniposide, theophylline, vinorelbine, warfarin, zidovudine
*Additive compatibilities:* Amino acids or sodium bicarbonate, metronidazole

### Patient/family education
• Teach patient to report sore throat, bruising, bleeding, joint pain; may indicate blood dyscrasias (rare)
• Advise patient to contact prescriber if vaginal itching, loose foul-smelling stools, furry tongue occur; may indicate superinfection
• Advise patient to notify prescriber of diarrhea with blood or pus, may indicate pseudomembranous colitis
• Cefditoren can be taken with oral contraceptives

### Evaluation
**Positive therapeutic outcome**
• Absence of signs/symptoms of infection (WBC <10,000/mm³, temp WNL, absence of red draining wounds, earache)
• Reported improvement in symptoms of infection
• Negative C&S

**Treatment of anaphylaxis:** EpINEPHrine, antihistamines, resuscitate if needed

---

## cephradine
*See cephalosporins—1st generation*

---

## cetirizine (Rx)
(se-tear'i-zeen)
Zyrtec
*Func. class:* Antihistamine, peripherally selective (2nd generation)
*Chem. class.:* Piperazine, $H_1$ histamine antagonist

**Pregnancy category B**

**Do not confuse:**
Zyrtec/Xanax/Zantac

**Action:** Acts on blood vessels, GI, respiratory system by competing with histamine for $H_1$-receptor site; decreases allergic response by blocking pharmacologic effects of histamine; minimal anticholinergic action

**Therapeutic outcome:** Absence of allergy symptoms, rhinitis, and chronic idiopathic urticaria

**Uses:** Rhinitis, allergy symptoms, and chronic idiopathic urticaria

### Dosage and routes
*Adult and child ≥6 yr:* PO 5-10 mg daily
*Child 2-5 yr:* PO 2.5 mg daily, may increase to 5 mg daily or 2.5 mg bid
*Child 1-2 yr:* PO 2.5 mg daily, may increase to 2.5 mg g12hr
*Child 6-11 mo:* PO 2.5 mg daily
*Geriatric:* PO 5 mg daily, may increase to 10 mg/day

*Renal dose*
*Adult:* PO CCr 11-31 ml/min 5 mg daily

*Hemodialysis*
*Adult:* PO 5 mg/day

*Hepatic dose*
*Adult:* PO 5 mg daily

**Available forms:** Tabs 5, 10 mg; syr 5 mg/5 ml

### Adverse effects
*CNS: Headache,* stimulation, *drowsiness,* sedation, *fatigue,* confusion, blurred vision, tinnitus, restlessness, tremors, parodoxical excitation in children or geriatric
*GI: Dry mouth,* increased liver function tests, constipation
*INTEG:* Rash, eczema, photosensitivity, urticaria
*RESP: Thickening of bronchial secretions;* dry nose, throat

**Contraindications:** Hypersensitivity to this product or hydrOXYzine, breastfeeding, newborn or premature infants, severe hepatic disease

**Precautions:** Pregnancy **B**, children, geriatric, respiratory disease, angle-closure glaucoma, prostatic hypertrophy, bladder neck obstruction, asthma

| Pharmacokinetics | |
|---|---|
| Absorption | Well absorbed, rapid |
| Distribution | Protein binding 93% |
| Metabolism | Liver |
| Excretion | Kidneys |
| Half-life | 8.3 hr, decreased in children, increased in renal/hepatic disease |

| Pharmacodynamics | |
|---|---|
| Onset | ½ hr |
| Peak | 1-2 hr |
| Duration | 24 hr |

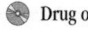

## Interactions
*Individual drugs*
Alcohol: increased CNS depression
*Drug classifications*
CNS depressants, opioids, sedative/hypnotics:
increased CNS depression
MAOIs: increased anticholinergic effect
*Drug/herb*
Corkwood: increased anticholinergic effect
Hops, Jamaican dogwood, kava, senna,
valerian: increased effects
*Drug/food*
Prolongs absorption by 1.7 hr
*Drug/lab test*
False negative: skin allergy tests (discontinue
antihistamine 3 days before testing)

## NURSING CONSIDERATIONS
### Assessment
• Assess respiratory status: rate, rhythm;
increase in bronchial secretions, wheezing,
chest tightness; provide fluids to 2 L/day to
decrease secretion thickness
• Assess for allergy symptoms: pruritus,
urticaria, watering eyes, baseline and during
treatment

### Nursing diagnoses
• Airway clearance, ineffective (uses)
• Injury, risk for (side effects)
• Knowledge, deficient (teaching)
• Noncompliance (teaching overuse)

### Implementation
• Give without regard to meals
• Store in tight, light-resistant container

### Patient/family education
• Teach all aspects of product uses; to notify
prescriber if confusion, sedation, hypotension
occur; to avoid driving or other hazardous
activity if drowsiness occurs; to avoid alcohol
or other CNS depressants that may potentiate
effect
• Instruct patient to take without regard to
meals
• Instruct patient not to exceed recommended
dose; dysrhythmias may occur
• Advise patient to avoid using if breastfeeding
• Advise patient to avoid exposure to sunlight;
burns may occur
• Advise patient to use sugarless gum, candy,
frequent sips of water to minimize dry mouth
• Advise patient to avoid alcohol, OTC antihistamines, other CNS depressants

### Evaluation
**Positive therapeutic outcome**
• Absence of runny or congested nose, rashes

**Treatment of overdose:**
Lavage, diazepam, vasopressors, barbiturates
(short acting)

C

### cetrorelix (Rx)
(set-roe-ree'lix)
Cetrotide
*Func. class.:* Gonadotropin-releasing hor-
mone antagonist
*Chem. class.:* Synthetic decapeptide
**Pregnancy category  X**

**Action:** Inhibitor of pituitary gonadotropin
secretion; initially increases LH and FSH,
induces a rapid suppression of gonadotropin
secretion

**Therapeutic outcome:** Pregnancy

**Uses:** For inhibition of premature LH surges
in women undergoing controlled ovarian
hyperstimulation

### Dosage and routes
*Single-dose regimen*
*Adult:* SUBCUT 3 mg when serum estradiol
level is at appropriate stimulation response,
usually on stimulation day 7; if hCG has not
been given within 4 days after inj of 3 mg
cetrorelix, give 0.25 mg daily until day of hCG
administration

*Multiple-dose regimen*
*Adult:* SUBCUT 0.25 mg is given on stimulation day 5 (either morning or evening) or 6
(morning) and continued daily until day hCG
is given

**Available forms:** Inj 0.25, 3 mg

### Adverse effects
*CNS:* Headache
*CV:* Edema
*ENDO:* Ovarian hyperstimulation syndrome,
abdominal pain (gyn)
*GI:* Nausea, vomiting, diarrhea
*INTEG:* Pain on inj; local site reactions,
bruising, pruritus
*OTHER:* Rapid weight gain
*RESP:* Shortness of breath
**SYST: Fetal death**

**Contraindications:** Pregnancy **X,** breastfeeding, hypersensitivity, latex allergy, renal
disease

**Precautions:** Geriatric

## Pharmacokinetics

| | |
|---|---|
| **Absorption** | Unknown |
| **Distribution** | Protein binding 86% |
| **Metabolism** | Liver to metabolites |
| **Excretion** | Feces/urine |
| **Half-life** | Depends on dosage |

## Pharmacodynamics

Unknown

## NURSING CONSIDERATIONS
### Assessment
• Assess for suspected pregnancy; product should not be used
• Assess for latex allergy; product should not be used
• Monitor ALT, AST, GGT, alkaline phosphatase, serum progesterone, LH; ovarian ultrasound days 7-14

### Nursing diagnoses
• Knowledge, deficient (teaching)

### Implementation
• Give SUBCUT using abdomen, 1 inch away from navel or upper thigh, swab inj area with disinfectant, clean a 2-in circle and allow to dry, pinch up area between thumb and finger, insert needle at 45-90 degrees to surface; if blood is drawn into the syringe, reposition needle without removing it; rotate inj sites
• Do not administer if patient is pregnant
• Protect from light

### Patient/family education
• Instruct to report abdominal pain, vaginal bleeding, nausea, vomiting, diarrhea, shortness of breath, peripheral edema
• Teach self-administration technique if needed

### Evaluation
**Positive therapeutic outcome**
• Pregnancy

---

## cetuximab (Rx)
(se-tux'i-mab)
Erbitux
*Func. class.:* Antineoplastic—miscellaneous, monoclonal antibody
*Chem. class.:* Epidermal growth factor receptor inhibitor

### Pregnancy category C

**Action:** Not fully understood; binds to epidermal growth factor receptors (EGFR); inhibits phosphorylation and activation of receptor associated kinase resulting in inhibition of cell growth

**Therapeutic outcome:** Decrease in tumor size

**Uses:** Alone or in combination with irinotecan for EGFR expressing metastatic colorectal carcinoma

### Dosage and routes
*Adult:* **IV** INF 400 mg/m² loading dose given over 120 min, max infusion rate 5 ml/min, weekly maintenance dose (all other infusions) is 250 mg/m² given over 60 min, max infusion rate 5 ml/min; premedicate with an H₁ antagonist (diphenhydrAMINE 50 mg **IV**); dosage adjustments are made for infusion reactions or dermatologic toxicity

**Available forms:** Inj 50 ml, single-use vial with 100 mg of cetuximab (2 mg/ml)

### Adverse effects
*CNS: Headache, insomnia, depression*
*GI: Nausea, diarrhea, vomiting, anorexia, mouth ulceration, dehydration, constipation, abdominal pain*
*HEMA: Leukepenia, anemia*
*INTEG: Rash, pruritus, acne, dry skin,* **toxic epidermal neurolysis, angioedema,** *blepharitis, cheilitis, cellulitis, cysts, alopecia, skin/nail disorder*
*MISC: Conjunctivitis, asthma, malaise, fever,* **renal failure**
*MS: Back pain*
*RESP: Interstitial lung disease, cough, dyspnea,* **pulmonary embolus,** *peripheral edema*
*SYST: Anaphylaxis, sepsis, infection*

**Contraindications:** Hypersensitivity to this product or murine proteins

**Precautions:** Pregnancy C, breastfeeding, child, geriatric, renal/hepatic disease, ocular, pulmonary disorders

## Pharmacokinetics

| | |
|---|---|
| **Absorption** | Unknown |
| **Distribution** | Unknown |
| **Metabolism** | Unknown |
| **Excretion** | Unknown |
| **Half-life** | 114 hrs |

## Pharmacodynamics

| | |
|---|---|
| **Onset** | Unknown |
| **Peak** | 168-235 g/ml, trough 41-85 g/ml |
| **Duration** | Steady state by 3rd weekly infusion |

---

 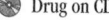

## NURSING CONSIDERATIONS
### Assessment
⊕ Monitor pulmonary changes: lung sounds, cough, dyspnea; interstitial lung disease may occur, may be fatal; discontinue therapy if confirmed
⊕ Assess for toxic epidermal necrosis, angioedema, anaphylaxis
• Assess GI symptoms: frequency of stools, dehydration, abdominal pain, stomatitis

### Nursing diagnoses
• Body image, disturbed (adverse reactions)
• Infection, risk for (adverse reactions)
• Injury, risk for (adverse reactions)
• Knowledge, deficient (teaching)

### Implementation
#### IV infusion route
• Administer by **IV** infusion only, do not give by **IV** push or bolus
• Do not shake or dilute
• Infusion pump: draw up volume of a vial using appropriate syringe/needle (a vented spike or other appropriate transfer device); fill Erbitux into sterile evacuated container/bag, repeat until calculated volume has been put into the container. Use a new needle for each vial; give through in-line filter (low protein binding 0.22-micrometer); affix infusion line and prime before starting infusion, max rate 5 ml/min; flush line at end of infusion with 0.9% NaCl
• Syringe pump: Draw up volume of a vial using appropriate syringe/needle (a vented spike); place syringe into syringe driver of a syringe pump and set rate; use an in-line filter 0.22 micrometer (low protein binding); connect infusion line and start infusion after priming; repeat until calculated volume has been given.
• Use a new needle and filter for each vial, max 5 ml/min rate; use 0.9% NaCl to flush line after infusion
• Do not piggyback to patient infusion line
• Observe patient for adverse reactions for 1 hr after infusion
• Infusion reactions: if mild (Grade 1 or 2) reduce all doses by 50%; if severe (Grade 3 or 4) permanently discontinue
• Store refrigerated 36°-46° F, discard unused portions

### Patient/family education
• Instruct patient to report adverse reactions immediately: SOB, severe abdominal pain, skin eruptions
• Explain reason for treatment, expected results

• Instruct patient to use contraception during treatment
• Advise patient to wear sunscreen and hats to limit sun exposure. Sun exposure can exacerbate any skin reactions

### Evaluation
#### Positive therapeutic outcome
• Decrease growth, spread of EGFR expressing metastatic colorectal carcinoma

## charcoal, activated (OTC)
Actidose-Aqua, Actidose with Sorbitol, CharAid-G, CharcoAid, Charcoal Plus DS, Charcocaps, EZ Char, Inst-Char, Liqu-Char
*Func. class.:* Antiflatulent/antidote

### Pregnancy category D

**Action:** Binds poisons, toxins, irritants; increases adsorption in GI tract; inactivates toxins and binds until excreted

**Therapeutic outcome:** Prevention of toxicity and death resulting from absorption of products

**Uses:** Poisoning, overdose

**Unlabeled uses:** Diarrhea, flatulence

### Dosage and routes
#### Poisoning
Children should not get more than 1 dose of products with sorbitol
*Adult and child:* PO 30-100 g or 1 g/kg, minimum dosage 30 g/250 ml of water; may give 20-40 g q6hr for 1-2 days in severe poisoning; take plenty of water

**Available forms:** Powder 15, 25 ✦, 30, 40, 120, 125, 240 g/container; oral susp 12.5 g/60 ml, 15 g/72 ml, 15 g/120 ml, 25 g/120 ml, 30 g/120 ml, 50 g/240 ml; ✦ 15 g/120 ml, 25 g/125 ml, 50 g/225 ml, 50 g/250 ml; tabs/caps should not be used in poisonings

### Adverse effects
*GI: Nausea, black stools,* vomiting, constipation, diarrhea, abdominal pain
*OTHER:* **Pulmonary aspiration**

**Contraindications:** Pregnancy **D,** hypersensitivity to this product, unconsciousness, semiconsciousness, poisoning of cyanide, mineral acids, alkalis, gag reflex, depression, ethanol intoxication, intestinal obstruction, absent bowel sounds

## Pharmacokinetics

| | |
|---|---|
| **Absorption** | None |
| **Distribution** | None |
| **Metabolism** | None |
| **Excretion** | Feces (unchanged) |
| **Half-life** | Unknown |

## Pharmacodynamics

| | |
|---|---|
| **Onset** | 1 min |
| **Peak** | Unknown |
| **Duration** | 4-12 hr |

### Interactions
**Individual drugs**
Acetylcysteine: inactivation

### NURSING CONSIDERATIONS
### Assessment
• Assess neurologic status including LOC, pupil reactivity, cough reflex, gag reflex, and swallowing ability before administration; do not give if neurologic status is impaired; aspiration may occur unless a protected airway is present
• Assess toxin, poison ingested, time of ingestion, and amount
• Monitor respiration, pulse, B/P to determine charcoal effectiveness if taken for barbiturate/opioid poisoning, serum electrolytes

### Nursing diagnoses
• Injury, risk for (uses)
• Knowledge, deficient (teaching)
• Poisoning, risk for (uses)

### Implementation
• Give after inducing vomiting unless vomiting contraindicated (i.e., cyanide or alkalis); mix with 8 oz of water or fruit juice to form thick syrup; do not use dairy products to mix charcoal; repeat dose if vomiting occurs soon after dose
• Space at least 2 hr before or after other products, or absorption will be decreased; use a laxative to promote elimination; constipation occurs often
• If patient unable to swallow, dilute to a less thick sol; keep container tightly closed to prevent absorption of gases
• Give through a nasogastric tube if patient unable to swallow

### Patient/family education
• Tell patient stools will be black
• Teach patient about overdose/poison prevention and about keeping poison control chart available

### Evaluation
**Positive therapeutic outcome**
• Alert, PERL (poisoning)
• Absence of distention
• Absence of odor in wounds

### chloral hydrate (Rx)
(klor'al hye'drate)
Aquachloral, chloral hydrate, Novo-Chlorhydrate ♣, PMS-Chloral Hydrate, Somnote
*Func. class.*: Sedative/hypnotic, non-barbiturate
*Chem. class.*: Chloral derivative

**Pregnancy category C**

**Controlled substance schedule IV (USA), schedule F (Canada)**

**Action:** Reduced to product trichloroethanol, which produces mild cerebral depression, causing sleep; generalized CNS depression

**Therapeutic outcome:** Ability to sleep, sedation

**Uses:** Sedation, short-term treatment of insomnia, preoperative reduction of anxiety, alcohol withdrawal, anxiety

### Dosage and routes
**Sedation**
*Adult:* PO/RECT 250 mg tid after meals; max 2 g/day
*Child:* PO 25-50 mg/kg tid, max 500 mg tid

**Alcohol withdrawal**
*Adult:* PO/RECT 500 mg-1 g q6hr, max 2 g/day

**Postop pain adjunct**
*Adult:* PO 250 mg tid, after meals, max 2 g/day

**Procedure sedation**
*Child:* PO/RECT 25-50 mg/kg, max 100 mg/kg or 2 g

**Insomnia**
*Adult:* PO/RECT 500 mg-1 g 30 min before bedtime; max 2 g/day
*Child:* PO/RECT 50-75 mg/kg (one dose)

**Renal disease**
*Adult:* PO/RECT CCr <50 ml/min avoid use

**Available forms:** Caps 500 mg; syr 250, 500 mg/5 ml; supp 325, 650 mg

### Adverse effects
*CNS: Drowsiness,* dizziness, stimulation, nightmares, ataxia, hangover (rare), light-

headedness, headache, paranoia, hallucinations
*CV:* Hypotension, **dysrhythmias**
*GI: Nausea, vomiting, flatulence, diarrhea,* unpleasant taste, **gastric necrosis,** abdominal pain
*HEMA:* **Eosinophilia, leukopenia**
*INTEG:* Rash, urticaria, **angioedema,** fever, purpura, eczema
*RESP:* **Depression**

**Contraindications:** Hypersensitivity to this product or triclofos, severe renal/hepatic disease, GI disorders (oral forms), gastritis

**Precautions:** Pregnancy **C,** breastfeeding, geriatric, severe cardiac disease, depression, suicidal individuals, asthma, intermittent porphyria, esophagitis, gastric/duodenal ulcers, gastritis

### Pharmacokinetics

| | |
|---|---|
| **Absorption** | Well absorbed (PO, RECT) |
| **Distribution** | Widely distributed; crosses placenta |
| **Metabolism** | Liver to trichloroethanol |
| **Excretion** | Kidneys (inactive metabolite), feces, breast milk |
| **Half-life** | 8-10 hr; active metabolite |

### Pharmacodynamics

| | PO | RECT |
|---|---|---|
| **Onset** | ½-1 hr | Slow |
| **Peak** | Unknown | Unknown |
| **Duration** | 4-8 hr | 4-8 hr |

### Interactions
*Individual drugs*
Alcohol: increased action of both products
Furosemide: increased action of furosemide
Phenytoin: decreased effect of phenytoin
*Drug classifications*
Anticoagulants (oral): increased action of anticoagulants
CNS depressants: increased action of both products
*Drug/herb*
Catnip, chamomile, clary, cowslip, hops, kava, lavender, mistletoe, nettle, pokeweed, poppy, Queen Anne's lace, senega, valerian: increased sedative effect
Black cohosh: increased hypotension
*Drug/lab test*
Interferences: urine catecholamines, urinary 17-OHCS

## NURSING CONSIDERATIONS
### Assessment
• Assess patient's sleep pattern and note physical (sleep apnea, obstructed airway, pain/discomfort, urinary frequency) and psychologic (fear, anxiety) circumstances that interrupt sleep
• Assess patient's bedtime routine, presleep cues/props
• Assess potential for abuse; this product may lead to physical and psychologic dependency; amount of product should be limited
• Monitor blood studies: Hct, Hgb, RBCs, serum folate (if on long-term therapy), pro-time in patients receiving anticoagulants since action of anticoagulant may be increased
• Monitor mental status: mood, sensorium, affect, memory (long, short)
• Monitor physical dependency: more frequent requests for medication, shakes, anxiety, pinpoint pupils
• Monitor respiratory dysfunction: respiratory depression, character, rate, rhythm; hold product if respirations are <10/min or if pupils are dilated (rare)
• Assess for blood dyscrasias: fever, sore throat, bruising, rash, jaundice, epistaxis (rare)
• Assess previous history of substance abuse, cardiac disease, or gastritis

### Nursing diagnoses
• Anxiety (uses)
• Knowledge, deficient (teaching)
• Noncompliance (teaching)
• Sleep deprivation (uses)

### Implementation
• Regulate environmental stimuli (light, noise, temperature), remove foods and fluids that interfere with sleep
• Place side rails up after giving medication for hypnotic; remove cigarettes/matches from patient's environment to prevent fires
**PO route**
• Do not break, crush, or chew caps
• Give ½-1 hr before bedtime for sleeplessness; give on empty stomach with full glass of water or juice for best absorption and to decrease corrosion (do not chew); after meals to decrease GI symptoms if used for sedation; dilute syr in 4 oz water or juice
◆ Check dose of syrup carefully, fatal overdoses have occurred
**Rectal route**
• Store supp in dark container, in refrigerator; remove outer wrapper before insertion

Adverse effects: *italic* = common, **bold** = life-threatening

### Patient/family education

• Caution patient to avoid driving and other activities requiring alertness; to avoid alcohol ingestion or CNS depressants; serious CNS depression may result plus tachycardia, flushing, headache, hypotension
• Instruct patient not to discontinue medication quickly after long-term use; product should be tapered over 1-2 wk, delirium may occur; that benefits may take 2 nights to be noticed; withdrawal symptoms include tremors, anxiety, hallucinations, delirium
• Teach patient alternative measures to improve sleep (reading, exercise several hours before bedtime, warm bath, warm milk, TV, self-hypnosis, deep breathing)
• Instruct the patient about factors that contribute to sleep pattern disturbances (lifestyle, shift work, long work hours, environmental factors, frequent napping)
• Teach patient to take product as prescribed, not to double doses
• Avoid breastfeeding

### Evaluation
**Positive therapeutic outcome**
• Ability to sleep at night
• Decreased amount of early morning awakening if taking product for insomnia
• Sedation

**Treatment of overdose:** Lavage, activated charcoal; monitor electrolytes, VS

---

## chlorambucil (Rx)
(klor-am′byoo-sil)
Leukeran
*Func. class.:* Antineoplastic alkylating agent
*Chem. class.:* Nitrogen mustard

**Pregnancy category D**

### Do not confuse:
Leukeran/leucovorin/Leukine

**Action:** Alkylates DNA, RNA; inhibits enzymes that allow synthesis of amino acids in proteins; activity is not cell cycle phase specific

**Therapeutic outcome:** Prevention of rapidly growing malignant cells

**Uses:** Chronic lymphocytic leukemia, non-Hodgkin's/Hodgkin's disease, other lymphomas, nephrotic syndrome, choreocarcinoma

**Unlabeled uses:** Macroglobulinemia, ovarian, testicular carcinoma, non-Hodgkin's lymphoma, Behçet's syndrome

### Dosage and routes
*Adult:* PO 0.1-0.2 mg/kg/day × 3-6 wk initially, then 4-10 mg/day maintenance
*Geriatric:* PO initially ≤2-4 mg/day
*Child:* PO 0.1-0.2 mg/kg/day (4.5 mg/m$^2$/day) in divided doses or 4.5 mg/m$^2$/day as 1 dose or in divided doses × 3-6 wk

**Nephrotic syndrome**
*Child:* PO 0.1-0.2 mg/kg daily with predniSONE × 8-12 wk

**Intractable idiopathic uveitis, Behçet's syndrome (unlabeled)**
*Adult:* PO 0.2 mg/kg

**Macroglobulinemia (unlabeled)**
*Adult:* PO 2-10 mg daily × 9 days, or 8 mg/m$^2$ daily with predniSONE × 10 days, repeat q6-8 wk as needed

**Available forms:** Tabs 2 mg

### Adverse effects
*CNS:* **Seizures,** tremors, confusion, agitation, ataxia
*GI: Nausea, vomiting, diarrhea, weight loss,* **hepatotoxicity,** *jaundice*
*GU:* Hyperuremia
*HEMA:* **Thrombocytopenia, leukopenia, pancytopenia** (prolonged use), **permanent bone marrow suppression**
*INTEG:* Alopecia (rare), dermatitis, rash, **Stevens-Johnson syndrome**
*RESP:* **Fibrosis, pneumonitis**

**Contraindications:** Pregnancy **D**, breastfeeding, radiation therapy within 1 mo, chemotherapy within 1 mo, thrombocytopenia, recent smallpox vaccination

**Precautions:** *Pneumococcus* vaccination, children

#### Pharmacokinetics

| | |
|---|---|
| **Absorption** | Rapidly, completely absorbed |
| **Distribution** | Crosses placenta |
| **Metabolism** | Liver, extensively |
| **Excretion** | Kidneys |
| **Half-life** | 2 hr |

#### Pharmacodynamics
Unknown

### Interactions
*Individual drugs*
Radiation: increased toxicity, bone marrow suppression
*Drug classifications*
Anticoagulants, salicylates: increased risk of bleeding

---

Antineoplastics: increased bone marrow suppression; increased toxicity

## NURSING CONSIDERATIONS
### Assessment
• Monitor CBC, differential, platelet count weekly; withhold product if WBC is <2000/mm³ or granulocyte count <1000/mm³ notify prescriber of results if WBC <20,000/mm³, platelets <50,000/mm³
• Monitor pulmonary function tests, chest x-ray films before, during therapy; chest film should be obtained q2 wk during treatment; check for dyspnea, crackles, unproductive cough, chest pain, tachypnea
• Assess for increased uric acid levels, swelling, joint pain primarily in extremities; patient should be well hydrated to prevent urate deposits
• Monitor renal function studies: BUN, serum uric acid, urine CCr before, during therapy; I&O ratio; report fall in urine output of 30 ml/hr; monitor for decreased hyperuricemia
• Assess for jaundice of skin, sclera, dark urine, clay-colored stools, itchy skin, abdominal pain, fever, diarrhea
• Monitor for cold, fever, sore throat (may indicate beginning infection); identify edema in feet, joint, stomach pain, shaking; prescriber should be notified
• Assess for bleeding: hematuria, guaiac, bruising or petechiae, mucosa or orifices q8hr, no rectal temp

### Nursing diagnoses
• Body image, disturbed (adverse reactions)
• Infection, risk for (adverse reactions)
• Injury, risk for (adverse reactions)
• Knowledge, deficient (teaching)

### Implementation
• Give 1 hr before or 2 hr after meals to lessen nausea and vomiting or antacid before oral agent, give product after evening meal, before bedtime or 1 hr before breakfast; antiemetic 30-60 min before giving product to prevent vomiting
• Give allopurinol to maintain uric acid levels, alkalinization of urine; increase fluid intake to 2-3 L/day to prevent urate deposits, calculus formation
• Antibiotics for prophylaxis of infection may be prescribed, since infection potential is high
• Give all products PO if possible, avoid IM inj when platelets <100,000/mm³
• Store in tight container

### Patient/family education
• Teach patient to avoid use of products containing aspirin or ibuprofen, razors, commercial mouthwash, since bleeding may occur; to report symptoms of bleeding (hematuria, tarry stools)
• Instruct patient to report signs of anemia (fatigue, headache, irritability, faintness, shortness of breath)
• Instruct patient to report any changes in breathing or coughing even several mo after treatment; to avoid crowds and persons with respiratory tract or other infections
• Advise patient hair loss is common; discuss the use of wigs or hairpieces
• Instruct patient to drink 2-3 L of fluid daily unless contraindicated
• Caution patient not to have any vaccinations without the advice of the prescriber; serious reactions can occur
• Advise patient contraception is needed during treatment and for several months after the completion of therapy, may cause irreversible gonadal suppression

### Evaluation
#### Positive therapeutic outcome
• Decreased size of tumor
• Decreased spread of malignancy
• Improved blood values
• Absence of sweating at night
• Increased appetite, increased weight

## chloramphenicol (Rx)
(klor-am-fen′i-kole)
chloramphenicol, Chloromycetin, Pentamycetin ✦
*Func. class.:* Antiinfective—miscellaneous
*Chem. class.:* Dichloroacetic acid derivative

### Pregnancy category C

**Action:** Binds to 50S ribosomal subunit, which interferes with or inhibits protein synthesis

**Therapeutic outcome:** Bactericidal for *Haemophilus influenzae, Salmonella typhi, Rickettsia, Neisseria, Staphylococcus, Streptococcus, Escherichia coli* mycoplasma

**Uses:** Meningitis, bacteremia, abdominal, skin, soft tissue infections

### Dosage and routes
*Adult and child:* PO/**IV** 50-75 mg/kg/day in divided doses q6hr; 100 mg/kg/day (for meningitis only); max 4 g/day
*Premature infant and neonate:* **IV** 25 mg/kg/day in divided doses q12-24hr

**Available forms:** Inj **IV** 1 g; caps 250 mg

Adverse effects: *italic* = common, **bold** = life-threatening

## Adverse effects

*CNS:* Headache, *depression,* confusion, peripheral neuritis

*CV:* **Gray syndrome in newborns: failure to feed, pallor, cyanosis, abdominal distention, irregular respiration, vasomotor collapse**

*EENT:* Optic neuritis, blindness

*GI:* *Nausea, vomiting, diarrhea,* abdominal pain, xerostomia, glossitis, colitis, pruritus ani

*HEMA:* **Anemia, thrombocytopenia, aplastic anemia, granulocytopenia, leukopenia, acute generalized exanthematous pustulosis (aged)** (rare)

*INTEG:* Itching, urticaria, contact dermatitis, rash

**Contraindications:** Hypersensitivity, severe renal/hepatic disease, minor infections

**Precautions:** Pregnancy **C**, breastfeeding, infants, children, renal/hepatic disease, bone marrow depression (product-induced)

### Pharmacokinetics

| | |
|---|---|
| **Absorption** | Well absorbed (PO), Completely absorbed (**IV**) |
| **Distribution** | Wide |
| **Metabolism** | Liver |
| **Excretion** | Kidneys, unchanged |
| **Half-life** | 1½-4 hr |

### Pharmacodynamics

| | PO | IV |
|---|---|---|
| **Onset** | 15 min | Rapid |
| **Peak** | 1-2 hr | Inf end |
| **Duration** | Unknown | Unknown |

## Interactions

### Individual drugs

Folic acid: decreased action of folic acid
Hydantoins: increased action of hydantoins
Iron: increased action of iron
Rifampin: decreased action of rifampin
Vitamin $B_{12}$: decreased action of vit $B_{12}$

### Drug classifications

Anticoagulants: increased PTT
Antidiabetics: increased action of antidiabetics
Barbiturates: increased levels of barbiturates
Penicillins: decreased action of penicillins

### Drug/herb

Acidophilus: do not use with antiinfectives; separate by several hours

## NURSING CONSIDERATIONS
### Assessment

• Assess patient for previous sensitivity reaction to other antiinfectives; cross-sensitivity between penicillins and cephalosporins is common

• Assess patient for signs and symptoms of infection including characteristics of wounds, sputum, urine, stool, WBC >10,000/mm$^3$, fever; obtain baseline information and during treatment

• Perform C&S testing before starting product therapy to identify if correct treatment has been initiated

• Monitor product level in impaired renal/hepatic systems; peak 15-20 mg/ml 3 hr after dose, trough 5-10 mg/ml before next dose

• Monitor blood studies: platelets q2 days, CBC

• Assess bowel pattern daily; if severe diarrhea occurs, product should be discontinued

• Monitor for bleeding: ecchymosis, bleeding gums, hematuria, stool guaiac daily if on long-term therapy

• Assess for overgrowth of infection: perineal itching, fever, malaise, redness, pain, swelling, drainage, rash, diarrhea, change in cough, sputum

### Nursing diagnoses

• Diarrhea (adverse reaction)
• Infection, risk for (uses)
• Injury, risk for (side effects)
• Knowledge, deficient (teaching)
• Noncompliance (teaching)

### Implementation
#### PO route

◆ Do not break, crush, or chew caps

• Give oral form on empty stomach with full glass of water

• Store cap in airtight container at room temperature

#### IV route

• Give after diluting 1 g/10 ml of sterile $H_2O$ for inj or $D_5W$ (10% sol); give >1 min

• May be further diluted in 50-100 ml of $D_5W$; give through Y-tube, 3-way stopcock, or additive infusion set; run over ½-1 hr; store reconstituted sol at room temperature for up to 30 days

**Syringe compatibilities:** Ampicillin, cloxacillin, heparin, methicillin, penicillin G sodium

**Y-site compatibilities:** Acyclovir, cyclophosphamide, enalaprilat, esmolol, foscarnet, hydromorphone, labetalol, magnesium sulfate, meperidine, morphine, perphenazine, tacrolimus

*Y-site incompatibilities:* Fluconazole
*Additive compatibilities:* Amikacin,
aminophylline, ascorbic acid, calcium
chloride/gluconate, cephalothin, cephapirin,
colistimethate, corticotropin, cyanocobalamin,
dimenhyDRINATE, DOPamine, epHEDrine,
heparin, hydrocortisone, kanamycin, lidocaine, magnesium sulfate, metaraminol,
methicillin, methyldopate, methylPREDNISolone, metronidazole, nafcillin, oxacillin,
oxytocin, penicillin G potassium, penicillin G
sodium, pentobarbital, phenylephrine, phytonadione, plasma protein fraction, potassium
chloride, promazine, ranitidine, sodium
bicarbonate, thiopental, verapamil, vit B

## Patient/family education
• Teach patient all aspects of product therapy;
need to complete entire course of medication
to ensure organism death (10-14 days);
culture may be taken after complete course of
medication
• Advise patient to report sore throat, fever,
fatigue, unusual bleeding, or bruising; could
indicate bone marrow depression (may occur
weeks or months after termination of product)
• Tell patient that product must be taken at
regular intervals around the clock to maintain
blood levels

## Evaluation
**Positive therapeutic outcome**
• Decreased symptoms of infection

## chloramphenicol ophthalmic
*See Appendix D*

## chloramphenicol otic
*See Appendix D*

## chlordiazepoxide (Rx)
(klor-dye-az-e-pox'ide)
Apo-Chlordiazepoxide ♣, Librium,
Novopoxide ♣
*Func. class.:* Antianxiety
*Chem. class.:* Benzodiazepine, long-acting

**Pregnancy category D**
**Controlled substance schedule IV**

**Do not confuse:**
Librium/Librax

**Action:** Potentiates the actions of GABA, an
inhibitory neurotransmitter, especially in the
limbic system reticular formation, which
depresses the CNS

**Therapeutic outcome:** Decreased
anxiety, successful alcohol withdrawal, relaxation

**Uses:** Short-term management of anxiety,
acute alcohol withdrawal, preoperative relaxation

## Dosage and routes
*Mild anxiety*
*Adult:* PO 5-10 mg tid-qid
*Geriatric:* PO 5 mg bid initially, increase as
needed
*Child >6 yr:* PO 5 mg bid-qid, max 10 mg
bid-tid
*Severe anxiety*
*Adult:* PO 20-25 mg tid-qid, IM/**IV** 50-100
mg initially, then 25-50 mg tid or 25-50 mg
initially in geriatric
*Preoperatively*
*Adult:* PO 5-10 mg tid-qid on day before
surgery; IM 50-100 mg 1 hr before surgery
*Alcohol withdrawal*
*Adult:* PO/IM/**IV** 50-100 mg q4-6hr prn,
max 300 mg/day
*Renal disease*
*Adult:* PO CCr <10 ml/min give 50% dose
*Liver disease*
*Adult:* PO 5 mg bid-qid

**Available forms:** Caps 5, 25 mg; IM inj
100 mg ampule

**Adverse effects:**
*CNS: Dizziness, drowsiness,* confusion,
headache, anxiety, tremors, stimulation,
fatigue, depression, insomnia, hallucinations
*CV: Orthostatic hypotension,* **ECG changes,
tachycardia,** hypotension, edema
*EENT: Blurred vision,* tinnitus, mydriasis
*GI:* Constipation, dry mouth, nausea, vomiting,
anorexia, diarrhea

Adverse effects: *italic* = common, **bold** = life-threatening

*GU:* Irregular periods, decreased libido
*HEMA:* **Agranulocytosis**
*INTEG:* Rash, dermatitis, itching

**Contraindications:** Pregnancy **D**, child <6 yr, hypersensitivity to benzodiazepines, angle-closure glaucoma, psychosis

**Precautions:** Geriatric, debilitated, renal/hepatic disease, suicidal ideation

### Pharmacokinetics

| | |
|---|---|
| **Absorption** | Well absorbed (PO); slow, erratic (IM) |
| **Distribution** | Widely distributed; crosses placenta, blood-brain barrier |
| **Metabolism** | Liver extensively |
| **Excretion** | Kidneys, breast milk |
| **Half-life** | 5-30 hr (increased in geriatric) |

### Pharmacodynamics

| | PO | IM | IV |
|---|---|---|---|
| **Onset** | 30 min | 15-30 min | 1-5 min |
| **Peak** | Within 2 hr | Unknown | Unknown |
| **Duration** | 4-6 hr | Unknown | Up to 1 hr |

### Interactions
*Individual drugs*
Alcohol: increased CNS depression
Cimetidine, disulfiram, fluoxetine, isoniazid, ketoconazole, metoprolol, propranolol, valproic acid: increased action of chlordiazepoxide
Levodopa: decreased action of levodopa
*Drug classifications*
CNS depressants: increased CNS depression
Contraceptives (oral): increased effect of chlordiazepoxide
CYP3A4 inhibitors (barbiturates, protease inhibitors, rifamycins): decreased effect of chlordiazepoxide
*Drug/herb*
Cowslip, kava, Queen Anne's lace, St. John's wort, valerian: decreased effect
*Drug/lab test*
False increase: 17-OHCS
False positive: pregnancy test (some methods)

### NURSING CONSIDERATIONS
Assessment
• Assess anxiety reaction: inability to sleep, apprehension, dread, foreboding, or uneasiness related to unidentified source of danger
• Assess for previous product dependence or tolerance; if product dependent or tolerant, amount of medication should be restricted

• Monitor B/P (with patient lying, standing), pulse; if systolic B/P drops 20 mm Hg, hold product, notify prescriber
• Monitor blood studies: CBC during long-term therapy; blood dyscrasias have occurred rarely
• Monitor hepatic studies: AST, ALT, bilirubin, creatinine, LDH, alkaline phosphatase during long-term therapy
• Monitor mental status: mood, sensorium, affect, sleeping patterns, drowsiness, dizziness, suicidal tendencies

### Nursing diagnoses
• Anxiety (uses)
• Knowledge, deficient (teaching)
• Noncompliance (teaching)

### Implementation
PO route
• Give with food or milk for GI symptoms, crushed if patient unable to swallow medication whole; do not open capsules; provide sugarless gum, hard candy, frequent sips of water for dry mouth
IM route
• Reconstitute with diluent provided (2 ml); agitate slowly, do not shake; give deep in large muscle mass to prevent severe pain; do not use IM diluent for **IV** route
IV route
• Reconstitute 100 mg/5 ml sterile water for inj or 0.9% NaCl; give over at least 1 min to prevent cardiac arrest, apnea, bradycardia
• Keep powder from light; refrigerate, mix when ready to use
*Y-site compatibilities:* Heparin, hydrocortisone, potassium chloride, vit B with C
*Solution compatibilities:* D$_5$W, 0.9% NaCl

### Patient/family education
• Instruct patient that product may be taken with food; if dose is missed take as soon as remembered; do not double doses
• Tell patient to avoid OTC preparations unless approved by prescriber; to avoid alcohol ingestion or other psychotropic medications unless directed by a prescriber
• Caution patient to avoid driving and activities requiring alertness, since drowsiness may occur; until medication response is known, tell patient that drowsiness may worsen at beginning of treatment
• Instruct patient not to discontinue medication abruptly after long-term use, product should be tapered over 1 wk
• Caution patient to rise slowly or fainting may occur, especially in geriatric

- Advise patient that product should be avoided during pregnancy

## Evaluation
### Positive therapeutic outcome
- Increased well being
- Decreased anxiety, restlessness, sleeplessness, dread
- Successful alcohol withdrawal

**Treatment of overdose:** Lavage, VS, supportive care

---

### chloroquine 🌀 (Rx)
(klor'oh-kwin)
Aralen HCl, Aralen Phosphate, chloroquine phosphate
*Func. class.:* Antimalarial
*Chem. class.:* Synthetic 4-aminoquinoline derivative

### Pregnancy category C

**Action:** Inhibits parasite replications, transcription of DNA to RNA by forming complexes with DNA of parasite

**Therapeutic outcome:** Decreased symptoms of malaria, amebiasis

**Uses:** Malaria caused by *Plasmodium vivax, Plasmodium malariae, Plasmodium ovale, Plasmodium falciparum* (some strains), amebiasis

### Dosage and routes
*Malaria suppression*
*Adult and child:* PO 5 mg base/kg/wk on same day of week, not to exceed 300 mg base; treatment should begin 1-2 wk before exposure and for 8 wk after leaving endemic area; if treatment begins after exposure, 600 mg base for adult and 10 mg base/kg for children in 2 divided doses 6 hr apart

*Extraintestinal amebiasis*
*Adult:* IM 160-200 mg base daily × 10-12 days or PO (HCl) 600 mg base daily × 2 days, then 300 mg base daily × 2-3 wk (phosphate)
*Child:* PO/IM 10 mg/kg daily (HCl) × 2-3 wk, not to exceed 300 mg/day

**Available forms:** Tabs 250 mg (150 mg base), 500 mg (300 mg base) phosphate; inj 50 mg (40 mg base)/ml HCl

### Adverse effects
*CNS:* Headache, stimulation, fatigue, **seizure,** psychosis
*CV:* Hypotension, **heart block, asystole with syncope,** ECG changes

*EENT: Blurred vision, corneal changes, retinal changes, difficulty focusing,* tinnitus, vertigo, deafness, photophobia, corneal edema
*GI: Nausea, vomiting, anorexia,* diarrhea, cramps
*HEMA:* **Thrombocytopenia, agranulocytosis, hemolytic anemia, leukopenia**
*INTEG:* Pruritus, pigmentary changes, skin eruptions, lichen planus–like eruptions, eczema, **exfoliative dermatitis**

**Contraindications:** Hypersensitivity, retinal field changes

**Precautions:** Pregnancy **C,** breastfeeding, children, blood dyscrasias, severe GI disease, neurologic disease, alcoholism, hepatic disease, G6PD deficiency, psoriasis, eczema, seizures, preexisting auditory damage

### Pharmacokinetics

| | |
|---|---|
| **Absorption** | Well absorbed |
| **Distribution** | Widely |
| **Metabolism** | Liver |
| **Excretion** | Kidneys, feces |
| **Half-life** | 3-5 days |

### Pharmacodynamics

| | PO | IM |
|---|---|---|
| **Onset** | Rapid | Rapid |
| **Peak** | 1-3 hr | 30 min |
| **Duration** | 6-8 hr | Unknown |

### Interactions
*Individual drugs*
Cimetidine: decreased oral clearance, metabolism
Kaolin: decreased absorption
Magnesium: decreased action of chloroquine
*Drug classifications*
Antacids (aluminum): decreased absorption

## NURSING CONSIDERATIONS
### Assessment
- Monitor liver studies weekly: ALT, AST, bilirubin; renal status: before exposure, monthly thereafter: BUN, creatinine, urine output, specific gravity, urinalysis
- Assess mental status often: affect, mood, behavioral changes; psychosis may occur
- Assess hepatic status: decreased appetite, jaundice, dark urine, fatigue
- Assess for toxicity: blurring vision, difficulty focusing, headache, dizziness, decreased knee and ankle reflexes, product should be discontinued immediately

Adverse effects: *italic* = common, **bold** = life-threatening

## Nursing diagnoses
- Diarrhea (side effects)
- Infection, risk for (uses)
- Injury, risk for (side effects)
- Knowledge, deficient (teaching)
- Noncompliance (teaching)

## Implementation
**PO route**
- Give with meals to decrease GI symptoms; better to take on empty stomach 1 hr before or 2 hr after meals
- Give antiemetic if vomiting occurs
- Give after C&S is completed; monthly to detect resistance

**IM route**
- Give IM after aspirating to prevent inj into bloodstream

*Additive compatibility:* Promethazine

## Patient/family education
- Advise patient that compliance with dosage schedule, duration is necessary
- Instruct patient that scheduled appointments must be kept or relapse may occur
- Caution patient to avoid alcohol while taking product
- Instruct diabetic to use blood glucose monitor to obtain correct result
- Teach patient to report weakness, fatigue, loss of appetite, nausea, vomiting, yellowing of skin or eyes, tingling/numbness of hands/feet
- Advise patient that urine may turn rust brown color
- Instruct patient to use sunglasses in bright sunlight to prevent photophobia

## Evaluation
**Positive therapeutic outcome**
- Decreased symptoms of malaria

**Treatment of overdose:** Induce vomiting, gastric lavage, administer barbiturate (ultrashort-acting), vasopressor; tracheostomy may be necessary

---

**chlorothiazide** (Rx)
(klor-oh-thye'a-zide)
Diuril
*Func. class.:* Diuretic, antihypertensive
*Chem. class.:* Thiazide; sulfonamide derivative

**Pregnancy category** B

**Do not confuse:**
chlorothiazide/chlorproMAZINE/
chlorproPAMIDE/chlorthalidone

**Action:** Acts on the distal tubule and thick ascending limb of the loop of Henle in the kidney, increasing excretion of sodium, water, chloride, magnesium, potassium, and bicarbonate

**Therapeutic outcome:** Decreased BP, decreased edema in tissues peripherally, diuresis

**Uses:** Hypertension, diuresis

## Dosage and routes
*Hypertension*
*Adult:* PO/**IV** 500 mg-2 g daily; may divide bid

*Edema*
*Adult:* IV 250 mg q6-12hr
*Child >6 mo:* PO 10-20 mg/kg/day may divide bid
*Child <6 mo:* PO up to 40 mg/kg/day in 2 doses

**Available forms:** Tabs 250, 500 mg; oral susp 250 mg/5 ml; powder for inj 500 mg

## Adverse effects
*CNS:* Paresthesia, headache, *dizziness, fatigue*
*CV:* Irregular pulse, orthostatic hypotension, volume depletion
*EENT:* Blurred vision
*ELECT: Hypokalemia,* hypercalcemia, hyponatremia, hypochloremia
*GI:* Nausea, vomiting, anorexia, constipation, diarrhea, cramps, pancreatitis, GI irritation, ***hepatitis***
*GU: Frequency,* polyuria
*HEMA:* **Aplastic anemia, hemolytic anemia, leukopenia, agranulocytosis, thrombocytopenia, neutropenia**
*INTEG:* Rash, urticaria, purpura, photosensitivity, alopecia
*META:* Hyperglycemia, *hyperuricemia,* increased creatinine, BUN

**Contraindications:** Hypersensitivity to thiazides or sulfonamides, anuria, renal decompensation, breastfeeding, hepatic coma

**Precautions:** Pregnancy **B**, geriatric, hypokalemia, renal/hepatic disease, gout, COPD, LE, diabetes mellitus, hyperlipidemia

---

| Pharmacokinetics | |
|---|---|
| | PO |
| **Absorption** | GI tract (10%-20%) |
| **Distribution** | Extracellular spaces; crosses placenta |
| **Metabolism** | Liver |
| **Excretion** | Urine, unchanged; breast milk |
| **Half-life** | 1-2 hr |

| Pharmacodynamics | | |
|---|---|---|
| | PO | IV |
| **Onset** | 2 hr | 15 min |
| **Peak** | 4 hr | ½ hr |
| **Duration** | 6-12 hr | 2 hr |

## Interactions
### Individual drugs
Alcohol: increased hypotension

Allopurinol, digoxin, lithium: increased toxicity

Amphotericin, mezlocillin, piperacillin, ticarcillin: increased hypokalemia

Cholestyramine, colestipol: decreased absorption of thiazides

### Drug classifications
Antihypertensives: increased antihypertensive effect

Glucocorticoids: increased hypokalemia

Nitrates: increased hypotension

NSAIDs: decreased diuretic action

Nondepolarizing skeletal muscle relaxants: increased toxicity

### Drug/herb
Aloe, buckthorn, cascara sagrada, Chinese rhubarb, gossypol, licorice, nettle, senna: increased hypokalemia (chronic use)

Aloe, cucumber, dandelion, horsetail, pumpkin, Queen Anne's lace: increased diuretic effect

St. John's wort: increased severe photosensitivity

### Drug/lab test
Increased: calcium, amylase, parathyroid test, CPK

Decreased: PBI

False negative: phentolamine and tyramine tests

Interference: urine steroid tests

## NURSING CONSIDERATIONS
### Assessment
- Assess glucose in urine if patient is diabetic
- Monitor improvement in CVP q8hr
- Check for rashes, temp elevation daily
- Assess for confusion, especially in geriatric; take safety precautions if needed
- Monitor manifestations of hypokalemia; *RENAL:* acidic urine, reduced urine osmolality, nocturia; *CV:* hypotension, broad T wave, U wave, ectopy, tachycardia, weak pulse; *NEURO:* muscle weakness, altered LOC, drowsiness, apathy, lethargy, confusion, depression; *GI:* anorexia, nausea, cramps, constipation, distention, paralytic ileus; *RESP:* hypoventilation, respiratory muscle weakness
- Monitor for manifestations of hypomagnesemia; *CNS:* agitation, muscle twitching, paresthesias, hyperactive reflexes, positive Babinski's reflex, dysphagia, nystagmus, seizures, tetany; *GI:* nausea, vomiting, diarrhea, anorexia, abdominal distention; *CV:* ectopy, tachycardia, broad, flat, or inverted T waves, depressed ST segment, prolonged QT interval, decreased cardiac output, hypotension
- Monitor for manifestations of hyponatremia: *CV:* increased B/P, cold, clammy skin, hypovolemia or hypervolemia; *GI:* anorexia, nausea, vomiting, diarrhea, abdominal cramps; *NEURO:* lethargy, increased ICP, confusion, headache, seizures, coma, fatigue, tremors, hyperreflexia
- Monitor for manifestations of hyperchloremia: *NEURO:* weakness, lethargy, coma; *RESP:* coma, deep rapid breathing
- Assess fluid volume status: I&O ratios and record, count or weigh diapers as appropriate, weight, distended neck veins, crackles in lung, color, quality and specific gravity of urine, skin turgor, adequacy of pulses, moist mucous membranes, bilateral lung sounds, peripheral pitting edema; dehydration symptoms of decreasing output, thirst, hypotension, dry mouth and mucous membranes should be reported
- Monitor electrolytes: potassium, sodium, calcium, magnesium; also include BUN, blood pH, ABGs, uric acid, CBC, blood glucose
- Assess B/P before and during therapy with patient lying, standing, and sitting as appropriate; orthostatic hypotension can occur rapidly

### Nursing diagnoses
- Fluid volume, deficient
- Fluid volume, excess (uses)
- Knowledge, deficient (teaching)
- Urinary elimination, impaired (adverse reactions)

### Implementation
- Give in AM to avoid interference with sleep
- Potassium replacement if potassium level is 3.0 mg/dl

Adverse effects: *italic* = common, **bold** = life-threatening

• Give whole, or use oral sol; product may be crushed if patient is unable to swallow

**PO route**

• Give with food; if nausea occurs, absorption may be increased

**IV route**

• Do not use sol that is yellow, has a precipitate, or crystals

• Administer **IV** after diluting 0.5 g/18 ml or more of sterile water for inj; may be diluted further with dextrose or NaCl; give over 5 min; sol is stable at room temperature for 24 hr

*Additive compatibilities:* Cimetidine, lidocaine, nafcillin, sodium bicarbonate

*Additive incompatibilities:* Amikacin, blood, blood products, chlorproMAZINE, codeine, hydrALAZINE, insulin, levorphanol, methadone, morphine, multivitamins, norepinephrine, polymyxin B, procaine, prochlorperazine, promazine, promethazine, streptomycin, tetracycline, triflupromazine, vancomycin

**Patient/family education**

• Teach patient to take medication early in the day to prevent nocturia

• Instruct patient to take with food or milk if GI symptoms of nausea and anorexia occur

• Teach patient to maintain a weekly record of weight and notify prescriber of weight loss >5 lb

• Caution patient that this product causes a loss of potassium, so food rich in potassium should be added to the diet; refer to a dietitian for assistance in planning

• Caution patient not to exercise in hot weather or stand for prolonged periods, since orthostatic hypotension will be enhanced; to use sunscreen to prevent burning

• Teach patient not to use alcohol or any OTC medications without prescriber's approval; serious product reactions may occur

• Emphasize the need to contact prescriber immediately if muscle cramps, weakness, nausea, dizziness, or numbness occurs

• Teach patient to take own B/P and pulse and record

• Caution patient that orthostatic hypotension may occur; patient should rise slowly from sitting or reclining positions and lie down if dizziness occurs

• Teach patient to continue taking medication even if feeling better; this product controls symptoms but does not cure the condition

• Advise the patient with hypertension to continue other medical treatment (exercise, weight loss, relaxation techniques, cessation of smoking)

**Evaluation**

**Positive therapeutic outcome**

• Decreased edema

• Decreased B/P

• Increased diuresis

**Treatment of overdose:** Lavage if taken orally, monitor electrolytes; administer dextrose in saline; monitor hydration, CV, renal status

---

## chlorpheniramine (OTC, Rx)

(klor-fen-ir′a-meen)

Aller-Chlor, Allergy, Chlo-Amine, Chlorate, chlorpheniramine maleate, Chlor-Trimeton, Chlor-Tripolon ♣, Gen-Allerate, Novo-Pheniram ♣, PediaCare Allergy Formula, Phenetron, Telachor, Teldrin

*Func. class.:* Antihistamine (1st generation, nonselective)

*Chem. class.:* Alkylamine, $H_1$-receptor antagonist

**Pregnancy category  B**

**Do not confuse:**
Teldrin/Tedral

**Action:** Acts on blood vessels, GI, respiratory system by competing with histamine for $H_1$-receptor site; decreases allergic response by blocking histamine

**Therapeutic outcome:** Absence of allergy symptoms and rhinitis

**Uses:** Allergy symptoms, rhinitis, conjunctivitis (allergic)

**Dosage and routes**

*Adult/child ≥12 yr:* PO 2-4 mg tid-qid, not to exceed 24 mg/day; TIME REL 8-12 mg bid-tid, not to exceed 24 mg/day; IM/SUBCUT/**IV** 5-40 mg/day, max 40 mg/day

*Child 6-12 yr:* PO 2 mg q4-6hr, not to exceed 12 mg/day; SUS REL 8 mg at bedtime or daily; SUS REL not recommended for child <6 yr; SUBCUT 87.5 mcg/kg or 2.5 mg/m² q6hr

*Child 2-5 yr:* PO 1 mg q4-6hr, not to exceed 4 mg/day

**Available forms:** Chewable tabs 2 mg; tabs 4, 8, 12 mg; ext rel tabs 8, 12 mg; ext rel caps 8, 12 mg; syr 1, 2, 2.5 mg/5 ml; inj 10, 100 mg/ml

**Adverse effects**

*CNS: Dizziness, drowsiness,* poor coordination, fatigue, anxiety, euphoria, confusion, paresthesia, neuritis

---

*EENT:* Blurred vision, dilated pupils, tinnitus, nasal stuffiness, dry nose, throat, mouth
*GI:* Nausea, anorexia, diarrhea
*GU: Retention,* dysuria, frequency
*HEMA:* **Thrombocytopenia, agranulocytosis, hemolytic anemia**
*INTEG:* Photosensitivity
*RESP:* Increased thick secretions, wheezing, chest tightness

**Contraindications:** Hypersensitivity to H$_1$-receptor antagonists, acute asthma attack, lower respiratory tract disease, stenosed peptic ulcers, bladder neck obstruction, angle-closure glaucoma, newborns/neonates

**Precautions:** Pregnancy **B**, breastfeeding, geriatric, increased intraocular pressure, renal/cardiac disease, hypertension, bronchial asthma, seizure disorder, hyperthyroidism, prostatic hypertrophy

| Pharmacokinetics | |
|---|---|
| Absorption | Well absorbed (PO, SUBCUT, IM, **IV**) |
| Distribution | Widely distributed; crosses blood-brain barrier |
| Metabolism | Liver, mostly |
| Excretion | Kidneys, metabolite; breast milk (minimal) |
| Half-life | 12-15 hr |

| Pharmacodynamics | | | | | |
|---|---|---|---|---|---|
| | PO | PO-ER | SUBCUT | IM | IV |
| Onset | 15-30 min | Unknown | Unknown | Unknown | Immediate |
| Peak | 1-2 hr | Unknown | Unknown | Unknown | Unknown |
| Duration | 4-12 hr | 8-24 hr | 4-12 hr | 4-12 hr | 4-12 hr |

### Interactions
*Individual drugs*
Alcohol: increased CNS depression
Atropine, haloperidol, quinidine: increased anticholinergic reactions
*Drug classifications*
CNS depressants, opiates, sedative/hypnotics, barbiturates, tricyclics: increased CNS depression
MAOIs: increased effect of chlorpheniramine
Phenothiazines: increased anticholinergic reactions
*Drug/herb*
Corkwood, henbane leaf: increased anticholinergic effect

Hops, Jamaican dogwood, kava, khat, senega: increased sedative effect
*Drug/lab test*
False negative: skin allergy tests (discontinue antihistamines 3 days before testing)

### NURSING CONSIDERATIONS
**Assessment**
• Assess respiratory status: rate, rhythm, increase in bronchial secretions, wheezing, chest tightness; provide fluids to 2 L/day to decrease secretion thickness
• Monitor I&O ratio: be alert for urinary retention, frequency, dysuria, especially geriatric; product should be discontinued if these occur
• **IV** administration may result in rapid drop in B/P, sweating, dizziness, especially in geriatric

**Nursing diagnoses**
• Airway clearance, ineffective (uses)
• Injury, risk for (side effects)
• Knowledge, deficient (teaching)
• Noncompliance (teaching, overuse)

**Implementation**
**PO route**
• Swallow time rel tabs and caps whole
• Do not break, crush, chew, or open time rel tabs
• Chewable tabs should be chewed and not swallowed whole
• May give with food to decrease GI upset
• Store in tight, light-resistant container
**IM/SUBCUT route**
• Use only 20 and 100 mg/ml strengths; does not need to be reconstituted or diluted
**IV route**
Give undiluted by direct **IV** (10 mg/ml strength only); administer 10 mg over 1 min or more
*Additive incompatibilities:* Calcium chloride, kanamycin, norepinephrine, pentobarbital

**Patient/family education**
• Teach all aspects of product use; to notify prescriber if confusion, sedation, hypotension, or difficulty voiding occurs; to avoid driving and other hazardous activity if drowsiness occurs; to avoid alcohol and other CNS depressants that may potentiate effect
• Teach patient not to exceed recommended dosage; dysrhythmias may occur
• Advise patient hard candy, gum, frequent rinsing of mouth may be used for dryness

Adverse effects: *italic* = common, **bold** = life-threatening

## Evaluation
**Positive therapeutic outcome**
• Absence of running or congested nose, rashes, conjunctivitis

**Treatment of overdose:** Administer lavage, diazepam, vasopressors, barbiturates (short acting)

---

**\*chlorproMAZINE** **(Rx)**
(klor-proe'ma-zeen)
chlorproMAZINE HCl, Chlorpromanyl ✦, Largactil ✦, Novo-Chlorpromazine ✦, Thorazine, Thor-Prom
*Func. class.:* Antipsychotic/neuroleptic/antiemetic
*Chem. class.:* Phenothiazine, aliphatic

**Pregnancy category C**

**Do not confuse:**
chlorproMAZINE/chlorothiazide/chlorproPAMIDE/chlorthalidone/prochlorperazine

**Action:** Depresses cerebral cortex, hypothalamus, limbic system, which control activity, aggression; blocks neurotransmission produced by dopamine at synapse; exhibits a strong α-adrenergic, anticholinergic blocking action; mechanism for antipsychotic effects is unclear

**Therapeutic outcome:** Decreased signs and symptoms of psychosis; control of nausea, vomiting, intractable hiccups, decreased anxiety preoperatively

**Uses:** Psychotic disorders, Tourette's syndrome, mania, schizophrenia, anxiety, intractable hiccups (adults), nausea, vomiting, preoperative relaxation, acute intermittent porphyria, behavioral problems in children, nonpsychotic patients with dementia

**Unlabeled uses:** Vascular headache

## Dosage and routes
*Psychosis*
**Adult:** PO 10-50 mg q1-4hr initially, then increase up to 2 g/day if necessary; IM 10-50 mg q1-4hr, usual dose 300-800 mg/day
**Geriatric:** PO 10-25 mg daily-bid, increased by 10-25 mg/day q4-7 days, max 800 mg/day
**Child >6 mo:** PO 0.5 mg/kg q4-6hr; IM 0.5 mg/kg q6-8hr; RECT 1 mg/kg q6-8hr

*Nausea and vomiting*
**Adult:** PO 10-25 mg q4-6hr prn; IM 25-50 mg q3hr prn; RECT 50-100 mg q6-8hr prn, not to exceed 400 mg/day; **IV** 25-50 mg daily-qid

**Child ≥6 mo:** PO 0.55 mg/kg q4-6hr; IM q6-8hr; RECT 1.1 mg/kg q6-8hr, max IM ≤5 yr or ≤22.7 kg 40 mg; max IM 5-10 yr or 22.7-45.5 kg 75 mg

*Intractable hiccups*
**Adult:** PO 25-50 mg tid-qid; IM 25-50 mg (used only if PO dose does not work); **IV** 25-50 mg in 500-1000 ml saline (only for severe hiccups)

**Available forms:** Tabs 10, 25, 50, 100, 200 mg; sus rel caps 30, 75, 150, 200, 300 mg; syr 10, 25, 100 mg/5 ml; conc 30, 40, 100 mg/ml; supp 25, 100 mg; inj 25 mg/ml

## Adverse effects
*CNS:* **Neuroleptic malignant syndrome,** dizziness, *extrapyramidal symptoms: pseudoparkinsonism, akathisia, dystonia, tardive dyskinesia,* **seizures,** *headache*
*CV: Orthostatic hypotension,* hypertension, **cardiac arrest,** ECG changes, **tachycardia**
*EENT:* Blurred vision, glaucoma, dry eyes
*GI: Dry mouth, nausea, vomiting, anorexia, constipation,* diarrhea, jaundice, weight gain
*GU:* Urinary retention, enuresis, impotence, amenorrhea, gynecomastia, breast engorgement
*HEMA:* Anemia, **leukopenia, leukocytosis, agranulocytosis**
*INTEG: Rash,* photosensitivity, dermatitis
*RESP:* **Laryngospasm,** dyspnea, **respiratory depression**

**Contraindications:** Hypersensitivity, circulatory collapse, liver damage, cerebral arteriosclerosis, coronary disease, severe hypo/hypertension, blood dyscrasias, coma, child <6 mo, brain damage, bone marrow depression, alcohol and barbiturate withdrawal, angle-closure glaucoma

**Precautions:** Pregnancy **C,** breastfeeding, geriatric, seizure disorders, hypertension, hepatic/cardiac disease, prostate enlargement, pulmonary/Parkinson's disease

| Pharmacokinetics | |
|---|---|
| **Absorption** | Variable (PO); well absorbed (IM) |
| **Distribution** | Widely distributed; crosses placenta |
| **Metabolism** | Liver, GI mucosa extensively |
| **Excretion** | Kidneys |
| **Half-life** | 30 hr |

## Pharmacodynamics

|          | PO      | RECT    | IM      | IV      |
|----------|---------|---------|---------|---------|
| Onset    | ½-1 hr  | 12 hr   | Unknown | Rapid   |
| Peak     | Unknown | Unknown | Unknown | Unknown |
| Duration | 4-6 hr* | 3-4 hr  | 4-8 hr  | Unknown |

*Duration PO ext rel is 10-12 hr.

## Interactions
### Individual drugs
Alcohol: increased effects of both products, oversedation

Aluminum hydroxide, magnesium hydroxide: decreased absorption

Bromocriptine, levodopa: decreased antiparkinsonian activity

Epinephrine: increased toxicity

Lithium: decreased chlorproMAZINE levels

Valproic acid: increased valproic acid level

Warfarin: decreased anticoagulant effect

### Drug classifications
Antacids: decreased absorption

Anticholinergics, antidepressants, antiparkinsonian agents: increased anticholinergic effects

Anticonvulsants: decreased seizure threshold

Antidepressants, antihistamines, barbiturate anesthetics, general anesthetics, MAOIs, opioids, sedative/hypnotics: increased CNS depression

Antithyroid agents: increased agranulocytosis

Barbiturates: decreased serum chlorproMAZINE

β-Adrenergic blockers: increased effect of both products

### Drug/herb
Cola tree, hops, nettle, nutmeg: increased action

Henbane leaf: increased anticholinergic effect

Betel palm, kava: increased EPS

### Drug/lab test
Increased: liver function tests, cardiac enzymes, cholesterol, blood glucose, prolactin, bilirubin, PBI, cholinesterase I, alkaline phosphatase, leukocytes, granulocytes, platelets, [131]I

Decreased: hormones (blood and urine)

False positive: pregnancy tests, PKU, urine

False negative: urinary steroids, 17-OHCS

## NURSING CONSIDERATIONS
### Assessment
• Assess mental status: orientation, mood, behavior, presence of hallucinations, and type before initial administration and monthly; this product should significantly reduce psychotic behavior

• Assess any potentially reversible cause of behavior problems in geriatric before and during therapy

• Check for swallowing of PO medication; check for hoarding or giving of medication to other patients

• Monitor I&O ratio; palpate bladder if low urinary output occurs, especially in geriatric; urinalysis recommended before, during prolonged therapy

• Monitor bilirubin, CBC, liver function studies monthly

• Assess affect, orientation, LOC, reflexes, gait, coordination, sleep pattern disturbances

• Monitor B/P with patient sitting, standing, and lying; take pulse and respirations q4hr during initial treatment; establish baseline before starting treatment; report drops of 30 mm Hg; obtain baseline ECG, Q wave, and T wave changes

• Check for dizziness, faintness, palpitations, tachycardia on rising; severe orthostatic hypotension is common

⚠ Identify for neuroleptic malignant syndrome: hyperpyrexia, muscle rigidity, increased CPK, altered mental status; product should be discontinued

• Assess for EPS including akathisia (inability to sit still, no pattern to movements), tardive dyskinesia (bizarre movements of the jaw, mouth, tongue, extremities), pseudoparkinsonism (rigidity, tremors, pill rolling, shuffling gate); an antiparkinsonian product should be prescribed

• Assess for constipation, urinary retention daily; if these occur, increase bulk, water in diet

### Nursing diagnoses
• Coping, ineffective (uses)
• Knowledge, deficient (teaching)
• Noncompliance (teaching)
• Thought processes, disturbed (uses)

### Implementation
#### PO route
⚠ Do not break, crush, or chew time rel caps

• Give product in liquid form mixed in glass of juice or cola if hoarding is suspected

• Periodically attempt dosage reduction in patients with behavioral problems

• Give with full glass of water, milk; or give with food to decrease GI upset

• Store in tight, light-resistant container, oral sol in amber bottle

#### IM route
• Inject in deep muscle mass; do not give SUBCUT; may be diluted with 0.9% NaCl, 2% procaine as prescribed; do not administer sol with a precipitate

Adverse effects: *italic* = common, **bold** = life-threatening

- Remain lying down after IM inj for at least 30 min

**Rectal route**
- Give after placing in refrigerator for 30 min if too soft to insert; this route is used for nausea, vomiting, hiccups

**IV route**
- Give by direct **IV** by diluting with 0.9% NaCl to a concentration of 1 mg/1 ml; administer at a rate of 1 mg/2 min
- Give by cont inf after diluting 50 mg/500-1000 ml of $D_5W$, $D_{10}W$, 0.9% NaCl, 0.45% NaCl, LR, Ringer's or combinations (used for intractable hiccups)

**Syringe compatibilities:**
Atropine, benztropine, butorphanol, diphenhydrAMINE, doxapram, droperidol, fentanyl, glycopyrrolate, hydromorphone, hydrOXYzine, meperidine, metoclopramide, midazolam, morphine, pentazocine, perphenazine, prochlorperazine, promazine, promethazine, scopolamine

**Syringe incompatibilities:**
Cimetidine, dimenhyDRINATE, heparin, pentobarbital, thiopental

**Y-site compatibilities:**
Amsacrine, cisatracurium, cisplatin, cladribine, cyclophosphamide, cytarabine, DOXOrubicin, DOXOrubicin liposome, famotidine, filgrastim, fluconazole, granisetron, heparin, hydrocortisone, ondansetron, potassium chloride, propofol, teniposide, thiotepa, vinorelbine

**Additive compatibilities:**
Ascorbic acid, ethacrynate, netilmicin, theophylline, vit B/C

**Additive incompatibilities:**
Aminophylline, amphotericin B, ampicillin, chloramphenicol, chlorothiazide, methicillin, methohexital, penicillin G, phenobarbital

**Patient/family education**
- Teach patient to use good oral hygiene; frequent rinsing of mouth, sugarless gum, candy, or ice chips for dry mouth
- Caution patient to avoid hazardous activities until product response is determined; dizziness, blurred vision may occur
- Inform patient that orthostatic hypotension occurs often and to rise from sitting or lying position gradually, to remain lying down after IM inj for at least 30 min; tell patient to avoid hot tubs, hot showers, tub baths, since hypotension may occur; tell patient that in hot weather heat stroke may occur; take extra precautions to stay cool
- Advise patient to avoid abrupt withdrawal of this product, or extrapyramidal symptoms may

result; product should be withdrawn slowly
- Teach patient to avoid OTC preparations (cough, hay fever, cold) unless approved by prescriber, since serious product interactions may occur; avoid use with alcohol, CNS depressants, since increased drowsiness may occur
- Caution patient to use sunscreen and sunglasses to prevent burns
- Teach patient about extrapyramidal symptoms and necessity of meticulous oral hygiene, since oral candidiasis may occur
- Instruct patient to take antacids 2 hr before or after taking this product
- Instruct patient to report sore throat, malaise, fever, bleeding, mouth sores; if these occur, CBC should be drawn and product discontinued
- Teach that urine may turn pink or reddish-brown
- Teach patient to use contraceptive measures

**Evaluation**
**Positive therapeutic outcome**
- Decrease in emotional excitement, hallucinations, delusions, paranoia
- Reorganization of patterns of thought, speech
- Increase in target behaviors

**Treatment of overdose:** Lavage if orally ingested; provide airway, *do not induce vomiting or use epINEPHrine*

## chlorthalidone (Rx)
(klor-tha'li-doan)
Apo-Chlorthalidone ✦, chlorthalidone, Hygroton, Thalitone, Uridon ✦
*Func. class.:* Diuretic, antihypertensive
*Chem. class.:* Thiazide-like phthalimindine derivative

**Pregnancy category  B**

**Do not confuse:**
chlorthalidone/chlorothiazide/chlorproMAZINE/chlorproPAMIDE, Hygroton/Regroton, Uridon ✦/Vicodin

**Action:** Acts on the distal tubule and thick ascending limb of the loop of Henle in the kidney, increasing excretion of sodium, water, chloride, magnesium, potassium, and bicarbonate, possible arteriolar dilatation

**Therapeutic outcome:** Decreased B/P, decreased edema in lung tissues and peripherally, diuresis

**Uses:** Edema in congestive heart failure, nephrotic syndrome; may be used alone or as adjunct with antihypertensives; also for edema in corticosteroid, estrogen therapy

## Dosage and routes
### Hypertension
*Adult:* PO 25-200 mg/day or 100 mg 3× wk
### Edema
*Adult:* PO 50-100 mg/day or 100 mg on alternate days, max 200 mg/day
*Geriatric:* PO 12.5 mg daily or every other day

**Available forms:** Tabs 25, 50, 100 mg

## Adverse effects
*CV:* Hypertension, orthostatic hypotension, palpitations, volume depletion
*CNS:* Paresthesia, headache, *dizziness, fatigue, weakness,* fever
*EENT:* Blurred vision
*ELECT: Hypokalemia,* hypercalcemia, hyponatremia, hypochloremia, hypomagnesemia
*GI: Nausea, vomiting, anorexia,* constipation, diarrhea, cramps, pancreatitis, GI irritation
*GU: Frequency,* polyuria, **uremia,** glucosuria, impotence
*HEMA:* **Aplastic anemia, hemolytic anemia, leukopenia, agranulocytosis, thrombocytopenia, neutropenia**
*INTEG:* Rash, urticaria, purpura, photosensitivity
*META: Hyperglycemia, hyperuricemia,* increased creatinine, BUN, gout

**Contraindications:** Hypersensitivity to thiazides or sulfonamides, anuria, renal decompensation, breastfeeding

**Precautions:** Pregnancy **B,** geriatric, hypokalemia, renal/hepatic disease, gout, diabetes mellitus, hyperlipidemia, SLE, hypotension

### Pharmacokinetics
| | |
|---|---|
| Absorption | Well absorbed |
| Distribution | Extracellular spaces; crosses placenta |
| Metabolism | Liver |
| Excretion | Urine, unchanged (30%-60%) |
| Half-life | 40 hr |

### Pharmacodynamics
| | |
|---|---|
| Onset | 2 hr |
| Peak | 6 hr |
| Duration | 24-72 hr |

## Interactions
### Individual drugs
Alcohol: increased hypotensive effect
Allopurinol, lithium: increased toxicity
Amphotericin B: increased hypokalemia
Cholestyramine, colestipol: decreased absorption of thiazides
Diazoxide: increased hyperglycemia, hypotension
### Drug classifications
Glucocorticoids: increased hypokalemia
Nondepolarizing skeletal muscle relaxants: increased toxicity
### Drug/herb
Buckthorn, cascara sagrada, Chinese rhubarb, gossypol, licorice, nettle, senna: increased hypokalemia
Cucumber, dandelion, horsetail, khella, pumpkin, Queen Anne's lace: increased hypotension
St. John's wort: severe photosensitivity
### Drug/lab test
Increased: triglycerides, calcium, amylase, cholesterol, bilirubin, creatinine, low-density lipoproteins, serum/urine glucose (diabetics), uric acid
Decreased: PBI, parathyroid test, magnesium, potassium, sodium, urinary calcium

## NURSING CONSIDERATIONS
### Assessment
• Monitor manifestations of hypokalemia; *CV:* hypotension, broad T wave, U wave, ectopy, tachycardia, weak pulse; *GI:* anorexia, nausea, cramps, constipation, distention, paralytic ileus; *NEURO:* muscle weakness, altered LOC, drowsiness, apathy, lethargy, confusion, depression; *RENAL:* acidic urine, reduced urine, osmolality, nocturia; *RESP:* hypoventilation, respiratory muscle weakness
• Monitor for manifestations of hypomagnesemia; *CNS:* agitation, muscle twitching, paresthesias, hyperactive reflexes, positive Babinski's reflex, dysphagia, nystagmus, seizures, tetany; *CV:* ectopy, tachycardia, broad, flat or inverted T waves, depressed ST segment, prolonged QT, decreased cardiac output, hypotension; *GI:* nausea, vomiting, diarrhea, anorexia, abdominal distention
• Monitor for manifestations of hyponatremia; *CV:* increased B/P, cold, clammy skin, hypovolemia or hypervolemia; *GI:* anorexia, nausea, vomiting, diarrhea, abdominal cramps; *NEURO:* lethargy, increased ICP, confusion, headache, seizures, coma, fatigue, tremors, hyperreflexia

---

Adverse effects: *italic* = common, **bold** = life-threatening

- Monitor for manifestations of hyperchloremia; *NEURO:* weakness, lethargy, coma; *RESP:* coma, deep rapid breathing
- Assess fluid volume status: I&O ratios and record, count or weigh diapers as appropriate, weight, distended red veins, crackles in lung, color, quality and specific gravity of urine, skin turgor, adequacy of pulses, moist mucous membranes, bilateral lung sounds, peripheral pitting edema; dehydration symptoms of decreasing output, thirst, hypotension, dry mouth, and mucous membranes should be reported
- Monitor electrolytes: potassium, sodium, calcium, magnesium; also include BUN, blood pH, ABGs, uric acid, CBC, blood glucose
- Assess B/P before and during therapy with patient lying, standing, and sitting as appropriate; orthostatic hypotension can occur rapidly

## Nursing diagnoses
- Fluid volume, deficient (adverse reactions)
- Fluid volume, excess (uses)
- Knowledge, deficient (teaching)
- Urinary elimination, impaired (side effect)

## Implementation
- Brand names Thalitone/Hygroton should not be used interchangeably
- Give in AM to avoid interference with sleep
- Provide potassium replacement if potassium level is 3.0 mg/dl; give whole, or use oral solutions lightly; product may be crushed if patient is unable to swallow
- Give with food if nausea occurs; may crush tab and mix with fluids or applesauce for swallowing

## Patient/family education
- Teach patient to take the medication early in the day to prevent nocturia
- Instruct patient to take with food or milk if GI symptoms of nausea and anorexia occur
- Teach patient to maintain weekly record of weight and notify prescriber of weight loss >5 lb
- Caution patient that this product causes a loss of potassium, so foods rich in potassium should be added to the diet; refer to a dietitian for assistance in planning
- Caution the patient not to exercise in hot weather or stand for prolonged periods, since orthostatic hypotension will be enhanced; to use sunscreen to prevent burns
- Teach patient not to use alcohol, or any OTC medications without prescriber's approval; serious product reactions may occur

- Emphasize the need to contact prescriber immediately if muscle cramps, weakness, nausea, dizziness, or numbness occurs
- Teach patient to take own B/P and pulse and record
- Caution patient that orthostatic hypotension may occur; patient should rise slowly from sitting or reclining positions and lie down if dizziness occurs
- Teach patient to continue taking medication even if feeling better; this product controls symptoms but does not cure the condition
- Advise patient with hypertension to continue other medical treatment (exercise, weight loss, relaxation techniques, cessation of smoking)

## Evaluation
**Positive therapeutic outcome**
- Decreased edema
- Decreased B/P
- Increased diuresis

**Treatment of overdose:** Lavage if taken orally, monitor electrolytes; administer dextrose in saline; monitor hydration, CV, renal status

## cholecalciferol
*See vitamin D*

## cholestyramine (Rx)
(koe-less-tear'a-meen)
LoCHOLEST, LoCHOLEST Light, Prevalite, Questran, Questran Light
*Func. class.:* Antilipemic
*Chem. class.:* Bile acid sequestrant
**Pregnancy category** C

**Action:** Absorbs, combines with bile acids to form an insoluble complex that is excreted through feces; loss of bile acids lowers cholesterol levels

**Therapeutic outcome:** Decreasing cholesterol levels and low-density lipoproteins, decreased pruritus

**Uses:** Primary hypercholesterolemia, pruritus associated with biliary obstruction

**Unlabeled uses:** Diarrhea caused by excess bile acid

## Dosage and routes
*Adult:* PO 4 g daily-bid, max 24 g/day
*Child:* PO 240 mg/kg/day in 3 divided doses; administer with food or drink, max 8 g/day

**Available forms:** Powder for susp 4 g/cholestyramine/packet or scoop; tab 1 g

**Adverse effects**

*CNS:* Headache, dizziness, drowsiness, vertigo, tinnitus, anxiety

*GI: Constipation, abdominal pain, nausea,* fecal impaction, hemorrhoids, flatulence, vomiting, steatorrhea, peptic ulcer

*HEMA:* **Bleeding,** increased pro-time

*INTEG:* Rash, irritation of perianal area, tongue, skin

*META:* Decreased vit A, D, K, red cell folate content, **hyperchloremic acidosis**

*MS:* Muscle, joint pain

**Contraindications:** Hypersensitivity; biliary obstruction; hyperlipidemia III, IV, V

**Precautions:** Pregnancy **C,** breastfeeding, children

| Pharmacokinetics | |
|---|---|
| Absorption | Not absorbed |
| Distribution | Not distributed |
| Metabolism | Not metabolized; LDL lowered in 4-7 days, serum cholesterol lowered in 1 mo |
| Excretion | Binds with bile acids, feces |
| Half-life | Unknown |

| Pharmacodynamics | |
|---|---|
| Onset | 24-48 hr |
| Peak | 1-3 wk |
| Duration | 2-4 wk |

**Interactions**

*Individual drugs*

Acetaminophen, amiodarone, clindamycin, clofibrate, gemfibrozil, glipizide, penicillin G, phenytoin, propranolol, iron, thyroid hormones, warfarin: decreased absorption of each specific product

*Drug classifications*

Cardiac glycosides, corticosteroids, tetracyclines, thiazides, vit A, D, E, K: decreased absorption

*Drug/herb*

Glucomannan: increased effect
Gotu kola: decreased effect

*Drug/lab test*

Increased: AST, ALT, alkaline phosphatase
Decreased: Na, K
Interference: cholecystography

**NURSING CONSIDERATIONS**

**Assessment**

• Assess nutrition: fat, protein, carbohydrates, nutritional analysis should be completed by dietitian

• Assess skin integrity after patient has been receiving product; itching, pruritus often occur from bile deposits on skin

• Monitor cardiac glycoside level if both products are being administered; cardiac glycoside levels will be decreased

• Monitor for signs of vit A, D, E, K deficiency; fasting LDL, HDL, total cholesterol, triglyceride levels, electrolytes if on extended therapy

• Monitor bowel pattern daily; increase bulk, water in diet if constipation develops

**Nursing diagnoses**

• Constipation (adverse reactions)
• Knowledge, deficient (teaching)
• Noncompliance (teaching)

**Implementation**

• Give product daily-bid, at bedtime; give all other medications 1 hr before cholestyramine or 4-6 hr after cholestyramine to avoid poor absorption; do not take dry; mix product with applesauce or stir into beverage (2-6 oz); let stand for 2 min; do not mix with carbonated beverages; avoid inhaling powder

• Provide supplemental doses of vit A, D, E, K, if levels are low

**Patient/family education**

⬥ Teach patient symptoms of hypoprothrombinemia: bleeding mucous membranes, dark tarry stools, hematuria, petechiae; report immediately

• Teach patient importance of compliance

• Teach patient that risk factors should be decreased: high-fat diet, smoking, alcohol consumption, absence of exercise

• Have patient mix product with 6 oz of milk, water, fruit juice; do not mix with carbonated beverages; rinse glass to make sure all medication is taken or may mix product in applesauce; allow to stand for 2 min before mixing

**Evaluation**

**Positive therapeutic outcome**

• Decreased cholesterol level (hyperlipidemia)

• Decreased diarrhea, pruritus (excess bile acids)

**choline salicylate** (Rx)
(koe'leen sa-lis'ih-late)
Arthropan
**choline/magnesium salicylates** (Rx)
CMT, Tricosal, Trilisate
*Func. class.:* Nonopioid analgesic
*Chem. class.:* Salicylate

**Pregnancy category C**

**Action:** Blocks pain impulses in CNS that occur in response to inhibition of prostaglandin synthesis; antipyretic action results from inhibition of hypothalamic heat-regulating center to produce vasodilatation to allow heat dissipation

**Therapeutic outcome:** Decreased pain, inflammation, fever

**Uses:** Mild to moderate pain or fever including arthritis, juvenile rheumatoid arthritis

**Dosage and routes**
435 mg of choline salicylate = 325 mg of aspirin

*Choline salicylate*
*Adult and child>12 yr:* PO 870-1740 mg qid; max 6×/day

*Pain/fever*
*Adult:* PO 435-870 mg q3-4hr prn

*Choline/magnesium salicylates*
*Adult:* PO 1500 mg bid
*Child>37 kg:* PO 2.2 g of salicylate/day divided bid
*Child<37 kg:* PO 50 mg of salicylate/kg/day divided bid

**Available forms:** Choline salicylate liquid 870 mg/5 ml; choline/magnesium salicylate tabs 500, 750, 1000 mg; liquid 500 mg/5 ml

**Adverse effects**
*CNS:* Stimulation, drowsiness, dizziness, confusion, **seizure**, headache, flushing, hallucinations, **coma**
*CV:* Rapid pulse, pulmonary edema
*EENT:* Tinnitus, hearing loss
*ENDO:* Hypoglycemia, hyponatremia, hypokalemia
*GI:* Nausea, vomiting, GI bleeding, diarrhea, heartburn, anorexia, **hepatitis, hepatotoxicity**
*HEMA:* Thrombocytopenia, **agranulocytosis, leukopenia, neutropenia, hemolytic anemia,** increased pro-time
*INTEG:* Rash, urticaria, bruising, sweating
*RESP:* Wheezing, hyperpnea, hyperventilation

**Contraindications:** Hypersensitivity to salicylates, GI bleeding, bleeding disorders, children <3 yr, vit K deficiency, children with flulike symptoms, Reye's syndrome

**Precautions:** Pregnancy **C**, breastfeeding, anemia, renal/hepatic disease, Hodgkin's disease

| Pharmacokinetics | |
|---|---|
| **Absorption** | Well absorbed |
| **Distribution** | Widely distributed; crosses placenta |
| **Metabolism** | Liver, extensively |
| **Excretion** | Kidney, active metabolites; breast milk |
| **Half-life** | 2-3 hr (low doses); 9-17 hr (high doses) |

| Pharmacodynamics | |
|---|---|
| **Onset** | 15-30 min |
| **Peak** | 1-3 hr |
| **Duration** | 3-6 hr |

**Interactions**
*Individual drugs*
Alcohol, aspirin, heparin, plicamycin: increased bleeding
Ammonium chloride, nizatidine: increased salicylate levels
Insulin, methotrexate, penicillins, phenytoin, valproic acid, warfarin: increased effects
Probenecid, spironolactone, sulfinpyrazone: decreased effects
*Drug classifications*
Antacids (high doses), corticosteroids, steroids, urinary alkalizers: decreased effects of choline salicylate
Anticoagulants, hypoglycemics (oral), sulfonamides, thrombolytics: increased effects
Antiinflammatories, NSAIDs, steroids: increased gastric ulcers
β-Blockers, NSAIDS, sulfonamides: decreased effects
Urinary acidifiers: increased salicylate levels
*Drug/herb*
Bilberry, bogbean, chondroitin, horse chestnut, Irish moss, kelpware, pansy: increased bleeding risk
*Drug/lab test*
Increased: coagulation studies, liver function studies, serum uric acid, amylase, $CO_2$, urinary protein
Decreased: serum potassium, cholesterol
Interference: VMA, TSH, 5-HIAA

## NURSING CONSIDERATIONS
### Assessment
- Monitor pain: location, duration, type, intensity, before dose and 1 hr after
- Monitor musculoskeletal status: ROM before dose
- Identify fever, length of time and related symptoms
- Monitor liver function studies: AST, ALT, bilirubin, creatinine if patient is on long-term therapy
- Monitor renal function studies: BUN, urine creatinine if patient is on long-term therapy; check I&O ratio; decreasing output may indicate renal failure
- Monitor blood studies: CBC, Hct, Hgb, protime if patient is on long-term therapy
- ⬥ Assess hepatotoxicity: dark urine, clay-colored stools, yellowing of the skin and sclera, itching, abdominal pain, fever, diarrhea if patient is on long-term therapy
- Assess for allergic reactions: rash, urticaria; if these occur, product may have to be discontinued
- Assess for ototoxicity: tinnitus, ringing, roaring in ears; audiometric testing needed before, after long-term therapy
- Check edema in feet, ankles, legs
- Identify prior product history; there are many product interactions

### Nursing diagnoses
- Injury, risk for (side effects)
- Knowledge, deficient (teaching)
- Mobility, impaired physical (uses)
- Pain, acute (uses)
- Pain, chronic (uses)

### Implementation
- Administer to patient crushed or whole
- Give with food or milk to decrease gastric symptoms; give 30 min before or 2 hr after meals; absorption may be slowed; sit upright for 30 min after dose
- Give antacids 1-2 hr after enteric products

### Patient/family education
- Teach patient to report any symptoms of hepatotoxicity, renal toxicity, visual changes, ototoxicity, allergic reactions, bleeding (long-term therapy)
- Advise patient to take with 8 oz of water
- Caution patient not to exceed recommended dosage; acute poisoning may result
- Caution patient to read label on other OTC products; many contain aspirin products
- Inform patient that the therapeutic response takes 2 wk (arthritis)
- Teach patient to report tinnitus, confusion, diarrhea, sweating, hyperventilation
- Caution patient to avoid alcohol ingestion; GI bleeding may occur
- Teach patient that patients who have allergies may develop allergic reactions
- Caution patient to avoid buffered or effervescent products
- Teach patient not to give to children; Reye's syndrome may develop

### Evaluation
**Positive therapeutic outcome**
- Decreased pain
- Decreased inflammation
- Decreased fever
- Increased mobility

**Treatment of overdose:** Lavage, activated charcoal, monitor electrolytes, VS

### cidofovir (Rx)
(si-doh-foh′veer)
Vistide
*Func. class.:* Antiviral
*Chem. class.:* Nucleotide analog
**Pregnancy category C**

**Action:** Suppresses cytomegalovirus (CMV) replication by selective inhibition of viral DNA synthesis

**Therapeutic outcome:** Decreased symptoms of CMV

**Uses:** CMV retinitis in patients with HIV, used with probenecid

### Dosage and routes
*Adult:* **IV** 5 mg/kg qwk × 2 wk; then 3 mg/kg q2 wk, give with probenecid

*Renal dose*
*Adult:* **IV** CCr ≤55 ml/min, do not use; SCr increase of 0.3-0.4 mg/dl above baseline, decrease dose to 3 mg/kg; SCr increase of ≥0.5 mg/dl above baseline or ≥2+ proteinuria, discontinue

**Available forms:** Inj 75 mg/ml

### Adverse effects
*CNS: Fever, chills,* **coma,** confusion, abnormal thought, *dizziness,* bizarre dreams, *headache,* psychosis, tremors, somnolence, paresthesia, *amnesia, anxiety, insomnia,* **seizures**
*CV:* **Dysrhythmias,** hypo/hypertension
*EENT:* Retinal detachment in CMV retinitis
*GI:* Abnormal liver function tests, *nausea, vomiting, anorexia, diarrhea,* abdominal pain, **hemorrhage**

Adverse effects: *italic* = common, **bold** = life-threatening

*GU:* **Hematuria,** increased creatinine, BUN, **nephrotoxicity**
*HEMA:* **Granulocytopenia, thrombocytopenia, irreversible neutropenia, anemia, eosinophilia**
*INTEG: Rash, alopecia, pruritus, acne,* urticaria, pain at inj site, phlebitis
*RESP:* Dyspnea

**Contraindications:** Hypersensitivity to this product or probenecid; sulfa products; renal failure

**Precautions:** Pregnancy **C,** breastfeeding, children <6 mo, geriatric, preexisting cytopenias, renal function impairment, platelet count <25,000/mm³

### Pharmacokinetics

| | |
|---|---|
| **Absorption** | Unknown |
| **Distribution** | Unknown |
| **Metabolism** | Unknown |
| **Excretion** | Unknown |
| **Half-life** | Terminal 2.6 hr |

### Pharmacodynamics
Unknown

### Interactions
*Individual drugs*
Amphotericin B, foscarnet, pentamidine **IV:** increased nephrotoxicity; wait 7 days after use to begin cidofovir
*Drug classifications*
Aminoglycosides, NSAIDs, salicylates: increased nephrotoxicity; wait 7 days after use to begin cidofovir

### NURSING CONSIDERATIONS
**Assessment**
• Obtain culture before treatment is initiated; cultures of blood, urine, and throat may all be taken; CMV is not confirmed by this method; the diagnosis is made by an ophthalmic exam
• Monitor renal, liver function, increased hematopoietic studies and BUN; serum creatinine, AST, ALT, creatinine, CCr, A-G ratio, baseline and drip treatment, blood counts should be done q2 wk; watch for decreasing granulocytes, Hgb; if low, therapy may have to be discontinued and restarted after hematologic recovery; blood transfusions may be required
• Assess for GI symptoms: severe nausea, vomiting, diarrhea; severe symptoms may necessitate discontinuing product
• Assess electrolytes and minerals: calcium, phosphorous, magnesium, sodium, potassium;

watch closely for tetany during first administration
• Assess for symptoms of blood dyscrasias (anemia, granulocytopenia); bruising, fatigue, bleeding, poor healing
• Assess allergic reactions: flushing, rash, urticaria, pruritus
• Assess for leukopenia, neutropenia, thrombocytopenia: WBCs, platelets q2 days during 2×/day dosing and qwk thereafter; check for leukopenias, with daily WBC count in patients with prior leukopenia, with other nucleoside analogs, or for whom leukopenia counts are <1000 cells/mm³ at start of treatment
• Monitor serum creatinine or CCr at least q2 wk; give only to those with creatinine levels ≤1.5 mg/dl, CCr >55 ml/min, urine protein <100 mg/dl

**Nursing diagnoses**
• Infection, risk for (uses)

**Implementation**
• Dilute in 100 ml 0.9% NaCl sol before administration; probenecid must be given PO 2 g 3 hr before the cidofovir INF and 1 g at 2 and 8 hr after ending the cidofovir INF; give 1 L of 0.9% NaCl sol **IV** with each INF of cidofovir, give saline INF over 1-2 hr period immediately before cidofovir; patient should be given a second L if the patient can tolerate the fluid load (second L given at time of cidofovir or immediately afterward and should be given over a 1-3 hr period)
• Mix under strict aseptic conditions using gloves, gown, and mask, and using precautions for antineoplastics
• Administer after diluting in 100 ml of 0.9% NaCl
• Give slowly; do not give by BOL **IV, IV,** SUBCUT inj
• Use diluted sol within 12 hr, do not refrigerate or freeze; do not use sol with particulate matter or discoloration
• Refrigerate up to 24 hr; allow to warm to room temperature before using

**Patient/family education**
• Advise to notify prescriber if sore throat, swollen lymph nodes, malaise, fever occur; may indicate other infections
• Advise to report perioral tingling, numbness in extremities, and paresthesias
• Teach that serious product interactions may occur if OTC products are ingested; check first with prescriber
• Teach that product is not a cure, but will control symptoms

 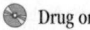

- Advise that regular ophthalmic exams must be continued
- Advise that major toxicities may necessitate discontinuing product
- Advise to use contraception during treatment and that infertility may occur; men should use barrier contraception for 90 days after treatment

### Evaluation
**Positive therapeutic outcome**
- Decreased symptoms of CMV

**Treatment of overdose:** Discontinue product; use hemodialysis, and increase hydration

---

### cilastatin
*See imipenem/cilastatin*

---

### cilostazol (Rx)
(sih-los'tah-zol)
Pletal
*Func. class.:* Platelet aggregation inhibitor
*Chem. class.:* Quinolinone derivative

**Pregnancy category** C

### Do not confuse:
Pletal/Plendil

**Action:** Reversibly inhibits cellular phosphodiesterase; inhibits platelet aggregation induced by thrombin, ADP, collagen, arachidonic acid, epINEPHrine, stress

**Therapeutic outcome:** Increased walking distance

**Uses:** Intermittent claudication

### Dosage and routes
*Adult:* PO 100 mg bid taken ≥30 min before or 2 hr after breakfast and dinner or 50 mg bid, if using products that inhibit CYP3A4 and CYP2C19; 12 wk of treatment may be needed for beneficial effect

**Available forms:** Tabs 50, 100 mg

### Adverse effects
*CNS: Dizziness,* headache
*CV: Palpitations, tachycardia,* **nodal dys-rhythmia,** postural hypotension
*EENT:* Blindness, diplopia, ear pain, tinnitus, retinal hemorrhage
*GI: Nausea, vomiting, diarrhea, GI disorder,* colitis, cholelithiasis, ulcer, esophagitis, gastritis, anorexia, *flatulence, dyspepsia*
*GU:* Cystitis, frequency, vaginitis, **vaginal hemorrhage,** hematuria

*HEMA:* **Bleeding (epistaxis, hematuria, retinal hemorrhage, GI bleeding), thrombocytopenia,** anemia, polycythemia
*INTEG: Rash,* urticaria, dry skin
*MISC: Back pain, infection, myalgia, peripheral edema,* chills, fever, malaise, diabetes mellitus
*RESP: Cough, pharyngitis, rhinitis,* asthma, pneumonia

**Contraindications:** Hypersensitivity, CHF, acute MI, active bleeding conditions, hemostatic conditions

**Precautions:** Pregnancy C, breastfeeding, children, geriatric, past liver disease, renal/cardiac disease, increased bleeding risk, low platelet count, platelet dysfunction, active bleeding

| Pharmacokinetics | |
|---|---|
| Absorption | Unknown |
| Distribution | 95%-98% protein binding |
| Metabolism | Hepatic extensively by CYP450 enzymes |
| Excretion | Urine (74%), feces (20%) |
| Half-life | 11-13 hr |

| Pharmacodynamics |
|---|
| Unknown |

### Interactions
*Individual drugs*
Abciximab, eptifibatide, ticlopidine, tirofiban: increased bleeding tendencies
Diltiazem, erythromycin, omeprazole, verapamil: increased cilostazol levels
Fluconazole, fluoxetine, fluvoxamine, itraconazole, ketoconazole, voriconazole: may increase cilostazol levels; exercise caution when coadministering and reduce dose to 50 mg bid

*Drug classifications*
Anticoagulants, NSAIDs, thrombolytics: may increase bleeding tendencies
Protease inhibitors: increased cilostazol levels

*Drug/herb*
Agrimony, alfalfa, angelica, anise, bilberry, black haw, bogbean, buchu, chondroitin, dong quai, fenugreek, feverfew, garlic, ginger, ginkgo, ginseng, green tea, horse chestnut, Irish moss, kelp, kelpware, khella, lovage, lungwort, meadowsweet, motherwort, mugwort, nettle, papaya, parsley (large amounts), pau d'arco, pineapple, poplar, prickly ash, safflower, saw palmetto, tonka bean, turmeric, wintergreen, yarrow: increased risk of bleeding

Adverse effects: *italic* = common, **bold** = life-threatening

Chamomile, coenzyme Q10, flax, glucomannan, goldenseal: decreased anticoagulant effect

***Drug/food***
Grapefruit juice: do not use; toxicity may occur

## NURSING CONSIDERATIONS
### Assessment
• Assess for underlying CV disease since cardiovascular risk is great; for severe headache, signs of toxicity
• Assess for CV lesions with repeated oral administration
• Assess for CHF
• Monitor blood studies: CBC, Hct, Hgb, pro-time if patient is on long-term therapy; thrombocytopenia, neutropenia may occur

### Nursing diagnoses
• Injury, risk for (uses)
• Knowledge, deficient (teaching)

### Implementation
• Give bid ≥1 hr before or 2 hr after meals; do not give with grapefruit juice

### Patient/family education
• Advise patient to report any unusual bleeding to prescriber
• Caution patient to report side effects such as diarrhea, skin rashes, subcutaneous bleeding
• Teach patient that effects may take 2-4 wk, treatment of up to 12 wk may be required for necessary effect
• Teach patients with CHF about potential risks
• Advise patient to take ≥1 hr before or 2 hr after meals
• Advise patient that reading patient package insert is necessary
• Advise patient to discontinue tobacco use

### Evaluation
**Positive therapeutic outcome**
• Increased walking distance and duration
• Decreased pain

---

**cimetidine**    (OTC, Rx)
(sye-met'i-deen)
Apo-Cimetidine ♣, cimetidine, Major Acid Reducer, Novocimetine ♣, Peptol ♣, Tagamet, Tagamet HB
*Func. class.:* H₂-receptor antagonist
*Chem. class.:* Imidazole derivative

**Pregnancy category B**

**Action:** Inhibits histamine at H₂-receptor site in the gastric parietal cells, which inhibits gastric acid secretion

---

**Therapeutic outcome:** Healing of duodenal or gastric ulcers; prevention of duodenal ulcers; decreases symptoms of gastroesophageal reflux disease (GERD) and Zollinger-Ellison syndrome

**Uses:** Short-term treatment of duodenal and gastric ulcers and maintenance; management of GERD, Zollinger-Ellison syndrome; prevention of upper GI bleeding; prevent, relieve heartburn, acid indigestion, upper GI bleeding

**Unlabeled uses:** Prevention of aspiration pneumonitis, stress ulcers

### Dosage and routes
***Treatment of active ulcers***
***Adult and child:*** PO 300 mg qid with meals, at bedtime × 8 wk or 400 mg bid, 800 mg at bedtime; after 8 wk give at bedtime dose only; IV BOL 300 mg/20 ml 0.9% NaCl over 1-2 min q6hr; IV INF 300 mg/50 ml D₅W over 15-20 min; IM 300 mg q6hr, not to exceed 2400 mg
***Child:*** PO 20-40 mg/kg/day; IM/IV 5-10 mg/kg q6-8hr

***Prophylaxis of duodenal ulcer***
***Adult and child >16 yr:*** 400 mg at bedtime

***GERD***
***Adult:*** PO 800-1600 mg/day in divided doses

***Hypersecretory conditions (Zollinger-Ellison syndrome)***
***Adult:*** PO/IM/IV 300-600 mg q6hr; may increase to 12 g/day if needed

***Upper GI bleeding prophylaxis***
***Adult:*** IV 50 mg/hr; lowered in renal disease

***Aspiration pneumonitis prophylaxis (unlabeled)***
***Adult:*** IM/IV 300 mg IM 1 hr before anesthesia, then 300 mg IV q4hr until patient is alert, max 2400 mg/day

***Warts***
***Adult:*** PO 400-800 mg tid × 12 wk or 30-40 mg/kg/day given tid × 3 mo

***Renal dose***
***Adult:*** PO CCr 20-40 ml/min 300 mg q8hr; CCr <20 ml/min 300 mg q12hr

**Available forms:** Tabs 100, 200, 300, 400, 800 mg; liquid 200, 300 mg/5 ml; inj 300 mg/2 ml, 300 mg/50 ml 0.9% NaCl

---

 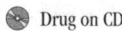

## Adverse effects

*CNS: Confusion, headache,* depression, dizziness, anxiety, weakness, psychosis, tremors, **seizures**

*CV:* Bradycardia, tachycardia, **dysrhythmias**

*GI: Diarrhea,* abdominal cramps, **paralytic ileus,** *jaundice*

*GU:* Gynecomastia, galactorrhea, impotence, increase in BUN, creatinine

*HEMA:* **Agranulocytosis, thrombocytopenia, neutropenia, aplastic anemia, increase in pro-time**

*INTEG:* Urticaria, rash, alopecia, sweating, flushing, **exfoliative dermatitis**

**Contraindications:** Hypersensitivity

**Precautions:** Pregnancy **B**, breastfeeding, child <16 yr, geriatric, organic brain syndrome, renal/hepatic disease

### Pharmacokinetics

| | |
|---|---|
| **Absorption** | Well absorbed (PO, IM); completely absorbed (**IV**) |
| **Distribution** | Widely distributed; crosses placenta |
| **Metabolism** | Liver (30%) |
| **Excretion** | Kidneys, unchanged (70%); breast milk |
| **Half-life** | 1½-2 hr; increased in renal disease |

### Pharmacodynamics

| | PO | IM/IV |
|---|---|---|
| **Onset** | ½ hr | 10 min |
| **Peak** | 45-90 min | ½ hr |
| **Duration** | 4-5 hr | 4-5 hr |

## Interactions
### Individual drugs
Carbamazepine, chloroquine, lidocaine, metronidazole, moricizine, phenytoin, quinidine, quinine, valproic acid, warfarin: increased toxicity (CYP450 pathway)

Itraconazole: decreased absorption of itraconazole

Ketoconazole: decreased absorption of ketoconazole

Sucralfate: decreased cimetidine absorption

### Drug classifications
Antacids: decreased absorption of cimetidine

Antidepressants (tricyclic), benzodiazepines, β-adrenergic blockers, calcium channel blockers, phenytoins, sulfonylureas, theophyllines: increased toxicity (CYP450 pathway)

### Drug/lab test
Increased: alkaline phosphatase, AST, creatinine, prolactin

False positive: Hemoccult, Gastroccult tests

False negative: TB skin tests

## NURSING CONSIDERATIONS
### Assessment
- Assess patient with ulcers or suspected ulcers: epigastric or abdominal pain, hematemesis, occult blood in stools, blood in gastric aspirate before and/or throughout treatment; monitor gastric pH (5 or > should be maintained)
- Monitor I&O ratio, BUN, creatinine, CBC with differential periodically

### Nursing diagnoses
- Knowledge, deficient (teaching)
- Pain, acute (uses)

### Implementation
**PO route**
- Give with meals for lengthened product effect; antacids 1 hr before or 1 hr after cimetidine

**IV route**
- Give by direct **IV** after diluting 300 mg/20 ml of 0.9% NaCl for inj; give over 5 min or more
- Give intermittent **IV** by diluting 300 mg/50 ml of $D_5W$; run over 15-20 min
- Give by cont inf after using total daily dose (900 mg) diluted in 100-1000 ml $D_5W$ given over 24 hr
- Store diluted sol at room temperature up to 48 hr

*Syringe compatibilities:* Atropine, butorphanol, cephalothin, diazepam, diphenhydrAMINE, doxapram, droperidol, fentanyl, glycopyrrolate, heparin, hydromorphone, hydrOXYzine, lorazepam, meperidine, midazolam, morphine, nafcillin, nalbuphine, penicillin G sodium, pentazocine, perphenazine, prochlorperazine, promazine, promethazine, scopolamine

*Syringe incompatibilities:* Cefamandole, cefazolin, chlorproMAZINE, pentobarbital, secobarbital

*Y-site compatibilities:* Acyclovir, amifostine, aminophylline, inamrinone, atracurium, aztreonam, cisatracurium, cisplatin, cladribine, cyclosphosphamide, cytarabine, diltiazem, DOXOrubicin, DOXOrubicin liposome, enalaprilat, esmolol, filgrastim, fluconazole, fludarabine, foscarnet, gallium, granisetron, haloperidol, heparin, hetastarch, idarubicin, labetalol, melphalan, meropenem, methotrexate, midazolam, ondansetron, paclitaxel, pancuronium, piperacillin/tazobactam, propofol, sargramostim, tacrolimus, teniposide, theophylline, thiotepa, tolazoline, vecuronium, vinorelbine, zidovudine

*Y-site incompatibilities:* Amsacrine

*Additive compatibilities:* Acetazolamide, amikacin, aminophylline, atracurium, cefoperazone, cefoxitin, chlorothiazide, clindamycin, colistimethate, dexamethasone, digoxin, epINEPHrine, erythromycin, ethacrynate, floxacillin, flumazenil, furosemide, gentamicin, insulin, isoproterenol, lidocaine, lincomycin, meropenem, metaraminol, methylPREDNISolone, norepinephrine, penicillin G potassium, phytonadione, polymyxin B, potassium chloride, protamine, quinidine, tacrolimus, tetracycline, vancomycin, verapamil, vit B complex, vit B/C
*Additive incompatibilities:* Amphotericin B

## Patient/family education
• Advise patient that any gynecomastia or impotence that develops is reversible after treatment is discontinued
• Caution patient to avoid driving, other hazardous activities until stabilized on this medication; drowsiness or dizziness may occur
• Advise patient to avoid black pepper, caffeine, alcohol, harsh spices, extremes in temperature of food; tell patient to avoid OTC preparations: aspirin, cough, cold preparations; condition may worsen
• Advise patient that smoking decreases the effectiveness of the product; smoking cessation should be considered
• Teach patient that product must be continued for prescribed time to be effective and taken exactly as prescribed; doses are not to be doubled; to take missed dose when remembered up to 1 hr before next dose
• Instruct patient to report bruising, fatigue, malaise; blood dyscrasias may occur
• Have patient report to prescriber immediately any diarrhea, black tarry stools, sore throat, dizziness, confusion, or delirium

## Evaluation
**Positive therapeutic outcome**
• Decreased pain in abdomen
• Healing of ulcers
• Absence of gastroesophageal reflux
• Gastric pH of ≥5

## cinacalcet (Rx)
(sin-a-kal'set)
Sensipar
*Func. class.:* Calcium receptor agonist
*Chem. class.:* Polypeptide hormone

**Pregnancy category** C

**Action:** Directly lowers PTH levels by increasing sensitivity of calcium sensing receptors to extracellular calcium

**Therapeutic outcome:** Decreased symptoms of hypercalcemia

**Uses:** Hypercalcemia in parathyroid carcinoma, secondary hyperparathyroidism in chronic kidney disease on dialysis, primary hyperparathyroidism

### Dosage and routes
*Parathyroid carcinoma*
**Adult:** PO 30 mg bid, titrate q2-4wk, with sequential doses of 30 mg bid, 60 mg bid, 90 mg bid, 90 mg tid-qid to normalize calcium levels

*Secondary hyperparathyroidism*
**Adult:** PO 30 mg daily, titrate no more frequently than 2-4 wks with sequential doses of 30, 60, 90, 120, 180 mg daily

**Available forms:** Tabs 30, 60, 90 mg

### Adverse effects
*CNS:* Dizziness, asthenia
*CV:* Hypertension
*GI:* Nausea, diarrhea, vomiting, anorexia
*MISC:* Access infection, noncardiac chest pain, hypocalcemia
*MS:* Myalgia

**Contraindications:** Hypersensitivity

**Precautions:** Pregnancy **C**, breastfeeding, children, seizure disorders, hepatic disease, hypocalcemia

| Pharmacokinetics | |
|---|---|
| Absorption | 93%-97% bound to plasma |
| Distribution | Unknown |
| Metabolism | Proteins metabolized by CYP3A4, 2D6, 1A2 |
| Excretion | Renal (80% renal, 15% feces) |
| Half-life | 30-40 hr |

| Pharmacodynamics | |
|---|---|
| Unknown | |

## Interactions
### Individual drugs
Ketoconazole, erythromycin, itraconazole (products metabolized by CYP3A4); flecainide, vinBLAStine, thioridazine: adjustments may be necessary
### Drug classifications
Tricyclics (metabolized by CYP2D6): adjustments may be necessary
### Drug/food
High-fat meal: increased action

## NURSING CONSIDERATIONS
### Assessment
• Assess for hypocalcemia: cramping, seizures, tetany, myalgia, paresthesia
• Monitor calcium, phosphorous within 1 wk and iPTH 1-4 wk after initiation or dosage adjustment when maintenance is established; measure calcium, phosphorus monthly; iPTH q1-3 mo, target range 150-300 pg/ml for iPTH level; biochemical markers of bone formation/resorption, radiologic evidence of fracture
• If calcium < 8.4 mg/dl, do not start therapy

### Nursing diagnoses
• Injury, risk for (uses)
• Knowledge, deficient (teaching)

### Implementation
• Swallow tabs whole; do not break, crush, chew, or divide tabs
• Can be used alone or in combination with vit D sterols and/or phosphate binders
• Take with food or shortly after meal
### Secondary hyperthyroidism
• Titrate q2-4 wk to target iPTH consistent with National Kidney Foundation-Kidney Disease Outcomes Quality Initiative (NKF-K/DOQI) for chronic kidney disease patient on dialysis of 150-300 pg/ml; if iPTH drops below 150-300 pg/ml, reduce dose of cinacalcet and/or vit D sterols or discontinue treatment
• Store at <77° F (25° C)

### Patient/family education
• Instruct patient to take with food or shortly after a meal
• Instruct patient to immediately report cramping, seizures, muscle pain, tingling, tetany

### Evaluation
**Positive therapeutic outcome**
• Calcium levels 9-10 mg/dl, decreasing symptoms of hypercalcemia

---

## ciprofloxacin (Rx)
(sip-ro-floks'a-sin)
Cipro, Cipro XR, ProQuinXR
*Func. class.:* Urinary antiinfectives, broad-spectrum
*Chem. class.:* Fluoroquinolone
**Pregnancy category C**

**Do not confuse:**
ciprofloxacin/cephalexin

**Action:** Interferes with conversion of intermediate DNA fragments into high-molecular-weight DNA in bacteria; DNA gyrase inhibitor

**Therapeutic outcome:** Bactericidal action against the following: gram-positive organisms *Staphylococcus epidermidis,* methicillin-resistant strains of *Staphylococcus aureus, Streptococcus pyogenes, Streptococcus pneumoniae;* gram-negative organisms *Escherichia coli, Klebsiella* species, *Enterobacter, Salmonella, Shigella, Proteus vulgaris, Providencia stuartii, Providencia rettgeri, Morganella morganii, Pseudomonas aeruginosa, Serratia, Haemophilus, Acinetobacter, Neisseria gonorrhoeae, Neisseria meningitidis, Branhamella catarrhalis, Yersinia, Vibrio, Brucella, Campylobacter, Aeromonas*

**Uses:** Adult urinary tract infections (including complicated); chronic bacterial prostatitis; acute sinusitis; lower respiratory, skin, bone, joint infections; infectious diarrhea; typhoid fever; complicated intraabdominal infections; nosocomial pneumonia; exposure to inhalation anthrax; conjunctivitis, corneal ulcers (ophthalmic)

### Dosage and routes
#### Uncomplicated urinary tract infections
*Adult:* PO 250 mg q12hr × 3 days or 500 mg q24hr × 3 days

#### Complicated/severe urinary tract infections
*Adult:* PO 500 mg q12hr or 1000 mg q24hr × 7-14 days; **IV** 400 mg q12hr

#### Respiratory, bone, skin, joint infections
*Adult:* PO 500-750 mg q12hr × 7-14 days; **IV** 400 mg q12hr

#### Corneal ulcers, conjunctivitis
*Adult:* Ophth 1-2 gtt q15-30 min until infection is controlled, then 1-2 gtt 4-6 times daily

---

Adverse effects: *italic* = common, **bold** = life-threatening

*Nosocomial pneumonia*
**Adult: IV** 400 mg q8hr × 10-14 days

*Intraabdominal infections, complicated*
**Adult:** PO 500 mg q12hr × 7-14 days, **IV** 400 mg q12hr × 7-14 days, usually given with metronidazole

*Acute sinusitis, mild/moderate*
**Adult:** PO 500 mg q12hr × 10 days; **IV** 400 mg q12hr × 10 days

*Inhalational anthrax (postexposure)*
**Adult:** PO 500 mg q12hr × 60 days; **IV** 400 mg q12hr × 60 days
**Child:** PO 15 mg/kg/dose, max 500 mg/dose; **IV** max 400 mg/dose × 60 days

*Infectious diarrhea*
**Adult:** PO 500 mg q12hr × 5-7 days

*Chronic bacterial prostatitis*
**Adult:** PO 500 mg q12hr × 28 days; **IV** 400 mg q12hr × 28 days

*Pyelonephritis, acute uncomplicated*
**Adult:** PO 1000 mg × q24hr × 7-14 days

*Renal dose*
**Adult:** PO CCr 30-50 ml/min PO 250-500 mg q12hr; CCr 5-29 ml/min PO 250-500 mg q18hr; **IV** 200-400 mg q18-24hr

**Available forms:** Tabs 100, 250, 500, 750 mg; ext rel tabs (XR) 500, 1000 mg; inj 200 mg/20 ml, 400 mg/40 ml, 200 mg/100 ml $D_5$, 400 mg/200 ml $D_5$; oral susp 250, 500 mg/5 ml

**Adverse effects**
*CNS: Headache,* dizziness, fatigue, insomnia, depression, *restlessness,* **seizures,** confusion
*GI: Nausea,* increased ALT, AST, flatulence, heartburn, *vomiting, diarrhea,* oral candidiasis, dysphagia, **pseudomembranous colitis,** dry mouth
*INTEG: Rash,* pruritus, urticaria, photosensitivity, flushing, fever, chills, **toxic epidermal necrolysis**
*MISC:* **Anaphylaxis, Stevens-Johnson syndrome,** visual impairment, QT prolongation
*MS:* Tremor, arthralgia, tendon rupture

**Contraindications:** Hypersensitivity to quinolones

**Precautions:** Pregnancy **C,** breastfeeding, children, geriatric, renal disease, epilepsy, QT prolongation, tendon pain, hypokalemia

## Pharmacokinetics

| | |
|---|---|
| **Absorption** | Well absorbed (75%) (PO) |
| **Distribution** | Widely distributed |
| **Metabolism** | Liver (15%) |
| **Excretion** | Kidneys (40%-50%) |
| **Half-life** | 3-4 hr; increased in renal disease |

## Pharmacodynamics

| | PO | IV |
|---|---|---|
| **Onset** | Rapid | Immediate |
| **Peak** | 1 hr | Infusion's end |

## Interactions
*Individual drugs*
Astemizole, droperidol, probucol: increased QT prolongation
Calcium, enteral feeding, sucralfate, zinc sulfate, iron: decreased ciprofloxacin absorption
CycloSPORINE: increased nephrotoxicity
Probenecid: increased blood levels of ciprofloxacin, increased toxicity
Theophylline: increased theophylline levels, monitor blood levels
Warfarin: increased warfarin effect, monitor blood levels
*Drug classifications*
Antacids (containing magnesium, aluminum), iron salts: decreased absorption of ciprofloxacin
*Drug/herb*
Acidophilus: do not use with antiinfectives; separate by several hours
Caffeine: increased caffeine levels
Fennel: decreased antiinfective effect
Yerba maté: increased toxicity
*Drug/food*
Dairy products, food: decreased absorption
*Drug/lab test*
Increased: AST, ALT, bilirubin, BUN, creatinine, alkaline phosphatase, LDH, glucose, proteinuria, albuminuria
Decreased: WBC, glucose

## NURSING CONSIDERATIONS
### Assessment
• Assess patient for previous sensitivity reaction
• Assess patient for signs and symptoms of infection including characteristics of wounds, sputum, urine, stool, WBC >10,000/mm³, fever; obtain baseline information before and during treatment
• Obtain C&S before beginning product therapy to identify if correct treatment has been initiated

- Assess for anaphylaxis: rash, urticaria, dyspnea, pruritus, chills, fever, joint pain; may occur a few days after therapy begins; epI-NEPHrine and resuscitation equipment should be available for anaphylactic reaction
- Identify urine output; if decreasing, notify prescriber (may indicate nephrotoxicity); also check for increased BUN, creatinine
- Monitor blood studies: AST, ALT, CBC, Hct, bilirubin, LDH, alkaline phosphatase, Coombs' test monthly if patient is on long-term therapy
- Monitor electrolytes: potassium, sodium, chloride monthly if patient is on long-term therapy
- Assess bowel pattern daily; if severe diarrhea occurs, product should be discontinued
- Monitor for bleeding: ecchymosis, bleeding gums, hematuria, stool guaiac daily if on long-term therapy
- Assess for overgrowth of infection: perineal itching, fever, malaise, redness, pain, swelling, drainage, rash, diarrhea, change in cough, sputum

### Nursing diagnoses
- Diarrhea (side effects)
- Infection, risk for (uses)
- Injury, risk for (side effects)
- Knowledge, deficient (teaching)
- Noncompliance (teaching)

### Implementation
**PO route**
- Give around the clock to maintain proper blood levels
- Administer 2 hr before or 2 hr after antacids, zinc, iron, calcium

**IV route**
- Check for irritation, extravasation, phlebitis daily
- For intermittent inf, dilute to 1-2 mg/ml of $D_5W$, 0.9% NaCl; give over 60 min; it will remain stable under refrigeration for 2 wk

*Y-site compatibilities:* Amifostine, amino acids, aztreonam, calcium gluconate, ceftazidime, cisatracurium, digoxin, diltiazem, diphenhydrAMINE, DOBUTamine, DOPamine, DOXOrubicin liposome, gallium, gentamicin, granisetron, hydrOXYzine, lidocaine, lorazepam, metoclopramide, midazolam, midodrine, piperacillin, potassium acetate, potassium chloride, potassium phosphates, predniso-LONE, promethazine, propofol, ranitidine, remifentanil, Ringer's, sodium chloride, tacrolimus, teniposide, thiotepa, tobramycin, verapamil

*Y-site incompatibilities:* Heparin, mezlocillin

*Additive compatibilities:* Amikacin, aztreonam, ceftazidime, cycloSPORINE, gentamicin, metronidazole, netilmicin, piperacillin, potassium acetate, potassium chloride, potassium phosphates, prednisoLONE, promethazine, propofol, ranitidine, Ringer's, sodium chloride, tobramycin, vit B/C

*Additive incompatibilities:* Aminophylline, amoxicillin, clindamycin, floxacillin, mezlocillin

### Patient/family education
- Teach patient to report sore throat, bruising, bleeding, joint pain; may indicate blood dyscrasias (rare)
- Teach patient to contact prescriber if adverse reaction occurs or if inflammation or pain in tendon occurs
- Advise patient to contact prescriber if vaginal itching, loose foul-smelling stools, furry tongue occur; may indicate superinfection; report itching, rash, pruritus, urticaria
- Instruct patient to take all medication prescribed for the length of time ordered; product must be taken around the clock to maintain blood levels; do not give medication to others
- Advise patient to notify prescriber of diarrhea with blood or pus
- Advise patient to rinse mouth frequently, use sugarless candy or gum for dry mouth

### Evaluation
**Positive therapeutic outcome**
- Absence of signs/symptoms of infection (WBC <10,000/mm$^3$, temp WNL, absence of red draining wounds)
- Reported improvement in symptoms of infection

---

### ciprofloxacin ophthalmic
*See Appendix D*

---

### cisatracurium  (Rx)
(sis-a-tra-cyoor'ee-um)
Nimbex
*Func. class.:* Neuromuscular blocker (nondepolarizing)

**Pregnancy category B**

**Action:** Inhibits transmission of nerve impulses by binding with cholinergic receptor sites, antagonizing action of acetylcholine

**Therapeutic outcome:** Paralysis of body for administration of anesthesia

---

Adverse effects: *italic* = common, **bold** = life-threatening

**Uses:** Facilitation of endotracheal intubation, skeletal muscle relaxation during mechanical ventilation surgery, or general anesthesia

### Dosage and routes
*Adult:* **IV** 0.15 and 0.2 mg/kg depending on desired time to intubate and length of surgery: use peripheral nerve stimulation to evaluate dosage
*Child 2-12 yr:* **IV** 0.1 mg/kg over 5-10 sec with halothane or opioid anesthesia

### Available forms: Inj 2, 10 mg/ml

### Adverse effects
*CV:* Bradycardia, tachycardia; increased, decreased B/P
*EENT:* Increased secretions
*INTEG:* Rash, flushing, pruritus, urticaria
*RESP:* **Prolonged apnea, bronchospasm, cyanosis, respiratory depression**

**Contraindications:** Hypersensitivity

**Precautions:** Pregnancy **B**, breastfeeding, children <2 yr, electrolyte imbalances, dehydration, cardiac/neuromuscular/respiratory disease

| Pharmacokinetics |
| --- |
| Unknown |

| Pharmacodynamics | |
| --- | --- |
| **Onset** | 1-3 min |
| **Peak** | 2-5 min |
| **Duration** | 30-40 min |

### Interactions
*Individual drugs*
Carbamazepine, phenytoin: decreased duration of neuromuscular blockade
Isoflurane, lithium: increased neuromuscular blockade
Succinylcholine: decreased neuromuscular blockade
*Drug classifications*
Aminoglycosides, antibiotics (polymix), β-adrenergic blockers, opioids: increased neuromuscular blockade

### NURSING CONSIDERATIONS
**Assessment**
• Assess for electrolyte imbalances (K, Mg), may lead to increased action of this product
• Assess vital signs (B/P, pulse, respirations, airway) until fully recovered; rate, depth, pattern of respirations; strength of handgrip
• Assess I&O ratio: check for urinary retention, frequency, hesitancy
• Assess recovery: decreased paralysis of face, diaphragm, legs, arms, rest of body

• Assess allergic reactions: rash, fever, respiratory distress, pruritus; product should be discontinued

### Nursing diagnoses
• Breathing pattern, ineffective (uses)
• Communication, impaired verbal (adverse reactions)
• Knowledge, deficient (teaching)

### Implementation
**IV route**
• Use nerve stimulator by anesthesiologist to determine neuromuscular blockade
• Give anticholinesterase to reverse neuromuscular blockade
• Give by slow **IV** only by qualified person, do not administer IM
• Store in light-resistant area
• Reassure if communication is difficult during recovery from neuromuscular blockage

### Evaluation
**Positive therapeutic outcome**
• Paralysis of jaw, eyelid, head, neck, rest of body

**Treatment of overdose:** Edrophonium or neostigmine, atropine, monitor VS; mechanical ventilation

---

### ! HIGH ALERT

## cisplatin (Rx)
(sis'pla-tin)
Platinol, Platinol-AQ
*Func. class.:* Antineoplastic alkylating agent
*Chem. class.:* Inorganic heavy metal

**Pregnancy category D**

**Do not confuse:**
cisplatin/carboplatin, Platinol/Paraplatin

**Action:** Alkylates DNA, RNA; inhibits enzymes that allow synthesis of amino acids in proteins; activity is not cell cycle phase specific

**Therapeutic outcome:** Prevention of rapidly growing malignant cells

**Uses:** Advanced bladder cancer; adjunctive in metastatic testicular cancer and metastatic ovarian cancer; osteosarcoma; soft tissue sarcomas; head, neck, esophageal, prostatic, lung, and cervical cancer; lymphoma

### Dosage and routes
Dosage protocols may vary

*Metastatic testicular cancer*
*Adult:* **IV** 20 mg/m$^2$ daily × 5 days, repeat q3 wk for 3 cycles or more, depending on response

*Advanced bladder cancer*
*Adult:* **IV** 50-70 mg/m$^2$ q3-4 wk

*Metastatic ovarian cancer*
*Adult:* **IV** 100 mg/m$^2$ q4 wk or 75 mg/m$^2$ q3 wk with cyclophosphamide therapy; mix with 2 L of NaCl and 37.5 g mannitol over 6 hr

**Available forms:** Inj 0.5 mg/ml ✦, 1 mg/ml; powder for inj 10, 50 mg vials

**Adverse effects**
*CNS:* **Seizures,** peripheral neuropathy
*CV:* Cardiac abnormalities
*EENT:* *Tinnitus, hearing loss, vestibular toxicity,* blurred vision, altered color perception
*GI:* *Severe nausea, vomiting, diarrhea, weight loss*
*GU:* **Renal tubular damage,** renal insufficiency, impotence, sterility, amenorrhea, gynecomastia, hyperuremia
*HEMA:* **Thrombocytopenia, leukopenia, pancytopenia**
*INTEG:* *Alopecia,* dermatitis
*META:* Hypomagnesemia, hypocalcemia, hypokalemia, hypophosphatemia
*RESP:* **Fibrosis**
*SYST:* **Anaphylaxis**

**Contraindications:** Pregnancy **D**, breastfeeding, radiation therapy within 1 mo, chemotherapy within 1 mo, thrombocytopenia, recent smallpox vaccination, aluminum products used to prepare or administer cisplatin

**Precautions:** Pneumococcal vaccination

**Pharmacokinetics**

| | |
|---|---|
| **Absorption** | Complete |
| **Distribution** | Widely distributed, accumulates in body tissues for several months |
| **Metabolism** | Liver |
| **Excretion** | Kidneys |
| **Half-life** | 30-100 hr |

**Pharmacodynamics**
Unknown

**Interactions**
*Individual drugs*
Alcohol, aspirin: increased risk of bleeding
Bumetanide, ethacrynic acid, furosemide: ototoxicity
Phenytoin: decreased phenytoin effect

*Drug classifications*
Aminoglycosides, diuretics (loop): increased nephrotoxicity
Myelosuppressive agents, radiation: increased myelosuppression
NSAIDs: increased risk of bleeding

Vaccines, live virus: decreased antibody response
*Drug/lab test*
Increased: uric acid, BUN, creatinine
Decreased: CCr, calcium, phosphate, potassium, magnesium
Positive: Coombs' test

**NURSING CONSIDERATIONS**
**Assessment**
• Monitor for bone marrow depression: CBC, differential, platelet count weekly; withhold product if WBC count is <4000/mm$^3$ or platelet count is <100,000/mm$^3$; notify prescriber of results if WBC <20,000/mm$^3$, platelets <150,000/mm$^3$
• Monitor renal function studies: BUN, creatinine, serum uric acid, urine CCr before and during therapy; I&O ratio; report fall in urine output to <30 ml/hr; dose should not be given if BUN <25 mg/dl; creatinine <1.5 mg/dl
• Assess for anaphylaxis: wheezing, tachycardia, facial swelling, fainting; discontinue product and report to prescriber, resuscitation equipment should be nearby
• Monitor temp q4hr (may indicate beginning of infection)
• Monitor liver function tests before and during therapy (bilirubin, AST, ALT, LDH) as needed or monthly; note yellowing of skin or sclera, dark urine, clay-colored stools, itchy skin, abdominal pain, fever, diarrhea
• Assess for increased uric acid levels, swelling, joint pain primarily in extremities; patient should be well hydrated to prevent urate deposits
• Assess for bleeding: hematuria, stool guaiac, bruising or petechiae, mucosa or orifices q8hr; note inflammation of mucosa, breaks in skin
• Identify dyspnea, crackles, nonproductive cough, chest pain, tachypnea
• Identify effects of alopecia on body image; discuss feelings about body changes
• Identify edema in feet, joint pain, stomach pain, shaking; prescriber should be notified

**Nursing diagnoses**
• Body image, disturbed (adverse reactions)
• Infection, risk for (adverse reactions)
• Injury, risk for (adverse reactions)
• Knowledge, deficient (teaching)

**Implementation**
• Hydrate patient with 0.9% NaCl over 8-12 hr before treatment
• Give all medications PO, if possible; avoid IM inj when platelets <100,000/mm$^3$

• Give epINEPHrine, antihistamines, corticosteroids for hypersensitivity reaction; antiemetic 30-60 min before giving product to prevent vomiting, and prn; allopurinol or sodium bicarbonate to maintain uric acid level, alkalinization of urine; antibiotics for prophylaxis of infection; diuretic (furosemide 40 mg **IV**) or mannitol after infusion

• After diluting 10 mg/10 ml or 50 mg/50 ml sterile water for inj; withdraw prescribed dose, dilute ½ dose with 1000 ml D₅ 0.2 NaCl or D₅ 0.45 NaCl with 37.5 g mannitol; **IV** inf is given over 3-4 hr; use a 0.45 µm filter; total dose 2000 ml over 6-8 hr; check site for irritation, phlebitis; do not use equipment containing aluminum

• Prepare in biologic cabinet using gown, gloves, mask; do not allow product to come in contact with skin, use soap and water if contact occurs

*Syringe compatibilities:* Bleomycin, cyclophosphamide, doxapram, DOXOrubicin, droperidol, fluorouracil, furosemide, heparin, leucovorin, methotrexate, metoclopramide, mitomycin, vinBLAStine, vinCRIStine

*Y-site compatibilities:* Allopurinol, aztreonam, bleomycin, chlorproMAZINE, cimetidine, cladribine, cyclophosphamide, dexamethasone, diphenhydrAMINE, doxapram, DOXOrubicin, DOXOrubicin liposome, droperidol, famotidine, filgrastim, fludarabine, fluorouracil, furosemide, ganciclovir, granisetron, heparin, hydromorphone, leucovorin, lorazepam, melphalan, methotrexate, methylPREDNISolone, metoclopramide, mitomycin, morphine, ondansetron, paclitaxel, prochlorperazine, promethazine, propofol, ranitidine, sargramostim, teniposide, vinBLAStine, vinCRIStine, vinorelbine

*Additive compatibilities:* Carboplatin, cyclophosphamide with etoposide, etoposide, etoposide with floxuridine, floxuridine, floxuridine with leucovorin, hydrOXYzine, ifosfamide, ifosfamide with etoposide, leucovorin, magnesium sulfate, mannitol, ondansetron

*Additive incompatibilities:* Fluorouracil, mesna, thiotepa

*Solution compatibilities:* D₅/0.225% NaCl, D₅/0.45% NaCl, D₅/0.9% NaCl, D₅/0.45% NaCl with mannitol 1.875%, D₅/0.33% NaCl with mannitol 1.875%, D₅/0.33% NaCl with KCl 20 mEq and mannitol 1.875%, 0.9% NaCl, 0.45% NaCl, 0.3% NaCl, 0.225% NaCl, water

*Solution incompatibilities:* Sodium bicarbonate 5%, 0.1% NaCl, water

## Patient/family education

• Teach patient to avoid use of products containing aspirin or ibuprofen, NSAIDs, alcohol (may cause GI bleeding), razors, commercial mouthwash; to report symptoms of bleeding (hematuria, tarry stools, bruising, petechiae)

• Advise patient to report numbness, tingling in face or extremities, poor hearing or joint pain, swelling

• Instruct patient to report signs of anemia (fatigue, headache, irritability, faintness, shortness of breath)

• Instruct patient to report any changes in breathing or coughing even several months after treatment; to avoid crowds and persons with respiratory tract or other infections

• Advise patient that hair may be lost during treatment; a wig or hair piece may make patient feel better; new hair may be different in color, texture

• Tell patient not to have any vaccinations without the advice of the prescriber; serious reactions can occur

• Caution patient contraception is needed during treatment and for several months after the completion of therapy

## Evaluation

**Positive therapeutic outcome**

• Prevention of rapid division of malignant cells

## citalopram (Rx)
(sigh-tal'oh-pram)
Celexa
*Func. class.:* Antidepressant
*Chem class.:* Selective serotonin reuptake inhibitor (SSRI)

**Pregnancy category** C

**Do not confuse:**
Celexa/Celebrex/Cerebyx/Cerebra

**Action:** Inhibits CNS neuron uptake of serotonin but not of norepinephrine; weak inhibitor of CYP450 enzyme system, making it more appealing than other products

**Therapeutic outcome:** Decreased symptoms of depression after 2-3 wk

**Uses:** Major depressive disorder

**Unlabeled uses:** Premenstrual disorders, panic disorder, social phobia, impulsive aggression in children, obsessive-compulsive disorder in adolescents, treatment of psychotic symptoms in nondepressed, demented patients, anxiety, hot flashes, menopause

## Dosage and routes
### Depression
*Adult:* PO 20 mg daily AM or PM, may increase if needed to 40 mg/day after 1 wk; maintenance: after 6-8 wk of initial treatment, continue for 24 wk (32 wk total), reevaluate long-term usefulness (max 60 mg/day)

### Hepatic dose/geriatric
*Adult:* PO 20 mg/day, may increase to 40 mg/day if no response

### Panic disorder (unlabeled)
*Adult:* PO 20-60 mg/day

### Premenstrual dysphoria, social phobia (unlabeled)
*Adult:* PO 20-40 mg/day used intermittently in premenstrual dysphoria

**Available forms:** Tabs 10, 20, 40 mg; oral sol 10 mg /5 ml; orally disintegrating tabs 10, 20, 40 mg

## Adverse effects
*CNS: Headache, nervousness, insomnia, drowsiness, anxiety, tremor, dizziness, fatigue, sedation, poor concentration, abnormal dreams, agitation,* **seizures,** apathy, euphoria, hallucinations, delusions, psychosis, **suicidal attempts**
*CV: Hot flashes, palpitations,* angina pectoris, **hemorrhage,** hypertension, 1st-degree tachycardia, 1st-degree AV block, bradycardia, MI, thrombophlebitis
*GI: Nausea, diarrhea, dry mouth, anorexia, dyspepsia, constipation, cramps, vomiting, taste changes, flatulence, decreased appetite*
*GU: Dysmenorrhea, decreased libido, urinary frequency, urinary tract infection,* amenorrhea, cystitis, impotence, urine retention
*INTEG: Sweating, rash, pruritus,* acne, alopecia, urticaria
*MS: Pain,* arthritis, twitching
*RESP: Infection, pharyngitis, nasal congestion, sinus headache, sinusitis, cough, dyspnea, bronchitis,* asthma, hyperventilation, pneumonia
*SYST: Asthenia, viral infection, fever, allergy, chills*

**Contraindications:** Hypersensitivity

**Precautions:** Pregnancy **C,** breastfeeding, children, geriatric, suicidal ideation, renal/hepatic disease, seizure disorder

### Pharmacokinetics
| | |
|---|---|
| **Absorption** | Well absorbed |
| **Distribution** | Unknown |
| **Metabolism** | Liver, by CYP1A2, CYP2D6 |
| **Excretion** | Kidneys, steady state 28-35 days |
| **Half-life** | Unknown |

### Pharmacodynamics
Unknown

## Interactions
### Individual drugs
Alcohol: increased CNS depression
Carbamazepine: decreased citalopram levels
Lithium: increased serotonergic effects
Pimoside, ziprasidone: increased QTc interval; do not use together
### Drug classifications
Anticoagulants, NSAIDs, salicylates, thrombolytics: increased risk of bleeding
Antidepressants, (tricyclics): increased effect, use cautiously
Antifungals (azole), macrolides: increased citalopram levels
Barbiturates, benzodiazepines, CNS depressants, sedative/hypnotics: increased CNS depression
β-Adrenergic blockers: increased plasma levels of β-blockers
MAOIs: hypertensive crisis, seizures, fatal reactions, do not use together
Quinolones: increased QTc interval; do not use together
### Drug/herb
SAM-e, St. John's wort: serotonin syndrome, do not use with citalopram, fatal reaction may occur
Yohimbe: increased CNS stimulation
### Drug/lab test
Increased: serum bilirubin, blood glucose, alkaline phosphatase
Decreased: VMA, 5-HIAA
False increase: increased urinary catecholamines

## NURSING CONSIDERATIONS
### Assessment
• Monitor B/P (lying, standing), pulse q4hr; if systolic B/P drops 20 mm Hg, hold product and notify prescriber; take vital signs q4hr in patients with cardiovascular disease
• Monitor blood studies: CBC, leukocytes, differential, cardiac enzymes if patient is receiving long-term therapy; check platelets, bleeding can occur
• Monitor hepatic studies: AST, ALT, bilirubin
• Check weight qwk; appetite may increase with product

Adverse effects: *italic* = common, **bold** = life-threatening

- Assess ECG for flattening of T wave, bundle branch block, AV block, dysrhythmias in cardiac patients
- Assess EPS primarily in geriatric: rigidity, dystonia, akathisia
- Assess mental status: mood, sensorium, affect, suicidal tendencies; increase in psychiatric symptoms: depression, panic
- Monitor urinary retention, constipation; constipation is more likely to occur in children or geriatric
⬥ Assess for withdrawal symptoms: headache, nausea, vomiting, muscle pain, weakness; usually do not occur unless product is discontinued abruptly
- Identify patient's alcohol consumption; if alcohol is consumed, hold dose until AM

### Nursing diagnoses
- Coping, ineffective (uses)
- Injury, risk for (side effects)
- Knowledge, deficient (teaching)
- Noncompliance (teaching)

### Implementation
- Give with food or milk for GI symptoms
- Give dosage at bedtime if oversedation occurs during day
- Leave orally disintegrating tabs on tongue and allow to dissolve before swallowing
- Store at room temperature; do not freeze

### Patient/family education
- Teach patient that therapeutic effects may take 4-6 wk
- Instruct patient to use caution in driving or other activities requiring alertness because of drowsiness, dizziness, blurred vision; to avoid rising quickly from sitting to standing, especially geriatric patients
- Advise that suicidal ideas, behavior may occur in children or young adults
- Caution patient to avoid alcohol ingestion, other CNS depressants
- Advise patient not to discontinue medication quickly after long-term use: may cause nausea, headache, malaise
- Instruct patient to increase fluids, bulk in diet if constipation, urinary retention occur, especially geriatric
- Advise patient to take gum, hard sugarless candy, or frequent sips of water for dry mouth
- Teach patient how to use orally disintegrating tabs

### Evaluation
**Positive therapeutic outcome**
- Decreased in depression
- Absence of suicidal thoughts

**clarithromycin** (Rx)
(clare-i-thro-mye′sin)
Biaxin, Biaxin XL
*Func. class.:* Antiinfective
*Chem. class.:* Macrolide

**Pregnancy category** C

**Action:** Binds to 50S ribosomal subunits of susceptible bacteria and suppresses protein synthesis

**Therapeutic outcome:** Bactericidal action against the following: *Streptococcus pneumoniae, Streptococcus pyogenes, Mycoplasma pneumoniae, Corynebacterium diphtheriae, Bordetella pertussis, Listeria monocytogenes, Haemophilus influenzae, Staphylococcus aureus, Mycobacterium avium (MAC), Mycobacterium intracellulare, Legionella pneumophila, Moxarella catarrhalis, Neisseria gonorrhoeae,* complex infections in AIDS patients, *Helicobacter pylori* in combination with omeprazole

**Uses:** Mild to moderate infections of the upper respiratory tract, lower respiratory tract; uncomplicated skin and skin structure infections

### Dosage and routes
***Acute exacerbation of chronic bronchitis***
*Adult:* PO 250-500 mg q12hr × 7-14 days or 1000 mg/day × 7 days (XL)

***Pharyngitis/tonsillitis***
*Adult:* PO 250 mg q12hr × 10 days

***Renal dose***
*Adult:* PO CCr <30 ml/min 250 mg/day × bid, may use an initial dose of 500 mg
*Child:* PO CCr <30 ml/min reduce dose by 50%

***Community-acquired pneumonia***
*Adult:* PO 250 mg q12hr × 7-14 days or 1000 mg/day × 7 days (XL)

***Endocarditis prophylaxis***
*Adult:* PO 500 mg 1 hr before procedure

***MAC prophylaxis/treatment***
*Adult:* PO 500 mg bid, will require an additional antiinfective for active infection

***H. pylori*** *infection*
*Adult:* PO 500 mg/day plus omeprazole 2 × 20 mg q AM (days 1-14), then omeprazole 20 mg q AM (days 15-28)

***Acute maxillary sinusitis***
*Adult:* PO 500 mg q12hr × 14 days

**Most infections**
*Child:* PO 7.5 mg/kg q12hr × 10 days, max 500 mg/dose for MAC

**Available forms:** Tabs 250, 500 mg; oral susp 125, 250 mg/5 ml; ext rel tab (XL) 500 mg

**Adverse effects**
*CV:* **Ventricular dysrhythmias**
*GI:* Nausea, vomiting, diarrhea, **hepatotoxicity,** abdominal pain, stomatitis, heartburn, anorexia, abnormal taste, **pseudomembranous colitis**
*GU:* Vaginitis, moniliasis
*HEMA:* Leukopenia, thrombocytopenia, increased INR
*INTEG:* Rash, urticaria, pruritus, **Stevens-Johnson syndrome, toxic epidermal necrolysis**
*MISC:* Headache, hearing loss

**Contraindications:** Hypersensitivity to this product or other macrolides

**Precautions:** Pregnancy **C**, breastfeeding, geriatric, renal/hepatic disease, QT prolongation

| Pharmacokinetics | |
|---|---|
| **Absorption** | 50% |
| **Distribution** | Widely distributed |
| **Metabolism** | Liver |
| **Excretion** | Kidneys, unchanged (20%-30%) |
| **Half-life** | 4-6 hr |

| Pharmacodynamics | |
|---|---|
| **Onset** | Unknown |
| **Peak** | 2 hr |
| **Duration** | Unknown |

**Interactions**
*Individual drugs*
Alprazolam, busPIRone, carbamazepine, cycloSPORINE, digoxin, disopyramide, felodipine, fluconazole, omeprazole, tacrolimus, theophylline: increased levels, increased toxicity
Carbamazepine: increased toxicity, from increased levels of carbamazepine, increased oral anticoagulants effect
Cisapride, pimozide: increased effect, increased dysrhythmias
Digoxin: increased blood levels of digoxin, increased digoxin effects, increased oral anticoagulants effect
Fluconazole: increased clarithromycin levels
Rifabutin, rifampin: decreased levels

Theophylline: increased toxicity from increased levels of theophylline, increased oral anticoagulants effect
Zidovudine: increased or decreased action
*Drug classifications*
All products metabolized by CYP3A enzyme system: increased action, risk of toxicity
Class IA, III antidysrhythmics: increased QT prolongation
HMG-CoA reductase inhibitors: increased levels
Oral anticoagulants: increased effects of oral anticoagulants
*Drug/herb*
Acidophilus: do not use with antiinfectives; separate by several hours
*Drug/lab test*
Increased: 17-OHCS/17-KS, AST, ALT, BUN, creatinine, LDH, total bilirubin
Decreased: folate assay, WBC

**NURSING CONSIDERATIONS**
**Assessment**
• Assess patient for signs and symptoms of infection including characteristics of wounds, sputum, urine, stool, WBC >10,000/mm$^3$, earache, fever; obtain baseline information before and during treatment
• Obtain C&S before beginning product therapy to identify if correct treatment has been initiated
• Monitor blood studies: AST, ALT, CBC, Hct, bilirubin, LDH, alkaline phosphatase, Coombs' test monthly if patient is on long-term therapy
• Assess bowel pattern daily; if severe diarrhea occurs, product should be discontinued
• Assess for overgrowth of infection: perineal itching, fever, malaise, redness, pain, swelling, drainage, rash, diarrhea, change in cough, sputum

**Nursing diagnoses**
• Diarrhea (side effects)
• Infection, risk for (uses)
• Knowledge, deficient (teaching)
• Noncompliance (teaching)

**Implementation**
• Do not break, crush, or chew ext rel tab
• Ensure adequate fluid intake (2 L) during diarrhea episodes
• Give q12hr to maintain serum level

**Patient/family education**
• Advise patient to contact physician if vaginal itching, loose foul-smelling stools, furry tongue occur; may indicate superinfection
• Instruct patient to take all medication prescribed for the length of time ordered

Adverse effects: *italic* = common, **bold** = life-threatening

- Advise prescriber if pregnancy is planned or suspected

### Evaluation
**Positive therapeutic outcome**
- Absence of signs/symptoms of infection (WBC <10,000/mm$^3$, temp WNL, absence of red draining wounds)
- Reported improvement in symptoms of infection

## clavulanate
*See amoxicillin/clavulanate, ticarcillin/clavulanate*

## clindamycin HCl (Rx)
(klin-dah-my'sin)
Cleocin HCl
## clindamycin palmitate (Rx)
Cleocin Pediatric, Dalacin C Palmitate
## clindamycin phosphate (Rx)
Cleocin Phosphate, Dalacin C, Dalacin C Phosphate
*Func. class.:* Antiinfective—miscellaneous
*Chem. class.:* Lincomycin derivative

**Pregnancy category    B**

**Action:** Binds to 50S subunit of bacterial ribosomes; suppresses protein synthesis

**Therapeutic outcome:** Absence of infection

**Uses:** Infections caused by staphylococci, streptococci, *Rickettsia, Fusobacterium, Actinomyces, Peptococcus, Bacteroides, Pneumocystis jiroveci*

### Dosage and routes
*Adults:* PO 150-450 mg q6hr, max 1.8 g/day; IM/**IV** 1.2-1.8 g/day in 2-4 divided doses q6-12hr, not to exceed 4800 mg/day
*Child <1 mo:* 15-20 mg/kg/day divided q6-8hr
*Child >1 mo:* PO 8-25 mg/kg/day in divided doses q6-8hr; IM/**IV** 20-40 mg/kg/day in divided doses q6-8hr in 3-4 equal doses

**PID**
*Adult:* **IV** 600 mg qid plus gentamicin or 900 mg q8hr

**Bacterial endocarditis prophylaxis**
*Adult:* 600 mg 1 hr before procedure

**P. jiroveci *pneumonia (unlabeled)***
*Adult:* PO 1200-1800 mg/day in divided doses with 15-30 mg primaquine/day

**Available forms:** Phosphate: inj 150, 300, 600 mg base/4 ml; 900 mg base/ml; inj inf in D$_5$ 300, 600, 900 mg; HCl: caps 75, 150, 300 mg; palmitate: oral sol 75 mg/5 ml

### Adverse effects
***GI:*** *Nausea, vomiting, abdominal pain, diarrhea,* **pseudomembranous colitis,** *anorexia, weight loss,* increased AST, ALT, bilirubin, alkaline phosphatase, jaundice
***GU:*** *Vaginitis,* urinary frequency
***HEMA:*** **Leukopenia, eosinophilia, agranulocytosis, thrombocytopenia, polyarthritis**
***INTEG:*** Rash, urticaria, pruritus, erythema, pain, abscess at inj site
***SYST:*** **Stevens-Johnson syndrome, exfoliative dermatitis**

**Contraindications:** Hypersensitivity to this product or lincomycin, tartrazine dye, ulcerative colitis/enteritis

**Precautions:** Pregnancy **B**, breastfeeding, geriatric, renal/liver/GI disease, tartrazine sensitivity, asthma, allergy

| Pharmacokinetics | |
|---|---|
| **Absorption** | Well absorbed (PO, IM), minimal (TOP) |
| **Distribution** | Widely distributed; crosses placenta |
| **Metabolism** | Liver, extensively |
| **Excretion** | Kidneys, breast milk |
| **Half-life** | 2½ hr |

| Pharmacodynamics | | | |
|---|---|---|---|
| | PO | IM | IV |
| **Onset** | Rapid | Rapid | Rapid |
| **Peak** | ½-1 hr | 1½ hr | Infusion's end |

### Interactions
*Individual drugs*
Erythromycin, chloramphenicol: decreased action of clindamycin
Kaolin: decreased absorption
*Drug classifications*
Neuromuscular blockers: increased neuromuscular blockade
*Drug/herb*
Acidophilus: do not use with antiinfectives; separate by several hours
*Drug/lab test*
Increased: alkaline phosphatase, bilirubin, CPK, AST, ALT

---

## NURSING CONSIDERATIONS
### Assessment

- Assess any patient with compromised renal system; product is excreted slowly in poor renal system function; toxicity may occur rapidly
- Assess patient for signs and symptoms of infection including characteristics of wounds, sputum, urine, stool, WBC >10,000/mm$^3$, fever; obtain baseline information before and during treatment
- Complete C&S testing before beginning product therapy; this will identify if correct treatment has been initiated
- Assess for allergic reactions: rash, urticaria, pruritus, chills, fever, joint pain; may occur a few days after therapy begins; epINEPHrine and resuscitation equipment should be available in case of an anaphylactic reaction
- Identify urine output; if decreasing, notify prescriber (may indicate nephrotoxicity); also look for increased BUN and creatinine levels
- Monitor blood studies: AST, ALT, CBC, Hct, bilirubin, LDH, alkaline phosphatase, Coombs' test monthly if patient is on long-term therapy
- Monitor electrolytes: potassium, sodium, chloride monthly if patient is on long-term therapy
- Assess bowel pattern daily; if severe diarrhea occurs, product should be discontinued; may indicate pseudomembranous colitis
- Monitor for bleeding: ecchymosis, bleeding gums, hematuria, stool guaiac daily if on long-term therapy
- Assess for overgrowth of infection: perineal itching, fever, malaise, redness, pain, swelling, drainage, rash, diarrhea, change in cough, sputum

### Nursing diagnoses

- Diarrhea (adverse reactions)
- Infection, risk for (uses)
- Injury, risk for (adverse reaction)
- Knowledge, deficient (teaching)
- Noncompliance (teaching)

### Implementation
#### PO route

- Do not break, crush, or chew caps
- Give with 8 oz of water; give with meals for GI symptoms
- Shake liquids well
- Do not refrigerate oral preparations; stable at room temperature for 2 wk

#### IM route

- If more than 600 mg must be given, divide into 2 inj
- Give deeply in large muscle mass; rotate sites

#### IV route

- Give by inf only; do not administer BOL dose; dilute 300 mg or more/50 ml or more of D$_5$W, 0.9% NaCl
- May be further diluted in greater amounts of D$_5$W, 0.9% NaCl and given as a cont inf in acute PID; give first dose 10 mg/min over ½ hr, then 0.75 mg/min; increased rates may be used to keep serum blood levels higher; run over >10 min; no more than 1200 mg in a 1 hr inf

*Syringe compatibilities:* Amikacin, aztreonam, gentamicin, heparin
*Syringe incompatibilities:* Tobramycin
*Y-site compatibilities:* Amifostine, amiodarone, amphotericin B cholesteryl, amsacrine, aztreonam, cisatracurium, cyclophosphamide, diltiazem, DOXOrubicin liposome, enalaprilat, esmolol, fludarabine, foscarnet, granisetron, heparin, hydromorphone, labetolol, magnesium sulfate, melphalan, meperidine, midazolam, morphine, multivitamins, odansetron, perphenazine, piperacillin/tazobactam, propofol, remifentanil, sargramostim, tacrolimus, teniposide, theophylline, thiotepa, vinorelbine, vit B/C, zidovudine
*Y-site incompatibilities:* Idarubicin
*Additive compatibilities:* Amikacin, ampicillin, aztreonam, cefamandole, cefazolin, cefepine, cefonicid, cefoperazone, cefotaxime, cefoxitin, ceftazidime, ceftizoxime, cefuroxime, cephalothin, cimetidine, fluconazole, heparin, hydrocortisone, kanamycin, methylPREDNISolone, metoclopramide, metronidazole, netilmicin, ofloxacin, penicillin G, pipercillin, potassium chloride, sodium bicarbonate, tobramycin, verapamil, vit B/C
*Additive incompatibilities:* Ciprofloxacin

### Patient/family education

- Tell patient to take oral product with full glass of water; may take with food if GI symptoms occur; antiperistaltic products may worsen diarrhea
- Teach patient aspects of product therapy: need to complete entire course of medication to ensure organism death (10-14 days); culture may be taken after medication course has been completed
- Advise patient to report sore throat, fever, fatigue; may indicate superimposed infection
- Advise patient that product must be taken at equal intervals around clock to maintain blood levels

Adverse effects: *italic* = common, **bold** = life-threatening

## Evaluation
**Positive therapeutic outcome**
• Decreased temp, negative C&S

## Treatment of hypersensitivity:
Withdraw product; maintain airway; administer epINEPHrine, aminophylline, O$_2$, **IV** corticosteroids

## clindamycin topical
*See Appendix D*

## clobetasol topical
*See Appendix D*

## *clomiPHENE (Rx)
(kloe'mi-feen)
Clomid, clomiPHENE citrate, Serophene
*Func. class.:* Ovulation stimulant
*Chem. class.:* Nonsteroidal antiestrogenic

**Pregnancy category  X**

### Do not confuse:
clomiPHENE/clomiPRAMINE

**Action:** Increases LH, FSH release from the pituitary, which increases maturation of ovarian follicle, ovulation, development of corpus luteum

**Therapeutic outcome:** Pregnancy

**Uses:** Female infertility (ovulatory failure)

### Dosage and routes
*Adult:* PO 50-100 mg daily × 5 days or 50-100 mg daily beginning on day 5 of cycle; may be repeated until conception occurs or 3 cycles of therapy have been completed

**Available forms:** Tabs 50 mg

### Adverse effects
*CNS: Headache, depression,* restlessness, anxiety, nervousness, fatigue, insomnia, dizziness, flushing
*CV:* Vasomotor flushing, phlebitis, **deep vein thrombosis**
*EENT:* Blurred vision, diplopia, photophobia
*GI: Nausea, vomiting, constipation,* abdominal pain, bloating
*GU:* Polyuria, frequency of urination, **birth defects, spontaneous abortions,** multiple ovulation, breast pain, oliguria, abnormal uterine bleeding, ovarian cyst, hypertrophy of ovary
*INTEG: Rash, dermatitis,* urticaria, alopecia

**Contraindications:** Pregnancy **X,** hypersensitivity, hepatic disease, undiagnosed uterine bleeding, uncontrolled thyroid or adrenal dysfunction, intracranial lesion, ovarian cysts, endometrial carcinoma

**Precautions:** Hypertension, depression, seizures, diabetes mellitus, abnormal ovarian enlargement, ovarian hyperstimulation

### Pharmacokinetics
| | |
|---|---|
| **Absorption** | Well distributed |
| **Distribution** | Unknown |
| **Metabolism** | Liver, extensively |
| **Excretion** | Feces |
| **Half-life** | 5 days |

### Pharmacodynamics
Unknown

## Interactions
*Drug/lab test*
Increased: FSH/LH, BSP, thyroxine, TBG

## NURSING CONSIDERATIONS
### Assessment
• Determine liver function tests before therapy: AST, ALT, alkaline phosphatase
• Monitor serum progesterone, urinary excretion of pregnanediol to identify occurrence of ovulation
• Pelvic examination should be done to determine ovarian size, cervical condition
• Endometrial biopsy may be done in women over 35 to rule out endometrial carcinoma

### Nursing diagnoses
• Knowledge, deficient (teaching)
• Sexual dysfunction (uses)

### Implementation
• Give after discontinuing estrogen therapy
• Give at same time daily to maintain product level; begin on 5th day of menstrual cycle

### Patient/family education
• Advise patient that multiple births are common after product is taken
• Instruct patient to notify prescriber immediately if low abdominal pain occurs; may indicate ovarian cyst, cyst rupture
• Advise patient to notify prescriber of photophobia, blurred vision, diplopia, abnormal bleeding, hot flashes, nausea, vomiting, headache
• Teach patient if dose is missed, double at next time; if more than one dose is missed, call prescriber
• Instruct patient that response usually occurs 4-10 days after last day of treatment

- Teach patient method for taking, recording basal body temp to determine whether ovulation has occurred; if ovulation can be determined (there is a slight decrease in temp, then a sharp increase for ovulation), to attempt coitus 3 days before and every other day until after ovulation
- Teach patient if pregnancy is suspected, to notify prescriber immediately

## Evaluation
**Positive therapeutic outcome**
- Fertility

---

**\*clomiPRAMINE** (Rx)
(klom-ip'ra-meen)
Anafranil
*Func. class.:* Tricyclic antidepressant
*Chem. class.:* Tertiary amine
**Pregnancy category** C

**Do not confuse:**
clomiPRAMINE/clomiPHENE/desipramine/norpramin

**Action:** Potentiates serotonin and norepinephrine uptake; also increases dopamine metabolism

**Therapeutic outcome:** Decreased signs and symptoms of obsessive-compulsive disorder, decreased depression

**Uses:** Obsessive-compulsive disorder, dysphoria, anxiety, agoraphobia and other phobias

## Dosage and routes
*Obsessive-compulsive disorder*
*Adult:* PO 25 mg at bedtime; increase gradually over 4 wk to a dosage of 75-250 mg/day in divided doses
*Child 10-18 yr:* PO 25-50 mg/day gradually increased or 3 mg/kg/day, whichever is smaller; max 200 mg/day

**Available forms:** Caps 25, 50, 75 mg

## Adverse effects
*CNS: Dizziness, tremors, mania,* **seizures,** aggressiveness, drowsiness, headache, EPS, **neuroleptic malignant syndrome,** mania
*CV:* Hypotension, tachycardia, **cardiac arrest**
*EENT:* Blurred vision
*ENDO:* Galactorrhea, hyperprolactinemia
*GI: Constipation, dry mouth, nausea, dyspepsia,* weight gain, **hepatic toxicity**
*GU: Delayed ejaculation, anorgasmia,* retention, decreased libido
*HEMA:* **Agranulocytosis, neutropenia, pancytopenia**

*INTEG:* Diaphoresis, photosensitivity
*META:* Hyponatremia
*SYST:* **Suicide in children/adolescents**

**Contraindications:** Hypersensitivity, immediately after MI

**Precautions:** Pregnancy C, breastfeeding, geriatric, seizures, suicidal patients, cardiac disease, suicidal ideation, glaucoma

### Pharmacokinetics
| | |
|---|---|
| Absorption | Well absorbed |
| Distribution | Widely distributed |
| Metabolism | Liver, extensively |
| Excretion | Kidneys, breast milk |
| Half-life | 19-37 hr; steady state 1-2 wk |

### Pharmacodynamics
| | |
|---|---|
| Onset | ≥2 wk |
| Peak | 2-6 hr |
| Duration | Unknown |

## Interactions
*Individual drugs*
Alcohol: increased CNS depression
Carbamazepine: decreased clomiPRAMINE action
Cimetidine, fluoxetine, fluvoxamine, sertraline: increased clomiPRAMINE level; do not use together
Clonidine, epINEPHrine, norepinephrine: severe hypertension; avoid use
Clonidine, haloperidol, levodopa: decreased effect of these products
Phenytoin: decreased clomiPRAMINE action
*Drug classifications*
Barbiturates: decreased clomiPRAMINE levels
CNS depressants, general anesthetics: increased effects; do not use together
Other tricyclics, phenothiazines: QT prolongation
MAOIs: hypertensive crisis, seizures; do not use together
Skeletal muscle relaxants, opiates: decreased action of these products
*Drug/herb*
SAM-e, St. John's wort: serotonin syndrome, do not use together
Belladonna, corkwood, henbane leaf, jimsonweed: increased anticholinergic effect
Hops, kava, lavender: increased sedative effect
Scopolia: increased clomiPRAMINE effect
*Drug/lab test*
Increased: prolactin, TBG, serum thyroid hormones

Adverse effects: *italic* = common, **bold** = life-threatening

## NURSING CONSIDERATIONS
### Assessment
- Monitor B/P (with patient lying, standing), pulse q4hr; if systolic B/P drops 20 mm Hg hold product, notify prescriber; take VS q4hr in patients with cardiovascular disease
- Monitor blood studies: CBC, leukocytes, differential, cardiac enzymes if patient is receiving long-term therapy
- Monitor hepatic studies: AST, ALT, bilirubin
- Check weight weekly; appetite may increase with product
- Assess ECG for flattening of T wave, QTc prolongation bundle branch block, AV block, dysrhythmias in cardiac patients
- Assess for EPS primarily in geriatric: rigidity, dystonia, akathisia
- Assess mental status: mood, sensorium, affect, suicidal tendencies; increase in psychiatric symptoms: depression, panic, frequency of obsessive-compulsive behaviors
- Monitor urinary retention, constipation; constipation is more likely to occur in children or geriatric
- Assess for withdrawal symptoms: headache, nausea, vomiting, muscle pain, weakness; do not usually occur unless product was discontinued abruptly
- Identify alcohol consumption; if alcohol is consumed, hold dose until morning

### Nursing diagnoses
- Coping, ineffective (uses)
- Injury, risk for physical (side effects)
- Knowledge, deficient (teaching)
- Noncompliance (teaching)

### Implementation
- Do not break, crush, or chew caps
- Give with food or milk for GI symptoms
- Store at room temperature; do not freeze

### Patient/family education
- Teach patient that therapeutic effects may take 4-6 wk
- Teach patient to use caution in driving or other activities requiring alertness because of drowsiness, dizziness, blurred vision; to avoid rising quickly from sitting to standing, especially geriatric
- Teach patient to avoid alcohol ingestion, other CNS depressants
- Teach patient not to discontinue medication quickly after long-term use: may cause nausea, headache, malaise
- Teach patient to wear sunscreen or large hat, since photosensitivity occurs
- Teach patient to increase fluids, bulk in diet if constipation, urinary retention occur, especially geriatric
- Teach patient to take gum, hard sugarless candy, or frequent sips of water for dry mouth
- Advise patient to notify prescriber if pregnancy is planned or suspected
- Teach patient that suicidal ideas, behavior may occur in children/young adults

### Evaluation
#### Positive therapeutic outcome
- Decrease in depression
- Absence of suicidal thoughts

**Treatment of overdose:** ECG monitoring, induce emesis, lavage, activated charcoal, administer anticonvulsant

## clonazepam (Rx)
(kloe-na′zi-pam)
Apo-Clonazepam ♣, Gen-Clonazepam ♣, Klonopin, Novo-Clonazepam ♣, Nu-Clonazepam ♣, PMS-Clonazepam, Rivotril
*Func. class.:* Anticonvulsant
*Chem. class.:* Benzodiazepine derivative

**Pregnancy category** D
**Controlled substance schedule** IV

### Do not confuse:
clonazepam/lorazepam/clorazepate, Klonopin/clonidine

**Action:** Inhibits spike, wave formation in absence seizures (petit mal), decreases amplitude, frequency, duration, spread of discharge in minor motor seizures

**Therapeutic outcome:** Decreased frequency, severity of seizures

**Uses:** Absence, atypical absence, akinetic, myoclonic seizures, Lennox-Gastaut syndrome, panic disorder

### Dosage and routes
*Adult:* PO not to exceed 1.5 mg/day in 3 divided doses; may be increased 0.5-1 mg q3 days until desired response; not to exceed 20 mg/day; RECT 0.02 mg/kg
*Child<10 yr or 30 kg:* PO 0.01-0.03 mg/kg/day in divided doses q8hr, not to exceed 0.05 mg/kg/day; may be increased 0.25-0.5 mg q3 days until desired response; max 0.1-0.2 mg/kg/day; RECT 0.05-0.1 mg/kg
*Geriatric:* PO 0.25 daily bid initially, increase by 0.25 daily q7-14 days as needed

**Available forms:** Tabs 0.5, 1, 2 mg; orally disintegrating tabs 0.125, 0.25, 0.5, 1, 2 mg

## Adverse effects

*CNS: Drowsiness,* dizziness, confusion, behavioral changes, tremors, insomnia, headache, **suicidal tendencies,** slurred speech
*CV:* Palpitations, bradycardia, tachycardia
*EENT: Increased salivation, nystagmus, diplopia,* abnormal eye movements
*GI: Nausea, constipation,* polyphagia, anorexia, xerostomia, diarrhea, gastritis, sore gums
*GU:* Dysuria, enuresis, nocturia, retention, libido changes
*HEMA:* **Thrombocytopenia, leukocytosis, eosinophilia**
*INTEG:* Rash, alopecia, hirsutism
*RESP:* **Respiratory depression,** dyspnea, congestion

**Contraindications:** Pregnancy **D,** hypersensitivity to benzodiazepines, acute angle-closure glaucoma, psychosis, severe liver disease

**Precautions:** Open-angle glaucoma, chronic respiratory disease, renal/hepatic disease, breastfeeding, geriatric

### Pharmacokinetics

| | |
|---|---|
| **Absorption** | Well absorbed |
| **Distribution** | Crosses blood-brain barrier, placenta |
| **Metabolism** | Liver, protein binding 85% |
| **Excretion** | Kidneys |
| **Half-life** | 18-50 hr |

### Pharmacodynamics

| | |
|---|---|
| **Onset** | ½-1 hr |
| **Peak** | 1-2 hr |
| **Duration** | 6-12 hr |

## Interactions
### Individual drugs

Alcohol: increased CNS depression
Carbamazepine: decreased effectiveness
Cimetidine, diltiazem, erythromycin, fluoxetine: increased clonazepam effect
Phenobarbitol: decreased clonazepam effect
Phenytoin: decreased clonazepam levels
### Drug classifications

Antidepressants, anticonvulsants, barbiturates, general anesthetics, opiates, sedative/hypnotics: increased CNS depression
Azoles, oral contraceptives: increased clonazepam effect
CYP3A4 inducers: decreased clonazepam effect
### Drug/herb

Ginkgo, melatonin: increased clonazepam effect

Ginseng, santonica, St. John's wort: decreased clonazepam effect
Kava: increased sedative effect
### Drug/lab test

Increased: AST, alkaline phosphatase

## NURSING CONSIDERATIONS
### Assessment

• Assess mental status: mood, sensorium, affect, memory (long, short), especially geriatric
• Assess for blood dyscrasias: fever, sore throat, bruising, rash, jaundice, epistaxis (long-term treatment only)
• Assess seizure activity including type, location, duration, and character; provide seizure precaution
• Assess renal studies: urinalysis, BUN, urine creatinine
• Monitor blood studies: RBCs, Hct, Hgb, reticulocyte counts weekly for 4 wk then monthly
• Monitor hepatic studies: ALT, AST, bilirubin, creatinine
• Monitor product levels during initial treatment
• Assess for signs of physical withdrawal if medication suddenly discontinued
• Assess eye problems: need for ophthalmic examinations before, during, after treatment (slit lamp, fundoscopy, tonometry)
• Assess allergic reaction: red raised rash; if this occurs, product should be discontinued
• Monitor for toxicity: bone marrow depression, nausea, vomiting, ataxia, diplopia, cardiovascular collapse

### Nursing diagnoses

• Injury, risk for (side effects)
• Knowledge, deficient (teaching)

### Implementation
**PO route**
• Give on empty stomach for best absorption
**Rectal route**
• **IV** sol may be used rectally, 1 ml syringe inserted 3 cm into rectum
• Oral susp may be used rectally (1 mg/ml of product with 1 ml of water), use plastic tube (volume 2.2-3.3 ml)

### Patient/family education

• Teach patient to carry/wear emergency ID card stating patient's name, products taken, condition, physician's name, phone number
• Caution patient to avoid driving, other activities that require alertness
• Caution patient to avoid alcohol ingestion or CNS depressants; increased sedation may occur

Adverse effects: *italic* = common, **bold** = life-threatening

- Teach patient not to discontinue medication quickly after long-term use; taper off over several weeks

### Evaluation
**Positive therapeutic outcome**
- Decreased seizure activity

**Treatment of overdose:** Lavage, activated charcoal, VS, flumazenil, monitor electrolytes

---

**clonidine** 🔵 **(Rx)**
(klon'i-deen)
Apo-Clonidine ✤, Catapres, Catapres-TTS, clonidine HCl, Dixarit ✤, Duraclon, Novo-Clonidine ✤, Nu-Clonidine ✤
*Func. class.:* Antihypertensive, centrally acting analgesic
*Chem. class.:* Centrally acting α-adrenergic agonist

**Pregnancy category** C

**Do not confuse:**
clonidine/Klonopin/clonazepam, Catapres/Cataflam/catarase

**Action:** Inhibits sympathetic vasomotor center in CNS, which reduces impulses in sympathetic nervous system; B/P, pulse rate, cardiac output decreased; prevents pain signal transmission in CNS by α-adrenergic receptor stimulation of the spinal cord

**Therapeutic outcome:** Decreased B/P in hypertension

**Uses:** Mild to moderate hypertension, used alone or in combination; severe pain in cancer patients (epidural)

**Unlabeled uses:** Opioid withdrawal, prevention of vascular headaches, treatment of menopausal symptoms, dysmenorrhea, attention deficit hyperactivity disorder (ADHD), autism, cycloSPORINE nephrotoxicity prophylaxis, diabetic neuropathy, ethanol withdrawal, Tourette's syndrome

**Dosage and routes**
*Hypertension*
*Adult:* PO/TD 0.1 mg bid, then increase by 0.1-0.2 mg/day at weekly intervals, until desired response; range 0.2-0.6 mg/day in divided doses
*Geriatric:* PO 0.1 mg at bedtime, may increase gradually
*Child:* PO 5-10 mcg/kg/day in divided doses q8-12hr, max 0.9 mg/day

*Opioid withdrawal (unlabeled)*
*Adult:* PO 0.3-1.2 mg/day; may decrease by 50% × 3 days then decrease by 0.1-0.2 mg/day or discontinue

*Severe pain*
*Adult:* CONT EPIDURAL INF 30 mcg/hr
*Child:* CONT EPIDURAL INF 0.5 mcg/kg/hr, then titrate to response

*Menopausal symptoms (unlabeled)*
*Adult:* TD 0.1 mg patch q1 wk; PO 0.05-0.4 mg daily

*ADHD/tic disorders in children/ autism (unlabeled)*
*Child:* PO 0.05 mg/kg/day in 3-4 divided doses × 8 wk, max 0.3 mg/day

**Available forms:** Tabs 0.025 ✤, 0.1, 0.2, 0.3 mg; transdermal sys 2.5, 5, 7.5 mg delivering 0.1, 0.2, 0.3 mg/24 hr, respectively; inj 100, 500 mcg/ml

**Adverse effects**
*CNS: Drowsiness, sedation, headache, fatigue,* nightmares, insomnia, mental changes, anxiety, depression, hallucinations, delirium
*CV: Orthostatic hypotension, palpitations,* **CHF,** ECG abnormalities
*EENT:* Taste change, parotid pain
*ENDO:* Hyperglycemia
*GI: Nausea, vomiting, malaise,* constipation, *dry mouth*
*GU:* Impotence, dysuria, *nocturia,* gynecomastia
*INTEG: Rash,* alopecia, facial pallor, pruritus, hives, edema, burning papules, excoriation (TD patches)
*MISC: Withdrawal symptoms*
*MS:* Muscle, joint pain, leg cramps

**Contraindications:** Hypersensitivity; (epidural) bleeding disorders, anticoagulants

**Precautions:** Pregnancy C, breastfeeding, child <12 yr (transdermal), geriatric, MI (recent), diabetes mellitus, chronic renal failure, Raynaud's disease, thyroid disease, depression, COPD, asthma, noncompliant patients

**Pharmacokinetics**

| | |
|---|---|
| **Absorption** | Well absorbed (PO, TD) |
| **Distribution** | Widely distributed; crosses blood-brain barrier |
| **Metabolism** | Liver, extensively |
| **Excretion** | Kidneys, unchanged (30%) |
| **Half-life** | 12-21 hr |

---

## Pharmacodynamics

|  | PO | TD |
|---|---|---|
| **Onset** | ½-1 hr | 3 days |
| **Peak** | 2-4 hr | Unknown |
| **Duration** | 8-12 hr | 8 hr (after removal) |

## Interactions
### Individual drugs
Alcohol: increased CNS depression
Levodopa: decreased levodopa effect
Prazosin: decreased hypotensive effects
Verapamil: AV block
### Drug classifications
Amphetamines, appetite suppressants, MAOIs, tricyclics: decreased hypotensive effects
Anesthetics, opiates, sedatives/hypnotics: increased CNS depression
Antidepressants (tricyclic), β-adrenergic blockers: life-threatening increase in B/P
Diuretics, nitrates: increased hypotensive effects
### Drug/herb
Aconite: increased toxicity, death
Astragalus, capsicum peppers, cola tree, coltsfoot, guarana, khat, licorice: decreased antihypertensive effect
Barberry, betony, black catechu, black cohosh, bloodroot, broom, burdock, cat's claw, dandelion, goldenseal, Irish moss, Jamaican dogwood, kelp, khella, mistletoe, parsley, Queen Anne's lace, rue: increased antihypertensive effect
### Drug/lab test
Increased: blood glucose
Decreased: VMA, urinary catecholamines, aldosterone

## NURSING CONSIDERATIONS
### Assessment
• Assess pain: location, intensity, character, alleviating, aggravation factors, baseline and frequency
• Perform blood studies: neutrophils, decreased platelets
• Perform renal studies: protein, BUN, creatinine; watch for increased levels that may indicate nephrotic syndrome: polyuria, oliguria, frequency
• Monitor baselines for renal/liver function tests before therapy begins; check potassium levels, although hyperkalemia rarely occurs
• Monitor B/P, pulse if the product is being used for hypertension; notify prescriber of changes
• Assess for opiate withdrawal in patients receiving the product for opioid withdrawal, including fever, diarrhea, nausea, vomiting, cramps, insomnia, shivering, dilated pupils, weakness
• Check for edema in feet, legs daily; monitor I&O; check for decreasing output
• Note allergic reaction: rash, fever, pruritus, urticaria; product should be discontinued if antihistamines fail to help
• Note allergic reaction from patches: rash, urticaria, angioedema; should not continue to use
• Assess for symptoms of CHF: edema, dyspnea, wet crackles, B/P, weight gain, report significant changes

### Nursing diagnoses
• Injury, risk for physical (side effects)
• Knowledge, deficient (teaching)
• Noncompliance (teaching)

### Implementation
**PO route**
• Give last dose at bedtime
**Transdermal route**
• Apply patch weekly; remove old patch and wash off residue; apply to site without hair; best absorption over chest or upper arm; rotate sites with each application; clean site before application; apply firmly, especially around edges
• Store patches in cool environment, tabs in tight container

### Patient/family education
• Instruct patient not to discontinue product abruptly, or withdrawal symptoms may occur: anxiety, increased B/P, headache, insomnia, increased pulse, tremors, nausea, sweating
• Caution patient not to use OTC (cough, cold, or allergy) products unless directed by prescriber
• Teach patient to comply with dosage schedule even if feeling better; product controls symptoms, does not cure
• Caution patient to change position slowly, to rise slowly to sitting or standing position to minimize orthostatic hypotension, especially geriatric
• Instruct patient to notify physician of mouth sores, sore throat, fever, swelling of hands or feet, irregular heartbeat, chest pain, signs of angioedema, increased weight
• Teach patient about excessive perspiration, dehydration, vomiting; diarrhea may lead to fall in B/P; consult prescriber if these occur
• Tell patient that product may cause dizziness, fainting; light-headedness may occur during first few days of therapy; use hard candy, saliva product, or frequent rinsing of mouth for dry mouth

Adverse effects: *italic* = common, **bold** = life-threatening

- Advise patient that compliance is necessary; not to skip or stop product unless directed by prescriber
- Teach patient that product may cause skin rash or impaired perspiration
- Teach patient that response may take 2-3 days if product is given TD; instruct on administration of patch; return demonstration
- Teach patient to avoid hazardous activities, since product may cause drowsiness, dizziness
- Teach patient to administer 1 hr before meals

### Evaluation
**Positive therapeutic outcome**
- Decrease in B/P in hypertension
- Decrease in withdrawal symptoms
- Decrease in pain
- Decrease in vascular headaches
- Decrease in dysmenorrhea
- Decrease in menopausal symptoms

**Treatment of overdose:** Supportive treatment; administer tolazoline, atropine, DOPamine prn

---

## clopidogrel (Rx)
(klo-pid'oh-grel)
Plavix
*Func. class.:* Platelet aggregation inhibitor
*Chem. class.:* Thienopyridine derivative

**Pregnancy category** B

**Action:** Inhibits first and second phases of ADP-induced effects in platelet aggregation

**Therapeutic outcome:** Decreased possibility of stroke, MI by decreasing platelet aggregation

**Uses:** Reducing the risk of stroke, MI, peripheral arterial disease in high-risk patients, acute coronary syndrome, transient ischemic attack (TIA), unstable angina

### Dosage and routes
*Recent MI, stroke, peripheral arterial disease*
*Adult:* PO 75 mg daily with or without aspirin

*Acute coronary syndrome*
*Adult:* PO 300 mg then 75 mg daily

**Available forms:** Tabs 75 mg

### Adverse effects
*CNS:* Headache, dizziness, depression, syncope, hyperesthesia, neuralgia
*CV:* Edema, hypertension

*GI:* Nausea, vomiting, diarrhea, GI discomfort, **GI bleeding, pancreatitis**
*GU:* **Glomerulonephritis**
*HEMA:* *Epistaxis,* purpura, **bleeding, neutropenia, aplastic anemia**
*INTEG:* Rash, pruritus
*MISC:* UTI, hypercholesterolemia, chest pain, fatigue, **intracranial hemorrhage, toxic epidermal necrolysis, Stevens-Johnson syndrome**
*MS:* Arthralgia, back pain
*RESP:* Upper respiratory tract infection, dyspnea, rhinitis, bronchitis, cough, **bronchospasm**

**Contraindications:** Hypersensitivity, active bleeding

**Precautions:** Pregnancy **B,** breastfeeding, children, past liver disease, increased bleeding risk, neutropenia, agranulocytosis, renal disease

### Pharmacokinetics
| | |
|---|---|
| **Absorption** | Rapidly absorbed |
| **Distribution** | Unknown |
| **Metabolism** | Liver, extensively, protein binding 95% |
| **Excretion** | Kidneys, unchanged product |
| **Half-life** | 8 hr |

### Pharmacodynamics
| | |
|---|---|
| **Onset** | Unknown |
| **Peak** | 1-3 hr |
| **Duration** | Unknown |

### Interactions
*Individual drugs*
Abciximab, aspirin, eptifibatide, ticlopidine, tirofiban: increased bleeding tendencies
Fluvastatin, phenytoin, tamoxifen, TOLBUTamide, torsemide, warfarin: increased action of each specific product
*Drug classifications*
Anticoagulants, NSAIDs, thrombolytics: increased bleeding tendencies
NSAIDs: increased action of some NSAIDs
*Drug/herb*
Arginine: increased gastric irritation
Bilberry, saw palmetto: decreased clopidogrel effect
Bogbean, dong quai, feverfew, garlic, ginger, ginkgo biloba, green tea, horse chestnut: increased clopidogrel effect
*Drug/lab test*
Increased: AST, ALT, bilirubin, uric acid, total cholesterol, nonprotein nitrogen (NPN)

---

## NURSING CONSIDERATIONS
### Assessment
- Assess for symptoms of stroke, MI during treatment
- Monitor liver function tests: AST, ALT, bilirubin, creatinine if patient is on long-term therapy (4 mo or more)
- Monitor blood studies: CBC, Hct, Hgb, protime, cholesterol if patient is on long-term therapy; thrombocytopenia, neutropenia may occur

### Nursing diagnoses
- Injury, risk for (uses)
- Knowledge, deficient (teaching)

### Implementation
- Give with food to decrease gastric symptoms

### Patient/family education
- Advise patient that blood work will be necessary during treatment
- Advise patient to report any unusual bleeding to prescriber, that it may take longer to stop bleeding
- Instruct patient to take with food or just after eating to minimize GI discomfort
- Caution patient to report diarrhea, skin rashes, subcutaneous bleeding, chills, fever, sore throat
- Teach patient to tell all health care providers that clopidogrel is used

### Evaluation
**Positive therapeutic outcome**
- Absence of stroke

---

## clorazepate (Rx)
(klor-az′e-pate)
APO-Clorazepate ✦, clorazepate, Novo-Clopate ✦, Gen-XENE, Tranxene, Tranxene-SD, Tranxene-SD Half Strength, Tranxene T-tab
*Func. class.:* Antianxiety, anticonvulsant, sedative/hypnotic
*Chem. class.:* Benzodiazepine, long-acting

**Pregnancy category  D**
**Controlled substance schedule  IV**

**Do not confuse:**
clorazapate/clonazepam

**Action:** Potentiates the actions of GABA; especially in limbic system, reticular formation has anticonvulsant effects

**Therapeutic outcome:** Decreased anxiety, restlessness, insomnia

**Uses:** Anxiety, acute alcohol withdrawal, adjunct in seizure disorders

**Unlabeled uses:** Insomnia

### Dosage and routes
*Anxiety*
*Adult:* PO 15-60 mg/day in divided doses or 7.5 mg tid; EXT REL 11.25-22.5 mg at bedtime, do not use EXT REL to initiate therapy
*Geriatric:* PO 7.5 mg daily bid

*Alcohol withdrawal*
*Adult:* PO 30 mg then day 1, 30-60 mg in divided doses; day 2, 45-90 mg in divided doses; day 3, 22.5-45 mg in divided doses; day 4, 15-30 mg in divided doses; then gradually reduce daily dose to 7.5-15 mg

*Seizure disorders*
*Adult and child>12 yr:* PO 7.5 mg tid; may increase by 7.5 mg/wk or less, max 90 mg/day
*Child 9-12 yr:* PO 3.75-7.5 mg bid; may increase by 3.75 mg/wk or less, max 60 mg/day

*Insomnia (unlabeled)*
*Adult:* PO 7.5-15 mg at bedtime
*Geriatric:* PO 3.75-7.5 mg at bedtime, max 15 mg at bedtime

**Available forms:** Tabs 3.75, 7.5, 15 mg; ext rel tab (Tranxene SD Half Strength) 11.25 mg, (Tranxene SD) 22.5 mg

### Adverse effects
*CNS: Dizziness, drowsiness,* confusion, headache, anxiety, tremors, stimulation, fatigue, depression, insomnia, hallucinations, lethargy
*CV: Orthostatic hypotension,* **ECG changes, tachycardia,** hypotension, chest pain
*EENT: Blurred vision,* tinnitus, mydriasis
*GI:* Constipation, dry mouth, nausea, vomiting, anorexia, diarrhea
*INTEG:* Rash, dermatitis, itching

**Contraindications:** Pregnancy **D**, breastfeeding, children <9 yr, hypersensitivity to benzodiazepines, angle-closure glaucoma, psychosis

**Precautions:** Geriatric, debilitated, renal/hepatic disease, suicidal ideation, dependency problems

### Pharmacokinetics

| | |
|---|---|
| **Absorption** | Well absorbed |
| **Distribution** | Widely distributed, crosses placenta, 97% protein binding |
| **Metabolism** | Liver |
| **Excretion** | Kidneys, breast milk |
| **Half-life** | 30-200 hr |

Adverse effects: *italic* = common, **bold** = life-threatening

| Pharmacodynamics | |
|---|---|
| **Onset** | 1 hr |
| **Peak** | 1-2 hr |
| **Duration** | Up to 24 hr |

## Interactions
### Individual drugs
Alcohol: increased CNS depression

Cimetidine, disulfiram, fluoxetine, isoniazid, ketoconazole, propoxyphene, valproic acid: increased effects of clorazepate

Rifampin: decreased action of clorazepate

### Drug classifications
Antidepressants, β-blockers (some), CYP3A4 inhibitors, MAOIs, oral contraceptives: increased clorazepate action

Barbiturates: decreased clorazepate effect

CNS depressants: increased CNS depression

### Drug/herb
Catnip, chamomile, clary, cowslip, kava, mistletoe, nettle, pokeweed, poppy, senega, Queen Anne's lace, St. John's wort, valerian: increased CNS depression

Black cohosh: increased hypotension

### Drug/lab test
Increased: AST/ALT

Decreased: HCT

## NURSING CONSIDERATIONS
### Assessment
• Assess seizures: duration, location, intensity, aura

• Monitor B/P (with patient lying, standing), pulse; if systolic B/P drops 20 mm Hg, hold product, notify prescriber

• Monitor blood studies: CBC during long-term therapy; blood dyscrasias have occurred rarely

• Monitor hepatic studies: AST, ALT, bilirubin, creatinine, LDH, alkaline phosphatase

• Monitor I&O; may indicate renal dysfunction

• Monitor mental status: mood, sensorium, affect, sleeping pattern, drowsiness, dizziness, physical dependency; withdrawal symptoms: headache, nausea, vomiting, muscle pain, weakness after long-term use; suicidal tendencies

### Nursing diagnoses
• Coping, ineffective (uses)

• Knowledge, deficient (teaching)

• Noncompliance (teaching)

### Implementation
• Give with food or milk for GI symptoms

• Give crushed if patient cannot swallow whole (tab only)

• Do not use Tranxene SD to start treatment

• Use sugarless gum, hard candy, frequent sips of water for dry mouth

• Check to see PO medication has been swallowed

### Patient/family education
• Teach patient that product may be taken with food

• Teach patient not to use for everyday stress or longer than 4 mo, unless directed by a prescriber; not to take more than prescribed amount; may be habit forming

• Caution patient to avoid OTC preparations unless approved by a prescriber

• Caution patient to avoid driving, activities that require alertness; drowsiness may occur, especially in geriatric

• Advise patient to avoid alcohol ingestion or other psychotropic medications, unless prescribed

• Advise patient not to discontinue medication abruptly after long-term use; restlessness, insomnia, irritability may occur

• Advise patient to rise slowly or fainting may occur

• Teach patient that drowsiness may worsen at beginning of treatment

### Evaluation
**Positive therapeutic outcome**
• Decreased anxiety, restlessness

• Decreased seizure activity

**Treatment of overdose:** Lavage, VS, supportive care, flumazenil

## clotrimazole topical
*See Appendix D*

## clotrimazole vaginal antifungal
*See Appendix D*

## clozapine (Rx)
(kloz′a-peen)
clozapine, Clozaril, Fazaclo
*Func. class.:* Antipsychotic
*Chem. class.:* Tricyclic dibenzodiazepine derivative

**Pregnancy category B**

**Do not confuse:**
Clozaril/Clinoril/Colazal

**Action:** Interferes with dopamine receptor binding with lack of EPS and tardive dyskinesia; also acts as an adrenergic, cholinergic, histaminergic, serotonergic antagonist

**Therapeutic outcome:** Decreased psychotic behavior

**Uses:** Management of psychotic symptoms in schizophrenic patients for whom other antipsychotics have failed, recurrent suicidal behavior; orally disintegrating tabs are not used for recurrent suicidal behavior

**Unlabeled uses:** Agitation, bipolar disorder, dementia, tremor in Parkinson's disease

**Dosage and routes**
*Adult:* PO 12.5 mg daily or bid; may increase by 25-50 mg/day; normal range 300-450 mg/day after 2 wk; do not increase dosage more than 2 times/wk; do not exceed 900 mg/day; use lowest dosage to control symptoms

*Tremor in Parkinson's disease (unlabeled)*
*Adult:* PO 40 mg at bedtime

*Dementia with multiple behavioral disturbances (unlabeled)*
*Geriatric:* PO 12.5 mg, may increase by 12.5 mg every other day; max 50 mg/day

**Available forms:** Tabs 12.5, 25, 50, 100, 200 mg; orally disintegrating tabs 25, 100 mg

**Adverse effects**
*CNS: Sedation, salivation, dizziness, headache, tremors, sleep problems, akinesia, fever,* **seizures,** *sweating, akathisia, confusion, fatigue, insomnia, depression, slurred speech, anxiety,* **neuroleptic malignant syndrome,** agitation
*CV: Tachycardia, hypo/hypertension,* chest pain, ECG changes, orthostatic hypotension
*EENT:* Blurred vision
*GI: Drooling or excessive salivation, constipation, nausea, abdominal discomfort, vomiting, diarrhea,* anorexia, weight gain, dry mouth, heartburn, dyspepsia, gastroesophageal reflux
*GU: Urinary abnormalities,* incontinence, ejaculation dysfunction, frequency, urgency, retention, dysuria
*HEMA:* **Leukopenia, neutropenia, agranulocytosis, eosinophilia**
*MS:* Weakness; pain in back, neck, legs; spasm; rigidity
*RESP:* Dyspnea, nasal congestion
*OTHER:* Diaphoresis

**Contraindications:** Hypersensitivity, myeloproliferative disorders, severe granulocytopenia (WBC <3500/mm$^3$ before therapy), CNS depression, coma, uncontrolled epilepsy

**Precautions:** Pregnancy **B,** breastfeeding, children <16 yr, geriatric, renal/hepatic/cardiac/CV/pulmonary disease, seizures, prostatic enlargement, angle-closure glaucoma

**C**

### Pharmacokinetics

| | |
|---|---|
| **Absorption** | Well absorbed |
| **Distribution** | Widely distributed; crosses blood-brain barrier, placenta; 95% bound to plasma proteins |
| **Metabolism** | Liver |
| **Excretion** | Kidneys, feces (metabolites) |
| **Half-life** | 8-12 hr |

### Pharmacodynamics

| | |
|---|---|
| **Onset** | Unknown |
| **Peak** | Steady state 7-10 days |
| **Duration** | 4-12 hr |

### Interactions
*Individual drugs*
Alcohol: increased CNS depression
Carbamazepine, omeprazole, phenobarbital, rifampin: decreased clozapine level
Caffeine, citalopram, erythromycin, fluoxetine, fluvoxamine, ketoconazole, risperidone, ritonavir, sertraline: increased clozapine levels
Digoxin: increased plasma concentration of digoxin
Warfarin: increased plasma concentrations
*Drug classifications*
Benzodiazepines: increased hypotension, respiratory, cardiac arrest, collapse
CNS depressants, psychoactives: increased CNS depression
CYP1A2 inducers: decreased clozapine levels
CYP1A2 inhibitors, CYP3A4 inhibitors: increased clozapine level
Highly protein-bound products: increased plasma concentrations
*Drug/herb*
Kava, St. John's wort: increased CNS depression
Cola tree, hops, nettle, nutmeg: increased clozapine action
Betel palm, kava: increased EPS
*Drug/food*
Caffeine: increased clozapine levels
*Drug/lab test*
Increased: liver function tests, cardiac enzymes, cholesterol, blood glucose, bilirubin, PBI, cholinesterase, $^{131}$I
False positive: pregnancy tests, PKU
False negative: urinary steroids, 17-OHCS

Adverse effects: *italic* = common, **bold** = life-threatening

## NURSING CONSIDERATIONS
### Assessment

• Assess mental status: orientation, mood, behavior, presence of hallucinations, and type before initial administration and monthly; this product should significantly reduce psychotic behavior

• Check for swallowing of PO medication; check for hoarding or giving of medication to other patients

• Monitor I&O ratio, palpate bladder if low urinary output occurs, especially in geriatric; urinalysis recommended before, during prolonged therapy

• Monitor bilirubin, CBC, liver function test monthly; discontinue treatment if WBC <3000/mm³ or if ANC <1500/mm³; test qwk; may resume when normal; if WBC <2000/mm³ or ANC <1000/mm³, discontinue

• Assess affect, orientation, LOC, reflexes, gait, coordination, sleep pattern disturbances

• Monitor B/P with patient sitting, standing, and lying; take pulse and respirations q4hr during initial treatment; establish baseline before starting treatment; report drops of 30 mm Hg

• Check for dizziness, faintness, palpitations, tachycardia on rising

• Assess for neuroleptic malignant syndrome: hyperpyrexia, muscle rigidity, increased CPK, altered mental status; product should be discontinued

• Assess for EPS including akathisia (inability to sit still, no pattern to movements), tardive dyskinesia (bizarre movements of the jaw, mouth, tongue, extremities), pseudoparkinsonism (rigidity, tremors, pill rolling, shuffling gate)

• Assess for constipation, urinary retention daily; if these occur, increase bulk, water in diet

### Nursing diagnoses
• Coping, ineffective (uses)
• Knowledge, deficient (teaching)
• Noncompliance (teaching)
• Thought processes, disturbed (uses)

### Implementation
• Decrease dosage in geriatric since metabolism is slowed

• Give with full glass of water, milk; or give with food to decrease GI upset

• Store in tight, light-resistant container; oral sol in amber bottle

• Patient-specific registration is required before administration; if WBC <3500 cells/mm³ or ANC <2000 cells/mm², therapy should not be started

### Patient/family education
• Teach patient to use good oral hygiene; frequent rinsing of mouth, sugarless gum for dry mouth

• Caution patient to avoid hazardous activities until product response is determined

• Inform patient that orthostatic hypotension occurs often and to rise from sitting or lying position gradually

• Caution patient to avoid hot tubs, hot showers, tub baths, since hypotension may occur

• Teach patient to avoid OTC preparations (cough, hay fever, cold) unless approved by prescriber, since serious product interactions may occur; avoid use with alcohol, CNS depressants; increased drowsiness may occur

• Teach patient about EPS and necessity of meticulous oral hygiene, since oral candidiasis may occur

• Teach patient to report sore throat, malaise, fever, bleeding, mouth sores; if these occur, CBC should be performed and product discontinued

• Advise patient that in hot weather, heat stroke may occur; take extra precautions to stay cool

• Teach patient symptoms of agranulocytosis and need for blood test qwk for 6 mo, then q2 wk; report flulike symptoms

### Evaluation
**Positive therapeutic outcome**
• Decrease in emotional excitement, hallucinations, delusions, paranoia
• Reorganization of patterns of thought, speech

### Treatment of anaphylaxis: Withdraw product, maintain airway; if diabetic, check blood glucose levels

---

## codeine ⊚ (Rx)
(koe'deen)
Paveral ✦
*Func. class.:* Opiate, phenanthrene derivative

### Pregnancy category  C
### Controlled substance schedule II, III, IV, V (depends on route)

### Do not confuse:
codeine/Lodine/Iodine/Cardene

### Action: Depresses pain impulse transmission at the spinal cord level by interacting with opioid receptors; decreases cough reflex, GI motility

---

 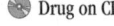

**Therapeutic outcome:** Pain relief, decreased cough, decreased diarrhea depending on route

**Uses:** Moderate to severe pain, nonproductive cough

**Unlabeled uses:** Diarrhea

**Dosage and routes**
*Pain*
*Adult:* PO 15-60 mg q4hr prn; IM/SUBCUT 15-60 mg q4hr prn
*Child:* PO 3 mg/kg/day in divided doses q4hr prn

*Cough*
*Adult:* PO 10-20 mg q4-6hr, not to exceed 120 mg/day
*Child:* PO 1-1.5 mg/kg/day in 4 divided doses, not to exceed 60 mg/day

*Renal dose*
*Adult:* PO CCr 10-50 ml/min 75% of dose; CCr <10 ml/min 50% of dose

*Diarrhea (unlabeled)*
*Adult:* PO 30 mg; may repeat qid prn

**Available forms:** Inj tab 30, 60 mg; tabs 15, 30, 60 mg; inj 15, 30 mg/ml

**Adverse effects**
*CNS: Drowsiness, sedation,* dizziness, agitation, dependency, lethargy, restlessness, euphoria, **seizures,** hallucinations, headache, confusion
*CV:* Bradycardia, palpitations, orthostatic hypotension, tachycardia, **circulatory collapse**
*GI: Nausea, vomiting, anorexia, constipation,* dry mouth
*GU:* Urinary retention
*INTEG:* Flushing, rash, urticaria, pruritus
*RESP:* **Respiratory depression, respiratory paralysis,** dyspnea
*SYST:* Anaphylaxis

**Contraindications:** Hypersensitivity to opiates, respiratory depression, increased intracranial pressure, seizure disorders, severe respiratory disorders, breastfeeding

**Precautions:** Pregnancy **C,** geriatric, cardiac dysrhythmias, prostatic hypertrophy, bowel impacton

**Pharmacokinetics**

| | |
|---|---|
| **Absorption** | Bioavailability 60%-90% |
| **Distribution** | Widely distributed; crosses placenta |
| **Metabolism** | Liver, extensively |
| **Excretion** | Kidneys (up to 15%), breast milk |
| **Half-life** | 3-4 hr |

**Pharmacodynamics**

| | PO | IM | SUBCUT |
|---|---|---|---|
| **Onset** | 30-60 min | 30-60 min | 15-30 min |
| **Peak** | 1-2 hr | 30-60 min | Unknown |
| **Duration** | 4 hr | 4 hr | 4 hr |

**Interactions**
*Individual drugs*
Alcohol: increased CNS depression
*Drug classifications*
Antipsychotics, CYP2D6, opiates, sedative/hypnotics, skeletal muscle relaxants: increased CNS depression
MAOIs: increased toxicity; use cautiously
*Drug/herb*
Corkwood: increased anticholinergic effects
Gotu kola, Jamaican dogwood, kava, lavender, mistletoe, nettle, pokeweed, poppy, senega, valerian: increased CNS depression
St. John's wort: decreased codeine level
*Drug/lab test*
Increased: amylase, lipase

**NURSING CONSIDERATIONS**
**Assessment**
• Assess pain: intensity, type, alleviating factors
• Assess GI function: nausea, vomiting, constipation
• Assess cough: type, duration, ability to raise secretion; for productive cough; do not use to suppress a productive cough
• Monitor VS after parenteral route; note muscle rigidity, product history, renal/hepatic function tests, respiratory dysfunction: respiratory depression, character, rate, rhythm; notify prescriber if respirations are <10/min
• Monitor CNS changes: dizziness, drowsiness, hallucinations, euphoria, LOC, pupil reaction
• Monitor allergic reactions: rash, urticaria

**Nursing diagnoses**
• Breathing pattern, ineffective (adverse reactions)
• Knowledge, deficient (teaching)
• Pain, acute (uses)
• Sensory perception, disturbed (adverse reactions)

**Implementation**
• Give with antiemetic if nausea, vomiting occur
• Administer when pain is beginning to return, determine dosage interval by patient response; continuous dosing of medication is more effective given prn; explain analgesic effect

Adverse effects: *italic* = common, **bold** = life-threatening

- Medication should be slowly withdrawn after long-term use to prevent withdrawal symptoms
- Store in light-resistant container at room temp

**PO route**
- May be given with food or milk to lessen GI upset

**IM/SUBCUT route**
- Do not give if cloudy, or a precipitate has formed

**IV route**
- Give slowly by direct inj

*Syringe compatibilities:* Glycopyrrolate, hydrOXYzine

*Y-site compatibilities:* Cefmetazole

*Additive incompatibilities:* Aminophylline, amobarbital, chlorothiazide, heparin, methicillin, pentobarbital, phenobarbital, phenytoin, secobarbital, thiopental

**Patient/family education**
- Teach patient to report any symptoms of CNS changes, allergic reactions; to avoid CNS depressants: alcohol, sedative/hypnotics for at least 24 hr after taking this product
- Discuss with patient that dizziness, drowsiness, and confusion are common
- Advise patient to avoid getting up without assistance
- Discuss in detail with patient all aspects of the product
- Advise patient not to breastfeed

**Evaluation**
**Positive therapeutic outcome**
- Decreased pain
- Decreased cough
- Decreased diarrhea

**Treatment of overdose:** Naloxone 0.4 ampule diluted in 10 ml 0.9% NaCl and given by direct IV push 0.02 mg q2min (adult)

---

**colchicine** 🔵 (Rx)
(kol'chi-seen)
Colsalide
*Func. class.:* Antigout agent
*Chem. class.: Colchicum autumnale* alkaloid

**Pregnancy category**
C **(PO),** D **(IV)**

**Action:** Inhibits microtubule formation of lactic acid in leukocytes, which decreases phagocytosis and inflammation in joints

**Therapeutic outcome:** Decreased pain, inflammation of joints

**Uses:** Gout, gouty arthritis (prevention, treatment); to arrest progression of neurologic disability in multiple sclerosis

**Unlabeled uses:** Hepatic cirrhosis, familial Mediterranean fever, pericarditis, amyloidosis, Behçet's syndrome, biliary cirrhosis, dermatitis herpetiformis, idiopathic thrombocytopenic purpura, Paget's disease, pseudogout, pulmonary fibrosis

**Dosage and routes**
*Gout prevention*
*Adult:* PO 0.6-1.8 mg daily depending on severity; **IV** 0.5-1 mg daily-bid

*Gout treatment*
*Adult:* PO 0.6-1.2 mg, then 0.5-1.2 mg q1hr, until pain decreases or side effects occur; **IV** 2 mg, then 0.5 mg q6hr, not to exceed 4 mg/24 hr

*Renal dose*
*Adult:* PO/**IV** CCr 10-50 ml/min, reduce by 50%

**Available forms:** Tabs 0.5, 0.6, 1 🍁 mg; inj 0.5 mg/ml in 2 ml ampule

**Adverse effects**
*GI:* Nausea, vomiting, anorexia, malaise, metallic taste, cramps, peptic ulcer, diarrhea
*GU:* Hematuria, **oliguria, renal damage**
*HEMA:* **Agranulocytosis, thrombocytopenia, aplastic anemia, pancytopenia**
*INTEG:* Chills, dermatitis, pruritus, purpura, erythema
*MISC:* Myopathy, alopecia, reversible azoospermia, peripheral neuritis

**Contraindications:** Pregnancy **D (IV)**, hypersensitivity; serious GI disorders, severe renal/hepatic/cardiac disorders

**Precautions:** Pregnancy **C** (PO), breastfeeding, children, geriatric, blood dyscrasias, hepatic disease

| Pharmacokinetics | |
|---|---|
| **Absorption** | Well absorbed |
| **Distribution** | WBCs |
| **Metabolism** | Deacetylates in liver |
| **Excretion** | Feces (metabolites/active product) |
| **Half-life** | 4.4 hr |

| Pharmacodynamics | |
|---|---|
| | PO |
| **Onset** | Unknown |
| **Peak** | ½-2 hr |
| **Duration** | Unknown |

## Interactions
### Individual drugs
CycloSPORINE, radiation: increased bone marrow depression

Clarithromycin, cycloSPORINE, erithromycin: toxicity

Ethanol: increased GI effects

Vitamin $B_{12}$: decreased action of vit $B_{12}$; may cause reversible malabsorption

### Drug classifications
Bone marrow depressants: increased bone marrow depression

NSAIDs: increased GI effects

### Drug/lab test
Increased: alkaline phosphatase, AST

False positive: urine, RBC, Hgb

Interference: urinary 17-hydroxycorticosteroids

## NURSING CONSIDERATIONS
### Assessment
• Assess pain and mobility of joints, uric acid levels returning to normal

• Monitor I&O ratio; observe for decrease in urinary output; CBC, platelets, reticulocytes before, during therapy (q3 mo), may cause aplastic anemia, agranulocytosis, decreased platelets

• Assess for toxicity: weakness, abdominal pain, nausea, vomiting, diarrhea

### Nursing diagnoses
• Knowledge, deficient (teaching)
• Mobility, impaired physical (uses)
• Pain, chronic (uses)

### Implementation
**PO route**
• Give with food for GI symptoms

**IV route**
• Give **IV** undiluted or diluted 1 mg/10-20 ml normal saline or sterile water for inj; give over 2-5 min; avoid surrounding area as tissue damage may occur

• Do not give IM or SUBCUT

• Do not dilute in $D_5W$ or change in **IV** line that is running or contains $D_5W$

• Wait ≥1 wk after giving a full course of **IV** colchicine before giving more doses

### Patient/family education
• Caution patient to avoid alcohol, OTC preparations that contain alcohol

• Instruct patient to report any pain, redness, or hard area, usually in legs; rash, sore throat, fever, bleeding, bruising, weakness, numbness, tingling

• Teach patient importance of complying with medical regimen (diet, weight loss,

product therapy); bone marrow depression may occur

### Evaluation
**Positive therapeutic outcome**
• Decreased stone formation on x-ray
• Decreased pain in kidney region
• Absence of hematuria
• Decreased pain in joints

**Treatment of overdose:** D/C medication, may need opioids to treat diarrhea

---

### colesevelam (Rx)
(coal-see-vel'am)

Welchol

*Func. class.:* Antilipemic
*Chem. class.:* Bile acid sequestrant

**Pregnancy category** C

**Action:** Absorbs, combines with bile acids to form insoluble complex that is excreted through feces; loss of bile acids lowers cholesterol levels

**Therapeutic outcome:** Decreasing LDL cholesterol

**Uses:** Elevated LDL cholesterol, alone or in combination with HMG-CoA reductase inhibitor

### Dosage and routes
*Monotherapy*
*Adult:* PO 3 625 mg tabs bid with meals or 6 tabs daily with a meal; may increase to 7 tabs if needed

*Combination therapy*
*Adult:* PO 3 tabs bid with meals or 6 tabs daily with a meal given with an HMG-CoA reductase inhibitor

**Available forms:** Tabs 625 mg

### Adverse effects
*CNS:* Headache, dizziness, drowsiness, vertigo, tinnitus

*GI: Constipation, abdominal pain, nausea,* fecal impaction, hemorrhoids, flatulence, vomiting, steatorrhea, peptic ulcer

*HEMA:* Decreased red cell folate content; **bleeding,** decreased pro-time

*INTEG:* Rash, irritation of perianal area, tongue, skin

*META:* Decreased vit A, D, K, **hyperchloremic acidosis**

*MS:* Muscle, joint pain

**Contraindications:** Hypersensitivity, biliary obstruction; dysphagia, bowel disease, primary biliary cirrhosis, triglycerides >300 mg/dl, fat-soluble vitamin deficiency

**Precautions:** Pregnancy **C**, breastfeeding, children

Pharmacokinetics

| | |
|---|---|
| **Absorption** | Unknown |
| **Distribution** | Unknown |
| **Metabolism** | Unknown |
| **Excretion** | Feces |
| **Half-life** | Unknown |

Pharmacodynamics
LDL decreased in 4-7 days

## Interactions
*Individual drugs*
Clindamycin, digoxin, diltiazem, gemfibrozil, glipiZIDE, iron, mycophenolate, penicillin G, phenytoin, propanolol, warfarin: decreased absorption of each specific product
Corticosteroid: decreased corticosteroid action
Thyroid hormones: decreased absorption of thyroid
*Drug classifications*
Tetracyclines: decreased absorption of tetracyclines
Thiazides: decreased absorption of thiazides
Vitamins (fat-soluble): decreased absorption of fat-soluble vitamins
*Drug/herb*
Glucomannan: increased effect
Gotu kola: decreased effect
*Drug/lab test*
Increased: liver function tests

## NURSING CONSIDERATIONS
### Assessment
• Assess cardiac glycoside level if both products are being administered
• Assess for signs of vit A, D, K deficiency
• Monitor fasting LDL, HDL, total cholesterol, triglyceride levels, electrolytes if on extended therapy
• Monitor bowel pattern daily; increase bulk, $H_2O$ in diet for constipation

### Nursing diagnoses
• Constipation (adverse reactions)
• Knowledge, deficient (teaching)
• Noncompliance (teaching)

### Implementation
• Give product daily; bid with meals; give all other medications 1 hr before colesevelam or 4 hr after colesevelam to avoid poor absorption, take with liquid

• Give supplemental doses of vit A, D, K, if levels are low

### Patient/family education
◆ Teach the symptoms of hypoprothrombinemia: bleeding mucous membranes, dark tarry stools, hematuria, petechiae; report immediately
• Teach the importance of compliance; toxicity may result if doses missed
• Teach that risk factors should be decreased: high-fat diet, smoking, alcohol consumption, absence of exercise
• Advise not to discontinue suddenly

### Evaluation
**Positive therapeutic outcome**
• Decreased cholesterol level (hyperlipidemia); diarrhea, pruritus (excess bile acids)

## colestipol (Rx)
(koe-les'ti-pole)
Colestid
*Func. class.:* Antilipemic
*Chem. class.:* Bile acid sequestrant

**Pregnancy category B**

**Action:** Absorbs, combines with bile acids to form an insoluble complex that is excreted through feces; loss of bile acids lowers cholesterol levels

**Therapeutic outcome:** Decreasing cholesterol levels and low-density lipoproteins, decreased pruritus

**Uses:** Primary hypercholesterolemia, xanthomas

**Unlabeled uses:** Digoxin toxicity/overdose, pruritus, diarrhea due to increased bile acids after surgery

### Dosage and routes
*Adult:* PO tabs 2 g daily-bid, may increase by 1 g/mo, max 16 g/day; GRANULES 5 g daily-bid, may increase qmo, max 30 g/day

**Available forms:** Granules 300, 450 g, 500 g bottles; 5 g colestipol/7.5 g powder; tabs 1 g

### Adverse effects
*GI: Constipation, abdominal pain, nausea,* fecal impaction, hemorrhoids, flatulence, vomiting, steatorrhea, peptic ulcer
*HEMA:* **Bleeding, increased pro-time**
*INTEG: Rash,* irritation of perianal area, tongue, skin

*META:* Decreased vit A, D, E, K, red folate content; **hyperchloremic acidosis**

**Contraindications:** Hypersensitivity, biliary obstruction

**Precautions:** Pregnancy **B,** breastfeeding, children, bleeding disorders

Pharmacokinetics

| | |
|---|---|
| **Absorption** | Not absorbed |
| **Distribution** | Not distributed |
| **Metabolism** | Not metabolized |
| **Excretion** | Binds with bile acids, feces |
| **Half-life** | Unknown |

Pharmacodynamics

| | |
|---|---|
| **Onset** | 24-48 hr |
| **Peak** | 30 days |
| **Duration** | 30 days |

### Interactions
*Individual drugs*
Clindamycin, digoxin, gemfibrozil, glipiZIDE, iron, penicillin G, propranolol, tetracycline, thyroid agents, warfarin: decreased action of each specific product
Phenytoin, TOLBUTamide: decreased effect of each specific product
*Drug classifications*
Diuretics (thiazide): decreased absorption
Corticosteroids: decreased corticosteroid action
Vitamins A, D, E, K: decreased absorption
*Drug/herb*
Glucomannan: increased effect
Gotu kola: decreased effect
*Drug/lab test*
Increased: Cl, $PO_4$, AST, ALT, alkaline phosphatase
Decreased: Na, K, Ca

### NURSING CONSIDERATIONS
**Assessment**
• Assess nutrition: fat, protein, carbohydrates; nutritional analysis should be completed by dietitian
• Assess skin integrity after patient has been receiving product; itching, pruritus often occur from bile deposits on skin
• Monitor cardiac glycoside level, if both products are being administered; cardiac glycoside levels will be decreased
• Monitor for signs of vit A, D, E, K deficiency; check serum cholesterol, triglyceride levels, electrolytes if on extended therapy
• Monitor bowel pattern daily; increase bulk, water in diet if constipation develops

### Nursing diagnoses
• Constipation (adverse reactions)
• Knowledge, deficient (teaching)
• Noncompliance (teaching)

### Implementation
• Swallow tabs whole; do not break, crush, or chew
• Give product daily or bid; give all other medications 1 hr before or 4 hr after colestipol to avoid poor absorption; give product mixed with applesauce or stirred into beverage (2-6 oz), let stand for 2 min; rinse glass to make sure all medication is taken; do not take dry
• Provide supplemental doses of vit A, D, E, K, if levels are low

### Patient/family education
◗ Teach patient symptoms of hypoprothrombinemia: bleeding mucous membranes, dark, tarry stools, hematuria, petechiae; report immediately
• Teach patient importance of compliance, not to miss or double doses
• Teach patient that risk factors should be decreased: high-fat diet, smoking, alcohol consumption, absence of exercise
• Tell patient to mix product with 6 oz of milk, water, fruit juice; may be mixed with carbonated beverages; rinse glass to make sure all medication is taken or may mix product in applesauce; allow to stand for 2 min before mixing

### Evaluation
**Positive therapeutic outcome**
• Decreased cholesterol level (hyperlipidemia)

---

**conivaptan** (Rx)
(kon-ih-vap'-tan)
Vaprisol
*Func. class.:* Vasopressin receptor antagonist

**Pregnancy category C**

**Action:** Dual arginine vasopressin (AVP) antagonist with affinity for $V_{1A}$, $V_2$ receptors; level of circulating AVP in circulating blood is critical for regulation of water, electrolyte balance and is usually elevated in euvolemic/hypervolemic hyponatremia

**Therapeutic outcome:** Correct serum sodium levels

---

Adverse effects: *italic* = common, **bold** = life-threatening

**Uses:** Euvolemia hyponatremia in those hospitalized, not indicated for CHF, hypervolemia, hyponatremia

## Dosage and routes
*Adult:* **IV** INF loading dose 20 mg given over 30 min, then CONT **IV** over 24 hr; after 1 day, give for an additional 1-3 days as a CONT INF of 20 mg/day total, can be titrated up to 40 mg/day if serum sodium is not rising at the desired rate; max time 4 days

**Available forms:** 5 mg/ml (20 mg) in single use ampule

## Adverse effects
*CNS:* Headache, confusion, insomnia
*CV:* **Atrial fibrillation,** hypo/hypertension, orthostatic hypotension, phlebitis
*GI:* Nausea, vomiting, constipation, dry mouth
*GU:* Hematuria, polyuria, UTI, pollakiuria
*HEMA:* Anemia
*INTEG:* Erythema, inj site reaction
*META:* Dehydration, hypo/hyperglycemia, hypokalemia, hypomagnesia, hyponatremia
*MISC:* Oral candidiasis, pain, peripheral edema, pneumonia

**Contraindications:** Hypersensitivity, hypovolemia

**Precautions:** Pregnancy **C,** breastfeeding, orthostatic/renal disease

### Pharmacokinetics
| | |
|---|---|
| **Absorption** | Unknown |
| **Distribution** | Protein binding 99% |
| **Metabolism** | By CYP3A4 |
| **Excretion** | Unknown |
| **Half-life** | Terminal 5 hr |

### Pharmacodynamics
Unknown

## Interactions
*Individual drugs*
Digoxin: decreased plasma concentration of conivaptan
*Drug classifications*
CYP3A4 inhibitors: increased plasma concentrations of conivaptan

## NURSING CONSIDERATIONS
### Assessment
• Monitor renal/hepatic function
• Assess frequent sodium volume status; overly rapid correction of sodium concentration (>12 mEq/L per 24 hr) may result in osmotic demyelination syndrome
• Assess neurologic status: confusion, headache

• Assess CV status: atrial fibrillation, hyper/hypotension, orthostatic hypotension; monitor B/P, pulse
• Monitor other electrolytes (magnesium and potassium)

### Nursing diagnoses
• Injury, risk for (uses)
• Knowledge, deficient (teaching)

### Implementation
**IV route**
• Withdraw 4 ml (20 mg) of conivaptan, add to 100 ml D$_5$W, gently invert several times to mix, give over 30 min
**Continuous IV infusion route**
• Withdraw 4 ml (20 mg) of conivaptan, add to 250 ml D$_5$W, gently invert several times to mix, give over 24 hr; or 40 mg in 250 ml D$_5$W, gently invert several times to mix, give over 24 hr

### Patient/family education
• Advise patient to avoid pregnancy, breastfeeding while taking this product
• Advise patient to report neurologic changes: headache, insomnia, confusion
• Teach patient administration procedure and expected result
• Advise patient to report inj site pain, redness, swelling

### Evaluation
**Positive therapeutic outcome**
• Correction of serum sodium levels

---

## CONTRACEPTIVES, HORMONAL

### MONOPHASIC, ORAL
**ethinyl estradiol/
desogestrel** (Rx)
Apri, Cesia, Desogen, Kariva, Mircette, Ortho-Cept, Reclipsen, Solia, Velivet
**ethinyl estradiol/
drospirenone** (Rx)
Yasmin, Yaz 28
**ethinyl estradiol/
ethynodiol** (Rx)
Demulen, Demulen 1/35, Kelnor 1/35, Zovia
**ethinyl estradiol/
levonorgestrel** (Rx)
Alesse, Aviane-28, Enpresse, Jolessa, Lessina, Levlen, Levlite, Levora, Lutera, Nordette, Portia, Quasense, Seasonique, Sronyx

---

 Alert     Canada Only    🝆 Drug on CD    * "Tall Man" lettering (See Preface)

C

**ethinyl estradiol/ norethindrone** (Rx)
Brevicon, Genora 0.5/35, Genora 1/35, Junel 21 1/20, Junel 21 1.5/20, Loestrin 21 1.5/30, Loestrin 21 1/20, Microgestin, Modicon, N.E.E 1/35, Nelova 0.5/35E, Nelova 1/35E, Norcept-E 1/35, Norethin 1/35E, Norinyl 1+35, Norlestrin 1/50, Norlestrin 2.5/50, Nortrel, Ortho-Novum 1/35, Ovcon 35, Ovcon 50

**ethinyl estradiol/ norgestimate** (Rx)
MonoNessa, Ortho-Cyclen, Previfem, Sprintec

**ethinyl estradiol/ norgestrel** (Rx)
Cryselle, Lo/Ovral, Low-Ogestrel, Ogestrel, Ovral

**mestranol/ norethindrone** (Rx)
Genora 1/50, Nelova 1/50m, Norethin 1/50m, Norinyl 1+50, Ortho-Novum 1/50

## BIPHASIC, ORAL
**ethinyl estradiol/ norethindrone** (Rx)
Nelova 10/11, Ortho-Novum 10/11

## TRIPHASIC, ORAL
**ethinyl estradiol/ desogestrel** (Rx)
Cyclessa

**ethinyl estradiol/ norethindrone** (Rx)
Necor 7/7/7, Nortrel 7/7/7, Ortho-Novum 7/7/7, Tri-Norinyl

**ethinyl estradiol/ norgestimate** (Rx)
Ortho Tri-Cyclen, Ortho Tri-Cyclen Lo

**ethinyl estradiol/ levonorgestrel** (Rx)
Enpresse, Portia, Tri-Levlen, Triphasil

## EXTENDED CYCLE, ORAL
**ethinyl estradiol/ levonorgestrel** (Rx)
Seasonale

## PROGESTIN, ORAL
**norethindrone** (Rx)
Errin, Ortho Micronor, Camila, Jolivette, Nor-Q D

## PROGRESSIVE ESTROGEN, ORAL
**ethinyl estradiol/ norethindrone acetate** (Rx)
Estrostep, Estrostep Fe

## EMERGENCY
**levonorgestrel/ethinyl estradiol** (Rx)
Preven
**levonorgestrel** (Rx)
Plan B
**medroxyprogesterone** (Rx)
Depo-Provera

## INTRAUTERINE
**levonorgestrel** (Rx)
Mirena

## IMPLANT
**etonogestrel** (Rx)
Implanon

## VAGINAL RING
**ethinyl estradiol/ etonogestrel** (Rx)
Nuva Ring

## TRANSDERMAL
**ethinyl estradiol/ norelgestromin** (Rx)
Ortho Evra

**Action:** Prevents ovulation by suppressing FSH, LH; *monophasic:* estrogen/progestin (fixed dose) used during a 21-day cycle; ovulation is inhibited by suppression of FSH and LH; thickness of cervical mucus and endometrial lining prevents pregnancy; *biphasic:* ovulation is inhibited by suppression of FSH and LH; alteration of cervical mucus, endometrial lining prevents pregnancy; *triphasic:* ovulation is inhibited by suppression of FSH and LH; change of cervical mucus, endometrial lining prevents pregnancy; variable doses of estrogen/progestin combinations may be similar to natural hormonal fluctuations; *extended cycle:* estrogen/progestin continuous for 84 days, off for 7 days, result 4 menstrual periods/yr; *progressive estrogen:* constant progestin with 3 progressive doses of estrogen; *progestin-only pill, implant, intrauterine:* change of cervical mucus and endometrial lining prevents pregnancy; ovulation may be suppressed

Adverse effects: *italic* = common, **bold** = life-threatening

**Therapeutic outcome:** Prevention of pregnancy, decreased severity of endometriosis, hypermenorrhea

**Uses:** To prevent pregnancy, regulation of menstrual cycle, treatment of acne in women over 14 yr that other treatment has failed, emergency contraception; *injection:* inhibits gonadotropin secretion, ovulation, follicular maturation; *emergency:* inhibits ovulation and fertilization, decreases transport of sperm and egg from fallopian tube to uterus; *vaginal ring, transdermal:* inhibits ovulation, prevents sperm entry into uterus; *antiacne:* may decrease sex hormone binding globulin, results in decreased testosterone

## Dosage and routes
### Monophasic
*Adult:* PO Take first tab on Sunday after start of menses × 21 days; skip 7 days; then repeat cycle; start on 1st day of menses × 21 days; skip 7 days, then repeat cycle; may contain 7 placebo tabs, where 1 tab is taken daily

### Biphasic
*Adult:* PO Take 10 days of small progestin, then large progestin; estrogen is the same during cycle; skip 7 days, then repeat cycle; may contain 7 placebo tabs, where 1 tab is taken daily

### Triphasic
*Adult:* PO Estrogen dose remains constant, progestin changes throughout 21 day cycle, some products contain 28 tabs per month

### Extended cycle
*Adult:* PO Start taking on first day of menses; continue for 84 days of active tab, then 7 days of placebo; repeat cycle

### Progestin
*Adult:* PO Start on 1st day of menses, then daily and continuously

### Progressive estrogen
*Adult:* PO Progestin dose remains constant, estrogen increases q7days throughout 21-day cycle, may include 7 placebo tabs for 28-day cycle

### Emergency
*Adult and adolescent:* Give within 72 hr of intercourse, repeat 12 hr later; Plan B 1 tab, then 1 tab 12 hr later; Preven 2 tab, then 2 tab 12 hr later; Ovral (unlabeled) 2 white tabs; Lo/Ovral (unlabeled) 4 white tabs; Levlen (unlabeled), Nordette (unlabeled) 4 orange tabs; Triphasil (unlabeled), Tri-Levlen (unlabeled) 4 yellow tabs

### Injectable
*Adult:* IM (Depo-Provera) 150 mg within 5 days of start of menses, or within 5 days postpartum (must not be breastfeeding); if breastfeeding, give 6 wk postpartum, repeat q3 mo

### Intrauterine
*Adult:* To be inserted using the levonorgestrel releasing intrauterine system (LRIS) by those trained in procedure; inserted into uterine cavity within 7 days of the onset of menstruation; use should not exceed 5 years per implant

### Vaginal ring
*Adult:* VAG Insert 1 ring on or prior to day 5 of cycle, leave in place 3 wk; remove for 1 wk, then repeat

### Transdermal
*Adult:* TRANSDERMAL Apply patch within 7 days of menses, change weekly × 3 wk; no patch wk 4, repeat cycle

### Implant
*Adult:* SUBDERMAL In inner side of upper arm on days 1-5 of menses, replace q3 yr

### Acne
*Adult:* PO (Ortho Tri-Cyclen) Take daily × 21 days, off 7 days

## Adverse effects
*CNS:* Depression, fatigue, dizziness, nervousness, anxiety, headache
*CV:* Increased B/P, **cerebral hemorrhage, thrombosis, pulmonary embolism,** fluid retention, edema
*EENT:* Optic neuritis, retinal thrombosis, cataracts
*ENDO:* Decreased glucose tolerance, increased TBG, PBI, $T_4$, $T_3$
*GI:* *Nausea,* vomiting, cramps, diarrhea, bloating, constipation, change in appetite, **cholestatic jaundice**
*GU:* Breakthrough bleeding, amenorrhea, spotting, dysmenorrhea, galactorrhea, endocervical hyperplasia, vaginitis, cystitis-like syndrome, breast change
*HEMA:* Increased fibrinogen, clotting factor
*INTEG: Chloasma, melasma,* acne, rash, urticaria, erythema, pruritus, hirsutism, alopecia, photosensitivity

**Contraindications:** Pregnancy **X**, breastfeeding, women 40 yr and over, reproductive cancer, thrombophlebitis, MI, hepatic tumors, hepatic disease, CAD, CVA

**Precautions:** Depression, hypertension, renal disease, seizure disorders, lupus erythematosus, rheumatic disease, migraine headache, amenorrhea, irregular menses, breast cancer (fibrocystic), gallbladder disease, diabetes mellitus, heavy smoking, acute mononucleosis, sickle cell disease

### Pharmacokinetics

| | |
|---|---|
| **Absorption** | Unknown |
| **Distribution** | Unknown |
| **Metabolism** | Unknown |
| **Excretion** | Breast milk |
| **Half-life** | Unknown |

### Pharmacodynamics
Unknown

## Interactions
### Individual drugs
Griseofulvin, rifampin: decreased effectiveness of oral contraceptive
### Drug classifications
Analgesics, antibiotics, anticonvulsants, antihistamines: decreased action of oral contraceptives
Anticoagulants (oral): decreased action of oral anticoagulants
### Drug/herb
Alfalfa, black cohosh, chaste tree: altered action
Saw palmetto, St. John's wort: decreased oral contraceptive effect
### Drug/food
Grapefruit juice: increased peak level
### Drug/lab test
Increased: pro-time; clotting factors VII, VIII, IX, X; TBG, PBI, $T_4$, platelet aggregation, BSP, triglycerides, bilirubin, AST, ALT
Decreased: $T_3$, antithrombin III, folate, metyrapone test, GTT, 17-OHCS

## NURSING CONSIDERATIONS
### Assessment
• Assess for reproductive changes: change in breasts, tumors, positive Pap smear; product should be discontinued if changes occur
• Monitor glucose, thyroid function, liver function tests, B/P

### Nursing diagnoses
• Body image, disturbed (adverse reactions)
• Injury, risk for (adverse reactions)
• Knowledge, deficient (teaching)
• Noncompliance (teaching)

### Implementation
#### PO route
• If GI symptoms occur, medication may be taken with food; take at same time each day

#### Implant route
• Inject 6 cap subdermally
• Implant is effective for 5 yr, should be removed after that
#### IM route
• Administer inj deep in large muscle mass after shaking susp well; ensure pregnancy has not occurred if inj are 2 wk or more apart

### Patient/family education
• Teach patient about detection of clots using Homans' sign; teach monitoring technique for heat, redness, pain, swelling
• Teach patient to use sunscreen or to avoid sunlight; photosensitivity can occur
• Teach patient to take at same time each day to ensure equal product level; to take another tab as soon as possible if one is missed
• Teach patient that after product is discontinued, pregnancy may not occur for several mo
• Instruct patient to report GI symptoms that occur after 4 mo
• Advise patient to use another birth control method during first 3 wk of oral contraceptive use
• Teach patient to report abdominal pain, change in vision, shortness of breath, change in menstrual flow, spotting, breakthrough bleeding, breast lumps, swelling, headache, severe leg pain, mental changes; that continuing medical care is needed: Pap smear and gynecologic exam q6 mo
• Teach patient to notify physicians and dentist of oral contraceptive use

### Evaluation
#### Positive therapeutic outcome
• Absence of pregnancy
• Decreased severity of endometriosis
• Decreased severity of hypermenorrhea

---

## cortisone  (Rx)
(kor'ti-sone)
Cortone ✦, cortone acetate
*Func. class.:* Corticosteroid, synthetic
*Chem. class.:* Short-acting glucocorticoid
**Pregnancy category D**

---

**Action:** Decreases inflammation by suppression of migration of polymorphonuclear leukocytes, fibroblasts, reversal of increased capillary permeability, and lysosomal stabilization; suppresses adrenal function with long-term use

**Therapeutic outcome:** Replacement of cortisol in adrenal insufficiency

**Uses:** Inflammation, severe allergy, adrenal insufficiency, collagen disorders, respiratory and dermatologic, rheumatic disorders

### Dosage and routes
*Adult:* PO 25-300 mg daily or q2 days, titrated to patient response
*Child:* PO 0.7-10 mg/kg/day

### Available forms: Tabs 25 mg

### Adverse effects
*CNS: Depression, flushing, sweating,* headache, mood changes
*CV: Hypertension,* **circulatory collapse, thrombophlebitis, embolism,** tachycardia, **necrotizing angiitis, CHF,** edema
*EENT:* Fungal infections, increased intraocular pressure, blurred vision, cataracts, glaucoma
*GI: Diarrhea, nausea, abdominal distention,* **GI hemorrhage,** increased appetite, **pancreatitis,** ulcerative esophagitis
*HEMA:* **Thrombocytopenia**
*INTEG:* Acne, poor wound healing, ecchymosis, bruising, petechiae, hirsutism
*META:* Sodium fluid retention; potassium loss, diabetes
*MS:* Fractures, osteoporosis, weakness, loss of muscle mass

**Contraindications:** Pregnancy **D**, child <2 yr, psychosis, hypersensitivity, idiopathic thrombocytopenia, acute glomerulonephritis, amebiasis, fungal infections, nonasthmatic bronchial disease, AIDS, TB

**Precautions:** Breastfeeding, diabetes mellitus, glaucoma, osteoporosis, seizure disorders, ulcerative colitis, CHF, myasthenia gravis, renal/hepatic disease, esophagitis, peptic ulcer

### Pharmacokinetics

| | |
|---|---|
| **Absorption** | Slowly IM |
| **Distribution** | Widely, crosses placenta |
| **Metabolism** | Liver |
| **Excretion** | Unknown |
| **Half-life** | 8-12 hr |

### Pharmacodynamics

| | PO |
|---|---|
| **Onset** | Unknown |
| **Peak** | 2 hr |
| **Duration** | 1½ days |

### Interactions
*Individual drugs*
Alcohol: increased side effects
Indomethacin: increased GI symptoms, increased side effects, increased action of cortisone
Ketoconazole: increased cortisone action
Phenobarbital, phenytoin: decreased effectiveness of cortisone
Rifampin, theophylline: decreased cortisone action

*Drug classifications*
Acetylcholinesterases, barbiturates: decreased cortisone action
Anticoagulants: decreased anticoagulant effect
Antidiabetics: decreased antidiabetic effect
Antiinfectives (macrolide), estrogens: increased cortisone action
Contraceptives (oral): increased action of cortisone
Diuretics (potassium-wasting), salicylates: increased side effects
NSAIDs: increased GI symptoms
Salicylates: increased GI symptoms, increased cortisone effects, increased side effects; decreased salicylate effect
Toxoids: decreased toxoid effect
Vaccines: decreased vaccine effect

*Drug/herb*
Aloe, buckthorn bark/berry, cascara sagrada bark, Chinese rhubarb, rhubarb root, senna leaf/fruits: increased potassium deficiency
Aloe, licorice, perilla: increased steroid effect

*Drug/lab test*
Increased: cholesterol, sodium, blood glucose, uric acid, calcium, urine glucose
Decreased: calcium, potassium, $T_4$, $T_3$, thyroid $^{131}I$ uptake test, urine 17-OHCS, 17-KS
False negative: skin allergy tests

### NURSING CONSIDERATIONS
**Assessment**
• Assess for adrenal insufficiency symptoms: weakness, nausea, vomiting, confusion, anxiety, restlessness, decreased B/P, weight loss; check before and during treatment
• Monitor potassium, blood glucose for patient on long-term therapy; hypokalemia and hyperglycemia can occur
• Check B/P, pulse q4hr; notify prescriber if chest pain occurs
• Monitor I&O ratio and weight daily; be alert for decreasing urinary output and increasing edema with bilateral crackles, dyspnea, weight gain
• Monitor plasma cortisol levels during long-term therapy (normal level: 138-635 nmol/L if checked at 8 AM)

- Assess for symptoms of infection: increased temp, WBC even after withdrawal of medication; product masks symptoms of infection
- Monitor for potassium depletion: paresthesias, fatigue, nausea, vomiting, depression, polyuria, dysrhythmias, weakness, edema, hypertension, cardiac symptoms, weight daily; notify prescriber of weekly gain >5 lb
- Assess for mental changes: affect, mood, behavioral changes, aggression; depression, psychosis may occur

## Nursing diagnoses
- Infection, risk for (adverse reactions)
- Injury, risk for (adverse reactions)
- Knowledge, deficient (teaching)

## Implementation
**PO route**
- Administer in AM with food or milk to decrease GI symptoms

## Patient/family education
- Advise patient to carry/wear emergency ID as steroid user at all times
- Instruct patient to notify prescriber if therapeutic response decreases; dosage adjustment may be needed; teach not to discontinue this medication abruptly or adrenal crisis can result; teach all aspects of product usage, including cushingoid symptoms
- Caution patient to avoid all OTC products: salicylates, potassium, alcohol in cough products, cold preparations unless directed by prescriber; avoid high-sodium foods
- Teach patient symptoms of adrenal insufficiency: nausea, anorexia, fatigue, dizziness, dyspnea, weakness, joint pain, tarry stools, bruising, blurred vision
- Advise patient to avoid persons with known infections; report probable infection rapidly; product masks infection
- Caution patient that diet modification is necessary if on long-term treatment: increased calcium, potassium, and protein; also low sodium and carbohydrates
- Advise the patient to avoid exposure to chickenpox, measles
- Advise the patient to take PO dose in AM with food or fluid (milk)

## Evaluation
**Positive therapeutic outcome**
- Decreased inflammation

## cotrimoxazole
*See trimethoprim/sulfamethoxazole*

## cyclobenzaprine (Rx)
(sye-kloe-ben′za-preen)
Amrix, cyclobenzaprine HCl, Cycloflex, Fexmid, Flexeril
*Func. class.:* Skeletal muscle relaxant, central acting
*Chem. class.:* Tricyclic amine salt
**Pregnancy category B**

**Do not confuse:**
cyclobenzaprine/cyproheptadine

**Action:** Reduction of tonic muscle activity at the brain stem; may be related to antidepressant effects

**Therapeutic outcome:** Relaxation of skeletal muscle

**Uses:** Adjunct for relief of muscle spasm and pain in musculoskeletal conditions

**Unlabeled uses:** Fibromyalgia

## Dosage and routes
*Musculoskeletal disorders*
*Adult:* PO 5 mg tid × 1 wk, max 30 mg/day × 3 wk

*Geriatric:* PO 5 mg tid

*Fibromyalgia (unlabeled)*
*Adult:* PO 10 mg at bedtime, titrated up

**Available forms:** Tabs 5, 10 mg; ext rel tab 15, 30 mg

## Adverse effects
*CNS: Dizziness, weakness, drowsiness,* headache, tremor, depression, insomnia, confusion, paresthesia, nervousness
*CV:* Postural hypotension, tachycardia, **dysrhythmias**
*EENT:* Diplopia, temporary loss of vision
*GI: Nausea,* vomiting, hiccups, dry mouth, constipation, hepatitis
*GU:* Urinary retention, frequency, change in libido
*INTEG:* Rash, pruritus, fever, facial flushing, sweating

**Contraindications:** Acute recovery phase of MI, dysrhythmias, heart block, CHF, hypersensitivity, child <12 yr, intermittent porphyria, thyroid disease

**Precautions:** Pregnancy **B**, breastfeeding, geriatric, renal/hepatic disease, addictive personality

## Pharmacokinetics

| | |
|---|---|
| **Distribution** | Well |
| **Metabolism** | Liver, partially |
| **Excretion** | Kidney (unchanged) |
| **Half-life** | 1-3 days |

## Pharmacodynamics

| | |
|---|---|
| **Onset** | 1 hr |
| **Peak** | 3-8 hr |
| **Duration** | 12-24 hr |

## Interactions
### Individual drugs
Alcohol: increased CNS depression
Erythromycin, levaquin: increased QT interval
Tramadol: do not use within 14 days
### Drug classifications
Antidepressants (tricyclic), barbiturates, opiates, sedative/hypnotics: increased CNS depression
MAOIs: do not use within 14 days
### Drug/herb
Kava: increased CNS depression

## NURSING CONSIDERATIONS
### Assessment
• Assess pain periodically: location, duration, mobility, stiffness, baseline
• Monitor ECG in epileptic patients; poor seizure control has occurred in patients taking this product
• Check for allergic reactions: rash, fever, respiratory distress
• Check for severe weakness, numbness, in extremities
• Assess for CNS depression: dizziness, drowsiness, psychiatric symptoms

### Nursing diagnoses
• Injury, risk for (adverse reactions)
• Knowledge, deficient (teaching)
• Mobility, impaired physical (uses)

### Implementation
• Give without regard to meals
• Store in airtight container at room temperature

### Patient/family education
• Teach patient not to discontinue medication quickly; insomnia, nausea, headache, spasticity, tachycardia will occur; product should be tapered off over 1-2 wk
• Caution patient not to take with alcohol, other CNS depressants
• Advise to avoid altering activities while taking this product
• Caution patient to avoid hazardous activities if drowsiness/dizziness occurs
• Caution patient to avoid using OTC medication: cough preparations, antihistamines, unless directed by prescriber
• Teach patient to use gum, frequent sips of water for dry mouth

### Evaluation
**Positive therapeutic outcome**
• Decreased pain, spasticity; muscle spasms of acute, painful musculoskeletal conditions are generally short term; long-term therapy is seldom warranted

**Treatment of overdose:** Empty stomach with emesis, gastric lavage, then administer activated charcoal; use anticonvulsants if indicated; monitor cardiac function

---

## cyclopentolate ophthalmic
*See Appendix D*

---

**!HIGH ALERT**

## cyclophosphamide 🕲 (Rx)
(sye-kloe-foss'fa-mide)
Cytoxan, Procytox ✦
*Func. class.:* Antineoplastic alkylating agent
*Chem. class.:* Nitrogen mustard
**Pregnancy category D**

**Do not confuse:**
cyclophosphamide/cycloSPORINE, Cytoxan/Cytosar/Cytotec/centoxin/Cytarabine

**Action:** Alkylates DNA, RNA; inhibits enzymes that allow synthesis of amino acids in proteins; is also responsible for cross-linking DNA strands; activity is not cell cycle phase specific

**Therapeutic outcome:** Prevention of rapidly growing malignant cells

**Uses:** Hodgkin's disease, lymphomas, leukemia, multiple myeloma, neuroblastoma, retinoblastoma, Ewing's sarcoma, cancer of female reproductive tract, breast, lung, prostate

### Dosage and routes
*Adult:* PO initially 1-5 mg/ kg over 2-5 days; maintenance 1-5 mg/kg; **IV** initially 40-50 mg/kg in divided doses over 2-5 days; maintenance 10-15 mg/kg q7-10 days, or 3-5 mg/kg q3 days
*Child:* PO/**IV** 2-8 mg/kg or 60-250 mg/m² in divided doses × 6 or more days; maintenance **IV** 10-15 mg/kg q7-10 days or 30 mg/kg q3-4 wk; dose should be reduced by half when bone marrow suppression occurs

---

**Available forms:** Inj **IV** 100, 200, 500 mg, 1, 2 g; tabs 25, 50 mg

### Adverse effects

*CNS:* Headache, dizziness

*CV:* **Cardiotoxicity (high doses), myocardial fibrosis**

*ENDO:* Syndrome of inappropriate antidiuretic hormone (SIADH), gonadal suppression

*GI: Nausea, vomiting, diarrhea, weight loss,* colitis, **hepatotoxicity**

*GU:* **Hemorrhagic cystitis,** hematuria, neoplasms, amenorrhea, azoospermia, sterility, ovarian fibrosis

*HEMA:* **Thrombocytopenia, leukopenia, pancytopenia, myelosuppression**

*INTEG: Alopecia,* dermatitis

*META:* Hyperuricemia

*MISC:* Secondary neoplasms, **anaphylaxis**

*RESP:* **Pulmonary fibrosis**

**Contraindications:** Pregnancy **D**, breastfeeding, severely depressed bone marrow function, hypersensitivity

**Precautions:** Radiation therapy

#### Pharmacokinetics

| | |
|---|---|
| **Absorption** | Well absorbed (PO) |
| **Distribution** | Widely distributed; crosses placenta, blood-brain barrier (50%) |
| **Metabolism** | Liver to active product |
| **Excretion** | Kidneys, unchanged (30%) |
| **Half-life** | 4-6½ hr |

#### Pharmacodynamics

Unknown

### Interactions
*Individual drugs*

Allopurinol: increased bone marrow suppression

Chloramphenicol: decreased cyclophosphamide effect

Digoxin: decreased digoxin levels

Insulin: increased hypoglycemia

Succinylcholine: increased neuromuscular blockade

Warfarin: increased warfarin action

*Drug classifications*

Diuretics (thiazides): increased bone marrow suppression

Barbiturates: increased toxicity of cyclophosphamide

Corticosteroids: decreased cyclophosphamide effect

Live virus vaccines: decreased antibody reaction

### Drug/lab test

Increased: uric acid

Decreased: pseudocholinesterase

False positive: Pap smear

False negative: PPD, mumps trichophytin, *Candida, Trichophyton,* Pap smear

### NURSING CONSIDERATIONS
#### Assessment

◆ Assess symptoms indicating severe allergic reaction: rash, pruritus, urticaria, purpuric skin lesions, inflammation, flushing

• Assess for tachypnea, ECG changes, dyspnea, edema, fatigue

• Monitor CBC, differential, platelet count weekly; withhold product if WBC count is <2500/mm$^3$ or platelet count is <75,000/mm$^3$; notify prescriber of results

• Assess for hemorrhagic cystitis: renal function studies including BUN, creatinine, serum uric acid, urine CCr before and during therapy; I&O ratio; report fall in urine output to <30 ml/hr

• Monitor temp q4hr (elevated temp may indicate beginning of infection)

• Monitor liver function tests before and during therapy (bilirubin, AST, ALT, LDH) as needed or monthly; note jaundice of skin or sclera, dark urine, clay-colored stools, itchy skin, abdominal pain, fever, diarrhea

• Assess for bleeding: hematuria, stool guaiac, bruising or petechiae, mucosa or orifices q8hr

• Identify dyspnea, crackles, unproductive cough, chest pain, tachypnea

• Identify effects of alopecia on body image; discuss feelings about body changes

#### Nursing diagnoses

• Body image, disturbed (adverse reactions)
• Infection, risk for (adverse reactions)
• Injury, risk for (adverse reactions)
• Knowledge, deficient (teaching)

#### Implementation

• Give fluids **IV** or PO before chemotherapy to hydrate patient

• Give antacid before oral agent, after PM meals, before bedtime; antiemetic 30-60 min before giving product to prevent vomiting and prn; antibiotics for prophylaxis of infection

• Give top or syst analgesics for pain; give in AM so product can be eliminated before bedtime

**IV route**

• Give **IV** after diluting 100 mg/5 ml of sterile or bacteriostatic water; shake; let stand until clear; may be further diluted in up to 250 ml D$_5$ 0.9% NaCl, 0.45% NaCl, LR, Ringer's; give

100 mg or less/min through 3-way stopcock of glucose or saline inf

• Use 21-, 23-, or 25-G needle; check site for irritation, phlebitis

*Syringe compatibilities:* Bleomycin, cisplatin, doxapram, DOXOrubicin, droperidol, fluorouracil, furosemide, heparin, leucovorin, methotrexate, metoclopramide, mitomycin, mitoxantrone, vinBLAStine, vinCRIStine

*Y-site compatibilities:* Amifostine, amikacin, ampicillin, azlocillin, aztreonam, bleomycin, cefamandole, cefazolin, cefepime, cefoperazone, cefotaxime, cefoxitin, cefuroxime, cephalothin, cephapirin, chloramphenicol, chlorproMAZINE, cimetidine, cisplatin, cladribine, clindamycin, dexamethasone, diphenhydrAMINE, DOXOrubicin, doxycycline, droperidol, erythromycin, famotidine, filgrastim, fludarabine, fluorouracil, furosemide, gallium, ganciclovir, gentamicin, granisetron, heparin, hydromorphone, idarubicin, kanamycin, leucovorin, lorazepam, melphalan, methotrexate, methylPREDNISolone, metoclopramide, metronidazole, mezlocillin, minocycline, mitomycin, moxalactam, nafcillin, ondansetron, oxacillin, paclitaxel, penicillin G potassium, piperacillin, piperacillin/tazobactam, prochlorperazine, promethazine, propofol, ranitidine, sargramostim, sodium bicarbonate, teniposide, tetracycline, thiotepa, ticarcillin, ticarcillin-clavulanate, tobramycin, trimethoprim-sulfamethoxazole, vancomycin, vinBLAStine, vinCRIStine, vinorelbine

*Additive compatibilities:* Cisplatin with etoposide, hydrOXYzine, methotrexate, methotrexate with fluorouracil, mitoxantrone, ondansetron

*Solution compatibilities:* Amino acids 4.25%/$D_{25}$, $D_5$/0.9% NaCl, $D_5$W, 0.9% NaCl

**Patient/family education**

• Teach patient to avoid use of products containing aspirin or ibuprofen, razors, commercial mouthwash, since bleeding may occur; to report symptoms of bleeding (hematuria, tarry stools, bruising)

• Instruct patient to report signs of anemia (fatigue, headache, irritability, faintness, shortness of breath)

• Teach patient to report any changes in breathing or coughing even several months after treatment

• Advise patient that hair may be lost during treatment; a wig or hairpiece may make patient feel better; new hair may be different in color, texture

• Teach patient not to have any vaccinations without the advice of the prescriber; serious reactions can occur

• Advise patient contraception is needed during treatment and for several months after the completion of therapy

**Evaluation**

**Positive therapeutic outcome**

• Prevention of rapid division of malignant cells

• Increased appetite, increased weight

---

**\*cycloSPORINE (Rx)**
(sye-kloe-spor′een)
Gengraf, Neoral, Pulminiq, Sandimmune
*Func. class.:* Immunosuppressant
*Chem. class.:* Fungus-derived peptide

**Pregnancy category C**

**Do not confuse:**
cycloSPORINE/CycloSERINE/cyclophosphamide

**Action:** Produces immunosuppression by inhibiting T lymphocytes

**Therapeutic outcome:** Absence of transplant rejection

**Uses:** Organ transplants (liver, kidney, heart) to prevent rejection, rheumatoid arthritis, psoriasis

**Unlabeled uses:** Recalcitrant ulcerative colitis, aplastic anemia, Crohn's disease, GVHD, thrombocytopenia purpura, lupus, nephritis, myasthenia gravis, psoriatic arthritis

**Dosage and routes**
*Prevention of transplant rejection*
*Adult and child:* PO 15 mg/kg several hr before surgery, daily for 2 wk, reduce dosage by 2.5 mg/kg/wk to 5-10 mg/kg/day; **IV** 5-6 mg/kg several hr before surgery, daily, switch to PO form as soon as possible

*Rheumatoid arthritis (Neoral/Gengraf)*
*Adult:* PO 2.5 mg/kg/day divided bid, may increase 0.5-0.75 mg/kg/day after 8-12 wk, max 4 mg/kg/day

*Psoriasis (Neoral/Gengraf)*
*Adult:* PO 2.5 mg/kg/day divided bid × 4 wk, then increase by 0.5 mg/kg/day q2 wk, max 4 mg/kg/day

*Idiopathic thrombocytopenia purpura (unlabeled)*
*Adult:* PO 1.25-2.5 mg/kg bid

---

### Severe aplastic anemia (unlabeled)
*Adult and child:* PO 12 mg/kg/day or 15 mg/kg/day (child) with antithymocyte globulin (ATG)

**Available forms:** Oral sol (Neoral) 100 mg/ml; soft gel cap 25, 50, 100 mg; inj 50 mg/ml; sol for inh 300 mg/4.8 ml

### Adverse effects
***CNS:*** *Tremors, headache,* **seizures,** confusion
***GI:*** Nausea, vomiting, diarrhea, *oral Candida, gum hyperplasia,* **hepatotoxicity,** pancreatitis
***GU:*** **Albuminuria, hematuria, proteinuria, renal failure**
***INTEG:*** Rash, acne, *hirsutism*
***META:*** Hyperkalemia, hypomagnesemia, hyperlipidemia, hyperuricemia
***MISC:*** *Infection*

**Contraindications:** Hypersensitivity to polyxyethylated castor oil (inj only), psoriasis or rheumatoid arthrits in renal disease (Neoral/Gengraf), uncontrolled, malignant hypertension; Gengraf/Neoral used with PUVA/UVB; methotrexate, coal tar, radiation in psoriasis, breastfeeding

**Precautions:** Pregnancy **C,** geriatric, severe renal/hepatic disease

#### Pharmacokinetics
| | |
|---|---|
| Absorption | Poorly absorbed (PO) |
| Distribution | Crosses placenta |
| Metabolism | Liver to mercaptopurine |
| Excretion | Kidney, minimal |
| Half-life | Biphasic 1.2 hr, 25 hr |

#### Pharmacodynamics
| | PO |
|---|---|
| Onset | Unknown |
| Peak | 4 hr |
| Duration | Unknown |

### Interactions
*Individual drugs*
Allopurinol, amiodarone, amphotericin B, bromocriptine, carvedilol, cimetidine, colchicine, foscarnet, imipenem-cilastatin, melphalan, metoclopramide: increased action, cycloSPORINE toxicity
Digoxin: increased digoxin level
Etoposide: increased etoposide level
Methotrexate: increased methotrexate level
Nafcillin, orlistat, phenobarbital, phenytoin, probucol terbinafine, ticlodipine,
trimethoprim/sulfamethoxazole: decreased cycloSPORINE action
Sirolimus: increased sirolimus level
Tacrolimus: increased tacrolimus level
*Drug classifications:*
Androgens, antifungals (azole), β-blockers, calcium channel blockers, contraceptives (oral), corticosteroids, fluoroquinolones, macrolides, NSAIDs, selective serotonin reuptake inhibitors: increased cycloSPORINE levels, toxicity
Anticonvulsants, rifamycins: decreased cycloSPORINE levels
HMG-CoA reductase inhibitors, diuretics (potassium-sparing): increased effects of each product
Live virus vaccines: decreased antibody reaction
*Drug/herb*
Ginseng, maitake, mistletoe, schisandra, St. John's wort, turmeric: decreased effect
Safflower: increased effect
*Drug/food*
Grapefruit juice, food: increased slowed metabolism of product

### NURSING CONSIDERATIONS
#### Assessment
• Monitor renal studies: BUN, creatinine at least monthly during treatment, 3 mo after treatment
• Monitor liver function studies: alkaline phosphatase, AST, ALT, bilirubin
• Monitor product blood levels during treatment
• Assess for hepatotoxicity: dark urine, jaundice, itching, light-colored stools; product should be discontinued
• Assess for nephrotoxicity: 6 wk postop, CyA trough level >200 ng/ml, intracapsular pressure <40 mm Hg, rise in creatinine 0.15 mg/dl/day

#### Nursing diagnoses
• Infection, risk for (uses)
• Knowledge, deficient (teaching)
• Mobility, impaired physical (uses)

#### Implementation
**PO route**
• Do not break, crush, or chew caps
• Use pipette provided to draw up oral sol; may mix with milk or juice, wipe pipette, do not wash
• Give for several days before transplant surgery with corticosteroids
• Microemulsion products (Neoral) and other products are not interchangeable

Adverse effects: *italic* = common, **bold** = life-threatening

- Give with meals for GI upset or place product in chocolate milk
- Give with oral antifungal for *Candida* infections

**IV route**

- Give **IV** after diluting each 50 mg/20-100 ml of 0.9% NaCl or D$_5$W; run over 2-6 hr; use an inf pump, glass inf bottles only; may give as cont inf over 24 hr

*Additive compatibilities:* Ciprofloxacin

*Y-site compatibility:* Cefmetazole, propofol, sargramostim

*Solution compatibilities:* D$_5$W, NaCl 0.9%

- Give for several days before transplant surgery
- Give with corticosteroids

**Patient/family education**

- Advise patient to report fever, rash, severe diarrhea, chills, sore throat, fatigue, since serious infections may occur; also to report clay-colored stools, cramping (may indicate hepatotoxicity); tremors, bleeding gums, increased B/P
- Advise patient to limit UV exposure
- Caution patient to use contraceptive measures during treatment and for 12 wk after ending therapy; product is teratogenic
- Caution patient to avoid crowds and persons with known infections to reduce risk of infection

**Evaluation**

**Positive therapeutic outcome**

- Absence of graft rejection

---

## cyproheptadine (Rx)

(si-proe-hep′ta-deen)
cyproheptadine HCl, PMS-Cyproheptadine
*Func. class.:* Antihistamine, H$_1$-receptor antagonist
*Chem. class.:* Piperidine

**Pregnancy category B**

**Do not confuse:**
cyproheptadine/cyclobenzaprine

**Action:** Acts on blood vessels, GI, respiratory system by competing with histamine for H$_1$-receptor site; decreases allergic response by blocking histamine; blocks serotonin to increase appetite and relieve vascular headaches

**Therapeutic outcome:** Absence of allergy symptoms and rhinitis

**Uses:** Allergy symptoms, rhinitis, pruritus, common cold, urticaria

**Unlabeled uses:** Appetite stimulant, management of vascular headache, nightmares, posttraumatic stress disorder

**Dosage and routes**
*Adult:* PO 4 mg tid-qid, not to exceed 0.5 mg/kg/day
*Geriatric:* PO 4 mg bid, may increase if needed
*Child 6-14 yr:* PO 4 mg bid-tid, not to exceed 16 mg/day
*Child 2-6 yr:* PO 2 mg bid-tid, not to exceed 12 mg/day

*Nightmares, posttraumatic stress disorder (unlabeled)*
*Adult:* PO 4-12 mg nightly, max 32 mg

**Available forms:** Tabs 4 mg; syr 2 mg/5 ml

**Adverse effects**
*CNS: Dizziness, drowsiness,* poor coordination, fatigue, anxiety, euphoria, confusion, paresthesia, neuritis
*CV:* Hypotension, palpitations, tachycardia
*EENT: Blurred vision,* dilated pupils; tinnitus; nasal stuffiness; dry nose, throat, mouth
*GI: Constipation, dry mouth,* nausea, vomiting, anorexia, diarrhea, weight gain, increased appetite
*GU: Urinary retention,* dysuria, urinary frequency
*HEMA:* **Hemolytic anemia, leukopenia, thrombocytosis, agranulocytosis**
*INTEG:* Rash, urticaria, photosensitivity
*MISC:* **Anaphylaxis**
*RESP:* Increased thick secretions, wheezing, chest tightness

**Contraindications:** Hypersensitivity to H$_1$-receptor antagonist, acute asthma attack, lower respiratory tract disease

**Precautions:** Pregnancy **B**, breastfeeding, geriatric, increased intraocular pressure, renal/cardiac disease, hypertension, bronchial asthma, seizure disorder, stenosed peptic ulcers, hyperthyroidism, prostatic hypertrophy, bladder neck obstruction

| Pharmacokinetics | |
|---|---|
| Absorption | Well absorbed |
| Distribution | Unknown |
| Metabolism | Liver, complete |
| Excretion | Kidneys, (65%-75%); feces (25%-35%) |
| Half-life | Unknown |

 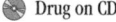

| Pharmacodynamics | |
| --- | --- |
| **Onset** | 15-60 min |
| **Peak** | 1-2 hr |
| **Duration** | 8 hr |

## Interactions
### Individual drugs
Alcohol: increased CNS depression
### Drug classifications
Antidepressants (tricyclics), barbiturates, CNS depressants, opiates, sedative/hypnotics: increased CNS depression

MAOIs: increased anticholinergic effect
### Drug/herb
Corkwood, henbane leaf: increased anticholinergic effect

Hops, Jamaican dogwood, kava, khat, senega: increased CNS depression
### Drug/lab test
False negative: skin allergy tests (discontinue antihistamine 3 days before testing)

## NURSING CONSIDERATIONS
### Assessment
• Assess respiratory status: rate, rhythm, increase in bronchial secretions, wheezing, chest tightness; provide fluids to 2 L/day to decrease secretion thickness
• Monitor I&O ratio: be alert for urinary retention, frequency, dysuria, especially geriatric; product should be discontinued if these occur; monitor food intake, weight if using as an appetite stimulant

### Nursing diagnoses
• Airway clearance, ineffective (uses)
• Injury, risk for (side effects)
• Knowledge, deficient (teaching)
• Noncompliance (teaching, overuse)

### Implementation
• May give with food to decrease GI upset
• Syrup may be used for patients with difficulty swallowing or children
• Store in tight, light-resistant container

### Patient/family education
• Teach all aspects of product uses; tell patient to notify prescriber if confusion, sedation, hypotension occur; to avoid driving and other hazardous activity if drowsiness occurs; to avoid alcohol and other CNS depressants that may potentiate effect
• Caution patient not to exceed recommended dosage; dysrhythmias may occur
• Teach patient hard candy, gum, frequent rinsing of mouth may be used for dryness
• Advise patient to avoid breastfeeding

## Evaluation
### Positive therapeutic outcome
• Absence of runny or congested nose, rashes

**Treatment of overdose:** Administer lavage, diazepam, vasopressors, barbiturates (short acting)

---

### ⚠ HIGH ALERT

### cytarabine (Rx)
(sye-tare′a-been)
Ara-C, Cytosar ✤, Cytosar-U, cytosine arabinoside, Depo Cyt
*Func. class.:* Antineoplastic, antimetabolite
*Chem. class.:* Pyrimidine nucleoside

### Pregnancy category D

**Do not confuse:**
Cytosar ✤/Cytovene/Cytoxan

**Action:** Competes with physiologic substrate of DNA synthesis, thus interfering with cell replication in the S phase of the cell cycle (before mitosis)

**Therapeutic outcome:** Prevention of rapidly growing malignant cells

**Uses:** Acute myelocytic leukemia, acute lymphocytic leukemia, chronic myelocytic leukemia, lymphomatous meningitis (IT)

**Unlabeled uses:** Hodgkin's, non-Hodgkin's lymphoma

### Dosage and routes
#### Acute nonlymphocytic/lymphocytic
*Adult:* IV INF 200 mg/m$^2$/day × 5 days q2 wk as single agent or 2-6 mg/kg/day (100-200 mg/m$^2$/day) as single dose or 2-3 divided doses for 5-10 days until remission, used in combination; maintenance 70-200 mg/m$^2$/day for 2-5 days qmo; SUBCUT maintenance 1 mg/kg 1-2×/wk

#### Meningeal leukemia
*Adult and child:* IT 5-75 mg/m$^2$ variable daily × 4 days to q 2-7 days

#### Refractory acute Hodgkin's/refractory non-Hodgkin's lymphoma (unlabeled)
*Adult:* IV 2 g/m$^2$/day; on day 5 q21 days, with etoposide, methylPREDNISolone, and cisplatin

**Available forms:** Powder for inj 100, 500 mg, 1, 2 g; sus rel (Depo Cyt) liposomal for IT use 10 mg/ml

C

Adverse effects: *italic* = common, **bold** = life-threatening

## Adverse effects

*CNS:* Neuritis, dizziness, headache, cerebellar syndrome, personality changes, ataxia, mechanical dysphasia, **coma; chemical arachnoiditis** (IT)

*CV:* Chest pain, **cardiopathy**

*CYTARABINE SYNDROME:* Fever, myalgia, bone pain, chest pain, rash, conjunctivitis, malaise (6-12 hr after administration)

*EENT:* Sore throat, conjunctivitis

*GI:* Nausea, vomiting, anorexia, diarrhea, stomatitis, **hepatotoxicity,** abdominal pain, hematemesis, **GI hemorrhage**

*GU:* Urinary retention, **renal failure, hyperuricemia**

*HEMA:* **Thrombophlebitis, bleeding, thrombocytopenia, leukopenia, myelosuppression, anemia**

*INTEG:* Rash, fever, freckling, cellulitis

*META:* Hyperuricemia

*RESP:* Pneumonia, dyspnea, **pulmonary edema** (high doses)

*SYST:* **Anaphylaxis**

**Contraindications:** Pregnancy **D**, hypersensitivity, infants

**Precautions:** Renal/hepatic disease, breastfeeding

### Pharmacokinetics

| | |
|---|---|
| **Absorption** | Complete |
| **Distribution** | Widely distributed; crosses blood-brain barrier, placenta |
| **Metabolism** | Liver, extensively |
| **Excretion** | Kidneys |
| **Half-life** | 1-3 hr; IT 100-236 hr |

### Pharmacodynamics

Unknown

### Interactions
*Individual drugs*

Digoxin oral: decreased digoxin effects

Radiation: increased toxicity, bone marrow suppression

*Drug classifications*

Antineoplastics: increased toxicity, bone marrow suppression

## NURSING CONSIDERATIONS
### Assessment

• Assess buccal cavity q8hr for dryness, sores or ulceration, white patches, pain, bleeding, dysphagia; obtain prescription for viscous lidocaine (Xylocaine)

• Assess symptoms indicating anaphylaxis: rash, pruritus, urticaria, purpuric skin lesions, itching, flushing; resuscitation equipment should be nearby

 Assess for chemical arachnoiditis (IT): headache, nausea, vomiting, fever; neck rigidity/pain, meningism, CSF pleocytosis; may be decreased by dexamethasone

• Assess tachypnea, dyspnea, edema, fatigue; identify dyspnea, crackles, unproductive cough, chest pain, tachypnea; pulmonary edema may be fatal (rare)

 Assess for cytarabine syndrome 6-12 hr after infusion: fever, myalgia, bone pain, chest pain, rash, conjunctivitis, malaise; corticosteroid may be ordered

• Monitor CBC, differential, platelet count weekly; withhold product if WBC count is <1000/mm$^3$ or platelet count is <50,000/mm$^3$

• Assess for increased uric acid levels, swelling, joint pain primarily in extremities; patient should be well hydrated to prevent urate deposits

• Monitor renal function studies: BUN, creatinine, serum uric acid, urine CCr before and during therapy; I&O ratio; report fall in urine output to <30 ml/hr

• Monitor temp q4hr (may indicate beginning of infection)

• Monitor liver function tests before and during therapy (bilirubin, AST, ALT, LDH) as needed or monthly; note yellowing of skin or sclera, dark urine, clay-colored stools, pruritus, abdominal pain, fever, diarrhea; an antispasmodic may be used for GI symptoms

• Assess for bleeding: hematuria, stool guaiac, bruising or petechiae, mucosa or orifices q8hr; identify inflammation of mucosa, breaks in skin

### Nursing diagnoses

• Body image, disturbed (adverse reactions)
• Infection, risk for (adverse reactions)
• Injury, risk for (adverse reactions)
• Knowledge, deficient (teaching)

### Implementation

• Avoid contact with skin; very irritating; wash completely to remove

• Give fluids **IV** or PO before chemotherapy to hydrate patient

• Give antiemetic 30-60 min before giving product to prevent vomiting, and prn; antibiotics for prophylaxis of infection

• Increase fluids to 3 L/day

• Give top or syst analgesics for pain

• Give in AM so product can be eliminated before bedtime

• Give **IV** direct after diluting 100 mg/5 ml of sterile water for inj; give by direct **IV** over 1-3 min through free-flowing tubing

**IM/SUBCUT route**

• Reconstitute 100 mg/5 ml or 500 mg/10 ml with bacteriostatic water for inj with benzyl alcohol 0.9%; do not use sol with precipitate; stable for 48 hr

**Intrathecal route**

• Liposomal: withdraw product immediately before use; use within 4 hr, do not save unused portions, or use in-line filter; give directly into CSF by intraventricular reservoir or by direct inj into lumbar site

• Give slowly over 1-5 min, follow with lumbar puncture, instruct patient to lie flat, give dexamethasone 4 mg bid PO or **IV** × 5 days beginning on day of liposomal inj

**IV infusion route**

• May be further diluted in 50-100 ml 0.9% NaCl or D₅W and given over 30 min to 24 hr depending on dosage; may be given by cont inf also

*Syringe compatibilities:* Metoclopramide

*Y-site compatibilities:* Amifostine, amsacrine, aztreonam, cefepime, chlorproMAZINE, cimetidine, cladribine, dexamethasone, diphenhydrAMINE, droperidol, famotidine, filgrastim, fludarabine, gentamicin, granisetron, heparin, hydrocortisone, hydromorphone, idarubicin, lorazepam, melphalan, methotrexate, methylPREDNISolone, metoclopramide, morphine, ondansetron, paclitaxel, piperacillin/tazobactam, prochlorperazine, promethazine, propofol, ranitidine, sargramostim, sodium bicarbonate, teniposide, thiotepa, vinorelbine

*Additive compatibilities:* Corticotropin, DAUNOrubicin with etoposide, etoposide, hydrOXYzine, lincomycin, mitoxantrone, potassium chloride, prednisoLONE, ondansetron, sodium bicarbonate, vinCRIStine

*Additive incompatibilities:* Carbenicillin, fluorouracil, heparin, regular insulin, nafcillin, oxacillin, penicillin G sodium

*Solution compatibilities:* Amino acids, 4.25%/D₂₅, D₅/LR, D₅/0.2% NaCl, D₅/0.9% NaCl, D₁₀/0.9% NaCl, D₅W, invert glucose 10% in electrolyte #1, Ringer's LR, 0.9% NaCl, sodium lactate 1/6 mol/L, TPN #57

**Patient/family education**

• Advise patient that contraceptive measures are recommended during and 4 mo after therapy

• Teach patient to avoid use of products containing aspirin or ibuprofen, NSAIDs, razors, commercial mouthwash, since bleeding may occur; to report symptoms of bleeding (hematuria, tarry stools)

• Advise that fever, headache, nausea, vomiting are likely to occur, but to continue using dexamethasone with IT administration

• Provide liquid diet: carbonated beverages; gelatin may be added if patient is not nauseated or vomiting

• Provide rinsing of mouth tid-qid with water, club soda; brushing of teeth bid-qid with soft brush or cotton-tipped applicators for stomatitis; use unwaxed dental floss

• Advise patient to report signs of anemia (fatigue, headache, irritability, faintness, shortness of breath)

• Advise patient to avoid foods with citric acid, hot or rough texture if stomatitis is present, use sponge brush and rinse with water after each meal; to report stomatitis: any bleeding, white spots, ulcerations in mouth; tell patient to examine mouth daily, report any symptoms

• Instruct patient to report any changes in breathing or coughing even several months after treatment; to avoid crowds and persons with respiratory tract or other infections; neurotoxicity

• Caution patient not to have any vaccinations without the advice of the prescriber; serious reactions can occur

• Advise patient to take fluids 3 L/day to prevent renal damage

**Evaluation**

**Positive therapeutic outcome**

• Prevention of rapid division of malignant cells

**⚠ HIGH ALERT**

**dacarbazine** (Rx)

(da-kar′ba-zeen)

dacarbazine, DTIC ✦, DTIC-Dome

*Func. class.:* Antineoplastic—miscellaneous agent

*Chem. class.:* Imidazole

**Pregnancy category C**

**Action:** Alkylates DNA, RNA; inhibits enzymes that allow synthesis of amino acids in proteins; also responsible for cross-linking DNA strands; activity is not cell cycle phase specific

**Therapeutic outcome:** Prevention of rapidly growing malignant cells

**Uses:** Hodgkin's disease, sarcomas, neuroblastoma, malignant melanoma

**Unlabeled uses:** Malignant pheochromocytoma in combination with cyclophosphamide

Adverse effects: *italic* = common, **bold** = life-threatening

and vinCRIStine, metastatic soft tissue sarcoma in combination with other agents, carcinoma meningitis, neuroblastoma

## Dosage and routes
### Metastatic malignant melanoma
**Adult: IV** 2-4.5 mg/kg daily × 10 days or 250 mg/m$^2$ daily × 5 days; repeat q3 wk depending on response

### Hodgkin's disease
**Adult: IV** 150 mg/m$^2$ daily × 5 days with other agents, repeat q4 wk or 375 mg/m$^2$ on day 1 when given in combination, repeat q15 days

### Osteogenic sarcoma (unlabeled)
**Adult and child: IV** 250 mg/m$^2$/day as a cont inf × 4 days q28 days

### Soft tissue sarcoma (unlabeled)
**Adult and child: IV** 250-300 mg/m$^2$/day as a cont inf × 3 days q21-28 days

### Carcinoma meningitis (unlabeled)
**Adult:** INTRATHECAL 5-30 mg in a fixed dose 2-3 × wk until disease controlled

**Available forms:** Powder for inj 100, 200 mg

## Adverse effects
*CNS:* Facial paresthesia, flushing, fever, malaise, confusion, headache, **seizures**, blurred vision (high doses)
*GI:* Nausea, anorexia, vomiting, **hepatotoxicity** (rare)
*HEMA:* **Thrombocytopenia, leukopenia,** anemia
*INTEG:* Alopecia, dermatitis, pain at inj site, photosensitivity, severe sun reactions (high doses)
*MISC:* Flulike symptoms, malaise, fever, myalgia
*SYST:* **Anaphylaxis**

**Contraindications:** Breastfeeding

**Precautions:** Pregnancy **C** (1st trimester), radiation therapy

| Pharmacokinetics | |
|---|---|
| **Absorption** | Complete bioavailability (**IV**) |
| **Distribution** | Widely distributed; concentrates in liver |
| **Metabolism** | Liver (50%, 5% protein bound) |
| **Excretion** | Kidneys, unchanged (50%) |
| **Half-life** | Initial 35 min, terminal 5 hr |

| Pharmacodynamics | |
|---|---|
| Unknown | |

## Interactions
### Individual drugs
Phenobarbital, phenytoin: increased metabolism; decreased dacarbazine effect
Radiation: bone marrow suppression, toxicity
### Drug classifications
Aminoglycosides: increased nephrotoxicity
Anticoagulants, salicylates: increased risk of bleeding
Antineoplastics, bone marrow–suppressing products: increased toxicity, bone marrow suppression
Diuretics, loop: increased ototoxicity
Live virus vaccines: increased adverse reactions; decreased antibody reaction

## NURSING CONSIDERATIONS
### Assessment
• Assess symptoms indicating severe allergic reaction: rash, pruritus, urticaria, purpuric skin lesions, itching, flushing; product should be discontinued
• Monitor CBC, differential, platelet count weekly; withhold product if WBC is <4000/mm$^3$ or platelet count is <100,000/mm$^3$
• Monitor renal function tests: BUN, creatinine, urine CCr before and during therapy; I&O ratio; report fall in urine output to <30 ml/hr
• Monitor temp q4hr (may indicate beginning of infection)
• Monitor liver function tests before and during therapy (bilirubin, AST, ALT, LDH) as needed or monthly; note jaundice of skin or sclera, dark urine, clay-colored stools, itchy skin, abdominal pain, fever, diarrhea; hepatotoxicity can be serious and fatal
• Assess for bleeding: hematuria, stool guaiac, bruising or petechiae, mucosa or orifices q8hr; check for inflammation of mucosa, breaks in skin
• Identify effects of alopecia on body image; discuss feelings about body changes

### Nursing diagnoses
• Body image, disturbed (adverse reactions)
• Infection, risk for (adverse reactions)
• Injury, risk for (adverse reactions)
• Knowledge, deficient (teaching)

### Implementation
• Give fluids **IV** or PO before chemotherapy to hydrate patient
• Give antiemetic 30-60 min before giving product to prevent vomiting, and prn; antibiotics for prophylaxis of infection
• Provide liquid diet: carbonated beverages; gelatin may be added if patient is not nauseated or vomiting

---

- After diluting 100 mg/9.9 ml of sterile water for inj (10 mg/ml), give by direct **IV** over 1 min through Y-tube or 3-way stopcock
- May be further diluted in 50-250 ml of D₅W or normal saline for inj and given over 30 min
- Watch for extravasation; give 3-5 ml of mixture of 4 ml sodium thiosulfate 10% plus 5 ml of sterile water SUBCUT as prescribed

*Y-site compatibilities:*
Amifostine, aztreonam, filgrastim, fludarabine, granisetron, melphalan, ondansetron, paclitaxel, sargramostim, teniposide, thiotepa, vinorelbine

*Additive compatibilities:*
Bleomycin, carmustine, cyclophosphamide, cytarabine, dactinomycin, DOXOrubicin, fluorouracil, mercaptopurine, methotrexate, ondansetron, vinBLAStine

*Additive incompatibilities:*
Hydrocortisone sodium succinate, cysteine

## Patient/family education
- Teach patient to avoid use of products containing aspirin or ibuprofen, razors, commercial mouthwash, since bleeding may occur; to report symptoms of bleeding (hematuria, tarry stools)
- Instruct patient to report signs of anemia (fatigue, headache, irritability, faintness, shortness of breath)
- Advise patient that hair may be lost during treatment; a wig or hairpiece may make patient feel better; new hair may be different in color, texture
- Caution patient not to have any vaccinations without the advice of prescriber; serious reactions can occur
- Advise patient contraception is needed during treatment and for several months after the completion of therapy; product has teratogenic properties

## Evaluation
**Positive therapeutic outcome**
- Prevention of rapid division of malignant cells

---

## ! HIGH ALERT

# daclizumab (Rx)
(dah-kliz′uh-mab)
Zenapax
*Func. class.:* Immunosuppressant
*Chem class.:* Humanized IgGl monoclonal antibody

**Pregnancy category** C

**D**

**Action:** Binds to the IL-2 receptor antagonist

**Therapeutic outcome:** Prevention of graft rejection

**Uses:** Acute allograft rejection in renal transplant patients

## Dosage and routes
*Adult:* **IV** 1 mg/kg as part of a regimen that includes cycloSPORINE and corticosteroids, mix calculated vol with 50 ml of 0.9% NaCl and give via peripheral/central vein over 15 min; do not admix

**Available forms:** Inj 5 mg/ml

## Adverse effects
*CNS: Chills, tremors, dizziness, insomnia,* headache, prickly sensation
*CV:* Hypertension, **tachycardia, thrombosis, bleeding,** chest pain
*GI: Vomiting, nausea, diarrhea, constipation, abdominal pain, pyrosis*
*GU:* Oliguria, dysuria, **renal tubular necrosis, renal damage, hydronephrosis**
*INTEG:* Impaired wound healing, acne
*MISC: Edema, peripheral edema, allergic reaction*
*RESP: Dyspnea, wheezing,* **pulmonary edema,** coughing, atelectasis, congestion, hypoxia

**Contraindications:** Hypersensitivity

**Precautions:** Pregnancy **C**, breastfeeding, child <11 mo, geriatric

Pharmacokinetics
Unknown

Pharmacodynamics
Unknown

## Interactions
*Drug/herb*
Ginseng, maitake, mistletoe, schisandra, St. John's wort, turmeric: decreased immunosuppressant effect
Safflower: increased immunosuppressant effect

---

Adverse effects: *italic* = common, **bold** = life-threatening

## NURSING CONSIDERATIONS
### Assessment
- Monitor blood studies: Hgb, WBC, platelets during treatment qmo; if leukocytes are <3000/mm$^3$, product should be discontinued
- Monitor liver function tests: alkaline phosphatase, AST, ALT, bilirubin
- Assess for hepatotoxicity: dark urine, jaundice, itching, light-colored stools; product should be discontinued
- Assess for anaphylaxis: have corticosteroids, epINEPHrine available

### Nursing diagnoses
- Injury, risk for (uses)
- Knowledge, deficient (teaching)

### Implementation
- Give all other medications PO if possible; avoid IM inj, since infection may occur

**IV route**
- Solution compatibilities 0.9% NaCl
- Protect undiluted sol from direct light; should be used with product for immunosuppression

### Patient/family education
- Teach patient to report fever, chills, sore throat, fatigue, since serious infection may occur
- Instruct patient to use contraception (women), before, during, and for 4 mo after treatment
- Advise patient to avoid vaccinations during treatment
- Advise patient to drink fluids during treatment

### Evaluation
**Positive therapeutic outcome**
- Absence of graft rejection

---

## ⚠ HIGH ALERT

### dactinomycin (Rx)
(dak-ti-noe-mye'sin)
Cosmegen
*Func. class.:* Antineoplastic, antibiotic

**Pregnancy category C**

**Action:** Inhibits DNA, RNA, protein synthesis; derived from *Streptomyces parvulus;* replication is decreased by binding to DNA, which causes strand splitting; cell cycle nonspecific; a vesicant

**Therapeutic outcome:** Prevention of rapidly growing malignant cells, immunosuppression

**Uses:** Sarcomas, melanomas, trophoblastic tumors in women, testicular cancer, Wilms' tumor, rhabdomyosarcoma

**Unlabeled uses:** Kaposi's sarcoma, malignant melanoma, osteogenic sarcoma, ovarian cancer, soft tissue sarcoma

### Dosage and routes
*Adult:* **IV** 500 mcg/m$^2$/day × 5 days; stop product for 2-4 wk; then repeat cycle
*Child:* **IV** 15 mcg/kg/day × 5 days, not to exceed 500 mcg/day; stop product until bone marrow recovery, then repeat cycle

**Available forms:** Inj 0.5 mg/vial

### Adverse effects
*CNS:* Malaise, fatigue, lethargy, fever
*EENT:* Cheilitis, dysphagia, esophagitis
*GI: Nausea, vomiting, anorexia, stomatitis,* **hepatotoxicity,** abdominal pain, diarrhea
*HEMA:* **Thrombocytopenia, leukopenia, aplastic anemia**
*INTEG:* **Rash,** alopecia, pain at inj site, folliculitis, acne, desquamation, **extravasation**
*MS:* Myalgia

**Contraindications:** Hypersensitivity, herpes infections, child <6 mo

**Precautions:** Pregnancy **C,** breastfeeding, renal/hepatic disease, bone marrow suppression

### Pharmacokinetics

| | |
|---|---|
| **Absorption** | Complete bioavailability |
| **Distribution** | Widely distributed; crosses placenta |
| **Metabolism** | Unknown |
| **Excretion** | Bile; feces, unchanged (50%); kidneys (10%) |
| **Half-life** | 36 hr |

### Pharmacodynamics
Unknown

### Interactions
*Individual drugs*
Radiation: increased toxicity
*Drug classifications*
Antineoplastics: increased toxicity
*Drug/lab test*
Increased: uric acid

## NURSING CONSIDERATIONS
### Assessment
- Assess buccal cavity q8hr for dryness, sores or ulceration, white patches, pain, bleeding, dysphagia; obtain prescription for viscous lidocaine (Xylocaine)

---

⚠ Assess symptoms indicating severe allergic reaction: rash, pruritus, urticaria, purpuric skin lesions, itching, flushing; product should be discontinued

• Monitor CBC, differential, platelet count weekly; withhold product if WBC is <4000/mm³ or platelet count is <100,000/mm³; notify prescriber of results if WBC <20,000/mm³, platelets <150,000/mm³

• Monitor renal function studies: BUN, creatinine, serum uric acid, urine CCr before and during therapy; I&O ratio; report fall in urine output to <30 ml/hr

• Monitor temp q4hr (may indicate beginning of infection)

• Monitor liver function tests before and during therapy (bilirubin, AST, ALT, LDH) as needed or monthly; note jaundice of skin or sclera, dark urine, clay-colored stools, itchy skin, abdominal pain, fever, diarrhea

• Assess for bleeding: hematuria, stool guaiac, bruising or petechiae, mucosa or orifices q8hr; check for inflammation of mucosa, breaks in skin

• Identify effects of alopecia on body image; discuss feelings about body changes

## Nursing diagnoses
• Body image, disturbed (adverse reactions)
• Infection, risk for (adverse reactions)
• Injury, risk for (adverse reactions)
• Knowledge, deficient (teaching)
• Oral mucous membranes, impaired (adverse reactions)

## Implementation
• Provide antacid before oral agent; give product after meals PM, before bedtime; antiemetic 30-60 min before giving product to prevent vomiting, and prn; antibiotics for prophylaxis of infection

• Provide liquid diet: carbonated beverages; gelatin may be added if patient is not nauseated or vomiting

• Help patient rinse mouth tid-qid with water, club soda, brush teeth bid-qid with soft brush or cotton-tipped applicators for stomatitis, use unwaxed dental floss

• Drug should be prepared by experienced personnel using proper precautions

• Give after diluting 0.5 mg/1.1 ml of sterile water for inj without preservative; use 2.2 ml (0.25 mg/ml), give by direct **IV** at 0.5 mg or less/min through Y-tube or 3-way stopcock of inf in progress

• Increase fluids to 3 L/day

**Intermittent IV infusion route**
• May be further diluted in 50 ml of D₅W or 0.9% NaCl for inf; run over 10-15 min

• Give hydrocortisone, sodium thiosulfate to infiltration area, and ice compress after stopping inf

• Store in darkness in cool environment

*Y-site compatibilities:* Allopurinol, amifostine, aztreonam, cefepime, fludarabine, granisetron, melphalan, ondansetron, sargramostim, teniposide, thiotepa, vinorelbine

## Patient/family education
• Teach patient to avoid use of products containing aspirin or ibuprofen, razors, commercial mouthwash, since bleeding may occur; to report symptoms of bleeding (hematuria, tarry stools)

• Instruct patient to report signs of anemia (fatigue, headache, irritability, faintness, shortness of breath)

• Advise patient that hair may be lost during treatment; a wig or hairpiece may make patient feel better; new hair may be different in color, texture

• Caution patient not to have any vaccinations without the advice of the prescriber, serious reactions can occur

• Advise patient that contraception is needed during treatment and for several months after the completion of therapy

• Advise patient to increase fluids to 3 L/day

## Evaluation
**Positive therapeutic outcome**
• Prevention of rapid division of malignant cells

---

**⚠ HIGH ALERT**

### dalteparin (Rx)
(dahl'ta-pear-in)
Fragmin
*Func. class.:* Anticoagulant
*Chem. class.:* Low-molecular-weight heparin

**Pregnancy category B**

**Action:** Inhibits factor Xa/IIa (thrombin) resulting in anticoagulation

**Therapeutic outcome:** Absence of deep vein thrombosis

**Uses:** Unstable angina/non-Q-wave MI; prevention of deep vein thrombosis in abdominal surgery, hip replacement patients, or those with restricted mobility during acute illness; pulmonary embolism

**Unlabeled uses:** Antiphospholipid antibody, arterial thromboembolism, cerebral thromboembolism

Adverse effects: *italic* = common, **bold** = life-threatening

## Dosage and routes
### Hip replacement surgery/ DVT prophylaxis
*Adult:* SUBCUT 2500 international units 2 hr before surgery and 2nd dose in the evening the day of surgery, then 5000 international units SUBCUT 1st postop day and daily 5-10 days

### Unstable angina/ non-Q-wave MI
*Adult:* SUBCUT 120 international units/kg × 5-8 days; do not exceed 10,000 international units q12hr × 5-8 days with concurrent aspirin, continue until stable

### Deep vein thrombosis, prophylaxis for abdominal surgery
*Adult:* SUBCUT 2500 international units daily, evening prior to abdominal surgery and repeat daily × 5-10 days; in high-risk patients 5000 international units should be used

**Available forms:** Prefilled syringes, 2500, 5000 international units/0.2 ml; 7500 international units/0.3 ml, 10,000 international units/ml

## Adverse effects
*CNS:* **Intracranial bleeding**
*HEMA:* **Thrombocytopenia**
*INTEG:* Pruritus, superficial wound infection
*SYST:* Hypersensitivity, **hemorrhage, anaphylaxis** possible

**Contraindications:** Hypersensitivity to this product, heparin, pork products, benzyl alcohol; active major bleeding, hemophilia, leukemia with bleeding, thrombocytopenic purpura, cerebrovascular hemorrhage, cerebral aneurysm, those undergoing regional anesthesia for unstable angina, non-Q-wave MI

**Precautions:** Pregnancy **B**, recent childbirth, breastfeeding, child, geriatric, hepatic disease, severe renal/cardiac disease, blood dyscrasias, subacute bacterial endocarditis, acute nephritis, peptic ulcer disease, pericarditis, pericardial effusion, recent lumbar puncture, vasculitis, other diseases where bleeding is possible, uncontrolled hypertension; recent brain, spine, eye surgery; congenital or acquired disorders, hemorrhagic stroke, history of HIT

### Pharmacokinetics

| | |
|---|---|
| **Absorption** | 87% |
| **Distribution** | Unknown |
| **Metabolism** | Liver |
| **Excretion** | Kidney |
| **Half-life** | 3-5 hr elimination |

### Pharmacodynamics

| | |
|---|---|
| **Onset** | Unknown |
| **Peak** | 4 hr |
| **Duration** | Unknown |

## Interactions
### Drug classifications
Anticoagulants, NSAIDs, platelet inhibitors, salicylates, thrombolytics: increased risk of bleeding
### Drug/herb
Agrimony, alfalfa, angelica, anise, bilberry, black haw, bogbean, bromelain, buchu, chondroitin, cinchona bark, dong quai, fenugreek, feverfew, garlic, ginger, ginkgo, ginseng, horse chestnut, Irish moss, kelp, kelpware, khella, lovage, lungwort, meadowsweet, motherwort, mugwort, nettle, papaya, parsley (large amounts), pau d'arco, pineapple, poplar, prickly ash, safflower, saw palmetto, senega, tonka bean, turmeric, wintergreen, yarrow: increased risk of bleeding
Chamomile, coenzyme Q10, flax, glucomannan, goldenseal, guar gum: decreased anticoagulant effect

## NURSING CONSIDERATIONS
### Assessment
• Assess for bleeding (Hct, occult blood in stools) during treatment since bleeding can occur
◆ Assess for bleeding gums, petechiae, ecchymosis, black tarry stools, hematuria, epistaxis, decrease in Hct, B/P; may indicate bleeding, possible hemorrhage; notify prescriber immediately, product should be discontinued
• Assess for hypersensitivity: fever, skin rash, urticaria; notify prescriber immediately
• Assess for needed dosage change q1-2 wk; dose may need to be decreased if bleeding occurs

### Nursing diagnoses
• Injury, risk for (uses, adverse reactions)
• Knowledge, deficient (teaching)
• Tissue perfusion, ineffective (uses)

### Implementation
**SUBCUT route**
• Cannot be used interchangeably (unit for unit with unfractionated heparin or LMWHs)
• Do not give IM or **IV** product route; approved in SUBCUT only; do not mix with other inj or sol
• Give by SUBCUT only; have patient sit or lie down; SUBCUT inj may be 2 in from umbilicus

in a U-shape, upper outer side of thigh, around navel, or upper outer quadrangle of the buttocks; rotate inj sites

• Changing needles is not recommended; change inj site daily, use at same time of day

### Patient/family education

• Advise patient to avoid OTC preparations that contain aspirin, other anticoagulants; serious product interaction may occur

• Advise patient to use soft-bristle toothbrush to avoid bleeding gums, avoid contact sports, use electric razor, avoid IM inj

• Instruct patient to report any signs of bleeding: gums, under skin, urine, stools; unusual bruising

### Evaluation

**Positive therapeutic outcome**

• Absence of deep vein thrombosis

**Treatment of overdose:** Protamine sulfate 1% given **IV**; 1 mg protamine/100 anti-Xa international units of dalteparin given

---

### dantrolene (Rx)

(dan'troe-leen)

Dantrium

*Func. class.:* Skeletal muscle relaxant, direct acting

*Chem. class.:* Hydantoin

**Pregnancy category** C

### Do not confuse:

Dantrium/danazol

**Action:** Interferes with intracellular release from the sarcoplasmic reticulum of calcium necessary to initiate contraction; slows catabolism in malignant hyperthermia

**Therapeutic outcome:** Decreased muscle spasticity; absence of malignant hyperthermia

**Uses:** Spasticity in multiple sclerosis, stroke, spinal cord injury, cerebral palsy, prevention and treatment of malignant hyperthermia

**Unlabeled uses:** Neuroleptic malignant syndrome

### Dosage and routes

*Spasticity*

*Adult:* PO 25 mg/day; may increase to 25-100 mg bid-qid, max 400 mg/day

*Child:* PO 1 mg/kg/day given in divided doses bid; may increase gradually, not to exceed 400 mg daily

*Malignant hyperthermia*

*Adult and child:* **IV** 1 mg/kg; may repeat to total dose of 10 mg/kg; PO 4-8 mg/kg/day in 4 divided doses × 3 days to prevent further hyperthermia; postcrisis follow-up 4-8 mg/kg/day for 1-3 days

*Prevention of malignant hyperthermia*

*Adult and child:* PO 4-8 mg/kg/day in 3-4 divided doses × 1-2 days before procedures; give last dose 4 hr preoperatively; **IV** 2.5 mg/kg prior to anesthesia

*Neuroleptic malignant syndrome (unlabeled)*

*Adult:* PO 100-300 mg/day in divided doses, **IV** 1.25-1.5 mg/kg

**Available forms:** Caps 25, 50, 100 mg; powder for inj 20 mg/vial

### Adverse effects

*CNS: Dizziness, weakness, fatigue, drowsiness,* headache, disorientation, insomnia, paresthesias, tremors, **seizures**

*CV:* Hypotension, chest pain, palpitations

*EENT:* Nasal congestion, blurred vision, mydriasis

*GI:* **Hepatic injury,** *nausea,* constipation, vomiting, increased AST and alkaline phosphatase, abdominal pain, dry mouth, anorexia, hepatitis, dyspepsia

*GU:* Urinary frequency, nocturia, impotence, crystalluria

*HEMA:* **Eosinophilia,** aplastic anemia, leukopenia

*INTEG:* Rash, pruritus, photosensitivity

*RESP:* Pleural effusion

**Contraindications:** Hypersensitivity, compromised pulmonary function, active hepatic disease, impaired myocardial function

**Precautions:** Pregnancy **C**, breastfeeding, geriatric, peptic ulcer disease, renal/cardiac/hepatic disease, stroke, seizure disorder, diabetes mellitus, ALS

| Pharmacokinetics | |
|---|---|
| **Absorption** | PO (30%-35%), poor |
| **Distribution** | Unknown |
| **Metabolism** | Liver, extensively |
| **Excretion** | Kidney |
| **Half-life** | 9 hr |

| Pharmacodynamics | | |
|---|---|---|
| | PO | IV |
| **Onset** | Unknown | Immediate |
| **Peak** | 5 hr | 5 hr |
| **Duration** | Dose related | Dose related |

Adverse effects: *italic* = common, **bold** = life-threatening

### Interactions
• Considered incompatible in sol or syringe; compatibility unknown
*Individual drugs*
Alcohol: increased CNS depression
Verapamil: increased dysrhythmias
*Drug classifications*
Antidepressants (tricyclic), antihistamines, barbiturates, opiates, sedative/hypnotics: increased CNS depression
Estrogens, hepatotoxic agents: increased hepatotoxicity

### NURSING CONSIDERATIONS
**Assessment**
• Monitor I&O ratio; check for urinary retention, frequency, hesitancy, especially geriatric
• Monitor ECG in epileptic patients; poor seizure control has occurred with patients taking this product; assess for increased seizure activity in epilepsy patient
• Monitor hepatic function by frequent determination of AST, ALT, bilirubin, alkaline phosphatase, GGTP, renal function studies, CBC
• Assess for allergic reactions: rash, fever, respiratory distress
• Monitor for severe weakness, numbness in extremities
• Assess for CNS depression: dizziness, drowsiness, psychiatric symptoms
◆ Assess for signs of hepatotoxicity: jaundice, yellow sclera, pain in abdomen, nausea, fever; product should be discontinued if these signs and symptoms occur

**Nursing diagnoses**
• Injury, risk for (adverse reactions)
• Knowledge, deficient (teaching)
• Mobility, impaired physical (uses)
• Pain, chronic (uses)

**Implementation**
*PO route*
• Do not crush or chew caps; caps may be opened and mixed with juice and swallowed; drink immediately after mixing
• Give with meals for GI symptoms
• Store in airtight container at room temperature
*IV route*
• Administer **IV** after reconstituting 20 mg/60 ml sterile water for inj without bacteriostatic agent (333 mcg/ml); shake until clear; give by rapid **IV** push through Y-tube or 3-way stopcock; follow by prescribed doses immediately; may also give by intermittent inf

over 1 hr before anesthesia; assess site for extravasation, phlebitis
• Protect diluted sol from light; use reconstituted sol within 6 hr
• Considered incompatible in sol or syringe, compatibility unknown

### Patient/family education
• Notify prescriber of abdominal pain, jaundiced sclera, clay-colored stools, change in color of urine, rash, itching
• Caution patient not to take with alcohol, other CNS depressants; severe CNS depression can occur; avoid using OTC medication (cough preparations, antihistamines, alcohol, other CNS depressants), unless directed by prescriber
• Tell patient that if improvement does not occur within 6 wk, prescriber may discontinue
• Caution patient to avoid hazardous activities if drowsiness, dizziness, blurred vision occurs; wait several days to identify patient response to medication
• Teach patient to use sunscreen, protective clothing for photosensitivity
• Instruct patient to take medication as prescribed; do not double doses; take missed dose within 1 hr of scheduled time

**Evaluation**
*Positive therapeutic outcome*
• Decreased pain, spasticity
• Absence or decreased symptoms of malignant hyperthermia

**Treatment of overdose:** Activated charcoal, supportive care

### dapiprazole ophthalmic
*See Appendix D*

### daptomycin (Rx)
(dap'toe-mye-sin)
Cubicin
*Func. class.:* Antiinfective—miscellaneous
*Chem. class.:* Lipopeptides
**Pregnancy category B**

**Action:** New class of antiinfective; binds to the bacterial membrane and results in a rapid depolarization of the membrane potential, leading to inhibition of DNA, RNA, and protein synthesis

**Therapeutic outcome:** Absence of infections

**Uses:** Complicated skin, skin structure infections caused by *Staphylococcus aureus,* including methicillin-resistant strains, *Streptococcus pyogenes, S. agalactiae, S. dysgalactiae, Enterococcus faecalis* (vancomycin-susceptible strains only)

### Dosage and routes
*Adult:* **IV** INF 4 mg/kg over ½ hr diluted in 0.9% NaCl, give q24hr ×7-14 days

### Renal dose
*Adult:* **IV** INF CCr >30 ml/min 4 mg/kg q24hr; CCr <30 ml/min; hemodialysis, CAPD 4 mg/kg q48hr

**Available forms:** lyophilized powder for inj 250, 500 mg

### Adverse effects
*CNS:* Headache, insomnia, dizziness
*CV:* Hypo/hypertension, increased CPK
*GI:* Nausea, constipation, diarrhea, vomiting, dyspepsia, **pseudomembranous colitis**
*GU:* **Nephrotoxicity: increased BUN, creatinine, albumin**
*INTEG:* Rash, pruritus
*MISC:* Fungal infections, UTI, anemia
*MS:* Muscle pain or weakness, arthralgia, pain

**Contraindications:** Hypersensitivity

**Precautions:** Pregnancy **B**, breastfeeding, children, geriatrics, renal disease

#### Pharmacokinetics
| | |
|---|---|
| **Absorption** | Unknown |
| **Distribution** | Protein binding 92% |
| **Metabolism** | Unknown |
| **Excretion** | Unknown |
| **Half-life** | Unknown |

#### Pharmacodynamics
Unknown

### Interactions
*Drug classifications*
HMG-CoA reductase inhibitors: myopathy

### NURSING CONSIDERATIONS
#### Assessment
• Monitor I&O ratio: report hematuria, oliguria; nephrotoxicity may occur
◆ Monitor any patient with compromised renal system, toxicity may occur; BUN, creatinine
• Monitor blood tests: CBC
• Monitor C&S, product may be given as soon as culture is taken
• Monitor B/P during administration; hypo/hypertension may occur
• Assess signs of infection

• Assess respiratory status: rate, character, wheezing
• Identify allergies before treatment, reaction of each medication

#### Nursing diagnoses
• Infection, risk for (uses)
• Knowledge, deficient (teaching)

#### Implementation
**IV route**
• Give after reconstitution with 5 ml 0.9% NaCl (250 mg/5 ml) or 10 ml 0.9% NaCl (500 mg/10 ml), further dilution is needed with 0.9% NaCl, infuse over ½ hr

**Solution compatibilities:** 0.9% NaCl, LR

#### Patient/family education
• Teach all aspects of product therapy
• Advise to report sore throat, fever, fatigue; could indicate superinfection

#### Evaluation
**Positive therapeutic outcome**
• Negative culture

### darbepoetin (Rx)
(dar'bee-poh'-eh-tin)
Aranesp
*Func. class.:* Hematopoietic agent
*Chem. class.:* Recombinant human erythropoietin
**Pregnancy category C**

**Action:** Stimulates erythropoiesis by the same mechanism as endogenous erythropoietin; in response to hypoxia, erythropoietin is produced in the kidney and released into the bloodstream, where it interacts with progenitor stem cells to increase red cell production

**Therapeutic outcome:** Decreased anemia with increased RBCs

**Uses:** Anemia associated with chronic renal failure in patients on and not on dialysis and anemic in nonmyeloid malignancies receiving coadministered chemotherapy

### Dosage and routes
*Correction of anemia*
*Adult:* SUBCUT/**IV** 0.45 mcg/kg as a single inj, titrate not to exceed a target Hgb of 12 g/dl

*Epoetin alfa to darbepoetin conversion*
*Adult:* SUBCUT/**IV** (epoetin alfa <2500 units/wk) 6.25 mcg/wk; (epoetin alfa 2500-4999 units/wk) 12.5 mcg/wk; (epoetin alfa 5000-10,999 units/wk) 25 mcg/wk; (epoetin

alfa 11,000-17,999 units/wk) 40 mcg/wk; (epoetin alfa 18,000-33,999 units/wk) 60 mcg/wk; (epoetin alfa 34,000-89,999 units/wk) 100 mcg/wk; (epoetin alfa >90,000 units/wk) 200 mcg/wk

**Available forms:** Sol for inj 25, 40, 60, 100, 150, 200, 300, 500 mcg/ml

### Adverse effects

*CNS:* **Seizures**, sweating, dizziness, **stroke**
*CV:* *Hypo/hypertension,* **cardiac arrest,** *angina pectoris,* **thrombosis, CHF, acute MI, dysrhythmias,** chest pain, transient ischemic attacks, edema
*GI: Diarrhea, vomiting, nausea, abdominal pain, constipation*
*HEMA:* **Red cell aplasia**
*MISC: Infection, fatigue, fever,* **death,** *fluid overload,* **vascular access hemorrhage,** dehydration, sepsis
*MS: Bone pain, myalgia, limb pain, back pain*
*RESP: Upper respiratory infection, dyspnea, cough, bronchitis,* **pulmonary embolism**
*SYST:* Allergic reactions, **anaphylaxis**

**Contraindications:** Hypersensitivity to mammalian cell–derived products or human albumin, uncontrolled hypertension, red cell aplasia

**Precautions:** Pregnancy **C**, breastfeeding, children, seizure disorder, porphyria, hypertension, sickle cell disease, vit $B_{12}$ folate deficiency, chronic renal failure, dialysis, Hgb >12 g/dl

### Pharmacokinetics

| | |
|---|---|
| **Absorption** | Slow, rate-limiting (SUBCUT) |
| **Distribution** | Vascular space |
| **Metabolism** | Metabolized in body (**IV**), extent unknown |
| **Excretion** | Unknown |
| **Half-life** | 49 hr |

### Pharmacodynamics

| | |
|---|---|
| **Onset** | Onset of increased reticulocyte count 1-6 wk |
| **Peak** | 34 hr |
| **Duration** | Unknown |

### Interactions

*Individual drugs*
◆ Do not use epoetin alfa with this product
*Drug classifications*
Androgens: increased darbepoetin alfa effect
*Drug/lab test*
Increased: WBC, platelets
Decreased: bleeding time

## NURSING CONSIDERATIONS

### Assessment

- Assess for serious allergic reactions: rash, urticaria; if anaphylaxis occurs, stop product, administer emergency treatment (rare)
- Assess blood studies: ferritin, transferrin monthly; transferrin sat ≥20%, ferritin ≥100 ng/ml; Hgb 2×/wk until stabilized in target range (30%-33%) then at regular intervals; those with endogenous erythropoietin levels of <500 units/L respond to this agent
- Assess renal studies: urinalysis, protein, blood, BUN, creatinine
- Assess B/P, Hct; check for rising B/P as Hct rises, antihypertensives may be needed
◆ Assess CV status: hypertension may occur rapidly leading to hypertensive encephalopathy; Hgb >12 g/dl may lead to death
- Assess I&O ratio; report drop in output to <50 ml/hr
- Assess for seizures if Hgb is increased within 2 wk by 4 pts
- Assess CNS symptoms: cold sensation, sweating, pain in long bones
- Assess dialysis patients for thrill, bruit of shunts; monitor for circulation impairment

### Nursing diagnoses

- Activity intolerance (uses)
- Fatigue (uses)
- Knowledge, deficient (teaching)

### Implementation

**IV/SUBCUT**
- Do not shake, do not dilute, do not mix with other products or solutions
- Check for discoloration, particulate matter; do not use if present, discard unused portion, do not pool unused portion

### Patient/family education

- Caution patient to avoid driving or hazardous activity during beginning of treatment
- Advise patient to monitor B/P
- Advise patient to take iron supplements, vit $B_{12}$, folic acid as directed
- Advise patient to report side effects to prescriber, to comply with treatment regimen
- Teach home administration and review information for patients and caregivers if home administration is deemed appropriate

### Evaluation

**Positive therapeutic outcome**
- Increased reticulocyte count, Hgb/Hct
- Increased appetite
- Enhanced sense of well-being

**Treatment of overdose:** If polycythemia occurs, discontinue product temporarily; perform phlebotomy if clinically indicated

---

 Alert      ✦ Canada Only       Drug on CD      * "Tall Man" lettering (See Preface)

## darunavir (Rx)

(dar-ue'na-vir)

Prezista

*Func. class.:* Antiretroviral

*Chem. class.:* Protease inhibitor

**Pregnancy category B**

**D**

**Action:** Inhibits human immunodeficiency virus (HIV-1) protease; this prevents maturation of virus

**Therapeutic outcome:** Decrease viral load, increase in CD4 counts

**Uses:** HIV-1 in combination with ritonavir and other antiretrovirals

### Dosage and routes

Reduce dose in mild/moderate hepatic impairment and ketaconazole coadministration

*Adult:* PO 600 mg bid; if given with ritonavir 100 mg bid with food

**Available forms:** Tabs 300 mg

### Adverse effects

*CNS: Headache, insomnia,* dizziness, somnolence

*GI: Diarrhea, abdominal pain, nausea, vomiting,* anorexia, dry mouth

*GU:* Nephrolithiasis

*INTEG:* Rash

*MS:* Pain

*OTHER:* Asthenia, **insulin-resistant hyperglycemia,** hyperlipidemia, **ketoacidosis,** lipodystrophy

**Contraindications:** Hypersensitivity

**Precautions:** Pregnancy **B,** breastfeeding, children, renal/hepatic disease, history of renal stones, diabetes, hypercholesterolemia

### Pharmacokinetics

| | |
|---|---|
| **Absorption** | Unknown |
| **Distribution** | Protein binding 95% |
| **Metabolism** | By CYP3A |
| **Excretion** | Feces 79.5%, urine 13.9% |
| **Half-life** | Terminal 15 hr |

### Pharmacodynamics

| | |
|---|---|
| **Onset** | Unknown |
| **Peak** | 2.5-4 hr |
| **Duration** | Unknown |

### Interactions

*Individual drugs*

Atorvastatin, lovastatin, simvastatin: increased myopathy

Delavirdine, itracinazole, ketoconazole: increased darunavir levels

Clarithromycin, zidovudine: increased levels of both products

Efavirenz, fluconazole, nevirapine: decreased darunavir levels

Isoniazid: increased levels of isoniazid

◆Midazolam, pimozide, rifampin, triazolam: life-threatening dysrhythmias

*Drug classifications*

Anticonvulsants: decreased both products

◆Ergots: life-threatening dysrhythmias; do not use concurrently

Oral contraceptives: increased levels of oral contraceptives

Rifamycins: decreased darunavir levels

*Drug/herb*

St. John's wort: decreased darunavir levels; avoid concurrent use

*Drug/food*

Darunavir: increased absorption

### NURSING CONSIDERATIONS
Assessment

• Assess for complaints of lower back, flank pain; indicates kidney stones

• Assess for signs of infection, anemia, the presence of other STDs

• Monitor liver function tests: ALT, AST, bilirubin, amylase; all may be elevated

• Monitor viral load, CD4 during treatment; viral load should be decreasing, CD4 increasing

• Assess bowel pattern before, during treatment; if severe abdominal pain with bleeding occurs, product should be discontinued; monitor hydration

• Assess skin eruptions: rash, urticaria, itching

• Assess allergies before treatment, reaction of each medication; place allergies on chart

### Nursing diagnoses

• Infection, risk for (uses)

• Knowledge, deficient (teaching)

• Noncompliance (teaching)

### Implementation

• Give with food and ritonavir

• Give water to 1.5 L/day minimum to prevent nephrolithiasis

### Patient/family education

• Instruct patient to take as prescribed; if dose is missed, take as soon as remembered up to 1 hr before next dose; do not double dose

• Advise patient that product must be taken in equal intervals around the clock to maintain blood levels for duration of therapy

Adverse effects: *italic* = common, **bold** = life-threatening

⚡ Advise patient that hyperglycemia may occur; watch for increased thirst, weight loss, hunger, dry, itchy skin; notify prescriber
• Teach patient to increase fluids to prevent kidney stones; if stone formation occurs, treatment may need to be interrupted
• Teach patient that product does not cure AIDS, only controls symptoms; do not donate blood

## Evaluation
**Positive therapeutic outcome**
• Decreased viral load, increased CD4 counts

---

## dasatinib (Rx)
(da-si'ti-nib)
Sprycel
*Func. class.:* Miscellaneous antineoplastic
*Chem. class.:* Protein-tyrosine kinase inhibitor

**Pregnancy category D**

**Action:** Inhibits BCR-ABL, SRC, LCK, YES, FYN, C-KIT, EPHA$_2$, and PDGFR-β tyrosine kinase created in chronic myeloid leukemia (CML)

**Therapeutic outcome:** Decrease in number of leukemic cells or size of tumor

**Uses:** Treatment of chronic myeloid leukemia (CML), accelerated blast crisis, or chronic phase, and acute lymphoblastic leukemia (ALL)

**Dosage and routes**
*Adult:* PO 70 mg bid

**Available forms:** Tabs 20, 50, 70 mg

**Adverse effects**
*CNS:* **CNS hemorrhage,** headache, dizziness, insomnia, neuropathy, asthenia
*CV:* Dysrhythmias, chest pain, CHF, pericardial effusion
*GI:* Nausea, **vomiting,** *anorexia, abdominal pain,* constipation, diarrhea, GI bleeding, muscositis, stomatitis
*HEMA:* **Neutropenia, thrombocytopenia, bleeding**
*INTEG:* *Rash, pruritus*
*META:* Fluid retention, edema
*MISC:* Increased/decreased weight
*MS:* Pain, arthralgia, myalgia
*RESP:* Cough, dyspnea, pulmonary edema/hypertension, pneumonia, URI

**Contraindications:** Pregnancy **D,** hypersensitivity

**Precautions:** Breastfeeding, children, geriatric

| Pharmacokinetics | |
|---|---|
| **Absorption** | Unknown |
| **Distribution** | Protein binding 96% |
| **Metabolism** | By CYP3A4 |
| **Excretion** | Feces 85%, urine 4% |
| **Half-life** | Terminal 1.3-5 hr |

| Pharmacodynamics | |
|---|---|
| **Onset** | 0.5-6 hr |
| **Peak** | Unknown |
| **Duration** | Unknown |

## Interactions
*Individual drugs*
Clarithromycin, erythromycin, itraconazole, ketoconazole, nefazodine, telithromycin: increased dasatinib concentrations
*Drug classifications*
CYP3A4 inducers (dexamethasone, phenytoin, carbamazepine, rifampin, phenobarbital), H$_2$ blockers (famotidine), proton pump inhibitors (omeprazole): decreased dasatinib concentrations
CYP3A4 substrates (alfentanil, cycloSPORINE, ergots, fentanyl, pimozide, quinidine, sirolimus, tacrolimus): altered action
Protease inhibitors: increased dasatinib concentrations
Simvastatin: increased concentrations of this product
*Drug/herb*
St. John's wort: decreased dasatinib concentration

## NURSING CONSIDERATIONS
**Assessment**
• Monitor ANC and platelets; in chronic phase if ANC <1 × 10$^9$/L and/or platelets <50 ×10$^9$/L, stop until ANC >1.5 × 10$^9$/L and platelets >75 × 10$^9$/L; in accelerated phase/blast crisis if ANC <0.5 × 10$^9$/L and/or platelets <10 × 10$^9$/L, determine whether cytopenia is related to biopsy/aspirate, if not, reduce dose by 200 mg, if cytopenia continues, reduce dose by another 100 mg; if cytopenia continues for 4 wk, stop product until ANC ≥1 × 10$^9$/L
• Assess for renal toxicity: if bilirubin >3 × IULN, withhold until bilirubin levels return to <1.5 × IULN
• Assess for hepatotoxicity: monitor liver function tests, before treatment and qmo; if liver transaminases >5 × IULN, withhold until transaminase levels return to <2.5 × IULN

---

• Monitor CBC, differential, platelet count weekly; withhold product if WBC is <3500/mm$^3$, or platelet count <100,000/mm$^3$; notify prescriber of these results; product should be discontinued

• Monitor for signs of fluid retention, edema: weigh, monitor lung sounds, assess for edema, some fluid retention is dose dependent

### Nursing diagnoses
• Infection, risk for (adverse reactions)
• Knowledge, deficient (teaching)
• Nutrition: less than body requirements, imbalanced (adverse reactions)

### Implementation
• Do not break, crush, or chew tab
• Give after meal and with large glass of water
• Give nutritious diet with iron, vitamin supplement
• Store at 25° C (77° F)

### Patient/family education
• Instruct patient to report adverse reactions immediately: SOB, swelling of extremities, bleeding
• Teach patient reason for treatment, expected result

### Evaluation
**Positive therapeutic outcome**
• Decrease in number of leukemic cells

---

! HIGH ALERT

\***DAUNOrubicin** (Rx)
(daw-noe-roo'bi-sin)
Cerubidine

\***DAUNOrubicin citrate liposome** (Rx)
DaunoXome
*Func. class.:* Antineoplastic, antibiotic
*Chem. class.:* Anthracycline glycoside
**Pregnancy category D**

**Do not confuse:**
DAUNOrubicin/DOXOrubicin

**Action:** Inhibits DNA synthesis, primarily; derived from *Streptomyces coeruleorubidus;* replication is decreased by binding to DNA, which causes strand splitting; cell cycle specific (S phase); a vesicant

**Therapeutic outcome:** Prevention of rapidly growing malignant cells; immunosuppression

**Uses:** Myelogenous, monocytic leukemia, acute nonlymphocytic leukemia, Ewing's sarcoma, rhabdomyosarcoma; DAUNOrubicin citrate liposome: advanced Kaposi's sarcoma in HIV

### Dosage and routes
Use decreased dose for those >60 yr

*DAUNOrubicin*
*Single agent*
*Adult:* **IV** 60 mg/m$^2$/day × 3-5 day q4 wk

*In combination*
*Adult:* **IV** 45 mg/m$^2$/day × 3 days, then 2 days of subsequent courses in combination
*Child:* **IV** 25-60 mg/m$^2$ depending on cycle

*DAUNOrubicin citrate liposome*
*Adult:* **IV** 40 mg/m$^2$ q2 wk

*Renal dose*
*Adult:* **IV** serum Cr >3 mg/dl reduce dose by 50%

*Hepatic dose*
*Adult:* **IV** serum bilirubin 1.2-3 mg/dl reduce dose by 25%; bilirubin >3 mg/dl reduce dose by 50%

**Available forms:** Inj 20 mg powder/vial, sol for inj 5 mg/ml (DaunoXome); liposome: dispersion for inj 2 mg/ml

### Adverse effects
*DAUNOrubicin*
*CNS:* Fever, chills
*CV:* **Dysrhythmias, CHF, pericarditis, myocarditis,** peripheral edema
*GI: Nausea, vomiting, anorexia, mucositis,* **hepatotoxicity**
*GU:* Impotence, sterility, amenorrhea, gynecomastia, hyperuricemia
*HEMA:* **Thrombocytopenia, leukopenia, anemia**
*INTEG: Rash, extravasation,* dermatitis, reversible alopecia, cellulitis, thrombophlebitis at inj site
*MISC:* **Anaphylaxis**

*DAUNOrubicin citrate liposome*
*CNS:* Fatigue, headache, depression, insomnia, dizziness, malaise, neuropathy
*CV:* Chest pain, edema
*GI:* Abdominal pain, nausea, vomiting, *diarrhea,* constipation, stomatitis
*INTEG: Alopecia,* sweating, *pruritus*
*MS: Rigors,* arthralgia, back pain
*RESP: Cough, dyspnea, rhinitis, sinusitis*

**Contraindications:** Pregnancy **D,** breastfeeding, hypersensitivity, systemic infections, cardiac disease, bone marrow depression

**Precautions:** Renal/hepatic disease, gout

---

Adverse effects: *italic* = common, **bold** = life-threatening

## Pharmacokinetics

| | |
|---|---|
| **Absorption** | Complete |
| **Distribution** | Widely distributed; crosses placenta |
| **Metabolism** | Liver, extensively |
| **Excretion** | Biliary (40%-50%) |
| **Half-life** | 18½ hr, liposome 55½ hr |

## Pharmacodynamics

Unknown

## Interactions
### Individual drugs
Cyclophosphamide, radiation: increased toxicity
### Drug classifications
Antineoplastics: increased toxicity
Live virus vaccines: decreased antibody reaction
NSAIDs, salicylates: increased risk of bleeding
### Drug/lab test
Increased: uric acid

## NURSING CONSIDERATIONS
### Assessment
• Assess buccal cavity q8hr for dryness, sores or ulceration, white patches, pain, bleeding, dysphagia; obtain prescription for viscous lidocaine (Xylocaine)
• Assess symptoms indicating severe allergic reaction: rash, pruritus, urticaria, purpuric skin lesions, itching, flushing; product should be discontinued
• Assess chest x-ray, echocardiography, radionuclide angiography, ECG; watch for ST-T wave changes, low QRS and T, possible dysrhythmias (sinus tachycardia, heart block, PVCs); watch for CHF (jugular vein distention, weight gain, edema, crackles), may occur after 2-6 mo of treatment
• Monitor CBC, differential, platelet count weekly, leukocyte nadir within 2 wk after administration, recovery within 3 wk; do not administer if absolute granulocyte count is <750/mm³ (liposome)
• Assess for increased uric acid levels, swelling, joint pain primarily in extremities; patient should be well hydrated to prevent urate deposits
• Monitor renal function tests: BUN, creatinine, serum uric acid, urine CCr baseline and before each dose; I&O ratio; report fall in urine output to <30 ml/hr
• Monitor temp q4hr (may indicate beginning of infection)
• Monitor liver function tests baseline and before each dose (bilirubin, AST, ALT, LDH) as

needed or monthly; note jaundice of skin or sclera, dark urine, clay-colored stools, itchy skin, abdominal pain, fever, diarrhea; hepatotoxicity can be severe
• Assess for bleeding: hematuria, stool guaiac, bruising or petechiae, mucosa or orifices q8hr; check for inflammation of mucosa, breaks in skin
• Identify effects of alopecia on body image; discuss feelings about body changes

### Nursing diagnoses
• Body image, disturbed (adverse reactions)
• Cardiac output, decreased (adverse reactions)
• Infection, risk for (adverse reactions)
• Injury, risk for (adverse reactions)
• Knowledge, deficient (teaching)

### Implementation
• Avoid contact with skin; very irritating; wash completely to remove
• Give fluids **IV** or PO before chemotherapy to hydrate patient; give antiemetic 30-60 min before giving product to prevent vomiting, and prn; antibiotics for prophylaxis of infection
• Provide liquid diet: carbonated beverages; gelatin may be added if patient is not nauseated or vomiting
• Help patient rinse mouth tid-qid with water, club soda, brush teeth bid-qid with soft brush or cotton-tipped applicators for stomatitis, use unwaxed dental floss
• Product should be prepared by experienced personnel using proper precautions

### Cerubidine
**IV route**
• Give after diluting 20 mg/4 ml sterile water for inj (5 mg/ml); rotate; further dilute in 10-15 ml 0.9% NaCl; give over 3-5 min by direct **IV** through Y-tube or 3-way stopcock of inf of $D_5W$ or 0.9% NaCl
**Intermittent IV infusion route**
• Dilute further in 50-100 ml 0.9% NaCl, LR, $D_5W$; give over 15 min (50 ml), 30 min (100 ml)
**Y-site compatibilities:** Amifostine, filgrastim, granisetron, melphalan, methotrexate, ondansetron, sodium bicarbonate, teniposide, thiotepa, vinorelbine
**Y-site incompatibilities:** Fludarabine
**Additive compatibilities:** Cytarabine with etoposide, hydrocortisone; not recommended for admixing
**Additive incompatibilities:** Dexamethasone, heparin
**Solution compatibilities:** $D_{3.3}$/0.3% NaCl, $D_5W$, Normosol-R, Ringer's, 0.9% NaCl

### *DaunoXome*
**IV route**

• Dilute with $D_5W$ (1 mg/ml), give over 60 min, do not use in-line filter, reconstituted sol may be stored ≤6 hr refrigerated; do not admix

### Patient/family education

• Teach patient to avoid use of products containing aspirin or ibuprofen, razors, commercial mouthwash, since bleeding may occur; to report symptoms of bleeding (hematuria, tarry stools)
• Instruct patient to report signs of anemia (fatigue, headache, irritability, faintness, shortness of breath); signs of infection; bleeding, bruising, shortness of breath, swelling, change in heart rate; to avoid crowds, those with known infections
• Advise patient that hair may be lost during treatment; a wig or hairpiece may make patient feel better; new hair may be different in color, texture
• Caution patient not to have any vaccinations without the advice of the prescriber; serious reactions can occur
• Advise patient that contraception is needed during treatment and for 4 mo after the completion of therapy
• Advise patient to avoid alcohol, aspirin, NSAIDs

### Evaluation
**Positive therapeutic outcome**

• Prevention of rapid division of malignant cells

---

### decitabine (Rx)
(de-sit′-a-been)
Dacogen
*Func. class.:* DNA demethylation agent
*Chem. class.:* Cytosine analog

**Pregnancy category  D**

**Action:** Incorporated into DNA and inhibits DNA methylation, halting growth of rapid proliferation of blasts

**Therapeutic outcome:** Decreasing blast count

**Uses:** Treatment of naïve and experienced myelodysplasic syndrome

### Dosage and routes
*Adult:* CONT **IV** First treatment cycle: 15 mg/m$^2$ over 3 hr, q8hr × 3 days; subsequent treatment cycles: repeat above cycle q6 wk for at least 4 cycles; a partial or complete response may take more than 4 cycles

**Available forms:** Powder for injection, lyophilized 50 mg, in single dose vial

### Adverse effects
*CNS: Headache, anxiety, dizziness, hypoesthesia, insomnia,* confusion
*CV: Edema, murmur, hypotension*
*GI: Nausea, anorexia, vomiting, diarrhea, constipation, stomatitis,* abdominal pain, dyspepsia
**HEMA: Neutropenia, thrombocytopenia, leukopenia, anemia**
*INTEG: Alopecia, ecchymosis, erythema, pallor, petechiae, pruritus, rash, swelling face, urticaria,* hematoma, cellulitis
*META: Decreased potassium, sodium, magnesium, albumin; increased bilirubin, increased/decreased glucose*
*MS: Myalgia, arthralgia, back pain, chest wall pain, pain in limbs*
*RESP: Cough, crackles, hypoxia, pharyngitis, pneumonia, pulmonary edema*

**Contraindications:** Pregnancy **D**, breastfeeding, children, hypersensitivity to this product, severe neurotoxicity, severe blood dyscrasias

**Precautions:** Severe renal/hepatic disease, men (men should not father a child while receiving treatments or for 2 months after treatment ends)

| Pharmacokinetics | |
|---|---|
| Absorption | Unknown |
| Distribution | Protein binding <1% |
| Metabolism | Liver, granulocytes, intestinal epithelium, whole blood |
| Excretion | Unknown |
| Half-life | Terminal 0.2-0.8 hr |

| Pharmacodynamics |
|---|
| Unknown |

### Interactions
*Drug classifications*
Do not use with live virus vaccines

### NURSING CONSIDERATIONS
### Assessment

• Monitor CBC (RBC, Hct, Hgb), differential, platelet count weekly; withhold product if WBC <4000/mm$^3$, platelets <75,000/mm$^3$, or RBC, Hct, Hgb is low; notify prescriber of results
• Monitor renal studies: BUN, serum uric acid, urine CCr, electrolytes before and during therapy
• Monitor temp q4hr; fever may indicate beginning infection; no rectal temps

Adverse effects: *italic* = common, **bold** = life-threatening

- Monitor hepatic studies before and during treatment: bilirubin, AST, ALT, alkaline phosphatase, as needed or monthly
- Assess for bleeding: hematuria, heme-positive stools, bruising or petechiae, mucosa or orifices daily; blood dyscrasias can occur
- Assess for dyspnea, crackles, unproductive cough, chest pain, tachypnea, fatigue, increased pulse, pallor, lethargy, personality changes
- Assess buccal cavity daily for dryness, ulceration, white patches, oral pain, bleeding, dysphagia
- Assess GI symptoms: frequency of stools, cramping; if severe diarrhea occurs, electrolytes may need to be given

## Nursing diagnoses
- Injury, risk for (uses)
- Knowledge, deficient (teaching)

## Implementation
- Use procedures for handling and disposal of products
- Rinse mouth tid-qid with water or club soda; brush teeth tid with soft toothbrush or cotton-tipped applicator for stomatitis; use unwaxed dental floss
- Store at room temperature, away from light

## Patient/family education
- Advise patient to report bleeding; not to use commercial mouthwashes, razors
- Teach patient to report signs of infection: increased temp, sore throat, flulike symptoms
- Teach patient to report signs of anemia: fatigue, headache, faintness, shortness of breath, irritability
- Advise patient to avoid citric acid, rough-textured foods, if stomatitis is present
- Teach patient to notify prescriber if pregnancy is suspected or planned; use contraception while taking this product
- Teach patient to avoid breastfeeding while taking this product
- Instruct patient not to operate machinery or perform other hazardous activities while taking this product
- Teach patient that men should not father a child while taking this product, pregnancy category **D**
- Teach patient to inform prescriber of kidney or liver disease
- Teach patient not to receive vaccinations while taking this product

## Evaluation
**Positive therapeutic outcome**
- Decreased blast count

# delavirdine (Rx)
(de-la-veer'deen)
Rescriptor
*Func. class.:* Antiretroviral
*Chem. class.:* Nonnucleoside reverse transcriptase inhibitor (NNRII)

**Pregnancy category** C

**Action:** Binds directly to reverse transcriptase and blocks RNA, DNA causing a disruption of the enzyme's site

**Therapeutic outcome:** Improvement of HIV-1 infection

**Uses:** HIV-1 in combination with other antiretrovirals

**Dosage and routes**
*Adult and child ≥16 yr:* PO 400 mg tid; max 1200 mg/day

**Available forms:** Tabs 100, 200 mg

**Adverse effects**
*CNS:* Headache, fatigue, anxiety, insomnia, fever
*GI:* Diarrhea, anorexia, abdominal pain, nausea, vomiting, dyspepsia, **hepatotoxicity**
*GU:* **Nephrotoxicity**
*HEMA:* **Neutropenia, leukopenia, thrombocytopenia, anemia, granulocytopenia**
*INTEG:* Rash, pruritis
*MISC:* Cough
*MS:* Pain, myalgia
*SYST:* **Stevens-Johnson syndrome**

**Contraindications:** Hypersensitivity to this product or atevirdine

**Precautions:** Pregnancy **C**, breastfeeding, children, renal/hepatic disease, myelosuppression

## Pharmacokinetics
| | |
|---|---|
| **Absorption** | Well |
| **Distribution** | 98% protein bound |
| **Metabolism** | Liver, extensively |
| **Excretion** | Kidneys, feces |
| **Half-life** | 2-11 hr |

## Pharmacodynamics
| | |
|---|---|
| **Onset** | Unknown |
| **Peak** | 1 hr |
| **Duration** | 8 hr |

## Interactions
*Individual drugs*
Alprazolam, amprenavir, atorvastatin, clarithromycin, dapsone, felodipine, indinavir, lovastatin, midazolam, NIFEdipine,

saquinavir, simvastatin: increased level of each specific product

Cisapride, pimozide, sildenafil: life-threatening reactions; do not combine

Clarithromycin, quinidine, warfarin: increased level of both products

Didanosine: decreased action of didanosine

Fluoxetine, ketoconazole: increased level of delavirdine

*Drug classifications*

Amphetamines, antidysrhythmics, benzodiazepines, calcium channel blockers, ergots, sedative/hypnotics: increased serious life-threatening adverse reaction

Antacids, anticonvulsants, protease inhibitors, rifamycins: decreased delavirdine levels

Antidysrhythmics, sedative/hypnotics: life-threatening reactions; do not combine

Contraceptives (oral): decreased action of oral contraceptives

Ergots: increased levels of ergots

**NURSING CONSIDERATIONS**
**Assessment**
• Assess signs of infection, anemia
• Assess liver function tests: ALT, AST; renal studies
• Assess C&S before product therapy; product may be taken as soon as culture is taken; repeat C&S after treatment; determine the presence of other STDs
• Assess bowel pattern before, during treatment; if severe abdominal pain with bleeding occurs, product should be discontinued; monitor hydration
• Assess skin eruptions; rash, urticaria, itching
• Assess allergies before treatment, reaction to each medication; place allergies on chart
• Assess plasma delavirdine concentrations (trough 10 μm)
• Assess CBC, blood chemistry, plasma HIV RNA, absolute $CD4^+/CD8^+$/cell counts/%, serum $\beta_2$ microglobulin, serum ICD+24 antigen levels
• Assess for signs of delavirdine toxicity: severe nausea, vomiting, maculopapular rash

**Nursing diagnoses**
• Diarrhea (side effects)
• Infection, risk for (uses)
• Knowledge, deficient (teaching)

**Implementation**
• Add 4 tabs/3-4 oz of water, let stand, stir, swallow, rinse glass, swallow; use only 100 mg tabs for dispersion
• Do not give within 1 hr of antacids or didanosine
• Take in equal intervals around the clock

**Patient/family education**
• Advise patient to take as prescribed; if dose is missed, take as soon as remembered up to 1 hr before next dose; do not double dose
• Advise patient that product must be taken in equal intervals around the clock to maintain blood levels for duration of therapy
• Advise patient that tabs may be dissolved, drink right away, rinse cup with water, and drink that to get all medication
• Instruct patient to make sure health care provider knows of all the medications being taken
• Advise patient that if severe rash, mouth sores, swelling, aching muscles/joints, or eye redness occur, stop taking and notify health care provider
• Advise patient not to breastfeed if taking this product
• Teach patient that this product is not a cure, only controls symptoms

**Evaluation**
**Positive therapeutic outcome**
• Increased $CD4^+$ cell count
• Decreased viral load
• Improvement in symptoms of HIV

**demecarium ophthalmic**
*See Appendix D*

**denileukin diftitox** (Rx)
(den-ih-loo'kin dif'tih-tox)
Ontak
*Func. class.:* Antineoplastic—miscellaneous agent

**Pregnancy category** C

**Action:** A recombinant DNA-derived cytotoxic protein; inhibits cellular protein synthesis

**Therapeutic outcome:** Prevention of rapidly growing malignant cells

**Uses:** Cutaneous T-cell lymphoma that expresses CD25 component of the IL-2 receptor

**Unlabeled uses:** Non-Hodgkin's lymphoma, psoriasis

**Dosage and routes**
*Adult:* **IV** 9-18 mcg/kg/day given for 5 days q21 days, give over ≥15 min

**Available forms:** Sol for inj, frozen 150 mcg/ml

### Adverse effects
***CNS:*** *Dizziness, paresthesia, nervousness, confusion, insomnia*
***CV:*** *Hypo/hypertension, vasodilatation, tachycardia, thrombosis, dysrhythmia*
***GI:*** *Nausea, anorexia, vomiting, diarrhea, constipation, dyspepsia, dysphagia*
***GU:*** *Hematuria*, albuminuria, pyuria, creatinine increase
***HEMA:*** **Thrombocytopenia, leukopenia,** anemia
***INTEG:*** *Rash, pruritus, sweating*
***META:*** Hypoalbuminemia, edema, hypocalcemia, weight decrease, dehydration, hypokalemia
***MISC:*** *Fever, chills, asthenia, infection, pain, headache, chest pain,* flulike symptoms
***MS:*** Myalgia, arthralgia
***RESP:*** *Dyspnea, cough, pharyngitis, rhinitis*

**Contraindications:** Hypersensitivity to denileukin, diphtheria toxin, interleukin-2

**Precautions:** Pregnancy **C**, breastfeeding, children, geriatric, radiation therapy

#### Pharmacokinetics
| | |
|---|---|
| **Absorption** | Complete bioavailability (**IV**) |
| **Distribution** | Widely distributed; concentrates in liver/kidneys |
| **Metabolism** | Proteolytic degradation |
| **Excretion** | Unknown |
| **Half-life** | Unknown |

#### Pharmacodynamics
Unknown

### Interactions
#### Drug classifications
Antineoplastics, bone marrow-suppressing products, radiation: increased bone marrow suppression
Live virus vaccines: increased adverse reactions; decreased antibody reaction

### NURSING CONSIDERATIONS
#### Assessment
• Assess symptoms indicating severe allergic reaction: rash, pruritus, urticaria, purpuric skin lesions, itching, flushing; product should be discontinued
• Assess for vascular leak syndrome after 2 wk of treatment: hypotension, edema, hypoalbuminemia; monitor weight, B/P, serum albumin, edema
• Obtain CD25 expression on skin biopsy samples
• Monitor CBC, differential, platelet count weekly; withhold product if WBC count is <4000/mm$^3$ or platelet count is <100,000/mm$^3$
• Monitor renal function studies: BUN, creatinine, urine CCr before and during therapy; I&O ratio; report fall in urine output to <30 ml/hr
• Monitor temp q4hr (may indicate beginning of infection)
• Monitor liver function tests before and during therapy (bilirubin, AST, ALT, LDH) as needed or monthly; note jaundiced skin or sclera, dark urine, clay-colored stools, itchy skin, abdominal pain, fever, diarrhea; hepatotoxicity can be serious and fatal
• Assess for bleeding: hematuria, stool guaiac, bruising or petechiae, mucosa or orifices q8hr; check for inflammation of mucosa, breaks in skin

#### Nursing diagnoses
• Body image, disturbed (adverse reactions)
• Infection, risk for (adverse reactions)
• Injury, risk for (adverse reactions)
• Knowledge, deficient (teaching)

#### Implementation
• Give fluids **IV** or PO before chemotherapy to hydrate patient
• Give antiemetic 30-60 min before giving product to prevent vomiting, and prn; antibiotics for prophylaxis of infection
• Provide liquid diet: carbonated beverages; gelatin may be added if patient is not nauseated or vomiting
• Prepare and hold sol in plastic syringes or soft plastic **IV** bags only
• Draw calculated dose from vial, inject into empty **IV** infusion bag, for each 1 ml of product removed from vial, no more than 9 ml of sterile saline without preservative should be added to **IV** bag; infuse over ≥15 min; do not give by BOL; do not admix with other products; do not use a filter
• Use within 6 hr, discard unused portions
• Watch for extravasation; give 3-5 ml of mixture of 4 ml sodium thiosulfate 10% plus 5 ml sterile water SUBCUT as prescribed

#### Patient/family education
• Teach patient to avoid use of products containing aspirin or NSAIDs, razors, commercial mouthwash, since bleeding may occur; to report symptoms of bleeding (hematuria, tarry stools)
• Instruct patient to report signs of anemia (fatigue, headache, irritability, faintness, shortness of breath)
• Caution patient not to have any vaccinations without the advice of prescriber; serious reactions can occur

- Advise patient contraception is needed during treatment and for several months after the completion of therapy; product has teratogenic properties

**Evaluation**

**Positive therapeutic outcome**

- Prevention of rapid division of malignant cells

## desipramine (Rx)
(dess-ip′ra-meen)
Apo-Desipramine ✦, desipramine HCl, Norpramin, Pertofrane ✦
*Func. class.:* Antidepressant, tricyclic
*Chem. class.:* Dibenzazepine, secondary amine

**Pregnancy category C**

**Action:** Blocks reuptake of norepinephrine, serotonin into nerve endings, increasing action of norepinephrine, serotonin in nerve cells

**Therapeutic outcome:** Decreased depression

**Uses:** Depression

**Unlabeled uses:** Chronic pain, ADHD, bulimia, diabetic neuropathy, panic disorder, social phobia

**Dosage and routes**
*Adult:* PO 100-200 mg/day in a single dose or in divided doses; max 300 mg/day
*Geriatric:* PO 25-50 mg/day, may increase to 150 mg/day
*Child >12 yr:* PO 25-50 mg/day in divided doses, max 100 mg/day
*Child 6-12 yr:* PO 10-30 mg/day or 1-5 mg/kg/day in divided doses, give >3 mg/kg/day with close medical monitoring

**Available forms:** Tabs 10, 25, 50, 75, 100, 150 mg

**Adverse effects**
*CNS: Dizziness, drowsiness,* confusion, headache, anxiety, tremors, stimulation, weakness, insomnia, nightmares, EPS (geriatric), increased psychiatric symptoms, paresthenia, suicidal ideation
*CV: Orthostatic hypo/hypertension, ECG changes, tachycardia, palpitations*
*EENT: Blurred vision,* tinnitus, mydriasis, ophthalmoplegia
*GI: Diarrhea, dry mouth,* nausea, vomiting, **paralytic ileus,** increased appetite, cramps, epigastric distress, jaundice, **hepatitis,** stomatitis, constipation
*GU: Retention,* **acute renal failure**

*HEMA:* **Agranulocytosis, thrombocytopenia, eosinophilia, leukopenia**
*INTEG:* Rash, urticaria, sweating, pruritus, photosensitivity

**Contraindications:** Hypersensitivity to tricyclics, angle-closure glaucoma, thyroid disease

**Precautions:** Pregnancy **C,** breastfeeding, geriatric, suicidal patients, severe depression, increased intraocular pressure, seizure disorder, CV disease, prostatic hypertrophy

### Pharmacokinetics

| | |
|---|---|
| **Absorption** | Well |
| **Distribution** | Widely, protein binding 92% |
| **Metabolism** | Extensively, liver |
| **Excretion** | Unknown |
| **Half-life** | 12-24 hr |

### Pharmacodynamics
Unknown

**Interactions**
*Individual drugs*
Alcohol: increased CNS depression
Cimetidine, fluvoxamine, fluoxetine, paroxetine, sertraline: increased desipramine level
Clonidine: increased life-threatening B/P elevations, do not use concurrently
EpINEPHrine, norepinephrine: increased hypertension
*Drug classifications*
Barbiturates, opioids, CNS depressants: increased CNS depression
MAOIs: increased hyperpyrexia, seizures, excitation, do not use within 14 days of MAOIs
Tricyclic antidepressants: increased QT interval
*Drug/herb*
Evening primrose oil: may lower seizure threshold, do not use concurrently
Chamomile, hops, kavan, valerian: increased CNS depression
St. John's wort, SAM-e: may increase serotonin syndrome; avoid concurrent use
*Drug/lab test*
Increase: serum bilirubin, blood glucose, alkaline phosphatase

**NURSING CONSIDERATIONS**
**Assessment**
- Monitor B/P (lying, standing), pulse q4hr; if systolic B/P drops 20 mm Hg, hold product, notify prescriber; take vital signs q4hr in patients with CV disease

---

Adverse effects: *italic* = common, **bold** = life-threatening

- Monitor blood studies: CBC, leukocytes, differential, cardiac enzymes if patient is receiving long-term therapy
- Monitor hepatic studies: AST, ALT, bilirubin
- Check weight qwk; appetite may increase with this product
- Monitor ECG for flattening T wave, bundle branch block, AV block, dysrhythmias in cardiac patients
- Assess for EPS primarily in geriatric: rigidity, dystonia, akathisia
- Assess for seizure activity in those with a history of seizures
- Assess mental status: mood, sensorium, affect, suicidal tendencies, increase in psychiatric symptoms: depression, panic
- Assess for urinary retention, constipation; constipation most likely in children
- Assess for withdrawal symptoms: headache, nausea, vomiting, muscle pain, weakness; not usual unless product discontinued abruptly
- Assess for alcohol consumption; if consumed, hold dose until morning

## Nursing diagnoses
- Coping, ineffective (uses)
- Knowledge, deficient (teaching)
- Noncompliance (teaching)

## Implementation
- Increase fluids, bulk in diet for constipation, especially in geriatric
- Take with food or milk for GI symptoms
- Crush if patient is unable to swallow medication whole
- Give dosage at bedtime if oversedation occurs during day; may take entire dose at bedtime; geriatric may not tolerate once a day dosing
- Give gum, hard candy, frequent sips of water for dry mouth
- Store at room temperature
- Provide assistance with ambulation during beginning of therapy for drowsiness/dizziness
- Provide safety measures, primarily in the geriatric
- Check to see that PO medication is swallowed

## Patient/family education
- Advise patient that therapeutic effects may take 2-3 wk
- Teach patient that suicidal thoughts and behavior may occur
- Advise patient to use caution in driving, other activities requiring alertness because of drowsiness, dizziness, blurred vision
- Teach patient to avoid alcohol ingestion, other CNS depressants

- Teach patient not to discontinue medication quickly after long-term use; may cause nausea, headache, malaise
- Teach patient to wear sunscreen or large hat, since photosensitivity occurs

## Evaluation
**Positive therapeutic outcome**
- Decreased depression

**Treatment of overdose:** ECG monitoring; induce emesis; lavage, activated charcoal; administer anticonvulsant

## desloratadine (Rx)
(des-lor-at'ah-deen)
Clarinex, Clarinex RediTabs
*Func. class.:* Antihistamine, 2nd generation
*Chem. class.:* Selective histamine ($H_1$-) receptor antagonist

### Pregnancy category C

**Action:** Binds to peripheral histamine receptors, providing antihistamine action without sedation

**Therapeutic outcome:** Decreased nasal stuffiness, itching, swollen eyes

**Uses:** Seasonal allergic rhinitis, chronic idiopathic urticaria

## Dosage and routes
*Adult and child ≥12 yr:* PO 5 mg daily
*Child 6-11 yr:* PO 2.5 mg daily
*Child 1-5 yr:* PO 1.25 mg daily
*Child 6-11 mo:* PO 1 mg daily

*Renal/hepatic dose*
*Adult:* PO 5 mg every other day

**Available forms:** Tabs 5 mg; orally disintegrating (Reditabs) 2.5 mg; syr 0.5 mg/ml

## Adverse effects
*CNS:* Sedation (more common with increased doses), headache, psychomotor hyperactivity, **seizures,** fatigue
*GI:* **Hepatitis,** nausea, dry mouth
*MISC:* Flulike symptoms

**Contraindications:** Hypersensitivity, acute asthma attacks, lower respiratory tract disease

**Precautions:** Pregnancy C, bronchial asthma, renal/hepatic impairment

## Pharmacokinetics

| | |
|---|---|
| **Absorption** | Unknown |
| **Distribution** | Bound to plasma proteins (82%-87%) |
| **Metabolism** | Liver (active metabolites) |
| **Excretion** | Urine, feces (metabolites) |
| **Half-life** | 8½-28 hr |

## Pharmacodynamics

| | |
|---|---|
| **Onset** | 1 hr, relief in 1 day |
| **Peak** | 1½ hr |
| **Duration** | 24 hr |

## Interactions
### Drug/food
Food may prolong time to peak with orally disintegrating tabs

## NURSING CONSIDERATIONS
### Assessment
• Assess for allergy: hives, rash, rhinitis; monitor respiratory status; test interaction, antigen skin test

### Nursing diagnoses
• Airway clearance, ineffective (uses)
• Knowledge, deficient (teaching)
• Noncompliance (teaching, overuse)

### Implementation
• May administer without regard to meals
• Store in airtight container at room temperature

### Patient/family education
• Advise patient to avoid driving, other hazardous activities if drowsiness occurs; to observe caution until product's effects are known
• Advise patient that product may cause photosensitivity; use sunscreen or stay out of the sun to prevent burns
• Caution patient to avoid use of other CNS depressants
• Teach not to remove Reditabs from blister until ready to use; to place Reditabs directly on tongue, may take with or without water

### Evaluation
**Positive therapeutic outcome**
• Absence of running or congested nose, other allergy symptoms

---

## desmopressin (Rx)
(des-moe-press'in)
DDAVP, Minirin, Octostim, Stimate
*Func. class.:* Pituitary hormone
*Chem. class.:* Synthetic antidiuretic hormone

### Pregnancy category B

D

**Action:** Promotes reabsorption of water by action on renal tubular epithelium in the kidney; causes smooth muscle constriction and increase in plasma factor VIII levels, which increases platelet aggregation resulting in vasopressor effect; similar to vasopressin

**Therapeutic outcome:** Prevention of nocturnal enuresis, decreased bleeding in hemophilia A, von Willebrand's disease type 1, control and stabilization of water in diabetes insipidus

**Uses:** Hemophilia A, von Willebrand's disease type 1, nonnephrogenic diabetes insipidus, symptoms of polyuria/polydipsia caused by pituitary dysfunction, nocturnal enuresis

### Dosage and routes
#### Primary nocturnal enuresis
***Adult and child ≥6 yr:*** INTRANASAL 20 mcg (10 mcg in each nostril) at bedtime may increase to 40 mcg; PO 0.2 mg at bedtime, may be increased to max 0.6 mg at bedtime

#### Diabetes insipidus
***Adult:*** INTRANASAL 0.1-0.4 ml daily in divided doses (1-4 sprays with pump); SUBCUT/**IV** 0.5-1 ml daily in divided doses
***Child 3 mo-12 yr:*** INTRANASAL 0.05-0.3 ml daily in divided doses

#### Hemophilia/von Willebrand's disease
***Adult and child >3 mo:*** **IV** 0.3 mcg/kg in NaCl over 15-30 min; may repeat if needed

#### Antihemorrhagic
***Adult and child >3 mo:*** **IV** 0.3 mcg/kg
***Adult and child <50 kg:*** INTRANASAL 1 spray in one nostril
***Adult and child >50 kg:*** 1 spray each nostril

**Available forms:** Inj 4, 15 mcg/ml, Rhinal Tube del 2.5 mg/vial (0.1 mg/ml); tabs 0.1, 0.2 mg; nasal spray pump 10 mcg/spray (0.1 mg/ml); nasal sol 1.5 mg/ml (150 mcg/dose)

### Adverse effects
***CNS:*** Drowsiness, headache, lethargy, flushing
***CV:*** Increased B/P, palpitations, tachycardia
***EENT:*** Nasal irritation, congestion, rhinitis

---

Adverse effects: *italic* = common, **bold** = life-threatening

*GI:* Nausea, heartburn, cramps
*GU: Vulval pain*
*META:* Hyponatremia
*SYST:* Anaphylaxis **(IV)**

**Contraindications:** Hypersensitivity, nephrogenic diabetes insipidus, severe renal disease

**Precautions:** Pregnancy **B,** breastfeeding, CAD, hypertension, cystic fibrosis, thrombus

### Pharmacokinetics

| | |
|---|---|
| **Absorption** | Nasal (up to 20%) |
| **Distribution** | Unknown |
| **Metabolism** | Unknown |
| **Excretion** | Unknown; breast milk |
| **Half-life** | 8 min (initial), 76 min (terminal) |

### Pharmacodynamics

| | PO | INTRANASAL | SUBCUT/IV |
|---|---|---|---|
| **Onset** | 1 hr | 1 hr | Rapid |
| **Peak** | 4-7 hr | 1-4 hr | 15-30 min |
| **Duration** | Unknown | 8-20 hr | 3 hr |

### Interactions
*Individual drugs*
Carbamazepine, chlorpropamide, clofibrate: increased antidiuretic action
Demeclocycline, epINEPHrine (large doses), alcohol, heparin, lithium: decreased antidiuretic action

### NURSING CONSIDERATIONS
#### Assessment
• Monitor I&O ratio, urine osmolality, specific gravity, weight daily; check for edema in extremities; if water retention is severe, diuretic may be prescribed; check pulse, B/P when giving product **IV** or SUBCUT
• Assess for water intoxication: lethargy, behavioral changes, disorientation, neuromuscular excitability, dehydration, poor skin turgor, severe thirst, dry skin, tachycardia
• Assess intranasal use: nausea, congestion, cramps, headache; usually decreased with decreased dosage
• Monitor for enuresis during treatment (nocturnal enuresis)
• Assess for allergic reaction including anaphylaxis **(IV** route)
• Assess for nasal mucosa changes: congestion, edema, discharge, scarring (nasal route)
• Monitor urine volume osmolality and plasma osmolality (diabetes insipidus)
• Monitor factor VIII coagulant activity before using for hemostasis

#### Nursing diagnoses
• Fluid volume, deficient (uses)
• Fluid volume, excess (side effects)
• Knowledge, deficient (teaching)

#### Implementation
• Draw medication into tube, insert tube into nostril to instill product and blow on other end to deliver sol into nasal cavity; rinse after use
• Store in refrigerator or cool environment
**IV, direct route**
• Give undiluted over 1 min in diabetes insipidus or **IV** for hemophilia
**Intermittent IV infusion route**
• Give single dose diluted in 50 ml of 0.9% NaCl (adult and child >10 kg); a single dose/10 ml as an **IV** inf over 15-30 min in von Willebrand's disease or hemophilia A

#### Patient/family education
• Use demonstration, return demonstration to teach technique for nasal instillation
• Teach patient to notify prescriber of dyspnea, vomiting, cramping, drowsiness, headache, nasal congestion
• Caution patient to avoid OTC products (cough, hay fever), since these preparations may contain epINEPHrine and decrease product response; do not use with alcohol
• Advise patient to carry/wear emergency ID or other identification specifying disease and medication used
• Advise patient if dose is missed, take when remembered up to 1 hr before next dose; do not double doses
• Teach patient to report upper respiratory infection, nasal congestion

#### Evaluation
**Positive therapeutic outcome**
• Absence of severe thirst
• Decreased urine output, osmolality
• Absence of bleeding (hemophilia)

---

### desonide topical
*See Appendix D*

### desoximetasone topical
*See Appendix D*

### desoxyephedrine nasal agent
*See Appendix D*

---

 Alert     Canada Only    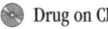 Drug on CD    * "Tall Man" lettering (See Preface)

## desoxyribonuclease
*See fibrinolysin/desoxyribonuclease*

## dexamethasone (Rx)
(dex-ah-meth'ah-sone)
Decadron, Deronil ✦, Dexasone ✦, Dexon, Hexadrol, Mymethasone

## dexamethasone acetate (Rx)
Dalalone DP, Dalalone LA, Decadron-LA, Decaject-LA, Dexacen LA-8, Dexasone-LA, Dexone LA, Solurex-LA

## dexamethasone sodium phosphate (Rx)
Dalalone, Decadron Phosphate, Decaject, Dexacen-4, Dexone, Hexadrol Phosphate, Solurex

*Func. class.:* Corticosteroid, synthetic
*Chem. class.:* Glucocorticoid, long-acting

**Pregnancy category** C

**Do not confuse:**
Decadron/Percodan

**Action:** Decreases inflammation by suppression of migration of polymorphonuclear leukocytes, fibroblasts, reversal of increased capillary permeability and lysosomal stabilization

**Uses:** Inflammation, allergies, neoplasms, cerebral edema, septic shock, collagen disorders

**Dosage and routes**
*Inflammation*
*Adult:* PO 0.75-9 mg/day, in divided doses q6-12hr; or phosphate IM 0.5-9 mg/day divided q6-12hr; or acetate IM 4-16 mg q1-3 wk
*Child:* PO 0.024-0.34 mg/kg/day in divided doses q6-12hr

*Shock*
*Adult:* **IV** (phosphate) single dose 1-6 mg/kg or **IV** 40 mg q2-6hr as needed up to 72 hr

*Cerebral edema*
*Adult:* **IV** (phosphate) 10 mg, then 4-6 mg IM q6hr × 2-4 days, then taper over 1 wk
*Child:* PO/IM/**IV** loading dose 1-2 mg/kg, then 1-1.5 mg/kg/day, max 16 mg/day divided q4-6hr for 2-4 days, then taper down qwk

*Adrenocortical insufficiency*
*Adult:* PO 0.5-9 mg/day in divided doses
*Child:* PO 0.03-0.3 mg/kg/day divided in 2-4 doses

*Suppression test*
*Adult:* PO 1 mg at 11 PM or 0.5 mg q6hr × 48 hr

*Croup (unlabeled)*
*Child:* PO 0.024-0.34 mg/kg/day or 0.66-10 mg/m$^2$/day in 2-4 divided doses; a single dose of 0.6 mg/kg has been used for mild to moderate croup; IM/**IV** 0.06-0.3 mg/kg/day or 1.2-10 mg/m$^2$/day in divided doses q6-12hr; a single dose of 0.6 mg/kg IM has been used for severe croup

**Available forms:** Dexamethasone: tabs 0.25, 0.5, 0.75, 1, 1.5, 2, 4, 6 mg; elix 0.5 mg/5 ml; oral sol 0.5 mg/5 ml, 1 mg/1 ml; inj phosphate 4, 10, 20, 24 mg/ml; inj dexamethasone acetate 8, 16 mg/ml

**Adverse effects**
*CNS: Depression, flushing, sweating,* headache, mood changes, euphoria, psychosis, **seizures,** insomnia
*CV: Hypertension,* **circulatory collapse, thrombophlebitis, embolism,** tachycardia, edema, cardiomyopathy
*EENT: Fungal infections, increased intraocular pressure, blurred vision, cataracts, glaucoma*
*ENDO: Hypothalmic-pituitary-adrenal axis suppression, hyperglycemia, sodium, fluid retention*
*GI: Diarrhea, nausea, abdominal distention,* **GI hemorrhage,** *increased appetite,* **pancreatitis**
*HEMA:* **Thrombocytopenia,** transient leukocytosis
*INTEG: Acne, poor wound healing, ecchymosis, petechiae, hirsutism*
*META: Hypokalemia*
*MS: Fractures, osteoporosis, weakness, arthralgia, myopathy*

**Contraindications:** Psychosis, hypersensitivity, idiopathic thrombocytopenia, acute glomerulonephritis, amebiasis, fungal infections, nonasthmatic bronchial disease, child <2 yr, AIDS, TB

**Precautions:** Pregnancy C, breastfeeding, diabetes mellitus, glaucoma, osteoporosis, seizure disorders, ulcerative colitis, CHF, myasthenia gravis, renal disease, peptic ulcer, esophagitis

| Pharmacokinetics | |
|---|---|
| **Absorption** | Unknown |
| **Distribution** | Unknown |
| **Metabolism** | Liver |
| **Excretion** | Kidneys |
| **Half-life** | 36-54 hr |

Adverse effects: *italic* = common, **bold** = life-threatening

| Pharmacodynamics | | |
|---|---|---|
| | PO | IM |
| **Onset** | 1 hr | Unknown |
| **Peak** | 1-2 hr | 8 hr |
| **Duration** | 2½ days | 6 days-3 wk |

## Interactions
### Individual drugs
Alcohol, amphotericin B, cycloSPORINE, digoxin, indomethacin: increased side effects

Ambemonium, isoniazid, neostigmine, sometrem: decreased effects of each specific product

Cholestyramine, colestipol, epHEDrine, phenytoin, rifampin, theophylline: decreased action of dexamethasone

Indomethacin, ketoconazole: increased action of dexamethasone

### Drug classifications
Antacids, barbiturates: decreased action of dexamethasone

Antibiotics (macrolide), contraceptives (oral), estrogens, salicylates: increased action of dexamethasone

Anticholinesterases, anticoagulants, anticonvulsants, antidiabetics, salicylates, toxoids/vaccines: decreased effects of each specific product

Diuretics, salicylates: increased side effects

### Drug/herb
Aloe, buckthorn bark/berry, cascara sagrada, Chinese rhubarb, senna pod/leaf: increased hypokalemia

Aloe, licorice, perilla: increased corticosteroid effect

### Drug/lab test
Increased: cholesterol, Na, blood glucose, uric acid, Ca, urine glucose

Decreased: Ca, K, $T_4$, $T_3$, thyroid $^{131}$I uptake test, urine 17-OHCS, 17-KS, PBI

False negative: skin allergy tests

## NURSING CONSIDERATIONS
### Assessment
• Monitor K, blood, urine glucose while on long-term therapy; hypokalemia and hyperglycemia

• Monitor weight daily; notify prescriber of weekly gain >5 lb

• Monitor B/P q4hr, pulse; notify prescriber of chest pain

• Monitor I&O ratio; be alert for decreasing urinary output, increasing edema

• Monitor plasma cortisol levels during long-term therapy (normal: 138-635 nmol/L SI units when assessed at 8 AM), prolonged use can cause Cushingoid symptoms

• Assess infection: fever, WBC even after withdrawal of medication; product masks infection

• Assess potassium depletion: paresthesias, fatigue, nausea, vomiting, depression, polyuria, dysrhythmias, weakness

• Assess edema, hypertension, cardiac symptoms

• Assess mental status: affect, mood, behavioral changes, aggression

### Nursing diagnoses
• Infection, risk for (adverse reaction)
• Knowledge, deficient (teaching)
• Mobility, impaired physical (uses)

### Implementation
#### PO route
• Give with food or milk to decrease GI symptoms

• Provide assistance with ambulation in patient with bone tissue disease to prevent fractures

#### IM route
• IM inj deep in large muscle mass; rotate sites; avoid deltoid; use 21-G needle

• In one dose in AM to prevent adrenal suppression; avoid SUBCUT administration, may damage tissue

#### IV route
• **IV** undiluted direct over 1 min or less or diluted with 0.9% NaCl or $D_5W$ and give as an **IV** inf at prescribed rate

• After shaking susp (parenteral); do not give susp **IV**

• Titrated dose; use lowest effective dose

### Dexamethasone sodium phosphate
**Syringe compatibilities:** Granisetron, metoclopramide, ranitidine, sufentanil

**Y-site compatibilities:** Acyclovir, allopurinol, amifostine, amikacin, amphotericin B cholesteryl, amsacrine, aztreonam, cefepime, cisatracurium, cisplatin, cladribine, cyclophosphamide, cytarabine, DOXOrubicin, DOXOrubicin liposome, famotidine, filgrastim, fluconazole, fludarabine, foscarnet, heparin, melphalan, meperidine, meropenem, morphine, ondansetron, paclitaxel, piperacillin/tazobactam, potassium chloride, propofol, remifentanil, sargramostim, sodium bicarbonate, sufentanil, tacrolimus, teniposide, theophylline, vinorelbine, vit B/C, zidovudine

**Additive compatibilities:** Aminophylline, bleomycin, cimetidine, floxacillin, furosemide, lidocaine, meropenem, nafcillin, netilmicin, ondansetron, prochlorperazine, ranitidine, verapamil

## Patient/family education
• Advise that emergency ID as steroid user should be carried or worn
• Teach to notify prescriber if therapeutic response decreases; dosage adjustment may be needed
• Teach not to discontinue abruptly or adrenal crisis can result
• Teach to avoid OTC products: salicylates, alcohol in cough products, cold preparations unless directed by prescriber
• Instruct patient to contact prescriber if surgery, trauma, stress occurs, dose may need to be adjusted
• Teach patient all aspects of product usage, including cushingoid symptoms
• Instruct patient to notify prescriber of infection
• Teach symptoms of adrenal insufficiency: nausea, anorexia, fatigue, dizziness, dyspnea, weakness, joint pain
• Advise patient to avoid exposure to chickenpox or measles, persons with infections

## Evaluation
**Positive therapeutic outcome**
Decreased inflammation

## dexamethasone ophthalmic
*See Appendix D*

## dexamethasone topical
*See Appendix D*

## dexmedetomidine (Rx)
(deks-med-ee-tome′a-dine)
Precedex
*Func. class.:* Sedative, $\alpha_2$-adrenoceptor agonist

**Pregnancy category C**

**Action:** Produces $\alpha_2$-agonist activity as seen at low and moderate doses; also, $\alpha_1$ at high doses

**Uses:** Sedation in mechanically ventilated, intubated patients in ICU

## Dosage and routes
*Adult:* **IV** Loading dose of 1 mcg/kg over 10 min, then 0.2-0.7 mcg/kg/hr, do not use for more than 24 hr

**Available forms:** Inj 100 mcg/ml

## Adverse effects
*CV: Bradycardia, hypo/hypertension,* **atrial fibrillation, infarction, cardiac arrest**

*GI: Nausea,* thirst
*GU:* Oliguria
*HEMA:* Leukocytosis, anemia
*MISC:* Hyperkalemia
*RESP:* **Pulmonary edema, pleural effusion, hypoxia,** respiratory acidosis

**Contraindications:** Hypersensitivity, chronic hypertension

**Precautions:** Pregnancy **C,** breastfeeding, children, geriatric, respiratory depression, severe respiratory disorders, cardiac dysrhythmias, hypovolemia, diabetes, CV/renal/hepatic disease

### Pharmacokinetics

| | |
|---|---|
| **Absorption** | Unknown |
| **Distribution** | Unknown |
| **Metabolism** | Unknown |
| **Excretion** | Unknown |
| **Half-life** | 8 min |

### Pharmacodynamics
Unknown

## Interactions
*Individual drugs*
Alcohol: increased CNS depression
*Drug classifications*
Anesthetics (inhalational), antipsychotics, opiates, sedative/hypnotics, skeletal muscle relaxants: increased CNS depression
Antihypertensives: increased hypotension

## NURSING CONSIDERATIONS
### Assessment
• Assess inj site: phlebitis, burning, stinging
• Monitor ECG for changes: atrial fibrillation; monitor geriatric more closely
• Assess CNS changes: movement, jerking, tremors, dizziness, LOC, pupil reaction
• Assess respiratory dysfunction: respiratory depression, character, rate, rhythm; notify prescriber if respirations are <10/min
• Assess cardiac status: B/P, heart rate

### Nursing diagnoses
• Injury, risk for (uses)

### Implementation
**IV route**
• Give after diluting with $D_5W$, 0.9% NaCl; withdraw 2 ml of product and add to 48 ml of 0.9% NaCl to a total of 50 ml; shake to mix well; use controlled infusion device
• Give only with resuscitative equipment available
• Give only by qualified persons trained in management of ICU sedation

*Adverse effects:* *italic* = common, **bold** = life-threatening

*Solution compatibilities:* LR, D$_5$W, 0.9% NaCl, 20% mannitol

*Additive compatibilities:* Atracurium, atropine, etomidate, fentanyl, glycopyrrolate, midazolam, mivacurium, morphine, pancuronium, phenylephrine, succinylcholine, thiopental, vecuronium

• Provide safety measures: side rails, nightlight, call bell within easy reach

### Evaluation
**Positive therapeutic outcome**

• Induction of sedation

---

## dexmethylphenidate (Rx)
(dex'meth-ul-fen'ih-dayt)
Focalin, Focalin XR
*Func. class.:* Central nervous system (CNS) stimulant, psychostimulant

**Pregnancy category C**

**Controlled substance schedule II**

**Action:** Increases release of norepinephrine and dopamine into the extraneuronal space, also blocks reuptake of norepinephrine and dopamine into the presynaptic neuron; mode of action in treating attention deficit hyperactivity disorder (ADHD) is unknown

**Therapeutic outcome:** Increased alertness, decreased fatigue, ability to stay awake (narcolepsy), increased attention span, decreased hyperactivity (ADHD)

**Uses:** ADHD, adjunctive treatment

### Dosage and routes
*Adult:* PO ext rel 10 mg/day, may adjust to 20 mg/day in 10 mg increments
*Child >6 yr:* PO 2.5 mg bid with doses at least 4 hr apart, gradually increase to a max of 20 mg/day (10 mg bid); for those taking methylphenidate, use ½ of methylphenidate dose initially, then increase as needed to a maximum of 20 mg/day; EXT REL 5 mg/day, may adjust to 20 mg/day in 5 mg increments

**Available forms:** Tabs 2.5, 5, 10 mg; ext rel caps (Focalin XR) 5, 10, 20 mg

### Adverse effects
*CNS:* Dizziness, headache, drowsiness, nervousness, insomnia, **toxic psychosis, neuroleptic malignant syndrome (rare)**, Gilles de la Tourette's syndrome
*CV:* Palpitations, B/P changes, angina, **dysrhythmias, tachycardia**
*GI:* *Nausea, anorexia*, abnormal liver function, **hepatic coma**, *abdominal pain*

*HEMA:* **Leukopenia, anemia, thrombocytopenic purpura**
*INTEG:* **Exfoliative dermatitis**, urticaria, rash, erythema multiforme
*MISC:* *Fever*, arthralgia, scalp hair loss

**Contraindications:** Hypersensitivity to methylphenidate, anxiety, history of Gilles de la Tourette's syndrome; children <6 yr, glaucoma, concurrent treatment with MAOIs or within 14 days of discontinuing treatment with MAOIs, breastfeeding, tics, psychosis

**Precautions:** Pregnancy **C,** hypertension, depression, seizures, product abuse, CV disorders, alcoholism

### Pharmacokinetics

| | |
|---|---|
| **Absorption** | Readily absorbed |
| **Distribution** | Unknown |
| **Metabolism** | Liver |
| **Excretion** | Kidneys |
| **Half-life** | 2.2 hr |

### Pharmacodynamics

| | PO | EXT REL |
|---|---|---|
| **Onset** | ½-1 hr | Unknown |
| **Peak** | 1-1 ½ hr | 4 hr |
| **Duration** | 4 hr | 8 hr |

### Interactions
*Drug classifications*
Anticoagulants (coumarin) (e.g., warfarin), anticonvulsants, selective serotonin reuptake inhibitors, tricyclics: increased effects
Antihypertensives: decreased effects
Decongestants, vasoconstrictors: increased sympathomimetic effect
MAOIs: hypertensive crisis if coadministered or given within 14 days
Vasopressors: hypertensive crisis
*Drug/herb*
Horsetail, yohimbe: increased stimulant effect
Melatonin: increased synergistic effect

### NURSING CONSIDERATIONS
**Assessment**

• Assess VS, B/P; may reverse antihypertensives; check patients with cardiac disease more often for increased B/P
• Assess CBC, differential, platelet counts during long-term therapy, urinalysis; in diabetes: blood/urine glucose; insulin changes may have to be made, since eating will decrease
• Assess height, growth rate q3 mo in children; growth rate may be decreased
• Assess mental status: mood, sensorium, affect, stimulation, insomnia, aggressiveness

---

◆ Assess withdrawal symptoms: headache, nausea, vomiting, muscle pain, weakness
• Assess appetite, sleep, speech patterns
• Assess for attention span, decreased hyperactivity in persons with ADHD

## Nursing diagnoses
• Coping, disabled family (uses)
• Coping, ineffective (uses)
• Knowledge, deficient (teaching)
• Thought processes, disturbed (uses, adverse reactions)

## Implementation
• Do not break, crush, or chew ext rel caps
• Twice daily at least 4 hr apart; ext rel once a day
• Without regard to meals

## Patient/family education
• Advise patient to decrease caffeine consumption (coffee, tea, cola, chocolate); may increase irritability, stimulation
• Advise patient to avoid OTC preparations unless approved by prescriber
• Caution patient to taper off product over several wk to avoid depression, increased sleeping, lethargy
• Caution patient to avoid alcohol ingestion
• Caution patient to avoid hazardous activities until stabilized on medication
• Advise patient to get needed rest; patients will feel more tired at end of day
• Notify all health providers including school nurse of medication and schedule
• Discuss information instructions provided in patient information section

## Evaluation
**Positive therapeutic outcome**
• Decreased hyperactivity or ability to stay awake

**Treatment of overdose:** Administer fluids; hemodialysis or peritoneal dialysis; antihypertensive for increased B/P; administer short-acting barbiturate before lavage

---

**dextroamphetamine** (Rx)
(dex-troe-am-fet´a-meen)
Dextroamphetamine, Dextrostat
*Func. class.:* Cerebral stimulant
*Chem. class.:* Amphetamine

**Pregnancy category** C
**Controlled substance schedule** II

**Action:** Increases release of norepinephrine, dopamine in cerebral cortex to reticular activating system

**Therapeutic outcome:** Increased alertness, decreased fatigue, ability to stay awake (narcolepsy); increased attention span, decreased hyperactivity (ADHD)

**Uses:** Narcolepsy, attention deficit disorder with hyperactivity

**Unlabeled use:** Obesity

## Dosage and routes
*Narcolepsy*
*Adult:* PO 5-60 mg daily in divided doses
*Child >12 yr:* PO 10 mg daily increasing by 10 mg/day at weekly intervals
*Child 6-12 yr:* PO 5 mg daily increasing by 5 mg/wk (max 60 mg/day)

*ADHD*
*Adult:* PO 5-60 mg/day in divided doses
*Child >6 yr:* PO 5 mg daily-bid increasing by 5 mg/day at weekly intervals
*Child 3-6 yr:* PO 2.5 mg daily increasing by 2.5 mg/day at weekly intervals

**Available forms:** Tabs 5, 10 mg

## Adverse effects
*CNS: Hyperactivity, insomnia, restlessness, talkativeness,* dizziness, headache, chills, stimulation, dysphoria, irritability, aggressiveness, tremor, dependence, addiction
*CV: Palpitations,* **tachycardia,** hypertension, decrease in heart rate, **dysrhythmias**
*GI: Anorexia,* dry mouth, diarrhea, constipation, weight loss, metallic taste
*GU:* Impotence, change in libido
*INTEG:* Urticaria

**Contraindications:** Hypersensitivity to sympathomimetic amines, hyperthyroidism, hypertension, glaucoma, severe arteriosclerosis, drug abuse, CV disease, anxiety, anorexia nervosa, tartrazine dye hypersensitivity

**Precautions:** Pregnancy C, breastfeeding, child <3 yr, Gilles de la Tourette's disorder, depression

### Pharmacokinetics

| | |
|---|---|
| **Absorption** | Well absorbed |
| **Distribution** | Widely distributed; crosses placenta |
| **Metabolism** | Liver |
| **Excretion** | Kidneys, pH dependent: increased pH, increased reabsorption |
| **Half-life** | 10-30 hr; increased when urine is alkaline |

### Pharmacodynamics

| | |
|---|---|
| **Onset** | ½ hr |
| **Peak** | 1-3 hr |
| **Duration** | 4-10 hr |

Adverse effects: *italic* = common **bold** = life-threatening

## Interactions
### Individual drugs
AcetaZOLAMIDE, sodium bicarbonate: increased effect of dextroamphetamine

Ammonium chloride, ascorbic acid: decreased effect of dextroamphetamine

Haloperidol: increased CNS effect

Phenytoin: decreased absorption of phenytoin

### Drug classifications
Adrenergic blockers: decreased adrenergic blocking effect

Antacids: increased effect of dextroamphetamine

Antidepressants (tricyclic), phenothiazines: increased CNS effect

Antidiabetics: decreased antidiabetic effect

Barbiturates: decreased absorption of barbiturate

MAOIs: hypertensive crisis if used within 14 days

### Drug/herb
Eucalyptus: decreased stimulant effect

Khat: increased stimulant effect

St. John's wort: increased serotonin syndrome

### Drug/food
Caffeine: increased amine effect

## NURSING CONSIDERATIONS
### Assessment
• Monitor VS, B/P, since this product may reverse antihypertensives; check patients with cardiac disease more often for increased B/P

• Monitor CBC, urinalysis; for diabetic patients monitor blood, urine glucose; insulin changes may be required, since eating will decrease

• Monitor height and weight q3 mo since growth rate in children may be decreased; appetite is suppressed so weight loss is common during the first few months of treatment

• Monitor mental status: mood, sensorium, affect, stimulation, insomnia; aggressiveness may occur; depression with crying spells may occur after product has worn off

• Assess for physical dependency; should not be used for extended time except in ADHD; dosage should be decreased gradually to prevent withdrawal symptoms

• Assess for narcoleptic symptoms before medication and after; ability to stay awake should increase significantly

• In children or adults with ADHD, monitor for improved organizational skills, attention span, attending to tasks, impulse control, socialization, and ability to get along better with others

• Assess for withdrawal symptoms: headache, nausea, vomiting, muscle pain, weakness; product tolerance develops after long-term use; dosage should not be increased if tolerance develops; this medication has a high abuse potential

### Nursing diagnoses
• Coping, compromised family (uses)
• Coping, ineffective (uses)
• Knowledge, deficient (teaching)
• Thought processes, disturbed (uses, adverse reactions)

### Implementation
• Give at least 6 hr before bedtime to avoid sleeplessness; titrate to patient's response; lowest dosage should be used to control symptoms

• Give gum, hard candy, frequent sips of water for dry mouth at beginning of treatment; these symptoms tend to lessen with time

### Patient/family education
• Advise patient to decrease caffeine consumption (coffee, tea, cola, chocolate), which may increase irritability and stimulation; to avoid OTC preparations unless approved by prescriber; to avoid alcohol ingestion; these may cause serious drug interactions

• Advise patient to take before meals (obesity)

• Caution patient to taper off product over several weeks, or depression, increased sleeping, lethargy may occur

• Caution patient to avoid hazardous activities until patient is stabilized on medication

• Instruct patient not to double doses if medication is missed; prescriber may suggest product holidays (ADHD) during the school year to assess progress and determine continued product necessity

• Instruct patient/family to notify prescriber if significant side effects occur: tremors, insomnia, palpitations, restlessness, product changes may be needed

• Inform patient that if dry mouth occurs, to use frequent sips of water, sugarless gum, hard candy during beginning therapy; dry mouth lessens with continued treatment

• Advise patient to get needed rest; patients will feel more tired at end of day; to give last dose at least 6 hr before bedtime to avoid insomnia

### Evaluation
**Positive therapeutic outcome**
• Decreased activity in ADHD
• Absence of sleeping during day in narcolepsy

**Treatment of overdose:** Administer fluids, hemodialysis, peritoneal dialysis, antihypertensives for increased B/P; ammonium chloride for increased excretion

## dextromethorphan (OTC)
(dex-troe-meth-or'fan)
Balminil DM ✦, Benylin DM, Broncho-Grippol-DM ✦, Children's Hold, Creo-Terpin, Delsym, dextromethorphan, Hold DM, Koffex ✦, Neo-DM ✦, Ornex-DM ✦, Pertussin, Pertussin ES, Robidex ✦, Robitussin Cough Calmers, Robitussin Pediatric, Sedatuss ✦, St. Joseph Cough Suppressant, Scot-Tussin DM, Sucrets Cough Control, Suppress, Vicks Formula 44
*Func. class.:* Antitussive, nonopioid
*Chem. class.:* Levorphanol derivative

**Pregnancy category** C

**Action:** Depresses cough center in medulla by direct effect related to levorphanol

**Therapeutic outcome:** Absence of cough

**Uses:** Nonproductive cough carried by minor respiratory tract infections or irritants that might be inhaled

**Unlabeled uses:** Neuropathy

**Dosage and routes**
*Adult and child ≥12 yr:* PO 10-20 mg q4hr, or 30 mg q6-8hr, not to exceed 120 mg/day; SUS REL LIQUID 60 mg q12hr, not to exceed 120 mg/day
*Child 6-12 yr:* PO 5-10 mg q4hr; SUS REL LIQUID 30 mg bid, not to exceed 60 mg/day; LOZENGE 5-10 mg q1-4hr, max 60 mg/day
*Child 2-6 yr:* PO 2.5-5 mg q4hr, or 7.5 mg q6-8hr, not to exceed 30 mg/day

*Neuropathy (unlabeled)*
*Adult:* PO doses vary widely

**Available forms:** Loz 2.5, 5, 7.5, 15 mg; liquid 3.5 mg, 7.5, 15 mg/5 ml, 3.5, 5, 7.5, 10, 15 mg/5 ml; syr 15 mg/15 ml, 10 mg/5 ml; sus action liquid equivalent to 30 mg/5 ml; caps 30 mg; ext rel susp 30 mg/5 ml; gel caps 15 mg

**Adverse effects**
*CNS: Dizziness,* sedation, confusion, ataxia, fatigue
*GI: Nausea*

**Contraindications:** Hypersensitivity, asthma/emphysema, productive cough

**Precautions:** Pregnancy **C**, nausea/vomiting, increased temp, persistent headache, hepatic disease

### Pharmacokinetics
| | |
|---|---|
| **Absorption** | Rapid (PO); slow (SUS REL) |
| **Distribution** | Unknown |
| **Metabolism** | Liver |
| **Excretion** | Kidneys |
| **Half-life** | Terminal 11 hr |

### Pharmacodynamics
| | PO | PO-SUS |
|---|---|---|
| **Onset** | 15-30 min | Unknown |
| **Peak** | Unknown | Unknown |
| **Duration** | 3-6 hr | 12 hr |

**Interactions**
*Individual drugs*
Alcohol: increased CNS depression
Amiodarone, fluoxetine, quinidine, sibutramine: increased adverse reactions
Furazolidone, linezolide, procarbazine: increased hypotension, hyperpyrexia
*Drug classifications*
Antihistamines, antidepressants, opiates, sedative/hypnotics: increased CNS depression
MAOIs: increased hypotension, hyperpyrexia, do not give within 2 wk of MAOI

**NURSING CONSIDERATIONS**
**Assessment**
• Assess cough: type, frequency, character including sputum; provide adequate hydration to 2 L/day to decrease viscosity of secretions

**Nursing diagnoses**
• Airway clearance, ineffective (uses)
• Knowledge, deficient (teaching)

**Implementation**
• Administer decreased dosage to geriatric patients; their metabolism may be slowed; do not provide water within 30 min of administration because it dilutes product
• Shake susp before administration

**Patient/family education**
• Caution patient to avoid driving or other hazardous activities until stabilized on this medication; may cause drowsiness, dizziness in some individuals
• Advise patient to avoid smoking, smoke-filled rooms, perfumes, dust, environmental pollutants, cleaners, which increase cough; may use gum, hard candy to prevent dry mouth
• Advise patient to avoid alcohol or other CNS depressants while taking this medication; drowsiness will be increased

Adverse effects: *italic* = common, **bold** = life-threatening

• Caution patient that any cough lasting over a few days should be assessed by prescriber

## Evaluation
**Positive therapeutic outcome**
• Absence of dry, irritating cough

---

## dextrose (D-glucose) (Rx)
Glucose, Glutose, Insta-Glucose
*Func. class.:* Caloric agent

**Action:** Needed for adequate utilization of amino acids; decreases protein, nitrogen loss; prevents ketosis

**Therapeutic outcome:** Provides calories, prevents severe hypoglycemia

**Uses:** Increases intake of calories; increases fluids in patients unable to take adequate fluids, calories orally; 2.5%-11.5% forms provide calories, increased hydration; 20%-70% forms used to treat severe hypoglycemia

### Dosage and routes
*Adult and child:* **IV**, depends on individual requirements

**Available forms:** Inj **IV** 2.5%, 5%, 10%, 20%, 25% 30%, 38.5%, 40%, 50%, 60%, 70%; oral gel 40%; chewable tabs 5 g

### Adverse effects
*CNS:* Confusion, **loss of consciousness,** dizziness
*CV:* Hypertension, **CHF, pulmonary edema, intracranial hemorrhage**
*ENDO:* Hyperglycemia, rebound hypoglycemia, hyperosmolar syndrome, hyperglycemic nonketolytic syndrome, aluminum toxicity, hypokalemia, hypomagnesium
*GI:* Nausea
*GU:* Glycosuria, osmotic diuresis
*INTEG:* Chills, flushing, warm feeling, rash, urticaria, extravasation necrosis
*RESP:* Pulmonary edema

**Contraindications:** Hyperglycemia, delirium tremens, hemorrhage (cranial/spinal), CHF, anuria, allergy to corn products

**Precautions:** Renal/liver/cardiac disease, diabetes mellitus, carbohydrate intolerance

### Pharmacokinetics

| Absorption | Well absorbed (PO); completely absorbed (**IV**) |
|---|---|
| Distribution | Widely distributed |
| Metabolism | Unknown |
| Excretion | Unknown |
| Half-life | Unknown |

### Pharmacodynamics

| | PO | IV |
|---|---|---|
| **Onset** | Rapid | Immediate |
| **Peak** | Rapid | Immediate |
| **Duration** | Rapid | Immediate |

### Interactions
*Drug classifications*
Corticosteroids: increased fluid retention/ electrolyte excretion

## NURSING CONSIDERATIONS
### Assessment
• Assess I&O, skin turgor, edema, electrolytes (potassium, sodium, calcium, chloride, magnesium), blood glucose, ammonia, phosphate
• Monitor inj site for extravasation: redness along vein, edema at site, necrosis, pain, hard tender area; site should be changed immediately
• Monitor temp q4hr for increased fever, indicating infection; if infection suspected, inf is discontinued and tubing, bottle, catheter tip cultured
• Monitor serum glucose in patients receiving hypertonic glucose 5% and over
• Assess nutritional status: calorie count by dietitian; GI system function

### Nursing diagnoses
• Fluid volume, excess (adverse reactions)
• Knowledge, deficient (teaching)
• Nutrition, less than body requirements, imbalanced (uses)

### Implementation
**PO route**
• Oral glucose preparations (gel, chewable tabs) are to be used for conscious patients only; serum blood glucose should be monitored after first oral dose; if glucose has not increased by 20 mg/100 ml in 20-30 min, dose should be repeated and serum glucose checked again
**IV route**
• Give only protein (4%) and dextrose (up to 12.5%) via peripheral vein; stronger sol requires central **IV** administration
• May be given undiluted via prepared sol; give 10% sol (5 ml/15 sec), 20% sol (1000 ml/3 hr or more), 50% sol (500 ml/30-60 min); too rapid **IV** administration may cause fluid overload and hyperglycemia
• After changing **IV** catheter, change dressing q24hr with aseptic technique

---

⬥ Alert    ♣ Canada Only    🔵 Drug on CD    * "Tall Man" lettering (See Preface)

#### Patient/family education
- Teach patient reason for dextrose infusion
- Provide literature and information on when and how to use oral products for hypoglycemia
- Review hypo/hyperglycemia symptoms
- Review blood glucose monitoring procedure

#### Evaluation
**Positive therapeutic outcome**
- Increased weight
- Blood glucose level at normal limits for patient
- Adequate hydration

---

### diazepam (Rx)
(dye-az'e-pam)
Apo-Diazepam ✦, Diastat, diazepam, Diazepam Intensol, Diazemuls ✦, Novo-Diapam ✦, PMS-Diazepam ✦, Valium, Vivol ✦
*Func. class.:* Antianxiety, anticonvulsant, skeletal muscle relaxant, central acting
*Chem. class.:* Benzodiazepine, long-acting

**Pregnancy category D**
**Controlled substance schedule IV**

**Do not confuse:**
diazepam/Ditropan/lorazepam

**Action:** Potentiates the actions of GABA, especially in limbic system, reticular formation; enhances presympathetic inhibition, inhibits spinal polysynaptic afferent paths

**Therapeutic outcome:** Decreased anxiety, restlessness, insomnia

**Uses:** Anxiety, acute alcohol withdrawal, adjunct in seizure disorders; preoperative skeletal muscle relaxation; rectally for acute repetitive seizures

#### Dosage and routes
*Anxiety/convulsive disorders*
*Adult:* PO 2-10 mg bid-qid; IM/IV 2-10 mg q3-4hr
*Geriatric:* PO 1-2 mg daily-bid, increase slowly as needed
*Child >6 mo:* IM/IV 0.04-0.3 mg/kg/dose q2-4hr, max 0.6 mg/kg in an 8-hr period

*Precardioversion*
*Adult:* IV 5-15 mg 5-10 min precardioversion

*Preendoscopy*
*Adult:* IV 2.5-20 mg, IM 5-10 mg ½ hr preendoscopy

*Muscle relaxation*
*Adult:* PO 2-10 mg tid-qid or ext rel 15-30 mg daily; IM/IV 5-10 mg repeat in 2-4 hr
*Geriatric:* PO 2-5 mg bid-qid; IM/IV 2-5 mg, may repeat in 2-4 hr

*Tetanic muscle spasms*
*Child >5 yr:* IM/IV 5-10 mg q3-4hr prn
*Infants >30 days:* IM/IV 1-2 mg q3-4hr prn

*Status epilepticus*
*Adult:* IM/IV 5-10 mg, 2 mg/min, may repeat q10-15 min, not to exceed 30 mg; may repeat in 2-4 hr if seizures reappear
*Child >5 yr:* IV 1 mg slowly; IM 1 mg q2-5 min
*Child 1 mo-5 yr:* IV 0.2-0.5 mg slowly; IM 0.2-0.5 mg slowly q2-5 min up to 5 mg; may repeat in 2-4 hr prn

*Seizures other than status epilepticus*
*Adult:* RECT 0.2 mg/kg, may repeat 4-12 hr later
*Child 6-11 yr:* RECT 0.3 mg/kg, may repeat 4-12 hr later
*Child 2-5 yr:* RECT 0.5 mg/kg, may repeat 4-12 hr later

*Alcohol withdrawal*
*Adult:* IV 10 mg initially, then 5-10 mg q3-4hr prn

**Available forms:** Tabs 2, 5, 10 mg; inj 5 mg/ml; oral sol 5 mg/5 ml, 5 mg/ml; gel, rectal delivery system 10 mg, twin packs; ext rel cap 15 mg

#### Adverse effects
*CNS: Dizziness, drowsiness,* confusion, headache, anxiety, tremors, stimulation, fatigue, depression, insomnia, hallucinations, ataxia, fatigue
*CV: Orthostatic hypotension,* **ECG changes, tachycardia,** hypotension
*EENT: Blurred vision,* tinnitus, mydriasis, nystagmus
*GI:* Constipation, dry mouth, nausea, vomiting, anorexia, diarrhea
*HEMA:* **Neutropenia**
*INTEG:* Rash, dermatitis, itching
*RESP:* **Respiratory depression**

**Contraindications:** Pregnancy **D**, breast-feeding, hypersensitivity to benzodiazepines, angle-closure glaucoma, psychosis, coma, respiratory depression, untreated open-angle glaucoma

**Precautions:** Geriatric, debilitated, renal/hepatic disease, addiction, child <6 mo

Adverse effects: *italic* = common, **bold** = life-threatening

## Pharmacokinetics

| | |
|---|---|
| **Absorption** | Rapid (PO); erratic (IM) |
| **Distribution** | Widely distributed; crosses blood-brain barrier, placenta; protein binding 99% |
| **Metabolism** | Liver, extensively, CYP2C19, CYP3A4 |
| **Excretion** | Kidneys, breast milk |
| **Half-life** | 20-80 hr |

## Pharmacodynamics

| | PO | IM | IV |
|---|---|---|---|
| **Onset** | ½ hr | 15 min | Immediate |
| **Peak** | 1-2 hr | ½-1½ hr | 15 min |
| **Duration** | 2-3 hr | 1-1½ hr | 15 min-1 hr |

## Interactions
### Individual drugs
Alcohol: increased CNS depression

Cimetidine, valproic acid: increased toxicity

CYP3A4 inducers (carbamazepine, ethetoin, phenytoins, rifampin): decreased diazepam effect

Disulfiram, isoniazid, propranolol, valproic acid: decreased metabolism of diazepam

### Drug classifications
Barbiturates, CNS depressants, CYP3A4 inhibitors, selective serotonin reuptake inhibitors: increased toxicity

CNS depressants: increased CNS depression

CYP3A4 inducers (barbiturates): decreased diazepam effect

Oral contraceptives: decreased metabolism of diazepam

### Drug/herb
Cowslip, goldenseal, kava, melatonin, mistletoe, pokeweed, poppy, Queen Anne's lace, valerian: increased diazepam effect

Cola tree, St. John's wort: decreased diazepam effect

### Drug/lab test
Increased: AST/ALT, serum bilirubin

Decreased: radioactive iodine uptake

False increase: 17-OHCS

## NURSING CONSIDERATIONS
### Assessment
• Assess degree of anxiety; what precipitates anxiety and whether product controls symptoms; other signs of anxiety: dilated pupils, inability to sleep, restlessness, inability to focus

• Assess for alcohol withdrawal symptoms, including hallucinations (visual, auditory), delirium, irritability, agitation, fine to coarse tremors

• Monitor B/P (with patient lying, standing), pulse, respiratory rate; if systolic B/P drops 20 mm Hg, hold product, notify prescriber; monitor respirations q5-15 min if given **IV**

• Monitor blood studies: CBC during long-term therapy; blood dyscrasias have occurred (rarely); hepatic studies: ALT, AST

• Monitor for seizure control; type, duration, and intensity of seizures; what precipitates seizures

• Monitor hepatic studies: AST, ALT, bilirubin, creatinine, LDH, alkaline phosphatase

• Assess mental status: mood, sensorium, affect, sleeping pattern, drowsiness, dizziness, suicidal tendencies, and ability of product to control these symptoms; check for tolerance, withdrawal symptoms: headache, nausea, vomiting, muscle pain, weakness after long-term use

• Assess for muscle spasms, pain relief

### Nursing diagnoses
• Anxiety (uses)
• Coping, ineffective (uses)
• Injury, risk for (uses, adverse reactions)
• Knowledge, deficient (teaching)
• Noncompliance (teaching)

### Implementation
#### PO route
• Give with food or milk for GI symptoms

• Crush tab if patient is unable to swallow medication whole

• Use sugarless gum, hard candy, frequent sips of water for dry mouth

• Reduce opioid dosage by one third if given concomitantly with diazepam

• Check to see PO medication has been swallowed

• Concentrate: use calibrated dropper only; mix with water, juice, pudding, applesauce; consume immediately

#### Rectal route
• Do not use more than 5×/mo or for an episode q5 days

#### IV route
• Administer **IV** into large vein; do not dilute or mix with any other product; give **IV** 5 mg or less/1 min or total dose over 3 min or more (children, infants); CONT INF is not recommended; inject closest vein insertion as possible; do not dilute or mix with other products

• Check **IV** site for thrombosis or phlebitis, which may occur rapidly

#### Sterile emulsion for injection route
• Use **IV** only, within 6 hr, flush line after use and after 6 hr

**Syringe compatibilities:** Cimetidine

*Syringe incompatibilities:* Benzquina-mide, doxapram, glycopyrrolate, heparin, nalbuphine

*Y-site compatibilities:* Cefmetazole, DOBUTamine, nafcillin, quinidine, sufentanil

*Y-site incompatibilities:* Hydromor-phone, fluconazole, foscarnet, heparin, pancuronium, potassium chloride, vecuronium, vit B with C

*Additive compatibilities:* Netilmicin, verapamil

## Patient/family education

• Advise patient that product may be taken with food; that product is not to be used for everyday stress or used longer than 4 mo unless directed by prescriber; take no more than prescribed amount; may be habit forming
• Caution patient to avoid OTC preparations unless approved by a prescriber; to avoid alcohol, other psychotropic medications unless prescribed; that smoking may decrease diazepam effect by increasing diazepam metabolism; not to discontinue medication abruptly after long-term use, gradually taper
• Inform patient to avoid driving, activities that require alertness; drowsiness may occur; to rise slowly or fainting may occur, especially in geriatric
• Advise patient not to become pregnant while using this product
• Inform patient that drowsiness may worsen at beginning of treatment

## Evaluation

**Positive therapeutic outcome**
• Decreased anxiety, restlessness, insomnia

**Treatment of overdose:** Lavage, VS, supportive care, flumazenil

---

**diazoxide** (Rx)

(dye-az-ox'ide)

Hyperstat IV, diazoxide parenteral

*Func. class.:* Antihypertensive

*Chem. class.:* Vasodilator

**Pregnancy category C**

---

**Action:** Vasodilates arteriolar smooth muscle by direct relaxation; a reduction in blood pressure with concomitant increases in heart rate, cardiac output; reduces release of insulin from the pancreas

**Therapeutic outcome:** Decreased B/P, increased blood glucose

**Uses:** Hypertensive crisis when urgent decrease of diastolic pressure required (**IV**);

increase blood glucose levels in hyperinsulinism

## Dosage and routes

### Hypoglycemia

**Adult and child:** PO 3-8 mg/kg/day in 2-3 divided doses q8-12hr

**Infant and neonate:** PO 8-15 mg/kg/day in 2-3 divided doses 8-12hr

### Hypertension

**Adult:** **IV** BOL 1-3 mg/kg rapidly up to a max of 150 mg in a single inj; dose may be repeated at 5-15 min intervals until desired response is achieved; give **IV** in 30 sec or less

**Child:** **IV** BOL 1-2 mg/kg rapidly: administration same as adult, not to exceed 150 mg

**Available forms:** Caps 50 mg; oral susp 50 mg/ml; inj 15 mg/ml, 300 mg/20 ml

## Adverse effects

***CNS:*** Headache, weakness, anxiety, dizziness, **seizures, cerebral ischemia, paralysis,** sleepiness, euphoria, anxiety, EPS, confusion, tinnitus, blurred vision

***CV:*** Palpitations, hypotension, **shock, MI,** T-wave changes, angina pectoris, **supraventricular tachycardia, edema,** rebound hypertension

***ENDO:*** Hyperglycemia in diabetics, transient hyperglycemia in nondiabetics, increased uric acid

***GI:*** Nausea, vomiting, dry mouth

***GU:*** Breast tenderness, increased BUN, fluid, electrolyte imbalances, Na, water retention

***HEMA:*** **Thrombocytopenia,** decreased Hgb, Hct

***INTEG:*** Rash

**Contraindications:** Hypersensitivity to this product or thiazides, sulfonamides, hypertension of aortic coarctation or AV shunt, pheochromocytoma, dissecting aortic aneurysm

**Precautions:** Pregnancy **C**, breastfeeding, children, tachycardia, fluid/electrolyte imbalances, impaired cerebral or cardiac circulation

| Pharmacokinetics | |
|---|---|
| **Absorption** | Well absorbed (PO); completely absorbed (**IV**) |
| **Distribution** | Crosses blood-brain barrier, placenta, protein binding >90% |
| **Metabolism** | Liver (50%) |
| **Excretion** | Kidneys, unchanged (50%) |
| **Half-life** | 20-36 hr |

---

| Pharmacodynamics | | |
|---|---|---|
| | PO | IV |
| **Onset** | 1 hr | 1-2 min |
| **Peak** | 8-12 hr | 5 min |
| **Duration** | 8 hr | 3-12 hr |

## Interactions
### Drug classifications
Antihypertensives: severe hypotension
Diuretics (thiazides): increased hyperuricemic, antihypertensive effects of diazoxide
Hydantoins: decreased anticonvulsant effect
NSAIDs, salicylates: decreased antihypertensive effect
Sulfonylureas: increased hyperglycemia
### Drug/herb
Aconite: increased toxicity, death

## NURSING CONSIDERATIONS
### Assessment
- Assess for allergies to sulfonamide; cross-sensitivity may occur
- Assess B/P q5 min until stabilized
- Monitor electrolytes, blood studies: potassium, sodium, chloride, carbon dioxide, CBC, serum glucose
- Monitor weight daily, I&O; edema in feet, legs daily; check skin turgor, dryness of mucous membranes for hydration status
- Assess for crackles, dyspnea, orthopnea; peripheral edema, fatigue, weight gain, jugular vein distention (CHF)
- Assess for signs of hyperglycemia: acetone breath, increased urinary output, severe thirst, lethargy, dizziness

### Nursing diagnoses
- Cardiac output, decreased (adverse reactions)
- Injury, risk for (side effects)
- Knowledge, deficient (teaching)

### Implementation
**PO route**
- Shake susp before using
- Store protected from light and heat
**IV route**
- Give by direct **IV** over 30 sec or less; may repeat q5-15 min until desired response; do not administer dark solution
- Give to patient in recumbent position; keep in that position for 1 hr after
**Syringe compatibility:** Heparin
**Y-site incompatibilities:** Hydralazine, propranolol

### Evaluation
**Positive therapeutic outcome**
- Decreased B/P in hypertension

**Treatment of overdose:** Administer levarterenol, DOPamine, or norepinephrine for hypotension, dialysis

---

## dibucaine topical
*See Appendix D*

---

## diclofenac ophthalmic
*See Appendix D*

---

## diclofenac potassium (Rx)
(dye-kloe'fen-ak)
Voltaren Rapide ✤
## diclofenac sodium (Rx)
Apo-Dilo ✤, Novo-Difenac ✤, Voltaren
*Func. class.:* Nonsteroidal antiinflammatory (NSAIDs), nonopioid analgesic
*Chem. class.:* Phenylacetic acid

### Pregnancy category C

**Action:** Inhibits prostaglandin synthesis by decreasing enzyme needed for biosynthesis; analgesic, antiinflammatory, antipyretic properties

**Therapeutic outcome:** Decreased pain, inflammation

**Uses:** Acute, chronic rheumatoid arthritis, osteoarthritis, ankylosing spondylitis, analgesia, primary dysmenorrhea

### Dosage and routes
*Osteoarthritis*
*Adult:* PO 100-150 mg/day in 2-3 divided doses
*Geriatric:* PO 50 mg bid-tid

*Rheumatoid arthritis*
*Adult:* PO 100-200 mg/day in 2-4 divided doses (potassium); 50 mg tid-qid, then reduce to lowest dose needed (25 mg tid) (sodium)
*Geriatric:* PO 50 mg bid-tid

*Ankylosing spondylitis*
*Adult:* PO 100-125 mg/day in 4-5 divided doses; give 25 mg qid and 25 mg at bedtime if needed (potassium)

*Postcataract surgery*
*Adult:* Ophth 1 gtt of 0.1% sol qid × 2 wk postsurgery

*Analgesia/primary dysmenorrhea*
*Adult:* PO 50 mg tid, max 150 mg/day (potassium)

---

**Available forms:** Potassium: tabs 50 mg; sodium: delayed rel tabs (enteric-coated) 25, 50, 75 mg

## Adverse effects

*CNS: Dizziness, headache,* drowsiness, fatigue, tremors, confusion, insomnia, anxiety, depression, nervousness, paresthesia, muscle weakness

*CV:* **CHF,** tachycardia, peripheral edema, palpitations, dysrhythmias, hypo/hypertension, fluid retention, **MI, stroke**

*EENT:* Tinnitus, hearing loss, blurred vision, **laryngeal edema**

*GI:* Nausea, anorexia, vomiting, diarrhea, jaundice, **cholestatic hepatitis,** constipation, flatulence, cramps, dry mouth, peptic ulcer, GI bleeding, **hepatotoxicity**

*GU:* **Nephrotoxicity: dysuria, hematuria, oliguria, azotemia, cystitis, UTI**

*HEMA:* **Blood dyscrasias,** epistaxis, bruising

*INTEG:* Purpura, rash, pruritus, sweating, erythema, petechiae, photosensitivity, alopecia

*RESP:* Dyspnea, hemoptysis, pharyngitis, **bronchospasm,** rhinitis, shortness of breath

*SYST:* **Anaphylaxis**

**Contraindications:** Hypersensitivity to aspirin, iodides, other NSAIDs; asthma, serious CV disease

**Precautions:** Pregnancy **C** (1st trimester), not recommended in 2nd half of pregnancy, breastfeeding, children, bleeding disorders, GI/cardiac disorders, hypersensitivity to other antiinflammatory agents, CCr <30 ml/min

### Pharmacokinetics

| | |
|---|---|
| **Absorption** | Well absorbed (PO, ophth) |
| **Distribution** | Crosses placenta; 99% bound to plasma proteins |
| **Metabolism** | Liver (50%) |
| **Excretion** | Breast milk |
| **Half-life** | 2.5 hr |

### Pharmacodynamics

| | PO | OPHTH |
|---|---|---|
| **Onset** | Unknown | Unknown |
| **Peak** | 2-3 hr | Unknown |
| **Duration** | Unknown | Unknown |

## Interactions

### Individual drugs

Aspirin: increased GI side effects

CycloSPORINE, lithium, methotrexate, phenytoin: increased toxicity

### Drug classifications

Anticoagulants: increased risk of bleeding

Antidiabetics: increased need for dosage adjustment

β-blockers, diuretics: decreased antihypertensive effect

Diuretics (potassium-sparing): hyperkalemia

NSAIDs: increased GI side effects

### Drug/herb

Arginine, gossypol: increased gastric irritation

Bearberry, bilberry: increased NSAIDs effect

Bogbean, chondroitin, saw palmetto, turmeric: increased bleeding risk

St. John's wort: increased severe photosensitivity

## NURSING CONSIDERATIONS

### Assessment

• Assess for pain of rheumatoid arthritis, osteoarthritis, ankylosing spondylitis; check ROM, inflammation of joints, characteristics of pain

• Assess ophthalmic patients for pain, inflammation, redness, swelling

◆ Monitor blood counts during therapy; watch for decreasing platelets; if low, therapy may need to be discontinued, restarted after hematologic recovery

• Assess for asthma, aspirin hypersensitivity, nasal polyps; may develop hypersensitivity

• Monitor liver function tests (may be elevated) and uric acid (may be decreased—serum; increased—urine) periodically; also BUN, creatinine, electrolytes (may be elevated)

◆ Monitor for blood dyscrasias (thrombocytopenia): bruising, fatigue, bleeding, poor healing

### Nursing diagnoses

• Injury, risk for (side effects)

• Knowledge, deficient (teaching)

• Mobility, impaired physical (uses)

• Pain, chronic (uses)

### Implementation

**PO route**

• Do not break, crush, chew, or dissolve enteric-coated or ext rel tabs

• Administer with food or milk to decrease gastric symptoms

• Remain upright for ½ hr

**Ophthalmic route**

• Administer with patient recumbent or tilting head back; pull down on lower lid; when conjunctival sac is exposed, instill 1 drop; wait a few minutes before instilling other drops

### Patient/family education

• Teach patient that product must be continued for prescribed time to be effective; to avoid aspirin, NSAIDs, acetaminophen, or other OTC medications unless approved by

Adverse effects: *italic* = common, **bold** = life-threatening

prescriber, alcoholic beverages; to contact prescriber before surgery regarding when to discontinue this product

• Caution patient to report bleeding, bruising, fatigue, malaise, since blood dyscrasias do occur

• Advise patient to report hepatotoxicity: flulike symptoms, nausea, vomiting, jaundice, pruritus, lethargy

• Instruct patient to use sunscreen to prevent photosensitivity

• Teach patient to avoid use in 3rd trimester of pregnancy

• Instruct patient to use caution when driving; drowsiness, dizziness may occur

• Teach patient to take with a full glass of water to enhance absorption; remain upright for ½ hr; if dose is missed, take as soon as remembered within 2 hr if taking 1-2 ×/day, do not double doses

### Evaluation
**Positive therapeutic outcome**

• Decreased pain in arthritic conditions

• Decreased inflammation in arthritic conditions

• Decreased ocular irritation

---

## dicloxacillin (Rx)
(dye-klox-a-sill'in)

dicloxacillin sodium, Dycill, Dynapen, Pathocil

*Func. class.:* Antiinfective

*Chem. class.:* Penicillinase-resistant penicillin

**Pregnancy category** B

**Do not confuse:**
Pathocil/Bactocil

**Action:** Interferes with cell wall replication of susceptible organisms; osmotically unstable cell wall swells, bursts from osmotic pressure

**Therapeutic outcome:** Bactericidal effects for the following: gram-positive cocci *Staphylococcus aureus, Streptococcus pyogenes, Streptococcus viridans, Streptococcus faecalis, Streptococcus bovis, Streptococcus pneumoniae;* infections caused by penicillinase-producing *Staphylococcus* organisms

**Uses:** Penicillinase-producing staphylococci, streptococci; respiratory tract, skin, skin structure infections; sinusitis

### Dosage and routes
*Adult and child ≥40 kg:* PO 125-250 mg q6hr, max 4 g/day

*Child ≤40 kg:* PO 12.5-25 mg/kg in divided doses q6hr, max 4 g/day

**Available forms:** Caps 250, 500 mg

### Adverse effects
*CNS:* Lethargy, hallucinations, anxiety, depression, twitching, **coma, seizures**

*GI: Nausea, vomiting, diarrhea,* increased AST, ALT, abdominal pain, glossitis, **pseudomembranous colitis, GI bleeding**

*GU:* Oliguria, proteinuria, hematuria, *vaginitis, moniliasis,* **glomerulonephritis**

*HEMA:* Anemia, increased bleeding time, **bone marrow depression, granulocytopenia, neutropenia**

*SYST:* Anaphylaxis, **Stevens-Johnson syndrome**

**Contraindications:** Hypersensitivity to penicillins; neonates

**Precautions:** Pregnancy **B,** breastfeeding, hypersensitivity to cephalosporins, severe renal/hepatic/GI disease, asthma

| Pharmacokinetics | |
|---|---|
| **Absorption** | Rapid, incomplete (35%-75%) |
| **Distribution** | Widely distributed; crosses placenta |
| **Metabolism** | Liver (6%-10%) |
| **Excretion** | Kidneys, unchanged (60%); breast milk |
| **Half-life** | ½-1 hr, increased in hepatic renal disease |

| Pharmacodynamics | |
|---|---|
| **Onset** | ½ hr |
| **Peak** | ½-2 hr |
| **Duration** | Unknown |

### Interactions
*Individual drugs*
Probenecid: increased dicloxacillin levels

*Drug classifications*
Oral anticoagulants: decreased anticoagulant effects

*Drug/herb*
Acidophilus: do not use with antiinfectives; separate by several hours

Khat: decreased absorption; separate by 2 hr

*Drug/food*
Food, citrus fruit juices: decreased absorption

*Drug/lab test*
False positive: urine glucose, urine protein

---

 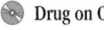

## NURSING CONSIDERATIONS
### Assessment
- Assess patient for previous sensitivity reaction to penicillins or other cephalosporins; cross-sensitivity between penicillins and cephalosporins is common
- Assess patient for signs and symptoms of infection including characteristics of wounds, sputum, urine, stool, WBC >10,000/mm$^3$, fever; obtain baseline information and during treatment
- Obtain C&S before beginning product therapy to identify if correct treatment has been initiated
- Assess for anaphylaxis: rash, urticaria, pruritus, chills, fever, joint pain may occur a few days after therapy begins; epINEPHrine and resuscitation equipment should be available for anaphylactic reaction
- ⬤ Identify urine output; if decreasing, notify prescriber (may indicate nephrotoxicity); check for increased BUN, creatinine
- Monitor blood studies: AST, ALT, CBC, Hct, bilirubin, LDH, alkaline phosphatase, Coombs' test monthly if patient is on long-term therapy
- Monitor electrolytes: potassium, sodium, chloride monthly if patient is on long-term therapy
- Assess bowel pattern daily; if severe diarrhea occurs, product should be discontinued; may indicate pseudomembranous colitis
- Monitor for bleeding: ecchymosis, bleeding gums, hematuria, stool guaiac daily if on long-term therapy
- Assess for overgrowth of infection: perineal itching, fever, malaise, redness, pain, swelling, drainage, rash, diarrhea, change in cough, sputum

### Nursing diagnoses
- Diarrhea (side effects)
- Infection, risk for (uses)
- Injury, risk for (side effects)
- Knowledge, deficient (teaching)
- Noncompliance (teaching)

### Implementation
- Do not break, crush, or chew caps
- Give in even doses around the clock; if GI upset occurs, give with food; product must be given for 10-14 days to ensure organism death and prevent superinfection; store in airtight container

### Patient/family education
- Teach patient to report sore throat, bruising, bleeding, joint pain; may indicate blood dyscrasias (rare)
- Advise patient to contact prescriber if vaginal itching, loose, foul-smelling stools, furry tongue occur; may indicate superinfection
- Instruct patient to take all medication prescribed for the length of time ordered, carry/wear emergency ID if allergic to penicillins
- Advise patient to notify prescriber of diarrhea with blood or pus, which may indicate pseudomembranous colitis

### Evaluation
**Positive therapeutic outcome**
- Absence of signs/symptoms of infection (WBC <10,000/mm$^3$, temp WNL, absence of red draining wounds)
- Reported improvement in symptoms of infection

**Treatment of anaphylaxis:** Withdraw product, maintain airway, administer epINEPHrine, aminophylline, $O_2$, **IV** corticosteroids

---

## didanosine (Rx)
(dye-dan'oh-seen)
ddI, dideoxyinosine, Videx, Videx EC
*Func. class.:* Antiretroviral
*Chem. class.:* Synthetic purine nucleoside reverse transcriptase inhibitor
### Pregnancy category B

**Action:** Nucleoside analog incorporating into cellular DNA by viral reverse transcriptase, thereby terminating the cellular DNA chain that prevents viral replication

**Therapeutic outcome:** Antiviral against the retroviruses, primarily HIV-1

**Uses:** HIV-1 infection in combination with other antiretrovirals

### Dosage and routes
*Adult:* PO >60 kg, 200 mg bid tabs, del rel caps 400 mg daily; <60 kg, 125 mg bid tabs, del rel caps 250 mg daily
*Child:* PO tabs 90-120 mg/m$^2$ q12hr; PO (child BSA 1.1-1.4 m$^2$) tab 100 mg q8-12hr; reconstituted pediatric powder 125 mg q8-12hr; PO (child BSA 0.8-1 m$^2$) tabs 75 mg q8-12hr; reconstituted pediatric powder 94 mg q8-12hr; PO (child BSA 0.5-0.7 m$^2$) tabs 50 mg q8-12hr; reconstituted pediatric powder 62 mg q8-12hr; PO (child BSA <0.4 m$^2$)

---

Adverse effects: *italic* = common, **bold** = life-threatening

tabs 25 mg q8-12hr; reconstituted pediatric powder 31 mg q8-12hr

### Videx EC cap
**Adult >60 kg:** PO CCr 30-59 ml/min 200 mg/day; CCr 10-29 ml/min 125 mg/day; CCr <10 ml/min 125 mg/day
**Adult <60 kg:** PO CCr 30-59 ml/min 125 mg/day; CCr 10-29 ml/min 125 mg/day; CCr <10 ml/min, avoid use

### Renal dose
**Adult:** PO reduce dosage CCr <60 ml/min

**Available forms:** Powder for oral sol 10 mg/ml; del rel caps 125, 200, 250, 400

### Adverse effects
***CNS:*** **Peripheral neuropathy, seizures,** confusion, *anxiety,* hypertonia, abnormal thinking, asthenia, *insomnia, CNS depression,* pain, dizziness, chills, fever
***CV:*** Hypertension, vasodilatation, **dysrhythmia,** syncope, **CHF,** palpitations
***EENT:*** Ear pain, otitis, photophobia, visual impairment, retinal depigmentation
***GI:*** Pancreatitis, *diarrhea, nausea,* vomiting, *abdominal pain,* constipation, stomatitis, dyspepsia, liver abnormalities, flatulence, taste perversion, dry mouth, oral thrush, melena, increased ALT, AST, alkaline phosphatase, amylase, **hepatic failure**
***GU:*** Increased bilirubin, uric acid
***HEMA:*** **Leukopenia, granulocytopenia, thrombocytopenia, anemia**
***INTEG:*** *Rash, pruritus,* alopecia, ecchymosis, hemorrhage, petechiae, sweating
***MS:*** Myalgia, arthritis, myopathy, muscular atrophy
***RESP:*** Cough, pneumonia, dyspnea, asthma, epistaxis, hypoventilation, sinusitis
***SYST:*** **Lactic acidosis, anaphylaxis**

**Contraindications:** Hypersensitivity, lactic acidosis, pancreatitis, phenylketonuria

**Precautions:** Pregnancy **B**, breastfeeding, children, renal/hepatic disease, sodium-restricted diets, elevated amylase, preexistent peripheral neuropathy, hyperuricemia

| Pharmacokinetics | |
|---|---|
| Absorption | Rapidly absorbed (up to 40%) |
| Distribution | Unknown |
| Metabolism | Not metabolized |
| Excretion | Kidneys (55%)/feces |
| Half-life | 0.8-1.6 hr, shorter in children |

| Pharmacodynamics | |
|---|---|
| Onset | Unknown |
| Peak | Up to 1 hr, del rel 2 hr |
| Duration | Unknown |

### Interactions
#### Individual drugs
Allopurinol, tenofovir: increased didanosine level
Dapsone, ketoconazole: decreased absorption of each specific product
Itraconazole: decreased concentrations
Methadone: decreased didanosine level
#### Drug classifications
Antacids, magnesium, aluminum: increased side effects
Antiretrovirals, other: decreased concentration
Fluoroquinolones, tetracyclines: decreased concentrations of each specific product
#### Drug/food
Do not use with acidic juices
Decreased: absorption 50%

## NURSING CONSIDERATIONS
### Assessment
- Assess for peripheral neuropathy: tingling or pain in hands and feet, distal numbness; onset usually occurs 2-6 mo after beginning treatment, if these occur during therapy, product may be decreased or discontinued
- Assess for pancreatitis: abdominal pain, nausea, vomiting, elevated liver enzymes; product should be discontinued, since condition can be fatal
- Assess children by dilated retinal examination q6 mo to rule out retinal depigmentation
- Monitor CBC, differential, platelet count monthly; withhold product if WBC is <4000/mm$^3$ or platelet count is <75,000 mm$^3$, viral load, CD4$^+$ count; notify prescriber of results
- Monitor renal function studies: BUN, serum uric acid, urine CCr before, during therapy; these may be elevated throughout treatment
- Assess for anaphylaxis, lactic acidosis
- Monitor temp q4hr; may indicate beginning of infection
- Monitor liver function tests before, during therapy (bilirubin, AST, ALT, amylase, alkaline phosphatase) as needed or monthly

### Nursing diagnoses
- Infection, risk for (uses)
- Injury, risk for (adverse reactions)
- Knowledge, deficient (teaching)

### Implementation
- Give on empty stomach 1 hr before or 2 hr after meals q12hr; food decreases effectiveness of product; adjust dose in renal impairment

- Patient should chew tabs; may be crushed and mixed with water
- Pediatric powder for oral sol should be prepared in the pharmacy; shake before using
- Packets for oral sol must be mixed with ½ glass of water, not fruit juice; stir until dissolved; drink immediately
- Store tabs, caps in tightly closed bottle at room temperature; store oral sol after dissolving at room temperature ≤4 hr
- Do not take dapsone at same time as ddI

### Patient/family education

- Advise patient to take on empty stomach; not to mix powder with fruit juice; to chew tab or crush and dissolve in water; to drink powder immediately after mixing; to use exactly as prescribed
- Instruct patient to report signs of infection: increased temp, sore throat, flulike symptoms; to avoid crowds and those with known infections
- Instruct patient to report signs of anemia: fatigue, headache, faintness, shortness of breath, irritability
- Advise patient to report numbness/tingling in extremities
- Instruct patient to report bleeding; avoid use of razors and commercial mouthwash
- Advise patient that hair may be lost during therapy; a wig or hairpiece may make patient feel better
- Caution patient to avoid OTC products and other medications without approval of prescriber; to avoid alcohol
- Teach patient not to have any sexual contact without use of a condom; needles should not be shared; blood from infected individual should not come in contact with another's mucous membranes

### Evaluation

**Positive therapeutic outcome**
- Absence of opportunistic infection, symptoms of HIV

---

### difenoxin with atropine
*See diphenoxylate with atropine*

---

**! HIGH ALERT**

**digoxin** 🔵 **(Rx)**
(di-jox′in)
digoxin, Lanoxicaps, Lanoxin
*Func. class.:* Inotropic antidysrhythmic, cardiac glycoside
*Chem. class.:* Digitalis preparation
**Pregnancy category** C

**Do not confuse:**
Lanoxin/Lasix/Lonox/Lomotil/Xanax/Levoxine

**Action:** Inhibits sodium-potassium ATPase, which makes more calcium available for contractile proteins, resulting in increased cardiac output; increases force of contraction (positive inotropic effect); decreases heart rate (chronotropic effect); decreases AV conduction speed

**Therapeutic outcome:** Decreased edema, pulse, respiration, crackles

**Uses:** Rapid digitalization in acute and chronic CHF, atrial fibrillation, atrial flutter, atrial tachycardia; cardiogenic shock, paroxysmal atrial tachycardia

### Dosage and routes

*Adult:* **IV** *digitalizing dose* 0.6-1.0 mg given as 50% of the dose initially, additional fractions given at 4-8 hr intervals; PO *digitalizing dose* 0.75-1.25 mg given as 50% of the dose initially, additional fractions given at 4-8 hr intervals; *maintenance* 0.125-0.5 mg/day (tabs), or 0.350-0.5 mg/day (gelatin cap)
*Child >10 yr:* **IV** *digitalizing dose* 8-12 mcg/kg given as 50% of the dose initially, additional fractions given at 4-8 hr intervals; PO *digitalizing dose* 0.01-0.015 mg/kg given as 50% of the dose initially, additional fractions given at 6-8 hr intervals; maintenance 25%-35% of the loading dose daily as a single dose
*Child 5-10 yr:* **IV** *digitalizing dose* 0.015-0.03 mg/kg given as 50% of the dose initially, additional fractions given at 4-8 hr intervals; PO *digitalizing dose* 0.02-0.035 mg/kg given as 50% of the dose initially, additional fractions given at 6-8 hr intervals; *maintenance* 25%-35% of the loading dose daily in 2 divided doses
*Child 2-5 yr:* **IV** *digitalizing dose* 0.025-0.035 mg/kg given as 50% of the dose initially, additional fractions given at 4-8 hr intervals; PO *digitalizing dose* 0.03-0.04 mg/kg given as 50% of the dose initially, additional fractions given at 6-8 hr intervals; *maintenance* 25%-35% of the loading dose daily in 2 divided doses

Adverse effects: *italic* = common, **bold** = life-threatening

**Child 1-2 yr:** IV *digitalizing dose* 0.03-0.05 mg/kg given as 50% of the dose initially, additional fractions given at 4-8 hr intervals; PO *digitalizing dose* 0.035-0.06 mg/kg given as 50% of the dose initially, additional fractions given at 4-8 hr intervals; *maintenance* 25%-35% of the loading dose daily in 2 divided doses

**Infant:** IV *digitalizing dose* 0.02-0.03 mg/kg given as 50% of the dose initially, additional fractions given at 4-8 hr intervals; PO *digitalizing dose* 0.025-0.035 mg/kg given as 50% of the dose initially, additional fractions given at 6-8 hr intervals; *maintenance* 25%-35% of the loading dose daily in 2 divided doses

**Premature infant:** IV *digitalizing dose* 0.015-0.025 mg/kg given as 50% of the dose initially, additional fractions given at 4-8 hr intervals; PO *digitalizing dose* 0.02-0.03 mg/kg given as 50% of the dose initially, additional fractions given at 6-8 hr intervals; *maintenance* 20%-30% of the loading dose daily in 2 divided doses

**Available forms:** Caps 0.05, 0.1, 0.2 mg; elix 0.05 mg/ml; tabs 0.125, 0.25, 0.5 mg; inj 0.5 ♣, 0.25 mg/ml; pediatric inj 0.1 mg/ml

### Adverse effects

*CNS:* **Headache,** drowsiness, apathy, confusion, disorientation, fatigue, depression, hallucinations
*CV:* **Dysrhythmias,** hypotension, bradycardia, **AV block**
*EENT:* Blurred vision, yellow-green halos, photophobia, diplopia
*GI:* Nausea, vomiting, anorexia, abdominal pain, diarrhea

**Contraindications:** Hypersensitivity to digoxin, ventricular fibrillation, ventricular tachycardia, carotid sinus syndrome, 2nd- or 3rd-degree heart block

**Precautions:** Pregnancy **C,** breastfeeding, geriatric, renal disease, acute MI, AV block, severe respiratory disease, hypothyroidism, sinus nodal disease, hypokalemia

### Pharmacokinetics

| | |
|---|---|
| **Absorption** | Unknown |
| **Distribution** | Widely distributed; 20%-25% protein bound |
| **Metabolism** | Liver, small amount; also intestinal bacteria |
| **Excretion** | Urine |
| **Half-life** | 1½ days |

### Pharmacodynamics

| | PO | IV |
|---|---|---|
| **Onset** | ½-1½ hr | 5-30 min |
| **Peak** | 2-6 hr | 1-5 hr |
| **Duration** | After steady state | 6-8 days |

### Interactions

*Individual drugs*
Amiodarone, diltiazem, NIFEdipine, propantheline, quinidine, verapamil: increased digoxin levels
Amphotericin B, carbenicillin, ticarcillin: increased hypokalemia, increased toxicity
Calcium IV: increased hypercalcemia, hypomagnesemia, digoxin toxicity
Cholestyramine, colestipol, metoclopramide, thyroid hormones: decreased digoxin levels
Kaolin/pectin: decreased absorption

*Drug classifications*
Antacids: decreased digoxin absorption
Anticholinergics: increased digoxin blood levels
Antidysrhythmics, β-adrenergic blockers: increased bradycardia
Diuretics (thiazide) corticosteroids: increased hypokalemia, hypercalcemia, hypomagnesemia, digoxin toxicity
Sympathomimetics: increased cardiac dysrhythmia risk

*Drug/herb*
Aconite, hawthorn, horsetail: increased toxicity
Aloe, betel palm, broom, buckthorn, cascara sagrada castor, Chinese rhubarb, figwort, fumitory, hawthorn, khat, kudzu, licorice, lily of the valley, Mayapple, mistletoe, motherwort, night blooming cereus, oleander, pheasant's eye, purple foxglove, Queen Anne's lace, rhubarb, rue, senna, Siberian ginseng, squill, yellow dock: increased digoxin action
Bethroot, goldenseal, St. John's wort: decreased digoxin effect
Blackroot: forms insoluble complex
Cocoa, coffee, cola, guarana, horsetail, licorice, yerba maté: increased hypokalemia
Indian snakeroot: increased bradycardia
Psyllium: decreased digoxin absorption

*Drug/lab test*
Increased: CPK

### NURSING CONSIDERATIONS
**Assessment**
• Assess and document apical pulse for 1 min before giving product; if pulse <60 in adult or <90 in an infant or is significantly different,

take again in 1 hr; if <60 in adult, call prescriber; note rate, rhythm, character
• Monitor electrolytes: potassium, sodium, chloride, magnesium, calcium; renal function studies: BUN, creatinine; other blood studies: ALT, AST, bilirubin, Hct, Hgb, product levels (therapeutic level 0.5-2 ng/ml) before initiating treatment and periodically thereafter
• Monitor I&O ratio, daily weights; monitor turgor, lung sounds, edema
• Monitor cardiac status: apical pulse, character, rate, rhythm; resolution of atrial dysrhythmias by ECG; if tachydysrhythmia develops, hold product; delay cardioversion while product levels are determined
• Monitor ECG continuously during parenteral loading doses and for patients with suspected toxicity; provide hemodynamic monitoring for patients with heart failure or administer multiple cardiac products

## Nursing diagnoses
• Cardiac output, decreased (uses)
• Gas exchange, impaired (adverse reactions)
• Knowledge, deficient (teaching)

## Implementation
• Do not give at same time as antacids or other products that decrease absorption
**PO route**
• Give PO with or without food; may crush tabs
• Take medication at same time each day
• Give potassium supplements if ordered for potassium levels <3, or give foods high in potassium: bananas, orange juice
**IV route**
• Give **IV** undiluted or 1 ml of product/4 ml sterile water, D₅ or 0.9% NaCl; give over >5 min through Y-tube or 3-way stopcock; during digitalization, close monitoring is necessary
• Store protected from light
*Syringe compatibilities:* Heparin, milrinone
*Syringe incompatibility:* Doxapram
*Y-site compatibilities:* Amrinone, cefmetazole, ciprofloxacin, cisatracurium, diltiazem, famotidine, meperidine, meropenem, midazolam, milrinone, morphine, potassium chloride, propofol, remifentanil, tacrolimus, vit B/C
*Y-site incompatibilities:* Fluconazole, foscarnet
*Additive compatibilities:* Bretylium, cimetidine, floxacillin, furosemide, lidocaine, ranitidine, verapamil
*Additive incompatibility:* DOBUTamine

## Patient/family education
• Caution patient to avoid OTC medications including cough, cold, allergy preparations, antacids, since many adverse product interactions may occur; do not take antacid at same time
• Instruct patient to notify prescriber of any loss of appetite, lower stomach pain, diarrhea, weakness, drowsiness, headache, blurred or yellow-green vision, rash, depression; teach toxic symptoms of this product and when to notify prescriber
• Advise patient to maintain a sodium-restricted diet as ordered; to take potassium supplements as ordered to prevent toxicity
• Instruct patient to report shortness of breath, difficulty breathing, weight gain, edema, persistent cough
• Teach patient purpose of product is to regulate the heart's functioning
• Teach patient as outpatient to check and record pulse for 1 min before taking dose; if there is a change of >15 bpm from usual pulse, prescriber should be notified
• Teach patient to take medication at the same time each day, take missed doses within 12 hr; do not double doses; notify prescriber if doses are missed for 2 days or more; how to monitor heart rate
• Advise patient to carry/wear emergency ID describing dosage and reason for digoxin

## Evaluation
**Positive therapeutic outcome**
• Decreased weight, edema, pulse, respiration, crackles
• Increased urine output
• Serum digoxin level 0.5-2 ng/ml

**Treatment of overdose:** Discontinue product, administer potassium, monitor ECG, administer an adrenergic blocking agent, digoxin immune Fab

## digoxin immune FAB (ovine) ⊛ (Rx)
(di-jox'in)
Digibind, DigiFab
*Func. class.:* Antidote, digoxin specific
**Pregnancy category** C

**Action:** Antibody fragments bind to free digoxin or to reverse toxicity by not allowing digoxin or digitoxin to bind to sites of action

**Therapeutic outcome:** Correction of digoxin toxicity

Adverse effects: *italic* = common, **bold** = life-threatening

**Uses:** Reversal of life-threatening digoxin or digitoxin toxicity, including severe bradycardia, ventricular tachycardia/fibrillation, severe hypertension

## Dosage and routes
1 (38 mg) vial binds 0.5 mg digoxin

### Digoxin toxicity (known amount) (tabs, oral sol, IM)
**Adult and child: IV** dose (mg) = dose ingested (mg) × 0.8/1000 × 38; if ingested amount is unknown, give 760 mg **IV**

### Toxicity (known amount) (cap, IV)
**Adult and child: IV** dose = dose ingested (mg)/0.5 × 38

### Toxicity (known amount) by serum digoxin concentrations (SDCs)
**Adult and child: IV** SDC (nanograms/ml) × kg of weight/100 × 38

### Digoxin toxicity (unknown amount)
**Adult and child >20 kg: IV** 228 mg (6 vials)
**Infant and child <20 kg: IV** 38 mg (1 vial)

### Acute ingestion
**Adult: IV** 10 vials (380 mg)

### Life-threatening ingestion
**Adult: IV** 20 vials (760 mg)

### Skin test
**Adult:** ID 9.5 mcg

**Available forms:** Inj 38 mg/vial (binds 0.5 mg of digoxin), 40 mg/vial (binds 0.5 mg digoxin)

## Adverse effects
**CV:** **CHF,** *ventricular rate increase,* **atrial fibrillation,** *low cardiac output,* hypotension
**INTEG:** *Hypersensitivity,* allergic reactions, facial swelling, redness, phlebitis
**META:** *Hypokalemia*
**MISC:** **Anaphylaxis** (rare)
**RESP:** **Impaired respiratory function, rapid respiratory rate**

**Contraindications:** Mild digoxin toxicity, hypersensitivity to this product or papain

**Precautions:** Pregnancy **C,** breastfeeding, children, geriatric, cardiac/renal disease, hypocalcemia, heart failure, allergy to ovine proteins

| Pharmacokinetics | |
|---|---|
| **Absorption** | Complete |
| **Distribution** | Widely distributed into plasma, interstitial fluids |
| **Metabolism** | Unknown |
| **Excretion** | Kidneys |
| **Half-life** | Biphasic (14-20 hr); increased in renal disease |

| Pharmacodynamics | |
|---|---|
| **Onset** | 30 min (variable) |
| **Peak** | Unknown |
| **Duration** | Unknown |

## Interactions
### Individual drugs
Considered incompatible with all products in syringe or sol
### Drug/lab test
Interference: immunoassay (digoxin)

## NURSING CONSIDERATIONS
### Assessment
• Assess for hypokalemia: ST depression, flat T waves, presence of U wave, ventricular dysrhythmias
• Obtain information on previous allergies: previous exposure to sheep (ovine) proteins; scratch test may be performed before use of this product; hypersensitive reactions are more common in persons with previous exposure
• Monitor VS before, during, and after infusion
• Monitor heart rate, B/P q10 min during inf and after completion until stabilized; hemodynamic monitoring is used for unstable or hypotensive patients; check potassium levels until toxicity is resolved
• Assess for oxygen or perfusion deficit: hypotension, chest pain, dizziness, loss of consciousness
• Assess respiratory status: auscultate lung fields for bibasilar crackles in patients with advanced CHF, B/P, volume overload

### Nursing diagnoses
• Injury, risk for (uses)
• Knowledge, deficient (teaching)

### Implementation
• Test doses have proven to be ineffective in the general population; only use test dose in those with known allergies or those previously treated with digoxin immune FAB
• For test dose dilute 0.1 ml or reconstituted product (9.5 mg/ml) in 9.9 ml sterile isotonic saline, inj 0.1 ml (1:100 dilution) ID and observe for wheal with erythema; read in 20 min

• For scratch test, place 1 drop of sol on skin and make a scratch through the drop with a sterile needle; read in 20 min

• Give after diluting 40 mg/4 ml of sterile water (10 mg/ml), mix gently; may be further diluted with 0.9% NaCl; sol should be clear, colorless

• Give by BOL if cardiac arrest is imminent or **IV** over 30 min using a 0.22-μm filter

• Store reconstituted sol for up to 4 hr in refrigerator; do not freeze DigiFab

### Patient/family education

• ˙Teach that purpose of medication is to bind excess digoxin and reduce high blood levels

• Instruct patients to report fever, chills, itching, sweating, dyspnea, delayed hypersensitivity

• Advise other prescribers that this medication has been used previously

### Evaluation
**Positive therapeutic outcome**

• Correction of digoxin toxicity

• Digoxin blood level 0.5-2 ng/ml

• Digitoxin blood level 9-25 ng/ml

---

## dihydroergotamine
*See ergotamine*

---

## dihydrotachysterol (Rx)
(dye-hye-droh-tak-iss′ter-ole)
DHT Intensol ✤, Hytakerol
*Func. class.:* Parathyroid agent (calcium regulator)
*Chem. class.:* Vitamin D analog

**Pregnancy category C**

**Action:** Increases intestinal absorption of calcium, increases renal tubular absorption of phosphorus; is able to regulate calcium levels by regulation of calcitonin, parathyroid hormone

**Therapeutic outcome:** Prevention of continued calcium loss in bones

**Uses:** Renal osteodystrophy, hypoparathyroidism, pseudohypoparathyroidism, familial hypophosphatemia, postoperative tetany

### Dosage and routes
*Hypophosphatemia*
*Adult and child:* PO 0.5-2 mg daily, maintenance 0.2-1.5 mg daily

*Hypoparathyroidism/*
*pseudohypoparathyroidism*
*Adult:* PO 0.8-2.4 mg daily × 4 days, maintenance 0.2-2 mg daily regulated by serum calcium levels
*Neonate:* PO 0.05-0.1 mg/day
*Infant and young child:* PO 0.1-0.5 mg/day
*Older child:* PO 0.5-1 mg/day

*Renal osteodystrophy*
*Adult:* PO 0.25-0.375 mg/day
*Child:* PO 0.125-0.5 mg/day

*Rickets (vit D resistant)*
*Child:* PO 0.25-1 mg/day

**Available forms:** Tabs 0.125, 0.2, 0.4 mg; caps 0.125 mg; oral sol 0.2, 0.25 mg/5 ml, 0.2 mg/ml ✤ (Intensol)

### Adverse effects
*CNS:* Drowsiness, headache, vertigo, fever, lethargy, depression
*CV:* **Dysrhythmias,** hypertension
*EENT:* Tinnitus
*GI:* Nausea, diarrhea, vomiting, jaundice, anorexia, dry mouth, constipation, cramps, metallic taste, thirst
*GU:* **Polyuria,** hypercalciuria, hyperphosphatemia, **hematuria,** nocturia, renal calculi
*MS:* Myalgia, arthralgia, decreased bone development, weakness, ataxia

**Contraindications:** Hypersensitivity, renal disease, hyperphosphatemia, hypercalcemia

**Precautions:** Pregnancy **C,** breastfeeding, renal calculi, CV disease

### Pharmacokinetics

| | |
|---|---|
| **Absorption** | Well absorbed from small intestine |
| **Distribution** | Liver, fat |
| **Metabolism** | Liver |
| **Excretion** | Feces (inactive, active metabolites) |
| **Half-life** | Unknown |

### Pharmacodynamics

| | |
|---|---|
| **Onset** | 2 wk |
| **Peak** | 2 wk |
| **Duration** | 2 wk |

### Interactions
*Individual drugs*
Cholestyramine, colestipol, mineral oil: decreased absorption of dihydrotachysterol
Phenytoin: decreased effect of dihydrotachysterol
Verapamil: increased dysrhythmias

Adverse effects: *italic* = common, **bold** = life-threatening

## Drug classifications

Barbiturates, corticosteroids: decreased effect of dihydrotachysterol
Calcium supplements, diuretics (thiazide): increased hypercalcemia
Cardiac glycosides: increased dysrhythmias

### Drug/lab test
False increase: cholesterol

## NURSING CONSIDERATIONS
### Assessment
• Monitor BUN, urinary calcium, AST, ALT, cholesterol, alkaline phosphatase, creatinine, uric acid, chloride, magnesium, electrolytes, urine pH, phosphate; may increase calcium; should be kept at 9-10 mg/dl; keep vit D at 50-135 international units/dl, phosphate at 70 mg/dl; these tests should be checked before and throughout treatment
• Monitor for increased blood level, since toxic reaction may occur rapidly
• Monitor for dry mouth, metallic taste, polyuria, bone pain, muscle weakness, headache, fatigue, tinnitus, change in LOC, irregular pulse, dysrhythmias, increased respirations, anorexia, nausea, vomiting, cramps, diarrhea, constipation; may indicate hypercalcemia; if these occur, discontinue product, give laxatives, low-calcium diet
• Monitor renal status: decreased urinary output (oliguria, anuria), edema in extremities, weight gain >5 lb, periorbital edema
• Assess nutritional status; check diet for sources of vit D (milk, some seafood), calcium (dairy products, dark green vegetables); phosphates (dairy products) must be avoided

### Nursing diagnoses
• Knowledge, deficient (teaching)
• Nutrition: less than body requirements, imbalanced (uses)

### Implementation
• Do not break, crush, or chew caps
• May be increased q4 wk depending on blood level; give with meals for GI symptoms
• Store in tight, light-resistant containers at room temperature
• Restrict sodium, potassium if required
• Restriction of fluids may be required for chronic renal failure

### Patient/family education
• Teach symptoms of hypercalcemia and when to report symptoms to prescriber
• Teach patient about foods rich in calcium, vit D; provide list of calcium-rich foods; renal failure patients are given a renal diet
• Caution patient not to double doses, take exactly as prescribed

### Evaluation
**Positive therapeutic outcome**
• Prevention of bone deficiencies
• Calcium, phosphorus at normal levels

## ⚠ HIGH ALERT

### diltiazem (Rx)
(dil-tye′a-zem)
Apo-Diltiaz ♣, Cardizem, Cardizem LA, Dilacor-XR, Diltia XR, Diltiaz, diltiazem, Syn-Diltiazem ♣, Tiazac
*Func. class.:* Calcium channel blocker, antianginal
*Chem. class.:* Benzothiazepine
**Pregnancy category C**

**Do not confuse:**
Cardizem/Cardene

**Action:** Inhibits calcium ion influx across cell membrane during cardiac depolarization, produces relaxation of coronary vascular smooth muscle, dilates coronary arteries, slows SA/AV node conduction times, dilates peripheral arteries

**Therapeutic outcome:** Decreased angina pectoris, dysrhythmias, B/P

**Uses**
*Oral:* Angina pectoris due to coronary insufficiency, hypertension, coronary artery spasm
*Parenteral:* Atrial fibrillation, flutter; paroxysmal supraventricular tachycardia

**Dosage and routes**
*Hypertension*
*Adult:* PO 60-120 mg bid (sus rel) (Cardizem SR), max 540 mg/day, or 180-240 mg (ext rel) daily

*Prinzmetal's or variant angina, chronic stable angina*
*Adult:* PO 30 mg qid, increasing dose gradually to 180-360 mg/day in divided doses or 60-120 mg bid; may increase to 240-360 mg/day or 120 or 180 mg ext rel (LA, CD, XT, XR products) PO daily

*Atrial fibrillation, flutter, paroxysmal supraventricular tachycardia*
*Adult:* IV 0.25 mg/kg as BOL over 2 min initially, then 0.35 mg/kg may be given after 15 min; if no response, may give CONT INF 5-15 mg/hr for up to 24 hr

**Available forms:** Tabs 30, 60, 90, 120 mg; ext rel tab 120, 180, 240, 300, 360, 420

mg; ext rel caps 60, 90, 120, 180, 240, 300, 360, 420 mg; sus rel caps 60, 90, 120 mg; inj 5 mg/ml (5, 10 ml); powder for inj 25 mg

### Adverse effects

*CNS: Headache, fatigue, drowsiness,* dizziness, depression, weakness, insomnia, tremor, paresthesia

*CV: Dysrhythmia, edema,* **CHF,** bradycardia, hypotension, palpitations, **heart block**

*GI: Nausea,* vomiting, diarrhea, gastric upset, *constipation,* increased liver function tests

*GU:* Nocturia, polyuria, **acute renal failure**

*INTEG: Rash,* pruritus at inj site, flushing, photosensitivity, burning

*RESP:* Rhinitis, dyspnea, pharyngitis

**Contraindications:** Sick sinus syndrome, 2nd- or 3rd-degree heart block, hypotension less than 90 mm Hg systolic, acute MI, pulmonary congestion, intracranial surgery, bleeding aneurysms, severe hypotension (systolic <90 mm Hg or diastolic <60 mg Hg)

**Precautions:** Pregnancy **C,** breastfeeding, children, CHF, hypotension, hepatic injury, renal disease

#### Pharmacokinetics

| | |
|---|---|
| **Absorption** | Well absorbed |
| **Distribution** | Not known |
| **Metabolism** | Liver, extensively |
| **Excretion** | Metabolites (96%) |
| **Half-life** | 3½-9 hr |

#### Pharmacodynamics

| | PO | PO–SUS REL | IV |
|---|---|---|---|
| **Onset** | ½ hr | Unknown | Unknown |
| **Peak** | 2-3 hr | Unknown | Unknown |
| **Duration** | 6-8 hr | 12 hr | Unknown |

### Interactions

*Individual drugs*

Carbamazepine, lithium, lovastatin, methylPREDNISolone: increased effects of each specific product

Cimetidine: increased effects of diltiazem

CycloSPORINE: increased cycloSPORINE effect

Digoxin: increased digoxin effect

Theophylline: increased effect, toxicity

*Drug classifications*

Anesthetics: increased effects of anesthetics

β-Adrenergic blockers: increased bradycardia, CHF, increased β-blocker effect

Benzodiazepines: increased effect of benzodiazepines

HMG-CoA reductase inhibitors: increased effects

*Drug/herb*

Barberry, betel palm, burdock, goldenseal, khat, khella, lily of the valley, plantain: increased diltiazem effect

Yohimbe: decreased diltiazem effect

*Drug/food*

Grapefruit juice: increased hypotension

### NURSING CONSIDERATIONS

#### Assessment

• Assess fluid volume status: I&O ratio and record, weight, distended red veins, crackles in lung, color, quality, and specific gravity of urine, skin turgor, adequacy of pulses, moist mucous membranes, bilateral lung sounds, peripheral pitting edema; dehydration symptoms of decreasing output, thirst, hypotension, dry mouth and mucous membranes should be reported

• Monitor B/P and pulse, respiration, ECG and intervals (PR, QRS, QT); PCWP, CVP often during infusion; if B/P drops 30 mm Hg, stop infusion and call prescriber

• Monitor ALT, AST, bilirubin daily; if these are elevated, hepatotoxicity is suspected

• If platelets are <150,000/mm³, product is usually discontinued and another product started

• Assess for extravasation: change site q48hr

#### Nursing diagnoses

• Cardiac output, decreased (uses)

• Knowledge, deficient (teaching)

#### Implementation

**PO route**

• Do not break, crush, or chew sus rel caps

• Give with meals for GI symptoms; may be crushed and mixed with food/fluids for swallowing difficulty; may sprinkle (reg tab) on applesauce

• Give Dilacor-XR on an empty stomach

• Store in airtight container at room temperature

**IV route**

• Give direct **IV** undiluted over 2 min

• For continuous inf dilute 125 mg/100 ml (1.25 mg/ml) or 250 mg/250 ml (1 mg/ml) or 250 mg/500 ml (0.5 mg/ml) of $D_5W$, 0.9% NaCl, $D_5$/0.45% NaCl; give 10 mg/hr; may increase by 5 mg/hr to 15 mg/hr; may continue inf up to 24 hr

*Y-site compatibilities:* Albumin, amikacin, amphotericin B, aztreonam, bretylium, bumetanide, cefazolin, cefotaxime, cefotetan, cefoxitin, ceftazidime, ceftriaxone, cefuroxime, cimetidine, ciprofloxacin, clindamycin, digoxin, DOBUTamine, DOPamine, doxycycline, epINEPHrine, erythromycin, esmolol, fentanyl,

---

Adverse effects: *italic* = common, **bold** = life-threatening

fluconazole, gentamicin, hetastarch, hydromorphone, imipenem-cilastatin, labetalol, lidocaine, lorazepam, meperidine, metoclopramide, metronidazole, midazolam, milrinone, morphine, multivitamins, niCARdipine, nitroglycerin, norepinephrine, oxacillin, penicillin G potassium, pentamidine, piperacillin, potassium chloride, potassium phosphates, ranitidine, sodium nitroprusside, theophylline, ticarcillin, ticarcillin/clavulanate, tobramycin, trimethoprim-sulfamethoxazole, vancomycin, vecuronium

### Patient/family education
• Caution patient to avoid hazardous activities until stabilized on product and dizziness is no longer a problem
• Instruct patient to limit caffeine consumption; to avoid grapefruit juice; to avoid alcohol and OTC products unless directed by prescriber
◆ Tell patient to comply in all areas of medical regimen; diet, exercise, stress reduction, product therapy; to notify prescriber of irregular heart beat, shortness of breath, swelling of feet and hands, pronounced dizziness, constipation, nausea, hypotension
• Teach patient to use as directed even if feeling better; may be taken with other cardiovascular products (nitrates, β-blockers); how to take pulse, B/P before taking product

### Evaluation
**Positive therapeutic outcome**
• Decreased anginal pain
• Decreased B/P
• Absence of dysrhythmias

**Treatment of overdose:** Atropine for AV block, vasopressor for hypotension

---

**\*dimenhyDRINATE** (OTC, Rx)
(dye-men-hye′dri-nate)
Apo-Dimenhydrinate ✤, Calm-X, Children's Dramamine, dimenhyDRINATE, Dimetabs, Dramamine, Dramanate, Dymenate, Gravol ✤, Gravol L/A ✤, Nauseatol ✤, Novo-Dimenate ✤, PMS-Dimenhydrinate ✤, Travamine ✤
*Func. class.:* Antiemetic, antihistamine, anticholinergic
*Chem. class.:* H₁-receptor antagonist, ethanolamine derivative

**Pregnancy category** B

**Do not confuse:**
dimenhyDRINATE/diphenhydrAMINE

**Action:** Vestibular stimulator is decreased; anticholinergic, antiemetic, antihistamine response; competes with histamine for H₁ receptors in GI tract, blood vessels, respiratory tract; central anticholinergic activity, which results in decreased vestibular stimulation and blockade of chemorecepter trigger zone

**Therapeutic outcome:** Absence of motion sickness

**Uses:** Motion sickness, nausea, vomiting, vertigo

### Dosage and routes
*Adult:* PO 50-100 mg q4hr; IM/**IV** 50 mg q4hr as needed ✤
*Child 6-12 yr:* PO 25-50 mg q6-8hr prn, max 150 mg/day
*Child 2-5 yr:* PO 12.5-25 mg q6-8hr, max 75 mg/day

**Available forms:** Tab 50 mg; inj 50 mg/ml ✤; elix 15 mg/5 ml ✤; chew tab 50 mg

### Adverse effects
***CNS:*** *Drowsiness,* restlessness, headache, dizziness, insomnia, confusion, nervousness, tingling, vertigo
***CV:*** Hypertension, *hypotension,* palpitations
***EENT:*** Dry mouth, blurred vision, diplopia, nasal congestion, photosensitivity
***GI:*** Nausea, anorexia, vomiting, *constipation*
***INTEG:*** Rash, urticaria, fever, chills, flushing
***MISC:*** Anaphylaxis

**Contraindications:** Hypersensitivity

**Precautions:** Pregnancy **B**, breastfeeding, children, geriatric, cardiac dysrhythmias, asthma, prostatic hypertrophy, bladder neck obstruction, angle-closure glaucoma, stenosing peptic ulcer, pyloroduodenal obstruction

### Pharmacokinetics
| | |
|---|---|
| **Absorption** | Well absorbed (PO, IM) |
| **Distribution** | Unknown; crosses placenta |
| **Metabolism** | Liver |
| **Excretion** | Kidneys, breast milk |
| **Half-life** | Unknown |

### Pharmacodynamics
| | PO | IM | IV |
|---|---|---|---|
| **Onset** | 15-60 min | 30 min | Immediate |
| **Peak** | 1-2 hr | 1-2 hr | Unknown |
| **Duration** | 4-6 hr | 4-6 hr | 4-6 hr |

### Interactions
*Individual drugs*
Alcohol: increased effect

*Drug classifications*
CNS depressants, anticholinergics, tricyclics, opiates, sedative/hypnotics, MAOIs: increased effects
*Drug/herb*
Corkwood, henbane leaf, jimsonweed, scopolia: increased anticholinergic effect
Hops, Jamaican dogwood, khat, senega: increased effect
*Drug/lab test*
False negative: skin allergy tests (discontinue antihistamines 3 days before testing)

## NURSING CONSIDERATIONS
### Assessment
• Assess for signs of toxicity to other products or masking of symptoms of disease (brain tumor, intestinal obstruction); monitor GI symptoms including nausea, vomiting, abdominal pain, increased bowel sounds
• Monitor VS, B/P; check patients with cardiac disease more often
• Monitor I&O; check for dehydration (poor skin turgor, increased specific gravity, tachycardia, severe thirst) especially in the geriatric

### Nursing diagnoses
• Injury, risk for (side effects)
• Knowledge, deficient (teaching)

### Implementation
**PO route**
• Tabs may be swallowed whole, chewed, or allowed to dissolve; give 1-2 hr before activity that may cause motion sickness; use measuring device for liquid for correct dosing
**IM route**
• Give IM inj in large muscle mass; aspirate to avoid **IV** administration; massage
**IV route**
• Give **IV** directly after diluting 50 mg/10 ml or NaCl inj; give 50 mg or less over 2 min
*Syringe compatibilities:* Atropine, diphenhydrAMINE, droperidol, fentanyl, heparin, hydromorphone, meperidine, metoclopramide, morphine, pentazocine, perphenazine, ranitidine, scopolamine
*Syringe incompatibilities:* Butorphanol, chlorproMAZINE, glycopyrrolate, hydrOXYzine, midazolam, pentobarbital, prochlorperazine, promazine, promethazine, thiopental
*Y-site compatibilities:* Acyclovir
*Y-site incompatibilities:* Aminophylline, heparin, hydrocortisone sodium succinate, hydrOXYzine, phenobarbital, phenytoin, predniSOLONE, prochlorperazine, promazine, promethazine

*Additive compatibilities:* Amikacin, calcium gluconate, chloramphenicol, corticotropin, erythromycin, heparin, hydrOXYzine, methicillin, norepinephrine, penicillin G potassium, pentobarbital, phenobarbital, potassium chloride, prochlorperazine, vancomycin, vit B/C
*Additive incompatibilities:* Tetracycline, thiopental

### Patient/family education
• Teach all aspects of product uses; to notify prescriber if confusion, sedation, hypotension occur; to avoid driving and other hazardous activity if drowsiness occurs; to avoid alcohol and other CNS depressants that may potentiate effect
• Tell patient not to exceed recommended dosage
• Inform patient hard candy, gum, frequent rinsing of mouth may be used for dryness
• Advise patient that a false negative result may occur with skin testing; these procedures should not be scheduled until 4 days after discontinuing use
• Caution patient to avoid hazardous activities, activities requiring alertness; dizziness may occur; instruct patient to request assistance with ambulation

### Evaluation
**Positive therapeutic outcome**
• Absence of motion sickness
• Absence of nausea, vomiting

---

## dinoprostone (Rx)
(dye-noe-prost'one)
Cervidil Vaginal Insert, Prepidil, Endocervical Gel, Prostin E Vaginal Suppository
*Func. class.:* Oxytocic, abortifacient
*Chem. class.:* Prostaglandin $E_2$

**Pregnancy category  C**

**Do not confuse:**
Prepidil/bepridil

**Action:** Stimulates uterine contractions similar to labor by myometrium stimulation, causing abortion; acts within 30 hr for complete abortion; GI smooth muscle stimulation, effacement, dilatation of the cervix

**Therapeutic outcome:** Beginning of labor, fetal expulsion

**Uses:** Abortion during 2nd trimester, benign hydatidiform mole, expulsion of uterine contents in fetal deaths to 28 wk, missed abortion, cervical effacement and dilatation in term pregnancy when they have not occurred spontaneously

## Dosage and routes
### Abortifacient
*Adult:* VAG SUPP 20 mg; repeat q3-5hr until abortion occurs; max dose is 240 mg

### Cervical ripening
*Adult:* GEL Warm to room temperature; choose correct length shielded catheter (10 or 20 mm); fill catheter by pushing plunger; have patient recumbent for 15-30 min; insert one 10 mg insert

**Available forms:** Vag supp 20 mg; gel 0.5 mg/3 g (prefilled syringe); vag insert 10 mg

## Adverse effects
*CNS: Headache,* dizziness, chills, fever
*CV:* Hypotension, **dysrhythmias**
*EENT:* Blurred vision
*GI: Nausea, vomiting, diarrhea*
*GU:* Vaginitis, vaginal pain, vulvitis, vaginismus
*INTEG:* Rash, skin color changes
*MS: Leg cramps, joint swelling,* weakness
**Insert:** Uterine hyperstimulation, fever, nausea, vomiting, diarrhea, abdominal pain
**Gel:** Uterine contractile abnormality, GI side effects, back pain, fever
**Fetal:** Bradycardia (i.e., deceleration)
**Suppository: Uterine rupture, anaphylaxis**

**Contraindications:** Hypersensitivity, uterine fibrosis, cervical stenosis, pelvic surgery, PID, respiratory disease

**Precautions:** Pregnancy **C,** renal/hepatic/cardiac disease, asthma, anemia, jaundice, diabetes mellitus, seizure disorders, hypo/hypertension, glaucoma

| Pharmacokinetics | |
|---|---|
| **Absorption** | Rapidly absorbed |
| **Distribution** | Unknown |
| **Metabolism** | Enzymes |
| **Excretion** | Kidneys |
| **Half-life** | Unknown |

| Pharmacodynamics | | |
|---|---|---|
| | GEL | SUPP |
| **Onset** | Rapid | 10 min |
| **Peak** | 30-45 min | Unknown |
| **Duration** | Unknown | 2-3 hr |

## Interactions
### Individual drugs
Alcohol: decreased oxytoxic effect

### Drug classifications
Other oxytocics: increased effect

## NURSING CONSIDERATIONS
### Assessment
• Assess dilatation and effacement of the cervix, uterine contractions, fetal heart tones; watch for contractions lasting over 1 min, hypertonus, fetal distress; product should be slowed or discontinued
• Assess for fever that occurs approximately 30 min after supp insertion (abortion)
• Monitor for nausea, vomiting, diarrhea; these may require medication
• Assess for hypersensitivity reaction: dyspnea, rash, chest discomfort
• Assess respiratory rate, rhythm, depth; notify prescriber of abnormalities, in pulse, B/P
• Check vaginal discharge; itching, irritation indicates vaginal infection

### Nursing diagnoses
• Injury, risk for (side effects)
• Knowledge, deficient (teaching)

### Implementation
#### Suppository route
• Warm supp by running warm water over package; insert high in vagina, wear gloves to prevent absorption; have patient recumbent for at least 10 min
#### Gel route
• Do not allow to come in contact with skin; use soap and water to wash after use
• Gel should be at room temperature
• Place patient in dorsal or lithotomy position to insert gel into cervical canal; remove catheter; discard all items after use; keep supine 15-30 min

### Patient/family education
• Teach patient all aspects of treatment including purpose of medication and expected results
• Tell patient that gel may produce warmth in her vagina
• Caution patient that if contractions are longer than 1 min to notify nurse or prescriber
• Advise patient to notify prescriber of cramping, pain, increased bleeding, chills, increased temp, or foul-smelling discharge; these symptoms may indicate uterine infection
• Advise patient to remain supine 10-15 min after insertion of suppository; 2 hr after insert, 15-30 min after gel

### Evaluation
**Positive therapeutic outcome**
• Progression of labor
• Abortion

## *diphenhydrAMINE (OTC, Rx)
(dye-fen-hye'dra-meen)

Allerdryl ✦, AllerMax, Allermed, Banophen, Benadryl, Benadryl 25, Benadryl Kapseals, Benahist 10, Benahist 50, Ben-Allergin-50, Benoject-10, Benoject-50, Benylin Cough, Bydramine, Compoz, Diphenadryl, Diphen Cough, Diphenhist, diphenhydrAMINE HCl, Dormin, Genahist, Hydramine, Hydramyn, Hydril, Hyrexin-50, Insomnal ✦, Nidryl, Nighttime Sleep Aid, Nordryl, Nordryl Cough, Nytol, Phendry, Siladril, Sleep-Eze 3, Sominex 2, Tusstat, Twilite, Uni-Bent Cough, Wehdryl

*Func. class.:* Antihistamine (1st generation, nonselective), antitussive
*Chem. class.:* Ethanolamine derivative, $H_1$-receptor antagonist

**Pregnancy category B**

**Do not confuse:**
diphenhydrAMINE/dicyclomine/dimenhyDRINATE

**Action:** Acts on blood vessels, GI, respiratory system by competing with histamine for $H_1$-receptor site; decreases allergic response by blocking histamine

**Therapeutic outcome:** Absence of allergy symptoms and rhinitis, decreased dystonic symptoms, absence of motion sickness, absence of cough, ability to sleep

**Uses:** Allergy symptoms, rhinitis, motion sickness, antiparkinsonism, nighttime sedation, infant colic, nonproductive cough

### Dosage and routes
*Adult and child >12 yr:* PO 25-50 mg q4-6hr, not to exceed 400 mg/day; IM/**IV** 10-50 mg, not to exceed 400 mg/day
*Child <12 yr:* PO/IM/**IV** 5 mg/kg/day in 4 divided doses, not to exceed 300 mg/day

*Nighttime sleep aid*
*Adult and child ≥12 yr:* PO 25-50 mg at bedtime

*Antitussive (syrup only)*
*Adult and child ≥12 yr:* 25 mg q4hr, max 100 mg/24 hr
*Child 6-12 yr:* 12.5 mg q4hr, max 75 mg/24 hr
*Child 2-6 yr:* 6.25 mg q4hr, max 37.5 mg/24 hr

*Renal dose*
*Adult:* PO CCr >50 ml/min give dose q6hr; CCr 10-50 ml/min dose q6-12hr; CCr <10 ml/min dose q12-18hr

**Available forms:** Caps 25, 50 mg; tabs 25, 50 mg; chew tabs 12.5 mg; elix 12.5 mg/5 ml; syr 12.5 mg/5 ml; inj 10, 50 mg/ml; orally disintegrating tabs 12.5 mg

**Adverse effects**
*CNS: Dizziness, drowsiness,* poor coordination, fatigue, anxiety, euphoria, confusion, paresthesia, neuritis, **seizures**
*CV:* Hypotension, palpitations
*EENT:* Blurred vision, dilated pupils, tinnitus, nasal stuffiness, dry nose, throat, mouth
*GI:* Nausea, anorexia, diarrhea
*GU: Retention,* dysuria, frequency
*HEMA:* **Thrombocytopenia, agranulocytosis, hemolytic anemia**
*INTEG:* Photosensitivity
*MISC:* **Anaphylaxis**
*RESP:* Increased thick secretions, wheezing, chest tightness

**Contraindications:** Hypersensitivity to $H_1$-receptor antagonist, acute asthma attack, lower respiratory tract disease

**Precautions:** Pregnancy **B**, breastfeeding, increased intraocular pressure, renal/cardiac disease, hypertension, bronchial asthma, seizure disorder, stenosed peptic ulcers, hyperthyroidism, prostatic hypertrophy, bladder neck obstruction

### Pharmacokinetics
| | |
|---|---|
| Absorption | Well absorbed (PO, IM); completely absorbed (**IV**) |
| Distribution | Widely distributed; crosses placenta |
| Metabolism | Liver (95%) |
| Excretion | Kidneys, breast milk |
| Half-life | 2½-7 hr |

### Pharmacodynamics
| | PO | IM | IV |
|---|---|---|---|
| Onset | 15-60 min | 30 min | Immediate |
| Peak | 1-4 hr | 1-4 hr | Unknown |
| Duration | 4-8 hr | 4-8 hr | 4-8 hr |

**Interactions**
*Individual drugs*
Alcohol: increased CNS depression
*Drug classifications*
Antidepressants (tricyclic), barbiturates, CNS depressants, opiates, sedative/hypnotics: increased CNS depression
MAOIs: increased effect of diphenhydrAMINE
*Drug/herb*
Corkwood, henbane leaf: increased anticholinergic effect

Adverse effects: *italic* = common, **bold** = life-threatening

Hops, Jamaican dogwood, khat, senega: increased effect

*Drug/lab test*

False negative: skin allergy tests (discontinue antihistamines 3 days before testing)

## NURSING CONSIDERATIONS
### Assessment

- Assess respiratory status: rate, rhythm, increase in bronchial secretions, wheezing, chest tightness; provide fluids to 2 L/day to decrease secretion thickness
- Monitor I&O ratio: be alert for urinary retention, frequency, dysuria, especially geriatric; product should be discontinued if these occur
- Monitor CBC during long-term therapy; blood dyscrasias may occur but are rare
- If giving for dystonic reactions, assess type of involuntary movements and evaluate response to this medication
- Assess cough characteristics including type, frequency, thickness of secretions, and evaluate response to this medication if using for cough

### Nursing diagnoses
- Injury, risk for (side effects)
- Knowledge, deficient (teaching)
- Sleep deprivation (uses)

### Implementation
- Give 20 min before bedtime if using for sleep aid

**PO route**
- Give with meals if GI symptoms occur; absorption rate may be slightly decreased; cap may be opened and product mixed with food/fluids for patients with swallowing difficulties

**IM route**
- Give IM inj in large muscle mass; aspirate to avoid **IV** administration; rotate sites

**IV route**
- Give **IV** undiluted 25 mg/min; may be diluted with 0.9% NaCl, $D_5W$, $D_{10}W$, 0.45% NaCl, $D_5$/0.9% NaCl, $D_5$/0.45% NaCl, $D_5$/0.25% NaCl, LR, Ringer's, give 25 mg/min or less

*Syringe compatibilities:* Atropine, butorphanol, chlorproMAZINE, cimetidine, cisatracurium, dimenhyDRINATE, DOXOrubicin liposome, droperidol, fentanyl, fluphenazine, glycopyrrolate, hydromorphone, hydrOXYzine, meperidine, metoclopramide, midazolam, morphine, nalbuphine, pentazocine, perphenazine, prochlorperazine, promazine, promethazine, ranitidine, remifentanil, scopolamine, sufentanil, thiothixene

*Syringe incompatibilities:* Pentobarbital, phenytoin, thiopental

*Y-site compatibilities:* Acyclovir, aldesleukin, amifostine, amsacrine, aztreonam, ciprofloxacin, cisplatin, cladribine, cyclophosphamide, cytarabine, DOXOrubicin, famotidine, filgrastim, fluconazole, fludarabine, gallium, granisetron, heparin, hydrocortisone, idarubicin, melphalan, meperidine, meropenem, methotrexate, ondansetron, paclitaxel, piperacillin/tazobactam, potassium chloride, propofol, sargramostim, sufentanil, tacrolimus, teniposide, thiotepa, vinorelbine, vit B/C

*Y-site incompatibilities:* Foscarnet

*Additive compatibilities:* Amikacin, aminophylline, ascorbic acid, bleomycin, cephapirin, erythromycin, hydrocortisone, lidocaine, methicillin, methyldopate, nafcillin, netilmicin, penicillin G potassium, penicillin G sodium, polymyxin B, vit B/C

*Additive incompatibilities:* Amobarbital, cephalothin, thiopental

### Patient/family education
- Tell patient that a false-negative result may occur with skin testing; these procedures should not be scheduled until 3 days after discontinuing use
- Caution patient to avoid hazardous activities and activities requiring alertness, since dizziness may occur; instruct patient to request assistance with ambulation
- Teach patient to use sunscreen to prevent photosensitivity
- Advise patient to avoid alcohol, other depressants; may potentiate effect; CNS depression may occur
- Teach all aspects of product uses; to notify prescriber if confusion, sedation, hypotension occur; to avoid driving and other hazardous activity if drowsiness occurs; to avoid alcohol or other CNS depressants that may potentiate effect
- Teach patient to avoid breastfeeding

### Evaluation
**Positive therapeutic outcome**
- Absence of motion sickness
- Absence of nausea, vomiting
- Ability to sleep
- Absence of cough
- Decrease in involuntary movements

### Treatment of overdose:
- Administer lavage, diazepam, vasopressors, barbiturates (short acting)

## diphenoxylate with atropine (Rx)
(dye-fen-ox'i-late)
Logen, Logene, Lomanate, Lomotil, Lonox, Lo-Trol, Low-Quel

## difenoxin/atropine (Rx)
(dye-fen-ox'in/a'troe-peen)
Motofen

*Func. class.:* Antidiarrheal
*Chem. class.:* Phenylpiperidine derivative, opiate agonist

**Pregnancy category** C

**Controlled substance schedule V**
diphenoxylate/atropine; **IV**
difenoxin/atropine (US)

**Do not confuse:**
Lomotil/Lamictal/Lamasil/Lanoxin/Lasix

**Action:** Inhibits gastric motility by acting on mucosal receptors responsible for peristalsis; related to opioid analgesics as adjunct

**Therapeutic outcome:** Decreased loose stools

**Uses:** Diarrhea (cause undetermined)

## Dosage and routes
*diphenoxylate/atropine*
**Adult:** PO 2.5-5 mg qid, titrated to patient response, not to exceed 8 tabs/24 hr
**Child 2-12 yr:** PO (liquid only) 0.3-0.4 mg/kg/day in divided doses

*difenoxin/atropine*
**Adult:** PO Initially 2 tabs, then 1 tab after each loose stool or q3-4hr prn, max 8 tabs/day

**Available forms:** diphenoxylate/atropine: tab 2.5 mg diphenoxylate/0.025 mg atropine; liq 2.5 mg diphenoxylate/0.025 mg atropine/5 ml; difenoxin/atropine: tabs 1 mg difenoxin/ 0.025 atropine

## Adverse effects
*CNS: Dizziness, drowsiness, light-headedness, headache,* fatigue, nervousness, insomnia, confusion
*EENT:* Blurred vision, burning eyes
*GI: Nausea, vomiting, dry mouth, epigastric distress,* constipation, **paralytic ileus**
*MISC:* **Anaphylaxis, angioedema**
*RESP:* **Respiratory depression**

**Contraindications:** Hypersensitivity, pseudomembranous enterocolitis, jaundice, glaucoma, child <2 yr, severe electrolyte imbalances, diarrhea associated with organisms that penetrate intestinal mucosa

**Precautions:** Pregnancy **C**, breastfeeding, renal/hepatic disease, ulcerative colitis, severe hepatic disease

### Pharmacokinetics
| | |
|---|---|
| **Absorption** | Well absorbed |
| **Distribution** | Unknown |
| **Metabolism** | Liver, active metabolite |
| **Excretion** | Kidneys |
| **Half-life** | 2½ hr |

### Pharmacodynamics
| | |
|---|---|
| **Onset** | 45-60 min |
| **Peak** | 2 hr |
| **Duration** | 3-4 hr |

## Interactions
*Individual drugs*
Alcohol: increased action of alcohol
*Drug classifications*
Anticholinergics: increased anticholinergic effect
Barbiturates: increased action of barbiturates
CNS depressants: increased action of CNS depressants
MAOIs: hypertensive crisis; do not use together
Opiates: increased action of opioids
*Drug/herb*
Nutmeg: increased antidiarrheal effect

## NURSING CONSIDERATIONS
### Assessment
• Monitor electrolytes (potassium, sodium, chloride) if on long-term therapy; fluid status, skin turgor
• Assess bowel pattern before, during treatment; check for rebound constipation after termination of medication; check bowel sounds
• Check response after 48 hr; if no response, product should be discontinued and other treatment initiated
• Assess for abdominal distention and toxic megacolon, which may occur in ulcerative colitis
• Assess hepatic function if on long-term therapy

### Nursing diagnoses
• Constipation (adverse reactions)
• Diarrhea (uses)
• Knowledge, deficient (teaching)
• Noncompliance (teaching)

### Implementation
• Give for 48 hr only; tabs may be given with food, crushed and mixed with fluids; liquid should be measured accurately

Adverse effects: *italic* = common, **bold** = life-threatening

### Patient/family education
- Advise patient to avoid alcohol and OTC products unless directed by prescriber; may cause increased CNS depression
- Caution patient not to exceed recommended dosage; that product may be habit forming
- Advise patient that product may cause drowsiness; to avoid hazardous activities until response to product is determined
- Teach patient that dry mouth can be decreased by frequent sips of water, hard candy, sugarless gum

### Evaluation
**Positive therapeutic outcome**
- Decreased diarrhea

---

### dipivefrin ophthalmic
*See Appendix D*

---

### dipyridamole (Rx)
(dye-peer-id´a-mole)
Apo-Dipyridamole ✤, dipyridamole, Novo-Dipiradol ✤, Persantine, Persantine IV
*Func. class.:* Coronary vasodilator, antiplatelet agent
*Chem. class.:* Nonnitrate

**Pregnancy category B**

**Action:** Inhibits adenosine uptake, which produces coronary vasodilatation; increases oxygen saturation in coronary tissues, coronary blood flow; acts on small vessels with little effect on vascular resistance; may increase development of collateral circulation; decreased platelet aggregation by the inhibition of phosphodiesterases (enzymes)

**Therapeutic outcome:** Inhibition of platelet aggregation; absence of ischemic attacks, reinfarction

**Uses:** Prevention of transient ischemic attacks, inhibition of platelet adhesion to prevent myocardial reinfarction, thromboembolism, with warfarin in prosthetic heart valves, prevention of coronary bypass graft occlusion with aspirin; **IV** form used to evaluate coronary artery disease; used as alternative to exercise in thallium myocardial perfusion imaging to evaluate coronary artery disease

### Dosage and routes
*Transient ischemic attacks*
**Adult:** PO 50 mg tid, 1 hr before meals, not to exceed 400 mg daily

*Inhibition of platelet adhesion*
**Adult:** PO 50-75 mg qid in combination with aspirin or warfarin

*Thallium myocardial perfusion imaging*
**Adult: IV** 570 mcg/kg

**Available forms:** Tabs 25, 50, 75 mg; inj 10 mg/2 ml

### Adverse effects
*CNS: Headache, dizziness, weakness, fainting, syncope;* **IV**: transient cerebral ischemia, weakness
*CV: Postural hypotension;* **IV**: MI
*GI: Nausea, vomiting,* anorexia, diarrhea
*INTEG: Rash,* flushing
*RESP:* **IV: Bronchospasm**

**Contraindications:** Hypersensitivity

**Precautions:** Pregnancy **B,** breastfeeding, hypotension

#### Pharmacokinetics
| | |
|---|---|
| **Absorption** | 30%-50% (PO) |
| **Distribution** | Widely distributed; crosses placenta |
| **Metabolism** | Liver |
| **Excretion** | Bile, undergoes enterohepatic recirculation; enters breast milk |
| **Half-life** | 10 hr |

#### Pharmacodynamics
| | PO | IV |
|---|---|---|
| **Onset** | Unknown | Unknown |
| **Peak** | 1.25 hr | 6 min |
| **Duration** | 6 hr | ½ hr |
| **Therapeutic effect** | Several mo | |

### Interactions
*Individual drugs*
Aspirin, cefamandole, cefotetan, cefoperazone, plicamycin, sulfinpyrazone, valproic acid: increased risk of bleeding
Theophylline: prevention of coronary vasodilation
*Drug classifications*
Anticoagulants, NSAIDs, salicylates, thrombolytics: increased risk of bleeding
*Drug/herb*
Arginine: increased gastric irritation
Bilberry, saw palmetto: decreased antiplatelet effect
Bogbean, dong quai, feverfew, garlic, ginger, ginkgo, grapeseed, primrose: increased antiplatelet effect

---

## NURSING CONSIDERATIONS
### Assessment
- Monitor B/P, pulse baseline and during treatment until stable; take B/P with patient lying, standing; orthostatic hypotension is common
- Assess cardiac status: chest pain, what aggravates or ameliorates condition
- If using by **IV** route, monitor VS before, during, and after infusion; monitor for chest pain, bronchospasm; use ECG for identifying dysrhythmias; use aminophylline up to 250 mg **IV** for bronchospasm and chest pain; if chest pain is unrelieved with the 250 mg dose of aminophylline, give SL dose of nitroglycerin

### Nursing diagnoses
- Cardiac output, decreased (uses)
- Knowledge, deficient (teaching)
- Pain, acute (uses)

### Implementation
**PO route**
- Give with 8 oz of water; to improve absorption give on an empty stomach; if GI symptoms occur may give with meals
- Tabs may be crushed, mixed with food or fluids for swallowing difficulty or swallowed whole
- Store at room temperature
**Intermittent IV infusion route**
- Give by **IV** after diluting to at least 1:2 ratio using $D_5W$, 0.45% NaCl, or 0.9% NaCl; 20-50 ml should be given; give over 4 min; do not give undiluted

### Patient/family education
- Teach patient that this medication is not a cure; that product may have to be taken continuously in evenly spaced doses only as directed; if a dose is missed, take one when remembered up to 4 hr; do not double doses
- Advise patient to rise slowly from sitting or lying down to prevent orthostatic hypotension
- Caution patient not to use alcohol or OTC medication unless approved by prescriber
- Caution patient to avoid hazardous activities until stabilized on medication; dizziness may occur

### Evaluation
**Positive therapeutic outcome**
- Absence of reinfarction, ischemic attacks

**Treatment of overdose:** Administer **IV** phenylephrine

---

## disopyramide (Rx)
(dye-soe-peer′a-mide)
disopyramide, Norpace, Norpace CR, Rhythmodan ✦, Rythmodan-LA ✦
*Func. class.:* Antidysrhythmic (class IA)
*Chem. class.:* Nonnitrate

**Pregnancy category  C**

**D**

**Action:** Prolongs action potential duration and effective refractory period; reduces disparity in refractory period between normal and infarcted myocardium; prevents increased myocardial excitability and conduction contractility

**Therapeutic outcome:** Suppression of supraventricular dysrhythmias

**Uses:** PVCs, ventricular tachycardia, supraventricular tachycardia

**Unlabeled uses:** Atrial flutter, fibrillation

### Dosage and routes
*Adult:* PO 100-200 mg q6hr; SUS REL cap 200-400 mg q12hr
*Child 12-18 yr:* PO 6-15 mg/kg/day, in divided doses q6hr
*Child 4-12 yr:* PO 10-15 mg/kg/day in divided doses q6hr
*Child 1-4 yr:* PO 10-20 mg/kg/day in divided doses q6hr
*Child <1 yr:* PO 10-30 mg/kg/day, in divided doses q6hr

*Renal dose*
*Adult:* PO CCr >40 ml/min 100 mg q6hr; CCr 30-40 ml/min dose q8hr; CCr 15-30 ml/min dose q12hr; CCr <15 ml/min dose q24hr

**Available forms:** Caps 100, 150 mg; cont rel caps 100, 150 mg; sus rel tabs 150 mg ✦

### Adverse effects
*CNS: Headache, dizziness,* psychosis, fatigue, depression, paresthesias, insomnia
*CV: Hypotension, bradycardia,* angina, PVCs, tachycardia, increases in QRS and QT segments, **cardiac arrest,** edema, weight gain, AV block, **CHF,** syncope, chest pain
*EENT: Blurred vision, dry nose, throat, eyes,* angle-closure glaucoma
*GI: Dry mouth, constipation,* nausea, anorexia, flatulence, diarrhea, vomiting
*GU: Retention, hesitancy,* impotence
*HEMA:* **Thrombocytopenia, agranulocytosis,** anemia (rare), decreased Hgb, Hct
*INTEG:* Rash, pruritus, urticaria
*META:* Hypoglycemia, hypokalemia
*MS:* Weakness, pain in extremities

---

Adverse effects: *italic* = common, **bold** = life-threatening

**Contraindications:** Hypersensitivity, 2nd- or 3rd-degree heart block, cardiogenic shock, CHF (uncompensated), sick sinus syndrome, QT prolongation

**Precautions:** Pregnancy **C**, breastfeeding, children, diabetes mellitus, renal/hepatic disease, myasthenia gravis, angle-closure glaucoma, cardiomyopathy, conduction abnormalities, potassium imbalance

### Pharmacokinetics

| | |
|---|---|
| **Absorption** | Well absorbed |
| **Distribution** | Widely distributed |
| **Metabolism** | Liver |
| **Excretion** | Kidneys |
| **Half-life** | 4-10 hr |

### Pharmacodynamics

| | PO | PO–SUS REL |
|---|---|---|
| **Onset** | ½-3½ hr | Unknown |
| **Peak** | 2 hr | Unknown |
| **Duration** | 1½-8 hr | 12 hr |

### Interactions
**Individual drugs**
Atenolol, erythromycin, lidocaine, procainamide, propranolol, quinidine: increased effects of disopyramide
Phenobarbital, phenytoin, rifampin: decreased effects of disopyramide
**Drug classifications**
Anticholinergics: increased side effects, urinary retention
Antidysrhythmics: increased disopyramide effect
**Drug/herb**
Aconite: increased toxicity, death
Aloe, broom, buckthorn (chronic use), cascara sagrada (chronic use), Chinese rhubarb, figwort, fumitory, goldenseal, kudzu, licorice, senna: increased effect
Coltsfoot: decreased effect
Horehound: increased serotonin effect
**Drug/lab test**
Increased: liver enzymes, lipids, BUN, creatinine
Decreased: Hgb/Hct, blood glucose

### NURSING CONSIDERATIONS
**Assessment**
• Assess respiratory status: auscultate lung fields for bibasilar crackles in patients with advanced CHF
• Monitor I&O ratio and electrolytes: potassium, sodium, chloride; watch for decreasing urinary output, possible retention

• Monitor liver function tests: AST, ALT, bilirubin, alkaline phosphatase
• Monitor ECG to determine product effectiveness, measure PR, QRS, QT intervals; check for PVCs, other dysrhythmias; monitor B/P for hypotension; check for prolonged widening QT intervals, QRS complex; if QT or QRS increase by 50% or more, withhold next dose, notify prescriber
• Monitor for dehydration or hypovolemia
• Monitor for CNS symptoms: psychosis, numbness, depression; if these occur, product should be discontinued

**Nursing diagnoses**
• Cardiac output, decreased (uses)
• Knowledge, deficient (teaching)

**Implementation**
• Do not break, crush, or chew sus rel tabs
• Give 1 hr before or 2 hr after meals
• If changing from regular release to sus rel cap, give sus rel 6 hr after last dose of regular release

**Patient/family education**
• Teach patient to report side effects immediately to prescriber; to take exactly as prescribed; if dose is missed take when remembered if within 3-4 hr of next dose; do not double doses
• Teach patient to complete follow-up appointment with prescriber including pulmonary function tests, chest x-ray
• Instruct patient that dry mouth may be relieved by frequent sips of water, hard candy, sugarless gum
• Caution patient to make position changes from lying to standing slowly to prevent orthostatic hypotension

**Evaluation**
**Positive therapeutic outcome**
• Decreased PVCs, ventricular tachycardia

**Treatment of overdose:** Administer $O_2$, artificial ventilation, ECG; administer DOPamine for circulatory depression; administer diazepam or thiopental for seizures, isoproterenol

---

**divalproex sodium**
*See valproate*

---

D

## *DOBUTamine (Rx)
(doe-byoo'ta-meen)
DOBUTamine, Dobutrex
*Func. class.:* Adrenergic direct-acting
$\beta_1$-agonist, inotropic agent, cardiac stimulant
*Chem. class.:* Catecholamine

**Pregnancy category B**

**Do not confuse:**
DOBUTamine/DOPamine, Dobutrex/Diamox

**Action:** Causes increased contractility,
increased cardiac output without marked
increase in heart rate by acting on $\beta_1$-
receptors in heart; minor $\alpha/\beta_2$ effects

**Therapeutic outcome:** Cardiac output
increased with decreased fatigue and dyspnea

**Uses:** Cardiac decompensation due to
organic heart disease or cardiac surgery

**Unlabeled uses:** Cardiogenic shock in
children, congenital heart disease in children
undergoing cardiac catherization

**Dosage and routes**
*Adult and child:* IV INF 2.5-10 mcg/kg/
min; may increase to 40 mcg/kg/min if needed

**Available forms:** Inj 12.5 mg/ml

**Adverse effects**
*CNS: Anxiety,* headache, dizziness, fatigue
*CV:* Palpitations, tachycardia, hypo/
hypertension, PVCs, angina
*GI:* Heartburn, nausea, vomiting
*MS:* Muscle cramps (leg)
*RESP:* Dyspnea

**Contraindications:** Hypersensitivity,
idiopathic hypertrophic subaortic stenosis

**Precautions:** Pregnancy **B,** breastfeeding,
children, hypertension, CAD, MI, hypovolemia,
dysrhythmias

| Pharmacokinetics | |
|---|---|
| **Absorption** | Complete |
| **Distribution** | Unknown |
| **Metabolism** | Liver |
| **Excretion** | Kidneys |
| **Half-life** | 2 min |

| Pharmacodynamics | |
|---|---|
| **Onset** | 1-5 min |
| **Peak** | 10 min |
| **Duration** | <10 min |

## Interactions
*Individual drugs*
Atomoxetine: increased pressor effect, dys-
rhythmias
Bretylium, oxytocin: increased dysrhythmias
Guanethidine: increased severe hypertension
Oxytocin: increased pressor effects
*Drug classifications*
Anesthetics: increased dysrhythmias
Antidepressants (tricyclic), COMT inhibitors,
MAOIs, oxytocics: increased pressor re-
sponse, dysrhythmias
$\beta$-Blockers: decreased action of DOBUTamine

## NURSING CONSIDERATIONS
**Assessment**
• Assess for hypovolemia; if present, correct
before beginning treatment with DOBUTamine;
avoid use in patients with atrial fibrillation
before digitalization
• Monitor ECG for dysrhythmias, ischemia
during treatment; some patients may not need
continuous ECG monitoring; also monitor
PCWP, CVP, $CO_2$, urinary output; notify prescriber if <30 ml/hr
• Assess for heart failure: bibasilar crackles,
$S_3$ gallop, dyspnea, neck vein distention in
patients with cardiomyopathy or CHF
• Assess for oxygenation or perfusion deficit:
decreased B/P, chest pain, dizziness, loss of
consciousness
• Monitor B/P and pulse q5 min during
infusion; if B/P drops 30 mm Hg, stop infusion
and call prescriber
• Monitor ALT, AST, bilirubin daily
• Monitor for sulfite sensitivity, which may be
life threatening

**Nursing diagnoses**
• Cardiac output, decreased (uses)
• Knowledge, deficient (teaching)

**Implementation**
**IV route**
• Reconstitute 250 mg/10 ml of $D_5W$ or sterile
water for inj; may add another 10 ml to
dissolve completely if needed, then dilute in 50
ml or more of $D_5W$, 0.9% NaCl, 0.45% NaCl,
$D_5$/0.45% NaCl, $D_5$/0.9% NaCl, $D_5$/LR, LR;
titrate to patient response; use infusion pump
for correct dose
• Use a CVP catheter or large peripheral vein,
use infusion pump, titrate to patient response
• Change **IV** site q48hr
*Syringe compatibilities:* Heparin,
ranitidine
*Syringe incompatibility:* Doxapram
*Y-site compatibilities:* Amifostine,
inamrinone, atracurium, aztreonam, brety-

Adverse effects: *italic* = common, **bold** = life-threatening

lium, calcium chloride, calcium gluconate, ciprofloxacin, cladribine, diazepam, diltiazem, DOPamine, enalaprilat, epINEPHrine, famotidine, fentanyl, fluconazole, granisetron, haloperidol, hydromorphone, regular insulin, labetalol, lidocaine, lorazepam, magnesium sulfate, meperidine, milrinone, morphine, niCARdipine, nitroglycerin, norepinephrine, pancuronium, potassium chloride, propofol, ranitidine, sodium nitroprusside, streptokinase, tacrolimus, theophylline, thiotepa, tolazoline, vecuronium, verapamil, zidovudine

*Y-site incompatibilities:* Acyclovir, alteplase, aminophylline, foscarnet, phytonadione

*Additive compatibilities:* Amiodarone, atracurium, atropine, DOPamine, enalaprilat, epINEPHrine, flumazenil, hydrALAZINE, isoproterenol, lidocaine, meperidine, meropenem, metaraminol, morphine, nitroglycerin, norepinephrine, phentolamine, phenylephrine, procainamide, propranolol, ranitidine, verapamil

*Additive incompatibilities:* Acyclovir, aminophylline, bumetanide, calcium gluconate, diazepam, digoxin, furosemide, insulin, magnesium sulfate, phenytoin, potassium phosphate, sodium bicarbonate

### Patient/family education
• Teach patient reason for medication and expected results, reason for all monitoring and procedures
• Advise patient to report dyspnea, headache, **IV** site discomfort, chest pain, numbness of extremities

### Evaluation
**Positive therapeutic outcome**
• Increased cardiac output
• Decreased PCWP, adequate CVP
• Decreased dyspnea, fatigue, edema, ECG
• Increased urine output

**Treatment of overdose:** Discontinue product, support circulation

---

### docetaxel (Rx)
(doe-se-tax'el)
Taxotere
*Func. class.:* Antineoplastic—miscellaneous
**Pregnancy category** D

**Do not confuse:**
Taxotere/Taxol

**Action:** Inhibits the reorganization of the microtubule network needed for interphase and mitotic cellular functions; also causes abnormal bundles of microtubules during cell cycle and multiple esters of microtubules during mitosis

**Therapeutic outcome:** Prevention of rapidly growing malignant cells

**Uses:** Locally advanced or metastatic breast cancer, non–small-cell lung cancer, androgen independent metastatic prostate cancer, postsurgery operable node-positive breast cancer, induction treatment of locally advanced squamous cell cancer of the head/neck

### Dosage and routes
*Locally advanced or metastatic breast cancer after failure of other chemotherapy*
*Adult:* **IV** 60-100 mg/m$^2$ given over 1 hr q3 wk; if neutrophil count is <500/mm$^3$ for >1 wk, reduce dose by 25%

*Locally advanced or metastatic non–small-cell lung cancer after failure of cisplatin chemotherapy*
*Adult:* **IV** 75 mg/m$^2$ over 1 hr q3 wk; if neutrophil count is <500/mm$^3$ for >1 wk, reduce dose to 55 mg/m$^2$; if patient develops grade 3 peripheral neuropathy, stop product

*Unresectable, locally advanced or metastatic non–small-cell lung cancer previously treated with chemotherapy*
*Adult:* **IV** 75 mg/m$^2$ over 1 hr, then cisplatin 75 mg/m$^2$ **IV** given over 30-60 min q3 wk; reduce dose to 65 mg/m$^2$ in those with hematologic or nonhematologic toxicities

*Androgen-independent metastatic prostate cancer*
*Adult:* **IV** 75 mg/m$^2$ given over 1 hr q3 wk, with 5 mg predniSONE PO bid continuously; give dexamethasone 8 mg PO at 12 hr, 3 and 1 hr prior to docetaxel; if neutrophil count is <500 cells/mm$^3$ for more than 1 wk or other toxicities occur, reduce dose to 60 mg/m$^2$

*Adjuvant postsurgery treatment of operable node-positive breast cancer*
*Adult:* **IV** 75 mg/m$^2$ over 1 hr, given 1 hr after DOXOrubicin 50 mg/m$^2$, cyclophosphamide 500 mg/m$^2$ q3 wk × 6 cycles

*Squamous cell cancer of head/neck*
*Adult:* **IV** 75 mg/m$^2$ over 1 hr, then cisplatin 75 mg/m$^2$ over 1 hr on day 1, then 5-FU 750 mg/m$^2$/day CONT INF ×5 days, repeat cycle q3 wk

**Available forms:** Inj 20, 80 mg in single dose vials

### Adverse effects
**CV:** *Hypotension,* fluid retention, peripheral edema, flushing
**GI:** *Nausea, vomiting, diarrhea,* **hepatotoxicity**
**HEMA:** **Neutropenia, leukopenia, thrombocytopenia, anemia,** bleeding, infections, **myelosuppression**
**INTEG:** *Alopecia,* nail pain, rash, skin eruptions
**MS:** *Arthralgia, myalgia,* back pain
**NEURO:** *Peripheral neuropathy*
**RESP:** Dyspnea, **pulmonary edema**
**SYST:** *Hypersensitivity reactions,* **death**

**Contraindications:** Pregnancy **D,** hypersensitivity to this product or other products with polysorbate 80, neutropenia (neutrophils <1500/mm$^3$), severe hepatic disease, bilirubin exceeding upper normal limit, or severely elevated ALT, AST, alkaline phosphatase

**Precautions:** Children, CV disease, pulmonary disorders, bone marrow depression, herpes zoster, pleural effusion

#### Pharmacokinetics
| | |
|---|---|
| **Absorption** | Completely absorbed |
| **Distribution** | Unknown |
| **Metabolism** | Liver, extensively |
| **Excretion** | Fecal |
| **Half-life** | 11.1 hr |

#### Pharmacodynamics
| | |
|---|---|
| **Onset** | Rapid |
| **Peak** | Unknown |
| **Duration** | Unknown |

### Interactions
*Individual drugs*
CycloSPORINE, erythromycin, ketoconazole, troleadomycin: altered metabolism of docetaxel
*Drug classifications*
Anineoplastics, radiation: increased myelosuppression
Live virus vaccines: decreased immune response

### NURSING CONSIDERATIONS
#### Assessment
• Assess CNS changes: confusion, paresthesias, dysethenia, pain, weakness: if severe, product should be discontinued
• Check buccal cavity q8hr for dryness, sores or ulceration, white patches, oral pain, bleeding, dysphagia; obtain prescription for viscous lidocaine (Xylocaine) to use in mouth
• Assess symptoms indicating severe allergic reaction, anaphylaxis: rash, pruritus, urticaria, purpuric skin lesions, itching, flushing
• Monitor CBC, differential, platelet count weekly; withhold product if WBC is <1500/mm$^3$ or platelet count is <100,000/mm$^3$, notify prescriber of results
• Monitor renal function tests: BUN, creatinine, serum uric acid, urine CCr before and during therapy; check I&O ratio; report fall in urine output to <30 ml/hr
• Monitor temp q4hr (may indicate beginning of infection)
• Monitor liver function tests before and during therapy (bilirubin, AST, ALT, LDH) as needed or monthly; check for jaundice of skin and sclera, dark urine, clay-colored stools, itchy skin, abdominal pain, fever, diarrhea
• Assess for bleeding: hematuria, stool guaiac, bruising or petechiae, mucosa or orifices q8hr; check for inflammation of mucosa, breaks in skin
• Assess effects of alopecia on body image; discuss feelings about body changes

#### Nursing diagnoses
• Body image, disturbed (adverse reactions)
• Infection, risk for (adverse reactions)
• Injury, risk for (adverse reactions)
• Knowledge, deficient (teaching)

#### Implementation
• Give top or systemic analgesics for pain to lessen effects of stomatitis
• Give liquid diet: carbonated beverages; gelatin may be added if patient is not nauseated or vomiting
**IV route**
• Use gloves and cytotoxic handling precautions
• Allow vials to warm to room temperature, withdraw all diluent and inject in vial of docetaxel, rotate gently to mix, allow to stand to decrease foaming, then withdraw the required amount (10 mg/ml) and inject in 250 ml of 0.9% NaCl or D$_5$W, mix gently, give over 1 hr
*Y-site compatibilities:* Acyclovir, amikacin, aminophylline, ampicillin/sulbactam, butorphanol, calcium gluconate, cefepime, cefotetan, ceftazidime, ceftriaxone, cimetidine, diphenhydrAMINE, droperidol, famotidine, fluconazole, furosemide, ganciclovir, gentamicin, granisetron, haloperidol, heparin, hydrocortisone, hydromorphone, lorazepam, magnesium sulfate, mannitol, meperidine, mesna, metoclopramide, morphine, ondansetron, potassium chloride,

prochlorperazine, ranitidine, sodium bicarbonate, vancomycin, zidovudine

## Patient/family education
• Inform patient that nonhormonal contraceptive measures are recommended during therapy and >4 mo after; teratogenic effects are possible
• Teach patient to avoid use of products containing aspirin or ibuprofen, razors, commercial mouthwash, since bleeding may occur; to report symptoms of bleeding (hematuria, tarry stools)
• Instruct patient to report signs of anemia (fatigue, headache, irritability, faintness, shortness of breath) and CNS reactions (confusion, psychosis, nightmares, seizures, severe headaches)
• Inform patient that hair may be lost during treatment; a wig or hairpiece may make patient feel better; new hair may be different in color and texture
• Inform patient that receiving vaccinations during therapy may cause serious reactions
• Instruct patient to rinse mouth tid-qid with water, club soda; brush teeth bid-qid with soft brush or cotton-tipped applicators for stomatitis; use unwaxed dental floss

## Evaluation
**Positive therapeutic outcome**
• Prevention of rapid division of malignant cells

---

## docosanol topical
*See Appendix D*

---

## docusate calcium (OTC)
(dok'yoo-sate)
DC Softgels, Dioctocal, Pro-Cal-Sof, Sulfalax, Surfak
## docusate sodium (OTC)
Colace, Correctol Extra Gentle, Diocto, Docu, DOK, DOS, DSS, Dulcolax Stool Softener, Ex-Lax, Fleet Sof-Lax, Modane, Regulex ✦, Silace, Therevac SB
*Func. class.:* Laxative, emollient
*Chem. class.:* Anionic surfactant

**Pregnancy category** C

**Action:** Increases water, fat penetration in intestine; allows for easier passage of stool; increases electrolyte, water secretion in colon

**Therapeutic outcome:** Passage of softened stool, absence of constipation

**Uses:** To soften stools, prevent constipation, soften fecal impaction (rectal route)

## Dosage and routes
*Adult:* PO 50-300 mg/day (docusate sodium) or 240 mg (docusate calcium or docusate potassium) prn; ENEMA 4 ml (docusate sodium)
*Child >12 yr:* ENEMA 2 ml (docusate sodium)
*Child 6-12 yr:* PO 40-150 mg/day (docusate sodium) in divided doses
*Child 3-6 yr:* PO 20-60 mg/day (docusate sodium) in divided doses
*Child <3 yr:* PO 10-40 mg/day (docusate sodium) in divided doses

**Available forms:** Docusate calcium: caps 240 mg; docusate sodium: caps 50, 100, 250 mg; tabs 100 mg; syr 20 mg/5 ml, 50 mg/15 ml, 100 mg/30 ml, 150 mg/15 ml; oral sol 10, 50 mg/ml; enema 283 mg/3.9 g cap

## Adverse effects
*EENT:* Bitter taste, throat irritation
*GI:* Nausea, anorexia, cramps, diarrhea
*INTEG:* Rash

**Contraindications:** Hypersensitivity, obstruction, fecal impaction, nausea/vomiting

**Precautions:** Pregnancy C, breastfeeding

### Pharmacokinetics
| | |
|---|---|
| **Absorption** | Minimal (PO) |
| **Distribution** | Unknown |
| **Metabolism** | Not metabolized |
| **Excretion** | Bile |
| **Half-life** | Unknown |

### Pharmacodynamics
| | PO | RECT |
|---|---|---|
| **Onset** | 24-72 hr | 4-6 hr |
| **Peak** | Unknown | Unknown |
| **Duration** | Unknown | Unknown |

## Interactions
*Individual drugs*
Mineral oil: toxicity
*Drug/herb*
Flax, senna: increased laxative action

## NURSING CONSIDERATIONS
### Assessment
• Assess cramping, rectal bleeding, nausea, vomiting; if these symptoms occur, product should be discontinued; identify cause of constipation; identify whether fluids, bulk, or exercise is missing from lifestyle

---

## Nursing diagnoses
- Constipation (uses)
- Diarrhea (side effects)
- Knowledge, deficient (teaching)
- Noncompliance (teaching)

## Implementation
**PO route**
- Dilute oral sol in juice or other fluid to disguise taste
- Give tabs or caps with 8 oz of liquid; give on empty stomach for increased absorption, results

## Patient/family education
- Discuss with patient that adequate fluid consumption is as necessary as bulk, exercise for adequate bowel function
- Teach patient that normal bowel movements do not always occur daily
- Advise patient not to use in presence of abdominal pain, nausea, vomiting; tell patient to notify prescriber if unrelieved constipation or if symptoms of electrolyte imbalance occur: muscle cramps, pain, weakness, dizziness, excessive thirst
- Advise patient that product may take up to 3 days to soften stools
- Instruct patient to take oral preparation with a full glass of water and increase fluid intake unless on fluid restrictions
- Caution patients with heart disease to avoid using the Valsalva maneuver to expedite evacuation

## Evaluation
**Positive therapeutic outcome**
- Decreased constipation within 3 days

## dofetilide
(doff-ee-till'-lide)
Tikosyn
*Func. class.:* Antidysrhythmic (Class III)
**Pregnancy category** C

**Action:** Blocks cardiac ion channel carrying the rapid component of delayed potassium current, no effect on sodium channels

**Therapeutic outcome:** Absence of atrial fibrillation

**Uses:** Atrial fibrillation, flutter, maintenance of normal sinus rhythm

## Dosage and routes
*Adult:* PO 125-500 mcg bid depending on CCr; may be adjusted q2-3hr to get appropriate increase in QTc

*Renal dose:* PO Initial dose for CCr >60 mg/ml 500 mcg bid; CCr 40-60 mg/min 250 mcg bid; CCr 20-39 mg/min 125 mcg bid; CCr <20 mg/min do not use

**Available forms:** Caps 125, 250, 500 mcg

## Adverse effects
*CNS: Syncope, dizziness,* headache
*CV: Hypotension, postural hypotension, bradycardia,* angina, PVCs, substernal pressure, precipitation of angina, transient hypertension
*GI: Nausea, vomiting,* severe diarrhea, anorexia

**Contraindications:** Hypersensitivity, digoxin toxicity, aortic stenosis, pulmonary hypertension, children, QT syndromes, severe renal disease

**Precautions:** Pregnancy **C**, breastfeeding, renal disease

### Pharmacokinetics
| | |
|---|---|
| Absorption | >90% |
| Distribution | Steady state 2-3 days |
| Metabolism | Not metabolized |
| Excretion | Kidneys 80% |
| Half-life | 10 hr |

### Pharmacodynamics
Unknown

## Interactions
*Individual drugs*
Amiloride, cimetidine, ketoconazole, megestrol, metformin, prochlorperazine, triamterene, trimethoprim/sulfamethoxazole, verapamil: do not use together
Diuretics, potassium depletion: increased hypokalemia
*Drug/herb*
◆Aconite: toxicity, death
Aloe, broom, buckthorn (chronic use), cascara sagrada (chronic use), Chinese rhubarb, figwort, fumitory, goldenseal, kudzu, licorice: increased effect
Coltsfoot: decreased effect
Horehound: increased serotonin effect

## NURSING CONSIDERATIONS
### Assessment
- Monitor ECG continuously to determine product effectiveness; measure PR, QRS, QT intervals; check for PVCs, other dysrhythmias; monitor B/P continuously; this product is available only to facilities that have been

Adverse effects: *italic* = common, **bold** = life-threatening

educated in its administration; patient must be hospitalized
• Before administration, QTc must be determined using an average of 5-10 beats, if the QTc >440 msec or 500 msec in ventricular conduction abnormalities, do not use; do not use if heart rate <60 bpm
• Before dosing, identify CCr, using CCr to determine dosing

### Nursing diagnoses
• Cardiac output, decreased (uses)
• Gas exchange, impaired (adverse reactions)
• Knowledge, deficient (teaching)

### Implementation
• Give for 3 days with patient hospitalized
• Give dofetilide after withholding class I or III antidysrhythmic for 3 half-lives of dofetilide before starting dofetilide

### Patient/family education
• Notify prescriber if fast heartbeats with fainting or dizziness occur
• Notify all prescribers of all medications and supplements taken
• Teach patient that if a dose is missed, do not double, take next dose at usual time

### Evaluation
**Positive therapeutic outcome**
• Increased control in atrial fibrillation

---

## dolasetron (Rx)
(do-la′se-tron)
Anzemet
*Func. class.:* Antiemetic
*Chem. class.:* 5-HT receptor antagonist

**Pregnancy category B**

**Action:** Prevents nausea, vomiting by blocking serotonin peripherally, centrally, and in the small intestine

**Therapeutic outcome:** Control of nausea, vomiting

**Uses:** Prevention of nausea, vomiting associated with cancer chemotherapy and prevention of postoperative nausea, vomiting

**Unlabeled uses:** Radiotherapy-induced nausea/vomiting

### Dosage and routes
*Prevention of nausea/vomiting associated with cancer chemotherapy*
*Adult and child 2-16 yr:* **IV** 1.8 mg/kg as a single dose ½ hr before chemotherapy

*Adult:* PO 100 mg 1 hr before chemotherapy
*Child 2-16 yr:* PO 1.8 mg/kg 1 hr before chemotherapy, max 100 mg

*Prevention of postoperative nausea/vomiting*
*Adult:* **IV** 12.5 mg as a single dose 15 min before cessation of anesthesia; PO 100 mg 2 hr before surgery (prevention only)
*Child 2-16 yr:* **IV** 0.35 mg/kg as a single dose 15 min before cessation of anesthesia; PO 1.2 mg/kg within 2 hr before surgery (prevention only)

**Available forms:** Tabs 50, 100 mg; inj 20 mg/ml (12.5 mg/0.625 ml)

**Adverse effects**
*CNS: Headache,* dizziness, fatigue, drowsiness
*CV: Dysrhythmias,* ECG changes, hypo/hypertension, tachycardia, bradycardia
*GI: Diarrhea,* constipation, increased AST, ALT, abdominal pain, anorexia
*GU:* Urinary retention, oliguria
*MISC:* Rash, **bronchospasm**

**Contraindications:** Hypersensitivity

**Precautions:** Pregnancy **B**, breastfeeding, children, geriatric, hypokalemia, electrolyte imbalances, granisetron, ondansetron hypersensitivity

| Pharmacokinetics | |
|---|---|
| **Absorption** | Completely absorbed |
| **Distribution** | Unknown |
| **Metabolism** | Liver, extensively |
| **Excretion** | Kidneys |
| **Half-life** | Unknown |

| Pharmacodynamics |
|---|
| Unknown |

### Interactions
*Individual drugs*
Cimetidine: increased dolasetron levels
Rifampin: decreased dolasetron levels
*Drug classifications*
Antidysrhythmics: increased dysrhythmias
Loop diuretics, thiazide: increased QT prolongation

### NURSING CONSIDERATIONS
**Assessment**
• Assess for absence of nausea, vomiting during chemotherapy
• Assess for hypersensitivity reaction: rash, bronchospasm

---

- Assess for cardiac conditions, electrolyte imbalances or dysrhythmias

### Nursing diagnoses
- Knowledge, deficient (teaching)
- Noncompliance (teaching)

### Implementation
**IV route**
- Administer by inj 100 mg/30 sec or less or diluted in 50 ml of compatible sol; give over 15 sec
- Store at room temperature for 24 hr after dilution

### Patient/family education
- Instruct patient to report diarrhea, constipation, rash, or changes in respirations; may cause headache, use analgesic
- Teach patient reason for medication and expected results

### Evaluation
**Positive therapeutic outcome**
- Absence of nausea, vomiting during cancer chemotherapy

---

### donepezil (Rx)
(don-ep-ee′zill)
Aricept, Aricept ODT
*Func. class.:* Reversible cholinesterase inhibitor

**Pregnancy category** C

**Action:** Elevates acetylcholine concentrations (cerebral cortex) by slowing degradation of acetylcholine released in cholinergic neurons; does not alter underlying dementia

**Therapeutic outcome:** Decreased symptoms of Alzheimer's disease

**Uses:** Treatment of mild to severe dementia in Alzheimer's disease

**Unlabeled uses:** Vascular dementia

### Dosage and routes
*Adult:* PO 5 mg/day at bedtime; may increase to 10 mg/day after 4-6 wk

**Available forms:** Tabs 5, 10 mg; oral sol 1 mg/ml; orally disintegrating tabs 5, 10 mg (Aricept ODT)

### Adverse effects
*CNS:* Dizziness, insomnia, somnolence, headache, fatigue, abnormal dreams, syncope, **seizures**, drowsiness, agitation, depression
*CV:* Atrial fibrillation, hypo/hypertension, **sinus bradycardia, AV block**
*GI: Nausea, vomiting,* anorexia, *diarrhea,* abdominal pain, weight loss, **GI bleeding**

*GU:* Frequency, UTI, incontinence
*INTEG:* Rash, flushing, diaphoresis
*MS:* Cramps, arthritis, arthralgia
*RESP:* Rhinitis, URI, cough, pharyngitis

**Contraindications:** Hypersensitivity to this product or piperidine derivatives

**Precautions:** Pregnancy **C**, breastfeeding, children, sick sinus syndrome, history of ulcers, GI bleeding, hepatic disease, bladder obstruction, asthma, seizures, asthma, COPD

D

#### Pharmacokinetics
| | |
|---|---|
| **Absorption** | Well |
| **Distribution** | Unknown |
| **Metabolism** | Liver to metabolites |
| **Excretion** | Unknown |
| **Half-life** | 10 hr (single dose) |

#### Pharmacodynamics
Unknown

---

### Interactions
*Individual drugs*
Carbamazepine, dexamethasone, phenobarbital, phenytoin, rifampin: decreased donepezil effect
Succinylcholine: synergistic effects
*Drug classification*
Anticholinergics: decreased activity
Cholinergic agonists, cholinesterase inhibitors: synergistic effects
NSAIDs: increased gastric acid secretions

### NURSING CONSIDERATIONS
**Assessment**
- Monitor B/P, heart rate: hypo/hypertension
- Assess mental status: affect, mood, behavioral changes, depression, complete suicide assessment
- Assess GI status: nausea, vomiting, anorexia, diarrhea
- Assess GU status: urinary frequency, incontinence

### Nursing diagnoses
- Confusion, chronic (uses)
- Memory, impaired (uses)

### Implementation
- Give between meals; may be given with meals for GI symptoms
- Administer dosage adjusted to response no more than q4-6 wk
- Provide assistance with ambulation during beginning therapy; dizziness, ataxia may occur
- Oral solution: measure with calibrated oral syringe or other calibrated device

Adverse effects: *italic* = common, **bold** = life-threatening

• Orally disintegrating tabs: allow to dissolve on tongue before swallowing

## Patient/family education
• Advise patient to report side effects: twitching, nausea, vomiting, sweating, dizziness; indicates overdose
• Advise patient to use product exactly as prescribed
• Advise patient to notify prescriber of nausea, vomiting, diarrhea (dose increase or beginning treatment), or rash
• Advise patient not to increase or abruptly decrease dose, serious consequences may result
• Instruct patient that product is not a cure

## Evaluation
**Positive therapeutic outcome**
• Decrease in confusion; improved mood

---

### ! HIGH ALERT

## *DOPamine (Rx)
(doe'pa-meen)
DOPamine HCl, Intropin, Revimine ♣
*Func. class.:* Agonist, vasopressor, inotropic agent
*Chem. class.:* Catecholamine

**Pregnancy category** C

## Do not confuse:
DOPamine/DOBUTamine

**Action:** Causes increased cardiac output; acts on β₁- and α-receptors, causing vasoconstriction in blood vessels; when low doses are administered, causes renal and mesenteric vasodilatation; β₁ stimulation produces inotropic effects with increased cardiac output

**Therapeutic outcome:** Increased B/P, cardiac output

**Uses:** Shock; to increase perfusion; hypotension

**Unlabeled uses:** COPD, RDS in infants, severe CHF

## Dosage and routes
*Shock*
*Adult:* **IV** INF 2-5 mcg/kg/min, not to exceed 50 mcg/kg/min; titrate to patient's response
*Child:* **IV** 5-20 mcg/kg/min adjust depending on response

*COPD*
*Adult:* **IV** 4 mcg/kg/min

*CHF*
*Adult:* **IV** 3-10 mcg/kg/min

*RDS*
*Infant:* **IV** 5 mcg/kg/min

**Available forms:** Inj 40, 80, 160 mg/ml; conc for **IV** inf 0.8, 1.6, 3.2 mg/ml in 250, 500 ml D₅W

## Adverse effects
*CNS:* Headache
*CV: Palpitations,* **tachycardia,** *hypertension,* **ectopic beats,** *angina,* **wide QRS complex,** peripheral vasoconstriction, hypotension
*GI: Nausea, vomiting, diarrhea*
*INTEG:* Necrosis, tissue sloughing with extravasation, **gangrene**
*RESP:* Dyspnea

**Contraindications:** Hypersensitivity, ventricular fibrillation, tachydysrhythmias, pheochromocytoma, hypovolemia

**Precautions:** Pregnancy **C,** breastfeeding, geriatric, arterial embolism, peripheral vascular disease

### Pharmacokinetics
| | |
|---|---|
| **Absorption** | Complete |
| **Distribution** | Widely |
| **Metabolism** | Liver |
| **Excretion** | Kidney, plasma |
| **Half-life** | 2 min |

### Pharmacodynamics
| | |
|---|---|
| **Onset** | 2-5 min |
| **Peak** | Unknown |
| **Duration** | <10 min |

## Interactions
*Individual drugs*
Phenytoin: bradycardia, hypotension
*Drug classifications*
α-Adrenergic blockers, β-adrenergic blockers: decreased action of DOPamine
Anesthetics (general): increased dysrhythmias
Antidepressants (tricyclic): increased pressor response
Ergots: severe hypertension
MAOIs: increased hypertension (severe), do not use within 2 wk, increased pressor effect
Oxytocics: increased B/P
*Drug/lab test*
Increased: urinary catecholamine, serum glucose

## NURSING CONSIDERATIONS
### Assessment
• Monitor ECG for dysrhythmias, ischemia during treatment; some patients may not need continuous ECG monitoring; also monitor

PCWP, CVP, $CO_2$, urinary output; notify prescriber if <30 ml/hr

• Assess for heart failure: bibasilar crackles, $S_3$ gallop, dyspnea, neck vein distention in patients with cardiomyopathy or CHF

• Assess for oxygenation or perfusion deficit: decreased B/P, chest pain, dizziness, loss of consciousness

• Monitor B/P and pulse q5 min during inf; if B/P drops 30 mm Hg, stop inf and call prescriber

• Check for extravasation: change site q48hr

### Nursing diagnoses
• Cardiac output, decreased (uses)
• Fluid volume, excess (uses)
• Knowledge, deficient (teaching)
• Tissue perfusion, ineffective (uses)

### Implementation
**Continuous infusion route**
• Dilute 200-400 mg/250-500 ml of $D_5W$, 0.9% NaCl, $D_5$/LR, $D_5$/0.45% NaCl, $D_5$/0.9% NaCl, LR; do not use discolored sol; sol is stable for 24 hr; give 0.5-5 mcg/kg/min; may increase by 1-4 mcg/kg/min q15-30 min until desired patient response; use infusion pump

*Syringe compatibilities:* Doxapram, heparin, ranitidine

*Y-site compatibilities:* Aldesleukin, amifostine, amiodarone, inamrinone, atracurium, aztreonam, cefmetazole, cefpirome, ciprofloxacin, cladribine, diltiazem, DOBUTamine, enalaprilat, epINEPHrine, esmolol, famotidine, fentanyl, fluconazole, foscarnet, granisetron, haloperidol, heparin, hydrocortisone, hydromorphone, labetalol, lidocaine, lorazepam, meperidine, methylPREDNISolone, metronidazole, midazolam, milrinone, morphine, niCARDipine, nitroglycerin, norepinephrine, ondansetron, pancuronium, piperacillin/tazobactam, potassium chloride, propofol, ranitidine, sargramostim, sodium nitroprusside, streptokinase, tacrolimus, theophylline, thiotepa, tolazoline, vecuronium, verapamil, vit B/C, warfarin, zidovudine

*Additive compatibilities:* Aminophylline, atracurium, bretylium, calcium chloride, cephalothin, chloramphenicol, DOBUTamine, enalaprilat, flumazenil, heparin, hydrocortisone, kanamycin, lidocaine, meropenem, methylPREDNISolone, nitroglycerin, oxacillin, potassium chloride, ranitidine, verapamil

### Patient/family education
• Teach patient reason for medication, expected results, reason for all monitoring, and procedures
• Advise patient to report all side effects

### Evaluation
**Positive therapeutic outcome**
• Increased cardiac output

**Treatment of overdose:** Discontinue product, support circulation; give a short-acting α-blocker

## doripenem
Doribax
*See Appendix A, Selected New Drugs*

## dorzolamide ophthalmic
*See Appendix D*

## doxapram (Rx)
(dox'a-pram)
Dopram
*Func. class.:* Analeptic (respiratory/cerebral stimulant)
**Pregnancy category  B**

**Action:** Respiratory stimulation through activation of peripheral carotid chemoreceptor in low dosages; with higher dosages medullary respiratory centers are stimulated, with progressive general CNS stimulation

**Therapeutic outcome:** Ease of breathing, ABGs at normal limits

**Uses:** COPD, postanesthesia CNS and respiratory depression, prevention of acute hypercapnia, product-induced CNS depression

**Unlabeled uses:** Treatment of apnea in premature infants when methylxanthines have failed

### Dosage and routes
*Postanesthesia stimulation*
*Adult:* **IV** INJ 0.5-1 mg/kg, not to exceed 1.5 mg/kg total as a single inj; **IV** INF 250 mg in 250 ml sol, not to exceed 4 mg/kg; run at 1-3 mg/min

*Drug-induced CNS depression*
*Adult:* **IV** Priming dose of 2 mg/kg, repeated in 5 min; repeat q1-2hr until patient awakens; **IV** INF priming dose 2 mg/kg at 1-3 mg/min, not to exceed 3 g/day

*COPD (hypercapnia)*
*Adult:* **IV** INF 1-2 mg/min, not to exceed 3 mg/min for no longer than 2 hr

Adverse effects: *italic* = common, **bold** = life-threatening

*Apnea of premature infant (unlabeled)*

*Infant:* **IV** 1-1.5 mg/kg/hr loading dose followed by inf of 0.5-2.5 mg/kg/hr

## Available forms: Inj **IV** 20 mg/ml

## Adverse effects

*CNS:* **Seizures** (clonus/generalized), *headache*, restlessness, dizziness, confusion, paresthesias, flushing, sweating, bilateral Babinski's sign, rigidity, depression
*CV:* *Chest pain, hypertension, change in heart rate,* lowered T waves, tachycardia, dysrhythmias
*EENT:* Pupil dilation, sneezing
*GI:* Nausea, vomiting, diarrhea, desire to defecate
*GU:* Retention, incontinence, elevation of BUN, albuminuria
*INTEG:* Pruritus, irritation at inj site
*RESP:* **Laryngospasm, bronchospasm,** rebound hypoventilation, dyspnea, cough, tachypnea, hiccups

**Contraindications:** Hypersensitivity, seizure disorders, severe hypertension, severe bronchial asthma, severe dyspnea, severe cardiac disorders, flail chest, pneumothorax, pulmonary embolism, severe respiratory disease

**Precautions:** Pregnancy **B**, breastfeeding, children, bronchial asthma, pheochromocytoma, severe tachycardia, dysrhythmias, hypertension, hyperthyroidism

### Pharmacokinetics

| | |
|---|---|
| **Absorption** | Complete |
| **Distribution** | Unknown |
| **Metabolism** | Liver |
| **Excretion** | Kidneys, metabolites |
| **Half-life** | 2.5-4 hr |

### Pharmacodynamics

| | |
|---|---|
| **Onset** | 20-40 sec |
| **Peak** | 1-2 min |
| **Duration** | 5-10 min |

## Interactions
### Individual drugs

Cyclopropane, enflurane, halothane: increased dysrhythmias; delay use of doxapram for 10 min after inhalation anesthetics
### Drug classifications

MAOIs, sympathomimetics: synergistic pressor effect

## NURSING CONSIDERATIONS
### Assessment

• Monitor B/P, heart rate, deep tendon reflexes, level of consciousness, ABGs before administration q30 min; check for $Po_2$, $Pco_2$, $O_2$ saturation during treatment
• Monitor ECG; watch for hypertension, increased pulse, increased pulmonary artery pressures
• Monitor for hypertension: dysrhythmias, tachycardia, dyspnea, skeletal muscle hyperactivity; may indicate overdosage; discontinue if these occur
• Assess for respiratory stimulation: increased respiratory rate, depth, abnormal rhythm; check for patent airway; elevate head of bed to 45 degrees or higher, position patient on side
• Check for extravasation: redness, inflammation, pain; may cause phlebitis; change **IV** site q48hr

### Nursing diagnoses

• Breathing pattern, ineffective (uses)
• Gas exchange, impaired (uses)
• Knowledge, deficient (teaching)

### Implementation

• May give **IV** diluted with equal parts of sterile water for inj; may be diluted 250 mg/250 ml (1 mg/ml) of $D_5W$, $D_{10}W$ (dilute 400 mg/180 ml of compatible **IV** sol [2 mg/ml] and run as inf over 2 hr)
• Give **IV** undiluted over 5 min; **IV** inf at 1-3 mg/min; adjust for desired respiratory response, using infusion pump **IV**; if an inf is used after initial dose, start at 1-3 mg/min; adjust for desired respiratory response, using infusion pump **IV**; if an inf is used after initial dose, start at 1-3 mg/min depending on patient response; discontinue after 2 hr; wait 1-2 hr and repeat
• Give only after adequate airway is established; ensure $O_2$, **IV** barbiturates, resuscitative equipment available
• Discontinue inf if side effects occur; narrow margin of safety
**Syringe compatibilities:** Amikacin, bumetadine, chlorproMAZINE, cimetidine, cisplatin, cyclophosphamide, DOPamine, doxycycline, epINEPHrine, hydrOXYzine, imipramine, isoniazid, lincomycin, methotrexate, netilmicin, phytonadione, pyridoxine, terbutaline, thiamine, tobramycin, vinCRIStine
**Syringe incompatibilities:** Aminophylline, ascorbic acid, cefoperazone, cefotaxime, cefotetan, cefuroxime, dexamethasone, diazepam, digoxin, DOBUTamine, folic acid, furosemide, hydrocortisone, ketamine, methylPREDNISolone, minocycline, thiopental, ticarcillin

### Patient/family education
- Teach all aspects of product, purpose, expected reactions
- Caution patient if difficulty breathing or shortness of breath occurs to notify nurse or prescriber

### Evaluation
**Positive therapeutic outcome**
- Increased breathing capacity
- ABGs WNL for patient

---

## doxazosin (Rx)
(dox-ay′zoe-sin)
Cardura
*Func. class.:* Peripheral α-adrenergic blocker, antihypertensive
*Chem. class.:* Quinazoline

**Pregnancy category C**

### Do not confuse:
Cardura/Coumadin/Cardene/Ridaura

**Action:** Peripheral blood vessels are dilated, peripheral resistance lowered; reduction in B/P results from peripheral α-adrenergic receptors being blocked

**Therapeutic outcome:** Decreased B/P, decreased symptoms of benign prostatic hypertrophy (BPH)

**Uses:** Hypertension alone or as an adjunct, urinary outflow obstruction, symptoms of benign prostatic hyperplasia

**Unlabeled uses:** BPH with finesteride

### Dosage and routes
*BPH*
*Adult:* PO 1 mg/day, increase in stepwise manner to 2, 4, 8 mg/day as needed at 1-2 wk intervals, max 8 mg

*Hypertension*
*Adult:* PO 1 mg/day, increasing up to 16 mg daily if required; usual range 4-16 mg/day
*Geriatric:* PO 0.5 mg nightly, gradually increase

**Available forms:** Tabs 1, 2, 4, 8 mg; ext rel tabs 4, 8 mg

### Adverse effects
*CNS: Dizziness,* headache, drowsiness, anxiety, depression, vertigo, weakness, fatigue, asthenia
*CV:* Palpitations, *orthostatic hypotension,* **tachycardia,** edema, **dysrhythmias,** chest pain
*EENT:* Epistaxis, tinnitus, dry mouth, red sclera, pharyngitis, rhinitis

*GI:* Nausea, vomiting, diarrhea, constipation, abdominal pain
*GU:* Incontinence, polyuria, priapism

**Contraindications:** Hypersensitivity to quinazolines

**Precautions:** Pregnancy **C,** breastfeeding, children, hepatic disease

### Pharmacokinetics
| | |
|---|---|
| **Absorption** | Well absorbed |
| **Distribution** | Not known; 98% plasma protein bound |
| **Metabolism** | Liver, extensively (<63%) |
| **Excretion** | Kidneys |
| **Half-life** | 22 hr |

### Pharmacodynamics
| | |
|---|---|
| **Onset** | 2 hr |
| **Peak** | 2-6 hr |
| **Duration** | 6-12 hr |

### Interactions
*Individual drugs*
Alcohol, sildenafil, vardenafil: increased hypotensive effects
Clonidine: decreased antihypertensive effect
*Drug classifications*
Other antihypertensives, nitrates: increased hypotensive effects
*Drug/herb*
Angelica, hawthorn: increased doxazosin effect
Butcher's broom, capsicum peppers: decreased doxazosin effect
Yohimbe: increased toxicity

### NURSING CONSIDERATIONS
**Assessment**
- Monitor B/P (lying, standing) and pulse, syncope; check for edema in feet, legs daily; I&O; monitor for weight daily; notify prescriber of changes
- Assess skin turgor, dryness of mucous membranes for hydration status
- Assess for orthostatic hypotension; tell patient to rise slowly from sitting or lying position; assess pulse, jugular venous distention q4hr, crackles, dyspnea, orthopnea with B/P

**Nursing diagnoses**
- Cardiac output, decreased (uses)
- Injury, risk for (side effects)
- Knowledge, deficient (teaching)
- Noncompliance (teaching)

**Implementation**
- Store in tight container at 86° F (30° C) or less

Adverse effects: *italic* = common, **bold** = life-threatening

- May be used in combination with other antihypertensives
- May be given with food to prevent GI symptoms

### Patient/family education

- Teach patient not to discontinue product abruptly; emphasize the importance of complying with dosage schedule, even if feeling better; if dose is missed take as soon as remembered; take at same time each day
- Instruct patient to take 1st dose at bedtime to decrease orthostatic B/P changes
- Teach patient not to use OTC products (cough, cold, allergy) unless directed by prescriber; also to avoid large amounts of caffeine
- Emphasize the need to rise slowly to sitting or standing position to minimize orthostatic hypotension
- Teach patient to notify prescriber of mouth sores, sore throat, fever, swelling of hands or feet, irregular heartbeat, chest pain
- Caution patient to report excessive perspiration, dehydration, vomiting, diarrhea; may lead to fall in B/P
- Caution patient that product may cause dizziness, fainting, light-headedness; may occur during 1st few days of therapy; to avoid hazardous activities
- Teach patient how to take B/P, and normal readings for age-group; to take B/P q7 days

### Evaluation

**Positive therapeutic outcome**

- Decreased B/P in hypertension
- Decreased symptoms of BPH

**Treatment of overdose:** Administer volume expanders or vasopressors; discontinue product; place in supine position

---

### doxepin (Rx)

(dox'e-pin)

doxepin HCl, Novo-Doxepin ♣, Prudoxin Cream, Sinequan, Triadapin ♣, Zonolon Topical Cream

*Func. class.:* Antidepressant, tricyclic; antianxiety

*Chem. class.:* Dibenzoxepin, tertiary amine

**Pregnancy category**
B (Topical)
C (PO)

---

### Do not confuse:

Sinequan/Serentil/Sarafem

**Action:** Blocks reuptake of norepinephrine, serotonin into nerve endings, increasing action

of norepinephrine, serotonin in nerve cells; has anticholinergic effects

**Therapeutic outcome:** Decreased symptoms of depression after 2-3 wk

**Uses:** Major depression, anxiety, insomnia, migraine prophylaxis; topical: lichen simplex, atopic dermatitis, eczema

**Unlabeled uses:** Topical: pruritus

### Dosage and routes
*Depression/anxiety*
*Adult:* PO 25-75 mg/day, may increase to 300 mg/day for severely ill, give in divided doses if >150 mg/day
*Geriatric:* PO 10-25 mg at bedtime, increase qwk by 10-25 mg to desired dose, max 150 mg/day

*Pruritus*
*Adult:* PO 10 mg at bedtime, may increase to 25 mg at bedtime; TOP apply a thin film qid ≥3 hr apart

**Available forms:** Caps 10, 25, 50, 75, 100, 150 mg; oral conc 10 mg/ml; cream 5%

### Adverse effects

*CNS: Dizziness, drowsiness,* confusion, headache, anxiety, tremors, stimulation, weakness, insomnia, nightmares, EPS (geriatric), increased psychiatric symptoms, paresthesia, suicidal ideation
*CV: Orthostatic hypotension, ECG changes,* **tachycardia,** *hypertension,* palpitations, **dysrhythmias**
*EENT: Blurred vision,* tinnitus, mydriasis, ophthalmoplegia, glossitis
*GI: Diarrhea, dry mouth,* nausea, vomiting, **paralytic ileus,** increased appetite, cramps, epigastric distress, jaundice, **hepatitis,** stomatitis, constipation
*GU: Retention,* **acute renal failure**
*HEMA:* **Agranulocytosis, thrombocytopenia, eosinophilia, leukopenia,** pancytopenia, purpuric disorder
*INTEG:* Rash, urticaria, sweating, pruritus, photosensitivity

**Contraindications:** Hypersensitivity to tricyclics, urinary retention, angle-closure glaucoma, prostatic hypertrophy

**Precautions:** Pregnancy **C** (PO), **B** (topical), breastfeeding, geriatric, suicidal patients, seizures

## Pharmacokinetics

| | |
|---|---|
| **Absorption** | Well absorbed |
| **Distribution** | Widely distributed; crosses placenta |
| **Metabolism** | Liver, extensively |
| **Excretion** | Kidneys, breast milk |
| **Half-life** | 8-24 hr |

## Pharmacodynamics

Unknown

## Interactions
### Individual drugs
Alcohol: increased CNS depression

Cimetidine, fluoxetine, sertraline: increased doxepin effect

Clonidine: epINEPHrine, norepinephrine: increased hypertensive action
### Drug classifications
Barbiturates, benzodiazepines, CNS depressants, sedative/hypnotics: increased CNS depression

MAOIs: hypertensive crisis, seizures, hyperpyretic crisis
### Drug/herb
Belladonna, corkwood, henbane, jimsonweed: increased anticholinergic effect

Hops, kava, lavender, scopolia: increased action of doxepin

SAM-e, St. John's wort: increased serotonin syndrome

Yohimbe: increased hypertension
### Drug/lab test
Increased: serum bilirubin, blood glucose, alkaline phosphatase

## NURSING CONSIDERATIONS
### Assessment
• Monitor B/P (with patient lying, standing), pulse q4hr; if systolic B/P drops 20 mm Hg, hold product, notify prescriber; take VS q4hr in patients with CV disease

• Monitor blood studies: CBC, leukocytes, differential, cardiac enzymes if patient is receiving long-term therapy

• Monitor liver function tests: AST, ALT, bilirubin

• Check weight weekly; appetite may increase with product

• Assess ECG for flattening of T wave, bundle branch block, AV block, dysrhythmias in cardiac patients; product should be discontinued gradually several days before surgery

• Assess for EPS primarily in geriatric: rigidity, dystonia, akathisia

• Assess mental status: mood, sensorium, affect, suicidal tendencies; increase in psychiatric symptoms: depression, panic

• Monitor urinary retention, constipation; constipation is more likely to occur in children or geriatric

• Assess for withdrawal symptoms: headache, nausea, vomiting, muscle pain, weakness; do not usually occur unless product was discontinued abruptly

• Identify alcohol consumption; if alcohol is consumed, hold dose until AM

### Nursing diagnoses
• Coping, ineffective (uses)
• Injury, risk for (side effects)
• Knowledge, deficient (teaching)

### Implementation
• Oral conc should be diluted with 120 ml of water, milk, or orange, grapefruit, tomato, prune, pineapple juice; do not mix with grape juice

• Give with food or milk for GI symptoms; do not give with carbonated beverages

• Give dosage at bedtime if oversedation occurs during day; may take entire dose at bedtime; geriatric may not tolerate once/day dosing

• Store at room temperature; do not freeze

• Provide safety measures, primarily for geriatric

### Patient/family education
• Tell patient that therapeutic effects of decreased depression may take 2-3 wk, antianxiety effects sooner; to use caution in driving and other activities requiring alertness because of drowsiness, dizziness, blurred vision

• Advise patient to avoid rising quickly from sitting to standing, especially geriatric

• Teach patient to avoid alcohol ingestion, other CNS depressants, may potentiate effects; not to discontinue medication quickly after long-term use: may cause nausea, headache, malaise

• Teach patient to wear sunscreen or large hat, since photosensitivity occurs

• Teach patient that clinical worsening and suicidal ideation may occur

• Teach patient to increase fluids, bulk in diet if constipation occurs, especially geriatric; to take gum, hard sugarless candy, or frequent sips of water for dry mouth

• Teach patient to report urinary retention immediately

### Evaluation
**Positive therapeutic outcome**
• Decrease in depression
• Absence of suicidal thoughts

Adverse effects: *italic* = common, **bold** = life-threatening

**Treatment of overdose:** ECG monitoring, induce emesis, lavage, activated charcoal, administer anticonvulsant

## doxercalciferol (Rx)
(dox-er-kal'-cif-er-ol)
Hectorol
*Func. class.:* Parathyroid agent (calcium regulator)
*Chem. class.:* Vitamin D hormone

**Pregnancy category C**

**Action:** Synthetic vit D analog, reduces parathyroid hormone

**Therapeutic outcome:** Calcium at normal level

**Uses:** To lower high parathyroid hormone levels in patients undergoing chronic kidney dialysis and those in stages 3/4 of chronic renal disease prior to dialysis

### Dosage and routes
*Adult:* PO iPTH level >400 pg/ml 10 mcg 3×/wk at dialysis; dose titration iPTH level decreased by <50% and >300 pg/ml increase by 2.5 mcg at 8 wk intervals as necessary; iPTH level 150-300 pg/ml maintain; iPTH levels <100 pg/ml suspend for 1 wk, then resume at a dose that is at least 2.5 mcg lower
*Adult:* IV BOL initial iPTH level >400 pg/ml 4 mcg 3×/wk at the end of dialysis, or approximately every other day; dose titration iPTH level decreased by <50% and >300 pg/ml increase by 1-2 mcg at 8 wk intervals; iPTH level 150-300 pg/ml maintain; iPTH level <100 pg/ml suspend for 1 wk, then resume at a dose that is at least 1 mcg lower

**Available forms:** Caps 2.5 mcg; inj 2 mcg/ml

### Adverse effects
*CNS:* Drowsiness, headache, lethargy
*GI:* Nausea, diarrhea, vomiting, anorexia, dry mouth, constipation, cramps, metallic taste
*GU:* Polyuria, hypercalciuria, hyperphosphatemia, hematuria
*MS:* Myalgia, arthralgia, decreased bone development
*RESP:* Shortness of breath

**Contraindications:** Hypersensitivity, hyperphosphatemia, hypercalcemia, vit D toxicity

**Precautions:** Pregnancy **C**, breastfeeding, renal calculi, CV disease

### Pharmacokinetics
| | |
|---|---|
| **Absorption** | Unknown |
| **Distribution** | Unknown |
| **Metabolism** | Liver |
| **Excretion** | Unknown |
| **Half-life** | 96 hr, Terminal |

### Pharmacodynamics
Unknown

### Interactions
*Individual drugs*
Cholestyramine, magnesium antacids, mineral oil: decreased doxercalciferol levels, do not use together

### NURSING CONSIDERATIONS
**Assessment**
• Assess GI symptoms, polyuria, flushing, head swelling, tingling, headache; may indicate hypercalcemia
• Identify nutritional status; check diet for sources of vit D (milk, some seafood), calcium (dairy products, dark green vegetables), phosphates
• Monitor BUN, creatinine, uric acid, chloride electrolytes, urine pH, urinary calcium, magnesium, phosphate, urinalysis (calcium should be kept at 9-10 mg/dl; vit D 50-135 international units/dl), alkaline phosphatase baseline and q3-6 mo
⊕ Assess for increased product level, since toxic reactions occur rapidly; have calcium chloride on hand if calcium level drops too low; check for tetany

**Nursing diagnoses**
• Injury, risk for (adverse reactions)
• Knowledge, deficient (teaching)
• Pain, chronic (uses)

**Implementation**
• Do not break, crush, or chew caps
• Give with meals for GI symptoms

**Patient/family education**
• Teach patient the symptoms of hypercalcemia and about foods rich in calcium
• Advise patient to avoid products with sodium: cured meats, dairy products, cold cuts, olives, beets, pickles, soups, meat tenderizers in chronic renal failure
• Advise patient to avoid products with potassium: oranges, bananas, dried fruit, peas, dark green leafy vegetables, milk, melons, beans in chronic renal failure
• Advise patient to avoid OTC products containing calcium, potassium, sodium, or antacids in chronic renal failure

- Instruct patient to avoid all preparations containing vit D
- Instruct patient to monitor weight weekly

## Evaluation
**Positive therapeutic outcome**
- Calcium levels 9-10 mg/dl

### ⚠ HIGH ALERT

**\*DOXOrubicin** (Rx)
(dox-oh-roo'bi-sin)
Adriamycin PFS, Adriamycin RDF, Rubex
**\*DOXOrubicin liposome** (Rx)
Doxil
*Func. class.:* Antineoplastic, antibiotic
*Chem. class.:* Anthracycline glycoside

**Pregnancy category** D

**Do not confuse:**
DOXOrubicin/DAUNOrubicin/idarubicin/idamycin, Adriamycin/Aredia/Idamycin

**Action:** Inhibits DNA synthesis primarily; derived from *Streptomyces peucetius;* replication is decreased by binding to DNA, which causes strand splitting; active throughout entire cell cycle; a vesicant

**Therapeutic outcome:** Prevention of rapidly growing malignant cells

**Uses:** Wilms' tumor; bladder, breast, liver, lung, ovarian, prostatic, stomach, testicular, thyroid cancer; Hodgkin's disease; acute lymphoblastic leukemia; myeloblastic leukemia; neuroblastomas; lymphomas; sarcomas; *Doxil:* AIDS-related Kaposi's sarcoma, metastatic ovarian carcinoma

## Dosage and routes
*DOXOrubicin*
**Adult:** IV 60-75 mg/m² q3 wk, or 30 mg/m² on days 1-3 of 4-wk cycle, not to exceed 550 mg/m² cumulative dose
**Child:** IV 30 mg/m²/day × 3 days, may repeat q4 wk

*Hepatic dose*
**Adult:** IV bilirubin 1.2-3 mg/dl give 50% of dose, bilirubin 3.1-5 mg/dl give 25% of dose

*DOXOrubicin liposome*
*Kaposi's sarcoma*
**Adult:** IV 20 mg/m² q3 wk

*Ovarian cancer (DOXOrubicin liposomal)*
**Adult:** IV 50 mg/m² (doxorubicin equivalent) given 1 mg/min if no adverse reactions, may increase to finish inf in 1 hr

**Available forms:** Inj 10, 20, 50, 100, 150 mg; liposomal dispersion for inj (Doxil) 20 mg/ml, 50 mg /30 ml

**Adverse effects**
*CV:* Increased B/P, **sinus tachycardia, PVCs,** chest pain, **bradycardia, extrasystole**
*GI:* Nausea, vomiting, anorexia, mucositis, **hepatotoxicity**
*GU:* Impotence, sterility, amenorrhea, gynecomastia, hyperuricemia
*HEMA:* **Thrombocytopenia, leukopenia, anemia**
*INTEG:* Rash, necrosis at inj site, dermatitis, reversible alopecia, cellulitis, thrombophlebitis at inj site

**Contraindications:** Pregnancy **D** (1st trimester), breastfeeding, hypersensitivity, systemic infections, cardiac disorders

**Precautions:** Renal/hepatic/cardiac disease, gout, bone marrow suppression (severe)

### Pharmacokinetics
| | |
|---|---|
| **Absorption** | Complete bioavailability |
| **Distribution** | Widely distributed; crosses placenta |
| **Metabolism** | Liver, extensively |
| **Excretion** | Bile (40%-50%) |
| **Half-life** | 12 min; 3½ hr; 29⅔ hr |

### Pharmacodynamics
Unknown

### Interactions
*Individual drugs*
Cyclophosphamide: increased cardiotoxicity, increased hemorrhagic cystitis risk
Mercaptopurine, radiation: increased toxicity, hypersensitivity
Radiation: increased toxicity
*Drug classifications*
Antineoplastics: increased toxicity, bone marrow suppression
Live virus vaccines: decreased antibody response
*Drug/lab test*
Increased: uric acid

### NURSING CONSIDERATIONS
**Assessment**
- Monitor ECG; watch for ST-T wave changes, low QRS and T; possible dysrhythmias (sinus tachycardia, heart block, PVCs); signs of irreversible cardiomyopathy
- Assess buccal cavity q8hr for dryness, sores or ulceration, white patches, pain, bleeding, dysphagia; obtain prescription for viscous lidocaine (Xylocaine)

Adverse effects: *italic* = common, **bold** = life-threatening

- Assess symptoms indicating severe allergic reaction: rash, pruritus, urticaria, purpuric skin lesions, itching, flushing; product should be discontinued
- Assess tachypnea, ECG changes, dyspnea, edema, fatigue
- Monitor CBC, differential, platelet count weekly; withhold product if WBC is <4000/mm³ or platelet count is <100,000/mm³; notify prescriber of results if WBC <20,000/mm³, platelets <150,000/mm³
- Assess for increased uric acid levels, swelling, joint pain, primarily extremities; patient should be well hydrated to prevent urate deposits
- Monitor renal function studies: BUN, creatinine, serum uric acid, urine CCr before and during therapy; I&O ratio; report fall in urine output to <30 ml/hr
- Monitor temp q4hr (may indicate beginning of infection)
- Monitor liver function tests before and during therapy (bilirubin, AST, ALT, LDH) as needed or monthly; note jaundice of skin or sclera, dark urine, clay-colored stools, itchy skin, abdominal pain, fever, diarrhea
- Assess for bleeding: hematuria, stool guaiac, bruising or petechiae, mucosa or orifices q8hr; inflammation of mucosa, breaks in skin
- Identify effects of alopecia on body image; discuss feelings about body changes

### Nursing diagnoses

- Body image, disturbed (adverse reactions)
- Infection, risk for (adverse reactions)
- Injury, risk for (adverse reactions)
- Knowledge, deficient (teaching)

### Implementation

- Avoid contact with skin; very irritating; wash completely to remove; give fluids **IV** or PO before chemotherapy to hydrate patient
- Give antiemetic 30-60 min before giving product to prevent vomiting and prn; give antibiotics for prophylaxis of infection
- Provide liquid diet: carbonated beverages; gelatin may be added if patient is not nauseated or vomiting
- Product should be prepared by experienced personnel using proper precautions
- Do not interchange DOXOrubicin with DOXOrubicin liposome
- Give **IV** after diluting 10 mg/5 ml of NaCl for inj; another 5 ml of diluent/10 mg is recommended; shake; give over 3-5 min; give through Y-tube or 3-way stopcock through free-flowing D₅ inf or 0.9% NaCl

- **IV** liposome inj (Doxil): dilute dose up to 90 mg/250 ml of D₅W, give over ½ hr; do not admix with other solution medications
- Use hydrocortisone, dexamethasone, or sodium bicarbonate (1 mEq/1 ml) for extravasation: apply ice compress
- Dose modifications for HFS: Toxicity Grade 1, redose unless patient has experienced previous grade 3 or 4; Grade 2, delay dosing up to 2 wk, or until resolved to grades 0 or 1; Grade 3 delay dosing up to 2 wk or until resolved to grades 0 or 1; resume dose at 25% decrease, return to original dosing after interval; Grade 4 delay dosing up to 2 wk or until grades 0 or 1; resume dose at 25% decrease, then return to original dose; if after 2 wk there is no resolution, discontinue

*Syringe compatibilities:* Bleomycin, cisplatin, cyclophosphamide, droperidol, fluorouracil, leucovorin, methotrexate, metoclopramide, mitomycin, vinCRIStine

*Syringe incompatibilities:* Furosemide, heparin

*Y-site compatibilities:* Amifostine, aztreonam, bleomycin, chlorproMAZINE, cimetidine, cisplatin, cladribine, cyclophosphamide, dexamethasone, diphenhydrAMINE, droperidol, famotidine, filgrastim, fludarabine, fluorouracil, granisetron, hydromorphone, leucovorin calcium, lorazepam, melphalan, methotrexate, methylPREDNISolone, metoclopramide, mitomycin, morphine, ondansetron, paclitaxel, prochlorperazine, promethazine, propofol, ranitidine, sargramostim, sodium bicarbonate, teniposide, thiotepa, vinBLAStine, vinCRIStine, vinorelbine

*Y-site incompatibilities:* Furosemide, heparin

*Additive compatibilities:* Ondansetron

*Additive incompatibilities:* Aminophylline, cephalothin, dexamethasone, diazepam, fluorouracil, hydrocortisone

### Patient/family education

- Help patient to rinse mouth tid-qid with water or club soda, brush teeth bid-qid with soft brush or cotton-tipped applicators for stomatitis, use unwaxed dental floss
- Advise patient to add 2-3 L of fluids unless contraindicated prior to and for 24-48 hr after, to decrease possible hemorrhagic cystitis
- Tell patient that urine and other body fluids may be red-orange for 48 hr; contraceptive measures are recommended during and 4 mo after therapy; product is teratogenic to fetus
- Advise patient to avoid use of products containing aspirin or ibuprofen, razors, commercial mouthwash, since bleeding may

occur; to report symptoms of bleeding (hematuria, tarry stools)

• Instruct patient to report signs of anemia (fatigue, headache, irritability, faintness, shortness of breath)

• Inform patient that hair may be lost during treatment; a wig or hairpiece may make patient feel better; new hair may be different in color, texture

• Caution patient not to have any vaccinations without the advice of the prescriber; serious reactions can occur

### Evaluation
**Positive therapeutic outcome**
• Prevention of rapid division of malignant cells

---

### doxycycline (Rx)
(dox-i-sye′kleen)
Adoxa, Apo-Doxy ✷, Doryx, Doxy, Doxycaps, Doxycin ✷, doxycycline, Monodox, Novodoxyclin ✷, Periostat, Vibramycin, Vibra-Tabs
*Func. class.:* Antiinfective
*Chem. class.:* Tetracycline

**Pregnancy category D**

**Do not confuse:**
doxycycline/doxepin

**Action:** Inhibits protein synthesis, phosphorylation in microorganisms by binding to 30S ribosomal subunits, reversibly binding to 50S ribosomal subunits; bacteriostatic

**Therapeutic outcome:** Bactericidal action against the following: gram-positive pathogens *Bacillus anthracis, Clostridium perfringens, Clostridium tetani, Listeria monocytogenes, Nocardia, Propionibacterium acnes, Actinomyces israelii;* gram-negative pathogens *Haemophilus influenzae, Legionella pneumophila, Yersinia enterocolitica, Yersinia pestis, Neisseria gonorrhoeae, Neisseria meningitidis, Mycoplasma, Chlamydia*

**Uses:** Syphilis, gonorrhea, *Chlamydia, Rickettsia,* lymphogranuloma venereum, uncommon gram-negative or -positive organisms, malaria prophylaxis, acne, anthrax, chronic periodontitis, Lyme disease

**Unlabeled uses:** Traveler's diarrhea, prevention of chronic bronchitis

### Dosage and routes
*Most infections*
*Adult:* PO/**IV** 100 mg q12hr on day 1, then 100 mg/day; **IV** 200 mg in 1-2 inf on day 1, then 100-200 mg/day
*Child >8 yr (>45 kg):* PO/**IV** 2.2-4.4 mg/kg/day in divided doses q12hr

*Gonorrhea (uncomplicated) (patients allergic to penicillin)*
*Adult:* PO 100 mg q12hr × 7 days, or 300 mg followed 1 hr later by another 300 mg

*Malaria prophylaxis*
*Adult:* 100 mg/day 1-2 days prior to travel, daily during travel, and 4 wk after return

*Chlamydia trachomatis*
*Adult:* PO 100 mg bid × 7days

*Syphilis*
*Adult:* PO 100 mg/bid × 14 days

*Anthrax*
*Adult and child >45 kg:* **IV** 100 mg q12hr, change to PO when able × 60 days
*Child ≤45 kg:* PO 2.2 mg/kg bid × 60 days; **IV** 100 mg q12hr, change to PO when able × 60 days

*Lyme disease*
*Adult:* PO 100 mg bid

*Periodontitis*
*Adult:* 20 mg bid after sealing and root planing for ≤9 mo; give close to meal AM or PM

**Available forms:** Tabs 100 mg; caps 50, 100 mg; syr 50 mg/5 ml; powder for inj 100, 200 mg; powder for oral susp 25 mg/5 ml; mouth products: tabs 20 mg; inj 42.5 mg

### Adverse effects
*CNS:* Fever
*CV:* Pericarditis
*EENT:* Dysphagia, glossitis, decreased calcification of deciduous teeth, oral candidiasis, tooth discoloration
*GI: Nausea, abdominal pain, vomiting, diarrhea,* anorexia, enterocolitis, **hepatotoxicity,** flatulence, abdominal cramps, gastric burning, stomatitis
*GU: Increased BUN*
*HEMA:* **Eosinophilia, neutropenia, thrombocytopenia, hemolytic anemia**
*INTEG:* Rash, urticaria, photosensitivity, increased pigmentation, **exfoliative dermatitis,** pruritus
*SYST:* **Stevens-Johnson syndrome, angioedema**

**Contraindications:** Pregnancy **D**, children <8 yr, esophageal ulceration, hypersensitivity to tetracyclines

Adverse effects: *italic* = common, **bold** = life-threatening

**Precautions:** Hepatic disease, breastfeeding

## Pharmacokinetics

| | |
|---|---|
| **Absorption** | Well absorbed |
| **Distribution** | Widely distributed, crosses placenta |
| **Metabolism** | Some hepatic recycling |
| **Excretion** | Bile, feces; kidneys unchanged (20%-40%), enters breast milk |
| **Half-life** | 14-17 hr; increased in severe renal disease |

## Pharmacodynamics

| | PO | IV |
|---|---|---|
| **Onset** | 1½-4 hr | Immediate |
| **Peak** | 1½-4 hr | Infusion's end |

## Interactions
### Individual drugs
Bismuth, carbamazepine, cimetidine, cholestyramine, colestipol, kaolin/pectin, NaHCO₃, phenytoin, rifampin, sucralfate: decreased effect of doxycycline
Digoxin: decreased effect of digoxin
Iron: forms chelates, decreased absorption
Penicillins: decreased effects of penicillins
Warfarin: increased effect of warfarin
### Drug classifications
Alkali products, antacids, barbiturates: decreased effect of doxycycline
Anticoagulants (oral): increased effect of anticoagulants
Contraceptives (oral): decreased effect of oral contraceptive
### Drug/herb
Acidophilus: do not use with antiinfectives; separate by several hours
Bromelain: increased action
### Drug/food
Decreased: absorption with dairy products
### Drug/lab test
Increased: BUN, alkaline phosphatase, bilirubin, amylase, ALT, AST
False increase: urinary catecholamines, ALT, AST

## NURSING CONSIDERATIONS
### Assessment
• Assess patient for previous sensitivity reaction
• Assess patient for signs and symptoms of infection including characteristics of wounds, sputum, urine, stool, WBC >10,000/mm³, fever; obtain baseline information before and during treatment
• Obtain C&S before beginning product therapy to identify if correct treatment has been initiated
• Assess for allergic reactions: rash, urticaria, pruritus, chills, fever, joint pain; angioedema may occur a few days after therapy begins
• Assess bowel pattern daily; if severe diarrhea occurs, product should be discontinued
• Monitor for bleeding: ecchymosis, bleeding gums, hematuria, stool guaiac daily if on long-term therapy; blood dyscrasias may occur
• Assess for overgrowth of infection: perineal itching, fever, malaise, redness, pain, swelling, drainage, rash, diarrhea, change in cough, sputum

### Nursing diagnoses
• Diarrhea (side effects)
• Infection, risk for (uses)
• Injury, risk for (side effects)
• Knowledge, deficient (teaching)
• Noncompliance (teaching)

### Implementation
#### PO route
• Do not break, crush, or chew caps
• Give around the clock to maintain proper blood levels; give with food to increase absorption of product; do not give within 3 hr of other agents; product reactions may occur
• Give with 8 oz of water, 1 hr before bedtime to prevent ulceration
• Shake liquid preparation well before giving; use calibrated device for proper dosing
• Do not give with iron, calcium, magnesium products or antacids, which decrease absorption and form insoluble chelate
#### IV route
• Check for irritation, extravasation, phlebitis daily; change site q72hr
• For intermittent inf, dilute each 100 mg/10 ml of 0.9% NaCl, sterile water for inj; further dilute in at least 100 ml of 0.9% NaCl, D₅W, Ringer's, LR, D₅/LR; protect from direct light; keep at room temperature; give over 1-4 hr; **IV** sol stable for 12 hr at room temperature, 72 hr refrigerated, discard if precipitate forms
*Syringe compatibilities:* Doxapram
*Y-site compatibilities:* Acyclovir, amifostine, amiodarone, aztreonam, cyclophosphamide, diltiazem, filgrastim, fludarabine, granisetron, hydromorphone, magnesium sulfate, melphalan, meperidine, morphine, ondansetron, perphenazine, propofol, sargramostim, tacrolimus, teniposide, theophylline, thiotepa, vinorelbine
*Y-site incompatibilities:* Hetastarch
*Additive compatibilities:* Ranitidine

## Patient/family education

• Teach patient to report sore throat, bruising, bleeding, joint pain; may indicate blood dyscrasias (rare)
• Advise patient to contact prescriber if vaginal itching, loose foul-smelling stools, furry tongue occur; may indicate superinfection; report itching, rash, pruritus, urticaria
• Instruct patient to take all medication prescribed for the length of time ordered; product must be taken around the clock to maintain blood levels; do not give medication to others
• Advise patient to notify prescriber of diarrhea with blood or pus

## Evaluation

**Positive therapeutic outcome**
• Absence of signs/symptoms of infection (WBC <10,000/mm$^3$, temp WNL, absence of red draining wounds)
• Reported improvement in symptoms of infection

---

**⚠ HIGH ALERT**

## droperidol (Rx)
(droe-per′i-dole)
droperidol, Inapsine
*Func. class.:* Neuroleptic, tranquilizer, antiemetic
*Chem. class.:* Butyrophenone derivative

**Pregnancy category C**

**Action:** Acts on CNS at subcortical levels, producing tranquilization, sleep; antiemetic; mild α-blockade

**Therapeutic outcome:** Maintenance of anesthesia

**Uses:** Premedication for surgery; induction, maintenance in general anesthesia; postoperatively for nausea and vomiting

## Dosage and routes
*Induction, adjunct*
*Adult:* **IV**/IM 1.25-2.5 mg, may give additional 1.25 mg
*Child 2-12 yr:* **IV** 0.05-0.1 mg/kg titrate to response
*Premedication*
*Adult:* IM 2.5-10 mg ½-1 hr before surgery, may give 1.25-2.5 mg additionally
*Child 2-12 yr:* IM 0.05-0.1 mg/kg
**Available forms:** Inj 2.5 mg/ml

## Adverse effects

*CNS:* EPS: Dystonia, akathisia, flexion of arms, fine tremors; dizziness, anxiety, drowsiness, restlessness, hallucinations, depression, **seizures,** extrapyramidal symptoms, **neuroleptic malignant syndrome**
*CV:* **Tachycardia,** *hypotension,* prolonged QT
*EENT:* Upward rotation of eyes, oculogyric crisis
*INTEG: Chills, facial sweating, shivering*
*RESP:* **Laryngospasm, bronchospasm**

**Contraindications:** Hypersensitivity, breastfeeding, child <2 yr

**Precautions:** Pregnancy C, geriatric, CV disease (hypotension, bradydysrhythmias), renal/hepatic disease, Parkinson's disease, pheochromocytoma

| Pharmacokinetics | |
|---|---|
| **Absorption** | Well absorbed (IM) |
| **Distribution** | Crosses blood-brain barrier, placenta |
| **Metabolism** | Liver |
| **Excretion** | Kidneys, unchanged (10%) |
| **Half-life** | 2-3 hr |

| Pharmacodynamics | |
|---|---|
| | IM/IV |
| **Onset** | 3-10 min |
| **Peak** | 30 min |
| **Duration** | 3-6 hr |

## Interactions
*Individual drugs*
Alcohol: increased CNS depression
Lithium: increased side effects of lithium
*Drug classifications*
Antihistamines, antipsychotics, barbiturates, CNS depressants, opiates: increased CNS depression
Antihypertensives, nitrates: increased hypotension
*Drug/herb*
Kava: increased action

## NURSING CONSIDERATIONS
**Assessment**
◆ Check VS q10 min during **IV** administration, q30 min after IM dose; for increasing heart rate or decreasing B/P, notify prescriber at once; do not place patient in Trendelenburg's position, sympathetic blockade may occur, causing respiratory arrest
• Assess extrapyramidal reactions: dystonia, akathisia, extended neck, restlessness, tremors; if these occur, an anticholinergic should be given

Adverse effects: *italic* = common, **bold** = life-threatening

- If given for nausea or vomiting, monitor for significant loss of fluids, bowel sounds before and during administration
- ECG prior to and 2-3 hr after administration for serious arrhythmias

## Nursing diagnoses
- Injury, risk for (adverse reactions)
- Knowledge, deficient (teaching)

## Implementation
- Protect from light

**IM route**
- Give deeply in large muscle mass

**IV route**
- Give direct **IV** undiluted; give through Y-tube or 3-way stopcock at 10 mg or less/min; titrate to patient response
- Intermittent inf may be given by adding dose to 250 ml of LR, $D_5W$, 0.9% NaCl; give slowly, titrate to patient response
- Give anticholinergics (benztropine, diphenhydrAMINE) for extrapyramidal reaction
- Give only with resuscitative equipment nearby

*Syringe compatibilities:* Atropine, bleomycin, butorphanol, chlorproMAZINE, cimetidine, cisplatin, cyclophosphamide, dimenhyDRINATE, diphenhydrAMINE, DOXOrubicin, fentanyl, glycopyrrolate, hydrOXYzine, meperidine, metoclopramide, midazolam, mitomycin, morphine, nalbuphine, pentazocine, perphenazine, prochlorperazine, promazine, promethazine, scopolamine, vinBLAStine, vinCRIStine

*Syringe incompatibilities:* Fluorouracil, furosemide, heparin, leucovorin, methotrexate, pentobarbital

*Y-site compatibilities:* Amifostine, aztreonam, bleomycin, cisatracurium, cisplatin, cladribine, cyclophosphamide, cytarabine, DOXOrubicin, DOXOrubicin liposome, famotidine, filgrastim, fluconazole, fludarabine, granisetron, hydrocortisone sodium succinate, idarubicin, melphalen, meperidine, metoclopramide, mitomycin, ondansetron, paclitaxel, potassium chloride, propofol, remifentanil, sargramostim, teniposide, thiotepa, vinBLAStine, vinCRIStine, vinorelbine, vit B/C

*Y-site incompatibilities:* Fluorouracil, foscarnet, furosemide, leucovorin, methotrexate, nafcillin

*Additive incompatibilities:* Barbiturates

## Patient/family education
- Advise patient that orthostatic hypotension is common; to rise from lying or sitting position slowly; to avoid ambulation without assistance

- Caution patient that drowsiness may occur; to call for assistance for ambulation

## Evaluation
**Positive therapeutic outcome**
- Decreased anxiety
- Absence of vomiting during and after surgery

---

## drotrecogin alfa (Rx)
(droh′treh-koh-jin al′fah)
Xigris
*Func. class.:* Thrombolytic agent
*Chem. class.:* Recombinant human activated protein C

**Pregnancy category  C**

**Action:** Activated protein C exerts an antithrombotic effect by inhibiting factor Va/VIIIa

**Therapeutic outcome:** Reduction of mortality in adult patients with severe sepsis who have a high risk of death

**Uses:** Severe sepsis (sepsis associated with acute organ dysfunction)

## Dosage and routes
*Adult:* **IV** INF 24 mcg/kg/hr × 96 hr; based on actual body weight

**Available forms:** Powder for inj, lyophilized, 5 mg, 20 mg

## Adverse effects
*HEMA:* Decreased Hct, **bleeding**
*SYST:* GI, GU, **intracranial, intraabdominal, intrathoracic, retroperitoneal bleeding; surface bleeding**

**Contraindications:** Hypersensitivity, internal active bleeding, intraspinal surgery, CNS neoplasms, ulcerative colitis, enteritis, hepatic disease, hypocoagulation, hemorrhagic stroke, epidural catheter in place, cerebral embolism/thrombosis/hemorrhage, recent major surgery, trauma

**Precautions:** Pregnancy **C**, breastfeeding, children, recent GI bleeding, prothrombin time −INR >3, use >96 hr

| Pharmacokinetics | |
|---|---|
| **Absorption** | Rapid |
| **Distribution** | Plasma |
| **Metabolism** | Unknown |
| **Excretion** | Unknown |
| **Half-life** | Unknown |

---

## Pharmacodynamics

| | |
|---|---|
| **Onset** | Within 2 hr of beginning infusion |
| **Peak** | 96 hr |
| **Duration** | 2 hr postinfusion |

## Interactions
### Individual drugs
Asprin, indomethacin, phenylbutazone: increased bleeding risk
### Drug classifications
Anticoagulants, glycoprotein IIb/IIIa inhibitors, thrombolytics: increased bleeding risk

## NURSING CONSIDERATIONS
### Assessment
⬥ Assess for bleeding during treatment; hematuria, hematemesis, bleeding from mucous membranes, epistaxis, ecchymosis; may require transfusion (rare), continue to assess for bleeding
• Assess blood studies (Hct, platelets, PTT, pro-time, TT, APTT) before starting therapy; pro-time or APTT must be less than 2× control before starting therapy; PTT or pro-time q3-4hr during treatment
• Assess VS, B/P, pulse, respirations, neurologic signs, temp at least q4hr; temp >104° F (40° C) indicates internal bleeding; systolic pressure increase >25 mm Hg should be reported to prescriber
⬥ Assess for neurologic changes that may indicate intracranial bleeding
⬥ Assess for retroperitoneal bleeding: back pain, leg weakness, diminished pulses

### Nursing diagnoses
• Knowledge, deficient (teaching)

### Implementation
• Store in refrigerator at 2°-8° C (36°-46° F); do not freeze
• Protect unreconstituted vials from light; keep in carton until time of use
**IV route**
• Reconstitute 5 mg vial/2.5 ml; 20 mg vial/10 ml sterile water for inj to a concentration of 2 mg/ml; slowly add sterile water for inj; do not shake or invert, gently swirl until dissolved
• Further dilute with 0.9% NaCl, slowly withdraw prescribed amount and add to bag of 0.9% NaCl, direct stream to side of bag, gently invert bag; do not transport infusion bag between locations using mechanical delivery systems
• Use immediately after reconstituting, may be held for only 3 hr at controlled room temperature 59°-86° F and must complete inf within 12 hr after preparation

• Do not use if discolored or if particulate is present
• If using an infusion pump, usual concentration is 100-200 mcg/ml; if using a syringe pump, usual concentration is 100-1000 mcg/ml
• Use a dedicated **IV** line, or dedicated lumen of central venous catheter, may use only 0.9% NaCl, LR, dextrose, or dextrose/saline mixtures through same line
• Do not expose to heat or direct sunlight
• Discontinue 2 hr prior to invasive surgery or procedures introducing risk of bleeding

### Evaluation
**Positive therapeutic outcome**
• Decreasing symptoms of sepsis, lack of mortality

## duloxetine (Rx)
(du-lox'uh-teen)
Cymbalta
*Func. class.:* Antidepressant— miscellaneous
*Chem. class:* Serotonin, norepinephrine reuptake inhibitor

### Pregnancy category C

**Action:** Unknown, may potentiate serotonergic, noradrenergic activity in the CNS. In studies duloxetine is a potent inhibitor of neuronal serotonin and norepinephrine reuptake

**Therapeutic outcome:** Decreased depression, decreased neuropathic pain

**Uses:** Major depressive disorder (MDD), neuropathic pain associated with diabetic neuropathy, generalized anxiety disorder

### Dosage and routes
#### Depression
*Adult:* PO 20 mg bid, may increase to 30 mg bid if needed
#### Diabetic neuropathy
*Adult:* PO 60 mg q day
#### Generalized anxiety disorder
*Adult:* PO 60 mg/day, may start with 30 mg/day × 1 wk, then increase to 60 mg/day
#### Renal dose
*Adult:* PO Start with 20 mg, gradually increase; avoid use in severe renal disease

**Available forms:** Caps 20, 30, 60 mg

### Adverse effects

*CNS:* Insomnia, anxiety, dizziness, tremor, fatigue, decreased appetite, decreased weight, agitation diaphoresis, hallucinations
*CV:* Thrombophlebitis, peripheral edema, palpitations
*EENT: Abnormal vision*
*GI:* Constipation, diarrhea, dysphagia, nausea, vomiting, anorexia, dry mouth, colitis, gastritis, abdominal pain
*GU:* Abnormal ejaculation, urinary hesitation, ejaculation delayed, erectile dysfunction, urinary frequency
*INTEG:* Photosensitivity, bruising, sweating
*SYST:* **Anaphylaxis, angioedema (rare)**

**Contraindications:** Hypersensitivity, angle-closure glaucoma

**Precautions:** Pregnancy **C**, breastfeeding, children, geriatric, mania, hypertension, cardiac/renal/hepatic disease, seizures, hepatotoxicity

---

#### Pharmacokinetics

| | |
|---|---|
| **Absorption** | Well absorbed |
| **Distribution** | 90% protein binding |
| **Metabolism** | Extensively metabolized (CYP 2D6, CYP 1A2) in the liver to an active metabolite |
| **Excretion** | 70% of product recovered in urine, 20% in feces |
| **Half-life** | 12 hr |

#### Pharmacodynamics

Unknown

---

### Interactions
*Individual drugs*
Alcohol: increased ALT, bilirubin
*Drug classifications*
 MAOIs: coadministration is contraindicated or within 14 days of MAOIs use: hyperthermia, rigidity, rapid fluctuations of VS, mental status changes, neuroleptic malignant syndrome
Opioids, antihistamines, sedative/hypnotics: increased CNS depression
CYP1A2 inhibitors (fluvoxamine, quinolone antiinfectives); CYP2D6 inhibitors (fluoxetine, quinidine, paroxetine): increased action of duloxetine
CYP2D6 extensively metabolized products (flecainide, phenothiazines, propafenone, tricyclics, thioridazine): narrow therapeutic index
*Drug/herb*
Chamomile, hops, kava, lavender, skullcap, valerian: increased CNS depression

Corkwood, jimsonweed: increased anticholinergic effect
SAM-e, St. John's wort: serotonin syndrome
Yohimbe: increased hypertension

### NURSING CONSIDERATIONS
#### Assessment
• Assess B/P lying, standing; pulse q4hr; if systolic B/P drops 20 mm Hg, hold product, notify prescriber; take VS q4hr in patients with CV disease
• Monitor hepatic studies: AST, ALT, bilirubin
• Monitor weight qwk; weight loss or gain; appetite may increase; peripheral edema may occur
• Offer sugarless gum, hard candy, frequent sips of water for dry mouth
• Assess mental status: mood, sensorium, affect, suicidal tendencies, increase in psychiatric symptoms; depression, panic
• Assess for withdrawal symptoms: headache, nausea, vomiting, muscle pain, weakness; not usual unless product is discontinued abruptly

#### Nursing diagnoses
• Injury, risk for (uses)
• Knowledge, deficient (teaching)
• Noncompliance (teaching)

#### Implementation
• Swallow caps whole; do not break, crush, or chew; do not sprinkle on food or mix with liquid
• Give without regard to food
• Store in tight container at room temperature; do not freeze
• Provide assistance with ambulation during beginning therapy, since drowsiness, dizziness occur
• Check to see if PO medication was swallowed

#### Patient/family education
• Advise that product is dispensed in small amounts because of suicide potential, especially in the beginning of therapy
• Teach patient/family to use caution when driving or other activities requiring alertness because of drowsiness, dizziness, blurred vision
• Advise patient to avoid alcohol ingestion, MAOIs, other CNS depressants
• Advise patient not to discontinue medication quickly after long-term use; may cause nausea, headache, malaise
• Advise patient to wear sunscreen or large hat, since photosensitivity may occur
• Advise patient to notify prescriber if pregnancy is planned or suspected, or if breastfeeding

---

• Tell patient that improvement may occur in 4-8 wk
• Advise that clinical worsening and suicide risk may occur

### Evaluation
**Positive therapeutic outcome**
• Decreased depression

---

## dutasteride (Rx)
(doo-tass'ter-ide)
Avodart
*Func. class.:* Sex hormone, 5α-reductase inhibitor
*Chem. class.:* Synthetic 4-azasteroid compound

**Pregnancy category** X

**Action:** Inhibits both types 1 and 2 forms of a steroid enzyme that converts testosterone to 5 μ-dihydrotestosterone (DHT), which is responsible for the initial growth of prostatic tissue

**Therapeutic outcome:** Decreased symptoms of benign prostatic hyperplasia (BPH)

**Uses:** Treatment of symptomatic BPH in men with an enlarged prostate gland

**Unlabeled uses:** Alopecia

### Dosage and routes
*Adult:* PO 0.5 mg/day

**Available forms:** Caps 0.5 mg

### Adverse effects
*GU:* Decreased libido, impotence, gynecomastia, ejaculation disorders (rare), mastalgia, teratogenesis

**Contraindications:** Pregnancy **X**, breastfeeding, children, women, hypersensitivity

**Precautions:** Hepatic disease

| Pharmacokinetics | |
|---|---|
| Absorption | Absolute bioavailability ~60% |
| Distribution | Protein binding 99% |
| Metabolism | Liver (CYP3A4) |
| Excretion | Feces |
| Half-life | 5 wk at steady state |

| Pharmacodynamics | |
|---|---|
| Onset | Rapid |
| Peak | 2-3 hr |
| Duration | Levels detectable 4-6 mo posttreatment |

### Interactions
*Individual drugs*
Cimetidine, ciprofloxacin, diltiazem, ketoconazole, ritonavir, verapamil: increased dutasteride concentrations
*Drug classifications*
Antiretroviral protease inhibitors or other CYP3A4-metabolized products: increased dutasteride concentrations
*Drug/lab test*
Increased: TSH
Decreased: PSA

### NURSING CONSIDERATIONS
### Assessment
• Assess for decreasing symptoms in BPH: decreasing urinary retention, frequency, urgency, nocturia
• Assess PSA levels, digital rectal exam, urinary obstruction; determine the absence of urinary cancer before starting treatment
• Assess liver function tests: ALT, AST, bilirubin

### Nursing diagnoses
• Body image, disturbed (adverse reactions)
• Knowledge, deficient (teaching)

### Implementation
• Swallow caps whole: do not break, crush, chew, or open
• May be given without regard to meals

### Patient/family education
• Advise patient to notify prescriber if therapeutic response decreases, if edema occurs
• Caution patient not to discontinue product abruptly
• Inform patient about changes in sex characteristics
• Caution patient not to donate blood for at least 6 mo after last dose to prevent possible blood administration to pregnant female
• Advise patient and family that caps should not be handled by pregnant women since this product can be absorbed through the skin
• Inform patient that ejaculate volume may decrease during treatment, that product rarely interferes with sexual function
• Advise patient to read patient information leaflet before starting therapy and reread it upon prescription renewal

### Evaluation
**Positive therapeutic outcome**
• Decreased levels of DHT (5 α-dihydrotestosterone)
• Decreased urinary frequency
• Decreased urinary retention
• Decreased urinary urgency
• Decreased nocturia

---

Adverse effects: *italic* = common, **bold** = life-threatening

## dyphylline (Rx)

(dye′fi-lin)

Dilor, Dyflex-200, Dylline, dyphylline, Lufyllin, Neothylline

*Func. class.:* Bronchodilator, phosphodiesterase inhibitor

*Chem. class.:* Xanthine, theophylline derivative

**Pregnancy category C**

**Action:** Relaxes smooth muscle of respiratory system by blocking phosphodiesterase, which increases cyclic AMP; cyclic AMP results in positive inotropic, chronotropic effects, bronchodilatation, stimulation of CNS

**Therapeutic outcome:** Bronchodilatation with ease of breathing

**Uses:** Bronchial asthma, bronchospasm in chronic bronchitis and emphysema, COPD

**Dosage and routes**

*Adult and child >6 yr:* PO 15 mg/kg/dose, max 60 mg/kg/day

*Renal dose*

*Adult:* PO CCr 50-80 ml/min 75% of original dose; CCr 10-50 ml/min 50% of original dose; CCr <10 ml/min 25% of original dose

**Available forms:** Tabs 200, 400 mg; elix 33.3, 53.3 mg/5 ml

**Adverse effects**

*CNS: Anxiety, restlessness, insomnia, dizziness, seizures,* headache, light-headedness, muscle twitching

*CV: Palpitations, sinus tachycardia,* hypotension, flushing, **dysrhythmias, circulatory failure**

*GI: Nausea,* diarrhea, *vomiting, anorexia,* dyspepsia, epigastric pain, rectal irritation, bleeding, reflux

*INTEG:* Flushing, urticaria

*OTHER:* Fever, dehydration, **albuminuria,** hyperglycemia, increased diuresis

*RESP:* Tachypnea, **respiratory arrest**

**Contraindications:** Hypersensitivity to xanthines

**Precautions:** Pregnancy **C,** breastfeeding, children, geriatric, CHF, cor pulmonale, diabetes mellitus, hypertension, renal/hepatic disease, glaucoma, hyperthyroidism, peptic ulcer, seizure disorder

### Pharmacokinetics

| | |
|---|---|
| **Absorption** | Well absorbed (PO) |
| **Distribution** | Unknown |
| **Metabolism** | Liver |
| **Excretion** | Kidneys (85%), breast milk |
| **Half-life** | 2 hr; increased in renal disease |

### Pharmacodynamics

| | PO | IM |
|---|---|---|
| **Onset** | Unknown | Unknown |
| **Peak** | 1 hr | Unknown |
| **Duration** | 6 hr | Unknown |

### Interactions

*Individual drugs*

Cimetidine, erythromycin, propranolol, probenecid: increased action of dyphylline

Phenytoin: decreased levels of phenytoin, increased metabolism of dyphylline

*Drug classifications*

Barbiturates: increased metabolism of dyphilline

β-Adrenergic blockers: increased cardiotoxicity

Uricosurics: decreased elimination of dyphylline

### NURSING CONSIDERATIONS

**Assessment**

• Monitor dyphylline blood levels (therapeutic level is <20 mcg/ml); toxicity (dysrhythmias, seizures, diuresis, flushing, headache) may occur with small increase above 20 mcg/ml, especially geriatric; determine whether theophylline was given recently (24 hr)

• Monitor I&O; an increase in diuresis occurs; dehydration may result in geriatric or children

• Assess respiratory rate, rhythm, depth; before and during treatment auscultate lung fields bilaterally; notify prescriber of abnormalities

• Assess for allergic reactions: rash, urticaria; if these occur, product should be discontinued

• Assess for product toxicity: nausea, vomiting, anorexia, cramping, diarrhea, confusion

**Nursing diagnoses**

• Activity intolerance (uses)

• Airway clearance, ineffective (uses)

• Injury, risk for (uses, adverse reactions)

• Knowledge, deficient (teaching)

**Implementation**

**PO route**

• Give around the clock to maintain blood levels, daily dose each AM

• Give 1 hr before or 2 hr after meals to increase absorption; elix should be measured accurately
• Take with 8 oz of water and food if GI upset occurs
• Increased fluids to 2 L/day
**IM route**
• Inject slowly; do not give by **IV** route; do not administer if cloudy or a precipitate occurs, avoid this route, do not give **IV**

## Patient/family education
• Teach patient to take doses as prescribed, not to skip doses or double dose; patient should check OTC medications and current prescription medications for epHEDrine, which increases CNS stimulation; tell patient not to drink alcohol or caffeine products (tea, coffee, chocolate, colas) or CV effects may occur, not to change brands
• Advise patient to avoid hazardous activities; dizziness may occur
• Caution patient if GI upset occurs, to take product with 8 oz of water and food
• Teach patient to notify prescriber of change in smoking habit; a change in dosage may be required
• Instruct patient to report nausea, vomiting, insomnia, tachycardia, dysrhythmias, seizures, or restlessness; can indicate toxicity
• Teach patient to increase fluids to 2 L/day to decrease viscosity of secretions
• Advise patient to obtain product level q6-12 mo

## Evaluation
**Positive therapeutic outcome**
• Decreased dyspnea
• Clear lung fields bilaterally

### econazole topical
*See Appendix D*

### ecothiophate ophthalmic
*See Appendix D*

### eculizumab
Soliris
*See Appendix A, Selected New Drugs*

## edrophonium (Rx)
(ed-roe-fone'ee-yum)
Enlon, Reversol, Tensilon
*Func. class.:* Cholinergics, anticholinesterase
*Chem. class.:* Quaternary ammonium compound

**Pregnancy category C**

**Action:** Inhibits destruction of acetylcholine, which increases concentration at sites where acetylcholine is released; this facilitates transmission of impulses across myoneural junction

**Therapeutic outcome:** Reversal of nondepolarizing neuromuscular blockers; absence of difficulty with muscular function in myasthenia gravis

**Uses:** Diagnosis of myasthenia gravis; curare antagonist; differentiation of myasthenic crisis from cholinergic crisis; reversal of nondepolarizing neuromuscular blockers

**Dosage and routes**
*Tensilon test (myasthenia gravis diagnosis)*
*Adult:* **IV** 1-2 mg over 15-30 sec, then 8 mg if no response; IM 10 mg; if cholinergic reaction occurs, retest after ½ hr with 2 mg IM
*Child >34 kg:* **IV** 2 mg; if no response in 45 sec, then 1 mg q45 sec, not to exceed 10 mg; IM 5 mg
*Child <34 kg:* **IV** 1 mg; if no response in 45 sec, then 1 mg q45 sec, not to exceed 5 mg; IM 2 mg
*Infant:* **IV** 0.5 mg

*Reversal of nondepolarizing neuromuscular blockers*
*Adult:* **IV** 10 mg over 30-45 sec, may repeat, not to exceed 40 mg

*Differentiation of myasthenic crisis from cholinergic crisis*
*Adult:* **IV** 1 mg, if no response in 1 min, may repeat

**Available forms:** Inj 10 mg/ml

**Adverse effects**
*CNS:* Dizziness, headache, sweating, weakness, **seizures**, uncoordination, **paralysis**, drowsiness, **loss of consciousness**
*CV:* Dysrhythmias, bradycardia, hypotension, **AV block**, ECG changes, **cardiac arrest**, syncope
*EENT:* Miosis, blurred vision, lacrimation, visual changes

Adverse effects: *italic* = common, **bold** = life-threatening

*GI:* *Nausea, diarrhea, vomiting, cramps, increased salivary and gastric secretions, dysphagia, increased peristalsis*
*GU:* Frequency, incontinence, urgency
*INTEG:* Rash, urticaria
*RESP:* **Respiratory depression, bronchospasm, constriction, laryngospasm, respiratory arrest,** dyspnea, increased bronchial secretions

**Contraindications:** Obstruction of intestine, renal system, hypersensitivity

**Precautions:** Pregnancy **C**, seizure disorders, bronchial asthma, coronary occlusion, hyperthyroidism, dysrhythmias, peptic ulcer, megacolon, poor GI motility, bradycardia, hypotension

Pharmacokinetics
Unknown

Pharmacodynamics

|  | IM | IV |
|---|---|---|
| **Onset** | 2-10 min | 30-60 sec |
| **Peak** | Unknown | Unknown |
| **Duration** | 12-45 min | 6-25 min |

**Interactions**
*Individual drugs*
Atropine, procainamide, quinidine: decreased action of edrophonium
Digoxin: increased bradycardia
*Drug classifications*
Muscle relaxants, depolarizing: prolonged action of muscle relaxant
Parasympathomimetics: increased edrophonium effects; avoid giving concurrently

**NURSING CONSIDERATIONS**
**Assessment**
• Assess VS, respiration during test
• Monitor diabetic patient carefully, this product lowers blood glucose

**Nursing diagnoses**
• Breathing pattern, ineffective (uses)
• Knowledge, deficient (teaching)

**Implementation**
**IV route**
• Administer undiluted 2 mg or less over 15-30 sec, or give as continuous inf in myasthenia crisis
⬥ Give only after ensuring that atropine sulfate is available for cholinergic crisis
• Give only after all other cholinergics have been discontinued
• Store at room temperature

*Y-site compatibilities:* Heparin, hydrocortisone, potassium chloride, vit B/C

**Patient/family education**
• Instruct patient to carry/wear emergency ID specifying myasthenia gravis and products taken

**Evaluation**
**Positive therapeutic outcome**
• Increased muscle strength, hand grasp; improved gait; absence of labored breathing (if severe)

**Treatment of overdose:** Respiratory support, atropine 1-4 mg (**IV**)

**efavirenz** (Rx)
(ef-ah-veer'enz)
Sustiva
*Func. class.:* Antiretroviral
*Chem. class.:* Nonnucleoside reverse transcriptase inhibitor (NNRTI)

**Pregnancy category D**

**Action:** Binds directly to reverse transcriptase and blocks RNA, DNA causing a disruption of the enzyme's site

**Therapeutic outcome:** Improvement of HIV-1 infection

**Uses:** HIV-1 in combination with other antiretrovirals

**Dosage and routes**
Given in combination with protease inhibitor or nucleoside analog reverse transcriptase inhibitors (NRTIs)
*Adult and child >40 kg:* PO 600 mg/day at bedtime
*Child:*
10-15 kg: PO 200 mg/day at bedtime
15-20 kg: PO 250 mg/day at bedtime
20-25 kg: PO 300 mg/day at bedtime
25-32.5 kg: PO 350 mg/day at bedtime
32.5-40 kg: PO 400 mg/day at bedtime

**Available forms:** Caps 50, 100, 200, 600 mg; tabs 600 mg

**Adverse effects**
*CNS:* Headache, dizziness, fatigue, impaired cognition, insomnia, abnormal dreams, depression, anxiety, drowsiness
*GI:* *Diarrhea,* abdominal pain, *nausea,* hyperlipidemia, constipation, increased liver function tests
*GU:* Hematuria, kidney stones
*INTEG:* *Rash,* **erythema multiforme, Stevens-Johnson syndrome, toxic epidermal necrolysis**

**Contraindications:** Pregnancy **D**, hypersensitivity

**Precautions:** Liver disease, breastfeeding, children <3 yr, renal disease, myelosuppression, depression, seizures

| Pharmacokinetics | |
|---|---|
| Absorption | Well |
| Distribution | Highly protein bound (99%) |
| Metabolism | Liver |
| Excretion | Kidneys, feces |
| Half-life | Terminal 52-76 hr |

| Pharmacodynamics | |
|---|---|
| Onset | Unknown |
| Peak | 3-5 hr |
| Duration | Unknown |

### Interactions
*Individual drugs*
Alcohol: increased CNS depression
Carbamazepine: decreased efavirenz levels
Cisapride, midazolam, triazolam: do not give together
Clarithromycin, indinavir, methadone, saquinavir: decreased level of each specific product
Midazolam, triazolam, warfarin: increased level of each specific product
Ritonavir: increased levels of both products
*Drug classifications*
Anticonvulsants, ergots, statins (except pravastatin, fluvastatin): increased levels of each specific product
Antidepressants, antihistamines, opioids: increased CNS depression
Benzodiazepines, ergots: do not give together
Estrogens: increased level of both products
Rifamycins: decreased efavirenz action
*Drug/herb*
St. John's wort: decreased efavirenz level; do not use together
*Drug/food*
Increased: absorption of high-fat foods
*Drug/lab test*
Increased: ALT
False positive: cannabinoids

### NURSING CONSIDERATIONS
**Assessment**
• Assess signs of infection, anemia
• Assess liver studies: ALT, AST; renal tests
• Assess bowel pattern before, during treatment; if severe abdominal pain with bleeding occurs, product should be discontinued; monitor hydration

• Assess skin eruptions; rash, urticaria, itching
• Assess allergies before treatment, reaction to each medication
• Assess CBC, blood chemistry, plasma HIV RNA, absolute CD4⁺/CD8⁺/cell counts/%, serum $\beta_2$ microglobulin, serum ICD+24 antigen levels, cholesterol, hepatic enzymes
• Assess for signs of toxicity: severe nausea/vomiting, maculopapular rash

**Nursing diagnoses**
• Diarrhea (side effects)
• Infection, risk for (uses)
• Knowledge, deficient (teaching)

**Implementation**
• Give at bedtime to decrease CNS side effects, give on empty stomach

**Patient/family education**
• Inform patient that product does not cure disease but controls symptoms; HIV still can be transmitted to others
• Advise patient to take as prescribed; if dose is missed, take as soon as remembered; do not double dose, take on empty stomach with water/juice
• Instruct patient to make sure health care provider knows of all the medications being taken, supplements, herbs, OTC products
• Advise patient that if severe rash occurs, stop taking and notify health care provider
• Advise patient not to breastfeed or become pregnant (serious birth defects have occurred) if taking this product
• Advise patient that adverse reactions: rash, dizziness, abnormal dreams, insomnia, lessen after a month
• Teach patient to avoid hazardous activities if dizziness, drowsiness occurs

**Evaluation**
**Positive therapeutic outcome**
• Increased CD4, cell counts
• Decreased viral load
• Improvement in symptoms and progression of HIV-1 infection

---

**eletriptan** (Rx)
(el-ee-trip′tan)
Relpax
*Func. class.:* Antimigraine agent
**Pregnancy category** C

**Action:** Binds selectively to the vascular 5-HT$_1$-receptor subtype, exerts antimigraine effect; causes vasoconstriction in cranial arteries

Adverse effects: *italic* = common, **bold** = life-threatening

**Therapeutic outcome:** Decreased severity of migraine

**Uses:** Acute treatment of migraine with or without aura

**Dosage and routes**
*Adult:* **PO** 20 mg, may increase if needed, max 40 mg (single dose); may repeat in 2 hr if headache improves but returns, max 80 mg/24 hr

**Available forms:** Tabs 20, 40 mg

**Adverse effects**
*CNS: Dizziness,* headache, anxiety, paresthesia, asthenia, somnolence, flushing, fatigue, hot/cold sensation
*CV:* Chest pain, palpitations, hypertension
*GI:* Nausea, dry mouth
*MS: Weakness*
*RESP:* Chest tightness, pressure

**Contraindications:** Concurrent use of ergotamine-containing preparations, uncontrolled hypertension, hypersensitivity, basilar or hemiplegic migraine, ischemic bowel disease, severe renal/hepatic disease, coronary artery vasospasm, peripheral vascular disease, heart disease

**Precautions:** Pregnancy **C**, breastfeeding, children, geriatric, postmenopausal women, men >40 yr, risk factors of CAD, MI, or other cardiac disease, hypercholesterolemia, obesity, diabetes, impaired renal/hepatic function

**Pharmacokinetics**

| | |
|---|---|
| **Absorption** | Unknown |
| **Distribution** | Unknown |
| **Metabolism** | Liver |
| **Excretion** | Urine, feces |
| **Half-life** | Unknown |

**Pharmacodynamics**

| | |
|---|---|
| **Onset** | Of pain relief 2 hr |
| **Peak** | Unknown |
| **Duration** | Unknown |

**Interactions**
*Individual drugs*
Clarithromycin, erythromycin, itraconazole, ketoconazole, nelfinavir, propranolol, ritonavir: increased plasma concentration of eletriptan
*Drug classifications*
CYP3A4 inhibitors: increased concentration of eletriptan
*Drug/herb*
Butterbur: increased effect

**NURSING CONSIDERATIONS**
**Assessment**
• Monitor B/P; signs/symptoms of coronary vasospasms
• Assess for tingling, hot sensation, burning, feeling of pressure, numbness, flushing
• Assess stress level, activity, recreation, coping mechanisms
• Assess neurologic status: LOC, blurring vision, nausea, vomiting, tingling in extremities preceding headache
• Identify ingestion of tyramine foods (pickled products, beer, wine, aged cheese), food additives, preservatives, colorings, artificial sweeteners, chocolate, caffeine, which may precipitate these types of headaches

**Nursing diagnoses**
• Knowledge, deficient (teaching)
• Pain, acute (uses)

**Implementation**
• Swallow tabs whole; do not break, crush, or chew
• Provide quiet, calm environment with decreased stimulation from noise, bright light, excessive talking

**Patient/family education**
• Have patient report any side effects to prescriber
• Teach patient to use contraception while taking product
• Teach patient to have dark, quiet environment
• Teach patient that product does not prevent or reduce number of migraine attacks

**Evaluation**
**Positive therapeutic outcome**
• Decreased severity of migraine

**emedastine ophthalmic**
*See Appendix D*

**emtricitabine** (Rx)
(em-tri-sit'uh-bean)
Emtriva
*Func. class.:* Antiretroviral
*Chem. class.:* Nucleoside reverse transcriptase inhibitor (NRTI)

**Pregnancy category B**

**Action:** Synthetic nucleoside analog of cytosine; inhibits replication of HIV virus by competing with the natural substrate and then becoming incorporated into cellular DNA by viral reverse transcriptase, thereby terminating cellular DNA chain

**Therapeutic outcome:** Decreasing symptoms of HIV

**Uses:** HIV-1 infection with other antiretrovirals

**Unlabeled uses:** HBV (hepatitis B virus) infection

**Dosage and routes**
*Adult:* PO 200 mg/day; oral sol 240 mg (24 ml) daily

*Child 3 mo-17 yr:* PO (caps) 200 mg/day; oral sol 6 mg/kg/day, max 240 mg (24 ml)

*Renal dose*
*Adult:* PO CCr 30-49 ml/min 200 mg q48hr, sol 120 mg q24hr; CCr 15-29 ml/min 200 mg q72hr, sol 80 mg q24hr; CCr <15 ml/min 200 mg q96hr, sol 40 mg q24hr

**Available forms:** Caps 200 mg; oral sol 10 mg/ml; oral cap and sol are not interchangeable

**Adverse effects**
*CNS:* Headache, abnormal dreams, depression, dizziness, insomnia, neuropathy, paresthesia, *asthenia*
*GI: Nausea, vomiting, diarrhea, anorexia, abdominal pain, dyspepsia,* **hepatomegaly with stenosis (may be fatal)**
*INTEG:* Rash, skin discoloration
*MS:* Arthralgia, myalgia
*RESP:* Cough
*SYST:* Change in body fat distribution, **lactic acidosis**

**Contraindications:** Hypersensitivity

**Precautions:** Pregnancy **B**, breastfeeding, children, geriatric, renal disease, hepatic insufficiency, chronic hepatitis B virus (HBV) infection

**Pharmacokinetics**

| | |
|---|---|
| Absorption | Rapidly, extensively absorbed |
| Distribution | Protein binding <4% |
| Metabolism | Unknown |
| Excretion | Excreted unchanged in urine (86%), feces (14%) |
| Half-life | 10 hr |

**Pharmacodynamics**

| | |
|---|---|
| Onset | Unknown |
| Peak | 1-2 hr |
| Duration | Unknown |

## NURSING CONSIDERATIONS
**Assessment**
• Monitor liver, renal function tests: AST, ALT, bilirubin, amylase, lipase, triglycerides periodically during treatment
◆ Assess for lactic acidosis, severe hepatomegaly with steatosis; if lab reports confirm these conditions, discontinue treatment

**Nursing diagnoses**
• Infection, risk for (uses)
• Injury, risk for (adverse reactions)
• Knowledge, deficient (teaching)

**Implementation**
• Give without regard to meals
• Store at 25° C (77° F)
• Take at same time every day
• Oral cap and solution are not interchangeable

**Patient/family education**
• Teach that GI complaints resolve after 3-4 wk of treatment
• Advise not to breastfeed while taking this product
• Instruct that product must be taken at same time of day to maintain blood level
• Advise that product will control symptoms, but is not a cure for HIV; patient is still infectious, may pass HIV virus on to others
• Instruct that other products may be necessary to prevent other infections
• Advise that changes in body fat distribution may occur

**Evaluation**
**Positive therapeutic outcome**
• Decrease in signs/symptoms of HIV

**enalapril/enalaprilat** (Rx)
(e-nal′april/e-nal′a-pril-at)
Vasotec, Vasotec IV
*Func. class.:* Antihypertensive
*Chem. class.:* Angiotensin-converting enzyme (ACE) inhibitor
**Pregnancy category D**

**Do not confuse:**
enalapril/Eldepryl/ramipril/Anafranil

**Action:** Selectively suppresses renin-angiotensin-aldosterone system; inhibits ACE; prevents conversion of angiotensin I to angiotensin II, resulting in dilation of arterial and venous vessels

**Therapeutic outcome:** Decreased B/P in hypertension; decreased preload, afterload in CHF

**Uses:** Hypertension, CHF, left ventricular dysfunction

## Dosage and routes
### Hypertension
*Adult:* PO 5 mg/day, may increase or decrease to desired response, range 10-40 mg/day; **IV** 0.625-1.25 mg q6hr over 5 min
*Child:* PO 0.08 mg/kg/day in 1-2 divided doses, max 0.58 mg/kg/day; **IV** 5-10 mcg/kg/dose q8-24hr

### Patients on diuretics
*Adult:* **IV** 0.625 mg over 5 min, may give additional doses of 1.25 mg q6hr

### CHF
*Adult:* PO 2.5-20 mg/day in 2 divided doses, max 40 mg/day in divided doses

### Renal dose
*Adult:* PO CCr <30 ml/min 2.5 mg/day, increase gradually; **IV** CCr >30 ml/min 1.25 mg q6hr; CCr <30 ml/min 0.625 mg as one-time dose, increase as per B/P

**Available forms:** Enalapril: tabs 2.5, 5, 10, 20 mg; enalaprilat: inj 1.25 mg/ml

## Adverse effects
*CNS: Insomnia, dizziness,* paresthesias, headache, fatigue, anxiety
*CV: Hypotension,* chest pain, tachycardia, **dysrhythmias,** syncope, angina, **MI,** orthostatic hypotension
*EENT: Tinnitus,* visual changes, sore throat, double vision, dry burning eyes
*GI:* Nausea, vomiting, colitis, cramps, diarrhea, constipation, flatulence, dry mouth, loss of taste
*GU:* **Proteinuria, renal failure,** increased frequency of polyuria or oliguria
*HEMA:* **Agranulocytosis, neutropenia**
*INTEG:* Rash, purpura, alopecia, hyperhidrosis, photosensitivity
*META:* Hyperkalemia
*RESP:* Dyspnea, dry cough, crackles, **angioedema**

**Contraindications:** Pregnancy **D,** hypersensitivity, history of angioedema

**Precautions:** Breastfeeding, renal disease, hyperkalemia, hepatic failure, dehydration, bilateral renal artery stenosis

## Pharmacokinetics
| | |
|---|---|
| **Absorption** | Well absorbed (PO), complete (**IV**) |
| **Distribution** | Unknown |
| **Metabolism** | Liver (active metabolite—enalaprilat) |
| **Excretion** | Kidneys (60%—enalaprilat, 20%—enalapril) |
| **Half-life** | Enalaprilat 11 hr, increased in renal disease |

## Pharmacodynamics
| | PO | IV |
|---|---|---|
| **Onset** | 1 hr | 15 min |
| **Peak** | 4-6 hr | 1-4 hr |
| **Duration** | 24 hr | 6 hr |

## Interactions
### Individual drugs
Alcohol: increased hypotension (large amounts)
Allopurinol: increased hypersensitivity
CycloSPORINE, indomethacin: increased potassium levels
Digoxin, lithium: increased serum levels
Rifampin: decreased effects of enalapril
### Drug classifications
Antacids: decreased effects of enalapril
Diuretics, general anesthesia, nitrates, other antihypertensives, phenothiazines: increased hypotension
Diuretics (potassium-sparing), potassium supplements, salt substitutes: increased potassium levels
### Drug/herb
Arginine: fatal hypokalemia
Pill-bearing spurge: increased effect
Pineapple, yobimbe: decreased effect
St. John's wort: severe photosensitivity
### Drug/lab test
Increased: ALT, AST, bilirubin, alkaline phosphatase, glucose, uric acid
False positive: ANA titer

## NURSING CONSIDERATIONS
### Assessment
• Monitor blood studies: neutrophils, decreased platelets with differential baseline and q3 mo if neutrophils <1000/mm³, discontinue treatment
• Monitor B/P, orthostatic hypotension, syncope; if changes occur, dosage change may be required; obtain peak/trough levels
• Monitor electrolytes: K, Na, Cl during 1st 2 wk of therapy
• Monitor renal studies: protein, BUN, creatinine; increased levels may indicate nephrotic syndrome and renal failure

- Monitor renal symptoms: polyuria, oliguria, frequency, dysuria
- Establish baselines in renal, liver function tests before therapy begins and 1 wk into therapy
- Check potassium levels throughout treatment, although hyperkalemia rarely occurs
- Check for edema in feet, legs daily
- Assess for allergic reactions: rash, fever, pruritus, urticaria; product should be discontinued if antihistamines fail to help

## Nursing diagnoses
- Cardiac output, decreased (uses)
- Injury, risk for (adverse reactions)
- Knowledge, deficient (teaching)
- Noncompliance (teaching)

## Implementation
### PO route
- Store in air-tight container at 86° F (30° C) or less
- Severe hypotension may occur after 1st dose of this medication; decreased hypotension may be prevented by reducing or discontinuing diuretic therapy 3 days before beginning benazepril therapy
- Give by IV inf of 0.9% NaCl (as ordered) to expand fluid volume if severe hypotension occurs

### IV route
- Give IV direct over 5 min
- Dilute in 50 ml of 0.9% NaCl, D₅W, D₅/0.9% NaCl, D₅/LR; diluted solution may be used for 24 hr

*Y-site compatibilities:* Allopurinol, amifostine, amikacin, aminophylline, ampicillin, ampicillin/sulbactam, aztreonam, butorphanol, calcium gluconate, cefazolin, cefoperazone, ceftazidime, ceftizoxime, chloramphenicol, cimetidine, cladribine, clindamycin, dextran 40, DOBUTamine, DOPamine, erythromycin lactobionate, esmolol, famotidine, fentanyl, filgrastim, ganciclovir, gentamicin, granisetron, heparin, hetastarch, hydrocortisone, labetalol, lidocaine, magnesium sulfate, melphalan, meropenem, methylPREDNISolone, metronidazole, morphine, nafcillin, niCARdipine, penicillin G potassium, phenobarbital, piperacillin, piperacillin/tazobactam, potassium chloride, potassium phosphate, propofol, ranitidine, teniposide, thiotepa, tobramycin, trimethoprim/sulfamethoxazole, vancomycin, vinorelbine

*Y-site incompatibilities:* Amphotericin B, phenytoin

*Additive compatibilities:* DOBUTamine, DOPamine, heparin, meropenem, nitroglycerin, nitroprusside, potassium chloride

## Patient/family education
- Advise patient not to discontinue product abruptly; advise patient to tell all persons associated with health care that product is being taken
- Teach patient not to use OTC products (cough, cold, allergy medications) unless directed by physician, to avoid potassium, salt substitutes; serious side effects can occur; xanthines, such as coffee, tea, chocolate, cola can prevent action of product
- Instruct patient on the importance of complying with dosage schedule, even if feeling better; to continue with medical regimen to decrease B/P: exercise, cessation of smoking, decreasing stress, diet modifications
- Emphasize the need to rise slowly to sitting or standing position to minimize orthostatic hypotension; not to exercise in hot weather, which can cause increased hypotension
- Advise patient to notify prescriber of mouth sores, sore throat, fever, swelling of hands or feet, irregular heartbeat, chest pain, coughing, shortness of breath
- Caution patient to report excessive perspiration, dehydration, vomiting, diarrhea; may lead to fall in B/P
- Caution patient that product may cause skin rash or impaired perspiration; that angioedema may occur and to discontinue if it occurs
- Caution patient that product may cause dizziness, fainting, light-headedness; may occur during 1st few days of therapy; to avoid activities that may be hazardous
- Teach patient how to take B/P, and normal readings for age-group

## Evaluation
### Positive therapeutic outcome
- Decreased B/P in hypertension

**Treatment of overdose:** Lavage, **IV** atropine for bradycardia; **IV** theophylline for bronchospasm, digoxin, O₂; diuretic for cardiac failure, hemodialysis

## enfuvirtide (Rx)
(en-fyoo'vir-tide)
Fuzeon
*Func. class.:* Antiretroviral
*Chem. class.:* Fusion inhibitor

**Pregnancy category B**

**Action:** Inhibitor of the fusion of HIV-1 with CD4+ cells

**Therapeutic outcome:** Decreasing symptoms of HIV

**Uses:** Treatment of HIV-1 infection in combination with other antiretrovirals

### Dosage and routes
*Adult:* SUBCUT 90 mg (1 ml) bid
*Child 6-16 yr:* SUBCUT 2 mg/kg bid, max 90 mg bid

**Available forms:** Powder for inj, lyophilized 108 mg (90 mg/ml when reconstituted)

### Adverse effects
*CNS:* Anxiety, peripheral neuropathy, taste disturbance, **Guillain-Barré syndrome,** insomnia, depression
*GI:* Abdominal pain, anorexia, constipation, pancreatitis
*GU:* **Glomerulonephritis, renal failure**
*HEMA:* **Thrombocytopenia, neutropenia**
*INTEG:* Inj site reactions
*MISC:* Influenza, cough, conjunctivitis, lymphadenopathy, myalgias, hyperglycemia, pneumonia, rhinitis, fatigue

**Contraindications:** Breastfeeding, hypersensitivity

**Precautions:** Pregnancy **B**, children <6 yr, liver disease, myelosuppression, infections

### Pharmacokinetics
| | |
|---|---|
| **Absorption** | Well |
| **Distribution** | 92% protein binding |
| **Metabolism** | Undergoes catabolism |
| **Excretion** | Unknown |
| **Half-life** | Terminal 3.8 hr |

### Pharmacodynamics
| | |
|---|---|
| **Onset** | Unknown |
| **Peak** | 8 hrs |
| **Duration** | Unknown |

### NURSING CONSIDERATIONS
**Assessment**
• Assess for signs of infection, inj site reactions
• Monitor renal studies: BUN, creatinine, renal failure may occur
• Monitor bowel pattern before, during treatment; if severe abdominal pain or constipation occurs, notify prescriber; monitor hydration
• Assess skin eruptions, rash, urticaria, itching
• Identify allergies before treatment, reaction to each medication
• CBC, blood chemistry, plasma HIV RNA, absolute CD4+/CD8+ cell counts/%, serum $\beta_2$ microglobulin, serum ICD+24 antigen levels, cholesterol

**Nursing diagnoses**
• Infection, risk for (uses)
• Injury, risk for (adverse reactions)
• Knowledge, deficient (teaching)

**Implementation**
• Give SUBCUT, bid; rotate sites; preferred sites are upper arm, anterior thigh, abdomen

**Patient/family education**
• Instruct to notify prescriber if pregnancy is suspected, or if breastfeeding
• Advise that pneumonia may occur, to contact prescriber if cough, fever occur
• Teach that hypersensitive reactions may occur, rash, pruritus; stop product, contact prescriber
• Teach that this product is not a cure for HIV-1 infection but controls symptoms, HIV-1 can still be transmitted to others
• Teach that this product is to be used in combination only with other antiretrovirals

**Evaluation**
**Positive therapeutic outcome**
• Increased CD4 cell counts; decreased viral load; slowing progression of HIV-1 infection

## ! HIGH ALERT

## enoxaparin (Rx)
(ee-nox'a-par-in)
Lovenox
*Func. class.:* Anticoagulant, antithrombotic
*Chem. class.:* Unfractionated porcine heparin (low-molecular-weight heparin)

**Pregnancy category B**

**Do not confuse:**
enoxaparin/enoxacin, Lovenox/Lotronex

**Action:** Prevents conversion of fibrinogen to fibrin and prothrombin to thrombin by enhancing inhibitory effects of antithrombin III; produces higher ratio of anti-factor Xa to anti-factor IIa

 Alert      Canada Only      Drug on CD          * "Tall Man" lettering (See Preface)

**Therapeutic outcome:** Prevention of deep vein thrombosis

**Uses:** Prevention of DVT, pulmonary emboli in hip and knee replacement, abdominal surgery at risk for thrombosis; unstable angina/non–Q-wave MI

## Dosage and routes
### DVT prevention before hip/knee surgery
*Adult:* SUBCUT 30 mg bid given 12-24 hr postoperatively for 7-10 days until DVT risk is diminished

### DVT prevention before hip replacement
*Adult:* SUBCUT 40 mg/day started 9-15 hr preop or 30 mg bid started 12-24 hr postop, continued until DVT risk is diminished or is adequately an anticoagulant

### DVT prophylaxis before abdominal surgery
*Adult:* SUBCUT 40 mg/day × 7-10 days to prevent thromboembolic complications, start 24 hr before surgery

### Treatment of DVT/PE
*Adult:* SUBCUT (outpatient without PE) 1 mg/kg q12hr or 1.5 mg/kg/day (outpatient/inpatient); warfarin should be started within 72 hr and continued until INR is 2-3 (usually 7 days)

### Prevention of ischemic complications in unstable angina/non–Q-wave MI with aspirin
*Adult:* SUBCUT/**IV** 1 mg/kg q12hr until stable with aspirin 100-325 mg/day × ≥2 days

**Available forms:** Prefilled syringes/inj 30 mg/0.3 ml, 40 mg/0.4 ml, 60 mg/0.6 ml, 80 mg/0.8 ml, 100 mg/1 ml, 120 mg/0.8 ml, 150 mg/ml; multidose vials 100 mg/ml (3 ml)

## Adverse effects
*CNS:* Fever, confusion
*GI:* Nausea
***HEMA:*** **Hemorrhage, hypochromic anemia, thrombocytopenia,** bleeding
***INTEG:*** Ecchymosis, inj site hematoma
***SYST:*** Edema, peripheral edema

**Contraindications:** Hypersensitivity to this product, benzyl alcohol, heparin, or pork; hemophilia; leukemia with bleeding; peptic ulcer disease; thrombocytopenic purpura, heparin-induced thrombocytopenia, increased risk of bleeding

**Precautions:** Pregnancy **B**, breastfeeding, children, geriatric, severe renal/hepatic disease, blood dyscrasias, severe hypertension,

subacute bacterial endocarditis, acute nephritis, recent burn, spinal surgery, indwelling catheters, low-weight men (<57 kg), women (<45 kg)

### Pharmacokinetics
| | |
|---|---|
| **Absorption** | Well absorbed (90%) |
| **Distribution** | Unknown |
| **Metabolism** | Unknown |
| **Excretion** | Kidneys |
| **Half-life** | 4½ hr |

### Pharmacodynamics
| | |
|---|---|
| **Onset** | Unknown |
| **Peak** | 3-5 hr |
| **Duration** | Unknown |

## Interactions
### Drug classifications
Anticoagulants, antiplatelets, NSAIDs, salicylates, thrombolytics: increased bleeding
### Drug/herb
Agrimony, alfalfa, angelica, anise, basil, bay, bilberry, black haw, bogbean, bromelain, buchu, cat's claw, chondroitin, cinchona bark, dong quai, evening primrose, fenugreek, feverfew, fish oils, garlic, ginger, ginkgo, ginseng, horse chestnut, Irish moss, kava, kelp, kelpware, khella, licorice, lovage, lungwort, meadowsweet, motherwort, mugwort, nettle, papaya, parsley (large amounts), pau d'arco, pineapple, poplar, prickly ash, red clover, safflower, saw palmetto, skullcap, tonka bean, turmeric, wintergreen, yarrow: increased risk of bleeding
Chamomile, coenzyme Q10, flax, glucomannan, goldenseal, guar gum: decreased anticoagulant effect
### Drug/lab test
Increased: AST/ALT
Decreased: platelets

## NURSING CONSIDERATIONS
### Assessment
• Monitor blood studies (Hct, CBC, coagulation studies, occult blood in stools), anti-Xa levels q3 mo; platelet count q2-3 days; thrombocytopenia may occur
• Assess patient for bleeding gums, petechiae, ecchymosis, black tarry stools, hematuria, epistaxis, decrease in B/P; indicate bleeding and possible hemorrhage; notify prescriber immediately
• Assess for neurosymptoms in patients who have received spinal anesthesia

Adverse effects: *italic* = common, **bold** = life-threatening

## Nursing diagnoses
- Injury, risk for (uses, adverse reactions)
- Knowledge, deficient (teaching)
- Tissue perfusion, ineffective (uses)

## Implementation
- Give at same time each day to maintain steady blood levels

**SUBCUT route**
- Administer SUBCUT deeply; do not give IM, begin 1 hr before surgery, do not aspirate, do not expel bubble from syringe before administration; sol is clear to yellow; do not use sol with precipitate; apply gentle pressure for 1 min
- Give to recumbent patient, rotate sites (left/right anterolateral, left/right posterolateral abdominal wall)
- Leave vascular access sheath in place for 6 hr after dose, then give next dose, 6 hr after sheath removed

**IV route**
- Use multidose vial for **IV** administration; use TB syringe or other graduated syringe to measure dose; give **IV** BOL through IV line; flush after
- If withdrawing from multidose vial, use TB syringe for proper measurement
- Prefilled syringes (30, 40 mg) are not graduated; do not use for partial doses
- Do not mix with other products or infusion fluids
- ◆ Give only this product when ordered; not interchangeable with heparin or LMWHs

## Patient/family education
- Warn patient to avoid OTC preparations unless directed by prescriber because they could cause serious product interactions
- Instruct patient to use soft-bristled toothbrush to avoid bleeding gums; to avoid contact sports; to use electric razor; to avoid IM inj
- Advise patient to report any signs of bleeding, bruising: gums, under skin, urine, stools

## Evaluation
**Positive therapeutic outcome**
- Absence of DVT

---

**entacapone** (Rx)
(en-ta′-ka-pone)
Comtan
*Func. class.:* Antiparkinsonian agent
*Chem. class.:* COMT

**Pregnancy category** c

**Action:** Inhibits COMT (catechol *O*-methyltransferase) and alters the plasma pharmacokinetics of levodopa; given with levodopa/carbidopa

**Therapeutic outcome:** Decreased symptoms of Parkinson's disease (involuntary movements)

**Uses:** Parkinsonism in those experiencing end of dose, decreased effect as an adjunct to levodopa/carbidopa

## Dosage and routes
*Adult:* PO 200 mg given with carbidopa/levodopa, max 1600 mg/day

**Available forms:** Tabs 200 mg film coated

## Adverse effects
*CNS: Involuntary choreiform movements, dyskinesia, hypokinesia, hyperkinesia, hand tremors, fatigue, headache, anxiety, twitching, numbness, weakness, confusion, agitation, nightmares,* psychosis, hallucinations, hypomania, severe depression, dizziness, **neuroleptic malignant syndrome**
*CV: Orthostatic hypotension*
*GI: Nausea, vomiting, anorexia, abdominal distress, dry mouth, flatulence, dyspepsia,* gastritis, GI disorder, *diarrhea, constipation,* bitter taste
*INTEG:* Rash, sweating, alopecia
*MISC:* Dark urine and other body fluids, back pain, dyspnea, purpura, fatigue, asthenia, infection-bacterial, **rhabdomyolysis**

**Contraindications:** Hypersensitivity

**Precautions:** Pregnancy **C**, breastfeeding, children, renal/hepatic disease, affective disorders, psychosis

| Pharmacokinetics | |
|---|---|
| **Absorption** | Well absorbed |
| **Distribution** | Protein binding 98% |
| **Metabolism** | Liver extensively |
| **Excretion** | Kidneys, feces; breast milk |
| **Half-life** | 0.5 hr initial, 2.5 hr second |

| Pharmacodynamics | |
|---|---|
| **Onset** | Unknown |
| **Peak** | Unknown |
| **Duration** | ≤8 hr |

## Interactions
*Individual drugs*
Ampicillin, chloramphenicol, erythromycin, probenecid, rifampin: decreased excretion of entacapone
Bitolterol, DOBUTamine, DOPamine, epINEPHrine, isoetharine, methyldopa,

norepinephrine: increased CV reactions; avoid use

*Drug classifications*
MAOIs: prevents catecholamine metabolism, do not use together

*Drug/herb*
Kava: decreased effect

## NURSING CONSIDERATIONS
### Assessment
- Assess for neuroleptic malignant syndrome: high temp, increased CPK, rigidity, change in consciousness
- Monitor B/P, respiration during initial treatment; hypotension should be reported
- Assess mental status: affect, mood, behavioral changes, depression; complete suicide assessment
- Monitor liver function enzymes: AST, ALT, alkaline phosphatase; also check LDH, bilirubin, CBC
- Assess for involuntary movements in parkinsonism: akinesia, tremors, staggering gait, muscle rigidity, drooling; these symptoms should improve with therapy when given with levodopa/carbidopa

### Nursing diagnoses
- Injury, risk for (uses)
- Knowledge, deficient (teaching)
- Mobility, impaired physical (uses)
- Noncompliance (teaching)

### Implementation
- Adjust dosage to patient response
- Give with meals to decrease GI upset; limit protein taken with product
- Give only after MAOIs have been discontinued for 2 wk

### Patient/family education
- Advise patient that hallucinations, mental changes, nausea, dyskinesia can occur
- Caution patient to change positions slowly to prevent orthostatic hypotension; not to drive or operate machinery until stabilized on medication and mental performance is not affected
- Instruct patient to use product exactly as prescribed
- Inform patient that urine, sweat may darken
- Inform patient to notify prescriber if pregnancy is suspected; if breastfeeding, product is excreted in breast milk

### Evaluation
**Positive therapeutic outcome**
- Decreased akathisia, other involuntary movements when used with levodopa/carbidopa
- Increased mood when used with levodopa/carbidopa

---

## entecavir (Rx)
(en-te′ka-veer)
Baraclude
*Func. class.:* Antiviral
*Chem. class.:* Guanosine nucleoside analog
**Pregnancy category C**

**Action:** Inhibits hepatitis B virus DNA polymerase by competing with natural substrates and by causing DNA termination after its incorporation into viral DNA; causes viral DNA death

**Therapeutic outcome:** Improved liver function tests in chronic hepatitis B (HBV)

**Uses:** Chronic hepatitis B (HBV)

**Dosage and routes**
*Chronic hepatitis B (nucleoside treatment–naive)*
*Adult and adolescent ≥16 yr:* PO 0.5 mg/day

*Chronic hepatitis B while receiving lamivudine or known lamivudine resistance mutations*
*Adult and adolescent ≥16 yr:* PO 1 mg/day

*Renal dose*
*Adult:* PO CCr ≥50 ml/min 0.5 mg/day; CCr 30-49 ml/min 0.25 mg daily, 0.5 mg/day for lamivudine refractory patient; CCr 10-29 ml/min 0.15/day, 0.3 for lamivudine refractory patient; CCr <10 ml/min 0.05 mg PO/day, 0.1 mg for lamivudine refractory patient

**Available forms:** Tabs, film coated 0.5, 1 mg; oral sol 0.05 mg/ml

**Adverse effects**
*CNS: Headache*, fatigue, dizziness, insomnia
*GI: Dyspepsia*, nausea, vomiting, diarrhea
***SYST: Lactic acidosis, severe hepatomegaly with stenosis***

**Contraindications:** Hypersensitivity

**Precautions:** Pregnancy **C**, breastfeeding, child, geriatric, severe renal disease

### Pharmacokinetics
| | |
|---|---|
| **Absorption** | 100% |
| **Distribution** | Extensively to tissues, protein binding 13% |
| **Metabolism** | Unknown |
| **Excretion** | Unchanged 62%-73% via kidneys |
| **Half-life** | Terminal 128-149 hr |

E

---

Adverse effects: *italic* = common, **bold** = life-threatening

| Pharmacodynamics | |
|---|---|
| **Onset** | Unknown |
| **Peak** | 0.5-1.5 hr |
| **Duration** | Unknown |

## Interactions
### Drug/lab test
Increased: ALT, AST, total bilirubin, amylase, lipase, creatinine, blood glucose, urine glucose
Decreased: platelets, albumin

## NURSING CONSIDERATIONS
### Assessment
• Assess for nephrotoxicity: increasing CCr, BUN
• Assess for HIV before beginning treatment because HIV resistance may occur in patients with chronic hepatitis B infection
◆ Assess for lactic acidosis, severe hepatomegaly with stenosis
• Monitor geriatric patients more carefully; may develop renal, cardiac symptoms more rapidly
• Assess for exacerbations of hepatitis after discontinuing treatment, monitor liver function tests

### Nursing diagnoses
• Infection, risk for (uses)
• Injury, risk for (uses, adverse reactions)

### Implementation
• Give by mouth on empty stomach 2 hr before or after food
• Store in cool environment; protect from light

### Patient/family education
• Teach patient not to take with food
• Teach patient to take exactly as prescribed
• Advise patient not to stop medication without approval of prescriber
• Advise that optimal duration of treatment is unknown
• Teach patient to avoid use with other medications unless approved by prescriber
• Teach patient to notify prescriber of decreased urinary output, blood in urine
• Teach patient symptoms of lactic acidosis: muscle pain, severe tiredness, weakness, trouble breathing, stomach pain with nausea/vomiting, coldness in arms/legs, fast/irregular heartbeat, dizziness
• Teach patient symptoms of hepatotoxicity: eyes/skin turns yellow, dark urine, light bowel movements, no appetite for days, nausea, stomach pain

• Advise patient that product does not cure, but lowers the amount of HBV in body
• Teach patient that product does not stop the spreading of HBV to others by sex, sharing needles, or being exposed to blood

### Evaluation
**Positive therapeutic outcome**
• Decreased symptoms of chronic hepatitis B, improving liver function tests

## ! HIGH ALERT

## *epHEDrine (Rx, OTC)
(e-fed′rin)
epHEDrine sulfate, Pretz-D
*Func. class.:* Bronchodilator, nonselective, adrenergic, mixed direct and indirect effects; bronchodilator, nasal decongestant, vasopressor
*Chem. class.:* Phenylisopropylamine

**Pregnancy category** C

**Do not confuse:**
epHEDrine/epINEPHrine

**Action:** Increases contractility and heart rate by acting on β-receptors in the heart; also acts on α-receptors, causing vasoconstriction in blood vessels

**Therapeutic outcome:** Decreased nasal congestion, bronchodilatation, stimulation, increased B/P

**Uses:** Shock; increased perfusion; hypotension, bronchodilatation; nasal congestion; orthostatic hypotension, depression, narcolepsy; vasopressor

### Dosage and routes
#### Bronchodilator
*Adult and child >12 yr:* PO 12.5-50 mg q3-4hr prn, max 150 mg/24 hr; NASAL 2-3 sprays in each nostril q4hr
*Child 2-12 yr:* PO 2-3 mg/kg or 100 mg/m²/day in 4-6 divided doses

#### Nasal decongestant
*Adult:* Fill dropper to the level marked, then use in each nostril q4hr or less

#### Hypotension
*Adult:* PO 25 mg daily-qid; IM/SUBCUT 25-50 mg; **IV** 10-25 mg max 150 mg/24 hr
*Child:* SUBCUT/**IV** 25-100 mg/m²/day in 4-6 divided doses

**Available forms:** Inj 25, 30, 50 mg/ml; caps 25, 50 mg

## Adverse effects
*CNS: Tremors, anxiety,* insomnia, sweating, headache, dizziness, confusion, hallucinations, **seizures, CNS depression, cerebral hemorrhage,** weakness, drowsiness
*CV:* Palpitations, tachycardia, hypertension, chest pain, **dysrhythmias**
*GI: Anorexia, nausea, vomiting*
*GU:* Dysuria, urinary retention
*RESP: Dyspnea*

**Contraindications:** Hypersensitivity to sympathomimetics, angle-closure glaucoma, nonanaphylactic shock during general anesthesia, diabetes mellitus, hypertension

**Precautions:** Pregnancy **C,** breastfeeding, cardiac disorders, hyperthyroidism, prostatic hypertrophy, angina

### Pharmacokinetics

| | |
|---|---|
| **Absorption** | Well absorbed (PO/IM/SUBCUT), complete (**IV**) |
| **Distribution** | Unknown |
| **Metabolism** | Liver |
| **Excretion** | Kidneys—unchanged |
| **Half-life** | 3-5 hr |

### Pharmacodynamics

| | PO | SUBCUT | IM | IV | NASAL |
|---|---|---|---|---|---|
| **Onset** | ¼-1 hr | Unkn | 15-30 min | 5 min | Unkn |
| **Peak** | Unkn | Unkn | Unkn | Unkn | Unkn |
| **Dura-tion** | 2-4 hr | 1 hr | 1 hr | 2 hr | 6 hr |

## Interactions
### Individual drugs
Guanethidine: decreased effect of guanethidine
Levodopa: increased dysrhythmias
Methyldopa: decreased effect of epHEDrine
### Drug classifications
α-Adrenergic blockers, antidepressants (tricyclic), diuretics, rauwolfia alkaloids, urinary acidifiers: decreased effect of epHEDrine
Anesthetics (halothane), cardiac glycosides: increased dysrhythmias
Ergots: hypertensive crisis
MAOIs: increased chance of hypertensive crisis, do not use together
Oxytoxics: increased severe hypertension
Sympathomimetics: increased adrenergic side effects
Urinary alkalizers: increased effect of epHEDrine

## NURSING CONSIDERATIONS
### Assessment
• Monitor respiratory function: vital capacity, forced expiratory volume, ABGs, lung sounds, heart rate, baseline rhythm (bronchodilator)
• Monitor for evidence of allergic reactions; paradoxical bronchospasm; withhold dose; notify prescriber
• Monitor ECG, B/P, pulse, q5 min when using **IV** route (shock)
• Assess for paresthesias and coldness of extremities; peripheral blood flow may decrease; long-term use may produce pseudo anxiety state requiring sedatives, increased lactic acid with severe metabolic acidosis
• Assess nasal congestion to identify factors contributing to ongoing congestion (nasal use)
• Assess mental status and sleeping patterns; mood, sensorium, ability to stay awake

### Nursing diagnoses
• Airway clearance, ineffective (uses)
• Gas exchange, impaired (uses)
• Knowledge, deficient (teaching)
• Sleep deprivation (uses)

### Implementation
**PO route**
• Administer several hr (up to 6 hr) before bedtime to prevent sleeplessness
**IV route**
• Give **IV** directly undiluted using 3-way stopcock or Y-site; give 10-25 mg slowly, may repeat in 5-10 min
• Use clear sol without precipitate; unused sol should be discarded, protect from light
*Syringe compatibilities:* Pentobarbital
*Y-site compatibilities:* Etomidate, propofol
*Additive compatibilities:* Chloramphenicol, lidocaine, metaraminol, nafcillin, penicillin G potassium
*Solution compatibilities:* 0.9% NaCl, 0.45% NaCl, $D_5W$, $D_{10}W$, Ringer's, LR

### Patient/family education
• Advise patient to avoid use of OTC medications; extra stimulation may occur, and not to use alcohol

### Evaluation
**Positive therapeutic outcome**
• Increased B/P (vasopressor)
• Ability to stay awake (absence of narcolepsy) or improved mood (absence of depression)
• Absence of bronchospasm
• Decreased nasal congestion

E

Adverse effects: *italic* = common, **bold** = life-threatening

---

### *epHEDrine nasal agent
*See Appendix D*

---

### epinastine ophthalmic
*See Appendix D*

---

### ⚠ HIGH ALERT

### *epINEPHrine (Rx, OTC)
(ep-i-nef′rin)
Adrenalin, Ana-Guard, AsthmaHaler Mist, AsthmaNefrin (racepinephrine), Bronitin Mist, Bronkaid Mist, epINEPHrine, Epinal, Epitrate, Eppy/N, Epinephrine Pediatric, EpiPen, EpiPen Jr., Medihaler, microNefrin, Nephron, Primatene Mist, S-2, Sus-Phrine, Vaponefrin (racepinephrine)
*Func. class.:* Bronchodilator, nonselective adrenergic agonist, cardiac stimulant, vasopressor
*Chem. class.:* Catecholamine

**Pregnancy category** C

**Do not confuse:**
epINEPHrine/ePHEDrine

**Action:** $\beta_1$- and $\beta_2$-agonist causing increased levels of cyclic AMP producing bronchodilatation, cardiac and CNS stimulation; large doses cause vasoconstriction via α-receptors; small doses can cause vasodilation via $\beta_2$-vascular receptors

**Therapeutic outcome:** Vasoconstrictor, cardiac stimulator, bronchodilator, decreased aqueous humor

**Uses:** Acute asthmatic attacks, hemostasis, bronchospasm, anaphylaxis, allergic reactions, cardiac arrest, adjunct in anesthesia, shock

**Dosage and routes**
*Asthma*
*Adult and child:* INH 1-2 puffs of 1:100 or 2.25% racemic q15 min

*Bronchodilator*
*Adult:* SUBCUT/IM 0.3-0.5 mg (1:1000 sol) q10-15 min-4 hr, max 1 mg/dose

*Anaphylactic reaction/asthma*
*Adult:* SUBCUT/IM 0.3-0.5 mg, repeat q10-15 min, not to exceed 1 mg/dose; epINEPHrine susp 0.5 mg SUBCUT, may repeat 0.5-1.5 mg q6hr
*Child:* SUBCUT 0.01 mg/kg, repeat q15 min × 2 doses, then q4hr as needed, up to 0.5 mg/dose; epINEPHrine susp 0.025 mg/kg SUBCUT, may repeat q6hr, max 0.75 mg in child ≤30 kg

*Cardiac arrest (ACLS)*
*Adult:* IV 1 mg q3-5 min; ENDOTRACHEAL 2-25 mg; IC 0.3-0.5 mg

*Symptomatic bradycardia/pulseless arrest (PALS)*
*Child:* IV 0.01 mg/kg, may repeat q3-5 min; ENDOTRACHEAL give 2-10 × IV dose diluted to a volume of 3-5 mg of 0.9% NaCl, followed by positive pressure ventilation

**Available forms:** Aerosol 0.16, 0.2, 0.25 mg/spray, inj 1:1000 (1 mg/ml), 1:200 (5 mg/ml), 0.01 mg/ml (1:100,000), 0.1 mg/ml (1:10,000), 0.5 mg/ml (1:2,000); sol for nebulization 1:100, 1.25% 2.25% (base)

**Adverse effects**
*CNS: Tremors, anxiety,* insomnia, headache, dizziness, weakness, drowsiness, confusion, hallucinations, **cerebral hemorrhage**
*CV: Palpitations, tachycardia,* hypertension, *dysrhythmias,* increased T-wave
*GI: Anorexia, nausea, vomiting*
*MISC:* Sweating, dry eyes
*RESP:* Dyspnea

**Contraindications:** Hypersensitivity to sympathomimetics, angle-closure glaucoma, nonanaphylactic shock during general anesthesia

**Precautions:** Pregnancy C, breastfeeding, cardiac disorders, hyperthyroidism, diabetes mellitus, prostatic hypertrophy, hypertension, organic brain syndrome, local anesthesia of certain areas, labor, cardiac dilation, coronary insufficiency, cerebral arteriosclerosis, organic heart disease

**Pharmacokinetics**

| | |
|---|---|
| **Absorption** | Well absorbed (PO), complete (**IV**) |
| **Distribution** | Unknown, crosses placenta |
| **Metabolism** | Liver |
| **Excretion** | Breast milk |
| **Half-life** | Unknown |

**Pharmacodynamics**

| | SUBCUT | IM | IV | INH |
|---|---|---|---|---|
| **Onset** | 3-5 min | 5-10 min | Immediate | 1 min |
| **Peak** | Unknown | Unknown | Unknown | Unknown |
| **Duration** | 1-4 hr | 1-4 hr | Unknown | 1-4 hr |

---

 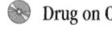

## Interactions
### Drug classifications
α-Adrenergic blockers: decreased hypertensive effects

Antidepressants (tricyclics): increased chance of hypertensive crisis; do not use together

MAOIs: increased chance of hypertensive crisis, do not use together

Other sympathomimetics: toxicity

## NURSING CONSIDERATIONS
### Assessment
- Monitor respiratory function: vital capacity, forced expiratory volume, ABGs, lung sounds, heart rate, rhythm (baseline); amount, color of sputum
- Monitor ECG during administration continuously; if B/P increases, product should be decreased; check B/P, pulse q5 min after parenteral route; CVP, PCWP, SVR; inadvertent high arterial B/P can result in angina, aortic rupture, cerebral hemorrhage
- Check inj site for tissue sloughing; if this occurs, administer phentolamine mixed with 0.9% NaCl
- Monitor for evidence of allergic reactions, paradoxical bronchospasm, withhold dose, notify prescriber; sulfite sensitivity, which may be life threatening

### Nursing diagnoses
- Airway clearance, ineffective (uses)
- Cardiac output, decreased (uses)
- Gas exchange, impaired (uses)
- Knowledge, deficient (teaching)
- Sensory perception, disturbed, visual (uses) (ophth)

### Implementation
- Check for correct concentration, route, dosage before administration
- Use this medication before other medications and allow at least 5 min between each to prevent overstimulation

**IM/SUBCUT route**
- Rotate inj sites, massage well, do not use gluteal (IM) site
- Shake susp before using

**Inhalation route**
- Use 2.25% sol diluted in nebulizer/respirator
- Rinse mouth after inh
- 10 gtt of a 1% sol should be placed in nebulizer
- Dilute racepinephrine 2.25% sol

**Endotracheal route**
- Only used in intubated patient; use **IV** dose that should be injected by endotracheal tube into bronchi

**IV route**
- Give after diluting 1 mg of 1:1000 sol/10 ml or more; 0.9% NaCl yields 1:10,000 sol, give 1 mg/min
- Give by continuous inf after further diluting in 0.9% NaCl, $D_5W$, $D_{10}W$, $D_5/LR$, LR via 3-way stopcock; for Y-site, use infusion pump, protect from light; increase dose of insulin in diabetic patients

**Syringe compatibilities:** Doxapram, heparin, milrinone

**Y-site compatibilities:** Amrinone, atracurium, calcium chloride, calcium gluconate, diltiazem, DOBUTamine, DOPamine, famotidine, fentanyl, furosemide, heparin, hydrocortisone sodium succinate, hydromorphone, labetalol, lorazepam, midazolam, milrinone, morphine, niCARdipine, nitroglycerin, norepinephrine, pancuronium, phytonadione, potassium chloride, propofol, ranitidine, vecuronium, vit B/C

**Y-site incompatibilities:** Ampicillin

**Additive compatibilities:** Amikacin, cimetidine, DOBUTamine, floxacillin, furosemide, metaraminol, ranitidine, verapamil

**Additive incompatibilities:** Aminophylline, mephentermine, sodium bicarbonate, warfarin

### Patient/family education
- Tell patient not to use OTC medications; extra stimulation may occur; to use this medication before other medications and allow at least 5 min between each, to prevent overstimulation
- Teach patient that paradoxical bronchospasm may occur and to stop product immediately and notify prescriber; to limit caffeine products such as chocolate, coffee, tea, and colas
- Patient should rinse mouth after inhalation
- Patient should report blurred vision, irritation with ophth preparations

### Evaluation
**Positive therapeutic outcome**
- Absence of dyspnea, wheezing
- Improved airway exchange, improved ABGs
- Decreased aqueous humor
- Stabilization of heart rate and cardiac output

**Treatment of overdose:** Administer a $\beta_2$-adrenergic blocker, vasodilators, α-blocker

---

**\*epINEPHrine/epinephryl borate ophthalmic**
*See Appendix D*

---

Adverse effects: *italic* = common, **bold** = life-threatening

## *epINEPHrine nasal agent
*See Appendix D*

---

! HIGH ALERT

### epirubicin (Rx)
(ep-i-roo'-bi-sin)
Ellence
*Func. class.:* Antineoplastic, antibiotic
*Chem. class.:* Anthracycline

**Pregnancy category D**

**Action:** Inhibits DNA synthesis primarily; replication is decreased by binding to DNA, which causes strand splitting; maximum cytotoxic effects at S and $G_2$ phases; a vesicant

**Therapeutic outcome:** Prevention of rapidly growing malignant cells

**Uses:** Breast cancer as an adjuvant therapy, with axillary node involvement, after resection

**Unlabeled uses:** Used in combination for treatment of advanced forms of cancer

### Dosage and routes
*Adult:* **IV** INF 100-120 mg/m² initially given with other antineoplastics (cyclophosphamide, 5-fluorouracil); given in repeated cycles; 3-4 wk cycles

### Epirubicin dosage adjustments
*Adult:* **IV** 100 mg/m² on day 1 of each cycle; toxicity nadir platelet counts <50,000 mm³, ANC 250 mm³, neutropenic fever or grade 3 or 4 nonhematologic toxicity; next cycle give 75% of day 1 dose; delay next cycle until platelets are ≥100,000 mm³, ANC >1500 mm³, and nonhematologic toxicities have recovered to < grade 1

### Hepatic dose
*Adult:* **IV** Bilirubin 1.2-3 mg/dl or AST 2-4 × normal upper limit, 50% of starting dose; bilirubin >3 mg/dl or AST >4 × normal upper limit, 25% of starting dose

**Available forms:** Inj 2 mg/ml

### Adverse effects
*CV:* Increased B/P, **sinus tachycardia, PVCs,** chest pain, **bradycardia, extrasystole, CHF; confirm for doses >900 mg/m²**
*GI:* Nausea, vomiting, diarrhea, anorexia, mucositis
*GU: Hot flashes, amenorrhea, hyperuricemia*
*HEMA:* **Thrombocytopenia, leukopenia, anemia, neutropenia, secondary AML**
*INTEG: Rash, necrosis, pain at inj site, reversible alopecia*

*MISC:* Infection, febrile neutropenia, lethargy, fever, conjunctivitis

**Contraindications:** Pregnancy **D**, breastfeeding, hypersensitivity to this product, anthracyclines, anthracenediones, systemic infections, severe hepatic disease, baseline neutrophil count <1500 cell/mm³, severe myocardial insufficiency, recent MI

**Precautions:** Children, geriatric, renal/hepatic/cardiac disease, gout, bone marrow suppression (severe)

### Pharmacokinetics
| | |
|---|---|
| **Absorption** | Complete bioavailability |
| **Distribution** | Widely distributed, crosses placenta |
| **Metabolism** | Liver, extensively |
| **Excretion** | Bile (60%) |
| **Half-life** | 3 min; 2.5 hr; 33 hr |

### Pharmacodynamics
Unknown

### Interactions
*Individual drugs*
Cimetidine, radiation: increased toxicity
*Drug classifications*
Antineoplastics: increased toxicity
Live virus vaccines: decreased antibody response

### NURSING CONSIDERATIONS
**Assessment**
• Monitor left ventricular ejection fraction, multigated acquisition scan or echocardiogram, ECG; watch for ST-T wave changes, low QRS and T; possible dysrhythmias (sinus tachycardia, heart block, PVCs) may occur; assess tachypnea, ECG changes, dyspnea, edema, fatigue; cardiac status: B/P, pulse, character, rhythm, rate, ABGs
• Assess for bone marrow depression, infection
• Assess symptoms indicating severe allergic reaction: rash, pruritus, urticaria, purpuric skin lesions, itching, flushing; product should be discontinued
• Monitor CBC, differential, platelet count weekly; withhold product if baseline neutrophil count is <1500/mm³; notify prescriber of results if WBC <20,000/mm³, platelets <150,000/mm³; leukocyte nadir occurs 10-14 days after administration, recovery by 21st day
• Assess for increased uric acid levels, swelling, joint pain, primarily extremities; patient should be well hydrated to prevent urate deposits

---

 Alert ♣ Canada Only 🌀 Drug on CD * ''Tall Man'' lettering (See Preface)

- Monitor renal function studies: BUN, creatinine, serum uric acid, urine CCr before and during therapy; I&O ratio; report fall in urine output to <30 ml/hr; dosage adjustment is needed if serum creatinine >5 mg/dl
- Monitor liver function tests before and during therapy (bilirubin, AST, ALT, LDH) as needed or monthly; note jaundice of skin or sclera, dark urine, clay-colored stools, itchy skin, abdominal pain, fever, diarrhea
- Assess for bleeding: hematuria, stool guaiac, bruising or petechiae, mucosa or orifices q8hr; inflammation of mucosa, breaks in skin
- Identify effects of alopecia on body image; discuss feeling about body changes

### Nursing diagnoses
- Body image, disturbed (adverse reactions)
- Infection, risk for (adverse reactions)
- Injury, risk for (adverse reactions)
- Knowledge, deficient (teaching)

### Implementation
- Avoid contact with skin; very irritating; wash completely to remove; give fluids **IV** or PO before chemotherapy to hydrate patient
- Give antiemetic 30-60 min before giving product to prevent vomiting and prn
- Administer prophylactic antibiotic with a fluoroquinolone or trimethoprim/sulfamethoxazole if dose of epirubicin is 120 mg/m²
- Provide liquid diet: carbonated beverages; gelatin may be added if patient is not nauseated or vomiting
- Product should be prepared by experienced personnel using proper precautions
- Give into tubing of free-flowing **IV** inf 0.9% NaCl or $D_5$ over 3-5 min; do not admix with other products in syringe
- Use hydrocortisone, dexamethasone, or sodium bicarbonate (1 mEq/1 ml) for extravasation: apply ice compress

### Patient/family education
- Advise patient to avoid use of products containing aspirin or NSAIDs, razors, commercial mouthwash, since bleeding may occur; to report symptoms of bleeding (hematuria, tarry stools)
- Instruct patient to report signs of anemia (fatigue, headache, irritability, faintness, shortness of breath)
- Inform patient that hair may be lost during treatment; a wig or hairpiece may make patient feel better; new hair may be different in color, texture
- Caution patient not to have any vaccinations without the advice of the prescriber; serious reactions can occur

- Advise patient to use contraception during treatment and 4 mo afterward
- Advise patient that urine may appear red for 2 days
- Instruct patient to avoid crowds, persons with known infection
- Caution patient to avoid OTC medications, supplements unless approved by prescriber

### Evaluation
**Positive therapeutic outcome**
- Prevention of rapid division of malignant cells

E

### eplerenone (Rx)
(ep-ler-ee′known)
Inspra
*Func. class.:* Antihypertensive

**Pregnancy category B**

**Action:** Binds to mineralocorticoid receptor and blocks the binding of aldosterone, a component of the renin-angiotensin-aldosterone system (RAAS)

**Therapeutic outcome:** Absence of hypertension

**Uses:** Hypertension, alone or in combination with thiazide diuretics, CHF, post-MI

### Dosage and routes
*Adult:* PO 50 mg/day initially, may increase to 50 mg bid after 4 wk; start dose at 25 mg/day if patient is taking CYP3A4 inhibitors

### CHF/post-MI
*Adult:* PO 25 mg/day initially, may increase to 50 mg/day max

**Available forms:** Tabs 25, 50, 100 mg

### Adverse effects
*CNS:* Headache, dizziness, fatigue
*CV:* Angina, **MI**
*GI:* Increased GGT diarrhea, abdominal pain, increased ALT
*GU:* Increased BUN, creatinine, gynecomastia, mastodynia (males), abnormal vaginal bleeding
*META:* Hyperkalemia, hyponatremia, hypercholesteremia, hypertriglyceridemia, increased uric acid
*RESP:* Cough

**Contraindications:** Breastfeeding, children, hypersensitivity, increased serum creatinine >2 mg/dl (male) or >1.8 mg/dl (female), potassium >5.5 mEq/L, type 2 diabetes with microalbuminuria, hepatic disease, CCr <30 ml/min, CCr <50 ml/min in hypertension

**Precautions:** Pregnancy **B**, breastfeeding, geriatric, impaired renal/hepatic function, hyperkalemia

### Pharmacokinetics

| | |
|---|---|
| **Absorption** | Unknown |
| **Distribution** | Protein binding 50% |
| **Metabolism** | Liver (CYP3A4 inhibitor) |
| **Excretion** | Urine |
| **Half-life** | 4-6 hr |

### Pharmacodynamics

| | |
|---|---|
| **Onset** | Unknown |
| **Peak** | 1½ hr |
| **Duration** | Unknown |

### Interactions
#### Individual drugs
Erythromycin, fluconazole, itraconazole, ketoconazole, saquinavir, verapamil: increased levels of eplerenone, reduce dose of eplerenone
Lithium: increased serum lithium levels
#### Drug classifications
ACE inhibitors, angiotensin II antagonists, diuretics (potassium-sparing), NSAIDs, potassium supplements: increased hyperkalemia
CYP3A4 inhibitors: increased levels of eplerenone, reduce dose of eplerenone
NSAIDs: decreased antihypertensive effect
#### Drug/herb
Aconite: increased toxicity, death
Astragalus, cola tree: increased or decreased antihypertensive effect
Barberry, betony, black catechu, black cohosh, bloodroot, broom, burdock, cat's claw, dandelion, goldenseal, hawthorn, Irish moss, Jamaican dogwood, kelp, khella, mistletoe, parsley: increased antihypertensive effect
Coltsfoot, guarana, khat, licorice, yohimbe: decreased antihypertensive effect
St. John's wort: decreased levels of eplerenone
#### Drug/food
Grapefruit juice: increased product level by 25%

### NURSING CONSIDERATIONS
#### Assessment
• Monitor B/P at peak/trough level of product, orthostatic hypotension, syncope when used with diuretic

• Monitor renal studies: protein, BUN, creatinine; increased liver function tests; uric acid may be increased
• Monitor potassium levels, hyperkalemia may occur

#### Nursing diagnoses
• Cardiac output, decreased (uses)
• Diarrhea (side effects)
• Knowledge, deficient (teaching)
• Noncompliance (teaching)
• Tissue perfusion, ineffective (uses)

#### Implementation
• Store in tight container at 86° F (30° C) or less

#### Patient/family education
• Advise not to discontinue product abruptly
• Advise not to use OTC products (cough, cold, allergy) unless directed by prescriber; do not use salt substitutes containing potassium without consulting prescriber
• Teach the importance of complying with dosage schedule, even if feeling better
• Teach that product may cause dizziness, fainting, light-headedness; may occur during first few days of therapy
• Teach how to take B/P, and normal readings for age-group

#### Evaluation
**Positive therapeutic outcome**
• Decreased in B/P

---

### epoetin (Rx)
(ee-poe′e-tin)
Epogen, EPO, Eprex ✦, Procrit
*Func. class.:* Antianemic, biologic modifier, hormone
*Chem. class.:* Amino acid polypeptide
#### Pregnancy category C

**Action:** Erythropoietin is one factor controlling rate of red cell production; product is developed by recombinant DNA technology

**Therapeutic outcome:** Decreased anemia with increased RBCs

**Uses:** Anemia caused by reduced endogenous erythropoietin production, primarily end-stage renal disease; to correct hemostatic defect in uremia; anemia caused by AZT (zidovudine) treatment in HIV-positive patients; anemia caused by chemotherapy; reduction of allogeneic blood transfusion in surgery patients

**Unlabeled uses:** Pruritus, anemia in premature preterm infants, anemia in myelodysplastic syndrome, anemia in chronic inflammatory disorders

## Dosage and routes
### Anemia secondary to chemotherapy
*Adult:* SUBCUT 150 units/kg 3×/wk, may increase after 2 mo up to 300 units/kg 3×/wk

### Anemia in chronic renal failure
*Adult:* SUBCUT/**IV** 50-100 units/kg 3×/wk, then adjust to maintain the target Hct of 30%-36%
*Child:* **IV**/SUBCUT 50 units/kg 3×/wk

### Anemia secondary to zidovudine treatment
*Adult:* SUBCUT/**IV** 100 units/kg 3×/wk × 2 mo; may increase by 50-100 units/kg q1-2 mo, up to 300 units/kg 3×/wk

### Surgery
*Adult:* SUBCUT 300 units/kg/day × 10 days before surgery, the day of surgery and for 4 days postsurgery or 600 units/kg 3, 2, 1 wk before and on day of surgery

**Available forms:** Inj 2000, 3000, 4000, 10,000, 20,000, 40,000 units/ml

## Adverse effects
*CNS:* **Seizures,** coldness, sweating, headache
*CV:* *Hypertension,* **hypertensive encephalopathy, CHF**
*MISC:* Iron deficiency
*MS:* Bone pain

**Contraindications:** Hypersensitivity to mammalian cell-derived products, or human albumin, uncontrolled hypertension

**Precautions:** Pregnancy **C,** breastfeeding, children <1 mo, seizure disorder, porphyria, Hgb >12 g/dl, CV disease, hemodialysis, latex allergy, surgery, hypertension, history of CABG, multidose preserved formulation contains benzyl alcohol and should not be used in premature infants

### Pharmacokinetics

| | |
|---|---|
| **Absorption** | Well absorbed (SUBCUT), completely absorbed (**IV**) |
| **Distribution** | Increased RBC count 2-6 wk |
| **Metabolism** | Unknown |
| **Excretion** | Unknown |
| **Half-life** | 5-14 hr |

### Pharmacodynamics

| | SUBCUT/IV |
|---|---|
| **Onset** | Unknown |
| **Peak** | Immediate |
| **Duration** | Unknown |

## Interactions
### Drug classifications
Anticoagulants: need for increased heparin during hemodialysis

## NURSING CONSIDERATIONS
### Assessment
• Monitor renal studies: urinalysis, protein, blood, BUN, creatinine; I&O; report drop in output to <50 ml/hr

◆ Monitor blood studies: ferritin, transferrin monthly, transferrin sat ≥20%; ferritin ≥100 ng/ml; Hct 2×/wk until stabilized in target range (30%-36%) then at regular intervals; those with endogenous erythropoietin levels of <500 units/L respond to this agent; check for symptoms of anemia: fatigue, pallor, dyspnea; monitor Hct 2×/wk in chronic renal failure; those being treated with zidovudine or cancer patients should be monitored weekly, then periodically after stabilization; death may occur in Hgb >12 g/dl

• Assess for CNS symptoms: coldness, sweating, pain in long bones

• Assess CV status: B/P before and during treatment; hypertension may occur rapidly leading to hypertension encephalopathy, antihypertensives may be needed

• Assess patient during hemodialysis for bruits, thrills, or shunts; product prevents severe anemia in chronic renal failure; clotting may need to be treated with increased anticoagulant

• Assess for seizures if Hct is increased within 2 wk by 4 pts

• Monitor serum iron levels, ferritin, transferrin levels; iron therapy may be needed to prevent recurring anemia

• Monitor B/P, check for rising B/P as Hct rises

• Monitor blood studies: BUN, creatinine, uric acid, platelets, WBC, phosphorus, potassium, bleeding time; Hct, Hgb, RBCs, reticulocytes should be checked in chronic renal failure

• For hypersensitivity reactions: Skin rashes, urticaria (rare), antibody development does not occur

◆ For pure cell aplasia (PRCA) in absence of other causes, evaluate by testing sera for recombinant erythropoietin antibodies; any loss of response to epoetin should be evaluated

### Nursing diagnoses
• Activity intolerance (uses)
• Fatigue (uses)
• Knowledge, deficient (teaching)

Adverse effects: *italic* = common, **bold** = life-threatening

## Implementation
**SUBCUT route**
- Before injecting, preservative-free, single-dose formulation may be admixed by using 0.9% NaCl, USP, with benzyl alcohol 0.9% at a 1:1 ratio to reduce injection site discomfort

**IV route**
- Administer by direct route at end of dialysis by venous line, do not shake vial
- If Hct increases by 4% in 2 wk, decrease dose by 25 units/kg; increase dose if Hct does not increase by 5-6 pts after 8 wk of therapy, suggested target Hct range 30%-36%
- Give additional heparin to lower chance of clots

*Solution compatibilities:* Do not dilute or administer with other solutions

## Patient/family education
- Teach patient how to take B/P
- Advise patients to take iron supplements, vit B$_{12}$, folic acid as directed
- Teach patient to avoid driving or hazardous activity during treatment
- Teach patients with renal disease to include high-iron and low-potassium foods in their diets (meat, dark green leafy vegetables, eggs, enriched breads)
- Teach patient the reason for treatment, expected results
- Advise patient to use contraception

## Evaluation
**Positive therapeutic outcome**
- Increased appetite
- Enhanced sense of well-being
- Increased in reticulocyte count in 2-6 wk, Hgb, Hct

---

## eprosartan (Rx)
(ep-roh-sar'tan)
Teveten
*Func. class.:* Antihypertensive
*Chem. class.:* Angiotensin II receptor antagonist (Subtype AT$_1$)

**Pregnancy category**
C (1st trimester),
D (2nd/3rd trimesters)

**Action:** Blocks the vasoconstrictor and aldosterone-secreting effects of angiotensin II; selectively blocks the binding of angiotensin II to the AT$_1$ receptor found in tissues

**Therapeutic outcome:** Decreased B/P

**Uses:** Hypertension, alone or in combination with other antihypertensives

## Dosage and routes
*Adult:* PO 600 mg/day; dose may be divided and given bid with total daily doses ranging from 400-800 mg

**Available forms:** Tabs 400, 600 mg

**Adverse effects**
*CNS:* *Dizziness*, depression, fatigue, headache
*CV:* Chest pain
*EENT:* Sinusitis
*GI:* *Diarrhea, dyspepsia,* abdominal pain
*GU:* UTI
*META:* Hypertriglyceridemia
*MS:* Myalgia, arthralgia
*RESP:* *Cough, upper respiratory infection,* rhinitis, pharyngitis, viral infection

**Contraindications:** Pregnancy **D** (2nd/3rd trimesters), hypersensitivity

**Precautions:** Pregnancy **C** (1st trimester), breastfeeding, children, geriatric, hypersensitivity to ACE inhibitors, renal/hepatic disease, angioedema

| Pharmacokinetics | |
|---|---|
| **Absorption** | Absolute bioavailability ~13%; food delays absorption |
| **Distribution** | Protein binding 98% |
| **Metabolism** | Moderate renal impairment increases product levels by 30%, hepatic impairment increases levels by 40% |
| **Excretion** | Urine, feces |
| **Half-life** | 5-9 hr |

| Pharmacodynamics | |
|---|---|
| **Onset** | Unknown |
| **Peak** | 1-2 hr |
| **Duration** | Unknown |

## Interactions
*Drug classifications*
NSAIDs, salicylates: decreased antihypertensive effect
*Drug/herb*
Aconite: increased toxicity, death
Astragalus, cola tree: increased or decreased antihypertensive effect
Barberry, betony, black catechu, black cohosh, bloodroot, broom, burdock, cat's claw, dandelion, goldenseal, Irish moss, Jamaican dogwood, kelp, khella, mistletoe, parsley: increased antihypertensive effect
Coltsfoot, guarana, khat, licorice, yohimbe: decreased antihypertensive effect
*Drug/lab test*
Increased: ALT, AST, alkaline phosphatase
Decreased: Hgb

---

## NURSING CONSIDERATIONS
### Assessment
- Assess B/P with position changes, pulse q4hr; note rate, rhythm, quality
- Assess electrolytes: K, Na, Cl
- Assess baselines in renal, liver function tests before therapy begins
- Assess for edema in feet, legs daily
- Assess skin turgor, dryness of mucous membranes for hydration status

### Nursing diagnoses
- Fluid volume, deficient (adverse reactions)
- Injury, risk for (adverse reactions)
- Knowledge, deficient (teaching)
- Noncompliance (teaching)

### Implementation
- May be given without regard to meals

### Patient/family education
- Advise patient to comply with dosage schedule, even if feeling better
- Advise patient to notify prescriber of fever, swelling of hands or feet, chest pain
- Inform patient that excessive perspiration, dehydration, diarrhea may lead to fall in blood pressure; consult prescriber if these occur
- Inform patient that product may cause dizziness; advise to avoid hazardous activities until effect is known
- Advise patient not to take this medication if pregnant or breastfeeding, or if allergic reaction to this product has occurred
- Advise patient to take missed dose as soon as possible, unless within 1 hr of next dose

### Evaluation
**Positive therapeutic outcome**
- Decreased B/P

---

**⁄ HIGH ALERT**

## eptifibatide (Rx)
(ep-tih-fib'ah-tide)
Integrilin
*Func. class.:* Antiplatelet agent
*Chem. class.:* Glycoprotein IIb/IIIa inhibitor

**Pregnancy category B**

**Action:** Platelet glycoprotein antagonist; reversibly prevents fibrinogen, von Willebrand's factor from binding to the glycoprotein IIb/IIIa receptor, inhibiting platelet aggregation

**Therapeutic outcome:** Decreased platelets

**Uses:** Acute coronary syndrome including those undergoing percutaneous coronary intervention (PCI)

### Dosage and routes
*Acute coronary syndrome*
**Adult:** IV BOL 180 mcg/kg as soon as diagnosed, max 22.6 mg; then **IV** CONT INF 2 mcg/kg/min until discharge or coronary artery bypass graft (CABG) up to 72 hr, max 15 mg/hr

*PCI in patients without acute coronary syndrome*
**Adult:** IV BOL 180 mcg/kg given immediately before PCI; then 2 mcg/kg/min × 18 hr and a second 180 mcg/kg BOL, 10 min after 1st BOL; continue inf for up to 18-24 hr at a rate of 1 mcg/kg/min

*Renal dose*
**Adult:** IV BOL CCr <50 ml/min 2-4 mg/dl same loading dose, then ½ usual inf dose

**Available forms:** Sol for inj 2 mg/ml (10 ml), 0.75 mg/ml (100 ml)

### Adverse effects
*CV:* **Stroke,** hypotension
*GU:* Hematuria
***HEMA:*** **Thrombocytopenia**
*SYST:* **Bleeding, anaphylaxis**

**Contraindications:** Hypersensitivity, active internal bleeding; history of bleeding, stroke within 2 yr; major surgery with severe trauma, severe hypertension, history of intracranial bleeding, current or planned use of another parenteral GPIIb/IIIa inhibitor, dependence on renal dialysis, coagulopathy, AV malformation, aneurysm

**Precautions:** Pregnancy **B,** breastfeeding, children, geriatric, bleeding, renal function impairment

| Pharmacokinetics | |
|---|---|
| **Absorption** | Unknown |
| **Distribution** | Unknown |
| **Metabolism** | Limited |
| **Excretion** | Kidneys |
| **Half-life** | 1.5-2 hr |

| Pharmacodynamics |
|---|
| Unknown |

### Interactions
*Individual drugs*
Abciximab, aspirin, clopidogrel, dipyridamole, heparin, ticlopidine, valproate: increased bleeding

Adverse effects: *italic* = common, **bold** = life-threatening

*Drug classifications*
Anticoagulants, NSAIDs, thrombolytics: increased bleeding
Platelet receptor inhibitors IIb, IIIa: do not give together

## NURSING CONSIDERATIONS
### Assessment
• Monitor platelets, Hgb, Hct, creatinine, pro-time/APTT baseline, INR, within 6 hr of loading dose and daily thereafter; patients undergoing PCI should have ACT monitored; maintain APTT 50-70 sec unless PCI is to be performed; during PCI, ACT should be 200-300 sec; if platelets drop <100,000/mm³, obtain additional platelet counts; if thrombocytopenia is confirmed, discontinue product; also draw Hct, Hgb, serum creatinine
• Assess for bleeding: gums, bruising, ecchymosis, petechiae; from GI, GU tract, cardiac catheter sites, IM inj sites

### Nursing diagnoses
• Knowledge, deficient (teaching)
• Tissue perfusion, ineffective (uses)

### Implementation
• Aspirin and heparin may be given with this product; check for bleeding
• Discontinue heparin before removing femoral artery sheath after PCI
**IV route**
• After withdrawing the BOL dose from 10-ml vial, give **IV** push over 1-2 min; follow BOL dose with cont inf using infusion pump, give product undiluted directly from the 100-ml vial, spike the 100-ml vial with a vented infusion set, use caution when centering the spike on the circle of the stopper top
• Do not use discolored sol or those with particulate
*Y-site compatibilities:* Alteplase, atropine, DOBUTamine, heparin, lidocaine, meperidine, metoprolol, midazolam, morphine, nitroglycerin, verapamil
*Solution compatibilities:* 0.9% NaCl, D₅/0.9% NaCl
• Discontinuing product before CABG
• Give all medications PO if possible, avoid IM inj and catheters

### Patient/family education
• Teach patient to report bruising, bleeding, chest pain immediately
• Inform patient of reason for medication and expected results

### Evaluation
**Positive therapeutic outcome**
• Decreased platelets

---

## ergocalciferol
*See vitamin D*

---

## ergonovine (Rx)
(er-goe-noe′veen)
Ergometrine, ergotrate
*Func. class.:* Oxytocic
*Chem. class.:* Ergot alkaloid
**Pregnancy category** UK

**Action:** Stimulates uterine and vascular smooth muscle contractions, decreases bleeding

**Therapeutic outcome:** Uterine contraction, decreases bleeding

**Uses:** Treatment of postpartum or postabortion hemorrhage

**Unlabeled uses:** Variant angina diagnosis

**Dosage and routes**
*Oxytoxic*
*Adult:* PO/SL 0.2-0.4 mg q6-12hr; IM 0.2 mg q2-4hr, not to exceed 5 doses; **IV** 0.2 mg given over 1 min

*Variant angina diagnosis (unlabeled)*
*Adult:* **IV** 50 mg q5 min up to 400 mcg or until chest pain occurs

**Available forms:** Inj 0.2, 0.25 ♣ mg/ml; tab 0.2 mg

**Adverse effects**
*CNS: Headache, dizziness,* fainting
*CV:* Hypertension, chest pain
*EENT:* Tinnitus
*GI: Nausea, vomiting,* diarrhea
*GU:* Cramping
*INTEG:* Sweating
*RESP:* Dyspnea

**Contraindications:** Hypersensitivity to ergot medication, augmentation of labor, before delivery of placenta, spontaneous abortion (threatened), PID

**Precautions:** Renal/cardiac/hepatic disease, asthma, anemia, seizure disorders, hypertension, glaucoma, obliterative vascular disease

### Pharmacokinetics
| | |
|---|---|
| **Absorption** | Well absorbed (IM), completely absorbed (**IV**) |
| **Distribution** | Unknown |
| **Metabolism** | Liver |
| **Excretion** | Kidneys |
| **Half-life** | Unknown |

---

 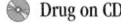

## Pharmacodynamics

|  | IM | IV |
|---|---|---|
| **Onset** | 2-5 min | Immediate |
| **Peak** | Unknown | Unknown |
| **Duration** | 3 hr | 45 min |

## Interactions
### Drug classifications
Ergots, sympathomimetics: increased hypertension
### Drug/herb
Horehound: increased serotonin effect

## NURSING CONSIDERATIONS
### Assessment
• Monitor B/P, pulse; watch for change that may indicate hemorrhage; check respiratory rate, rhythm, depth; notify prescriber of abnormalities
• Assess fundal tone, nonphasic contractions; check for relaxation or severe cramping
• Assess for ergotism or overdose: nausea, vomiting, weakness, muscular pain, insensitivity to cold, paresthesia of extremities; product should be decreased or infusion discontinued
• Before administering ergonovine, calcium levels should be checked; if hypocalcemia is present, correction should be made to increase effectiveness of this product
• Monitor prolactin levels and decreased breast milk production

### Nursing diagnoses
• Injury, risk for (adverse reactions)
• Knowledge, deficient (teaching)
• Tissue perfusion, ineffective (uses)

### Implementation
#### IM route
• Contractions begin in 2-5 min, product is given q2-4hr for contractions to continue; give deeply in large muscle mass; rotate inj sites if additional doses are given
#### IV route
• Give **IV** directly after dilution with 5 ml of 0.9% NaCl, give over >1 min through Y-site of free-running **IV** of 0.9% NaCl or D₅W
#### Additive compatibilities: Amikacin, cephapirin, sodium bicarbonate

### Patient/family education
• Advise patient to report increased blood loss, increased temp or foul-smelling lochia; need for pad count
• Inform patient that cramping is normal; pad count should be done to determine amount of bleeding
• Tell patient not to smoke during treatment to prevent excessive vasoconstriction

### Evaluation
**Positive therapeutic outcome**
• Absence of severe bleeding
**Treatment of overdose:** Stop product; give vasodilators, heparin, dextran

## ergotamine (Rx)
(er-got'a-meen)
Ergostat, Ergomar ✦, Gynergen
## dihydroergotamine
(dy-hy'droh-er-got'ah-meen)
DHE 45, Dihydroergotamine Sandoz ✦, Migranal
*Func. class.:* α-Adrenergic blocker, vascular headache suppressant
*Chem. class.:* Ergot alkaloid–amino acid
### Pregnancy category X

**Action:** Constricts smooth muscle in peripheral, cranial blood vessels; relaxes uterine muscle; blocks serotonin release

**Therapeutic outcome:** Absence of headache

**Uses:** Vascular headache (migraine, histamine, cluster)

### Dosage and routes
#### Ergotamine
*Adult:* SL 1 tab (2 mg), may use q30 min, max 3 tabs (6 mg)/24 hr or 10 mg/wk

#### Dihydroergotamine
*Adult:* SUBCUT/IM 1 mg, may repeat in 1 hr to 3 mg, max 3 mg/day or 6 mg/ wk; **IV** 0.5 mg, may repeat in 1 hr, max 2 mg/day or 6 mg/wk; INTRANASAL 1 spray in each nostril, repeat in 15 min, max 3 mg/24 hr, 4 mg/wk
*Child ≥6 yr:* SUBCUT/IM 0.5 mg, may repeat in 1 hr; **IV** 0.25 mg, may repeat in 1 hr

#### Severe acute migraine
*Child 12-16 yr:* **IV** 0.25-0.5 mg, may repeat q20 min for 1-2 doses

**Available forms:** Ergotamine: SL tab 2 mg; tabs 1 mg; dihydroergotamine: inj 1 mg/ml; nasal spray 4 mg/ml

### Adverse effects
*CNS: Numbness in fingers, toes,* headache, weakness
*CV:* Transient tachycardia, chest pain, bradycardia, edema, claudication, increase or decrease in B/P, **MI,** peripheral vascular ischemia
*GI:* Nausea, vomiting, diarrhea, abdominal cramps
*MS:* Muscle pain

Adverse effects: *italic* = common, **bold** = life-threatening

**Contraindications:** Pregnancy **X,** hypersensitivity to ergot preparations, occlusion (peripheral, vascular), CAD, renal/hepatic disease, peptic ulcer, hypertension, Raynaud's disease, peripheral vascular disease, intermittent claudication, glaucoma, angina, CVA

**Precautions:** Breastfeeding, children, geriatric, anemia, basilar/hemiplagic migraine

## Pharmacokinetics

| | |
|---|---|
| **Absorption** | Erratic (PO), poor (SL), rapidly (SUBCUT, IM) |
| **Distribution** | Crosses blood-brain barrier |
| **Metabolism** | Liver—extensively |
| **Excretion** | Kidneys (metabolites) |
| **Half-life** | Biphasic 2.7 hr, 21 hr |

## Pharmacodynamics

| | PO | SL | IM/SUBCUT | IV |
|---|---|---|---|---|
| **Onset** | 1-2 hr | Unknown | Unknown | Unknown |
| **Peak** | ½-3 hr | Unknown | Unknown | ¼-2 hr |
| **Duration** | Unknown | Unknown | 8 hr | 8 hr |

## Interactions
### Individual drugs
Nicotine: increased vasoconstriction
### Drug classifications
β-Blockers, contraceptives (oral), vasoconstrictors, other migraine agents: increased vasoconstriction

CYP450384 inhibitors (protease inhibitors, some macrolides, azole antifungals): increased ergot toxicity, do not use together
### Drug/herb
Horehound: increased serotonin effect

## NURSING CONSIDERATIONS
### Assessment
• Assess characteristics of pain: duration, intensity, location, frequency, alleviating factors; also identify if halos, nausea, vomiting, blurred vision occur with headache; assess before and during treatment
• Assess for ergotism or overdose: nausea, vomiting, weakness, muscular pain, insensitivity to cold, paresthesia of extremities; product should be decreased or infusion discontinued
• Check for hypertension: B/P, pulse, monitor all peripheral pulses; if hypertension occurs, notify prescriber; also check for tachycardia or bradycardia

### Nursing diagnoses
• Injury, risk for (adverse reactions)
• Knowledge, deficient (teaching)
• Pain, acute (uses)
### Implementation
#### SL route
• Do not break, crush, chew or swallow SL tab
• Place tab under tongue, do not drink, eat, or smoke until tab has dissolved
#### Inhalation route
• Teach patient how to use inhaler, protect ampules from heat/light
#### IV route
• Give dihydroergotamine undiluted over 1 min

### Patient/family education
• Caution patient not to smoke during treatment to prevent excessive vasoconstriction
• Advise patient to avoid alcohol or OTC medications unless approved by prescriber
• Tell patient to inform prescriber if pregnancy occurs

### Evaluation
#### Positive therapeutic outcome
• Decreasing headache

**Treatment of overdose:** Stop product, give vasodilators, heparin, dextran

## erlotinib (Rx)
(er-loe'tye-nib)
Tarceva
*Func. class.:* Misc. antineoplastic
*Chem. class.:* Epidermal growth factor receptor inhibitor

### Pregnancy category D

**Action:** Not fully understood. Inhibits intracellular phosphorylation of cell surface receptors associated with epidermal growth factor receptors.

**Therapeutic outcome:** Decrease in tumor size

**Uses:** Nonsmall cell lung cancer (NSCLC), pancreatic cancer

**Unlabeled uses:** Squamous cell, head and neck cancer

**Dosage and routes**
*CYP3A4 inducers concurrently (such as rifampin or phenytoin)*
Dosage increase is advised

*CYP3A4 inhibitors (atazanavir, clarithromycin, indinavir, itraconazole, ketoconazole, telithromycin, ritonavir, saquinavir, troleandomycin, nelfinavir)*
Dosage reduction may be needed.

*Non–small cell lung cancer (NSCLC)*
*Adult:* PO 150 mg/day

*Pancreatic cancer*
*Adult:* PO 100 mg/day

Available forms: Tabs 25, 100, 150 mg

Adverse effects
*GI: Nausea, diarrhea, vomiting, anorexia, mouth ulceration*
*INTEG: Rash*
*MISC: Conjunctivitis, eye pain, fatigue, infection*
**RESP: Interstitial lung disease,** *cough, dyspnea*

*Pancreatic cancer*
*CNS:* **CVA,** anxiety, depression, headache, rigors
*CV:* **MI/ischemia**
*GI: Nausea, diarrhea, vomiting, anorexia, mouth ulceration*
**HEMA: DVT**
*INTEG: Rash*
*MISC: Conjunctivitis, eye pain, fatigue, infection*
**RESP: Interstitial lung disease,** *cough, dyspnea*

Contraindications: Pregnancy **D**, breastfeeding, hypersensitivity

Precautions: Renal, hepatic, ocular, pulmonary disorders, children, geriatric

### Pharmacokinetics
| | |
|---|---|
| **Absorption** | Slowly absorbed |
| **Distribution** | Unknown |
| **Metabolism** | Metabolized by CYP3A4 |
| **Excretion** | Feces (86%), urine (<4%) |
| **Half-life** | 36 hr |

### Pharmacodynamics
| | |
|---|---|
| **Onset** | Unknown |
| **Peak** | 3-7 hr |
| **Duration** | Unknown |

Interactions
*Individual drugs*
Warfarin, metoprolol: increased plasma concentrations

*Drug classifications*
CYP3A4 inhibitors (clarithromycin, erythromycin, itraconazole, ketoconazole, telithromycin): increased erlotinib concentrations
CYP3A4 inducers (phenytoin, rifampin, carbamazepine, phenobarbital): decreased erlotinib levels
*Drug/herb*
St. John's wort: decreased erlotinib levels

### NURSING CONSIDERATIONS
Assessment
⬧ Assess for pulmonary changes: lung sounds, cough, dyspnea; interstitial lung disease may occur, may be fatal; discontinue therapy if confirmed
• Assess for ocular changes: eye irritation, corneal erosion/ulcer, aberrant eyelash growth
• Assess for GI symptoms: frequency of stools, if diarrhea is poorly tolerated, therapy may be discontinued for up to 14 days

Nursing diagnoses
• Body image, disturbed (adverse reactions)
• Infection, risk for (adverse reactions)
• Injury, risk for (adverse reactions)
• Knowledge, deficient (teaching)

Implementation
• Administer 1 hr before or 2 hr after food

Patient/family education
⬧ Teach patient to report adverse reactions immediately: SOB, severe abdominal pain, persistent diarrhea or vomiting, ocular changes, skin eruptions
• Explain reason for treatment, expected results
• Advise patient to use contraception during treatment

Evaluation
**Positive therapeutic outcome**
• Decrease non–small cell lung cancer cells

## ertapenem (Rx)
(er-tah-pen'em)
Invanz
*Func. class.:* Antiinfective—miscellaneous
*Chem. class.:* Carbapenem
**Pregnancy category B**

Do not confuse:
Invanz/Aninza

Action: Interferes with cell wall replication of susceptible organisms; osmotically unstable cell wall swells, bursts from osmotic pressure

Adverse effects: *italic* = common, **bold** = life-threatening

**Therapeutic outcome:** Bactericidal action against the following organisms: *Bacteroides fragilis, Bacteroides distasonis, Bacteroides ovatus, Bacteroides thetaiotaomicron, Bacteroides uniformis; Clostridium clostridioforme, Escherichia coli, Eubacterium lentum, Haemophilus influenzae* (β lactamase–negative), *Klebsiella pneumoniae, Moraxella catarrhalis, Peptostreptococcus* sp., *Porphyromonas asaccharolytica, Prevotella bivia, Staphylococcus aureus* (methicillin-susceptible); *Streptococcus agalactiae, Streptococcus pneumoniae* (penicillin-susceptible), *Streptococcus pyogenes*

**Uses:** Adult patients with moderate to severe intraabdominal infections, complicated skin/skin structure infections, community-acquired pneumonia, complicated UTI, acute pelvic infections, infection prophylaxis prior to elective colorectal surgery

### Dosage and routes
*Complicated intraabdominal infections*
*Adult:* **IV**/IM 1 g/day × 5-14 days
*Child 3 mo-12 yr:* **IV**/IM 15 mg/kg bid × 5-14 days

*Complicated skin/skin structure infections*
*Adult:* **IV**/IM 1 g/day × 7-14 days
*Child 3 mo-12 yr:* **IV**/IM 15 mg/kg bid × 7-14 days

*Community-acquired pneumonia*
*Adult:* **IV**/IM 1 g/day × 10-14 days
*Child 3 mo-12 yr:* **IV**/IM 15 mg/kg bid × 10-14 days

*Complicated UTI*
*Adult:* **IV**/IM 1 g/day × 10-14 days
*Child 3 mo-12 yr:* **IV**/IM 15 mg/kg bid × 10-14 days

*Acute pelvic infections*
*Adult:* **IV**/IM 1 g/day × 3-10 days
*Child 3 mo-12 yr:* **IV**/IM 15 mg/kg bid × 3-10 days

*Surgical infection prophylaxis*
*Adult:* **IV** 1 g as a single dose 1 hr prior to surgical incision

**Available forms:** Powder, lyophilized, 1 g

### Adverse effects
*CNS:* Insomnia, **seizures**, dizziness, *headache*
*CV:* **Tachycardia**
*GI:* *Diarrhea, nausea, vomiting,* **pseudomembranous colitis**
*GU:* *Vaginitis*

*INTEG:* *Rash*, urticaria, *pruritus,* pain at inj site, *infused vein complication, phlebitis/thrombophlebitis,* erythema at inj site
*RESP:* Dyspnea, cough, pharyngitis, crackles, respiratory distress
*SYST:* **Anaphylaxis**

**Contraindications:** Hypersensitivity to this product or its components, to amide-type local anesthetics (IM only); anaphylactic reactions to β-lactams

**Precautions:** Pregnancy **B,** breastfeeding, children, geriatric, renal/hepatic/GI disease

| Pharmacokinetics | |
|---|---|
| **Absorption** | Almost completely absorbed (IM); completely (**IV**) |
| **Distribution** | 85%-95% plasma protein bound |
| **Metabolism** | Liver (IM, **IV**) |
| **Excretion** | Urine (80%), feces (10%), breast milk (IM, **IV**) |
| **Half-life** | 4 hr (**IV**) |

| Pharmacodynamics | | |
|---|---|---|
| | IM | IV |
| **Onset** | Unknown | Immediate |
| **Peak** | 2.3 hr | Dose-dependent |
| **Duration** | Unknown | Unknown |

### Interactions
*Individual drugs*
Probenecid: increased ertapenem plasma levels; do not coadminister
*Drug/herb*
Acidophilus: do not use with antiinfectives; separate by several hours
*Drug/lab test*
Increased: hepatic enzymes

### NURSING CONSIDERATIONS
**Assessment**
• Assess for sensitivity to carbapenem antibiotics, other β-lactam antibiotics, penicillins
• Assess for renal disease: lower dose may be required
• Assess bowel pattern daily: if severe diarrhea occurs, product should be discontinued; may indicate pseudomembranous colitis
• Assess for infection: temp, sputum, characteristics of wound before, during, after treatment
◆ Assess for allergic reactions, anaphylaxis: rash, urticaria, pruritus; may occur a few days after therapy begins
• Assess for overgrowth of infection: perineal itching, fever, malaise, redness, pain, swelling, drainage, rash, diarrhea, change in cough or sputum

---

◆ Alert      ♣ Canada Only      🔵 Drug on CD      * "Tall Man" lettering (See Preface)

## Nursing diagnoses
• Diarrhea (adverse reaction)
• Infection, risk for (uses)
• Injury, risk for (adverse reactions)
• Knowledge, deficient (teaching)
• Noncompliance (teaching)

## Implementation
• Administer by **IV** or IM
• Give after C&S is taken
**IM route**
• Reconstitute 1 g vial of ertapenem with 3.2 ml of 1% lidocaine HCl without epINEPHrine, shake well
• Withdraw contents, administer deep IM in large muscle mass, use within 1 hr
**IV route**
• Do not co-infuse or mix with other medications; do not use diluents containing dextrose
• Reconstitute 1 g vial of ertapenem with either 10 ml of water for inj, 0.9% NaCl, or bacteriostatic water for inj
• Shake well to dissolve, transfer contents of reconstituted vial to 50 ml 0.9% NaCl inj
• Complete infusion within 6 hr

## Patient/family education
• Advise patient to report severe diarrhea; may indicate pseudomembranous colitis
• Advise patient to report overgrowth of infection: black, furry tongue, vaginal itching, foul-smelling stools
• Caution patient to avoid breastfeeding; product is excreted in breast milk

## Evaluation
**Positive therapeutic outcome**
• Negative C&S, absence of signs and symptoms of infection

**Treatment of overdose:** Administer epINEPHrine, antihistamines; resuscitate if needed (anaphylaxis)

## erythromycin base (Rx)
(eh-rith-roh-my'sin)
Apo Erythro ✦, E-base, E-Mycin, Eramycin, Erybid ✦, Eryc, Ery-Tab, Erythromid ✦, Erythromycin Base Filmtab, Erythromycin Delayed-Release, Novo-Rythro Encap ✦, PCE
## erythromycin estolate (Rx)
Ilosone, Novo-Rythro ✦
## erythromycin ethylsuccinate (Rx)
Apo-Erythro-ES ✦, EES, Ery Ped, Novo-Rythro ✦
## erythromycin gluceptate (Rx)
## erythromycin lactobionate (Rx)
Erythrocin
## erythromycin stearate (Rx)
Apo-Erythro-s ✦, Novo-Rythro ✦
*Func. class.:* Antiinfective
*Chem. class.:* Macrolide

**Pregnancy category** B

**Do not confuse:**
erythromycin/azithromycin

**Action:** Binds to 50S ribosomal subunits of susceptible bacteria and suppresses protein synthesis

**Therapeutic outcome:** Bactericidal action against the following organisms: *Neisseria gonorrhoeae, Streptococcus pneumoniae, Mycoplasma pneumoniae, Corynebacterium diphtheriae, Bordetella pertussis, Borrelia burgdorferi, Listeria monocytogenes;* syphilis, Legionnaire's disease; streptococci, staphylocci; gram-positive bacilli: *Clostridium, Corynebacterium;* gram-negative pathogens: *Neisseria, Haemophilus influenzae* (when used with sulfonamides), *Legionella pneumophila, Mycoplasma, Chlamydia trachomatis, Entamoeba histolytica*

**Uses:** Mild to moderate respiratory tract, skin, soft tissue infections

## Dosage and routes
*Soft tissue infections*
*Adult:* PO 250-500 mg q6hr (base, estolate, stearate); PO 400-800 mg q6hr (ethylsuccinate); **IV** INF 15-20 mg/kg/day (lactobionate) divided q6hr
*Child:* PO 30-50 mg/kg/day in divided doses q6hr (salts); **IV** 20-40 mg/kg/day in divided doses q6hr (lactobionate), max adult dose

Adverse effects: *italic* = common, **bold** = life-threatening

## N. gonorrhoeae/*PID*
*Adult:* **IV** 500 mg q6hr × 3 days (gluceptate, lactobionate), then PO 250 mg (base,
estolate, stearate) or 400 mg (ethylsuccinate)
q6hr × 1 wk

## Syphilis
*Adult:* PO 500 mg qid × 14 days

## Chlamydia
*Adult:* PO 500 mg q6hr × 1 wk or 250 mg
qid × 2 wk
*Infant:* PO 50 mg/kg/day in 4 divided
doses × 3 wk or more
*Newborn:* PO 50 mg/kg/day in 4 divided
doses × 2 wk or more

## Intestinal amebiasis
*Adult:* PO 250 mg q6hr × 10-14 days (base,
estolate, stearate)
*Child:* PO 30-50 mg/kg/day in divided
doses q6hr × 10-14 days (base, estolate,
stearate)

**Available forms:** Base: enteric-coated tab
250, 333, 500 mg; film-coated tab 250,
500 mg; enteric-coated caps, 250, 333 mg;
estolate: tabs 500 mg; caps 125, 250 mg;
drops 100 mg/ml; susp 125, 250 mg/5 ml;
stearate: film-coated tabs, 250 mg;
ethylsuccinate: chewable tabs 200 mg; susp
100 mg/2.5 ml, 200, 400 mg/5 ml; powder for
inj 500 mg, 1 g (lactobionate); 1 g (as gluceptate)

## Adverse effects
*CV:* **Dysrhythmias,** QT prolongation
*EENT:* Hearing loss, tinnitus
*GI:* *Nausea, vomiting, diarrhea,* **hepatotox-
icity,** abdominal pain, stomatitis, heartburn,
anorexia, pruritus ani, **pseudomembranous
colitis**
*GU:* *Vaginitis, moniliasis*
*INTEG:* Rash, urticaria, pruritus, thrombo-
phlebitis (**IV** site)
*SYST:* **Anaphylaxis**

**Contraindications:** Hypersensitivity,
preexisting liver disease (estolate)

**Precautions:** Pregnancy **B**, breastfeeding,
geriatric, hepatic/GI disease, QT prolongation,
seizure disorder

### Pharmacokinetics

| | |
|---|---|
| **Absorption** | Well absorbed (PO) |
| **Distribution** | Widely distributed; minimally distrib-uted (CSF); crosses placenta |
| **Metabolism** | Liver, partially |
| **Excretion** | Bile, unchanged; kidneys (minimal), unchanged |
| **Half-life** | 1-3 hr |

### Pharmacodynamics

| | PO | IV |
|---|---|---|
| **Onset** | 1 hr | Rapid |
| **Peak** | 4 hr | Infusion's end |
| **Duration** | Unknown | Unknown |

## Interactions
### Individual drugs
Alfentanil, alprazolam, bromocriptine, bus-
PIRone, carbamazepine, cilostazol, clindamycin, clopazine, cycloSPORINE, diazepam,
digoxin, dihydropyridine, disopyramide,
felodipine lovastatin, methylPREDNISolone,
midazolam, quinidine, rifabutin, sildenafil,
simvastatin, tacrolimus, tadalafil, theophylline, triazolam, vardenafil, vinBLAStine,
warfarin: increased toxicity, increased action
Diltiazem, itraconazole, ketoconazole, nefazodone, pimozide, sparfloxacin, verapamil:
increased serious dysrhythmias, do not use
together
### Drug classifications
Ergots: increased action, toxicity
HMG-CoA reductase inhibitors: increased
action, toxicity
Protease inhibitors: serious dysrhythmias
### Drug/herb
Acidophilus: do not use with antiinfectives
### Drug/lab test
Increased: AST/ALT
Decreased: folate assay
False increase: 17-OHCS/17-KS

## NURSING CONSIDERATIONS
### Assessment
• Assess patient for previous sensitivity reaction
• Assess patient for signs and symptoms of
infection including characteristics of wounds,
sputum, urine, stool, WBC >10,000/mm$^3$,
earache, fever; obtain baseline information
before and during treatment
• Obtain C&S test results before beginning
product therapy to identify if correct treatment
has been initiated
• Assess for allergic reactions: rash, urticaria
may occur a few days after therapy begins
• Identify urine output; if decreasing, notify
prescriber (may indicate nephrotoxicity); also
monitor increases in BUN, creatinine
• Monitor blood studies: AST, ALT, CBC, Hct,
bilirubin, LDH, alkaline phosphatase, Coombs'
test monthly if patient is on long-term therapy
• Monitor electrolytes: potassium, sodium,
chloride monthly if patient is on long-term
therapy

- Assess bowel pattern daily; if severe diarrhea occurs, product should be discontinued
- Assess for overgrowth of infection: perineal itching, fever, malaise, redness, pain, swelling, drainage, rash, diarrhea, change in cough, sputum

## Nursing diagnoses
- Diarrhea (adverse reactions)
- Infection, risk for (uses)
- Injury, risk for (adverse reactions)
- Knowledge, deficient (teaching)
- Noncompliance (teaching)

## Implementation
**PO route**
- Give around the clock on an empty stomach, at least 1 hr before or 2 hr after meals; may be taken with food if GI upset occurs; do not take with juices; take dose with a full glass of water: use calibrated measuring device for drops or susp; shake well
- Store susp in refrigerator
- Chewable tab may be crushed or chewed, not swallowed whole
- Do not crush or chew enteric-coated tab

**IV route**
- Add 10 ml of sterile water for inj without preservatives to 250- or 500-mg vials and 20 ml to 1-g vial; sol is stable for 1 wk after reconstitution if refrigerated

**Intermittent IV infusion**
- Dilute further in 100-250 ml of 0.9% NaCl or D$_5$W
- Give over 20-60 min to avoid phlebitis; assess for pain along vein; slow inf if pain occurs; apply ice to site and notify prescriber if unable to relieve pain

**Continuous infusion**
- May also be administered as an infusion in a dilution of 1 g/L of 0.9% NaCl, D$_5$W, over 4 hr

*Syringe incompatibilities:* Heparin
*Additive compatibilities:* Calcium gluconate, hydrocortisone, lidocaine, methicillin, penicillin G potassium, potassium chloride, sodium bicarbonate
*Additive incompatibilities:* Aminophylline, cephapirin, pentobarbital, secobarbital, streptomycin, tetracycline

## Erythromycin lactobionate
*Syringe compatibilities:* Methicillin
*Syringe incompatibilities:* Ampicillin, heparin
*Y-site compatibilities:* Acyclovir, amiodarone, cyclophosphamide, enalaprilat, esmolol, famotidine, foscarnet, hydromorphone, idarubicin, labetalol, lorazepam, magnesium sulfate, merperidine, midazolam, morphine, multivitamins, perphenazine, vit B/C, zidovudine
*Y-site incompatibilities:* Fluconazole
*Additive compatibilities:* Aminophylline, ampicillin, cimetidine, diphenhydrAMINE, hydrocortisone, lidocaine, methicillin, penicillin G potassium, penicillin G sodium, pentobarbital, polymyxin B, potassium chloride, prednisoLONE, prochlorperazine, promazine, ranitidine, sodium bicarbonate, verapamil
*Additive incompatibilities:* Cephalothin, colistimethate, floxacillin, furosemide, heparin, metaraminol, metoclopramide, tetracycline, vit B/C

## Patient/family education
- Teach patient to report sore throat, bruising, bleeding, joint pain; may indicate blood dyscrasias (rare)
- Advise patient to contact prescriber if vaginal itching, loose foul-smelling stools, furry tongue occur; may indicate superimposed infection
- Instruct patient to take all medication prescribed for the length of time ordered

## Evaluation
**Positive therapeutic outcome**
- Absence of signs/symptoms of infection (WBC <10,000/mm$^3$, temp WNL, absence of red, draining wounds, earache)
- Reported improvement in symptoms of infection

**Treatment of overdose:** Withdraw product, maintain airway, administer epINEPHrine, aminophylline, O$_2$, **IV** corticosteroids

---

## erythromycin ophthalmic
*See Appendix D*

---

## erythromycin topical
*See Appendix D*

---

## escitalopram (Rx)
(es-sit-tal'oh-pram)
Lexapro
*Func. class.:* Antidepressant, selective serotonin reuptake inhibitor
**Pregnancy category** C

**Action:** Inhibits CNS neuron uptake of serotonin but not of norepinephrine

**Therapeutic outcome:** Decreased symptoms of depression

Adverse effects: *italic* = common, **bold** = life-threatening

**Uses:** General anxiety disorder, major depressive disorder, social phobia

**Unlabeled uses:** Panic disorder

## Dosage and routes
*Adult:* PO 10 mg/day in AM or PM; after 1 wk if no clinical improvement is noted, dose may be increased to 20 mg/day PM; maintenance 10-20 mg/day; reassess to determine need for treatment

*Geriatric/hepatic dose:* PO 10 mg/day

**Available forms:** Tabs 5, 10, 20 mg; oral sol 5 mg (as base)/5 ml

## Adverse effects
*CNS: Headache, nervousness, insomnia, drowsiness, anxiety, tremor, dizziness, fatigue, sedation, poor concentration, abnormal dreams, agitation,* **seizures,** apathy, euphoria, hallucinations, delusions, psychosis

*CV: Hot flashes, palpitations,* angina pectoris, **hemorrhage,** hypertension, **tachycardia,** 1st-degree AV block, **bradycardia, MI, thrombophlebitis,** postural hypotension

*EENT:* Visual changes, ear/eye pain, photophobia, tinnitus

*GI: Nausea, diarrhea, dry mouth, anorexia, dyspepsia, constipation, cramps, vomiting, taste changes, flatulence, decreased appetite*

*GU: Dysmenorrhea, decreased libido, urinary frequency, UTI,* amenorrhea, cystitis, impotence, urine retention

*INTEG: Sweating, rash, pruritus,* acne, alopecia, urticaria, photosensitivity

*MS: Pain,* arthritis, twitching

*RESP: Infection, pharyngitis, nasal congestion, sinus headache, sinusitis, cough, dyspnea, bronchitis,* asthma, hyperventilation, pneumonia

*SYST: Asthenia, viral infection, fever, allergy, chills*

**Contraindications:** Hypersensitivity

**Precautions:** Pregnancy **C,** breastfeeding, children, geriatric, renal/hepatic disease, history of seizures

### Pharmacokinetics
| | |
|---|---|
| **Absorption** | Unknown |
| **Distribution** | Unknown |
| **Metabolism** | Liver |
| **Excretion** | Urine |
| **Half-life** | Unknown |

### Pharmacodynamics
Unknown

## Interactions
### Individual drugs
Alcohol: increased CNS depression

Amantadine, bromocriptine, busPIRone, lithium, tryptophan: increased serotonin syndrome

BusPIRone: increased symptoms of OCD

Carbamazepine, lithium, phenytoin, warfarin: increased levels or toxicity of each specific product

Cyproheptadine: decreased escitalopram effect

Diazepam: increased half-life of diazepam

Haloperidol: increased effect of haloperidol

### Drug classifications
Antidepressants, amphetamines: increased serotonin syndrome

Antidepressants, opioids, sedatives: increased CNS depression

Antipsychotics, antidysrhythmics: increased levels, toxicity

Highly protein-bound products: increased side effects of escitalopram

MAOIs: do not use with or 14 days before escitalopram

Phenothiazines: increased levels of phenothiazines

Tricyclics: increased levels of tricyclics

### Drug/herb
Corkwood, jimsonweed: increased anticholinergic effect

Hops, kava, lavender: increased CNS effect

SAM-e, St. John's wort: do not use together

Yohimbe: increased hypertension

### Drug/lab test
Increased: serum bilirubin, blood glucose, alkaline phosphatase

Decreased: VMA, 5-HIAA

False increase: urinary catecholamines

## NURSING CONSIDERATIONS
### Assessment
• Assess mental status: mood, sensorium, affect, suicidal tendencies, increase in psychiatric symptoms, depression, panic

• Assess appetite in bulimia nervosa, weight daily, increase nutritious foods in diet, watch for bingeing and vomiting

• Assess allergic reactions: itching, rash, urticaria; product should be discontinued, may need to give antihistamine

• Monitor B/P (lying/standing), pulse q4hr; if systolic B/P drops 20 mm Hg, hold product, notify prescriber; take VS q4hr in patients with cardiovascular disease

• Monitor blood studies: CBC, leukocytes, differential, cardiac enzymes if patient is receiving long-term therapy; check platelets; bleeding can occur

- Montior liver function tests: AST, ALT, bilirubin, creatinine
- Monitor weight qwk; appetite may decrease with product
- Monitor ECG for flattening of T wave, bundle branch, AV block, dysrhythmias in cardiac patients
- Monitor alcohol consumption; if alcohol is consumed, hold dose until AM

## Nursing diagnoses
- Coping, ineffective (uses)
- Injury, risk for (uses/adverse reactions)
- Knowledge, deficient (teaching)

## Implementation
- Give with food or milk for GI symptoms
- Give crushed if patient is unable to swallow medication whole
- Give dosage at bedtime if oversedation occurs during the day
- Give gum, hard candy, frequent sips of water for dry mouth
- Store at room temperature; do not freeze
- Provide assistance with ambulation during therapy, because drowsiness, dizziness occur
- Provide safety measures primarily in geriatric
- Check to see if PO medication swallowed

## Patient/family education
- Teach that therapeutic effect may take 1-4 wk
- Advise to use caution in driving, other activities requiring alertness because of drowsiness, dizziness, blurred vision
- Advise to use sunscreen to prevent photosensitivity
- Advise to avoid alcohol ingestion, other CNS depressants
- Advise patient to notify prescriber if pregnant or plan to become pregnant or breastfeed
- Advise patient to change positions slowly, orthostatic hypotension may occur
- Teach to avoid all OTC products unless approved by prescriber
- Teach patient to report immediately signs of urinary retention
- Teach patient that clinical worsening and suicide risk may occur

## Evaluation
**Positive therapeutic outcome**
- Decreased depression

**Treatment of overdose:** Activated charcoal, supportive care

## esmolol (Rx)
(ez'moe-lole)
Brevibloc
*Func. class.:* β-Adrenergic blocker (antidysrhythmic II)

**Pregnancy category** C

### Do not confuse:
esmolol/Osmitrol, Brevibloc/Brevital

**Action:** Competitively blocks stimulation of β$_1$-adrenergic receptors in the myocardium; produces negative chronotropic, inotropic activity (decreases rate of SA node discharge, increases recovery time), slows conduction of AV node, decreases heart rate, decreases O$_2$ consumption in myocardium; also decreases renin-aldosterone-angiotensin system at high doses; inhibits β$_2$-receptors in bronchial system at higher doses

**Therapeutic outcome:** Decreased supraventricular tachycardia

**Uses:** Supraventricular tachycardias, noncompensatory sinus tachycardia, hypertensive crisis, intraoperative and postoperative tachycardia and hypertension

### Dosage and routes
*Adult:* **IV** Loading dose 500 mcg/kg/min over 1 min; maintenance 50 mcg/kg/min for 4 min; if no response in 5 min, give 2nd loading dose; then increase inf to 100 mcg/kg/min for 4 min; if no response, repeat loading dose, then increase maintenance inf by 50 mcg/kg/min (max of 200 mcg/kg/min); titrate to patient response
*Child:* **IV** 50 mcg/kg/min, may increase q10 min, max 300 mcg/kg/min

**Available forms:** Inj 10 mg, 250 mg/ml

### Adverse effects
*CNS:* Confusion, light-headedness, paresthesia, somnolence, fever, dizziness, fatigue, headache, depression, anxiety, **seizures**
*CV:* Hypotension, bradycardia, chest pain, peripheral ischemia, shortness of breath, CHF, conduction disturbances 1st-, 2nd-, 3rd-degree heart block
*GI:* Nausea, vomiting, anorexia, gastric pain, flatulence, constipation, heartburn, bloating
*GU:* Urinary retention, impotence, dysuria
*INTEG: Induration, inflammation at inj site,* discoloration, edema, erythema, burning, pallor, flushing, rash, pruritus, dry skin, alopecia
*RESP:* **Bronchospasm,** dyspnea, cough, wheezing, nasal stuffiness

E

Adverse effects: *italic* = common, **bold** = life-threatening

**Contraindications:** Heart block (2nd- or 3rd-degree), cardiogenic shock, CHF, cardiac failure, hypersensitivity

**Precautions:** Pregnancy **C,** breastfeeding, hypotension, peripheral vascular disease, diabetes, hypoglycemia, thyrotoxicosis, renal disease

### Pharmacokinetics

| | |
|---|---|
| **Absorption** | Complete |
| **Distribution** | Unknown |
| **Metabolism** | Liver |
| **Excretion** | Kidneys |
| **Half-life** | 9 min |

### Pharmacodynamics

| | |
|---|---|
| **Onset** | Rapid |
| **Peak** | Unknown |
| **Duration** | 1-2 min |

### Interactions
*Individual drugs*
Amphetamine, epHEDrine, epINEPHrine, norepinephrine, phenylephrine, pseudoephedrine: increased α-adrenergic stimulation
Digoxin: increased digoxin levels
Thyroid hormones: decreased effect of esmolol, decreased action of thyroid hormone
*Drug classifications*
MAOIs: avoid use
*Drug/herb*
Aloe, buckthorn, cascara sagrada, senna: increased hypokalemia
Betel palm, butterbur, cola tree, figwort, fumitory, guarana, hawthorn, lily of the valley, motherwort, plantain: increased β-blocking effect
Coenzyme Q10, yohimbe: decreased β-blocking effect
Jamborandi tree: increased CV reactions
*Drug/lab test*
Interference: glucose/insulin tolerance test

### NURSING CONSIDERATIONS
**Assessment**
• Monitor B/P during beginning treatment, periodically thereafter; pulse q4hr; note rate, rhythm, quality; apical/radial pulse before administration; notify prescriber of any significant changes (pulse <50 bpm)
• Check for baselines in renal, liver function tests before therapy begins
• Assess for edema in feet, legs daily, monitor I&O, daily weight; check for jugular vein distention, crackles bilaterally, dyspnea (CHF)
• Monitor skin turgor, dryness of mucous membranes for hydration status, especially geriatric

**Nursing diagnoses**
• Cardiac output, decreased (uses)
• Injury, risk for (adverse reactions)
• Knowledge, deficient (teaching)
• Noncompliance (teaching)

**Implementation**
• Give by intermittent inf after diluting 5 g/500 ml of D₅W, 0.9% NaCl, D₅/0.45% NaCl, D₅/LR, D₅/0.9% NaCl, 0.45% NaCl, LR (10 mg/ml)
• Give loading dose over 1 min, then maintenance dose over 4 min, may repeat loading dose q5 min with increased maintenance dose; maintenance dose should not be >200 mcg/kg/min and be administered up to 48 hr; dosage should be tapered at a rate of 25 mcg/kg/min
• Store at room temperature for 24 hr; sol should be clear
*Y-site compatibilities:* Amikacin, aminophylline, ampicillin, amiodarone, atracurium, butorphanol, calcium chloride, cefazolin, cefmetazole, cefoperazone, ceftazidime, ceftizoxime, chloramphenicol, cimetidine, cisatracurium, clindamycin, diltiazem, DOPamine, enalaprilat, erythromycin, famotidine, fentanyl, gentamicin, heparin, hydrocortisone, regular insulin, labetalol, magnesium sulfate, methyldopate, metronidazole, midazolam, morphine, nafcillin, nitroglycerin, norepinephrine, nitroprusside, pancuronium, penicillin G potassium, phenytoin, piperacillin, polymyxin B, potassium chloride, potassium phosphate, propofol, ranitidine, remifentanil, streptomycin, tacrolimus, tobramycin, trimethoprim/sulfamethoxazole, vancomycin, vecuronium
*Y-site incompatibilities:* Furosemide
*Additive compatibilities:* Aminophylline, atracurium, bretylium, heparin
*Additive incompatibilities:* Diazepam, procainamide, sodium bicarbonate, thiopental

**Patient/family education**
• Teach patient need for medication and expected results
• Caution patient to rise slowly to prevent orthostatic hypotension
• Advise patient to notify if pain, swelling occurs at **IV** site

**Evaluation**
**Positive therapeutic outcome**
• Absence of dysrhythmias

**Treatment of overdose:** Defibrillation, vasopressor for hypotension

## esomeprazole (Rx)
(es'oh-mep'rah-zohl)
Nexium
*Func. class.:* Anti-ulcer, proton pump inhibitor
*Chem. class.:* Benzimidazole

**Pregnancy category B**

**Action:** Suppresses gastric secretion by inhibiting hydrogen/potassium ATPase enzyme system in the gastric parietal cell; characterized as gastric acid pump inhibitor, since it blocks final step of acid production

**Therapeutic outcome:** Absence of duodenal ulcers; decreased gastroesophageal reflux

**Uses:** Gastroesophageal reflux disease (GERD), severe erosive esophagitis; treatment of active duodenal ulcers in combination with antiinfectives for *Helicobacter pylori* infection; long-term use in hypersecretory conditions

**Dosage and routes**
*Active duodenal ulcers associated with* **H. pylori**
*Adult:* PO 40 mg/day × 10 days in combination with clarithromycin 500 mg bid × 10 days and amoxicillin 1000 mg bid × 10 days

*Hepatic dose*
*Adult:* PO/**IV** max 20 mg/day (severe hepatic disease)

*GERD*
*Adult:* PO 20 or 40 mg/day × 4-8 wk; no adjustment needed in renal, liver failure, geriatric; **IV** 20 or 40 mg/day
*Child and adolescent 12-17 yr:* PO 20-40 mg/day 1 hr before meals up to 8 wk

**Available forms:** Del rel caps 20, 40 mg; powder for **IV** inj 20, 40 mg/vial; del rel powder for oral suspension 20, 40 mg

**Adverse effects**
*CNS: Headache, dizziness*
*GI: Diarrhea, flatulence,* abdominal pain, constipation, dry mouth, **hepatic failure, hepatitis**
*INTEG: Rash,* dry skin
*MISC:* **Heart failure**
*RESP: Cough*
*SYST:* **Stevens-Johnson syndrome, toxic epidermal necrolysis, exfoliative dermatitis**

**Contraindications:** Hypersensitivity

**Precautions:** Pregnancy **B**, breastfeeding, children, geriatric

### Pharmacokinetics
| | |
|---|---|
| **Absorption** | Unknown |
| **Distribution** | 97% plasma protein bound |
| **Metabolism** | Liver (metabolites) |
| **Excretion** | Urine (metabolites), feces (metabolites); in geriatric, elimination rate decreased, bioavailability increased |
| **Half-life** | 1-1½ hr |

### Pharmacodynamics
| | |
|---|---|
| **Onset** | Unknown |
| **Peak** | 1½ hr |
| **Duration** | Unknown |

### Interactions
*Individual drugs*
Calcium carbonate, dapsone, indinavir, iron, itraconazole, ketoconazole, vitamin $B_{12}$: decreased effect
Diazepam, digoxin, penicillins: increased effect, toxicity

### NURSING CONSIDERATIONS
**Assessment**
• Assess GI system: bowel sounds q8hr, abdomen for pain, swelling, anorexia
• Assess hepatic enzymes: AST, ALT, alkaline phosphatase during treatment

**Nursing diagnoses**
• Knowledge, deficient (teaching)
• Pain, acute (uses)
• Pain, chronic (uses)

**Implementation**
• Swallow caps whole; do not break, crush, or chew
• Administer at least 1 hr before eating

**Patient/family education**
• Instruct patient to report severe diarrhea; product may have to be discontinued
• Advise diabetic patients that hypoglycemia may occur
• Advise patient to avoid hazardous activities; dizziness may occur
• Advise patient to avoid alcohol, salicylates, ibuprofen; may cause GI irritation

**Evaluation**
**Positive therapeutic outcome**
• Absence of epigastric pain, swelling, fullness

E

## estradiol (Rx)
(ess-tra-dye′ole)
Estrace

## estradiol cypionate (Rx)
depGynogen, Depo-Estradiol, Depogen, Dura-Estrin, E-Cypionate, Estragyn LAS, Estro-Cyp, Estrofem, Estroject-LA, Estro-L.A.

## estradiol topical emulsion (Rx)
Estrasorb

## estradiol valerate (Rx)
Clinagen LA, Delestrogen, Dioval, Duragan, Estra-L, Estro-span, Femogex ✤, Gynogen LA, Menaval, Valergen

## estradiol transdermal system (Rx)
Alora, Climara, Esclim, Estraderm, FemPatch, Vivelle

## estradiol vaginal tablet (Rx)
Vagifem

## estradiol vaginal ring (Rx)
Estring

## estradiol gel (Rx)
Divigel, Elestrin

## estradiol spray (Rx)
Evamist
*Func. class.:* Estrogen, progestin
*Chem. class.:* Nonsteroidal synthetic estrogen

**Pregnancy category X**

**Action:** Needed for adequate functioning of female reproductive system; affects release of pituitary gonadatropins, inhibits ovulation, promotes adequate calcium use in bone structure

**Therapeutic outcome:** Decreased tumor size in prostatic cancer; increased estrogen levels in menopause, female hypogonadism

**Uses:** Vasomotor symptoms associated with menopause, inoperable breast cancer (selected cases), prostatic cancer, atrophic vaginitis, kraurosis vulvae, hypogonadism, primary ovarian failure, prevention of osteoporosis, castration

**Dosage and routes**
*Hormone replacement/menopause symptoms*
*Adult:* TRANSDERMAL 0.05-0.1 mg/24 hr apply 2×/wk; GEL apply entire unit dose packet to 5 × 7-inch area of upper thigh daily, alternate thighs; SPRAY 1 spray to inner surface of forearm daily in AM

*Menopause/hypogonadism/castration/ovarian failure*
*Adult:* PO 1-2 mg/day 3 wk on, 1 wk off or 5 days on, 2 days off; IM 1-5 mg q3-4 wk (cypionate), 10-20 mg q4 wk (valerate); TOP Estraderm 0.05 mg/24 hr applied 2×/wk, Climara 0.05 mg/hr applied 1×/wk in a cyclic regimen, women with hysterectomy may use continuously

*Prostatic cancer*
*Adult:* IM 30 mg q1-2 wk (valerate); PO 1-2 mg tid (oral estradiol)

*Breast cancer*
*Adult:* PO 10 mg tid × 3 mo or longer

*Atropic vaginitis/kraurosis vulvae*
*Adult:* VAG Cream 2-4 g/day × 1-2 wk, then 1 g 1-3 ×/wk cycled; VAG tab 1/day × 2 wk, maintenance 1 tab 2×/wk; VAG ring inserted and left in place continuously for 3 mo

*Vasomotor symptoms*
*Adult:* TOP After cleaning and drying skin on left thigh, calf, rub in contents of pouch using both hands until completely absorbed, wash hands

**Available forms:** Estradiol: tabs 0.5, 1, 2 mg; valerate: inj 10, 20, 40 mg/ml; transdermal 0.025, 0.0375, 0.05, 0.075, 0.1 mg/24-hr release rate; vag cream 100 mcg/g; vag ring 2 mg/90 days; vag tab 25 mcg; topical emulsion: 2.5 mg; gel 0.1% (Divigel); spray (Evamist) 1.53 mg/acuation

**Adverse effects**
*CNS:* Dizziness, headache, migraine, depression, **seizures**
*CV:* Hypotension, thrombophlebitis, edema, **thromboembolism, stroke, pulmonary embolism, MI**
*EENT:* Contact lens intolerance, increased myopia, astigmatism
*GI:* Nausea, vomiting, diarrhea, anorexia, pancreatitis, cramps, constipation, increased appetite, increased weight, **cholestatic jaundice, hepatic adenoma**
*GU:* Amenorrhea, cervical erosion, breakthrough bleeding, dysmenorrhea, vaginal candidiasis, breast changes, *gynecomastia, testicular atrophy, impotence,* **increased risk of breast, endometrial cancer,** changes in libido
*INTEG:* Rash, urticaria, acne, hirsutism, alopecia, oily skin, seborrhea, purpura, melasma

---

⬥ Alert ✤ Canada Only 🔵 Drug on CD ✳ "Tall Man" lettering (See Preface)

**META:** Folic acid deficiency, hypercalcemia, hyperglycemia

**Contraindications:** Pregnancy **X**, breast-feeding, breast cancer, thromboembolic disorders, reproductive cancer, genital bleeding (abnormal, undiagnosed)

**Precautions:** Hypertension, asthma, blood dyscrasias, gallbladder disease, CHF, diabetes mellitus, bone disease, depression, migraine headache, seizure disorders, renal/hepatic disease, family history of cancer of breast or reproductive tract, smoking, uterine fibroids, vaginal irritation infection

### Pharmacokinetics

| | |
|---|---|
| **Absorption** | Well absorbed |
| **Distribution** | Widely distributed, crosses placenta |
| **Metabolism** | Unknown |
| **Excretion** | Unknown |
| **Half-life** | Unknown |

### Pharmacodynamics

| | PO | IM | IV |
|---|---|---|---|
| **Onset** | Rapid | Slow | Rapid |
| **Peak** | Unknown | Unknown | Unknown |
| **Duration** | Unknown | Unknown | Unknown |

### Interactions
#### Individual drugs
Calcium, phenylbutazone, rifampin: decreased estradiol action
CycloSPORINE, dantrolene: increased toxicity
Tamoxifen: decreased tamoxifen action
#### Drug classifications
Anticoagulants: decreased action of anticoagulants
Anticonvulsants, barbiturates: decreased estradiol action
Corticosteroids: increased action of corticosteroids
Hypoglycemics (oral): decreased action of hypoglycemics
#### Drug/herb
Alfalfa, hops: increased estrogen effect
Saw palmetto: decreased estrogen effect
Black cohosh, DHEA: altered estrogen effect
#### Drug/food
Grapefruit juice: increased estrogen level
#### Drug/lab test
Increased: BSP retention test; PBI; $T_4$; serum sodium; platelet aggregation; thyroxine-binding globulin (TBS); prothrombin; factors VII, VIII, IX, X; triglycerides
Decreased: serum folate, serum triglyceride, $T_3$ resin uptake test, glucose tolerance test, antithrombin III, pregnanediol, metyrapone test
False positive: LE prep, ANA titer

## NURSING CONSIDERATIONS
### Assessment
• Monitor blood glucose in patient with diabetes; hyperglycemia may occur
• Monitor B/P q4hr; watch for increase caused by water and sodium retention
• Monitor I&O ratio; be alert for decreasing urinary output and increasing edema; monitor weight daily; notify prescriber if weekly weight gain is >5 lb; if increased, diuretic may be ordered
• Obtain liver function tests baseline, periodically, including AST, ALT, bilirubin, alkaline phosphatase, periodic folic acid level
• Assess edema, hypertension, cardiac symptoms, jaundice
• Assess mental status: affect, mood, behavioral changes, aggression; depression may occur, product may need to be discontinued
• Assess female patient for intact uterus, if so, progesterone should be added to estrogen therapy to decrease risk of endometrial cancer

### Nursing diagnoses
• Injury, risk for (adverse reactions)
• Sexual dysfunction (uses)

### Implementation
**PO route**
• Give titrated dose, use lowest effective dose
• Give with food or milk to decrease GI symptoms
**IM route**
• Administer deeply in large muscle mass; product is painful
• Rotate syringe to mix oil and medication
**Transdermal route**
• Apply to area free of hair to ensure adhesion on trunk of body 2×/wk; press firmly and hold in place for 10 sec to ensure good contact
• Start transdermal dose 7 days before last PO dose if routes are to be changed
**Topical route spray (Evamist)**
• Use daily; spray to inner upper arm; may increase to 2-3 times/day based on response; let dry for 2 min
**Vaginal route**
• Place cream in applicator by attaching tube to applicator; squeeze cream into tube to mark; insert with patient reclining
• Applicator should be washed after each use

### Patient/family education
• Tell patient to take exactly as prescribed; do not double doses

Adverse effects: *italic* = common, **bold** = life-threatening

◆ Advise patient that increased weight gain and symptoms of fluid retention should be reported to prescriber: edema of feet, ankles, sacral area; abnormal vaginal bleeding; breast lumps; hepatic disease (dark urine, clay-colored stools, jaundice of skin, sclera, pruritus)

◆ Caution patient that thromboembolic symptoms should be reported: tenderness in legs, chest pain, dyspnea, headaches, blurred vision

• Inform patient to use sunscreen and protective clothing because sunburns may occur

• Advise patient to stop smoking; smokers have a greater chance of thromboembolic disorder

• Tell patient to use nonhormonal birth control and to notify prescriber if pregnancy is suspected

### Evaluation
**Positive therapeutic outcome**
• Reversal of menopausal symptoms
• Decrease in tumor size in prostatic or breast cancer
• Decrease in itching, inflammation of vagina
• Absence of symptoms of osteoporosis

### estrogens, conjugated
(Rx)
Cenestin, C.E.S ♥, Congest, Premarin, Premphase

### estrogens, conjugated synthetic B (Rx)
Enjuvia

**Pregnancy category X**

**Do not confuse:**
Premarin/Provera

**Action:** Needed for adequate functioning of female reproductive system; affects release of pituitary gonadotropins; inhibits ovulation; promotes adequate calcium use in bone structures

**Therapeutic outcome:** Decreased tumor size in prostatic cancer; increased estrogen levels in menopause, female hypogonadism

**Uses:** Symptoms associated with menopause, inoperable breast cancer, prostatic cancer, abnormal uterine bleeding, hypogonadism, castration, primary ovarian failure, prevention of osteoporosis

### Dosage and routes
*Estrogens, conjugated*
*Menopause*
*Adult:* PO 0.3-1.25 mg/day 3 wk on, 1 wk off

*Prevention of osteoporosis*
*Adult:* PO 0.625 mg/day or in a cycle

*Atrophic vaginitis*
*Adult:* VAG 2-4 g cream/day × 21 days, off 7 days, repeat

*Prostatic cancer*
*Adult:* PO 1.25-2.5 mg tid

*Advanced inoperable breast cancer*
*Adult:* PO 10 mg tid × 3 mo or longer

*Abnormal uterine bleeding*
*Adult:* **IV**/IM 25 mg, repeat in 6-12 hr

*Ovariectomy/primary ovarian failure/castration*
*Adult:* PO 1.25 mg/day 3 wk on, 1 wk off

*Hypogonadism*
*Adult:* PO 2.5-7.5 mg/day × 20 days/mo

*Estrogens, conjugated synthetic B*
*Menopause*
*Adult:* PO 0.625 mg/day initially, may increase based on response

**Available forms:** Tabs 0.3, 0.45, 0.625, 0.9, 1.25, 2.5 mg; inj 25 mg/vial; vag cream 0.625 mg/g; synthetic B: tabs 0.625, 1.25 mg

**Adverse effects**
***CNS:*** Dizziness, headache, migraine, depression, **seizures,** mood disturbances
***CV:*** Hypotension, thrombophlebitis, edema, **thromboembolism, stroke, pulmonary embolism, MI**
***EENT:*** Contact lens intolerance, increased myopia, astigmatism
***GI:*** *Nausea,* vomiting, diarrhea, anorexia, pancreatitis, cramps, constipation, increased appetite, **cholestatic jaundice, hepatic adenoma,** weight gain/loss
***GU:*** Amenorrhea, cervical erosion, breakthrough bleeding, dysmenorrhea, vaginal candidiasis, breast changes, *gynecomastia, testicular atrophy, impotence,* **increased risk of breast, endometrial cancer,** libido changes
***INTEG:*** Rash, urticaria, acne, hirsutism, alopecia, oily skin, seborrhea, purpura, melasma
***META:*** Folic acid deficiency, hypercalcemia, hyperglycemia

**Contraindications:** Pregnancy X, breastfeeding, thromboembolic disorders, reproductive cancer, genital bleeding (abnormal, undiagnosed), hypersensitivity

**Precautions:** Hypertension, asthma, blood dyscrasias, gallbladder disease, CHF, diabetes mellitus, bone disease, depression, migraine headache, seizure disorders, renal/hepatic disease, family history of cancer of breast or reproductive tract, smoking, dementia, hypothyroidism, obesity, SLE

### Pharmacokinetics

| | |
|---|---|
| **Absorption** | Well absorbed (PO), completely absorbed **(IV)** |
| **Distribution** | Widely distributed, crosses placenta |
| **Metabolism** | Liver—exclusively; hepatic recirculation |
| **Excretion** | Kidney |
| **Half-life** | Unknown |

### Pharmacodynamics

| | PO | IM | IV |
|---|---|---|---|
| **Onset** | Rapid | Slow | Immediate |
| **Peak** | Unknown | Unknown | Unknown |
| **Duration** | Unknown | Unknown | Unknown |

### Interactions
#### Individual drugs
CycloSPORINE, dantrolene: increased toxicity
Phenylbutazone, rifampin: decreased action of estrogens
Tamoxifen: decreased tamoxifen action
#### Drug classifications
Anticoagulants: decreased action of anticoagulants
Anticonvulsants, barbiturates: decreased action of estrogens
Corticosteroids: increased action of corticosteroids
Oral hypoglycemics: decreased action of hypoglycemics
#### Drug/herb
Alfalfa, hops: increased estrogen level
Black cohosh, DHEA: altered estrogen effect
Saw palmetto: decreased estrogen level
#### Drug/food
Grapefruit juice: increased estrogen level
#### Drug/lab test
Increased: BSP retention test; PBI, $T_4$; serum sodium; platelet aggregation; thyroxine-binding globulin (TBG); prothrombin; factors VII, VIII, IX, X; triglycerides
Decreased: serum folate, serum triglyceride, $T_3$ resin uptake test, glucose tolerance test, antithrombin III, pregnanediol, metyrapone test
False positive: LE prep, ANA titer

### NURSING CONSIDERATIONS
#### Assessment
• Monitor blood glucose in patient with diabetes; hyperglycemia may occur
• Monitor B/P q4hr; watch for increase caused by water and sodium retention
• Monitor I&O ratio; be alert for decreasing urinary output and increasing edema; monitor weight daily; notify prescriber if weekly weight gain is >5 lb; if increased, diuretic may be ordered
• Obtain liver function tests, including AST, ALT, bilirubin, alkaline phosphatase
• Assess edema, hypertension, cardiac symptoms, jaundice
• Assess mental status: affect, mood, behavioral changes, aggression; depression may occur, product may need to be discontinued
• Assess female patient for intact uterus; if so, progesterone should be added to estrogen therapy to decrease risk of endometrial cancer; abnormal uterine bleeding, breast exam

#### Nursing diagnoses
• Injury, risk for (adverse reactions)
• Sexual dysfunction (uses)

#### Implementation
**PO route**
• Give titrated dose, use lowest effective dose
• Give in 1 dose in AM for prostatic cancer, vaginitis, hypogonadism
• Give with food or milk to decrease GI symptoms
**IM route**
• Reconstitute after withdrawing at least 5 ml of air from container and inject sterile diluent on vial side, rotate to dissolve
• Give IM inj deeply in large muscle
**Vaginal route**
• Place cream in applicator by attaching tube to applicator, squeeze cream into tube to mark, insert with patient recumbent
• Applicator should be washed after each use
**IV, direct route**
• Reconstitute as for IM, inject into distal port of running **IV** line of $D_5W$, 0.9% NaCl, LR, at a rate of 5 mg/min or less
**Y-site compatibilities:** Heparin/hydrocortisone, potassium chloride, vit B/C

#### Patient/family education
• Caution patient to take exactly as prescribed and not to double doses
◆ Advise patient that increased weight gain and symptoms of fluid retention should be reported to prescriber: edema of feet, ankles, sacral area; abnormal vaginal bleeding; breast lumps; hepatic disease (dark urine, clay-

Adverse effects: *italic* = common, **bold** = life-threatening

colored stools, jaundice of skin, sclera, pruritus)

⬥ Caution patient that thromboembolic symptoms should be reported: pain, redness, tenderness in legs; chest pain, dyspnea, headaches, blurred vision

• Inform patient that sunburns may occur and to use sunscreen and protective clothing

• Advise patient to stop smoking; smokers have a greater chance of thromboembolic disorder

• Tell patient to use nonhormonal birth control, and to notify prescriber if pregnancy is suspected

• Tell patient that vasomotor symptoms improve in 2 wk, max relief 8 wk

### Evaluation
**Positive therapeutic outcome**
• Reversal of menopause symptoms
• Decrease in tumor size in prostatic, breast cancer
• Decrease in itching, inflammation of vagina
• Absence of symptoms of osteoporosis

## eszopiclone (Rx)
(es-zop'i-klone)
Lunesta
*Func. class.:* Sedative/hypnotic, non-benzodiazepine
*Chem. class.:* Cyclopyrrolone

**Pregnancy category** C
**Controlled substance schedule** IV

**Action:** Interacts with GABA receptors

**Therapeutic outcome:** Ability to sleep and stay asleep throughout the night

**Uses:** Insomnia

### Dosage and routes
*Adult:* PO 2 mg immediately before bed, may increase to 3 mg if needed

*Hepatic dose/CYP3A4 inhibitors*
*Adult:* PO 1 mg immediately before bed

**Available forms:** Tabs 1, 2, 3 mg

### Adverse effects
*CNS:* Depression, hallucinations, headache, daytime drowsiness
*CV:* Peripheral edema, chest pain
*GI:* Dry mouth, bitter taste (dysgeusia)
*INTEG:* Rash

**Contraindications:** Hypersensitivity, ethanol intoxication

**Precautions:** Pregnancy **C**, breastfeeding, children, geriatric, severe hepatic disease

### Pharmacokinetics
| | |
|---|---|
| **Absorption** | Unknown |
| **Distribution** | Unknown |
| **Metabolism** | Extensively in the liver by CYP3A4, CYP2E1 |
| **Excretion** | Via kidneys |
| **Half-life** | 6 hr |

### Pharmacodynamics
| | |
|---|---|
| **Onset** | Rapid |
| **Peak** | 1 hr |
| **Duration** | 6 hr |

### Interactions
*Drug classifications*
CNS depressants: increased CNS depression
CYP3A4 inhibitors (clarithromycin, itraconazole, ketoconazole, nefazodone, nelfinavir, ritonavir, troleandomycin): increased toxicity due to decreased eszopiclone elimination
*Drug/food*
High-fat meal: decreased product action

## NURSING CONSIDERATIONS
### Assessment
• Assess sleep pattern: ability to go to sleep, stay asleep; early morning awakenings; conservative methods used
• Monitor for abuse of this or other products

### Nursing diagnoses
• Injury, risk for (adverse reactions)
• Knowledge, deficient (teaching)
• Sleep deprivation (uses)

### Implementation
• Do not break, crush, or chew tab
• Give immediately before bedtime
• Avoid use with a high fat meal

### Patient/family education
• Caution patient that daytime drowsiness may occur; not to engage in hazardous activities until effect is known
• Advise patient that all other medications and supplements should be avoided unless approved by prescriber
• Advise patient to notify prescriber if pregnancy is suspected or planned

### Evaluation
**Positive therapeutic outcome**
• Ability to sleep and stay asleep throughout the night

## etanercept (Rx)

(eh-tan'er-sept)

Enbrel

*Func. class.:* Antirheumatic agent (disease-modifying)

**Pregnancy category B**

**Action:** Binds to tumor necrosis factor (TNF), which decreases inflammation and immune response

**Therapeutic outcome:** Decreased pain, inflammation

**Uses:** Acute, chronic rheumatoid arthritis that has not responded to other disease-modifying agents; polyarticular course juvenile rheumatoid arthritis (JRA), ankylosing spondylitis, plaque psoriasis, psoriatic arthritis

**Unlabeled uses:** Crohn's disease

**Dosage and routes**
*Rheumatoid/psoriatic arthritis, ankylosing spondylitis*
*Adult:* SUBCUT 50 mg qwk
*Child 4-17 yr:* SUBCUT 0.8 mg/kg/wk, max 25 mg/dose

*Plaque psoriasis*
*Adult:* SUBCUT 50 mg 2×/wk

**Available forms:** Powder for inj 25 mg; inj 50 mg/ml; auto injector, single use

**Adverse effects**
*CNS:* Headache, asthenia, dizziness
*GI:* Abdominal pain, dyspepsia
*HEMA:* Pancytopenia
*INTEG:* Rash, *inj site reaction*
*RESP:* Pharyngitis, rhinitis, *cough, URI,* non-URI sinusitis
*SYST:* **Serious infections, sepsis, death, malignancies**

**Contraindications:** Hypersensitivity, sepsis, active infections

**Precautions:** Pregnancy **B**, breastfeeding, children <4 yr, geriatric, malignancies, latex allergy

### Pharmacokinetics

| | |
|---|---|
| **Absorption** | Rapidly (60%) |
| **Distribution** | Unknown |
| **Metabolism** | Unknown |
| **Excretion** | Unknown |
| **Half-life** | 115 hr |

### Pharmacodynamics
Unknown

**Interactions**
*Individual drugs*
Anakinra, cyclophosphamide: avoid use
*Drug classifications*
Immunizations: should be brought up to date before treatment
Immunizations, vaccines: do not give concurrently

## NURSING CONSIDERATIONS
### Assessment
• Assess for pain of rheumatoid arthritis; check ROM, inflammation of joints, characteristics of pain
• Assess inj site for pain, swelling, usually occurs after 2 inj (4-5 days)

### Nursing diagnoses
• Injury, risk for (side effects)
• Knowledge, deficient (teaching)
• Mobility, impaired physical (uses)
• Pain, chronic (uses)

### Implementation
• Administer after reconstituting 1 ml of supplied diluent, slowly inject diluent into vial, swirl contents, do not shake, sol should be clear/colorless, do not use if cloudy or discolored
• Do not admix with other sol or medications; do not use filter
• May be injected SUBCUT into upper arm, abdomen, thigh; rotate inj sites

### Patient/family education
• Teach patient that product must be continued for prescribed time to be effective; to avoid aspirin, alcoholic beverages
• Instruct patient to use caution when driving; dizziness may occur
• Teach patient about self-administration, if appropriate: inj should be made in thigh, abdomen, upper arm; rotate sites at least 1 in from old site

### Evaluation
**Positive therapeutic outcome**
• Decreased pain in arthritic conditions
• Decreased inflammation in arthritic conditions

E

## ethambutol (Rx)

(e-tham'byoo-tole)

Etibi ✦, Myambutol

*Func. class.:* Antitubercular

*Chem. class.:* Diisopropylethylene diamide derivative

**Pregnancy category B**

**Do not confuse:**

ethambutol/Ethmozine

**Action:** Inhibits RNA synthesis, decreases tubercle bacilli replication

**Therapeutic outcome:** Resolution of TB infection

**Uses:** Pulmonary TB, as an adjunct, other mycobacterial infections

**Dosage and routes**

*Adult and child >13 yr:* PO 15-25 mg/kg/day as a single dose or 50 mg/kg 2×/wk or 25-30 mg/kg 3×/wk

*Renal dose*

*Adult:* PO CCr 10-50 ml/min dose q24-36hr; CCr <10 ml/min dose q48hr

*Retreatment*

*Adult:* PO 25 mg/kg/day as single dose × 2 mo with at least 1 other product, then decrease to 15 mg/kg/day as single dose, max 2.5 g/day

*Child:* PO 15 mg/kg/day

**Available forms:** Tabs 100, 400 mg

**Adverse effects**

*CNS: Headache, confusion,* fever, malaise, dizziness, *disorientation,* hallucinations

*EENT:* Blurred vision, optic neuritis, photophobia, decreased visual acuity

*GI: Abdominal distress, anorexia, nausea, vomiting*

*INTEG:* Dermatitis, pruritus, **toxic epidermal necrolysis**

*META: Elevated uric acid, acute gout,* liver function impairment

*MISC:* **Thrombocytopenia,** joint pain, bloody sputum, **anaphylaxis**

**Contraindications:** Hypersensitivity, optic neuritis, child <13 yr

**Precautions:** Pregnancy **B**, breastfeeding, renal disease, diabetic retinopathy, cataracts, ocular defects, hepatic and hematopoietic disorders

### Pharmacokinetics

| | |
|---|---|
| **Absorption** | Rapidly absorbed |
| **Distribution** | Widely distributed, crosses blood-brain barrier, placenta |
| **Metabolism** | Liver |
| **Excretion** | Kidneys—unchanged |
| **Half-life** | 3 hr, increased in liver, kidney disease |

### Pharmacodynamics

| | |
|---|---|
| **Onset** | Rapid |
| **Peak** | 2-4 hr |
| **Duration** | Unknown |

### Interactions

*Drug classifications*

Antacids, aluminum: decreased absorption

Neurotoxic agents, other: increased neurotoxicity

### NURSING CONSIDERATIONS

**Assessment**

- Obtain C&S tests including sputum tests before initiating treatment; monitor qmo to detect resistance
- Monitor liver function tests qwk × 2 wk, then q2 mo: ALT, AST, bilirubin; renal studies: before, qmo: BUN, creatinine, output, specific gravity, urinalysis, uric acid
- Assess patient's mental status often: affect, mood, behavioral changes; psychosis may occur with hallucinations, confusion
- Assess patient's hepatic status: decreased appetite, jaundice, dark urine, fatigue
- Assess patient for visual disturbance that may indicate optic neuritis: blurred vision, change in color perception; may lead to blindness

**Nursing diagnoses**

- Diarrhea (adverse reactions)
- Infection, risk for (uses)
- Knowledge, deficient (teaching)
- Noncompliance (teaching)
- Sensory perception, disturbed (adverse reactions)

**Implementation**

- Give with meals to decrease GI symptoms, at same time each day to maintain blood level
- Give 2 hr before antacids
- Give antiemetic if vomiting occurs

**Patient/family education**

- Advise patient that compliance with dosage schedule and duration is necessary to eradicate disease; to keep scheduled appointments including ophthalmic appointments or relapse may occur

- Caution patient to report weakness, fatigue, loss of appetite, nausea, vomiting, yellowing of skin or eyes, tingling/numbness of hands/feet, weight gain, or decreased urine output
- Instruct patient to report any visual changes; rash; hot, swollen, painful joints; numbness or tingling of extremities to physician
- Caution patient to inform prescriber if pregnancy is suspected

### Evaluation
**Positive therapeutic outcome**
- Decreased symptoms of TB
- Decrease in acid-fast bacteria

---

## etidronate (Rx)
(eh-tih-droe′nate)
Didronel, Didronel IV
*Func. class.:* Bone resorption inhibitor
*Chem. class.:* Bisphosphonate

**Pregnancy category C**

**Do not confuse:**
etidronate/etomidate/etretinate

**Action:** Decreases bone resorption and new bone development (accretion)

**Therapeutic outcome:** Decreased bone reabsorption, calcium levels WNL

**Uses:** Paget's disease, heterotopic ossification, hypercalcemia of malignancy

### Dosage and routes
*Paget's disease*
**Adult:** PO 5-10 mg/kg/day, 2 hr before meals with water, not to exceed 20 mg/kg/day, max 6 mo or 11-20 mg/kg/day for max of 3 mo

*Heterotopic ossification*
**Adult:** PO 20 mg/kg/day × 2 wk, then 10 mg/kg/day for 10 wk, total 12 wk

*Hypercalcemia*
**Adult:** IV 7.5 mg/kg/day × 3 days, then 20 mg/kg/day (PO)

*Heterotopic ossification/hip replacement*
**Adult:** PO 20 mg/kg/day × 4 wk before and 3 mo after surgery (4 months total)

**Available forms:** Tabs 200, 400 mg; inj 50 mg/ml

### Adverse effects
*CNS:* Headache
*GI:* Nausea, constipation, metallic taste, diarrhea(**IV**), gastritis, esophagitis
*GU:* **Nephrotoxicity**
*MISC:* Dyspnea; low magnesium, phosphorus, alopecia, **Stevens-Johnson syndrome**

*MS:* *Bone pain,* hypocalcemia, decreased mineralization of nonaffected bones, **osteonecrosis of the jaw,** arthralgia, leg cramps

**Contraindications:** Pathologic fractures, clinically overt osteomalacia, severe renal disease with creatinine >5 mg/dl, poor dentition

**Precautions:** Pregnancy **C,** breastfeeding, children, renal disease, restricted vit D, calcium, enterocolitis

### Pharmacokinetics

| | |
|---|---|
| **Absorption** | Poorly absorbed (PO), completely absorbed (**IV**) |
| **Distribution** | 50% bond to crystals in osteogenesis |
| **Metabolism** | None |
| **Excretion** | Feces (unabsorbed), kidney (unchanged) |
| **Half-life** | 5-7 hr; in bone >3 mo |

### Pharmacodynamics

| | PO | IV |
|---|---|---|
| **Onset** | 4 wk | 24 hr |
| **Peak** | Unknown | 3-4 days |
| **Duration** | Up to 1 yr | 10-12 days |

### Interactions
*Individual drugs*
Warfarin: increased protime
*Drug classifications*
Antacids, mineral supplements with magnesium, calcium, iron products, or aluminum: decreased absorption of etidronate
*Drug/food*
Dairy products: decreased absorption of etidronate

### NURSING CONSIDERATIONS
**Assessment**
- Assess for GI symptoms, polyuria, flushing, head swelling, tingling, headache, may indicate hypercalcemia; nervousness, irritability, twitching, seizures, spasm, paresthesia indicates hypocalcemia at start of treatment
- Identify nutritional status; evaluate diet for sources of vit D (milk, some seafood), calcium (dairy products, dark green vegetables), phosphates
- Monitor BUN, creatinine, uric acid, chloride, electrolytes, urine pH, urinary calcium, magnesium, phosphate, urinalysis (calcium: should be kept at 9-10 mg/dl), albumin, alkaline phosphatase baseline and q3-6 mo; check urine sediment for casts throughout treatment

Adverse effects: *italic* = common, **bold** = life-threatening

- Assess for increased product level; toxic reactions occur rapidly; have calcium chloride or gluconate on hand if calcium level drops too low; check for tetany
- Assess for dental health

### Nursing diagnoses
- Injury, risk for (adverse reactions)
- Knowledge, deficient (teaching)
- Pain, chronic (uses)

### Implementation
**PO route**
- Administer on empty stomach to improve absorption (2 hr before meals)

**IV route**
- Used in hypercalcemias; give by intermittent inf after diluting 300 mg/250 ml or more 0.9% NaCl; run over 2-3 hr, therapy should not last >6 mo

### Patient/family education
- Teach method of inj if patient will be responsible for self-medication
- Caution patient to notify prescriber if hypercalcemia recurs: renal calculi, nausea, vomiting, thirst, lethargy, deep bone or flank pain, heat over bone, restricted mobility
- Teach patient that warmth and flushing occur and last 1 hr
- Teach patient to follow a low-calcium diet as prescribed (Paget's disease, hypercalcemia)
- Advise patient to notify prescriber of diarrhea, nausea; dose may be divided to lessen these symptoms
- Inform patient that metallic taste may occur with **IV** dosing

### Evaluation
**Positive therapeutic outcome**
- Calcium levels 9-10 mg/dl
- Decreasing symptoms of Paget's disease including pain
- Decreased bone loss in osteoporosis

---

## etodolac (Rx)
(ee-toe-doe'lak)
Lodine, Lodine XL
*Func. class.:* Nonsteroidal antiinflammatory, nonopioid analgesic

**Pregnancy category** C

**Do not confuse:**
Lodine/codeine/iodine

**Action:** Inhibits prostaglandin synthesis by decreasing enzyme needed for biosynthesis; analgesic, antiinflammatory properties

**Therapeutic outcome:** Decreased pain, inflammation

**Uses:** Mild to moderate pain, osteoarthritis

### Dosage and routes
*Osteoarthritis*
*Adult:* PO 800-1200 mg/day in divided doses q6-8hr initially, then adjust to 600-1200 mg/day in divided doses; do not exceed 1200 mg/day; patients <60 kg not to exceed 20 mg/kg

*Analgesia*
*Adult:* PO 200-400 mg q6-8hr prn for acute pain; do not exceed 1200 mg/day; patients <60 kg not to exceed 20 mg/kg

**Available forms:** Caps 200, 300 mg; tabs 400, 500 mg; ext rel tabs 400, 600 mg

### Adverse effects
*CNS:* Dizziness, headache, drowsiness, fatigue, tremors, confusion, insomnia, anxiety, depression, light-headedness, vertigo
*CV:* Tachycardia, peripheral edema, fluid retention, palpitations, dysrhythmias, CHF
*EENT:* Tinnitus, hearing loss, blurred vision, photophobia
*GI: Nausea, anorexia,* vomiting, diarrhea, jaundice, **cholestatic hepatitis,** constipation, flatulence, cramps, dry mouth, peptic ulcer, dyspepsia, **GI bleeding**
*GU:* **Nephrotoxicity, dysuria, hematuria, oliguria, azotemia, cystitis, UTI**
*HEMA:* **Blood dyscrasias**
*INTEG:* Erythema, urticaria, purpura, rash, pruritus, sweating, **Stevens-Johnson syndrome**
*SYST:* **Angioedema, anaphylaxis**

**Contraindications:** Hypersensitivity; patients in whom aspirin, iodides, or other NSAIDs have produced asthma, rhinitis, urticaria, nasal polyps, angioedema, bronchospasm; avoid in 2nd half of pregnancy

**Precautions:** Pregnancy **C**, breastfeeding, children, geriatric, bleeding, GI/cardiac/renal/hepatic disorders

| Pharmacokinetics | |
|---|---|
| **Absorption** | Well absorbed |
| **Distribution** | Highly bound to plasma protein |
| **Metabolism** | Unknown |
| **Excretion** | Unknown |
| **Half-life** | 7 hr |

| Pharmacodynamics | |
|---|---|
| **Onset** | ½ hr |
| **Peak** | 1-2 hr |
| **Duration** | 4-12 hr |

---

## Interactions
*Individual drugs*
Aspirin: may increase GI toxicity
CycloSPORINE, digoxin, lithium, methotrexate, phenytoin: increased toxicity
*Drug classifications*
Antacids: delayed etodolac effect
β-Adrenergic blockers: decreased effect
Diuretics: decreased effectiveness of diuretics
*Drug/herb*
Arginine, gossypol: increased gastric irritation
Bearberry, bilberry: increased NSAIDs action
Bogbean, chondroitin, saw palmetto, turmeric: increased bleeding risk
St. John's wort: severe photosensitivity

## NURSING CONSIDERATIONS
### Assessment
• Assess pain: location, frequency, characteristics; relief after medication
• Assess for GI bleeding: black stools, hematemesis
• Assess for asthma, aspirin hypersensitivity, nasal polyps that may be hypersensitive to etodolac
• Monitor blood counts during therapy; watch for decreasing platelets; if low, therapy may need to be discontinued, then restarted after hematologic recovery; watch for blood dyscrasia (thrombocytopenia): bruising, fatigue, bleeding, poor healing

### Nursing diagnoses
• Injury, risk for (adverse reactions)
• Knowledge, deficient (teaching)
• Mobility, impaired physical (uses)
• Pain, acute (uses)
• Pain, chronic (uses)

### Implementation
• Do not break, crush, or chew ext rel tabs
• Administer with full glass of water to enhance absorption
• Administer with food or milk to decrease gastric symptoms; food will slow absorption slightly, will not decrease absorption

### Patient/family education
• Inform patient that product must be continued for prescribed time to be effective; to avoid aspirin, alcoholic beverages, NSAIDs
• Caution patient to report bleeding, bruising, fatigue, malaise because blood dyscrasias can occur
• Instruct patient to use caution when driving; drowsiness, dizziness may occur
• Teach patient to take with a full glass of water to enhance absorption

### Evaluation
**Positive therapeutic outcome**
• Decreased pain
• Decreased inflammation
• Increased mobility

---

### ⚠ HIGH ALERT

## etoposide (Rx)
(e-toe′poe-side)
VePesid, VP-16
## etoposide phosphate (Rx)
Etopophos
*Func. class.:* Antineoplastic—miscellaneous
*Chem. class.:* Semisynthetic podophyllotoxin

**Pregnancy category D**

**Do not confuse:**
VePesid/Versed

**Action:** Inhibits mitotic activity through metaphase to mitosis; also inhibits cells from entering mitosis, depresses DNA, RNA synthesis, cell cycle specific S and $G_2$

**Therapeutic outcome:** Prevention of rapid growth of malignant cells

**Uses:** Leukemias, small cell carcinoma of the lung, testicular cancer, lymphomas, neuroblastoma, melanoma

**Unlabeled uses:** Lymphomas

**Dosage and routes**
*Testicular cancer*
*Adult:* **IV** 50-100 mg/m²/day × 5 days given q3-5 wk or 200-250 mg/m²/wk, or 125-140 mg/m²/day 3 × wk, q5 wk

*Small cell carcinoma of the lung*
*Adult:* **PO** 70 mg/m²/day × 4 days, repeated q3-4 wk; **IV** 35 mg/m²/day × 4 days, up to 50 mg/m²/day × 5 day q3-4 wk

**Available forms:** Inj 20 mg/ml, caps 50 mg

**Adverse effects**
*CNS:* Headache, *fever,* peripheral neuropathy, paresthesia, confusion
*CV: Hypotension,* **MI,** dysrhythmia
*GI: Nausea, vomiting, anorexia,* **hepatotoxicity,** dyspepsia, diarrhea, constipation
*GU:* **Nephrotoxicity**
*HEMA:* **Thrombocytopenia, leukopenia, myelosuppression, anemia**
*INTEG: Rash, alopecia,* phlebitis at **IV** site, radiation recall
*RESP:* **Bronchospasm,** pleural effusion
*SYST:* **Anaphylaxis**

---

Adverse effects: *italic* = common, **bold** = life-threatening

**Contraindications:** Pregnancy **D**, breast-feeding, hypersensitivity, bone marrow depression, severe renal/hepatic disease, bacterial infection, viral infection

**Precautions:** Children, renal/hepatic disease, gout

### Pharmacokinetics

| | |
|---|---|
| **Absorption** | Variably absorbed |
| **Distribution** | Rapidly absorbed, 97% protein binding, crosses placenta |
| **Metabolism** | Liver—some |
| **Excretion** | Kidneys, unchanged 50%, breast milk |
| **Half-life** | 3 hr initially, 15 hr terminally |

### Pharmacodynamics

Unknown

### Interactions
*Individual drugs*
Radiation: increased bone marrow depression
*Drug classifications*
Antineoplastics: increased bone marrow depression
Live virus vaccines: increased adverse reactions

### NURSING CONSIDERATIONS
**Assessment**
• Monitor B/P (baseline and q15 min) during administration
• Monitor CBC, differential, platelet count weekly; withhold product if WBC is <4000/mm$^3$ or platelet count is <75,000/mm$^3$; notify prescriber of results; recovery will take 3 wk
• Monitor renal function tests: BUN, urine CCr before, during therapy; I&O ratio; report fall in urine output of 30 ml/hr; for decreased hyperuricemia
• Monitor for cold, fever, sore throat (may indicate beginning of infection); notify prescriber if these occur
• Assess for bleeding: hematuria, guaiac, bruising or petechiae, mucosa or orifices q8hr: no rectal temp; avoid IM inj; use pressure to venipuncture sites
• Identify nutritional status: an antiemetic may need to be prescribed
◆ Assess for symptoms indicating severe allergic reactions: rash, pruritus, urticaria, itching, flushing, bronchospasm, hypotension; epINEPHrine and crash cart should be nearby

**Nursing diagnoses**
• Body image, disturbed (adverse reactions)
• Infection, risk for (adverse reactions)
• Injury, risk for (adverse reactions)
• Knowledge, deficient (teaching)

### Implementation
**PO route**
• Caps need to be refrigerated
**IV route**
• Give by intermittent inf
• Sol should be prepared by qualified personnel and only under controlled conditions
• Use Luer-Lok tubing to prevent leakage; do not let sol come in contact with skin; if contact occurs, wash well with soap and water
• Give after diluting 100 mg/250 ml or more D$_5$W or NaCl to a concentration of 0.2-0.4 mg/ml; infuse over 30-60 min; phosphate may be given over 5 min-3½ hr; may dilute further to 0.1 mg/ml in 0.9% NaCl, D$_5$W
• Give hyaluronidase 150 units/ml to 1 ml NaCl to infiltration area; ice compress for treatment of vesicant activity
*Y-site compatibilities:* Allopurinol, amifostine, aztreonam, cladribine, fludarabine, granisetron, melphalan, ondansetron, paclitaxel, piperacillin/tazobactam, sargramostim, sodium bicarbonate, teniposide, thiotepa, vinorelbine
*Y-site incompatibility:* Idarubicin
*Additive compatibilities:* Carboplatin, cisplatin, cytarabine, floxuridine, fluorouracil, hydrOXYzine, ifosfamide, ondansetron

### Patient/family education
• Teach patient to avoid use of products containing aspirin or ibuprofen, razors, commercial mouthwash because bleeding may occur; to report symptoms of bleeding (hematuria, tarry stools)
• Instruct patient to report signs of anemia (fatigue, headache, irritability, faintness, shortness of breath)
• Teach patient to report any changes in breathing or coughing even several months after treatment
• Advise patient that contraception will be necessary during treatment because teratogenesis may occur
• Caution patient that hair loss may occur during treatment; a wig or hairpiece may make patient feel better; new hair will be different in color, texture
• Advise patient to avoid vaccinations during treatment because serious reactions may occur
• Teach patient to report signs/symptoms of infection; fever, chills, sore throat; patient should avoid crowds and persons with known infections

## Evaluation
**Positive therapeutic outcome**
• Decreased spread of malignant, leukemic cells

---

## exemestane (Rx)
(x-ee-mes'-tane)
Aromasin
*Func. class.:* Antineoplastic
*Chem. class.:* Aromatase inhibitor

**Pregnancy category D**

**Action:** Lowers serum estradiol concentrations; many breast cancers have strong estrogen receptors

**Therapeutic outcome:** Prevention of rapidly growing malignant cells

**Uses:** Advanced breast carcinoma that has not responded to other therapy in estrogen receptor–positive patients (postmenopausal)

**Dosage and routes**
*Adult:* PO 25 mg/day after meals

**Available forms:** Tabs 25 mg

**Adverse effects**
*CNS:* Headache, fatigue, depression, insomnia, anxiety
*CV:* Hypertension
*GI:* Nausea, vomiting, increased appetite, diarrhea, constipation, abdominal pain, hot flashes
***HEMA:*** *Lymphopenia*
*RESP:* Cough, dyspnea

**Contraindications:** Pregnancy **D**, hypersensitivity, premenopausal women

**Precautions:** Breastfeeding, children, geriatric, renal/hepatic disease

### Pharmacokinetics
| | |
|---|---|
| **Absorption** | Rapidly absorbed |
| **Distribution** | Unknown |
| **Metabolism** | Liver |
| **Excretion** | Feces, urine |
| **Half-life** | 24 hr |

### Pharmacodynamics
Unknown

## Interactions
*Drug classifications*
CYP3A4 inducers, estrogens: decreased exemestane action

---

## NURSING CONSIDERATIONS
### Assessment
• Assess B/P, hypertension may occur

### Nursing diagnoses
• Injury, risk for (adverse reactions)
• Knowledge, deficient (teaching)

### Implementation
• Give with food or fluids for GI upset
• Store in light-resistant container at room temperature

### Patient/family education
• Instruct patient to report any complaints, side effects to prescriber; if dose is missed, do not double next dose
• Advise patient that hot flashes can occur, and are reversible after discontinuing treatment
• Inform patient about who should be told about therapy

### Evaluation
**Positive therapeutic outcome**
• Decreased spread of malignant cells in breast cancer

---

## exenatide (Rx)
(ex-en'a-tide)
Byetta
*Func. class.:* Antidiabetic
*Chem. class.:* Incretin mimetic

**Pregnancy category C**

**Action:** Binds and activates known human GLP-1 receptor, mimics natural physiology for self-regulating glycemic control

**Therapeutic outcome:** Decreased polyuria, polydipsia, polyphagia; improved A1c

**Uses:** Type 2 diabetes mellitus given in combination with metformin or a sulfonylurea

**Dosage and routes**
*Adult:* SUBCUT 5 mcg bid 1 hr before morning and evening meal; may increase to 10 mcg bid after 1 mo of therapy

**Available forms:** Inj 250 mcg/ml pen injector

**Adverse effects**
*CNS:* Headache, *dizziness,* feeling jittery, restlessness, weakness
***ENDO:*** **Hypoglycemia**
*GI:* Nausea, vomiting, diarrhea, dyspepsia, anorexia, gastroesophageal reflux, weight loss

**Contraindications:** Hypersensitivity

---

Adverse effects: *italic* = common, **bold** = life-threatening

**Precautions:** Pregnancy **C**, geriatric, severe renal/hepatic/GI disease

| Pharmacokinetics | |
|---|---|
| **Absorption** | Unknown |
| **Distribution** | Unknown |
| **Metabolism** | Unknown |
| **Excretion** | Glomerular filtration |
| **Half-life** | Unknown |

| Pharmacodynamics | |
|---|---|
| **Onset** | Unknown |
| **Peak** | 2.1 hr |
| **Duration** | Unknown |

## Interactions
### Individual drugs
Acetaminophen: may increase the effect of acetaminophen

Acetaminophen (elixir), digoxin, lovastatin: decreased action of these products

Alcohol, disopyramide: increased hypoglycemia

Dextrothyroxine, niacin, triamterene: decreased hypoglycemia

Erythromycin, metoclopramide: do not use with exenatide

Exenatide: increased action

### Drug classifications
ACE inhibitors, anabolic steroids, androgens, corticosteroids, fibric acid derivatives: increased hypoglycemia

Estrogens, MAOIs, oral contraceptives, progestins, thiazide diuretics: decreased hypoglycemia

Phenothiazines: increased hyperglycemia

## NURSING CONSIDERATIONS
### Assessment
• Monitor fasting blood, glucose, A1c levels, postprandial glucose during treatment to determine diabetes control
• Assess for hypo/hyperglycemic reaction that can occur soon after meals; for severe hypoglycemia give **IV** D$_{50}$W, then **IV** dextrose solution

### Nursing diagnoses
• Injury, risk for (uses)
• Knowledge, deficient (teaching)
• Noncompliance (teaching)

### Implementation
• Give 1 hr before meals; if patient is NPO, may need to hold dose to prevent hypoglycemia
• Store in refrigerator

## Patient/family education
• Teach patient symptoms of hypo/hyperglycemia, what to do about each; to have glucagon emergency kit available; to carry a glucose source (candy, sugar cube) to treat hypoglycemia
• Advise patient that product must be continued on daily basis; explain consequences of discontinuing product abruptly
• Teach patient that diabetes is a lifelong illness; product will not cure disease
• Advise that all food in diet plan must be eaten to prevent hypoglycemia
• Advise patient to carry emergency ID with prescriber and medications
• Advise patient to continue weight control, dietary restrictions, exercise, hygiene
• Inform patient that regular blood glucose monitoring and A1c testing is needed
• Advise patient to notify prescriber if pregnant or intend to become pregnant
• Advise patient to read "Information for the Patient" and "Pen User Manual"

## Evaluation
**Positive therapeutic outcome**
• Decrease in polyuria, polydipsia, polyphagia, clear sensorium; improved A1c, weight; absence of dizziness, stable gait

---

## ezetimibe (Rx)
(ehz-eh-tim'bee)
Zetia
*Func. class.:* Antilipemic
**Pregnancy category C**

**Action:** Inhibits absorption of cholesterol by the small intestine

**Therapeutic outcome:** Decreased cholesterol levels

**Uses:** Hypercholesterolemia, homozygous familial hypercholesterolemia (HoFH), homozygous sitosterolemia

**Dosage and routes**
*Adult:* **PO** 10 mg/day; may be given with HMG-CoA reductase inhibitor at same time; may be given with bile acid sequestrant; give ezetimibe 2 hr before or 4 hr after the bile acid sequestrant

**Available forms:** Tabs 10 mg

**Adverse effects**
*CNS:* Fatigue, dizziness, headache
*GI:* Diarrhea, abdominal pain
*MISC:* Chest pain

---

*MS: Myalgias, arthralgias,* back pain
*RESP:* Pharyngitis, sinusitis, cough, URI

**Contraindications:** Hypersensitivity, severe hepatic disease

**Precautions:** Pregnancy **C**, breastfeeding, children, hepatic disease

### Pharmacokinetics

| | |
|---|---|
| **Absorption** | Unknown |
| **Distribution** | Unknown |
| **Metabolism** | Small intestine, liver |
| **Excretion** | Urine (11%), feces (78%) |
| **Half-life** | Unknown |

### Pharmacodynamics
Unknown

### Interactions
*Individual drugs*
Cholestyramine: decreased ezetimibe action
CycloSPORINE: increased action of ezetimibe
*Drug classifications*
Antacids: decreased action of ezetimibe
Fibric acid derivatives: increased ezetimibe action
*Drug/herb*
Glucomannan: increased effect
Gotu kola: decreased effect

### NURSING CONSIDERATIONS
**Assessment**
• Monitor lipid levels, liver function tests baseline and periodically during treatment

**Nursing diagnoses**
• Knowledge, deficient (teaching)
• Noncompliance (teaching)

**Implementation**
• Give without regard to meals

**Patient/family education**
• Teach patient that compliance is needed
• Advise that risk factors should be decreased: high-fat diet, smoking, alcohol consumption, absence of exercise
• Advise patient to notify prescriber if pregnancy is suspected or planned

**Evaluation**
**Positive therapeutic outcome**
• Decreased cholesterol

---

## factor VIIa, recombinant (Rx)
NovoSeven
*Func. class.:* Antihemophilic

**Pregnancy category  C**

**Action:** Promotes hemostasis by activating the intrinsic pathway of coagulation

**Therapeutic outcome:** Prevention of hemorrhage

**Uses:** Bleeding in hemophilia A or B, with inhibitors to factor VIII or IX, acquired hemophilia, factor VII deficiency

**Unlabeled uses:** Coumarin toxicity

**Dosage and routes**
*Bleeding prophylaxis or hemophilic with inhibitors to factor VIII/IX*
*Adult:* IV BOL 90 mcg/kg q2hr until hemostasis occurs, or until therapy is deemed to be inadequate; posthemostatic doses q3-6hr may be required

*Bleeding prophylaxis factor VII deficiency*
*Adult:* IV BOL 15-30 mcg/kg over 2-5 min q4-6hr

**Available forms:** Lyophilized powder 1.2 mg/vial (1200 mcg/vial), 2.4 mg/vial (2400 mcg/vial), 4.8 mg/vial (4800 mcg/vial) recombinant human coagulation factor VIIa (rFVIIa)

**Adverse effects**
*CNS:* Fever, headache, **cerebral artery occlusion**
*CV:* **Ischemic heart disease, MI**
*INTEG:* Pain, redness at inj site, pruritus, purpura, rash
*SYST:* **Hemorrhage not otherwise specified, hemarthrosis, fibrinogen plasma decreased,** hypertension, bradycardia, **DIC, coagulation disorder, thrombosis, acute renal failure**

**Contraindications:** Hypersensitivity to this product or mouse, hamster, or bovine products

**Precautions:** Pregnancy **C**, breastfeeding, children, DIC, septicemia, intracranial hemorrhage

---

Adverse effects: *italic* = common, **bold** = life-threatening

## Pharmacokinetics

| | |
|---|---|
| **Absorption** | Unknown |
| **Distribution** | Unknown |
| **Metabolism** | Unknown |
| **Excretion** | Unknown |
| **Half-life** | 2-3 hr |

## Pharmacodynamics

Unknown

## Interactions
### Individual drugs
Activated prothrombin complex concentrate, prothrombin complex concentrate: do not use together

## NURSING CONSIDERATIONS
### Assessment
- Assess VS, B/P, pulse, respirations, neurologic signs, temp at least q4hr, temp 104° F (40° C) or indicators of internal bleeding, cardiac rhythm
- Monitor pro-time, APTT, plasma FVII clotting
- Monitor for thrombosis, dose should be reduced or stopped

### Nursing diagnoses
- Injury, risk for (uses, adverse reactions)
- Tissue perfusion, ineffective (uses)

### Implementation
**IV route**
- Bring to room temperature; for 1.2 mg vial/2.2 ml sterile water for inj; 4.8 mg vial/8.5 ml sterile water for inj; remove caps from stopper, cleanse stopper with alcohol, allow to dry, draw back plunger of sterile syringe and allow air into syringe, insert needle of syringe into sterile water for inj, inject the air and withdraw amount required, insert syringe needle with diluent into product vial, aim to side so liquid runs down vial wall, gently swirl until dissolved, use within 3 hr, give by BOL over 3-5 min
- Do not admix, keep refrigerated until ready to use, avoid sunlight

### Evaluation
**Positive therapeutic outcome**
- Therapeutic response: hemostasis

## ! HIGH ALERT

### factor IX complex (human)
BeneFIX, Konyne 80, Profilnine/Alpha Nine, Proplex T, Proplex SX-T, Alpha Nine SD, Mononine
*Func. class.:* Hemostatic
*Chem. class.:* Factors II, VII, IX, X
**Pregnancy category C**

**Action:** Causes an increase in blood levels of clotting factors II, VII, IX, X; factor IX (human) has IX activity only

**Therapeutic outcome:** Replacement of factors II, VII, IX, X

**Uses:** Hemophilia B (Christmas disease), factor IX deficiency, anticoagulant reversal, control of bleeding in patients with factor VIII inhibitors; reversal of overdose of anticoagulants in emergencies

### Dosage and routes
*Bleeding in hemophilia A and inhibitors of factor VIII (Proplex T, Konyne 80)*
*Adult and child:* 75 units/kg, repeat in 12 hr

*Factor IX complex (human) bleeding in hemophilia B*
*Adult and child:* **IV** Establish 25% of normal factor IX activity or 60-75 units/kg then 10-20 units/kg/day × 1-2 wk

*Prophylaxis of bleeding in hemophilia B*
*Adult and child:* **IV** 10-20 units/kg 1-2 × wk

*Reversal of oral anticoagulant*
*Adult and child:* 15 units/kg

*Factor VII deficiency (use Proplex T only)*
*Adult and child:* 0.5 units/kg × body weight (kg) × desired factor IX increase (in % of normal); repeat q4-6hr if needed

*Factor IX (human) minor to moderate hemorrhage*
Use only Alpha Nine, Alpha Nine SD
*Adult and child:* **IV** Dose to increase plasma factor IX level to 20%-30% in one dose

*Serious hemorrhage*
*Adult and child:* **IV** Dose to increase plasma factor IX level to 30%-50% given as daily inf

*Minor hemorrhage (Mononine only)*
*Adult and child:* **IV** Dose to increase plasma factor IX level to 15%-25% (20-30 units/kg), may repeat in 24 hr if needed

## Major hemorrhage
**Adult and child: IV** Dose to increase plasma factor IX level to 25%-50% (75 units/kg) q18-30hr for up to 10 days

**Available forms:** Inj (number of units noted on label)

## Adverse effects
*CNS: Headache, dizziness,* malaise, paresthesia, *lethargy, chills, fever, flushing*
*CV: Hypotension,* tachycardia, **MI, venous thrombosis, pulmonary embolism**
*GI:* Nausea, vomiting, abdominal cramps, jaundice, **viral hepatitis**
*HEMA:* **Thrombosis, hemolysis, AIDS, DIC**
*INTEG:* Rash, flushing, *urticaria*
*RESP:* **Bronchospasm**

**Contraindications:** Hypersensitivity to mouse protein, hepatic disease, DIC, elective surgery, mild factor IX deficiency

**Precautions:** Pregnancy **C,** neonates, infants

### Pharmacokinetics

| | |
|---|---|
| **Absorption** | 40% (PO), complete (**IV**) |
| **Distribution** | Unknown |
| **Metabolism** | Rapidly cleared from plasma, liver 30% |
| **Excretion** | Kidneys—70% unchanged |
| **Half-life** | 24 hr |

### Pharmacodynamics
Unknown

## Interactions
### Individual drugs
Aminocaproic acid: increased risk of thrombosis; do not use together
Warfarin: decreased effect of warfarin
### Drug classifications
Incompatible with protein products

## NURSING CONSIDERATIONS
### Assesment
• Monitor blood studies (coagulation factor assays by % normal: 5% prevents spontaneous hemorrhage, 30%-50% for surgery, 80%-100% for severe hemorrhage); check for bleeding q15-30 min, immobilize and apply ice to affected joints
• Monitor for increased B/P, pulse
• Monitor I&O; if urine becomes orange or red, notify prescriber
• Assess for allergic or pyrogenic reaction: fever, chills, rash, itching; slow inf rate if not severe

⬦ Assess for DIC: bleeding, ecchymosis, hypersensitivity, changes in coagulation tests

### Nursing diagnoses
• Injury, risk for (uses)
• Knowledge, deficient (teaching)
• Tissue perfusion, ineffective (uses)

### Implementation
**IV route**
• Give hepatitis B vaccine before administration
• Give **IV** after warming to room temperature 3 ml/min or less, with plastic syringe only; do not admix
• Give after dilution with provided diluent, 50 or 25 units/ml; give so as not to exceed 10 ml/min; decrease rate if fever, headache, flushing, tingling occur
• Give after crossmatch is completed if patient has blood type A, B, AB, to determine incompatibility with factor
• Store reconstituted sol for 3 hr at room temperature or up to 2 yr if refrigerated (powder); check expiration date
• Incompatible with protein products
**BeneFIX**
• Allow vials of concentrate/diluent to warm to room temperature
• After removing flip-top cap from vial, wipe top of vial with alcohol swab; let dry
• Peel back cover from vial adapter package; do not remove
• Place vial adapter over vial; press firmly until snaps; attach plunger rod to diluent syringe and break plastic tip cap from diluent syringe
• Lift the package away from the adapter and connect diluent syringe; depress plunger; swirl contents

### Patient/family education
• Advise patient to report any signs of bleeding: gums, under skin, urine, stools, emesis
• Caution patient about risk of viral hepatitis, AIDS; that immunization for hepatitis B may be given first; to be tested q2-3 mo for HIV, even though the risk is low
• Tell patient to carry/wear emergency ID identifying disease and treatment; avoid salicylates, NSAIDs, to inform other health professionals about condition

### Evaluation
**Positive therapeutic outcome**
• Prevention of hemorrhage

Adverse effects: *italic* = common, **bold** = life-threatening

## famciclovir (Rx)
(fam-sye-klo′vir)
Famvir
*Func. class.:* Antiviral
*Chem. class.:* Guanosine nucleoside

**Pregnancy category B**

**Action:** Inhibits DNA polymerase and viral DNA synthesis by the conversion of this guanosine nucleoside to penciclovir

**Therapeutic outcome:** Decreasing size and number of lesions

**Uses:** Treatment of acute herpes zoster (shingles), genital herpes, recurrent mucocutaneous herpes simplex virus (HSV) in HIV patients, initial episodes of herpes genitalis

### Dosage and routes
*Herpes zoster*
*Adult:* PO 500 mg q8hr × 7 days

*Renal dose*
*Adult:* PO CCr ≥ 60 ml/min 500 mg q8hr; 40-59 ml/min 500 mg q12hr; 20-39 ml/min 500 mg q24hr; CCr <20 ml/min 250 mg q24hr

*Recurrent HSV*
*Adult:* PO 125 mg q12hr × 5 days

*Renal dose*
*Adult:* PO CCr <39 ml/min 125 mg q24hr × 5 days

*Suppression of recurrent HSV*
*Adult:* PO 250 mg q12hr up to 1 yr

*Renal dose*
*Adult:* PO CCr 20-39 ml/min 125 mg q12hr × 5 days; CCr <20 ml/min 125 mg q24hr × 5 days

*Genital herpes (recurrent)*
*Adult:* PO 125 mg bid × 5 days; begin treatment at first sign of recurrence

*Suppression of recurrent genital herpes*
*Adult:* PO 250 mg bid for up to a year

*Herpes genitalis initial episodes*
*Adult:* PO 250 mg tid × 7-10 days

**Available forms:** Tabs 125, 250, 500 mg

### Adverse effects
***CNS:*** *Headache, fatigue, dizziness,* paresthesia, somnolence, fever
***GI:*** Nausea, vomiting, diarrhea, constipation, abdominal pain, anorexia
***GU:*** Decreased sperm count
***INTEG:*** *Pruritus*
***MS:*** Back pain, arthralgia
***RESP:*** Pharyngitis, sinusitis

**Contraindications:** Hypersensitivity to this product, penciclovir, acyclovir, ganciclovir, valacyclovir, or valganciclovir

**Precautions:** Pregnancy **B**, breastfeeding, renal disease, hypersensitivity to acyclovir, ganciclovir

### Pharmacokinetics
| | |
|---|---|
| **Absorption** | Well absorbed, 77% |
| **Distribution** | Protein binding 20% |
| **Metabolism** | Intestinal tissue, blood, liver |
| **Excretion** | Breast milk, kidney, bile |
| **Half-life** | Terminal 2-3 hr |

### Pharmacodynamics
| | |
|---|---|
| **Onset** | Unknown |
| **Peak** | 1 hr |
| **Duration** | 8 hr |

### Interactions
*Individual drugs*
Cimetidine: decreased metabolism
Digoxin, probenecid, theophylline: decreased renal excretion

### NURSING CONSIDERATIONS
**Assessment**
• Assess amount and distribution of lesions; also burning, itching, or pain (early symptoms of herpes infection); neuralgia during and after treatment
• Monitor renal function tests: urine CCr, BUN before and during treatment if patient has decreased renal function; dose may need to be lowered
• Monitor bowel pattern before, during treatment; diarrhea may occur

**Nursing diagnoses**
• Infection, risk for (uses)
• Knowledge, deficient (teaching)

**Implementation**
• Give with or without meals; absorption does not appear to be lowered when taken with food
• Give within 72 hr of the appearance of rash in herpes zoster

**Patient/family education**
• Teach patient how to recognize signs of beginning of infection
• Teach patient how to prevent the spread of infection to others
• Teach patient reason for medication and expected results
• Advise patient that this medication does not prevent spread of disease to others, that condoms should be used

---

 Alert　　 Canada Only　　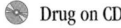 Drug on CD　　\* "Tall Man" lettering (See Preface)

• Advise women with genital herpes to have yearly Pap smears, cervical cancer is more likely

## Evaluation

**Positive therapeutic outcome**
• Decreased size and spread of lesions

---

## famotidine (Rx, OTC)
(fa-moe'to-deen)
Maximum Strength Pepcid, Mylanta AR, Pepcid, Pepcid AC, Pepcid AC Acid Controller, Pepcid RPD ✦
*Func. class.:* H$_2$-histamine receptor antagonist, antiulcer agent

**Pregnancy category B**

**Action:** Inhibits histamine at H$_2$-receptor site in gastric parietal cells, which inhibits gastric acid secretion

**Therapeutic outcome:** Healing of duodenal ulcers or gastric ulcers; prevention of duodenal ulcers; decreases symptoms of gastroesophageal reflux disease or Zollinger-Ellison syndrome, heartburn

**Uses:** Short-term treatment of active duodenal ulcer, maintenance therapy for duodenal ulcer, Zollinger-Ellison syndrome, multiple endocrine adenomas, gastric ulcers, heartburn, gastroesophageal reflux disease

**Unlabeled uses:** GI disorders in those taking NSAIDs, urticaria, prevention of stress ulcers, aspiration pneumonitis, inactivation of oral pancreatic enzymes in pancreatic disorders, prevention of paclitaxel hypersensitivity reactions

### Dosage and routes
*Active ulcer*
*Adult:* PO 40 mg/day at bedtime × 4-8 wk, then 20 mg/day at bedtime if needed (maintenance); **IV** 20 mg q12hr if unable to take PO
*Child 1-16 yr:* PO 0.5 mg/kg/day at bedtime or divided bid, max 40 mg/day

*Hypersecretory conditions*
*Adult:* PO 20 mg q6hr; may give 160 mg q6hr if needed; **IV** 20 mg q12hr if unable to take PO
*Child 1-16 yr:* PO 1 mg/kg/day divided bid, max 40 mg bid

*Paclitaxel hypersensitivity reactions*
*Adult:* **IV** 20 mg ½ hr before inf

*Heartburn relief/prevention*
*Adult:* PO 10 mg with water or 1 hr before eating

*Renal dose*
*Adult:* PO CCr <10 ml/min 20 mg at bedtime or dose q36-48hr

**Available forms:** Tabs 10, 20, 40 mg; powder for oral susp 40 mg/5 ml; inj 10 mg/ml, 20 mg/50 ml 0.9% NaCl; orally disintegrating tabs (RPD) 20, 40 mg; chew tabs 10 mg; gel cap 10 mg

**Adverse effects:**
*CNS: Headache, dizziness,* paresthesia, depression, anxiety, somnolence, insomnia, fever
*CV:* **Dysrhythmias**
*EENT:* Taste change, tinnitus, orbital edema
*GI: Constipation,* nausea, vomiting, anorexia, cramps, abnormal liver enzymes, diarrhea
*HEMA:* **Thrombocytopenia, aplastic anemia**
*INTEG:* Rash
*MS:* Myalgia, arthralgia

**Contraindications:** Hypersensitivity

**Precautions:** Pregnancy **B**, breastfeeding, children <12 yr, geriatric, severe renal/hepatic disease

| Pharmacokinetics | |
|---|---|
| **Absorption** | 50% absorbed (PO) |
| **Distribution** | Plasma, protein binding (15%-20%) |
| **Metabolism** | Liver (30% active metabolizing) |
| **Excretion** | Kidneys (70%) |
| **Half-life** | 2½-3½ hr |

| Pharmacodynamics | | |
|---|---|---|
| | PO | IV |
| **Onset** | 30-60 min | Immediate |
| **Peak** | 1-3 hr | ½-3 hr |
| **Duration** | 6-12 hr | 8-15 hr |

### Interactions
*Individual drugs*
Ketoconazole: decreased absorption of ketoconazole
*Drug classifications*
Antacids: decreased absorption of famotidine

### NURSING CONSIDERATIONS
**Assessment**
• Assess patient with ulcers or suspected ulcers: epigastric, abdominal pain, hematemesis, occult blood in stools, blood in gastric aspirate before treatment; throughout treat-

---

Adverse effects: *italic* = common, **bold** = life-threatening

ment, monitor gastric pH (5 should be maintained)
• Monitor I&O ratio, BUN, creatinine, CBC with differential monthly

## Nursing diagnoses
• Knowledge, deficient (teaching)
• Pain, acute (uses)

## Implementation
**PO route**
• Give antacids 1 hr before or 2 hr after famotidine; may be given with foods or liquid
• Administer oral susp after shaking well; discard unused sol after 1 mo
**IV route**
• Give **IV** direct after diluting 2 ml of product (10 mg/ml) in 0.9% NaCl to total volume of 5-10 ml; inject over 2 min to prevent hypotension
• Administer **IV** intermittent inf after diluting 20 mg of product in 100 ml of LR, 0.9% NaCl, $D_5W$, $D_{10}W$; run over 15-30 min
• Store in cool environment (oral); **IV** solution is stable for 48 hr at room temperature; do not use discolored sol
*Y-site compatibilities:* Acyclovir, allopurinol, amifostine, aminophylline, amphotericin, ampicillin, ampicillin/sulbactam, inamrinone, amsacrine, atropine, aztreonam, bretylium, calcium gluconate, cefazolin, cefoperazone, cefotaxime, cefotetan, cefoxitin, ceftazidime, ceftizoxime, ceftriaxone, cefuroxime, cephalothin, cephapirin, chlorproMAZINE, cisplatin, cladribine, cyclophosphamide, cytarabine, dexamethasone, dextran 40, digoxin, diphenhydrAMINE, DOBUTamine, DOPamine, DOXOrubicin, droperidol, enalaprilat, epINEPHrine, erythromycin lactobionate, esmolol, filgrastim, fluconazole, fludarabine, folic acid, gentamicin, granisetron, haloperidol, heparin, hydrocortisone, hydromorphone, hydrOXYzine, imipenem/cilastatin, regular insulin, isoproterenol, labetalol, lidocaine, lorazepam, magnesium sulfate, melphalan, meperidine, methotrexate, methylPREDNISolone, metoclopramide, mezlocillin, midazolam, morphine, nafcillin, nitroglycerin, nitroprusside, norepinephrine, ondansetron, oxacillin, paclitaxel, perphenazine, phenylephrine, phenytoin, phytonadione, piperacillin, potassium chloride, potassium phosphate, procainamide, propofol, sargramostim, sodium bicarbonate, teniposide, theophylline, thiamine, thiotepa, ticarcillin, ticarcillin/clavulanate, verapamil, vinorelbine
*Additive compatibilities:* Cefazolin, cefmetazole, flumazenil

## Patient/family education
• Caution patient to avoid driving, other hazardous activities until stabilized on this medication; dizziness may occur
• Advise patient to avoid black pepper, caffeine, alcohol, harsh spices, extremes in temperature of food; tell patient to avoid OTC preparations: aspirin, cough, cold preparations; condition may worsen
• Advise patient to avoid taking the OTC and the prescription preparations of this product concurrently
• Tell patient that smoking decreases the effectiveness of the product; that smoking cessation should be considered
• Instruct patient that product must be continued for prescribed time to be effective and taken exactly as prescribed; doses are not to be doubled; take missed dose when remembered up to 1 hr before next dose
• Tell patient to report bruising, fatigue, malaise; blood dyscrasias may occur
• Tell patient to report diarrhea, black tarry stools, sore throat, rash, dizziness, confusion, or delirium to prescriber immediately

## Evaluation
**Positive therapeutic outcome**
• Decreased pain in abdomen
• Healing of ulcers

---

## fat emulsions (Rx)
(fat ee-mul'shuns)
Intralipid 10%, Intralipid 20%, Liposyn II 10%, Liposyn II 20%, Liposyn III 10%, Liposyn III 20%, Soyacal 20%
*Func. class.:* Caloric
*Chem. class.:* Fatty acid, long chain
### Pregnancy category C

**Action:** Needed for energy, heat production; consists of neutral triglycerides, primarily unsaturated fatty acids

**Therapeutic outcome:** Increased available calories and fatty acids

**Uses:** Increase calorie intake, prevent fatty acid deficiency

## Dosage and routes
*Deficiency*
*Adult and child:* **IV** 8%-10% of required calorie intake (intralipid)

*Adjunct to TPN*
*Adult:* **IV** 1 ml/min over 15-30 min (10%) or 0.5 ml/min over 15-30 min (20%); may increase to 500 ml over 4-8 hr if no adverse reactions occur; not to exceed 2.5 g/kg

---

 Alert   ♣ Canada Only    Drug on CD           * "Tall Man" lettering (See Preface)

*Child:* **IV** 0.1 ml/min over 10-15 min (10%) or 0.05 ml/min over 10-15 min (20%); may increase to 1 g/kg over 4 hr if no adverse reactions occur; not to exceed 4 g/kg

**Prevention of deficiency**
*Adult:* **IV** 500 ml 2 × wk (10%), given 1 ml/min for 30 min, not to exceed 500 ml over 6 hr
*Child:* **IV** 5-10 ml/kg/day (10%), given 0.1 ml/min for 30 min, not to exceed 100 ml/hr

**Available forms:** Inj 10% (50, 100, 200, 250, 500 ml), 20% (50, 100, 200, 250, 500 ml)

**Adverse effects**
*CNS:* Dizziness, headache, drowsiness, **focal seizures**
*CV:* **Shock**
*GI:* Nausea, vomiting, **hepatomegaly**
*HEMA:* **Hyperlipemia, hypercoagulation, thrombocytopenia, leukopenia, leukocytosis**
*RESP:* Dyspnea, **fat in lung tissue**

**Contraindications:** Hypersensitivity to this product, eggs, soybeans, or legumes; hyperlipemia; lipid necrosis; acute pancreatitis accompanied by hyperlipemia; hyperbilirubinemia of the newborn; renal insufficiency; hepatic damage

**Precautions:** Pregnancy **C**, term newborns, severe liver disease, diabetes mellitus, thrombocytopenia, gastric ulcers, premature, sepsis

**Pharmacokinetics**

| | |
|---|---|
| **Absorption** | Completely absorbed |
| **Distribution** | Intravascular space |
| **Metabolism** | Conversion to triglycerides, to free fatty acids |
| **Excretion** | Unknown |
| **Half-life** | Unknown |

**Pharmacodynamics**
Unknown

**NURSING CONSIDERATIONS**
**Assessment**
• Monitor triglycerides, free fatty acid levels, platelet counts daily to prevent fat overload, thrombocytopenia
• Monitor liver function tests: AST, ALT, Hct, Hgb; notify prescriber if abnormal
• Assess nutritional status: calorie count by dietitian; monitor weight daily

**Nursing diagnoses**
• Knowledge, deficient (teaching)
• Nutrition: less than body requirements, imbalanced (uses)

**Implementation**
• Administer using infusion pump at prescribed rate; do not use in-line filter sized for lipid emulsion; clogging will occur
• Do not use mixed sol that looks oily or is not separated; discard unused sol
• Change **IV** tubing at each inf: infection may occur with old tubing
• Give by intermittent inf at a rate of 10% sol (1 ml/min); 20% sol (0.5 ml/min) initially for 15-30 min; may be increased to 10% sol (120 ml/hr) or 20% sol (62.5 ml/hr) if no adverse reactions occur; do not give more than 500 ml during the first day; children should be given 10% (0.1 mg/ ml) or 20% (0.05 ml/min) initially for 15-30 min, may be increased 1 g/kg/4 hr, do not give more than 10% (100 ml/hr) or 20% (50 ml/hr)

**Y-site compatibilities:** Ampicillin, cefamandole, cefazolin, cefoxitin, cephapirin, clindamycin, digoxin, DOPamine, erythromycin, furosemide, gentamicin, IL-2, isoproterenol, lidocaine, kanamycin, norepinephrine, oxacillin, penicillin G potassium, ticarcillin, tobramycin

**Y-site incompatibilities:** Amikacin, tetracycline

**Additive compatibilities:** Cefamandole, chloramphenicol, cimetidine, cycloSPORINE, diphenhydrAMINE, famotidine, heparin, hydrocortisone, multivitamins, nizatidine, penicillin G potassium

**Patient/family education**
• Teach patient reason for use of lipids and expected results

**Evaluation**
**Positive therapeutic outcome**
• Increased weight
• Fatty acids at adequate levels

**felodipine** (Rx)
(feh-loh′dih-peen)
Plendil, Renedil ♦
*Func. class.:* Calcium-channel blocker, antihypertensive, antianginal
*Chem. class.:* Dihydropyridine
**Pregnancy category C**

**Do not confuse:**
Plendil/pindolol/Prinivil/Prilosec/Pletal

**Action:** Inhibits calcium ion influx across cell membrane, resulting in inhibition of excitation/contraction

**Therapeutic outcome:** Decreased B/P in hypertension

Adverse effects: *italic* = common, **bold** = life-threatening

**Uses:** Essential hypertension, alone or with other antihypertensives, angina pectoris, Prinzmetal's angina (vasospastic)

## Dosage and routes

*Adult:* PO 5 mg/day initially, usual range 5-10 mg/day; max 10 mg/day; do not adjust dosage at intervals of <2 wk

*Geriatric:* PO 2.5 mg/day

## Hepatic dose

*Adult:* PO 2.5-5 mg/day, max 10 mg/day

**Available forms:** Ext rel tabs 2.5, 5, 10 mg

## Adverse effects

*CNS:* Headache, fatigue, drowsiness, dizziness, anxiety, depression, nervousness, insomnia, light-headedness, paresthesia, tinnitus, psychosis, somnolence

*CV:* **Dysrhythmias,** edema, **CHF,** hypotension, palpitations, **MI, pulmonary edema,** tachycardia, syncope, AV block, angina

*GI:* Nausea, vomiting, diarrhea, gastric upset, constipation, increased liver function studies, dry mouth

*GU:* Nocturia, polyuria

*HEMA:* Anemia

*INTEG:* Rash, pruritus

*MISC:* Flushing, sexual difficulties, cough, nasal congestion, shortness of breath, wheezing, epistaxis, respiratory infection, chest pain, **Stevens-Johnson syndrome,** gingival hyperplasia

**Contraindications:** Hypersensitivity, sick sinus syndrome, 2nd- or 3rd-degree heart block, hypotension <90 mm Hg systolic

**Precautions:** Pregnancy **C,** breastfeeding, children, geriatric, CHF, hepatic injury, renal disease

### Pharmacokinetics

| | |
|---|---|
| **Absorption** | Well absorbed |
| **Distribution** | Unknown; protein binding >99% |
| **Metabolism** | Liver, extensively |
| **Excretion** | Kidneys |
| **Half-life** | 11-16 hr |

### Pharmacodynamics

| | |
|---|---|
| **Onset** | 2-3 hr |
| **Peak** | 2½-5 hr |
| **Duration** | <24 hr |

## Interactions

### Individual drugs

Alcohol, fentanyl, quinidine: increased hypotension

Digoxin, disopyramide, phenytoin: increased bradycardia, increased CHF

Erythromycin, ketoconazole, itraconazole, propanolol: increased toxicity

### Drug classifications

β-Adrenergic blockers: increased bradycardia, CHF

NSAIDs: decreased antihypertensive effects

### Drug/herb

Aconite: increased toxicity, death

Astragalus, cola tree: increased or decreased antihypertensive effect

Barberry, betony, black catechu, black cohosh, bloodroot, broom, burdock, cat's claw, dandelion, goldenseal, Irish moss, Jamaican dogwood, kelp, khella, mistletoe, parsley: increased antihypertensive effect

Coltsfoot, guarana, khat, licorice: decreased antihypertensive effect

### Drug/food

Grapefruit juice: increased felodipine level

## NURSING CONSIDERATIONS
### Assessment

- Assess fluid volume status: I&O ratio and record; weight; skin turgor; adequacy of pulses; moist mucous membranes; bilateral lung sounds; peripheral pitting edema; dehydration symptoms of decreasing output, thirst, hypotension, dry mouth, and mucous membranes should be reported; for CHF: weight gain, crackles, dyspnea, edema, jugular venous distention
- Monitor ALT, AST, bilirubin daily if these are elevated
- Monitor cardiac status: B/P, pulse, respiration, ECG, periodically
- Assess for anginal pain: duration, intensity, ameliorating, aggravating factors

### Nursing diagnoses

- Cardiac output, decreased (uses)
- Knowledge, deficient (teaching)

### Implementation

- Do not break, crush, or chew ext rel tabs
- Give once a day with food for GI symptoms

### Patient/family education

- Caution patient to avoid hazardous activities until stabilized on product, and dizziness is no longer a problem
- Instruct patient to limit caffeine consumption; to avoid alcohol and OTC products unless directed by prescriber
- Urge patient to comply in all areas of medical regimen: diet, exercise, stress reduction, product therapy; to notify prescriber of irregular heartbeat, shortness of breath, swelling of feet and hands, pronounced dizziness, constipation, nausea, hypotension

 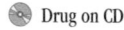

- Advise patient to use protective clothing, sunscreen to prevent photosensitivity
- Teach patient to change positions slowly to prevent orthostatic hypotension
- Advise patient to obtain correct pulse, to contact prescriber if pulse is <50 bpm
- Teach patient to use as directed even if feeling better; may be taken with other CV products (nitrates, β-blockers), that capsules may appear in stools but are insignificant

## Evaluation
### Positive therapeutic outcome
- Decreased B/P
- Decreased anginal attacks
- Increase in activity tolerance

---

## fenofibrate (Rx)
(fen-oh-fee' brate)
Antara, Lofibra, Tricor, Triglide
*Func. class.:* Antilipemic
*Chem. class.:* Fibric acid derivative

### Pregnancy category C

**Action:** Increases lipolysis and elimination of triglyceride-rich particles from plasma by activating lipoprotein lipase, resulting in triglyceride change in size and composition of LDL, leading to rapid breakdown of LDL; mobilizes triglycerides from tissue; increases excretion of neutral sterols

**Therapeutic outcome:** Decreasing cholesterol levels and low-density lipoproteins, decreased pruritus

**Uses:** Patients with types IV, V hyperlipidemia who do not respond to other treatment and who are at risk for pancreatitis Fredrickson type IIa, IIb, hypertriglyceridemia

**Unlabeled uses:** Polymetabolic syndrome X

### Dosage and routes
*Hypertriglyceridemia*
*Adult:* PO (Antara) 43-130 mg/day; (Lofibra) 67-200 mg/day; (Tricor) 48-145 mg/day; (Triglide) 50-160 mg/day

*Primary hypercholesterolemia/ mixed hyperlipidemia*
*Adult:* PO (Antara) 130 mg/day; (Lofibra) 200 mg/day; (Tricor) 145 mg/day; (Triglide) 160 mg/day

*Renal dose*
*Geriatric:* PO (Antara) 43 mg/day; (Lofibra) 67 mg/day; (Tricor) 48 mg/day

**Available forms:** Tabs (Triglide) 50, 160 mg; (Tricor) 48, 145 mg; micronized cap (Antara) 45, 87, 130 mg; (Lofibra) 67, 134, 200 mg

### Adverse effects
*CNS:* Fatigue, weakness, drowsiness, dizziness, insomnia, depression, vertigo
*CV:* Angina, **dysrhythmias**, hypertension
*GI:* Nausea, vomiting, dyspepsia, increased liver enzymes, flatulence, hepatomegaly, gastritis
*GU:* Dysuria, proteinuria, oliguria, urinary frequency
*HEMA:* Anemia, **leukopenia**, ecchymosis
*INTEG:* Rash, urticaria, pruritus
*MISC:* Polyphagia, weight gain
*MS:* Myalgias, arthralgias, myopathy
*RESP:* Pharyngitis, bronchitis, cough

**Contraindications:** Hypersensitivity, severe renal/hepatic disease, primary biliary cirrhosis, preexisting gallbladder disease

**Precautions:** Pregnancy **C**, breastfeeding, geriatric, peptic ulcer, pancreatitis, renal/ hepatic disease

### Pharmacokinetics
| | |
|---|---|
| Absorption | Unknown |
| Distribution | Protein binding 99% |
| Metabolism | Liver |
| Excretion | Urine 60% |
| Half-life | 20 hr |

### Pharmacodynamics
| | |
|---|---|
| Onset | Unknown |
| Peak | 6-8 hr |
| Duration | Unknown |

### Interactions
*Drug classifications*
Anticoagulants (oral): increased effect of anticoagulants
Bile acid sequestrants: decreased absorption
CycloSPORINE: increased nephrotoxicity
HMG-CoA reductase inhibitors: do not use together/ rhabdomyolysis may occur
*Drug/herb*
Glucomannan: increased effect
Gotu kola: decreased effect
*Drug/food*
Increased absorption

### NURSING CONSIDERATIONS
### Assessment
- Assess lipid levels, liver function tests, baseline and periodically during treatment;

---

CPK if muscle pain occurs, CBC, Hct, Hgh, pro-time with anticoagulant therapy
• Assess for pancreatitis, cholelithiasis, renal failure, rhabdomyolysis, (when combined with HMG-CoA reductase inhibitors) myositis, product should be discontinued
• Assess nutrition: fat, protein, carbohydrates, nutritional analysis should be completed by dietitian
• Assess skin integrity after patient has been receiving product; itching, pruritus often occur from bile deposits on skin
• Monitor cardiac glycoside level if both products are being administered; cardiac glycoside levels will be decreased
• Monitor for signs of vit A, D, K deficiency; serum cholesterol, triglyceride levels, electrolytes if on extended therapy
• Monitor bowel pattern daily; increase bulk, water in diet if constipation develops

### Nursing diagnoses
• Knowledge, deficient (teaching)
• Noncompliance (teaching)

### Implementation
• Do not break, crush, or chew tabs
• Give with evening meal; if dose is increased, take with breakfast and evening meal
• Store in cool environment in tight, light-resistant container

### Patient/family education
• Inform patient that compliance is needed
• Teach patient that risk factors—high-fat diet, smoking, alcohol consumption, absence of exercise—should be decreased
• Caution patient to notify prescriber if pregnancy is planned or suspected
• Teach patient to notify prescriber if the GI symptoms of diarrhea, abdominal or epigastric pain, nausea, or vomiting occur
• Instruct patient to report GU symptoms: dysuria, proteinuria, oliguria, decreased libido, impotence
• Advise patient to notify prescriber of muscle pain, weakness, fever, fatigue, epigastric pain

### Evaluation
**Positive therapeutic outcome**
• Decrease in cholesterol to desired level after 8 wk

---

# fenoldopam (Rx)
(fen-nahl'doh-pam)
Corlopam
*Func. class.:* Antihypertensive, vasodilator
**Pregnancy category B**

**Action:** Agonist at $D_1$-like dopamine receptors; binds to $\alpha_2$-adrenoreceptors; increases renal blood flow

**Therapeutic outcome:** B/P, decreased

**Uses:** Hypertensive crisis, malignant hypertension

**Unlabeled uses:** Prevention of contrast agent-associated nephrotoxicity

### Dosage and routes
*Adult:* **IV** 0.01-1.6 mcg/kg/min
*Child:* CONT **IV** 0.2 mcg/kg/min with effects within 5 min; may increase dose to 0.3-0.5 mcg/kg/min q20-30 min depending on response

**Available forms:** Inj conc 10 mg/ml in single-use ampules; inj 10 mg/ml

### Adverse effects
*CNS: Headache,* anxiety, dizziness, insomnia
*CV: Hypotension,* ST-T-wave changes, angina pectoris, palpitations, **MI, ischemic heart disease,** *flushing*
*GI:* Nausea, vomiting, constipation, diarrhea
*HEMA:* **Leukocytosis, bleeding**
*INTEG:* Sweating
*META:* Increased BUN, glucose, LDH, creatinine, hypokalemia

**Contraindications:** Hypersensitivity, sulfite sensitivity

**Precautions:** Pregnancy **B,** breastfeeding, children, tachycardia, intraocular pressure, hypokalemia

#### Pharmacokinetics
| | |
|---|---|
| **Absorption** | Unknown |
| **Distribution** | Steady state 20 min |
| **Metabolism** | Unknown |
| **Excretion** | Unknown |
| **Half-life** | 5 min (elimination) |

#### Pharmacodynamics
Unknown

### Interactions
*Drug classifications*
β-Adrenergic blockers: increased hypotension
*Drug/herb*
Aconite: increased toxicity, death

---

Astragalus, cola tree: increased or decreased antihypertensive effect

Barberry, betony, black catechu, black cohosh, bloodroot, broom, burdock, cat's claw, dandelion, goldenseal, Irish moss, Jamaican dogwood, kelp, khella, mistletoe, parsley: increased antihypertensive effect

Coltsfoot, guarana, khat, licorice: decreased antihypertensive effect

## NURSING CONSIDERATIONS
### Assessment
• Monitor B/P q5 min until stabilized, then q1hr × 2 hr, then q4hr; pulse, jugular venous distention q4hr
• Monitor electrolytes, blood studies: K, Na, Cl, $CO_2$, CBC, serum glucose
• Assess skin turgor, dryness of mucous membranes for hydration status
• Assess **IV** site for extravasation, rate

### Nursing diagnoses
• Knowledge, deficient (teaching)
• Noncompliance (teaching)
• Tissue perfusion, ineffective (uses)

### Implementation
**IV route**
• Administer after diluting contents of ampules in 0.9% NaCl, or 5% dextrose inj (40 mcg/ml); then add 4 ml of conc (40 mg of product/1000 ml); 2 ml of conc (20 mg of product/500 ml); 1 ml of conc (10 mg of product/250 ml); do not admix
• Give to patient in recumbent position; keep in that position for 1 hr after administration
• Diluted sol is stable in normal light/ temperature for 24 hr

### Patient/family education
• Teach patient reason for medication and expected results
• Instruct patient to report dyspnea, chest pain, bleeding

### Evaluation
**Positive therapeutic outcome**
• Decreased B/P

---

## ! HIGH ALERT

### fentanyl (Rx)
(fen'ta-nill)
fentanyl, Fentanyl Fentora, Sublimaze
### fentanyl transdermal (Rx)
Duragesic
*Func. class.:* Opioid analgesic
*Chem. class.:* Synthetic phenylpiperidine derivative

**Pregnancy category** C
**Controlled substance schedule** II

F

**Do not confuse:**
fentanyl/Sufenta

**Action:** Inhibits ascending pain pathways in CNS, increases pain threshold, alters pain perception by binding to opiate receptors

**Therapeutic outcome:** Relief of pain, supplement to anesthesia

**Uses:** Controls moderate to severe pain; preoperatively, postoperatively; adjunct to general anesthetic, adjunct to regional anesthesia; Fentanyl: for anesthesia as pre-medication, conscious sedation; Actiq: for breakthrough cancer pain

### Dosage and routes
*Fentanyl*
*Anesthetic*
*Adult:* **IV** 25-100 mcg (0.7-2 mcg/kg) q2-3 min prn

*Anesthesia supplement*
*Adult and child >12 yr:* IM/**IV** 2-20 mcg/kg **IV** INF 0.025-0.25 mcg/kg/min

*Induction and maintenance*
*Adult:* **IV** BOL 5-40 mcg/kg
*Child 2-12 yr:* **IV** 2-3 mcg/kg

*Preoperatively*
*Adult and child >12 yr:* IM/**IV** 0.05-0.1 mg q30-60 min before surgery

*Postoperatively*
*Adult:* IM 0.05-0.1 mg q1-2hr prn

*Sedation/analgesia*
*Adult and child >12 yr:* **IV** 0.5-1 mcg/kg/dose; may repeat after 30-60 min
*Child 1-12 yr:* **IV** BOL 1-2 mcg/kg/dose; may repeat after 30-60 min intervals; CONT **IV** 1-5 mcg/kg/hr after **IV** BOL dose
*Neonate:* **IV** BOL 0.5-3 mcg/kg/dose; CONT **IV** 0.5-2 mcg/kg/hr after **IV** BOL

*Actiq*
*Adult:* TRANSMUCOSAL 200 mcg, redose if needed 15 min after completion of 1st dose,

---

Adverse effects: *italic* = common, **bold** = life-threatening

do not give more than 2 doses during titration period

**Fentora**
*Adult:* PO BUCCAL 100 mg placed above rear molar

**Fentanyl transdermal**
*Adult:* 25 mcg/hr; may increase until pain relief occurs; apply patch to flat surface on upper torso and wear for 72 hr; apply new patch to different site for continued relief

**Available forms:** Inj 0.05 mg/ml; lozenges 100, 200, 300, 400 mcg; lozenges on a stick 200, 400, 600, 800, 1200, 1600 mcg; buccal tab 100, 200, 400, 600, 800 mcg; transdermal patch 12.5, 25, 50, 75, 100 mcg/hr

**Adverse effects**
***CNS:*** Dizziness, delirium, euphoria, sedation
***CV:*** **Bradycardia, cardiac arrest,** hypo/hypertension
***EENT:*** Blurred vision, miosis
***GI:*** Nausea, vomiting, constipation
***GU:*** Urinary retention
***INTEG:*** Rash, diaphoresis
***MS:*** Muscle rigidity
***RESP:*** **Respiratory depression, arrest, laryngospasm**

**Contraindications:** Hypersensitivity to opiates, myasthenia gravis

**Precautions:** Pregnancy **C**, breastfeeding, geriatric, respiratory depression, increased ICP, seizure disorders, severe respiratory disorders, cardiac dysrhythmias

#### Pharmacokinetics

| Absorption | Well absorbed (IM), completely absorbed (**IV**) |
|---|---|
| Distribution | Unknown, crosses placenta |
| Metabolism | Extensively—liver, 80% bound to plasma proteins |
| Excretion | Kidneys—up to 25% unchanged, breast milk |
| Half-life | 1½-6 hr; 17 hr after removal of patch (TD) |

#### Pharmacodynamics

| | IM | IV | TD |
|---|---|---|---|
| Onset | 7-8 min | Rapid | 6 hr |
| Peak | 30 min | 3-5 min | 12-24 hr |
| Duration | 1-2 hr | ½-1 hr | 72 hr |

**Interactions**
*Individual drugs*
Alcohol: increased respiratory depression, hypotension, increased sedation

*Drug classifications*
Antipsychotics, opioids, skeletal muscle relaxants: effects increased
CNS depressants, sedative/hypnotics: increased respiratory depression, hypotension
CYP3A4 inducers (carbamazepine, phenobarbital, phenytoin, rifampin): decreased fentanyl effect
*Drug/herb*
Corkwood: increased anticholinergic effect
Gotu kola, Jamaican dogwood, kava, lavender, mistletoe, nettle, pokeweed, poppy, senaga, St. John's wort, valerian: increased fentanyl action
*Drug/lab test*
Increased: amylase, lipase

**NURSING CONSIDERATIONS**
**Assessment**
• Monitor VS after parenteral route (B/P, pulse, respiration); note muscle rigidity; take product history before administering product; check renal/liver function tests; assess for respiratory dysfunction: respiratory depression, character, rate, rhythm; notify prescriber if respirations are <10/min
• Monitor CNS changes: dizziness, drowsiness, hallucinations, euphoria, LOC, pupil reaction
• Monitor allergic reactions: rash, urticaria; product should be discontinued
• Assess for pain: intensity, location, duration, type, before and 15 min after IM route or 3-5 min after **IV** route

**Nursing diagnoses**
• Breathing pattern, ineffective (adverse reactions)
• Knowledge, deficient (teaching)
• Pain, acute (uses)
• Sensory perception, disturbed: visual, auditory (adverse reactions)

**Implementation**
• Give by inj (IM, **IV**), only with resuscitative equipment available; give slowly to prevent rigidity
• Store in light-resistant area at room temperature
**Transmucosal route**
• Remove foil just before administration; instruct patient to place between cheek and lower gum, moving it back and forth and suck, not chew (Actiq); place above rear molar (Fentora); all products not used or partially used should be flushed down the toilet
**Transdermal route**
• Apply patch to chest on a flat area with skin intact; for skin preparation, use clear water with no soap; clip hair, skin should be dry

 **Alert**    **Canada Only**    **Drug on CD**   * "Tall Man" lettering (See Preface)

before applying patch; apply immediately after removing from package and press firmly in place with palm of hand; flush old patch down toilet immediately upon removal

**Use pain dosing**

• Dosage is titrated based on patient's report of pain; dosage is determined by calculating the previous 24-hr requirement and converting to equianalgesic morphine dose

• To convert to another opioid analgesic, remove transdermal patch and begin treatment with half the equal pain-controlling dose of the new analgesic in 12-18 hr

**IV route**

• Give **IV** undiluted by anesthesiologist or diluted with 5 ml or more sterile water or 0.9% NaCl given through Y-tube or 3-way stopcock given at 0.1 mg or less/1.2 min

*Syringe compatibilities:* Atracurium, atropine, bupivacaine/ketamine, butorphanol, chlorproMAZINE, cimetidine, clonidine/lidocaine, dimenhyDRINATE, diphenhydrAMINE, droperidol, heparin, hydromorphone, hydrOXYzine, meperidine, metoclopramide, midazolam, morphine, pentazocine, perphenazine, prochlorperazine, promazine, promethazine, ranitidine, scopolamine

*Syringe incompatibilities:* Pentobarbital

*Y-site compatibilities:* Amphotericin B cholesteryl, atracurium, cisatracurium, diltiazem, dobutamine, DOPamine, enalaprilat, epINEPHrine, esmolol, etomidate, furosemide, heparin, hydrocortisone, hydromorphone, labetalol, lorazepam, midazolam, milrinone, morphine, nafcillin, niCARdipine, nitroglycerin, norepinephrine, pancuronium, potassium chloride, propofol, ranitidine, remifentanil, sargramostim, thiopental, vecuronium, vit B/C

*Additive compatibilities:* Bupivacaine, sodium bicarbonate

*Additive incompatibilities:* Methohexital, pentobarbital, thiopental

*Solution compatibilities:* $D_5W$, 0.9% NaCl

**Patient/family education**

• Advise patient to report any symptoms of CNS changes, allergic reactions

• Instruct patient to avoid CNS depressants: alcohol, sedative/hypnotics for at least 24 hr after taking this product

• Teach patient that dizziness, drowsiness, confusion are common, and to avoid getting up without assistance

• Discuss in detail with patient all aspects of the product

• Teach patient CNS changes: physical dependence; not to use with alcohol, other CNS depressants

**Transdermal route**

• Discuss with patient that excessive heat may increase absorption; excessive perspiration may alter adhesiveness

• Discuss with patient that hair may need to be clipped before applying

• Teach patient how to dispose of patch: place sticky sides together and flush in toilet

**Evaluation**

**Positive therapeutic outcome**

• Maintenance of anesthesia

• Decreased pain

**Treatment of overdose:** Naloxone 0.2-0.8 **IV**, $O_2$, **IV** fluids, vasopressors

---

**ferrous fumarate** (Rx, OTC)
(fer'us fyu'-muh-rāt)
Femiron, Feostat, Feostat Drops, Hemocyte, Ircon, Nephro-Fer, Novofumar ✦, Palafer ✦, Span-FF

**ferrous gluconate** (Rx, OTC)
Fergon, Fertinic ✦, Novoferrogluc ✦

**ferric gluconate complex** (Rx, OTC)
Ferrlecit

**ferrous sulfate** (Rx, OTC)
Apo-Ferrous Sulfate ✦, ED-INSOL, Feosol, Fer-gen-sol, Fer-Iron Drops, Fero-Grad, Mol-Iron

**ferrous sulfate, dried** (Rx, OTC)
$Fe^{50}$, Feosol, Feratab, Novoferrosulfa ✦, PMS-Ferrous Sulfate, Slow Fe

**iron, carbonyl** (OTC)
(kar'boh-nil)
Feosol

**iron polysaccharide** (OTC)
(pah-lee-sack'ah-ride)
Hytinic, Niferex, Nu-Iron, Nu-Iron 150
*Func. class.:* Hematinic
*Chem. class.:* Iron preparation

**Pregnancy category** B, C

**Action:** Replaces iron stores needed for red blood cell development, energy and $O_2$ transport, utilization; fumarate contains 33% elemental iron; gluconate, 12%; sulfate, 20%; iron, 30%; ferrous sulfate exsiccated

F

Adverse effects: *italic* = common, **bold** = life-threatening

**Therapeutic outcome:** Prevention and correction of iron deficiency

**Uses:** Iron deficiency anemia, prophylaxis for iron deficiency in pregnancy

## Dosage and routes
### Fumarate
*Adult:* PO 50-100 mg tid
*Child 2-12 yr:* PO 3 mg/kg/day (elemental iron) tid-qid
*Child 6 mo-2 yr:* PO Up to 6 mg/kg/day (elemental iron) tid-qid
*Infant:* PO 10-25 mg/day (elemental iron) in 3-4 divided doses, max 15 mg/day

### Gluconate
*Adult:* PO 200-600 mg daily-tid
*Child 6-12 yr:* PO 300-900 mg/day
*Child <6 yr:* PO 100-300 mg/day

### Sulfate
*Adult:* PO 0.750-1.5 g/day in divided doses tid
*Child 6-12 yr:* 600 mg/day in divided doses

### Pregnancy
*Adult:* PO 300-600 mg/day in divided doses

### Complex
*Adult:* **IV** INF (125 mg) 10 ml/100 ml of NaCl for inj given over 1 hr

### Iron polysaccharide
*Adult:* 100-200 mg tid
*Child:* PO 4-6 mg/kg/day in 3 divided doses

**Available forms:** Fumarate: tabs 63, 195, 200, 324, 325 mg; chewable tabs 100 mg; controlled-release tabs 300 mg; oral susp 100 mg/5 ml, 45 mg/0.6 ml; gluconate: tabs 300, 320, 325 mg; caps 86, 325, 435 mg; film-coated tabs 300 mg; elix 300 mg/5 ml; sulfate: tabs 195, 300, 325 mg; enteric-coated tabs 325 mg; ext rel tabs, time-rel caps 525 mg; dried: tabs 200 mg; ext rel tabs 160 mg; ext rel caps 160 mg; complex: inj 62.5 mg/5 ml (12.5 mg/ml); iron polysaccharide: tabs 50 mg; caps 150 mg; sol 100 mg/5 ml

## Adverse effects
*GI: Nausea, constipation, epigastric pain, black and red tarry stools,* vomiting, diarrhea
*INTEG:* Temporarily discolored tooth enamel and eyes
*SYST:* **Hypersensitivity reactions (Ferrlecit)**

**Contraindications:** Hypersensitivity, ulcerative colitis/regional enteritis, hemosiderosis/hemochromatosis, peptic ulcer disease, hemolytic anemia, cirrhosis

**Precautions:** Pregnancy **B** (ferric gluconate complex), **C** (iron dextran, oral products); anemia (long-term)

### Pharmacokinetics
| | |
|---|---|
| **Absorption** | Up to 30% |
| **Distribution** | Bound to transferrin, crosses placenta |
| **Metabolism** | Recycled |
| **Excretion** | Feces, urine, skin, breast milk |
| **Half-life** | Unknown |

### Pharmacodynamics
Unknown

## Interactions
### Individual drugs
Chloramphenicol, vit C: increased absorption of iron products
Cholestyramine: decreased absorption of iron
L-Thyroxine: decreased L-thyroxine absorption
Levodopa: decreased absorption of levodopa
Methyldopa: decreased absorption of methyldopa
Penicillamine: decreased absorption of penicillamine
Tetracycline: decreased absorption of tetracycline
Vit E: decreased absorption of iron preparations

### Drug classifications
Antacids, $H_2$ antagonists, proton pump inhibitors: decreased absorption of iron preparations
Fluoroquinolones: decreased absorption of fluoroquinolone

### Drug/herb
Allspice, bilberry, condurango, elderberry, eye bright (PO), gentian, ground ivy, marshmallow, meadowsweet, mistletoe, motherwort, nettle, raspberry, valerian, tea made with artichoke, hawthorn, horse chestnut, lady mantle, lemon balm, oak bark, plantain, poplar, prickly ash, sage: decreased iron absorption
Anise: increased iron effect
Black catechu: forms insoluble complex

### Drug/food
Caffeine, dairy products, eggs: decreased absorption

### Drug/lab test
False positive: occult blood

## NURSING CONSIDERATIONS
### Assessment
• Monitor blood studies: Hct, Hgb, reticulocytes, bilirubin before treatment, at least monthly; iron studies (Fe, TIBC, ferritin)

• Assess for toxicity: nausea, vomiting, diarrhea (green, then tarry stools,) hematemesis, pallor, cyanosis, shock, coma
• Assess bowel elimination; if constipation occurs, increase water, bulk, activity before laxatives are required
• Assess nutrition: amount of iron in diet (meat, dark green leafy vegetables, dried beans, dried fruits, eggs); provide referral to dietitian if indicated
• Identify cause of iron loss or anemia, including salicylates, sulfonamides, antimalarials, quinidine

### Nursing diagnoses
• Fatigue (uses)
• Knowledge, deficient (teaching)
• Nutrition, less than body requirements, imbalanced (uses)

### Implementation
• Swallow all tabs whole; do not break, crush, or chew
• Give between meals for best absorption; may give with juice; do not give with antacids or milk, delay at least 1 hr; if GI symptoms occur, give after meals even if absorption is decreased; eggs, milk products, chocolate, caffeine interfere with absorption; ferrous gluconate is less GI irritating than ferrous sulfate
• Give liquid preparations through plastic straw to avoid discoloration of tooth enamel; dilute thoroughly
• Give at least 1 hr before bedtime because corrosion may occur in stomach
• Give for <6 mo for anemia
• Store in airtight, light-resistant container

### Patient/family education
• Advise patient that iron will make stools black or dark green; that iron poisoning may occur if increased beyond recommended level
• Keep out of reach of children
• Caution patient not to substitute one iron salt for another; elemental iron content differs (e.g., 300 mg ferrous fumarate contains about 100 mg elemental iron, whereas 300 mg ferrous gluconate contains only about 30 mg elemental iron)
• Caution patient to avoid reclining position for 15-30 min after taking product to avoid esophageal corrosion; to follow diet high in iron
• Caution patient to avoid taking iron, dairy products, calcium supplements together, vit C; they compete for absorption

### Evaluation
**Positive therapeutic outcome**
• Decreased fatigue, weakness
• Improvement in Hct, Hgb, reticulocytes

**Treatment of overdose:** Induce vomiting; give eggs, milk until lavage can be done

---

### fexofenadine (Rx)
(fex-oh-fin'a-deen)
Allegra
*Func. class.:* H$_1$-Histamine antagonist
*Chem. class:* Piperidine, peripherally selective

**Pregnancy category** C

**Do not confuse:**
Allegra/Viagra

**Action:** Acts on blood vessels, GI, respiratory system by competing with histamine for H$_1$-receptor site; decreases allergic response by blocking pharmacologic effects of histamine; less sedation rate than with other antihistamines; causes increased heart rate, vasodilatation, increased secretions

**Therapeutic outcome:** Absence of allergy symptoms and rhinitis

**Uses:** Rhinitis, allergy symptoms, chronic idiopathic urticaria

### Dosage and routes
*Adult and child >12 yr:* PO 60 mg bid or 180 mg/day
*Child 6-11 yr:* PO 30 mg bid; ORALLY DISINTEGRATING TAB 30 mg bid dissolved on tongue
*Renal dose*
*Adult and child ≥12 yr:* PO CCr <80 ml/min 60 mg/day

**Available forms:** Caps 60 mg; tabs 30, 60, 180 mg; oral suspension, orally disintegrating tab 30 mg

### Adverse effects
*CNS:* Headache, stimulation, drowsiness, sedation, fatigue, confusion, blurred vision, tinnitus, restlessness, tremors, paradoxical excitation in children or geriatric
*CV:* Hypotension, palpitations, bradycardia, tachycardia, **dysrhythmias (rare)**
*GI:* Nausea, diarrhea, abdominal pain, vomiting, constipation
*GU:* Frequency, dysuria, urinary retention, impotence
*HEMA:* **Hemolytic anemia, thrombocyto-**

---

Adverse effects: *italic* = common, **bold** = life-threatening

**penia, leukopenia, agranulocytosis, pancytopenia**
*INTEG:* Rash, eczema, photosensitivity, urticaria
*RESP:* Thickening of bronchial secretions; dry nose, throat

**Contraindications:** Breastfeeding, newborn or premature infants, hypersensitivity, severe hepatic disease

**Precautions:** Pregnancy **C**, children, geriatric, respiratory disease, angle-closure glaucoma, prostatic hypertrophy, bladder neck obstruction, asthma

### Pharmacokinetics

| | |
|---|---|
| **Absorption** | Well absorbed |
| **Distribution** | Unknown |
| **Metabolism** | Liver |
| **Excretion** | Kidneys |
| **Half-life** | Unknown |

### Pharmacodynamics

| | |
|---|---|
| **Onset** | 1 hr |
| **Peak** | 2-3 hr |
| **Duration** | 12-24 hr |

### Interactions
*Drug classifications*
Aluminum, antacids, magnesium: decreased fexofenadine effect
*Drug/herb*
Corkwood, henbane leaf: increased anticholinergic effect
Hops, Jamaican dogwood, khat, senega: increased sedation
*Drug/food*
Apple, orange, grapefruit juice: decreased absorption
*Drug/lab test*
False negative: skin allergy tests (discontinue antihistamine 3 days before testing)

### NURSING CONSIDERATIONS
**Assessment**
• Assess respiratory status: rate, rhythm, increase in bronchial secretions, wheezing, chest tightness; provide fluids to 2 L/day to decrease secretion thickness
• Monitor I&O ratio: be alert for urinary retention, frequency, dysuria, especially geriatric; product should be discontinued if these occur

**Nursing diagnoses**
• Airway clearance, ineffective (uses)
• Injury, risk for (side effects)
• Knowledge, deficient (teaching)
• Noncompliance (teaching, overuse)

**Implementation**
• Give on an empty stomach 1 hr before or 2 hr after meals to facilitate absorption, with food or milk for GI symptoms, do not take with juice
• Orally disintegrating tab: allow to dissolve, swallow
• Store in tight, light-resistant container

**Patient/family education**
• Teach all aspects of product uses; to notify prescriber if confusion, sedation, hypotension occur; to avoid driving or other hazardous activity if drowsiness occurs; to avoid alcohol or other CNS depressants that may potentiate effect
• Instruct patient to take 1 hr before or 2 hr after meals to facilitate absorption
• Instruct patient not to exceed recommended dose; dysrhythmias may occur
• Teach patient that hard candy, gum, frequent rinsing of mouth may be used for dryness

**Evaluation**
**Positive therapeutic outcome**
• Absence of running or congested nose, rashes

**Treatment of overdose:** Administer lavage, diazepam, vasopressors, barbiturates (short acting)

## filgrastim (Rx)
(fill-gras′stim)
G-CSF, granulocyte colony stimulator, Neupogen
*Func. class.:* Biologic modifier
*Chem. class.:* Granulocyte colony-stimulating factor

**Pregnancy category C**

**Action:** Stimulates proliferation and differentiation of neutrophils; a glycoprotein

**Therapeutic outcome:** Absence of infection

**Uses:** To decrease infection in patients receiving antineoplastics that are myelosuppressive; to increase WBC in patients with product-induced neutropenia; bone marrow depression

**Unlabeled uses:** Neutropenia in HIV infection, aplastic anemia, ganciclovir-induced neutropenia, zidovudine-induced neutropenia

**Dosage and routes**
*After myelosuppressive chemotherapy*
*Adult and child:* **IV**/SUBCUT 5 mcg/kg/day in a single dose × 14 days; may increase

by 5 mcg/kg in each chemotherapy cycle; give daily for up to 2 wk until ANC has reached 10,000/mm$^3$; response to G-CSF is much greater with SUBCUT than **IV** therapy

### After bone marrow transplantation
*Adult:* **IV**/SUBCUT 10 mcg/kg as an inf (**IV**) over 4 or 24 hr, begin 24 hr after chemotherapy and 24 hr after bone marrow transplantation

### Peripheral blood progenitor cell collection/therapy
*Adult:* 10 mcg/kg/day as a BOL or CONT INF × 4 days or more before leukapheresis, continue to last leukapheresis, may alter dose if WBC >100,000/mm$^3$

### Severe neutropenia (chronic)
*Adult:* SUBCUT 5 mcg/kg daily-bid

**Available forms:** Inj 300 mcg/ml, 480 mcg/1.6 ml, 480 mcg/0.8 ml, 3000 mcg/0.5 ml

### Adverse effects
*CNS:* Fever
*GI:* Nausea, vomiting, diarrhea, mucositis, anorexia
*HEMA:* **Thrombocytopenia,** excessive leukocytosis
*INTEG:* Alopecia, exacerbation of skin conditions, urticaria, vasculitis
*MS:* Osteoporosis, skeletal pain
*OTHER:* Chest pain
*RESP:* **Respiratory distress syndrome,** wheezing

**Contraindications:** Hypersensitivity to proteins of *Escherichia coli*

**Precautions:** Pregnancy **C,** breastfeeding, children, cardiac conditions, myeloid malignancies, radiation therapy, sepsis, sickle cell disease, chemotherapy, respiratory disease

### Pharmacokinetics
| Absorption | Well absorbed (SUBCUT), completely absorbed (**IV**) |
|---|---|
| Distribution | Unknown |
| Metabolism | Unknown |
| Excretion | Unknown |
| Half-life | Unknown |

### Pharmacodynamics
| | IV | SUBCUT |
|---|---|---|
| Onset | 5-60 min | 5-60 min |
| Peak | 24 hr | 2-8 hr |
| Duration | up to 1 wk | up to 1 wk |

### Interactions
*Individual drugs*
Lithium: do not use concurrently
*Drug classifications*
Antineoplastics: increased neutrophils, do not use together 24 hr before or after antineoplastics
*Drug/lab test*
Increased: uric acid, lactate dehydrogenase, alkaline phosphatase

## NURSING CONSIDERATIONS
### Assessment
• Monitor blood studies: CBC, platelet count before treatment and twice weekly; neutrophilcounts (ANC) may be increased for 2 days after therapy, but treatment should continue until ANC >10,000/mm$^3$
• Assess for bone pain: frequency, intensity, duration; analgesics may be given; opiates should not be used
• Check B/P, heart rate, respiration, baseline and during treatment

### Nursing diagnoses
• Infection, risk for (uses)
• Knowledge, deficient (teaching)
• Pain, acute (adverse reaction)

### Implementation
**IV route**
• Give 300 mcg/ml or 480 mcg/1.6 ml; allow to warm to room temperature; give single dose over 1 min or less through Y-tube or medport
• Use single-use vials; after dose is withdrawn, do not reenter vial
• Give for 2 wk or until ANC = 10,000/mm$^3$ after the expected chemotherapy neutrophil nadir
• Store in refrigerator; do not freeze; may store at room temperature for up to 6 hr; avoid shaking
**Y-site compatibilities:** Acyclovir, allopurinol, amikacin, aminophylline, ampicillin, ampicillin/sulbactam, aztreonam, bleomycin, bumetanide, buprenorphine, butorphanol, calcium gluconate, carboplatin, carmustine, cefazolin, cefotetan, ceftazidime, chlorproMAZINE, cimetidine, cisplatin, cyclophosphamide, cytarabine, dacarbazine, DAUNOrubicin, dexamethasone, diphenhydrAMINE, DOXOrubicin, doxycycline, droperidol, enalaprilat, famotidine, floxuridine, fluconazole, fludarabine, gallium, ganciclovir, granisetron, haloperidol, hydrocortisone, hydromorphone, hydrOXYzine, idarubicin, ifosfamide, leucovorin, lorazepam, mechlorethamine, melphalan, meperidine, mesna, methotrexate, metoclopramide, miconazole, minocycline, mitoxantrone,

**F**

Adverse effects: *italic* = common, **bold** = life-threatening

morphine, nalbuphine, netilmicin, ondansetron, plicamycin, potassium chloride,
promethazine, ranitidine, sodium bicarbonate,
streptozocin, ticarcillin, ticarcillin/clavulanate,
tobramycin, trimethoprim-sulfamethoxazole,
vancomycin, vinBLAStine, vinCRIStine, vinorelbine, zidovudine

## Patient/family education
• Teach patient technique for self-
administration: dose, side effects, disposal of
containers and needles; provide instruction
sheet

## Evaluation
**Positive therapeutic outcome**
• Absence of infection

---

## finasteride (Rx)
(fin-ass'te-ride)
Propecia, Proscar
*Func. class.:* Androgen hormone inhibitor,
hair stimulant
*Chem. class.:* 5-α-Reductase inhibitor
**Pregnancy category** X

**Do not confuse:**
Proscar/Prosom/Prozac

**Action:** Inhibits 5-α-reductase and reduction in dihydrotestosterone (DHT); DHT
induces androgenic effects by binding to
androgen receptors in the cell nuclei of the
prostate gland, liver, skin; prevents development of benign prostatic hypertrophy (BPH)

**Therapeutic outcome:** Reduced prostate size

**Uses:** Symptomatic BPH; male-pattern
baldness (Propecia)

## Dosage and routes
*BPH*
*Adult:* PO 5 mg/day × 6-12 mo
*Male pattern baldness*
*Adult:* PO 1 mg/day for 3 mo or more for
results

**Available forms:** Tabs (Propecia) 1 mg,
(Proscar) 5 mg

## Adverse effects
*GU:* Impotence, decreased libido, decreased
volume of ejaculate
*INTEG:* Rash
*MISC:* Breast tenderness

**Contraindications:** Pregnancy X, breastfeeding, children, women who are pregnant or
may become pregnant should not handle tabs,
hypersensitivity

**Precautions:** Large residual urinary
volume, severely diminished urinary flow, liver
function abnormalities

| Pharmacokinetics | |
|---|---|
| **Absorption** | 63%, readily |
| **Distribution** | Plasma protein binding, crosses blood-brain barrier |
| **Metabolism** | Liver |
| **Excretion** | Kidneys—metabolites (39%), feces (57%) |
| **Half-life** | 6-15 hr |

| Pharmacodynamics | |
|---|---|
| **Onset** | Immediate |
| **Peak** | 1-2 hr |
| **Duration** | 14 days |

## Interactions
*Drug classifications*
Anticholinergics, bronchodilators (adrener-
gic), theophylline: decreased effect of
finasteride
*Drug/lab test*
Decreased: PSA levels (finasteride)

## NURSING CONSIDERATIONS
### Assessment
• Assess urinary patterns, residual urinary
volume, severely diminished urinary flow; PSA
levels and digital rectal exam results before
initiating therapy and periodically thereafter
• Monitor liver function tests before initiating
treatment; extensively metabolized in liver

### Nursing diagnoses
• Knowledge, deficient (teaching)
• Urinary elimination, impaired (uses)

### Implementation
• Administer without regard to meals; give for
a minimum of 6 mo; not all patients will
respond
• Store at temp <86° F (30° C); protect from
light; keep container tightly closed

### Patient/family education
• Advise patient that pregnant women or
women who may become pregnant should not
touch crushed tab or come into contact with
semen of a patient taking this product; may
adversely affect development of male fetus
• Inform patient that volume of ejaculate may
be decreased during treatment; impotence and
decreased libido may also occur
• Inform patient that Propecia results may not
occur for 3 mo
• Inform patient that Proscar results may not
occur for 6-12 mo

---

 Alert     Canada Only    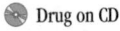 Drug on CD    * "Tall Man" lettering (See Preface)

## Evaluation
**Positive therapeutic outcome**
- Decreased postvoiding dribbling, frequency, nocturia
- Increased urinary flow
- Regression of prostate size
- Hair growth within 3-6 mo

---

## flavocoxid (Rx)
(flav-uh-kox'id)
Limbrel
*Func. class.:* Oral nutritional supplement
**Pregnancy category** UK

**Action:** Exhibits anti-inflammatory, analgesic properties, thought to be due to inhibition of prostaglandin synthesis via inhibition of cyclooxygenase

**Therapeutic outcome:** Decreased pain, inflammation in osteoarthritis

**Uses:** For dietary management of osteoarthritis

### Dosage and routes
*Adult:* PO 250 mg q12hr

**Available forms:** Caps 250 mg

### Adverse effects
*MISC:* Hypertension, increase in varicose veins, psoriasis
*MS:* Fluid accumulation in the knees

**Contraindications:** Hypersensitivity

**Precautions:** Pregnancy UK, breastfeeding, children <18 yr, history of stomach ulcers

| Pharmacokinetics | |
|---|---|
| Absorption | Unknown |
| Distribution | Unknown |
| Metabolism | Primarily via glucuronidation and sulfation |
| Excretion | Unknown |
| Half-life | Unknown |

| Pharmacodynamics |
|---|
| Unknown |

## NURSING CONSIDERATIONS
### Assessment
- Assess for pain of rheumatoid arthritis, osteoarthritis; check ROM, inflammation of joints, characteristics of pain

### Nursing diagnoses
- Injury, risk for (uses)
- Knowledge, deficient (teaching)

### Implementation
- Administer 1 hr before or after meals

### Patient/family education
- Teach patient that product does not take the place of other products including corticosteroids for osteoarthritis
- Advise patient to notify prescriber if pregnancy is planned or suspected

### Evaluation
**Positive therapeutic outcome**
- Decreased pain, inflammation in arthritic conditions

---

## flecainide (Rx)
(flek'a-nide)
Tambocor
*Func. class.:* Antidysrhythmic (Class IC)
**Pregnancy category** C

**Action:** Decreases conduction in all parts of the heart, with greatest effect on the His-Purkinje system, which stabilizes the cardiac membrane

**Therapeutic outcome:** Absence of dysrhythmias

**Uses:** Life-threatening ventricular dysrhythmias, sustained ventricular tachycardia; supraventricular tachydysrhythmias, paroxysmal atrial fibrillation/flutter associated with disabling symptoms

**Unlabeled uses:** Atrial fibrillation, single dose

### Dosage and routes
*PSVTT/PAT*
*Adult:* PO 50-100 mg q12hr; may increase every 4 days by 50 mg q12hr to desired response, not to exceed 300 mg/day

*Life-threatening ventricular dysrhythmias*
*Adult:* PO 100 mg q12hr, may increase by 50 mg q12hr q4 days, max 400 mg/day

*Renal dose*
*Adult:* PO CCr <35 ml/min dose 50%-75%

**Available forms:** Tabs 50, 100, 150 mg

### Adverse effects
*CNS: Headache, dizziness,* involuntary movement, confusion, psychosis, restlessness, irritability, paresthesias, ataxia, flushing, somnolence, depression, anxiety, malaise, fatigue, asthenia, tremors
*CV: Hypotension,* **bradycardia,** angina, PVCs, **heart block, cardiovascular collapse,**

*Adverse effects: italic = common, **bold** = life-threatening*

**arrest, dysrhythmias, CHF, fatal ventricular tachycardia**
***EENT:*** Tinnitus, *blurred vision,* hearing loss
***GI:*** Nausea, vomiting, anorexia, constipation, abdominal pain, flatulence, change in taste
***GU:*** Impotence, decreased libido, polyuria, urinary retention
***HEMA:*** Leukopenia, thrombocytopenia
***INTEG:*** Rash, urticaria, edema, swelling
***RESP:*** Dyspnea, **respiratory depression**

**Contraindications:** Hypersensitivity, severe heart block, cardiogenic shock, non-sustained ventricular dysrhythmias, frequent PVCs, non–life-threatening dysrhythmias

**Precautions:** Pregnancy **C,** breastfeeding, children, renal/hepatic disease, CHF, respiratory depression, myasthenia gravis

### Pharmacokinetics

| | |
|---|---|
| **Absorption** | Well absorbed |
| **Distribution** | Widely distributed |
| **Metabolism** | Liver |
| **Excretion** | 30% kidneys, unchanged |
| **Half-life** | 14 hr |

### Pharmacodynamics

| | |
|---|---|
| **Onset** | Unknown |
| **Peak** | 3 hr |
| **Duration** | Unknown |

### Interactions
*Individual drugs*
Amiodarone, cimetidine, ritonavir: increased level of flecainide
Digoxin: increased digoxin levels
Disopyramide, verapamil: increased CV depressant action
Propanolol: increased both products
*Drug classifications*
Acidifying agents, alkalizing agents: increased or decreased effect
β-Adrenergic blockers: increased CV depressant action
*Drug/herb*
Aconite: increased toxicity, death
Aloe, broom, buckthorn (chronic use), cascara sagrada (chronic use), Chinese rhubarb, figwort, fumitory, goldenseal, kudzu, licorice: increased effect
Coltsfoot: decreased effect
Horehound: increased serotonin effect
*Drug/lab test*
Increased: CPK

## NURSING CONSIDERATIONS
### Assessment
• Monitor ECG continuously to determine product effectiveness; measure PR, QRS, QT intervals; check for PVCs, other dysrhythmias; monitor B/P continuously for hypo/hypertension, and rebound hypertension (after 1-2 hr); check for dehydration or hypovolemia
• Monitor I&O ratio; electrolytes: (K [potassium], Na [sodium]), Cl (chloride); check weight daily and for signs of CHF or pulmonary toxicity: dyspnea, fatigue, cough, fever, chest pain, jugular vein distention, crackles; if these occur, product should be discontinued
• Monitor liver function studies: AST, ALT, bilirubin, alkaline phosphatase
• Assess patient for CNS symptoms: confusion, psychosis, numbness, depression, involuntary movements; if these occur, product should be discontinued
• Monitor cardiac rate, respiration: rate, rhythm, character, chest pain; watch for ventricular tachycardia, supraventricular tachycardia, or fibrillation

### Nursing diagnoses
• Cardiac output, decreased (uses)
• Knowledge, deficient (teaching)

### Implementation
• Give reduced dosage slowly with ECG monitoring; do not increase dose fewer than 4 days apart
• Give with meals if GI upset occurs

### Patient/family education
• Instruct patient to report side effects immediately to prescriber
• Instruct patient to complete follow-up appointment with health care provider including pulmonary function tests, chest x-ray
• Teach patient to change position slowly from lying or sitting to standing to minimize orthostatic hypotension
• Advise patient not to skip or double doses
• Advise patient to carry/wear emergency ID with disorder, medications taken
• Advise patient to avoid hazardous activities that require alertness until response is known

### Evaluation
**Positive therapeutic outcome**
• Absence of dysrhythmias

**fluconazole** (Rx)

(floo-kon′a-zole)

Diflucan

*Func. class.:* Antifungal

**Pregnancy category** B

**Do not confuse:**

Diflucan/Diprivan

**Action:** Inhibits ergosterol biosynthesis, causes direct damage to membrane phospholipids in the cell wall of fungi

**Therapeutic outcome:** Fungistatic fungicidal against the following susceptible organisms: *Candida, Cryptococcus neoformans*

**Uses:** Oropharyngeal esophageal candidiasis in AIDS patients, chronic mucocutaneous candidiasis, urinary candidiasis, cryptococcal meningitis, prevention of candidiasis in bone marrow transplant

**Dosage and routes**

*Renal dose*

*Adult:* PO CCr 11-50 ml/min dose 50%

*Vaginal candidiasis*

*Adult:* PO 150 mg as a single dose

*Serious fungal infections*

*Adult:* PO/**IV** 50-400 mg initially, then 200 mg once daily for 4 wk

*Child:* 6-12 mg/kg/day

*Oropharyngeal candidiasis*

*Adult:* PO 200 mg initially, then 100 mg/day for at least 2 wk

*Child:* 3 mg/kg/day

*Prevention of candidiasis in bone marrow transplant*

*Adult:* PO/**IV** 400 mg/day

**Available forms:** Tabs 50, 100, 150, 200 mg; inj 2 mg/ml; powder for oral susp 50, 200 mg/ml

**Adverse effects**

*CNS:* Headache

*GI:* Nausea, vomiting, diarrhea, cramping, flatus, increased AST, ALT, **hepatotoxicity**

*INTEG:* **Stevens-Johnson syndrome**

**Contraindications:** Hypersensitivity to this product or azoles

**Precautions:** Pregnancy **B**, breastfeeding, renal/hepatic disease

**Pharmacokinetics**

| | |
|---|---|
| **Absorption** | Well absorbed (PO) |
| **Distribution** | Widely distributed (peritoneum, CSF) |
| **Metabolism** | <10%—liver |
| **Excretion** | 80% kidneys (unchanged) |
| **Half-life** | 30 hr, increased in renal disease |

**Pharmacodynamics**

| | PO | IV |
|---|---|---|
| **Onset** | Unknown | Immediate |
| **Peak** | 2-4 hr | Infusion's end |
| **Duration** | Unknown | Unknown |

**Interactions**

*Individual drugs*

CycloSPORINE, phenytoin, rifabutin, tacrolimus, theophylline: increased plasma concentrations

Warfarin: increased anticoagulation

Zidovudine: increased effect

*Drug classification*

Contraceptives (oral): decreased effect

Oral antidiabetics: hypoglycemia

*Drug/herb*

Gossypol: increased nephrotoxicity

**NURSING CONSIDERATIONS**

**Assessment**

• Assess for signs and symptoms of infection: clearing of CSF culture during treatment, obtain C&S baseline and during treatment, product may be started as soon as culture is taken

• Monitor for hepatotoxicity: increased AST, ALT, alkaline phosphatase, bilirubin; product will be discontinued if hepatotoxicity occurs

**Nursing diagnoses**

• Infection, risk for (uses)

• Injury, risk for (adverse reactions)

• Knowledge, deficient (teaching)

**Implementation**

• Take with food to reduce GI effects

**PO route**

• Shake oral susp before each use

**IV route**

• Give after diluting according to package directions; run at 200 mg/hr or less; do not use plastic containers in connections

• Do not admix

• Administer **IV** using an in-line filter, using distal veins; check for extravasation and necrosis q2hr

• Give product only after C&S confirms organism, product needed to treat condition

• Store protected from moisture and light, diluted sol is stable for 24 hr

Adverse effects: *italic* = common, **bold** = life-threatening

*Y-site compatibilities:* Acyclovir, aldesleukin, allopurinol, amifostine, amikacin, aminophylline, ampicillin/sulbactam, aztreonam, benztropine, cefazolin, cefepime, cefotetan, cefoxitin, chlorproMAZINE, cimetidine, dexamethasone, diphenhydrAMINE, DOBUTamine, DOPamine, droperidol, famotidine, filgrastim, fludarabine, foscarnet, gallium, ganciclovir, gentamicin, granisetron, heparin, hydrocortisone, immune globulin, leucovorin, lorazepam, melphalan, meperidine, meropenem, metoclopramide, metronidazole, midazolam, morphine, nafcillin, nitroglycerin, ondansetron, oxacillin, paclitaxel, pancuronium, penicillin G, potassium, phenytoin, piperacillin/tazobactam, prochlorperazine, promethazine, propofol, ranitidine, sargramostim, sulfamethoxazole, tacrolimus, teniposide, theophylline, thiotepa, ticarcillin/clavulanate, tobramycin, vancomycin, vecuronium, vinorelbine, zidovudine

*Y-site incompatibilities:* Amphotericin B, ampicillin, calcium gluconate, cefotaxime, ceftriaxone, ceftazidime, cefuroxime, chloramphenicol, clindamycin, diazepam, digoxin, erythromycin lactobionate, furosemide, haloperidol, hydrOXYzine, imipenem/cilastatin, pentamidine, ticarcillin, trimethoprim/sulfamethoxazole

*Additive compatibilities:* Acyclovir, amikacin, amphotericin B, cefazolin, ceftazidime, clindamycin, gentamicin, heparin, meropenem, metronidazole, morphine, piperacillin, potassium chloride, theophylline

### Patient/family education

• Caution patient that long-term therapy may be needed to clear infection; to take entire course of medication; take in equal intervals (PO)
• Teach patient the signs and symptoms of hepatotoxicity: nausea, vomiting, clay-colored stools, dark urine, anorexia, fatigue, jaundice; prescriber should be notified immediately
• Inform patient that medication may be taken with food to reduce GI effects
• Advise patient to consider using alternative contraception if using oral contraceptives

### Evaluation

**Positive therapeutic outcome**
• Decreasing oral candidiasis, fever, malaise, rash
• Negative C&S for infecting organism

---

## fludrocortisone (Rx)
(floo-droe-kor'ti-sone)
Florinef
*Func. class.:* Corticosteroid, synthetic
*Chem. class.:* Mineralocorticoid

### Pregnancy category C

**Action:** Promotes increased reabsorption of sodium and loss of potassium, water, hydrogen from the distal renal tubules

**Therapeutic outcome:** Treatment of adrenal insufficiency symptoms

**Uses:** Adrenal insufficiency, salt-losing adrenogenital syndrome

**Unlabeled uses:** Renal tubular acidosis (type IV), idiopathic orthostatic hypertension

### Dosage and routes
*Adult:* PO 0.1-0.2 mg/day
*Child:* PO 0.05-0.1 mg/day

*Idiopathic hypotension (unlabeled)*
*Adult:* PO 50-100 mcg/day

**Available forms:** Tabs 0.1 mg

### Adverse effects
*CNS: Flushing, sweating,* headache, paralysis, dizziness, **seizures**
*CV: Hypertension,* **circulatory collapse, thrombophlebitis, embolism,** tachycardia, **CHF,** edema
*ENDO:* Weight gain, adrenal suppression, hyperglycemia
*META: Hypokalemia*
*MISC:* Hypersensitivity, cataracts, GI ulcers, **anaphylaxis**
*MS:* Fractures, osteoporosis, weakness

**Contraindications:** Hypersensitivity, acute glomerulonephritis, amebiasis, psychoses, Cushing's syndrome, fungal infections, child <2 yr

**Precautions:** Pregnancy **C,** breastfeeding, child >2 yr, osteoporosis, CHF, hypertension, diabetes

| Pharmacokinetics | |
|---|---|
| **Absorption** | Well absorbed |
| **Distribution** | Widely |
| **Metabolism** | Liver |
| **Excretion** | Kidneys, breast milk |
| **Half-life** | 3½ hr |

| Pharmacodynamics | |
|---|---|
| **Onset** | Unknown |
| **Peak** | 1.5 hr |
| **Duration** | Unknown |

---

 Alert    ♣ Canada Only    🔘 Drug on CD    * "Tall Man" lettering (See Preface)

## Interactions
### Individual drugs
Amphotericin B, mezlocillin, piperacillin: increased hypokalemia
Phenytoin: decreased action of fludrocortisone
Rifampin: decreased effect of fludrocortisone
### Drug classifications
Barbiturates: decreased action of fludrocortisone
Diuretics (loop), thiazides, potassium-wasting products: decreased potassium levels
### Drug/herb
Aloe, buckthorn, cascara sagrada, Chinese rhubarb, senna: increased hypokalemia
Aloe, licorice, perilla: increased corticosteroid effect
### Drug/food
Increased salt/sodium ingestion: increased B/P
### Drug/lab test
Increased: potassium, sodium
Decreased: hematocrit

## NURSING CONSIDERATIONS
### Assessment
• Monitor patient for fluid retention: weigh daily, notify prescriber of weekly gain >5 lb; B/P q4hr, pulse; notify prescriber if chest pain occurs; I&O ratio; be alert for decreasing urinary output and increasing edema
• Check for potassium depletion: paresthesias, fatigue, nausea, vomiting, depression, polyuria, dysrhythmias, weakness; also sodium, chloride

### Nursing diagnoses
• Fluid volume, deficient (uses)
• Fluid volume, excess (adverse reactions)
• Knowledge, deficient (teaching)
### Implementation
• Administer titrated dose; use lowest effective dose; scored tab may be broken if lower dose is necessary
• Give with food or milk to decrease GI symptoms

### Patient/family education
• Advise patient to carry/wear emergency ID as steroid user at all times during diagnosis and treatment
• Caution patient not to discontinue this medication abruptly; Addisonian crisis may occur
• Counsel patient to follow dietary regimen recommended by prescriber; should include high potassium and, possibly, low sodium
• Advise patient to report weight gain >5 lb; edema in legs, hands; abdominal cramping; muscle cramps; nausea; vomiting; anorexia; dizziness or weakness, infection, trauma, stress
• Advise patient not to breastfeed
• Tell patient to avoid exposure to disease, trauma
### Evaluation
**Positive therapeutic outcome**
• Correction of adrenal insufficiency
• Electrolytes and fluids in normal range

## flumazenil (Rx)
(flu-maz'e-nil)
Anexate ♣, Romazicon
*Func. class.:* Benzodiazepine receptor antagonist
*Chem. class.:* Imidazobenzodiazepine derivative
### Pregnancy category C

**Action:** Antagonizes the actions of benzodiazepines on the CNS, competitively inhibits the activity at the benzodiazepine receptor complex

**Therapeutic outcome:** Reversed benzodiazepine toxic effects

**Uses:** Reversal of the sedative effects of benzodiazepines

### Dosage and routes
#### Reversal of conscious sedation or in general anesthesia
**Adult:** IV 0.2 mg (2 ml) given over 15 sec; wait 45 sec, then give 0.2 mg (2 ml) if consciousness does not occur; may be repeated at 60-sec intervals as needed (max 3 mg/hr)
**Child:** IV 10 mcg (0.01 mg)/kg; cumulative dose of 1 mg or less

#### Management of suspected benzodiazepine overdose
**Adult:** IV 0.2 mg (2 ml) given over 30 sec; wait 30 sec, then give 0.3 mg (3 ml) over 30 sec if consciousness does not occur; further doses of 0.5 mg (5 ml) can be given over 30 sec at intervals of 1 min up to cumulative dose of 3 mg
**Child:** IV 10 mcg (0.01 mg/kg); cumulative dose of less than 1 mg

**Available forms:** Inj 0.1 mg/ml
### Adverse effects
*CNS:* Dizziness, agitation, emotional lability, confusion, **seizures,** somnolence, panic attacks
*CV:* Hypertension, palpitations, cutaneous vasodilatation, **dysrhythmias,** bradycardia, tachycardia, chest pain

Adverse effects: *italic* = common, **bold** = life-threatening

*EENT:* Abnormal vision, blurred vision, tinnitus
*GI:* Nausea, vomiting, hiccups
*SYST:* Headache, inj site pain, increased sweating, fatigue, rigors

**Contraindications:** Hypersensitivity to this product or benzodiazepines, serous tricyclic overdose, patients given benzodiazepine for control of life-threatening condition

**Precautions:** Pregnancy **C**, breastfeeding, children, geriatric, ambulatory patients, renal/hepatic disease, status epilepticus, head injury, labor and delivery, hypoventilation, panic disorder, product and alcohol dependency

### Pharmacokinetics

| | |
|---|---|
| **Absorption** | Complete |
| **Distribution** | Unknown |
| **Metabolism** | Liver |
| **Excretion** | Unknown |
| **Half-life** | 41-79 min |

### Pharmacodynamics

| | |
|---|---|
| **Onset** | 1-2 min |
| **Peak** | 10 min |
| **Duration** | Unknown |

### Interactions
*Individual drugs*
Zaleplon, zolpidem: antagonize action
*Drug classifications*
Benzodiazepines: antagonize action
Toxicity: mixed product overdosage

### NURSING CONSIDERATIONS
**Assessment**
- Assess cardiac status using continuous monitoring
- Assess for seizures, protect patient from injury; most likely in those who usually experience withdrawal from sedatives
- Assess for GI symptoms: nausea, vomiting; place in side-lying position to prevent aspiration
- Assess for allergic reactions: flushing, rash, urticaria, pruritus

**Nursing diagnoses**
- Injury, risk for (uses)
- Poisoning, risk for (uses)

**Implementation**
- Give directly undiluted or diluted in 0.9% NaCl, D₅W, or LR; give over 15 sec into running **IV**
- Use large vein

- Check airway and **IV** access before administration
- Stable for 24 hr if drawn into a syringe or mixed with other solutions
*Additive compatibilities:* Aminophylline, cimetidine, DOBUTamine, DOPamine, famotidine, heparin, lidocaine, procainamide, ranitidine

**Patient/family education**
- Caution patient that amnesia may continue
- Instruct patient to avoid any hazardous activities for 18-24 hr after discharge
- Inform patient not to take any alcohol or nonprescription products for 18-24 hr; serious reactions may occur

**Evaluation**
**Positive therapeutic outcome**
- Decreased sedation, respiratory depression
- Absence of toxicity

---

**flunisolide nasal agent**
*See Appendix D*

---

**fluocinolone topical**
*See Appendix D*

---

**fluorometholone ophthalmic**
*See Appendix D*

---

⚠ HIGH ALERT

**fluorouracil** (Rx)
(flure-oh-yoor'a-sil)
5-FU, Adrucil, Efudex, Fluoroplex
*Func. class.:* Antineoplastic, antimetabolite
*Chem. class.:* Pyrimidine antagonist
**Pregnancy category D**

**Do not confuse:**
fluorouracil/flucytosine

**Action:** Inhibits DNA, RNA synthesis; interferes with cell replication by competitively inhibiting thymidylate synthesis, cell cycle–specific (S phase), a vesicant

**Therapeutic outcome:** Prevention of rapidly growing malignant cells

**Uses:** *Systemic:* cancer of breast, colon, rectum, stomach, pancreas; *Topical:* superficial basal cell carcinoma; multiple actinic keratoses

---

 Alert     Canada Only    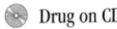 Drug on CD    * "Tall Man" lettering (See Preface)

### Dosage and routes
#### Advanced colorectal cancer
*Adult:* **IV** 370 mg/m² given after leucovorin or 425 mg/m² given after leucovorin daily × 5 days; repeat q4-5wk

#### Other cancer
*Adult:* **IV** 12 mg/kg/day × 4 days, not to exceed 800 mg/day; may repeat with 6 mg/kg on day 6, 8, 10, 12; maintenance is 10-15 mg/kg/wk as a single dose, not to exceed 1 g/wk

#### Actinic/solar keratoses
*Adult:* TOP 1% cream/sol 1-2×/day

#### Superficial basal cell carcinoma
*Adult:* TOP 5% sol 2×/day × 3-12 wk

**Available forms:** Inj 50 mg/ml; cream 1, 5%; sol 1, 2, 5%

### Adverse effects
#### Systemic use
*CNS:* Lethargy, malaise, weakness, acute cerebellar dysfunction
*CV:* Myocardial ischemia, angina
*EENT:* Epistaxis
*GI: Anorexia, stomatitis,* diarrhea, nausea, vomiting, **hemorrhage, enteritis, glossitis**
*HEMA:* **Thrombocytopenia, leukopenia, myelosuppression, anemia, agranulocytosis**
*INTEG: Rash,* fever, photosensitivity

**Contraindications:** Pregnancy **D**, breastfeeding, hypersensitivity, myelosuppression, poor nutritional status, serious infections, major surgery within 1 mo

**Precautions:** Children, renal/hepatic disease, bone marrow depression, angina

#### Pharmacokinetics
| | |
|---|---|
| **Absorption** | Completely bioavailable (**IV**), minimal (topical) |
| **Distribution** | Widely distributed, concentration in tumor |
| **Metabolism** | Liver—converted to active metabolite |
| **Excretion** | Lungs (60%-80%), kidneys (up to 15%) |
| **Half-life** | 20 hr terminal |

#### Pharmacodynamics
Unknown

### Interactions
#### Individual drugs
Radiation: increased toxicity, bone marrow suppression

#### Drug classifications
Antineoplastics: increased toxicity, bone marrow depression
Live virus vaccines: decreased antibody response

#### Drug/lab test
Increased: AST, ALT, LDH, serum bilirubin, Hct, Hgb, WBC, platelets, 5-HIAA
Decreased: albumin

### NURSING CONSIDERATIONS
#### Assessment
• Monitor ECG; watch for ST-T wave changes, low QRS and T, possible dysrhythmias (sinus tachycardia, heart block, PVCs)
• Assess buccal cavity q8hr for dryness, sores or ulceration, white patches, oral pain, bleeding, dysphagia; obtain prescription for viscous lidocaine (Xylocaine)
• Assess tachypnea, ECG changes, dyspnea, edema, fatigue; identify dyspnea, crackles, unproductive cough, chest pain, tachypnea
• Monitor CBC, differential, platelet count daily (**IV**); withhold product if WBC is <4000/mm³ or platelet count is <100,000/mm³; notify prescriber of results if WBC <20,000/mm³, platelets <50,000/mm³; nadir of leukopenia within 2 wk, recovery 1 mo
• Monitor renal function studies: BUN, creatinine, serum uric acid, urine CCr before and during therapy; I&O ratio; report fall in urine output to <30 ml/hr
• Monitor temp q4hr (may indicate beginning of infection)
• Monitor liver function tests before and during therapy (bilirubin, AST, ALT, LDH) as needed or monthly; jaundice of skin, sclera, dark urine, clay-colored stools, itchy skin, abdominal pain, fever, diarrhea
• Assess for bleeding: hematuria, stool guaiac, bruising or petechiae, mucosa or orifices q8hr; inflammation of mucosa, breaks in skin

#### Nursing diagnoses
• Body image, disturbed (adverse reactions)
• Infection, risk for (adverse reactions)
• Injury, risk for (adverse reactions)
• Knowledge, deficient (teaching)

#### Implementation
• Avoid contact with skin (very irritating); wash completely to remove
• Give fluids **IV** or PO before chemotherapy to hydrate patient
• Give antiemetic 30-60 min before giving product to prevent vomiting, and prn for several days thereafter; antibiotics for prophylaxis of infection

F

Adverse effects: *italic* = common, **bold** = life-threatening

- Provide liquid diet: carbonated beverages; gelatin may be added if patient is not nauseated or vomiting
- Provide rinsing of mouth tid-qid with water, club soda; brushing of teeth bid-qid with soft brush or cotton-tipped applicators for stomatitis; use unwaxed dental floss

**Topical route**
- Wear gloves when applying; may use with a loose dressing, use a plastic or wooden applicator

**IV route**
- Prepare in biologic cabinet using gloves, gown, mask
- **IV** undiluted; may inject through Y-tube or 3-way stopcock; give over 1-3 min
- May be diluted in 0.9% NaCl, $D_5W$, given over 2-8 hr as an **IV** inf

*Syringe compatibilities:* Bleomycin, cisplatin, cyclophosphamide, furosemide, heparin, leucovorin, methotrexate, metoclopramide, mitomycin, vinBLAStine, vinCRIStine

*Syringe incompatibilities:* Droperidol

*Y-site compatibilities:* Allopurinol, amifostine, aztreonam, bleomycin, cefepime, cisplatin, cyclophosphamide, DOXOrubicin, fludarabine, furosemide, granisetron, heparin, hydrocortisone, leucovorin, mannitol, melphalan, methotrexate, metoclopramide, mitomycin, paclitaxel, piperacillin/tazobactam, potassium chloride, propofol, sargramostin, thiotepa, thiposide, vinBLAStine, vinCRIStine, vit B/C

*Y-site incompatibilities:* Droperidol, vinorelbine

*Additive compatibilities:* Bleomycin, cephalothin, cyclophosphamide, etoposides, floxuridine, hydromorphone, ifosfamide, leucovorin, methotrexate, mitoxantrone, prednisoLONE, vinCRIStine

*Additive incompatibilities:* Carboplatin, cisplatin, cytarabine, diazepam, DOXOrubicin

*Solution compatibilities:* Amino acids 4.25%/$D_{25}$, $D_5$/LR, $D_{3.3}$/0.3% NaCl, $D_5W$, 0.9% NaCl, TPN #23

**Patient/family education**
- Caution patient that contraceptive measures are recommended during therapy
- Teach patient to avoid using aspirin, NSAIDs, or ibuprofen-containing products, razors, commercial mouthwash because bleeding may occur; to report symptoms of bleeding (hematuria, tarry stools)
- Instruct patient to report signs of anemia (fatigue, headache, irritability, faintness, shortness of breath)

- Instruct patient to report signs of stomatitis (bleeding, white spots, ulcerations in the mouth); tell patient to examine mouth daily, to report symptoms; viscous lidocaine (Xylocaine) may be used
- Teach patient to avoid crowds, persons with known infections
- Advise patient to avoid vaccinations during therapy, to use sunscreen or stay out of the sun to prevent burns; about hair loss, explore use of wigs or other products until hair regrowth occurs

**Evaluation**
**Positive therapeutic outcome**
- Prevention of rapid division of malignant cells

---

**fluoxetine** (Rx)
(floo-ox′uh-teen)
Prozac, Prozac Weekly, Sarafem
*Func. class.:* Antidepressant, selective serotonin reuptake inhibitor

**Pregnancy category C**

**Do not confuse:**
Prozac/Proscar/Prilosec/Prosom, Sarafem/Serophene

**Action:** Inhibits CNS neuron uptake of serotonin, but not of norepinephrine

**Therapeutic outcome:** Decreased symptoms of depression after 2-3 wk

**Uses:** Major depressive disorder, obsessive-compulsive disorder (OCD), bulimia nervosa; Sarafem: premenstrual dysphoric disorder (PMDD), panic disorder

**Unlabeled uses:** Alcoholism, anorexia nervosa, attention deficit hyperactivity disorder, bipolar II affective disorder, borderline personality disorder, cataplexy, narcolepsy, kleptomania, migraine, obesity, posttraumatic stress disorder, schizophrenia, Gilles de la Tourette's syndrome, trichotillomania, levodopa-induced dyskinesia, social phobia

**Dosage and routes**
*Depression/OCD*
*Adult:* PO 20 mg/day AM; after 4 wk if no clinical improvement is noted, dose may be increased to 20 mg bid in AM, afternoon; not to exceed 80 mg/day; PO 90 mg weekly
*Geriatric:* PO 5-10 mg/day, increase as needed
*Child 5-18 yr:* PO 5-10 mg/day, max 20 mg/day

---

*Bulimia nervosa*
*Adult:* PO 60 mg/day in AM

*ADHD (unlabeled)*
*Adult:* PO 20-60 mg/day

*Alcoholism (unlabeled)*
*Adult:* PO 20-80 mg/day

*Anorexia nervosa (unlabeled)*
*Adult:* PO 10 mg every other day-20 mg/day

*Bipolar II affective disorder (unlabeled)*
*Adult:* PO 10 mg every other day-20 mg/day

*Borderline personality disorder (unlabeled)*
*Adult:* PO 20 mg/day

*Kleptomania (unlabeled)*
*Adult:* PO 60-80 mg/day

*Migraine, chronic daily headaches (unlabeled)*
*Adult:* PO 10-80 mg/day

*Narcolepsy (unlabeled)*
*Adult:* PO 20-40 mg/day

*Posttraumatic stress disorder (unlabeled)*
*Adult:* PO 10-80 mg/day

*Premenstrual dysphoric disorder (Sarafem)*
*Adult:* PO 20 mg/day, may be taken daily 14 days before menses

*Schizophrenia (unlabeled)*
*Adult:* PO 20-60 mg/day

**Available forms:** Caps 10, 20, 40 mg; tabs 10, 20 mg; oral sol 20 mg/5 ml; del rel caps (Prozac Weekly) 90 mg

**Adverse effects**
*CNS: Headache, nervousness, insomnia, drowsiness, anxiety, tremor, dizziness, fatigue, sedation, poor concentration, abnormal dreams, agitation,* **seizures,** apathy, euphoria, hallucinations, delusions, psychosis, **suicidal ideation**
*CV: Hot flashes, palpitations,* angina pectoris, **hemorrhage,** hypertension, **tachycardia,** 1st-degree AV block, **bradycardia, MI, thrombophlebitis**
*EENT: Visual changes, ear/eye pain, photophobia, tinnitus*
*GI: Nausea, diarrhea, dry mouth, anorexia, dyspepsia, constipation, cramps, vomiting, taste changes, flatulence, decreased appetite*
*GU: Dysmenorrhea, decreased libido, urinary frequency, urinary tract infection,* amenorrhea, cystitis, impotence, urine retention

*INTEG: Sweating, rash, pruritus,* acne, alopecia, urticaria
*MS: Pain,* arthritis, twitching
*RESP: Infection, pharyngitis, nasal congestion, sinus headache, sinusitis, cough, dyspnea, bronchitis,* asthma, hyperventilation, pneumonia
*SYST: Asthenia, viral infection, fever, allergy, chills,* hyponatremia

**Contraindications:** Hypersensitivity

**Precautions:** Pregnancy **C,** breastfeeding, children, geriatric, diabetes mellitus

## Pharmacokinetics

| | |
|---|---|
| **Absorption** | Well absorbed |
| **Distribution** | Crosses blood-brain barrier |
| **Metabolism** | Liver, extensively to norfluoxetine |
| **Excretion** | Kidneys, unchanged (12%), metabolite (7%); steady state 28-35 days, protein binding 94% |
| **Half-life** | 1-3 days metabolite up to 1 wk |

## Pharmacodynamics

| | |
|---|---|
| **Onset** | Unknown |
| **Peak** | 6-8 hr |
| **Duration** | Unknown |

## Interactions
### Individual drugs
Alcohol: increased CNS depression
BusPIRone: increased worsening of OCD
Carbamazepine, digoxin, lithium, phenytoin, warfarin: increased toxicity
Cyproheptadine: decreased fluoxetine effect
Diazepam: increased half-life of diazepam
Haloperidol: increased haloperidol effect
Thioridazine: do not use, or use within 5 wk of discontinuing fluoxetine
### Drug classifications
Antidepressants, opioids, sedative/hypnotics: increased CNS depression
Highly protein-bound products: increased side effects
MAOIs: hypertensive crisis, seizures; do not use with or 14 days prior to fluoxetine
Phenothiazines, tricyclics: increased levels
Serotonin precursors (tryptophan): do not use together
### Drug/herb
Corkwood, jimsonweed: increased anticholinergic effect
Hops, kava, lavender: increased CNS effect
St. John's wort, SAM-e: do not use together; increased risk of serotonin syndrome
### Drug/lab test
Increased: serum bilirubin, blood glucose, alkaline phosphatase

Adverse effects: *italic* = common, **bold** = life-threatening

Decreased: VMA, 5-HIAA
False increase: urinary catecholamines

## NURSING CONSIDERATIONS
### Assessment
• Monitor B/P (lying, standing), pulse q4hr; if systolic B/P drops 20 mm hg, hold product and notify prescriber; take VS q4hr in patients with CV disease
• Monitor blood studies: CBC, leukocytes, differential, cardiac enzymes if patient is receiving long-term therapy; check platelets, bleeding can occur
• Monitor hepatic studies: AST, ALT, bilirubin
• Check weight qwk; appetite may increase with product
• Assess ECG for flattening of T wave, bundle branch block, AV block, dysrhythmias in cardiac patients
• Assess mental status: mood, sensorium, affect, suicidal tendencies; increase in psychiatric symptoms: depression, panic; monitor for seizures; seizure potential is increased
• Monitor urinary retention, constipation; constipation is more likely to occur in children or geriatric
• Identify patient's alcohol consumption; if alcohol is consumed, hold dose until AM
• Assess appetite in bulimia nervosa, weight daily, increase nutritious foods in diet, watch for bingeing and vomiting
• Assess allergic reactions: itching, rash, urticaria, product should be discontinued; may need to give antihistamine

### Nursing diagnoses
• Coping, ineffective (uses)
• Injury, risk for (side effects)
• Knowledge, deficient (teaching)
• Noncompliance (teaching)

### Implementation
• Give with food or milk for GI symptoms
• Give dosage at bedtime if oversedation occurs during day; may take entire dose at bedtime; geriatric may not tolerate once/day dosing, crushed if patient unable to swallow whole (tabs only)
• Prozac weekly: Give on same day each week
• Store at room temperature; do not freeze

### Patient/family education
• Teach patient that therapeutic effects may take 1-4 wk
• Instruct patient to use caution in driving or other activities requiring alertness because of drowsiness, dizziness, blurred vision; to avoid rising quickly from sitting to standing, especially geriatric; to use sunscreen to prevent photosensitivity
• Caution patient to avoid alcohol ingestion, other CNS depressants
• Advise patient not to discontinue medication quickly after long-term use: may cause nausea, headache, malaise
• Instruct patient to increase fluids, bulk in diet if constipation, urinary retention occur, especially geriatric
• Advise patient to take gum, hard sugarless candy, or frequent sips of water for dry mouth
• Teach patient to avoid all OTC products unless approved by prescriber
• Advise patient to change positions slowly, orthostatic hypotension may occur
• Teach that suicidal thoughts, behavior may occur in young adults, children

### Evaluation
**Positive therapeutic outcome**
• Decrease in depression
• Absence of suicidal thoughts
• Decreased symptoms of OCD

**Treatment of overdose:** Activated charcoal, supportive care

## fluphenazine decanoate (Rx)
(floo-fen'ah-zeen)
Modecate ✦, Modecate Concentrate, Prolixin Decanoate
## fluphenazine enanthate (Rx)
Moditen Enanthate ✦, Proloxin Enanthate
## fluphenazine hydrochloride (Rx)
Apo-Fluphenazine ✦, Moditen HCL ✦, Moditen HCl-H.P. ✦, Permitil ✦, Prolixin
*Func. class.:* Antipsychotic/neuroleptic
*Chem. class.:* Phenothiazine, piperazine

**Pregnancy category C**

**Do not confuse:**
Prolixin/Proloid

**Action:** Depresses cerebral cortex, hypothalamus, limbic system, which control activity and aggression; blocks neurotransmission produced by dopamine at synapse; exhibits strong α-adrenergic and anticholinergic blocking action; mechanism for antipsychotic effects is unclear

**Therapeutic outcome:** Decreased signs and symptoms of psychosis

**Uses:** Psychotic disorders, schizophrenia

## Dosage and routes
### Decanoate
*Adult and child >16 yr:* IM/SUBCUT 12.5-25 mg q1-3 wk, may increase slowly
*Child 12-16 yr:* IM/SUBCUT 6.25-18.75 mg, then repeat q1-3 wk, then increase slowly, max 25 mg
*Child 5-12 yr:* IM/SUBCUT 3.125-12.5 mg, then repeat q1-3 wk, increase slowly

### Enanthate
*Adult:* IM/SUBCUT 25 mg q1-3 wk, max 100 mg/dose

### HCl
*Adult:* PO 2.5-10 mg, in divided doses q6-8hr, max 40 mg/day; IM initially 1.25 mg then 2.5-10 mg in divided doses q6-8hr
*Child:* PO 0.25-3.5 mg/day in divided doses q4-6hr, max 10 mg/day

**Available forms:** HCl: tabs 1, 2.5, 5, 10 mg; elixir 2.5 mg/5 ml; inj 2.5 mg/ml; decanoate: inj 25 mg/ml; enanthate: inj 25 mg/ml

## Adverse effects
*CNS: EPS, pseudoparkinsonism, akathisia, dystonia, tardive dyskinesia, drowsiness, headache,* **seizures, neuroleptic malignant syndrome**
*CV: Orthostatic hypotension,* hypertension, **cardiac arrest,** ECG changes, **tachycardia**
*EENT:* Blurred vision, glaucoma, dry eyes
*GI: Dry mouth, nausea, vomiting, anorexia, constipation,* diarrhea, jaundice, weight gain, **paralytic ileus, hepatitis,** cholecystic jaundice
*GU:* Urinary retention, urinary frequency, enuresis, impotence, amenorrhea, gynecomastia
*HEMA:* Anemia, **leukopenia, leukocytosis, agranulocytosis, aplastic anemia, thrombocytopenia**
*INTEG: Rash,* photosensitivity, dermatitis
*RESP:* **Laryngospasm,** dyspnea, **respiratory depression**

**Contraindications:** Hypersensitivity, circulatory collapse, liver damage, cerebral arteriosclerosis, coronary disease, severe hypo/hypertension, blood dyscrasias, coma, brain damage, bone marrow depression, alcohol and barbiturate withdrawal, angle-closure glaucoma

**Precautions:** Pregnancy **C**, breastfeeding, children <12 yr, geriatric, seizure disorders, hypertension, hepatic/cardiac disease

## Pharmacokinetics

| | |
|---|---|
| **Absorption** | Well absorbed (PO, IM) |
| **Distribution** | Widely absorbed, crosses blood-brain barrier, placenta |
| **Metabolism** | Liver, extensively, not dialyzable |
| **Excretion** | Kidneys (metabolites) |
| **Half-life** | HCl-4.7-15.3 hr, enanthate 3½-4 days, decanoate 6.8-14.3 days |

## Pharmacodynamics

| | PO/IM HCl | IM Enanthate | IM Decanoate |
|---|---|---|---|
| **Onset** | 1 hr | 1-2 days | 1-3 days |
| **Peak** | 1½-2 hr | 2-3 days | 1-2 days |
| **Duration** | 6-8 hr | 1-3 wk | >4 wk |

## Interactions
### Individual drugs
Alcohol: increased effects of both products, oversedation
Epinephrine: increased toxicity
Levodopa: decreased antiparkinson activity
Lithium: decreased effects of lithium
### Drug classifications
Anticholinergics: increased anticholinergic effects
Barbiturates: decreased effect of fluphenazine, oversedation
CNS depressants: oversedation
Smoking: decreased effects of fluphenazine
### Drug/herb
Betel palm, kava: increased EPS
Cola tree, hops, kava, nettle, nutmeg: possible increased action
Henbane leaf: increased anticholinergic effect
### Drug/lab test
Increased: liver function tests, cardiac enzymes, cholesterol, blood glucose, prolactin, bilirubin, cholinesterase
Decreased: hormones (blood and urine)
False positive: pregnancy tests, PKU, urinary steroids, 17-OHCS

## NURSING CONSIDERATIONS
### Assessment
• Assess mental status: orientation, mood, behavior, presence of hallucinations, and type before initial administration and monthly; this product should significantly reduce psychotic behavior
• Check for swallowing of PO medication; check for hoarding or giving of medication to other patients
• Monitor I&O ratio, palpate bladder if low urinary output occurs, especially in geriatric; urinalysis recommended before, during prolonged therapy

Adverse effects: *italic* = common, **bold** = life-threatening

- Monitor bilirubin, CBC, liver function tests monthly
- Assess affect, orientation, LOC, reflexes, gait, coordination, sleep pattern disturbances
- Monitor B/P with patient sitting, standing, and lying down; take pulse and respirations q4hr during initial treatment; establish baseline before starting treatment; report drops of 30 mm Hg; obtain baseline ECG, Q-wave and T-wave changes
- Check for dizziness, faintness, palpitations, tachycardia on rising; severe orthostatic hypotension is common
- ◆ Assess for neuroleptic malignant syndrome: hyperpyrexia, muscle rigidity, increased CPK, altered mental status; product should be discontinued
- Assess for EPS including akathisia (inability to sit still, no pattern to movements), tardive dyskinesia (bizarre movements of the jaw, mouth, tongue, extremities), pseudoparkinsonism (rigidity, tremors, pill rolling, shuffling gait), an antiparkinson product should be prescribed
- Assess for constipation, urinary retention daily; if these occur, increase bulk, water in diet

### Nursing diagnoses
- Coping, ineffective (uses)
- Knowledge, deficient (teaching)
- Noncompliance (teaching)
- Thought processes, disturbed (uses)

### Implementation
**PO route**
- Give product in liquid form mixed in glass of juice or cola if hoarding is suspected; do not mix in caffeine drinks, tannics, or pectinates; decrease dose in geriatric
- Give PO with full glass of water, milk; or give with food to decrease GI upset
- Take antacids 2 hr before or after this product
- Store in tight, light-resistant container, oral sol in amber bottle
**SUBCUT route**
- May be given by this route; however, it is painful
**IM route**
- Inject in deep muscle mass, use a 21-G needle into dorsal gluteal site, keep patient recumbent for ½ hr to prevent orthostatic hypotension
- Patient should remain lying down after IM inj for at least 30 min
*Syringe compatibilities:* Benztropine, diphenhydrAMINE, hydrOXYzine

### Patient/family education
- Teach patient to use good oral hygiene; frequent rinsing of mouth, sugarless gum for dry mouth
- Caution patient to avoid hazardous activities until product response is determined; dizziness, blurred vision may occur
- Inform patient that orthostatic hypotension occurs often and to rise from sitting or lying position gradually; tell patient to avoid hot tubs, hot showers, tub baths because hypotension may occur; tell patient that in hot weather, heat stroke may occur; extra precautions are necessary to stay cool
- Instruct patient to avoid abrupt withdrawal of this product, or EPS may result; product should be withdrawn slowly
- Teach patient to avoid OTC preparations (cough, hay fever, cold) unless approved by physician because serious product interactions may occur; avoid use with alcohol, CNS depressants; increased drowsiness may occur
- Instruct patient to use a sunscreen and sunglasses to prevent burns
- Teach patient about EPS and necessity of meticulous oral hygiene because oral candidiasis may occur
- Instruct patient to take antacids 2 hr before or after this product
- Advise patient to report sore throat, malaise, fever, bleeding, mouth sores; if these occur, CBC should be performed and product discontinued

### Evaluation
**Positive therapeutic outcome**
- Decrease in emotional excitement, hallucinations, delusions, paranoia
- Reorganization of patterns of thought, speech

**Treatment of overdose:** Lavage if orally ingested; provide airway; *do not induce vomiting or use epiNEPHrine*

### flurandrenolide topical
*See Appendix D*

---

# flurazepam (Rx)

(flure-az'e-pam)

Apo-flurazepam ✦, Dalmane, flurazepam, Novoflupam ✦, Somnol ✦

*Func. class.:* Sedative-hypnotic
*Chem. class.:* Benzodiazepine derivative, long-acting

## Pregnancy category X

## Controlled substance schedule IV (USA), Targeted (CDSA IV) (Canada)

### Do not confuse:
flurazepam/temazepam

**Action:** Produces CNS depression at the limbic, thalamic, hypothalamic levels of CNS; may be mediated by neurotransmitter γ-aminobutyric acid (GABA); results are sedation, hypnosis, skeletal muscle relaxation, anticonvulsant activity, anxiolytic action

**Therapeutic outcome:** Ability to sleep, relaxation

**Uses:** Insomnia, short term

### Dosage and routes
*Adult:* PO 15-30 mg at bedtime; may repeat dose once if needed
*Geriatric:* PO 15 mg at bedtime; may increase if needed

*Hepatic dose*
*Adult:* PO 5 mg at bedtime

**Available forms:** Caps 15, 30 mg

### Adverse effects
*CNS: Lethargy, drowsiness, daytime sedation,* dizziness, confusion, light-headedness, headache, anxiety, irritability, complex sleep-related reactions (sleep driving, sleep eating)
*CV:* Chest pain, pulse changes, palpitations
*GI:* Nausea, vomiting, diarrhea, heartburn, abdominal pain, constipation
*HEMA:* **Leukopenia, granulocytopenia (rare)**
*MISC:* Physical, psychologic dependence, blurred vision, **apnea**

**Contraindications:** Pregnancy **X**, breastfeeding, intermittent porphyria, uncontrolled pain, sleep apnea, hypersensitivity to this product or benzodiazepines

**Precautions:** Anemia, renal/hepatic disease, suicidal individuals, drug abuse, geriatric, psychosis, children <15 yr, angioedema, pulmonary disease

## Pharmacokinetics

| | |
|---|---|
| Absorption | Well absorbed |
| Distribution | Widely absorbed, crosses blood-brain barrier, crosses placenta, protein binding 97% |
| Metabolism | Liver to active, inactive metabolites |
| Excretion | Kidneys, breast milk |
| Half-life | 2½ hr, 30-200 hr active metabolites |

## Pharmacodynamics

| | |
|---|---|
| Onset | 15-30 min |
| Peak | ½-1 hr |
| Duration | 7-8 hr |

F

## Interactions
### Individual drugs
Alcohol: increased CNS depression
Cimetidine, disulfiram, fluoxetine, isoniazid, ketoconazole, propranolol, valproic acid: increased action of flurazepam
Probenecid: increased effects of flurazepam
Rifampin: increased action of flurazepam
Theophylline: decreased effect of flurazepam
### Drug classifications
Barbiturates: decreased effect of flurazepam
CNS depressants: increased CNS depression
CYP3A4 inhibitors, oral contraceptives: increased effect of flurazepam
### Drug/herb
Black cohosh: increased hypotension
Catnip, chamomile, clary, cowslip, kava, lavender, mistletoe, nettle, pokeweed, poppy, Queen Anne's lace, senega, valerian: increased effect
St. John's wort: decreased flurazepam effect
### Drug/lab test
Increased: AST, ALT, serum bilirubin
Decreased: radioactive iodine uptake
False increase: urinary 17-OHCS

## NURSING CONSIDERATIONS
### Assessment
• Assess anxiety reaction: inability to sleep, apprehension, dread, foreboding, or uneasiness related to unidentified source of danger
• Assess for previous product dependence or tolerance; if product dependent or tolerant, amount of medication should be restricted
• Monitor B/P (lying, standing), pulse; if systolic B/P drops 20 mm Hg, hold product, notify prescriber; I&O, may indicate renal dysfunction
• Monitor blood studies: CBC during long-term therapy; blood dyscrasias have occurred rarely
• Monitor hepatic studies: AST, ALT, bilirubin, creatinine, LDH, alkaline phosphatase

Adverse effects: *italic* = common, **bold** = life-threatening

- Monitor patient's mental status: mood, sensorium, affect, sleeping patterns, drowsiness, dizziness, suicidal tendencies
- Assess for withdrawal signs if discontinued abruptly
- Assess for excessive sedation, impaired coordination, especially in the geriatric

## Nursing diagnoses
- Knowledge, deficient (teaching)
- Noncompliance (teaching)
- Sleep pattern, disturbed (uses)

## Implementation
- Give after removing cigarettes to prevent fires
- Give after trying conservative measures for insomnia
- Give ½-1 hr before bedtime for sleeplessness; caps may be opened and mixed with food; give after meals to decrease GI symptoms if used for sedation
- Provide assistance with ambulation after receiving dose
- Provide safety measures: nightlight, call bell within easy reach
- Check to see if PO medication has been swallowed
- Store in tight container in cool environment

## Patient/family education
- Inform patient that product may be taken with food; if dose is missed take as soon as remembered; do not double doses
- Advise patient to avoid OTC preparations unless approved by a physician, to avoid alcohol ingestion or other psychotropic medications unless approved by prescriber, that 1-2 wk of therapy may be required before therapeutic effects occur
- Caution patient to avoid driving, activities requiring alertness, drowsiness may occur; until medication response is known, tell patient that drowsiness may worsen at beginning of treatment
- Instruct patient not to discontinue medication abruptly after long-term use
- Caution patient to rise slowly or fainting may occur, especially in geriatric
- Inform patient that hangover is common in geriatric
- Teach patients to use contraceptives, pregnancy category **X**

## Evaluation
**Positive therapeutic outcome**
- Increased well-being
- Decreased anxiety, restlessness, sleeplessness, dread

**Treatment of overdose:** Lavage, activated charcoal; monitor electrolytes, VS

---

## flurbiprofen ophthalmic
*See Appendix D*

---

## flutamide (Rx)
(floo'ta-mide)
Apo-Flutamide ✦, Eulexin, Novo-Flutamide ✦
*Func. class.:* Antineoplastic hormone
*Chem. class.:* Antiandrogen
**Pregnancy category D**

**Do not confuse:**
Eulexin/Edecrin

**Action:** Interferes with testosterone uptake in the nucleus or testosterone activity in target tissues; arrests tumor growth in androgen-sensitive tissue (i.e., prostate gland)

**Therapeutic outcome:** Prevention of rapidly growing malignant cells

**Uses:** Metastatic prostatic carcinoma, stage $D_2$ in combination with LHRH agonist analogs (leuprolide)

## Dosage and routes
*Adult:* PO 250 mg q8hr tid, for a daily dosage of 750 mg

**Available forms:** Caps 125, 250 ✦ mg

## Adverse effects
*CNS: Hot flashes,* drowsiness, confusion, depression, anxiety, paresthesia
*GI: Diarrhea, nausea, vomiting,* increased liver function studies, **hepatitis,** anorexia, **hepatotoxicity**
*GU: Decreased libido, impotence, gynecomastia*
*HEMA:* **Leukopenia, thrombocytopenia, hemolytic anemia**
*INTEG:* Irritation at site, rash, photosensitivity
*MISC:* Edema, neuromuscular and pulmonary symptoms, hypertension

**Contraindications:** Pregnancy **D**, hypersensitivity

| Pharmacokinetics | |
|---|---|
| **Absorption** | Well absorbed |
| **Distribution** | Unknown |
| **Metabolism** | Liver |
| **Excretion** | Unknown |
| **Half-life** | 6 hr |

---

## Pharmacodynamics
Unknown

## Interactions
*Individual drugs*
Leuprolide: decreased flutamide action
Warfarin: increased PT

## NURSING CONSIDERATIONS
### Assessment
• Monitor CBC, bilirubin, creatinine, AST, ALT, alkaline phosphatase, which may be elevated, product may need to be discontinued
• Identify CNS symptoms: drowsiness, confusion, depression, anxiety

### Nursing diagnoses
• Body image, disturbed (adverse reactions)
• Infection, risk for (adverse reactions)
• Injury, risk for (adverse reactions)
• Knowledge, deficient (teaching)
• Sexual dysfunction (adverse reactions)

### Implementation
• Used in combination with LHRH agonist (leuprolide)
• May be given with food or fluids

### Patient/family education
• Tell the patient to report side effects: decreased libido, impotence, breast enlargement, hot flashes, diarrhea, which occur when the two products are given together; also nausea, vomiting; jaundice in eyes, skin; dark urine, clay-colored stools, hepatotoxicity may occur
• Inform patient that this product is taken with leuprolide for medical castration, do not change dosing

### Evaluation
**Positive therapeutic outcome**
• Prevention of rapid division of malignant cells

---

## fluticasone (Rx)
(floo-tic′a-sone)
Flonase, Flovent HFA, Flovent Diskus ✦
*Func. class.:* Corticosteroids, inhalation; antiasthmatic

**Pregnancy category** C

**Action:** Decreases inflammation by inhibiting mast cells, macrophages, and leukotrienes; antiinflammatory and vasoconstrictor properties

**Therapeutic outcome:** Decreased severity of asthma

**Uses:** Prevention of chronic asthma during maintenance treatment in those requiring oral corticosteroids; nasal symptoms of seasonal/perennial and allergic/nonallergic rhinitis

## Dosage and routes
*Prevention of chronic asthma during maintenance treatment in those requiring oral corticosteroids*
*Flovent HFA*
*Adult and child ≥12 yr:* INH 88-660 mcg bid (in those previously taking bronchodilators alone); INH 88-220 mcg bid, max 440 mcg bid (in those previously taking inhaled corticosteroids); INH 440 mcg bid, max 880 mcg bid (in those previously taking oral corticosteroids)
*Flovent Diskus*
*Adult and child ≥12 yr:* INH 100 mcg bid, max 500 mcg (in those previously taking bronchodilators alone); INH 100-250 mcg bid, max 500 mcg bid (in those previously taking inhaled corticosteroids); INH 500-1000 mcg bid, max 1000 mcg bid (in those previously taking oral corticosteroids)
*Child 4-11 yr:* INH Initially 50 mcg bid, max 100 mcg bid (in those previously taking bronchodilators alone or inhaled corticosteroids)

*Nasal symptoms of seasonal/perennial rhinitis*
*Flonase*
*Adult:* NASAL SPRAY 2 sprays (100 mcg) in each nostril daily or 1 spray (50 mcg) in each nostril bid; when symptoms are controlled, decrease to 1 spray (50 mcg) in each nostril every day
*Adolescent and child ≥4 yr:* NASAL SPRAY 1 spray (50 mcg) in each nostril daily; may increase to 2 sprays (100 mcg) in each nostril daily; max 2 sprays in each nostril daily

**Available forms:** Nasal spray 50 mcg/metered spray; oral inh aerosol 44, 110, 220 mcg; oral inh powder 50, 100, 250 mcg

## Adverse effects
*CNS:* Fever, headache, nervousness, dizziness, migraines, numbness in fingers
*EENT: Pharyngitis,* sinusitis, rhinitis, laryngitis, hoarseness, dry eyes, cataracts, nasal discharge, epistaxis
*GI:* Diarrhea, abdominal pain, nausea, vomiting, *oral candidiasis,* gastroenteritis
*GU:* UTI
*INTEG:* Urticaria, dermatitis
*META:* Hyperglycemia, growth retardation in children, cushingoid features

Adverse effects: *italic* = common, **bold** = life-threatening

*MISC:* Influenza, **eosinophilic conditions, angioedema, Churg-Strauss syndrome**
*MS:* Osteoporosis, muscle soreness, joint pain
*RESP:* *Upper respiratory infection,* dyspnea, cough, bronchitis, **bronchospasm**

**Contraindications:** Hypersensitivity, primary treatment in status asthmaticus

**Precautions:** Pregnancy C, breastfeeding, active infections, glaucoma, diabetes, immuno-compromised patients

### Pharmacokinetics

| | |
|---|---|
| **Absorption** | 30% aerosol, 13.5% powder |
| **Distribution** | Protein binding 91% |
| **Metabolism** | In liver after absorption in lung |
| **Excretion** | <5% in urine and feces |
| **Half-life** | 7.8 hr |

### Pharmacodynamics

| | NASAL INH | ORAL INH |
|---|---|---|
| **Onset** | 12 hr | 24 hr |
| **Peak** | Several days | Several days |
| **Duration** | 1-2 wk | 1-2 wk |

### Interactions
*Drug classifications*
CYP450 3A4 inhibitors (ketoconazole): increased fluticasone levels
*Drug/lab test*
Increased: urine/serum glucose

### NURSING CONSIDERATIONS
### Assessment
• Assess respiratory status: lung sounds, pulmonary function tests during and several months after change from systemic to inhalation corticosteroids
• Assess for withdrawal symptoms from oral corticosteroids: depression, pain in joints, fatigue
◆ Monitor adrenal insufficiency: nausea, weakness, fatigue, hypotension, hypoglycemia, anorexia; may occur when changing from systemic to inhalation corticosteroids; may be life-threatening
• Monitor growth rate in children
• Monitor adrenal function tests periodically: hypothalamic–pituitary-adrenal axis suppression in long-term treatment

### Nursing diagnoses
• Airway clearance, ineffective (uses)
• Noncompliance (teaching)

### Implementation
• Give at 1 min intervals
• Decrease dose to lowest effective dose after

desired effect; decrease dose at 2 to 4-wk intervals

### Patient/family education
• Advise patient to use bronchodilator first before using inhalation, if taking both
• Caution patient not to use for acute asthmatic attack; for acute asthma, may require oral corticosteroids
• Advise patient to avoid smoking, smoke-filled rooms, those with URIs, those not immunized against chickenpox or measles

### Evaluation
**Positive therapeutic outcome**
• Decreased severity of asthma

---

### fluticasone nasal agent
*See Appendix D*

---

### fluticasone topical
*See Appendix D*

---

### fluvastatin (Rx)
(flu′vah-stay-tin)
Lescol, Lescol XL
*Func. class.:* Antilipidemic
*Chem. class.:* HMG-CoA reductase inhibitor

**Pregnancy category X**

**Action:** Inhibits HMG-CoA reductase enzyme, which reduces cholesterol synthesis

**Therapeutic outcome:** Decreased cholesterol levels and LDLs, increased HDLs

**Uses:** As an adjunct in primary hypercholesterolemia (types Ia, Ib), coronary atherosclerosis in CAD; to reduce the risk of undergoing coronary revascularization in patients with CAD

### Dosage and routes
*Adult:* PO 20-40 mg/day in PM initially, usual range 20-80, not to exceed 80 mg; may be given in 2 doses (40 mg AM, 40 mg PM); dosage adjustments may be made in 4-wk intervals or more

**Available forms:** Caps 20, 40 mg; ext rel tab 80 mg

### Adverse effects
*CNS:* Headache, dizziness, insomnia
*EENT:* Lens opacities
*GI:* Nausea, constipation, diarrhea, abdominal pain, cramps, dyspepsia, flatus, liver dysfunction, pancreatitis

---

*HEMA:* **Thrombocytopenia, hemolytic anemia, leukopenia**
*INTEG:* Rash, pruritus
*MISC:* Fatigue, influenza, photosensitivity
*MS:* Myalgia, *arthritis, arthralgia,* myositis, **rhabdomyolysis**
*RESP:* Upper respiratory infection, rhinitis, cough, pharyngitis, sinusitis

**Contraindications:** Pregnancy **X,** breastfeeding, hypersensitivity, active liver disease

**Precautions:** Past liver disease, alcoholism, severe acute infections, trauma, hypotension, uncontrolled seizure disorders, severe metabolic disorders, electrolyte imbalance

### Pharmacokinetics

| | |
|---|---|
| **Absorption** | Unknown |
| **Distribution** | Steady state 4-5 wk |
| **Metabolism** | Liver |
| **Excretion** | Feces, kidneys |
| **Half-life** | 1-6 days |

### Pharmacodynamics
Unknown

### Interactions
*Individual drugs*
Alcohol, cimetidine, lithium, ranitidine, omeprazole, saquinavir: increased fluvastatin effect
Clofibrate, cycloSPORINE, erythromycin, gemfibrozil, niacin: increased myalgia, myositis
Clozapine, methadone, propranolol, theophylline, tricyclics: increased levels of these products
Digoxin, warfarin: increased action
Pimozide, thioridazine: increased QTc interval
Tramadol: increased serotonin syndrome
*Drug classifications:*
Azole antiinfectives given with clofibrate: increased myalgia, increased myositis
MAOIs: increased serotonin syndrome
*Drug/herb*
Glucomannan: increased effect
Gotu kola, St. John's wort: decreased effect
*Drug/food*
Grapefruit juice: possible increased fluvastatin toxicity
Oat bran, high fat: decreased absorption

### NURSING CONSIDERATIONS
Assessment
• Assess nutrition: fat, protein, carbohydrates; nutritional analysis should be completed by dietitian before treatment

• Monitor bowel pattern daily; diarrhea may be a problem
• Assess fasting lipid profile (cholesterol, LDL, HDL, triglycerides) q8 wk, then q3-6 mo when stable
• Monitor liver function studies q1-2 mo during the first 1½ yr of treatment; AST, ALT, liver function test results may be increased
• Monitor renal studies in patients with compromised renal system: BUN, I&O ratio, creatinine
• Obtain ophth exam before, 1 mo after treatment begins, annually; lens opacities may occur

F

### Nursing diagnoses
• Diarrhea (adverse reactions)
• Knowledge, deficient (teaching)
• Noncompliance (teaching)

### Implementation
• Give with evening meal; if dosage is increased, take with breakfast and evening meal
• Store in cool environment in airtight, light-resistant container

### Patient/family education
• Inform patient that compliance is needed for positive results to occur, not to double doses
• Advise patient to notify prescriber if GI symptoms of diarrhea, abdominal or epigastric pain, nausea, vomiting, or if chills, fever, sore throat occur; also muscle pain, weakness, tenderness
• Advise patient that treatment is chronic
• Advise patient that blood studies and eye exam will be necessary during treatment
• Instruct patient to report suspected pregnancy, not to use during pregnancy
• Advise patient that previously prescribed regimen will continue, including diet, exercise, smoking cessation
• Advise patient to use sunscreen or stay out of the sun to prevent burns
• Instruct patient to notify all health care providers of products taken

### Evaluation
**Positive therapeutic outcome**
• Decreased LDL, VLDL, total cholesterol levels
• Improved ratio of HDLs

Adverse effects: *italic* = common, **bold** = life-threatening

## folic acid (vitamin B₉) (PO, OTC; IM/IV, Ph)

(foe-lik a'sid)

Apo-Folic ♣, Folate, Folvite, Novofolacid ♣, Vitamin B₉

*Func. class.:* Vitamin B-complex group
*Chem. class.:* Supplement

**Pregnancy category A**

**Action:** Needed for erythropoiesis; increases RBC, WBC, and platelet formation in megaloblastic anemias

**Therapeutic outcome:** Absence of macrocytic, megaloblastic anemias

**Uses:** Megaloblastic or macrocytic anemia caused by folic acid deficiency; liver disease; alcoholism; hemolysis; intestinal obstruction; pregnancy; to reduce risk of neural tube defect

**Dosage and routes**
*RDA*
*Adult (pregnant/breastfeeding):* PO 400 mcg/day
*Adult and child ≥14 yr:* PO 200 mcg
*Child 9-13 yr:* PO 300 mcg
*Child 4-8 yr:* PO 200 mcg
*Child 1-3 yr:* PO 150 mcg
*Infant 6 mo-1 yr:* PO 80 mcg
*Neonate and infant <6 mo:* PO 65 mcg

*Megaloblastic/macrocytic anemia due to folic acid or nutritional deficiency*
*Pregnant:* PO 600 mcg
*Breastfeeding:* PO 500 mcg

*Therapeutic dose*
*Adult and child:* PO/IM/SUBCUT/**IV** Up to 1 mg/day

*Maintenance dose*
*Adult and child >4 yr:* PO/IM/**IV**/SUBCUT 0.4 mg/day
*Child <4 yr:* PO/IM/**IV**/SUBCUT Up to 0.3 mg/day
*Infant:* PO/IM/**IV**/SUBCUT Up to 0.1 mg/day

*Pregnant and/or lactating:*
PO/IM/**IV**/SUBCUT 0.8 mg/day

*Prevention of neural tube defects during pregnancy*
*Adult:* PO 0.4 mg/day

*Prevention of megaloblastic anemia during pregnancy*
*Adult:* PO/IM/SUBCUT up to 1 mg/day during pregnancy

*Tropical sprue*
*Adult:* PO 3-15 mg/day

**Available forms:** Tabs 0.1, 0.4, 0.8, 1, 5 mg; inj 5, 10 mg/ml

**Adverse effects**
*INTEG:* Flushing
*RESP:* Bronchospasm

**Contraindications:** Hypersensitivity, anemias other than megaloblastic/macrocytic anemia, vit B₁₂ deficiency anemia, uncorrected pernicious anemia

**Precautions:** Pregnancy **A**

| Pharmacokinetics | |
|---|---|
| **Absorption** | Well absorbed |
| **Distribution** | Liver, crosses placenta |
| **Metabolism** | Liver (converted to active metabolite) |
| **Excretion** | Kidneys (unchanged) |
| **Half-life** | Unknown |

| Pharmacodynamics | |
|---|---|
| **Onset** | Unknown |
| **Peak** | ½-1 hr |
| **Duration** | Unknown |

**Interactions**
*Individual drugs*
Carbamazepine: increased need for folic acid
Fosphenytoin: decreased fosphenytoin levels, may increase seizures
Methotrexate, sulfasalazine: decreased action of folic acid
Phenytoin: decreased phenytoin levels, may increase seizures
*Drug classifications*
Estrogens, glucocorticoids, hydantoins: increased need for folic acid
Sulfonamides: decreased action of folic acid

**NURSING CONSIDERATIONS**
**Assessment**
• Assess patient for fatigue, dyspnea, weakness, shortness of breath, activity intolerance (signs of megaloblastic anemia)
• Monitor Hgb, Hct, and reticulocyte count; folate levels: 6-15 mcg/ml baseline and throughout treatment
• Assess nutritional status: bran, yeast, dried beans, nuts, fruits, fresh vegetables, asparagus; if high folic acid foods are missing from the diet, a referral to a dietitian may be indicated
• Identify products currently taken: alcohol, oral contraceptives, estrogens, glucocorticoids, carbamazepine, hydantoins, trimethoprim; these products may cause

increased folic acid use by the body and contribute to deficiency

## Nursing diagnoses
- Activity intolerance (uses)
- Fatigue (uses)
- Knowledge, deficient (teaching)
- Nutrition: less than body requirements, imbalanced (uses)

## Implementation
### IV route
- Give **IV** directly, undiluted 5 mg or less over 1 min or more, or may be added to most **IV** sol or TPN
- Store in light-resistant container

*Y-site compatibilities:* Famotidine
*Solution compatibilities:* $D_{20}W$
*Solution incompatibilities:* $D_{40}W$, $D_{50}W$, calcium gluconate

## Patient/family education
- Advise patient to take product exactly as prescribed; not to double doses, toxicity may occur
- Instruct patient to notify prescriber of side effects; rash or fever may indicate hypersensitivity
- Advise patient that urine may become more yellow
- Instruct patient to increase intake of foods rich in folic acid in diet as recommended by dietitian or health care provider
- Teach patient to avoid breastfeeding

## Evaluation
### Positive therapeutic outcome
- Absence of fatigue, weakness, dyspnea
- Absence of symptoms of megaloblastic anemia
- Increase in reticulocyte count within 5 days
- Absence of neural tube defect

---

## fondaparinux (Rx)
(fon-dah-pair'ih-nux)
Arixtra
*Func. class.:* Anticoagulant, antithrombotic
*Chem. class.:* Synthetic, selective factor Xa inhibitor
### Pregnancy category B

### Do not confuse:
Arixtra/Anti-Xa

**Action:** Acts by antithrombin III (ATIII)-mediated selective inhibition of factor Xa; neutralization of factor Xa interrupts blood coagulation and inhibits thrombin formation;

does not inactivate thrombin (activated factor II) or affect platelets

**Therapeutic outcome:** Prevention of deep vein thrombosis

**Uses:** Prevention of deep vein thrombosis, pulmonary emboli in hip and knee replacement, hip fracture surgery

## Dosage and routes
### Deep vein thrombosis/PE
*Adult <50 kg:* SUBCUT 5 mg/day × 5 days or more until INR is 2-3; may give warfarin within 72 hr of fondaparinux
*Adult 50-100 kg:* SUBCUT 7.5 mg/day × 5 days or more until INR is 2-3; may give warfarin within 72 hr of fondaparinux
*Adult >100 kg:* SUBCUT 10 mg/day × 5 days or more until INR is 2-3; may give warfarin within 72 hr of fondaparinux

### Prevention of deep vein thrombosis
*Adult:* SUBCUT 2.5 mg/day, given 6 hr after surgery; continue for 5-9 days; hip surgery up to 32 days; abdominal surgery up to 24 days

**Available forms:** Inj 2.5 mg/0.5 ml, 5 mg/0.4 ml, 7.5 mg/0.6 ml, 10 mg/0.8 ml prefilled syringes

## Adverse effects
*CNS: Fever,* confusion, headache, dizziness, *insomnia*
*GI: Nausea, vomiting,* diarrhea, dyspepsia, *constipation,* increased AST, ALT
*GU:* UTI, urinary retention
*HEMA: Anemia,* minor bleeding, purpura, hematoma, **thrombocytopenia, major bleeding (intracranial, cerebral, retroperitoneal hemorrhage), postoperative hemorrhage**
*INTEG:* Local reaction—*rash,* pruritus, inj site bleeding, increased wound drainage, bullous eruption
*META:* Hypokalemia
*MISC:* Hypotension, pain, *edema*

**Contraindications:** Hypersensitivity to this product; hemophilia, leukemia with bleeding, peptic ulcer disease, hemorrhagic stroke, surgery, thrombocytopenic purpura, weight <50 kg, severe renal disease (CCr <30 ml/min), active major bleeding, bacterial endocarditis

**Precautions:** Pregnancy **B,** breastfeeding, children, geriatric, alcoholism, hepatic disease (severe), blood dyscrasias, heparin-induced thrombocytopenia, uncontrolled severe hypertension, subacute bacterial endocarditis, acute nephritis, mild-moderate renal disease

Adverse effects: *italic* = common, **bold** = life-threatening

## Pharmacokinetics

| | |
|---|---|
| **Absorption** | Rapidly, completely absorbed |
| **Distribution** | Blood; does not bind to plasma proteins except 94% to ATIII |
| **Metabolism** | Unknown |
| **Excretion** | Eliminated unchanged in 72 hr in normal renal function |
| **Half-life** | 17-21 hr |

## Pharmacodynamics

| | |
|---|---|
| **Onset** | Unknown |
| **Peak** | 3 hr |
| **Duration** | Unknown |

## Interactions

Before starting fondaparinux, discontinue use of other products that may increase the risk of hemorrhage; monitor closely if coadministration is essential

### Individual drugs

Abciximab, clopidogrel, dipyridamole, eptifibatide, quinidine, tirofiban, valproic acid: increased risk of bleeding

### Drug classifications

NSAIDs, salicylates: increased risk of bleeding

### Drug/herb

Agrimony, alfalfa, angelica, anise, basil, bay, bilberry, black haw, bogbean, bromelain, buchu, chondroitin, cinchona bark, dong quai, fenugreek, feverfew, garlic, ginger, ginkgo, ginseng, horse chestnut, Irish moss, kelp, kelpware, khella, lovage, lungwort, meadowsweet, motherwort, mugwort, nettle, papaya, parsley (large amounts), paud'arco, pineapple, poplar, prickly ash, safflower, saw palmetto, tonka bean, turmeric, wintergreen, yarrow: increased risk of bleeding

Chamomile, coenzyme Q10, flax, glucomannan, goldenseal, guar gum: decreased anticoagulant effect

## NURSING CONSIDERATIONS

### Assessment

• Assess blood studies (Hct, CBC, coagulation studies, platelets, occult blood in stools), anti-Xa; thrombocytopenia may occur
• Assess for bleeding: gums, petechiae, ecchymosis, black tarry stools, hematuria; notify prescriber
• Assess for neurologic symptoms in patients who have received spinal anesthesia

### Nursing diagnoses

• Injury, risk for (uses, adverse reactions)
• Knowledge, deficient (teaching)
• Tissue perfusion, ineffective (uses)

## Implementation

• Do not mix with other products or solutions; cannot be used interchangeably (unit to unit) with other anticoagulants
• Administer for 5-9 days
• Give only after screening patient for bleeding disorders
• Administer SUBCUT only; do not give IM
• Store at 77° F (25° C); do not freeze

### SUBCUT route

• Check for discolored sol or sol with particulate; if present, do not give
• Begin 2 hr prior to surgery
• Administer to recumbent patient, rotate inj sites (left/right anterolateral, left/right posterolateral abdominal wall)
• Wipe surface of inj site with alcohol swab, twist plunger cap and remove, remove rigid needle guard by pulling straight off needle, do not aspirate, do not expel air bubble from surface
• Insert whole length of needle into skin fold held with thumb and forefinger
• When product is injected, a soft click may be felt or heard
• Give at same time each day to maintain steady blood levels
• Avoid all IM inj that may cause bleeding
 Administer only this product when ordered; not interchangeable with heparin

### Patient/family education

• Advise patient to use soft-bristle toothbrush to avoid bleeding gums, to use electric razor
• Advise patient to report any signs of bleeding: gums, under skin, urine, stools
• Caution patient to avoid OTC products containing aspirin

## Evaluation

### Positive therapeutic outcome

• Absence of deep vein thrombosis

---

## formoterol (Rx)

(for-moh'ter-ahl)

Foradil Aerolizer, Perforomist

*Func. class.:* β-Adrenergic agonist

*Chem. class.:* Sympathomimetic catecholamine

### Pregnancy category C

**Do not confuse:**

Foradil/Toradol

**Action:** Has β₁ and β₂ action; relaxes bronchial smooth muscle and dilates the trachea and main bronchi by increasing levels of cAMP, which relaxes smooth muscles;

causes increased contractility and heart rate by acting on β-receptors in the heart

**Therapeutic outcome:** Bronchodilation, increased heart rate and cardiac output from action on β-receptors in heart

**Uses:** Maintenance, treatment of asthma, COPD, prevention of exercise-induced bronchospasm

## Dosage and routes
*Maintenance, treatment of asthma*
*Adult and child ≥5 yr:* INH AM and PM long-term, 1 cap q12hr using aerolizer inhaler

*Maintenance of COPD*
*Adult:* INH 12 mcg q12hr

*Prevention of exercise-induced bronchospasm*
*Adult and child ≥12 yr:* prn occasionally 1 cap (12 mcg) at least 15 min before exercise

**Available forms:** INH powder in cap 12 mcg

## Adverse effects
*CNS:* Tremors, *anxiety*, insomnia, headache, dizziness, stimulation
*CV:* Palpitations, tachycardia, hypertension
*GI:* Nausea, vomiting, xerostomia
*RESP:* Bronchial irritation, dryness of oropharynx, **bronchospasms (overuse)**; infection, inflammatory reactions (child)

**Contraindications:** Hypersensitivity to sympathomimetics, angle-closure glaucoma

**Precautions:** Pregnancy **C**, geriatric, cardiac disorders, hyperthyroidism, diabetes mellitus, prostatic hypertrophy, hypertension

### Pharmacokinetics
| | |
|---|---|
| **Absorption** | Rapid (INH) |
| **Distribution** | Plasma protein binding 61%-64% at concentrations of 0.1-100 ng/mL; 31%-38% at concentrations of 5-500 ng/mL |
| **Metabolism** | Liver, lungs, GI tract |
| **Excretion** | Urine, feces |
| **Half-life** | 10 hr mean terminal elimination half-life |

### Pharmacodynamics
| | |
|---|---|
| **Onset** | Unknown |
| **Peak** | 5 min (INH) |
| **Duration** | Unknown |

## Interactions
*Drug classifications*
β-Blockers: decreased action of formoterol
MAOIs, antidepressants (tricyclics): serious dysrhythmias
Sympathomimetics: increased action of both products

## NURSING CONSIDERATIONS
### Assessment
• Assess respiratory function: B/P, pulse, lung sounds
• Assess I&O ratio; check for urinary retention, frequency, hesitancy
• Assess for paresthesias and coldness of extremities; peripheral blood flow may decrease

### Nursing diagnoses
• Airway clearance, ineffective (uses)
• Gas exchange, impaired (uses)
• Knowledge, deficient (teaching)

### Implementation
• Store at room temperature, protect from heat, moisture
• Do not use discolored solution
• Rinse mouth after use

### Patient/family education
• Review package insert with patient and inform about all aspects of product
• Teach correct use of inhaler
• Teach use of spacer device in children or geriatric
• Advise patient to avoid getting aerosol in eyes
• Instruct patient to rinse mouth after use
• Advise patient to wash inhaler in warm water and dry daily
• Advise patient to avoid smoking, smoke-filled rooms, persons with respiratory infections

### Evaluation
**Positive therapeutic outcome**
• Absence of dyspnea, wheezing
• Improved airway exchange
• Improved ABGs

**Treatment of overdose:** Administer β-blocker

## fosamprenavir (Rx)
(fos-am-pren'a-veer)
Lexiva
*Func. class.:* Antiretroviral
*Chem. class.:* Protease inhibitor

**Pregnancy category** C

**Action:** Prodrug of amprenavir; inhibits human immunodeficiency virus (HIV) protease, which prevents maturation of the infectious virus

**Therapeutic outcome:** Decreasing symptoms of HIV

**Uses:** HIV-1 infection in combination with antiretrovirals

### Dosage and routes
*Therapy-naïve patients*
*Adult:* PO 1400 mg bid without ritonavir, or fosamprenavir 1400 mg/day and ritonavir 200 mg/day, or fosamprenavir 700 mg bid and ritonavir 100 mg bid

*Protease-experienced patients (PI)*
*Adult:* PO 700 mg bid and ritonavir 100 mg bid

*Combination with efavirenz*
*Adult:* PO Add another 100 mg/day of ritonavir for a total of 300 mg/day when all three products are given

*Hepatic dose*
*Adult:* PO (Child-Pugh 5-9) 700 mg bid; (Child-Pugh 10-12) 350 mg bid

**Available forms:** Tabs 700 mg (equivalent to 600 mg amprenavir)

### Adverse effects
*CNS:* Headache, fatigue, depression, oral paresthesia
*GI: Nausea, diarrhea, vomiting, abdominal pain*
*INTEG:* Rash, pruritus
*MISC:* Redistribution or accumulation of body fat, hyperglycemia, **Stevens-Johnson syndrome**

**Contraindications:** Hypersensitivity to protease inhibitors

**Precautions:** Pregnancy **C**, breastfeeding, geriatric, liver disease, hemolytic anemia, diabetes, sulfa sensitivity

### Pharmacokinetics
| | |
|---|---|
| **Absorption** | Unknown |
| **Distribution** | 90% protein binding |
| **Metabolism** | In the liver by CYP4503AY (CYP3A4) |
| **Excretion** | Excretion of unchanged product is minimal |
| **Half-life** | Unknown |

### Pharmacodynamics
| | |
|---|---|
| **Onset** | Unknown |
| **Peak** | 1½-4 hr |
| **Duration** | Unknown |

### Interactions
*Individual drugs*
◆Amiodarone, flecainide, lidocaine, midazolam, pimozide, propafenone, triazolam: serious life-threatening reactions
Carbamazepine, delavirdine, phenobarbital, phenytoin, rifampin: avoid use; may lose virologic response and possibly lead to resistance to fosamprenavir
Carbamazepine, efavirenz, nevirapine, phenytoin, ranitidine, saquinavir: decreased fosamprenavir levels
Itraconazole, ketoconazole, rifbutin, sildenafil, vardenafil: increased effect
Methadone: decreased effect
Warfarin: may affect coagulation
*Drug classifications*
Antacids: decreased fosamprenavir levels
◆Calcium channel blockers, ergots: serious life-threatening reactions
Contraceptives (oral): decreased effect
Estrogens, H$_2$ receptor antagonists, oral contraceptives, proton pump inhibitors: avoid use; may lose virologic response and possibly lead to resistance of fosamprenavir
HMG-CoA reductase inhibitors: increased toxicity
*Drug/herb*
Avoid use with St. John's wort because may lose virologic response and possibly lead to resistance of fosamprenavir
*Drug/lab test*
Increased: serum glucose, AST, ALT, triglycerides

### NURSING CONSIDERATIONS
**Assessment**
• Assess bowel pattern before, during treatment; monitor hydration
• Assess skin eruptions, rash, urticaria, itching
• Monitor viral load, CD4 cell counts baseline and throughout treatment

### Nursing diagnoses
• Infection, risk for (uses)
• Injury, risk for (adverse reactions)
• Knowledge, deficient (teaching)

### Implementation
• Administer without regard to food
• Patients receiving phosphodiesterase type 5 inhibitors may be at increased risk for PDE5 inhibitor adverse effects

### Patient/family education
• Advise to avoid taking with other medications unless directed by provider
• Teach that product does not cure, but does manage symptoms; that product does not prevent transmission of HIV to others
• Advise to use nonhormonal form of birth control while taking this product
• Instruct if dose is missed, take as soon as remembered up to 1 hr before next dose; do not double dose
• Instruct not to alter dose or stop therapy without talking to physician
• Advise physician if patient has a sulfa allergy
• Advise to report all medications, including herbal supplements, to physician

### Evaluation
**Positive therapeutic outcome**
• Decreasing symptoms of HIV

---

### foscarnet (Rx)
(foss-kar′net)
Foscavir
*Func. class.:* Antiviral
*Chem. class.:* Inorganic pyrophosphate organic analog

**Pregnancy category C**

---

**Action:** Antiviral activity is produced by selective inhibition at the pyrophosphate binding site on virus-specific DNA polymerases and reverse transcriptases at concentrations that do not affect cellular DNA polymerases

**Therapeutic outcome:** Virostatic agents against CMV retinitis

**Uses:** Treatment of CMV, retinitis, herpes simplex virus (HSV) infections; used with ganciclovir for relapsing patients

### Dosage and routes
*CMV retinitis*
**Adult:** **IV** INF 60 mg/kg given over at least 1 hr, q8hr × 2-3 wk initially, or 90 mg/kg q12hr, usually given with at least 750-1000 ml of 0.9% NaCl daily

*HSV*
**Adult:** **IV** 40 mg/kg q8-12hr × 2-3 wk
*Renal dose*
**Adult: IV**
**Male:**

$$\frac{140 - age}{72 \times serum\ creatinine\ (mg/dl)} = CCr$$

**Female:** 0.85 × above value; dose based on table provided in package insert

**Available forms:** Inj 6000 mg/250 ml,12,000 mg/500 ml (24 mg/ml)

### Adverse effects
*CNS:* Fever, dizziness, *headache,* **seizures,** *fatigue,* neuropathy, tremor, ataxia, dementia, stupor, EEG abnormalities, vertigo, **coma,** abnormal gait, hypertonia, extrapyramidal disorders, hemiparesis, **paralysis,** hyperreflexia, paraplegia, **tetany,** hyporeflexia, neuralgia, neuritis, **cerebral edema,** *paresthesia,* depression, *confusion, anxiety,* insomnia, somnolence, amnesia, hallucinations, agitation
*CV:* Hypertension, palpitations, ECG abnormalities, 1st-degree AV block, nonspecific ST-T segment changes, hypotension, cerebrovascular disorder, cardiomyopathy, **cardiac arrest,** bradycardia, **dysrhythmias**
*EENT:* Visual field defects, vocal cord paralysis, speech disorders, taste perversion, eye pain, conjunctivitis, tinnitus, otitis
*GI:* Nausea, vomiting, diarrhea, anorexia, abdominal pain, constipation, dysphagia, rectal hemorrhage, dry mouth, melena, flatulence, ulcerative stomatitis, pancreatitis, enteritis, enterocolitis, glossitis, proctitis, stomatitis, increased amylases, gastroenteritis, **pseudomembranous colitis,** duodenal ulcer, **paralytic ileus, esophageal ulceration,** abnormal A-G ratio, increased AST, ALT, cholecystitis, **hepatitis,** dyspepsia, tenesmus, hepatosplenomegaly, jaundice
*GU:* **Acute renal failure,** decreased CCr and increased serum creatinine, **glomerulonephritis, toxic nephropathy, nephrosis, renal tubular disorders, pyelonephritis, uremia, hematuria, albuminuria,** dysuria, polyuria
*HEMA:* Anemia, **granulocytopenia, leukopenia, thrombocytopenia, platelet abnormalities, thrombosis, pulmonary embolism, coagulation disorders, decreased prothrombin, hypochromic anemia, pancytopenia, hemolysis, leukocytosis,** lymphadenopathy, epistaxis, lymphopenia
*INTEG:* Rash, sweating, pruritus, skin ulceration, seborrhea, SKIN discoloration, alopecia, acne, dermatitis, pain/inflammation at injec-

---

Adverse effects: *italic* = common, **bold** = life-threatening

tion site, facial edema, dry skin, urticaria
*MS:* Arthralgia, myalgia
*RESP: Coughing, dyspnea,* pneumonia, sinusitis, pharyngitis, **pulmonary infiltration,** stridor, **pneumothorax, hemoptysis, bronchospasm,** bronchitis, **respiratory depression, pleural effusion, pulmonary hemorrhage,** rhinitis
*SYST: Hypokalemia, hypocalcemia, hypomagnesemia,* increased alkaline phosphatase, LDH, BUN, acidosis, hypophosphatemia, hyperphosphatemia, dehydration, glycosuria, increased creatine phosphokinase, hypervolemia, infection, **sepsis, death, ascites,** hyponatremia, hypochloremia, hypercalcemia

**Contraindications:** Hypersensitivity, CCr <0.4 ml/min/kg

**Precautions:** Pregnancy **C,** breastfeeding, children, geriatric, renal disease, seizure disorders, electrolyte/mineral imbalances, severe anemia

### Pharmacokinetics

| | |
|---|---|
| **Absorption** | Complete (**IV**) |
| **Distribution** | 14%-17% plasma protein binding |
| **Metabolism** | Not metabolized |
| **Excretion** | Kidneys (79%-92%) unchanged, breast milk |
| **Half-life** | 18-88 hr; increased in renal disease |

### Pharmacodynamics

| | |
|---|---|
| **Onset** | 48 hr |
| **Peak** | 2 wk |
| **Duration** | Unknown |

### Interactions
#### Individual drugs
Amphotericin B, cycloSPORINE, lithium: increased nephrotoxicity
Pentamide: increased hypocalcemia
#### Drug classifications
Aminoglycosides, NSAIDs: increased nephrotoxicity

### NURSING CONSIDERATIONS
#### Assessment
• Culture should be done before treatment with foscarnet is begun; cultures of blood, urine, and throat may all be taken; CMV is not confirmed by this method; the diagnosis is made by an ophth exam
• Assess kidney and liver function; increased hemopoietic studies: BUN, serum creatinine, creatinine clearance, if CCr <0.4 ml/min/kg, discontinue product; AST, ALT, A-G ratio, baseline and during treatment; blood counts

should be done q2 wk; watch for decreasing granulocytes, Hgb; if low, therapy may have to be discontinued and restarted after hematologic recovery; blood transfusions may be required
• Assess for GI symptoms: severe nausea, vomiting, diarrhea; severe symptoms may necessitate discontinuing product
• Monitor electrolytes and minerals: calcium, phosphorous, magnesium, sodium, potassium; watch closely for tetany during first administration
◆ Assess for symptoms of blood dyscrasias (anemia, granulocytopenia); bruising, fatigue, bleeding, poor healing
• Assess for symptoms of allergic reactions: flushing, rash, urticaria, pruritus

#### Nursing diagnoses
• Infection, risk for (uses)
• Injury, risk for (adverse reactions)
• Knowledge, deficient (teaching)

#### Implementation
**IV route**
• Administer increased fluids before and during product administration to induce diuresis and minimize renal toxicity
• Administer via infusion pump, at no more than 1 mg/kg/min; do not give by rapid or bolus **IV;** give by central venous line or peripheral vein; standard 24 mg/ml sol may be used without dilution if using by central line; dilute the 24 mg/ml sol to 12 mg/ml with $D_5W$ or 0.9% NaCl if using peripheral vein
• Monitor patient closely during therapy; if tingling, numbness, paresthesias occur, stop inf and obtain lab sample for electrolytes
*Y-site compatibilities:* Aldesleukin, aminophylline, amikacin, ampicillin, aztreonam, benzquinamide, cefazolin, cefoperazone, cefoxitin, ceftazidime, ceftizoxime, ceftriaxone, cefuroxime, chloramphenicol, cimetidine, clindamycin, dexamethasone, DOPamine, erythromycin, fluconazole, flucytosine, furosemide, gentamicin, heparin, hydrocortisone, hydromorphone, hydrOXYzine, imipenem-cilastatin, metoclopramide, metronidazole, miconazole, morphine, nafcillin, oxacillin, penicillin G potassium, phenytoin, piperacillin, ranitidine, ticarcillin/clavulanate, tobramycin
*Y-site incompatibilities:* Acyclovir, amphotericin B, calcium, cotrimoxazole, diazepam, digoxin, gancyclovir, haloperidol, leucovorin, midazolam, pentamidine, phenytoin, prochlorperazine, vancomycin

---

### Patient/family education

- Advise patient to notify prescriber if sore throat, swollen lymph nodes, malaise, fever occur, may indicate presence of other infections
- Advise patient to report perioral tingling, numbness in extremities, and paresthesias; infusion should be stopped and electrolytes should be requested
- Caution patient that serious product interactions may occur if OTC products are ingested; check first with prescriber
- Inform patient that product is not a cure, but will control symptoms
- Advise patient that ophth exams must be continued

### Evaluation
**Positive therapeutic outcome**
- Improvement in CMV retinitis

---

### fosinopril (Rx)
(foss-in-o'pril)
Monopril
*Func. class.:* Antihypertensive
*Chem. class.:* Angiotensin-converting enzyme (ACE) inhibitor

**Pregnancy category  D**

**Do not confuse:**
Monopril/minoxidil/Accupril/Monoket

**Action:** Selectively suppresses renin-angiotensin-aldosterone system; inhibits ACE; prevents conversion of angiotensin I to angiotensin II; results in dilatation of arterial, venous vessels

**Therapeutic outcome:** Decreased B/P in hypertension

**Uses:** Hypertension, alone or in combination with thiazide diuretics, systolic CHF

### Dosage and routes
*Hypertension*
*Adult:* PO 10 mg/day initially, then 20-40 mg/day divided bid or daily, max 80 mg/day

*CHF*
*Adult:* PO 10 mg/day, then up to 40 mg/day, increased over several weeks; use lower dose in those undergoing diuresis before fosinopril

**Available forms:** Tabs 10, 20, 40 mg

### Adverse effects
*CNS: Insomnia, paresthesia, headache, dizziness,* fatigue, memory disturbance, tremor, mood change

*CV: Hypotension,* chest pain, palpitations, angina, orthostatic hypotension, dysrhythmias, tachycardia
*GI: Nausea,* constipation, vomiting, diarrhea
*GU:* **Proteinuria,** increased BUN, creatinine, decreased libido
*HEMA:* Decreased Hct, Hgb, **eosinophilia, leukopenia, neutropenia**
*INTEG:* **Angioedema,** rash, flushing, sweating, photosensitivity, pruritus
*META:* Hyperkalemia
*MS:* Arthralgia, myalgia
*RESP:* Cough, sinusitis, dyspnea, **bronchospasm**

**Contraindications:** Pregnancy **D**, breastfeeding, children, hypersensitivity to ACE inhibitors

**Precautions:** Geriatric, impaired liver function, hypovolemia, blood dyscrasias, CHF, COPD, asthma, angioedema, hyperkalemia, renal artery stenosis, renal disease

### Pharmacokinetics
| | |
|---|---|
| **Absorption** | 30% |
| **Distribution** | Crosses placenta |
| **Metabolism** | Liver—converted to fosinoprilate |
| **Excretion** | 50% kidneys (metabolites), 50% feces |
| **Half-life** | 12 hr—fosinoprilat |

### Pharmacodynamics
| | |
|---|---|
| **Onset** | 1 hr |
| **Peak** | 2-6 hr |
| **Duration** | 24 hr |

### Interactions
*Individual drugs*
Alcohol (acute ingestion): increased hypotension (large amounts)
Allopurinol: increased hypersensitivity
Digoxin, hydralazine, lithium, prazosin: increased toxicity
Indomethacin: decreased antihypertensive effect

*Drug classifications*
Adrenergic blockers, antihypertensives, diuretics, ganglionic blockers, nitrates, phenothiazines: increased hypotension
Antacids: decreased absorption
Diuretics (potassium-sparing), sympathomimetics, vasodilators: increased toxicity
NSAIDs, salicylates: decreased antihypertensive effect

*Drug/herb*
⬥Arginine: fatal hypokalemia
Hawthorn, pill-bearing spurge: increased antihypertensive effect

Adverse effects: *italic* = common, **bold** = life-threatening

Pineapple, yohimbe: decreased antihypertensive effect

St. John's wort: severe photosensitivity

*Drug/lab test*

Increased: AST, ALT, alkaline phosphatase, glucose, bilirubin, uric acid

Positive: ANA titer

False positive: urine acetone

## NURSING CONSIDERATIONS
### Assessment

• Monitor blood studies: neutrophils, decreased platelets; obtain WBC with differential baseline and qmo × 6 mo, then q2-3 mo × 1 yr; if neutrophils <1000/mm³, discontinue

• Monitor B/P, check for orthostatic hypotension, syncope; if changes occur, dosage change may be required

• Monitor renal studies: protein, BUN, creatinine; watch for increased levels that may indicate nephrotic syndrome and renal failure; monitor urine daily for protein; monitor renal symptoms: polyuria, oliguria, frequency, dysuria

• Establish baselines in renal, liver function tests before therapy begins

• Check potassium levels throughout treatment although hyperkalemia rarely occurs

• Check for edema in feet, legs daily, monitor weight daily

• Assess for allergic reactions: rash, fever, pruritus, urticaria; product should be discontinued if antihistamines fail to help

### Nursing diagnoses

• Cardiac output, decreased (uses)
• Injury, risk for (side effects)
• Knowledge, deficient (teaching)
• Noncompliance (teaching)

### Implementation

• Store in airtight container at 86° F (30° C) or less

• Severe hypotension may occur after 1st dose of this medication; hypotension may be prevented by reducing or discontinuing diuretic therapy 3 days before beginning benzapril therapy

### Patient/family education

• Advise patient not to discontinue product abruptly; warn patient to tell all persons associated with his or her care

• Teach patient not to use OTC products (cough, cold, allergy) unless directed by prescriber because serious side effects can occur; xanthines such as coffee, tea, chocolate, cola can prevent action of product

• Teach patient the importance of complying with dosage schedule, even if feeling better; to continue with medical regimen to decrease

B/P: exercise, smoking cessation, decreasing stress, diet modifications

• Emphasize the need to rise slowly to sitting or standing position to minimize orthostatic hypotension; not to exercise in hot weather or increased hypotension can occur

• Teach patient to notify prescriber of mouth sores, sore throat, fever, swelling of hands or feet, irregular heartbeat, chest pain, coughing, shortness of breath

• Instruct patient to report excessive perspiration, dehydration, vomiting, diarrhea; may lead to fall in B/P

• Caution patient that product may cause dizziness, fainting, light-headedness; may occur during 1st few days of therapy; to avoid activities that may be hazardous

• Teach patient how to take B/P, and normal readings for age-group

• Advise patient to notify prescriber if pregnancy is planned or suspected

### Evaluation
**Positive therapeutic outcome**

• Decreased B/P in hypertension

**Treatment of overdose:** 0.9% NaCl **IV** inf, hemodialysis

---

## fosphenytoin (Rx)
(foss-fen′i-toy-in)
Cerebyx
*Func. class.:* Anticonvulsant
*Chem. class.:* Hydantoin
**Pregnancy category D**

**Action:** Inhibits spread of seizure activity in motor cortex by altering ion transport; increases AV conduction; prodrug of phenytoin

**Therapeutic outcome:** Decreased seizures, absence of dysrhythmias

**Uses:** Generalized tonic-clonic seizures, status epilepticus, partial seizures

**Dosage and routes**
All doses in PE (phenytoin sodium equivalent)

*Status epilepticus*
*Adult and child >1 mo:* **IV** 15-18 mg PE/kg
*Neonate:* **IV** 15-20 mg PE/kg

*Nonemergency/maintenance dosing*
*Adult and adolescent >16 yr:* **IM/IV** 10-20 mg PE/kg 10 mg dose; 4-6 mg PE/kg/day (maintenance); start maintenance 12 hr after loading dose; give in 2-3 divided doses

---

*Child 10-16 yr:* IM/**IV** 6-7 mg PE/kg/day
*Child 7-9 yr:* IM/**IV** 7-8 mg PE/kg/day
*Child 4-6 yr:* IM/**IV** 7.5-9 mg PE/kg/day
*Child 6 mo-3 yr:* IM/**IV** 8-10 mg PE/kg/day
*Infant:* IM/**IV** 5 mg PE/kg/day
*Neonate:* IM/**IV** 5-8 mg PE/kg/day

**Available forms:** Inj 150 mg (100 mg PE) 750 mg (500 mg PE), 50 mg/ml vials

### Adverse effects

*CNS:* Drowsiness, dizziness, insomnia, paresthesias, depression, suicidal tendencies, aggression, headache, confusion
*CV:* Hypotension, **ventricular fibrillation,** hypertension, **CHF, shock**
*EENT:* Nystagmus, diplopia, blurred vision
*GI:* Nausea, vomiting, diarrhea, constipation, anorexia, weight loss, **hepatitis,** jaundice, gingival hyperplasia
*HEMA:* **Agranulocytosis, leukopenia, aplastic anemia, thrombocytopenia, megaloblastic anemia**
*INTEG:* Rash, lupus erythematosus, **Stevens-Johnson syndrome,** hirsutism
*SYST:* Hyperglycemia, hypokalemia

**Contraindications:** Pregnancy **D,** hypersensitivity, psychiatric conditions, bradycardia, SA and AV block, Stokes-Adams syndrome

**Precautions:** Breastfeeding, allergies, renal/hepatic disease, myocardial insufficiency, hypoalbuminemia, hypothyroidism

#### Pharmacokinetics

| | |
|---|---|
| **Absorption** | Unknown |
| **Distribution** | Protein binding 99% |
| **Metabolism** | Liver |
| **Excretion** | Kidneys |
| **Half-life** | Unknown |

#### Pharmacodynamics
Unknown

### Interactions
*Individual drugs*
Alcohol: decreased effects of fosphenytoin (chronic use)
Amiodarone, carbamazepine, chloramphenicol, cimetidine, folic acid, reserpine, rifampin, theophylline, tramadol: decreased effects of fosphenytoin
*Drug classifications*
Antacids, antihistamines, antineoplastics, CYP1A2 inducers: decreased effects of fosphenytoin
Antidepressants (tricyclics), CYP1A2 inhibitors, estrogens, H$_2$-receptor antagonists,

phenothiazines, salicylates, sulfonamides: increased fosphenytoin level
*Drug/herb*
Ginseng, santonica, valerian: decreased anticonvulsant effect
Ginkgo: increased anticonvulsant effect
*Drug/lab test*
Increased: glucose, alkaline phosphatase
Decreased: dexamethasone, metyrapone test serum, urinary steroids

## NURSING CONSIDERATIONS
### Assessment
• Assess product level: toxic level 30-50 mcg/ml, wait at least 2 hr after dose before testing
• Assess seizure activity including type, location, duration, and character; provide seizure precaution
• Assess renal studies: urinalysis, BUN, urine creatinine
• Monitor hepatic studies: ALT, AST, bilirubin, creatinine
• Assess allergic reaction: red raised rash; if this occurs, product should be discontinued
• Monitor for toxicity: bone marrow depression, nausea, vomiting, ataxia, diplopia, cardiovascular collapse, slurred speech, confusion
• Assess product level: toxic level 30-50 mcg/ml
⚠ Assess for rash, discontinue as soon as rash develops, serious adverse reactions such as Stevens-Johnson syndrome can occur
• Assess mental status: mood, sensorium, affect, memory (long, short), especially geriatric
• Assess for blood dyscrasias: fever, sore throat, bruising, rash, jaundice, epistaxis (long-term treatment only)
• Monitor blood studies: RBC, Hct, Hgb, reticulocyte counts weekly for 4 wk then monthly; also check thyroid function tests, serum calcium, albumin, phosphorus

### Nursing diagnoses
• Injury, risk for (uses, adverse reactions)
• Knowledge, deficient (teaching)
• Noncompliance (teaching)

### Implementation
**IV route**
• Administer by direct **IV** after diluting with D$_5$ or 0.9% NaCl to 1.5-25 mg PE/ml
*Solution compatibilities:* D$_5$W, D$_{10}$W, amino acid inj 10%, D$_5$LR, D$_5$/0.9% NaCl, Plasmalyte A, LR, per sterile water for inj
*Additive compatibilities:* Potassium chloride

Adverse effects: *italic* = common, **bold** = life-threatening

## Patient/family education
- Teach patient the reason for and expected outcome of treatment
- Instruct patient not to use machinery or engage in hazardous activity; drowsiness, dizziness may occur
- Advise patient to carry/wear emergency ID identifying product used, name of prescriber
- Advise patient to notify prescriber of rash, bleeding, bruising, slurred speech, jaundice of skin or eyes, joint pain, nausea, vomiting, severe headache
- Advise patient to keep all medical appointments, including lab work, physical assessment
- Advise patient to notify prescriber if pregnancy is planned or suspected; to use contraception with this product

## Evaluation
**Positive therapeutic outcome**
- Decreased seizure activity

---

## frovatriptan (Rx)
(froh-vah-trip′tan)
Frova
*Func. class.:* Antimigraine agent
*Chem. class.:* 5-HT₁ receptor agonist

### Pregnancy category C

**Action:** Binds selectively to the vascular 5-HT$_{1B}$, 5-HT$_{1D}$ receptor subtypes, exerts antimigraine effect; binds to benzodiazepine receptor sites, causes vasoconstriction in cranium

**Therapeutic outcome:** Absence of migraines

**Uses:** Acute treatment of migraine with or without aura

### Dosage and routes
*Adult:* PO 2.5 mg, a 2nd dose may be taken after ≥2 hr; max 3 tabs/day (7.5 mg)

**Available forms:** Tabs 2.5 mg

### Adverse effects
***CNS:*** *Hot sensation,* paresthesia, *dizziness,* headache, fatigue, cold sensation
***CV:*** *Flushing,* chest pain, palpitation
***GI:*** Dry mouth, dyspepsia, abdominal pain, diarrhea, vomiting
***MS:*** Skeletal pain

**Contraindications:** Angina pectoris, history of MI, documented silent ischemia, Prinzmetal's angina, ischemic heart disease, concurrent ergotamine-containing preparations, uncontrolled hypertension, hypersensitivity, basilar or hemiplegic migraine; ischemic bowel disease; peripheral vascular disease, severe hepatic disease, prophylactic migraine treatment

**Precautions:** Pregnancy **C,** breastfeeding, children, geriatric, postmenopausal women, men >40 yr, risk factors for CAD, hypercholesterolemia, obesity, diabetes, impaired hepatic function, seizure disorder

### Pharmacokinetics
| | |
|---|---|
| **Absorption** | Absolute bioavailability of PO dose ~20% in males, 30% in females |
| **Distribution** | Protein binding 15%; reversibly bound to blood cells at equilibrium 60% |
| **Metabolism** | Liver |
| **Excretion** | Urine (32%), feces (62%) |
| **Half-life** | 25-29 hr |

### Pharmacodynamics
| | |
|---|---|
| **Onset** | 10 min-2 hr |
| **Peak** | 2-4 hr |
| **Duration** | Unknown |

### Interactions
*Individual drugs*
Estrogen, propranolol: increased effects of frovatriptan
*Drug classifications*
CYP1A2 inhibitors (cimetidine, ciprofloxacin, erythromycin), oral contraceptives: increased frovatriptan levels
Selective serotonin reuptake inhibitors, other serotonin agonists (dextromethorphan, tramadol, antidepressants): increased toxicity
*Drug/herb*
Butterbur: increased effect

### NURSING CONSIDERATIONS
**Assessment**
- Assess B/P; signs/symptoms of coronary vasospasms
- Assess for stress level, activity, recreation, coping mechanisms
- Assess neurologic status: LOC, paresthesia, hot/cold sensations, dizziness, headache, fatigue
- Assess for ingestion of tyramine-containing foods (pickled products, beer, wine, aged cheese), food additives, preservatives, colorings, artificial sweeteners, chocolate, caffeine, which may precipitate these types of headaches

### Nursing diagnoses
- Knowledge, deficient (teaching)
- Pain, acute (uses)

### Implementation
- Ensure that tablets are swallowed whole
- Provide quiet, calm environment with decreased stimulation from noise, bright light, excessive talking

### Patient/family education
- Instruct patient to report any side effects to prescriber
- Advise patient to use contraception while taking product
- Advise patient that photosensitivity may occur, to use sunscreen and wear protective clothing when outdoors
- Advise patient to have dark, quiet environment available

### Evaluation
**Positive therapeutic outcome**
- Decrease in frequency, severity of migraine

**Treatment of overdose:** No specific antidote; monitor patient closely for ≥48 hr, treat any symptoms as necessary

---

## fulvestrant (Rx)
(full-ves′trant)
Faslodex
*Func. class.:* Antineoplastic

**Pregnancy category** D

**Action:** Inhibits cell division by binding to cytoplasmic estrogen receptors; resembles normal cell complex but inhibits DNA synthesis and estrogen response of target tissue

**Therapeutic outcome:** Decreased tumor size, spread of malignancy

**Uses:** Advanced breast carcinoma in estrogen-receptor–positive patients (usually postmenopausal)

### Dosage and routes
*Adult:* IM 250 mg qmo

**Available forms:** Inj 50 mg/ml

### Adverse effects
*CNS: Headache,* depression, dizziness, insomnia, paresthesia, anxiety
*GI: Nausea, vomiting,* anorexia, constipation, diarrhea, abdominal pain
*INTEG: Rash,* sweating, hot flashes, inj site pain
*MS:* Bone pain, arthritis, back pain
*RESP:* Pharyngitis, dyspnea, cough

**Contraindications:** Pregnancy **D**, breastfeeding, children, hypersensitivity
**Precautions:** Hepatic disease

### Pharmacokinetics

| | |
|---|---|
| **Absorption** | Unknown |
| **Distribution** | Unknown |
| **Metabolism** | CYP3A4 |
| **Excretion** | Feces 90% |
| **Half-life** | 40 days |

### Pharmacodynamics
Unknown

F

### NURSING CONSIDERATIONS
### Assessment
- Monitor for side effects, report to prescriber

### Nursing diagnoses
- Infection, risk for (adverse reactions)
- Knowledge, deficient (teaching)
- Nutrition: less than body requirements, imbalanced (adverse reactions)

### Implementation
- Give IM 5 ml as a single inj or 2, 2.5 ml inj; give slowly in buttock
- Give antacid before oral agent; give product after evening meal, before bedtime
- Give antiemetic 30-60 min before giving product to prevent vomiting
- Provide liquid diet, if needed, including cola, Jell-O; dry toast or crackers may be added if patient is not nauseated or vomiting
- Provide nutritious diet with iron, vitamin supplements as ordered
- Increase fluids to 2 L/day unless contraindicated
- Store in refrigerator

### Patient/family education
- Advise patient to report any complaints, side effects to prescriber
- Teach patient to increase fluids to 2 L/day unless contraindicated
- Advise patient to report vaginal bleeding immediately
- Teach patient that tumor flare—increase in size of tumor, increased bone pain—may occur and will subside rapidly; may take analgesics for pain
- Teach that premenopausal women must use mechanical birth control because ovulation may be induced

### Evaluation
**Positive therapeutic outcome**
- Decreased tumor size, spread of malignancy

---

Adverse effects: *italic* = common, **bold** = life-threatening

## furosemide  (Rx)
(fur-oh'se-mide)

Apo-Furosemide ✽, Furoside ✽, Lasix, Lasix Special ✽, Myrosemide, Novosemide ✽, Uritol ✽

*Func. class.:* Loop diuretic
*Chem. class.:* Sulfonamide derivative

**Pregnancy category C**

**Do not confuse:**
furosemide/torsemide, Lasix/Lanoxin/Lomotil/Luvox

**Action:** Acts on the ascending loop of Henle in the kidney, inhibiting reabsorption of electrolytes sodium and chloride, causing excretion of sodium, calcium, magnesium, chloride, water, and some potassium; decreases reabsorption of sodium and chloride and increases excretion of potassium in the distal tubule of the kidney; responsible for slight antihypertensive effect and peripheral vasodilatation

**Therapeutic outcome:** Decreased edema in lung tissue, peripherally; decreased B/P

**Uses:** Edema in CHF, nephrotic syndrome, ascites, caused by hepatic disease, hepatic cirrhosis

**Unlabeled uses:** Hypercalcemia in malignancy

**Dosage and routes**
*Adult:* PO 20-80 mg/day in AM, may give another dose in 6 hr, up to 600 mg/day; IM/**IV** 20-40 mg, increased by 20 mg q2hr until desired response
*Child:* PO/IM/**IV** 2 mg/kg, may increase by 1-2 mg/kg/q6-8hr up to 6 mg/kg

*Acute pulmonary edema*
*Adult:* **IV** 40 mg given over several min, repeated in 1 hr; increase to 80 mg if needed

*Hypertensive crisis/acute renal failure*
*Adult:* **IV** 100-200 mg over 1-2 min

*Antihypercalcemia*
*Adult:* IM/**IV** 80-100 mg q1-4hr or PO 120 mg/day or divided bid
*Child:* IM/**IV** 25-50 mg, repeat q4hr if needed

**Available forms:** Tabs 20, 40, 80 mg; oral sol 8 mg/ml, 10 mg/ml; inj IM, **IV** 10 mg/ml

**Adverse effects**
*CNS:* Headache, fatigue, weakness, vertigo, paresthesias
*CV:* Orthostatic hypotension, chest pain, ECG changes, **circulatory collapse**
*EENT:* Loss of hearing, ear pain, tinnitus, blurred vision
*ELECT: Hypokalemia, hypochloremic alkalosis, hypomagnesemia, hyperuricemia, hypocalcemia, hyponatremia,* metabolic alkalosis
*ENDO: Hyperglycemia*
*GI: Nausea,* diarrhea, dry mouth, vomiting, anorexia, cramps, oral or gastric irritations, pancreatitis
*GU: Polyuria,* **renal failure,** *glycosuria*
*HEMA: Thrombocytopenia,* **agranulocytosis, leukopenia, neutropenia, anemia**
*INTEG: Rash, pruritus, purpura,* **Stevens-Johnson syndrome,** sweating, photosensitivity, urticaria
*MS:* Cramps, stiffness

**Contraindications:** Hypersensitivity to sulfonamides; anuria, hypovolemia, breast-feeding, infants, electrolyte depletion

**Precautions:** Pregnancy **C**, diabetes mellitus, dehydration, severe renal disease, cirrhosis, ascites

| Pharmacokinetics | | | |
|---|---|---|---|
| | PO | | |
| **Absorption** | GI tract (60%-70%) | | |
| | PO/IM/IV | | |
| **Distribution** | Crosses placenta | | |
| **Metabolism** | Liver (30%-40%) | | |
| **Excretion** | Breast milk, urine, feces | | |
| **Half-life** | ½-1 hr | | |

| Pharmacodynamics | | | |
|---|---|---|---|
| | PO | IM | IV |
| **Onset** | 1 hr | ½ hr | 5 min |
| **Peak** | 1-2 hr | Unknown | ½ hr |
| **Duration** | 6-8 hr | 4-8 hr | 2 hr |

**Interactions**
*Individual drugs*
Cisplatin, vancomycin: increased risk of ototoxicity
Digoxin: increased toxicity
Lithium: decreased renal clearance, causing increased toxicity
*Drug classifications*
Aminoglycosides: increased ototoxicity
Antihypertensives: increased antihypertensive effect
Nitrates: increased hypotensive action
Nondepolarizing skeletal muscle relaxants: increased toxicity

### Drug/herb
Aloe, cucumber, dandelion, horsetail, khella, pumpkin, Queen Anne's lace: increased diuretic effect
St. John's wort: severe photosensitivity

### Drug/lab test
Interference: GTT

## NURSING CONSIDERATIONS
### Assessment
• Assess patient for tinnitus, hearing loss, ear pain; periodic testing of hearing is needed when high doses of this product are given by **IV** route
• Monitor for renal, cardiac, neurologic, GI, pulmonary manifestations of hypokalemia: acidic urine, reduced urine osmolality, nocturia, polyuria and polydipsia; hypotension, broad T-wave, U-wave, ectopy, tachycardia, weak pulse; muscle weakness, altered LOC, drowsiness, apathy, lethargy, confusion, depression; anorexia, nausea, cramps, constipation, distention, paralytic ileus; hypoventilation, respiratory muscle weakness
• Monitor for CNS, GI, cardiovascular, integumentary, neurologic manifestations of hypocalcemia: personality changes, anxiety, disturbances, depression and psychosis; nausea, vomiting, constipation, abdominal pain from muscle spasm; decreased contractility, decreased cardiac output, hypotension, lengthened ST segment, prolonged QT interval; scaling eczema, alopecia, hyperpigmentation; tetany, muscle twitching, cramping, grimacing, seizure, altered deep tendon reflexes, spasm
• Monitor for CNS, neuromuscular, GI, cardiac manifestations of hypomagnesemia, agitation; muscle twitching, paresthesias, hyperactive reflexes, positive Babinski reflex, dysphagia, nystagmus, seizures, tetany; nausea, vomiting, diarrhea, anorexia, abdominal distention; ectopy, tachycardia, broad, flat or inverted T-waves, depressed ST segment, prolonged QT, decreased cardiac output, hypotension
• Monitor for CV, GI, neurologic manifestations of hyponatremia: increased B/P, cold, clammy skin, hypovolemia or hypervolemia; anorexia, nausea, vomiting, diarrhea, abdominal cramps; lethargy, increased ICP, confusion, headache, seizures, coma, fatigue, tremors, hyperreflexia
• Monitor for neurologic, respiratory manifestations of hyperchloremia: weakness, lethargy, coma; deep rapid breathing
• Assess fluid volume status: I&O ratios and record, count or weigh diapers as appropriate, weight, distended red veins, crackles in lung, color, quality and specific gravity of urine, skin turgor, adequacy of pulses, moist mucous membranes, bilateral lung sounds, peripheral pitting edema; dehydration symptoms of decreasing output, thirst, hypotension, dry mouth and mucous membranes should be reported
• Monitor electrolytes: potassium, sodium, calcium, magnesium; also include BUN, blood pH, ABGs, uric acid, CBC, blood glucose
• Assess B/P before and during therapy lying, standing, and sitting as appropriate; orthostatic hypotension can occur rapidly

### Nursing diagnoses
• Fluid volume, deficient (side effects)
• Fluid volume, excess (uses)
• Knowledge, deficient (teaching)

### Implementation
• Give in AM to avoid interference with sleep
• Potassium replacement if potassium level is <3.0 mg/dl, or use oral sol slightly, product may be crushed if patient is unable to swallow

**PO route**
• With food or milk if nausea occurs, absorption may be reduced

**IV route**
• Do not use sol that is yellow, has a precipitate, or crystals

**IV, direct route**
• Give undiluted through Y-tube on 3-way stopcock; give 20 mg or less/min

**Intermittent IV infusion route**
• May be added to 0.9% NaCl, $D_5W$, $D_{10}W$, $D_{20}W$; invert sugar 10% in electrolyte #1, LR, use within 24 hr to ensure compatibility; give through Y-tube or 3-way stopcock; give at 4 mg/min or less, use infusion pump

**Syringe compatibilities:** Bleomycin, cisplatin, cyclophosphamide, fluorouracil, heparin, leucovorin, methotrexate, mitomycin

**Syringe incompatibilities:** Doxapram, DOXOrubicin, droperidol, metaclopramide, milrinone

**Y-site compatibilities:** Allopurinol, amifostine, amikacin, aztreonam, bleomycin, cefepime, cefmetazole, cisplatin, cladribine, cyclophosphamide, cytarabine, dexamethasone, epINEPHrine, fentanyl, fludarabine, fluorouracil, foscarnet, gallium, granisetron, heparin, hydrocortisone, hydromorphone, indomethacin, kanamycin, leucovorin, lorazepam, melphalan, meropenem, methotrexate, mitomycin, morphine, nitroglycerin, norepinephrine, paclitaxel, piperacillin/tazobactam, potassium chloride, propofol, ranitidine, sargramostim, tacrolimus, teniposide, thio-

---

Adverse effects: *italic* = common, **bold** = life-threatening

tepa, tobramycin, tolazoline, vit B complex with C

*Y-site incompatibilities:* Amsacrine, bleomycin, DOXOrubicin, droperidol, esmolol, fluconazole, gentamicin, idarubicin, metoclopramide, milrinone, netilmicin, ondansetron, quinidine, vinBLAStine, vinCRIStine

*Additive compatibilities:* Amikacin, aminophylline, ampicillin, atropine, bumetanide, calcium gluconate, cefamandole, cefoperazone, cefuroxime, cimetidine, cloxacillin, dexamethasone, diamorphine, digoxin, epINEPHrine, heparin, isosorbide, kanamycin, lidocaine, meropenem, morphine, nitroglycerin, penicillin G, potassium chloride, ranitidine, scopolamine, sodium bicarbonate, theophylline, tobramycin, verapamil

*Additive incompatibilities:* Bleomycin, DOBUTamine, gentamicin, chlorproMAZINE, diazepam, erythromycin, isoproterenol, meperidine, metoclopramide, netilmicin, opium alkaloids, prochlorperazine, tetracycline

## Patient/family education

• Teach patient to take the medication early in the day to prevent nocturia
• Instruct the patient to take with food or milk if GI symptoms of nausea and anorexia occur
• Teach patient to maintain a record of weight on a weekly basis and notify physician of weight loss of >5 lb
• Caution the patient that this product causes a loss of potassium, that food rich in potassium should be added to the diet; refer to a dietitian for assistance in planning
• Caution the patient to rise slowly from sitting or reclining positions, not to exercise in hot weather or stand for prolonged periods of time because orthostatic hypotension will be enhanced; lie down if dizziness occurs
• Advise patient to wear protective clothing and sunscreen to prevent photosensitivity
• Teach patient not to use alcohol or any OTC medications without physician's approval, serious product reactions may occur
• Emphasize the need to contact physician immediately if muscle cramps, weakness, nausea, dizziness, or numbness occurs
• Teach patient to take and record own B/P and pulse
• Teach patient to continue taking medication even if feeling better, this product controls symptoms but does not cure the condition
• Advise the patient with hypertension to continue other medical treatment (exercise, weight loss, relaxation techniques, cessation of smoking)

## Evaluation

**Positive therapeutic outcome**

• Decreased edema
• Decreased B/P
• Lowered calcium level in malignancy
• Increased diuresis

## gabapentin (Rx)

(gab'a-pen-tin)

Neurontin

*Func. class.:* Anticonvulsant

**Pregnancy category** C

**Do not confuse:**

Neurontin/Noroxin/Neoral

**Action:** Mechanism unknown; may increase seizure threshold; structurally similar to GABA; gabapentin binding sites in neocortex, hippocampus

**Therapeutic outcome:** Decreased seizure activity

**Uses:** Adjunct treatment of partial seizures, with or without generalization in patients >12 yr; adjunct in partial seizures in children 3-12 yr, postherpetic neuralgia

**Unlabeled uses:** Tremors in multiple sclerosis, neuropathic pain, bipolar disorder, migraine prophylaxis, diabetic neuropathy

## Dosage and routes

*Adult and child >12 yr:* PO 900-1800 mg/day in 3 divided doses; may titrate by giving 300 mg on the first day, 300 mg bid on second day, 300 mg tid on third day; may increase to 1800 mg/day by adding 300 mg on subsequent days

*Child 5-12 yr:* PO 10-15 mg/kg/day in 3 divided doses, initially titrate dose upward over approximately 3 days; 25-35 mg/kg/day; all given in 3 divided doses

*Child 3-4 yr:* PO 10-15 mg/kg/day in 3 divided doses, initially titrate dose upward over approximately 3 days, 40 mg/kg/day; all given in 3 divided doses

*Postherpetic neuralgia*

*Adult:* PO 300 mg on day 1, 600 mg/day divided bid on day 2, 900 mg/day divided tid, may titrate to 1800 mg divided tid if needed

*Renal dose*

*Adult and child >12 yr:* CCr 30-60 ml/min 300 mg bid; CCr 15-30 ml/min 300 mg/day; CCr <15 ml/min 125 mg/day

---

◆ Alert    ♣ Canada Only    🐟 Drug on CD         * "Tall Man" lettering (See Preface)

**Available forms:** Caps 100, 300, 400 mg; tabs 600, 800 mg; oral sol 250 mg/5 ml

**Adverse effects**
*CNS: Drowsiness, confusion,* dizziness, fatigue, anxiety, somnolence, ataxia, amnesia, abnormal thinking, unsteady gait, depression; 3-12 yr old, emotional lability, aggression, thought disorder, hyperkinesia, hostility, **seizures**
*CV:* Vasodilatation, peripheral edema, hypotension
*EENT:* Dry mouth, blurred vision, diplopia, nystagmus
*GI:* Constipation, increased appetite, dental abnormalities, nausea, vomiting
*GU:* Impotence, bleeding, *UTI*
*HEMA:* **Leukopenia,** decreased WBC
*INTEG:* Pruritus, abrasion, **Stevens-Johnson syndrome**
*MS:* Myalgia
*RESP:* Rhinitis, pharyngitis, coughing

**Contraindications:** Hypersensitivity to this product

**Precautions:** Pregnancy **C,** breastfeeding, children <12 yr, geriatric, renal disease, hemodialysis

**Pharmacokinetics**

| | |
|---|---|
| **Absorption** | Unknown |
| **Distribution** | Unknown |
| **Metabolism** | None |
| **Excretion** | Urine unchanged |
| **Half-life** | 5-7 hr, 130 hr in ESRD |

**Pharmacodynamics**
Unknown

**Interactions**
*Individual drugs*
Alcohol: increased CNS depression
Sevelamer: decreased gabapentin levels
*Drug classifications*
Antacids: decreased gabapentin levels
Antihistamines, all other CNS depressants: increased CNS depression
*Drug/herb*
Chamomille, hops, kava, skullcap, valerian: increased CNS depression
*Drug/lab test*
False positive: urinary protein using Ames N-multistix SG

**NURSING CONSIDERATIONS**
**Assessment**
• Assess seizures: aura, location, duration, activity at onset
• Assess renal studies: urinalysis, BUN, urine creatinine q3 mo
• Assess mental status: mood, sensorium, affect, behavioral changes; if mental status changes, notify prescriber
• Assess eye problems, need for ophth exam before, during, after treatment (slit lamp, fundoscopy, tonometry)

**Nursing diagnoses**
• Knowledge, deficient (teaching)
• Noncompliance (teaching)

**Implementation**
• Do not break, crush, or chew caps
• Give at least 2 hr after meals with antacids, give without regard to meals
• Store at room temperature away from heat and light
• Provide assistance with ambulation during early part of treatment; dizziness occurs
• Provide seizure precautions: padded side rails; move objects that may harm patient

**Patient/family education**
• Advise patient to carry/wear emergency ID stating patient's name, products taken, condition, prescriber's name and phone number
• Teach patient to avoid driving, other activities that require alertness
• Teach patient not to discontinue medication quickly after long-term use, withdrawal-precipitated seizures may occur, not to double dose; if dose is missed, take if 2 hr or more before next dose
• Teach patient to gradually withdraw over 7 days; abrupt withdrawal may precipitate seizures
• Teach patient to use hard candy, gum, and frequent rinsing of mouth for dry mouth
• Teach patient to increase fluids, bulk in diet for constipation
• Advise patient to notify prescriber if pregnancy is planned or suspected, avoid breast feeding

**Evaluation**
**Positive therapeutic outcome**
• Decreased seizure activity; document on patient's chart

**Treatment of overdose:** Lavage, VS

Adverse effects: *italic* = common, **bold** = life-threatening

## galantamine (Rx)

(gah-lan'tah-meen)

Razadyne, Razadyne ER

*Func. class.:* Anti-Alzheimer's agent, cholinesterase inhibitor

**Pregnancy category** B

**Action:** Enhances cholinergic functioning by increasing acetylcholine

**Therapeutic outcome:** Decreased signs and symptoms of Alzheimer's dementia

**Uses:** Mild to moderate dementia of Alzheimer's disease, vascular dementia

### Dosage and routes

*Adult:* PO 4 mg bid with morning and evening meals; after 4 wk or more may increase to 8 mg bid; after another 4 wk may increase to 12 mg bid; usual dose 16-24 mg/day in 2 divided doses; EXT REL 8 mg/day in AM; may increase to 16 mg/day after 4 wk, and 24 mg/day after another 4 wk

### Hepatic dose

*Adult, Child-Pugh 7-9:* PO Max 16 mg/day

*Adult, Child-Pugh 10-15:* PO Avoid use

### Renal dose/moderate renal impairment: Max 16 mg/day

*CCr <9 ml/min:* PO Avoid use

**Available forms:** Tabs 4, 8, 12 mg; ext rel tabs 8, 16, 24 mg; oral sol 4 mg/ml

### Adverse effects

*CNS: Tremors, insomnia,* depression, dizziness, headache, somnolence, fatigue

*CV:* Bradycardia, chest pain

*GI: Nausea, vomiting, anorexia, abdominal distress, flatulence,* diarrhea

*GU:* Urinary incontinence, bladder outflow obstruction, hematuria

*HEMA:* Anemia

*META:* Weight decrease

*MS:* Asthenia

*RESP:* URI, rhinitis

**Contraindications:** Hypersensitivity to this product

**Precautions:** Pregnancy B, breastfeeding, children, renal/hepatic disease, respiratory disease, seizure disorder, peptic ulcer, asthma, bradycardia, heart block

### Pharmacokinetics

| | |
|---|---|
| **Absorption** | Rapidly and completely absorbed |
| **Distribution** | Unknown |
| **Metabolism** | P450 enzyme |
| **Excretion** | Kidneys; clearance decreased in geriatric, hepatic disease, females (20% lower) |
| **Half-life** | Elimination 7 hr |

### Pharmacodynamics
Unknown

### Interactions

*Individual drugs*

Amitriptyline, cimetidine, erythromycin, fluvoxamine, ketoconazole, paroxetine, quinidine: increased galantamine bioavailability

*Drug classifications*

Cholinesterase inhibitors, cholinomimetics: synergistic effect

*Drug/herb*

Jimsonweed, scopola: cholinergic antagonism

Pill-bearing spurge: increased effect

### NURSING CONSIDERATIONS

#### Assessment

- Assess liver function enzymes: AST, ALT, alkaline phosphatase, LDH, bilirubin, CBC
- Assess for severe GI effects: nausea, vomiting, anorexia, weight loss
- Assess B/P, heart rate, respiration during initial treatment
- Assess mental status: affect, mood, behavioral changes, depression

#### Nursing diagnoses

- Knowledge, deficient (teaching)
- Thought processes, disturbed

#### Implementation

- Give with meals, morning and evening
- Dose increase after minimum of 4 wk at prior dose; if dose is interrupted for several days, restart at lower dose, titrate to current dose
- Provide assistance with ambulation during beginning therapy
- Perform complete suicide assessment

#### Patient/family education

- Teach patient or caregiver correct procedure for giving oral solution, using instruction sheet provided
- Instruct patient or caregiver to notify prescriber of severe GI effects
- Instruct patient or caregiver to report hypo/hypertension, slow heart rate

## Evaluation
### Positive therapeutic outcome
- Decreased symptoms of dementia
- Increased coherence
- Improved cognitive performance (memory, orientation, attention, reasoning, language, praxis)

**Treatment of overdose:** Administer **IV** atropine titrated to effect at an initial dose of 0.5-1 mg, with subsequent doses based on clinical response; provide general supportive measures

---

# gallium (Rx)
(gal'ee-yum)
Ganite
*Func. class.:* Electrolyte modifier
*Chem. class.:* Hypocalcemic product

**Pregnancy category C**

**Action:** Lowers serum calcium levels by inhibiting calcium resorption from bone

**Therapeutic outcome:** Decrease calcium level to 5-9 mg/dl

**Uses:** Cancer-related hypercalcemia

### Dosage and routes
*Adult:* **IV** 100-200 mg/m²/day × 5 days; INF over 24 hr, rest period of 2-4 wk between courses, discontinue earlier if serum calcium is in normal range

**Available forms:** Inj 25 mg/ml

### Adverse effects
*CNS:* Confusion, hallucination, vivid dreams, encephalopathy, lethargy
*CV:* Tachycardia, hypotension
*EENT:* Blurred vision, optic neuritis, hearing loss
*GI:* Nausea, vomiting, diarrhea, constipation, mucositis, metallic taste
*GU:* **Nephrotoxicity,** increased BUN, creatinine
*HEMA:* **Anemia, leukopenia, thrombocytopenia**
*META:* *Hypophosphatemia,* hypocalcemia, decreased serum bicarbonate, hypomagnesemia
*RESP:* Dyspnea, **pleural effusion**

**Contraindications:** Hypersensitivity, hypocalcemia, renal failure, severe renal disease (specific gravity >2.5 mg/dl)

**Precautions:** Pregnancy **C,** breastfeeding, children, mild renal disease, dehydration

### Pharmacokinetics
| | |
|---|---|
| **Absorption** | Completely absorbed |
| **Distribution** | Unknown |
| **Metabolism** | Unknown |
| **Excretion** | Kidneys (unchanged) |
| **Half-life** | Unknown |

### Pharmacodynamics
| | |
|---|---|
| **Onset** | 12-48 hr |
| **Peak** | Unknown |
| **Duration** | 4-14 days |

### Interactions
*Individual drugs*
Amphotericin B, cisplatin, foscarnet, ganciclovir, vancomycin: increased nephrotoxicity
*Drug classifications*
Aminoglycosides, toxoids, vaccines: increased nephrotoxicity

### NURSING CONSIDERATIONS
#### Assessment
- Renal status: BUN, creatinine, urine output; if creatinine level is 2.5 mg/dl or more, product should be discontinued
- Monitor calcium, phosphate, bicarbonate; all levels may be decreased and supplements of phosphate may be needed; calcium daily, phosphate 2-3 ×/wk
- Assess for hypercalcemia: nausea, vomiting, fatigue, weakness, thirst, dehydration, dysrhythmias, headache, confusion, coma, decreased reflexes
- For hypocalcemia: dysrhythmias, hypotension, paresthesia; twitching, colic, laryngospasm; hypercalcemia: poor coordination, myalgia, hypotonia, shortened ST segment and QT interval, prolonged PR interval, cone-shaped T wave, sinus bradycardia; Trousseau's, Chvostek's sign: tremors, tetany, cramping, grimacing, seizures, altered deep tendon reflexes and spasms, personality changes including irritability, depression, psychosis
- Monitor for indications of hypophosphatemia: weakness, malaise, tremors, memory loss, inattention, confusion, decreased reflexes, aching bone pain, joint stiffness, rapid, shallow respiration, decreased tidal volume, nausea, vomiting, anorexia, portal hypertension

#### Nursing diagnoses
- Injury, risk for (uses)
- Knowledge, deficient (teaching)

#### Implementation
- Provide adequate hydration with **IV** saline, 2 L/day during treatment; saline increases the extracellular calcium

---

Adverse effects: *italic* = common, **bold** = life-threatening

- Give by cont **IV** inf after dilution of dose/1 L of 0.9% NaCl or D$_5$W, run over 24 hr, use infusion pump
- Store solution for 48 hr at room temperature or 1 wk in refrigerator

**Y-site compatibilities:** Acyclovir, allopurinol, aminophylline, ampicillin/sulbactam, amifostine, aztreonam, cefazolin, ceftazidime, ceftriaxone, cimetidine, ciprofloxacin, cladribine, cyclophosphamide, dexamethasone, diphenhydrAMINE, filgrastim, fluconazole, furosemide, granisetron, heparin, hydrocortisone, fosfamide, magnesium sulfate, mannitol, melphalan, meperidine, mesna, methotrexate, metoclopramide, ondansetron, piperacillin, piperacillin/tazobactam, potassium chloride, ranitidine, sodium bicarbonate, teniposide, thiotepa, ticarcillin/clavulanate, trimethoprim, sulfamethoxazole, vancomycin, vinorelbine

### Patient/family education

- Instruct patient to follow dietary guidelines given by prescriber, including avoiding calcium (dietary products, broccoli) and vit D (fortified milk, grain products, fish oil)
- Explain purpose of product and expected results

### Evaluation

**Positive therapeutic outcome**

- Decreased serum calcium levels to 5-9 mg/dl

---

### ganciclovir (Rx)

(gan-sye′kloe-vir)

Cytovene, Vitrasert

*Func. class.:* Antiviral

*Chem. class.:* Synthetic nucleoside analog

**Pregnancy category** C

**Do not confuse:**

Cytovene /Cytosar

**Action:** Inhibits replication of herpes viruses in vitro, competitively inhibits human cytomegalovirus (CMV) DNA polymerase and is incorporated, resulting in termination of DNA elongation

**Therapeutic outcome:** Decreased proliferation of virus responsible for CMV retinitis

**Uses:** CMV retinitis in immunocompromised persons, including those with AIDS, after indirect ophthalmoscopy confirms diagnosis, prophylaxis of CMV in transplantation

**Unlabeled uses:** CMV pneumonia in organ transplant patients, CMV gastroenteritis in patients with irritable bowel syndrome, CMV pneumonitis

### Dosage and routes

*Induction treatment*

*Adult:* **IV** 5 mg/kg/dose given over 1 hr q12hr × 2-3 wk

*Maintenance treatment*

*Adult:* **IV** INF 5 mg/kg/day given over 1 hr, daily × 7 days/wk; or 6 mg/kg/day × 5 days/wk; PO 1000 mg tid with food or 500 mg q3hr while awake; INTRAVITREAL 4.5-mg implant for 6 doses

*Prevention of CMV infection*

*Adult:* **IV** 5 mg/kg/dose over 1 hr q12hr × 1-2 wk, then 5 mg/kg/day × 7 days/wk then 6 mg/kg/day × 5 days/wk; PO 1000 mg tid

*Renal dose*

CCr <70 ml/min reduce dose

**Available forms:** Powder for inj 500 mg/vial, caps 250, 500 mg; implant, intravitreal 4.5 mg

### Adverse effects

***CNS:*** *Fever,* chills, **coma,** *confusion,* abnormal thoughts, dizziness, bizarre dreams, *headache,* psychosis, tremors, somnolence, *paresthesia, weakness,* **seizures,** peripheral neuropathy

***CV:*** Dysrhythmia, hypo/hypertension

***EENT:*** Retinal detachment in CMV retinitis, cataracts

***GI:*** *Abnormal liver function tests, nausea, vomiting, anorexia, diarrhea, abdominal pain,* **hemorrhage, perforation, pancreatitis**

***GU:*** *Hematuria, increased creatinine,* BUN

***HEMA:*** **Granulocytopenia, thrombocytopenia, irreversible neutropenia, anemia, eosinophilia, pancytopenia**

***INTEG:*** *Rash,* alopecia, *pruritus,* urticaria, pain at inj site, phlebitis, **Stevens-Johnson syndrome**

***RESP:*** Dyspnea

**Contraindications:** Hypersensitivity to acyclovir, famciclovir, penciclovir, valacyclovir, valganciclovir, or ganciclovir; ANC <500/mm$^3$, platelet count <25,000/mm$^3$

**Precautions:** Pregnancy **C,** breastfeeding, children <6 mo, geriatric, preexisting cytopenias, renal function impairment, radiation therapy, secondary malignancy, bone marrow suppression

---

## Pharmacokinetics

| | |
|---|---|
| **Absorption** | Completely absorbed |
| **Distribution** | Crosses blood-brain barrier, CSF |
| **Metabolism** | Not metabolized |
| **Excretion** | Kidneys (90%) unchanged, breast milk |
| **Half-life** | 3 hr |

## Pharmacodynamics

Unknown

## Interactions
### Individual drugs
Amphotericin B, adriamycin, cycloSPORINE, dapsone, DOXOrubicin, flucytosine, pentamidine, probenecid, trimethoprim/sulfa combinations, vinBLAStine, vinCRIStine: increased ganciclovir toxicity

Didanosine: decreased effect

Imipenem with cilastatin: increased chance of seizures

Probenecid: decreased renal clearance of ganciclovir

Radiation, zidovudine: severe granulocytopenia; do not give together

### Drug classifications
Antineoplastics: severe granulocytopenia; do not give together

Nucleoside analogs: increased toxicity

## NURSING CONSIDERATIONS
### Assessment
• Culture should be done before treatment with ganciclovir is initiated; cultures of blood, urine, and throat may all be taken; CMV is not confirmed by this method; the diagnosis is made by an ophthalmic exam

• Assess kidney, liver function; increases in hemopoietic studies: BUN, serum creatinine, AST creatinine clearance, ALT, A-G ratio, baseline, and drip treatment; blood counts should be done q2 wk; watch for decreasing granulocytes, Hgb; if low, therapy may have to be discontinued and restarted after hematologic recovery; blood transfusions may be required

• Assess for GI symptoms: severe nausea, vomiting, diarrhea; severe symptoms may necessitate discontinuing product

• Monitor electrolytes and minerals: calcium, phosphorus, magnesium, sodium, potassium; watch closely for tetany during 1st administration

• Assess for symptoms of blood dyscrasias (anemia, granulocytopenia); bruising, fatigue, bleeding, poor healing

• Assess for symptoms of allergic reactions: flushing, rash, urticaria, pruritus

• Monitor for leukopenia/neutropenia/thrombocytopenia: WBCs, platelets q2 days during 2 ×/day dosing and q1 wk thereafter; check for leukopenia with daily WBC count in patients with prior leukopenia with other nucleoside analogs or for whom leukopenia counts are <1000 cells/mm$^3$ at start of treatment

• Monitor serum creatinine or creatinine clearance at least q2 wk

• Assess for seizures, dysrhythmias

### Nursing diagnoses
• Infection, risk for (uses)
• Injury, risk for (uses, adverse reactions)
• Knowledge, deficient (teaching)

### Implementation
#### PO route
• Give with food
#### IV route
• Medicine should be mixed under strict aseptic conditions using gloves, gown, and mask, and using precautions for antineoplastics

#### Intermittent IV infusion route
• Administer **IV** after diluting 500 mg/10 ml of sterile water for inj (50 mg/ml); shake; further dilute in 100 ml of $D_5W$, 0.9% NaCl, LR, Ringer's and run over 1 hr; use infusion pump, in-line filter

• Give slowly; do not give by BOL **IV**, IM, SUBCUT inj

• Use reconstituted sol within 12 hr, do not refrigerate or freeze; infusion solution is stable for 14 days when refrigerated; do not use sol with particulate matter or discoloration, fludarabine, sargramostim

*Y-site compatibilities:* Allopurinol, cisplatin, cyclophosphamide, enalaprilat, etoposide, filgrastim, fluconazole, gatifloxacin, granisetron, linezolid, melphalan, methotrexate, paclitaxel, propofol, tacrolimus, teniposide, thiotepa

*Y-site incompatibilities:* Amsacrine, fludarabine, foscarnet, ondansetron, sargramostim, vinorelbine

### Patient/family education
• Advise patient to notify prescriber if sore throat, swollen lymph nodes, malaise, fever occur; may indicate other infections

• Advise patient to report perioral tingling, numbness in extremities, and paresthesias

• Caution patient that serious product interactions may occur if OTC products are ingested; check first with prescriber

G

---

Adverse effects: *italic* = common, **bold** = life-threatening

- Inform patient that product is not a cure, but will control symptoms
- Advise patient that regular blood tests, ophth exams must be continued
- Inform patient that major toxicities may necessitate discontinuing product
- Instruct patient to use contraception during treatment and that infertility may occur; men should use barrier contraception for 90 days after treatment
- Teach patient to take PO with food
- Teach patient to report infection: fever, chills, sore throat; blood dyscrasias: bruising, bleeding, petechiae
- Tell patient to avoid crowds, persons with respiratory infection
- Advise patient to use sunscreen to prevent burns

### Evaluation
**Positive therapeutic outcome**
- Decreased symptoms of CMV infection

### ganciclovir ophthalmic
*See Appendix D*

### ganirelix (Rx)
(gan-i-rell'-ex)
Antagon
*Func. class.:* Gonadotropin-releasing hormone antagonist
*Chem. class.:* Synthetic decapeptide

**Pregnancy category** X

**Action:** Inhibitor of pituitary gonadotropin secretion; initially increases LH and FSH, induces a rapid suppression of gonadotropin secretion

**Therapeutic outcome:** Pregnancy

**Uses:** For inhibition of premature LH surges in women undergoing controlled ovarian hyperstimulation

### Dosage and routes
*Adult:* SUBCUT 250 mcg/day during early to mid follicular phase; continue until day of hCG administration

**Available forms:** Inj 250 mcg/0.5 ml

### Adverse effects
*CNS:* Headache
*ENDO:* Ovarian hyperstimulation syndrome, abdominal pain (gynecologic)
*GI:* Nausea

*GU: Spotting, breakthrough bleeding,* decreased urine, **fetal death**
*INTEG:* Pain on inj
*SYST:* **Fetal death**

**Contraindications:** Pregnancy **X**, breastfeeding, hypersensitivity, latex allergy

#### Pharmacokinetics
| | |
|---|---|
| **Absorption** | Unknown |
| **Distribution** | Unknown |
| **Metabolism** | To metabolites |
| **Excretion** | Unknown |
| **Half-life** | 13-16 hr |

#### Pharmacodynamics
| | |
|---|---|
| **Onset** | Unknown |
| **Peak** | Unknown |
| **Duration** | Treatment length |

### NURSING CONSIDERATIONS
### Assessment
- Monitor reproductive tests: serum progesterone, LH, estradiol, ovarian ultrasound, pelvic exam, baseline and during treatment
- Assess for suspected pregnancy, product should not be used
- Assess for latex allergy, product should not be used

### Nursing diagnoses
- Knowledge, deficient (teaching)
- Sexual dysfunction (uses)

### Implementation
- Administer SUBCUT using abdomen, around navel or upper thigh, swab inj area with disinfectant, clean a 2-in circle and allow to dry, pinch up area between thumb and finger, insert needle at 45-90 degrees to surface, if positioned correctly, no blood will be drawn back into syringe, if blood is drawn into syringe, reposition needle without removing it, inject slowly
- Protect from light

### Patient/family education
- Teach patient to report abdominal pain, vaginal bleeding

### Evaluation
**Positive therapeutic outcome**
- Pregnancy

### gatifloxacin ophthalmic
*See Appendix D*

## gefitinib (Rx)
(ge-fi'tye-nib)
Iressa
*Func. class.:* Antineoplastic—miscellaneous
*Chem. class.:* Epidermal growth factor
receptor inhibitor
**Pregnancy category** D

**Action:** Not fully understood; inhibits
intracellular phosphorylation of cell surface
receptors associated with epidermal growth
factor receptors

**Therapeutic outcome:** Decreased
growth and spread of malignant cells

**Uses:** Advanced/metastatic non–small cell
lung cancer (NSCLC) in those who have not
responded to platinum or docetaxel products

**Dosage and routes**
*Adult:* PO 250 mg/day
*CYP3A4 inducers concurrently*
*(such as rifampin or phenytoin)*
*Adult:* PO 500 mg/day

**Available forms:** Tabs 250 mg

**Adverse effects**
*EENT:* Amblyopia, conjunctivitis, eye pain,
corneal erosion/ulcer
*GI:* Nausea, diarrhea, vomiting, anorexia,
**pancreatitis,** mouth ulceration
*INTEG:* Rash, pruritus, acne, dry skin, **toxic
epidermal neurolysis, angioedema**
*MISC:* Peripheral edema
*RESP:* **Interstitial lung disease,** cough,
dyspnea

**Contraindications:** Pregnancy **D,** breastfeeding, children, hypersensitivity

**Precautions:** Renal/hepatic/ocular/
pulmonary disorders, geriatric

### Pharmacokinetics
| | |
|---|---|
| **Absorption** | Slowly |
| **Distribution** | Unknown |
| **Metabolism** | Unknown |
| **Excretion** | In feces (86%), urine (<4%) |
| **Half-life** | Unknown |

### Pharmacodynamics
| | |
|---|---|
| **Onset** | Unknown |
| **Peak** | 3-7 hr |
| **Duration** | Unknown |

**Interactions**
*Individual drugs*
Cimetidine, phenytoin, ranitidine, rifampin,
sodium bicarbonate: decreased levels

Clarithromycin, erythromycin, itraconazole,
ketoconazole: increased concentration
Metoprolol, warfarin: increased plasma
concentration
*Drug/herb*
St. John's wort: decreased gefitinib levels

### NURSING CONSIDERATIONS
**Assessment**
⬥ Assess pulmonary changes: lung sounds,
cough, dyspnea; interstitial lung disease may
occur, may be fatal; discontinue therapy if
confirmed
• Assess ocular changes: eye irritation,
corneal erosion/ulcer, aberrant eyelash
growth
⬥ Assess for pancreatitis: abdominal pain,
levels of amylase, lipase
⬥ Assess for toxic epidermal necrosis, angioedema
• Monitor GI symptoms: frequency of stools; if
diarrhea is poorly tolerated, therapy may be
discontinued for up to 14 days

**Nursing diagnoses**
• Body image, disturbed (adverse reactions)
• Infection, risk for (adverse reactions)
• Injury, risk for (adverse reactions)
• Knowledge, deficient (teaching)

**Implementation**
• Give without regard to food

**Patient/family education**
• Teach to report adverse reactions
immediately: SOB, severe abdominal pain,
occular changes, skin eruptions
• Advise of reason for treatment, expected
results
• Advise to use contraception during treatment

**Evaluation**
**Positive therapeutic outcome**
• Decreased non–small cell lung cancer cells

## gemcitabine (Rx)
(gem-sit'a-been)
Gemzar
*Func. class.:* Antineoplastic—miscellaneous
*Chem. class.:* Nucleoside analog
**Pregnancy category** D

**Do not confuse:**
Gemzar/Zinecard

**Action:** Exhibits antitumor activity by killing
cells undergoing DNA synthesis (S phase) and
blocking $G_1$/S-phase boundary

Adverse effects: *italic* = common, **bold** = life-threatening

**Therapeutic outcome:** Prevention of growth of tumor

**Uses:** Adenocarcinoma of the pancreas (nonresectable stage II, III, or metastatic stage IV); in combination with cisplatin for inoperable, advanced, or metastatic non–small cell lung cancer; advanced breast cancer in combination with paclitaxel; with carboplatin for ovarian cancer

## Dosage and routes
### Pancreatic carcinoma
**Adult: IV** 1000 mg/m² given over ½ hr qwk × 7 wk, then 1 wk rest period; subsequent cycles should be infused once qwk × 3 wk out of every 4 wk

### Non–small cell lung cancer
**4 wk schedule**
**Adult: IV** 1000 mg/m² given over ½ hr on days 1, 8, 15 of each 28-day cycle; give cisplatin **IV** 100 mg/m² on day 1 after gemcitabine

**3 wk schedule**
**Adult: IV** 1250 mg/m² given over ½ hr on days 1, 8 of each 21-day cycle; give cisplatin 100 mg/m² after the INF of gemcitabine on day 1

### Advanced breast cancer
**Adult: IV** 1250 mg/m² over ½ hr on days 1 and 8 of a 21-day cycle; give paclitaxel on day 1, 175 mg/m² over 3 hr prior to gemcitabine

### Ovarian cancer
**Adult: IV** 1 g on days 1, 8 of a 21-day cycle

**Available forms:** Lyophilized powder for inj 20 mg/ml

## Adverse effects
***GI:*** Diarrhea, nausea, vomiting, anorexia, constipation, stomatitis
***GU:*** Proteinuria, hematuria
***HEMA: Leukopenia, anemia, neutropenia, thrombocytopenia***
***INTEG:*** Irritation at site, rash, alopecia
***MISC:*** Dyspnea, fever, ***hemorrhage***, infection, flulike syndrome, paresthesia, edema

**Contraindications:** Pregnancy **D**, breastfeeding, hypersensitivity

**Precautions:** Children, geriatric, myelosuppression, irradiation, renal/hepatic disease

### Pharmacokinetics

| | |
|---|---|
| **Absorption** | Unknown |
| **Distribution** | Crosses placenta |
| **Metabolism** | Unknown |
| **Excretion** | Unknown |
| **Half-life** | 42-379 min |

### Pharmacodynamics
Unknown

## Interactions
### Individual drug
Alcohol: increased bleeding
### Drug classifications
Anticoagulants, NSAIDs, salicylates: increased bleeding
Antineoplastics, radiation: increased myelosuppression, diarrhea
Live virus vaccines: decreased antibody response
### Drug/lab test
Increased: BUN, AST, ALT, alkaline phosphatase, bilirubin, creatinine

## NURSING CONSIDERATIONS
### Assessment
• Monitor CBC, differential, platelet count before each dose; absolute granulocyte count >1000/mm³, platelets >100,000/mm³, give complete dose; absolute granulocyte count 500-1000/mm³, platelets 50,000-100,000/mm³, give 75%; absolute granulocyte count <500/mm³, platelets <50,000/mm³, do not give
• Assess for blood dyscrasias: bruising, bleeding, petechiae
• Monitor I&O, nutritional intake
• Monitor renal/hepatic studies before and during treatment, may increase AST, ALT, alkaline phosphatase, bilirubin, BUN, creatinine
• Assess food preferences: list likes, dislikes
• Assess buccal cavity for dryness, sores or ulceration, white patches, oral pain, bleeding, dysphagia
• Assess GI symptoms: frequency of stools; cramping
• Assess signs of dehydration: rapid respirations, poor skin turgor, decreased urine output, dry skin, restlessness, weakness

### Nursing diagnoses
• Infection, risk for (adverse reactions)
• Nutrition: less than body requirements, imbalanced (adverse reaction)

### Implementation
• Give increased fluid intake to 2-3 L/day to prevent dehydration, unless contraindicated
**IV route**
• Prepare in biologic cabinet using gown, mask, gloves
• After reconstituting with 0.9% NaCl 5 ml/200 mg vial of product or 25 ml/1 g of product, shake (40 mg/ml); may be further

diluted with 0.9% NaCl to concentrate as low as 0.1 mg/ml; discard unused portion, give over ½ hr, do not admix

## Patient/family education
• Teach patient to rinse mouth tid-qid with water, club soda; brush teeth bid-tid with soft brush or cotton-tipped applicator for stomatitis; use unwaxed dental floss
• Advise patient to avoid foods with citric acid or hot or rough texture if stomatitis is present; to drink adequate fluids
• Advise patient to report stomatitis; any bleeding, white spots, ulcerations in mouth; tell patient to examine mouth daily, report symptoms
• Advise patient to report signs of anemia: fatigue, headache, faintness, shortness of breath, irritability; hematuria, dysuria
• Advise patient to use contraception during therapy and for 4 mo after
• Instruct patient to avoid use with NSAIDs, salicylates, alcohol; not to receive vaccinations during treatment

## Evaluation
**Positive therapeutic outcome**
• Decrease in tumor size, decrease in spread of cancer, symptom relief

## Treatment of overdose:
Induce vomiting, provide supportive care

## gemfibrozil (Rx)
(gem-fye'broe-zil)
gemfibrozil, Lopid
*Func. class.:* Antilipemic
*Chem. class.:* Fibric acid derivative
**Pregnancy category  C**

## Do not confuse:
Lopid/Levbid/Slo-bid

**Action:** Inhibits biosynthesis of VLDL, decreases triglycerides, increases HDLs

**Therapeutic outcome:** Decreased hepatic triglyceride production, VLDL; accelerates removal of cholesterol from liver

**Uses:** Type IIb, IV, V hyperlipidemia as adjunct with diet therapy

## Dosage and routes
*Adult:* PO 1200 mg in divided doses bid 30 min before meals

**Available forms:** Tabs 600 mg; caps 300 mg ✤

## Adverse effects
*CNS:* Fatigue, vertigo, headache, paresthesia, dizziness, somnolence
*GI:* Nausea, vomiting, *dyspepsia, diarrhea, abdominal pain*
**HEMA: Leukopenia, anemia, eosinophilia, thrombocytopenia**
*INTEG:* Rash, urticaria, pruritus
*MISC:* Task perversion

**Contraindications:** Severe renal/hepatic disease, preexisting gallbladder disease, primary biliary cirrhosis, hypersensitivity

**Precautions:** Pregnancy **C,** breastfeeding, monitor hematologic and hepatic function

G

### Pharmacokinetics
| | |
|---|---|
| **Absorption** | Well absorbed |
| **Distribution** | Unknown, plasma protein binding >90% |
| **Metabolism** | Liver—minimal |
| **Excretion** | Kidney—unchanged (70%), feces (6%) |
| **Half-life** | 1½ hr |

### Pharmacodynamics
| | |
|---|---|
| **Onset** | 1-2 hr |
| **Peak** | 1-2 hr |
| **Duration** | 2-4 months |

## Interactions
### Individual drugs
CycloSPORINE: decreased cycloSPORINE effect
### Drug classifications
Anticoagulants (oral): increased effect of anticoagulants
HMG-CoA reductase inhibitors: increased risk of myositis, myalgia
Sulfonylureas: increased hypoglycemic effect
### Drug/herb
Glucomannan: increased effect
Gotu kola: decreased effect
### Drug/lab test
Increased: liver function tests, CPK, BSP, thymol turbidity, glucose
Decreased: Hgb, Hct, WBC

## NURSING CONSIDERATIONS
### Assessment
• Assess nutrition: fat, protein, carbohydrates; nutritional analysis should be performed by dietitian before treatment is initiated
• Assess renal, liver function tests, CBC, blood glucose if patient is on long-term therapy; if liver function test results increase, product should be discontinued
• Monitor bowel pattern daily; diarrhea may be a problem

Adverse effects: *italic* = common, **bold** = life-threatening

• Monitor triglycerides, cholesterol, lipids baseline and during treatment; LDL and VLDL should be watched closely and if increased, product should be discontinued

## Nursing diagnoses
• Diarrhea (adverse reactions)
• Knowledge, deficient (teaching)
• Noncompliance (teaching)

## Implementation
• Give 30 min before AM and PM meals

## Patient/family education
• Inform patient that compliance is needed for positive results to occur; not to double doses; that product may be discontinued if no improvement in 3 mo
• Caution patient to decrease risk factors: high-fat diet, smoking, alcohol consumption, lack of exercise
• Advise patient to notify prescriber if GI symptoms of diarrhea, abdominal or epigastric pain, nausea, vomiting occur; or if chills, fever, sore throat occur; also occurrence of muscle cramps, abdominal cramps, severe flatulence

## Evaluation
**Positive therapeutic outcome**
• Decreased cholesterol levels, serum triglyceride and improved ratio with HDLs

---

## gemifloxacin (Rx)
(gem-ah-flox′a-sin)
Factive
*Func. class.:* Antiinfective
*Chem. class.:* Fluoroquinolone

**Pregnancy category C**

**Action:** Inhibits DNA gyrase, which is an enzyme involved in replication, transcription, and repair of bacterial DNA

**Therapeutic outcome:** Negative C&S, decreasing symptoms of infection

**Uses:** Acute bacterial exacerbation of chronic bronchitis caused by *Streptococcus pneumoniae, Haemophilus influenzae, H. parainfluenzae, Moraxella catarrhalis;* community-acquired pneumonia caused by *Streptococcus pneumoniae* including multiproduct-resistant strains, *H. influenzae, M. catarrhalis, Mycoplasma pneumoniae, Chlamydia pneumoniae, Klebsiella pneumoniae*

## Dosage and routes
*Adult:* PO 320 mg/day × 5-7 days depending on type of infection

**Renal dose**
*Adult:* PO CCr ≤40 ml/min 160 mg q24hr

**Available forms:** Tabs 320 mg

**Adverse effects**
*CNS: Dizziness, headache,* somnolence, depression, insomnia, nervousness, confusion, agitation, **seizures**
*EENT:* Visual disturbances
*GI:* Diarrhea, *nausea,* vomiting, anorexia, flatulence, heartburn, dry mouth; increased AST, ALT; constipation, abdominal pain, oral thrush, glossitis, stomatitis, pseudomembranous colitis
*INTEG:* Rash, pruritus, urticaria, *photosensitivity*
*SYST:* **Anaphylaxis, Stevens-Johnson syndrome**

**Contraindications:** Hypersensitivity to quinolones

**Precautions:** Pregnancy **C**, breastfeeding, children, geriatric, hypokalemia, hypomagnesemia, renal disease, seizure disorders, excessive exposure to sunlight, psychosis, increased intracranial pressure, history of QT interval prolongation

| Pharmacokinetics | |
|---|---|
| **Absorption** | Rapidly, bioavailability 71% |
| **Distribution** | Unknown |
| **Metabolism** | Unknown |
| **Excretion** | In urine as active product, metabolites |
| **Half-life** | 4-12 hr |

| Pharmacodynamics | |
|---|---|
| **Onset** | Unknown |
| **Peak** | 1-2 hr |
| **Duration** | Unknown |

## Interactions
*Individual drugs*
Probenecid: may increase toxicity
*Drug classifications*
Antacids containing aluminum, iron, magnesium, sucralfate, zinc: decreased absorption
Antiarrhythmics (amiodarone, disopyramide, procainamide, quinidine, sotalol), antidepressants (tricyclics): may decrease effect, resulting in life-threatening dysrhythmias, QT prolongation
*Drug/herb*
Do not use acidophilus with antiinfectives; separate by several hours

---

## NURSING CONSIDERATIONS
### Assessment

- Monitor renal, liver function tests: BUN, creatinine, AST, ALT
- Monitor I&O ratio; urine pH, <5.5 is ideal
- Assess CNS symptoms: insomnia, vertigo, headache, agitation, confusion
- ⬥ Assess allergic reactions and anaphylaxis: rash, flushing, urticaria, pruritus, chills, fever, joint pain; may occur a few days after therapy begins; epINEPHrine and resuscitation equipment should be available for anaphylactic reaction
- Monitor bowel pattern daily; if severe diarrhea occurs, product should be discontinued
- Assess for overgrowth of infection: perineal itching, fever, malaise, redness, pain, swelling, drainage, rash, diarrhea, change in cough, sputum

### Nursing diagnoses

- Infection, risk for (uses)
- Knowledge, deficient (teaching)
- Noncompliance (teaching)

### Implementation

- Give with or without food
- Theophylline should not be used with this product, toxicity may result
- Administer 2 hr before or 3 hr after antacids, iron, zinc, or buffered products; 2 hr before sucralfate

### Patient/family education

- Advise that fluids must be increased to 2 L/day to avoid crystallization in kidneys
- Instruct that if dizziness or light-headedness occurs, to ambulate, perform activities with assistance
- Instruct to complete full course of product therapy
- Teach to contact prescriber if adverse reactions occur
- Teach to avoid iron- or mineral-containing supplements or aluminum/magnesium antacids within 2 hr before or 3 hr after dosing
- Advise that photosensitivity may occur and sunscreen should be used
- Advise to use frequent rinsing of mouth, sugarless candy or gum for dry mouth
- Teach to avoid other medication unless approved by prescriber

### Evaluation
**Positive therapeutic outcome**

- Negative C&S, absence of signs/symptoms of infection

## ❗ HIGH ALERT

### gemtuzumab (Rx)
(gem-tue-zue'mab)
Mylotarg
*Func. class.:* Antineoplastic—miscellaneous
*Chem. class.:* Monoclonal antibody

**Pregnancy category  D**

**Action:** Composed of recombinant humanized $IgG_4$ κ antibody, binds to CD33 antigen that is released in myeloid cells

**Therapeutic outcome:** Decreasing signs/symptoms of leukemia

**Uses:** Acute myeloid leukemia (AML) in patients with first relapse who are 60 yr or older

### Dosage and routes
*Adult:* **IV** 9 m/m$^2$ as a 2 hr inf; before giving INF, give diphenhydrAMINE 50 mg PO, acetaminophen 650-1000 mg PO 1 hr; then use acetaminophen 650-1000 mg q1-4hr prn

**Available forms:** Powder for inj, lyophilized 5 mg

### Adverse effects

*CNS: Dizziness,* insomnia, depression, headache

*CV:* Hypertension, **hemorrhage,** tachycardia, hypotension

*HEMA:* **Prolonged neutropenia, thrombocytopenia**

*INTEG: Rash,* herpes simplex, local reaction, petechiae

*GI:* Anorexia, diarrhea, constipation, nausea, stomatitis, vomiting, **fatal liver toxicity**

*GU:* Hematuria, **vaginal hemorrhage**

*META:* Hypokalemia, hypomagnesemia

*MISC: Fever, myalgias, headache, chills,* peripheral edema

*RESP:* Cough, pneumonia, epistaxis, rhinitis, dyspnea

**Contraindications:** Pregnancy **D,** breastfeeding, hypersensitivity, severe myelosuppression

**Precautions:** Children, severe renal/hepatic disease, pulmonary disease

#### Pharmacokinetics

| | |
|---|---|
| **Absorption** | Unknown |
| **Distribution** | Unknown |
| **Metabolism** | Unknown |
| **Excretion** | Unknown |
| **Half-life** | 45, 100 hr, respectively |

Adverse effects: *italic* = common, **bold** = life-threatening

Pharmacodynamics
Unknown

## NURSING CONSIDERATIONS
### Assessment
- Assess for pulmonary symptoms: cough, dyspnea
- Monitor blood studies: BUN, creatinine, AST, ALT, electrolytes
- Assess for symptoms of infection; chills, fever, headache, may be masked by product
- Assess CNS reaction: LOC, mental status, dizziness, confusion
- Assess cardiac status: lung sounds; ECG before and during treatment, especially in those with cardiac disease
- Assess bone marrow depression: bruising, bleeding, blood in stools, urine, sputum, emesis

### Nursing diagnoses
- Infection, risk for (adverse reactions)
- Nutrition: less than body requirements, imbalanced (adverse reactions)
- Oral mucous membrane, impaired (adverse reactions)

### Implementation
- Do not give **IV** push or bolus
- Protect from light, use biologic safety hood, allow to come to room temperature
- Reconstitute each vial with 5 ml of sterile water for inj using sterile syringes, swirl each vial, check for discoloration or particulate matter, give over 2 hr, use a separate line with 1.2-micron terminal filter
- May be premedicated with methylPRED-NISolone
- Store reconstituted sol for ≤8 hr in refrigerator

### Patient/family education
- Advise patient to take acetaminophen for fever
- Instruct patient to avoid hazardous tasks, since confusion, dizziness may occur; avoid prolonged sunlight, use sunscreen
- Instruct patient to report signs of infection: sore throat, fever, diarrhea, vomiting
- Teach patient to avoid immunizations, crowds, people with known infections
- Teach patient that product is very toxic

### Evaluation
**Positive therapeutic outcome**
- Improvement in blood counts

## gentamicin (Rx)
(jen-ta-mye′sin)
Cidomycin ✚, G-mycin, Garamycin, Gentamicin Sulfate, Jenamicin
*Func. class.:* Antiinfective
*Chem. class.:* Aminoglycoside
**Pregnancy category  C**

**Do not confuse:**
Garamycin/kanamycin

**Action:** Interferes with protein synthesis in bacterial cell by binding to ribosomal subunit, causing misreading of genetic code; inaccurate peptide sequence forms in protein chain, causing bacterial death

**Therapeutic outcome:** Bactericidal effects for the following organisms: *Pseudomonas aeruginosa, Proteus, Klebsiella, Serratia, Escherichia coli, Enterobacter, Citrobacter, Staphylococcus, Shigella, Salmonella, Acinetobacter, Bacillus anthracis*

**Uses:** Severe systemic infections of CNS; respiratory, GI, and urinary tracts; bone; skin; soft tissues; acute PID caused by susceptible strains

### Dosage and routes
*Severe systemic infections*
*Adult:* **IV** INF 3-5 mg/kg/day in 3 divided doses q8hr; dilute in 50-200 ml 0.9% NaCl or $D_5W$ given over 30 min-1 hr; IM 3 mg/kg/day in divided doses q8hr
*Child:* **IV**/IM 2-2.5 mg/ kg q8hr
*Neonate and infant:* **IV**/IM 2.5 mg/kg q8-12hr
*Neonate <1 wk:* 2.5 mg/kg q12-24hr

*Once-daily dosing/extended interval dosing (unlabeled)*
*Adult:* **IV** 4-7 mg/kg q24hr adjust according to levels

*Renal dose*
*Adult:* IM/**IV** 1-1.7 mg/kg initially, then adjust according to CCr levels

**Available forms:** Inj 10, 40 mg/ml; premixed inj 40, 60, 70, 80, 100 mg/50 ml; 40, 60, 80, 90, 100, 120, 160, 180 mg/ml

### Adverse effects
*CNS:* Confusion, depression, numbness, tremors, **seizures,** muscle twitching, **neurotoxicity,** dizziness, vertigo
*CV:* Hypotension, hypertension, palpitations
*EENT:* Ototoxicity, deafness, visual disturbances, tinnitus

**GI:** *Nausea, vomiting, anorexia,* increased ALT, AST, bilirubin, hepatomegaly, **hepatic necrosis,** splenomegaly

**GU:** **Oliguria, hematuria, renal damage, azotemia, renal failure, nephrotoxicity,** proteinuria

**HEMA:** **Agranulocytosis, thrombocytopenia, leukopenia, eosinophilia,** anemia

**INTEG:** *Rash,* burning, urticaria, dermatitis, alopecia

**Contraindications:** Severe renal disease, hypersensitivity

**Precautions:** Pregnancy **C,** breastfeeding, geriatric, neonates, mild renal disease, hearing deficits, myasthenia gravis, Parkinson's disease

### Pharmacokinetics

| | |
|---|---|
| Absorption | Well absorbed (IM) |
| Distribution | Distributed in extracellular fluids, poorly distributed in CSF; crosses placenta |
| Metabolism | Liver, minimal |
| Excretion | Mostly unchanged (79%) kidneys |
| Half-life | 1-2 hr; infants 6-7 hr; increased in renal disease |

### Pharmacodynamics

| | IM | IV |
|---|---|---|
| Onset | Rapid | Rapid |
| Peak | ½-1½ hr | Infusion's end |
| Duration | Unknown | Unknown |

### Interactions
*Individual drugs*
Acyclovir, amphotericin B, cidofovir, cisplatin, ethacrynic acid, furosemide, mannitol, methoxyflurane, polymyxin, vancomycin: increased ototoxicity, neurotoxicity, nephrotoxicity

*Drug classifications*
Aminoglycosides, cephalosporins, penicillins: increased ototoxicity, neurotoxicity, nephrotoxicity

Nondepolarizing neuromuscular blockers: increased neuromuscular blockade, respiratory depression

*Drug/herb*
Do not use acidophilus with antiinfectives; separate by several hours

### NURSING CONSIDERATIONS
**Assessment**
• Assess patient for previous sensitivity reaction
• Assess patient for signs and symptoms of infection including characteristics of wounds, sputum, urine, stool, WBC >10,000/mm³,

fever; obtain baseline information and during treatment
• Complete culture and sensitivity before beginning product therapy; this will ensure that correct treatment has been initiated
• Assess for allergic reactions: rash, urticaria, pruritus, chills, fever, joint pain may occur a few days after therapy begins
• Identify urine output; if decreasing, notify prescriber (may indicate nephrotoxicity); also, increased BUN, creatinine, urine CCr <80 ml/min
• Monitor blood studies: AST, ALT, CBC, Hct, bilirubin, LDH, alkaline phosphatase, Coombs' test monthly if patient is on long-term therapy
• Monitor electrolytes: potassium, sodium, chloride, magnesium monthly if patient is on long-term therapy
• Monitor for bleeding: ecchymosis, bleeding gums, hematuria; assess stool guaiac daily if on long-term therapy
• Assess for overgrowth of infection: perineal itching, fever, malaise, redness, pain, swelling, drainage, rash, diarrhea, change in cough, sputum
• Obtain weight before treatment; calculation of dosage is usually based on ideal body weight but may be calculated on actual body weight
• Monitor I&O ratio; urinalysis daily for proteinuria, cells, casts; report sudden change in urine output
• Monitor VS during inf, watch for hypotension, change in pulse
• Assess **IV** site for thrombophlebitis including pain, redness, swelling q30 min, change site if needed; apply warm compresses to discontinued site
• Obtain serum peak, measured at 30-60 min after **IV** inf or 60 min after IM inj, trough level measured just before next dose; blood level should be 2-4 times bacteriostatic level
• Assess urine pH if product is used for UTI; urine should be kept alkaline
• Assess for deafness by audiometric testing, ringing, roaring in ears, vertigo; assess hearing before, during, after treatment
• Assess for dehydration: high specific gravity, decrease in skin turgor, dry mucous membranes, dark urine

**Nursing diagnoses**
• Diarrhea (side effects)
• Infection, risk for (uses)
• Injury, risk for (side effects)
• Knowledge, deficient (teaching)
• Noncompliance (teaching)

G

Adverse effects: *italic* = common, **bold** = life-threatening

## Implementation
**IM route**
• Give inj deeply in large muscle mass; rotate sites
**Topical route**
• Wash hands, wear gloves, clean skin before applying
**IV route**
• Give in even doses around the clock; product must be given for 10-14 days to ensure organism death and prevent superimposed infection
• Give by intermittent inf over ½-1 hr, flush with 0.9% NaCl or D₅W after inf
• Separate aminoglycosides and penicillins by ≥1 hr
• Store in tight container
*Syringe compatibilities:* Clindamycin, methicillin, penicillin G sodium
*Y-site compatibilities:* Acyclovir, amifostine, amiodarone, amsacrine, atracurium, aztreonam, cefpirome, ciprofloxacin, cyclophosphamide, cytarabine, diltiazem, enalaprilat, esmolol, famotidine, fluconazole, fludarabine, foscarnet, granisetron, hydromorphone, IL-2, insulin, labetalol, lorazepam, magnesium sulfate, melphalan, meperidine, meropenem, midazolam, morphine, multivitamins, ondansetron, paclitaxel, pancuronium, perphenazine, sargramostim, tacrolimus, teniposide, theophylline, thiotepa, tolazine, vecuronium, vinorelbine, vit B with C, zidovudine
*Y-site incompatibilities:* Idarubicin, indomethacin, zidovudine
*Additive compatibilities:* Atracurium, aztreonam, bleomycin, cefoxitin, cimetidine, ciprofloxacin, fluconazole, meropenem, methicillin, metronidazole, ofloxacin, penicillin G sodium, ranitidine, verapamil

## Patient/family education
• Teach patient to report sore throat, bruising, bleeding, joint pain; may indicate blood dyscrasias (rare)
• Advise patient to contact prescriber if vaginal itching, loose foul-smelling stools, furry tongue occur; may indicate superimposed infection

## Evaluation
**Positive therapeutic outcome**
• Absence of signs/symptoms of infection (WBC <10,000/mm³, temp WNL, absence of red, draining wounds)
• Reported improvement in symptoms of infection

**Treatment of overdose:** Withdraw product, hemodialysis

## gentamicin ophthalmic
*See Appendix D*

## gentamicin topical
*See Appendix D*

## glatiramer (Rx)
(glah-teer'a-mer)
Copaxone
*Func. class.:* Multiple sclerosis agent
**Pregnancy category  B**

**Action:** Unknown; may modify the immune responses responsible for multiple sclerosis

**Therapeutic outcome:** Decreased symptoms of multiple sclerosis

**Uses:** Reduction of the frequency of relapses in patients with relapsing-remitting multiple sclerosis

## Dosage and routes
*Adult:* SUBCUT 20 mg/day

**Available forms:** Inj premixed 20 mg/ml

## Adverse effects
*CNS:* Anxiety, hypertonia, tremor, vertigo, speech disorder, agitation, confusion
*CV:* Migraine, palpitations, syncope, tachycardia, vasodilatation, chest pain
*EENT:* Ear pain, blurred vision
*GI:* Nausea, vomiting, diarrhea, anorexia, gastroenteritis
*GU:* Urgency, dysmenorrhea, vaginal moniliasis
*HEMA:* Ecchymosis, lymphadenopathy
*INTEG:* Pruritus, rash, sweating, urticaria, erythema
*META:* Edema, weight gain
*MS:* Arthralgia, back pain, neck pain
*RESP:* Bronchitis, dyspnea, laryngismus, rhinitis

**Contraindications:** Hypersensitivity to this product or mannitol

**Precautions:** Pregnancy **B**, breastfeeding, children <18 yr, immune disorders, renal disease

Pharmacokinetics
Unknown

Pharmacodynamics
Unknown

# glimepiride/glipiZIDE   455

## NURSING CONSIDERATIONS
### Assessment
- Monitor blood, renal, liver function tests; before treatment
- Assess for CNS symptoms: anxiety, confusion, vertigo
- Assess GI status: diarrhea, vomiting, abdominal pain, gastroenteritis
- Assess cardiac status: tachycardia, palpitations, vasodilatation, chest pain

### Nursing diagnoses
- Knowledge, deficient (teaching)
- Noncompliance (teaching)

### Implementation
**SUBCUT route**
- Use a sterile syringe/needle to transfer the supplied diluent into the vial, rotate vial gently, do not shake; withdraw medication using a syringe with 27G needle; administer SUBCUT into hip, thigh, arm; discard unused portion
- Use SUBCUT route only; do not give IM or **IV**
- Do not use sol that contains precipitate or is discolored

### Patient/family education
- Give written, detailed instructions about the product; provide initial and return demonstrations on inj procedure; give information on use and disposal of product
- Advise patient that blurred vision, sweating may occur
- Advise patient that irregular menses, dysmenorrhea, or metrorrhagia, as well as breast pain may occur; use contraception during treatment
- Advise patient that if pregnancy is suspected or if nursing to notify prescriber
- Advise patient not to change dosing or to stop taking product without advice of prescriber

### Evaluation
**Positive therapeutic outcome**
- Decreased symptoms of multiple sclerosis

---

**glimepiride** (Rx)
(gly-meh'pih-ride)
Amaride
***glipiZIDE** (Rx)
(glip-i'zide)
Glucotrol, Glucotrol **XL**
*Func. class.:* Antidiabetic
*Chem. class.:* Sulfonylurea (2nd generation)

**Pregnancy category** C

**Do not confuse:**
glipiZIDE/glucotrol/glyBURIDE

**Action:** Causes functioning β-cells in pancreas to release insulin, leading to drop in blood glucose levels; may improve insulin binding to insulin receptors or increase the number of insulin receptors with prolonged administration; may also reduce basal hepatic glucose secretion; not effective if patient lacks functioning β-cells

**Therapeutic outcome:** Decrease in polyuria, polydipsia, polyphagia, clear sensorium, absence of dizziness, stable gait

**Uses:** Type 2 diabetes mellitus

### Dosage and routes
*Glimepiride*
*Adult:* PO 1-2 mg/day with breakfast, then increase q1-2 wk, max 8 mg/day
*Geriatric:* PO 1 mg/day, may increase if needed

*Renal dose*
*Adult:* CCr <20 ml/min; PO 1 mg/day with breakfast, may titrate upward as needed

*GlipiZIDE*
*Adult:* PO 5 mg initially before breakfast, then increase to desired response; max 40 mg/day in divided doses or 15 mg/dose; (XL) PO 5 mg/day with breakfast, may increase to 10 mg/day, max 20 mg/day
*Geriatric:* PO 2.5 mg/day, may increase if needed

*Hepatic dose*
*Adult:* PO 2.5 mg initially, then increase to desired response; max 40 mg/day in divided doses or 15 mg/dose

**Available forms:** Glimepiride: tabs 1, 2, 4 mg; glipiZIDE: tabs 5, 10 mg scored; ext rel tabs 2.5, 5, 10 mg

### Adverse effects
*CNS: Headache, weakness, dizziness, drowsiness,* tinnitus, fatigue, vertigo
*ENDO:* **Hypoglycemia**
*GI:* **Hepatotoxicity, cholestatic jaundice,** nausea, vomiting, diarrhea, heartburn

Adverse effects: *italic* = common, **bold** = life-threatening

*HEMA:* **Leukopenia, thrombocytopenia, agranulocytosis, aplastic anemia,** increased AST, ALT, alkaline phosphatase, **pancytopenia, hemolytic anemia**
*INTEG:* Rash, allergic reactions, pruritus, urticaria, eczema, photosensitivity, erythema

**Contraindications:** Hypersensitivity to sulfonylureas, type 1 diabetes, diabetic ketoacidosis

**Precautions:** Pregnancy **C**, geriatric, cardiac disease, severe renal/hepatic disease

### Pharmacokinetics

| | |
|---|---|
| **Absorption** | Completely absorbed GI tract |
| **Distribution** | Unknown |
| **Metabolism** | Liver |
| **Excretion** | Via kidneys |
| **Half-life** | 2-4 hr |

### Pharmacodynamics

| | |
|---|---|
| **Onset** | 1-1½ hr |
| **Peak** | 1-3 hr |
| **Duration** | 10-24 hr |

## Interactions
### Individual drugs
Charcoal, cholestyramine, diazoxide, isoniazid, rifampin: possible decreased action of glipiZIDE

Chloramphenicol, cimetidine, clofibrate, fenfluramine, gemfibrozil, guanethidine, insulin, methyldopa, phenylbutazone, probenecid, sulfinpyrizine: increased hypoglycemia

Digoxin: increased action of digoxin
### Drug classifications
Androgens, anticoagulants, $H_2$-antagonists, magnesium salts, MAOIs, NSAIDs, salicylates, sulfonamides, tricyclics, urinary acidifiers: increased hypoglycemia

β-Blockers: may mask symptoms of hypoglycemia

Diuretics (thiazide), hydantoins, urinary alkalinizers: possible decreased action of glipiZIDE

Glycosides: increased action of glycosides
### Drug/herb
Alfalfa, aloe, basil, bay, bilberry, bitter melon, black catechu, buchu, burdock, coriander, dandelion, eyebright (po), garlic, glucomannan, glucosamine, goat's rue, gymnema, horehound, horse chestnut, jambul, myrrh, myrtle: increased antidiabetic effect

Bee pollen, blue cohosh, broom, chromium, elecampane, eucalyptus, gotu kola: decreased antidiabetic effect

Broom, buchu, dandelion, glucosamine, juniper: decreased hypoglycemic effect

Chromium, coenzyme Q10, fenugreek, ginseng: increased or decreased hypoglycemic effect

Karela: increased glucose tolerance

## NURSING CONSIDERATIONS
### Assessment
• Assess for hypoglycemic/hyperglycemic reactions that can occur soon after meals; hypoglycemic reactions (sweating, weakness, dizziness, anxiety, tremors, hunger); hyperglycemic reactions

• Monitor CBC, A1c (baseline, q3 mo) during treatment; check liver function tests periodically: AST, LDH, and renal tests: BUN, creatinine during treatment

### Nursing diagnoses
• Injury, risk for (adverse reactions)
• Knowledge, deficient (teaching)
• Noncompliance (teaching)
• Nutrition: less than body requirements, imbalanced (adverse reactions)
• Nutrition: more than body requirements, imbalanced (uses)

### Implementation
• Do not break, crush, or chew ext rel tabs
• Convert from other oral hypoglycemic agents or insulin dosage of <40 units/day; change may be made without gradual dosage change.
• Patients taking >40 units/day of insulin convert gradually by receiving oral hypoglycemic agents and 50% of previous insulin dosage for 3-5 days
• Monitor serum or urine glucose and ketones 3 ×/day during conversion
• Give product 30 min before breakfast; if large dose is required, may be divided into 2 doses; give with meals to decrease GI upset and provide best absorption; if patient is NPO, may need to hold dose to prevent hypoglycemia
• Give tab crushed and mixed with meal or fluids for patients with difficulty swallowing
• For severe hypoglycemia give **IV** $D_{50}W$, then **IV** dextrose solution
• Store in tight container in cool environment

### Patient/family education
• Teach patient to check for symptoms of cholestatic jaundice: dark urine, pruritus, yellow sclera; if these occur, prescriber should be notified
• Teach patient to use capillary blood glucose test
• Teach patient symptoms of hypo/hyperglycemia, what to do about each

• Instruct patient that product must be continued on daily basis; explain consequence of discontinuing product abruptly
• Teach patient to take product in ᴀᴍ to prevent hypoglycemic reactions at night
• Caution patient to avoid OTC medications unless approved by a prescriber
• Teach patient that diabetes is a lifelong illness; that this product is not a cure
• Teach patient to avoid alcohol; inform about disulfiram reaction (nausea, headache, cramps, flushing, hypoglycemia)
• Instruct patient that all food included in diet plan must be eaten to prevent hypoglycemia
• Advise patient to use sunscreen or stay out of the sun to prevent burns
• Advise patient to carry/wear emergency ID and carry a glucagon emergency kit for emergency purposes; also prescriber name, phone number, and medications taken
• Teach patient ext rel tab may appear in stool

### Evaluation
**Positive therapeutic outcome**
• Decrease in polyuria, polydipsia, polyphagia; clear sensorium; absence of dizziness; stable gait
• Improved serum glucose, A1c

---

## *glyBURIDE (Rx)
(glye′byoor-ide)
Apo-Glyburide ✿, DiaBeta ✿, Euglucon ✿, Gen-Glybe ✿, Glynase PresTab, Micronase, novo-Glyburide ✿, nu-Glyburide ✿
*Func. class.:* Antidiabetic
*Chem. class.:* Sulfonylurea (2nd generation)
**Pregnancy category B**

### Do not confuse:
glyBURIDE/Glucotrol/glipiZIDE, DiaBeta/Zebeta

**Action:** Causes functioning β-cells in pancreas to release insulin, leading to drop in blood glucose levels; may improve insulin binding to insulin receptors and increase number of insulin receptors with prolonged administration; may also reduce basal hepatic glucose secretion; not effective if patient lacks functioning β-cells

**Therapeutic outcome:** Decrease in polyuria, polydipsia, polyphagia, clear sensorium, absence of dizziness, stable gait

**Uses:** Type 2 diabetes mellitus

### Dosage and routes
*DiaBeta/Micronase*
**Adult:** PO 1.25-5 mg initially, then increased to desired response at weekly intervals up to 20 mg/day, may be given as a single or divided dose
**Geriatric:** PO 1.25 mg initially, then increased to desired response; max 20 mg/day, maintenance 1.25-20 mg/day

*Glynase PresTab (micronized)*
**Adult:** PO 1.5-3 mg/day initially, may increase by 1.5 mg/wk, max 12 mg/day
**Geriatric:** PO 0.75-3 mg/day, may increase by 1.5 mg/wk

**Available forms:** Tabs (Diabeta) 1.25, 2.5, 5 mg; tabs micronized (Glynase PresTab) 1.5, 3, 6 mg

### Adverse effects
*CNS:* Headache, *weakness,* paresthesia, tinnitus, fatigue, vertigo
*ENDO:* **Hypoglycemia**
*GI:* Nausea, fullness, heartburn, **hepatoxicity, cholestatic jaundice,** vomiting, diarrhea
*HEMA:* **Leukopenia, thrombocytopenia, agranulocytosis, aplastic anemia,** increased AST, ALT, alkaline phosphatase
*INTEG:* Rash, allergic reactions, pruritus, urticaria, eczema, photosensitivity, erythema
*MS:* Joint pains

**Contraindications:** Hypersensitivity to sulfonylureas, type 1 diabetes, diabetic ketoacidosis, renal failure

**Precautions:** Pregnancy **B,** geriatric, cardiac/thyroid disease, severe renal/hepatic disease, severe hypoglycemic reactions

| Pharmacokinetics | |
|---|---|
| **Absorption** | Completely absorbed GI tract |
| **Distribution** | 99% plasma protein binding |
| **Metabolism** | Liver |
| **Excretion** | Urine, feces (metabolites), crosses placenta |
| **Half-life** | 10 hr |

| Pharmacodynamics | |
|---|---|
| **Onset** | 2-4 hr |
| **Peak** | 4 hr |
| **Duration** | 24 hr |

### Interactions
*Individual drugs*
Charcoal, cholestyramine, isoniazid, rifampin: decreased action of glyBURIDE
Chloramphenicol, fenfluramine, fluconazo¹ gemfibrozil, guanethidine, insulin, m⸍

G

Adverse effects: *italic* = common, **bold** = life-t⸍

dopa, phenylbutazone, probenecid, sulfinpyrazone: increased hypoglycemia

Diazoxide: both products may have action decreased

Digoxin: increased level

*Drug classifications*

Androgens, anticoagulants, antidepressants (tricyclics), H$_2$-antagonists, magnesium salts, MAOIs, NSAIDs, salicylates, sulfonamides, urinary acidifiers: increased hypoglycemia

β-Adrenergic blockers: increased masking of symptoms of hypoglycemia

Diuretics (thiazide), hydantoins, urinary alkalinizers: decreased action of glyBURIDE

*Drug/herb*

Alfalfa, aloe, basil, bay, bilberry, bitter melon, black catechu, buchu, burdock, coriander, dandelion, eyebright (po), garlic, glucomannan, glucosamine, goat's rue, gymnema, horehound, horse chestnut, jambul, myrrh, myrtle: increased antidiabetic effect

Bee pollen, blue cohosh, broom, chromium, elecampane, eucalyptus, gotu kola: decreased antidiabetic effect

Broom, buchu, dandelion, glucosamine, juniper: decreased hypoglycemic effect

Chromium, coenzyme Q10, fenugreek, ginseng: increased or decreased hypoglycemic effect

Karela: increased glucose tolerance

*Drug/lab test*

Increased: AST, ALT, LDH, BUN, creatinine

## NURSING CONSIDERATIONS
### Assessment

• Assess for hypo/hyperglycemic reactions that can occur soon after meals; hypoglycemic reactions (sweating, weakness, dizziness, anxiety, tremors, hunger); hyperglycemic reactions

• Monitor CBC, A1c (baseline, q3 mo) during treatment; check liver function tests periodically, AST, LDH, and renal studies: BUN, creatinine during treatment

### Nursing diagnoses

• Injury, risk for (adverse reactions)
• Knowledge, deficient (teaching)
• Noncompliance (teaching)
• Nutrition: less than body requirements, imbalanced (adverse reactions)
• Nutrition: more than body requirements, imbalanced (uses)

### Implementation

• Conversion from other oral hypoglycemic agents or insulin dosage of <40 units/day; change may be made without gradual dosage change

• Patients taking >40 units/day of insulin convert gradually by receiving oral hypoglycemic agents and 50% of previous insulin dosage for 3-5 days

• Monitor serum or urine glucose and ketones 3 ×/day during conversion

• Give product 30 min before breakfast; if large dose is required, may be divided into two; give with meals to decrease GI upset and provide best absorption, if patient is NPO, may need to hold dose to avoid hypoglycemia

• Give tab crushed and mixed with meal or fluids for patients with difficulty swallowing

• For severe hypoglycemia, give **IV** D$_{50}$W, then **IV** dextrose sol

• Store in tight container in cool environment

### Patient/family education

• Teach patient to check for symptoms of cholestatic jaundice: dark urine, pruritus, yellow sclera; if these occur, prescriber should be notified

• Teach patient to use capillary blood glucose test

• Teach patient symptoms of hypo/hyperglycemia, what to do about each

• Instruct patient that product must be continued on daily basis; explain consequence of discontinuing product abruptly

• Teach patient to take product in AM to prevent hypoglycemic reactions at night

• Caution patient to avoid OTC medications unless approved by a prescriber

• Teach patient that diabetes is a lifelong illness; that this product is not a cure

• Instruct patient that all food included in diet plan must be eaten to prevent hypoglycemia

• Advise patient to carry/wear emergency ID and carry a glucagon emergency kit for emergency purposes: have sugar packets available; also prescriber name, phone number, and medications

• Advise patient to use sunscreen or stay out of the sun to prevent burns

### Evaluation
**Positive therapeutic outcome**

• Decrease in polyuria, polydipsia, polyphagia; clear sensorium; absence of dizziness; stable gait

• Improved serum glucose, A1c

## glycopyrrolate (Rx)

(glye-koe-pye′roe-late)
glycopyrrolate, Robinul, Robinul-Forte
*Func. class.:* Cholinergic blocker
*Chem. class.:* Quaternary ammonium
compound

### Pregnancy category B

**Action:** Inhibits action of acetylcholine at
receptor sites in autonomic nervous system,
which controls secretions, free acids in stomach

**Therapeutic outcome:** Decreased
secretions in the respiratory tract, GI system

**Uses:** Decreased secretions before surgery,
reversal of neuromuscular blockade, peptic
ulcer disease, irritable bowel syndrome,
bradycardia, drooling

### Dosage and routes
*Preoperatively*
*Adult:* IM 4.4 mcg/kg ½-1 hr before surgery, max 0.1 mg
*Child:* IM 4.4-8.8 mcg/kg ½-1 hr before
surgery

*Intraoperative*
*Adult:* **IV** 0.1 mg; may repeat 2-3 min prn
*Child:* IM/**IV** 4 mcg/kg q2-3 min prn; max
0.1 mg/dose

*Reversal of neuromuscular
blockage*
*Adult and child:* **IV** 200 mcg for each 1
mg of neostigmine or 5 mg **IV** of pyridostigmine simultaneously

*GI disorders*
*Adult:* PO 1-2 mg bid-tid; IM/**IV** 100-200
mcg tid-qid, titrated to patient response

*Antidysrhythmic*
*Adult:* **IV** 100 mcg, may repeat q2 min
*Child:* **IV** 4.4 mcg/kg, may repeat q2 min,
max 100 mcg

*Secretion control*
*Child:* PO 40-100 mcg/kg/dose tid-qid;
IM/**IV** 4-10 mcg/kg/dose q3-4hr; max 0.2
mg/dose or 0.8 mg/24hr

**Available forms:** Tabs 1, 2 mg; inj 200
mcg 0.2 mg/ml

### Adverse effects
*CNS:* Confusion, anxiety, restlessness, irritability, delusions, hallucinations, headache,
sedation, depression, incoherence, dizziness,
lethargy, flushing, weakness
*CV:* Palpitations, tachycardia, postural hypotension, paradoxical bradycardia
*EENT:* Blurred vision, photophobia, dilated

pupils, difficulty swallowing, increased intraocular pressure, mydriasis, cycloplegia
*GI: Dryness of mouth, constipation,* nausea,
vomiting, abdominal distress, paralytic ileus,
altered taste perception
*GU:* Hesitancy, retention, impotence
*INTEG:* Urticaria, allergic reactions
*MISC:* Suppression of breastfeeding, nasal
congestion, decreased sweating
***SYST:* Anaphylaxis**

**Contraindications:** Children <3 yr,
hypersensitivity, angle-closure glaucoma,
myasthenia gravis, GI/GU obstruction, tachycardia, myocardial ischemia, hepatic disease,
ulcerative colitis, toxic megacolon, prostatic
hypertrophy

**Precautions:** Pregnancy **B,** breastfeeding,
geriatric, pulmonary/renal disease, CHF,
hyperthyroidism

### Pharmacokinetics
| | |
|---|---|
| **Absorption** | Well absorbed (PO, SUBCUT, IM) |
| **Distribution** | Unknown |
| **Metabolism** | Not metabolized |
| **Excretion** | Unchanged feces |
| **Half-life** | 2 hr |

### Pharmacodynamics
| | PO | IM | IV |
|---|---|---|---|
| **Onset** | Unknown | 15-30 min | Immediate |
| **Peak** | 1 hr | 30-45 min | 10-15 min |
| **Duration** | 8-12 hr | 2-7 hr | 2-7 hr |

### Interactions
*Individual drugs*
Alcohol, amantadine: increased anticholinergic
effect
*Drug classifications*
Antacids: decreased absorption of glycopyrrolate
Antidepressants (tricyclic), antihistamines,
phenothiazines: increased anticholinergic
effect
Antidiarrheals: decreased absorption of
glycopyrrolate

### NURSING CONSIDERATIONS
**Assessment**
• Monitor I&O ratio; retention commonly
causes decreased urinary output; check for
urinary hesitation; palpate bladder if retention
occurs
• Monitor ECG for ectopic ventricular beats,
PVC, tachycardia

Adverse effects: *italic* = common, **bold** = life-threatening

- Monitor for bowel sounds; check for constipation; increase fluids, bulk, exercise if constipation occurs
- Assess mental status: affect, mood, CNS depression, worsening of psychiatric symptoms during early therapy

### Nursing diagnoses
- Knowledge, deficient (teaching)

### Implementation
**PO route**
- Give PO with or after meals to prevent GI upset; may give with fluids other than water

**IM route**
- Give IM inj deeply in large muscle mass

**IV route**
- Administer **IV** undiluted, give at a rate of 0.2 mg or less over 5-15 min through Y-tube or 3-way stopcock; do not add to **IV** sol
- Administer parenteral dose with patient recumbent to prevent postural hypotension

*Syringe compatibilities:* Atropine, benzquinamide, chlorproMAZINE, cimetidine, codeine, diphenhydrAMINE, droperidol, droperidol/fentanyl, hydromorphone, hydrOXYzine, levorphanol, lidocaine, meperidine, meperidine/promethazine, midazolam, morphine, nalbuphine, neostigmine, oxymorphone, procaine, prochlorperazine, promazine, promethazine, pyridostigmine, ranitidine, scopolamine, triflupromazine, trimethobenzamide

*Y-site compatibilities:* Propofol
*Solution compatibilities:* $D_5W$, 0.9% NaCl, Ringer's $D_5$/0.45% NaCl

### Patient/family education
- Caution patient not to operate machinery or engage in hazardous activities if drowsiness, blurred vision occurs
- Advise patient not to take OTC products, cough, cold preparations with alcohol, antihistamines without approval of prescriber
- Teach patient to avoid hot temperature; since sweating is decreased, heat stroke is possible
- Advise patient to notify prescriber of eye pain, blurred vision, light sensitivity
- Caution patient not to discontinue this product abruptly; tapering should be done over 1 wk

### Evaluation
**Positive therapeutic outcome**
- Decreased secretions, bronchial, GI
- Decreased pain in GI disorders
- Reversal of neuromuscular blockade

## goserelin (Rx)
(goe'se-rel-lin)
Zoladex
*Func. class.:* Gonadotropin-releasing hormone, antineoplastic
*Chem. class.:* Synthetic decapeptide analog of LHRH

**Pregnancy category** D, X

**Action:** Inhibitor of pituitary gonadotropin secretion; initially increases LH and FSH, with increases in testosterone, reduction in sex steroid levels (substitute serum testosterone levels)

**Therapeutic outcome:** Decrease in tumor size and spread of malignant cells

**Uses:** Advanced prostate cancer (10.8 mg); endometriosis, advanced breast cancer, endometrial thinning (3.6 mg)

### Dosage and routes
*Adult:* SUBCUT 3.6 mg q4 wk (implant) or 10.8 mg q12 wk

### Endometrial thinning
*Adult:* SUBCUT 1-2 depot inj; usually 1 depot, surgery performed at 4 wk; if 2 depots, surgery performed 2-4 wk after 2nd depot

**Available forms:** Depot inj 3.6, 10.8 mg

### Adverse effects
*CNS:* Headaches, **spinal cord compression**, anxiety, depression, dizziness, insomnia, lethargy, hot flashes
*CV:* **Dysrhythmia, cerebrovascular accident,** hypertension, **MI**, chest pain, CHF
*ENDO:* Gynecomastia, breast tenderness, hot flashes
*GI:* Nausea, vomiting, constipation, diarrhea, ulcer
*GU:* *Spotting, breakthrough bleeding, decreased libido,* renal insufficiency, urinary obstruction, urinary tract infection, impotence
*INTEG:* Rash, pain on inj
*MS:* Osteoneuralgia
*RESP:* COPD, URI

**Contraindications:** Pregnancy **D** (breast cancer), **X** (endometriosis, breastfeeding, nondiagnosed vaginal bleeding), children, 10.8 mg dose in women, hypersensitivity to LHRH, LHRH-agonist analogs

**Precautions:** Spinal cord decompression, renal disease, bone mineral density loss

## Pharmacokinetics

| Absorption | Well absorbed |
|---|---|
| Distribution | Unknown |
| Metabolism | Unknown |
| Excretion | Unknown |
| Half-life | 4½ hr |

## Pharmacodynamics

| Onset | Unknown |
|---|---|
| Peak | 14-28 days |
| Duration | Treatment length |

## Interactions
### Drug/lab test
Increased: alkaline phosphatase, estradiol, FSH, LH, testosterone levels
Decreased: testosterone levels, progesterone

## NURSING CONSIDERATIONS
### Assessment
• Assess for relief of bone pain (back pain), change in motor function
• Monitor I&O ratios, palpate bladder for distention (urinary obstruction) at beginning of treatment; renal insufficiency and obstruction may occur
• Monitor acid phosphatase, PSA baseline and periodically
• Obtain pregnancy test prior to therapy

### Nursing diagnoses
• Knowledge, deficient (teaching)
• Sexual dysfunction (uses)

### Implementation
• Administer via implant inserted by qualified persons into upper subcutaneous tissue in abdominal wall q28 days or q12 wk (10.8 mg), do not attempt to remove air bubbles from syringe

### Patient/family education
• Caution patient that gynecomastia and postmenopausal symptoms may occur but will decrease after treatment is discontinued; that bone pain may increase, then decrease
• Teach patient to contact prescriber if difficulty urinating, hot flashes occur during treatment
• Advise patient not to breastfeed while taking product; use effective nonhormonal contraception

### Evaluation
**Positive therapeutic outcome**
• More normal levels of PSA, acid phosphatase, alkaline phosphatase; testosterone level of <25 mg/dl

## granisetron (Rx)
(grane-iss'e-tron)
Kytril
*Func. class.:* Antiemetic
*Chem. class.:* 5-HT$_3$ receptor antagonist
### Pregnancy category B

**Action:** Prevents nausea, vomiting by blocking serotonin peripherally, centrally, and in the small intestine

**Therapeutic outcome:** Absence of nausea and vomiting

**Uses:** Prevention of nausea, vomiting associated with cancer chemotherapy including high-dose cisplatin

**Unlabeled uses:** Acute nausea, vomiting after surgery

**Dosage and routes**
*Nausea, vomiting in chemotherapy*
*Adult and child ≥2 yr:* **IV** 10 mcg/kg over 5 min, 30 min before the start of cancer chemotherapy
*Adult:* PO 1 mg bid, give 1st dose 1 hr before chemotherapy and next dose 12 hr after 1st

*Nausea, vomiting in radiation therapy*
*Adult:* PO 2 mg/day 1 hr prior to radiation

**Available forms:** Inj 1 mg/ml; tabs 1 mg
**Adverse effects**
*CNS: Headache, asthenia,* anxiety, dizziness
*CV:* Hypertension
*GI:* Diarrhea, *constipation,* increased AST, ALT, *nausea*
**HEMA: Leukopenia,** anemia, **thrombocytopenia**
*MISC:* Rash, **bronchospasm**

**Contraindications:** Hypersensitivity

**Precautions:** Pregnancy **B,** breastfeeding, children, geriatric, ondansetron hypersensitivity

## Pharmacokinetics

| Absorption | Unknown |
|---|---|
| Distribution | Unknown |
| Metabolism | Liver |
| Excretion | Unknown |
| Half-life | 10-12 hr |

## Pharmacodynamics
Unknown

G

Adverse effects: *italic* = common, **bold** = life-threatening

### Interactions
**Drug classifications**
Antipsychotics: increased EPS

## NURSING CONSIDERATIONS
### Assessment
• Assess patient for absence of nausea, vomiting during chemotherapy
• Assess patient for hypersensitive reaction: rash, bronchospasm

### Nursing diagnoses
• Fluid volume, deficient (uses)
• Knowledge, deficient (teaching)

### Implementation
• Administer **IV**
• Dilute in 0.9% NaCl for inj or $D_5W$ (20-50 ml), give over 5-15 min
• Store at room temp for 24-hr dilution

**Y-site compatibilities:** Acyclovir, allopurinol, amifostine, amikacin, aminophylline, amphotericin B cholesteryl, ampicillin, ampicillin/sulbactam, amsacrine, aztreonam, bleomycin, bumetanide, buprenorphine, butorphanol, calcium gluconate, carboplatin, carmustine, cefazolin, cefepime, cefonicid, cefoperazone, cefotaxime, cefotetan, cefoxitin, ceftazidime, ceftizoxime, ceftriaxone, cefuroxime, chlorproMAZINE, cimetidine, ciprofloxacin, cisplatin, cladribine, clindamycin, cyclophosphamide, cytarabine, dacarbazine, dactinomycin, DAUNOrubicin, dexamethasone, diphenhydrAMINE, DOBUTamine, DOPamine, DOXOrubicin, DOXOrubicin liposome, doxycycline, droperidol, enalaprilat, etoposide, famotidine, filgrastim, floxuridine, fluconazole, fluorouracil, fludarabine, furosemide, gallium, ganciclovir, gentamicin, haloperidol, heparin, hydrocortisone, hydromorphone, hydrOXYzine, idarubicin, ifosfamide, imipenem-cilastatin, leucovorin, lorazepam, magnesium sulfate, melphalan, meperidine, mesna, methotrexate, methylPREDNISolone, metoclopramide, metronidazole, mezlocillin, miconazole, minocycline, mitomycin, mitoxantrone, morphine, nalbuphine, netilmicin, ofloxacin, paclitaxel, piperacillin, piperacillin/tazobactam, plicamycin, potassium chloride, prochlorperazine, promethazine, propofol, ranitidine, sargramostim, sodium bicarbonate, streptozocin, teniposide, thiotepa, ticarcillin, ticarcillin/clavulanate, tobramycin, trimethoprim/sulfamethoxazole, vancomycin, vinBLAStine, vinCRIStine, vinorelbine, zidovudine

**Y-site incompatibilities:** Fluorouracil, furosemide, sodium bicarbonate

**Additive compatibilities:** Dexamethasone, methylPREDNISolone

**Solution compatibilities:** $D_5W$, 0.9% NaCl

### Patient/family education
• Advise patient to report diarrhea, constipation, rash, or changes in respirations

### Evaluation
**Positive therapeutic outcome**
• Absence of nausea, vomiting during cancer chemotherapy

---

## guaifenesin (Rx, OTC)
(gwye-fen′e-sin)
All Fen Jr., Altarussin, Benylin-E ♣, Calmylin Expectorant ♣, Diabetic Tussin, Ganidin NR, guaifenesin, Guaifenesin NR, Guiatuss, Hytuss, Hytuss 2X, Mucinex, Naldecon Senior EX, Organidin NR, Pneumomist, Respa-GF, Resyl ♣, Robitussin, Scot-Tussin Expectorant, Siltussin DAS, Siltussin SA
*Func. class.:* Expectorant

**Pregnancy category C**

---

**Action:** Increases the volume and reduces the viscosity of secretions in the trachea and bronchi to facilitate secretion removal

**Therapeutic outcome:** Decreased cough

**Uses:** Productive and nonproductive cough

### Dosage and routes
**Adult and child ≥12 yr:** PO 200-400 mg q4hr, or EXT REL 600-1200 mg q12hr; max 2.4 g/day
**Child 6-12 yr:** PO 100-200 mg q4hr or EXT REL 600 mg q12hr; max 1.2 g/day
**Child 2-6 yr:** PO: 50-100 mg q4hr; max 600 mg/day
**Child 6 mo-<2 yr:** PO 25-50 mg q4hr, max 300 mg/day, individualized or 12 mg/kg/day in 6 divided doses

**Available forms:** Tabs 100, 200, 400 mg; ext rel tabs 600, 1200 mg; caps 200 mg; syr 100 mg/5 ml; oral sol 100, 200 mg/5 ml

### Adverse effects
**CNS:** Drowsiness, headache, dizziness
**GI:** Nausea, anorexia, vomiting

**Contraindications:** Hypersensitivity, chronic persistent cough

**Precautions:** Pregnancy **C**, breastfeeding, CHF, asthma, emphysema

---

◆ Alert    ♣ Canada Only    🔵 Drug on CD    * "Tall Man" lettering (See Preface)

## Pharmacokinetics

| Absorption | Well absorbed |
|---|---|
| Distribution | Unknown |
| Metabolism | Unknown |
| Excretion | Unknown |
| Half-life | 1 hr |

## Pharmacodynamics

| | PO | PO–EXT REL |
|---|---|---|
| Onset | ½ hr | Unknown |
| Peak | Unknown | Unknown |
| Duration | 4-6 hr | 12 hr |

## NURSING CONSIDERATIONS
### Assessment
• Assess cough: type, frequency, character, including characteristics of sputum; lung sounds bilaterally; fluids should be increased to 2 L/day to decrease secretion viscosity (thickness)

### Nursing diagnoses
• Airway clearance, ineffective (uses)
• Knowledge, deficient (teaching)

### Implementation
• Store at room temperature; provide room humidification to assist with liquefying secretions
• Avoid fluids for ½ hr after administration

### Patient/family education
• Caution patient to avoid driving, other hazardous activities if drowsiness occurs (rare)
• Advise patient to avoid smoking, smoke-filled rooms, perfumes, dust, environmental pollutants, cleansers
• Instruct patient to notify prescriber if dry, nonproductive cough lasts over 7 days

### Evaluation
**Positive therapeutic outcome**
• Absence of dry cough
• Thinner, more productive cough that raises secretions

## halcinonide topical
*See Appendix D*

---

# haloperidol (Rx)
(hal-oh-pehr'ih-dol)
Apo-Haloperidol ✦, Haldol, Novo-Peridol ✦, Peridol ✦
## haloperidol decanoate (Rx)
Haldol Decanoate, Haldol LA ✦
## haloperidol lactate (Rx)
Haldol, Haldol Concentrate, Haloperidol Intensol
*Func. class.:* Antipsychotic/neuroleptic
*Chem. class.:* Butyrophenone
**Pregnancy category C**

**Do not confuse:**
haloperidol/Halotestin, Haldol/Stadol

**Action:** Depresses cerebral cortex, hypothalamus, limbic system, which control activity and aggression; blocks neurotransmission produced by dopamine at synapse; exhibits strong α-adrenergic, anticholinergic blocking action; mechanism for antipsychotic effects unclear

**Therapeutic outcome:** Decreased signs and symptoms of psychosis

**Uses:** Psychotic disorders, control of tics, vocal utterances in Gilles de la Tourette syndrome, short-term treatment of hyperactive children showing excessive motor activity, prolonged parenteral therapy in chronic schizophrenia, organic mental syndrome with psychotic features, hiccups (short-term), emergency sedation of severely agitated or delirious patients

**Unlabeled uses:** Nausea, vomiting in surgery, autism, migraine headache

### Dosage and routes
*Psychosis*
*Adult:* PO 0.5-5 mg bid or tid initially depending on severity of condition; increase to desired dosage, max 100 mg/day; IM (lactate) 2-5 mg q4-8hr or bid-tid
*Geriatric:* 0.25-0.5 mg daily-bid, titrate q3-4 days by 0.25-0.5 mg/dose
*Child 3-12 yr:* PO/IM (lactate) 0.05-0.15 mg/kg/day

*Decanoate*
*Adult:* Initial dose IM is 10-15 mg × daily oral dose at 4-wk interval; do not administer **IV**; not to exceed 100 mg

*Chronic schizophrenia*
*Adult:* IM 50-100 mg q4 wk (decanoate)
*Child 3-12 yr:* PO/IM 0.05-0.15 mg/kg/day

### Tics/vocal utterances
**Adult:** PO 0.5-5 mg bid or tid, increased until desired response occurs
**Child 3-12 yr:** PO 0.05-0.075 mg/kg/day

### Hyperactive children
**Child 3-12 yr:** PO 0.05-0.075 mg/kg/day

**Available forms:** Tabs 0.5, 1, 2, 5, 10, 20 mg; lactate: conc 2 mg/ml; inj 5 mg/ml; decanoate: 50, 100 mg/ml

### Adverse effects
*CNS: EPS, pseudoparkinsonism, akathisia, dystonia, tardive dyskinesia, drowsiness, headache,* **seizures, neuroleptic malignant syndrome,** confusion
*CV: Orthostatic hypotension,* hypertension, **cardiac arrest,** ECG changes, **tachycardia, QT prolongation, sudden death**
*EENT:* Blurred vision, glaucoma, dry eyes
*GI: Dry mouth, nausea, vomiting, anorexia, constipation,* diarrhea, jaundice, weight gain, **ileus, hepatitis**
*GU:* Urinary retention, urinary frequency, dysuria, enuresis, impotence, amenorrhea, gynecomastia
*INTEG: Rash,* photosensitivity, dermatitis
*RESP:* **Laryngospasm,** dyspnea, **respiratory depression**

**Contraindications:** Children <3 yr, hypersensitivity, blood dyscrasias, coma, brain damage, bone marrow depression, alcohol and barbiturate withdrawal states, Parkinson's disease, angina, epilepsy, urinary retention, angle-closure glaucoma

**Precautions:** Pregnancy **C**, breastfeeding, geriatric, seizure disorders, hypertension, hepatic/cardiac/pulmonary disease

### Pharmacokinetics

| | |
|---|---|
| **Absorption** | Well absorbed (PO, IM); decanoate (IM) absorbed slowly |
| **Distribution** | High concentrations in liver, crosses placenta, protein binding 92% |
| **Metabolism** | Liver, extensively |
| **Excretion** | Kidneys, breast milk |
| **Half-life** | 21-24 hr |

### Pharmacodynamics

| | PO | IM | IM (decanoate) |
|---|---|---|---|
| **Onset** | Erratic | ½ hr | 3-9 days |
| **Peak** | 2-6 hr | 30-45 min | 4-11 days |
| **Duration** | 8-12 hr | 4-8 hr | 3 wk |

### Interactions
### Individual drugs
Alcohol: increased effects of both products, oversedation
Carbamazepine: decreased effects of haloperidol
EpINEPHrine: increased toxicity
Levodopa: decreased effects of levodopa
Lithium: increased toxicity; decreased effects of lithium
Phenobarbital: decreased effects of haloperidol

### Drug classifications
Anticholinergics: increased anticholinergic effects
Barbiturate anesthetics: oversedation
β-Adrenergic blockers: increased effects of both products
CNS depressants: oversedation

### Drug/herb
Chamomile, cola tree, hops, kava, nettle, nutmeg, skullcap, valerian: increased action
Betel palm, kava: increased EPS
Jimsonweed, scopolia: antagonist action

### Drug/lab test
Increased: liver function tests, cardiac enzymes, cholesterol, blood glucose, prolactin, bilirubin, PBI, cholinesterase, alkaline phosphatase
Decreased: hormones (blood and urine), protime
False positive: pregnancy tests, PKU
False negative: urinary steroids

## NURSING CONSIDERATIONS
### Assessment
• Assess mental status: orientation, mood, behavior, presence and type of hallucinations before initial administration and monthly; this product should significantly reduce psychotic behavior
• Check for swallowing of PO medication; check for hoarding or giving of medication to other patients
• Monitor I&O ratio; palpate bladder if low urinary output occurs, especially in geriatric; urinalysis is recommended before, during prolonged therapy
• Monitor bilirubin, CBC, liver function tests monthly
• Assess affect, orientation, LOC, reflexes, gait, coordination, sleep pattern disturbances
• Monitor B/P with patient sitting, standing, and lying; take pulse and respirations q4hr during initial treatment; establish baseline before starting treatment; report drops of 30 mm Hg; obtain baseline ECG, Q-wave and T-wave changes

---

- Check for dizziness, faintness, palpitations, tachycardia on rising; severe orthostatic hypotension is common
- Assess for neuroleptic malignant syndrome: hyperpyrexia, muscle rigidity, increased CPK, altered mental status; product should be discontinued immediately; if seizures, hypo/hypertension, tachycardia occur, notify prescriber immediately
- Assess for EPS including akathisia (inability to sit still, no pattern to movements), tardive dyskinesia (bizarre movements of the jaw, mouth, tongue, extremities), pseudoparkinsonism (ragged tremors, pill rolling, shuffling gate); an antiparkinsonian product should be prescribed
- Assess for constipation and urinary retention daily; if these occur, increase bulk, water in diet

### Nursing diagnoses
- Coping, ineffective (uses)
- Knowledge, deficient (teaching)
- Noncompliance (teaching)
- Thought processes, disturbed (uses)

### Implementation
**PO route**
- Give product in liquid form mixed in glass of juice or caffeine-free cola if hoarding is suspected; do not mix in caffeine drinks, tannics, pectins
- Give decreased dosage in geriatric because of slower metabolism
- Give PO with full glass of water, milk; or give with food to decrease GI upset
- Give antacids 2 hr before or after this product
- Store in tight, light-resistant container, oral sol in amber bottle

**IM route**
- Inject in deep muscle mass, do not give SUBCUT; use 21G 2-in needle; do not administer sol with a precipitate; give <3 ml per inj site; give slowly, may be painful
- Patient should remain lying down after IM inj for at least 30 min

**IV route**
- Give undiluted for psychotic episode at 5 mg/min
- Give by intermittent inf after dilution in 30-50 ml of $D_5W$, run over ½ hr

***Syringe compatibilities:*** Hydromorphone, sufentanil

***Y-site compatibilities:*** Amifostine, amsacrine, aztreonam, cimetidine, cisatracurium, cladribine, DOBUTamine, DOPamine, DOXOrubicin liposome, famotidine, filgrastim, fludarabine, granisetron, lidocaine, lorazepam, melphalan, midazolam, nitroglycerin, norepinephrine, ondansetron, paclitaxel, phenylephrine, propofol, remifentanil, sufentanil, tacrolimus, teniposide, theophylline, thiotepa, vinorelbine

***Y-site incompatibilities:*** Fluconazole, foscarnet, heparin, sargramostim

### Patient/family education
- Teach patient to use good oral hygiene; use frequent rinsing of mouth, sugarless gum for dry mouth; oral candidiasis may occur
- Advise patient to avoid hazardous activities until product response is determined; dizziness, blurred vision are common
- Inform patient that orthostatic hypotension occurs often and to rise from sitting or lying position gradually; tell patient to avoid hot tubs, hot showers, tub baths, since hypotension may occur; tell patient that in hot weather heat stroke may occur; take extra precautions to stay cool
- Instruct patient to avoid abrupt withdrawal of this product, or EPS may result; product should be withdrawn slowly
- Caution patient to avoid OTC preparations (cough, hay fever, cold) unless approved by prescriber, since serious product interactions may occur; avoid use with alcohol, CNS depressants since increased drowsiness may occur
- Advise patient to use a sunscreen and sunglasses to prevent burns
- Instruct patient to take antacids 2 hr before or after this product
- Tell patient to report sore throat, malaise, fever, bleeding, mouth sores; if these occur, CBC should be obtained and product discontinued

### Evaluation
**Positive therapeutic outcome**
- Decrease in emotional excitement, hallucinations, delusions, paranoia, reorganization of patterns of thought, speech; improvement in specific behaviors

**Treatment of overdose:** Lavage if orally ingested; provide airway; *do not induce vomiting*

## ! HIGH ALERT

**heparin** �*/* (Rx)
(hep'a-rin)
Calcilean 🍁, Calciparine, Hepalean 🍁,
heparin sodium, Heparin Leo 🍁, Hep-
Lock, Hep-Lock U/P
*Func. class.:* Anticoagulant, antithrombotic

### Pregnancy category C

### Do not confuse:
heparin/Hespan

**Action:** Prevents conversion of fibrinogen to
fibrin and prothrombin to thrombin by enhancing inhibitory effects of antithrombin III

**Therapeutic outcome:** Prevention of
thrombi

**Uses:** Prevention of deep vein thrombosis
(DVT) and pulmonary emboli (PE) (treatment
and prevention), MI, open heart surgery,
disseminated intravascular clotting syndrome,
atrial fibrillation with embolization, as an
anticoagulant in transfusion and dialysis
procedures, prevention of DVT/PE, to maintain
patency of indwelling venipuncture devices,
diagnosis, treatment of disseminated intravascular coagulation (DIC)

### Dosage and routes
*Deep vein thrombosis/MI*
**Adult:** **IV** BOL 5000-7000 units q4hr then
titrated to PTT or ACT level; **IV** INF after BOL
dose, then 1000 units/hr titrated to PTT or ACT
level
**Child:** **IV** INF 50 units/kg, maintenance 100
units/kg q4hr or 20,000 units/m² daily

*Anticoagulation*
**Adult:** SUBCUT 5000 units **IV** then 10,000-
20,000 units, then 8,000-10,000 units q8hr or
15,000-20,000 units q12hr; intermittent **IV**
BOL 10,000 units, then 5000-10,000 units
q4-6hr; CONT **IV** INF 5000 units (35-70
units/kg), then 20,000-40,000 units given over
24 hr
**Child >1 yr:** Intermittent **IV** BOL 50-100
units/kg, then 50-100 units/kg q4hr; CONT INF
75 units/kg, then 20 units/kg/hr, adjust to
maintain aPTT at 60-85 sec
**Neonates, infants <1 yr:** CONT **IV** INF
75 units/kg, then 28 units/kg/hr, adjust to
maintain aPTT at 60-85 sec

*Cardiovascular surgery*
**Adult:** **IV** INF 150-300 units/kg
**Child, infants, neonates:** IA 100
units/kg in artery prior to cardiac catheter

*Prophylaxis for DVT/PE*
**Adult:** SUBCUT 5000 units q8-12hr
*Heparin flush*
**Adult and child:** **IV** 10-100 units/ml
*Arterial line patency*
**Neonates:** IA 0.5-2 units/ml

**Available forms:** Sol for inj 10, 100,
1000, 5000, 7500, 10,000, 20,000, 40,000
units/ml; premixed 1000 units/500 ml, 2000
units/1000 ml, 12,500 units/250 ml, 25,000
units/250 ml, 25,000 units/500 ml; lock flush
preparations 10 units/ml

### Adverse effects
*CNS: Fever,* chills, headache
*GU:* **Hematuria**
*HEMA:* **Hemorrhage, thrombocytopenia,
anemia**
*INTEG: Rash,* dermatitis, urticaria, pruritus,
delayed transient alopecia, hematoma, cutane-
ous necrosis (SUBCUT)
*SYST:* **Anaphylaxis**

**Contraindications:** Hypersensitivity,
hemophilia, leukemia with bleeding, peptic
ulcer disease, severe thrombocytopenic
purpura, renal/hepatic disease (severe), blood
dyscrasias, severe hypertension, subacute
bacterial endocarditis, acute nephritis

**Precautions:** Pregnancy **C,** children,
geriatric, alcoholism, hyperlipidemia, diabetes,
renal disease

### Pharmacokinetics
| | |
|---|---|
| **Absorption** | Well absorbed (SUBCUT) |
| **Distribution** | Unknown |
| **Metabolism** | Partially in kidney, liver |
| **Excretion** | Lymph, spleen, in urine (<50% unchanged) |
| **Half-life** | 1½ hr |

### Pharmacodynamics
| | SUBCUT | IV |
|---|---|---|
| **Onset** | ½-1 hr | 5 min |
| **Peak** | 2 hr | 10 min |
| **Duration** | 8-12 hr | 2-6 hr |

### Interactions
*Individual drugs*
Dextran, dipyridole, ticlopidine: increased
  action of heparin
Diazepam: increased action of diazepam
Digoxin: decreased action of heparin
Streptokinase: resistance to heparin

## Drug classifications
Anticoagulants (oral), cephalosporins, NSAIDs, penicillins, platelet inhibitors, salicylates: increased action of heparin

Antihistamines, tetracyclines: decreased action of heparin

Corticosteroids: decreased action of corticosteroids

## Drug/herb
Agrimony, alfalfa, angelica, anise, basil, bay, bilberry, black haw, bogbean, bromelain, buchu, chondroitin, cinchona bark, dong quai, fenugreek, feverfew, garlic, ginger, ginkgo, ginseng, horse chestnut, Irish moss, kelp, kelpware, khella, lovage, lungwort, meadowsweet, motherwort, mugwort, nettle, papaya, parsley (large amounts), pau d'arco, pineapple, poplar, prickly ash, safflower, saw palmetto, tonka bean, turmeric, wintergreen, yarrow: increased risk of bleeding

Coenzyme Q10, flax, glucomannan, goldenseal, guar gum: decreased anticoagulant effect

## Drug/lab test
Increased: ALT, AST, INR, pro-time, PTT, potassium

Decreased: platelets, triglycerides, cholesterol, plasma free fatty acids

## NURSING CONSIDERATIONS
### Assessment
• Assess for blood studies (Hct, occult blood in stools) q3 mo if patient is on long-term therapy

• Monitor PPT, which should be 1½-2 × control, PTT; often done daily, APTT, ACT

• Monitor platelet count q2-3 days; thrombocytopenia may occur on fourth day of treatment and resolve, or continue to eighth day of treatment

◆ Assess for bleeding gums, petechiae, ecchymosis, black tarry stools, hematuria, epistaxis, decrease in Hct, B/P; may indicate bleeding and possible hemorrhage; notify prescriber immediately; HIT may occur after product discontinuation

• Monitor for hypersensitivity: fever, skin rash, urticaria; notify prescriber immediately

### Nursing diagnoses
• Injury, risk for (uses, adverse reactions)
• Knowledge, deficient (teaching)
• Tissue perfusion, ineffective (uses)

### Implementation
**SUBCUT route**
• Give SUBCUT with at least 25-G ⅜-in needle; do not massage area or aspirate fluid when giving SUBCUT inj; give in abdomen between pelvic bones, rotate sites; do not pull back on plunger, leave in for 10 sec; apply gentle pressure for 1 min

• Give at same time each day to maintain steady blood levels

• Changing needles is not recommended

**Heparin lock route**
• Do not mistake heparin sodium injection 10,000 units/ml and Hep-Lock U/P 10 units/ml; they have similar blue labeling

• Inject 10-100 units/0.5-1 ml after each inf or q8-12hr

**IV route**
• Cannot be used interchangeably (unit for unit) with LMWHs or heparinoids

• Give directly; **IV** loading dose over 1 min

• Give **IV** diluted in 0.9% NaCl, dextrose, Ringer's and by intermittent or cont inf; inf may run from 4-24 hr; use infusion pump

• When product is added to inf sol for cont **IV**, invert container at least 6× to ensure adequate mixing

*Syringe compatibilities:* Aminophylline, amphotericin B, ampicillin, atropine, azlocillin, bleomycin, cefamandole, cefazolin, cefoperazone, cefotaxime, cefoxitin, chloramphenicol, cimetidine, cisplatin, clindamycin, cyclophosphamide, diazoxide, digoxin, dimenhyDRINATE, DOBUTamine, DOPamine, epiNEPHrine, fentanyl, fluorouracil, furosemide, leucovorin, lidocaine, lincomycin, methotrexate, metoclopramide, mezlocillin, mitomycin, moxalactam, nafcillin, naloxone, neostigmine, nitroglycerin, norepinephrine, pancuronium, penicillin G, phenobarbital, piperacillin, sodium nitroprusside, succinylcholine, trimethoprim-sulfamethoxazole, verapamil, vinCRIStine

*Y-site compatibilities:* Acyclovir, aldesleukin, allopurinol, amifostine, aminophylline, ampicillin, ampicillin/sulbactam, atracurium, atropine, aztreonam, betamethasone, bleomycin, calcium gluconate, cefazolin, cefotetan, ceftazidime, ceftriaxone, cephalothin, cephapirin, chlordiazepoxide, chlorproMAZINE, cimetidine, cisplatin, cladribine, clindamycin, conjugated estrogens, cyanocobalamin, cyclophosphamide, cytarabine, dexamethasone, digoxin, diphenhydrAMINE, DOPamine, DOXOrubicin liposome, edrophonium, enalaprilat, epINEPHrine, erythromycin, esmolol, ethacrynate, famotidine, fentanyl, fluconazole, fludarabine, fluorouracil, foscarnet, furosemide, gallium, granisetron, hydrALAZINE, hydrocortisone, hydromorphone, regular insulin, isoproterenol, kanamycin, leucovorin, lidocaine, lorazepam, magnesium sulfate, melphalan, menadiol sodium, meperi-

H

dine, meropenem, methicillin, methotrexate, methoxamine, methyldopate, methylergonovine, metoclopramide, metronidazole, midazolam, milrinone, minocycline, mitomycin, morphine, nafcillin, neostigmine, nitroglycerin, nitroprusside, norepinephrine, ondansetron, oxacillin, oxytocin, paclitaxel, pancuronium, penicillin G potassium, pentazocine, phytonadione, piperacillin, piperacillin/ tazobactam, propofol, potassium chloride, prednisoLONE, procainamide, prochlorperazine, propofol, propranolol, pyridostigmine, ranitidine, remifentanil, sargramostim, scopolamine, sodium bicarbonate, streptokinase, succinylcholine, tacrolimus, teniposide, theophylline, thiopental, thiotepa, ticarcillin, ticarcillin/clavulanate, trimethobenzamide, vecuronium, vinBLAStine, vinorelbine, warfarin, zidovudine

*Y-site incompatibilities:* Alteplase, ciprofloxacin, dacarbazine, diazepam, DOBUTamine, DOXOrubicin, ergotamine, gentamicin, haloperidol, idarubicin, methotrimeprazine, phenytoin, promethazine, tobramycin, triflupromazine

*Additive compatibilities:* Aminophylline, amphotericin, ascorbic acid, bleomycin, calcium gluconate, cefepime, cephapirin, chloramphenicol, clindamycin, colistimethate, dimenhyDRINATE, doxacillin, DOPamine, enalaprilat, erythromycin, esmolol, floxacillin, fluconazole, flumazenil, furosemide, hydrocortisone, isoproterenol, lidocaine, lincomycin, magnesium sulfate, meropenem, methyldopate, methylPREDNISolone, metronidazole/ sodium bicarbonate, nafcillin, norepinephrine, octreotide, penicillin G, potassium chloride, prednisoLONE, promazine, ranitidine, sodium bicarbonate, verapamil, vit B complex, vit B complex with C

*Additive incompatibilities:* Amikacin, erythromycin lactobionate, gentamicin, kanamycin, meperidine, methadone, morphine, polymyxin B, streptomycin

### Patient/family education
• Advise patient to avoid OTC preparations that may cause serious product interactions unless directed by prescriber; may contain aspirin or other anticoagulants
• Tell patient that product may be held during active bleeding (menstruation), depending on condition
• Caution patient to use soft-bristle toothbrush to avoid bleeding gums; avoid contact sports; use electric razor; avoid IM inj
• Instruct patient to carry/wear emergency ID

or other identification identifying product taken and condition treated
• Advise patient to report any signs of bleeding: gums, under skin, urine, stools; or unusual bruising even after discontinuing product

### Evaluation
**Positive therapeutic outcome**
• Decrease of DVT
• PTT of 1.5-2.5 × control
• Free-flowing **IV**

**Treatment of overdose:** Withdraw product, give protamine sulfate 1 mg protamine/100 units heparin

## hepatitis B immune globulin (Rx)
(hep-a-tite′iss)
BayHep B, Nabi-HB
*Func. class.:* Immune globulin
**Pregnancy category** C

**Action:** Provides passive immunity to hepatitis B

**Therapeutic outcome:** Passive immunity to hepatitis B

**Uses:** Prevention of hepatitis B virus in exposed patients, including passive immunity in neonates born to HBsAg-positive mothers

### Dosage and routes
*Acute exposure to blood with HBsAg*
*Adult:* 2 doses, given after exposure and 1 mo later

*Perinatal exposure of infants born to HBsAg-positive mothers*
*Infant:* 1 dose at birth, then start hepatitis B vaccine series soon after birth

*Sexual exposure to HBsAg*
*Adult:* Administer 1 dose within 2 wk of exposure

**Available forms:** Sol for inj (Bay Hep B): 15%-18% protein; sol for inj (Nabi-HB): 5% ± 1% protein

### Adverse effects
*CNS:* Headache, dizziness, fever
*GI:* Nausea, vomiting
*INTEG:* Soreness at inj site, urticaria, erythema, swelling
*SYST:* Induration, **anaphylaxis, angioedema**

 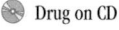

**Contraindications:** Hypersensitivity to immune globulins, coagulation disorders

**Precautions:** Pregnancy **C**, breastfeeding, children, geriatric, hemophilia, active infection, IgA deficiency

### Pharmacokinetics

| | |
|---|---|
| **Absorption** | Slowly absorbed |
| **Distribution** | Unknown |
| **Metabolism** | Unknown |
| **Excretion** | Unknown |
| **Half-life** | 3 wk |

### Pharmacodynamics

| | |
|---|---|
| **Onset** | 1-7 days |
| **Peak** | 3-10 days |
| **Duration** | 2-6 mo |

### Interactions
#### Drug classifications

MMR, varicella, rotavirus vaccines: do not use within 3 mo of hepatitis B immune globulin

### NURSING CONSIDERATIONS
#### Assessment

• Assess for history of allergies, skin conditions (eczema, psoriasis, dermatitis), reactions to vaccinations

• Assess for skin reactions: rash, induration, urticaria

• Assess for sneezing, pruritus, angioedema, dysphagia, vomiting, abdominal pain

◆ Assess for anaphylaxis: inability to breathe, bronchospasm, hypotension, wheezing, diaphoresis, fever, flushing; epINEPHrine and emergency equipment should be available

#### Nursing diagnoses

• Infection, risk for (uses)
• Knowledge, deficient (teaching)

#### Implementation

• Give after rotating vial; do not shake
• Give in deltoid (adult) or anterolateral thigh for better protection; give 2-ml dose in two different sites; do not give **IV**
• Refrigerate unused portion; sol should be clear, light amber, and thick

#### Patient/family education

• Teach patient purpose of medication and expected results
• Give patient a list of adverse reactions that need to be reported immediately: wheezing, vomiting, sneezing, abdominal pain, sweating, tightness in chest
• Advise patient that pain, rash, swelling at inj site can be expected
• Give patient written record of immunization

### Evaluation
#### Positive therapeutic outcome
• Prevention of hepatitis B

---

### homatropine ophthalmic
*See Appendix D*

---

### *hydrALAZINE (Rx)
(hye-dral'a-zeen)
Apresoline, Novo-Hylazin ✦, hydrALAZINE HCl
*Func. class.:* Antihypertensive, direct-acting peripheral vasodilator
*Chem. class.:* Phthalazine
### Pregnancy category  C

**Do not confuse:**
hydrALAZINE/hydrOXYzine, Apresoline/allopurinol

**Action:** Vasodilates arterioles in smooth muscle by direct relaxation; reduces B/P with reflex increases in heart rate, stroke volume, cardiac output

**Therapeutic outcome:** Decreased B/P in hypertension, decreased afterload in CHF

**Uses:** Essential hypertension, severe essential hypertension

**Unlabeled uses:** CHF

### Dosage and routes
#### Hypertension
*Adult:* PO 10 mg qid 2-4 days, then 25 mg for rest of 1st wk, then 50 mg qid individualized to desired response, not to exceed 300 mg/day
*Child:* PO 0.75-3 mg/kg/day in 4 divided doses; max 7.5 mg/kg/24 hr

#### Hypertensive crisis
*Adult:* **IV** BOL 20-40 mg q4-6hr; administer PO as soon as possible; IM 20-40 mg q4-6hr
*Child:* **IV** BOL 0.1-0.6 mg/kg q4-6hr; IM 0.1-0.6 mg/kg q4-6hr

#### CHF
*Adult:* PO 10-25 mg bid, max 75 mg tid

**Available forms:** Inj 20 mg/ml; tabs 10, 25, 50, 100 mg

### Adverse effects
*CNS: Headache, tremors, dizziness, anxiety,* peripheral neuritis, depression, fever, chills
*CV: Palpitations, reflex tachycardia, angina,* **shock,** rebound hypertension
*GI: Nausea, vomiting, anorexia, diarrhea,* constipation, paralytic ileus

H

---

Adverse effects: *italic* = common, **bold** = life-threatening

*GU:* Urinary retention
*HEMA:* **Leukopenia, agranulocytosis,** anemia, **thrombocytopenia**
*INTEG:* Rash, pruritus, urticaria
*MISC:* Nasal congestion, muscle cramps, *lupuslike symptoms,* flushing, edema, dyspnea

**Contraindications:** Hypersensitivity to hydrALAZINEs, mitral valvular rheumatic heart disease, dissecting aortic aneurysm

**Precautions:** Pregnancy **C**, breastfeeding, geriatric, CVA, advanced renal disease, CAD, liver disease, SLE

### Pharmacokinetics

| | |
|---|---|
| **Absorption** | Rapidly absorbed (PO); well absorbed (IM); completely absorbed (**IV**) |
| **Distribution** | Widely distributed; crosses placenta |
| **Metabolism** | GI mucosa, liver extensively |
| **Excretion** | Kidneys, urine (12%-14%) |
| **Half-life** | 2-8 hr |

### Pharmacodynamics

| | PO | IM | IV |
|---|---|---|---|
| **Onset** | ½ hr | 10-30 min | 5-20 min |
| **Peak** | 1-2 hr | 1 hr | 10-80 min |
| **Duration** | 6-12 hr | 4-6 hr | 4-6 hr |

### Interactions
*Individual drugs*
Alcohol: increased hypotension
Indomethacin: decreased effects of hydrALAZINE

*Drug classifications*
MAOIs: severe hypotension
β-Adrenergic blockers: increased effects
Other antihypertensives: increased hypertension
Sympathomimetics (epINEPHrine, norepinephrine): increased tachycardia, angina

*Drug/herb*
Aconite: increased toxicity, death
Astragalus, cola tree: increased or decreased antihypertensive effect
Barberry, betony, black catechu, black cohosh, bloodroot, broom, burdock, cat's claw, dandelion, goldenseal, Irish moss, Jamaican dogwood, kelp, khella, mistletoe, parsley: increased antihypertensive effect
Coltsfoot, guarana, khat, licorice: decreased antihypertensive effect

### NURSING CONSIDERATIONS
#### Assessment
• Assess B/P q5 min for 2 hr, then q1hr for 2 hr, then q4hr; pulse, jugular venous distention q4hr
• Monitor electrolytes, blood studies: potassium, sodium, chloride, carbon dioxide, CBC, serum glucose; LE prep, ANA titer before starting treatment
• Monitor weight daily, I&O; edema in feet, legs daily; check skin turgor, dryness of mucous membranes for hydration status
• Assess for crackles, dyspnea, orthopnea; peripheral edema, fatigue, weight gain, jugular vein distention (CHF)
• For fever, joint pain, rash, sore throat (lupuslike symptoms), notify prescriber

#### Nursing diagnoses
• Cardiac output, decreased (adverse reactions)
• Injury, risk for (side effects)
• Knowledge, deficient (teaching)

#### Implementation
**PO route**
• Give with meals to enhance absorption
• Store protected from light and heat
**IV route**
• Give by **IV** undiluted through Y-tube or 3-way stopcock, give each 10 mg over 1 min or more
• Administer with patient in recumbent position; keep in that position for 1 hr after administration
*Y-site compatibilities:* Heparin, hydrocortisone, potassium chloride, verapamil, vit B/C
*Y-site incompatibilities:* Aminophylline, ampicillin, diazoxide, furosemide, paclitaxel
*Additive incompatibilities:* Aminophylline, ampicillin, chlorothiazide, edetate calcium disodium, ethacrynate, hydrocortisone, melphalan, mephentermine, methohexital, nitroglycerin, phenobarbital, verapamil, vinorelbine
*Additive compatibilities:* DOBUTamine

#### Patient/family education
• Teach patient to take with food to increase bioavailability (PO)
• Teach patient to avoid OTC preparations unless directed by prescriber
• Advise patient to notify prescriber if chest pain, severe fatigue, fever, muscle or joint pain occur
• Advise patient to rise slowly to prevent orthostatic hypertension

- Advise patient to notify prescriber if pregnancy is suspected

## Evaluation
### Positive therapeutic outcome
- Decreased B/P in hypertension

**Treatment of overdose:** Administer vasopressors, volume expanders for shock; PO, lavage or give activated charcoal, digitalization

## hydrochlorothiazide
(Rx)

(hye-droe-klor-oh-thye'a-zide)
Apo-Hydrol ✣, Esidrix, HCTZ, Hydro-Chlor, hydrochlorothiazide, Hydro-D, HydroDIURIL, Microzide, Neo-Codema ✣, Novohydrazide ✣, Oretic, Urozide ✣
*Func. class:* Diuretic, antihypertensive
*Chem. class:* Thiazide, sulfonamide derivative

### Pregnancy category B

**Action:** Acts on the distal tubule in the kidney, increasing excretion of sodium, water, chloride, magnesium, potassium, and bicarbonate

**Therapeutic outcome:** Decreased B/P, decreased edema in lung tissues peripherally

**Uses:** Edema in CHF, nephrotic syndrome; edema in corticosteroid, estrogen, NSAID therapy; idiopathic lower extremity edema; may be used alone or as adjunct with antihypertensives

### Dosage and routes
*Adult:* PO 12.5-100 mg/day
*Geriatric:* PO 12.5 mg/day, initially
*Child >6 mo:* PO 2 mg/kg/day in divided doses
*Child <6 mo:* PO Up to 4 mg/kg/day in divided doses

**Available forms:** Tabs 25, 50, 100 mg; caps 12.5 mg; oral sol 10 mg/5 ml, 100 mg/ml

### Adverse effects
*CNS:* Drowsiness, paresthesia, depression, headache, *dizziness, fatigue, weakness,* fever
*CV:* Irregular pulse, orthostatic hypotension, palpitations, volume depletion, allergic myocarditis
*EENT:* Blurred vision
*ELECT: Hypokalemia,* hypercalcemia, hyponatremia, hypochloremia, hypomagnesemia
*GI: Nausea, vomiting, anorexia,* constipation, diarrhea, cramps, pancreatitis, GI irritation, **hepatitis**

*GU: Frequency,* polyuria, **uremia,** glucosuria, hyperuricemia
***HEMA:* Aplastic anemia, hemolytic anemia, leukopenia, agranulocytosis, thrombocytopenia, neutropenia**
*INTEG: Rash,* urticaria, purpura, photosensitivity, alopecia, erythema multiforme
*META: Hyperglycemia, hyperuricemia,* increased creatinine, BUN

**Contraindications:** Hypersensitivity to thiazides or sulfonamides, anuria, renal decompensation, hypomagnesemia

**Precautions:** Pregnancy **B,** breastfeeding, hypokalemia, renal/hepatic disease, gout, COPD, lupus erythematosus, diabetes mellitus, hyperlipidemia, CCr <25 ml/min

### Pharmacokinetics
| | |
|---|---|
| **Absorption** | Variable |
| **Distribution** | Extracellular spaces; crosses placenta |
| **Metabolism** | Excreted unchanged in urine |
| **Excretion** | Breast milk |
| **Half-life** | 6-15 hr |

### Pharmacodynamics
| | |
|---|---|
| **Onset** | 2 hr |
| **Peak** | 4 hr |
| **Duration** | 6-12 hr |

## Interactions
### Individual drugs
Amphotericin B: increased hypokalemia
Cholestyramine, colestipol: decreased absorption of hydrochlorothiazide
Diazoxide: increased hyperglycemia, hyperuricemia, hypotension
Lithium: increased toxicity
### Drug classifications
Antidiabetics: decreased effect of antidiabetic agent
Cardiac glycosides, nondepolarizing skeletal muscle relaxants: increased toxicity
Diuretics (loop): increased effects of diuretic
Glucocorticoids: increased hypokalemia
NSAIDs: increased risk of renal failure
### Drug/herb
Aloe, buckthorn, cascara sagrada, Chinese rhubarb, gossypol, licorice, nettle, senna: increased hypokalemia
Cucumber, dandelion, ginkgo, horsetail, khella, licorice, nettle, pumpkin, Queen Anne's lace: increased effect
St. John's wort: severe photosensitivity

### Drug/lab test

Increased: retention, amylase, parathyroid test

## NURSING CONSIDERATIONS
### Assessment

- Monitor glucose in urine if patient is diabetic
- Assess improvement in CVP q8hr
- Check for rashes, temp elevation daily
- Assess for confusion, especially in geriatric; take safety precautions if needed
- Monitor manifestations of hypokalemia: acidic urine, reduced urine, osmolality, nocturia; hypotension, broad T wave, U wave, ectopy, tachycardia, weak pulse; muscle weakness, altered LOC, drowsiness, apathy, lethargy, confusion, depression; anorexia, nausea, cramps, constipation, distention, paralytic ileus; hypoventilation, respiratory muscle weakness
- Monitor for manifestations of hypo-magnesemia: agitation, muscle twitching, paresthesias, hyperactive reflexes, positive Babinski reflex, dysphagia, nystagmus, seizures, tetany; nausea, vomiting, diarrhea, anorexia, abdominal distention; ectopy, tachycardia, broad, flat, or inverted T waves, depressed ST segment, prolonged QT interval, decreased cardiac output, hypotension
- Monitor for manifestations of hyponatremia: increased B/P, cold, clammy skin, hypovolemia or hypervolemia; anorexia, nausea, vomiting, diarrhea, abdominal cramps; lethargy, increased ICP, confusion, headache, seizures, coma, fatigue, tremors, hyperreflexia
- Monitor for manifestations of hyper-chloremia: weakness, lethargy, coma, deep rapid breathing
- Assess fluid volume status: I&O ratios, record, count, or weigh diapers as appropriate; weight; distended red veins; crackles in lungs; color, quality, and specific gravity of urine; skin turgor; adequacy of pulses; moist mucous membranes; bilateral lung sounds; peripheral pitting edema; assess for dehydration: symptoms of decreasing output, thirst, hypotension; dry mouth and mucous membranes should be reported
- Monitor electrolytes: potassium, sodium, calcium, magnesium; also include BUN, blood pH, ABGs, uric acid, CBC, blood glucose, renal function
- Assess B/P before and during therapy with patient lying, standing, and sitting as appropriate; orthostatic hypotension can occur rapidly

### Nursing diagnoses

- Fluid volume, deficient (side effects)
- Fluid volume, excess (uses)
- Knowledge, deficient (teaching)
- Urinary elimination, impaired (side effects)

### Implementation

- Give in AM to avoid interference with sleep
- Provide potassium replacement if potassium level is ≤3.0 mg/dl; give whole tab or use oral sol lightly; product may be crushed if patient is unable to swallow
- Administer with food; if nausea occurs, absorption may be increased

### Patient/family education

- Teach patient to take the medication early in the day to prevent nocturia
- Instruct patient to take with food or milk if GI symptoms of nausea and anorexia occur
- Teach patient to maintain a weekly record of weight and notify prescriber of weight loss >5 lb
- Caution patient that this product causes a loss of potassium and that food rich in potassium should be added to the diet; refer to a dietitian for assistance in planning
- Caution patient to rise slowly from sitting or reclining positions, not to exercise in hot weather or stand for prolonged periods since orthostatic hypotension will be enhanced; lie down if dizziness occurs
- Teach patient not to use alcohol or any OTC medications without prescriber's approval; serious product reactions may occur
- Emphasize the need to contact prescriber immediately if muscle cramps, weakness, nausea, dizziness, or numbness occurs
- Teach patient to take own B/P and pulse and record findings
- Teach patient to continue taking medication even if feeling better; this product controls symptoms but does not cure the condition
- Advise patient with hypertension to continue other medical treatment (exercise, weight loss, relaxation techniques, cessation of smoking)

### Evaluation
**Positive therapeutic outcome**

- Decreased edema
- Decreased B/P
- Increased diuresis

### Treatment of overdose: 
Lavage if taken orally, monitor electrolytes, administer dextrose in saline, monitor hydration, CV, renal status

## hydrocodone (Rx)
(hye-droe-koe'done)
Hycodan ✤, Robidone ✤, Tussigon
## hydrocodone/ acetaminophen (Rx)
Anexsia, Bancap HC, Ceta-Plus, Co-Gesic, Dolacet, Dolagesic, Duocet, Hycomed, Hyco-Pap, Hydrocet, Hydrogesic, Lorcet, Lortab, Onset, Pancet, Panlor, Polygesic, Stagesic, T-Gesic, Ugesic, Vanacet, Vandone, Vicodin, Zydone
## hydrocodone/aspirin (Rx)
Alor, Azdone, Damason-P, Lortab ASA, Panasol
## hyprocodone/ibuprofen (Rx)
Vicoprofen
*Func. class.:* Antitussive opioid analgesic/ nonopioid analgesic

**Pregnancy category** C
**Controlled substance schedule** III

**Do not confuse:**
hydrocodone/hydrocortisone, Hycodan/ Vicodin

**Action:** Acts directly on cough center in medulla to suppress cough; binds to opiate receptors in the CNS to reduce pain

**Therapeutic outcome:** Pain relief, decreased cough, decreased diarrhea

**Uses:** Hyperactive and nonproductive cough, mild to moderate pain

**Dosages and routes**
*Analgesic*
*Adult:* PO 2.5-10 mg q3-6hr prn
*Child:* PO 0.15-0.2 mg/kg q3-6hr prn

*Antitussive*
*Adult:* PO 5 mg q4-6hr prn

**Available forms:** Hydrocodone: tabs 5 mg (Hycodan); syr 5 mg/ml (Hycodan, Robidone ✤; hydrocodone/acetaminophen: tabs 2.5 mg hydrocodone/500 mg acetamino-phen (Lortabs 2.5/500), 5 mg hydrocodone/ 400 mg acetaminophen (Zydone), 5 mg hydrocodone/500 mg acetaminophen (Anexsia 5/500, Co-Gesic, Dolacet, Hydrocet, Hydroge-sic, Hy-Phen, Loracet, Loratab 5/500, Maragesic-H, Panacet 5/500, Stagesic, T-Gesic, Vicodin); 7.5 mg hydrocodone/400 mg acet-aminophen (Zydone), 7.5 mg hydrocodone/ 500 mg acetaminophen (Loratab) 7.5/500, 7.5 mg hydrocodone/650 mg acetaminophen (Anexsia 7.5/650, Loracet Plus), 7.5 mg hydrocodone/750 mg acetaminophen (Vicodin ES), 10 mg hydrocodone/325 mg acetamino-phen (Norco), 10 mg hydrocodone/500 mg acetaminophen (Lortab 10/500), 10 mg hydrocodone/650 mg acetaminophen (Loracet 10/650, Vicodin HP), 10 mg hydrocodone/660 mg acetaminophen (Anexia 10/660); caps 5 mg hydrocodone/500 mg acetaminophen (Bancap-HC, Dolacet, Hydrocet, Hydrogesic, Loracet-HD, Maragesic-H, Stragesic, T-Gesic, Zydone); elixir or oral solution 2.5 mg hydrocodone/167 mg acetaminophen/5 ml; hydrocodone/aspirin: tabs 5 mg hydrocodone/ 500 mg aspirin (Alor 5/500, Azdone, Damason-P, Loratab ASA, Panasal 5/500); hydrocodone/ibuprofen: tabs 7.5 mg hydrocodone/200 mg ibuprofen (Vicoprofen)

**Adverse effects**
*CNS: Drowsiness,* dizziness, light-headedness, confusion, headache, sedation, euphoria, dysphoria, weakness, hallucinations, disorien-tation, mood changes, dependence, **seizures**
*CV:* Palpitations, tachycardia, bradycardia, change in B/P, **circulatory depression,** syncope
*EENT:* Tinnitus, blurred vision, miosis, diplopia
*GI: Nausea, vomiting, anorexia, constipa-tion,* cramps, dry mouth, ulcers
*GU:* Increased urinary output, dysuria, urinary retention
*INTEG:* Rash, urticaria, flushing, pruritus
*RESP:* **Respiratory depression**

**Contraindications:** Hypersensitivity, addiction (opioid)

**Precautions:** Pregnancy **C,** breastfeeding, addictive personality, increased ICP, MI (acute), severe heart disease, respiratory depression, renal/hepatic disease, bowel impaction, urinary retention

| Pharmacokinetics | |
|---|---|
| **Absorption** | Well absorbed |
| **Distribution** | Unknown; crosses placenta |
| **Metabolism** | Liver, extensively |
| **Excretion** | Kidneys |
| **Half-life** | 3½-4½ hr |

| Pharmacodynamics | | |
|---|---|---|
| | PO (analgesic) | PO (antitussive) |
| **Onset** | 10-20 min | Unknown |
| **Peak** | 30-60 min | Unknown |
| **Duration** | 4-6 hr | 4-6 hr |

**Interactions**
*Individual drugs*
Alcohol: increased CNS depression

H

### Drug classifications
Antidepressants (tricyclics), CNS depressants, general anesthetics, opioids, phenothiazines, sedative/hypnotics, skeletal muscle relaxants: increased CNS depression
### Drug/herb
Corkwood: increased anticholinergic effect
Jamacian dogwood, lavender, mistletoe, nettle, pokeweed, poppy, senega, valerian: increased CNS depression
### Drug/lab test
Increased: amylase, lipase

## NURSING CONSIDERATIONS
### Assessment
• Assess pain: intensity, type, location, duration, precipitating factor
• Monitor VS after parenteral route; note muscle rigidity; product history; liver; renal function tests; cough; and respiratory dysfunction: respiratory depression, character, rate, rhythm; notify prescriber if respirations are <10/min
• Monitor CNS changes: dizziness, drowsiness, hallucinations, euphoria, LOC, pupil reaction
• Monitor allergic reactions: rash, urticaria
• Obtain history of ulcers if using ibuprofen combination product

### Nursing diagnoses
• Breathing pattern, ineffective (adverse reactions)
• Knowledge, deficient (teaching)
• Pain, acute (uses)
• Sensory perception, disturbed: visual, auditory (adverse reactions)

### Implementation
• Do not break, crush, or chew tabs; only scored tabs can be broken
• Give with antiemetic if nausea, vomiting occur
• Give when pain is beginning to return; determine dosage interval by patient response; continuous dosing of medication is more effective given prn
• Medication should be slowly withdrawn after long-term use to prevent withdrawal symptoms
• Do not exceed 4 g acetaminophen with combination product
• Store in light-resistant container at room temperature
• May be given with food or milk to lessen GI upset

### Patient/family education
• Instruct patient to report any symptoms of CNS changes, allergic reactions; to avoid CNS depressants: alcohol, sedative/hypnotics for at least 24 hr after taking this product
• Teach patient that dizziness, drowsiness, and confusion are common and to avoid getting up without assistance, driving, or other hazardous activities
• Discuss in detail all aspects of the product

### Evaluation
**Positive therapeutic outcome**
• Decreased pain
• Decreased cough

**Treatment of overdose:** Naloxone HCl (Narcan) 0.2-0.8 **IV**, O$_2$, **IV** fluids, vasopressors

---

## hydrocortisone (Rx)
(hy-droh-kor'tih-sone)
Cortef, Cortenema, Hydrocortone
## hydrocortisone acetate (Rx)
Cortifoam, Hydrocortone Acetate
## hydrocortisone cypionate (Rx)
Cortef
## hydrocortisone sodium phosphate (Rx)
Hydrocortone Phosphate
## hydrocortisone sodium succinate (Rx)
A-hydroCort, Solu-Cortef
*Func. class.:* Short-acting glucocorticoid
*Chem. class.:* Natural nonfluorinated, group IV potency (valerate), group VI potency (acetate and plain)

### Pregnancy category C

**Do not confuse:**
hydrocortisone/hydrocodone

**Action:** Decreases inflammation by suppressing migration of polymorphonuclear leukocytes and fibroblasts and reversing increased capillary permeability and lysosomal stabilization (systemic); antipruritic, antiinflammatory (topical)

**Therapeutic outcome:** Decreased inflammation

**Uses:** Severe inflammation, septic shock, adrenal insufficiency, ulcerative colitis, collagen disorders (systemic), psoriasis, eczema, contact dermatitis, pruritus (topical)

---

## Dosage and routes
### Adrenal insufficiency/ inflammation
*Adult:* PO 5-30 mg bid-qid; IM/**IV** 100-250 mg (succinate), then 50-100 mg IM as needed; IM/**IV** 15-240 mg q12hr (phosphate)

### Shock
*Adult:* IM/**IV** 500 mg-2 g q2-6hr (succinate)
*Child:* IM/**IV** 0.186-1 mg/kg bid-tid (succinate)

### Colitis
*Adult:* Enema 100 mg nightly for 21 days

### Topical route
*Adult and child >2 yr:* Apply to affected area daily-qid

**Available forms:** Tabs 5, 10, 20 mg; inj 25, 50 mg/ml; acetate: inj 25 ✿, 50 mg/ml ✿, enema 10% aerosol foam, supp 25 mg; cypionate: oral susp 10 mg/5 ml; phosphate: inj 50 mg/ml; succinate: inj 100 mg ✿, 250 mg ✿, 500 mg ✿, 1000 mg/vial ✿

## Adverse effects
*CNS:* Depression, flushing, sweating, headache, mood changes
*CV:* Hypertension, **circulatory collapse, thrombophlebitis, embolism,** tachycardia, edema
*EENT:* Fungal infections, increased intraocular pressure, blurred vision
*GI:* Diarrhea, nausea, abdominal distention, **GI hemorrhage,** increased appetite, pancreatitis
*HEMA:* **Thrombocytopenia**
*INTEG:* Acne, poor wound healing, ecchymosis, petechiae
*MS:* Fractures, osteoporosis, weakness

**Contraindications:** Children <2 yr, psychosis, hypersensitivity, idiopathic thrombocytopenia (IM), acute glomerulonephritis, amebiasis, fungal infections, nonasthmatic bronchial disease, AIDS, TB, recent MI (associated with left-ventricular rupture)

**Precautions:** Pregnancy **C,** breastfeeding, diabetes mellitus, glaucoma, osteoporosis, seizure disorders, ulcerative colitis, CHF, myasthenia gravis, renal disease, esophagitis, peptic ulcer, metastatic carcinoma

### Pharmacokinetics
| | |
|---|---|
| **Absorption** | Well absorbed (PO); systemic (topical) |
| **Distribution** | Crosses placenta |
| **Metabolism** | Liver, extensively |
| **Excretion** | Kidney |
| **Half-life** | 3-5 hr, adrenal suppression 3-4 days |

### Pharmacodynamics
| | PO | IM | IV | TOPICAL |
|---|---|---|---|---|
| **Onset** | 1-2 hr | 20 min | Rapid | Min to hr |
| **Peak** | 1 hr | 4-8 hr | Unkn | Hr to days |
| **Duration** | 1½ days | 1½ days | 1½ days | Hr to days |

## Interactions
### Individual drugs
Alcohol, amphotericin B, cycloSPORINE, digoxin: increased side effects
Cholestyramine, colestipol, ePHEDrine, phenytoin, rifampin, theophylline: decreased action of hydrocortisone

### Drug classifications
Anticoagulants, calcium supplements, toxoids, vaccines: decreased action of anticoagulant
Anticonvulsants: decreased effects of anticonvulsant
Antidiabetics: decreased effects of antidiabetics
Barbiturates: decreased action of hydrocortisone
Diuretics: increased side effects
NSAIDs, salicylates: increased risk of GI bleeding

### Drug/herb
Aloe, buckthorn, cascara sagrada, cat's claw, Chinese rhubarb, echinacea, senna, St. John's wort: increased hyokalemia
Aloe, licorice, perilla: increased corticosteroid effect

### Drug/lab test
Increased: cholesterol, sodium, blood glucose, uric acid, calcium, urine glucose
Decreased: calcium, potassium, $T_4$, $T_3$, thyroid [131]I uptake test, urine 17-OHCS, 17-KS
False negative: skin allergy tests

## NURSING CONSIDERATIONS
### Assessment
• Monitor potassium, blood glucose, urine glucose while patient is on long-term therapy; hypokalemia and hyperglycemia may occur
• Monitor I&O ratio; be alert for decreasing urinary output and increasing edema; weigh daily; notify prescriber of weekly gain >5 lb or edema, hypertension, cardiac symptoms
• Monitor plasma cortisol levels during long-term therapy (normal level is 138-635 nmol/L when obtained at 8 AM); check adrenal

function periodically for hypothalamic-pituitary-adrenal axis suppression
• Assess for infection: increased temp, WBC even after withdrawal of medication; product masks infection symptoms; if fever develops, product should be discontinued
• Check for potassium depletion: paresthesias, fatigue, nausea, vomiting, depression, polyuria, dysrhythmias, weakness
• Assess mental status: affect, mood, behavioral changes, aggression
• Check nasal passages during long-term treatment for changes in mucus (nasal)
• Assess for systemic absorption: increased temp, inflammation, irritation (topical)

### Nursing diagnoses
• Infection, risk for (adverse reactions)
• Knowledge, deficient (teaching)
• Noncompliance (teaching) (topical/nasal preparation)

### Implementation
**PO route**
• Give with food or milk to decrease GI symptoms
**Rectal route**
• Use applicator provided
• Clean applicator after each use
**Topical route**
• Apply only to affected areas; do not get in eyes
• Cleanse and dry area before applying medication, then cover with occlusive dressing (only if prescribed); seal to normal skin; change q12hr; systemic absorption may occur; use only on dermatoses; do not use on weeping, denuded, or infected area
• Use for a few days after area has cleared
• Store at room temperature
**Nasal route**
• Patient should clear nasal passages before administration; use decongestant if needed; shake inhaler, invert, tilt head backward, insert nozzle into nostril, away from septum; hold other nostril closed and depress activator, inhale through nose, exhale through mouth
**IV route**
• Give only sodium phosphate product **IV**; reconstitute with sol provided; give 100 mg over >1 min
• May be given by intermittent inf in compatible sol
• Give titrated dose; use lowest effective dosage

### Sodium phosphate preparations
*Syringe compatibilities:* Fluconazole, fludarabine, metoclopramide

*Additive compatibilities:* Amikacin, amphotericin B, bleomycin, cephapirin, metaraminol, sodium bicarbonate, verapamil
*Y-site compatibilities:* Allopurinol, amifostine, aztreonam, cefepime, cladribine, famotidine, filgrastim, fluconazole, fludarabine, granisetron, melphalan, ondansetron, paclitaxel, piperacillin/tazobactam, teniposide, thiotepa, vinorelbine

### Sodium succinate preparations
*Syringe compatibilities:* Metoclopramide, thiopental
*Y-site compatibilities:* Acyclovir, allopurinol, amifostine, aminophylline, ampicillin, amphotericin B cholesteryl, inamrinone, amsacrine, atracurium, atropine, aztreonam, betamethasone, calcium gluconate, cefepime, cefmetazole, cephalothin, cephapirin, chlordiazepoxide, chlorproMAZINE, cisatracurium, cladribine, cyanocobalamin, cytarabine, dexamethasone, digoxin, diphenhydrAMINE, DOPamine, DOXOrubicin liposome, droperidol, edrophonium, enalaprilat, epINEPHrine, esmolol, conjugated estrogens, ethacrynate, famotidine, fentanyl, fentanyl/droperidol, filgrastim, fludarabine, fluorouracil, foscarnet, furosemide, gallium, granisetron, heparin, hydrALAZINE, regular insulin, isoproterenol, kanamycin, lidocaine, lorazepam, magnesium sulfate, melphalan, menadiol, meperidine, methicillin, methoxamine, methylergonovine, minocycline, morphine, neostigmine, norepinephrine, ondansetron, oxacillin, oxytocin, paclitaxel, pancuronium, penicillin G potassium, pentazocine, phytonadione, piperacillin/tazobactam, prednisoLONE, procainamide, prochlorperazine, propofol, propranolol, pyridostigmine, remifentanil, scopolamine, sodium bicarbonate, succinylcholine, tacrolimus, teniposide, theophylline, thiotepa, trimethaphan, trimethobenzamide, vecuronium, vinorelbine
*Y-site incompatibilities:* Diazepam, ergotamine tartrate, idarubicin, phenytoin, sargramostim
*Additive compatibilities:* Amikacin, aminophylline, amphotericin B, calcium chloride, calcium gluconate, cephalothin, cephapirin, chloramphenicol, clindamycin, cloxacillin, corticotropin, DAUNOrubicin, diphenhydrAMINE, DOPamine, erythromycin, floxacillin, lidocaine, magnesium sulfate, mephentermine, metronidazole/sodium bicarbonate, mitomycin, mitoxantrone, netilmicin, netilmicin/potassium chloride, norepinephrine, penicillin G potassium/sodium, piperacillin, polymyxin B, potassium

chloride, sodium bicarbonate, theophylline, thiopental, vancomycin, verapamil, vit B/C
*Additive incompatibilities:* Bleomycin, DOXOrubicin

## Patient/family education

- Teach patient all aspects of product usage, including cushingoid symptoms
- Advise patient to carry/wear emergency ID as steroid user; not to discontinue abruptly; adrenal crisis can result
- Instruct patient to notify prescriber if therapeutic response decreases; dosage adjustment may be needed
- Instruct patient to notify prescriber of signs of infection
- Teach patient that product can mask infections; hypoglycemia (diabetic)
- Teach patient to avoid live-virus vaccines if using steroids long term
- Caution patient to avoid OTC products unless directed by prescriber: salicylates, alcohol in cough products, cold preparations
- Teach patient symptoms of adrenal insufficiency: nausea, anorexia, fatigue, dizziness, dyspnea, weakness, joint pain, and when to notify prescriber
- Advise patient that long-term therapy may be needed to resolve infection (1-2 mo depending on type of infection)

**Nasal route**

- Instruct patient to clear nasal passages if sneezing attack occurs, then repeat dose; to continue using product even if mild nasal bleeding occurs; bleeding is usually transient
- Teach method of instillation after providing written instruction from manufacturer on instillation

## Evaluation

**Positive therapeutic outcome**

- Decrease in runny nose (nasal)
- Decreased inflammation
- Absence of severe itching, patches on skin, flaking (top)
- Decreased GI symptoms

---

## hydrocortisone topical
*See Appendix D*

---

## hydromorphone (Rx)
(hye-droe-mor'fone)
Dilaudid, Dilaudid-HP, Hydromorphone HCl, Hydrostat IR, PMS Hydromorphone
*Func. class.:* Antitussive, opioid analgesic agonist
*Chem. class.:* Phenanthrene derivative, guaifenesin

**Pregnancy category** C
**Controlled substance schedule** II

**Do not confuse:**
hydromorphone/meperidine/morphine,
Dilaudid/Demerol

**Action:** Inhibits ascending pain pathways in CNS, increases pain threshold, alters pain perception

**Therapeutic outcome:** Decreased cough, decreased pain

**Uses:** As an antitussive to suppress cough; moderate to severe pain

## Dosage and routes
*Antitussive*
*Adult:* PO 1 mg q3-4hr prn
*Child 6-12 yr:* PO 0.5 mg q3-4hr

*Analgesic*
*Adult:* PO 1-6 mg q4-6hr prn; SUBCUT/IM/**IV** 1-2 mg q4-6hr prn; may be increased; RECT 3 mg q4-6hr prn
*Geriatric:* PO 1-2 mg q4-6hr
*Child:* PO 0.03-0.08 mg/kg q4-6hr, max 5 mg/dose

**Available forms:** Inj 1, 2, 3, 4, 10 mg/ml; tabs 1, 2, 3, 4, 8 mg; oral sol 5 mg/5 ml; syr 1 mg/5 ml supp 3 mg

## Adverse effects
*CNS:* Dizziness, drowsiness, *sedation, confusion,* headache, euphoria, mood changes, **seizures**
*CV:* *Hypotension, bradycardia,* palpitations, change in B/P, tachycardia, peripheral vasodilation
*EENT:* Miosis, diplopia, blurred vision, tinnitus
*GI:* *Nausea, constipation, vomiting, anorexia,* dry mouth, cramps, paralytic ileus
*GU:* Increased urinary output, dysuria, urinary retention
*INTEG:* Urticaria, rash, flushing, bruising, diaphoresis, pruritus
***RESP:* Respiratory depression,** dyspnea

**Contraindications:** Hypersensitivity, opiate addiction

---

Adverse effects: *italic* = common, **bold** = life-threatening

**Precautions:** Pregnancy **C**, breastfeeding, children <18 yr, increased ICP, addictive personality, renal/hepatic disease, MI (acute), severe heart disease, respiratory depression, bowel impaction

### Pharmacokinetics

| | |
|---|---|
| **Absorption** | Well absorbed (PO), complete (**IV**) |
| **Distribution** | Unknown; crosses placenta |
| **Metabolism** | Liver, extensively |
| **Excretion** | Kidneys |
| **Half-life** | 2-3 hr |

### Pharmacodynamics

| | PO/IM/SUBCUT | IV | RECT |
|---|---|---|---|
| **Onset** | 15-30 min | 10-15 min | 15-30 min |
| **Peak** | 30-60 min | 15-30 min | 30-90 min |
| **Duration** | 4-5 hr | 2-3 hr | 4-5 hr |

### Interactions
#### Individual drugs
Alcohol: increased respiratory depression, hypotension, sedation
#### Drug classifications
Antipsychotics, opiates, sedative/hypnotics, skeletal muscle relaxants: increased effects
#### Drug/herb
Chamomile, hops, Jamaican dogwood, kava, lavender, mistletoe, nettle, pokeweed, poppy, senega, skullcap, St. John's wort, valerian: increased action
Corkwood: increased anticholinergic effect
#### Drug/lab test
Increased: amylase

### NURSING CONSIDERATIONS
#### Assessment
• Assess pain control, sedation by scoring on 0-10 scale, around-the-clock dosing is best for pain control
• Monitor VS after parenteral route; note muscle rigidity; product history, renal, liver function tests; respiratory dysfunction: respiratory depression, character, rate, rhythm; notify prescriber if respirations are <10/min
• Monitor CNS changes: dizziness, drowsiness, hallucinations, euphoria, LOC, pupil reaction
• Monitor allergic reactions: rash, urticaria; bowel function, constipation

#### Nursing diagnoses
• Breathing pattern, ineffective (adverse reactions)
• Knowledge, deficient (teaching)
• Pain, acute (uses)
• Sensory perception, disturbed: visual, auditory (adverse reactions)

### Implementation
• Give with antiemetic if nausea, vomiting occur
• Give when pain is beginning to return; determine dosage interval by patient response; continuous dosing of medication is more effective given prn; explain analgesic effect
• Withdraw medication slowly after long-term use to prevent withdrawal symptoms
• Store in light-resistant container at room temperature
#### PO route
• May be given with food or milk to lessen GI upset
#### IM/SUBCUT route
• Do not give if sol is cloudy or a precipitate has formed; rotate inj sites
#### IV route
• Give by direct **IV** after diluting with 5 ml or more of sterile water or 0.9% NaCl for inj
• Give slowly at 2 mg over 3-5 min or less through Y-connector or 3-way stopcock
*Syringe compatibilities:* Atropine, bupivacaine, ceftazidime, chlorproMAZINE, cimetidine, dimenhyDRINATE, diphenhydrA-MINE, fentanyl, glycopyrrolate, haloperidol, hydrOXYzine, lorazepam, midazolam, penta-zocaine, pentobarbital, prochlorperazine, promethazine, ranitidine, scopolamine, tetracaine, thiethylperazine, trimetho-benzamide
*Y-site compatibilities:* Acyclovir, allopurinol, amifostine, amikacin, amsacrine, aztreonam, cefamandole, cefepime, cef-metazole, cefoperazone, cefotaxime, cefoxitin, ceftazidime, ceftizoxime, cefuroxime, ce-phalothin, cephapirin, chloramphenicol, cisplatin, cladribine, clindamycin, cyclophos-phamide, cytarabine, diltiazem, DOBUTamine, DOPamine, DOXOrubicin, doxycycline, epINEPHrine, erythromycin lactobionate, famotidine, fentanyl, filgrastim, fludarabine, foscarnet, furosemide, gentamicin, granis-etron, heparin, kanamycin, labetalol, loraze-pam, magnesium sulfate, melphalan, methotrexate, metronidazole, mezlocillin, midazolam, milrinone, morphine, moxalac-tam, nafcillin, niCARdipine, nitroglycerin, norepinephrine, ondansetron, oxacillin, paclitaxel, penicillin G potassium, piperacillin, piperacillin/tazobactam, propofol, ranitidine, teniposide, thiotepa, ticarcillin, tobramycin, trimethoprim/sulfamethoxazole, vancomycin, vecuronium, vinorelbine
*Y-site incompatibilities:* Ampicillin, diazepam, minocycline, phenobarbital, phe-nytoin, sargramostim

*Additive compatibilities:* Bupivacaine, fluorouracil, midazolam, ondansetron, promethazine, verapamil
*Additive incompatibilities:* Sodium bicarbonate, thiopental
*Solution compatibilities:* D₅W, D₅/0.45% NaCl, D₅/0.9% NaCl, D₅/LR, D₅/Ringer's, 0.45% NaCl, 0.9% NaCl, Ringer's and lactated Ringer's

## Patient/family education
• Instruct patient to report any symptoms of CNS changes, allergic reactions; to avoid CNS depressants: alcohol, sedative/hypnotics for at least 24 hr after taking this product
• Advise patient that dizziness, drowsiness, and confusion are common and to avoid getting up without assistance, driving, or other hazardous activities
• Discuss in detail all aspects of the product

## Evaluation
**Positive therapeutic outcome**
• Decreased pain
• Decreased cough

**Treatment of overdose:** Naloxone HCl (Narcan) 0.2-0.8 **IV**, O₂, **IV** fluids, vasopressors

---

## hydroxychloroquine (Rx)
(hye-drox-ee-klor'oh-kwin)
Plaquenil
*Func. class.:* Antimalarial, antirheumatic (DMARDs)
*Chem. class.:* 4-Aminoquinoline derivative
**Pregnancy category C**

**Action:** Inhibits parasite replications, transcription of DNA to RNA by forming complexes with DNA in parasite

**Therapeutic outcome:** Resolution of infection

**Uses:** Malaria caused by *Plasmodium vivax, P. malariae, P. ovale, P. falciparum* (some strains): LE, rheumatoid arthritis

## Dosage and routes
*Malaria*
*Adult:* PO Suppression or prevention 200 mg qwk, begin 1-2 wk before travel, continue 4 wk after returning; treatment 400 mg, then 200 mg at 6, 24, 48 hr after 1st dose
*Child:* PO Suppression or prevention 5 mg/kg qwk, begin 1-2 wk before travel, continue 4 wk after returning; treatment 10 mg/kg, then 5 mg/kg at 6, 24, 48 hr after 1st dose

*Lupus erythematosus*
*Adult:* PO 400 mg daily-bid; length depends on patient response; maintenance 200-400 mg/day

*Rheumatoid arthritis*
*Adult:* PO 400-600 mg/day for 4-12 wk; then 200-300 mg/day after good response
*Child:* PO 3-5 mg/kg/day max 400 mg/day

**Available forms:** Tabs 200 mg

## Adverse effects
***CNS:*** Headache, stimulation, fatigue, irritability, **seizures**, bad dreams, dizziness, confusion, psychosis, decreased reflexes
***CV:*** Hypotension, heart block, **asystole with syncope**
***EENT:*** *Blurred vision, corneal changes, retinal changes, difficulty focusing,* tinnitus, vertigo, deafness, photophobia, corneal edema
***GI:*** *Nausea, vomiting, anorexia,* diarrhea, cramps
***HEMA:*** **Thrombocytopenia, agranulocytosis, leukopenia, aplastic anemia**
***INTEG:*** Pruritus, pigmentation changes, skin eruptions, lichen planus–like eruptions, eczema, **exfoliative dermatitis**, alopecia

**Contraindications:** Hypersensitivity, retinal field changes, children (long-term)

**Precautions:** Pregnancy **C**, breastfeeding, blood dyscrasias, severe GI disease, neurologic disease, alcoholism, hepatic disease, G6PD deficiency, psoriasis, eczema

### Pharmacokinetics
| | |
|---|---|
| **Absorption** | Well absorbed |
| **Distribution** | Widely distributed, crosses placenta |
| **Metabolism** | Liver |
| **Excretion** | Urine/feces |
| **Half-life** | 3-5 day |

### Pharmacodynamics
| | |
|---|---|
| **Onset** | Rapid |
| **Peak** | 1-2 hr |
| **Duration** | Days-weeks |

## Interactions
*Individual products*
Magnesium, aluminum products: decreased malarial action
Digoxin: increased levels
Rabies vaccine: increased antibody titer

## NURSING CONSIDERATIONS
**Assessment**
• Assess for lupus erythematosus, malaria symptoms

Adverse effects: *italic* = common, **bold** = life-threatening

- Assess for rheumatoid arthritis: pain, swelling, ROM, temperature of joints
- Assess ophthalmic exam baseline and q6 mo if long-term treatment or product dosage >150 mg/day
- Assess hepatic studies qwk: AST, ALT, bilirubin
- Assess blood studies: CBC, platelets; WBC, RBC, platelets may be decreased; if severe, product should be discontinued
- Assess for decreased reflexes: knee, ankle
- Assess ECG during therapy
- Assess for depression of T waves, widening of QRS complex
- Assess allergic reactions: pruritus, rash, urticaria
- Assess blood dyscrasias: malaise, fever, bruising, bleeding (rare)
- Assess for ototoxicity (tinnitus, vertigo, change in hearing); audiometric testing should be done before, after treatment

◆ Assess for toxicity: blurring vision, difficulty focusing, headache, dizziness, knee, ankle reflexes; product should be discontinued immediately

### Nursing diagnoses
- Infection, risk for (uses)
- Knowledge, deficient (teaching)
- Pain, chronic (uses)

### Implementation
- Give before or after meals with milk, at same time each day to maintain product level
- Tabs may be crushed and mixed with food, fluids
- Malaria prophylaxis should be started 2 wk prior to exposure and 4-6 wk after leaving exposure area
- Store in tight, light-resistant container at room temperature

### Patient/family education
- Teach patient to use sunglasses in bright sunlight to decrease photophobia
- Teach patient that urine may turn rust or brown
- Teach patient to report hearing, visual problems, fever, fatigue, bruising, bleeding, which may indicate blood dyscrasias

### Evaluation
**Positive therapeutic outcome**
- Decreased symptoms of malaria, LE, rheumatoid arthritis

### Treatment of overdose: Induce vomiting; gastric lavage; administer barbiturate (ultra–short-acting), vasopressor, ammonium chloride; tracheostomy may be necessary

## hydroxyurea (Rx)
(hye-drox-ee-yoo-ree'ah)
Droxia, Hydrea
*Func. class.:* Antineoplastic, antimetabolite
*Chem. class.:* Synthetic urea analog

### Pregnancy category D

**Action:** Acts by inhibiting DNA synthesis without interfering with RNA or protein synthesis; incorporates thymidine into DNA, causing direct damage to DNA strands; cell cycle specific (S phase)

**Therapeutic outcome:** Prevention of rapidly growing malignant cells

**Uses:** Melanoma, chronic myelogenous leukemia, recurrent or metastatic ovarian cancer, squamous cell carcinoma of the head and neck, sickle cell anemia, psoriasis

### Dosage and routes
*Solid tumors*
*Adult:* PO 80 mg/kg as a single dose q3 days or 20-30 mg/kg as a single dose daily

*In combination with radiation*
*Adult:* PO 80 mg/kg as a single dose q3 days; should be started 7 days before irradiation

*Resistant chronic myelogenous leukemia*
*Adult:* PO 10-30 mg/kg/day as a single daily dose

*Sickle cell anemia*
*Adult:* PO 15 mg/kg/day, may increase by 5 mg/kg/day, max 35 mg/kg/day

*Renal dose*
*Adult:* CCr 10-50 ml/min dose 50%; CCr <10 ml/min PO dose 20%

**Available forms:** Caps 200, 300, 400, 500 mg

### Adverse effects
*CNS:* Headache, confusion, hallucinations, dizziness, **seizures**
*CV:* Angina, ischemia
*GI:* Nausea, vomiting, anorexia, diarrhea, stomatitis, constipation, **hepatotoxicity**
*GU:* Increased BUN, uric acid, creatinine, temporary renal function impairment
*HEMA:* **Leukopenia, anemia, thrombocytopenia, megaloblastic erythropoiesis**
*INTEG: Rash,* urticaria, pruritus, dry skin, facial erythema
*MISC:* Fever, chills, malaise, secondary cancers

**Contraindications:** Pregnancy **D**, breastfeeding, hypersensitivity, leukopenia (<2500/

mm$^3$), thrombocytopenia (<100,000/mm$^3$), anemia (severe)

**Precautions:** Renal disease (severe)

| Pharmacokinetics | |
|---|---|
| Absorption | Well absorbed |
| Distribution | Crosses blood-brain barrier |
| Metabolism | Liver (50%) |
| Excretion | Kidneys, unchanged (50%), eliminated as $CO_2$ |
| Half-life | Terminal 3.5-4.5 hr |

| Pharmacodynamics | |
|---|---|
| Onset | Unknown |
| Peak | 1-4 hr |
| Duration | Unknown |

### Interactions
*Individual drugs*
Radiation: increased toxicity
*Drug classifications*
Anticoagulants, NSAIDs: increased bleeding
Antineoplastics: increased toxicity
*Drug/lab test*
Increased: renal function tests

### NURSING CONSIDERATIONS
**Assessment**
• Assess buccal cavity q8hr for dryness, sores or ulceration, white patches, oral pain, bleeding, dysphagia; obtain prescription for viscous lidocaine (Xylocaine)
• Assess symptoms indicating severe allergic reaction: rash, pruritus, urticaria, purpuric skin lesions, itching, flushing
• Monitor CBC, differential, platelet count weekly; withhold product if WBC is <2500/mm$^3$ or platelet count is <100,000/mm$^3$; notify prescriber of results if WBC <20,000/mm$^3$, platelets <150,000/mm$^3$
• Assess for increased uric acid levels, swelling, joint pain primarily in extremities; patient should be well hydrated to prevent urate deposits
• Monitor renal function studies: BUN, creatinine, serum uric acid, urine CCr before and during therapy; I&O ratio; report fall in urine output to <30 ml/hr
• Monitor temp (may indicate beginning of infection)
• Monitor liver function tests before and during therapy (bilirubin, AST, ALT, LDH) as needed or monthly
• Assess for bleeding: hematuria, stool guaiac, bruising or petechiae, mucosa or orifices

q8hr; check for inflammation of mucosa, breaks in skin
✦ Assess for tumor lysis syndrome

**Nursing diagnoses**
• Body image, disturbed (adverse reactions)
• Infection, risk for (adverse reactions)
• Injury, risk for (adverse reactions)
• Knowledge, deficient (teaching)

**Implementation**
• Do not crush or chew caps; for difficulty swallowing, caps can be opened and contents mixed with water
• Avoid contact with skin, very irritating; wash completely to remove
• Give fluids **IV** or PO before chemotherapy to hydrate patient
• Give antiemetic 30-60 min before giving product and prn to prevent vomiting; antibiotics for prophylaxis of infection
• Provide liquid diet: carbonated beverages; gelatin may be added if patient is not nauseated or vomiting

**Patient/family education**
• Advise patient that contraceptive measures are recommended during therapy
• Teach patient to avoid use of products containing aspirin or ibuprofen, razors, commercial mouthwash, since bleeding may occur; instruct patient to report symptoms of bleeding (hematuria, tarry stools)
• Teach patient to rinse mouth tid-qid with water, club soda; brush teeth bid-qid with soft brush or cotton-tipped applicators for stomatitis; use unwaxed dental floss
• Instruct patient to report signs of anemia (fatigue, headache, irritability, faintness, shortness of breath)
• Advise patient to report any changes in breathing or coughing even several mo after treatment; to avoid crowds and persons with respiratory tract or other infections
• Caution patient not to have any vaccinations without the advice of the prescriber, serious reactions can occur

**Evaluation**
**Positive therapeutic outcome**
• Prevention of rapid division of malignant cells

H

## *hydrOXYzine (Rx)
(hye-drox'i-zeen)
Apo-hydroxyzine ✦, Atarax, hydroxyzine,
Hyzine-50, Multipax ✦,
Novohydroxyzine ✦, Vistaril
*Func. class.:* Antianxiety, sedative, hypnotic,
antihistamine, antiemetic
*Chem. class.:* Piperazine derivative

**Pregnancy category** C

### Do not confuse:
hydrOXYzine/hydrALAZINE, Atarax/amoxicillin/
Ativan, Vistaril/Versed

**Action:** Depresses subcortical levels of CNS,
including limbic system, reticular formation;
anticholinergic, antiemetic, antihistaminic
responses; competes with $H_1$-receptor sites

**Therapeutic outcome:** Absence of
allergy symptoms, rhinitis, pruritus, absence of
nausea/vomiting, sedation, absence of anxiety

**Uses:** Anxiety preoperatively, postoperatively
to prevent nausea, vomiting; to potentiate
opioid analgesics; sedation; pruritus; prevention of alcohol, product withdrawal

### Dosage and routes
*Anxiety*
**Adult:** PO 25-100 mg tid-qid, max 600
mg/day; IM 50-100 mg q4-6hr
**Child >6 yr:** PO 50-100 mg/day in divided
doses
**Child <6 yr:** PO 50 mg/day in divided doses

*Alcohol withdrawal*
**Adult:** IM 50-100 mg, then q4-6hr

*Preoperatively/postoperatively*
**Adult:** IM 25-100 mg q4-6hr
**Child:** IM 0.5-1.1 mg/kg q4-6hr

*Pruritus*
**Adult:** PO 25 mg tid-qid
**Geriatric:** PO 10 mg tid-qid, max 50 mg/day

*Antiemetic*
**Adult:** IM 25-100 mg/dose q4-6hr prn

**Available forms:** Tabs 10, 25, 50, 100
mg; caps 10, 25, 50, 100 mg; oral susp 5 mg/5
ml; inj 25, 50 mg/ml

### Adverse effects
*CNS: Dizziness, drowsiness,* confusion, head-
ache, tremors, fatigue, depression, **seizures**
*CV:* Hypotension
*GI:* Dry mouth, nausea, diarrhea, increased
appetite, weight gain

**Contraindications:** Pregnancy (1st
trimester), breastfeeding, acute asthma,
hypersensitivity to this product or cetirizine

**Precautions:** Pregnancy C (2nd/3rd
trimesters), geriatric, debilitated patients,
renal/hepatic disease, angle-closure glaucoma,
COPD, prostatic hypertrophy, asthma

### Pharmacokinetics
| | |
|---|---|
| **Absorption** | Well absorbed |
| **Distribution** | Not known |
| **Metabolism** | Liver, completely |
| **Excretion** | Feces, urine, bile |
| **Half-life** | 3 hr |

### Pharmacodynamics
| | PO/IM |
|---|---|
| **Onset** | 15-60 min |
| **Peak** | 2-4 hr |
| **Duration** | 4-6 hr |

### Interactions
*Individual drugs*
Alcohol: increased CNS depression
Atropine, disopyramide, haloperidol,
quinidine: increased anticholinergic reac-
tions
*Drug classifications*
Analgesics, barbiturates, CNS depressants,
opiates, sedative/hypnotics: increased CNS
depression
Antidepressants, antihistamines, MAOIs,
phenothiazines: increased anticholinergic
reactions
*Drug/herb*
Corkwood, henbane leaf, jimsonweed,
scopolia: increased anticholinergic effect
Chamomile, cowslip, hops, Jamaican dog-
wood, khat, kava, Queen Anne's lace, senega, skullcap, valerian: increased sedative
action
*Drug/lab test*
False increase: 17-OHCS

### NURSING CONSIDERATIONS
**Assessment**
• Assess mental status: mood, sensorium,
affect, behavior, increased sedation
• Assess respiratory status: rate, rhythm,
increase in bronchial secretions, wheezing,
chest tightness; provide fluids to 2 L/day to
decrease secretion thickness
• Monitor I&O ratio: be alert for urinary
retention, frequency, dysuria, especially in the
geriatric; product should be discontinued if
these occur
• Observe for drowsiness, dizziness
• Assess cough characteristics including type,
frequency, thickness of secretions; evaluate
response to this medication if using for cough

## Nursing diagnoses
- Anxiety (uses)
- Injury, risk for (side effects)
- Knowledge, deficient (teaching)

## Implementation
**PO route**
- Take 1 hr after or 2 hr before meals to facilitate absorption
- May crush tab if patient unable to swallow whole
- Give with meals if GI symptoms occur; absorption may be slightly decreased
- Caps may be opened and product mixed with food/fluids for patients with swallowing difficulties

**IM route**
- Give IM inj in large muscle mass; aspirate to prevent **IV** administration; use Z-track method; severe necrosis can result with improper technique; never give **IV**/SUBCUT

*Syringe compatibilities:* Atropine, atropine/meperidine, benzquinamide, bupivacaine, butorphanol, chlorproMAZINE, cimetidine, codeine, diphenhydrAMINE, doxapram, droperidol, fentanyl, fluphenazine, glycopyrrolate, hydromorphone, lidocaine, meperidine, meperidine/atropine, methotrimeprazine, metoclopramide, midazolam, morphine, nalbuphine, oxymorphone, pentazocine, perphenazine, procaine, prochlorperazine, promazine, promethazine, remifentanil, scopolamine, sufentanil, thiothixene

*Syringe incompatibilities:* Aminophylline, chloramphenicol, dimenhyDRINATE, heparin, penicillin G potassium, pentobarbital, phenobarbital, phenytoin

*Additive compatibilities:* Cisplatin, cyclophosphamide, cytarabine, dimenhyDRINATE, etoposide, lidocaine, mesna, methotrexate, nafcillin

## Patient/family education
- Caution patient to avoid hazardous activities and activities requiring alertness, since dizziness may occur; instruct patient to request assistance with ambulation
- Advise patient to avoid alcohol, other CNS depressants including cough, cold preparations; CNS depression may occur
- Teach all aspects of product use; to notify prescriber if confusion, sedation, hypotension occur; to avoid driving and other hazardous activity if drowsiness occurs
- Caution patient not to exceed recommended dosage; dysrhythmias may occur
- Tell patient hard candy, gum, frequent rinsing of mouth may be used for dryness

## Evaluation
**Positive therapeutic outcome**
- Absence of nausea, vomiting
- Decreased anxiety

**Treatment of overdose:** Lavage if orally ingested, VS, supportive care, **IV** norepinephrine for hypotension

### hyoscyamine (Rx)
(hye-oh-sye′a-meen)
Anaspaz, A-Spas S/L, Cystospaz, Cystospaz-M, Donnamar, ED-SPAZ, Gastrosed, Levsin, Levsinex, NuLev Timecaps
*Func. class.:* Anticholinergic/antispasmodics
*Chem. class.:* Belladonna alkaloid
**Pregnancy category  C**

**Action:** Inhibits muscarinic actions of acetylcholine at postganglionic parasympathetic neuroeffector sites, reduces rigidity, tremors, hyperhidrosis of parkinsonism

**Therapeutic outcome:** Absence of peptic ulcer after treatment

**Uses:** Treatment of peptic ulcer disease in combination with other products; other GI disorders, other spastic disorders, IBS, urinary incontinence

### Dosage and routes
*Adult:* PO/SL 0.125-0.25 mg tid-qid before meals, at bedtime; TIME REL 0.375 mg q12hr; IM/SUBCUT/IV 0.25-0.5 mg q6hr
*Child 2-12 yr:* PO (orally disintegrating tabs) 0.0625-0.125 mg (½-1 tab) q4hr, max 6×/day
*Child 34-36 kg:* PO 125-187 mcg q4hr prn
*Child 22.7-33 kg:* PO 94-125 mcg q4hr prn
*Child 13.6-22.6 kg:* PO 63 mcg q4hr prn
*Child 9.1-13.5 kg:* PO 31.3 mcg q4hr prn
*Child 6.8-9 kg:* PO 25 mcg q4hr prn
*Child 4.5-6.7 kg:* PO 18.8 mcg q4hr prn
*Child 3.4-4.4 kg:* PO 15.6 mcg q4hr prn
*Child 2.3-3.3 kg:* PO 12.5 mcg q4hr prn

**Available forms:** Tabs 0.125, 0.15 mg; time rel caps 0.375 mg; time rel tabs 0.375 ml; sol 0.125 mg/ml; elix 0.125 mg/ml; inj 0.5 mg/ml

### Adverse effects
*CNS: Confusion, stimulation in geriatric,* headache, insomnia, dizziness, drowsiness, anxiety, weakness, hallucination
*CV: Palpitations,* tachycardia

H

**EENT:** *Blurred vision*, photophobia, mydriasis, cycloplegia, increased ocular tension
**GI:** *Dry mouth, constipation, paralytic ileus*, heartburn, nausea, vomiting, dysphagia, absence of taste
**GU:** *Urinary hesitancy, retention*, impotence
**INTEG:** Urticaria, rash, pruritus, anhidrosis, fever, allergic reactions

**Contraindications:** Hypersensitivity to anticholinergics, angle-closure glaucoma, GI obstruction, myasthenia gravis, paralytic ileus, GI atony, toxic megacolon, prostatic hypertrophy

**Precautions:** Pregnancy **C**, geriatric, hyperthyroidism, CAD, dysrhythmias, CHF, ulcerative colitis, hypertension, hiatal hernia, renal/hepatic disease, urinary retention

### Pharmacokinetics

| | |
|---|---|
| **Absorption** | Well |
| **Distribution** | Cross blood-brain barrier, placenta |
| **Metabolism** | Liver |
| **Excretion** | Urine |
| **Half-life** | 3½ hr |

### Pharmacodynamics

| | PO | IM/**IV**/SUBCUT |
|---|---|---|
| **Onset** | 30 min | 2-3 min |
| **Peak** | Unknown | Unknown |
| **Duration** | 4-6 hr | 4-6 hr |

### Interactions
#### Individual products
Amantidine: increased anticholinergic effect
Levodopa, ketoconazole: decreased effects
#### Drug classifications
Antacids: decreased hyoscyamine effect
Antihistamines, H₁, antidepressants (tricyclics), MAOIs: increased anticholinergic effect
Phenothiazines: decreased effect of phenothiazines
#### Drug/herb
Black catechu: increased constipation
Butterbur, jimsonweed: increased anticholinergic effect
Jaborandi tree, pill-bearing spurge: decreased anticholinergic effect

### NURSING CONSIDERATIONS
#### Assessment
• Monitor VS, cardiac status: checking for dysrhythmias, increased rate, palpitations
• Monitor I/O ratio; check for urinary retention or hesitancy
• Monitor GI complaints: pain, bleeding (frank or occult), nausea, vomiting, anorexia

### Nursing diagnoses
• Constipation (adverse reactions)
• Injury, risk for (adverse reactions)
• Knowledge, deficient (teaching)

### Implementation
• Do not break, crush, or chew time rel caps
• Give ½ hour before meals for better absorption
• Give decreased dose to geriatric patients; metabolism may be slowed
• Store in tight container protected from light

### Patient/family education
• Teach patient to avoid driving, other hazardous activities until stabilized on medication
• Teach patient to avoid alcohol or other CNS depressants; will enhance sedating properties of this product
• Teach patient to avoid hot environments; heat stroke may occur; product suppresses perspiration
• Teach patient to use sunglasses when outside to prevent photophobia; may cause blurred vision
• Teach patient to use gum, hard candy, frequent rinsing of mouth for dryness of oral cavity
• Teach patient to increase fluids, bulk, exercise to decrease constipation

### Evaluation
**Positive therapeutic outcome**
• Absence of epigastric pain, bleeding, nausea, vomiting

### ibandronate (Rx)
(eye-ban'dro-nate)
Boniva
*Func. class.:* Bone-resorption inhibitor, electrolyte modifier
*Chem. class.:* Bisphosphonate
**Pregnancy category C**

**Action:** Inhibits bone resorption, apparently without inhibiting bone formation and mineralization; absorbs calcium phosphate crystals in bone and may directly block dissolution of hydroxyapatite crystals of bone; more potent than other products

**Therapeutic outcome:** Increased bone mineral density

**Uses:** Osteoporosis and prophylaxis

**Unlabeled uses:** Hypercalcemia, osteolytic metastases, Paget's disease

## Dosage and routes
### Postmenopausal osteoporosis
**Adult:** PO 150 mg qmo; **IV** BOL 3 mg q3 mo

### Prophylaxis
**Adult:** PO 2.5 mg/day or 150 mg qmo

### Paget's disease (unlabeled)
**Adult:** **IV** 2 mg as a single dose

### Osteolytic metastases (unlabeled)
**Adult:** **IV** 6 mg over 1 hr × 3 days, repeat q4 wk

### Hypercalcemia (unlabeled)
**Adult:** **IV** INF 2 mg over 2 hr

**Available forms:** Tabs 2.5, 150 mg; sol for inj 3 mg/ml

## Adverse effects
***CNS:*** Fever, insomnia, dizziness, headache
***CV:*** Hypertension
***EENT:*** Ocular pain/inflammation, uveitis
***GI:*** Constipation, nausea, vomiting, diarrhea, dyspepsia
***INTEG:*** Rash, inj site reaction
***META:*** *Hypomagnesemia, hypophosphatemia, hypocalcemia*
***MS:*** Bone pain, myalgia

**Contraindications:** Achalasia, esophageal stricture, hypocalcemia, intraarterial administration, renal failure, vitamin D deficiency, hypersensitivity to bisphosphonates

**Precautions:** Pregnancy **C**, breastfeeding, children, geriatric, anemia, chemotherapy, coagulopathy, dental disease, diabetes mellitus, dysphagia, GI/renal disease, GERD, hypertension, infection, multiple myeloma, phosphate hypersensitivity

| Pharmacokinetics | |
|---|---|
| **Absorption** | Poor |
| **Distribution** | Taken up primarily by bones, 86%-99% protein binding |
| **Metabolism** | Unknown |
| **Excretion** | Primarily by kidneys |
| **Half-life** | 5-60 hr |

| Pharmacodynamics | |
|---|---|
| **Onset** | Unknown |
| **Peak** | 0.5-2 hr |
| **Duration** | Up to 1 month |

## Interactions
### Individual drugs
Calcium, vitamin D: decreased ibandronate effect

CycloSPORINE, tacrolimus: possible increased neurotoxicity
Digoxin: hypomagnesemia, hypokalemia
### Drug classifications
Aminoglycosides, NSAIDs, radiopaque contrast agents: possible increased neurotoxicity
Loop diuretics: increased hypocalcemia

## NURSING CONSIDERATIONS
### Assessment
- Assess for blood studies: electrolytes, Ca, P, Mg; creatinine/BUN
- Assess for hypercalcemia: nausea, vomiting, constipation, thirst, dysrhythmias; hypocalcemia, paresthesia, twitching, laryngospasm, Chvostek's, Trousseau's signs
- Assess for bone pain; use analgesics
- Monitor DEXA scan for bone mineral density

### Nursing diagnoses
- Injury, risk for (uses)
- Knowledge, deficient (teaching)

### Implementation
#### IV route
- Use single-dose prefilled syringe; discard unused portion; give over 15-30 sec
- Store at room temperature

### Patient/family education
- Teach patient to report hypercalcemic relapse: nausea, vomiting, bone pain, thirst; unusual muscle twitching, muscle spasms, severe diarrhea, constipation
- Advise patient to continue with dietary recommendations, including calcium and vit D
- Instruct patient to obtain an analgesic from provider for bone pain
- Advise patient that if nausea/vomiting occur, small, frequent meals may help
- Teach patient to report vision symptoms: blurred vision, edema, inflammation; report to prescriber

### Evaluation
#### Positive therapeutic outcome
- Increased bone mineral density

## ibritumomab tiuxetan (Rx)
(ee-brit-u-moe'mab)
Zevalin
*Func. class.:* Radiopharmaceutical
**Pregnancy category D**

**Action:** High affinity for indium-111, yttrium-90; induces CD20$^+$ B-cell lines

**Therapeutic outcome:** Decrease in tumor size, spread of malignancy

---

Adverse effects: *italic* = common, **bold** = life-threatening

**Uses:** Non-Hodgkin's lymphoma, B-cell NHL

## Dosage and routes
*Adult:* Ritaximab 250 mg/m² given first; within 4 hr, give 5 mCi (1.6 mg total) over 10 min, then repeat 7-9 days later

**Available forms:** Inj 3.2 mg/2 ml

## Adverse effects
*CV:* **Cardiac dysrhythmias**
*GI: Nausea, vomiting, anorexia,* abdominal pain, diarrhea
*GU:* **Renal failure**
*HEMA:* **Leukopenia, neutropenia, thrombocytopenia,** anemia
*INTEG: Irritation at site, rash,* **fatal mucocutaneous infections (rare)**
*OTHER:* Fever, chills, asthenia, headache, **angioedema,** hypotension, myalgia, **bronchospasm, hemorrhage,** infections, cough, dyspnea, dizziness, anxiety
*SYST:* **Stevens-Johnson syndrome, secondary malignancies (AML, MDS), fatal infections**

**Contraindications:** Pregnancy **D**, hypersensitivity to this agent or murine proteins, neutropenia, thrombocytopenia, prior murine antibody exposure

**Precautions:** Breastfeeding, children, geriatric, cardiac conditions, immunizations after therapy

| Pharmacokinetics | |
|---|---|
| **Absorption** | Unknown |
| **Distribution** | Unknown |
| **Metabolism** | Unknown |
| **Excretion** | Unknown |
| **Half-life** | 30 hr |

| Pharmacodynamics |
|---|
| Unknown |

## NURSING CONSIDERATIONS
### Assessment
- Assess for infection, murine antibody titers
- ⬥ Assess for signs of fatal infusion reaction: hypoxia, pulmonary infiltrates, ARDS, MI, ventricular fibrillation, cardiogenic shock; most fatal infusion reactions occur with first infusion; potentially fatal
- Assess biodistribution: first image 2-24 hr, second image 48-72 hr, third image 90-120 hr (optimal)
- Assess for signs of severe mucocutaneous reactions: Stevens-Johnson syndrome, lichenoid dermatitis, toxic epidermal lysis; occur 1-13 wk after product was given

⬥ Assess for tumor lysis syndrome: acute renal failure requiring hemodialysis, hyperkalemia, hypocalcemia, hyperuricemia, hyperphosphatemia
- Monitor CBC, differential, platelet count weekly; withhold product if WBC is <3500/mm³ or platelet count <150,000/mm³; notify prescriber of these results
- Monitor GI symptoms: frequency of stools
- Assess for signs of dehydration: rapid respirations, poor skin turgor, decreased urine output, dry skin, restlessness, weakness

### Nursing diagnoses
- Infection, risk for (adverse reactions)
- Knowledge, deficient (teaching)
- Nutrition: less than body requirements, imbalanced (adverse reactions)

### Implementation
- Do not use as BOL or **IV** direct
- Provide increased fluid intake to 2-3 L/day to prevent dehydration, unless contraindicated

**IV infusion route**
- See manufacturer's product labeling for preparation
- Have emergency equipment nearby with epinephrine, antihistamines, corticosteroids

### Patient/family education
- Teach patient radiation safety precautions, disposal of body fluids
- Teach patient symptoms of infection
- Teach patient decreased blood count precautions
- Advise patient to report adverse reactions
- Advise patient to use contraception during and for 12 mo after therapy

### Evaluation
**Positive therapeutic outcome**
- Improvement in blood counts

## ibuprofen 🚱 (OTC)
(eye-byoo-proe'fen)

Actiprofen ✦, Advil, Advil Liqui-Gels, Advil Migraine, Apo-Ibuprofen ✦, Bayer Select Ibuprofen Pain Relief, Children's Advil, Children's Motrin, Excedrin IB, Genpril, Haltran, ibuprofen, IBU-TAB, Infant's Motrin, Junior Strength Advil, Medipren, Menadol, Midol Maximum Strength Cramp Formula, Motrin, Motrin IB, Motrin Junior Strength, Motrin Migraine Pain, Novoprofen ✦, Nu-Ibuprofen, Nuprin, PediaCare Children's Fever

*Func. class.:* Nonsteroidal antiinflammatory; nonopiate analgesic, antipyretic

*Chem. class.:* Propionic acid derivative

### Pregnancy category B

Do not confuse:
Nuprin/Lupron

Action: Inhibits prostaglandin synthesis by decreasing enzyme needed for biosynthesis; analgesic, antiinflammatory, antipyretic

Therapeutic outcome: Decreased pain, inflammation, fever

Uses: Rheumatoid arthritis, osteoarthritis, primary dysmenorrhea, gout, dental pain, musculoskeletal disorders, fever

### Dosage and routes
*Analgesia*
**Adult:** PO 200-400 mg q4-6hr, not to exceed 3.2 g/day
**Child:** PO 4-10 mg/kg/dose q6-8hr

*Dysmenorrhea*
**Adult:** PO 400 mg q4hr

*Antipyretic*
**Child 6 mo-12 yr:** PO 5 mg/kg (temp <102.5° F or 39.2° C), 10 mg/kg (temp >102.5° F), may repeat q4-6hr; max 40 mg/kg/day

*Antiinflammatory*
**Adult:** PO 300-800 mg tid-qid; max 3.2 g/day
**Child:** PO 30-40 mg/kg/day in 3-4 divided doses; max 50 mg/kg/day

Available forms: Tabs 100, 200, 300, 400, 600, 800 mg; liqui-gel caps 200 mg; oral susp 100 mg/2.5 ml, 100 mg/5 ml; liquid 100 mg/5 ml; chew tabs 50, 100 mg; drops 50 mg/1.25 ml

### Adverse effects
*CNS: Headache,* dizziness, drowsiness, fatigue, tremors, confusion, insomnia, anxiety, depression

*CV:* Tachycardia, peripheral edema, palpitations, dysrhythmias, **CV thrombotic events, MI, stroke**

*EENT:* Tinnitus, hearing loss, blurred vision

*GI: Nausea, anorexia,* vomiting, diarrhea, jaundice, **hepatitis,** constipation, flatulence, cramps, dry mouth, peptic ulcer, **GI bleeding**

*GU:* **Nephrotoxicity,** dysuria, hematuria, oliguria, azotemia

*HEMA:* **Blood dyscrasias,** increased bleeding time

*INTEG:* Purpura, rash, pruritus, sweating, urticaria, **necrotizing fasciitis**

*SYST:* **Anaphylaxis, Stevens-Johnson syndrome**

Contraindications: Avoid in 2nd/3rd trimester of pregnancy, hypersensitivity, asthma, severe renal/hepatic disease, perioperative pain in CABG

Precautions: Pregnancy **B** (1st trimester), breastfeeding, children, geriatric, bleeding disorders, GI disorders, cardiac disorders, hypersensitivity to other antiinflammatory agents, CHF, CCr <25 ml/min

| Pharmacokinetics | |
|---|---|
| **Absorption** | Well absorbed |
| **Distribution** | Not known; crosses placenta |
| **Metabolism** | Liver, extensively |
| **Excretion** | Kidneys, unchanged (10%) |
| **Half-life** | 1.8-2 hr |

| Pharmacodynamics | |
|---|---|
| **Onset** | ½ hr |
| **Peak** | 1-2 hr |
| **Duration** | 4-6 hr |

### Interactions
*Individual drugs*
Alcohol, aspirin: increased GI reactions
Aspirin: decreased ibuprofen action
Cefotetan, cefoperazone, valproic acid, warfarin: increased risk of bleeding
CycloSPORINE, digoxin, lithium, probenecid: increased toxicity
Furosemide: decreased effect of furosemide
Insulin: increased hypoglycemia
Radiation: increased risk of blood dyscrasias
*Drug classifications*
Anticoagulants, antiplatelet agents, thrombolytics: increased risk of bleeding
Anticoagulants (oral): increased toxicity
Antidiabetics (oral): increased hypoglycemia
Antihypertensives: decreased effect of antihypertensives

Adverse effects: *italic* = common, **bold** = life-threatening

Antineoplastics: increased risk of blood dyscrasias

Corticosteroids, NSAIDs: increased GI reactions

Diuretics: decreased effectiveness of diuretics (thiazides)

*Drug/herb*

Arginine, gossypol: increased gastric irritation

Arnica, bogbean, chamomile, chondroitin, clove, dong quai, fenugreek, feverfew, garlic, ginger, ginkgo, ginseng *(Panax):* increased risk of bleeding

Bearberry, bilberry: increased NSAIDs effect

*Drug/lab test*

Increased: bleeding time

## NURSING CONSIDERATIONS
### Assessment

- Assess for infection; may mask symptoms
- Assess pain: location, duration, type, intensity before dose and 1 hr after
- Assess musculoskeletal status: ROM before dose and 1 hr after
- Monitor liver function tests: AST, ALT, bilirubin, creatinine if patient is on long-term therapy
- Monitor renal function tests: BUN, urine creatinine if patient is on long-term therapy
- Assess cardiac status: edema (peripheral), tachycardia, palpitations; monitor B/P, pulse for character, quality, rhythm
- Monitor blood studies: CBC, Hct, Hgb, pro-time if patient is on long-term therapy
- Check I&O ratio; decreasing output may indicate renal failure if patient is on long-term therapy
- Assess hepatotoxicity: dark urine, clay-colored stools, jaundice of skin and sclera, itching, abdominal pain, fever, diarrhea if patient is on long-term therapy
- Assess for history of peptic ulcer disorder; asthma, aspirin, hypersensitivity, check closely for hypersensitivity reactions
- Assess for allergic reactions: rash, urticaria; if these occur, product may have to be discontinued
- Assess for ototoxicity: tinnitus, ringing, roaring in ears; audiometric testing needed before, after long-term therapy
- Assess for visual changes: blurring, halos; may indicate corneal, retinal damage
- Identify prior product history; there are many product interactions
- Identify fever: length of time in evidence and related symptoms

### Nursing diagnoses

- Injury, risk for (side effects)
- Knowledge, deficient (teaching)

- Mobility, impaired physical (uses)
- Pain, acute (uses)
- Pain, chronic (uses)

### Implementation

- Administer to patient crushed or whole; 800-mg tab may be dissolved in water
- Give with food or milk to decrease gastric symptoms; give 2 hr before or 30 min after meals; absorption may be slowed

### Patient/family education

- Teach patient to report any symptoms of hepatotoxicity, renal toxicity, visual changes, ototoxicity, allergic reactions, bleeding if patient is on long-term therapy
- Caution patient not to exceed recommended dosage; acute poisoning may result
- Advise patient to read label on other OTC products
- Inform patient that the therapeutic response takes 1 mo (arthritis)
- Caution patient to avoid alcohol ingestion, salicylates, NSAIDs; GI bleeding may occur
- Advise patient with allergies that allergic reactions may develop
- Advise patient to use sunscreen to prevent photosensitivity

### Evaluation
**Positive therapeutic outcome**

- Decreased pain
- Decreased inflammation
- Decreased fever
- Increased mobility

**Treatment of overdose:** Lavage, activated charcoal, induce diuresis

---

**⚠ HIGH ALERT**

### ibutilide (Rx)
(eye-byoo′te-lide)
Corvert
*Func. class.:* Antidysrhythmic (Class III)

**Pregnancy category** C

**Action:** Prolongs duration of action potential and effective refractory period

**Uses:** For rapid conversion of atrial fibrillation/flutter occurring within 1 wk of coronary artery bypass or valve surgery

### Dosage and routes
*Atrial fibrillation/flutter*
*Adult:* **IV** INF (≥60 kg) 1 vial (1 mg) given over 10 min, may repeat same dose in 10 min; **IV** INF (<60 kg) 0.01 mg/kg given over 10 min, may repeat same dose in 10 min

---

*Atrial fibrillation/flutter after
cardiac surgery*
**Adult ≥60 kg: IV** INF 0.5 mg; may repeat
1 time
**Adult <60 kg: IV** INF 0.005 mg/kg; may
repeat 1 time

**Available forms:** Inj 0.1 mg/ml

**Adverse effects**
*CNS: Headache*
*CV: Hypotension, bradycardia,* **sinus arrest,
CHF, dysrhythmias,** hypertension, extrasysto-
les, ventricular tachycardia, bundle branch
block, AV block, palpitations, supraventricular
extrasystoles, syncope
*GI:* Nausea

**Contraindications:** Hypersensitivity

**Precautions:** Pregnancy **C,** breastfeeding,
children <18 yr, geriatric, sinus node dysfunction, 2nd- or 3rd-degree AV block, electrolyte
imbalances, bradycardia, renal/hepatic disease

| Pharmacokinetics | |
|---|---|
| **Absorption** | Unknown |
| **Distribution** | Unknown |
| **Metabolism** | Liver |
| **Excretion** | Kidney |
| **Half-life** | 6 hr |

| Pharmacodynamics |
|---|
| Unknown |

**Interactions**
*Individual drugs*
Digoxin: masking of cardiotoxicity
*Drug classifications*
Antidepressants (tricyclics/tetracyclics):
    prodysrhythmia
Antihistamines, H$_2$-receptor antagonists,
    phenothiazines: increased prodysrhythmia
Class Ia antidysrhythmics (disopyramide,
    quinidine, procainamide), class III agents
    (amiodarone, sotalol): do not use within 5
    hr of ibutilide
*Drug/herb*
Aconite: increased toxicity, death
Aloe, broom, buckthorn (chronic use),
    cascara sagrada (chronic use), Chinese
    rhubarb, figwort, fumitory, goldenseal,
    kudzu, licorice: increased effect
Coltsfoot: decreased effect
Horehound: increased serotonin effect

**NURSING CONSIDERATIONS**
**Assessment**
• Monitor I&O ratio; monitor electrolytes:
potassium, sodium, chloride

• Monitor liver function tests: AST, ALT,
bilirubin, alkaline phosphatase
• Monitor ECG continuously to determine
product effectiveness; measure PR, QRS, QT
intervals; check for PVCs, other dysrhythmias;
monitor B/P continuously for hypo/
hypertension; check for rebound hypertension
after 1-2 hr; discontinue product when atrial
fibrillation/flutter ceases
• Monitor for dehydration or hypovolemia
• Assess for CNS symptoms: confusion,
psychosis, numbness, depression, involuntary
movements; if these occur product should be
discontinued
• Monitor cardiac rate, respiration; rate,
rhythm, character, chest pain, ventricular
tachycardia, supraventricular tachycardia or
fibrillation

**Nursing diagnoses**
• Cardiac output, decreased (uses)
• Gas exchange, impaired (adverse reactions)
• Knowledge, deficient (teaching)

**Implementation**
**IV route**
• Give reduced dosage slowly with ECG
monitoring only
• Give undiluted or diluted in 50 ml of 0.9%
NaCl or D$_5$W (0.017 mg/ml), give over 10 min
• Solution is stable for 48 hr refrigerated or
24 hr at room temperature
• Do not admix with other solution, products

**Patient/family education**
• Instruct patient to report side effects immediately to prescriber

**Evaluation**
**Positive therapeutic outcome**
• Decrease in atrial fibrillation/flutter

---

**⚠ HIGH ALERT**

**idarubicin** (Rx)
(eye-da-roo'bi-sin)
Idamycin, Idamycin PFS
*Func. class.:* Antineoplastic, antibiotic
*Chem. class.:* Anthracycline glycoside
**Pregnancy category** D

**Do not confuse:**
idarubicin/DOXOrubicin/DAUNOrubicin/
epirubicin, Idamycin/Adriamycin

**Action:** Non–cell cycle specific; topoisomerase II inhibitor, a vesicant

**Therapeutic outcome:** Prevention of
rapidly growing malignant cells

**Uses:** Used in combination with other antineoplastics for acute myelocytic leukemia in adults

**Unlabeled uses:** Breast cancer, liquid tumors

**Dosage and routes**
*Adult:* **IV** 8-12 mg/m²/day × 3 days in combination with cytarabine (induction)

*Renal/hepatic dose*
*Adult:* **IV** Reduce dose if bilirubin is 2.6-5 mg/dl; do not administer if bilirubin >5 mg/dl

**Available forms:** Inj 1 mg/ml

**Adverse effects**
*CNS:* Fever, chills, headache
*CV:* **Dysrhythmias, CHF, pericarditis, myocarditis,** peripheral edema, angina, **MI, myocardial toxicity**
*GI:* Nausea, vomiting, abdominal pain, mucositis, diarrhea, **hepatotoxicity**
*GU:* **Nephrotoxicity**
*HEMA:* **Thrombocytopenia, leukopenia, anemia**
*INTEG:* Rash, **extravasation**, dermatitis, reversible alopecia, urticaria, thrombophlebitis, tissue necrosis at inj site

**Contraindications:** Pregnancy **D,** breastfeeding, hypersensitivity, myelosuppression, bilirubin >5 mg/dl

**Precautions:** Children, renal/hepatic disease, gout, bone marrow depression, preexisting CV disease

| Pharmacokinetics | |
|---|---|
| **Absorption** | Complete bioavailability |
| **Distribution** | Rapidly distributed, protein binding 97% |
| **Metabolism** | Liver, extensively |
| **Excretion** | Bile |
| **Half-life** | 22 hr |

| Pharmacodynamics |
|---|
| Unknown |

**Interactions**
*Individual drugs*
Radiation: increased toxicity
*Drug classifications*
Antineoplastics: increased toxicity
Live virus vaccines: decreased antibody response
*Drug/lab test*
Increased: uric acid

**NURSING CONSIDERATIONS**
**Assessment**
• Assess symptoms indicating severe allergic reaction: rash, pruritus, urticaria, purpuric skin lesions, itching, flushing; product should be discontinued
• Assess for tachypnea, ECG changes, dyspnea, edema, fatigue
• Assess for cardiac toxicity: CHF, dysrhythmias, cardiomyopathy; cardiac studies should be done before and periodically during treatment; ECG, chest x-ray, MUGA
• Monitor CBC, differential, platelet count weekly; withhold product if WBC is <4000/mm³ or platelet count is <100,000/mm³; notify prescriber of results if WBC <20,000/mm³, platelets <150,000/mm³
• Monitor renal function studies: BUN, uric acid, urine CCr, electrolytes, before, during therapy
• Monitor temp (may indicate beginning of infection)
• Monitor liver function tests before and during therapy (bilirubin, AST, ALT, LDH) as needed or monthly; note jaundice of skin and sclera, dark urine, clay-colored stools, itchy skin, abdominal pain, fever, diarrhea; hepatoxicity can be severe
• Assess for bleeding: hematuria, stool guaiac, bruising or petechiae, mucosa or orifices, assess for inflammation of mucosa, breaks in skin
• Identify effects of alopecia on body image; discuss feelings about body changes
 Assess for local irritation, pain, burning at injection site, extravasation, a vesicant

**Nursing diagnoses**
• Body image, disturbed (adverse reactions)
• Cardiac output, decreased (adverse reactions)
• Infection, risk for (adverse reactions)
• Injury, risk for (adverse reactions)
• Knowledge, deficient (teaching)

**Implementation**
• Avoid contact with skin; very irritating; wash completely to remove
• Give fluids **IV** or PO before chemotherapy to hydrate patient
• Administer antiemetic 30-60 min before giving product and prn to prevent vomiting; administer antibiotics for prophylaxis of infection
• Give a liquid diet: carbonated beverages; gelatin may be added if patient is not nauseated or vomiting

- Product should be prepared by experienced personnel using proper precautions (biologic cabinet, wearing gown, gloves, mask)
- Give after reconstituting 5-mg vial with 5 ml of 0.9% NaCl (1 mg/1 ml); give over 10-15 min through Y-tube or 3-way stopcock of inf of $D_5$ or 0.9% NaCl; discard unused portion
- Apply ice compress after stopping inf (extravasation)
- Store at room temperature for 3 days after reconstituting or 7 days refrigerated

*Y-site compatibilities:* Amifostine, amikacin, aztreonam, cimetidine, cladribine, cyclophosphamide, cytarabine, diphenhydrA-MINE, droperidol, erythromycin, filgrastim, granisetron, imipenem/cilastatin, magnesium sulfate, mannitol, melphalan, metoclopromide, potassium chloride, ranitidine, sargramostim, thiotepa, vinorelbine

*Y-site incompatibilities:* Acyclovir, ampicillin/sulbactam, cefazolin, ceftazidine, clindamycin, dexamethasone, etoposide, furosemide, gentamicin, hydrocortisone, lorazepam, meperidine, methotrexate, mezlocillin, sargramostim, sodium bicarbonate, vancomycin, vinCRIStine

*Solution compatibilities:* $D_{3.3}$/0.3% NaCl, $D_5$/0.9% NaCl, $D_5$W, Ringer's, 0.9% NaCl, LR

## Patient/family education

- Teach patient to avoid use of products containing aspirin or ibuprofen, razors, commercial mouthwash, since bleeding may occur; to report symptoms of bleeding (hematuria, tarry stools)
- Instruct patient to report signs of anemia (fatigue, headache, irritability, faintness, shortness of breath)
- Advise patient that hair may be lost during treatment; a wig or hairpiece may make patient feel better; new hair may be different in color, texture
- Teach patient to rinse mouth tid-qid with water, club soda; brush teeth bid-qid with soft brush or cotton-tipped applicators for stomatitis; use unwaxed dental floss
- Tell patient not to have any vaccinations without the advice of the prescriber; serious reactions can occur
- Advise patient that contraception is needed during treatment and for several mo after the completion of therapy
- Teach patient to report signs of CHF, cardiac toxicity, beginning infection
- Advise patient to avoid crowds, those with upper respiratory illness

## Evaluation

**Positive therapeutic outcome**

- Prevention of rapid division of malignant cells

### ⚠ HIGH ALERT

**ifosfamide** 🔵 (Rx)
(i-foss'fa-mide)
Ifex
*Func. class.:* Antineoplastic alkylating agent
*Chem. class.:* Nitrogen mustard

**Pregnancy category D**

**Do not confuse:**
ifosfamide/cyclophosphamide

**Action:** Alkylates DNA, RNA; inhibits enzymes that allow synthesis of amino acids in proteins; also responsible for cross-linking DNA strands; activity is not cell cycle stage specific

**Therapeutic outcome:** Prevention of rapidly growing malignant cells

**Uses:** Testicular cancer

**Unlabeled uses:** Soft-tissue sarcoma, Ewing's sarcoma, non-Hodgkin's lymphoma, lung/pancreatic cancer, sarcoma

**Dosage and routes**
*Adult:* **IV** 1.2-2 g/m²/day × 5 days; repeat course q3 wk; give with mesna

*Renal dose*
*Adult:* **IV** CCr 31-60 ml/min give 75% of dose; CCr 10-30 ml/min give 50% of dose; CCr <10 ml/min, do not give

**Available forms:** Inj 1, 3 g vials

**Adverse effects**
*CNS:* Facial paresthesia, fever, malaise, somnolence, confusion, depression, hallucinations, dizziness, disorientation, **seizures, coma,** cranial nerve dysfunction
*GI:* Nausea, vomiting, anorexia, **hepatotoxicity,** stomatitis, constipation, diarrhea
*GU:* **Hematuria, nephrotoxicity, hemorrhagic cystitis,** dysuria, urinary frequency
*HEMA:* **Thrombocytopenia, leukopenia, anemia**
*INTEG:* Dermatitis, alopecia, pain at inj site, hyperpigmentation
*META:* Metabolic acidosis

**Contraindications:** Pregnancy **D,** hypersensitivity, bone marrow suppression

**Precautions:** Renal/hepatic disease, breastfeeding, children

Adverse effects: *italic* = common, **bold** = life-threatening

## Pharmacokinetics

| | |
|---|---|
| **Absorption** | Complete bioavailability |
| **Distribution** | Saturation at high dosages |
| **Metabolism** | Liver |
| **Excretion** | Breast milk |
| **Half-life** | 15 hr, depends on dose |

## Pharmacodynamics

Unknown

## Interactions
### Individual drugs
Allopurinol: increased toxicity
Radiation: increased bone marrow suppression

### Drug classifications
Anticoagulants, NSAIDs: increased bleeding risk
Antineoplastics: increased bone marrow suppression
CYP3A4 inducers, barbiturates: increased toxicity
CYP3A4 inhibitors: decreased ifosfamide effect
Live virus vaccines: decreased antibody response

## NURSING CONSIDERATIONS
### Assessment
 Monitor CBC, differential, platelet count weekly; withhold product if WBC is <2000 or platelet count is <50,000; notify prescriber of results if WBC <10,000/mm$^3$, platelets <100,000/mm$^3$, severe myelosuppression
• Monitor renal function studies: BUN, serum uric acid, urine CCr before, during therapy; I&O ratio; report fall in urine output of 30 ml/hr
• Monitor for cold, fever, sore throat (may indicate beginning of infection); identify edema in feet and joints, stomach pain, shaking; prescriber should be notified
• Assess for bleeding: hematuria, guaiac, bruising or petechiae, mucosa or orifices; no rec temp
• Monitor liver function tests before and during therapy (ALT, AST, LDH); jaundice of skin, sclera, dark urine, clay-colored stools, itching, abdominal pain, fever, diarrhea that may indicate liver involvement

### Nursing diagnoses
• Body image, disturbed (adverse reactions)
• Infection, risk for (adverse reactions)
• Injury, risk for (adverse reactions)
• Knowledge, deficient (teaching)

### Implementation
• Always give with mesna to prevent ifosfamide-induced hemorrhagic cystitis
• Give fluids **IV** or PO before and after chemotherapy to hydrate patient
• Give antiemetic 30-60 min before giving product and prn to prevent vomiting
• Provide liquid diet: carbonated beverages; gelatin may be added if patient is not nauseated or vomiting
• Give **IV** after diluting 1 g/20 ml of sterile or bacteriostatic water for inj with parabens or benzyl only; shake
• Give by intermittent inf after further diluting with D$_5$W, LR, 0.9% NaCl, sterile water for inj (1 g/20 ml = 50 mg/ml; 1 g/50 ml = 20 mg/ml; 1 g/200 ml = 5 mg/ml); give over ≥30 min; may also give as a cont inf over 72 hr
• Store powder at room temperature; always give with mesna, increase fluids to 3 L/day to prevent ifosfamide-induced hemorrhagic cystitis

**Syringe compatibilities:** Mesna
**Y-site compatibilities:** Allopurinol, amifostine, aztreonam, filgrastim, fludarabine, gallium, granisetron, melphalan, ondansetron, paclitaxel, piperacillin/tazobactam, propofol, sargramostim, teniposide, thiotepa, vinorelbine
**Additive compatibilities:** Carboplatin, cisplatin, etoposide, fluorouracil, mesna

### Patient/family education
• Teach patient to avoid use of products containing aspirin or NSAIDs, razors, commercial mouthwash, since bleeding may occur; to report symptoms of bleeding (hematuria, tarry stools)
• Instruct patient to report signs of anemia (fatigue, headache, irritability, faintness, shortness of breath)
• Advise patient to report any changes in breathing or coughing even several mo after treatment; to avoid crowds and persons with respiratory tract or other infections
• Teach patient that hair loss is common; discuss the use of wigs or hairpieces; that hair may be a different texture when regrowth occurs
• Caution patient not to have any vaccinations without the advice of the prescriber; serious reactions can occur
• Advise patient that contraception is needed during treatment and for several mo after completion of therapy
• Advise patient to report confusion, hallucinations, extreme drowsiness, numbness, tingling; avoid use of alcohol for ≥4 months after treatment

## Evaluation
**Positive therapeutic outcome**
- Prevention of rapid division of malignant cells
- Absence of swelling at night
- Increased appetite, increased weight

## imatinib (Rx)
(im-ah-tin'ib)
Gleevec
*Func. class.:* Antineoplastic—miscellaneous
*Chem. class.:* Protein-tyrosine kinase inhibitor

### Pregnancy category D

**Action:** Inhibits Bcr-Abl tyrosine kinase created in chronic myeloid leukemia (CML)

**Therapeutic outcome:** Decreased tumor size, prevention of spread of cancer

**Uses:** Treatment of chronic myeloid leukemia (CML), Philadelphia chromosome positive in blast cell crisis or chronic failure after treatment failure with interferon alfa, gastrointestinal stromal tumors (GIST), positive for KIT; chronic eosinophilic leukemia, acute lymphocytic leukemia, dermatofibrosarcoma protuberans, myelodysplastic syndrome

### Dosage and routes
*CML, chronic phase*
*Adult:* PO 400-600 mg/day
*Child:* PO 340 mg/m²/day

*Hepatic dose*
*Adult:* PO 300 mg/day, may increase to 400 mg/day
*Child ≥3 yr:* PO 200 mg/m²/day; may increase to 340 mg/m²/day in 1-2 divided doses

*CML, accelerated phase/blast crisis*
*Adult:* PO 600-800 mg/day

*GIST*
*Adult:* PO 400 or 600 mg/day

**Available forms:** Tabs 100, 400 mg

### Adverse effects
***CNS:*** **CNS hemorrhage,** headache, dizziness, insomnia
***CV:*** **Hemorrhage, heart failure**
***GI:*** *Nausea,* **hepatotoxicity,** *vomiting, dyspepsia,* **GI hemorrhage,** *anorexia,* abdominal pain
***HEMA:*** **Neutropenia, thrombocytopenia, bleeding**
***INTEG:*** *Rash, pruritus*
***META:*** Edema, fluid retention, hypokalemia
***MISC:*** Fatigue, epistaxis, pyrexia, night sweats, increased weight, flulike symptoms

***MS:*** Cramps, pain, arthralgia, myalgia
***RESP:*** Cough, dyspnea, nasopharyngitis, pneumonia, URI

**Contraindications:** Pregnancy **D,** hypersensitivity

**Precautions:** Breastfeeding, children, geriatric, cardiac/renal/hepatic disease

### Pharmacokinetics
| | |
|---|---|
| **Absorption** | Well absorbed; bound to plasma protein (98%) |
| **Distribution** | Unknown |
| **Metabolism** | Liver (metabolites) |
| **Excretion** | Feces, primarily (metabolites) |
| **Half-life** | 18-40 hr |

### Pharmacodynamics
| | |
|---|---|
| **Onset** | Unknown |
| **Peak** | 2-4 hr |
| **Duration** | 24 hr (imatinib), 40 hr (metabolite) |

### Interactions
*Individual drugs*
Acetaminophen: increased hepatotoxicity
CYP3A4 inducers (carbamazepine, dexamethasone, phenobarbital, phenytoin, rifampin): decreased imatinib concentrations
CYP3A4 inhibitors (clarithromycin, erythromycin, ketoconazole, itraconazole): increased imatinib concentrations
Simvastatin: increased plasma concentrations
Warfarin: increased plasma concentration of warfarin; avoid coadministration; use low-molecular-weight anticoagulants instead
*Drug classifications*
Calcium channel blockers, ergots: increased plasma concentrations
*Drug/herb*
St. John's wort: decreased imatinib concentration

### NURSING CONSIDERATIONS
### Assessment
- Assess ANC and platelets; in chronic phase if ANC <1 × 10⁹/L and/or platelets <50 × 10⁹/L, stop until ANC >1.5 × 10⁹/L and platelets >75 × 10⁹/L; in accelerated phase/blast crisis if ANC <0.5 × 10⁹/L and/or platelets <10 × 10⁹/L, determine whether cytopenia is related to biopsy/aspirate, if not, reduce dose by 200 mg, if cytopenia continues, reduce dose by another 100 mg; if cytopenia continues for 4 wk, stop product until ANC ≥1 × 10⁹/L
- Assess for hepatotoxicity: monitor liver function tests, before treatment and qmo
- Assess CBC, differential, platelet count weekly; withhold product if WBC is <3500/

Adverse effects: *italic* = common, **bold** = life-threatening

mm$^3$, or platelet count <100,000/mm$^3$; notify prescriber of these results
- Assess food preferences: list likes, dislikes
- Assess GI symptoms: frequency of stools
- Assess signs of fluid retention, edema: weigh, monitor lung sounds, assess for edema, 50-ml fluid retention is dose dependent

### Nursing diagnoses
- Injury, risk for (side effects)
- Knowledge, deficient (teaching)

### Implementation
- Give with meal and large glass of water to decrease GI symptoms
- Store at 25° C (77° F)

### Patient/family education
- Instruct patient to report adverse reactions immediately: shortness of breath, swelling of extremities, bleeding
- Teach patient reason for treatment, expected result
- Instruct patient to eat a nutritious diet with iron, vit supplement, low fiber, few dairy products

### Evaluation
**Positive therapeutic outcome**
- Decrease in leukemic cells, size of tumors

---

## imipenem/ cilastatin (Rx)
(i-me-pen'em sye-la-stat'in)
Primaxin IM, Primaxin IV
*Func. class.:* Antiinfective—miscellaneous penicillin
*Chem. class.:* Carbapenem

**Pregnancy category  C**

### Do not confuse:
imipenem/Omnipen, Primaxin/Premarin

**Action:** Interferes with cell wall replication of susceptible organisms; osmotically unstable cell wall swells and bursts from osmotic pressure; addition of cilastatin prevents renal inactivation that occurs with high urinary concentrations of imipenem

**Therapeutic outcome:** Bactericidal action against the following: *Streptococcus pneumoniae,* group A β-hemolytic streptococci, *Staphylococcus aureus,* enterococcus; gram-negative organisms: *Klebsiella, Proteus, Escherichia coli, Acinetobacter, Serratia, Pseudomonas aeruginosa; Salmonella, Shigella, Haemophilus influenzae, Listeria* sp.

**Uses:** Serious infections caused by gram-positive or gram-negative organisms

### Dosage and routes
*Adult:* **IV** 250-500 mg q6-8hr; severe infections may require 1 g q8hr; may give IM q12hr (total daily IM dose >1500 mg not recommended); mild to moderate infections
*Child:* **IV** 60-100 mg/kg/day in divided doses, max 4 g/day; IM 10-15 mg/kg q6hr

### Renal dose
*Adult:* **IV** CCr 30-70 ml/min give 50% dose q6-8hr; CCr 20-30 ml/min give 40% of dose q8-12hr; CCr 5-20 ml/min give 25% of dose q12hr

**Available forms: IV** inj 250, 500; IM inj 500, 750 mg

### Adverse effects
***CNS:*** Fever, somnolence, **seizures,** confusion, dizziness, weakness, myoclonia
***CV:*** Hypotension, palpitations, tachycardia
***GI:*** *Diarrhea, nausea, vomiting,* **pseudomembranous colitis, hepatitis,** glossitis
***HEMA:*** **Eosinophilia, neutropenia,** decreased Hgb, Hct
***INTEG:*** Rash, urticaria, pruritus, pain at inj site, phlebitis, erythema at inj site
***RESP:*** Chest discomfort, dyspnea, hyperventilation
***SYST:*** **Anaphylaxis, Stevens-Johnson syndrome**

**Contraindications:** Hypersensitivity, IM hypersensitivity to local anesthetics of the amide type

**Precautions:** Pregnancy **C**, breastfeeding, children, geriatric, hypersensitivity to penicillins, seizure disorders, renal disease, head trauma

### Pharmacokinetics
| | |
|---|---|
| Absorption | Complete bioavailability (**IV**) |
| Distribution | Widely distributed; crosses placenta |
| Metabolism | Liver |
| Excretion | Kidneys, unchanged (70%-80%); breast milk |
| Half-life | 1 hr; increased in renal disease |

### Pharmacodynamics
| | IM | IV |
|---|---|---|
| Onset | Unknown | Rapid |
| Peak | Unknown | ½-1 hr |

### Interactions
*Individual drugs*
Aminophylline, cycloSPORINE, ganciclovir, theophylline: increased risk of seizures
Probenecid: increased imipenem plasma levels

---

 Alert     Canada Only     Drug on CD    * "Tall Man" lettering (See Preface)

### Drug classifications
β-Lactam antibiotics: increased antagonistic effect
### Drug/herb
Do not use acidophilus with antiinfectives; separate by several hours
### Drug/lab test
Increased: AST, ALT, LDH, BUN, alkaline phosphatase, bilirubin, creatinine
False positive: direct Coombs' test

## NURSING CONSIDERATIONS
### Assessment
• Assess patient for previous penicillin sensitivity reaction, may have sensitivity to this product
• Assess patient for signs and symptoms of infection, including characteristics of wounds, sputum, urine, stool, WBC >10,000/mm$^3$, fever; obtain baseline information before and during treatment
• Complete C&S tests before beginning product therapy to identify if correct treatment has been initiated
• Assess for allergic reactions, anaphylaxis: rash, urticaria, pruritus, chills, wheezing, laryngeal edema, fever, joint pain; angioedema may occur a few days after therapy begins; epiNEPHrine, resuscitation equipment should be available for anaphylactic reaction
• Identify urine output; if decreasing, notify prescriber (may indicate nephrotoxicity); also check for increased BUN, creatinine
• Monitor blood studies: AST, ALT, CBC, Hct, bilirubin, LDH, alkaline phosphatase, Coombs' test monthly if patient is on long-term therapy
• Monitor electrolytes: potassium, sodium, chloride monthly if patient is on long-term therapy
• Assess bowel pattern daily; if severe diarrhea occurs, product should be discontinued; may indicate pseudomembranous colitis
• Monitor for bleeding: ecchymosis, bleeding gums, hematuria, stool guaiac daily if patient is on long-term therapy
• Assess for overgrowth of infection: perineal itching, fever, malaise, redness, pain, swelling, drainage, rash, diarrhea, change in cough, sputum

### Nursing diagnoses
• Diarrhea (adverse reactions)
• Infection, risk for (uses)
• Injury, risk for (adverse reactions)
• Knowledge, deficient (teaching)
• Noncompliance (teaching)

### Implementation
**IM route**
• Reconstitute 500 mg/2 ml or 750 mg/3 ml lidocaine without epiNEPHrine; shake well, withdraw and administer entire vial; give inj deep in large muscle mass, massage
**IV route**
• Reconstitute each 250 or 500 mg/10 ml of compatible diluent; shake well; transfer the resulting susp to not <100 ml of compatible diluent; add 10 ml to each previously reconstituted vial and shake to ensure all medication is used; transfer the remaining contents of the vial to the infusion container; do not administer susp by direct inj; reconstitute 120-ml infusion bottles/100 ml of a compatible diluent; shake until clear; may use 0.9% NaCl, D$_5$W, D$_{10}$W, D$_5$/0.2% sodium bicarbonate, D$_5$/0.9% NaCl, D$_5$/0.45% NaCl, D$_5$/0.225% NaCl, mannitol 2.5%, 5%, or 10%
• Give by intermittent inf: each 250- or 500-mg dose over 20-30 min, and each 1-g dose over 40-60 min; administer over 15-20 min for pediatric patients; do not administer direct **IV**; do not admix with other antibiotics
**Y-site compatibilities:** Acyclovir, amifostine, aztreonam, cefepime, diltiazem, famotidine, fludarabine, foscarnet, granisetron, idarubicin, regular insulin, melphalan, methotrexate, ondansetron, propofol, tacrolimus, teniposide, thiotepa, vinorelbine, zidovudine
**Y-site incompatibilities:** Fluconazole, meperidine, sargramostim
**Additive incompatibilities:** Fluconazole, meperidine, sargramostim

### Patient/family education
• Teach patient to report sore throat, bruising, bleeding, joint pain; may indicate blood dyscrasias (rare)
• Advise patient to contact prescriber if vaginal itching, loose foul-smelling stools, furry tongue occur; may indicate superinfection
• Advise patient to notify prescriber of diarrhea with blood or pus; may indicate pseudomembranous colitis

### Evaluation
**Positive therapeutic outcome**
• Absence of signs/symptoms of infection (WBC <10,000/mm$^3$, temp WNL, absence of red, draining wounds)
• Reported improvement in symptoms of infection

### Treatment of anaphylaxis: EpINEPHrine, antihistamines, resuscitate if needed

Adverse effects: *italic* = common, **bold** = life-threatening

## imipramine 🔵 (Rx)

(im-ip′ra-meen)
Apo-Imipramine ✦, Imipramine HCl,
Impril ✦, Norfranil, Novo Pramine ✦,
Tofranil, Tofranil PM, Tipramine
*Func. class.:* Antidepressant, tricyclic
*Chem. class.:* Dibenzazepine, tertiary amine

### Pregnancy category D

### Do not confuse:
imipramine/desipramine

**Action:** Blocks reuptake of norepinephrine and serotonin into nerve endings, increasing action of norepinephrine and serotonin in nerve cells; has anticholinergic effects

**Therapeutic outcome:** Decreased symptoms of depression after 2-3 wk; decreased bedwetting in children

**Uses:** Depression, enuresis in children

**Unlabeled uses:** Chronic pain, migraine headaches, cluster headaches as adjunct, incontinence

### Dosage and routes
*Adult:* PO 100 mg/day in divided doses; may increase by 25-50 mg up to 200 mg, max 300 mg/day; may give daily dose at bedtime
*Geriatric:* PO 25 mg at bedtime, may increase to 100 mg/day in divided doses
*Child:* PO 1.5 mg/kg/day in divided doses; max 100 mg/day

*Enuresis*
*Child 6-12 yr:* PO 10 mg at bedtime, max 75 mg

**Available forms:** Tabs 10, 25, 50 mg; caps 75, 100, 125, 150 mg

### Adverse effects
*CNS:* *Dizziness, drowsiness,* confusion, headache, anxiety, tremors, stimulation, weakness, insomnia, nightmares, EPS (geriatric), increased psychiatric symptoms, paresthesia, **seizures**
*CV:* *Orthostatic hypotension, ECG changes, tachycardia,* hypertension, palpitations, **dysrhythmias**
*EENT:* Blurred vision, tinnitus, mydriasis
*GI:* *Diarrhea, dry mouth,* nausea, vomiting, **paralytic ileus,** increased appetite, cramps, epigastric distress, jaundice, **hepatitis,** stomatitis, constipation, taste change
*GU:* *Retention,* **acute renal failure**
*HEMA:* **Agranulocytosis, thrombocytopenia, eosinophilia, leukopenia**
*INTEG:* Rash, urticaria, sweating, pruritus, photosensitivity

**Contraindications:** Pregnancy **D,** hypersensitivity to tricyclics, recovery phase of MI, seizure disorders, prostatic hypertrophy

**Precautions:** Suicidal patients, severe depression, increased intraocular pressure, angle-closure glaucoma, urinary retention, cardiac/hepatic disease, hyperthyroidism, electroshock therapy, elective surgery, breastfeeding, geriatric

### Pharmacokinetics
| | |
|---|---|
| **Absorption** | Well absorbed |
| **Distribution** | Widely distributed; crosses placenta |
| **Metabolism** | Liver, extensively |
| **Excretion** | Kidneys, breast milk |
| **Half-life** | 6-20 hr |

### Pharmacodynamics
| | PO | IM |
|---|---|---|
| **Onset** | 1 hr | 1 hr |
| **Peak** | Unknown | Unknown |
| **Duration** | Unknown | Unknown |

### Interactions
*Individual drugs*
Alcohol: increased effects
Clonidine: hyperpyretic crisis, seizures, hypertensive episode
Clonidine, guanethidine: decreased effects
Gatifloxacin, levofloxacin, moxifloxacin, ziprasidone: increased QT interval
*Drug classifications*
Barbiturates, benzodiazepines, CNS depressants: increased effects
MAOIs: hyperpyretic crisis, hypertensive episode, seizures
Selective serotonin reuptake inhibitors: increased toxicity, avoid concurrent use
Sympathomimetics (direct acting [epINEPHrine]), barbiturates, benzodiazepines, CNS depressants: increased effects
Sympathomimetics (indirect acting [epHEDrine]): decreased effects
Tricyclic antidepressants: increased QT interval
*Drug/herb*
Belladonna, corkwood, henbane, jimsonweed, scopolia: increased anticholinergic effect
Chamomile, hops, kava, lavender, skullcap, valerian: increased imipramine effect
SAM-e, St. John's wort: serotonin syndrome
Yohimbe: increased hypertension
*Drug/lab test*
Increased: serum bilirubin, blood glucose, alkaline phosphatase
Decreased: VMA, 5-HIAA, urinary catecholamines

# immune globulin IM 497

## NURSING CONSIDERATIONS
### Assessment
- Monitor B/P (with patient lying, standing), pulse q4hr; if systolic B/P drops 20 mm Hg, hold product, notify prescriber; take vital signs q4hr in patients with CV disease
- Monitor blood studies: CBC, leukocytes, differential, cardiac enzymes if patient is receiving long-term therapy
- Monitor hepatic studies: AST, ALT, bilirubin
- Check weight weekly; appetite may increase with product
- Assess ECG for flattening of T wave, bundle branch block, AV block, dysrhythmias in cardiac patients
- Assess for EPS primarily in geriatric: rigidity, dystonia, akathisia
- Assess mental status: mood, sensorium, affect, suicidal tendencies; increase in psychiatric symptoms: depression, panic
- Monitor urinary retention, constipation; constipation is more likely to occur in children or geriatric
- ◆ Assess for withdrawal symptoms: headache, nausea, vomiting, muscle pain, weakness, diarrhea, insomnia, restlessness; do not usually occur unless product was discontinued abruptly
- Identify alcohol consumption; if alcohol is consumed, hold dose until AM

### Nursing diagnoses
- Coping, ineffective (uses)
- Injury, risk for (side effects)
- Knowledge, deficient (teaching)
- Noncompliance (teaching)

### Implementation
#### PO route
- Do not break, crush, or chew caps
- Give with food or milk
- Store at room temperature; do not freeze
*Syringe compatibilities:* Doxapram
*Y-site compatibilities:* Cladribine

### Patient/family education
- Teach patient that therapeutic effects may take 2-3 wk
- Teach patient to use caution in driving and other activities requiring alertness because of drowsiness, dizziness, blurred vision; to avoid rising quickly from sitting position, especially geriatric; orthostatic hypotension may occur
- Teach patient to avoid alcohol ingestion, other CNS depressants during treatment
- Teach patient not to discontinue medication quickly after long-term use: may cause nausea, headache, malaise
- Teach patient to wear sunscreen or large hat, since photosensitivity occurs

- Teach patient to increase fluids, bulk in diet if constipation, urinary retention occur, especially geriatric
- Teach patient to take gum, hard sugarless candy, or frequent sips of water for dry mouth

### Evaluation
#### Positive therapeutic outcome
- Decreased depression
- Absence of suicidal thoughts
- Decreased enuresis in children
- Decreased pain

**Treatment of overdose:** ECG monitoring, lavage, activated charcoal, administer anticonvulsant

## immune globulin IM (Rx)
gamma globulin, IG, IGIM, Bay Gam
## immune globulin IV (IGIV) (Rx)
Carimune NF, Flebogamma 5%, Gamimune N, Gamma-Gard S/D, gamma globulin, Gammar-PIV, Gamunex, Iveegam, Iveegam EN, Octagam, Panglobulin NF, Polygam, Polygam SD, Sandoglobulin, Venoglobulin-I, Venoglobulin-S
*Func. class.:* Immune serum
*Chem. class.:* IgG
### Pregnancy category C

**Action:** Provides passive immunity to hepatitis A, measles, varicella, rubella, immune globulin deficiency; contains γ-globulin antibodies (IgG)

**Therapeutic outcome:** Absence of infection

**Uses:** Immunodeficiency syndrome, B-cell chronic lymphocytic leukemia, Kawasaki syndrome, bone marrow transplantation, pediatric HIV infection, agammaglobulinemia, hepatitis A, B exposure, measles exposure, measles vaccine complications, purpura, rubella exposure, chickenpox exposure

**Unlabeled uses:** IV posttransfusion purpura, Guillain-Barré syndrome, chronic inflammatory demyelinating polyneuropathy

### Dosage and routes
#### Primary immunodeficiency
*Adult and child:* IV (Carimune, Panglobulin NF) 200 mg/kg qmo, max 300 mg/kg qmo or give more frequently if needed; IV (Gamimune N) 100-200 mg/kg qmo, max 400 mg/kg; IV (Gammagard S/D) 200-400 mg qmo, minimum 100 mg/kg qmo; IV (Gamunex) 300-600 mg/kg q3-4wk; IV (Iveegam

Adverse effects: *italic* = common, **bold** = life-threatening

EN) 200 mg/kg qmo, max 800 mg/kg; **IV** (Octagam) 300-600 mg q3-4wk; **IV** (Polygam S/D) 200-400 mg/kg qmo

*Hepatitis A exposure (IGIM)*
*Adult and child:* IM 0.02-0.04 ml/kg

*Chickenpox exposure (IGIM)*
*Adult and child:* IM 0.6-1.2 ml/kg as soon as exposed

*Measles (postexposure) (IGIM)*
*Adult and child:* IM 0.25 ml/kg within 6 days

*B-cell chronic lymphocytic leukemia (CLL) (IGIV) (Gammagard S/D, Polygam S/D)*
*Adult:* **IV** 400 mg/kg q3-4 wk

*Idiopathic thrombocytopenia purpura*
*Adult and child:* **IV** 0.4 g/kg/day × 5 days or 1 g/kg/day × 1-2 days

*Kawasaki syndrome to prevent coronary artery aneurysm (IGIV) (Iveegam, Venoglobulin-S, Gammagard S/D, Polygam S/D)*
*Adult and child:* **IV** (Iveegam, Venglobulin-S 5% or 10%) 2000 mg/kg over 10-12 hr, may repeat; **IV** (Gammagard S/D, Polygam S/D) 1 g/kg as single dose

*Bone marrow transplantation (BMT) (IGIV) (Gamimune N)*
*Adult >20 yr:* **IV** 500 mg/kg 5% or 10% sol on days 2, 7 before transplant then qwk for 90 days thereafter

*Pediatric HIV (IGIV) (Gamimune N)*
*Child:* **IV** 400 mg/kg 5% or 10% sol q28 days

**Available forms:** IM (Bay Gam) inj 2, 10 ml vial; **IV** (Gamimune N, Venoglobulin-S) 5%, 10% sol; powder for inj (Carimune NF) 1-, 3-, 6-, 12-g vials; (Gammagard S/D) 50 mg protein/ml in 2.5-, 5-, 10-g vials; (Gammar-P IV) 1-, 2.5-, 5-, 10-g vials; (Iveegam) 500 mg, 1-, 2.5-, 5-g vials; (Panglobulin) 6-, 12-g vials; (Polygam S/D) 2.5-, 5-, 10-g vials; sol for inj (Gamunex) 1-, 2.5-, 5-, 10-, 20-g vials

**Adverse effects**
*CNS:* Headache, fatigue, malaise
*GI:* Abdominal pain
*INTEG:* Pain at inj site, rash, pruritus, chills
*MS:* Arthralgia, chest pain
*SYST:* Lymphadenopathy, **anaphylaxis**

**Contraindications:** Hypersensitivity
**Precautions:** Pregnancy **C**

### Pharmacokinetics

| | |
|---|---|
| **Absorption** | Well absorbed (IM); completely absorbed (**IV**) |
| **Distribution** | Rapidly |
| **Metabolism** | Liver, catabolism |
| **Excretion** | Kidneys |
| **Half-life** | 3-4 wk |

### Pharmacodynamics

| | IM | IV |
|---|---|---|
| **Onset** | Unknown | Rapid |
| **Peak** | Unknown | Unknown |
| **Duration** | Unknown | Unknown |

### Interactions
**Drug classifications**
Live virus vaccines: do not give within 3 mo
**Drug/lab test**
Interference: glucose testing system

### NURSING CONSIDERATIONS
**Assessment**
• Assess for exposure date: this product should be given within 6 days of measles, 1 wk of hepatitis B, 14 days of hepatitis A; if the date of exposure is outside these limits, immune globulin will not be effective
• Monitor blood studies in leukemia, idiopathic thrombocytopenic purpura: WBCs (leukemia), platelets
• Identify the number of inj of this product patient has received; multiple inj may lead to sensitization (diaphoresis, fever, chills, malaise)
• Assess for anaphylaxis in patient receiving **IV** immune globulin: diaphoresis, flushing, nausea, vomiting, wheezing, difficulty breathing, hypotension, chest tightness, fever, weakness, sneezing, abdominal pain; VS should be monitored during infusion and 1 hr after beginning infusion; emergency equipment should be available with epINEPHrine and antihistamines to treat anaphylaxis

**Nursing diagnoses**
• Infection, risk for (uses)
• Knowledge, deficient (teaching)

**Implementation**
**IM route**
• Give IM (IGIM) inj in deltoid or anterolateral thigh in adults or anterolateral thigh in young children; if large amounts are given, several injections may be needed
• Do not give the IM preparation **IV**, SUBCUT, or intradermally
• Sol should be transparent and clear or slightly colored

**IV route**

• Warm to room temperature before administration (diluent, powder for inj)
• A transfer device is provided by manufacturer; this product should not be agitated or shaken
• Do not give the **IV** preparation SUBCUT, IM, or intradermally
• Check for adverse reaction during inf; stop inf if adverse reactions are present

*Y-site compatibilities:* Fluconazole, sargramostim

**Gamimune N:** Dilute **IV** with D₅; give 0.01 ml/kg/min; may increase to 0.02-0.04 ml/min if no adverse reactions are present; may increase to 0.08 ml/kg/hr; sol should be refrigerated; do not freeze

**Gammagard S/D:** Reconstitute with sterile water for inj (50 mg protein/ml); give within 2 hr of reconstitution; give 0.5 ml/kg/hr; may increase to 4 ml/kg/hr if no adverse reactions occur; use inf set provided

**Gammar-P IV:** Give 0.01 ml/kg/min (50 mg/ml sol) over 15-30 min; may increase to 0.02 ml/kg/min; if adverse reactions are not present, may increase to 0.03-0.06 ml/kg/min; do not freeze; store at room temperature

**Iveegam (5%):** Give 1-2 ml/min; refrigerate, do not freeze

**Sandoglobulin:** **IV** diluted with provided diluent; give 0.5-1 ml/min over 15-30 min; may increase to 1.5-2.5 ml/min; other inf may be given 2-2.5 ml/min; store at room temperature

**Venoglobulin-I:** Give 50 mg/ml sol 0.01-0.02 ml/kg/min over 30 min if no adverse reactions; increase 0.04 ml/kg/min; store at room temperature

**Patient/family education**

• Advise patient that passive immunity is temporary; explain reason for and expected results of this product
• Advise patient that pain and tenderness may occur at inj site

**Evaluation**

**Positive therapeutic outcome**

• Prevention of infection
• Increased platelets

**Treatment of anaphylaxis:** EpINEPHrine, diphenhydrAMINE, O₂, vasopressors, corticosteroids

---

**❗ HIGH ALERT**

# inamrinone  (Rx)
(in-am'rih-nohn)
Inocor
*Func. class.:* Inotropic agent
*Chem. class.:* Bipyrimidine derivative

**Pregnancy category** C

**Do not confuse:**
inamrinone/amiodarone

**Action:** Positive inotropic agent with vasodilator properties; reduces preload and afterload by direct relaxation of vascular smooth muscle; increases myocardial contractility

**Therapeutic outcome:** Increased inotropic effect resulting in increased cardiac output

**Uses:** Short-term management of CHF that has not responded to other medication (diuretics, other vasodilators); can be used with digoxin

**Dosage and routes**
*Adult and child:* IV BOL 0.75 mg/kg given over 2-3 min; start INF of 5-10 mcg/kg/min; may give another BOL 30 min after start of therapy, max 10 mg/kg total daily dose
*Infants:* IV 3-4.5 mg/kg in divided doses, then give by INF 10 mcg/kg/min
*Neonates:* IV 3-4.5 mg/kg in divided doses, then give by INF 3-5 mcg/kg/min

**Available forms:** Inj 5 mg/ml

**Adverse effects**
*CV: Dysrhythmias, hypotension,* chest pain
*GI: Nausea, vomiting, anorexia,* abdominal pain, **hepatotoxicity (rare), ascites,** jaundice, hiccups
*HEMA:* **Thrombocytopenia**
*INTEG:* Allergic reactions, burning at inj site
*RESP:* Pleuritis, **pulmonary densities, hypoxemia**

**Contraindications:** Hypersensitivity to this product or bisulfites, severe aortic disease, severe pulmonic valvular disease, acute MI

**Precautions:** Pregnancy **C**, breastfeeding, children, geriatric, renal/hepatic disease, atrial flutter/fibrillation, asthma

| Pharmacokinetics | |
|---|---|
| **Absorption** | Complete bioavailability |
| **Distribution** | Unknown |
| **Metabolism** | Liver, 50% |
| **Excretion** | Kidney, metabolites (60%-90%) |
| **Half-life** | 4-6 hr, increased in CHF |

---

Adverse effects: *italic* = common, **bold** = life-threatening

| Pharmacodynamics | |
|---|---|
| **Onset** | 2-5 min |
| **Peak** | 10 min |
| **Duration** | Variable |

## Interactions

### Individual drugs
Disopyramide: increased hypotension

### Drug classifications
Antihypertensives: increased hypotension
Cardiac glycosides: increased additive effect

### Drug/herb
Aloe, buckthorn, cascara sagrada, senna: increased inamrinone action

### Drug/lab test
Increased: hepatic enzymes
Decreased: potassium

## NURSING CONSIDERATIONS
### Assessment
• Monitor manifestations of hypokalemia: *RENAL:* acidic urine, reduced urine, osmolality, nocturia; *CV:* hypotension, broad T wave, U wave, ectopy, tachycardia, weak pulse; *NEURO:* muscle weakness, altered LOC, drowsiness, apathy, lethargy, confusion, depression; *GI:* anorexia, nausea, cramps, constipation, distention, paralytic ileus; *RESP:* hypoventilation, respiratory muscle weakness
• Assess fluid volume status: CVP in geriatric, I&O ratio and record, weight, distended red veins, crackles in lung, color, quality, and specific gravity of urine, skin turgor, adequacy of pulses, moist mucous membranes, bilateral lung sounds, peripheral pitting edema; dehydration symptoms of decreasing output, thirst, hypotension, dry mouth, and mucous membranes should be reported
• Monitor electrolytes: potassium, sodium, calcium, magnesium; also include BUN, blood pH, ABGs
• Monitor B/P and pulse, PCWP, CVP, index, often during inf; if B/P drops 30 mm Hg, stop infusion and call prescriber
• Monitor ALT, AST, bilirubin daily; if these are elevated, hepatotoxicity is suspected
◆ If platelets are <150,000/mm$^3$, product is usually discontinued and another product started
• Assess for extravasation: change site q48hr

### Nursing diagnoses
• Cardiac output, decreased (uses)
• Fluid volume, excess (uses)
• Knowledge, deficient (teaching)

## Implementation
• Patients with low potassium levels (hypokalemia) should receive potassium supplements before inamrinone administration
• Administer potassium supplements if ordered for potassium levels <3.0 mg/dl, correct before using inamrinone

**IV route**
• Do not mix directly with dextrose sol; chemical reaction occurs over 24 hr; precipitate forms if inamrinone and furosemide come in contact

**IV, direct route**
• May inject into running dextrose inf through Y-connector or directly into tubing; may give undiluted over 2-3 min or dilute with 0.9%, 0.45% NaCl to concentration of 1-3 mg/ml; run at prescribed rate by cont inf; another loading dose may be given in 30 min

**Continous IV route**
• Give after diluting with 0.9% or 0.45% NaCl (1-3 mg/ml); do not dilute with dextrose sol; decomposition of product will occur; use infusion pump; use sol within 24 hr of dilution; titrate to patient response

### Syringe compatibilities: Propranolol, verapamil

### Y-site compatibilities: Aminophylline, atropine, bretylium, calcium chloride, cimetidine, cisatracurium, digoxin, DOBUTamine, DOPamine, epINEPHrine, famotidine, hydrocortisone, isoproterenol, lidocaine, metaraminol, methylPREDNISolone, nitroglycerin, nitroprusside, norepinephrine, phenylephrine, potassium chloride, procainamide, propranolol, remifentanil, verapamil

### Y-site incompatibilities: Furosemide, inamrinone, sodium bicarbonate

### Patient/family education
• Teach patient reason for medication and expected results
• Instruct patient to make position changes slowly; orthostatic hypotension may occur
• Teach patient signs and symptoms of hypersensitivity reactions and hypokalemia
• Advise patient that burning may occur at **IV** site

### Evaluation
**Positive therapeutic outcome**
• Increased cardiac output
• Decreased PCWP, adequate CVP
• Decreased dyspnea, fatigue, edema, ECG

**Treatment of overdose:** Discontinue product, support circulation

---

## indapamide (Rx)

(in-dap′a-mide)

indapamide, Lozide ✦, Lozol

*Func. class.:* Diuretic, thiazide-like, antihypertensive

*Chem. class.:* Thiazide-like sulfonamide derivative

**Pregnancy category** B

**Action:** Acts on proximal section of distal renal tubule by inhibiting reabsorption of sodium, may act by direct vasodilation caused by blocking of calcium channels

**Therapeutic outcome:** Decreased B/P, decreased edema in lung tissues, peripherally

**Uses:** Edema of CHF, hypertension, diuresis

### Dosage and routes
*Edema*
*Adult:* PO 2.5 mg/day in AM; may be increased to 5 mg/day if needed

*Antihypertensive*
*Adult:* PO 1.25-5 mg/day; may increase to 5 mg/day over 8 wks

**Available forms:** Tabs 1.25, 2.5 mg

### Adverse effects
*CNS:* Depression, *headache, dizziness, fatigue, weakness, nervousness, agitation,* extremity numbness
*CV:* Orthostatic hypotension, palpitations, volume depletion, PVCs, dysrhythmias
*EENT:* Blurred vision, nasal congestion, increased intraocular pressure
*ELECT: Hypokalemia, hypercalcemia, hyponatremia, hypochloremic alkalosis, hypomagnesemia,* hyperuricemia, hyperglycemia
*GI: Nausea,* vomiting, anorexia, constipation, diarrhea, cramps, abdominal pain, dry mouth
*GU: Frequency, polyuria, nocturia,* impotence
*INTEG:* Rash, *pruritus*
*MS:* Cramps

**Contraindications:** Hypersensitivity, anuria, hepatic coma

**Precautions:** Pregnancy **B**, breastfeeding, hypokalemia, severe renal disease, hepatic disease, ascites, dehydration, CCr <25 ml/min (not effective)

Pharmacokinetics

| | |
|---|---|
| **Absorption** | Well absorbed |
| **Distribution** | Widely distributed |
| **Metabolism** | Liver; 7% |
| **Excretion** | Unchanged (urine) |
| **Half-life** | 14-18 hr |

**Pharmacodynamics**

| | |
|---|---|
| **Onset** | 1-2 hr |
| **Peak** | 2 hr |
| **Duration** | Up to 36 hr |

### Interactions
*Individual drugs*
Amphotericin B: decreased potassium
Cholestyramine, colestipol: decreased absorption
Diazoxide: hyperglycemia
Digoxin, lithium: increased toxicity
Indomethacin: decreased hypotensive effect
*Drug classifications*
Anticoagulants, antidiabetics, antigout agents: decreased effects
Diuretics (other), steroids: decreased potassium
Muscle relaxants, steroids: increased toxicity
NSAIDs: decreased hypotensive effects
*Drug/herb*
Aloe, buckthorn, cascara sagrada, Chinese cucumber, licorice, senna: increased hypokalemia
Aloe, cucumber, dandelion, horsetail, pumpkin, Queen Anne's lace: increased diuretic effect
St. John's wort: severe photosensitivity
*Drug/lab test*
Increased: calcium, parathyroid test, glucose, uric acid

### NURSING CONSIDERATIONS
**Assessment**
• Check for rashes, temp elevation daily
• Monitor patients that receive cardiac glycosides for increased hypokalemia, toxicity
• Monitor manifestations of hypokalemia: acidic or reduced urine, osmolality, nocturia; hypotension, broad T-wave, U-wave, ectopy, tachycardia, weak pulse; muscle weakness, altered LOC, drowsiness, apathy, lethargy, confusion, depression; anorexia, nausea, cramps, constipation, distention, paralytic ileus; hypoventilation, respiratory muscle weakness
• Monitor for manifestations of hypomagnesemia: agitation, muscle twitching, paresthesias, hyperactive reflexes, positive Babinski reflex, dysphagia, nystagmus, seizures, tetany; nausea, vomiting, diarrhea, anorexia, abdominal distention; ectopy, tachycardia, broad, flat- or inverted T-waves, depressed ST segment, prolonged QT interval, decreased cardiac output, hypotension
• Monitor for manifestations of hyponatremia: increased B/P, cold, clammy skin, hypo/

hypervolemia; anorexia, nausea, vomiting, diarrhea, abdominal cramps; lethargy, increased ICP, confusion, headache, seizures, coma, fatigue, tremors, hyperreflexia
• Monitor for manifestations of hyperchloremia: weakness, lethargy, coma, deep rapid breathing
• Assess fluid volume status: I&O ratios and record, weight, distended red veins, crackles in lung, color, quality and specific gravity of urine, skin turgor, adequacy of pulses, moist mucous membranes, bilateral lung sounds, peripheral pitting edema; dehydration symptoms of decreasing output, thirst, hypotension, dry mouth and mucous membranes should be reported
• Monitor electrolytes: potassium, sodium, calcium, magnesium; also include BUN, blood pH, ABGs, uric acid, CBC, blood glucose
• Assess B/P before and during therapy with patient lying, standing, and sitting as appropriate; orthostatic hypotension can occur rapidly

## Nursing diagnoses
• Fluid volume, deficient (side effects)
• Fluid volume, excess (uses)
• Knowledge, deficient (teaching)
• Urinary elimination, impaired (side effect)

## Implementation
• Give in AM to avoid interference with sleep
• Provide potassium replacement if potassium level is <3.0 mg/dl; give whole
• Give with food and milk if nausea occurs, absorption may be increased

## Patient/family education
• Teach patient to take the medication early in the day to prevent nocturia
• Instruct the patient to take with food or milk if GI symptoms of nausea and anorexia occur
• Teach patient to maintain weekly record of weight and notify prescriber of weight loss >5 lb
• Caution the patient that this product causes a loss of potassium, so food rich in potassium should be added to the diet; refer to a dietitian for assistance in planning
• Caution the patient to rise slowly from sitting or reclining positions, not to exercise in hot weather or stand for prolonged periods, since orthostatic hypotension will be enhanced; lie down if dizziness occurs
• Teach patient not to use alcohol or any OTC medications without prescriber's approval; serious product reactions may occur
• Emphasize the need to contact prescriber immediately if muscle cramps, weakness, nausea, dizziness, or numbness occurs

• Teach patient to take own B/P and pulse and record findings
• Teach patient to continue taking medication even if feeling better; this product controls symptoms but does not cure the condition
• Advise the patient with hypertension to continue other medical treatment (exercise, weight loss, relaxation techniques, cessation of smoking)

## Evaluation
**Positive therapeutic outcome**
• Decreased edema
• Decreased B/P
• Increased diuresis

**Treatment of overdose:** Lavage, monitor electrolytes, administer **IV** fluids, monitor hydration, CV, renal status

---

## indinavir (Rx)
(en-den'a-veer)
Crixivan
*Func. class.:* Antiretroviral
*Chem. class.:* Protease inhibitor
**Pregnancy category** C

**Do not confuse:**
idinavir/Denavir

**Action:** Inhibits HIV-1 protease; this prevents maturation of the infectious virus

**Therapeutic outcome:** Decreased signs/symptoms of HIV-1 infection

**Uses:** HIV-1 in combination with other antiretrovirals

**Unlabeled uses:** Prevention of HIV-1 after exposure

## Dosage and routes
Reduce dose in mild/moderate hepatic impairment and ketoconazole coadministration
*Adult:* PO 800 mg q8hr; if given with didanosine, give 1 hr apart on empty stomach

**Available forms:** Caps 100, 200, 333, 400 mg

## Adverse effects
*CNS: Headache, insomnia,* dizziness, somnolence
*GI: Diarrhea, abdominal pain, nausea, vomiting,* anorexia, dry mouth
*GU:* Nephrolithiasis
*INTEG:* Rash
*MISC:* Asthenia, **insulin-resistant hyperglycemia,** hyperlipidemia, **ketoacidosis,** lipodystrophy
*MS:* Pain

 Alert     Canada Only    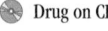 Drug on CD    * "Tall Man" lettering (See Preface)

**Contraindications:** Hypersensitivity

**Precautions:** Pregnancy **C**, breastfeeding, children, renal/hepatic disease, history of renal stones, diabetes, hypercholesterolemia, hemophilia

### Pharmacokinetics

| | |
|---|---|
| **Absorption** | Unknown |
| **Distribution** | Unknown |
| **Metabolism** | 60% protein binding; liver |
| **Excretion** | 20% unchanged, urine |
| **Half-life** | Terminal 1-2 hr |

### Pharmacodynamics
Unknown

### Interactions
*Individual drugs*
Atorvastatin, lovastatin, simvastatin: increased myopathy
Clarithromycin, zidovudine: increased levels of both products
Delavirdine, itraconazole, ketoconazole: increased indinavir level
Efavirenz, fluconazole, nevirapine: decreased indinavir level
Isoniazid: increased isoniazid level
Midazolam, rifampin, triazolam: increased life-threatening dysrhythmias
*Drug classifications*
Anticonvulsants: decreased effect of both products
Ergots: increased life-threatening dysrhythmias
Oral contraceptives: increased levels of oral contraceptives
Rifamycins: decreased indinavir levels
*Drug/herb*
St. John's wort: decreased indinavir level, avoid use
*Drug/food*
High fat, high protein, grapefruit juice: decreased absorption
*Drug/lab test*
Increased: AST, ALT, amylase, total bilirubin

### NURSING CONSIDERATIONS
**Assessment**
• Assess for lower back, flank pain, indicates kidney stones
• Monitor signs of infection, anemia
• Monitor liver studies: ALT, AST; total bilirubin, amylase; all may be elevated
• Determine the presence of other STDs
• Assess bowel pattern before, during treatment; if severe abdominal pain with bleeding occurs, product should be discontinued; monitor hydration
• Assess skin eruptions; rash, urticaria, itching

• Assess allergies before treatment, reaction of each medication; place allergies on chart
• Monitor viral load CD4 during treatment

**Nursing diagnoses**
• Infection, risk for (uses)
• Knowledge, deficient (teaching)

**Implementation**
• Do not break, crush, or chew caps
• Give with water, 1 hr before or 2 hr after meals; may be given with other liquids or small meal; do not give with high-fat, high-protein meals
• Give in equal intervals around the clock
• Dosage adjustment will need to be considered when given with efavirenz
• Give water to 1.5 L/day minimum, to prevent nephrolithiasis

**Patient/family education**
• Advise to take as prescribed; if dose is missed, take as soon as remembered up to 1 hr before next dose; do not double dose
• Advise that product must be taken in equal intervals around the clock to maintain blood levels for duration of therapy
• Instruct patient to increase fluids to prevent kidney stones; if stone formation occurs, treatment may need to be interrupted
• Inform patient that product does not cure AIDS, controls symptoms only; not to donate blood
• Advise patient that hyperglycemia may occur, watch for symptoms (thirst, hunger, dry, itchy skin); notify prescriber

**Evaluation**
**Positive therapeutic outcome**
• Decreased signs/symptoms of infection, HIV

### indomethacin (Rx)
(in-doe-meth′a-sin)
Apo-Indomethacin ✦, Indameth ✦, Indocid ✦, Indocin, Indocin IV, Indocin PDA ✦, Indocin SR, indomethacin, Indomethacin Extended-Release, Indomethacin SR, Novomethacin ✦, Nu-Indo ✦
*Func. class.:* NSAID (nonsteroidal antiinflammatory), antirheumatic
*Chem. class.:* Propionic acid derivative

**Pregnancy category**
B (1st trimester),
X (2nd/3rd trimesters)

**Action:** Inhibits prostaglandin synthesis by decreasing enzyme needed for biosynthesis; analgesic, antiinflammatory, antipyretic

Adverse effects: *italic* = common, **bold** = life-threatening

**Therapeutic outcome:** Decreased pain, inflammation; or closure of patent ductus arteriosus (premature infants)

**Uses:** Rheumatoid arthritis, ankylosing spondylitis, osteoarthritis, bursitis, tendinitis, acute gouty arthritis; closure of patent ductus arteriosus in premature infants (**IV**)

## Dosage and routes
### Arthritis/antiinflammatory
*Adult:* PO 25-50 mg bid-qid, max 200 mg/day; SUS REL 75 mg daily; may increase to 75 mg bid

### Acute arthritis
*Adult:* PO 100 mg initially, then 50 mg tid; use only for acute attack, then reduce dosage

### Patent ductus arteriosus
Longer or repeated treatment courses may be necessary for very premature infants
*Infant <2 days:* IV 0.2 mg/kg, then 0.1 mg/kg × 2 doses after 12, 24 hr
*Infant 2-7 days:* IV 0.2 mg/kg, then 0.2 mg/kg × 2 doses after 12, 24 hr
*Infant >7 days:* IV 0.2 mg/kg, then 0.25 mg/kg × 2 doses after 12, 24 hr

**Available forms:** Caps 25, 50 mg; sus rel caps 75 mg; oral susp 25 mg/5 ml; rectal supp 50 mg; inj 1-mg vials

## Adverse effects
***CNS:*** Dizziness, drowsiness, fatigue, tremors, confusion, insomnia, anxiety, depression, headache
***CV:*** Tachycardia, peripheral edema, palpitations, dysrhythmias, hypertension, **CV thrombotic events, MI, stroke**
***EENT:*** Tinnitus, hearing loss, blurred vision
***GI:*** *Nausea,* anorexia, *vomiting,* diarrhea, jaundice, **cholestatic hepatitis,** *constipation,* flatulence, cramps, dry mouth, peptic ulcer, **ulceration, perforation, GI bleeding**
***GU:*** **Nephrotoxicity (dysuria, hematuria, oliguria, azotemia)**
***HEMA:*** **Blood dyscrasias,** prolonged bleeding
***INTEG:*** Purpura, rash, pruritus, sweating

**Contraindications:** Pregnancy **X** (2nd/3rd trimesters) hypersensitivity, asthma, severe renal/hepatic disease, ulcer disease, perioperative pain in CABG

**Precautions:** Pregnancy **B** (1st trimester), breastfeeding, children, bleeding disorders, GI disorders, cardiac disorders, hypersensitivity to other antiinflammatory agents, depression

### Pharmacokinetics
| | |
|---|---|
| **Absorption** | Well absorbed (PO); erratic (RECT); complete (**IV**) |
| **Distribution** | Crosses blood-brain barrier; placenta, 99% plasma protein binding |
| **Metabolism** | Liver, extensively |
| **Excretion** | Breast milk |
| **Half-life** | 4.5 hr |

### Pharmacodynamics
| | PO | PO–EXT REL | IV |
|---|---|---|---|
| **Onset** | 1-2 hr | ½ hr | 2 day |
| **Peak** | 3 hr | Unknown | Unknown |
| **Duration** | 4-6 hr | 4-6 hr | Unknown |

## Interactions
### Individual drugs
Abciximab, cefamandole cefoperazone, cefotetan, clopidogrel, eptifibatide, plicamycin, ticlodipine, tirofiban, valproic acid: increased bleeding risk
CycloSPORINE, lithium, methotrexate, zidovudine: increased toxicity
Digoxin, penicillamine, phenyton: increased effect of each specific product

### Drug classifications
Aminoglycosides: increased effects of aminoglycosides
Anticoagulants, cephalosporins, thrombolytics: increased risk of bleeding
Antihypertensives: decreased effect of antihypertensives
Diuretics (potassium sparing): increased hyperkalemia

### Drug/herb
Anise, arnica, bogbean, chamomile, chondroitin, clove, dong quai, feverfew, garlic, ginger, ginkgo, ginseng *(Panax):* increased bleeding risk
Arginine, gossypol: increased gastric irritation
Bearberry, bilberry: increased NSAIDs effect

## NURSING CONSIDERATIONS
### Assessment
• Assess for patent ductus arteriosus: respiratory rate, character, heart sounds
• Assess for joint pain (duration, intensity, ROM), baseline and during treatment
• Assess for confusion, mood changes, hallucinations, especially in geriatric
• Assess renal, liver, blood studies: BUN, creatinine, AST, ALT, Hgb before treatment and periodically thereafter; if renal function decreases, do not give subsequent doses
• Assess for cardiac disease, CV, thrombotic events (MI, stroke) prior to administration

## Nursing diagnoses
- Knowledge, deficient (teaching)
- Mobility, impaired physical (uses)
- Pain, acute (uses)
- Pain, chronic (uses)

## Implementation
**PO route**
- Swallow sus rel cap whole; do not break, crush, or chew sus rel cap
- Give with food or milk to decrease gastric symptoms, and prevent ulceration
- Shake susp, do not mix with other liquids

**Rectal route**
- Have patient retain rectal supp for 1 hr after insertion

**IV route**
- Give after diluting 1-2 mg/ml or more normal saline or sterile water for inj without preservative; give over 5-10 sec to avoid dramatic shift in cerebral blood flow; avoid extravasation

*Y-site compatibilities:* Furosemide, insulin (regular), potassium chloride, sodium bicarbonate, sodium nitroprusside

## Patient/family education
- Advise patient to report change in vision, blurring, rash, tinnitus, black stools
- Tell patient not to use for any other condition than prescribed
- Advise patient to avoid use with OTC medications for pain unless approved by prescriber
- Advise patient to avoid hazardous activities, since dizziness or drowsiness can occur
- Instruct patient to use sunscreen to prevent photosensitivity

## Evaluation
**Positive therapeutic outcome**
- Decreased stiffness
- Increased joint mobility
- Decreased pain

---

## infliximab (Rx)
(in-fliks'ih-mab)
Remicade
*Func. class.:* Monoclonal antibody

**Pregnancy category B**

**Action:** Monoclonal antibody that neutralizes the activity of tumor necrosis factor α (TNFα) that has been found in Crohn's disease; decreased infiltration of inflammatory cells

**Therapeutic outcome:** Decreased cramping and blood in stools

**Uses:** Crohn's disease, fistulizing, moderate-severe; rheumatoid arthritis given with methotrexate

**Unlabeled uses:** Plaque psoriasis, ankylosing spondylitis, ulcerative colitis, psoriatic arthritis, psoriasis, Behçet syndrome, uveitis, juvenile arthritis

## Dosage and routes
*Crohn's disease (moderate-severe)*
*Adult:* **IV** INF 5 mg/kg × 1

*Crohn's disease (fistulizing)*
*Adult:* **IV** INF 5 mg/kg initially, then repeat dose 2, 6 wk after 1st dose

*Rheumatoid arthritis*
*Adult:* **IV** 3 mg/kg initially, and 2, 6 wk and q8 wk thereafter, given with methotrexate

**Available forms:** Powder for inj 100 mg

## Adverse effects
*CNS: Headache, dizziness, depression, vertigo, fatigue, anxiety, fever,* **seizures,** *chills, flulike symptoms*
*CV: Chest pain, hypo/hypertension, tachycardia,* **CHF**
*GI: Nausea, vomiting, abdominal pain, stomatitis, constipation, dyspepsia, flatulence*
*GU: Dysuria, frequency*
***HEMA: Anemia***
*INTEG: Rash, dermatitis, urticaria,* dry skin, sweating, flushing, hematoma, pruritus
*MS: Myalgia, back pain, arthralgia*
*RESP: URI, pharyngitis, bronchitis, cough, dyspnea, sinusitis*
***SYST: Anaphylaxis, fatal infections, sepsis, malignancies, immunogenicity***

**Contraindications:** Hypersensitivity to murines, moderate to severe CHF (NYHA class III/IV)

**Precautions:** Pregnancy **B,** breastfeeding, children, geriatric

## Pharmacokinetics
| | |
|---|---|
| **Absorption** | Unknown |
| **Distribution** | Vascular compartment |
| **Metabolism** | Unknown |
| **Excretion** | Unknown |
| **Half-life** | 9½ days |

## Pharmacodynamics
Unknown

## Interactions
### Drug classifications
Live virus vaccines: do not administer live
vaccines concurrently

## NURSING CONSIDERATIONS
### Assessment
- Assess GI symptoms: nausea, vomiting, abdominal pain
- Take periodic blood counts: CBC
- Assess CV status: B/P, pulse, chest pain
◆ Assess for allergic reaction, anaphylaxis: rash, dermatitis, urticaria, fever, chills, dyspnea, hypotension; discontinue if severe, administer epINEPHrine, corticosteroids; antihistamines; assess for allergy to murine proteins before starting therapy
- Fatal infections: discontinue if infection occurs, do not administer to patients with active infections
- Identify TB before beginning treatment; a TB test should be obtained; if present, TB should be treated prior to receiving infliximab

### Nursing diagnoses
- Diarrhea (uses)
- Injury, risk for (uses)
- Knowledge, deficient (teaching)

### Implementation
**IV infusion route**
- Administer immediately after reconstitution; reconstitute each vial with 10 ml of sterile water for inj, further dilute total dose/250 ml of 0.9% NaCl inj to a total conc of between 0.4 and 4 mg/ml; use 21G or smaller needle for reconstitution, direct sterile water at glass wall of vial, gently swirl
- Give over ≥2 hr, use polyethylene-lined infusion with in-line, sterile, low-protein-bind filter
- Do not admix
- Provide refrigerated storage, do not freeze

### Patient/family education
- Teach patient not to breastfeed while taking this product
- Advise patient to notify prescriber of GI symptoms, hypersensitivity reactions
- Advise patient not to operate machinery or drive if dizziness, vertigo occurs

### Evaluation
**Positive therapeutic outcome**
- Absence of blood in stool
- Reported improvement in comfort
- Weight gain

## ❗HIGH ALERT

## INSULINS

### RAPID ACTING
**insulin glulisine** (Rx)
Apidra
**insulin aspart** (Rx)
Novolog, Novolog Flexpen, Novolog PenFill
**insulin lispro** (Rx)
Humalog

### SHORT ACTING
**insulin, regular** 🔘 (OTC)
Humulin R ✦, Novolin R, Novolin R PenFill, Novolin R Prefilled
**insulin, regular concentrated** (Rx)
regular (concentrated)

### INTERMEDIATE ACTING
**insulin, isophane suspension (NPH)** 🔘 (OTC)
Humulin N, Novolin N, Novolin N PenFill, Novolin N Prefilled
**insulin, zinc suspension (Lente)** (OTC)
Novolin GE Lente ✦, Novolin L

### LONG ACTING
**insulin detemir** (Rx)
Levemir
**insulin glargine** (Rx)
Lantus

### MIXTURES
**insulin, isophane suspension and regular insulin** (Rx)
Humulin 70/30, Humalin 30/70 ✦, Novolin 70/30, Novolin 70/30 PenFill, Novolin 70/30 Prefilled, Novolin ge 30/70 ✦
**isophane insulin suspension (NPH) and insulin mixtures** (Rx)
Humulin 50/50, Novolin 50/50
**insulin lispro mixture** (Rx)
Humalog Mix 75/25
**insulin aspart mixture** (Rx)
Novolog Max 70/30
*Func. class.:* Antidiabetic, pancreatic hormone
*Chem. class.:* Modified structures of endogenous human insulin

**Pregnancy category** B, C

**Do not confuse:**
Lantus/lente, Novolin 70/30 PenFill/Novolin 70/30 Prefilled

**Action:** Decreases blood glucose; by transport of glucose into cells and the conversion of glucose to glycogen, indirectly increases blood pyruvate and lactate, decreases phosphate and potassium; insulin may be human (processed by recombinant DNA technologies)

**Therapeutic outcome:** Decreased blood glucose levels in diabetes mellitus

**Uses:** Type 1 diabetes mellitus, type 2 diabetes mellitus, gestational diabetes, insulin lispro may be used in combination with sulfonylureas in children >3 yr

### Dosage and routes
*Insulin glulisine*
*Adult:* SUBCUT Dosage individualized, give within 15 min before or 20 min after starting a meal; **IV** dilute to 1 unit/ml in infusion systems with 0.9% NaCl, using PVC Viaflex infusion bags and PVC tubing, use dedicated line

*Insulin aspart*
*Adult and child ≥6 yr:* 0.5-1 unit/kg/day divided in treatment, meal-related, highly individualized

*Insulin lispro*
*Adult:* SUBCUT 15 min before meals

*Human regular*
*Adult:* SUBCUT ½-1 hr before meals

*Insulin, isophane suspension*
*Adult:* SUBCUT Dosage individualized by blood, urine glucose; usual dose 7-26 units; may increase by 2-10 units/day if needed

*Insulin detemir*
*Adult:* SUBCUT 1 or 2 times/day; if 1 time, give with evening meal

*Insulin glargine*
*Adult and child ≥6 yr:* SUBCUT 10 international units/day, range 2-100 international units/day

*Regular insulin (ketoacidosis)*
*Adult:* **IV** 5-10 units, then 5-10 units/hr until desired response, then switch to SUBCUT dose; **IV**/INF 2-12 units (50 units/500 ml of normal saline)
*Child:* **IV** 0.1 units/kg

*Replacement*
*Adult and child:* SUBCUT 0.5-1 units/kg/day qid given 30 min before meals
*Adolescent:* SUBCUT 0.8-1.2 mg/kg/day; this dosage is used during rapid growth

**Available forms:** NPH Inj 100 units/ml; regular inj 100 units/ml, cartridges 100 units/ml; zinc susp 100 units/ml; insulin analog inj 100 units/ml; insulin zinc suspension, (lente) inj 100 units/ml; isophane insulin inj 100 units/ml, cartridges 100 units/ml; insulin lispro 100 units/ml, 1.5-ml cartridges, insulin lispro Humalog Pen sol for inj 100 units/ml; insulin glulisine inj 100 units/ml;

**Pharmacodynamics**

**Rapid acting**
Insulin glulisine — Onset 15-30 min, peak ½-1½ hr, duration 3-4 hr
Insulin aspart — Onset 10-20 min, peak 1-3 hr, duration 3-5 hr
Insulin lispro — Onset 15-30 min, peak ½-1½ hr, duration 3-4 hr

**Short acting**
Insulin regular — Onset 30 min, peak 2.5-5 hr, duration up to 6 hr

**Intermediate acting**
Insulin, isophane suspension (NPH) — Onset 1.5-4 hr, peak 4-12 hr, duration up to 24 hr
Insulin, zinc suspension (Lente) — Onset 3-4 hr, peak 6-12 hr, duration 12-18 hr

**Long acting**
Insulin detmir — Onset 0.8-2 hr, peak unknown, duration up to 24 hr
Insulin glargine — Onset 1.5 hr, no peak identified, duration ≥24 hr

**Mixtures**
Insulin, isophane suspension and regular insulin (70/30) — Onset 10-20 hr, peak 2.4 hr, duration up to 24 hr
Isophane insulin suspension (NPH) and insulin mixtures (50/50) — Onset ½-1 hr, peak dual, duration 10-16 hr

Adverse effects: *italic* = common, **bold** = life-threatening

insulin glargine inj 100 units/ml; insulin detemir inj 100 units/ml in 10 vials, 3-ml cartridges; insulin aspart inj 100 mg/ml (Flex Pen, Pen Fill)

### Adverse effects

*EENT:* Blurred vision, dry mouth
*INTEG:* Flushing, rash, urticaria, warmth, *lipodystrophy,* lipohypertrophy, swelling, redness
*META:* Hypoglycemia, rebound hyperglycemia (Somogyi effect 12-72 hr or longer)
*SYST:* **Anaphylaxis**

**Contraindications:** Hypersensitivity to protamine; creosol (aspart)

**Precautions:** Pregnancy **B** (lispro, aspart), **C** (all others)

| Pharmacokinetics | |
|---|---|
| **Absorption** | Rapidly absorbed (SUBCUT) |
| **Distribution** | Widely distributed |
| **Metabolism** | Liver, muscle, kidney |
| **Excretion** | Kidneys |
| **Half-life** | Regular 3-5 min; NPH 10 min |

### Interactions

*Individual drugs*
Alcohol: increased hypoglycemia
Dobutamine: increased insulin need
EpINEPHrine: decreased hypoglycemia
Fenfluramine, guanethedine, phenylbutazone, sulfinpyrazone, tetracycline: decreased insulin need

*Drug classifications*
Anabolic steroids, β-adrenergic blockers, hypoglycemics (oral), salicylates: increased hypoglycemia
Contraceptives (oral), corticosteroids, diuretics (thiazide), thyroid hormones: decreased hypoglycemia
Estrogens: increased insulin need
MAOIs: decreased insulin need

*Drug/herb*
Aceitilla, adiantam, agrimony, aloe gel, banana flowers/roots, banyan stem bark, bilberry, bitter melon, broom, bugleweed, burdock, carob, cumin, damiana, dandelion, eucalyptus, fenugreek, fo-ti, garlic, goat's rue, guar gum, horse chestnut, jambul, juniper, konjac, maitake, onion, psyllium, reishi: increased hypoglycemia
Alfalfa, aloe, basil, bay, bilberry, bitter melon, black catechu, buchu, burdock, coriander, dandelion, eyebright (po), fenugreek, garlic, ginseng, glucomannan, glucosamine, goat's rue, gymnema, horehound, horse chestnut,

jambul, myrrh, myrtle: increased antidiabetic effect
Annato, cocoa seeds, coffee beans, cola seeds, guarana, ma huang, rosemary, yerba maté: decreased hypoglycemic effect
Bee pollen, blue cohosh, broom, chromium, elecampane, eucalyptus, gotu kola: decreased antidiabetic effect
Chromium: increased or decreased hypoglycemia
Karela: increased glucose tolerance

*Drug/lab test*
Increased: VMA
Decreased: potassium, calcium
Interference: liver, thyroid function tests

### NURSING CONSIDERATIONS

**Assessment**
• Fasting blood glucose, 2 hr PP (80-150 mg/dl, normal fasting level; 70-130 mg/dl, normal 2 hr level); also A1c may be drawn to identify treatment effectiveness q3 mo
• Urine ketones during illness; insulin requirements may increase during stress, illness, surgery
• For hypoglycemic reaction that can occur during peak time (sweating, weakness, dizziness, chills, confusion, headache, nausea, rapid weak pulse, fatigue, tachycardia, memory lapses, slurred speech, staggering gait, anxiety, tremors, hunger)
• For hyperglycemia: acetone breath, polyuria, fatigue, polydipsia, flushed, dry skin, lethargy

**Nursing diagnoses**
• Injury, risk for (adverse reactions)
• Knowledge, deficient (teaching)
• Noncompliance (teaching)

**Implementation**
• Store at room temperature for <1 mo (some insulins); keep away from heat and sunlight; refrigerate all other supply; NPH, premixed insulins are cloudy; regular, rapid-acting analogs, long-acting analogs are clear; do not freeze—**IV** route, regular only
**SUBCUT route**
• Give after warming to room temperature by rotating in palms to prevent injecting cold insulin; use only insulin syringes with markings or syringe matching units/ml; rotate inj sites within one area: abdomen, upper back, thighs, upper arm, buttocks; keep record of sites
• Give increased dosages if tolerance occurs

- Premixed insulins and NPH are cloudy suspensions
- Regular human insulin, rapid-acting analogs, and long-acting analogs are clear; do not use if cloudy, thick, or discolored

**CONT SUBCUT route (insulin infusion CSII)**

- Do not mix with other insulins when using a pump
- Insulin lispro 3 ml cartridges are to be used in Disetronic H-TRON plus V100 pump using Disetronic rapid infusion sets; the infusion set and the cartridge adapter should be changed q48hr; replace 3 ml cartridge q7days

**IV route (insulin glulisine only)**

- Dilute to 1 international unit/ml in infusion systems with 0.9% NaCl using PVC viaflex infusion bags and PVC tubing; use dedicated line; do not admix

**IV route (regular only)**

- ◆ When regular insulin is administered IV, monitor glucose, potassium often to prevent fatal hypoglycemia, hypokalemia
- **IV** direct, undiluted via vein, Y-site, 3-way stopcock; give at 50 units/min or less
- Give by cont inf after diluting with **IV** sol and run at prescribed rate; use **IV** inf pump for correct dosing; give reduced dose at serum glucose level of 250 mg/100 ml

*Additive compatibilities:* Bretylium, cimetidine, lidocaine, meropenem, ranitidine, verapamil

*Additive incompatibilities:* Aminophylline, amobarbital, chlorothiazide, cytarabine, DOBUTamine, pentobarbital, phenobarbital, phenytoin, secobarbital, sodium bicarbonate, thiopental

*Syringe compatibilities:* Metoclopramide

*Y-site compatibilities:* Amiodarone, ampicillin, ampicillin/sulbactam, aztreonam, cefazolin, cefotetan, DOBUTamine, esmolol, famotidine, gentamicin, heparin, heparin/hydrocortisone, imipenem/cilastatin, indomethacin, magnesium sulfate, meperidine, meropenem, midazolam, morphine, nitroglycerin, oxytocin, pentobarbital, potassium chloride, propofol, ritodrine, sodium bicarbonate, sodium nitroprusside, tacrolimus, terbutaline, ticarcillin, ticarcillin/clavulanate, tobramycin, vancomycin, vit B/C

*Y-site incompatibilities:* Nafcillin

**Patient/family education**

- Advise patient that blurred vision occurs; not to change corrective lens until vision is stabilized 1-2 mo
- Advise patient to keep insulin, equipment available at all times; carry a glucagon kit, candy, or lump sugar to treat hypoglycemia
- Inform patient that product does not cure diabetes but controls symptoms
- Advise patient to carry emergency ID as diabetic
- Instruct patient to recognize hypoglycemia reaction: headache, tremors, fatigue, weakness
- Instruct patient to recognize hyperglycemia reaction: frequent urination, thirst, fatigue, hunger
- Teach patient the dosage, route, mixing instructions, if any diet restrictions, disease process
- Teach patient the symptoms of ketoacidosis: nausea, thirst, polyuria, dry mouth, decreased B/P, dry, flushed skin, acetone breath, drowsiness, Kussmaul respirations
- Advise patient that a plan is necessary for diet, exercise; all food on diet should be eaten; exercise routine should not vary
- Teach patient about blood glucose testing; make sure patient is able to determine glucose level
- Advise patient to avoid OTC products unless directed by prescriber

**Evaluation**

**Positive therapeutic outcome**

- Decrease in polyuria, polydipsia, polyphagia; clear sensorium; absence of dizziness; stable gait
- Blood glucose level under control

**Treatment of overdose:** Glucose 25 g **IV**, via dextrose 50% sol, 50 ml or glucagon 1 mg

---

**interferon alfa-2a (recombinant)** (Rx)
(in-ter-feer'on)
Roferon-A
**interferon alfa-2b (recombinant)** (Rx)
a-2-interferon, Intron-A
*Func. class.:* Antineoplastic—miscellaneous
*Chem. class.:* Protein product

**Pregnancy category** C

**Do not confuse:**
Roferon-A/Imferon

**Action:** Antiviral action inhibits viral replication by reprogramming virus; antitumor action suppresses cell proliferation; immunomodulating action phagocytizes target cells; may also inhibit virus replication

---

Adverse effects: *italic* = common, **bold** = life-threatening

**Therapeutic outcome:** Prevention of rapid growth of malignant cells; treatment of hepatitis non-A, non-B (liver function improvement)

**Uses:** Hairy cell leukemia in persons >18 yr; condylomata acuminata (alfa 2b); chronic hepatitis non-A, non-B (alfa 2b); chronic hepatitis C (alfa 2b); 2a only chronic myelogenous leukemia; 2b only hepatitis B, malignant melanoma

**Unlabeled uses:** Bladder tumors, carcinoid tumors, non-Hodgkin's lymphoma, essential thrombocytopenia, cytomegaloviruses, herpes simplex, human papilloma virus–associated diseases

## Dosage and routes
### Hairy cell leukemia (2a)
*Adult:* SUBCUT/IM 3 million international units/day × 16-24 wk, then 3 million international units 3 ×/wk maintenance

### Hairy cell leukemia (2b)
*Adult:* 3 million international units/$m^2$ 3 ×/wk; if severe adverse reactions occur, dose should be skipped or reduced by half

### Kaposi's sarcoma (2b)
*Adult:* SUBCUT/IM 30 million international units $m^2$ 3 ×/wk

### Condylomata acuminata (2a)
*Adult:* 1 million international units/lesion 3 ×/wk × 3 wk

### Chronic hepatitis B (2b)
*Adult:* SUBCUT/IM 3 million international units 3 ×/wk × 18-24 mo or 5 million international units/day or 10 million international units 3 ×/wk × 16 wk

**Available forms:** Alfa-2a: inj 3, 6, 36 million international units/ml; alfa-2b: inj 3, 5, 10, 18, 25 million units/vial, powder for inj 5, 10, 18, 25, 50 million units/vial

## Adverse effects
***CNS:*** *Dizziness, confusion, numbness, paresthesia,* hallucinations, **seizures, coma,** amnesia, anxiety, mood changes, depression, somnolence, paranoia, irritability, hostility, encephalopathy
***CV:*** *Edema, hypotension,* hypertension, chest pain, palpitations, dysrhythmias, **CHF, MI, CVA,** tachycardia, syncope
***GI:*** *Weight loss, taste changes,* nausea, anorexia, diarrhea, xerostomia
***GU:*** *Impotence*
***HEMA:*** **Neutropenia, thrombocytopenia**
***INTEG:*** *Rash, dry skin, itching, alopecia,* flushing, photosensitivity, **serious skin reaction**

***MISC:*** *Flulike symptoms: fever, fatigue, myalgias, headache, chills,* optic neuritis, **anaphylaxis, angioedema**

**Contraindications:** Hypersensitivity

**Precautions:** Pregnancy **C,** breastfeeding, children, severe hypotension, dysrhythmia, tachycardia, severe renal/hepatic disease, seizure disorder, autoimmune disorders, optic neuritis, ocular disease, thyroid/pulmonary/cardiac disease

### Pharmacokinetics
| | |
|---|---|
| **Absorption** | 80%-90% (SUBCUT/IM) |
| **Distribution** | Unknown |
| **Metabolism** | Renal tubular (degraded) |
| **Excretion** | Kidneys |
| **Half-life** | 3.7-8.5 hr (2a); 2-7 hr (2b) |

### Pharmacodynamics
| | |
|---|---|
| **Onset** | Unknown |
| **Peak** | 3-8 hr |
| **Duration** | Unknown |

## Interactions
### Individual drugs
Aminophylline: increased toxicity, blood levels
Clozapine, warfarin, zidovudine: increased neutropenia
### Drug/lab test
Interference: AST, ALT, LDH, alkaline phosphatase, WBC, platelets, granulocytes, creatinine

## NURSING CONSIDERATIONS
### Assessment
- Assess cardiac status: lung sounds, ECG before and during treatment, especially in those with cardiac disease, hypo/hypertension, MI, CHF, CVA may occur
- Assess bone marrow depression: bruising, bleeding, blood in stools, urine, sputum, emesis
- Assess mental status: depression, suicidal thoughts, hallucinations, amnesia
- Assess for symptoms of infection; may be masked by drug fever; fever, chills, headache, sore throat may occur 6 hr after dose; give acetaminophen for symptoms
- Assess liver, thyroid function tests
- In AIDS patients with Kaposi's sarcoma, assess characteristics of lesions during therapy; symptoms should decrease
- Assess for bleeding: hematuria, stool guaiac, bruising or petechiae, mucosa or orifices q8hr; check for inflammation of mucosa, breaks in skin; avoid IM inj, rectal temp, or any other procedures that break the skin

- Assess for CNS reaction: LOC, mental status, dizziness, confusion, poor coordination, difficulty speaking, behavior changes; notify prescriber (alfa-2b)

## Nursing diagnoses
- Body image, disturbed (adverse reactions)
- Infection, risk for (adverse reactions)
- Injury, risk for (adverse reactions)
- Knowledge, deficient (teaching)

## Implementation
- Sol should be prepared by qualified personnel only under controlled conditions in biologic cabinet using gown, gloves, and mask
- Use Luer-Lok tubing to prevent leakage; do not let sol come in contact with skin; if contact occurs, wash well with soap and water
- Give at bedtime to minimize side effects
- Give acetaminophen as ordered to alleviate fever and headache

**Alfa-2a**
- SUBCUT/IM after reconstituting 18 million units/3 ml of diluent provided (6 million units/ml)
- 36 million units/ml is used for Kaposi's sarcoma only
- Store reconstituted sol; must be used within 24 hr

**Alfa-2b**
- Give by IM/SUBCUT after reconstituting 3-5 million international units/1 ml, 10 million international units/2 ml, 25 million international units/5 ml, of diluent provided; mix gently, do not shake; each brand has different dilution directions; check patient insert

**Intralesional route (2b)**
- Give by intralesional route after reconstituting 10 million international units/1 ml of bacteriostatic water for inj; no more than 5 lesions can safely be treated at a time; using a 25G needle inject 0.1 ml into base at center

## Patient/family education
- Caution patient to avoid hazardous tasks, since confusion, dizziness may occur; fatigue is common; activity may have to be altered; to take at bedtime to minimize flulike symptoms; to take acetaminophen for fever; avoid prolonged sunlight
- Advise patient that brands of this product should not be changed; each form is different, with different dosages
- Caution patient not to become pregnant while taking product; possible mutagenic effects; impotence may occur during treatment but is temporary
- Advise patient to report signs of infection: sore throat, fever, diarrhea, vomiting; sores or white patches in mouth

- Advise patient that emotional lability is common; notify prescriber if severe or incapacitating

## Evaluation
**Positive therapeutic outcome**
- Improved leukocytes, Hgb, platelets
- Decreased amount of genital warts

## interferon alfacon-1 (Rx)
(in-ter-feer′on al′fa-kon)
Infergen
*Func. class.:* Recombinant type I interferon
**Pregnancy category C**

**Action:** Induces biologic responses and has antiviral, antiproliferative, and immunomodulatory effects

**Therapeutic outcome:** Decreased signs/symptoms of hepatitis C

**Uses:** Chronic hepatitis C infections in those 18 yr and older with compensated liver disease who have anti-HCV antibodies or HCV RNA

**Unlabeled uses:** Hairy cell leukemia when used with G-CSF

**Dosage and routes**
*Adult:* SUBCUT 9 mcg as a single inj 3×/wk × 24 wk

**Available forms:** Inj 9 mg/0.3 ml, 15 mg/0.5 ml

**Adverse effects**
*CNS:* Headache, fatigue, fever, rigors, insomnia, dizziness, depression, agitation
*CV:* Hypertension, palpitation
*EENT:* Tinnitus, earache, conjunctivitis, eye pain
*GI:* Abdominal pain, nausea, diarrhea, anorexia, dyspepsia, vomiting, constipation, flatulence, hemorrhoids, decreased salivation
*GU:* Dysmenorrhea, vaginitis, menstrual disorders
*HEMA:* **Granulocytopenia, thrombocytopenia, leukopenia,** ecchymosis, **aplastic anemia**
*INTEG:* Alopecia, pruritus, rash, erythema, dry skin
*MISC:* **Anaphylaxis, angioedema**
*MS:* Back, limb, neck, skeletal pain
*PSYCH:* Nervousness, depression, anxiety, lability, abnormal thinking
*RESP:* Pharyngitis, upper respiratory infection, cough, sinusitis, rhinitis, respiratory tract congestion, epistaxis, dyspnea, bronchitis

Adverse effects: *italic* = common, **bold** = life-threatening

**Contraindications:** Hypersensitivity to α-interferons, or products from *Escherichia coli*

**Precautions:** Pregnancy **C,** breastfeeding, children <18 yr, thyroid disorders, myelosuppression, hepatic/cardiac disease, alcoholism

| Pharmacokinetics | |
|---|---|
| Unknown | |

| Pharmacodynamics | |
|---|---|
| **Onset** | Unknown |
| **Peak** | 24-36 hr |
| **Duration** | Unknown |

### NURSING CONSIDERATIONS
**Assessment**
- Assess CBC, liver function tests, ECG, platelet counts, heme concentration, ANC, serum creatinine concentration, albumin, bilirubin, TSH, $T_4$
- Assess for myelosuppression, low dose if neutrophil count is <500 × 10-6/L or if platelets are <50 × 10-9/L
- Assess for hypersensitivity; discontinue immediately if hypersensitivity occurs

**Nursing diagnoses**
- Infection, risk for (uses)
- Knowledge, deficient (teaching)

**Patient/family education**
- Provide patient or family member with written, detailed instructions about the product
- Caution patient to use contraception during treatment

**Evaluation**
**Positive therapeutic outcome**
- Decreased hepatitis C signs/symptoms

---

**interferon beta-1a** (Rx)
(in-ter-feer′on)
Avonex, Rebif
**interferon beta-1b** (Rx)
Betaseron
*Func. class.:* Multiple sclerosis agent, immune modifier
*Chem. class.:* Interferon, *Escherichia coli* derivative
**Pregnancy category** C

---

**Action:** Antiviral, immunoregulatory; action not clearly understood; biologic response-modifying properties mediated through specific receptors on cells, inducing expression of interferon-induced gene products

**Therapeutic outcome:** Decreased symptoms of multiple sclerosis

**Uses:** Ambulatory patients with relapsing or remitting multiple sclerosis

**Unlabeled uses:** May be useful in treatment of AIDS, AIDS-related Kaposi's sarcoma, malignant melanoma, metastatic renal cell carcinoma, cutaneous T cell lymphoma, acute non-A/ non-B hepatitis

**Dosage and routes**
*Interferon beta-1a*
*Adult:* IM 30 mcg qwk

*Interferon beta-1b*
*Relapsing/remitting multiple sclerosis*
*Adult:* SUBCUT 0.0625 mg every other day for wk 1 and 2; then 0.125 mg every other day for wk 3 and 4; then 0.1875 mg every other day for wk 5 and 6; then 0.25 mg every other day thereafter

**Available forms:** Beta-1a: 33 mcg (6.6 million international units/vial); beta-1b: powder for inj 0.3 mg (9.6 m international units)

**Adverse effects**
*CNS: Headache, fever, pain, chills, mental changes,* hypertonia, **suicide attempts, seizures**
*CV: Migraine, palpitations, hypertension,* tachycardia, peripheral vascular disorders
*EENT:* Conjunctivitis, blurred vision
*GI: Diarrhea, constipation, vomiting, abdominal pain*
*GU: Dysmenorrhea, irregular menses, metorrhagia,* cystitis, breast pain
*HEMA:* **Decreased lymphocytes,** ANC, **WBC;** *lymphadenopathy,* anemia
*INTEG: Sweating, inj site reaction,*
*MS: Myalgia,* **myasthenia**
*RESP: Sinusitis,* dyspnea

**Contraindications:** Hypersensitivity to natural or recombinant interferon-beta or human albumin, hamster protein

**Precautions:** Pregnancy **C,** breastfeeding, children <18 yr, chronic progressive multiple sclerosis, depression, mental disorders, seizure disorders, latex allergy, autoimmune disorders, bone marrow suppression, hepatotoxicity, cardiac disease

## Pharmacokinetics

| | |
|---|---|
| **Absorption** | 50% is absorbed |
| **Distribution** | Unknown |
| **Metabolism** | Unknown |
| **Excretion** | Unknown |
| **Half-life** | 8 min-4½ hr (beta-1b), 8.6 hr (beta-1a) |

## Pharmacodynamics

| | BETA-1A | BETA-1B |
|---|---|---|
| **Onset** | Up to 12 hr | Rapid |
| **Peak** | 48 hr | 2-8 hr |
| **Duration** | 4 days | Unknown |

### Interactions
*Individual drugs*
Zidovudine: decreased clearance
*Drug classifications*
Antineoplastics: increased myelosuppression
*Drug/herb*
Astragalus, echinacea, melatonin: change in immunomodulation
*Drug/lab test*
Increased: liver function tests
Interference: vaccines, toxoids; avoid concurrent use

### NURSING CONSIDERATIONS
#### Assessment
• Monitor blood, renal, liver function tests: CBC, differential, platelet counts, BUN, creatinine, ALT, urinalysis; if neutrophil count is <750/mm$^3$, or if AST, ALT, is 10 × greater than upper normal limit, or if bilirubin is 5 × greater than upper normal limit; when neutrophil count exceeds 750/mm$^3$ and liver function or renal studies return to normal, treatment may resume at 50% original dosage
• Assess for CNS symptoms: headache, fatigue, depression; if depression occurs and is severe, product should be discontinued
• Assess for multiple sclerosis symptoms
• Assess mental status: depression, depersonalization, suicidal thoughts, insomnia
• Monitor GI status: diarrhea or constipation, vomiting, abdominal pain
• Monitor cardiac status: increased B/P, tachycardia

#### Nursing diagnoses
• Knowledge, deficient (teaching)
• Mobility, impaired physical (uses)

#### Implementation
• Reconstitute 0.3 mg (9.6 million international units)/1.2 ml of supplied diluent (0.2 mg or 8 million international units concentration); rotate vial gently, do not shake; withdraw 1 ml using a syringe with 27G needle; administer SUBCUT only into hip, thigh, arm; discard unused portion
• Products are not interchangeable
**Interferon beta-1a**
• Reconstitute with 1.1 ml of diluent, swirl, give within 6 hr
**Interferon beta-1b**
• Reconstitute by injecting diluent provided (1.2 ml) into vial, swirl (8 milli-international units/ml), use 27-G needle for inj
• Give acetaminophen for fever, headache; use SUBCUT route only; do not give IM or **IV**
• Store reconstituted sol in refrigerator; do not freeze; do not use sol that contains precipitate or is discolored

#### Patient/family education
• Provide patient or family member with written, detailed instructions about the product; provide initial and return demonstrations on inj procedure; give information on use and disposal of product
• Inform patient that blurred vision, sweating may occur
• Advise women patients that irregular menses, dysmenorrhea, or metorrhagia as well as breast pain may occur; use contraception during treatment; product may cause spontaneous abortion
• Teach patient to use sunscreen to prevent photosensitivity
• Instruct patient to notify prescriber if pregnancy is suspected
• Teach patient inj technique and care of equipment
• Instruct patient to notify prescriber of increased temp, chills, muscle soreness, fatigue

#### Evaluation
**Positive therapeutic outcome**
• Decreased symptoms of multiple sclerosis

## interferon gamma-1b (Rx)
(in-ter-feer'on)
Actimmune
*Func. class.:* Biologic response modifier
*Chem. class.:* Lymphokine, interleukin type
**Pregnancy category C**

**Action:** Species-specific protein synthesized in response to viruses; potent phagocyte-activating effects; capable of mediating the killing of *Staphylococcus aureus, Toxoplasma gondii, Leishmania donovani, Listeria monocytogenes, Mycobacterium* *avium-intracellulare;* enhances oxidative metabolism of macrophages; enhances antibody-dependent cellular cytotoxicity

**Therapeutic outcome:** Decreased signs/symptoms of infection (serious) in chronic granulomatous disease

**Uses:** Serious infections associated with chronic granulomatous disease, osteoporosis

**Unlabeled uses:** Osteoporosis, *Mycobacterium avium* complex (MAC), ovarian cancer, pulmonary fibrosis

**Dosage and routes**
*Adult:* SUBCUT 50 mcg/m$^2$ (1.5 million units/m$^2$) for patients with a surface area of >0.5 m$^2$; 1.5 mcg/kg/dose for patient with a surface area of <0.5/m$^2$; give on Monday, Wednesday, Friday for 3 ×/wk dosing

**Available forms:** Inj 100 mcg (3 million units)/single-dose vial

**Adverse effects**
*CNS:* *Headache, fatigue,* depression, fever, chills
*GI:* *Nausea, anorexia,* abdominal pain, weight loss, diarrhea, vomiting
*HEMA:* **Leukopenia, thrombocytopenia**
*INTEG:* Rash, pain at inj site
*MS:* Myalgia, arthralgia

**Contraindications:** Hypersensitivity to interferon γ, *Escherichia coli*–derived products

**Precautions:** Pregnancy **C**, breastfeeding, children <1 yr, cardiac disease, seizure/CNS disorders, myelosuppression

| Pharmacokinetics | |
| --- | --- |
| Absorption | Slowly absorbed 89% |
| Distribution | Unknown |
| Metabolism | Unknown |
| Excretion | Unknown |
| Half-life | 5.9 hr |

| Pharmacodynamics | |
| --- | --- |
| Onset | Unknown |
| Peak | 7 hr |
| Duration | Unknown |

**Interactions**
*Individual drugs*
Aminophylline, theophylline: increased levels
Fosphenytoin, phenytoin, warfarin: increased interference
*Drug classifications*
Myelosuppressive agents: increased myelosuppression

Toxoids, vaccines: interference with antibody reaction

**NURSING CONSIDERATIONS**
**Assessment**
• Monitor blood, renal, hepatic studies: CBC with differential, platelet count, BUN, creatinine, ALT, urinalysis before and q3 mo during treatment
• Assess for infection: headache, fever, chills, fatigue; these are common adverse reactions
• Monitor CNS symptoms: headache, fatigue, depression

**Nursing diagnoses**
• Infection, risk for (uses)
• Knowledge, deficient (teaching)

**Implementation**
• Give at bedtime to minimize adverse reactions; administer acetaminophen for fever, headache; use 50% of the dosage prescribed if severe reactions occur or discontinue treatment until reactions subside
• Give in right or left deltoid and anterior thigh; warm to room temperature before use; do not leave at room temperature over 12 hr (unopened vial); does not contain preservatives
• Store in refrigerator upon receipt; do not freeze; do not shake

**Patient/family education**
• Provide patient or family member with written, detailed instructions about the product; provide initial and return demonstrations on inj procedure; give information on use and disposal of product
• Caution patient to use contraception during treatment

**Evaluation**
**Positive therapeutic outcome**
• Decreased serious infections
• Improvement in existing infections and inflammatory conditions

**ipratropium** (Rx)
(i-pra-troe'pee-um)
Atrovent HFA
*Func. class.:* Anticholinergic, bronchodilator
*Chem. class.:* Synthetic quaternary ammonium compound

**Pregnancy category B**

**Do not confuse:**
Atrovent/Alupent

**Action:** Inhibits interaction of acetylcholine at receptor sites on the bronchial smooth muscle, resulting in decreased cyclic guanosine monophosphate (cGMP) and bronchodilatation

**Therapeutic outcome:** Bronchodilatation

**Uses:** Bronchodilatation during bronchospasm for patients with COPD; rhinorrhea in children 6-11 yr (nasal spray)

**Dosage and routes**
*Adult:* 1-4 INH qid, not to exceed 24 puffs/24 hr; sol 250-500 mcg (1 unit dose) given 3-4 ×/day
*Child:* INH 1-2 inhalations q6-8hr; NEB 125-250 mcg q4-6hr
*Child 5-12 yr:* NASAL 1 spray in each nostril

**Available forms:** Aerosol 18 mcg/actuation; nasal spray 0.03%, 0.06%; sol for inh 0.0125% ♣, 0.02%

**Adverse effects**
*CNS: Anxiety, dizziness, headache,* nervousness
*CV:* Palpitations
*EENT:* Dry mouth, blurred vision
*GI: Nausea, vomiting, cramps*
*INTEG:* Rash
*RESP: Cough, worsening of symptoms,* **bronchospasm**

**Contraindications:** Hypersensitivity to this product, atropine, soya lecithin

**Precautions:** Pregnancy **B**, breastfeeding, children <12 yr, angle-closure glaucoma, prostatic hypertrophy, bladder neck obstruction

| Pharmacokinetics | |
|---|---|
| Absorption | Minimal |
| Distribution | Does not cross blood-brain barrier |
| Metabolism | Liver, minimal |
| Excretion | Unknown |
| Half-life | 2 hr |

| Pharmacodynamics | |
|---|---|
| Onset | 5-15 min |
| Peak | 1-1½ hr |
| Duration | 3-6 hr |

**Interactions**
*Individual drugs*
Disopyramide: increased anticholinergic action

*Drug classifications*
Antihistamines, phenothiazines: increased anticholinergic action
Bronchodilators (other): increased toxicity
*Drug/herb*
Black catechu: increased constipation
Butterbur, jimsonweed: increased anticholinergic effect
Green tea (large amounts), guarana: increased bronchodilator effect
Jamborandi tree, pill-bearing spurge: decreased anticholinergic effect

**NURSING CONSIDERATIONS**
**Assessment**
• Monitor respiratory function: vital capacity, FEV, ABGs, lung sounds, heart rate, rhythm (baseline and during treatment); if severe bronchospasm is present, a more rapid medication is required
• Monitor for evidence of allergic reactions, paradoxic bronchospasm; withhold dose and notify prescriber; identify if patient is allergic to belladonna products or atropine; allergy to this product may occur

**Nursing diagnoses**
• Airway clearance, ineffective (uses)
• Gas exchange, impaired (uses)
• Knowledge, deficient (teaching)

**Implementation**
• Give after shaking container; have patient exhale, place mouthpiece in mouth, inhale slowly, hold breath, remove, exhale slowly; allow at least 1 min between inhalations
• Give this medication before other medications and allow at least 5 min between each
**Nebulizer route**
• Use solution in nebulizer with a mouthpiece rather than a face mask
**Nasal route**
• Prime pump, initially requires 7 actuations of the pump, priming again is not necessary if used regularly
• Store in light-resistant container; do not expose to temperature over 86° F (30° C)

**Patient/family education**
• Advise patient not to use OTC medications unless approved by prescriber; extra stimulation may occur; to use this medication before other medications and allow at least 5 min between each to prevent overstimulation
• Teach patient that compliance is necessary with number of inhalations/24 hr, or overdose may occur
• Instruct patient to use spacer device if geriatric

• Teach patient the proper use of the inhaler; review package insert with patient; to avoid getting aerosol in eyes; blurring may result; to wash inhaler in warm water daily and dry; to avoid smoking, smoke-filled rooms, persons with respiratory tract infections

• Teach patient if paradoxic bronchospasm occurs to stop product immediately and notify prescriber; to limit caffeine products such as chocolate, coffee, tea, and colas

• Instruct patient on administration of dose, not to use more than prescribed; serious side effects may occur; if dose is missed, take when remembered; space other doses on new time schedule; do not double doses

## Evaluation
**Positive therapeutic outcome**
• Absence of dyspnea, wheezing after 1 hr
• Improved airway exchange
• Improved ABGs

---

## irbesartan (Rx)
(er-be-sar′tan)
Avapro
*Func. class.:* Antihypertensive
*Chem. class.:* Angiotensin II receptor (Type AT$_1$)

**Pregnancy category**
C (1st trimester),
D (2nd/3rd trimesters)

**Do not confuse:**
Avapro/Anaprox

**Action:** Blocks the vasoconstrictor and aldosterone-secreting effects of angiotensin II; selectively blocks the binding of angiotensin II to the AT$_1$ receptor found in tissues

**Therapeutic outcome:** Decreased B/P

**Uses:** Hypertension, alone or in combination, nephropathy in type 2 diabetic patients

**Unlabeled uses:** Heart failure

## Dosage and routes
*Hypertension*
*Adult:* PO 150 mg/day; may be increased to 300 mg/day

*Nephropathy in type 2 diabetic patients*
*Adult:* PO maintenance dose 300 mg/day, start 75 mg/day
*Child 13-16 yr:* PO 150 mg/day, may increase to 300 mg/day
*Child 6-12 yr:* PO 75 mg/day may increase to 150 mg/day

*Volume and salt depleted patients*
*Adult:* PO 75 mg/day

**Available forms:** Tabs 75, 150, 300 mg

**Adverse effects**
*CNS:* Dizziness, anxiety, headache, fatigue
*CV:* Hypotension
*GI: Diarrhea, dyspepsia*
*MISC:* Edema, chest pain, rash, tachycardia, UTI, **angioedema**, hyperkalemia
*RESP: Cough, upper respiratory infection,* rhinitis, pharyngitis, sinus disorder

**Contraindications:** Pregnancy **D** (2nd/3rd trimesters), hypersensitivity

**Precautions:** Pregnancy **C** (1st trimester), breastfeeding, children, geriatric, renal/hepatic disease, renal artery stenosis, hypersensitivity to ACE inhibitors

### Pharmacokinetics
| | |
|---|---|
| **Absorption** | Well |
| **Distribution** | Bound to plasma proteins (90%) |
| **Metabolism** | Liver (minimal) |
| **Excretion** | Feces, urine |
| **Half-life** | 11-15 hr |

### Pharmacodynamics
Unknown

## Interactions
*Drug classifications*
CYP2C9 inhibitors: increased irbesartan level
Diuretics (potassium sparing), potassium salt substitutes: increased hyperkalemia
NSAIDs: decreased antihypertensive effect
*Drug/herb*
Aconite: increased toxicity, death
Astragalus, cola tree: increased or decreased antihypertensive effect
Barberry, betony, black catechu, black cohosh, bloodroot, broom, burdock, cat's claw, dandelion, goldenseal, Irish moss, Jamaican dogwood, kelp, khella, mistletoe, parsley: increased antihypertensive effect
Coltsfoot, guarana, khat, licorice: decreased antihypertensive effect

## NURSING CONSIDERATIONS
*Assessment*
• Assess B/P, pulse q4hr; note rate, rhythm, quality
• Monitor electrolytes: potassium, sodium, chloride
• Obtain baselines for renal, liver function tests before therapy begins
• Monitor for edema in feet, legs daily

---

 Alert     Canada Only     Drug on CD    * "Tall Man" lettering (See Preface)

- Assess for skin turgor, dryness of mucous membranes for hydration status

### Nursing diagnoses
- Fluid volume, deficient (side effects)
- Knowledge, deficient (teaching)
- Noncompliance (teaching)

### Implementation
- Administer without regard to meals

### Patient/family education
- Advise patient to comply with dosage schedule, even if feeling better
- Inform patient that product may cause dizziness, fainting; light-headedness may occur
- Caution patient to rise slowly to sitting or standing position to minimize orthostatic hypotension
- Advise patient to notify prescriber if pregnancy is suspected

### Evaluation
**Positive therapeutic outcome**
- Decreased B/P

---

### ! HIGH ALERT

## irinotecan (Rx)
(ear-een-oh-tee′kan)
Camptosar
*Func. class.:* Antineoplastic hormone
*Chem. class.:* Topoisomerase inhibitor

**Pregnancy category D**

**Action:** Cytotoxic by producing damage to single-strand DNA during DNA synthesis, binds to topoisomerase I

**Therapeutic outcome:** Prevention in growth of tumor size

**Uses:** Metastatic carcinoma of colon or rectum, or 1st line treatment in combination with fluorouracil (5-FU) and leucovorin for metastatic carcinoma of colon or rectum

### Dosage and routes
*Single agent*
*Adult:* **IV** 125 mg/m$^2$ given over 1½ hr qwk × 4 wk, then 2 wk rest period, may be repeated; 4 wk or 2 wk off, dosage adjustments may be made to 150 mg/m$^2$ (high) or 50 mg/m$^2$ (low); adjustments should be made in increments of 25-50 mg/m$^2$ depending on patient's tolerance

*Combination dosage schedule*
*Regimen 1:* Irinotecan 75-125 mg/m$^2$, leucovorin 20 mg/m$^2$, 5-FU 300-500 mg/m$^2$, depending on dosing levels

*Regimen 2:* Irinotecan 120-180 mg/m$^2$, leucovorin 200 mg/m$^2$, 5 FU-BOL 240-400 mg/m$^2$, 5 FU infusion 360-600 mg/m$^2$

**Available forms:** Inj 20 mg/ml

### Adverse effects
*CNS:* Fever, headache, chills, dizziness
*CV:* Vasodilation
*GI:* **Severe diarrhea,** nausea, vomiting, anorexia, constipation, cramps, flatus, stomatitis, dyspepsia, **hepatotoxicity**
*HEMA:* **Leukopenia,** anemia, **neutropenia**
*INTEG:* Irritation at site, rash, sweating, alopecia
*MISC:* Edema, asthenia, weight loss
*RESP:* Dyspnea, increased cough, rhinitis

**Contraindications:** Pregnancy **D,** hypersensitivity

**Precautions:** Breastfeeding, children, geriatric, myelosuppression, irradiation, hepatic disease

### Pharmacokinetics
| | |
|---|---|
| **Absorption** | Complete |
| **Distribution** | Widely, 30%-68% bound to plasma proteins, increased risk of toxicity in those homozygous for UGT1A128 |
| **Metabolism** | Unknown |
| **Excretion** | Urine/bile |
| **Half-life** | Unknown |

### Pharmacodynamics
Unknown

### Interactions
*Individual products*
Carbamazepine, phenobarbital, phenytoin: decreased irinotecan levels
Dexamethasone: increased lymphocytopenia
Ketoconazole: increased irinotecan levels
Prochlorperazine: increased akathisia
Radiation: increased myelosuppression, diarrhea
*Drug classifications*
Anticoagulants, NSAIDs: increased bleeding risk
Antineoplastics: increased myelosuppression, diarrhea
Diuretics: increased dehydration
*Drug/herb*
St. John's wort: decreased product level; avoid concurrent use

### NURSING CONSIDERATIONS
### Assessment
- Assess for CNS symptoms: fever, headache, chills, dizziness

• Assess CBC, differential, platelet count weekly; withhold product if WBC is <2000/mm³, or platelet count is <100,000/mm³, Hgb ≤ g/dl, neutrophils ≤1000/mm³; notify prescriber of these results, product should be discontinued and colony-stimulating factor given

• Assess buccal cavity for dryness, sores or ulceration, white patches, oral pain, bleeding, dysphagia

• Assess GI symptoms: frequency of stools; cramping; severe life-threatening diarrhea may occur with fluid and electrolyte imbalances

• Assess early diarrhea and other cholinergic symptoms, treat with atropine; late diarrhea must be treated promptly with loperimide, late diarrhea can be life threatening

• Assess signs of dehydration: rapid respirations, poor skin turgor, decreased urine output; dry skin, restlessness, weakness

• Assess for bone marrow depression: bruising, bleeding, blood in stools, urine, sputum, emesis

### Nursing diagnoses
• Infection, risk for (adverse reactions)
• Knowledge, deficient (teaching)

### Implementation
• Give antiemetics and dexamethasone 10 mg at least ½ hr before antineoplastics
• Give after preparing in biologic cabinet using gloves, mask, gown

**IV route**
• Give by intermittent inf after diluting with 0.9% NaCl or D₅W (0.12-1.1 mg/ml); give over 1½ hr
• Do not admix with other solutions or medications
• Provide increased fluid intake to 2-3 L/day to prevent dehydration, unless contraindicated
• Change **IV** site q48hr
• Provide rinsing of mouth tid-qid with water, club soda; brushing of teeth bid-tid with soft brush or cotton-tipped applicator for stomatitis; use unwaxed dental floss
• Provide nutritious diet with iron, low fiber, few dairy products; avoid raw fruits, vegetables, herbals
• Stable for 24 hr at room temperature, 48 hr if refrigerated

### Patient/family education
• Advise patient to avoid foods with citric acid or hot or rough texture if stomatitis is present; to drink adequate fluids
• Advise patient to report stomatitis; any bleeding, white spots, ulcerations in mouth; tell patient to examine mouth daily, report symptoms

• Advise patient to report signs of anemia: fatigue, headache, faintness, shortness of breath, irritability
• Advise patient to use contraception during therapy
• Advise patient to avoid vaccinations while taking this product
• Instruct patient to report diarrhea that occurs 24 hr after administration; severe dehydration can occur rapidly
• Teach patient to avoid salicylates, NSAIDs, alcohol; bleeding may occur

### Evaluation
**Positive therapeutic outcome**
• Decrease in tumor size, decrease in spread of cancer

**Treatment of overdose:** Induce vomiting, provide supportive care, prevent dehydration

---

### iron, carbonyl
*See ferrous fumarate*

---

### iron dextran (Rx)
DexFerrum, Imferon, InFed
*Func. class.:* Hematinic
*Chem. class.:* Ferric hydroxide complex with dextran

**Pregnancy category** C

**Do not confuse:**
Imferon/Imuran/Roferon-A

**Action:** Iron is carried by transferrin to the bone marrow, where it is incorporated into hemoglobin

**Therapeutic outcome:** Prevention and resolution of iron-deficiency anemia

**Uses:** Iron-deficiency anemia in patients who cannot take oral preparations

### Dosage and routes
*Adult and child:* IM 0.5 ml as a test dose by Z-track, then no more than the following per day:
*Adult <50 kg:* IM 100 mg
*Adult >50 kg:* IM 250 mg
*Child 5-9 kg:* IM 50 mg
*Infant <5 kg:* IM 25 mg
*Adult:* IV 0.5 ml (25 mg) test dose, then 100 mg/day after 2-3 days; give 25 mg test

---

dose, wait 5 min, then INF over 6-12 hr or follow equation:

$$\frac{0.3 \times weight\ (lb) \times 100\ Hgb\ (g/dl) \times 100}{14.8} = mg\ iron$$

Patients <30 lb (66 kg) should be given 80% of above formula dose

**Available forms:** Inj IM/**IV** 50 mg/ml; inj IM only 50 mg/ml (2 ml, 10 ml vials)

## Adverse effects

*CNS:* Headache, paresthesia, dizziness, shivering, weakness, **seizures**

*CV:* Chest pain, **shock**, hypotension, tachycardia

*GI: Nausea,* vomiting, metallic taste, abdominal pain

*HEMA:* Leukocytosis

*INTEG:* Rash, pruritus, urticaria, fever, sweating, chills, brown skin discoloration, pain at inj site, necrosis, sterile abscesses, phlebitis

*MISC:* **Anaphylaxis**

*RESP:* Dyspnea

**Contraindications:** Hypersensitivity, all anemias excluding iron-deficiency anemia, hepatic disease

**Precautions:** Pregnancy **C,** breastfeeding, infants <4 mo, children, acute renal disease, asthma, rheumatoid arthritis (**IV**)

| Pharmacokinetics | |
|---|---|
| **Absorption** | Well absorbed; lymphatics over wk or mo |
| **Distribution** | Crosses placenta |
| **Metabolism** | Slow; blood loss, desquamation |
| **Excretion** | Breast milk, feces, urine, bile |
| **Half-life** | 6 hr |

| Pharmacodynamics |
|---|
| Unknown |

## Interactions

### Individual drugs

Chloramphenicol: decreased reticulocyte response

Oral iron: do not use together, increased toxicity

### Drug/lab test

False increase: serum bilirubin

False decrease: serum calcium

False positive: $^{99m}$Tc diphosphate bone scan, iron test (large doses >2 ml)

## NURSING CONSIDERATIONS

### Assessment

- Observe for 1 hr after test dose
- Monitor blood studies: Hct, Hgb, reticulocytes, transferrin, plasma iron concentrations, ferritin, total iron-binding bilirubin before treatment, at least monthly
- Assess for allergic reaction and anaphylaxis; rash, pruritus, fever, chills, wheezing, notify prescriber immediately, keep emergency equipment available
- Assess cardiac status: anginal pain, hypotension, tachycardia
- Assess for nutrition: amount of iron in diet (meat, dark green leafy vegetables, dried fruits, eggs); cause of iron loss or anemia, including salicylates, sulfonamides
- Monitor pulse, B/P during **IV** administration
- Assess for toxicity: nausea, vomiting, diarrhea, fever, abdominal pain (early symptoms); cyanotic lips, nailbeds, seizures, CV collapse (late symptoms)

### Nursing diagnoses

- Activity intolerance (uses)
- Fatigue (uses)
- Knowledge, deficient (teaching)

### Implementation

#### IM route

- Discontinue oral iron before parenteral; give only after test dose of 25 mg by preferred route; wait at least 1 hr before giving remaining portion
- Give IM inj deep in large muscle mass; use Z-track method and 19-G, 20-G 2-, 3-inch needle; ensure needle is long enough to place product deep in muscle; change needles after withdrawing medication and injecting to prevent skin and tissue staining

#### IV route

- Give **IV** after flushing tubing with 10 ml of 0.9% NaCl; give undiluted; give 1 ml (50 mg) or less over 1 min or more; flush line after use with 10 ml of 0.9% NaCl; patient should remain recumbent for 30-60 min to prevent orthostatic hypotension
- **IV** inj requires single-dose vial without preservative; verify on label **IV** use is approved
- Give by cont inf after diluting in 50-250 ml of 0.9% NaCl for inf; administer over 4-5 hr
- Give only with epINEPHrine available in case of anaphylactic reaction during dose
- Store at room temperature in cool environment

*Additive compatibilities:* Netilmicin

---

## Patient/family education
• Caution patient that iron poisoning may occur if increased beyond recommended level; to not take oral iron preparation or vitamins containing iron unless approved by prescriber
• Advise patient that delayed reaction may occur 1-2 days after administration and last 3-4 days (**IV**) or 3-7 days (IM); report fever, chills, malaise, muscle, joint aches, nausea, vomiting, backache
• Advise patient to avoid breastfeeding
• Advise patient that stools may become dark

## Evaluation
**Positive therapeutic outcome**
• Increased serum iron levels, Hct, Hgb

## Treatment of overdose:
• Discontinue product, treat allergic reaction, give diphenhydrAMINE or epINEPHrine as needed for anaphylaxis; give iron-chelating product in acute poisoning

---

### iron polysaccharide
*See ferrous fumarate*

---

### iron sucrose (Rx)
Venofer
*Func. class.:* Hematinic
*Chem. class.:* Ferric hydroxide complex with dextran

**Pregnancy category B**

**Action:** Iron is carried by transferrin to the bone marrow, where it is incorporated into hemoglobin

**Therapeutic outcome:** Improved signs/symptoms of iron deficiency anemia; iron levels improved

**Uses:** Iron deficiency anemia

**Unlabeled uses:** Dystrophic epidermolysis bullosa (DEB)

## Dosage and routes
*Adult:* **IV** 5 ml (100 mg of elemental iron) given during dialysis, most will need 1000 mg of elemental iron over 10 dialysis sessions

**Available forms:** Inj 20 mg/ml

## Adverse effects
*CNS:* Headache, dizziness
*CV:* Chest pain, hypo/hypertension, hypervolemia
*GI: Nausea, vomiting, abdominal pain*
*INTEG:* Rash, pruritus, urticaria, fever, sweating, chills

*MISC:* **Anaphylaxis**
*RESP:* Dyspnea, pneumonia, cough

**Contraindications:** Hypersensitivity, all anemias excluding iron deficiency anemia, iron overload

**Precautions:** Pregnancy **B**, breastfeeding (**IV**), children, geriatric

| Pharmacokinetics | |
| --- | --- |
| **Absorption** | Unknown |
| **Distribution** | Unknown |
| **Metabolism** | Unknown |
| **Excretion** | Urine |
| **Half-life** | 6 hr |

| Pharmacodynamics |
| --- |
| Unknown |

## Interactions
*Individual drugs*
Iron (oral): increased toxicity, do not use together

## NURSING CONSIDERATIONS
### Assessment
• Monitor blood studies: Hct, Hgb, reticulocytes, transferrin, plasma iron concentrations, ferritin, total iron binding, bilirubin before treatment, at least monthly
• Assess for allergy: anaphylaxis, rash, pruritus, fever, chills, wheezing; notify prescriber immediately, keep emergency equipment available
• Assess cardiac status: hypotension, hypertension, hypervolemia
• Assess for toxicity: nausea, vomiting, diarrhea, fever, abdominal pain (early symptoms), cyanotic-looking lips and nailbeds, seizures, CV collapse (late symptoms)

### Nursing diagnoses
• Knowledge, deficient (teaching)
• Nutrition, less than body requirements, imbalanced (uses)

### Implementation
⬥ Give only with epINEPHrine, solu-medrol in case of anaphylactic reaction during dose
**IV route**
• Give directly in dialysis line by slow inj or inf; give by slow inj at 1 ml/min (5 min/vial); inf dilute each vial exclusively in a maximum of 100 ml of 0.9% NaCl, give at rate of 100 mg of iron/15 min, discard unused portions
• Store at room temperature in cool environment, do not freeze

---

## Patient/family education

• Teach patient that iron poisoning may occur if increased beyond recommended level; not to take oral iron preparations
• Teach patient to report itching, rash, chest pain, headache, vertigo, nausea, vomiting, abdominal pain, joint/muscle pain, numbness, tingling

## Evaluation

**Positive therapeutic outcome**

• Increased serum iron levels, Hct, Hgb

**Treatment of overdose:** Discontinue product, treat allergic reaction, give diphenhydrAMINE or epINEPHrine as needed, give iron-chelating product in acute poisoning

---

### isoflurophate ophthalmic
*See Appendix D*

---

### isoniazid 🛇 (Rx)
(eye-soe-nye′a-zid)
INH, isoniazid, Isotamine ✦, Laniazid, Nydrazid, PMS-Isoniazid ✦
*Func. class.:* Antitubercular
*Chem. class.:* Isonicotinic acid hydrazide

**Pregnancy category  C**

**Action:** Bactericidal interference with lipid, nucleic acid biosynthesis

**Therapeutic outcome:** Resolution of TB infection

**Uses:** Pulmonary TB as an adjunct; other infections caused by mycobacteria

## Dosage and routes
*Treatment*
**Adult:** PO/IM 300 mg/day or 15 mg/kg 2-3 ×/wk, max 900 mg 2-3 ×/wk
**Child and infant:** PO/IM 10-20 mg/kg/day in 1-2 divided doses; max 300 mg/day or 20-40 mg/kg, max 900 mg 2-3 ×/wk

**Available forms:** Tabs 50, 100, 300 mg; inj 100 mg/ml; powder 50 mg/5 ml; syr 50 mg/5 ml

## Adverse effects

**Hypersensitivity:** Fever, skin eruptions, lymphadenopathy, vasculitis
***CNS:*** *Peripheral neuropathy, dizziness,* memory impairment, **toxic encephalopathy, seizures,** psychosis, slurred speech
***EENT:*** Blurred vision, optic neuritis
***GI:*** *Nausea, vomiting,* epigastric distress, **jaundice, fatal hepatitis**

***HEMA:*** **Agranulocytosis, hemolytic anemia, aplastic anemia, thrombocytopenia, eosinophilia, methemoglobinemia**
***MISC:*** Dyspnea, vit $B_6$ deficiency, pellagra, hyperglycemia, metabolic acidosis, gynecomastia, rheumatic syndrome, systemic lupus erythematosus–like syndrome

**Contraindications:** Hypersensitivity, acute liver disease

**Precautions:** Pregnancy **C,** child <13 yr, diabetic retinopathy, cataracts, ocular defects, renal/hepatic disease

### Pharmacokinetics

| | |
|---|---|
| **Absorption** | Well |
| **Distribution** | Widely |
| **Metabolism** | Liver |
| **Excretion** | Kidneys |
| **Half-life** | 1-4 hr |

### Pharmacodynamics

| | PO | IM |
|---|---|---|
| **Onset** | Rapid | Rapid |
| **Peak** | 1-2 hr | 45-60 min |
| **Duration** | 6-8 hr | 6-8 hr |

## Interactions
*Individual drugs*
Alcohol, carbamazepine, cycloSERINE, ethionamide, meperidine, phenytoin, rifampin, warfarin: increased toxicity
BCG vaccine, ketoconazole: decreased effectiveness
*Drug classifications*
Antacids, aluminum: decreased absorption
Benzodiazepines: increased toxicity
*Drug/food*
Tyramine foods: increased toxicity

## NURSING CONSIDERATIONS
**Assessment**

• Obtain C&S tests, including sputum tests, before treatment; monitor every mo to detect resistance
• Monitor liver function tests weekly: ALT, AST, bilirubin, increased results may indicate hepatitis; renal studies during treatment and monthly: BUN, creatinine, output, specific gravity, urinalysis, uric acid
• Assess mental status often: affect, mood, behavioral changes; psychosis may occur with hallucinations, confusion
• Assess hepatic status: decreased appetite, jaundice, dark urine, fatigue
• Assess for visual disturbance that may indicate optic neuritis: blurred vision, change in color perception; may lead to blindness

---

Adverse effects: *italic* = common, **bold** = life-threatening

### Nursing diagnoses
- Diarrhea (adverse reactions)
- Infection, risk for (uses)
- Injury, risk for (adverse reactions)
- Knowledge, deficient (teaching)
- Noncompliance (teaching)

### Implementation
- Give antiemetic for vomiting
- Provide a list of foods to avoid while taking this product

**PO route**
- Give with meals to decrease GI symptoms; absorption is better when taken on empty stomach, 1 hr before or 2 hr after meals

**IM route**
- Give inj deep in large muscle mass, massage; rotate inj sites, warm inj to room temperature to dissolve crystals

### Patient/family education
- Instruct patient that compliance with dosage schedule for duration is necessary; not to skip or double doses; that scheduled appointments must be kept or relapse may occur
- Caution patient to avoid alcohol while taking product or hepatoxicity may result; to avoid ingestion of aged cheeses, fish or hypertensive crisis may result; give patient written directions on which foods to avoid while taking this medication
- Tell patient to report peripheral neuritis: weakness, tingling/numbness of hands/feet, fatigue; hepatoxicity: loss of appetite, nausea, vomiting, jaundice of skin or eyes

### Evaluation
**Positive therapeutic outcome**
- Decreased symptoms of TB
- Culture negative for TB

### Treatment of overdose:
Pyridoxine

---

### isosorbide dinitrate (Rx)
(eye-soe-sor'bide)
Apo-ISDN ♣, Cedocard-SR ♣, Coronex ♣, Dilatrate-SR, ISDN, Iso-Bid, Isonate, Isorbid, Isordil, Isosorbide dinitrate, Isotrate, Novosorbide ♣, Sorbitrate
### isosorbide mononitrate (Rx)
Imdur, ISMO, Isotrate ER, Monoket
*Func. class.:* Antianginal, vasodilator
*Chem. class.:* Nitrate

**Pregnancy category C**

**Do not confuse:**
Imdur/Imuran/Inderal/K-Dur, Monoket/
Monopril

**Action:** Relaxation of vascular smooth muscle, which leads to decreased preload, afterload, thus decreasing left ventricular end-diastolic pressure, systemic vascular resistance, and reducing cardiac $O_2$ demand

**Therapeutic outcome:** Relief and prevention of angina pectoris

**Uses:** Treatment, prevention of chronic stable angina pectoris; diffuse esophageal spasm

### Dosage and routes
***Dinitrate***
*Adult:* PO 5-40 mg qid; SL buccal tab 2.5-5 mg; may repeat q5-10min × 3 doses; CHEW TAB 5-10 mg prn or q2-3hr as prophylaxis; SUS REL CAP 40-80 mg q8-12hr

***Mononitrate***
*Adult:* PO (ISMO, Monoket) 10-20 mg bid, 7 hr apart; (Imdur) initiate at 30-60 mg/day as a single dose, increase q3 days as needed, may increase to 120 mg/day, max 240 mg/day

**Available forms:** Dinitrate: sus rel caps 40 mg; tabs 5, 10, 20, 30, 40 mg; SL tabs 2.5, 5, 10 mg; chew tabs 5, 10 mg; mononitrate: tabs (Monoket, ISMO) 10, 20 mg; ext rel tabs (Imdur, ER) 30, 60, 120 mg

### Adverse effects
*CNS: Vascular headache, flushing, dizziness,* weakness, faintness
*CV: Postural hypotension,* tachycardia, **collapse,** syncope, palpitations
*GI:* Nausea, vomiting, diarrhea
*INTEG:* Pallor, sweating, rash
*MISC:* Twitching, hemolytic anemia, **methemoglobinemia**

**Contraindications:** Hypersensitivity to this product or nitrates, severe anemia, increased ICP, cerebral hemorrhage, acute MI

**Precautions:** Pregnancy **C**, breastfeeding, children, postural hypotension, MI, CHF, severe renal/hepatic disease

| Pharmacokinetics | |
|---|---|
| **Absorption** | Well |
| **Distribution** | Unknown |
| **Metabolism** | Liver |
| **Excretion** | Urine, metabolites |
| **Half-life** | Dinitrate 1 hr, mononitrate 5 hr |

| Pharmacodynamics | | | |
|---|---|---|---|
| | **SUS REL** | **SL** | **PO** |
| **Onset** | Up to 4 hr | 2-5 min | 15-30 min |
| **Peak** | Unknown | Unknown | Unknown |
| **Duration** | 6-8 hr | 1-4 hr | 4-6 hr |

---

 Alert     Canada Only     Drug on CD    * "Tall Man" lettering (See Preface)

## Interactions
### Individual drugs
Alcohol: increased hypotension

◆Sildenafil, tadalafil, vardenafil: fatal hypotension
### Drug classifications
Antihypertensives, β-adrenergic blockers, calcium channel blockers, diuretics, phenothiazines: increased hypotension
### Drug/herb
Blue cohosh: decreased antianginal effect

## NURSING CONSIDERATIONS
### Assessment
• Assess for pain: duration, time started, activity being performed, character, intensity
• Monitor for orthostatic B/P, pulse at baseline and during treatment
### Nursing diagnoses
• Cardiac output, decreased (uses)
• Knowledge, deficient (teaching)
• Tissue perfusion, ineffective (uses)
### Implementation
**PO route**
• Swallow sus rel cap and ext rel tab whole; do not break, crush, or chew
• Do not swallow SL tab; tab should be dissolved under tongue
• Chew tab should be chewed thoroughly
• Give 1 hr before or 2 hr after meals with 8 oz of water
**SL route**
• Hold SL tab under tongue until dissolved (a few min); do not take anything PO when SL tab is in place
### Patient/family education
• Instruct patient to not skip or double doses; if dose is missed take when remembered if 2 hr before next dose (dinitrate), 6 hr before next dose (sus rel), or 8 hr before next dose (mononitrate)
• Caution patient to avoid alcohol and OTC medications unless approved by prescriber
• Inform patient that product may be taken before stressful activity: exercise, sexual activity
• Advise patient that SL tab may sting mucous membranes
• Caution patient to avoid driving and hazardous activities if dizziness occurs
• Advise patient to comply with complete medical regimen
• Caution patient to make position changes slowly to prevent orthostatic hypotension
### Evaluation
**Positive therapeutic outcome**
• Decrease in, prevention of anginal pain

## isradipine (Rx)
(is-ra'di-peen)
DynaCirc, DynaCirc CR
*Func. class.:* Calcium channel blocker, antihypertensive, antianginal
*Chem. class.:* Dihydropyridine
### Pregnancy category C

**Do not confuse:**
DynaCirc/Dynabac/Dynacin

**Action:** Inhibits calcium ion influx across cell membrane during cardiac depolarization; produces relaxation of coronary vascular smooth muscle and peripheral vascular smooth muscle; dilates coronary vascular arteries

**Therapeutic outcome:** Decreased B/P

**Uses:** Hypertension, angina pectoris, vasospastic angina

### Dosage and routes
*Adult:* PO 2.5 mg bid; increase at 2-4 wk intervals up to 10 mg bid or 5 mg/day; CONT REL may be increased q2-4 wk, max 20 mg/day

**Available forms:** Caps 2.5, 5 mg; cont rel tabs 5, 10 mg

### Adverse effects
*CNS:* Headache, fatigue, dizziness, fainting, sleep disturbances, weakness, depression, drowsiness
*CV:* Peripheral edema, tachycardia, hypotension, chest pain, **dysrhythmias,** syncope
*GI:* Nausea, vomiting, diarrhea, gastric upset, constipation, **hepatitis,** abdominal pain, distention, dry mouth
*GU:* Nocturia, urinary frequency
*HEMA:* **Leukopenia**
*INTEG:* Rash, pruritus, urticaria
*MISC:* Flushing

**Contraindications:** Sick sinus syndrome, 2nd- or 3rd-degree heart block, hypotension <90 mm Hg systolic, hypersensitivity

**Precautions:** Pregnancy **C,** breastfeeding, children, geriatric, CHF, hypotension, renal/hepatic disease

| Pharmacokinetics | |
|---|---|
| **Absorption** | Well absorbed |
| **Distribution** | High plasma protein binding (95%) |
| **Metabolism** | Liver, extensively and rapidly |
| **Excretion** | Kidney |
| **Half-life** | 8 hr |

Adverse effects: *italic* = common, **bold** = life-threatening

| Pharmacodynamics | |
|---|---|
| **Onset** | 1-2 hr |
| **Peak** | 1.5 hr (immediate rel), 7-18 hr (cont rel) |
| **Duration** | 12 hr |

## Interactions
### Individual drugs
Cimetidine, ranitidine: increased serum concentration of isradipine

Disopyramide: increased bradycardia, conduction effects

Fentanyl: increased hypotension

Flovastatin: decreased flovastatin concentration

Lovastatin: decreased lovastatin concentration

Rifampin: decreased serum concentration of isradipine

### Drug classifications
Antihypertensives, nitrates: increased hypotension

β-Adrenergic blockers: increased synergistic effect

CYP3A4 inducers: increased serum concentration of isradipine

CYP3A4 inhibitors: decreased serum concentration of isradipine

NSAIDs, salicylates: decreased antihypertensive action

### Drug/herb
Aconite: increased toxicity, death

Astragalus, cola tree: increased or decreased antihypertensive effect

Barberry, betony, black catechu, black cohosh, bloodroot, broom, burdock, cat's claw, dandelion, ginkgo, ginseng, goldenseal, hawthorn, Irish moss, Jamaican dogwood, kelp, khella, mistletoe, parsley: increased antihypertensive effect

Coltsfoot, guarana, khat, licorice, St. John's wort, yohimbe: decreased antihypertensive effect

## NURSING CONSIDERATIONS
### Assessment
• Assess fluid volume status: I&O ratio and record, weight, distended red veins, crackles in lung, color, quality, and specific gravity of urine, skin turgor, adequacy of pulses, moist mucous membranes, bilateral lung sounds, peripheral pitting edema; dehydration symptoms of decreasing output, thirst, hypotension, dry mouth and mucous membranes should be reported

• Monitor ALT, AST, bilirubin; if these are elevated, hepatotoxicity is suspected

• Assess renal, hepatic status, electrolytes before and during treatment

• Monitor cardiac status: B/P, pulse, respiration, ECG; assess anginal pain, precipitating, ameliorating factors

### Nursing diagnoses
• Cardiac output, decreased (uses)
• Knowledge, deficient (teaching)

### Implementation
• Do not break, crush, or chew caps, cont rel tabs
• Give once a day with full glass of water; with food for GI symptoms

### Patient/family education
• Instruct patient to avoid hazardous activities until stabilized on product and dizziness is no longer a problem
• Instruct patient to limit caffeine consumption; to avoid alcohol and OTC products unless directed by prescriber
• Advise patient to comply in all areas of medical regimen: diet, exercise, stress reduction, product therapy; to notify prescriber of irregular heartbeat, shortness of breath, swelling of feet and hands, pronounced dizziness, constipation, nausea, hypotension
• Teach patient to use as directed even if feeling better
• Teach patient to take with a full glass of water

### Evaluation
**Positive therapeutic outcome**
• Decreased B/P

**Treatment of overdose:** Defibrillation, atropine for AV block, vasopressor for hypotension

---

### itraconazole (Rx)
(it-tra-kon'a-zol)
Sporanox
*Func. class.:* Antifungal (systemic)
*Chem. class.:* Triazole derivative
**Pregnancy category** C

**Action:** Increases cell membrane permeability in susceptible organisms by binding sterols in fungal cell membrane; decreases potassium, sodium, and nutrients in cell

**Therapeutic outcome:** Fungistatic against *Histoplasma capsulatum, Blastomyces dermatitis, Cryptococcus neoformans, Aspergillus fumigatus, Candida*

**Uses:** Systemic candidiasis, chronic mucocandidiasis, oral thrush, candiduria, histoplasmosis, chromomycosis, paracoccidioidomycosis, blastomycosis (pulmonary and extrapulmonary)

**Unlabeled uses:** Dermatomycosis, chromoblastomycosis, coccidioidomycosis, pityriasis versicolor, sebopsoriasis, vaginal candidiasis, cryptococcal, subcutaneous mycoses, dimorphic infections, leishmaniasis, fungal keratitis, alternariosis, zygomycosis

### Dosage and routes
Dose varies with type of infection
*Adult:* PO 200 mg/day with food; may increase to 400 mg/day if needed; life-threatening infections may require a loading dose of 200 mg tid × 3 days; **IV** 200 mg bid × 4 doses, then 200 mg/day; give each dose over 1 hr, maintenance PO 100 mg/day
*Child:* PO 3-5 mg/kg/day

### Available forms: 
Caps 100 mg; oral sol 10 mg/ml; inj 10 mg/ml

### Adverse effects
*CNS:* Headache, dizziness, insomnia, somnolence, depression
*CV:* Hypertension
*GI:* Nausea, vomiting, anorexia, diarrhea, cramps, abdominal pain, flatulence, **GI bleeding, hepatotoxicity**
*GU:* Gynecomastia, impotence, decreased libido
*INTEG:* Pruritus, fever, rash, **toxic epidermal necrolysis**
*MISC:* Edema, fatigue, malaise, hypertension, hypokalemia, tinnitus, **rhabdomyolysis**

**Contraindications:** Hypersensitivity, fungal meningitis, onychomycosis, or dermatomycosis in cardiac dysfunction

**Precautions:** Pregnancy **C**, breastfeeding, children, cardiac/hepatic disease, achlorhydria or hypochlorhydria (product-induced)

### Pharmacokinetics
| | |
|---|---|
| Absorption | Variable |
| Distribution | Tissue, plasma, CSF, highly protein bound |
| Metabolism | Liver, extensively, inhibits CYP4503A enzyme |
| Excretion | Feces, breast milk |
| Half-life | 20-21 hr |

### Pharmacodynamics
| | |
|---|---|
| Onset | Unknown |
| Peak | 4 hr |
| Duration | Unknown |

### Interactions
*Individual drugs*
Busulfan, clarithromycin, cycloSPORINE, diazepam, digoxin, felodipine, fentanyl, indinavir, isradipine, niCARdipine, NIFEdipine, nimoldipine, phenytoin, ritonavir, saquinavir, tacrolimus, warfarin: increased toxicity
BusPIRone: increased busPIRone levels, toxicity
Didanosine: decreased antifungal action
Dofetilide, pimozide, quinidine: life-threatening CV reaction
Midazolam (oral): increased sedation
Quinidine: increased tinnitus, hearing loss, increased toxicity
Rifamycins: decreased action of itraconazole
Triazolam: increased sedation
*Drug classifications*
Antacids, H$_2$-receptor antagonists: decreased action of itraconazole
Calcium channel blockers: increased edema
Contraceptives (oral): decreased effect
Hepatotoxic products: hepatotoxicity
Oral hypoglycemics: increased effects of oral hypoglycemics
*Drug/herb*
Gossypol: nephrotoxicity
*Drug/food*
Increased: absorption

### NURSING CONSIDERATIONS
### Assessment
- Assess for infection: WBC, sputum baseline and periodically, may start treatment before obtaining results
- Monitor for hepatotoxicity: increasing AST, ALT, alkaline phosphatase, bilirubin
- Monitor for allergic reaction: dermatitis, rash; product should be discontinued, antihistamines (mild reaction) or epINEPHrine (severe reaction) administered; check inj site for thrombophlebitis
- Monitor for hypokalemia, check potassium level: anorexia, drowsiness, weakness, decreased reflexes, dizziness, increased urinary output, increased thirst, paresthesias; if these occur, product should be decreased or discontinued and potassium administered

### Nursing diagnoses
- Infection, risk for (uses)
- Injury, risk for (adverse reaction)
- Knowledge, deficient (teaching)

### Implementation
**PO route**
- Swallow caps whole; do not break, crush, or chew

Adverse effects: *italic* = common, **bold** = life-threatening

- Give caps after full meal to ensure absorption
- Give with food or milk to prevent nausea and vomiting
- Take 2 hr before administration of other products that increase gastric pH
- Store in tight container at room temperature
- Oral sol and caps are not interchangeable on a mg/mg basis
- Oral sol: patient should swish in mouth vigorously

**IV route**
- **IV** after adding full contents 25 ml to 50 ml of NaCl, mix gently, use flow control device, give over 1 hr; use separate line, flush after use

### Patient/family education
- Advise patient that long-term therapy may be needed to clear infection (1 wk-6 mo depending on type of infection)
- Teach patient side effects and when to notify prescriber
- Instruct patient to avoid hazardous activities if dizziness occurs
- Instruct patient to take 2 hr before administration of other products that increase gastric pH (antacids, H₂-blockers, omeprazole, sucralfate, anticholinergics)
- Teach patient importance of compliance with product regimen
- Instruct patient to notify prescriber of GI symptoms, signs of liver dysfunction (fatigue, nausea, anorexia, vomiting, dark urine, pale stools)

### Evaluation
**Positive therapeutic outcome**
- Decreased fever, malaise, rash
- Negative C&S for infectious organism

---

### ixabepilone (Rx)
(ix-ab-ep′i-lone)
Ixempra
*Func. class.:* Antineoplastic—miscellaneous
*Chem. class.:* Epothilone

**Pregnancy category D**

**Action:** Microtubule stabilizing agent; microtubles are needed for interphase and mitotic cellular functions

**Therapeutic outcome:** Decreased tumor size, spread of malignancy

**Uses:** Breast cancer

### Dosage and routes
*Breast cancer, metastatic or locally advanced given with capecitabine, and resistant to anthracycline, taxane*
Adult: **IV** INF 40 mg/m² over 3 hr, q3 wk plus capecitabine PO 2000 mg/m²/day in 2 divided doses on days 1-14 q21 days

*Breast cancer, metastatic or locally advanced resistant/refractory to anthracyclines, taxanes, capecitabine*
Adult: **IV** INF 40 mg/m² over 3 hr q3 wk

*Dosage reduction in those taking a strong CYP3A4 inhibitor*
Adult: **IV** INF 20 mg/m² over 3 hr q3 wk

**Available forms:** Powder for inj 15, 45 mg

### Adverse effects
*CV:* Bradycardia, *hypotension,* abnormal ECG, angina, atrial flutter, cardiomyopathy, chest pain, edema, MI, vasculitis
*GI:* Nausea, vomiting, diarrhea, abdominal pain, anorexia, colitis, constipation, coagulopathy, gastritis, jaundice, GERD, hepatic failure
*HEMA:* **Neutropenia, thrombocytopenia, anemia,** infections
*INTEG:* Alopecia, rash
*META:* Hypokalemia, metabolic acidosis
*MS:* Arthralgia, myalgia
*NEURO:* Peripheral neuropathy, chills, fatigue, fever, flushing, headache, insomnia, impaired cognition, asthenia
*RESP:* Bronchospasm, cough, dyspnea
*SYST:* Hypersensitivity reactions, **anaphylaxis,** dehydration

**Contraindications:** Pregnancy **D**, hypersensitivity to products with polyoxyethylated castor oil, breastfeeding

**Precautions:** Children, geriatric, neutropenia of <1500/mm³, alcoholism, bone marrow suppression, cardiac dysrhythmias, cardiac/renal/hepatic disease, diabetes mellitus, peripheral neuropathy, thrombocytopenia, ventricular dysfunction

| Pharmacokinetics | |
|---|---|
| **Absorption** | Unknown |
| **Distribution** | Unknown |
| **Metabolism** | Liver by P45CYP3A4 |
| **Excretion** | Feces 65%, urine 21% |
| **Half-life** | Terminal 52 hr |

| Pharmacodynamics | |
|---|---|
| Unknown | |

---

 Alert       Canada Only       Drug on CD      * "Tall Man" lettering (See Preface)

## Interactions
### Drug classifications
CYP3A4 inducers (aminoglutethimide, barbiturates, bexarotene, bosentan, carbamazepine, dexamethasone, efavirenz, griseofulvin, modafinil, nafcillin, nevirapine, oxcarbazepine, phenytoin, rifamycin, topiramate): decreased ixabepilone levels

CYP3A4 inhibitors (amiodarone, amprenavir, aprepitant, atazanavir, chloramphenicol, clarithromycin, conivaptan, cycloSPORINE, danazol, darunavir, dalforpristan, delavirdine, diltiazem, erythromycin, estradiol, fluconazole, fluvoxamine, fosamprenavir, imatinib, indinavir, isoniazid, itraconazole, ketoconazole, lopinavir, miconazole, nefazodone, nelfinavir, propoxyphene, ritonavir, RU-486, saquinavir, tamoxifen, telithromycin, troleandomycin, verapamil, voriconazole, zafirlukast): increased ixabepilone level

### Drug/herb
St. John's wort: avoid use
### Drug/food
Grapefruit products: avoid use

## NURSING CONSIDERATIONS
### Assessment
• Monitor CBC, differential, platelet count prior to and qwk; withhold product if WBC is <1500/mm$^3$ or platelet count is <100,000/mm$^3$, notify prescriber
• Monitor temp q4hr (may indicate beginning infection)
• Monitor liver function tests before, during therapy (bilirubin, AST, ALT, LDH) prn or qmo; check for jaundiced skin and sclera, dark urine, clay-colored stool, itchy skin, abdominal pain, fever, diarrhea
• Monitor VS during 1st hr of infusion; check IV site for signs of infiltration
◆ Assess for hypersensitive reactions, anaphylaxis including hypotension, dyspnea, angioedema, generalized urticaria; discontinue infusion immediately; keep emergency equipment available
• Assess effects of alopecia on body image; discuss feelings about body changes

### Nursing diagnoses
• Injury, risk for (uses, adverse reactions)
• Knowledge, deficient (teaching)

### Implementation
• Give antiemetic 30-60 min before giving product and prn
**IV route**
• Let kit stand at room temperature for 30 min; to reconstitute, withdraw supplied diluent

(8 ml for 15 mg vials, 23.5 ml for 45 mg vials); slowly inject solution into vial; gently swirl and invert to mix, final conc 2 mg/ml; further dilute in LR in DEHP free bags, final conc should be 0.2-0.6 mg/ml; after added, mix by manual rotation
• Diluted sol is stable for 6 hr at room temperature; infusion must be completed within 6 hr
• Use in-line filter 0.2-1.2 micron
• Give over 3 hr

### Patient/family education
• Teach patient to report signs of infection: fever, sore throat, flulike symptoms
• Teach patient to report signs of anemia: fatigue, headache, faintness, shortness of breath
• Teach patient to report any complaints or side effects to nurse or prescriber
• Caution patient that hair may be lost during treatment; a wig or hairpiece may make patient feel better; new hair may be different in color, texture
• Advise patient that pain in muscles and joints 2-5 days after infusion is common
• Advise patient to use nonhormonal type of contraception
• Instruct patient to avoid receiving vaccinations while on this product

### Evaluation
**Positive therapeutic outcome**
• Decreased tumor size, spread of malignancy

---

## ketoconazole (Rx)
(kee-toe-koe'na-zole)
Nizoral
*Func. class.:* Antifungal
*Chem. class.:* Imidazole derivative
**Pregnancy category C**

### Do not confuse:
Nizoral/Nasarel/Neoral

**Action:** Alters cell membrane and inhibits several fungal enzymes; prevents production of adrenal sterols; prevents fungal metabolism

**Therapeutic outcome:** Fungistatic/fungicidal against susceptible organisms: *Blastomycoses, Candida, Coccidioides, Cryptococcus, Histoplasma;* topical route: tinea cruris, tinea corporis, tinea versicolor, *Pityrosporum ovale*

**Uses:** Systemic candidiasis, chronic mucocandidiasis, oral thrush, candiduria, coccidioidomycosis, histoplasmosis, chromomycosis, paracoccidioidomycosis, blastomycosis, tinea cruris, tinea corporis, tinea versicolor, *Pityrosporum ovale*

**Unlabeled uses:** Cushing's syndrome, advanced prostatic cancer

### Dosage and routes
*Adult:* PO 200-400 mg once/day for 1-2 wk (candidiasis), 6 wk (other infections); 400 mg tid (prostate cancer, unlabeled)
*Children >2 yr:* 3.3-6.6 mg/kg/day as single daily dose

**Available forms:** Tabs 200 mg; oral susp ✦ 100 mg/5 ml topical (see Appendix D)

### Adverse effects
*CNS:* Headache, dizziness, somnolence
*GI:* Nausea, vomiting, anorexia, diarrhea, abdominal pain, **hepatotoxicity**
*GU:* Gynecomastia, impotence
*HEMA:* **Thrombocytopenia, leukopenia, hemolytic anemia**
*INTEG:* Pruritus, fever, chills, photophobia, rash, dermatitis, purpura, urticaria
*SYST:* **Anaphylaxis**

**Contraindications:** Breastfeeding, hypersensitivity, fungal meningitis; coadministration with terfenadine or products that prolong QTc interval

**Precautions:** Pregnancy **C**, children <2 yr, renal/hepatic disease, achlorhydria (product induced), other hepatotoxic agents including terfenadine, other products metabolized by CYP450

| Pharmacokinetics | |
|---|---|
| **Absorption** | pH dependent; decreased pH increased absorption |
| **Distribution** | Widely distributed; crosses placenta |
| **Metabolism** | Liver, partially |
| **Excretion** | Feces, bile, breast milk |
| **Half-life** | Biphasic: 2 hr, 8 hr |

| Pharmacodynamics | |
|---|---|
| **Onset** | Unknown |
| **Peak** | 1-3 hr |
| **Duration** | Unknown |

### Interactions
*Individual drugs*
Alcohol: increased hepatotoxicity
Alfentanil, alprazolam, amprenavir, atorvastatin, carbamazepine, cerivastatin, clarithromycin, cyclophosphamide, cycloSPORINE, donepezil, erythromycin, fentanyl, ifosfamide, indinavir, lovastatin, midazolam, nelfinavir, nisoldipine, quinidine, ritonavir, saquinavir, sildenafil, simvastatin, sufentanil, tamoxifen, triazolam, vinBLAStine, vinCRIStine, zolpidem: increased toxicity, inhibition of CYP450 3A4 pathway
Isoniazid, phenytoin, rifampin: decreased effect of ketoconazole
Paclitaxel: inhibited metabolism
Theophylline: decreased effectiveness
Warfarin: increased effects of warfarin
*Drug classifications*
Antacids, anticholinergics, gastric acid pump inhibitors, H₂-receptor agonists: decreased ketoconazole action
Anticoagulants (oral): increased effects of oral anticoagulants
Calcium channel blockers, corticosteroids, vinca alkaloids: increased toxicity, decreased CYP4503A4 pathway
Contraceptives (oral): decreased effect of oral contraceptives
Hepatotoxic agents: increased hepatotoxicity
*Drug/herb*
Gossypol: nephrotoxicity
Yew: decreased ketoconazole action

### NURSING CONSIDERATIONS
**Assessment**
• Assess for signs and symptoms of infection: drainage, sore throat, urinary pain, hematuria, fever
• Obtain cultures for C&S before beginning treatment; therapy may be started after culture is taken
◆ Monitor for hepatotoxicity: increased AST, ALT, alkaline phosphatase, bilirubin; product is discontinued if hepatotoxicity occurs

**Nursing diagnoses**
• Infection, risk for (uses)
• Injury, risk for (adverse reactions)
• Knowledge, deficient (teaching)

**Implementation**
*PO route*
• Give in the presence of acid products only; do not use alkaline products, proton pump inhibitors, H₂-antagonists, or antacids within 2 hr of product; may give coffee, tea, acidic fruit juices, cola; give with food to decrease GI symptoms; dissolve tab/4 ml of aqueous sol 0.2 N HCl, use straw to avoid contact with, rinse with water afterward and swallow
• Give with HCl if achlorhydria is present
• Store in tight container at room temperature

**Topical route**
• Use enough medication to cover fungally infected and surrounding area; rub in; do not use occlusive dressing; do not get in eyes

**Shampoo**
• Hair should be wet; apply shampoo, lather, rub gently into scalp and hair for 1 min; rinse; reapply × 3 min; continue treatment 2 ×/wk for 1 mo, no more than once q3 days

## Patient/family education
• Advise patient that long-term therapy may be needed to clear infection (1 wk-6 mo depending on infection)
• Advise patient to avoid hazardous activities if dizziness occurs
• Instruct patient to take 2 hr before administration of other products that increase gastric pH (antacids, H₂-blockers, omeprazole, sucralfate, anticholinergics)
• Stress the importance of compliance with product regimen
• Advise patient to notify prescriber of GI symptoms, signs of liver dysfunction (fatigue, nausea, anorexia, vomiting, dark urine, pale stools)
• Teach patient proper hygiene: hand washing, nail care, use of concomitant topical agents if prescribed
• Caution patient to avoid alcohol, since nausea, vomiting, hypertension may occur
• Advise patient to use sunscreen or avoid direct sunlight to prevent photosensitivity
• Advise patient to notify prescriber of sore throat, fever, skin rash, which may indicate superinfection
• Advise patient to use sunglasses to prevent photophobia

## Evaluation
**Positive therapeutic outcome**
• Decreased oral candidiasis, fever, malaise, rash
• Negative C&S for infectious organism
• Absence of dandruff, scaling

## ketoconazole topical
*See Appendix D*

---

## ketoprofen (OTC, Rx)
(ke-to-proe'fen)
Apo-Keto ✦, Apo-Keto-E ✦, Ketoprofen, Orudis-E ✦, Orudis-KT, Orudis-SR ✦, Oruvail, Rhodis ✦
*Func. class.:* NSAID; nonopioid analgesic, antirheumatic
*Chem. class.:* Propionic acid derivative

**Pregnancy category B**

**Do not confuse:**
Oruvail/Clinorill/Elavil

**Action:** Inhibits prostaglandin synthesis by decreasing enzyme needed for biosynthesis; analgesic, antiinflammatory, antipyretic

**Therapeutic outcome:** Decreased pain, inflammation

**Uses:** Mild to moderate pain; osteoarthritis; rheumatoid arthritis; dysmenorrhea; OTC relief of minor aches, pains

**Dosage and routes**
*Antiinflammatory*
*Adult:* PO 150-300 mg in divided doses tid-qid, not to exceed 300 mg/day or EXT REL 150-200 mg/day

*Analgesic*
*Adult:* PO 25-50 mg q6-8hr

**Available forms:** Caps 25, 50, 75 mg; ext rel caps 150, 200 mg; tabs 12.5 mg

**Adverse effects**
*CNS:* Dizziness, drowsiness, fatigue, tremors, confusion, insomnia, anxiety, depression, headache
*CV:* Tachycardia, peripheral edema, palpitations, dysrhythmias, hypertension, **CV thrombotic events, MI, stroke**
*EENT:* Tinnitus, hearing loss, blurred vision
*GI: Nausea, anorexia, vomiting, diarrhea,* jaundice, **hepatitis,** constipation, flatulence, cramps, dry mouth, peptic ulcer, **GI bleeding**
*GU:* **Nephrotoxicity: dysuria, hematuria, oliguria, azotemia**
*HEMA:* **Blood dyscrasias**
*INTEG:* Purpura, rash, pruritus, sweating
*SYST:* **Anaphylaxis**

**Contraindications:** Avoid in 2nd/3rd trimesters of pregnancy; hypersensitivity, asthma, severe renal/hepatic disease, ulcer disease, perioperative pain in CABG

**Precautions:** Pregnancy **B** (1st trimester), breastfeeding, children, geriatric, bleeding/GI/ cardiac disorders, hypersensitivity to other antiinflammatory agents

K

| Pharmacokinetics | |
|---|---|
| **Absorption** | Well absorbed |
| **Distribution** | Not known |
| **Metabolism** | Liver |
| **Excretion** | Kidneys |
| **Half-life** | 2-4 hr |

| Pharmacodynamics | |
|---|---|
| **Onset** | Unknown |
| **Peak** | 2 hr |
| **Duration** | Unknown |

## Interactions
### Individual drugs
Alcohol: increased adverse GI reactions, toxicity

Aspirin: increased ketoprofen levels, increased adverse GI reactions

Cefamandole, cefaperazone, cefotetan, clopidogrel, eptifibatide, plicamycin, ticlopidine, tirofiban, valproic acid: increased risk of bleeding

CycloSPORINE, digoxin, lithium, methotrexate, phenytoin: increased ketoprofen levels, increased toxicity

Insulin: increased hypoglycemia

Probenecid: increased ketocazole levels

Radiation: increased risk of hematologic toxicity

### Drug classifications
Anticoagulants, thrombolytics: increased risk of bleeding

Antihypertensives: decreased effect of antihypertensives

Corticosteroids: increased adverse GI reactions

Diuretics: decreased effectiveness of diuretics

Sulfonylureas: increased hypoglycemia

NSAIDs: increased adverse GI reactions

### Drug/herb
Anise, arnica, bogbean, chamomile, chondroitin, clove, dong quai, feverfew, garlic, ginger, ginkgo, ginseng *(Panax):* increased risk of bleeding

Arginine, gossypol: increased gastric irritation

Bearberry, bilberry: increased NSAIDs effect

### Drug/lab test
Increased: bleeding time, potassium, BUN, alkaline phosphatase, AST, ALT, creatinine, LDH

Decreased: blood glucose, Hct, Hgb, CCr, platelets, leukocytes

Interference: urine albumin, 17 KS, 17 hydroxycorticosteroids, bilirubin

## NURSING CONSIDERATIONS
### Assessment
- Assess for pain: type, location, intensity; ROM before and 1-2 hr after treatment
- Monitor renal, liver function tests: AST, ALT, bilirubin, creatinine, BUN, urine creatinine, CBC Hct, Hgb, pro-time if patient is on long-term therapy
- Check I&O ratio; decreasing output may indicate renal failure (long-term therapy)
- Assess hepatotoxicity: dark urine, clay-colored stools, jaundice of skin and sclera, itching, abdominal pain, fever, diarrhea if patient is on long-term therapy
- Assess for allergic reactions: rash, urticaria; if these occur, product may have to be discontinued
- Assess for ototoxicity: tinnitus, ringing, roaring in ears; audiometric testing needed before, after long-term therapy
- Assess for visual changes: blurring, halos; may indicate corneal, retinal damage
- Assess for GI bleeding: blood in sputum, emesis, stools
- Check edema in feet, ankles, legs
- Identify prior product history; there are many product interactions
- Monitor pain: location, duration, type, intensity, before dose and 1 hr after; ROM before dose and after
- Assess for CV thrombotic events: MI, stroke

### Nursing diagnoses
- Injury, risk for (adverse reactions)
- Knowledge, deficient (teaching)
- Mobility, physical impaired (uses)
- Pain, acute (uses)
- Pain, chronic (uses)

### Implementation
- Swallow whole; do not break, crush, chew, or open ext rel cap
- Give with 8 oz of water and sit upright for 30 min after dose to prevent ulceration
- Give with food or milk to decrease gastric symptoms; give 30 min before or 2 hr after meals; absorption may be slowed

### Patient/family education
- Teach patient to report any symptoms of hepatotoxicity, renal toxicity, visual changes, ototoxicity, allergic reactions, bleeding (long-term therapy)
- Advise patient to take with 8 oz of water and sit upright for 30 min after dose to prevent ulceration
- Caution patient not to exceed recommended dosage; acute poisoning may result; to take as prescribed; do not double dose

- Advise patient to read label on other OTC products; many contain other antiinflammatories
- Advise patient to use sunscreen to prevent photosensitivity
- Inform patient that the therapeutic response takes 2 wk (arthritis)
- Teach patient to report tinnitus, confusion, diarrhea, sweating, hyperventilation, blurred vision, fever, joint aches
- Caution patient to avoid alcohol ingestion; GI bleeding may occur

### Evaluation
**Positive therapeutic outcome**
- Decreased pain
- Decreased inflammation
- Increased mobility
- Decreased fever

---

## ketorolac (Rx)
(kee'toe-role-ak)
Acular, Toradol
*Func. class.:* NSAID, nonopioid analgesic
*Chem. class.:* Acetic acid

**Pregnancy category C**

### Do not confuse:
Toradol/Tegretol/Foradil/Inderal/Torecan/tramadol

**Action:** Inhibits prostaglandin synthesis by decreasing an enzyme needed for biosynthesis; analgesic, antiinflammatory, antipyretic effects

**Therapeutic outcome:** Decreased pain, inflammation, ocular itching

**Uses:** Mild to moderate pain (short term); decreased ocular itching in seasonal allergic conjunctivitis (ophthalmic)

### Dosage and routes
*Adult <65 yr:* PO 20 mg, then 10 mg q4-6hr prn, max 40 mg/day; IM (single dose) 60 mg; **IV** 30 mg; IM (multiple dosing) 15 mg q6hr, max 60 mg/day × 5 days combined either PO/IM/**IV**
*Adult >65 yr, renal disease, <50 kg:* PO 10 mg q4-6hr prn, max 40 mg/day; IM (single dose) 30 mg; **IV** 15 mg; IM/**IV** (multiple dosing) 15 mg q6hr, max 60 mg/day × 5 days combined either PO/IM/**IV**

### Ophthalmic route
*Adult:* 1 gtt (0.25 mg) qid × 7 days
*Child:* **IV** 1 mg/kg then 0.5 mg/kg q6hr

**Available forms:** Inj 15, 30 mg/ml (prefilled syringes); ophth 0.5% sol; tabs 10 mg

### Adverse effects
***CNS:*** Dizziness, *drowsiness,* tremors
***CV:*** Hypertension, flushing, syncope, pallor, edema, vasodilation, **CV thrombotic events, MI, stroke**
***EENT:*** Tinnitus, hearing loss, blurred vision
***GI:*** Nausea, anorexia, vomiting, diarrhea, constipation, flatulence, cramps, dry mouth, peptic ulcer, **GI bleeding, perforation,** taste change
***GU:*** **Nephrotoxicity: dysuria, hematuria, oliguria, azotemia**
***HEMA:*** **Blood dyscrasias,** prolonged bleeding
***INTEG:*** Purpura, rash, pruritus, sweating

**Contraindications:** Breastfeeding, hypersensitivity, asthma, severe renal/hepatic disease, peptic ulcer disease, labor and delivery, CV bleeding, perioperative pain in CABG prior to major surgery

**Precautions:** Pregnancy **C,** children, geriatric, bleeding disorders, GI/cardiac disorders, hypersensitivity to other antiinflammatory agents, CCr <25 ml/min

**K**

### Pharmacokinetics

| | |
|---|---|
| **Absorption** | Rapidly, completely absorbed |
| **Distribution** | Bound to plasma proteins (99%) |
| **Metabolism** | Liver (<50%) |
| **Excretion** | Kidney, metabolites (92%); breast milk (6%); feces |
| **Half-life** | 6 hr (IM); increased in renal disease |

### Pharmacodynamics

| | IM | OPHTH/PO |
|---|---|---|
| **Onset** | Up to 10 min | Unknown |
| **Peak** | 50 min IM; 2-3 hr PO | Unknown |
| **Duration** | 4-6 hr PO | Unknown |

### Interactions
*Individual drugs*
Alcohol, aspirin: increased GI effects
Aspirin: increased ketorolac levels, contraindicated
Cefamandole, cefoperazone, cefotetan, clopidogrel, eptifibatide, plicamycin, ticlopidine, tirofiban, valproic acid: increased risk of bleeding
CycloSPORINE, lithium, methotrexate: increased toxicity
*Drug classifications*
ACE inhibitors: increased renal impairment
Anticoagulants: increased effects

Adverse effects: *italic* = common, **bold** = life-threatening

Antihypertensives: decreased antihypertensive effect

Cephalosporins (some), salicylates, thrombolytics: increased risk of bleeding

Corticosteroids, NSAIDs, potassium products, steroids: increased GI effects

Diuretics: decreased diuretic effect

*Drug/herb*

Anise, arnica, bogbean, chamomile, chondroitin, clove, dong quai, feverfew, garlic, ginger, ginkgo, ginseng *(Panax)*: increased risk of bleeding

Arginine, gossypol: increased gastric irritation

Bearberry, bilberry: increased NSAIDs effect

*Drug/lab test*

Increased: AST, ALT, LDH, alkaline phosphatase, bleeding time, BUN, creatinine, potassium

Decreased: blood glucose, Hct/Hgb, platelets

## NURSING CONSIDERATIONS
### Assessment

⬥ Monitor blood counts during therapy; watch for decreasing platelets; if low, therapy may need to be discontinued and restarted after hematologic recovery; assess for blood dyscrasia (thrombocytopenia): bruising, fatigue, bleeding, poor healing

• Monitor for aspirin sensitivity, asthma; these patients may be more likely to develop hypersensitivity to NSAIDs

• Assess patient's eyes: redness swelling, tearing, itching

• Monitor for pain: type, location, intensity, ROM before and 1 hr after treatment

• Assess for GI bleeding: blood in sputum, emesis, stools

• Assess for CV thrombotic events: MI, stroke

### Nursing diagnoses

• Injury, risk for (adverse reactions)
• Knowledge, deficient (teaching)
• Mobility, impaired physical (uses)
• Pain, acute (uses)

### Implementation
**PO route**

• Administer to patient crushed or whole
• Do not exceed 5 days
• Give with full glass of water; give with food or milk to decrease gastric symptoms; give 30 min before or 2 hr after meals; absorption may be slowed

**IM/IV route**

• **IV** give undiluted ≥15 sec
• Give IM inj deeply into large muscle mass

*Y-site compatibilities:* Cisatracurium, remifentanil, sufentanil

*Syringe incompatibilities:* Morphine, meperidine, promethazine, hydrOXYzine

*Solution compatibilities:* $D_5W$, 0.9% NaCl, LR, $D_5$, plasmalate

### Patient/family education

• Teach patient that product must be continued for prescribed time to be effective; to avoid aspirin, alcoholic beverages, other NSAIDs, acetaminophen

• Caution patient to report bleeding, bruising, fatigue, malaise, since blood dyscrasias do occur

• Instruct patient to use caution when driving; drowsiness, dizziness may occur

• Teach patient to take with a full glass of water to enhance absorption

• Caution patient that this product may cause eye redness, burning if soft contact lenses are worn

### Evaluation
**Positive therapeutic outcome**

• Decreased pain
• Decreased inflammatory response
• Increased mobility
• Decreased ocular itching

## ketorolac ophthalmic
*See Appendix D*

## ketotifen ophthalmic
*See Appendix D*

## labetalol (Rx)
(la-bet'a-lole)

Normodyne, Trandate

*Func. class.:* Antihypertensive, antianginal

*Chem. class.:* α- and β-blocker

**Pregnancy category** C

**Do not confuse:**
Trandate/Tridate

**Action:** Competitively blocks stimulation of β-adrenergic receptor within vascular smooth muscle; produces chronotropic, inotropic activity (decreases rate of SA node discharge, increases recovery time), slows conduction of AV node, decreases heart rate, which decreases $O_2$ consumption in myocardium; also has α-adrenergic blocking activity

**Therapeutic outcome:** Decreased B/P

**Uses:** Mild to moderate hypertension; treatment of severe hypertension (**IV**)

**Unlabeled uses:** Hypertension in patients with pheochromocytoma, hypertension in clonidine withdrawal

## Dosage and routes
### Hypertension
*Adult:* PO 100 mg bid; may be given with a diuretic; may increase to 200 mg bid after 2 days; may continue to increase q1-3 days; max 2400 mg/day in divided doses

### Hypertensive crisis
*Adult:* **IV** INF 200 mg/160 ml D₅W, run at 2 ml/min; stop INF after desired response obtained; repeat q6-8hr as needed; **IV** BOL 20 mg over 2 min; may repeat 40-80 mg q10 min, not to exceed 300 mg

**Available forms:** Tabs 100, 200, 300 mg; inj 5 mg/ml in 20-ml ampules

## Adverse effects
*CNS:* Dizziness, mental changes, drowsiness, fatigue, headache, catatonia, depression, anxiety, nightmares, paresthesias, lethargy
*CV: Orthostatic hypotension,* **bradycardia, CHF,** chest pain, **ventricular dysrhythmias,** AV block, scalp tingling
*EENT: Tinnitus,* visual changes, sore throat, double vision, dry burning eyes
*GI: Nausea, vomiting, diarrhea,* dyspepsia, taste distortion
*GU:* Impotence, dysuria, ejaculatory failure
*HEMA:* **Agranulocytosis, thrombocytopenia, purpura** (rare)
*INTEG:* Rash, alopecia, urticaria, pruritus, fever
*RESP:* **Bronchospasm,** dyspnea, wheezing

**Contraindications:** Hypersensitivity to β-blockers, cardiogenic shock, heart block (2nd or 3rd degree), sinus bradycardia, CHF, bronchial asthma

**Precautions:** Pregnancy **C,** breastfeeding, geriatric, major surgery, diabetes mellitus, thyroid/renal/hepatic disease, COPD, well-compensated heart failure, CAD, nonallergic bronchospasm, peripheral vascular disease

### Pharmacokinetics
| | |
|---|---|
| **Absorption** | Bioavailability 25% (PO); complete (**IV**) |
| **Distribution** | Crosses placenta, CNS |
| **Metabolism** | Liver, extensively |
| **Excretion** | Breast milk, kidneys, bile |
| **Half-life** | 6-8 hr |

### Pharmacodynamics
| | PO | IV |
|---|---|---|
| **Onset** | 1-2 hr | 5 min |
| **Peak** | 2-4 hr | 15 min |
| **Duration** | 8-12 hr | 2-4 hr |

## Interactions
### Individual drugs
Alcohol (large amounts), cimetidine, nitroglycerin: increased hypotension
Glutethimide: decreased effect of labetalol
Indomethacin, lidocaine: decreased effect of each specific product
Verapamil: increased myocardial depression
### Drug classifications
Antihypertensives: increased hypotension
β-Blockers, bronchodilators, sympathomimetics, xanthines: decreased effects
Diuretics: increased hypotension
General anesthetics, hydantoins: increased myocardial depression
MAOIs: do not use within 2 wk
NSAIDs, salicylates: decreased antihypertensive effect
Theophyllines: decreased bronchodilation
### Drug/herb
Aconite: increased toxicity, death
Astragalus, cola tree: increased or decreased antihypertensive effect
Barberry, betony, black catechu, black cohosh, bloodroot, broom, burdock, cat's claw, dandelion, goldenseal, Irish moss, Jamaican dogwood, kelp, khella, mistletoe, parsley: increased antihypertensive effect
Coltsfoot, guarana, khat, licorice, yohimbe: decreased antihypertensive effect
### Drug/lab test
Increased: ANA titer, blood glucose, alkaline phosphatase, LDH, AST, ALT, BUN, potassium, triglycerides, uric acid
False increase: urinary catecholamines

## NURSING CONSIDERATIONS
### Assessment
• Monitor B/P at beginning of treatment, periodically thereafter; pulse q4hr; note rate, rhythm, quality: apical/radial pulse before administration; notify prescriber of any significant changes (pulse <50 bpm)
• Check for baselines in renal, liver function tests before therapy begins
• Assess for edema in feet, legs daily, monitor I&O, daily weight; check for jugular vein distention, crackles bilaterally, dyspnea (CHF)
• Monitor skin turgor, dryness of mucous membranes for hydration status, especially geriatric

Adverse effects: *italic* = common, **bold** = life-threatening

## Nursing diagnoses
- Cardiac output, decreased (uses)
- Injury, risk for (side effects)
- Knowledge, deficient (teaching)
- Noncompliance (teaching)

## Implementation
### PO route
- Given before meals, at bedtime, tab may be crushed or swallowed whole; give with food to prevent GI upset, increase absorption; reduce dosage in renal dysfunction
- Store protected from light, moisture; place in cool environment

### IV route
- Give **IV** undiluted 20 mg/2 min; may increase q10 min 40-80 mg until desired effect
- Give **IV** cont inf by diluting in LR, $D_5W$, $D_5$ in 0.2%, 0.9%, 0.33% NaCl or Ringer's; inf is titrated to patient response; 200 mg of product/160 ml sol (1 mg/ml); 300 mg of product/240 ml sol (1 mg/ml); 200 mg of product/250 ml sol (2 mg/3ml); use infusion pump
- Keep patient recumbent during and for 3 hr after inf, monitor VS q5-15 min

*Y-site compatibilities:* Amikacin, aminophylline, amiodarone, ampicillin, butorphanol, calcium gluconate, cefazolin, ceftazidime, ceftizoxime, chloramphenicol, cimetidine, clindamycin, diltiazem, DOBUTamine, DOPamine, enalaprilat, epINEPHrine, erythromycin, esmolol, famotidine, fentanyl, gentamicin, hydromorphone, lidocaine, lorazepam, magnesium sulfate, meperidine, metronidazole, midazolam, milrinone, morphine, niCARdipine, nitroglycerin, nitroprusside, norepinephrine, oxacillin, penicillin G potassium, piperacillin, potassium chloride, potassium phosphate, propofol, ranitidine, sodium acetate, tobramycin, trimethoprim/sulfamethoxazole, vancomycin, vecuronium

*Y-site incompatibilities:* Cefoperazone, nafcillin

*Solution compatibilities:* $D_5R$, $D_5LR$, $D_{2\frac{1}{2}}$/0.45% NaCl, $D_5$/0.2% NaCl, $D_5$/0.33% NaCl, $D_5$/0.9% NaCl, $D_5W$, Ringer's, LR

*Solution incompatibilities:* Sodium bicarbonate 5%

## Patient/family education
- Teach patient not to discontinue product abruptly, or precipitate angina might occur; taper over 2 wk
- Teach patient not to use OTC products containing α-adrenergic stimulants (such as nasal decongestants, cold preparations); to avoid alcohol, smoking and to limit sodium intake as prescribed
- Teach patient how to take pulse and B/P at home; advise when to notify prescriber
- Instruct patient to comply with weight control, dietary adjustments, modified exercise program
- Advise patient to carry/wear emergency ID to identify products being taken, allergies; that product controls symptoms but does not cure the condition
- Caution patient to avoid hazardous activities if dizziness, drowsiness are present
- Teach patient to report symptoms of CHF: difficulty breathing, especially on exertion or when lying down, night cough, swelling of extremities, bradycardia, dizziness, confusion, depression, fever
- Teach patient to take product as prescribed, not to double or skip doses; take any missed doses as soon as remembered if at least 4 hr until next dose

## Evaluation
### Positive therapeutic outcome
- Decreased B/P in hypertension (after 1-2 wk)
- Absence of dysrhythmias

**Treatment of overdose:** Lavage, **IV** atropine for bradycardia, **IV** theophylline for bronchospasm, digoxin, $O_2$, diuretic for cardiac failure, hemodialysis, **IV** glucose for hyperglycemia, **IV** diazepam (or phenytoin) for seizures

---

## lactulose (Rx)
(lak'tyoo-lose)
Cephulac, Cholac, Chronulac, Constilac, Constulose, Duphalac, Enulose, Evalose, Heptalac, Kristalose, Lactulax ♣, Lactulose PSE, Portalac
*Func. class.:* Laxative (hyperosmotic/ammonia detoxicant)
*Chem. class.:* Lactose synthetic derivative

**Pregnancy category B**

**Action:** Increases osmotic pressure; draws fluid into colon; prevents absorption of ammonia in colon; increases water in stool

**Therapeutic outcome:** Decreased constipation, decreased blood ammonia level

**Uses:** Chronic constipation, portal-systemic encephalopathy in patients with hepatic disease

## Dosage and routes
### Constipation
*Adult:* PO 15-30 ml/day (10-20 g), may increase to 60 ml/day prn
*Child (unlabeled):* PO 7.5 ml/day

---

 Alert     Canada Only    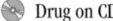 Drug on CD    * "Tall Man" lettering (See Preface)

### Encephalopathy
**Adult:** PO 30-45 ml tid or qid until stools are soft; retention enema 300 ml diluted
**Infant (unlabeled):** PO 2.5-10 ml/day in divided doses
**Child (unlabeled):** PO 40-90 ml/day in divided doses given 2-4 ×/day

**Available forms:** Syr 10 g/15 ml, single-use packets (Kristalose) 10, 20 g

### Adverse effects
*GI: Nausea, vomiting, anorexia, abdominal cramps, diarrhea,* flatulence, *distention, belching*

**Contraindications:** Hypersensitivity, low-galactose diet

**Precautions:** Pregnancy **B**, breastfeeding, geriatric and debilitated patient, diabetes mellitus

#### Pharmacokinetics

| | |
|---|---|
| Absorption | Poorly absorbed |
| Distribution | Not known |
| Metabolism | Colonic bacteria to acids |
| Excretion | Kidneys, unchanged |
| Half-life | Unknown |

#### Pharmacodynamics
Unknown

### Interactions
*Individual drugs*
Neomycin: decreased lactulose effect
*Drug classifications*
Antiinfectives (oral): decreased lactulose effect
Laxatives: do not use together
*Drug/herb*
Flax, senna: increased laxative effect

### NURSING CONSIDERATIONS
#### Assessment
• Monitor glucose levels in diabetic patients (increases)
• Monitor blood, urine, electrolytes if used often by patient; may cause diarrhea, hypokalemia, hypernatremia; check I&O ratio to identify fluid loss
• Assess cramping, rectal bleeding, nausea, vomiting; if these symptoms occur, product should be discontinued; identify cause of constipation; identify whether fluids, bulk, or exercise is missing from lifestyle
• Monitor blood ammonia level (30-70 mg/100 ml); monitor for clearing of confusion, lethargy, restlessness, irritability (hepatic encephalopathy); may decrease ammonia level by 50%

### Nursing diagnoses
• Constipation (uses)
• Diarrhea (adverse reactions)
• Knowledge, deficient (teaching)
• Noncompliance (teaching)

### Implementation
**PO route**
• Give with full glass of fruit juice, water, milk to increase palatability of oral form; increase fluids by 2 L/day; do not give with other laxatives; if diarrhea occurs, reduce dosage
**Rectal route**
• Administer retention enema by diluting 300 ml of lactulose/700 ml of water or of 0.9% NaCl; administer by rec balloon catheter; retain for 30-60 min; repeat if evacuated too quickly

### Patient/family education
• Discuss with patient that adequate fluid consumption is necessary
• Teach patient that normal bowel movements do not always occur daily
• Teach patient not to use in presence of abdominal pain, nausea, vomiting; tell patient to notify prescriber if constipation unrelieved or if symptoms of electrolyte imbalance occur: muscle cramps, pain, weakness, dizziness, excessive thirst
• Teach patient not to use laxatives for long-term therapy; bowel tone will be lost
• Do not give at bedtime as a laxative; may interfere with sleep
• Notify prescriber if diarrhea occurs; may indicate overdosage

### Evaluation
**Positive therapeutic outcome**
• Decreased constipation
• Decreased blood ammonia level
• Clearing of mental state

### lamivudine (Rx)
(lam-i'vue-dine)
Epivir, Epivir-HBV, 3TC
*Func. class.:* Antiretroviral
*Chem. class.:* Nucleoside reverse transcriptase inhibitor
#### Pregnancy category C

**Do not confuse:**
lamivudine/Lamotrigine

**Action:** Inhibits replication of HIV virus by incorporating into cellular DNA by viral reverse transcriptase, thereby terminating the cellular DNA chain

**Therapeutic outcome:** Improved symptoms of HIV infection

**Uses:** HIV infection in combination with other antiretrovirals; chronic hepatitis B (Epivir-HBV)

**Unlabeled uses:** Prophylaxis of HIV postexposure with indinavir and zidovudine

### Dosage and routes
#### HIV infection
**Adult and child >12 yr:** PO 150 mg bid or 300 mg/day

**Child 3 mo-12 yr:** PO 4 mg/kg bid; max 150 mg bid

#### Renal dose
**Adult:** PO CCr 30-49 ml/min 150 mg/day; CCr 15-29 ml/min 150 mg (1st dose), then 100 mg/day; CCr 5-14 ml/min 150 mg/day (1st dose), then 50 mg/day; CCr <5 ml/min 50 mg (1st dose), then 25 mg/day

#### Chronic hepatitis B
**Adult:** PO 100 mg/day

**Available forms:** Oral sol (Epivir) 10 mg/ml, tabs 150, 300/mg; oral sol (Epivir-HBV) 5 mg/ml, tabs 100 mg

### Adverse effects
**CNS:** Fever, headache, malaise, dizziness, insomnia, depression, fatigue, chills, **seizures**
**EENT:** Taste change, hearing loss, photophobia
**GI:** Nausea, vomiting, diarrhea, anorexia, cramps, dyspepsia, **hepatomegaly with steatosis, pancreatitis**
**HEMA:** Neutropenia, anemia, **thrombocytopenia**
**INTEG:** Rash
**MS:** Myalgia, arthralgia, pain
**RESP:** Cough
**SYST:** Lactic acidosis, anaphylaxis, Stevens-Johnson syndrome

**Contraindications:** Hypersensitivity, lactic acidosis

**Precautions:** Pregnancy **C**, breastfeeding, children, geriatric, granulocyte count <1000/mm$^3$ or Hgb <9.5 g/dl, renal disease, severe hepatic dysfunction, pancreatitis

#### Pharmacokinetics
| | |
|---|---|
| **Absorption** | Rapidly absorbed |
| **Distribution** | Extravascular space |
| **Metabolism** | Protein binding <36% |
| **Excretion** | Unchanged in urine |
| **Half-life** | Terminal half-life 5-7 hr |

#### Pharmacodynamics
Unknown

### Interactions
#### Individual drugs
Trimethoprim/sulfamethoxazole: increased level of lamivudine
Zalcitabine: decreased both products
Zidovudine: increased level
#### Drug/lab test
Increased: ALT, bilirubin
Decreased: Hgb, neutrophil, platelet count

### NURSING CONSIDERATIONS
#### Assessment
- Monitor blood counts q2 wk; watch for neutropenia, thrombocytopenia, Hgb, CD4, viral load, lipase, triglycerides periodically during treatment; if low, therapy may have to be discontinued and restarted after hematologic recovery; blood transfusions may be required
- Monitor liver function tests: AST, ALT, bilirubin; amylase
- Monitor children for pancreatitis: abdominal pain, nausea, vomiting
- Assess for lactic acidosis, severe hepatomegaly with steatosis: obtain baseline liver function tests; if elevated, discontinue treatment; discontinue even if liver function tests are normal and symptoms of lactic acidosis, severe hepatomegaly develop

#### Nursing diagnoses
- Infection, risk for (uses)
- Injury, risk for (adverse reactions)
- Knowledge, deficient (teaching)

#### Implementation
- Administer PO daily, bid without regard to meals
- Give with other antiretrovirals only
- Store in cool environment; protect from light

#### Patient/family education
- Teach patient that GI complaints and insomnia resolve after 3-4 wk of treatment
- Tell patient that product is not a cure for AIDS but will control symptoms
- Teach patient to notify prescriber of sore throat, swollen lymph nodes, malaise, fever; other infections may occur
- Teach patient that virus is still infective, may pass AIDS virus to others
- Encourage patient to continue follow-up visits since serious toxicity may occur; blood counts must be done q2 wk

- Teach patient that product must be taken as prescribed, even if feeling better
- Tell patient that other products may be necessary to prevent other infections
- Teach patient that product may cause fainting or dizziness

### Evaluation
**Positive therapeutic outcome**
- Absence of infection, symptoms of HIV infection

## lamotrigine (Rx)
(lam-o-trye′geen)
Lamictal, Lamictal Chewable Dispersible
*Func. class.:* Anticonvulsant—miscellaneous
*Chem. class.:* Phenyltriazine
**Pregnancy category** C

**Do not confuse:**
lamotrigine/lamivudine, Lamictal/Lamisil/Lomotil

**Action:** Unknown; may inhibit voltage-sensitive sodium channels

**Therapeutic outcome:** Decrease in intensity and amount of seizures

**Uses:** Adjunct in the treatment of partial, tonic-clonic seizures, children with Lennox-Gastaut syndrome, bipolar disorder

**Unlabeled uses:** Absence seizures

### Dosage and routes
*Seizures: monotherapy*
**Adult:** PO 50 mg/day for wk 1 and 2, then increase to 100 mg divided bid for wk 3 and 4; maintenance 300-500 mg/day
**Child:** PO 2 mg/kg/day in 2 divided doses × 2 wk, then 10 mg/kg/day, max 15 mg/kg/day or 400 mg/day

*Seizures: multiple therapy with valproate*
**Adult:** PO 25 mg every other day, then 25 mg/day wk 3-4, increase by 25-50 mg q1-2 wk; maintenance 100-400 mg/day
**Child:** PO 0.1-0.2 mg/kg/day initially, then increase q2 wk as needed to 2 mg/kg/day or 150 mg/day

*Hepatic dose*
**Adult (Child-Pugh grade B):** PO reduce by 25%
**Adult (Child-Pugh grade C):** PO reduce by 50%

*Bipolar disorder*
**Adult:** PO wk 1-2 25 mg/day; wk 3-4 50 mg/day; wk 5 100 mg/day; wk 6-7 200 mg/day;

for patients taking valproic acid: wk 1-2 25 mg every other day; wk 3-4 25 mg/day; wk 5 50 mg/day; wk 6 100 mg/day; wk 7 100 mg/day

**Available forms:** Tabs 25, 100, 150, 200 mg; chew tabs 2, 5, 25 mg

### Adverse effects
***CNS:*** Fever, insomnia, tremor, depression, anxiety, *dizziness,* ataxia, *headache*
***EENT:*** Nystagmus, *diplopia, blurred vision*
***GI:*** *Nausea, vomiting, anorexia,* abdominal pain, **hepatotoxicity**
***GU:*** *Dysmenorrhea*
***HEMA:*** Anemia, **DIC, leukopenia, thrombocytopenia**
***INTEG:*** **Rash (potentially life-threatening),** alopecia, photosensitivity
***SYST:*** **Stevens-Johnson syndrome, angioedema**

**Contraindications:** Hypersensitivity

**Precautions:** Pregnancy C, breastfeeding, children <16 yr, geriatric, renal/hepatic/cardiac disease, severe depression, suicidal, blood dyscrasias

| Pharmacokinetics | |
|---|---|
| **Absorption** | Well absorbed, rapid |
| **Distribution** | Protein binding 55% |
| **Metabolism** | Glucuronic acid |
| **Excretion** | Crosses placenta, excreted in breastmilk |
| **Half-life** | Varies, depending on dose |

| Pharmacodynamics | |
|---|---|
| **Onset** | Unknown |
| **Peak** | 1.4-2.3 hr |
| **Duration** | Unknown |

### Interactions
*Individual drugs*
Acetaminophen, carbamazepine, oxcarbazepine, phenobarbital, phenytoin, primidone: decreased lamotrigine serum concentration
Valproic acid: decreased metabolic clearance of lamotrigine
*Drug classifications*
CYP3A4 inhibitors: decreased metabolic clearance of lamotrigine
Contraceptives (oral), estrogens, succinimides, rifamycins: decreased lamotrigine serum concentration
*Drug/herb*
Ginkgo: increased anticonvulsant effect
Ginseng, santonica: decreased anticonvulsant effect

Adverse effects: *italic* = common, **bold** = life-threatening

## NURSING CONSIDERATIONS
### Assessment
🔶 Assess for rash (Stevens-Johnson syndrome or toxic epidermal necrolysis) in pediatric patients, product should be discontinued at first sign of rash
• Assess for seizure activity: duration, type, intensity, halo before seizure
• Assess for hypersensitive reactions

### Nursing diagnoses
• Injury, risk for (uses)
• Knowledge, deficient (teaching)

### Implementation
• Give in divided doses with or after meals to decrease adverse effects
• May be given with food or fluids
• Dispersible tabs should be swallowed whole, chewed, dispersed in water or diluted fruit juice; if chewed, a small amount of water should be taken

### Patient/family education
• Caution patient not to discontinue product abruptly; seizures may occur
• Caution patient to avoid hazardous activities until stabilized on product
• Advise patient to notify prescriber of skin rash or increased seizure activity
• Instruct patient to report to prescriber if pregnancy is suspected or planned
• Teach patient to use sunscreen and protective clothing, photosensitivity occurs
• Advise patient to carry/wear emergency ID stating product use

### Evaluation
**Positive therapeutic outcome**
• Decrease in severity of seizures

---

## lanreotide
Somatuline Depot
*See Appendix A, Selected New Drugs*

---

## lansoprazole (Rx)
(lan-soe'prah-zole)
Prevacid, Prevacid IV, Prevacid SoluTab
*Func. class.:* Anti-ulcer–proton pump inhibitor
*Chem. class.:* Benzimidazole

**Pregnancy category B**

### Do not confuse:
Prevacid/Pravachol/Prinivil

**Action:** Suppresses gastric secretion by inhibiting hydrogen/potassium ATPase enzyme system in gastric parietal cell; characterized as gastric acid pump inhibitor since it blocks final step of acid production

**Therapeutic outcome:** Reduction in gastric pain, swelling, fullness

**Uses:** Gastroesophageal reflux disease (GERD), severe erosive esophagitis, poorly responsive systemic GERD, pathologic hypersecretory conditions (Zollinger-Ellison syndrome, systemic mastocytosis, multiple endocrine adenomas); possibly effective for treatment of duodenal, gastric ulcers, maintenance of healed duodenal ulcers

### Dosage and routes
#### NG tube
*Adult:* Use intact granules mixed in 40 ml of apple juice injected through NG tube, then flush with apple juice

#### Duodenal ulcer
*Adult:* PO 15 mg/day before meals for 4 wk, then 15 mg/day to maintain healing of ulcers; ulcers associated with *Helicobacter:* 30 mg lansoprazole, 500 mg clarithromycin, 1 g amoxicillin bid × 14 days or 30 mg lansoprazole, 1 g amoxicillin tid × 14 days

#### Erosive esophagitis
*Adult:* **IV** 30 mg over 30 min or for up to 7 days; switch to PO as soon as patient can tolerate, for 6-8 wk

#### Pathologic hypersecretory conditions
*Adult:* PO 60 mg/day, may give up to 90 mg bid, administer doses of >120 mg/day in divided doses

#### GERD/esophagitis
*Child 1-11 yr (>30 kg):* PO 30 mg/day ≤12 wk
*Child 1-11 yr (≤30 kg):* 15 mg/day ≤12 wk

**Available forms:** Del rel caps 15, 30 mg; granules for oral susp 15, 30 mg/packet; orally disintegrating tabs 15, 30 mg; lyophilized powder for IV inj 30 mg/vial

### Adverse effects
*CNS:* Headache, dizziness, confusion, agitation, amnesia, depression
*CV:* Chest pain, angina, tachycardia, bradycardia, palpitations, **CVA**, hypo/hypertension, **MI**, **shock**, vasodilation
*EENT:* Tinnitus, taste perversion, deafness, eye pain, otitis media
*GI:* Diarrhea, abdominal pain, vomiting, nausea, constipation, flatulence, acid regurgitation, anorexia, irritable colon, microscopic colitis

---

*GU:* Hematuria, glycosuria, impotence, kidney calculus, breast enlargement
*HEMA:* **Hemolysis,** anemia
*INTEG:* Rash, urticaria, pruritus, alopecia
*META:* Weight gain/loss, gout
*RESP:* Upper respiratory infections, cough, epistaxis, asthma, bronchitis, dyspnea

**Contraindications:** Hypersensitivity

**Precautions:** Pregnancy **B,** breastfeeding, children

### Pharmacokinetics

| | |
|---|---|
| **Absorption** | Rapid after granules leave stomach |
| **Distribution** | Protein binding 97% |
| **Metabolism** | Liver extensively |
| **Excretion** | Urine, feces; clearance decreased in geriatric, renal/hepatic disease |
| **Half-life** | Plasma 1.5 hr |

### Pharmacodynamics

Unknown

### Interactions
*Individual products*

Calcium carbonate, indinavir, iron, itraconazole, ketoconazole: decreased absorption of each specific product

Sucralfate: delayed absorption of lansoprazole

### NURSING CONSIDERATIONS
**Assessment**

• Assess GI system; bowel sounds q8hr, abdomen for pain, swelling, anorexia
• Monitor liver enzymes (AST, ALT, alkaline phosphatase) during treatment

**Nursing diagnoses**

• Knowledge, deficient (teaching)
• Pain, chronic (uses)

**Implementation**

• Swallow del rel cap whole; do not break, crush, chew, or open
• Administer before eating

**Patient/family education**

• Instruct patient to report severe diarrhea; product may have to be discontinued
• Inform diabetic patient that hypoglycemia may occur
• Encourage patient to avoid hazardous activities; dizziness may occur
• Tell patient to avoid alcohol, salicylates, ibuprofen; may cause GI irritation

**Evaluation**
**Positive therapeutic outcome**

• Absence of gastric pain, swelling, fullness

---

## lapatinib (Rx)
(la-pa′tin-ib)
Tykerb
*Func. class.:* Antineoplastic—miscellaneous
*Chem. class.:* Biologic response modifier, signal transduction inhibitor (STIs)

**Pregnancy category  D**

**Action:** Reverses tyrosine kinase of both the epidermal growth factor receptor (ERbB1) and human epidermal receptor type 2 (HER2) (ERbB2)

**Therapeutic outcome:** Decrease in breast cancer progression

**Uses:** Advanced, metastatic breast cancer patients with tumor that overexpresses HER2 protein and who has received previous chemotherapy

### Dosage and routes
*Adult:* PO 1250 mg (5 tabs)/day 1 hr before or after food on days 1-21 plus capecitabine 2000 mg/m$^2$/day in 2 divided doses on days 1-14 in a repeating 21-day cycle; continue until therapeutic response or toxicity occurs

*Hepatic dose*
*Adult (Child-Pugh C):* PO 750 mg/day

**Available forms:** Tabs 250 mg

**Adverse effects**
*CNS:* Fatigue, insomnia
*CV:* **Heart failure,** palpitations, **QT prolongation**
*GI:* Anorexia, diarrhea, dyspepsia, mouth ulcerations, nausea, vomiting, xerosis
*HEMA:* **Anemia, neutropenia, thrombocytopenia**
*INTEG:* Rash
*NEURO:* Palmar-plantar erythrodysesthesia
*RESP:* Dyspnea

**Contraindications:** Pregnancy **D,** hypersensitivity, breastfeeding, torsade de pointes

**Precautions:** Geriatric, hepatic/cardiac disease, bradycardia, hypertension, hypokalemia, hypomagnesemia, QT prolongation

### Pharmacokinetics

| | |
|---|---|
| **Absorption** | Incomplete |
| **Distribution** | Steady state 6-7 days |
| **Metabolism** | Liver, extensively, by P450 enzymes CYP3A4, CYP3A5; >99% protein bound |
| **Excretion** | Unknown |
| **Half-life** | Elimination 24 hr; increased in hepatic disease |

L

---

## Pharmacodynamics

| | |
|---|---|
| **Onset** | Unknown |
| **Peak** | 4 hr |
| **Duration** | Unknown |

## Interactions
### Individual drugs
Arsenic trioxide, bepridil, chlorpromazine, chloroquine, grepafloxacin, halofantrine, haloperidol, levomethadyl, mesoridazine, pentamine, probucol, sparfloxacin, thioridazine: increased QT prolongation
### Drug classifications
CYP3A4 inhibitors (amiodarone, amprenavir, aprepitant, atazanavir, chloramphenicol, clarithromycin, conivaptan, dalfopristin, danazol, darunavir, delavirdine, diltiazem, efavirenz, erythromycin, estradiol, fluconazole, fluvoxamine, imatinib, indinavir, isoniazid, itraconazole, ketoconazole, miconazole, mifepristone, nefazodone, nelfinavir, propoxyphene, quinupristin, ritonavir, RU-486, saquinavir, telithromycin, troleandomycin, verapamil, voriconazole, zafirlukast): increased effect of lapatinib; avoid concurrent use
CYP3A4 inhibitors (amiodarone, clarithromycin, erythromycin, telithromycin, troleandomycin), class IA, III antidysrhythmics: increased QT prolongation
CYP3A4 substrates (methadone, pimozide, quetiapine, quinidine, risperidone, terfenadine, ziprasidone): increased effect of these products, QT prolongation

## NURSING CONSIDERATIONS
### Assessment
• Assess cardiac status: EEG for QT prolongation, ejection fraction; chest pain, palpitations, dyspnea
• Assess hepatic status: liver function tests; jaundice of sclera, skin; dose should be reduced in hepatic disease
• Assess for skin toxicities NCI CTC grade 2 or greater; discontinue use in those with decreased left ventricular ejection fraction (LVEF) or for a LVEF that drops below the institution's lower limit of normal; the product may be restarted after 2 wk if the LVEF recovers to normal at 1000 mg/day; restart at 1250 mg/day when toxicity improves to grade 1 or better

### Nursing diagnoses
• Injury, risk for (uses, adverse reactions)
• Knowledge, deficient (teaching)

### Implementation
• Give once a day, with water, on an empty stomach, 1 hr before or after food
• Do not use with grapefruit products
• Store at room temperature, away from heat

### Patient/family education
• Instruct patient to take with a full glass of water, once a day, 1 hr before or after food; do not take with food or grapefruit products
• Advise patient to take as directed only; if a dose is missed, take as soon as remembered; if it is close to the next dose, take only that dose; do not double
• Teach patient to report to prescriber: chest pain, difficulty breathing, fever, chills, sore throat, bleeding, bruising, yellow skin or eyes, severe fatigue, dizziness, palpitations
• Advise patient of other side effects that may occur, but do not need to be reported: nausea, diarrhea, heartburn, mouth sores, rash, numbness/pain in hands/feet
• Advise patient to use adequate contraception, as the fetus could be damaged from this product

### Evaluation
**Positive therapeutic outcome**
• Decrease in breast cancer progression

## latanoprost ophthalmic
See Appendix D

## leflunomide (Rx)
(leh-floo'noh-mide)
Arava
*Func. class.:* Antirheumatic (DMARDs)
*Chem. class.:* Immune modulator, pyrimidine synthesis inhibitor
### Pregnancy category X

**Action:** Inhibits an enzyme involved in pyrimidine synthesis and has antiproliferative, antiinflammatory effect

**Therapeutic outcome:** Decreased pain, joint swelling, increased mobility

**Uses:** Rheumatoid arthritis, to reduce disease process as well as symptoms

**Unlabeled uses:** Juvenile rheumatoid arthritis

**Dosage and routes**
*Adult:* **PO** Loading dose 100 mg/day × 3 days, maintenance 20 mg/day; may be decreased to 10 mg/day if not well tolerated

*Juvenile rheumatoid arthritis
(unlabeled)*
*Adolescent and child >40 kg:* PO
20 mg
*Adolescent and child 20-40 kg:* PO
15 mg
*Adolescent and child 10-19.9 kg:*
PO 10 mg

**Available forms:** Tabs 10, 20, 100 mg
**Adverse effects**
*CNS:* Dizziness, insomnia, depression, paresthesia, anxiety, migraine, neuralgia, headache
*CV:* Palpitations, hypertension, chest pain, angina pectoris, peripheral edema
*EENT:* Pharyngitis, oral candidiasis, stomatitis, dry mouth, blurred vision
*GI: Nausea, anorexia, vomiting, constipation, flatulence, diarrhea, increased liver function tests,* **hepatotoxicity**
*HEMA:* Anemia, ecchymosis, hyperlipidemia
*INTEG:* Rash, pruritus, alopecia, acne, hematoma, herpes infections
*RESP:* Pharyngitis, rhinitis, bronchitis, cough, respiratory infection, pneumonia, sinusitis

**Contraindications:** Pregnancy **X**, breastfeeding, hypersensitivity, jaundice, lactase deficiency, hepatic disease

**Precautions:** Children, renal disorders, vaccinations, infection, alcoholism, immunosuppression

### Pharmacokinetics

| | |
|---|---|
| **Absorption** | Unknown |
| **Distribution** | Unknown |
| **Metabolism** | Liver |
| **Excretion** | Kidneys |
| **Half-life** | Unknown |

### Pharmacodynamics
Unknown

### Interactions
*Individual drugs*
Activated charcoal, cholestyramine: decreased effect of leflunomide
Methotrexate: increased leflunomide side effects
Rifampin: increased rifampin levels
*Drug classifications*
Live virus vaccines: decreased antibody reaction
NSAIDs: increased NSAID effect
Hepatotoxic agents: increased side effects of leflunomide

### NURSING CONSIDERATIONS
**Assessment**
• Monitor liver function tests: if ALT elevations are >2 times baseline, reduce dose to 10 mg/day
• Assess arthritic symptoms: ROM, mobility, swelling of joints, baseline and during treatment

**Nursing diagnoses**
• Knowledge, deficient (teaching)
• Mobility, impaired physical (uses)
• Pain, chronic (uses)

**Implementation**
• Give with full glass of water to enhance absorption
• Give PO with food, milk, or antacids for GI upset
• To eliminate product give cholestyramine 8 g tid × 11 days, check levels

**Patient/family education**
• Teach patient that product must be continued for prescribed time to be effective
• Instruct patient to take with food, milk, or antacids to avoid GI upset
• Advise patient to use caution when driving; drowsiness, dizziness may occur
• Advise patient to take with a full glass of water to enhance absorption
• Advise patient to avoid pregnancy while taking this product
• Inform patient that hair may be lost, review alternatives
• Advise patient to avoid live virus vaccinations during treatment

**Evaluation**
**Positive therapeutic outcome**
• Increased joint mobility without pain
• Decreased joint swelling

### lenalidomide (Rx)
(len-a-lid'o-mide)
Revlimid
*Func. class.:* Antianemic, biologic response modifier, hormone
*Chem. class.:* Thalidomide derivative
**Pregnancy category X**

**Action:** Decreases secretion of inflammatory cytokines and increases secretion of antiinflammatory cytokines, also COX-2 inhibition

**Therapeutic outcome:** Increase in reticulocyte count

**Uses:** Transfusion-dependent anemia due to low or intermediate-1–risk myelodysplastic

Adverse effects: *italic* = common, **bold** = life-threatening

syndrome (MDS); multiple myeloma in combination with dexamethasone

## Dosage and routes
### Transfusion-dependent anemia
*Adult:* PO 10 mg/day

### Multiple myeloma
*Adult:* PO 25 mg/day on days 1-21, with dexamethasone 40 mg/day on days 1-4, 9-12, 17-20 of each 28-day cycle for first 4 therapy cycles; starting with cycle 5, leave lenalidomide the same, give dexamethasone 40 mg/day on days 1-4 of a 28-day cycle

### Treatment of patients with transfusion-dependent anemia due to low- or intermediate-1–risk MDS associated with a deletion 5q cytogenetic abnormality with or without additional cytogenetic abnormalities
*Adult:* PO 10 mg/day; continue/adjust based on clinical toxicity/lab findings

### Treatment of multiple myeloma in combination with dexamethasone in patients who have failed to respond to at least one prior therapy
*Adult:* PO 25 mg/day on days 1-21 along with dexamethasone 40 mg/day PO on days 1-4, 9-12, 17-20 of each 28-day cycle for the first 4 therapy cycles; starting with cycle 5, the lenalidomide dose stays the same, but only give dexamethasone 40 mg/day PO on days 1-4 q28 days; continue/adjust dosing based on clinical and laboratory findings

### Dosage adjustments of lenalidomide for hematologic toxicities associated with MDS
**Thrombocytopenia or neutropenia that develops within 4 wk of starting at 10 mg/day PO:** Reduce dose from 10 mg/day PO to 5 mg/day PO; withhold lenalidomide if platelet count <50,000/mm³ from a baseline of at least 100,000/mm³, if platelet count falls to 50% of the baseline value, if the baseline is <100,000/mm³, if absolute neutrophil count (ANC) <750/mm³ from a baseline of at least 1000/mm³, or if <500/mm³ from a baseline of <1000/mm³; the new dose of 5 mg/day PO may begin once the platelet count is at least 50,000/mm³ (30,000/mm³ if the baseline <60,000/mm³), and the ANC returns to at least 1000/mm³ or 500/mm³ for patients with a baseline <1000/mm³

**Thrombocytopenia or neutropenia that develops after 4 wk of starting at 10 mg/day PO:** Reduce dose from 10 mg/day PO to 5 mg/day PO; withhold lenalidomide if platelet count <30,000/mm³, if platelet count <50,000/mm³ and a platelet transfusion, if neutrophils <500/mm³ for at least 7 days, or if <500/mm³ and a temp of at least 38.5° C are present; the new dose of 5 mg/day PO may begin once the platelet count is at least 30,000/mm³ without hemostatic failure, and the ANC is at least 500/mm³

**Thrombocytopenia or neutropenia that develops while taking 5 mg/day PO:** Reduce dose from 5 mg/day PO to 5 mg PO every other day; withhold lenalidomide if platelet count <30,000/mm³, platelet count <50,000/mm³ and a platelet transfusion, neutrophils <500/mm³ for at least 7 days, or if <500/mm³ and a temp of at least 38.5° C are present; the new dose of 5 mg PO every other day may begin once the platelet count is at least 30,000/mm³ without hemostatic failure, and the ANC is at least 500/mm³

### Dosage adjustments of lenalidomide for toxicities associated with multiple myeloma
**Thrombocytopenia:** Reduce dose from 25 mg/day PO to 15 mg/day PO; withhold lenalidomide if platelet count <30,000/mm³; check CBC qwk; the new dose of 15 mg/day PO may begin once the platelet count is at least 30,000/mm³; withhold lenalidomide each time the platelet count is <30,000/mm³; a new dose of 5 mg less than the previous dose should be started once the platelet count is at least 30,000/mm³; do not dose below 5 mg/day PO

**Neutropenia without other toxicity:** Hold dose; withhold lenalidomide and add G-CSF if neutrophils <1000/mm³; check CBC weekly; resume lenalidomide at 25 mg/day PO once neutrophils are at least 1000/mm³, and neutropenia is the only toxicity

**Neutropenia with other toxicity:** Reduce dose from 25 mg/day PO to 15 mg/day PO; withhold lenalidomide and add G-CSF if neutrophils <1000/mm³; check CBC qwk; resume lenalidomide at 15 mg/day PO once neutrophils are at least 1000/mm³; withhold lenalidomide and add G-CSF each time the neutrophils are <1000/mm³; if other toxicity is present, a new dose of 5 mg less than the previous dose should be started once the neutrophils are at least 1000/mm³; do not dose below 5 mg/day PO

*Other grade 3 or 4 toxicity judged to be related to lenalidomide:*
Reduce dose from 25 mg/day PO to 15 mg/day PO; withhold lenalidomide and resume lenalidomide at 15 mg/day PO once the toxicity has resolved to grade 2 or less; withhold lenalidomide each time a grade 3 or 4 toxicity occurs; a new dose of 5 mg less than the previous dose should be started once the toxicity has resolved to grade 2 or less; do not dose below 5 mg/day PO

**Available forms:** Caps 5, 10, 15, 25 mg

**Adverse effects**
*CV:* Chest pain, hypotension, palpitations
*GI:* Abdominal pain, anorexia, constipation, diarrhea, nausea/vomiting, dysgeusia, xerosis
*HEMA:* Anemia, leukopenia, pancytopenia, thrombocytopenia
*META:* Hypokalemia, hypomagnesium
*MS:* Arthralgia, back pain, myalgia
*NEURO:* Depression, dizziness, fatigue, fever, headache, sweating, peripheral enuropathy
*RESP:* Cough, dyspnea, **pulmonary embolism**, epistaxis, rhinitis

**Contraindications:** Pregnancy **X**, breastfeeding, hypersensitivity

**Precautions:** Accidental exposure, bone marrow suppression, children, dental disease, uterine bleeding, geriatric, neutropenia/thrombocytopenia, females, fungal/viral infections

| Pharmacokinetics | |
|---|---|
| **Absorption** | Rapid |
| **Distribution** | Unknown |
| **Metabolism** | Unknown |
| **Excretion** | Unknown |
| **Half-life** | Elimination 3 hr |

| Pharmacodynamics |
|---|
| Unknown |

**Interactions**
*Drug classifications*
Anticoagulants, NSAIDs, platelet inhibitors, salicylates, thrombolytics: increased bleeding risk
Toxoids, vaccines: decreased immune response

**NURSING CONSIDERATIONS**
**Assessment**
• Monitor blood tests: HCT, Hgb, electrolytes
• Monitor B/P for hypotension
• Assess blood dyscrasias

• Assess for hypersensitivity reactions: skin rashes, urticaria (rare)

**Nursing diagnoses**
• Activity intolerance (uses)
• Knowledge, deficient (teaching)

**Implementation**
• Give PO, with dexamethasone for multiple myeloma

**Patient/family education**
• Advise patient to avoid driving or hazardous activity during beginning of treatment

**Evaluation**
**Positive therapeutic outcome**
• Increase in reticulocyte count

---

**⚠ HIGH ALERT**

**lepirudin** 🚫 (Rx)
(lep-ih-roo'din)
Refludan
*Func. class.:* Anticoagulant
*Chem. class.:* Thrombin inhibitor, hirudin

**Pregnancy category B**

**Action:** Direct inhibitor of thrombin that is highly specific

**Therapeutic outcome:** Absence of thrombocytopenia, stroke, MI, or other thromboembolic conditions

**Uses:** Heparin-induced thrombocytopenia (HIT) and other thromboembolic conditions

**Unlabeled uses:** Adjunct therapy in unstable angina, acute MI without ST elevation, prevention of DVT, PCI

**Dosage and routes**
*Heparin-induced thrombocytopenia (not receiving thrombolytic therapy concurrently)*
*Adult:* **IV** 0.4 mg/kg (≤110 kg) over 15-20 sec; then 0.15 mg/kg (≤110 kg/hr) as a CONT INF for 2-10 days or longer

*Concomitant use with thrombolytic therapy*
*Adult:* **IV** BOL 0.2 mg/kg initially
*Adult:* CONT **IV** INF 0.1 mg/kg/hr

*Renal dose*
*Adult:* **IV** BOL 0.2 mg/kg over 15-20 sec; CCr 45-60 ml/min 0.075 mg/kg/hr; CCr 30-44 ml/min 0.045 mg/kg/hr; CCr 15-29 ml/min 0.0225 mg/kg/hr

**Available forms:** Powder for inj 50 mg

L

### Adverse effects
*CNS:* *Fever*, **intracranial bleeding**
*CV:* **Heart failure, pericardial effusion, ventricular fibrillation**
*GI:* GI bleeding, abnormal liver function tests
*GU:* **Hematuria,** abnormal kidney function, vaginal bleeding
*HEMA:* **Hemorrhage, thrombocytopenia**
*INTEG:* Allergic skin reactions
*RESP:* Pneumonia
*SYST:* **Multiorgan failure, sepsis, anaphylaxis**

**Contraindications:** Hypersensitivity to hirudins

**Precautions:** Pregnancy **B,** breastfeeding, children, women, geriatric, intracranial bleeding, hepatic disease, recent major surgery, hemorrhagic diathesis, bacterial endocarditis, severe uncontrolled hypertension, advanced renal disease, recent active peptic ulcer, recent CVA, stroke, intracerebral surgery

### Pharmacokinetics
| | |
|---|---|
| **Absorption** | Unknown |
| **Distribution** | Unknown |
| **Metabolism** | Possibly by the release of amino acids during catabolism |
| **Excretion** | 50% unchanged in urine |
| **Half-life** | Unknown |

### Pharmacodynamics
Unknown

### Interactions
*Individual drugs*
Aspirin, cefamandole, cefoperazone, cefotetan, clopidogrel, dipyridamole, eptifibatide, plicamycin, ticlopidine, tirofiban, valproic acid: increased bleeding risk
*Drug classifications*
NSAIDs, thrombolytics, warfarin derivatives: increased bleeding risk
*Drug/herb*
Agrimony, alfalfa, angelica, anise, basil, bay, bilberry, black haw, bogbean, bromelain, buchu, chondroitin, cinchona bark, dong quai, fenugreek, feverfew, garlic, ginger, ginkgo, ginseng, horse chestnut, Irish moss, kelp, kelpware, khella, lovage, lungwort, meadowsweet, motherwort, mugwort, nettle, papaya, parsley (large amounts), paud'arco, pineapple, poplar, prickly ash, safflower, saw palmetto, tonka bean, turmeric, wintergreen, yarrow: increased risk of bleeding
Chamomile, coenzyme Q10, flax, glucomannan, goldenseal, guar gum: decreased anticoagulant effect

## NURSING CONSIDERATIONS
### Assessment
• Obtain baseline APTT before treatment; do not start treatment if APTT ratio is ≥2.5, then APTT 4 hr after initiation of treatment and at least daily thereafter; if APTT is above target, stop infusion for 2 hr, then restart at 50%, take APTT in 4 hr; if below target, increase inf rate by 20%, take APTT in 4 hr, do not exceed inf rate of 0.21 mg/kg/hr without checking for coagulation abnormalities
• Monitor APTT, which should be 1.5-2.5 × control
⬥ Assess bleeding gums, petechiae, ecchymosis, black tarry stools, hematuria/epistaxis, B/P, vaginal bleeding, puncture sites; may indicate bleeding and possible hemorrhage
• Assess fever, skin rash, urticaria
• Monitor Hgb, Hct, platelets, serum creatinine, urinalysis, stool guaiac

### Nursing diagnoses
• Injury, risk for (side effects)
• Knowledge, deficient (teaching)
• Tissue perfusion, ineffective (uses)

### Implementation
• Administer after reconstitution and further dilution under sterile conditions; use water for inj or 0.9% NaCl; for further dilution 0.9% NaCl or D₅; for rapid and complete reconstitution, inject 1 ml of diluent into vial and shake gently, use immediately, warm to room temperature before use
• Avoid all IM inj that may cause bleeding
**IV route**
• Administer **IV** bol: use sol with conc of 5 mg/ml, reconstitute 5 mg (1 vial)/1 ml of water for inj or 0.9% NaCl, use body weight for correct weight calculation
• Administer **IV** inf: use sol with a conc of 0.2 or 0.4 mg/ml; reconstitute 100 mg (2 vials) with 1 ml each (2 ml) water for inj or 0.9% NaCl, transfer to infusion bag with either 500 or 250 ml of 0.9% NaCl or D₅W

### Patient/family education
• Teach patient to use soft-bristle toothbrush to avoid bleeding gums, avoid contact sports, use electric razor, avoid IM inj
• Teach patient to report any signs of bleeding: gums, under skin, urine, stools

### Evaluation
**Positive therapeutic outcome**
• Absence of thrombocytopenia without significant bleeding

---

⬥ Alert     ♣ Canada Only     🔵 Drug on CD          * "Tall Man" lettering (See Preface)

## letrozole (Rx)
(let'tro-zohl)
Femara
*Func. class.:* Antineoplastic, nonsteroidal aromatase inhibitor

**Pregnancy category D**

**Action:** Binds to the heme group of aromatase; inhibits conversion of androgens to estrogens to reduce plasma estrogen levels

**Therapeutic outcome:** Decreased spread of malignancy

**Uses:** Early, advanced, or metastatic breast cancer in postmenopausal women

**Dosage and routes**
*Adult:* PO 2.5 mg/day

**Available forms:** Tabs 2.5 mg

**Adverse effects**
*CNS:* Somnolence, dizziness, depression, anxiety, *headache, lethargy*
*CV:* Angina, **MI, CVA, thromboembolic events,** peripheral edema, hypertension
*GI:* Nausea, vomiting, anorexia, constipation, heartburn, diarrhea
*GU:* **Endometrial cancer, vaginal bleeding, endometrial proliferation disorder**
*INTEG:* Rash, pruritus, alopecia, sweating
*MISC:* Hot flashes, night sweats, **second malignancies**
*MS:* Arthralgia, arthritis, bone fracture, myalgia, osteoporosis
*RESP:* Dyspnea, cough

**Contraindications:** Pregnancy **D**, hypersensitivity, premenopausal females

**Precautions:** Hepatic disease, respiratory disease, osteoporosis

### Pharmacokinetics
| | |
|---|---|
| Absorption | Well absorbed |
| Distribution | Widely |
| Metabolism | Liver |
| Excretion | Kidneys |
| Half-life | Terminal 48 hr |

### Pharmacodynamics
| | |
|---|---|
| Onset | Unknown |
| Peak | 2-6 wk |
| Duration | Unknown |

**NURSING CONSIDERATIONS**
**Assessment**
• Monitor temperature q4hr; may indicate beginning of infection

• Monitor liver function tests before, during therapy (bilirubin, AST, ALT, LDH) as needed or monthly

**Nursing diagnoses**
• Body image, disturbed (adverse reactions)
• Infection, risk for (adverse reactions)
• Injury, risk for (adverse reactions)
• Knowledge, deficient (teaching)

**Implementation**
• May administer biphosphates to increase bone density
• Give with food or fluids for GI upset
• Give in equal intervals q6hr

**Patient/family education**
• Advise patient to avoid use of alcohol, which potentiates this product
• Tell patient that product may be taken without regard to meals
• Teach patient to report vaginal bleeding, diarrhea, chest/bone pain
• Advise patient to use adequate contraception in perimenopausal, recently postmenopausal women

**Evaluation**
**Positive therapeutic outcome**
• Prevention of rapid division of malignant cells, postmenopausal cancer, prostate cancer

**Treatment of overdose:** Induce vomiting, provide supportive care

## leucovorin (Rx)
(loo-koe-vor'in)
Citrovorum Factor, Folinic Acid, leucovorin calcium
*Func. class.:* Vitamin/folic acid antagonist antidote
*Chem. class.:* Tetrahydrofolic acid derivative

**Pregnancy category C**

**Do not confuse:**
leucovorin/Leukeran/Leukine

**Action:** Needed for normal growth patterns; prevents toxicity during antineoplastic therapy by protecting normal cells

**Therapeutic outcome:** Reversal of severe toxic effects of folic acid antagonists

**Uses:** Megaloblastic or macrocytic anemia caused by folic acid deficiency, overdose of folic acid antagonist, methotrexate toxicity, toxicity caused by pyrimethamine or trimethoprim, pneumocystosis, toxoplasmosis

## Dosage and routes
### Megaloblastic anemia caused by enzyme deficiency
*Adult and child:* PO/IM/**IV** up to 6 mg/day

### Megaloblastic anemia caused by deficiency of folate
*Adult and child:* IM 1 mg or less/day until adequate response

### Advanced colorectal cancer
*Adult:* **IV** 200 mg/m$^2$, then 5-fluorouracil 370 mg/m$^2$; or leucovorin 20 mg/m$^2$, then 5-fluorouracil 425 mg/m$^2$; give daily × 5 days q4-5 wk

### Methotrexate toxicity—leucovorin rescue
*Adult and child:* PO/IM/**IV** (normal elimination) given 6-36 hr after dose of methotrexate 10 mg/m$^2$ until methotrexate is $<5 \times 10^{-8}$ m, CCr has increased 50% above prior level, or methotrexate level is $5 \times 10^{-8}$ m at 24 hr or at 48 hr level is $>9 \times 10^{-8}$ m; give leucovorin 100 mg/m$^2$ q3hr until level drops to $<10^{-8}$ m

### Pyrimethamine toxicity
*Adult and child:* PO/IM 5-15 mg/day

### Trimethoprim toxicity
*Adult and child:* PO/IM 400 mcg/day

**Available forms:** Tabs 5, 10, 15, 25 mg; inj 3, 5 mg/ml; powder for inj 10 mg/ml

## Adverse effects
***HEMA:*** Thrombocytosis (intraarterial)
***INTEG:*** Rash, pruritus, erythema, urticaria
***RESP:*** Wheezing

**Contraindications:** Hypersensitivity, anemias other than megaloblastic not associated with vit B$_{12}$ deficiency

**Precautions:** Pregnancy **C**

### Pharmacokinetics
| | |
|---|---|
| **Absorption** | Rapidly absorbed (PO); completely absorbed (**IV**) |
| **Distribution** | Widely distributed |
| **Metabolism** | Liver |
| **Excretion** | Kidney |
| **Half-life** | 3½ hr |

### Pharmacodynamics
| | PO/IM/IV |
|---|---|
| **Onset** | Up to 5 min |
| **Peak** | Unknown |
| **Duration** | 4-6 hr |

## Interactions
### Individual drugs
Chloramphenicol: decreased folate levels
Fluorouracil: increased toxicity
Phenobarbital: increased metabolism of phenobarbital
### Drug classifications
Hydantoins: increased metabolism of hydantoins

## NURSING CONSIDERATIONS
### Assessment
• Obtain CCr before leucovorin rescue and daily to detect nephrotoxicity, methotrexate level
• Monitor I&O, urine pH q6hr; maintain at >7 to prevent neurotoxicity; watch for nausea and vomiting; if vomiting occurs IM or **IV** route may be necessary
• Assess products currently taken: alcohol, hydantoins, trimethoprim may cause increased folic acid use by body
• Assess for allergic reactions: rash, dyspnea, wheezing
• Assess neurologic status (rescue), weakness, fatigue
• Monitor calcium levels
• Assess for megaloblastic anemia, plasma lactic acid, reticulocyte count, Hct, Hgb

### Nursing diagnoses
• Injury, risk for (uses)
• Knowledge, deficient (teaching)
• Nutrition: less than body requirements, imbalanced (uses)

### Implementation
• Instruct patient about leucovorin rescue; have patient drink 3 L of fluid each day of rescue
• Do not give concurrently with systemic methotrexate
**PO route**
• Use PO route only if patient is not vomiting
**IM route**
• Treatment of megaloblastic anemia uses IM dosing
• Give within 1 hr of folic acid antagonist, no reconstitution needed
• Give increased fluid intake if used to treat folic acid inhibitor overdose
• Provide protection from light and heat when storing ampules
**IV route**
• Reconstitute 50 mg/5 ml of bacteriostatic water or sterile water for inj (10 mg/ml) or 100 mg/10 ml; use immediately if sterile water for inj is used to reconstitute

- Give by direct **IV** over 160 mg/min or less (16 ml of 10 mg/ml sol/min)
- Give by intermittent inf after diluting in 100-500 ml of 0.9% NaCl, $D_5W$, $D_{10}W$, LR, Ringer's

*Syringe compatibilities:* Bleomycin, cisplatin, cyclophosphamide, DOXOrubicin, fluorouracil, furosemide, heparin, methotrexate, metoclopramide, mitomycin, vinBLAStine, vinCRIStine

*Y-site compatibilities:* Amifostine, aztreonam, bleomycin, cefepime, cisplatin, cladribine, cyclophosphamide, DOXOrubicin, filgrastim, fluconazole, fluorouracil, furosemide, granisetron, heparin, methotrexate, metoclopramide, mitomycin, piperacillin/tazobactam, tacrolimus, teniposide, thiotepa, vinBLAStine, vinCRIStine

*Additive compatibilities:* Cisplatin, cisplatin/floxuridine, floxuridine

### Patient/family education
- Advise patient to take product exactly as prescribed; to notify prescriber of side effects immediately
- Advise patient to report signs of hypersensitivity reaction immediately
- Advise patient with folic acid deficiency to eat folic acid–rich foods: bran, yeast, dried beans, nuts, fruits, fresh green leafy vegetables, asparagus
- Advise patient to avoid breastfeeding

### Evaluation
**Positive therapeutic outcome**
- Increased weight
- Improved orientation, well-being
- Absence of fatigue
- Reversal of toxicity: methotrexate, folic acid antagonist overdose

---

### ! HIGH ALERT

### leuprolide (Rx)
(loo-proe'lide)
Eligard, Leupron Depo PED, Lupron Depot, Lupron, Lupron Depot-4 month, Lupron Depot-4 month Viadur
*Func. class.:* Antineoplastic hormone
*Chem. class.:* Gonadotropin-releasing hormone

**Pregnancy category X**

**Do not confuse:**
Lupron/Lopurin/Nuprin

**Action:** Causes initial increase in circulating levels of LH, FSH; continuous administration results in decreased LH, FSH; in men testosterone is reduced to castration levels; in premenopausal women estrogen is reduced to menopausal levels

**Therapeutic outcome:** Prevention of rapidly growing malignant cells in prostate cancer, decreased pain in endometriosis, resolution of central precocious puberty (CPP)

**Uses:** Metastatic prostate cancer, management of endometriosis (depot), CPP, uterine leiomyomata (fibroids)

### Dosage and routes
*Prostate cancer*
*Adult:* SUBCUT 1 mg/day; IM 7.5 mg/dose qmo; Viadur implant (72 mg) qyr; or IM 22.5 mg q3 mo; or IM 30 mg q4mo

*Endometriosis/fibroids*
*Adult:* IM 3.75 mg qmo for 6 mo, 11.25 mg q3 mo for 6 mo, or IM 30 mg q4 mo

*Central precocious puberty*
*Child:* SUBCUT 50 mcg/kg/day; increase as needed by 10 mcg/kg/day
*Child >37.5 kg:* IM 15 mg q4 wk
*Child 25-37.5 kg:* IM 11.25 mg q4 wk
*Child ≤25 kg:* 7.5 mg q4 wk

**Available forms:** Inj 5 mg/ml; powder for inj, lyophilized 7.5 mg; microspheres for inj, lyophilized 3.75, 7.5, 11.25, 15, 22.5, 30 mg; implant 72 mg; depot 7.5, 22.5, 30, 45 mg; depot 3.75, 11.25 mg; intradermal kit 65 mg

### Adverse effects
*CNS:* Memory impairment, depression
*CV:* **MI, pulmonary emboli, dysrhythmias,** peripheral edema
*GI:* Anorexia, diarrhea, **GI bleeding,** nausea, vomiting
*GU:* Edema, hot flashes, impotence, decreased libido, amenorrhea, vaginal dryness, gynecomastia. profuse vaginal bleeding
*INTEG:* Alopecia
*MS:* Bone pain

**Contraindications:** Pregnancy **X,** breastfeeding, hypersensitivity to GnRH or analogs, thromboembolic disorders, undiagnosed vaginal bleeding, Viadur implant or Eligard should not be used in women or children

**Precautions:** Edema, hepatic disease, CVA, MI, seizures, hypertension, diabetes mellitus

L

## Pharmacokinetics

| | |
|---|---|
| **Absorption** | Rapidly absorbed (SUBCUT); slowly absorbed (IM depot) |
| **Distribution** | Unknown |
| **Metabolism** | Unknown |
| **Excretion** | Unknown |
| **Half-life** | 3-4 hr |

## Pharmacodynamics

Unknown

## Interactions
### Individual drugs
Flutamide, megestrol: increased antineoplastic action

## NURSING CONSIDERATIONS
### Assessment
• Assess for symptoms of endometriosis/fibroids including lower abdominal pain, excessive vaginal bleeding, bloating if product is given for the diagnosis of endometriosis
• If giving this product for CPP, the diagnosis should have been confirmed by development of secondary sex characteristics in children <9 yr; also included to confirm the diagnosis of CPP is estradiol/testosterone, GnRH test, tomography of head, adrenal steroid, chorionic gonadotropin, wrist x-ray, height, weight; patients diagnosed with CPP display the signs of testicular growth, facial, body hair (males), breast development, menses (females)
• Monitor liver function tests before, during therapy (bilirubin, AST, ALT, LDH) as needed or monthly; prostate-specific antigen in prostate cancer
• Monitor PSA in prostate cancer; calcium, testosterone, bone mineral density
• Monitor pituitary gonadotropic and gonadal function during therapy and 4-8 wk after therapy is decreased; check LH, FSH, acid phosphate at beginning of treatment
• Monitor worsening of signs and symptoms (normal during beginning therapy): fatigue, increased pulse, pallor, lethargy, edema in feet, joints, stomach pain, shaking
• Monitor renal status: I&O ratio, check for bladder distention daily during beginning therapy (renal obstruction)

### Nursing diagnoses
• Injury, risk for (adverse reactions)
• Knowledge, deficient (teaching)
• Sexual dysfunction (adverse reactions)

### Implementation
• Use syringe and product packaged together; give deep in large muscle mass; rotate sites
• Use depot only IM; never give SUBCUT

• Unused vials may be stored at room temperature
• Give monthly: reconstitute single-use vial with 1 ml of diluent, if multiple vials are used, withdraw 0.5 ml and inject into each vial (1 ml) withdraw all and inject
• Give 3 month: reconstitute microspheres using 1.5 ml of diluent and inject in vial, shake, withdraw and inject; 12-month: inserted into upper arm at the end of 12 months, implant must be removed

### Patient/family education
• Advise patient to notify prescriber if menstruation continues; menstruation should stop; to use a nonhormonal method of contraception during therapy
• Instruct patient to report any complaints, side effects to nurse or prescriber; hot flashes may occur; record weight, report gain of 2 lb/day
• Teach patient how to prepare, administer; to rotate sites for SUBCUT inj; to keep accurate records of dosing (prostate cancer)
• Instruct patient that tumor flare may occur: increase in size of tumor, increased bone pain; tell patient that bone pain disappears after 1 wk; may take analgesics for pain; premenopausal women must use mechanical birth control; ovulation may be induced
• Advise the patient not to breastfeed while taking this product
• Inform patient that voiding problems may increase in beginning of therapy, but will decrease in several weeks

### Evaluation
#### Positive therapeutic outcome
• Decreased size, spread of malignancy
• Decreased pain in endometriosis, fibroids
• Decreased signs of CPP
• Increased follicle maturation

## levalbuterol (Rx)
(lev-al-bute'er-ole)
Xopenex
*Func. class.:* Bronchodilator
*Chem. class.:* Adrenergic $\beta_2$-agonist
### Pregnancy category C

**Action:** Causes bronchodilatation by action on $\beta_2$ (pulmonary) receptors by increasing levels of cyclic adenosine monophosphate (cAMP), which relaxes smooth muscle; produces bronchodilatation; CNS, cardiac stimulation, increased diuresis, and increased gastric acid secretion; longer acting than isoproterenol

**Therapeutic outcome:** Increased ability to breathe because of bronchodilatation

**Uses:** Treatment or prevention of bronchospasm (reversible obstructive airway disease)

**Dosage and routes**
*Adult and child ≥12 yr:* INH 0.63 mg tid, q6-8hr by nebulization; may increase to 1.25 mg q8hr
*Child 6-11 yr:* INH 0.31 mg tid via nebulization, max 0.63 mg tid

**Available forms:** Sol, inh 0.63, 1.25 mg/3 ml

**Adverse effects**
*CNS: Tremors, anxiety,* insomnia, headache, dizziness, stimulation, *restlessness,* hallucinations, flushing, irritability
*CV:* Palpitations, tachycardia, hypertension, angina, hypotension, dysrhythmias, **QT prolongation**
*EENT:* Dry nose, irritation of nose and throat
*GI:* Heartburn, nausea, vomiting
*INTEG:* Rash
*META:* Hypokalemia, hyperglycemia
*MS:* Muscle cramps
*RESP:* Cough
*SYST:* **Anaphylaxis, angioedema**

**Contraindications:** Hypersensitivity to sympathomimetics, tachydysrhythmias, severe cardiac disease

**Precautions:** Pregnancy **C**, breastfeeding, cardiac disorders, hyperthyroidism, diabetes mellitus, hypertension, prostatic hypertrophy, angle-closure glaucoma, seizures, renal disease, QT prolongation

| Pharmacokinetics | |
| --- | --- |
| **Absorption** | Unknown |
| **Distribution** | Unknown |
| **Metabolism** | Liver extensively, tissues |
| **Excretion** | Unknown, breast milk |
| **Half-life** | Unknown |

| Pharmacodynamics | |
| --- | --- |
| | INH |
| **Onset** | 5-15 min |
| **Peak** | 1-1½ hr |
| **Duration** | 6-8 hr |

**Interactions**
*Drug classifications*
Adrenergics: increased levalbuterol action
Antidepressants (tricyclics): increased levalbuterol action

β-Adrenergic blockers: decreased levalbuterol action
Bronchodilators (aerosol): increased action of bronchodilator
MAOIs: increased levalbuterol action
*Drug/herb*
Cola nut, guarana, tea (black/green), coffee, yerba maté: increased stimulation

**NURSING CONSIDERATIONS**
**Assessment**
• Assess cardiac status: palpitations, increased or decreased B/P, dysrhythmias, QT prolongation
• Assess respiratory function: vital capacity, forced expiratory volume, ABGs, lung sounds, heart rate, rhythm (baseline and during therapy); character of sputum: color, consistency, amount
• Determine that patient has not received theophylline therapy before giving dose, to prevent additive effect; client's ability to self-medicate
• Monitor for evidence of allergic reactions; paradoxic bronchospasm, anaphylaxis, angioedema; withhold dose; notify prescriber

**Nursing diagnoses**
• Airway clearance, ineffective (uses)
• Gas exchange, impaired (uses)
• Knowledge, deficient (teaching)

**Implementation**
• Give by nebulization q6-8hr; wait at least 1 min between inhalation of aerosols
• Use this medication before other medications and allow 5 min between each to prevent overstimulation

**Patient/family education**
• Tell patient not to use OTC medications before consulting prescriber; extra stimulation may occur; instruct patient to use this medication before other medications and allow at least 5 min between each to prevent overstimulation; to limit caffeine products such as chocolate, coffee, tea, and cola or herbs such as cola nut, guarana, yerba maté
◆ Teach patient that if paradoxic bronchospasm occurs to stop product immediately and notify prescriber

**Evaluation**
**Positive therapeutic outcome**
• Absence of dyspnea and wheezing after 1 hr
• Improved airway exchange
• Improved ABGs

**Treatment of overdose:** Administer a β₁-adrenergic blocker

**L**

Adverse effects: *italic* = common, **bold** = life-threatening

## levetiracetam (Rx)
(lev-ee-tye'ra-see-tam)
Keppra
*Func. class.:* Anticonvulsant

**Pregnancy category C**

**Action:** Unknown; may inhibit nerve impulses by limiting influx of sodium ions across cell membrane in motor cortex

**Therapeutic outcome:** Absence of seizures

**Uses:** Adjunctive therapy in partial onset seizures, primary generalized tonic-clonic seizures

**Dosage and routes**
*Adjunctive treatment of partial seizures*
*Adult and adolescent ≥16 yr:* **IV** 500 mg bid, may titrate by 1000 mg/day q2 wk max 3000 mg/day in divided doses

*Myoclonic seizures/tonic-clonic seizures/partial seizures*
*Adult:* PO/**IV** 500 mg bid, may increase by 1000 mg/day q2 wk, max 3000 mg/day

**Available forms:** Tabs 1000 mg; oral sol 100 mg/ml; sol for inj 100 mg/ml

**Adverse effects**
*CNS:* Dizziness, somnolence, asthenia, psychosis, **suicidal ideation**
*HEMA:* Decreased Hct, Hgb, RBC, infection
*MISC:* Abdominal pain, pharyngitis, infection

**Contraindications:** Hypersensitivity

**Precautions:** Pregnancy **C**, breastfeeding, children, geriatric, cardiac/renal disease, psychosis

| Pharmacokinetics | |
|---|---|
| **Absorption** | Rapidly absorbed |
| **Distribution** | Widely distributed, not protein bound |
| **Metabolism** | Small amount liver |
| **Excretion** | Kidneys (66%) unchanged |
| **Half-life** | 6-8 hr or more in geriatric |

| Pharmacodynamics |
|---|
| Unknown |

**Interactions**
*Individual drugs*
Alcohol: avoid using
Carbamazepine: increased carbamazepine toxicity

Sevelamer: decreased levetiracetam absorption; separate by 1 hr before, 3 hr after sevelamer

**NURSING CONSIDERATIONS**
**Assessment**
• Monitor urine function tests (BUN, urine protein) periodically during treatments
• Assess seizure activity including type, location, duration, and character; provide seizure precautions

**Nursing diagnoses**
• Injury, risk for (side effects)
• Knowledge, deficient (teaching)

**Implementation**
**PO route**
• Give with food, milk to decrease GI symptoms (rare)
• Store at room temperature (PO); diluted preparation stable for 24 hr at room temperature in polyvinyl bags
**IV route**
• Single-use vials: dilute in 100 mg of 0.9% NaCl, $D_5$, LR; give over 15 min

**Patient/family education**
• Teach patient to carry/wear emergency ID stating patient's name, products taken, condition, prescriber's name, phone number
• Caution patient to avoid driving, other activities that require alertness until stabilized on medication
• Teach patient not to discontinue medication quickly after long-term use
• Teach patient to use a nonhormonal type of contraception to prevent harm to the fetus
• Teach patient to take exactly as prescribed, do not double or omit doses

**Evaluation**
**Positive therapeutic outcome**
• Decreased seizure activity

## levobetaxolol ophthalmic
*See Appendix D*

## levobunolol ophthalmic
*See Appendix D*

## levocabastine ophthalmic
*See Appendix D*

## levocetirizine (Rx)

(lee-voh-she-teer'ah-zeen)

Xyzal

*Func. class.:* Antihistamine, low sedating
*Chem. class.:* $H_1$-histamine blocker

**Pregnancy category B**

**Action:** Acts on blood vessels, GI, respiratory system by competing with histamine for $H_1$-receptor site; decreases allergic response by blocking pharmacologic effects of histamine; minimal anticholinergic action

**Therapeutic outcome:** Absence of running or congested nose or rashes

**Uses:** Perennial or seasonal rhinitis, allergy symptoms, chronic idiopathic urticaria

### Dosage and routes

*Adult and child ≥12 yr:* PO 2.5-5 mg/day in the evening
*Child 6-11 yr:* PO 2.5 mg/day in the evening
*Geriatric:* PO 2.5-5 mg/day in the evening

*Renal dose*
*Adult:* PO CCr 50-80 ml/min 2.5 mg/day; CCr 30-50 ml/min 2.5 mg every other day; CCr 10-30 ml/min 2.5 mg 2×/wk; CCr <10 ml/min, do not use

**Available forms:** Tabs 5 mg

### Adverse effects

*CNS: Drowsiness, fatigue,* asthenia
*GI:* Dry mouth, increased liver function tests
*INTEG:* Rash, transient

**Contraindications:** Breastfeeding; end-stage renal disease; dialysis; child 6-11 yr with renal disease; hypersensitivity to this product, cetrizine, hydroxyzine

**Precautions:** Pregnancy **B**

### Pharmacokinetics

| | |
|---|---|
| **Absorption** | Rapid |
| **Distribution** | Unknown |
| **Metabolism** | Protein binding 91%-92% |
| **Excretion** | Urine 85.4%, feces 12.9% |
| **Half-life** | 8 hr |

### Pharmacodynamics

| | |
|---|---|
| **Onset** | Unknown |
| **Peak** | 0.9 hr |
| **Duration** | Unknown |

### Interactions

*Individual drugs*
Alcohol: increased CNS depression

*Drug classifications*
MAOIs, phenothiazines, tricyclics: increased anticholinergic/sedative effect
Other CNS depressants: increased CNS depression

*Drug/herb*
Corkwood: increased anticholinergic effect
Hops, Jamaican dogwood, kava, senega, valerian: increased effect

*Drug/lab test*
False negative: skin allergy tests

### NURSING CONSIDERATIONS
### Assessment

• Allergy symptoms: pruritus, urticaria, watering eyes, baseline and during treatment
• Respiratory status: rate, rhythm, increase in bronchial secretions, wheezing, chest tightness
• Liver function tests, serum creatinine, BUN

### Nursing diagnoses

• Knowledge, deficient (teaching)
• Noncompliance (teaching)

### Implementation

• Give without regard to meals in the evening; tabs are scored and may be broken in half
• Store in tight, light-resistant container

### Patient/family education

• Teach patient all aspects of product use; to notify prescriber if confusion, sedation, hypotension occur
• Advise patient to avoid driving, other hazardous activities if drowsiness occurs
• Advise patient to avoid alcohol, other CNS depressants
• Inform patient that product is not recommended during breastfeeding

### Evaluation
**Positive therapeutic outcome**
• Absence of running or congested nose or rashes

**Treatment of overdose:** Administer diazepam, vasopressors, barbiturates (short-acting)

## levodopa ⬤ (Rx)

(lee'voe-doe-pa)

Dopar, Larodopa, L-Dopa

*Func. class.:* Antiparkinsonian agent
*Chem. class.:* Catecholamine, dopamine agonist

**Pregnancy category C**

**Do not confuse:**
L-dopa/methyldopa/levodopa

Adverse effects: *italic* = common, **bold** = life-threatening

**Action:** Decarboxylation to dopamine, which increases dopamine levels in brain

**Therapeutic outcome:** Decreased symptoms of Parkinson's disease (involuntary movements)

**Uses:** Parkinsonism

### Dosage and routes
*Adult:* PO 0.5-1 g/day divided bid-qid with meals; may increase by up to 0.75 g q3-7 days, max 8 g/day unless closely supervised

**Available forms:** Caps 100, 250, 500 mg; tabs 100, 250, 500 mg

### Adverse effects
*CNS: Involuntary choreiform movements, hand tremors, fatigue, headache, anxiety, twitching, numbness, weakness, confusion, agitation, insomnia, nightmares,* psychosis, hallucinations, hypomania, severe depression, dizziness
*CV: Orthostatic hypotension,* tachycardia, hypertension, palpitations
*EENT:* Blurred vision, diplopia, dilated pupils
*GI: Nausea, vomiting, anorexia, abdominal distress, dry mouth, flatulence, dysphagia,* bitter taste, diarrhea, constipation
*HEMA:* **Hemolytic anemia, leukopenia, agranulocytosis**
*INTEG:* Rash, sweating, alopecia
*MISC:* Urinary retention, incontinence, weight change, dark urine

**Contraindications:** Hypersensitivity, angle-closure glaucoma, undiagnosed skin lesions

**Precautions:** Pregnancy **C**, breastfeeding, children <12 yr, renal/cardiac/hepatic disease, respiratory disease, MI with dysrhythmias, seizures, peptic ulcer, asthma, endocrine disease, affective disorders, psychosis, peptic ulcer

| Pharmacokinetics | |
|---|---|
| **Absorption** | Well absorbed |
| **Distribution** | Widely distributed |
| **Metabolism** | Liver, GI tract, extensively |
| **Excretion** | Kidneys to metabolites; breast milk |
| **Half-life** | 1 hr |

| Pharmacodynamics | |
|---|---|
| **Onset** | 10-15 min |
| **Peak** | 1-3 hr |
| **Duration** | Up to 24 hr |

### Interactions
*Individual drugs*
Papaverine, pyridoxine: decreased effects of levodopa
*Drug classifications*
Antacids: increased levodopa effects
Anticholinergics, hydantoins: decreased effects of levodopa
MAOIs: hypertensive crisis
*Drug/herb*
Indian snakeroot: increased EPS; decreased levodopa effect
Kava: increased Parkinson's symptoms
*Drug/food*
Increased: protein food will decrease absorption
*Drug/lab test*
Decreased: VMA
False positive: urine ketones, urine glucose, Coombs' test
False negative: urine glucose (glucose oxidase)
False increase: uric acid, urine protein

### NURSING CONSIDERATIONS
### Assessment
• Monitor B/P, respiration during initial treatment; hypo/hypertension should be reported
• Assess mental status: affect, mood, behavioral changes, depression; complete suicide assessment
• Monitor liver function, renal function tests: AST, ALT, alkaline phosphatase; also check LDH, bilirubin, CBC, BUN, PBI
• Assess for involuntary movements in parkinsonism: akinesia, tremors, staggering gait, muscle rigidity, drooling; these symptoms should improve with levodopa therapy
⬥ Assess for levodopa toxicity: mental, personality changes, increased twitching, grimacing, tongue protrusion; these should be reported to prescriber

### Nursing diagnoses
• Injury, risk for (uses)
• Knowledge, deficient (teaching)
• Mobility, impaired physical (uses)
• Noncompliance (teaching)

### Implementation
• Levodopa/carbidopa should not be started until levodopa is withheld for 8 hr; toxicity may result if the two products are taken close together
• Give levodopa until NPO before surgery
• Adjust dosage to patient response
• Give with meals to decrease GI upset; limit protein taken with product

- Give only after MAOIs have been discontinued for 2 wk

## Patient/family education
- Advise patient that therapeutic effects may take several wk to a few months
- Caution patient to change positions slowly to prevent orthostatic hypotension
- Instruct patient to report side effects: twitching, eye spasms; indicate overdose
- Instruct patient to use product exactly as prescribed; if product is discontinued abruptly, parkinsonian crisis may occur
- Inform patient that urine, sweat may darken
- Advise patient to avoid vit $B_6$ preparations, vitamin-fortified foods containing $B_6$; these foods can reverse effects of levodopa; also OTC preparations should be avoided unless approved by prescriber

## Evaluation
**Positive therapeutic outcome**
- Decreased akathisia, other involuntary movements
- Improved mood

## levofloxacin (Rx)
(lev-o-floks'a-sin)
Levaquin
*Func. class.:* Antiinfective
*Chem. class.:* Fluoroquinolone antibacterial

**Pregnancy category** C

**Action:** Interferes with conversion of intermediate DNA fragments into high molecular weight DNA in bacteria; DNA gyrase inhibitor; inhibits topoisomerase **IV**

**Therapeutic outcome:** Bacterial action against the following: *Streptococcus pneumoniae, Haemophilus influenzae, Haemophilus parainfluenzae, Moraxella catarrhalis, Klebsiella pneumoniae, Mycoplasma pneumoniae, Escherichia coli, Serratia marcescens, Chlamydia pneumoniae, Legionella pneumophilia, Enterococcus faecalis, Staphylococcus epidermidis, Staphylococcus pyogenes*

**Uses:** Adult urinary tract infections (including complicated); lower respiratory, skin infection

**Unlabeled uses:** Gonococcal infections, disseminated; PID

## Dosage and routes
*Acute bacterial exacerbation of chronic bronchitis*
*Adult:* PO/**IV** 500 mg q24hr × 7 days

*Acute bacterial sinusitis*
*Adult:* PO 500 mg q24hr × 10-14 days or 750 mg q24hr × 5 days
*Acute pyelonephritis*
*Adult:* PO 250 mg q24hr × 10 days
*Chronic bacterial prostatitis*
*Adult:* PO 500 mg q24hr × 28 days
*Postexposure inhalational anthrax*
*Adult:* PO/**IV** 500 mg q24hr × 60 days
*Pneumonia, community acquired*
*Adult:* PO/**IV** 500 mg q24hr × 7-14 days or 750 mg q24hr × 5 days
*Pneumonia, nosocomial*
*Adult:* PO/**IV** 750 mg q24hr × 7-14 days
*SSSI, complicated*
*Adult:* PO/**IV** 750 mg q24hr × 7-14 days
*SSSI, uncomplicated*
*Adult:* PO 500 mg q24hr × 7-10 days
*UTI, complicated*
*Adult:* PO/**IV** 250 mg q24hr × 10 days
*UTI, uncomplicated*
*Adult:* PO 250 mg q24hr × 3 days
*Gonococcal infection, disseminated (unlabeled)*
*Adult:* **IV** 250 mg q24hr × 24-48 hr, then PO 500 mg/day x 7 days
*PID (unlabeled)*
*Adult:* **IV** 500 mg q24hr × 14 days
*Renal disease*
*Adult:* PO/**IV** CCr 20-49 ml/min initial 500 mg, then 250 mg q24hr; CCr 10-19 ml/min 250 or 500 mg, depending on condition, then 250 mg q48hr

**Available forms:** Single-use vials (500, 750 mg), premixed flexible container; 250 mg/50 ml $D_5W$, 500 mg/100 ml $D_5W$, 750 mg/150 ml $D_5W$; tabs 250, 500, 750 mg

**Adverse effects:**
*CNS:* Headache, dizziness, *insomnia,* anxiety, **seizures,** encephalopathy, paresthesia
*CV:* Chest pain, palpitations, vasodilatation, QT prolongation
*EENT:* Dry mouth, visual impairment
*GI: Nausea,* flatulence, *vomiting,* diarrhea, abdominal pain, **pseudomembranous colitis**
*GU:* Vaginitis, crystalluria
*HEMA:* Eosinophilia, **hemolytic anemia,** lymphophemia
*INTEG:* Rash, pruritus, photosensitivity, **epidermal necrolysis**
*MISC:* Hypoglycemia, hypersensitivity, tendon rupture

L

Adverse effects: *italic* = common, **bold** = life-threatening

**RESP:** Pneumonitis
**SYST: Anaphylaxis, multisystem organ
failure, Stevens-Johnson syndrome**

**Contraindications:** Hypersensitivity to
quinolones, photosensitivity

**Precautions:** Pregnancy **C**, breastfeeding,
children

### Pharmacokinetics

| | |
|---|---|
| **Absorption** | Unknown |
| **Distribution** | Unknown |
| **Metabolism** | Liver |
| **Excretion** | Kidneys unchanged |
| **Half-life** | 6-8 hr |

### Pharmacodynamics

| | |
|---|---|
| **Onset** | Immediate |
| **Peak** | Infusion's end |
| **Duration** | Unknown |

## Interactions
### Individual drugs
Calcium, iron, sucralfate, zinc: decreased
absorption of levofloxacin
Foscarnet: increased CNS stimulation, seizures
Magnesium: decreased levofloxacin
absorption; do not use in same **IV** line
Theophylline: decreased theophylline clear-
ance, toxicity may result
Warfarin: increased bleeding
### Drug classifications
Antacids (magnesium, aluminum): decreased
absorption of levofloxacin
NSAIDs: increased CNS stimulation, seizures
### Drug/herb
Acidophilus: do not use with antiinfectives;
separate by several hours
Cola tree: increased antiinfective effect
### Drug/lab test
Decreased: glucose, lymphocytes

## NURSING CONSIDERATIONS
### Assessment
• Assess patient for previous sensitivity reaction
• Assess patient for signs and symptoms of
infection including characteristics of wounds,
sputum, urine, stool, WBC >10,000/mm$^3$,
fever; baseline and during treatment
• Obtain C&S before beginning product
therapy to identify if correct treatment has
been initiated
• Assess for allergic reactions and
anaphylaxis: rash, urticaria, pruritus, chills,
fever, joint pain; may occur a few days after
therapy begins; epINEPHrine and resuscitation

equipment should be available for anaphylactic
reaction
• Determine urine output; if decreasing, notify
prescriber (may indicate nephrotoxicity); also
check for increased BUN, creatinine
• Monitor blood tests: AST, ALT, CBC, Hct,
bilirubin, LDH, alkaline phosphatase, Coombs'
test monthly if patient is on long-term therapy
• Monitor electrolytes: potassium, sodium,
chloride monthly if patient is on long-term
therapy
• Assess bowel pattern daily; if severe diarrhea occurs, product should be discontinued
• Monitor for bleeding: ecchymosis, bleeding
gums, hematuria, stool guaiac daily if on
long-term therapy
• Assess for overgrowth of infection: perineal
itching, fever, malaise, redness, pain, swelling,
drainage, rash, diarrhea, change in cough,
sputum

### Nursing diagnoses
• Diarrhea (side effects)
• Infection, risk for (uses)
• Injury, risk for (side effects)
• Knowledge, deficient (teaching)
• Noncompliance (teaching)

### Implementation
• Give PO 4 hr before or 2 hr after antacids,
iron, calcium, zinc
• Check for irritation, extravasation, phlebitis
daily
• Give product around the clock to maintain
blood levels
• Do not use theophylline with this product

### Patient/family education
• Teach patient to report sore throat, bruising,
bleeding, joint pain; may indicate blood
dyscrasias (rare)
• Advise patient to contact prescriber if
vaginal itching, loose foul-smelling stools,
furry tongue occur, may indicate
superinfection; report itching, rash, pruritus,
urticaria
• Instruct patient to take all medication
prescribed for the length of time ordered;
product must be taken around the clock to
maintain blood levels; do not give medication
to others
• Advise patient to notify prescriber of diarrhea with blood or pus
• Instruct patient to take 4 hr before antacids,
iron, calcium, zinc products
• Tell patient to complete full course of
therapy; to increase fluid intake to 2 L/day to
prevent crystalluria
• Advise patient to avoid hazardous activities
until response to product is known

- Instruct patient to rinse mouth frequently and use sugarless candy or gum for dry mouth
- Instruct patient to avoid taking other medications unless approved by prescriber
- Advise patient to avoid sun exposure or use sunscreen to prevent phototoxicity

## Evaluation
**Positive therapeutic outcome**
- Absence of signs/symptoms of infection (WBC <10,000/mm$^3$, temp WNL)
- Reported improvement in symptoms of infection

## levofloxacin ophthalmic
*See Appendix D*

## levothyroxine ⊛ (Rx)
(lee-voe-thye-rox′een)
Eltroxin ✦, Levo-T, Levothroid, levothyroxine sodium, Levoxyl, PMS-Levothyroxine Sodium ✦, Synthroid, T$_4$
*Func. class.:* Thyroid hormone
*Chem. class.:* Levoisomer of thyroxine
**Pregnancy category A**

**Do not confuse:**
Synthroid/Symmetrel

**Action:** Controls protein synthesis; increases metabolic rate, cardiac output, renal blood flow, O$_2$ consumption, body temp, blood volume, growth, development at cellular level, exact mechanism unknown

**Therapeutic outcome:** Correction of lack of thyroid hormone

**Uses:** Hypothyroidism, myxedema coma, thyroid hormone replacement, cretinism, thyrotoxicosis, congenital hypothyroidism, some types of thyroid cancer

## Dosage and routes
**Severe hypothyroidism**
*Adult:* PO 50 mcg/day, increase by 25 mcg q6-8 wk, average dose 100-200 mcg/day, max 200 mcg/day; IM/**IV** 50-100 mcg/day as a single dose or 50% of usual oral dosage
*Child >12 yr:* PO 2-3 mcg/kg/day given as a single dose AM
*Child 6-12 yr:* PO 4-5 mcg/kg/day given as a single dose AM
*Child 1-5 yr:* PO 5-6 mcg/kg/day given as a single dose AM
*Child 6-12 mo:* PO 6-8 mcg/kg/day given as a single dose AM

*Child to 6 mo:* PO 8-10 mcg/kg/day given as a single dose AM

**Myxedema coma**
*Adult:* **IV** 200-500 mcg; may increase by 100-300 mcg after 24 hr; give oral medication as soon as possible

**Available forms:** Powder for inj 200, 500 mcg/vial; tabs 0.025, 0.05, 0.075, 0.088, 0.1, 0.112, 0.125, 0.137, 0.15, 0.175, 0.2, 0.3 mg

## Adverse effects
***CNS:*** *Anxiety, insomnia, tremors,* headache, **thyroid storm**
***CV:*** *Tachycardia, palpitations, angina, dysrhythmias,* hypertension, **cardiac arrest**
***GI:*** Nausea, diarrhea, increased or decreased appetite, cramps
***MISC:*** Menstrual irregularities, weight loss, sweating, heat intolerance, fever, alopecia

**Contraindications:** Adrenal insufficiency, recent MI, thyrotoxicosis, hypersensitivity to beef, alcohol intolerance (inj only)

**Precautions:** Pregnancy **A**, breastfeeding, geriatric, angina pectoris, hypertension, ischemia, cardiac disease, diabetes

### Pharmacokinetics
| | |
|---|---|
| **Absorption** | Erratic (PO); complete (**IV**) |
| **Distribution** | Widely distributed |
| **Metabolism** | Liver; enterohepatic recirculation |
| **Excretion** | Feces via bile; breast milk (small amounts) |
| **Half-life** | 6-7 days |

### Pharmacodynamics
| | PO | IV |
|---|---|---|
| **Onset** | 3-5 days | 6-8 hr |
| **Peak** | 12-48 hr | 12-48 hr |
| **Duration** | Unknown | Unknown |

## Interactions
*Individual drugs*
Cholestyramine, colestipol, ferrous sulfate: decreased absorption of levothyroxine
Digoxin: decreased effect of digoxin
Insulin: increased requirement for insulin
*Drug classifications*
Anticoagulants (oral): increased anticoagulant effect
Antidepressants (tricyclics): increased tricyclic effect
epINEPHrine products: increased cardiac insufficiency risk
Estrogens: decreased thyroid hormone effects
Hypoglycemics: decreased hypoglycemic effect
Selective serotonin reuptake inhibitors: decreased levothyroxine effects

L

Adverse effects: *italic* = common, **bold** = life-threatening

Sympathomimetics: increased sympathomimetic effect

**Drug/herb**

Agar, bugleweed, carnitine, kelpware, soy, spirulina: decreased thyroid hormone effect

**Drug/lab test**

Increased: CPK, LDH, AST, PBI, blood glucose
Decreased: thyroid function tests

## NURSING CONSIDERATIONS
### Assessment

- Determine if the patient is taking anticoagulants, antidiabetic agents; document on chart
- Take B/P, pulse before each dose; monitor I&O ratio and weight every day in same clothing, using same scale, at same time of day
- Monitor height, weight, psychomotor development, and growth rate if given to a child
- Monitor $T_3$, $T_4$, which are decreased; radioimmunoassay of TSH, which is increased; radioactive iodine uptake (RAIU), which is increased if patient is on too low a dosage of medication
- Monitor pro-time (may require decreased anticoagulant); check for bleeding, bruising
- Assess for increased nervousness, excitability, irritability, which may indicate too high a dosage of medication, usually after 1-3 wk of treatment
- Assess cardiac status: angina, palpitations, chest pain, change in VS; the geriatric patient may have undetected cardiac problems and baseline ECG should be completed before treatment

### Nursing diagnoses

- Knowledge, deficient (teaching)
- Noncompliance (teaching)

### Implementation
**PO route**

- Give in AM if possible as a single dose to decrease sleeplessness; give at same time each day to maintain product level
- Give crushed and mixed with water, nonsoy formula, or breast milk for infants/children
- Give only for hormone imbalances; not to be used for obesity, male infertility, menstrual conditions, lethargy; give lowest dosage that relieves symptoms; lower dosage for the geriatric and in cardiac diseases
- Store in tight, light-resistant container
- Remove medication 4 wk before RAIU test

**IV route**

- Give **IV** after diluting with provided diluent (0.9% NaCl), 0.5 mg/5 ml; shake well; give through Y-tube or 3-way stopcock; give 0.1 mg or less over 1 min; do not add to **IV** inf; 0.1 mg = 1 ml; discard any unused portion

## Patient/family education

- Teach patient that product is not a cure but controls symptoms and treatment is long term
- Instruct patient to report excitability, irritability, anxiety, sweating, heat intolerance, chest pain, palpitations, which indicate overdose
- Advise patient not to switch brands unless approved by prescriber; bioavailability may differ; do not take with food; absorption will be decreased
- Teach patient that product may be discontinued after giving birth; thyroid panel will be evaluated after 1-2 mo
- Teach patient or parent that hyperthyroid child will show almost immediate behavior/personality change; that hair loss will occur in child but is temporary
- Caution patient that product is not to be taken to reduce weight
- Caution patient to avoid OTC preparations with iodine; read labels; other medications should not be used unless approved by prescriber
- Teach patient to avoid iodine-rich food: iodized salt, soybeans, tofu, turnips, high iodine seafood, some bread

### Evaluation
**Positive therapeutic outcome**

- Absence of depression
- Weight loss, increased diuresis, pulse, appetite
- Absence of constipation, peripheral edema, cold intolerance, pale, cool dry skin, brittle nails, alopecia, coarse hair, menorrhagia, night blindness, paresthesias, syncope, stupor, coma, rosy cheeks
- Improved levels of $T_3$, $T_4$ by laboratory tests
- Child: age-appropriate weight, height, and psychomotor development

**Treatment of overdose:** Withhold dose for up to 1 wk: acute overdose: gastric lavage or induced emesis, activated charcoal; provide supportive treatment to control symptoms

## ! HIGH ALERT

## lidocaine, parenteral
(Rx)
(lye'doe-kane)
Lidopen Auto-Injector, Xylocard ✦,
Xylocaine, Zingo
*Func. class.:* Antidysrhythmic (class IB)
*Chem. class.:* Aminoacyl amide

### Pregnancy category  B

**Action:** Increases electrical stimulation threshold of ventricle and His-Purkinje system, which stabilizes cardiac membrane and decreases automaticity; locally produces anesthesia by preventing initiation and conduction of nerve impulses

**Therapeutic outcome:** Decreased ventricular dysrhythmia; produces anesthesia locally

**Uses:** Ventricular tachycardia, ventricular dysrhythmias during cardiac surgery, MI, digoxin toxicity, cardiac catheterization; anesthesia locally

### Dosage and routes
*Adult:* **IV** BOL 50-100 mg (1 mg/kg) over 2-3 min; repeat q3-5 min, max 300 mg in 1 hr; begin **IV** INF 20-50 mcg/kg/min; IM 200-300 mg (4.3 mg/kg) in deltoid muscle, may repeat in 1-1½ hr if needed
*Child:* ID (Zingo) 0.5 mg applied 1-3 min prior to needle insertion

### CHF, reduced liver function
*Geriatric:* **IV** BOL ½ adult dose
*Child:* **IV** BOL 1 mg/kg, then **IV** INF 30 mcg/kg/min

**Available forms: IV** inf 0.2% (2 mg/ml), 0.4% (4 mg/ml), 0.8% (8 mg/ml); **IV** admixture 4% (40 mg/ml), 10% (100 mg/ml), 20% (200 mg/ml); **IV** direct 1% (10 mg/ml), 2% (20 mg/ml); IM 300 mg/3 ml; (Zingo) needle free (powder intradermal)

### Adverse effects
*CNS: Headache, dizziness,* involuntary movement, confusion, tremor, *drowsiness,* euphoria, **seizures**
*CV: Hypotension, bradycardia,* **heart block, cardiovascular collapse, arrest**
*EENT:* Tinnitus, blurred vision
*GI:* Nausea, vomiting, anorexia
*HEMA:* **Methemoglobinemia**
*INTEG:* Rash, urticaria, edema, swelling
*MISC:* Febrile response, phlebitis at inj site
*RESP:* Dyspnea, **respiratory depression**

**Contraindications:** Hypersensitivity to amides, severe heart block, supraventricular dysrhythmias, Adams-Stokes syndrome, Wolff-Parkinson-White syndrome

**Precautions:** Pregnancy **B**, breastfeeding, children, geriatric, renal/hepatic disease, CHF, respiratory depression, malignant hyperthermia, myasthenia gravis, weight <50 kg

### Pharmacokinetics
| | |
|---|---|
| **Absorption** | Complete bioavailability (**IV**) |
| **Distribution** | Erythrocytes, cardiovascular endothelium |
| **Metabolism** | Liver |
| **Excretion** | Kidneys |
| **Half-life** | Biphasic 8 min, 1-2 hr |

### Pharmacodynamics
| | IV | IM |
|---|---|---|
| **Onset** | 2 min | 5-15 min |
| **Peak** | Unknown | ½ hr |
| **Duration** | 20 min | 1½ hr |

### Interactions
*Individual drugs*
Cimetidine, metoprolol, phenytoin, propranolol: increased lidocaine effects
Tubocurarine: increased neuromuscular blockade
*Drug classifications*
Barbiturates: decreased lidocaine effects
Neuromuscular blockers: increased neuromuscular blockade
*Drug/herb*
Aconite: increased toxicity, death
Aloe, broom, buckthorn (chronic use), cascara sagrada (chronic use), Chinese rhubarb, figwort, fumitory, goldenseal, kudzu, licorice, senna: increased effect
Coltsfoot: decreased effect
Horehound: increased serotonin effect
*Drug/lab test*
Increased: CPK

### NURSING CONSIDERATIONS
Assessment
• Assess for oxygenation or perfusion deficit: decreased B/P, chest pain, dizziness, loss of consciousness
• Assess respiratory status: auscultate lung fields for bibasilar crackles in patients with advanced CHF
• Assess for urinary retention: check for pain, abdominal absorption, palpate bladder; check males with benign prostatic hypertrophy; anticholinergic reaction may cause retention

L

• Monitor I&O ratio, electrolytes (potassium, sodium, chloride); watch for decreasing urinary output, possible retention
• Monitor liver function tests: AST, ALT, bilirubin, alkaline phosphatase
• Monitor ECG continuously to determine product effectiveness, measure PR, QRS, QT intervals, check for PVCs, other dysrhythmias; monitor B/P continuously for hypo/hypertension; check for rebound hypertension after 1-2 hr, prolonged PR/QT intervals, QRS complex; if QT or QRS increases by 50% or more, withhold next dose, notify prescriber
• Monitor for CNS symptoms: confusion, numbness, depression, involuntary movements; if these occur, product should be discontinued
• Monitor blood levels (therapeutic level 1.5-5 mcg/ml), notify prescriber of abnormal results

### Nursing diagnoses
• Cardiac output, decreased (uses)
• Gas exchange, impaired (adverse reactions)
• Knowledge, deficient (teaching)

### Implementation
**IM route**
• Administer in deltoid, aspirate to prevent **IV** administration
• Check site daily for extravasation
**IV route**
• Give **IV** bolus undiluted (1%, 2% only); give 6 mg or less over 1 min; if using an **IV** line, use port near insertion site, flush with 0.9% NaCl (50 ml)
• Store at room temperature; sol should be clear
• Give by cont inf after adding 1 g/250-1000 ml of D$_5$W; give 1-4 mg/min; use infusion pump for correct dosage; pediatric inf is 120 mg of lidocaine/100 ml of D$_5$W; 1-2.5 ml/kg/hr = 20-50 mcg/kg/min; use only 1%, 2% sol
*Solution compatibilities:* D$_5$W, D$_5$/0.9% NaCl, D$_5$/0.45% NaCl, D$_5$/LR, LR, 0.9% NaCl, 0.45% NaCl
*Syringe compatibilities:* Cloxacillin, glycopyrrolate, heparin, hydrOXYzine, methicillin, metoclopramide, milrinone, moxalactam, nalbuphine
*Syringe incompatibilities:* Cefazolin
*Y-site compatibilities:* Alteplase, amiodarone, inamrinone, cefazolin, ciprofloxacin, diltiazem, DOBUTamine, DOPamine, enalaprilat, etomidate, famotidine, haloperidol, heparin, heparin with hydrocortisone, labetalol, meperidine, morphine, nitroglycerin, nitroprusside, potassium chloride, propofol, streptokinase, theophylline, vit B/C, warfarin

*Additive compatibilities:* Alteplase, aminophylline, amiodarone, atracurium, bretylium, calcium chloride, calcium gluceptate, calcium gluconate, chloramphenicol, chlorothiazide, cimetidine, dexamethasone, digoxin, diphenhydrAMINE, DOBUTamine, DOPamine, epHEDrine, erythromycin, floxacillin, flumazenil, furosemide, heparin, hydrocortisone, nafcillin, hydrOXYzine, regular insulin, mephentermine, metaraminol, nafcillin, nitroglycerin, penicillin G potassium, pentobarbital, phenylephrine, potassium chloride, procainamide, prochlorperazine, promazine, ranitidine, sodium bicarbonate, sodium lactate, theophylline, verapamil, vit B/C
*Additive incompatibilities:* Methohexital, phenytoin; do not admix with blood transfusions
*Infiltration*
Physician may order lidocaine with epINEPHrine to minimize systemic absorption and prolong local anesthesia

### Patient/family education
• Teach patient or family reason for use of medication and expected results
◆ Instruct patient in at-home use of Lidopen Auto-Injector; patient should call prescriber before use if heart attack is imminent

### Evaluation
**Positive therapeutic outcome**
• Decreased B/P, dysrhythmias
• Decreased heart rate
• Normal sinus rhythm

**Treatment of overdose:** Oxygen, artificial ventilation, ECG, administer DOPamine for circulatory depression, diazepam or thiopental for seizures, decreased product or discontinuation may be required

### lidocaine topical
*See Appendix D*

### lindane (OTC)
(lin-dane)
GBH ✦, G-Well, Hexit ✦, Kwell, lindane, PMS Lindane ✦, Scabene, Thionex
*Func. class.:* Scabicide/pediculicide
*Chem. class.:* Chlorinated hydrocarbon (synthetic)

### Pregnancy category  B

**Action:** Stimulates nervous system of arthropods, resulting in seizures, death of organism

**Therapeutic outcome:** Resolution of infestation

**Uses:** Scabies, lice (head/pubic/body), nits

## Dosage and routes
### Lice
*Adult and child:* TOP/CREAM/LOTION
Wash area with soap and water, remove visible crusts; apply to skin surfaces; remove with soap, water 8-12 hr after application; may reapply in 1 wk if needed; SHAMPOO using 30 ml work into lather, rub for 5 min, rinse, dry with towel; use fine-toothed comb to remove nits; most require 1 oz, max 2 oz

### Scabies
*Adult and child:* TOP Apply 1% cream/lotion to skin from neck to bottom of feet, toes; repeat in 1 wk if necessary; most require 1 oz, max 2 oz

**Available forms:** Lotion, shampoo, cream (1%)

## Adverse effects
*CNS:* Tremors, **seizures**, stimulation, dizziness (chronic inhalation of vapors), anxiety, **CNS toxicity**
*CV:* **Ventricular fibrillation** (chronic inhalation of vapors)
*GI: Nausea, vomiting, diarrhea,* liver damage (inhalation of vapors)
*GU:* **Kidney damage** (chronic inhalation of vapors)
*HEMA:* **Aplastic anemia** (chronic inhalation of vapors), myelosuppression
*INTEG: Pruritus, rash, irritation, contact dermatitis*

**Contraindications:** Hypersensitivity; premature neonate; patients with known seizure disorders; inflammation of skin, abrasions, or breaks in skin; Norwegian (crusted) scabies

**Precautions:** Pregnancy **B**, breastfeeding, infants, children <10 yr; avoid contact with eyes

| Pharmacokinetics | |
|---|---|
| Absorption | 20% |
| Distribution | Fat |
| Metabolism | Liver |
| Excretion | Kidneys |
| Half-life | 18 hr |

| Pharmacodynamics | |
|---|---|
| Onset | Rapid |
| Peak | Rapid |
| Duration | 3 hr |

## Interactions
Oil-based hair dressing: increased absorption; wash, rinse, and dry hair before using lindane

## NURSING CONSIDERATIONS
### Assessment
• Assess head, hair for lice and nits before and after treatment; if scabies are present, check all skin surfaces
• Identify source of infection: school, family members, sexual contacts

### Nursing diagnoses
• Knowledge, deficient (teaching)
• Skin integrity, impaired (uses)

### Implementation
• Apply to body areas, scalp only; do not apply to face, lips, mouth, eyes, any mucous membrane, anus, or meatus
• Give topical corticosteroids as ordered to decrease contact dermatitis; provide antihistamines
• Apply menthol or phenol lotions to control itching
• Give topical antibiotics for infection
• Provide isolation until areas on skin, scalp have cleared and treatment is completed
• Remove nits by using a fine-toothed comb rinsed in vinegar after treatment; use gloves

### Patient/family education
• Advise patient to wash all inhabitants' clothing, using insecticide; preventive treatment may be required for all persons living in same house, using lotion or shampoo to decrease spread of infection; use rubber gloves when applying product
• Instruct patient that itching may continue for 4-6 wk; that product must be reapplied if accidently washed off, or treatment will be ineffective; remove after specified time to prevent toxicity
• Advise patient not to apply to face; if accidental contact with eyes occurs, flush with water
• Advise patient that sexual contacts should be treated simultaneously
• Inform the patient of CNS toxicity: dizziness, cramps, anxiety, nausea, vomiting, seizures

### Evaluation
**Positive therapeutic outcome**
• Decreased crusts, nits, brownish trails on skin, itching papules in skinfolds
• Decreased itching after several wk

**Treatment of ingestion:** Gastric lavage, saline laxatives, **IV** diazepam (Valium) for seizures (if taken orally)

Adverse effects: *italic* = common, **bold** = life-threatening

## linezolid (Rx)

(lih-nee'zoh-lid)

Zyvox

*Func. class.*: Broad-spectrum antiinfective
*Chem. class.*: Oxazolidinone

**Pregnancy category** C

**Action:** Binds to bacterial 23S ribosomal RNA of the 50S subunit preventing formation of the bacterial translation process in primarily gram-positive organisms

**Therapeutic outcome:** Negative blood cultures, absence of signs/symptoms of infection

**Uses:** Vancomycin-resistant *Enterococcus faecium* infections, nosocomial pneumonia, uncomplicated or complicated skin and skin structure infections, community-acquired pneumonia

**Dosage and routes**
*Vancomycin-resistant E. faecium infections*
*Adult:* **IV**/PO 600 mg q12hr × 14-28 days, max 1200 mg/day

*Nosocomial pneumonia/complicated skin infections/community-acquired pneumonia/concurrent bacterial infection*
*Adult:* **IV**/PO 600 mg q12hr × 10-14 days, max 1200 mg/day

*Uncomplicated skin infections*
*Adult:* **IV**/PO 400 mg q12hr × 10-14 days; max 1200 mg/day
*Adolescent:* PO 600 mg q12hr × 10-14 days, max 1200 mg/day

**Available forms:** Tabs 600 mg; oral susp 100 mg/5 ml; inj 2 mg/ml

**Adverse effects**
*CNS: Headache,* dizziness
*GI: Nausea, diarrhea,* increased ALT, AST, *vomiting,* taste change, tongue color change, **pseudomembranous colitis**
*HEMA:* **Myelosuppression**
*MISC:* Vaginal moniliasis, fungal infection, oral moniliasis, **lactic acidosis**

**Contraindications:** Hypersensitivity

**Precautions:** Pregnancy **C,** breastfeeding, children, thrombocytopenia, bone marrow suppression

### Pharmacokinetics

| | |
|---|---|
| **Absorption** | Rapidly, excessively |
| **Distribution** | Protein binding 31% |
| **Metabolism** | Oxidation of the morpholine ring |
| **Excretion** | Unknown |
| **Half-life** | Unknown |

### Pharmacodynamics

Unknown

### Interactions
*Individual drugs*
Amoxapine, cyclobenzaprine, maprotiline, mirtazapine, trazodone: increased hypertensive crisis, seizures, coma
Levodopa: increased hypertensive crisis
*Drug classifications*
Adrenergic blockers: increased effects of adrenergics
Antidepressants (tricyclics): increased hypertensive crisis, seizures, coma
MAOIs or those that possess MAOI-like action (flurazolidone, isoniazid, INH, procarbazine): do not use together; hypertensive crisis may occur
Serotonergic agents: increased effect
*Drug/herb*
Acidophilus: do not use with antiinfectives; separate by several hours
Green tea: avoid use
*Drug/food*
Tyramine foods: avoid; increased pressor response

### NURSING CONSIDERATIONS
**Assessment**
- Assess CNS symptoms: headache, dizziness
- Monitor liver function tests: AST, ALT
- Monitor allergic reactions: fever, flushing, rash, urticaria, pruritus
- Assess for pseudomembranous colitis: severe diarrhea, cramping
- Monitor CBC weekly, assess for myelosuppression (anemia, leukopenia, pancytopenia, thrombocytopenia)

**Nursing diagnoses**
- Infection, risk for (uses)
- Knowledge, deficient (teaching)

**Implementation**
**PO route**
- Store reconstituted oral suspension at room temperature, use within 3 wk
**IV route**
- Give over 30-120 min; do not use **IV** infusion bag in series connections, do not use with additives in sol, do not use with another product, administer separately

**Y-site compatibilities:** Acyclovir, alfentanil, amikacin, aminophylline, ampicillin, aztreonam, bretylium, buprenorphine, butorphanol, calcium gluconate, carboplatin, cefazolin, cefoperazone, cefotetan, cefoxitin, ceftazidine, ceftizoxime, ceftriaxone, cefuroxime, cimetidine, ciprofloxacin, cisatracurium, cisplatin, clindamycin, cyclophosphamide, cycloSPORINE, cytarabine, hydromorphone, ifosfamide, labetalol, leucovorin, levofloxacin, lidocaine, lorazepam, magnesium sulfate, mannitol, meperidine, meropenem, mesna, methotrexate, methylPREDNISolone, metoclopramide, metronidazole, midazolam, minocycline, mitoxantrone, morphine, nalbuphine, naloxone, nitroglycerin, ofloxacin, ondansetron, paclitaxel, pentobarbital, piperacillin, potassium chloride, prochlorperazine, promethazine, propranolol, ranitidine, remifentanil, theophylline, ticarcillin, tobramycin, vancomycin, vecuronium, verapamil, vinCRIStine, zidovudine
**Solution compatibilities:** D$_5$, 0.9% NaCl, LR

### Patient/family education
• Advise patient if dizziness occurs, to ambulate, perform activities with assistance
• Advise patient to complete full course of product therapy
• Advise patient to contact prescriber if adverse reaction occurs
• Advise patient to avoid large amounts of tyramine-containing foods (give list)

### Evaluation
**Positive therapeutic outcome**
• Decreased symptoms of infection, blood cultures negative

---

## liothyronine (T$_3$) (Rx)
(lye-oh-thye'roe-neen)
Cytomel, I-Triiodothyronine, liothyronine sodium, Triostat, T$_3$
*Func. class.:* Thyroid hormone
*Chem. class.:* Synthetic T$_3$
**Pregnancy category   A**

**Action:** Controls protein synthesis; increases metabolic rates, cardiac output, renal blood flow, O$_2$ consumption, body temp, blood volume, growth, development at cellular level, exact mechanism unknown

**Therapeutic outcome:** Correction of lack of thyroid hormone

**Uses:** Hypothyroidism, myxedema coma, thyroid hormone replacement, nontoxic goiter, T$_3$ suppression test, congenital hypothyroidism

### Dosage and routes
*Adult:* PO 25 mcg/day, increased by 12.5-25 mcg q1-2 wk until desired response, maintenance dose 25-75 mcg/day; max 100 mcg/day
*Geriatric:* PO 5 mcg/day, increase by 5 mcg/day q1-2 wk, maintenance 25-75 mcg/day

### Congenital hypothyroidism
*Child >3 yr:* PO 50-100 mcg/day
*Child <3 yr:* PO 5 mcg/day, increase by 5 mcg q3-4 days titrated to response, maintenance 20 mcg/day

### Myxedema, severe hypothyroidism
*Adult:* PO 25-50 mcg then may increase by 5-10 mcg q1-2 wk; maintenance dose 50-100 mcg/day

### Myxedema coma/precoma
*Adult:* **IV** 25-50 mcg initially; 5 mcg in geriatric; 10-20 mcg in cardiac disease; give doses q4-12hr

### Nontoxic goiter
*Adult:* PO 5 mcg/day, increase by 12.5-25 mcg q1-2 wk; maintenance dose 75 mcg/day

### Suppression test (T$_3$)
*Adult:* PO 75-100 mcg daily × 1 wk; $^{131}$I is given before and after 1st wk dose

**Available forms:** Tabs 5, 25, 50 mcg; inj 10 mcg/ml

### Adverse effects
*CNS: Insomnia, tremors,* headache, **thyroid storm**
*CV: Tachycardia, palpitations, angina, dysrhythmias,* hypertension, **cardiac arrest**
*GI:* Nausea, diarrhea, increased or decreased appetite, cramps
*MISC:* Menstrual irregularities, weight loss, sweating, heat intolerance, fever, alopecia

**Contraindications:** Adrenal insufficiency, MI, thyrotoxicosis

**Precautions:** Pregnancy **A,** breastfeeding, geriatric, angina pectoris, hypertension, ischemia, cardiac disease, diabetes

| Pharmacokinetics | |
|---|---|
| **Absorption** | Well (PO); complete (**IV**) |
| **Distribution** | Widely distributed; does not cross placenta |
| **Metabolism** | Liver |
| **Excretion** | Feces via bile, breast milk |
| **Half-life** | 1-2 days |

L

Adverse effects: *italic* = common, **bold** = life-threatening

### Pharmacodynamics

|  | PO/IV |
|---|---|
| **Onset** | Unknown |
| **Peak** | 12-24 hr |
| **Duration** | 72 hr |

## Interactions
### Individual drugs
Cholestyramine, colestipol: decreased absorption of thyroid hormone

Digoxin: decreased effects of digoxin

Insulin: increased requirement for insulin

### Drug classifications
Amphetamines, anticoagulants (oral), antidepressants (tricyclics), decongestants, sympathomimetics, vasopressors: increased effect of each specific product

Estrogens: decreased effects of liothyronine

Hypoglycemics: decreased effect of each specific product

### Drug/herb
Agar, bugleweed, carnitine, kelpware, soy, spirulina: decreased thyroid hormone effect

### Drug/lab test
Increased: CPK, LDH, AST, PBI, blood glucose

Decreased: thyroid function tests

## NURSING CONSIDERATIONS
### Assessment
• Determine if the patient is taking anticoagulants, antidiabetic agents; document on patient record

• Take B/P, pulse before each dose; monitor I&O ratio and weight every day in same clothing, using same scale, at same time of day

• Monitor height, weight, psychomotor development, and growth rate if given to a child

• Monitor $T_3$, $T_4$, FTIs, which are decreased; radioimmunoassay of TSH, which is increased; radioactive iodine uptake, which is increased if medication dose is too low

• Monitor protime; may require decreased anticoagulant; check for bleeding, bruising

• Assess for increased nervousness, excitability, irritability, which may indicate too high a dose, usually after 1-3 wk of treatment

• Assess cardiac status: angina, palpitations, chest pain, change in VS; geriatric patients may have undetected cardiac problems, and baseline ECG should be completed before treatment

### Nursing diagnoses
• Knowledge, deficient (teaching)

• Noncompliance (teaching)

## Implementation
### PO route
• Give in AM if possible as a single dose to decrease sleeplessness; give at same time each day to maintain product level

• Do not take with food or absorption will be decreased

• Give only for hormone imbalances; not to be used for obesity, male infertility, menstrual conditions, lethargy; give lowest dose that relieves symptoms; give lower dose to the geriatric and those with cardiac diseases

• Store in airtight, light-resistant container

### IV route
• Administer **IV** for myxedema coma and precoma; do not give IM or SUBCUT; give q4-12hr; use PO dose as soon as feasible

## Patient/family education
• Teach patient that product is not a cure but controls symptoms, and treatment is long term

• Instruct patient to report excitability, irritability, anxiety, sweating, heat intolerance, chest pain, palpitations, which indicate overdose

• Advise patient not to switch brands unless approved by prescriber; bioavailability may differ

• Teach patient that product may be discontinued after giving birth; thyroid panel will be evaluated after 1-2 mo

• Teach patient that hyperthyroid child will show almost immediate behavior/personality change; that hair loss will occur in child but is temporary

• Caution patient that product is not to be taken to reduce weight

• Caution patient to avoid OTC preparations with iodine; read labels; other medications should not be used unless approved by prescriber

• Teach patient to avoid iodine-rich food: iodized salt, soybeans, tofu, turnips, high iodine seafood, some bread

## Evaluation
### Positive therapeutic outcome
• Absence of depression

• Weight loss

• Increased diuresis, pulse, appetite

• Absence of constipation, peripheral edema, cold intolerance, pale, cool dry skin, brittle nails, alopecia, coarse hair, menorrhagia, night blindness, paresthesias, syncope, stupor, coma, rosy cheeks

• Improved levels of $T_3$, $T_4$ by laboratory tests

• Child: age-appropriate weight, height, and psychomotor development

---

 Alert     Canada Only    🌀 Drug on CD    * "Tall Man" lettering (See Preface)

**Treatment of overdose:** Withhold dose for up to 1 wk; for acute overdose: gastric lavage or induce emesis, then activated charcoal; provide supportive treatment to control symptoms

## liotrix (Rx)
(lye'oh-trix)
T₃/T₄, Thyrolar
*Func. class.:* Thyroid hormone
*Chem. class.:* Levothyroxine/liothyronine (synthetic T₄, T₃)
**Pregnancy category A**

**Do not confuse:**
Thyrolar/Thyrar

**Action:** Controls protein synthesis; increases metabolic rates, cardiac output, renal blood flow, $O_2$ consumption, body temp, blood volume, growth, development at cellular level, exact mechanism unknown

**Therapeutic outcome:** Correction of lack of thyroid hormone

**Uses:** Hypothyroidism, thyroid hormone replacement

**Dosage and routes**
*Adult and child:* PO 50 mcg levothyroxine/12.5 mcg liothyronine daily, increased by 50 mcg levothyroxine/12.5 mcg liothyronine q2-3 wk until desired response; may increase by 15-30 mg q2 wk in child
*Geriatric:* PO 12.5-25 mcg levothyroxine/3.1-6.2 mcg liothyronine, may increase by 12.5-25 mcg levothyroxine/3.1-6.2 mcg liothyronine q6-8 wk until adequate response

**Available forms:** Tabs 12.5/3.1, 25/6.25, 50/12.5, 100/25, 150 mcg levothyroxine/37.5 mcg liothyronine

**Adverse effects**
*CNS: Insomnia, tremors,* headache, **thyroid storm**
*CV: Tachycardia, palpitations, angina, dysrhythmias,* hypertension, **cardiac arrest**
*GI:* Nausea, diarrhea, increased or decreased appetite, cramps
*MISC:* Menstrual irregularities, weight loss, sweating, heat intolerance, fever

**Contraindications:** Adrenal insufficiency, MI, thyrotoxicosis

**Precautions:** Pregnancy **A**, breastfeeding, geriatric, angina pectoris, hypertension, ischemia, cardiac disease, diabetes

### Pharmacokinetics
| | |
|---|---|
| Absorption | 50%-80% (T₄); 95% (T₃) |
| Distribution | Widely distributed; does not cross placenta |
| Metabolism | Liver, tissues |
| Excretion | Feces via bile; breast milk |
| Half-life | 6-7 days (T₄); 2 days (T₃) |

### Pharmacodynamics
| | PO (T₄) | PO (T₃) |
|---|---|---|
| Onset | Unknown | Unknown |
| Peak | Unknown | 24-72 hr |
| Duration | Unknown | 72 hr |

### Interactions
*Individual drugs*
Cholestyramine: decreased absorption of thyroid hormone
Colestipol: decreased absorption of liotrix
Digoxin: decreased effect of digoxin
Insulin: increased requirement for insulin
*Drug classifications*
Amphetamines, decongestants, vasopressors: increased effect of each specific product
Anticoagulants (oral): increased effect of anticoagulants
Antidepressants (tricyclics): increased tricyclic effect
Catecholamines: increased catecholamine effect
Estrogens: decreased liotrix effect
Hypoglycemics: decreased hypoglycemic effect
Sympathomimetics: increased sympathomimetic effect
*Drug/herb*
Agar, bugleweed, carnitine, kelpware, soy, spirulina: decreased thyroid hormone effect
*Drug/lab test*
Increased: CPK, LDH, AST, PBI, blood glucose
Decreased: thyroid function tests

### NURSING CONSIDERATIONS
**Assessment**
• Determine if the patient is taking anticoagulants, antidiabetic agents; document on chart
• Take B/P, pulse before each dose; monitor I&O ratio and weight every day in same clothing, using same scale, at same time of day
• Monitor height, weight, psychomotor development, and growth rate if given to a child
• Monitor T₃, T₄, FTIs, which are decreased; radioimmunoassay of TSH, which is increased; radioactive iodine uptake (RA international units), which is increased if medication dose is too low

- Monitor pro-time; may require decreased anticoagulant; check for bleeding, bruising
- Assess for increased nervousness, excitability, irritability, which may indicate too high a dose of medication, usually after 1-3 wk of treatment
- Assess cardiac status: angina, palpitations, chest pain, change in VS; the geriatric patient may have undetected cardiac problems, and baseline ECG should be completed before treatment

### Nursing diagnoses
- Knowledge, deficient (teaching)
- Noncompliance (teaching)

### Implementation
- Give in AM if possible as a single dose to decrease sleeplessness; give at same time each day to maintain product level
- Do not take with food or absorption will be decreased
- Give only for hormone imbalances; not to be used for obesity, male infertility, menstrual conditions, lethargy; give lowest dose that relieves symptoms; give lower dose to the geriatric and those with cardiac diseases
- Store in airtight, light-resistant container
- Remove medication 4 wk before RAIU test

### Patient/family education
- Teach patient that product is not a cure but controls symptoms, and treatment is long term
- Instruct patient to report excitability, irritability, anxiety, sweating, heat intolerance, chest pain, palpitations, which indicate overdose
- Advise patient not to switch brands unless approved by prescriber; bioavailability may differ
- Teach patient that product may be discontinued after giving birth; thyroid panel will be evaluated after 1-2 mo
- Teach patient that hyperthyroid child will show almost immediate behavior/personality change; that hair loss will occur in child but is temporary
- Caution patient that product is not to be taken to reduce weight
- Caution patient to avoid OTC preparations with iodine; read labels; other medications should not be used unless approved by prescriber
- Teach patient to avoid iodine-rich food: iodized salt, soybeans, tofu, turnips, high iodine seafood, some bread

### Evaluation
**Positive therapeutic outcome**
- Absence of depression
- Weight loss

- Increased diuresis, pulse, appetite
- Absence of constipation, peripheral edema, cold intolerance, pale, cool dry skin, brittle nails, alopecia, coarse hair, menorrhagia, night blindness, paresthesias, syncope, stupor, coma, rosy cheeks
- Improved levels of $T_3$, $T_4$ by laboratory tests
- Child: age-appropriate weight, height, and psychomotor development

**Treatment of overdose:** Withhold dose for up to 1 wk; acute overdose: gastric lavage or induce emesis, then activated charcoal; provide supportive treatment to control symptoms

---

## lisdexamfetamine (Rx)
(lis-dex′am-fet′a-meen)
Vyvanse
*Func. class.:* CNS stimulant
*Chem. class.:* Amphetamine

**Pregnancy category** C
**Controlled substance schedule** II

**Action:** Increases release of norepinephrine, dopamine in cerebral cortex to reticular activating system

**Therapeutic outcome:** Able to focus, decreased hyperactivity

**Uses:** Attention deficit disorder with hyperactivity (ADHD)

### Dosage and routes
*Child 6-12 yr:* PO 30 mg/day in the AM, may increase by 20 mg/day at weekly intervals, max 70 mg/day

**Available forms:** Caps 30, 50, 70 mg

### Adverse effects
*CNS: Hyperactivity, insomnia, restlessness, talkativeness,* dizziness, headache, dysphoria, irritability, aggressiveness, CNS tumor, dependence, addiction, mild euphoria, somnolence, lability
*CV: Palpitations, tachycardia,* hypertension, decrease in heart rate, **dysrhythmias,** MI, **cardiomyopathy**
*ENDO:* Growth inhibition
*GI: Anorexia,* dry mouth, diarrhea, weight loss
*GU:* Impotence, change in libido
*INTEG:* Urticaria, **angioedema, Stevens-Johnson syndrome, toxic epidermal necrolysis**

**Contraindications:** Hyperthyroidism, hypertension, glaucoma, severe arteriosclerosis, drug abuse, CV disease, anxiety, anorexia

---

 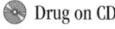

nervosa, breastfeeding, hypersensitivity to sympathomimetic amines

**Precautions:** Pregnancy **C**, children <3yr, Gilles de la Tourette's disorder, depression

### Pharmacokinetics
| | |
|---|---|
| **Absorption** | Unknown |
| **Distribution** | Crosses placenta, breast milk |
| **Metabolism** | Liver |
| **Excretion** | Urine pH dependent |
| **Half-life** | <1 hr |

### Pharmacodynamics
Unknown

### Interactions
#### Individual drugs
AcetaZOLAMIDE, sodium bicarbonate: increased lisdexamfetamine effect

Ascorbic acid, ammonium chloride: decreased lisdexamfetamine effect

Haloperidol, modafinil: increased CNS effect

Melatonin: increased CNS stimulation

Phenytoin: decreased absorption

#### Drug classifications
Adrenergic blockers, antidiabetics: decreased effect

Antacids: increased lisdexamfetamine effect

⚠MAOIs or within 14 days of MAOIs: hypertensive crisis

Phenothiazines, tricyclics: increased CNS effect

#### Drug/herb
Eucalyptus: decreased stimulant effect

Khat: increased stimulant effect

St. John's wort: serotonin syndrome

#### Drug/food
Caffeine: increased amine effect

### NURSING CONSIDERATIONS
#### Assessment
• Monitor VS, B/P; this product may reverse antihypertensives; check patients with cardiac disease often

• Monitor CBC, urinalysis; in diabetes: blood glucose; insulin changes may be required, since eating may decrease

• Monitor height, growth rate in children; growth rate may be decreased

• Assess mental status: mood, sensorium, affect, stimulation, insomnia, irritability

• Assess for tolerance or dependency: an increased amount may be used to get same effect; will develop after long-term use

• Assess for overdose: pain, fever, dehydration, insomnia, hyperactivity

### Nursing diagnoses
• Knowledge, deficient (teaching)
• Noncompliance (teaching)

### Implementation
• Give at least 6 hr before bedtime to avoid sleeplessness

• Provide gum, hard candy, frequent sips of water for dry mouth

### Patient/family education
• Advise patient to decrease caffeine consumption (coffee, tea, cola, chocolate); may increase irritability, stimulation

• Advise patient to avoid OTC preparations unless approved by prescriber

• Teach patient to taper product over several weeks; depression, increased sleeping, lethargy

• Caution patient to avoid alcohol ingestion

• Advise patient to avoid hazardous activities until stabilized on medication

• Instruct patient to get needed rest; patient will feel more tired at end of day

### Evaluation
#### Positive therapeutic outcome
• Ability to stay on task, decreased hyperactivity

**Treatment of overdose:** Administer fluids, hemodialysis, or peritoneal dialysis; antihypertensive for increased B/P, ammonium chloride for increased excretion

---

## lisinopril (Rx)
(lyse-in'oh-pril)
Prinivil, Zestril
*Func. class.:* Antihypertensive, angiotensin converting enzyme (ACE) inhibitor
*Chem. class.:* Enalaprilat lysine analog

### Pregnancy category
**C** (1st trimester),
**D** (2nd/3rd trimesters)

### Do not confuse:
lisinopril/Risperdal, Prinivil/Plendil/Prilosec/Proventil

**Action:** Selectively suppresses renin-angiotensin-aldosterone system; inhibits ACE; prevents conversion of angiotensin I to angiotensin II; results in dilatation of arterial, venous vessels

**Therapeutic outcome:** Decreased B/P in hypertension, decreased preload, afterload in CHF

**Uses:** Mild to moderate hypertension, adjunctive therapy of systolic CHF, acute MI

Adverse effects: *italic* = common, **bold** = life-threatening

## Dosage and routes
### Hypertension
**Adult:** PO 10-40 mg/day; may increase to 80 mg/day if required
**Geriatric:** PO 2.5-5 mg/day, increase q7 days

### CHF
**Adult:** PO 5 mg initially with diuretics/digoxin, range 5-20 mg

**Available forms:** Tabs 2.5, 5, 10, 20, 30 40 mg

## Adverse effects
**CNS:** *Vertigo,* depression, **stroke,** insomnia, paresthesias, *headache,* fatigue, asthenia, dizziness
**CV:** Chest pain, hypotension
**EENT:** Blurred vision, nasal congestion
**GI:** Nausea, vomiting, anorexia, constipation, flatulence, GI irritation, diarrhea
**GU: Proteinuria, renal insufficiency,** sexual dysfunction, impotence
**INTEG:** Rash, pruritus
**MISC:** Muscle cramps, hyperkalemia
**RESP:** Dry cough, dyspnea
**SYST: Angioedema**

**Contraindications:** Pregnancy **D** (2nd/3rd trimesters), hypersensitivity, angioedema

**Precautions:** Pregnancy **C** (1st trimester), breastfeeding, renal disease, hyperkalemia, renal artery stenosis, CHF

### Pharmacokinetics
| | |
|---|---|
| **Absorption** | Variable |
| **Distribution** | Unknown |
| **Metabolism** | Not metabolized |
| **Excretion** | Kidneys, unchanged |
| **Half-life** | 12 hr |

### Pharmacodynamics
| | |
|---|---|
| **Onset** | 1 hr |
| **Peak** | 6-8 hr |
| **Duration** | 24 hr |

## Interactions
### Individual drugs
Alcohol (large amounts), probenecid: increased hypotension
Allopurinol: increased hypersensitivity
Aspirin: decreased lisinopril effect
CycloSPORINE: increased hyperkalemia
Digoxin: increased serum levels, toxicity
Indomethacin: decreased antihypertensive effect
Lithium: increased levels of lithium, toxicity

## Drug classifications
Antihypertensives, diuretics, nitrates, phenothiazines: increased hypotension
Diuretics, potassium-sparing, potassium salt substitutes, potassium supplements: increased hyperkalemia
NSAIDs: decreased lisinopril effect
### Drug/herb
Aconite: increased toxicity, death
Astragalus, cola tree: increased or decreased antihypertensive effect
Barberry, betony, black catechu, black cohosh, bloodroot, broom, burdock, cat's claw, dandelion, goldenseal, Irish moss, Jamaican dogwood, kelp, khella, mistletoe, parsley: increased antihypertensive effect
Coltsfoot, guarana, khat, licorice, yohimbe: decreased antihypertensive effect
### Drug/food
High-potassium diet (bananas, orange juice, avocados, broccoli, nuts, spinach) should be avoided; hyperkalemia may occur
### Drug/lab test
Interference: glucose/insulin tolerance tests, ANA titer

## NURSING CONSIDERATIONS
### Assessment
• Assess blood studies: platelets, WBC with differential, baseline and periodically q3 mo; if neutrophils <1000/mm$^3$, discontinue treatment
• Monitor B/P, check for orthostatic hypotension, syncope; if changes occur, dosage change may be required
• Establish baselines in renal, liver function tests before therapy begins
• Monitor renal, liver function tests: protein, BUN, creatinine; watch for increased levels that may indicate nephrotic syndrome and renal failure; monitor renal symptoms: polyuria, oliguria, frequency, dysuria
• Check potassium levels throughout treatment, although hyperkalemia rarely occurs
• Check for edema in feet, legs daily
• Assess for allergic reactions: rash, fever, pruritus, urticaria; product should be discontinued if antihistamines fail to help

### Nursing diagnoses
• Cardiac output, decreased (uses)
• Injury, risk for (side effects)
• Knowledge, deficient (teaching)
• Noncompliance (teaching)

### Implementation
• Store in airtight container at 86° F (30° C) or less
• Severe hypotension may occur after 1st dose

 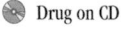

of this medication; may be prevented by reducing or discontinuing diuretic therapy 3 days before beginning lisinopril therapy

### Patient/family education
• Caution patient not to discontinue product abruptly; advise patient to inform all health care providers about taking this product
• Teach patient not to use OTC products (cough, cold, allergy) unless directed by prescriber; serious side effects can occur
• Teach patient the importance of complying with dosage schedule, even if feeling better; to continue with medical regimen to decrease B/P: exercise, cessation of smoking, decreasing stress, diet modifications
• Teach patient to notify prescriber of mouth sores, sore throat, fever, swelling of hands or feet, irregular heartbeat, chest pain, coughing, shortness of breath
• Caution patient to report excessive perspiration, dehydration, vomiting, diarrhea; may lead to fall in B/P
• Emphasize the need to rise slowly to sitting or standing position to minimize orthostatic hypotension; not to exercise in hot weather or increased hypotension can occur
• Caution patient that product may cause dizziness, fainting, light-headedness; may occur during 1st few days of therapy; to avoid activities that may be hazardous
• Teach patient how to take B/P, and normal readings for age-group; advise patient to take B/P regularly
• Instruct patient to avoid increasing potassium in the diet

### Evaluation
**Positive therapeutic outcome**
• Decreased B/P in hypertension
• Decreased CHF symptoms

**Treatment of overdose:** 0.9% NaCl **IV** inf, hemodialysis

---

### lithium (Rx)
(li'thee-um)
Carbolith ✦, Duralith ✦, Eskalith, Eskalith CR, lithium carbonate, Lithizine ✦, Lithobid, Lithonate, Lithotabs
*Func. class.:* Antimanic, antipsychotic
*Chem. class.:* Alkali metal ion salt
**Pregnancy category D**

**Action:** May alter sodium, potassium ion transport across cell membrane in nerve, muscle cells; may balance biogenic amines of norepinephrine, serotonin in CNS areas involved in emotional responses

**Therapeutic outcome:** Stable mood

**Uses:** Bipolar disorders (manic phase), prevention of bipolar manic-depressive psychosis

### Dosage and routes
*Adult:* PO 300-600 mg tid; maintenance 300 mg tid or qid; SLOW REL TAB 300 mg bid; dosage should be individualized to maintain blood levels at 0.5-1.5 mEq/L
*Geriatric:* PO 300 mg bid, increase q7 days by 300 mg to desired dose
*Child:* PO 15-20 mg/kg/day in 2-3 divided doses; increase as needed; do not exceed adult doses; maintain blood levels at 0.4-0.5 mEq/L

### Renal dose
*Adult:* PO CCr 10-50 ml/min 50-75% of dose; CCr <10 ml/min 25%-50% of dose

**Available forms:** Caps 150, 300, 600 mg; tabs 300 mg; ext rel tabs 300, 450 mg; syr 300 mg/5 ml (8 mEq/5 ml); slow rel caps 150, 300 mg ✦

### Adverse effects
*CNS: Headache, drowsiness, dizziness, tremors,* twitching, ataxia, **seizures,** slurred speech, restlessness, *confusion,* stupor, memory loss, clonic movements, *fatigue*
*CV: Hypotension,* ECG changes, **dysrhythmias, circulatory collapse, edema**
*EENT:* Tinnitus, blurred vision
*ENDO:* Hypothyroidism, goiter, hyperglycemia, hyperthyroidism, hyponatremia
*GI: Dry mouth, anorexia, nausea, vomiting, diarrhea,* incontinence, abdominal pain, metallic taste
*GU:* **Polyuria, glycosuria, proteinuria, albuminuria,** urinary incontinence, polydipsia
*HEMA:* **Leukocytosis**
*INTEG:* Drying of hair, alopecia, rash, pruritus, hyperkeratosis, *acneiform rash, folliculitis*
*MS: Muscle weakness*

**Contraindications:** Pregnancy **D**, breastfeeding, children <12 yr, hepatic disease, brain trauma, organic brain syndrome, schizophrenia, severe cardiac/renal disease, severe dehydration

**Precautions:** Geriatric, thyroid disease, seizure disorders, diabetes mellitus, systemic infection, urinary retention

L

## Pharmacokinetics

| | |
|---|---|
| **Absorption** | Completely absorbed |
| **Distribution** | Reabsorbed by renal tubules (80%); crosses blood-brain barrier; crosses placenta |
| **Metabolism** | Unknown |
| **Excretion** | Urine, unchanged |
| **Half-life** | 18-36 hr depending on age |

## Pharmacodynamics

| | |
|---|---|
| **Onset** | Rapid |
| **Peak** | ½-12 hr |
| **Duration** | Unknown |

## Interactions
### Individual drugs
Acetazolamide, aminophylline, mannitol, sodium bicarbonate: increased renal clearance

Calcium iodide, iodinated glycerol, potassium iodide: increased hypothyroid effect

Carbamazepine, fluoxetine, methyldopa, probenecid: increased lithium effect/toxicity

Haloperidol: increased neurotoxicity

Indomethacin, losartan: increased toxicity

Thioridazine: brain damage

Urea: decreased lithium effect

### Drug classifications
Antithyroid agents: increased hypothyroid effects

Neuromuscular blocking agents: increased effect of neuromuscular blocking effects

NSAIDs, thiazides: increased lithium toxicity

Phenothiazines: increased effect of phenothiazines

Theophyllines, urinary alkalinizers: decreased effect of lithium

### Drug/herb
Broom, buchu, dandelion, goldenrod, horsetail, juniper, nettle, parsley: increased lithium effect, increased toxicity

Coffee, cola nut, guarana, plantain, tea (black/green), yerba maté: decreased lithium effect

### Drug/food
Significant changes in sodium intake will alter lithium excretion

### Drug/lab test
Increased: potassium excretion, urine glucose, blood glucose, protein, BUN

Decreased: VMA, $T_3$, $T_4$, PBI, $^{131}I$

## NURSING CONSIDERATIONS
### Assessment
• Assess for minor lithium toxicity: vomiting, diarrhea, poor coordination, fine motor tremors, weakness, lassitude; major toxicity: coarse tremors, severe thirst, tinnitus, dilute urine

• Assess weight daily; check for edema in legs, ankles, wrists; report if present; check skin turgor at least daily

• Monitor sodium intake; decreased sodium intake with decreased fluid intake may lead to lithium retention; increased sodium and fluids may decrease lithium retention

• Monitor urine for albuminuria, glycosuria, uric acid during beginning treatment, q2 mo thereafter

• Assess neurologic status: LOC, gait, motor reflexes, hand tremors

• Monitor serum lithium levels weekly initially, then q2 mo (therapeutic level: 0.5-1.5 mEq/L); toxic level >1.5 mcg/L; toxicity and therapeutic levels are very close; toxicity may occur rapidly; blood levels are measured before the AM dose

### Nursing diagnoses
• Coping, ineffective (uses)
• Knowledge, deficient (teaching)
• Noncompliance (teaching)
• Thought processes, disturbed (uses)

### Implementation
• Do not break, crush, or chew caps and slow rel caps

• Administer reduced dosage to geriatric; give with meals to avoid GI upset

• Provide adequate fluids (2-3 L/day) to prevent dehydration during initial treatment, 1-2 L/day during maintenance

• Give list of products that interact with lithium

### Patient/family education
• Provide patient with written information on symptoms of minor toxicity: vomiting, diarrhea, poor coordination, fine motor tremors, weakness, lassitude; major toxicity: coarse tremors, severe thirst, tinnitus, dilute urine

• Advise patient to monitor urine specific gravity; emphasize need for follow-up care to determine lithium effects

• Advise patient that contraception is necessary, since lithium may harm fetus

• Caution patient not to operate machinery until lithium levels are stable and response determined; that beneficial effects may take 1-3 wk

• Provide to the patient a list of products that interact with lithium and discuss need for adequate, stable intake of salt and fluid

• Advise to have lithium levels monitored to ensure effectiveness

## Evaluation
### Positive therapeutic outcome
- Decrease in excitement, poor judgment, insomnia (manic phase)
- Decreased mood swings and lability

**Treatment of overdose:** Induce emesis or lavage, maintain airway, respiratory function; dialysis for severe intoxication

## Iodoxamide ophthalmic
*See Appendix D*

## lomustine (Rx)
(loe-mus′teen)
CCNU, CeeNU
*Func. class.:* Antineoplastic alkylating agent
*Chem. class.:* Nitrosourea

**Pregnancy category  D**

**Action:** Changes essential cellular ions to covalent bonding with resultant alkylation; this interferes with normal biologic function of DNA; activity is not phase specific; action is due to myelosuppression

**Therapeutic outcome:** Prevention of rapid growth of malignant cells in chronic myelocytic leukemia

**Uses:** Hodgkin's disease, malignant glioma

**Unlabeled uses:** Brain, breast, renal, GI tract, bronchogenic carcinoma; melanomas

### Dosage and routes
*Adult:* PO 100-130 mg/m² as a single dose q6 wk; titrate dosage to WBC level; do not give repeat dose unless WBCs are >4000/mm³, platelet count >100,000/mm³

**Available forms:** Caps 10, 40, 100 mg

### Adverse effects
*GI: Nausea, vomiting, anorexia, stomatitis,* **hepatotoxicity**
*GU:* **Azotemia, renal failure**
*HEMA:* **Thrombocytopenia, leukopenia, myelosuppression, anemia**
*RESP:* **Fibrosis, pulmonary infiltrate**

**Contraindications:** Pregnancy **D**, breastfeeding, "blastic" phase of chronic myelocytic leukemia, hypersensitivity, leukopenia, thrombocytopenia

**Precautions:** Radiation therapy, pulmonary disease

### Pharmacokinetics
| | |
|---|---|
| Absorption | Rapidly absorbed |
| Distribution | Widely |
| Metabolism | Liver |
| Excretion | Kidneys, breast milk |
| Half-life | 16-48 hr |

### Pharmacodynamics
Unknown

### Interactions
*Individual drugs*
Allopurinol: increased bone marrow suppression
Aspirin: increased bleeding
Cimetidine, chloral hydrate, phenytoin: increased toxicity
Phenobarbital: increased lomustine metabolism
Succinylcholine: increased lomustine effect
*Drug classifications*
Anticoagulants: increased bleeding
Barbiturates: increased toxicity
*Drug/lab test*
False positive: cytology tests for breast, bladder, cervix, lung

### NURSING CONSIDERATIONS
#### Assessment
◆ Monitor CBC, differential, platelet count weekly; withhold product if WBC is <4000/mm³ or platelet count is <100,000/mm³; notify prescriber of results if WBC <20,000/mm³, platelets <150,000/mm³; these may occur after 4-6 wk and with cumulative dose >600 mg
- Monitor pulmonary function tests, chest x-ray films before, during therapy; chest film should be obtained q2 wk during treatment; assess for dyspnea, crackles, unproductive cough, chest pain, tachypnea
- Monitor renal function tests: BUN, serum uric acid, urine CCr before, during therapy; I&O ratio; report fall in urine output of 30 ml/hr; check for decreased hyperuricemia
- Monitor for cold, fever, sore throat (may indicate beginning of infection), usually after 4 wk; identify edema in feet, joint and stomach pain, shaking; prescriber should be notified
- Assess for bleeding: hematuria, guaiac, bruising or petechiae, mucosa or orifices q8hr, no rectal temp

#### Nursing diagnoses
- Body image, disturbed (adverse reactions)
- Infection, risk for (adverse reactions)
- Injury, risk for (adverse reactions)
- Knowledge, deficient (teaching)

Adverse effects: *italic* = common, **bold** = life-threatening

## Implementation
- Give product after evening meal, before bedtime; administer antiemetic and dexamethasone 30-60 min before giving product to prevent vomiting; no food or drinks for ≥2 hr after administration
- Store in tight container

## Patient/family education
- Teach patient to avoid use of products containing aspirin or ibuprofen, razors, commercial mouthwash, since bleeding may occur; to report symptoms of bleeding (hematuria, tarry stools)
- Advise patient to report signs of anemia (fatigue, headache, irritability, faintness, shortness of breath)
- Caution patient to report any changes in breathing or coughing even several mo after treatment; to avoid crowds and persons with respiratory tract or other infections
- Caution patient not to have any vaccinations without the advice of prescriber; serious reactions can occur
- Tell patient contraception is needed during treatment and for several mo after the completion of therapy, avoid breastfeeding

## Evaluation
**Positive therapeutic outcome**
- Decreased tumor sizes
- Decreased spread of malignancy

## loperamide (OTC, Rx)
(loe-per'a-mide)
loperamide solution, Imodium, Imodium A-D, Imodium A-D Caplet, Loperamide, Kaopectate II Caplets, Maalox Antidiarrheal Caplets, Neo-Diaral, Pepto Diarrhea Control
*Func. class.:* Antidiarrheal
*Chem. class.:* Piperidine derivative

**Pregnancy category B**

**Action:** Direct action on intestinal muscles to decrease GI peristalsis; reduces volume, increases bulk; electrolytes are not lost

**Therapeutic outcome:** Absence of diarrhea

**Uses:** Diarrhea (cause undetermined), chronic diarrhea, to decrease amount of ileostomy discharge, traveler's diarrhea, IBD

## Dosage and routes
*Adult:* PO 4 mg, then 2 mg after each loose stool, max 16 mg/day
*Child 9-11 yr:* PO 2 mg, then 1 mg after each loose stool, max 6 mg/24 hr

*Child 2-5 yr:* PO 1 mg, then 0.1 mg/kg after each loose stool, max 4 mg/24 hr

**Available forms:** Caps 2 mg; liquid 1 mg/5 ml; tabs 2 mg

## Adverse effects
*CNS:* Dizziness, drowsiness, fatigue, fever
*GI: Nausea, dry mouth, vomiting, constipation,* abdominal pain, anorexia, **toxic megacolon,** bacterial enterocolitis
*INTEG:* Rash
*MISC:* Hyperglycemia

**Contraindications:** Hypersensitivity, severe ulcerative colitis, pseudomembranous colitis, acute diarrhea associated with *Escherichia coli,* bacterial enterocolitis

**Precautions:** Pregnancy **B**, breastfeeding, children <2 yr, hepatic disease, dehydration, bacterial disease, AIDS

### Pharmacokinetics
| | |
|---|---|
| **Absorption** | Poor |
| **Distribution** | Unknown |
| **Metabolism** | Liver |
| **Excretion** | Feces, unchanged; small amount in urine |
| **Half-life** | 9-14 hr |

### Pharmacodynamics
| | |
|---|---|
| **Onset** | ½-1 hr |
| **Peak** | Unknown |
| **Duration** | 4-5 hr |

## Interaction
*Individual drugs*
Alcohol: increased CNS depression
*Drug classifications*
Antihistamines, analgesics (opioids), sedative/hypnotics: increased CNS depression
*Drug/herb*
Chamomile, hops, kava, skullcap, valerian: increased CNS depression
Nutmeg: increased antidiarrheal effect

## NURSING CONSIDERATIONS
**Assessment**
- Monitor electrolytes (potassium, sodium, chloride) if patient is on long-term therapy; check fluid status, skin turgor
- Assess bowel pattern before, during treatment; check for rebound constipation after termination of medication; check bowel sounds
- Check response after 48 hr; if no response, product should be discontinued and other treatment initiated

- Assess for abdominal distention, toxic megacolon, which may occur in ulcerative colitis
- Assess for dehydration, CNS symptoms in children or those with hepatic disease

### Nursing diagnoses
- Constipation (adverse reactions)
- Diarrhea (uses)
- Knowledge, deficient (teaching)
- Noncompliance (teaching)

### Implementation
- Do not break, crush, or chew caps
- Store in airtight containers
- Do not mix oral sol with other sol

### Patient/family education
- Caution patient to avoid alcohol and OTC products unless directed by prescriber; may cause increased CNS depression
- Advise patient not to exceed recommended dosage; product may be habit forming; ileostomy patient may take this product for extended time
- Advise patient that product may cause drowsiness and to avoid hazardous activities until response to product is determined
- Teach patient that dry mouth can be decreased by frequent sips of water, hard candy, sugarless gum

### Evaluation
**Positive therapeutic outcome**
- Decreased diarrhea

---

### loracarbef
*See cephalosporins—2nd generation*

---

### loratadine (Rx, OTC)
(lor-a'ti-deen)
Alavert, Children's Loratadine, Children's ND Non-Drowsy Allergy, Claritin, Claritin Non-Drowsy Allergy, Clear-Atadine, Dimetapp, Tavist ND
*Func. class.:* Antihistamine (2nd generation)
*Chem. class.:* Selective histamine ($H_1$) receptor antagonist

**Pregnancy category B**

**Action:** Binds to peripheral histamine receptors, which provides antihistamine action without sedation

**Therapeutic outcome:** Decreased nasal stuffiness, itching, swollen eyes

**Uses:** Seasonal rhinitis, chronic idiopathic urticaria for those ≥2 yr

**Dosage and routes**
*Adult and child ≥6 yr:* PO 10 mg/day
*Child 2-5 yr:* PO 5 mg/day

*Renal dose*
*Adult:* PO CCr <30 ml/min 10 mg every other day

*Hepatic dose*
*Adult:* PO 10 mg every other day

**Available forms:** Tabs 10 mg; rapid-disintegrating tabs 10 mg; orally disintegrating tabs 10 mg; syr 1 mg/ml, susp 5 mg/ml

**Adverse effects**
*CNS:* Sedation (more common with increased dosages), headache

**Contraindications:** Hypersensitivity, acute asthma attacks, lower respiratory tract disease

**Precautions:** Pregnancy **B,** increased intraocular pressure, bronchial asthma

| Pharmacokinetics | |
|---|---|
| **Absorption** | Well absorbed |
| **Distribution** | Unknown |
| **Metabolism** | Liver, extensively, to active metabolite desloratadine |
| **Excretion** | Kidneys |
| **Half-life** | 17-28 hr |

| Pharmacodynamics | |
|---|---|
| **Onset** | 1-3 hr |
| **Peak** | 8-12 hr |
| **Duration** | > 24 hr |

### Interactions
*Individual drugs*
Alcohol: increased CNS depression
Cimetidine, ketoconazole: increased loratadine level
*Drug classifications*
Antidepressants, antihistamines (other), opiates, sedative/hypnotics: increased CNS depression
Macrolides (clarithromycin, erythromycin): increased loratadine level
MAOIs: increased antihistamine effects
*Drug/herb*
Chamomile, hops, Jamaican dogwood, kava, khat, senega, skullcap, valerian: increased CNS depression
Corkwood, henbane: increased anticholinergic effect

Adverse effects: *italic* = common, **bold** = life-threatening

*Drug/lab test*
False negative: skin allergy tests (discontinue antihistamine 3 days before testing)

## NURSING CONSIDERATIONS
### Assessment
• Assess allergy: hives, rash, rhinitis
• Assess respiratory status: rate, rhythm, increase in bronchial secretions, wheezing, chest tightness; provide fluids to 2 L/day to decrease secretion thickness

### Nursing diagnoses
• Airway clearance, ineffective (uses)
• Knowledge, deficient (teaching)
• Noncompliance (teaching, overuse)

### Implementation
• Give on an empty stomach, 1 hr before or 2 hr after meals to facilitate absorption
• Place rapidly disintegrating tabs on tongue, then swallow after disintegrated with or without water
• Use within 6 mo of opening pouch; immediately after opening blister pack
• Store in airtight, light-resistant container

### Patient/family education
• Teach all aspects of product uses; to notify prescriber if confusion, sedation, hypotension occur; to avoid driving and other hazardous activity if drowsiness occurs; to avoid alcohol and other CNS depressants that may potentiate effect
• Teach patient to take 1 hr before or 2 hr after meals to facilitate absorption
• Advise patient to use sunscreen or stay out of the sun to prevent burns
• Caution patient not to exceed recommended dosage; dysrhythmias may occur
• Teach patient that hard candy, gum, frequent rinsing of mouth may be used for dryness

### Evaluation
**Positive therapeutic outcome**
• Absence of runny or congested nose, other allergy symptoms

## lorazepam (Rx)
(lor-az'e-pam)
Apo-Lorazepam ✦, Ativan, lorazepam, Novo-Lorazem ✦, Nu-Loraz ✦
*Func. class.:* Sedative/hypnotic, antianxiety agent
*Chem. class.:* Benzodiazepine, short acting

**Pregnancy category D**

**Controlled substance schedule IV**

**Do not confuse:**
lorazepam /alprazolam/clonazepam

**Action:** Potentiates the actions of GABA, an inhibitory neurotransmitter, especially in the limbic system and reticular formation, which depresses the CNS

**Therapeutic outcome:** Decreased anxiety, relaxation

**Uses:** Anxiety, irritability in psychiatric or organic disorders, preoperatively, insomnia, adjunct in endoscopic procedures

**Unlabeled uses:** Antiemetic before chemotherapy, status epilepticus, rectal use

**Dosage and routes**
*Anxiety*
*Adult:* PO 2-6 mg/day in divided doses, not to exceed 10 mg/day
*Geriatric:* PO 0.5-1 mg/day in divided doses; or 0.5-1 mg at bedtime
*Child ≥12 yr:* PO 0.05 mg/kg/dose, q4-8 hr

*Insomnia*
*Adult:* PO 2-4 mg at bedtime; only minimally effective after 2 wk continuous therapy
*Geriatric:* PO 0.5-1 mg initially

*Preoperatively*
*Adult:* IM 50 mcg/kg 2 hr before surgery; **IV** 44 mcg/kg 15-20 min before surgery, max 2 mg 15-20 min prior to surgery
*Child ≥12 yr:* 0.05 mg/kg

*Status epilepticus*
*Neonate:* 0.05 mg/kg
*Child:* 0.1 mg/kg up to 4 mg/dose; RECT (unlabeled) 0.05-0.1 mg × 2; wait 7 min before giving 2nd dose

**Available forms:** Tabs 0.5, 1, 2 mg; inj 2, 4 mg/ml; conc sol 2 mg/ml

**Adverse effects**
*CNS: Dizziness, drowsiness,* confusion, headache, anxiety, tremors, stimulation, fatigue, depression, insomnia, hallucinations, weakness, unsteadiness

*CV: Orthostatic hypotension,* **ECG changes, tachycardia,** hypotension; **apnea, cardiac arrest (IV, rapid)**
*EENT: Blurred vision,* tinnitus, mydriasis
*GI:* Constipation, dry mouth, nausea, vomiting, anorexia, diarrhea
*INTEG:* Rash, dermatitis, itching
*MISC:* Acidosis

**Contraindications:** Pregnancy **D,** breast-feeding, hypersensitivity to benzodiazepines, angle-closure glaucoma, psychosis, history of drug abuse, COPD, sleep apnea

**Precautions:** Geriatric, debilitated patients, children <12 yr, renal/hepatic disease, addiction, suicidal ideation

### Pharmacokinetics

| | |
|---|---|
| **Absorption** | Well absorbed (PO); completely absorbed (IM) |
| **Distribution** | Widely distributed; crosses placenta, blood-brain barrier |
| **Metabolism** | Liver, extensively |
| **Excretion** | Kidneys, breast milk |
| **Half-life** | 14 hr |

### Pharmacodynamics

| | PO | IM | IV |
|---|---|---|---|
| **Onset** | ½ hr | 15-30 min | 5-15 min |
| **Peak** | 1-3 hr | 1-1½ hr | Unknown |
| **Duration** | 12-24 hr | 6-8 hr | 6-8 hr |

### Interactions
#### Individual drugs
Alcohol: increased CNS depression
Disulfiram: increased lorazepam effects
Smoking: increased metabolism, decreased effect
Valproic acid: decreased lorazepam effects
#### Drug classifications
CNS depressants, oral contraceptives: increased lorazepam effects
#### Drug/herb
Black cohosh: increased hypotension
Catnip, chamomile, clary, cowslip, hops, kava, lavender, mistletoe, nettle, pokeweed, poppy, Queen Anne's lace, senega, skullcap, valerian: increased CNS depression
#### Drug/lab test
Increased: AST, ALT, serum bilirubin
Decreased: radioactive iodine uptake
False increase: 17-OHCS

### NURSING CONSIDERATIONS
#### Assessment
• Assess degree of anxiety; what precipitates anxiety and whether product controls symptoms; other signs of anxiety: dilated pupils, inability to sleep, restlessness, inability to focus
• Assess for alcohol withdrawal symptoms, including hallucinations (visual, auditory), delirium, irritability, agitation, fine to coarse tremors
• Monitor B/P (with patient lying/standing), pulse, check respiratory rate; if systolic B/P drops 20 mm Hg, hold product, notify prescriber; respirations q5-15 min if given **IV**
• Monitor CBC during long-term therapy; blood dyscrasias have occurred (rarely)
• Monitor for seizure control; type, duration, and intensity of seizures; what precipitates seizures
• Monitor hepatic studies: AST, ALT, bilirubin, creatinine, LDH, alkaline phosphatase
• Assess mental status: mood, sensorium, affect, sleeping pattern, drowsiness, dizziness, suicidal tendencies, and ability of product to control these symptoms; check for tolerance, withdrawal symptoms: headache, nausea, vomiting, muscle pain, weakness after long-term use

#### Nursing diagnoses
• Coping, ineffective (uses)
• Knowledge, deficient (teaching)
• Noncompliance (teaching)
• Sleep deprivation (uses)

#### Implementation
##### PO route
• Give largest dose before bedtime if giving in divided dose
• Concentrate: use calibrated dropper; add to food/drink, consume immediately
• Give with food or milk for GI symptoms; crush tab if patient is unable to swallow medication whole; provide sugarless gum, hard candy, frequent sips of water for dry mouth
##### SUBCUT route
• Use by SL route for rapid response (investigational use)
##### IM route
• Give deep in muscle mass; if using for preoperative sedation, give 2 hr or more before surgical procedure
##### IV route
• Prepare immediately before use, short stability time
• Dilute with sterile water for inj, 0.9% NaCl, or $D_5W$ just before using; give by Y-site or 3-way stopcock at 2 mg/min
• Do not use sol that is discolored or contains a precipitate
*Syringe compatibilities:* Cimetidine, hydromorphone

L

*Y-site compatibilities:* Acyclovir, albumin, allopurinol, amifostine, amikacin, amoxicillin, amoxicillin/clavulanate, amsacrine, atracurium, bumetanide, cefepime, cefmetazole, cefotaxime, ciprofloxacin, cisatracurium, cisplatin, cladribine, clonidine, cyclophosphamide, cytarabine, dexamethasone, diltiazem, DOBUTamine, DOPamine, DOXOrubicin, epINEPHrine, erythromycin, etomidate, famotidine, fentanyl, filgrastim, fluconazole, fludarabine, furosemide, gentamicin, granisetron, haloperidol, heparin, hydrocortisone, hydromorphone, ketanserin, labetalol, melphalan, methotrexate, metronidazole, midazolam, milrinone, morphine, niCARdipine, nitroglycerin, norepinephrine, paclitaxel, pancuronium, piperacillin, piperacillin/tazobactam, potassium chloride, propofol, ranitidine, tacrolimus, teniposide, thiotepa, trimethoprim/sulfamethoxazole, vancomycin, vecuronium, vinorelbine, zidovudine

*Y-site incompatibilities:* Idarubicin, ondansetron, sargramostim

## Patient/family education

• Advise patient that product may be taken with food; that product is not to be used for everyday stress or used longer than 4 mo unless directed by a prescriber; to take no more than prescribed amount; may be habit forming

• Caution patient to avoid OTC preparations unless approved by prescriber; to avoid alcohol, other psychotropic medications unless prescribed by physician; not to discontinue medication abruptly after long-term use

• Inform patient to avoid driving and activities that require alertness; drowsiness may occur; to rise slowly or fainting may occur, especially in geriatric

• Inform patient that drowsiness may worsen at beginning of treatment

## Evaluation

**Positive therapeutic outcome**

• Decreased anxiety, restlessness, insomnia

**Treatment of overdose:** Lavage, VS, supportive care

---

## losartan (Rx)
(low-sar'tan)

Cozaar

*Func. class.:* Antihypertensive
*Chem. class.:* Angiotensin II receptor (type $AT_1$)

**Pregnancy category**
C (1st trimester),
D (2nd/3rd trimesters)

### Do not confuse:
losartan/valsartan, Cozaar/Zocor

**Action:** Blocks the vasoconstrictor and aldosterone-secreting effects of angiotensin II; selectively blocks the binding of angiotensin II to the $AT_1$ receptor found in tissues

**Therapeutic outcome:** Decreased B/P

**Uses:** Hypertension, alone or in combination; nephropathy in type 2 diabetes, hypertension with left ventricular hypertrophy

### Dosage and routes
*Hypertension*
**Adult:** PO 50 mg/day alone or 25 mg/day when used in combination with diuretic, maintenance 25-100 mg/day

*Hepatic dose*
**Adult:** PO 25 mg/day as starting dose

*Hypertension with left ventricular hypertrophy*
**Adult:** PO 50 mg/day, add hydrochlorothiazide 12.5 mg/day and/or increase losartan to 100 mg/day, then increase hydrochlorothiazide to 25 mg/day

*Nephropathy in type 2 diabetes patients*
**Adult:** PO 50 mg/day, may increase to 100 mg/day

**Available forms:** Tabs 25, 50, 100 mg

### Adverse effects
*CNS:* Dizziness, insomnia, anxiety, confusion, abnormal dreams, migraine, tremor, vertigo, headache
*CV:* Angina pectoris, 2nd-degree AV block, **CVA**, hypotension, **MI, dysrhythmias**
*EENT:* Blurred vision, burning eyes, conjunctivitis
*GI:* Diarrhea, dyspepsia, anorexia, constipation, dry mouth, flatulence, gastritis, vomiting
*GU:* Impotence, nocturia, urinary frequency, urinary tract infection, **renal failure**
*HEMA:* Anemia

---

*INTEG:* Alopecia, dermatitis, dry skin, flushing, photosensitivity, rash, pruritus, sweating
**angioedema**
*META:* Gout
*MS:* Cramps, myalgia, pain, stiffness
*RESP: Cough, upper respiratory infection,* congestion, dyspnea, bronchitis

**Contraindications:** Pregnancy **D** (2nd/3rd trimesters), hypersensitivity

**Precautions:** Pregnancy **C** (1st trimester) breastfeeding, children, geriatric, hypersensitivity to ACE inhibitors, hepatic disease, angioedema, renal artery stenosis

### Pharmacokinetics

| | |
|---|---|
| **Absorption** | Well |
| **Distribution** | Bound to plasma proteins |
| **Metabolism** | Extensive |
| **Excretion** | Feces, urine |
| **Half-life** | Biphasic, 2 hr, 6-9 hr |

### Pharmacodynamics
Unknown

## Interactions
### Individual drugs
Fluconazole: increased antihypertensive effect
Lithium: increased toxicity
Phenobarbital, rifamycin: decreased antihypertensive effect
### Drug classifications
ACE inhibitors, diuretics (potassium-sparing), potassium supplements: increased hyperkalemia
NSAIDs, salicylates: decreased antihypertensive effect
### Drug/herb
Aconite: increased toxicity, death
Astragalus, cola tree: increased or decreased antihypertensive effect
Barberry, betony, black catechu, black cohosh, bloodroot, broom, burdock, cat's claw, dandelion, goldenseal, Irish moss, Jamaican dogwood, kelp, khella, mistletoe, parsley: increased antihypertensive effect
Coltsfoot, guarana, khat, licorice, yohimbe: decreased antihypertensive effect

## NURSING CONSIDERATIONS
### Assessment
• Assess B/P with position changes, pulse q4hr; note rate, rhythm, quality
• Monitor electrolytes: potassium, sodium, chloride
• Obtain baselines for renal, liver function tests before therapy begins
• Monitor for edema in feet, legs daily
• Assess for skin turgor, dryness of mucous membranes for hydratio status

### Nursing diagnoses
• Fluid volume, deficient (side effects)
• Noncompliance (teaching)
• Knowledge, deficient (teaching)

### Implementation
• Administer without regard to meals

### Patient/family education
• Teach patient to avoid sunlight or wear sunscreen if in sunlight; photosensitivity may occur
• Advise patient to comply with dosage schedule, even if feeling better
• Teach patient to notify prescriber of mouth sores, fever, swelling of hands or feet, irregular heartbeat, chest pain
• Advise patient that excessive perspiration, dehydration, vomiting, diarrhea may lead to fall in blood pressure, consult prescriber if these occur
• Inform patient that product may cause dizziness, fainting; light-headedness may occur
• Caution patient to rise slowly to sitting or standing position to minimize orthostatic hypotension
• Advise patient to use contraception while taking this product

### Evaluation
**Positive therapeutic outcome**
• Decreased B/P

## loteprednol ophthalmic
*See Appendix D*

## lovastatin (Rx)
(loe'va-sta-tin)
Altocor, Altoprev, Mevacor
*Func. class.:* Antilipemic
*Chem. class.:* HMG-CoA reductase inhibitor
**Pregnancy category X**

**Do not confuse:**
lovastatin/Lotensin

**Action:** By inhibiting HMG-CoA reductase, inhibits biosynthesis of VLDL and LDL, which are responsible for cholesterol development

**Therapeutic outcome:** Decreased cholesterol levels and LDLs, increased HDLs

**Uses:** As an adjunct in primary hypercholesterolemia (types IIa, IIb), atherosclerosis, primary and secondary prevention of coronary events

## Dosage and routes
(Patient should first be consuming a cholesterol-lowering diet)
*Adult:* PO 20 mg/day with evening meal; may increase to 20-80 mg/day in single or divided doses; not to exceed 80 mg/day; dosage adjustments should be made monthly; reduce dose in renal disease; EXT REL 20-60 mg/day at bedtime

**Available forms:** Tabs 10, 20, 40 mg; ext rel tab (Altocor) 10, 20, 40, 60 mg

## Adverse effects
*CNS:* Dizziness, headache, tremor, insomnia, paresthesia
*EENT:* Blurred vision, lens opacities
*GI:* Nausea, constipation, diarrhea, dyspepsia, *flatus,* abdominal pain, heartburn, **liver dysfunction,** vomiting, acid regurgitation, dry mouth, dysgeusia
*HEMA:* **Thrombocytopenia, hemolytic anemia, leukopenia**
*INTEG:* Rash, pruritus, photosensitivity
*MS:* Muscle cramps, myalgia, **myositis, rhabdomyolysis,** leg, shoulder or localized pain

**Contraindications:** Pregnancy **X,** breast-feeding, hypersensitivity, active liver disease

**Precautions:** Past liver disease, alcoholism, severe acute infections, trauma, hypotension, uncontrolled seizure disorders, severe metabolic disorders, electrolyte imbalances, visual condition, children

### Pharmacokinetics
| | |
|---|---|
| **Absorption** | Poorly absorbed, erratic |
| **Distribution** | Crosses placenta, blood-brain barrier |
| **Metabolism** | Liver, extensively |
| **Excretion** | Feces (83%); kidneys, urine (10%) |
| **Half-life** | 3-4 hr |

### Pharmacodynamics
| | |
|---|---|
| **Onset** | Unknown |
| **Peak** | 2-4 hr |
| **Duration** | Unknown |

## Interactions
### Individual drugs
Bosentan, exonatide: decreased action of lovastatin

Clarithromycin, clofibrate, cycloSPORINE, dalfopristin, danazol, diltiazem, erythromycin, gemfibrozil, niacin, quinupristin, telithromycin, verapamil: increased myalgia, myositis

Digoxin: increased digoxin effect
Warfarin: increased bleeding

### Drug classifications
Azole antifungals, protease inhibitors: increased myositis, myalgia
Bile acid sequestrants: decreased lovastatin effects

### Drug/herb
Glucomannan: increased effect
Gotu kola, St. John's wort: decreased effect

### Drug/food
Increased levels of lovastatin with food, must be taken with food
Grapefruit juice: increased toxicity
Oat bran: decreased absorption

### Drug/lab test
Increased: CPK, liver function tests

## NURSING CONSIDERATIONS
### Assessment
- Assess nutrition: fat, protein, carbohydrates; nutritional analysis should be completed by dietitian before treatment
- Monitor bowel pattern daily; diarrhea may be a problem
- Monitor triglycerides, fasting cholesterol LDL, HDL at baseline and throughout treatment; watch LDL and VLDL closely; if increased, product should be discontinued
- Assess for muscle pain, tenderness, obtain CPK; if these occur, product may need to be discontinued

### Nursing diagnoses
- Diarrhea (adverse reactions)
- Knowledge, deficient (teaching)
- Noncompliance (teaching)

### Implementation
- Give with evening meal; if dosage is increased, take with breakfast and evening meal
- Store in cool environment in airtight, light-resistant container

### Patient/family education
- Inform patient that compliance is needed for positive results to occur; not to double doses
- Inform patient that blood work and ophthalmic exam will be necessary during treatment
- Teach patient that risk factors should be decreased: high-fat diet, smoking, alcohol consumption, absence of exercise
- Advise patient to report if pregnancy is suspected
- Advise patient to notify prescriber if the GI symptoms of diarrhea, abdominal or epigastric pain, nausea, vomiting occur; or if chills, fever,

sore throat, blurred vision, dizziness, headache, muscle pain, weakness occur

• Advise patient to stay out of the sun or use sunscreen to prevent burns

### Evaluation
**Positive therapeutic outcome**
• Decreased cholesterol, serum triglyceride levels
• Improved ratio of HDLs

---

## loxapine (Rx)
(lox'a-peen)
Loxapac ✿, loxapine succinate ✿, Loxitane IM, Loxitane, Loxitane-C
*Func. class.:* Antipsychotic/neuroleptic
*Chem. class.:* Dibenzoxazepine

**Pregnancy category** C

### Do not confuse:
Loxitane/Soriatane

**Action:** Depresses cerebral cortex, hypothalamus, limbic system, which control activity and aggression; blocks neurotransmission produced by DOPamine at synapse; exhibits strong α-adrenergic, anticholinergic blocking action; mechanism for antipsychotic effects is unclear

**Therapeutic outcome:** Decreased psychotic behavior

**Uses:** Psychotic disorders, nonpsychotic symptoms associated with dementia

**Unlabeled uses:** Depression, anxiety

### Dosage and routes
*Adult:* PO 10 mg bid-qid initially; may be rapidly increased depending on severity of condition; maintenance 60-100 mg/day; IM 12.5-50 mg q4-6hr or more until desired response, then start PO form; max 250 mg/day
*Geriatric:* PO 5-10 mg/day bid, increase q4-7 days by 5-10 mg, max 250 mg/day

**Available forms:** Caps 5, 10, 25, 50 mg; conc 25 mg/ml; inj 50 mg/ml; tabs 5, 10, 25, 50 mg

### Adverse effects
*CNS: EPS, pseudoparkinsonism, akathisia, dystonia, tardive dyskinesia, drowsiness, headache,* **seizures,** *confusion,* **neuroleptic malignant syndrome**
*CV: Orthostatic hypotension,* **cardiac arrest,** *ECG changes, tachycardia*
*EENT:* Blurred vision, glaucoma
*GI: Dry mouth, nausea, vomiting, anorexia, constipation, diarrhea, jaundice, weight gain*
*GU:* Urinary retention, urinary frequency, enuresis, impotence, amenorrhea, gynecomastia
*HEMA:* **Anemia, leukopenia, leukocytosis, agranulocytosis**
*INTEG: Rash,* photosensitivity, dermatitis
*RESP:* **Laryngospasm,** dyspnea, **respiratory depression**

**Contraindications:** Hypersensitivity, blood dyscrasias, coma, severe CNS depression, brain damage, bone marrow depression, alcohol and barbiturate withdrawal states, angle-closure glaucoma

**Precautions:** Pregnancy **C,** breastfeeding, children <16 yr, geriatric, seizure disorders, cardiac/renal/hepatic disease, prostatic hypertrophy, cardiac conditions

### Pharmacokinetics
| | |
|---|---|
| **Absorption** | Well absorbed (PO) |
| **Distribution** | Unknown |
| **Metabolism** | Liver, extensively |
| **Excretion** | Kidneys |
| **Half-life** | Biphasic 5 hr, 19 hr |

### Pharmacodynamics
| | PO | IM |
|---|---|---|
| **Onset** | ½ hr | 15-30 min |
| **Peak** | 2-4 hr | 15-20 min |
| **Duration** | 12 hr | 12 hr |

### Interactions
*Individual drugs*
Alcohol: increased CNS depression
EpINEPHrine: increased toxicity
Guanadrel, guanethidine, levodopa: decreased effects
*Drug classifications*
Antidepressants, MAOIs: increased CNS depression
Antipsychotics: increased EPS
*Drug/herb*
Betel palm, kava: increased EPS
Chamomile, cola tree, hops, kava, nettle, nutmeg, skullcap, valerian: increased CNS depression

### NURSING CONSIDERATIONS
**Assessment**
• Assess mental status: orientation, mood, behavior, presence and type of hallucinations before initial administration and monthly; this product should significantly reduce psychotic behavior
• Check for swallowing of PO medication; check for hoarding or giving of medication to other patients
• Monitor I&O ratio; palpate bladder if low

---

Adverse effects: *italic* = common, **bold** = life-threatening

urinary output occurs, especially in geriatric; urinalysis recommended before, during prolonged therapy, urinary retention may be cause
- Monitor bilirubin, CBC, liver function tests monthly
- Assess affect, orientation, LOC, reflexes, gait, coordination, sleep pattern disturbances
- Monitor B/P with patient sitting, standing, and lying; take pulse and respirations q4hr during initial treatment; establish baseline before starting treatment; report drops of 30 mm Hg
- Check for dizziness, faintness, palpitations, tachycardia on rising; severe orthostatic hypotension is common

 Identify for neuroleptic malignant syndrome: hyperpyrexia, muscle rigidity, increased CPK, altered mental status; product should be discontinued
- Assess for EPS, including akathisia (inability to sit still, no pattern to movements), tardive dyskinesia (bizarre movements of the jaw, mouth, tongue, extremities), pseudoparkinsonism (ragged tremors, pill rolling, shuffling gait); an antiparkinsonian product should be prescribed
- Assess for constipation, urinary retention daily; if these occur, increase bulk, water in diet

### Nursing diagnoses
- Coping, ineffective (uses)
- Knowledge, deficient (teaching)
- Noncompliance (teaching)
- Thought processes, disturbed (uses)

### Implementation
**PO route**
- Administer product in liquid form mixed in glass of juice or cola if hoarding is suspected; do not mix in caffeine drinks, tannics, pectins
- Administer lowered dose in geriatric, since metabolism is slowed
- Administer with full glass of water or milk; or give with food to decrease GI upset
- Give antacids 2 hr before or after taking this product
- Store in airtight, light-resistant container, oral sol in amber bottle

**IM route**
- Inject deep in muscle mass; do not give SUBCUT; do not administer sol with a precipitate; amber-colored sol can be used
- Patient should remain lying down after IM inj for at least 30 min

### Patient/family education
- Teach patient to use good oral hygiene; suggest frequent rinsing of mouth, sugarless gum for dry mouth; oral candidiasis can occur
- Caution patient to avoid hazardous activities until product response is determined; dizziness, blurred vision may occur
- Inform patient that orthostatic hypotension occurs often and to rise from sitting or lying position gradually; caution patient to avoid hot tubs, hot showers, tub baths, since hypotension may occur; tell patient that in hot weather heat stroke may occur; take extra precautions to stay cool
- Advise patient to avoid abrupt withdrawal of this product, or EPS may result; product should be withdrawn slowly
- Advise patient to avoid use with alcohol, CNS depressants; increased drowsiness may occur
- Advise patient to use a sunscreen and sunglasses to prevent burns
- Suggest patient take antacids 2 hr before or after taking this product
- Instruct patient to report sore throat, malaise, fever, bleeding, mouth sores; if these occur, CBC should be performed and product discontinued

### Evaluation
**Positive therapeutic outcome**
- Decrease in emotional excitement, hallucinations, delusions, paranoia
- Reorganization of patterns of thought, speech

**Treatment of overdose:** Lavage if orally ingested; barbiturates; provide airway, **IV** fluids; do not use epINEPHrine, which may increase hypotension

## lubiprostone (Rx)
(loo-bee-pros′-tone)
Amitiza
*Func. class.:* Miscellaneous gastrointestinal agent
**Pregnancy category** C

**Action:** Locally acting chloride channel activator, enhances a chloride-rich intestinal fluid secretion without altering other electrolytes; increases motility in the intestine, increasing softening and passage of stool

**Therapeutic outcome:** Decreased constipation

**Uses:** Chronic idiopathic constipation

### Dosage and routes
*Adult:* PO 24 mcg bid with food

**Available forms:** Caps 24 mcg

## Adverse effects

**CNS:** *Headache,* dizziness, depression, fatigue, insomnia
**CV:** Hypertension, chest pain
**GI:** *Nausea, abdominal pain, eructation,* abdominal distention, constipation, diarrhea, dry mouth, dyspepsia, flatulence, gastroenteritis viral, gastroesophageal reflux disease, vomiting, fecal incontinence, fecal urgency
**GU:** UTI
**MISC:** Chest pain, peripheral edema, influenza, pyrexia, viral infection
**MS:** Back pain, arthralgia, muscle cramps, pain in extremities
**RESP:** Bronchitis; cough, dyspnea, nasopharyngitis, sinusitis, URI

**Contraindications:** Hypersensitivity, GI obstruction

**Precautions:** Pregnancy **C**, breastfeeding, children, diarrhea, IBD

| Pharmacokinetics | |
|---|---|
| Absorption | Unknown |
| Distribution | Protein binding 94% |
| Metabolism | Rapid in stomach, jejunum |
| Excretion | Unknown |
| Half-life | 0.9-1.4 hr |

| Pharmacodynamics | |
|---|---|
| Onset | Unknown |
| Peak | 1.14 hr |
| Duration | Unknown |

## Interactions
### Individual drugs
Antidiarrheals, anticholinergics: decreased effects of lubiprostone

## NURSING CONSIDERATIONS
### Assessment
• Assess GI symptoms: nausea, abdominal pain
• Assess periodically, need for continued treatment

### Nursing diagnoses
• Constipation (uses)
• Knowledge, deficient (teaching)

### Implementation
• Give with foods, bid
• Store at room temperature

### Patient/family education
• Teach patient to notify prescriber of GI symptoms, diarrhea, hypersensitivity reactions

## Evaluation
**Positive therapeutic outcome**
• Decreased constipation

## lymphocyte immune globulin (anti-thymocyte) (Rx)
Atgam, Thymoglobulin
*Func. class.:* Immune globulin immunosuppressant

**Pregnancy category  C**

**Action:** Produces immunosuppression by inhibiting the function of T-lymphocytes

**Therapeutic outcome:** Absence of transplant rejection; hematologic remission (aplastic anemia)

**Uses:** Organ transplants to prevent rejection, aplastic anemia

**Unlabeled uses:** Multiple sclerosis, myasthenia gravis, immunosuppressant in liver, bone marrow, heart and other organ transplants, pure red cell aplasia, scleroderma

### Dosage and routes
#### Renal allograft
**Adult:** **IV** 10-30 mg/kg/day
**Child:** **IV** 5-25 mg/kg/day

#### Delay of renal allograft rejection
**Adult:** **IV** 15 mg/kg/day × 14 days, then every other day × 14 days for a total of 21 doses in 28 days

#### Aplastic anemia
**Adult:** **IV** 10-20 mg/kg/day × 8-14 days

**Available forms:** Inj 50 mg horse gamma globulin/ml

### Adverse effects
#### Renal transplant
**CNS:** Fever, chills, headache, dizziness, weakness, faintness, seizures
**CV:** Chest pain, hypertension, tachycardia
**GI:** Diarrhea, nausea, vomiting, epigastric pain, **GI bleeding**
**INTEG:** Rash, pruritus, urticaria, wheal
**SYST:** **Anaphylaxis**
#### Aplastic anemia
**CNS:** Fever, chills, headache, **seizures,** light-headedness, encephalitis, postviral encephalopathy
**CV:** Bradycardia, myocarditis, irregularity
**GI:** Nausea, liver function test abnormality

**Contraindications:** Hypersensitivity

**Precautions:** Pregnancy **C**, breastfeeding, children, severe renal/hepatic disease

L

Adverse effects: *italic* = common, **bold** = life-threatening

| Pharmacokinetics | |
|---|---|
| **Absorption** | Unknown |
| **Distribution** | Unknown |
| **Metabolism** | Unknown |
| **Excretion** | Unknown |
| **Half-life** | 5.7 days |

| Pharmacodynamics | |
|---|---|
| **Onset** | Rapid |
| **Peak** | Unknown |
| **Duration** | Unknown |

## NURSING CONSIDERATIONS
### Assessment
• Assess for infection; if infection occurs, evaluation will be needed to continue treatment
• Monitor renal function tests: BUN, creatinine at least monthly during treatment, 3 mo after treatment
• Monitor liver function tests: alkaline phosphatase, AST, ALT, bilirubin

### Nursing diagnoses
• Infection, risk for (uses)
• Knowledge, deficient (teaching)
• Mobility, impaired physical (uses)

### Implementation
**IV route**
• Do not infuse <4 hr
• Keep emergency equipment nearby for severe allergic reactions
• Skin testing must be completed before treatment; use intradermal inj of 0.1 ml of a 1:1000 dilution (5 mcg of horse IgG) in 0.9% NaCl, if a wheal or rash >10 mm or both, use caution during inf
• Dilute in saline sol before inf; invert **IV** bag, so undiluted product does not contact the air inside, concentration should not be >1 mg/ml

### Patient/family education
• Advise patient to report fever, rash, chills, sore throat, fatigue, since serious infections may occur
• Caution patient to use contraceptive measures during treatment and for 12 wk after ending therapy; product is teratogenic
• Caution patient to avoid crowds and persons with known infections to reduce risk of infection

### Evaluation
**Positive therapeutic outcome**
• Absence of graft rejection
• Hematologic recovery (aplastic anemia)

## mafenide topical
*See Appendix D*

## magaldrate (OTC)
(mag'al-drate)
Isopan, Losapan ♦, Riopan, Riopan Extra Strength ♦
*Func. class.:* Antacid
*Chem. class.:* Aluminum/magnesium hydroxide

### Pregnancy category C

**Action:** Neutralizes gastric acidity; product is dissolved in gastric contents; this product is a combination of aluminum and magnesium

**Therapeutic outcome:** Decreased pain of ulcers

**Uses:** Antacid, hiatal hernia, indigestion/heartburn, hyperacidity

**Unlabeled uses:** Duodenal and gastric ulcers, peptic ulcer disease (adjunct), reflex esophagitis

**Dosage and routes**
*Adult/child/geriatric:* SUSP 5-10 ml (480-1080 mg) with water between meals, at bedtime

**Available forms:** Susp 540 mg/5 ml

**Adverse effects**
*GI:* Constipation, diarrhea, anorexia
*META:* Hypermagnesemia, hypophosphatemia

**Contraindications:** Hypersensitivity to this product or aluminum products

**Precautions:** Pregnancy **C**, geriatric, fluid restriction, decreased GI motility, GI obstruction, dehydration, renal disease, sodium-restricted diets, bone disease, hypertension

| Pharmacokinetics | |
|---|---|
| **Absorption** | Not absorbed |
| **Distribution** | Not distributed |
| **Metabolism** | Not metabolized |
| **Excretion** | Kidneys |
| **Half-life** | Unknown |

| Pharmacodynamics | |
|---|---|
| **Onset** | Unknown |
| **Peak** | ½ hr |
| **Duration** | 1 hr |

### Interactions
*Individual drugs*
Chlordiazepoxide, cimetidine, isoniazid, ketoconazole, phenytoin, tetracycline:

decreased absorption of each specific product

Flecainide, quinidine: increased action when taken in large amounts

*Drug classifications*

Amphetamines: increased action when taken in large amounts

Anticholinergics, corticosteroids, fluoroquinolones, iron salts, phenothiazines, salicylates: decreased absorption of each specific product

Salicylates: decreased action when taken in large amounts

**NURSING CONSIDERATIONS**
**Assessment**
• Assess GI status: location of pain, intensity, characteristics, what aggravates, ameliorates pain; heartburn/indigestion; hematemesis
• Monitor serum magnesium, calcium, phosphate, potassium if using long term or with impaired renal function
• Assess for constipation: increase bulk in diet if needed or obtain order for stool softener

**Nursing diagnoses**
• Knowledge, deficient (teaching)
• Pain, acute (uses)

**Implementation**
• Take antacids 2 hr before or 2 hr after taking enteric-coated products
• Give laxatives or stool softeners if constipation occurs
• Give susp after shaking; give between meals and at bedtime
• Give when stomach is empty after meals and at bedtime

**Patient/family education**
• Advise patient to separate ingestion of enteric-coated products and antacid by 2 hr
• Advise patient to use 2 wk or less; product should not be used for long periods
• Teach patient to notify prescriber immediately if coffee-ground emesis, emesis with frank blood, or black tarry stools occur

**Evaluation**
**Positive therapeutic outcome**
• Absence of abdominal pain
• Decreased acidity

**magnesium salts** (OTC)
(mag-neez'ee-um)
**magnesium chloride** (Rx)
Chloromag, Slo-Mag
**magnesium citrate** (OTC)
Citrate of Magnesia, Citroma, Citromag ✦
**magnesium gluconate** (OTC)
Almoate Magonate, Magtrate  OTC
**magnesium hydroxide** (OTC)
Phillips Magnesia Tablets, Phillips Milk of Magnesia, MOM
**magnesium oxide** (OTC)
Mag-Ox 400, Maox, Uro-Mag
**magnesium sulfate** (OTC, Rx)
epsom salt, magnesium sulfate (**IV**)—
**HIGH ALERT**
*Func. class.:* Electrolyte; anticonvulsant, laxative, saline; antacid

**Pregnancy category** A, B

**Action:** Increases osmotic pressure, draws fluid into colon, neutralizes HCl

**Therapeutic outcome:** Magnesium levels WNL, absence of constipation

**M**

**Uses:** Constipation, bowel preparation before surgery or exam, electrolyte, anticonvulsant, in preeclampsia, eclampsia (magnesium sulfate), electrolyte

**Dosage and routes**
*Laxative*
*Adult:* PO 30-60 ml at bedtime (Milk of Magnesia)
*Adult and child >6 yr:* PO 15 g in 8 oz of H$_2$O (magnesium sulfate); PO 10-20 ml (Concentrated Milk of Magnesia); PO 5-10 oz at bedtime (magnesium citrate)
*Child 2-6 yr:* 5-15 ml/day (Milk of Magnesia)

*Prevention of magnesium deficiency*
*Adult and child ≥10 yr:* PO (male): 350-400 mg/day; (female): 280-300 mg/day; (breastfeeding): 335-350 mg/day; (pregnancy): 320 mg/day
*Child 8-10 yr:* PO 170 mg/day
*Child 4-7 yr:* PO 120 mg/day
*Infant to 4 yr:* 40-80 mg/day

*Magnesium sulfate deficiency*
*Adult:* PO 200-400 mg in divided doses tid-qid; IM 1 g q6hr × 4 doses; **IV** 5 g (severe)

Adverse effects: *italic* = common, **bold** = life-threatening

*Child 6-12 yr:* 3-6 mg/kg/day in divided doses tid-qid

*Preeclampsia/eclampsia magnesium sulfate*
*Adult:* IM/**IV** 4-5 g **IV** INF; with 5 g IM in each gluteus, then 5 g q4hr or 4 g **IV** inf, then 1-2 g/hr cont inf, max 40 g/day or 20 g/48 hr in severe renal disease

**Available forms:** Chloride: sus rel tabs 535 mg (64 mg Mg); enteric tabs 833 mg (100 mg Mg); hydroxide: liquid 400 mg/5 ml (164 mg Mg/5 ml); conc liquid 800 mg/5 ml (328 mg Mg/5 ml); chew tabs 300, 600 mg; oxide: tabs 400 mg (241.3 mg Mg); caps 140 mg (84.5 mg Mg); sulfate: powder for oral; bulk packages; (epsom salts) bulk packages; inj 10, 12.5, 25, 50%; citrate: oral sol 240, 296, 300 ml bottles (77 mEq/100 ml)

**Adverse effects**
*CNS:* Muscle weakness, flushing, sweating, confusion, sedation, depressed reflexes, **flaccid paralysis, hypothermia**
*CV:* Hypotension, heart block, **circulatory collapse,** vasodilation
*GI: Nausea, vomiting, anorexia, cramps*
*HEMA:* Prolonged bleeding time
*META:* Electrolyte, fluid imbalances
*RESP:* **Respiratory depression/paralysis**

**Contraindications:** Hypersensitivity, abdominal pain, nausea/vomiting, obstruction, acute surgical abdomen, rectal bleeding, heart block, myocardial damage

**Precautions:** Pregnancy **A, B** (magnesium sulfate), renal disease/cardiac disease

| Pharmacokinetics | |
| --- | --- |
| **Absorption** | Unknown |
| **Distribution** | Unknown |
| **Metabolism** | Unknown |
| **Excretion** | Kidneys |
| **Half-life** | Unknown |
| | effective anticonvulsant levels 2.5-7.5 mEq/L |

| Pharmacodynamics | | | |
| --- | --- | --- | --- |
| | PO | IM | IV |
| **Onset** | 3-6 hr | 1 hr | Unknown |
| **Peak** | Unknown | Unknown | Unknown |
| **Duration** | Unknown | 4 hr | ½ hr |

**Interactions**
*Individual products*
Digoxin: decreased effect of digoxin
Nitrofurantoin: decreased absorption

*Drug classifications*
Antihypertensives: increased hypotension
Antiinfectives (aminoquinolones), tetracyclines: decreased absorption
Neuromuscular blockers: increased effect

**NURSING CONSIDERATIONS**
**Assessment**
• Assess I&O ratio; check for decrease in urinary output
• Assess cause of constipation; lack of fluids, bulk, exercise
• Assess cramping, rectal bleeding, nausea, vomiting; product should be discontinued
◆ Assess Mg toxicity: thirst, confusion, decrease in reflexes
• Assess visual changes: blurring, halos, corneal and retinal damage
• Assess edema in feet, ankles, legs
• Assess prior product history; there are many product interactions

**Nursing diagnoses**
• Constipation (uses)
• Injury, risk for, physical
• Knowledge, deficient (teaching)

**Implementation**
**PO route**
• Administer with 8 oz of $H_2O$
• Refrigerate magnesium citrate before administration
• Shake susp before using
• Administer to patient crushed or whole; chewable tablets may be chewed
• Administer with food or milk to decrease gastric symptoms; give 30 min before or 2 hr after antacids
**IV route**
• Administer only when calcium gluconate available for magnesium toxicity
• Administer **IV** undiluted 1.5 ml of 10% sol over 1 min; may dilute to 20% sol, infuse over 3 hr
• Administer **IV** at less than 150 mg/min; circulatory collapse may occur
*Y-site compatibilities:* Acyclovir, aldesleukin, amifostine, amikacin, ampicillin, aztreonam, cefamandole, cefazolin, cefmetazole, cefoperazone, cefotaxime, cefoxitin, cephalothin, cephapirin, chloramphenicol, cisatracurium, DOBUTamine, doxycycline, DOXOrubicin liposome, enalaprilat, erythromycin, esmolol, famotidine, fludarabine, gallium, gentamicin, granisetron, heparin, hydromorphone, idarubicin, insulin, kanamycin, labetalol, meperidine, metronidazole, minocycline, morphine, moxalactam, nafcillin, ondansetron, oxacillin, paclitaxel, penicillin G

potassium, piperacillin, piperacillin/
tazobactam, potassium chloride, propofol,
remifentanil, sargramostim, thiotepa, ticarcillin, tobramycin, trimethoprim/
sulfamethoxazole, vancomycin, vit B
complex/C
**Additive compatibilities:** Cephalothin,
chloramphenicol, cisplatin, heparin, hydrocortisone, isoproterenol, meropenem, methyldopate, norepinephrine, penicillin G potassium,
potassium phosphate, verapamil

**Patient/family education**
• Inform patient to report any symptoms of
hepatotoxicity, renal toxicity, visual changes,
ototoxicity, allergic reactions, bleeding (long-
term therapy)
• Inform patient not to exceed recommended
dosage; acute poisoning may result
• Inform patient to read label on other OTC
products; many contain aspirin
• Inform patient that therapeutic response
takes 2 wk (arthritis)
• Inform patient to avoid alcohol ingestion; GI
bleeding may occur
• Inform patient that if anticoagulants are
given with this product, both should be discontinued 2 wk before surgery

**Evaluation**
**Positive therapeutic outcome**
• Decreased pain, fever

**Treatment of overdose:** Lavage,
activated charcoal, monitor electrolytes, VS

## mannitol (Rx)
(man'i-tole)
mannitol, Osmitrol, Resectisol
*Func. class.:* Diuretic-osmotic
*Chem. class.:* Hexahydric alcohol
**Pregnancy category** C

**Action:** Increases osmolarity of glomerular
filtrate, which raises osmotic pressure of fluid
in renal tubules; there is a decrease in reabsorption of water, electrolytes; increases in
urinary output, sodium, chloride, potassium,
calcium, phosphorus, uric acid, urea, magnesium

**Uses:** Edema; promote systemic diuresis in
cerebral edema, decrease intraocular pressure, improve renal function in acute renal
failure, chemical poisoning

**Dosage and routes**
**Oliguria, prevention**
*Adult:* **IV** 50-100 g of a 5%-25% sol, may
use test dose 0.2 g/kg over 3-5 min

**Oliguria, treatment**
*Adult:* **IV** 300-400 mg/kg of a 20%-25% sol
up to 100 g of a 15%-20% sol over 30-60 min
*Child:* **IV** 0.25-2 g/kg as a 15%-20% sol, run
over 2-6 hr

**Intraocular pressure/ICP**
*Adult:* **IV** 0.25-2 g/kg of a 15%-25% sol
over 30-60 min
*Child:* **IV** 1-2 g/kg (30-60 g/m$^2$) as a
15%-20% sol run over 2-6 hr

**Renal failure**
*Adult:* **IV** 50-200 g/24 hr, adjusting to
maintain output of 30-50 mg/hr

**Diuresis in product intoxication**
*Adult and child >12 yr:* 5%-10% sol
continuously up to 200 g **IV**, while maintaining 100-500 ml urine output/hr

**Available forms:** Inj 5%, 10%, 15%,
20%, 25%; GU irrigation 5%

**Adverse effects**
*CNS:* Dizziness, headache, **seizures, rebound increased ICP,** confusion
*CV:* Edema, hypotension, hypertension, **tachycardia, CHF,** thrombophlebitis, angina-like
chest pains, fever, chills, **circulatory overload**
*EENT:* Loss of hearing, blurred vision, nasal
congestion, decreased intraocular pressure
*ELECT:* Fluid, electrolyte imbalances, **acidosis,** electrolyte loss, dehydration, hyper/
hypokalemia
*GI:* Nausea, vomiting, dry mouth, diarrhea
*GU:* Marked diuresis, urinary retention, thirst
*RESP:* Pulmonary congestion

**Contraindications:** Active intracranial
bleeding, hypersensitivity, anuria, severe
pulmonary congestion, edema, severe dehydration, progressive heart disease, renal
failure

**Precautions:** Pregnancy **C,** breastfeeding,
dehydration, severe renal disease, CHF, electrolyte imbalances

| Pharmacokinetics | |
|---|---|
| Absorption | Complete |
| Distribution | Extracellular spaces |
| Metabolism | Minimal |
| Excretion | Renal |
| Half-life | 100 min |

M

| Pharmacodynamics | |
|---|---|
| **Onset** | ½-1 hr |
| **Peak** | 1 hr |
| **Duration** | 6-8 hr |

## Interactions
### Drug/food
Potassium foods: increased hyperkalemia
### Drug/lab test
Interference: inorganic phosphorus, ethylene glycol

## NURSING CONSIDERATIONS
### Assessment
• Assess neurologic status: LOC, ICP reading, pupil size and reaction when product is given for increased ICP

• Assess for visual changes or eye discomfort or pain before and during treatment; (increases intraocular pressure); neurologic checks, ICP during treatment (increased ICP)

• Assess patient for tinnitus, hearing loss, ear pain; periodic testing of hearing is needed when high doses of this product are given by **IV** route

• Monitor manifestations of hypokalemia: acidic urine, reduced urine osmolality, nocturia, polyuria, polydipsia; hypotension, broad T wave, U wave, ectopy, tachycardia, weak pulse; muscle weakness, altered LOC, drowsiness, apathy, lethargy, confusion, depression; anorexia, nausea, cramps, constipation, distention, paralytic ileus; hypoventilation, respiratory muscle weakness

• Monitor for manifestations of hyponatremia: increased B/P, cold, clammy skin, hypovolemia or hypervolemia; anorexia, nausea, vomiting, diarrhea, abdominal cramps; lethargy, increased ICP, confusion, headache, seizures, coma, fatigue, tremors, hyperreflexia

• Assess fluid volume status: check I&O ratios and record hourly urine values, CVP, breath sounds, weight, distended red veins, crackles in lung, color, quality and specific gravity of urine, skin turgor, adequacy of pulses, moist mucous membranes, bilateral lung sounds, peripheral pitting edema

• Assess for dehydration; symptoms of decreasing output, thirst, hypotension, dry mouth and mucous membranes should be reported

• Monitor electrolytes: potassium, sodium, calcium, magnesium; also include BUN, ABGs, CVP, PAP, CBC; regularly monitor serum and urine levels of sodium and potassium

• Assess B/P before and during therapy with patient lying, standing, and sitting as appropriate; orthostatic hypotension can occur rapidly

• Monitor for rebound ICP: headache, confusion

### Nursing diagnoses
• Fluid volume, deficient (adverse reactions)
• Fluid volume, excess (uses)
• Knowledge, deficient (teaching)
• Urinary elimination, impaired (adverse reactions)

### Implementation
• Administer potassium replacement if potassium level is <3 mg/ml

• Use an in-line filter for 15%, 20%, 25% give with infusion pump; check **IV** patency at infusion site before and during administration; do not use sol that is yellow or has a precipitate or crystals; to redissolve, run bottle under hot water and shake vigorously; cool to body temp before giving

• Run at 30-50 ml/hr in oliguria

• Run over 30-60 min in increased ICP

• Run over 30 min for intraocular pressure; 60-90 min after surgery

**Irrigation**
• Use 100 ml of 25%/900 ml of sterile water for inj (2.5% sol)

**Y-site compatibilities:** Allopurinol, amifostine, aztreonam, cladribine, fludarabine, fluorouracil, gallium, idarubicin, melphalan, ondansetron, paclitaxel, piperacillin, propofol, sargramostim, teniposide, thiotepa, vinorelbine

**Y-site incompatibilities:** Amsacrine, bleomycin, DOXOrubicin, fluconazole, gentamicin, quinidine, vinBLAStine, vinCRIStine

**Additive compatibilities:** Amikacin, bretylium, cefamandole, cefoxitin, cimetidine, cisplatin, DOPamine, fosphenytoin, furosemide, gentamicin, metoclopramide, netilmicin, nizatidine, ofloxacin, ondansetron, sodium bicarbonate, tobramycin, verapamil

**Additive incompatibilities:** Blood, blood products, imipenem-cilastatin, potassium chloride, sodium chloride

### Patient/family education
• Teach patient reason for and method of treatment

### Evaluation
**Positive therapeutic outcome**
• Decreased intraocular pressure
• Prevention of hypokalemia (diuretic use)
• Decreased edema
• Decreased ICP
• Increased diuresis of >30 ml/hr
• Increased excretion of toxic substances

**Treatment of overdose:** Discontinue infusion, correct fluid, electrolyte imbalances, hemodialysis, monitor hydration, CV, renal function

---

## maraviroc (Rx)
(mah-rav′er-rock)
Selzentry
*Func. class.:* Antiretroviral
*Chem. class.:* Fusion inhibitor
**Pregnancy category** B

**Action:** Interferes with entry into HIV-1 by inhibiting the fusion of the virus and cell membrane

**Therapeutic outcome:** Improvement in $CD_4$, viral load, T-cell count

**Uses:** CCR5-tropic HIV in combination with other antiretroviral agents in treating experienced patients

**Dosage and routes**
*Those not taking any CYP3A inducers/inhibitors*
*Adult:* PO 300 mg bid

*Those taking CYP3A4 inhibitors with/without a CYP3A inducer*
*Adult:* PO 150 mg bid

*Those taking CYP3A4 inducers without a strong CYP3A inhibitor*
*Adult:* PO 600 mg bid

**Available forms:** Tabs 150, 300 mg

**Adverse effects**
*CNS:* Dizziness, depression, **viral meningitis**, disturbances in consciousness, peripheral neuropathy, paresthesia, dysesthesia, fever
*CV:* **MI, cardiac ischemia, orthostatic hypotension**
*EENT:* Gingival hyperplasia
*GI:* Diarrhea, constipation, dyspepsia, **pseudomembranous colitis, hepatotoxicity**
*INTEG:* Rash, urticaria, pruritus, folliculitis
*MS:* Joint pain, leg pain, muscle cramps
*RESP:* Cough, URI, sinusitis, bronchitis, pneumonia, **bronchospasm, obstruction**
*SYST:* Herpes virus

**Contraindications:** Hypersensitivity

**Precautions:** Pregnancy **B**, breastfeeding, renal/hepatic disease, electrolyte imbalance, dehydration

**Pharmacokinetics**

| | |
|---|---|
| **Absorption** | Unknown |
| **Distribution** | Unknown |
| **Metabolism** | By P450 system, CYP3A metabolism |
| **Excretion** | Urine 20%, feces 76% |
| **Half-life** | Unknown |

**Pharmacodynamics**
Unknown

**Interactions**
*Drug classifications*
CYP3A inhibitors (amiodarone, aprepitant, chloramphenicol, clarithromycin, conivaptan, cycloSPORINE, dalfopristin, danazol, diltiazem, erythromycin, estradiol, fluconazole, fluvoxamine, imatinib, isoniazid, itraconazole, ketoconazole, miconazole, nefazodone, niCARdipine, propoxyphene, RU-486, tamoxifen, telithromycin, troleandomycin, verapamil, voriconazole, zafirlukast): increased maraviroc levels
*Drug/food*
High-fat meal: decreased absorption 33%

**NURSING CONSIDERATIONS**
**Assessment**
• Assess for signs of infection
• Monitor blood tests: $CD_4$, T-cell count, plasma HIV RNA
• Monitor renal tests: serum creatinine
• Monitor C&S before product therapy; product may be taken as soon as culture is taken; repeat C&S after treatment; determine the presence of other infections
• Assess bowel pattern before, during treatment
• Assess skin eruptions: rash, urticaria, itching
• Assess allergies before treatment and before each dose

**Nursing diagnoses**
• Injury, risk for (uses, adverse reactions)
• Knowledge deficient (teaching)

**Implementation**
• May give without regard to meals, with 8 oz of water
• Store at room temperature

**Patient/family education**
• Advise patient to take as prescribed; if dose is missed, take as soon as remembered up to 1 hr before next dose; do not double dose; that product does not cure the condition
• Teach patient that product does not cure infection, just controls symptoms and does not prevent infecting others

M

Adverse effects: *italic* = common, **bold** = life-threatening

◆ Teach patient to report sore throat, fever, fatigue (may indicate superinfection)
• Advise patient that product must be taken in equal intervals around the clock to maintain blood levels for duration of therapy
• Teach patient to notify prescriber of side effects

### Evaluation
**Positive therapeutic outcome**
• Improvement in CD4, viral load, T-cell count

---

## mebendazole (Rx)
(me-ben′da-zole)
Vermox
*Func. class.:* Anthelmintic
*Chem. class.:* Carbamate

**Pregnancy category C**

**Action:** Inhibits glucose uptake, degeneration of cytoplasmic microtubules in the cell; interferes with absorption, secretory function

**Therapeutic outcome:** Parasite, cyst, egg death

**Uses:** Infestation with pinworms, roundworms, hookworms, whipworms, threadworms, pork tapeworms, dwarf tapeworms, beef tapeworms; hydatid cyst

### Dosage and routes
*Adult and child >2 yr:* PO 100 mg as a single dose (pinworms) or bid × 3 days (whipworms, roundworms, or hookworms); course may be repeated in 3 wk if needed

**Available forms:** Chew tabs 100 mg

### Adverse effects
*CNS:* Dizziness, fever, headache, **seizures (rare)**
*GI:* Transient diarrhea, abdominal pain, nausea, vomiting, constipation, **hepatitis**
*INTEG:* Rash

**Contraindication:** Hypersensitivity

**Precautions:** Pregnancy **C** (1st trimester), breastfeeding, children <2 yr, Crohn's disease, hepatic disease, IBD, ulcerative colitis

| Pharmacokinetics | |
|---|---|
| **Absorption** | Minimal |
| **Distribution** | Highly bound to plasma proteins |
| **Metabolism** | Liver |
| **Excretion** | Feces in metabolites (>95%); urine, unchanged |
| **Half-life** | 2½-9 hr; increased in hepatic disease |

| Pharmacodynamics | |
|---|---|
| **Onset** | Unknown |
| **Peak** | ½-7 hr |
| **Duration** | Unknown |

### Interactions
*Individual drugs*
Carbamazepine: decreased effect of mebendazole
*Drug classifications*
Hydantoins: decreased effect of mebendazole
*Drug/food*
High-fat foods: increased absorption

### NURSING CONSIDERATIONS
**Assessment**
• Assess stools during entire treatment, also 1-3 wk after treatment is completed; specimens must be sent to lab while still warm; monitor for diarrhea during expulsion of worms; avoid self-contamination with patient's feces
• Assess for allergic reaction: rash (rare)
• Identify infestation in other family members, since transmission from person to person is common
• If pinworms are suspected, place a piece of cellophane tape over the anal area at night for 1 wk after treatment at night to identify ova; negative perianal swabs taken every AM for 3 days confirm that the patient is no longer infested
• Monitor blood tests: AST, ALT, alkaline phosphatase, BUN, CBC during treatment

**Nursing diagnoses**
• Infection, risk for (uses)
• Knowledge, deficient (teaching)

**Implementation**
• Tabs may be chewed or crushed and mixed with food if patient is unable to swallow whole
• Give PO after meals to avoid GI symptoms
• Give second course after 3 wk if needed; usually recommended (pinworms)
• Store in airtight container

**Patient/family education**
• Teach patient proper hygiene after bowel movements, including hand-washing technique; tell patient to avoid putting fingers in mouth; clean fingernails
• Advise patient that infested person should sleep alone; do not shake bed linen; wash bed linen daily in hot water; change and wash undergarments daily; that all members of the family should be treated (pinworms)
• Advise patient to clean toilet daily with disinfectant (green soap sol)

---

 Alert     Canada Only     Drug on CD    * "Tall Man" lettering (See Preface)

- Inform patient that compliance is needed with dosage schedule, duration of treatment
- Tell patient to wear shoes, wash all fruits and vegetables well before eating, use commercial fruit and vegetable cleaner solution
- Advise patient to report jaundice, liver pain

### Evaluation
**Positive therapeutic outcome**
- Expulsion of worms
- Three negative stool cultures after completion of treatment

---

## mecasermin (Rx)
(mec-a'sir-men)
Increlex
*Func. class.:* Biologic response modifier; insulin-like growth factor

**Pregnancy category C**

**Action:** Stimulates growth; IGF-1 is the principal hormonal mediator of statural growth. GH binds to its receptor in the liver and other tissues

**Therapeutic outcome:** Increased height

**Uses:** Growth failure in children with severe primary insulin-like growth factor-1 (IGF-1) deficiency (primary IGFD) or with growth hormone (GH) gene deletion who have developed neutralizing antibodies to GH

**Unlabeled uses:** ALS

### Dosage and routes
*Child:* SUBCUT 0.04-0.08 mg/kg (40-80 mcg/kg) bid; if well tolerated for 1 wk, may increase by 0.04 mg/kg/dose, max 0.12 mg/kg bid

**Available forms:** Inj 10 mg/ml

### Adverse effects
*CNS:* Headache, **seizures,** dizziness, cardiac valvulopathy
*CV:* Cardiac murmur
*EENT:* Ear pain, otitis media, abnormal tympanometry, papilledema, visual impairment
*ENDO:* **Hypoglycemia, ketosis, hypothyroidism**
*GU:* Vomiting
*HEMA:* Thymus hypertrophy
*META:* Hypoglycemia
*MISC:* Bruising, lipohypertrophy, hypersensitivity reactions
*MS:* Arthralgia, joint pain
*RESP:* Snoring, tonsillar hypertrophy, **apnea**
*SYST:* **Antibodies to growth hormone**

**Contraindications:** Hypersensitivity, benzyl alcohol, closed epiphyses, active/suspected neoplasia, **IV** use

**Precautions:** Pregnancy **C**, breastfeeding, children <2 yr, diabetes mellitus, hypothyroidism, increased ICP, malnutrition, scoliosis, sleep apnea

### Pharmacokinetics
| | |
|---|---|
| **Absorption** | Near 100% |
| **Distribution** | Unknown |
| **Metabolism** | Liver/kidneys |
| **Excretion** | Unknown |
| **Half-life** | 5.8 hr |

### Pharmacodynamics
Unknown

### Interactions
*Drug classifications*
Antidiabetics, corticosteroids: increased hypoglycemia

### NURSING CONSIDERATIONS
**Assessment**
- Monitor preprandial glucose at beginning of treatment and until well tolerated
- Monitor by funduscopic exam at beginning and periodically during treatment
- Assess for allergic reactions; if present, interrupt treatment and notify prescriber
- Assess growth rate of child at intervals during treatment

**Nursing diagnoses**
- Knowledge, deficient (teaching)

**Implementation**
**SUBCUT route**
- Rotate inj site; use sterile, disposable syringe/needles; use small-volume syringe for accurate measurement
- Give shortly before or after a meal or snack to lessen hypoglycemia
- Store in refrigerator before opening, avoid freezing; after opening, stable for 30 days after initial vial entry, store in refrigerator, do not use if particulate matter is present, avoid direct light, do not use after expiration date

**Patient/family education**
- Teach patient that treatment may continue for years; regular assessments are required
- Advise patient to avoid hazardous activities, driving within 2-3 hr of dosing
- Teach patient correct administration and needle disposal

M

## Evaluation
**Positive therapeutic outcome**
- Growth in children

---

## mechlorethamine (Rx)
(me-klor-eth'a-meen)
Mustargen, nitrogen mustard
*Func. class.:* Antineoplastic alkylating agent
*Chem. class.:* Nitrogen mustard

**Pregnancy category D**

**Action:** Alkylates DNA, RNA; inhibits enzymes that allow synthesis of amino acids in proteins; activity is not cell cycle phase specific; a vesicant

**Therapeutic outcome:** Prevention of rapidly growing malignant cells

**Uses:** Hodgkin's disease, lymphomas, leukemias, lymphosarcoma; ovarian, breast, lung carcinoma; neoplastic effusions

### Dosage and routes
*Adult:* IV 0.4 mg/kg or 6 mg/m² as 1 dose or 2-4 divided doses over 2-4 days; second course after 3 wk depending on blood cell count

### Neoplastic effusions
*Adult:* INTRACAVITY 0.4 mg/kg, may be 200-400 mcg/kg

**Available forms:** Inj 10 mg/vial

### Adverse effects
*CNS: Headache, dizziness, drowsiness, paresthesia,* peripheral neuropathy, **coma**
*EENT:* Tinnitus, hearing loss
*GI: Nausea, vomiting, diarrhea, stomatitis, weight loss,* colitis, **hepatotoxicity**
*HEMA:* **Thrombocytopenia, leukopenia, agranulocytosis,** anemia
*INTEG: Alopecia,* pruritus, herpes zoster, extravasation

**Contraindications:** Pregnancy **D**, breastfeeding, myelosuppression, acute herpes zoster

**Precautions:** Radiation therapy, chronic lymphocytic leukopenia

### Pharmacokinetics

| | |
|---|---|
| **Absorption** | Complete (**IV**) |
| **Distribution** | Unknown |
| **Metabolism** | Tissues/fluids |
| **Excretion** | Kidneys |
| **Half-life** | Unknown |

### Pharmacodynamics

| | IV |
|---|---|
| **Onset** | 1 day |
| **Peak** | 1-2 wk |
| **Duration** | 1-3 wk |

### Interactions
*Individual drugs*
Amphotericin B: increased blood dyscrasia
Aspirin: increased bleeding
Radiation: increased toxicity
*Drug classifications*
Anticoagulants, NSAIDs: increased bleeding
Antineoplastics: increased toxicity
Live virus vaccines: decreased antibody reaction

### NURSING CONSIDERATIONS
**Assessment**
- Monitor CBC, differential, platelet count weekly; withhold product if WBC is <1000/mm³ or platelet count is <75,000/mm³; notify prescriber of results if WBC <20,000/mm³, platelets <150,000/mm³; recovery of WBC platelets within 20 days
- Monitor pulmonary function tests, chest x-ray films before, during therapy; chest film should be obtained q2 wk during treatment; assess for dyspnea, crackles, unproductive cough, chest pain, tachypnea
- Assess for increased uric acid levels, swelling, joint pain primarily in extremities; patient should be well hydrated to prevent urate deposits
- Monitor renal function tests: BUN, serum uric acid, urine CCr before, during therapy; I&O ratio; report fall in urine output of 30 ml/hr; for decreased hyperuricemia
- Monitor for cold, fever, sore throat (may indicate beginning of infection); identify edema in feet, joint and stomach pain, shaking; prescriber should be notified
- Assess for bleeding: hematuria, guaiac, bruising or petechiae, mucosa or orifices; no rectal temp

**Nursing diagnoses**
- Body image, disturbed (adverse reactions)
- Infection, risk for (adverse reactions)
- Injury, risk for (adverse reactions)
- Knowledge, deficient (teaching)

**Implementation**
- Give fluids **IV** or PO before chemotherapy to hydrate patient
- Give antacid before oral agent; give product after evening meal, before bedtime; administer antiemetic 30-60 min and dexamethasone before giving product and prn to prevent

---

vomiting; give antibiotics for prophylaxis of infection
• Give topical or systemic analgesics for pain
• Give in AM so product can be eliminated before bedtime
• Use a liquid diet: carbonated beverages; gelatin may be added if patient is not nauseated or vomiting
**Intracavity route**
• Further dilute in 100 ml of 0.9% NaCl; administration is completed by prescriber
• Watch for infiltration; if infiltration occurs, infiltrate area with isotonic sodium thiosulfate; apply ice for 6-12 hr, a vesicant
**IV route**
• Give **IV** after diluting 10 mg/10 ml sterile water or 0.9% NaCl; leave needle in vial, shake, withdraw dose, give through Y-tube or 3-way stopcock or directly over 3-5 min into running **IV** of 0.9% NaCl
*Y-site compatibilities:* Amifostine, aztreonam, filgrastim, fludarabine, granisetron, melphalan, ondansetron, sargramostim, teniposide, vinorelbine
*Additive incompatibilities:* Methohexital
*Solution incompatibilities:* D$_5$W, 0.9% NaCl (**IV** only)
**Patient/family education**
• Teach patient to avoid use of products containing aspirin or ibuprofen, razors, commercial mouthwash, since bleeding may occur; to report symptoms of bleeding (hematuria, tarry stools)
• Teach patient to report signs of anemia (fatigue, headache, irritability, faintness, shortness of breath)
• Advise patient to report any changes in breathing or coughing even several months after treatment; to avoid crowds and persons with respiratory tract or other infections
• Tell patient hair loss is common; discuss the use of wigs or hairpieces
• Caution patient not to have any vaccinations without the advice of the prescriber, serious reactions can occur
• Advise patient that contraception is needed during treatment and for several months after the completion of therapy
• Have patient rinse mouth tid-qid with water, club soda; brush teeth bid-qid with soft brush or cotton-tipped applicators for stomatitis; use unwaxed dental floss
**Evaluation**
**Positive therapeutic outcome**
• Decreased size of tumor
• Decreased spread of malignancy

• Improved blood values
• Absence of sweating at night
• Increased appetite, increased weight

---

## meclizine (OTC, Rx)
(mek'li-zeen)
Antivert, Antrizine, Bonamine ✦, Bonine, Dramamine Less Drowsy Formula, meclizine HCl, Meni-D, Vergan
*Func. class.:* Antiemetic, antihistamine, anticholinergic
*Chem. class.:* H$_1$-Receptor antagonist, piperazine derivative

**Pregnancy category B**

**Action:** Acts centrally by blocking chemoreceptor trigger zone, which in turn acts on vomiting center

**Therapeutic outcome:** Decreased nausea in motion sickness; decreased vertigo

**Uses:** Vertigo, motion sickness

**Dosage and routes**
*Vertigo*
*Adult:* PO 25-100 mg/day in divided doses
*Motion sickness*
*Adult:* PO 25-50 mg 1 hr before traveling; repeat dose q12-24 hr prn

**Available forms:** Tabs 12.5, 25, 50 mg; chew tabs 25 mg; caps 25, 30 mg

**Adverse effects**
*CNS: Drowsiness,* fatigue, restlessness, headache, insomnia
*CV:* Hypotension
*EENT:* Dry mouth, blurred vision
*GI:* Nausea, anorexia, constipation, increased appetite
*GU:* Urinary retention

**Contraindications:** Hypersensitivity to cyclizines, shock

**Precautions:** Pregnancy **B**, breastfeeding, children, geriatric, angle-closure glaucoma, glaucoma, urinary retention, prostatic hypertrophy, CV disease, hypertension, seizure disorder

| Pharmacokinetics | |
|---|---|
| **Absorption** | Well |
| **Distribution** | Unknown |
| **Metabolism** | Unknown |
| **Excretion** | Unknown |
| **Half-life** | 6 hr |

M

| Pharmacodynamics | |
|---|---|
| Onset | 1 hr |
| Peak | Unknown |
| Duration | 8-24 hr |

## Interactions
*Individual drugs*
Alcohol: increased effects
*Drug classifications*
CNS depressants, opioids: increased CNS depression
*Drug/herb*
Corkwood, henbane leaf: increased anticholinergic effect
Hops, Jamaican dogwood, khat, senega: increased sedative effect
*Drug/lab test*
False negative: allergy skin testing

## NURSING CONSIDERATIONS
### Assessment
• Monitor VS, B/P
◆ Assess for signs of toxicity of other products or masking of symptoms of disease: brain tumor, intestinal obstruction
• Observe for drowsiness, dizziness, LOC

### Nursing diagnoses
• Injury, risk for (adverse reactions)
• Knowledge, deficient (teaching)

### Implementation
• Tabs may be swallowed whole, chewed, or allowed to dissolve; give with food to decrease GI upset
• Give lowest possible dose in geriatric, anticholinergic effects

### Patient/family education
• Teach patient that a false-negative result may occur with skin testing for allergies; these procedures should not be scheduled for 4 days after discontinuing use
• Teach patient to avoid hazardous activities, activities requiring alertness; dizziness may occur; instruct patient to request assistance with ambulation
• Teach patient to avoid alcohol, other depressants, breastfeeding

### Evaluation
**Positive therapeutic outcome**
• Absence of dizziness, vomiting

**\*medroxyPROGESTERone** (Rx)
(me-drox-ee-proe-jess'te-rone)
Amen, Curretab, Cycrin, Depo-Provera, medroxyPROGESTERone, Provera
*Func. class.:* Hormone—progestogen; contraceptive; antineoplastic
*Chem. class.:* Progesterone derivative

**Pregnancy category** X

**Do not confuse:**
medroxyPROGESTERone/methylPREDNISolone, Amen/Ambien, Provera/Premarin/Covera

**Action:** Inhibits secretion of pituitary gonadotropins, which prevents follicular maturation and ovulation; stimulates growth of mammary tissue; antineoplastic action against endometrial cancer

**Therapeutic outcome:** Decreased abnormal uterine bleeding, absence of amenorrhea

**Uses:** Uterine bleeding (abnormal), secondary amenorrhea, endometrial cancer, renal cancer, contraceptive, prevention of endometrial changes associated with estrogen replacement therapy (ERT)

**Unlabeled uses:** Pickwickian syndrome, sleep apnea

**Dosage and routes**
*Secondary amenorrhea*
*Adult:* PO 5-10 mg/day × 5-10 days

*Uterine bleeding*
*Adult:* PO 5-10 mg/day × 5-10 days starting on 16th or 21st day of menstrual cycle

*With ERT*
*Adult:* PO Monophasic 2.5 mg/day; biphasic 5 mg days 15-28 of cycle

*Contraceptive*
*Adult:* IM 150 mg q12 wk

**Available forms:** Tabs 2.5, 5, 10 mg; inj susp 50, 150, 400 mg/ml; 104 mg/0.65 ml

**Adverse effects**
*CNS:* Dizziness, headache, migraines, depression, fatigue, nervousness
*CV:* Hypotension, thrombophlebitis, edema, **thromboembolism, stroke, pulmonary embolism, MI**
*EENT:* Diplopia
*GI:* Nausea, vomiting, anorexia, cramps, increased weight, **cholestatic jaundice,** abdominal pain
*GU:* Amenorrhea, cervical erosion, breakthrough bleeding, dysmenorrhea, vaginal candidiasis, breast changes, *gynecomastia,*

*testicular atrophy, impotence,* endometri-
osis, **spontaneous abortion**
***INTEG:*** Rash, urticaria, acne, hirsutism,
alopecia, oily skin, seborrhea, purpura,
melasma, photosensitivity
***META:*** Hyperglycemia
***MS:*** Decreased bone density
***SYST:*** **Angioedema, anaphylaxis**

**Contraindications:** Pregnancy **X**, breast
cancer, hypersensitivity, thromboembolic
disorders, reproductive cancer, genital bleeding (abnormal, undiagnosed), missed abortion

**Precautions:** Breastfeeding, hypertension,
asthma, blood dyscrasias, gallbladder disease,
CHF, diabetes mellitus, bone disease, depression, migraine headache, seizure disorders,
renal/hepatic disease, family history of cancer
of breast or reproductive tract, bone mineral
density loss, ocular disorders

---

| Pharmacokinetics | | |
| --- | --- | --- |
| Unknown | | |

| Pharmacodynamics | | |
| --- | --- | --- |
| | PO | IM |
| **Onset** | Unknown | Unknown |
| **Peak** | Unknown | Unknown |
| **Duration** | 2-4 hr | Unknown |

---

**Interactions**
*Individual drugs*
Aminoglutethimide: decreased contraceptive
   effect
*Drug/lab test*
Increased: alkaline phosphatase, preg-
   nanediol, amino acids, sodium
Decreased: GTT, HDL

**NURSING CONSIDERATIONS**
**Assessment**
• Assess for symptoms indicating severe
allergic reaction, angioedema; have epINEPH-
rine and resuscitative equipment available
• Monitor B/P at beginning of treatment and
periodically; check weight daily; notify prescriber of weekly weight gain >5 lb; bone
mineral density
• Monitor I&O ratio: be alert for decreasing
urinary output, increasing edema, hypertension
• Assess liver function tests: ALT, AST, bilirubin, periodically during long-term therapy
• Assess for edema, hypertension, cardiac
symptoms, jaundice
• Assess mental status: affect, mood, behavioral changes, depression

**Nursing diagnoses**
• Injury, risk for (adverse reactions)
• Knowledge, deficient (teaching)
• Sexual dysfunction (uses)
• Tissue perfusion, ineffective (adverse
reactions)

**Implementation**
**PO route**
• Give with food or milk to decrease GI
symptoms
**IM route**
• Store in dark area
• Give titrated dosage; use lowest effective
dosage; give oil sol deep in large muscle mass
(IM); rotate sites; use after warming to dis-
solve crystals

**Patient/family education**
• Advise patients to avoid sunlight or use
sunscreen; photosensitivity and melasma
(brown patches on the face) can occur
• Teach patient about cushingoid symptoms:
weight gain, moon face, buffalo hump, acne
• Teach women patients to report breast
lumps, vaginal bleeding, edema, jaundice,
dark urine, clay-colored stools, dyspnea,
headache, blurred vision, abdominal pain,
sudden changes in speech/coordination,
numbness or stiffness in legs, chest pain; men
to report impotence or gynecomastia
• Teach patient to report suspected pregnancy
immediately; fertility returns in 6-12 mo after
discontinuing
• Teach patient that long-term use decreases
bone density; exercise, calcium supplements
can help lessen this

**Evaluation**
**Positive therapeutic outcome**
• Decreased abnormal uterine bleeding
• Absence of amenorrhea
• Prevention of pregnancy
• Arrested spread of malignant cells

---

**medrysone ophthalmic**
*See Appendix D*

M

---

Adverse effects: *italic* = common, **bold** = life-threatening

## megestrol (Rx)

(me-jess'trole)

Megace, Megace ES, megestrol

*Func. class.:* Antineoplastic hormone

*Chem. class.:* Progestin

### Pregnancy category
D (tabs),
X (susp)

### Do not confuse:
Megace/Reglan

**Action:** Affects endometrium by antiluteinizing effect; this is thought to bring about cell death

**Therapeutic outcome:** Prevention of rapidly growing malignant cells; weight gain, increased appetite in AIDS

**Uses:** Breast, endometrial, renal cell cancer; increase weight, decrease cachexia and anorexia associated with AIDS

**Unlabeled uses:** Hot flashes, prostate cancer

### Dosage and routes
*Endometrial/ovarian carcinoma*
*Adult:* PO 40-320 mg/day in divided doses

*Breast carcinoma*
*Adult:* PO 40 mg qid or 160 mg/day

*Anorexia (AIDS)*
*Adult:* PO 800 mg/day (oral susp) or 625 mg/day (ES)

*Hot flashes (unlabeled)*
*Adult:* PO 20 mg/day

**Available forms:** Tabs 20, 40 mg; oral susp 40, 125 mg/ml

### Adverse effects
*CNS:* Mood swings, insomnia
*CV:* **Thrombophlebitis, thromboembolism,** hypertension
*ENDO:* Adrenal insufficiency
*GI:* Nausea, vomiting, diarrhea, abdominal cramps, weight gain, flatus, indigestion
*GU:* Gynecomastia, fluid retention, hypercalcemia, vaginal bleeding, discharge, impotence, decreased libido
*INTEG:* Alopecia, rash, pruritus, purpura, itching, sweating

**Contraindications:** Pregnancy **X** (susp), **D** (tabs), hypersensitivity

**Precautions:** Diabetes, thrombosis, adrenal insufficiency

### Pharmacokinetics

| | |
|---|---|
| **Absorption** | Well absorbed; food increases oral sol |
| **Distribution** | Unknown |
| **Metabolism** | Liver, completely |
| **Excretion** | Unknown |
| **Half-life** | 1 hr |

### Pharmacodynamics

| | |
|---|---|
| **Onset** | Several wk-mo |
| **Peak** | Unknown |
| **Duration** | 1-3 days |

### Interactions
*Drug/lab test*
Increased: alkaline phosphatase, urinary pregnanediol, plasma amino acids, urinary sodium
Decreased: HDL, GTT
False positive: urine glucose

### NURSING CONSIDERATIONS
**Assessment**
• Monitor effects of alopecia on body image; discuss feelings about body changes
• In AIDS patients monitor calorie counts, weight, appetite
• Assess for thrombophlebitis: pain, redness, swelling in legs; notify prescriber immediately if these occur

**Nursing diagnoses**
• Knowledge, deficient (teaching)

**Implementation**
• Administer with meals for GI symptoms
• Oral susp is usually used for AIDS patients, shake well
• Give tablets for carcinoma

**Patient/family education**
• Teach patient to report any complaints or side effects to prescriber
• Advise patient that contraceptive measures must be used during and several mo after treatment; product is teratogenic
• Explore with patient the need for wig or a hairpiece for hair loss
• Caution patient to report vaginal bleeding to prescriber
• Review with patient the need to comply with dosage schedule, not to miss or double doses; missed doses may be taken up to 1 hr before next dose
• Teach patient how to recognize signs of fluid retention, thromboembolism and report immediately

 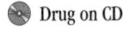

## Evaluation
**Positive therapeutic outcome**
- Decreased spread of malignant cells
- Weight gain, increased appetite in AIDS patients
- Resolved dysfunctional uterine bleeding

## meloxicam (Rx)
(mel-ox'i-kam)
Mobic
*Func. class.:* Nonsteroidal antiinflammatory/nonopioid analgesic (NSAIDs)
*Chem. class.:* Oxicam

**Pregnancy category**
C (1st trimester),
D (2nd/3rd trimesters)

**Action:** Inhibits prostaglandin synthesis by decreasing an enzyme needed for biosynthesis; analgesic, antiinflammatory, antipyretic effects

**Therapeutic outcome:** Decreased pain, swelling of joints; improved mobility

**Uses:** Osteoarthritis, rheumatoid arthritis, juvenile arthritis

**Dosage and routes**
*Adult:* PO 7.5 mg/day, may increase to 15 mg/day

**Available forms:** Tabs 7.5, 15 mg; susp 7.5 mg/5 ml

**Adverse effects**
*CNS:* Dizziness, drowsiness, tremors, headache, nervousness, malaise, fatigue, insomnia, depression, **seizures**
*CV:* Hypertension, angina, **cardiac failure, MI,** hypotension, palpitations, **dysrhythmias,** tachycardia, stroke
*EENT:* Tinnitus, hearing loss
*GI:* Pancreatitis, nausea, colitis, GERD, vomiting, diarrhea, constipation, flatulence, cramps, dry mouth, peptic ulcer, **GI bleeding, perforation**
*GU:* Nephrotoxicity: dysuria, hematuria, oliguria, azotemia
*HEMA:* **Blood dyscrasias,** anemia, prolonged bleeding
*INTEG:* Rash, urticaria, photosensitivity
*SYST:* Angioedema, anaphylaxis, **Stevens-Johnson syndrome, toxic epidermal necrosis**

**Contraindications:** Pregnancy **D** (2nd/3rd trimesters), labor and delivery, breastfeeding, hypersensitivity, asthma, severe renal/hepatic disease, peptic ulcer disease, CV bleeding, perioperative pain in CABG surgery

**Precautions:** Pregnancy **C** (1st trimester), children, geriatric, bleeding/GI/cardiac disorders, hypersensitivity to other antiinflammatory agents, CCr <25 ml/min

### Pharmacokinetics
| | |
|---|---|
| **Absorption** | Unknown |
| **Distribution** | Unknown |
| **Metabolism** | Liver <50% |
| **Excretion** | Breast milk, kidneys |
| **Half-life** | 6 hr |

### Pharmacodynamics
| | PO | IM |
|---|---|---|
| **Onset** | Unknown | Unknown |
| **Peak** | 4-5 hr | 50 min |
| **Duration** | Unknown | Unknown |

## Interactions
*Individual drugs*
Cholestyramine: decreased action of meloxicam
CycloSPORINE: increased nephrotoxicity
Phenytoin: increased action of meloxicam
*Drug classifications*
Aminoglycosides, anticoagulants, diuretics, hydantoins: increased action of each specific product
β-Adrenergic blockers: decreased action of β-blockers
Salicylates, sulfonamides: increased action of meloxicam
*Drug/herb*
Arginine, gossypol: increased gastric irritation
Bearberry, bilberry: increased NSAIDs effect
Bogbean, chondroitin: increased bleeding risk

## NURSING CONSIDERATIONS
### Assessment
- Monitor renal, liver, blood tests: BUN, creatinine, AST, ALT, Hgb before treatment, periodically thereafter
- Assess for bleeding times; check for bruising, bleeding; test for occult blood in urine
⬧ Assess for anaphylaxis and angioedema; emergency equipment should be nearby
⬧ Assess for hepatic dysfunction: jaundice, yellow sclera and skin, clay-colored stools
- Assess for audiometric, ophth exam before, during, after treatment
- Assess for GI condition, hypertension, cardiac conditions

### Nursing diagnoses
- Knowledge, deficient (teaching)
- Mobility, impaired physical (uses)
- Pain, chronic (uses)

Adverse effects: *italic* = common, **bold** = life-threatening

### Implementation
- May take without regard to meals, take with food for GI upset
- Take with full glass of water and sit upright for ½ hr
- Store at room temperature

### Patient/family education
- Advise patient to report blurred vision or ringing, roaring in ears (may indicate toxicity)
- Advise patient to avoid driving, other hazardous activities if dizziness or drowsiness occurs
- Teach patient to report change in urine pattern, weight increase, edema, pain increase in joints, fever, blood in urine (indicates nephrotoxicity); to report rash, black stools, or continuing headache
- Teach patient to not use alcohol, aspirin, acetaminophen without consulting prescriber

### Evaluation
**Positive therapeutic outcome**
- Decreased pain, stiffness, swelling in joints, able to move more easily

---

### ⚠ HIGH ALERT

## melphalan (Rx)
(mel'fa-lan)
Alkeran, L-Pam, phenylalanine mustard
*Func. class.:* Antineoplastic, alkylating agent
*Chem. class.:* Nitrogen mustard

**Pregnancy category D**

### Do not confuse:
melphalan/myleran

**Action:** Alkylates DNA, RNA; inhibits enzymes that allow synthesis of amino acids in proteins; activity is not cell cycle phase specific

**Therapeutic outcome:** Prevention of rapidly growing malignant cells

**Uses:** Multiple myeloma, malignant melanoma, advanced ovarian cancer

**Unlabeled uses:** Breast, testicular, prostate carcinoma; osteogenic sarcoma, chronic myelogenous leukemia, non-Hodgkin's lymphoma

### Dosage and routes
*Multiple myeloma*
**Adult:** PO 150 mcg/kg/day × 1 wk, then 21 days off, then 50 mcg/kg/day or 100-150 mcg/kg/day or 250 mcg/kg/day × 4 days for 2-3 wk, then 2-4 wk off, then 2-4 mg/day or 7 mg/m$^2$ × 5 days q5-6 wk

**Adult:** IV INF 16 mg/m$^2$; reduce in renal insufficiency; give over 15-20 min; give at 2-wk intervals × 4 doses, then at 4-wk intervals
*Ovarian carcinoma*
**Adult:** PO 200 mcg/kg/day × 5 days q4-5 wk

**Available forms:** Tabs 2 mg; inj 50 mg

### Adverse effects
*GI: Nausea, vomiting,* stomatitis, diarrhea, **hepatitis**
*GU:* Amenorrhea, hyperuricemia, gonadal suppression
*HEMA:* **Thrombocytopenia, neutropenia, leukopenia,** anemia
*INTEG:* Rash, urticaria, alopecia, pruritus
*RESP:* **Fibrosis, dysplasia**
*SYST:* **Anaphylaxis,** allergic reaction, **secondary malignancies**

**Contraindications:** Pregnancy **D,** breastfeeding, hypersensitivity to this product or other nitrogen mustards

**Precautions:** Children, radiation therapy, bone marrow depression, infection, renal disease

### Pharmacokinetics
| | |
|---|---|
| **Absorption** | Variable; incompletely absorbed |
| **Distribution** | Rapidly distributed, protein binding 80%-90% |
| **Metabolism** | Bloodstream |
| **Excretion** | Kidneys, unchanged (10%) |
| **Half-life** | 1½ hr |

### Pharmacodynamics
Unknown

### Interactions
*Individual drugs*
Carmustine: increased pulmonary toxicity
CycloSPORINE: increased renal failure risk
Nalidixic acid: increased enterocolitis risk
Radiation: increased toxicity
*Drug classifications*
Anticoagulants, NSAIDs: increased bleeding risk
Antineoplastics: increased toxicity
Live virus vaccines: increased adverse reactions; decreased antibody reaction
*Drug/lab test*
Increased: uric acid

### NURSING CONSIDERATIONS
**Assessment**
- Monitor CBC, differential, platelet count weekly; withhold product if WBC is <3000/mm$^3$ or platelet count is <100,000/mm$^3$; notify prescriber of results if WBC <20,000/

---

mm$^3$, platelets <100,000/mm$^3$; recovery usually occurs in 6 wk

• Monitor pulmonary function tests, chest x-ray films before, during therapy; chest film should be obtained q2 wk during treatment; check for dyspnea, crackles, unproductive cough, chest pain, tachypnea

• Assess for increased uric acid levels, swelling, joint pain primarily in extremities; patient should be well hydrated to prevent urate deposits

• Monitor renal function tests: BUN, serum uric acid, urine CCr before, during therapy; check I&O ratio; report fall in urine output of 30 ml/hr; check for decreased hyperuricemia; monitor AST, ALT

• Monitor for cold, fever, sore throat (may indicate beginning of infection); identify edema in feet, joint and stomach pain, shaking; prescriber should be notified

• Assess for bleeding: hematuria, guaiac, bruising or petechiae, from mucosa or orifices q8hr; no rectal temp

• Assess for symptoms indicating severe allergic reaction: rash, pruritus, urticaria, purpuric skin lesions, itching, flushing; assess allergy to chlorambucil, cross-sensitivity may occur

## Nursing diagnoses

• Body image, disturbed (adverse reactions)
• Infection, risk for (adverse reactions)
• Injury, risk for (adverse reactions)
• Knowledge, deficient (teaching)

## Implementation

• Give fluids **IV** or PO before chemotherapy to hydrate patient

• Give antacid before oral agent; give product after evening meal, before bedtime; provide antiemetic 30-60 min before giving product and prn to prevent vomiting; give antibiotics for prophylaxis of infection

• Give in AM so product can be eliminated before bedtime

• Use a liquid diet: carbonated beverages; gelatin may be added if patient is not nauseated or vomiting

**PO route**

• Give 1 hr before or 2 hr after meals to prevent nausea/vomiting

**Intermittent IV INF route**

• Use gloves during administration; if skin exposure occurs, wash immediately with soap and water

• Reconstitute with provided diluent (10 ml) to 5 mg/ml; shake until clear; further dilute with 0.9% NaCl to <0.45 mg/ml; give over 15 min, give within 1 hr

***Y-site compatibilities:*** Acyclovir, amikacin, aminophylline, ampicillin, aztreonam, bleomycin, bumetanide, buprenorphine, butorphanol, calcium gluconate, carboplatin, carmustine, cefazolin, cefepime, cefoperazone, cefotaxime, cefotetan, ceftazidime, ceftizoxime, ceftriaxone, cefuroxime, cimetidine, cisplatin, clindamycin, cyclophosphamide, cytarabine, dacarbazine, dactinomycin, DAUNOrubicin, dexamethasone, diphenhydrAMINE, DOXOrubicin, doxycycline, droperidol, enalaprilat, etoposide, famotidine, floxuridine, fluconazole, fludarabine, fluorouracil, furosemide, gallium, ganciclovir, gentamicin, granisetron, haloperidol, heparin, hydrocortisone sodium phosphate, hydromorphone, hydrOXYzine, idarubicin, ifosfamide, imipenem-cilastatin, lorazepam, mannitol, mechlorethamine, meperidine, mesna, methylPREDNISolone, metoclopramide, methotrexate, metronidazole, miconazole, minocycline, mitomycin, mitoxantrone, morphine, nalbuphine, netilmicin, ondansetron, pentostatin, piperacillin, plicamycin, potassium chloride, prochlorperazine, promethazine, ranitidine, sodium bicarbonate, streptozocin, teniposide, thiotepa, ticarcillin, ticarcillin/clavulanate, tobramycin, trimethoprim/sulfamethoxazole, vancomycin, vinBLAStine, vinCRIStine, vinorelbine, zidovudine

**M**

## Patient/family education

• Teach patient to avoid use of products containing aspirin or ibuprofen, razors, commercial mouthwash, since bleeding may occur; to report symptoms of bleeding (hematuria, tarry stools)

• Instruct patient to report signs of anemia (fatigue, headache, irritability, faintness, shortness of breath)

• Instruct patient to report any changes in breathing or coughing even several mo after treatment; to avoid crowds and persons with respiratory tract or other infections

• Tell patient hair loss is common; discuss the use of wigs or hairpieces

• Caution patient not to have any vaccinations without the advice of the prescriber, serious reactions can occur

• Advise patient that contraception is needed during treatment and for several mo after the completion of therapy

• Teach patient to rinse mouth tid-qid with water, club soda; brush teeth bid-qid with soft brush or cotton-tipped applicators for stomatitis; use unwaxed dental floss

Adverse effects: *italic* = common, **bold** = life-threatening

**Evaluation**

**Positive therapeutic outcome**
- Decreased size of tumor
- Decreased spread of malignancy

---

## memantine (Rx)
(me-man'teen)
Namenda
*Func. class.:* Anti-Alzheimer's disease agent
*Chem. class.:* NMDA receptor antagonist

**Pregnancy category B**

**Action:** Antagonist action of CNS NMDA receptors that may contribute to the symptoms of Alzheimer's disease

**Therapeutic outcome:** Improved mood, orientation, decreasing confusion

**Uses:** Treatment of moderate to severe dementia in Alzheimer's disease

**Unlabeled uses:** Vascular dementia

**Dosage and routes**
*Adult:* PO 5 mg/day, may increase dose in 5-mg increments ≥1-wk intervals; recommended target dose 20 mg/day

**Available forms:** Tabs 5, 10 mg; tab titration pak 5, 10 mg; oral sol 2 mg/ml, 10 mg/5 ml

**Adverse effects**
*CNS: Dizziness, confusion,* somnolence, headache, hallucinations
*CV:* Hypertension
*GI:* Vomiting, constipation
*INTEG:* Rash
*MISC:* Back pain, fatigue, pain
*RESP:* Coughing, dyspnea

**Contraindications:** Hypersensitivity, breastfeeding, children, renal failure

**Precautions:** Pregnancy **B**, renal disease, seizures, severe hepatic disease, GU conditions that raise urine pH

| Pharmacokinetics | |
|---|---|
| **Absorption** | Rapidly absorbed PO |
| **Distribution** | 44% protein binding |
| **Metabolism** | Very little |
| **Excretion** | 57%-82% excreted unchanged in urine |
| **Half-life** | Terminal elimination half-life 60-80 hr |

| Pharmacodynamics | |
|---|---|
| Unknown | |

**Interactions**
*Individual drugs*
Cimetidine, hydrochlorothiazide, nicotine, quinidine, ranitidine, triamterene: may alter levels of both products
*Drug classifications*
Drugs that make the urine alkaline (sodium bicarbonate, carbonic anhydrase inhibitors): decreased clearance

**NURSING CONSIDERATIONS**
**Assessment**
- Monitor B/P: hypertension; respiratory status: dyspnea
- Assess mental status: affect, mood, behavioral changes; hallucinations, confusion
- Assess GI status: vomiting, constipation, add bulk, increase fluids for constipation
- Assess GU status: urinary frequency

**Nursing diagnoses**
- Injury, risk for (uses)
- Knowledge, deficient (teaching)
- Noncompliance (teaching)
- Thought processes, disturbed (uses)

**Implementation**
- Can be taken without regard to meals
- Give twice a day if dose >5 mg
- Dosage is adjusted to response no more than ≥1 wk
- Provide assistance with ambulation during beginning therapy; dizziness may occur

**Patient/family education**
- Advise to report side effects: restlessness, psychosis, visual hallucinations, stupor, loss of consciousness; indicate overdose
- Advise to use product exactly as prescribed; product is not a cure

**Evaluation**
**Positive therapeutic outcome**
- Decrease in confusion, improved mood

---

## menotropins (Rx)
(men-oh-troe'pinz)
Humegon, Menopur, Pergonal, Repronex
*Func. class.:* Gonadotropin
*Chem. class.:* Exogenous gonadotropin

**Pregnancy category X**

**Action:** In women, increases follicular growth, maturation; in men, when given with hCG, stimulates spermatogenesis; contains FSH and LH

**Therapeutic outcome:** Pregnancy, ovulation

---

 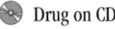

**Uses:** Infertility, anovulation in women; stimulates spermatogenesis in men; usually used with hCG

## Dosage and routes
*Infertility*
*Adult (men):* IM 1 ampule 3 times a wk with hCG 2000 units 2 times a wk × 4 mo
*Adult (women):* IM 75 international units of FSH, LH daily × 9-12 days, then 10,000 units of hCG 1 day after these products; repeat × 2 menstrual cycles, then increase to 150 international units of FSH, LH daily × 9-12 days, then 10,000 units of hCG 1 day after these products × 2 menstrual cycles

*Anovulation*
*Adult (women):* IM 75 international units FSH, LH daily × 9-12 days, then 10,000 units hCG 1 day after last dose of these products: repeat × 1-3 menstrual cycles

**Available forms:** Powder for inj lyophilized 75, 150 international units FSH, LH activity

## Adverse effects
*CNS:* Fever, hot flashes, dizziness
*CV:* **Hypovolemia,** tachycardia
*GI:* *Nausea,* vomiting, diarrhea, anorexia
*GU:* **Ovarian hyperstimulation syndrome (OHSS),** multiple births, abdominal distention, pain, sudden ovarian enlargement, ascites with or without pain, ectopic pregnancy, gynecomastia in men
*HEMA:* **Hemoperitoneum, arterial thromboembolism**
*INTEG:* Rash, swelling of inj site
*OTHER:* **Anaphylaxis**
*RESP:* **ARDS, pulmonary embolism, pulmonary infarction, pleural effusion,** atelectasis, dyspnea, tachypnea

**Contraindications:** Pregnancy **X,** primary ovarian failure, abnormal bleeding, thyroid/adrenal dysfunction, organic intracranial lesion, ovarian cysts, primary testicular failure, high FSH

### Pharmacokinetics

| | |
|---|---|
| **Absorption** | Well absorbed |
| **Distribution** | Unknown |
| **Metabolism** | Unknown |
| **Excretion** | Kidneys, unchanged (8%) |
| **Half-life** | 70 hr (FSH); 4 hr (LH) |

### Pharmacodynamics
Unknown

## NURSING CONSIDERATIONS
### Assessment
• Monitor weight daily; notify prescriber if weight gain increases rapidly
• Monitor estrogen excretion level; if >100 mcg/24 hr, product is withheld; serum progesterone, LH, estradiol level, pelvic exam, ovarian ultrasound; hyperstimulation syndrome may occur
• Monitor I&O ratio; be alert for decreasing urinary output
• Assess for ovarian enlargement, abdominal distention/pain; report symptoms immediately

### Nursing diagnoses
• Knowledge, deficient (teaching)
• Sexual dysfunction (uses)

### Implementation
• Give after reconstituting with 1-2 ml of sterile saline inj; use immediately

### Patient/family education
• Advise patient that multiple births are possible; if pregnancy occurs, it is usually 4-6 wk after start of treatment
• Instruct patient to keep daily appointment for 2 wk during treatment

### Evaluation
**Positive therapeutic outcome**
• Pregnancy

M

---

**⚠ HIGH ALERT**

## meperidine 😷 (Rx)
(me-per′i-deen)
Demerol, meperidine HCl, Pethidine
*Func. class.:* Opioid analgesic
*Chem. class.:* Phenylpiperidine derivative

**Pregnancy category B**
**Controlled substance schedule II**

**Do not confuse:**
meperidine/hydromorphone/meprobamate/morphine, Demerol/Dilaudid

**Action:** Depresses pain impulse transmission at the spinal cord level by interacting with opioid receptors; produces CNS depression

**Therapeutic outcome:** Relief of pain

**Uses:** Moderate to severe pain, preoperatively, postoperatively

**Unlabeled uses:** Rigors

## Dosage and routes
*Pain*
*Adult:* PO/SUBCUT/IM 50-150 mg q3-4hr prn; **IV** 15-35 mg/hr as a CONT INF; PCA 10

---

Adverse effects: *italic* = common, **bold** = life-threatening

mg, then 1-5 mg incremental dose; lockout interval 6-10 min
*Child:* PO/SUBCUT/IM 1.1-1.8 mg/kg q3-4hr prn, max 100 mg q4hr
*Preoperatively*
*Adult:* IM/SUBCUT 50-100 mg 30-90 min before surgery; dosage should be reduced if given **IV**
*Child:* IM/SUBCUT 1-2.2 mg/kg 30-90 min before surgery
*Renal dose*
*Adult:* CCr 10-50 ml/min 75% of dose; CCr <10 ml/min 50% of dose
*Labor analgesia*
*Adult:* SUBCUT/IM 50-100 mg given when contractions are regulary spaced, repeat q1-3hr prn

**Available forms:** Inj 10, 25, 50, 75, 100 mg/ml; tabs 50, 100 mg; syr 50 mg/5 ml

### Adverse effects
*CNS:* Drowsiness, dizziness, confusion, headache, sedation, euphoria, **increased ICP, seizures,** serotonin syndrome
*CV:* Palpitations, bradycardia, hypotension, change in B/P, tachycardia (**IV**)
*EENT:* Tinnitus, blurred vision, miosis, diplopia, depressed corneal reflex
*GI:* Nausea, vomiting, anorexia, constipation, cramps, biliary spasm, paralytic ileus
*GU:* Urinary retention, dysuria
*INTEG:* Rash, urticaria, bruising, flushing, diaphoresis, pruritus
*RESP:* **Respiratory depression**

**Contraindications:** Hypersensitivity, addiction (opiate)

**Precautions:** Pregnancy **B**, breastfeeding, child <18 yr, geriatric, addictive personality, increased ICP, MI (acute), severe heart disease, respiratory depression, renal/hepatic disease

| Pharmacokinetics | |
|---|---|
| **Absorption** | Well absorbed (IM, SUBCUT); 50% (PO) |
| **Distribution** | Widely distributed; crosses placenta; protein binding 65%-75% |
| **Metabolism** | Liver, extensively |
| **Excretion** | Kidneys; breast milk |
| **Half-life** | 3-4 hr |

| Pharmacodynamics | | | |
|---|---|---|---|
| | **PO** | **IM/ SUBCUT** | **IV** |
| **Onset** | 15 min | 10 min | Rapid |
| **Peak** | ½-1 hr | ½-1 hr | 5-7 min |
| **Duration** | 2-4 hr | 2-4 hr | 2-4 hr |

### Interactions
*Individual drugs*
Alcohol: increased respiratory depression, hypotension, sedation
Phenytoin: decreased meperidine effect
Procarbazine: fatal reaction, do not use together
*Drug classifications*
CNS depressants, opioids, sedative/hypnotics, antipsychotics, skeletal muscle relaxants: increased effects
MAOIs: do not use for 2 wk before taking meperidine; may cause fatal reaction
Protease inhibitor antiretrovirals: increased adverse reactions
*Drug/herb*
Chamomile, gotu kola, hops, Jamaican dogwood, kava, lavender, mistletoe, nettle, pokeweed, poppy, senega, skullcap, St. John's wort, valerian: increased CNS depression
Parsley: may promote serotonin syndrome, avoid concurrent medicinal use
*Drug/lab test*
Increased: amylase, lipase

### NURSING CONSIDERATIONS
**Assessment**
• Assess pain: location, duration, intensity before and 1 hr (IM, SUBCUT, PO) and 5-10 min (**IV**) after administration
• Assess renal function before initiating therapy; poor renal function can lead to accumulation of toxic metabolite and seizures
• Monitor VS after parenteral route; note muscle rigidity, product history, liver, kidney function tests, respiratory dysfunction: respiratory depression, character, rate, rhythm; notify prescriber if respirations are <10/min
• Monitor CNS changes: dizziness, drowsiness, hallucinations, euphoria, LOC, pupil reaction; these are due to metabolite produced; CNS stimulation occurs with chronic or high doses
• Monitor allergic reactions: rash, urticaria

**Nursing diagnoses**
• Breathing pattern, ineffective (adverse reactions)
• Injury, risk for (adverse reactions)
• Knowledge, deficient (teaching)
• Pain, acute (uses)
• Sensory perception, disturbed: visual, auditory (adverse reactions)

**Implementation**
• Give with antiemetic if nausea, vomiting occur

- Administer when pain is beginning to return; determine dosage interval by patient response; continuous dosing of medication is more effective given prn
- Medication should be slowly withdrawn after long-term use to prevent withdrawal symptoms
- Store in light-resistant container at room temperature

**PO route**
- May be given with food or milk to lessen GI upset
- Syr should be mixed with 4 oz of water

**IM/SUBCUT route**
- Do not give if cloudy or a precipitate has formed
- Patient should remain recumbent for 1 hr after administration

**IV route**
- Give by direct **IV** after diluting to 10 mg/ml with sterile water, 0.9% NaCl for inj; give slowly at 25 mg/1 min; rapid administration may cause respiratory depression, hypotension, circulatory collapse
- Give cont inf after diluting to 1 mg/ml with $D_5W$, $D_{10}W$, dextrose/saline combinations, dextrose/Ringer's, inj combinations, 0.45% NaCl, 0.9% NaCl, Ringer's, LR; give by infusion pump; titrate according to response

*Syringe compatibilities:* Atropine, benzquinamide, butorphanol, chlorproMA-ZINE, cimetidine, dimenhyDRINATE, diphenhydrAMINE, droperidol, fentanyl, glycopyrrolate, hydrOXYzine, ketamine, metoclopramide, midazolam, pentazocine, perphenazine, prochlorperazine, promazine, promethazine, ranitidine, scopolamine
*Syringe incompatibilities:* Heparin, morphine, pentobarbital
*Y-site compatibilities:* Amifostine, amikacin, ampicillin, atenolol, aztreonam, bumetanide, cefamandole, cefazolin, cefmetazole, cefotaxime, cefotetan, cefoxitin, ceftazidime, ceftizoxime, ceftriaxone, cefuroxime, cephalothin, cephapirin, chloramphenicol, cladribine, clindamycin, dexamethasone, diltiazem, diphenhydrAMINE, DOBUTamine, DOPamine, doxycycline, droperidol, erythromycin lactobionate, famotidine, filgrastim, fluconazole, fludarabine, gallium, gentamicin, granisetron, heparin, hydrocortisone, regular insulin, kanamycin, labetalol, lidocaine, magnesium sulfate, melphalan, methyldopate, methylPREDNISolone, metoclopramide, metoprolol, metronidazole, moxalactam, ondansetron, oxacillin, oxytocin, paclitaxel, penicillin G potassium, piperacillin, potassium chloride, propofol, propranolol, ranitidine,

sargramostim, teniposide, thiotepa, ticarcillin, ticarcillin/clavulanate, tobramycin, trimethoprim/sulfamethoxazole, vancomycin, verapamil, vinorelbine
*Y-site incompatibilities:* Cefoperazone, idarubicin, imipenem/cilastatin, mezlocillin, minocycline
*Additive compatibilities:* Cefazolin, DOBUTamine, ondansetron, scopolamine, succinylcholine, trifluopromazine, verapamil

**Patient/family education**
- Advise patients to avoid CNS depressants (alcohol, sedative/hypnotics) for at least 24 hr after taking this product
- Discuss with patient that dizziness, drowsiness, and confusion are common; to avoid getting up without assistance
- Discuss in detail with patient all aspects of the product, including its purpose and what to expect
- Caution patient to make position changes carefully to lessen orthostatic hypotension

**Evaluation**
**Positive therapeutic outcome**
- Decreased pain

**Treatment of overdose:** Naloxone 0.2-0.8 mg **IV**, $O_2$, **IV** fluids, vasopressors

**M**

## mercaptopurine (Rx)
(mer-kap-toe-pyoor'een)
6-MP, Purinethol
*Func. class.:* Antineoplastic, antimetabolite
*Chem. class.:* Purine analog
**Pregnancy category  D**

**Action:** Inhibits purine metabolism at multiple sites, which inhibits DNA and RNA synthesis S phase of cell cycle

**Therapeutic outcome:** Prevention of rapidly growing malignant cells

**Uses:** Chronic myelocytic leukemia, acute lymphoblastic leukemia in children

**Unlabeled uses:** Polycythemia vera, psoriatic arthritis, colitis, lymphoma, acute myelogenous leukemia

**Dosage and routes**
*Acute lymphocytic leukemia*
*Adult:* PO 2.5-5 mg/kg/day or 80-100 mg/m²/day, maintenance 1.5-2.5 mg/kg/day
*Child:* PO 2.5-5 mg/kg/day, maintenance 1.5-2.5 mg/kg/day or 70-100 mg/m²/day

**Available forms:** Tabs 50 mg

Adverse effects: *italic* = common, **bold** = life-threatening

## Adverse effects

*CNS:* Weakness
*GI: Nausea, vomiting, anorexia, diarrhea, stomatitis,* **hepatotoxicity** (with high doses), jaundice, gastritis
*GU:* **Renal failure,** hyperuricemia, **oliguria,** crystalluria, **hematuria**
*HEMA:* **Thrombocytopenia, leukopenia, myelosuppression, anemia**
*INTEG: Rash,* dry skin, urticaria

**Contraindications:** Pregnancy **D,** breastfeeding, patients with prior product resistance, leukopenia, thrombocytopenia, anemia

**Precautions:** Renal/hepatic disease

### Pharmacokinetics

| | |
|---|---|
| **Absorption** | Variable |
| **Distribution** | Widely—body water |
| **Metabolism** | Liver—extensively |
| **Excretion** | Kidneys unchanged (small amounts) |
| **Half-life** | Terminal 1-1.5 hr |

### Pharmacodynamics

| | |
|---|---|
| **Onset** | Unknown |
| **Peak** | 1-2 hr |
| **Duration** | Unknown |

## Interactions
### Individual products
Allopurinol, cotrimoxazole: increased bone marrow depression
Radiation: increased effects
Warfarin: increased effect of warfarin
### Drug classifications
Anticoagulants, NSAIDs, platelet inhibitors, thrombolytics: increased bleeding risk
Antineoplastics, immunosuppressants: increased effects
Live virus vaccines: decreased antibodies

## NURSING CONSIDERATIONS
### Assessment
• Assess buccal cavity for dryness, sores or ulceration, white patches, oral pain, bleeding, dysphagia; obtain prescription for viscous lidocaine (Xylocaine)
⬥ Assess symptoms indicating severe allergic reaction: rash, pruritus, urticaria, purpuric skin lesions, itching, flushing
• Monitor CBC, differential, platelet count weekly; withhold product if WBC is <4000/mm$^3$ or platelet count is <100,000/mm$^3$; notify prescriber of results if WBC <20,000/mm$^3$, platelets <150,000/mm$^3$

• Assess for increased uric acid levels, swelling, joint pain primarily in extremities; patient should be well hydrated to prevent urate deposits
• Monitor renal function tests: BUN, creatinine, serum uric acid, urine CCr before and during therapy; check I&O ratio; report fall in urine output to <30 ml/hr
• Monitor temp q4hr (may indicate beginning of infection)
• Monitor liver function tests before and during therapy (bilirubin, AST, ALT, LDH) as needed or monthly; check for yellowing of skin or sclera, dark urine, clay-colored stools, itchy skin, abdominal pain, fever, diarrhea
• Assess for bleeding: hematuria, stool guaiac, bruising or petechiae, mucosa or orifices q8hr; check for inflammation of mucosa, breaks in skin

### Nursing diagnoses
• Body image, disturbed (adverse reactions)
• Infection, risk for (adverse reactions)
• Injury, risk for (adverse reactions)
• Knowledge, deficient (teaching)

### Implementation
• Give fluids **IV** or PO before chemotherapy to hydrate patient
• Give antiemetic 30-60 min before giving product and prn to prevent vomiting
• Give in PM on empty stomach
• Give entire dose at one time
• Provide liquid diet: carbonated beverages; gelatin may be added if patient is not nauseated or vomiting
• Tab may be crushed and added to fluids or food to facilitate swallowing

### Patient/family education
• Encourage patient to rinse mouth tid-qid with water, club soda; brush teeth bid-qid with soft brush or cotton-tipped applicators for stomatitis; use unwaxed dental floss
• Advise patient that contraceptive measures are recommended during therapy; serious teratogenic effects may occur, to avoid breastfeeding
• Teach patient to avoid use of products containing aspirin or NSAIDs, razors, commercial mouthwash, since bleeding may occur; to report symptoms of bleeding (hematuria, tarry stools)
• Instruct patient to report signs of anemia (fatigue, headache, irritability, faintness, shortness of breath)
• Instruct patient to report any changes in breathing or coughing even several mo after

treatment; to avoid crowds and persons with respiratory tract or other infections

• Caution patient not to have any vaccinations without the advice of the prescriber; serious reactions can occur

• Advise patient to take entire dose at one time

### Evaluation

**Positive therapeutic outcome**

• Prevention of rapid division of malignant cells

---

### meropenem (Rx)
(mer-oh-pen′em)
Merrem **IV**
*Func. class.:* Antiinfective—miscellaneous
**Pregnancy category B**

**Action:** Interferes with cell wall replication of susceptible organisms; osmotically unstable cell wall swells and bursts from osmotic pressure

**Therapeutic outcome:** Bactericidal action against the following: *Streptococcus pneumoniae*, group A β-hemolytic streptococci, *viridans* group streptococci, enterococcus; gram-negative organisms *Klebsiella, Proteus, Escherichia coli, Pseudomonas aeruginosa, Bacteroides fragilis, Bacteroides thetaiotamicron*, bacterial meningitis (>3 mo old)

**Uses:** Serious infections caused by gram-positive or gram-negative organisms (appendicitis, peritonitis)

**Unlabeled uses:** Febrile neutropenic, community-acquired pneumonia

### Dosage and routes
*Adult:* **IV** 1 g q8hr, given over 15-30 min or as an **IV** BOL 5-20 ml given over 3-5 min
*Child ≥ 3 mo:* **IV** 20-40 mg/kg q8hr (max 2 g q8hr meningitis)
*Child >50 kg:* **IV** 1 g q8hr (intra-abdominal infection) or 2 g q8hr (meningitis) given over 15-30 min or as an **IV** BOL 5-20 ml over 3-5 min

*Renal dose*
*Adult:* **IV** CCr 26-50 ml/min 1 g q12hr; CCr 10-25 ml/min 500 mg q12hr; CCr <10 ml/min 500 mg q24hr

**Available forms:** Inj 500 mg, 1 g

### Adverse effects
*CNS:* Fever, somnolence, *seizures,* dizziness, weakness, *headache,* myoclonia, confusion

*CV:* Hypotension, palpitations, tachycardia
*GI:* Diarrhea, nausea, vomiting, **pseudomembranous colitis, hepatitis,** glossitis
*HEMA:* **Eosinophilia, neutropenia,** decreased Hgb, Hct, **agranulocytosis**
*INTEG:* *Rash,* urticaria, *pruritus,* pain at inj site, phlebitis, erythema at inj site
*RESP:* Chest discomfort, dyspnea, hyperventilation, **pulmonary embolism**
*SYST:* **Anaphylaxis, Stevens-Johnson syndrome,** angioedema

**Contraindications:** Hypersensitivity to meropenem or imipenem

**Precautions:** Pregnancy **B,** breastfeeding, geriatric, renal disease, seizure disorder

#### Pharmacokinetics

| | |
|---|---|
| **Absorption** | Complete bioavailability |
| **Distribution** | Widely distributed |
| **Metabolism** | Liver |
| **Excretion** | Kidneys |
| **Half-life** | 1 hr; increased in renal disease |

#### Pharmacodynamics

| | |
|---|---|
| **Onset** | Rapid |
| **Peak** | Dose dependent |
| **Duration** | Unknown |

M

### Interactions
*Individual drugs*
Probenecid: increased meropenem levels
Valproic acid: decreased effect of valproic acid
*Drug/herb*
Do not use acidophilus with antiinfectives; separate by several hours
*Drug/lab test*
Increased: AST, ALT, LDH, BUN, alkaline phosphatase, bilirubin, creatinine
False positive: direct Coombs' test

### NURSING CONSIDERATIONS
**Assessment**

• Assess patient for previous sensitivity reaction to carbapenem antiinfectives, penicillins

• Assess patient for signs and symptoms of infection, including characteristics of wounds, sputum, urine, stool, WBC >10,000/100 mm$^3$, fever; obtain baseline information before and during treatment

• Complete C&S tests before beginning product therapy to identify if correct treatment has been initiated

• Assess for allergic reactions, anaphylaxis: rash, urticaria, pruritus, chills, fever, joint pain; angioedema may occur a few days after therapy begins; epINEPHrine and resuscitation

---

Adverse effects: *italic* = common, **bold** = life-threatening

equipment should be available for anaphylactic reaction

• Identify urine output; if decreasing, notify prescriber (may indicate nephrotoxicity); also check for increased BUN, creatinine

• Monitor blood studies: AST, ALT, CBC, Hct, bilirubin, LDH, alkaline phosphatase, Coombs' test monthly if patient is on long-term therapy

• Monitor electrolytes: potassium, sodium, chloride monthly if patient is on long-term therapy

• Assess bowel pattern daily; if severe diarrhea occurs, product should be discontinued; may indicate pseudomembranous colitis

• Monitor for bleeding: ecchymosis, bleeding gums, hematuria, stool guaiac daily if on long-term therapy

• Assess for overgrowth of infection: perineal itching, fever, malaise, redness, pain, swelling, drainage, rash, diarrhea, change in cough, sputum

## Nursing diagnoses
• Diarrhea (adverse reactions)
• Infection, risk for (uses)
• Injury, risk for (adverse reactions)
• Knowledge, deficient (teaching)
• Noncompliance (teaching)

## Implementation
### IV route
• Reconstitute with 0.9% NaCl, D₅W, LR, dilute in 5-20 ml of compatible sol; give by direct **IV** over 3-5 min
• Give by intermittent inf, dilute in 5-20 ml of compatible sol, give over 15-30 min

*Y-site compatibilities:* Aminophylline, atenolol, atropine, cimetidine, dexamethasone, digoxin, diphenhydrAMINE, enalaprilat, fluconazole, furosemide, gentamicin, heparin, insulin (regular), metoclopramide, morphine, norepinephrine, phenobarbital, vancomycin

*Additive compatibilities:* Aminophylline, atropine, cimetidine, dexamethasone, DOBUTamine, DOPamine, enalaprilat, fluconazole, furosemide, gentamicin, heparin, insulin (regular), magnesium sulfate, metoclopramide, morphine, norepinephrine, phenobarbital, ranitidine, vancomycin

## Patient/family education
• Teach patient to report sore throat, bruising, bleeding, joint pain; may indicate blood dyscrasias (rare)
• Advise patient to contact prescriber if vaginal itching, loose foul-smelling stools, furry tongue occur; may indicate superinfection
• Advise patient to avoid breastfeeding, product is excreted in breast milk

• Advise patient to notify prescriber of diarrhea with blood or pus, may indicate pseudomembranous colitis

## Evaluation
### Positive therapeutic outcome
• Absence of signs/symptoms of infection (WBC <10,000/mm³, temp WNL, absence of red draining wounds)
• Reported improvement in symptoms of infection

## Treatment of anaphylaxis:
EpINEPHrine, antihistamines, resuscitate if needed

---

## mesalamine, 5-ASA (Rx)
(mez-al′a-meen)
Asacol, Lialda, Pentasa, Rowasa, Salofulk ✦
*Func class.:* GI antiinflammatory
*Chem class.:* 5-Aminosalicylic acid

### Pregnancy category B

### Do not confuse:
Asacol/Ansaid/Os-Cal

**Action:** May diminish inflammation by blocking cyclooxygenase, inhibiting prostaglandin production in colon, local action only

**Therapeutic outcome:** Decreased cramping, pain in GI conditions

**Uses:** Mild to moderate active distal ulcerative colitis, proctosigmoiditis, proctitis

**Unlabeled uses:** Crohn's disease

### Dosage and routes
*Adult:* RECT 60 ml (4 g) at bedtime, retained for 8 hr × 3-6 wk; PO 1000 mg qid for up to 8 wk; DEL REL TAB 1.2 g/day

**Available forms:** Enema 4 g/60 ml; del rel tabs 250 ✦, 400, 500 ✦ mg; ext rel tab 500 mg; ext rel cap 250 mg, 1 g; del rel tab (Lialda) 1.2 g

### Adverse effects
*CNS: Headache, fever, dizziness,* insomnia, asthenia, weakness, fatigue
*CV:* Pericarditis, myocarditis, chest pain, palpitations
*EENT:* Sore throat, cough, pharyngitis, rhinitis
*GI: Cramps, gas, nausea, diarrhea,* rectal pain, constipation
*INTEG: Rash, itching,* acne
*SYST: Flulike symptoms, malaise,* back pain, peripheral edema, leg and joint pain, arthralgia, dysmenorrhea, **anaphylaxis,** acute intolerance syndrome

---

**Contraindications:** Hypersensitivity to this product or salicylates

**Precautions:** Pregnancy **B**, breastfeeding, children, geriatric, renal disease, sulfite sensitivity, pyloric stenosis

### Pharmacokinetics

| | |
|---|---|
| **Absorption** | 20%-30% (PO), 10%-25% (RECT) |
| **Distribution** | Unknown |
| **Metabolism** | Unknown |
| **Excretion** | Feces |
| **Half-life** | 1 hr; metabolite 5-10 hr |

### Pharmacodynamics
Unknown

### Interactions
*Individual drugs*
Azathioprine: increased azathioprine action
Digoxin: decreased digoxin level
Lactulose: decreased mesalamine absorption
Omeprazole: increased mesalamine absorption
*Drug/lab test*
Increased: AST, ALT, alkaline phosphatase, LDH, GGTP, amylase, lipase

### NURSING CONSIDERATIONS
**Assessment**
• Assess for GI symptoms: cramping, gas, nausea, diarrhea, rectal pain, abdominal pain; if severe, the product should be discontinued
• Assess for allergy to salicylates, sulfonamides; if allergic reactions occur, discontinue product
• Assess renal function before and during treatment: BUN, creatinine
• Monitor I & O ratios, increase fluids to 1500 ml daily to prevent crystalluria

**Nursing diagnoses**
• Diarrhea (uses)
• Knowledge, deficient (teaching)
• Pain, chronic (uses)

**Implementation**
**PO route**
• Do not break, crush, or chew del rel tabs
• May give orally
**Rectal route (susp)**
• Give at bedtime, retained until AM; empty bowel before insertion
• Store at room temperature
• Usual course of therapy is 3-6 wk
• Give after shaking bottle well

**Patient/family education**
• Advise patient to notify prescriber if abdominal pain, cramping, diarrhea with blood,
headache, fever, rash, chest pain occur; product should be discontinued
• Teach correct administration for PO, or enema

### Evaluation
**Positive therapeutic outcome**
• Absence of pain, bleeding from GI tract

---

### metaproterenol (Rx)
(met-a-proe-ter'e-nole)
Alupent, Arm-a-Med, Dey-Lute
*Func. class.:* Selective $\beta_2$-agonist, bronchodilator

**Pregnancy category C**

**Do not confuse:**
Alupent/Atrovent

**Action:** Relaxes bronchial smooth muscle by direct action on $\beta_2$-adrenergic receptors, with increased levels of cAMP and increased bronchodilatation, diuresis, and cardiac and CNS stimulation

**Therapeutic outcome:** Bronchodilatation with ease of breathing

**Uses:** Bronchial asthma, bronchospasm

### Dosage and routes
*Adult and child >12 yr:* INH 2-3 puffs, may repeat q3-4hr, not to exceed 12 puffs/day; IPPB or NEB 0.2-0.3 ml of 5% sol diluted in 2.5 ml of ½ NS or NS, or 2.5 mil of 0.4, 0.6% sol q4hr prn
*Child 6-12 yr:* IPPB/NEB 0.1-0.2 ml of a 5% sol diluted in NS to a final volume of 3 ml q4hr prn
*Adult:* PO 20 mg q6-8hr
*Geriatric:* PO 10 mg tid-qid, initially
*Child >9 yr or >27 kg:* PO 20 mg q6-8hr or 0.4-0.9 mg/kg tid
*Child 6-9 yr or <27 kg:* PO 10 mg q6-8hr or 0.4-0.9 mg/kg tid
*Child 2-6 yr:* PO 1.3-2.6 mg/kg divided q6-8hr
*Child 1-2 yr:* PO 0.4 mg/kg q6-8hr

**Available forms:** Tabs 10, 20 mg; aerosol 0.65 mg/dose; syr 10 mg/5 ml; sol for inh 0.4%, 0.6%, 5%

### Adverse effects
*CNS: Tremors,* anxiety, insomnia, headache, dizziness, stimulation
*CV:* Palpitations, tachycardia, hypertension, **dysrhythmias, cardiac arrest** (high dose)
*GI:* Nausea, vomiting, dry mouth
*MISC:* Hypokalemia, pyrosis
*RESP:* **Paradoxical bronchospasm**

M

Adverse effects: *italic* = common, **bold** = life-threatening

**Contraindications:** Hypersensitivity to sympathomimetics, angle-closure glaucoma, cardiac dysrhythmias with tachycardia

**Precautions:** Pregnancy **C**, children <6 yr, (NEB), children <12 yr (INH), geriatric, cardiac disorders, hyperthyroidism, diabetes mellitus, prostatic hypertrophy, seizure disorder

| Pharmacokinetics | |
|---|---|
| **Absorption** | Well absorbed (PO) |
| **Distribution** | Unknown |
| **Metabolism** | Liver, tissues |
| **Excretion** | Unknown |
| **Half-life** | 2-4 hr |

| Pharmacodynamics | | |
|---|---|---|
| | PO | INH |
| **Onset** | 15 min | 5 min |
| **Peak** | 1 hr | 1 hr |
| **Duration** | 4 hr | 1-6 hr |

## Interactions
### Drug classifications
β-Adrenergic blockers: block therapeutic effect

Bronchodilators, aerosol: increased action of both products

MAOIs, antidepressants (tricyclics): increased chance of hypertensive crisis

Sympathomimetics: increased effects of both products

### Drug/herb
Coffee, cola nut, guarana, tea (black/green), yerba maté: increased effect

### Drug/lab test
Decreased: potassium

## NURSING CONSIDERATIONS
### Assessment
• Monitor respiratory function: vital capacity, FEV, ABGs, lung sounds, heart rate, rhythm (baseline)

• Determine that patient has not received theophylline therapy before giving dose; identify client's ability to self-medicate

• Monitor for evidence of allergic reactions; paradoxic bronchospasm; withhold dose; notify prescriber

### Nursing diagnoses
• Airway clearance, ineffective (uses)
• Gas exchange, impaired (uses)
• Knowledge, deficient (teaching)

## Implementation
• Give this medication before other medications and allow 5 min between each to prevent overstimulation

**PO route**
• Give PO with meals to decrease gastric irritation; syrup to children (no alcohol, sugar)

**Aerosol route**
• Give after shaking, exhale, place mouthpiece in mouth, inhale slowly, hold breath, remove, exhale slowly; allow at least 1 min between inhalations

• Store in light-resistant container, do not expose to temperature over 86° F (30° C)

• Provide spacer device for geriatric

## Patient/family education
• Advise patient not to use OTC medications; excess stimulation may occur; to use this medication before other medications and allow at least 5 min between each to prevent overstimulation

• Teach patient use of inhaler; review package insert with patient; teach patient to avoid getting aerosol in eyes, since blurring may result; to wash inhaler in warm water daily and dry; to avoid smoking, smoke-filled rooms, persons with respiratory tract infections

• Advise patient that paradoxic bronchospasm may occur and to stop product immediately and notify prescriber; to limit caffeine products such as chocolate, coffee, tea, and colas

• Instruct patient on administration of dose; not to use more than prescribed; serious side effects may occur

## Evaluation
### Positive therapeutic outcome
• Absence of dyspnea, wheezing after 1 hr
• Improved airway exchange
• Improved ABGs

**Treatment of overdose:** Administer a β₁-adrenergic blocker

**metformin** (Rx)
(met-for′min)
Fortamet, Glucophage, Glucophage XR, Novo-Metformin ✤, Riomet
*Func. class.:* Antidiabetic, oral
*Chem. class.:* Biguanide
### Pregnancy category B

**Action:** Inhibits hepatic glucose production and increases sensitivity of peripheral tissue to insulin

**Therapeutic outcome:** Blood glucose at normal levels

**Uses:** Type 2 diabetes mellitus

## Dosage and routes
### Diabetes mellitus
*Adult:* PO 500 mg bid initially, then increase to desired response 1-2 g; dosage adjustment q2-3 wk or 850 mg/day with morning meal with dosage increased every other week, max 2500 mg/day; EXT REL max 2550 mg/day
*Geriatric:* PO use lowest effective dose

**Available forms:** Tabs 500, 850, 1000 mg; ext rel tabs 500 mg; oral sol (Riomet) 500 mg/5 ml

## Adverse effects:
*CNS: Headache, weakness, dizziness, drowsiness,* tinnitus, fatigue, vertigo, *agitation*
*ENDO:* **Lactic acidosis,** hypoglycemia
*GI:* Nausea, vomiting, diarrhea, heartburn, anorexia, metallic taste
*HEMA:* **Thrombocytopenia,** decreased vit B$_{12}$ levels
*INTEG:* Rash

**Contraindications:** Hypersensitivity, hepatic disease, creatinine >1.5 mg/ml (males) ≥1.4 (females), alcoholism, cardiopulmonary disease, history of lactic acidosis, acidemia, acute MI, cardiogenic shock, diabetic ketoacidosis, metabolic acidosis

**Precautions:** Pregnancy **B**, geriatric, thyroid disease, previous hypersensitivity, CHF

| Pharmacokinetics | |
|---|---|
| **Absorption** | Unknown |
| **Distribution** | Unknown |
| **Metabolism** | Unknown |
| **Excretion** | Kidneys, unchanged (35%-50%) |
| **Half-life** | 1½-5, Terminal 6-20 hr |

| Pharmacodynamics | |
|---|---|
| **Onset** | Unknown |
| **Peak** | 1-3 hr |
| **Duration** | Unknown |

## Interactions
### Individual drugs
Acetazolamide: increased blood glucose levels
Cimetidine, digoxin, morphine, procainamide, quinidine, ranitidine, triamterene, vancomycin: increased metformin level
Cimetidine, phenytoin: increased hypoglycemia
Ethanol: increased risk of lactic acidosis

Radiologic contrast media: do not give together, may cause renal failure
### Drug classifications
Calcium channel blockers, contraceptives (oral), corticosteroids, diuretics, estrogens, phenothiazines, sympathomimetics: increased hypoglycemia
### Drug/herb
Alfalfa, aloe, basil, bay, bilberry, bitter melon, black catechu, buchu, burdock, coriander, dandelion, eyebright (po), fenugreek, garlic, ginseng, glucomannan, glucosamine, goat's rue, gymnema, horehound, horse chestnut, jambul, myrrh, myrtle, rue: increased antidiabetic effect
Bee pollen, blue cohosh, broom, chromium, elecampane, eucalyptus, gotu kola: decreased antidiabetic effect
Chromium, coenzyme Q10, fenugreek: increased hypoglycemia
Glucosamine: increased hyperglycemia
Quinine: increased metformin level

## NURSING CONSIDERATIONS
### Assessment
• Assess for hypoglycemic reactions (sweating, weakness, dizziness, anxiety, tremors, hunger), hyperglycemic reactions soon after meals; these occur rarely with this product
• Monitor CBC (baseline, q3 mo) during treatment; check liver function tests (AST, LDH) and renal tests (BUN, creatinine) periodically during treatment; glucose, A1c
◆ Monitor for lactic acidosis: malaise, myalgia, abdominal distress; risk increases with age, poor renal function; monitor electrolytes, lactate, pyruvate, blood pH, ketones, glucose

### Nursing diagnoses
• Knowledge, deficient (teaching)

### Implementation
• Do not break, crush, or chew ext rel tabs
• Conversion from other oral hypoglycemic agents; change may be made without gradual dosage change; monitor serum or urine glucose and ketones tid during conversion
• Give twice a day with meals to decrease GI upset and provide best absorption; may also be taken as a single dose; titrate slowly to therapeutic response, side effect tolerance
• Give in AM to prevent hypoglycemic reactions in PM
• Give immediate rel tabs crushed and mixed with meal or fluids for patients with difficulty swallowing
• Store in tight container in cool environment

M

### Patient/family education

• Teach patient to regularly self-monitor blood glucose using blood glucose meter
• Teach patient symptoms of hypo/hyperglycemia, what to do about each (rare)
• Advise patient that product must be continued on daily basis; explain consequence of discontinuing product abruptly
• Advise patient to take product in morning to prevent hypoglycemic reactions at night
• Advise patient to avoid OTC medications, alcohol unless approved by the prescriber
• Teach patient that diabetes is a lifelong illness; that this product controls symptoms, but does not cure the condition
• Teach patient symptoms of lactic acidosis: hyperventilation, fatigue, malaise, myalgia, chills, somnolence to notify prescriber immediately
• Teach patient to carry/wear emergency ID and glucagon emergency kit for emergencies
• Advise patient that glucophage XR tab may appear in stool
• Advise patient to take with first meal of the day

### Evaluation

**Positive therapeutic outcome**
• Decrease in polyuria, polydipsia, polyphagia; clear sensorium; absence of dizziness; stable gait; blood glucose, A1c at normal level

**Treatment of overdose:** Glucose 25 g **IV** via dextrose 50% sol, 50 ml or 1 mg glucagon

---

### ⚠ HIGH ALERT

### methadone (Rx)
(meth'a-done)
Dolophine, methadone, Methadose
*Func. class.:* Opioid analgesic
*Chem. class.:* Synthetic diphenylheptane derivative

**Pregnancy category C**

**Controlled substance schedule II**

**Do not confuse:**
methadone/methylphenidate

**Action:** Depresses pain impulse transmission at the spinal cord level by interacting with opioid receptors; produces CNS depression

**Therapeutic outcome:** Relief of pain; successful opioid withdrawal

**Uses:** Severe pain, opiate withdrawal

### Dosage and routes
*Severe pain*
**Adult:** PO/SUBCUT/IM 2.5-10 mg q8-12hr prn

*Opiate withdrawal*
**Adult:** PO 15-40 mg/day individualized initially, then 20-120 mg/day titrated to patient response
**Child:** 0.05-0.1 mg/kg/dose q6-12hr

*Renal dose*
**Adult:** PO CCr 10-50 ml/min dose q8hr; CCr <10 ml/min dose q8-12hr

**Available forms:** Inj 10 mg/ml; tabs 5, 10 mg; oral sol 5, 10 mg/5 ml; dispersible tabs 40 mg; oral conc 10 mg/ml; oral sol 5, 10 mg/5 ml, 10 mg/10 ml

### Adverse effects
*CNS: Drowsiness, dizziness, confusion, headache, sedation,* euphoria, **seizures**
*CV:* Palpitations, bradycardia, change in B/P, **cardiac arrest, shock,** hypotension, **torsade de pointes, QT prolongation**
*EENT:* Tinnitus, blurred vision, miosis, diplopia
*GI: Nausea, vomiting, anorexia, constipation, cramps,* biliary tract spasm
*GU:* Increased urinary output, dysuria, urinary retention, impotence
*INTEG: Rash,* urticaria, bruising, flushing, diaphoresis, pruritus
*RESP:* **Respiratory depression, respiratory arrest**

**Contraindications:** Hypersensitivity to this product, or hypersensitivity to chlorobutanol (inj route), addiction (opiate)

**Precautions:** Pregnancy **C,** breastfeeding, children <18 yr, geriatric, addictive personality, increased ICP, MI (acute), severe heart disease, respiratory depression, renal/hepatic disease, QT prolongation, respiratory insufficiency, torsade de pointes, pulmonary disease, COPD

| Pharmacokinetics | |
|---|---|
| Absorption | Well absorbed (PO, SUBCUT, IM) |
| Distribution | Widely distributed; crosses placenta, half as active PO, as Inj |
| Metabolism | Liver, extensively |
| Excretion | Kidneys, breast milk |
| Half-life | 8-59 hr; extended interval with continued dosing |

| Pharmacodynamics | | |
|---|---|---|
| | PO | IM/SUBCUT |
| Onset | ½-1 hr | 20 min |
| Peak | 1-1.5 hr | 1½-2 hr |
| Duration | 4-12 hr | 4-6 hr |

## Interactions
### Individual drugs
Alcohol: increased respiratory depression, hypotension, sedation

Nalbuphine, pentazine, phenytoin, rifampin: decreased analgesia

### Drug classifications
Antipsychotics, opiates, sedative/hypnotics, skeletal muscle relaxants: increased respiratory depression, hypotension

CYP3A4 inducers (barbiturates, bosentan, carbamazepine, efavirenz, phenytoins, nevirapine, rifabutin, rifampin): decreased methadone effect

CYP3A4 inhibitors (aprepitant, antiretroviral protease inhibitors, clarithromycin, danazol, delavirdine, diltiazem, erythromycin, fluconazole, fluoxetine, fluvoxamine, imatinib, ketoconazole, mibefradil, nefazodone, telithromycin, voriconazole): increased toxicity

MAOIs: do not use for 2 wk before taking methadone, unpredictable reactions

### Drug/herb
Chamomile, hops, Jamaican dogwood, kava, lavender, mistletoe, nettle, pokeweed, poppy, senega, skullcap, valerian: increased CNS depression

Corkwood: increased anticholinergic effect

St. John's wort: avoid use

### Drug/lab test
Increased: amylase, lipase

## NURSING CONSIDERATIONS
### Assessment
• Assess for pain: type, location, intensity, grimacing before and 1½-2 hr after administration; use pain scoring

• Monitor VS after parenteral route; note muscle rigidity, product history, liver, kidney function tests, respiratory dysfunction: respiratory depression, character, rate, rhythm; notify prescriber if respirations are <10/min

• Monitor CNS changes: dizziness, drowsiness, hallucinations, euphoria, LOC, pupil reaction

• Monitor allergic reactions: rash, urticaria

• Monitor opioid detoxification: no analgesia occurs, only prevention of withdrawal symptoms

• Monitor B/P, pulse, QT prolongation, hypotension, palpitations

• Monitor bowel changes, bulk, fluids, laxatives should be used for constipation

### Nursing diagnoses
• Breathing pattern, ineffective (adverse reactions)

• Knowledge, deficient (teaching)

• Pain, acute (uses)

• Sensory perception, disturbed: visual, auditory (adverse reactions)

### Implementation
• Medication should be slowly withdrawn after long-term use to prevent withdrawal symptoms

#### PO route
• May be given with food or milk to lessen GI upset

• Store in light-resistant container at room temperature

#### IM/SUBCUT route
• Do not give if cloudy or a precipitate has formed

• Give deeply in large muscle mass; rotate inj sites

### Patient/family education
• Instruct patient to report any symptoms of CNS changes, allergic reactions; to avoid CNS depressants: alcohol, sedative/hypnotics for at least 24 hr after taking this product

• Discuss with patient that dizziness, drowsiness, and confusion are common; to avoid getting up without assistance

• Discuss in detail with patient all aspects of the product

• Caution patient to make position changes slowly to prevent orthostatic hypotension

### Evaluation
#### Positive therapeutic outcome
• Decreased pain
• Successful opioid withdrawal

**Treatment of overdose:** Naloxone (Narcan) 0.2-0.8 mg **IV**, O₂, **IV** fluids, vasopressors

## methimazole (Rx)
(meth-im'a-zole)
Tapazole
*Func. class.:* Thyroid hormone antagonist (antithyroid)
*Chem. class.:* Thioamide

**Pregnancy category** D

**Do not confuse:**
methimazole/metoprolol/minoxidil

**Action:** Inhibits synthesis of thyroid hormones by decreasing iodine use in the manufacture of thyroglobin and iodothyronine; does not affect already formed hormones

**Therapeutic outcome:** Decreased T₄ levels, hyperthyroid symptoms

Adverse effects: *italic* = common, **bold** = life-threatening

**Uses:** Hyperthyroidism, preparation for thyroidectomy, thyrotoxic crisis, thyroid storm

## Dosage and routes
### Hyperthyroidism
*Adult:* PO 15 mg/day (mild hyperthyroidism); 30-40 mg/day (moderate-severe); 60 mg/day (severe); maintenance dosage 5-15 mg/day
*Child:* PO 0.4 mg/kg/day in divided doses q8hr; continue until euthyroid; maintenance dosage 0.2 mg/kg/day in divided doses q8hr, max 30 mg/24 hr

### Preparation for thyroidectomy
*Adult and child:* PO Same as above; iodine may be added for 10 days before surgery

### Thyrotoxic crisis
*Adult and child:* PO Same as hyperthyroidism with iodine and propranolol

**Available forms:** Tabs 5, 10 mg

## Adverse effects
*CNS: Drowsiness, headache, vertigo, fever,* paresthesias, neuritis
*ENDO: Enlarged thyroid*
*GI: Nausea, diarrhea, vomiting, jaundice,* **hepatitis,** loss of taste
*GU: Nephritis*
*HEMA:* **Agranulocytosis, leukopenia, thrombocytopenia, hypothrombinemia, lymphadenopathy,** bleeding, vasculitis
*INTEG: Rash, urticaria, pruritus, alopecia, hyperpigmentation,* lupus-like syndrome
*MS: Myalgia, arthralgia, nocturnal muscle cramps*

**Contraindications:** Pregnancy **D**, breastfeeding, hypersensitivity

**Precautions:** Infection, bone marrow depression, hepatic disease

### Pharmacokinetics
| | |
|---|---|
| **Absorption** | Rapidly absorbed |
| **Distribution** | Crosses placenta |
| **Metabolism** | Liver, extensively |
| **Excretion** | Kidneys, unchanged; breast milk |
| **Half-life** | 5-13 hr |

### Pharmacodynamics
| | |
|---|---|
| **Onset** | ½ hr |
| **Peak** | Unknown |
| **Duration** | 2-4 hr |

## Interactions
### Individual drugs
Amiodarone, potassium iodide: decreased effectiveness
Digoxin, warfarin: increased response
Radiation: increased bone marrow depression
### Drug classifications
Antineoplastics: increased bone marrow depression
Phenothiazines: increased agranulocytosis
### Drug/lab test
Increased: protime, AST, ALT, alkaline phosphatase

## NURSING CONSIDERATIONS
### Assessment
• Monitor pulse, B/P, temp; check I&O ratio; check for edema (puffy hands, feet, periorbititis); indicates hypothyroidism
• Check weight daily; same clothing, scale, time of day
• Monitor $T_3$, $T_4$, which are increased; serum TSH, which is decreased; free thyroxine index, which is increased if dosage is too low; discontinue product 3-4 wk before radioactive iodine uptake
 Monitor blood studies: CBC for blood dyscrasias (leukopenia, thrombocytopenia, agranulocytosis); if these occur, product should be discontinued and other treatment initiated; liver function tests
• Assess for hypersensitivity (rash, enlarged cervical lymph nodes); product may have to be discontinued
• Assess for hypoprothrombinemia (bleeding, petechiae, ecchymosis)
• Monitor clinical response: after 3 wk should include increased weight, pulse, decreased $T_4$
 Assess for bone marrow depression: sore throat, fever, fatigue

### Nursing diagnoses
• Knowledge, deficient (teaching)
• Noncompliance (teaching)

### Implementation
• Give with meals to decrease GI upset; give at same time each day to maintain product level
• Give lowest dosage that relieves symptoms
• Store in light-resistant container
• Increase fluids to 3-4 L/day, unless contraindicated

### Patient/family education
• Advise patient to abstain from breastfeeding after delivery; product appears in breast milk
• Instruct patient to take pulse daily; to keep graph of weight, pulse, mood
• Advise patient to report redness, swelling,

sore throat, mouth lesions, which indicate blood dyscrasias
• Caution patient to avoid OTC products that contain iodine; that seafood and other iodine-containing products may be restricted by prescriber
• Caution patient not to discontinue this medication abruptly; thyroid crisis may occur; stress patient compliance
• Advise patient that response may take several mo if thyroid is large
• Teach patient symptoms/signs of overdose: periorbital edema, cold intolerance, mental depression; notify prescriber at once
• Teach patient symptoms of inadequate dosage: tachycardia, diarrhea, fever, irritability; prescriber should be notified to adjust
• Teach patient to take medication exactly as prescribed, not to skip or double doses; missed doses should be taken when remembered up to 1 hr before next dose
• Instruct patient to carry ID describing medication taken and condition being treated

### Evaluation
**Positive therapeutic outcome**
• Decreased weight gain
• Decreased pulse
• Decreased $T_4$
• Decreased B/P

---

### methocarbamol (Rx)
(meth-oh-kar′ba-mole)
Carbacot, methocarbamol, Relaxin, Robaxin
*Func. class.:* Skeletal muscle relaxant, central acting
*Chem. class.:* Carbamate derivative

**Pregnancy category** C

**Action:** Depresses multisynaptic pathways in the spinal cord, causing skeletal muscle relaxation

**Therapeutic outcome:** Decreased pain, spasm, resolution of tetanic spasms

**Uses:** Adjunct for relief of spasm and pain in musculoskeletal conditions, tetanus

### Dosage and routes
*Pain of muscle spasm*
*Adult:* PO 1.5 g qid × 2-3 days, then 1 g qid; IM 500 mg in each gluteal region; may repeat q8hr; **IV** BOL 1-3 g/day max at 3 ml/min; **IV** INF 1 g/250 ml D$_5$W or 0.9% NaCl, not to exceed 3 g/day

*Geriatric:* PO 500 mg qid, titrate to needed dose

*Tetanus management*
*Adult:* **IV** DIRECT 1-2 g or **IV** INF 1-3 g q6hr
*Child:* **IV** 15 mg/kg q6hr prn

**Available forms:** Tabs 500, 750 mg; inj 100 mg/ml

### Adverse effects
*CNS: Dizziness, weakness, drowsiness,* headache, tremor, depression, insomnia; **seizures** (**IV**, IM only)
*CV:* Postural hypotension, *bradycardia*
*EENT:* Diplopia, temporary loss of vision, blurred vision, nystagmus
*GI: Nausea,* vomiting, hiccups, anorexia, metallic taste
*GU:* Brown, black, green urine
*HEMA:* Hemolysis, increased hemoglobin (**IV** only)
*INTEG:* Rash, pruritus, fever, facial flushing, urticaria, phlebitis
*MISC:* **Anaphylaxis** (IM, **IV**)

**Contraindications:** Hypersensitivity, children <12 yr, intermittent porphyria, renal disease (IM/**IV**)

**Precautions:** Pregnancy C, renal/hepatic disease, addictive personalities, myasthenia gravis, epilepsy

M

### Pharmacokinetics
| | |
|---|---|
| Absorption | Rapidly absorbed (PO) |
| Distribution | Widely distributed; crosses placenta |
| Metabolism | Liver, partially |
| Excretion | Kidney, unchanged |
| Half-life | 1-2 hr |

### Pharmacodynamics
| | PO | IM | IV |
|---|---|---|---|
| Onset | ½ hr | Rapid | Rapid |
| Peak | 1-2 hr | Unknown | Inf end |
| Duration | >8 hr | Unknown | Unknown |

### Interactions
*Individual drugs*
Alcohol: increased CNS depression
*Drug classifications*
Antidepressants (tricyclic), barbiturates, opioids, sedative/hypnotics: increased CNS depression
*Drug/herb*
Chamomile, hops, kava, skullcap, valerian: increased CNS depression
*Drug/lab test*
False increase: VMA, urinary 5-HIAA

---

Adverse effects: *italic* = common, **bold** = life-threatening

## NURSING CONSIDERATIONS
### Assessment
- Assess for pain and spasm: location, duration, intensity, range of motion
- Monitor during and after inj: CNS effects, rash, conjunctivitis, and nasal congestion may occur
- Monitor ECG in epileptic patients; poor seizure control has occurred in patients taking this product
- Assess allergic reactions: rash, fever, respiratory distress; check for severe weakness, numbness in extremities
- Assess for tolerance: increased need for medication, more frequent requests for medication, increased pain
- Assess for CNS depression: dizziness, drowsiness, psychiatric symptoms

### Nursing diagnoses
- Injury, risk for (adverse reactions)
- Knowledge, deficient (teaching)
- Mobility, impaired physical (uses)

### Implementation
- Methocarbamol incompatible with any product in sol or syringe
**PO route**
- Give with meals if GI symptoms occur
- Store in airtight container at room temperature
**IM route**
- Give inj deep in large muscle mass; rotate sites
- Do not give SUBCUT
**IV route**
- Give **IV** undiluted over 1 min or more; give 300 mg or less/1 min or longer; may be diluted in 250 ml or less D₅ or isotonic NaCl sol for slow **IV** inf
- Give by slow **IV** to prevent phlebitis; keep recumbent during and for 15 min after to prevent orthostatic hypotension; check for extravasation

### Patient/family education
- Advise patient not to discontinue medication quickly; insomnia, nausea, headache, spasticity, tachycardia will occur; product should be tapered off over 1-2 wk
- Inform patient that urine may turn green, black, or brown
- Caution patient not to take with alcohol, other CNS depressants; increased CNS depression can occur
- Advise patient to avoid altering activities while taking this product
- Caution patient to avoid hazardous activities if drowsiness, dizziness occur; driving should be avoided until product response is known
- Advise patient to avoid using OTC medications that are CNS depressants (cough preparations, antihistamines) unless directed by prescriber; CNS depression can occur

### Evaluation
**Positive therapeutic outcome**
- Decreased pain, spasticity

**Treatment of overdose:** Activated charcoal, dialysis; have epINEPHrine, antihistamines, and corticosteroids available, enhance elimination with osmotic diureses, **IV** fluids for hypotension

## ❗ HIGH ALERT

## methotrexate, (amethopterin, MTX)
### 💿 (Rx)
(meth-oh-trex′ate)
Methotrexate, Rheumatrex, Dose Pack, Trexall
*Func. class.:* Antineoplastic, antimetabolite
*Chem. class.:* Folic acid antagonist

**Pregnancy category** X

**Do not confuse:**
methotrexate/metolazone/mitoxantene

**Action:** Inhibits an enzyme that reduces folic acid, which is needed for nucleic acid synthesis in all cells; cell cycle specific (S phase); immunosuppressive

**Therapeutic outcome:** Prevention of rapidly growing malignant cells; immunosuppression

**Uses:** Acute lymphocytic leukemia, in combination for breast, lung, head, neck carcinoma, lymphosarcoma, gestational choriocarcinoma, hydatidiform mole, psoriasis, rheumatoid arthritis, mycosis fungoides, osteosarcoma

**Unlabeled uses:** Used investigationally to produce abortion

**Dosage and routes**
*Acute lymphocytic leukemia*
*Adult and child:* PO/IM/**IV** 3.3 mg/m²/day × 4-6 wk until remission, then 20-30 mg/m² PO/IM qwk in 2 divided doses or 2.5 mg/kg **IV** × 2 wk

*Burkitt's lymphoma (stages I, II, III)*
*Adult:* PO 10-25 mg/day × 4-8 days with 7-day rest period

*Lymphosarcoma (stage III)*
*Adult:* PO/IM/**IV** 0.625-2.5 mg/kg/day

---

🔺 Alert      ♣ Canada Only      💿 Drug on CD          * "Tall Man" lettering (See Preface)

### Meningeal leukemia
*Adult and child:* 12 mg/m$^2$ IT q2-5 days until CSF is normal, then one additional dose, max 15 mg

### Choriocarcinoma
*Adult and child:* PO/IM 15-30 mg/m$^2$/day × 5 days, then off 1 wk; may repeat

### Breast cancer
*Adult:* **IV** 40 mg/m$^2$ on days 1 and 8 with other antineoplastics

### Rheumatoid arthritis
*Adult:* PO 7.5 mg/wk or divided doses of 2.5 mg q12hr × 3 given qwk, max 20 mg/wk

### Polyarticular-course juvenile RA
*Child:* PO 10 mg/m$^2$ qwk

### Osteosarcoma
*Adult and child:* **IV** 12 g/m$^2$ given over 4 hr, then leucovorin rescue is given

### Mycosis fungoides
*Adult:* PO 2.5-10 mg/day until cleared (may be many mo); IM 50 mg qwk or 25 mg 2 ×/wk

### Psoriasis
*Adult:* PO/IM/**IV** 10-25 mg qwk or 2.5 mg PO q12hr × 3 doses; may increase to 25 mg qwk

**Available forms:** Tabs 2.5, 5, 7.5, 10, 15 mg; inj 25 mg/ml; powder for inj 20 mg, 1 g

### Adverse effects
*CNS:* Dizziness, **seizures,** headache, confusion, hemiparesis, malaise, fatigue, chills, fever, **leukoencephalopathy; arachnoiditis** (intrathecal)
*GI: Nausea, vomiting, anorexia, diarrhea, ulcerative stomatitis,* **hepatotoxicity,** cramps, ulcer, gastritis, **GI hemorrhage,** abdominal pain, hematemesis, **hepatic fibrosis, acute toxicity**
*GU:* Urinary retention, **renal failure,** menstrual irregularities, defective spermatogenesis, **hematuria, azotemia, uric acid nephropathy**
*HEMA:* **Leukopenia, thrombocytopenia, myelosuppression, anemia**
*INTEG: Rash, alopecia,* dry skin, urticaria, photosensitivity, folliculitis, vasculitis, petechiae, ecchymosis, acne, alopecia, **severe fatal skin reactions**
*RESP:* **Methotrexate-induced lung disease**
*SYST:* **Sudden death,** *Pneumocystis jiroveci* **pneumonia**

**Contraindications:** Pregnancy **X,** hypersensitivity, leukopenia (<3500/mm$^3$), thrombocytopenia (<100,000/mm$^3$), anemia,

psoriatic patients with severe renal/hepatic disease, alcoholism, HIV infection

**Precautions:** Renal disease, breastfeeding, children

### Pharmacokinetics

| | |
|---|---|
| **Absorption** | Well absorbed (GI) |
| **Distribution** | Widely distributed; crosses placenta |
| **Metabolism** | Not metabolized |
| **Excretion** | Kidneys, unchanged; breast milk (minimal) |
| **Half-life** | Terminal 10-12 hr; increased in renal disease |

### Pharmacodynamics

| | PO | IM/IV | IT |
|---|---|---|---|
| **Onset** | Unknown | Unknown | Unknown |
| **Peak** | 1-4 hr | ½-2 hr | Unknown |
| **Duration** | Unknown | Unknown | Unknown |

### Interactions
#### Individual drugs
Alcohol, phenylbutazone, probenecid, radiation, theophylline: increased toxicity
Digoxin (PO), fosphenytoin, phenytoin: decreased effect of each specific product
Folic acid: decreased effect of methotrexate
Radiation: increased bone marrow suppression

#### Drug classifications
Anticoagulants (oral): increased hypoprothrombinemia
Antineoplastics, NSAIDs, penicillins, salicylates, sulfa products: increased toxicity
Live virus vaccines: decreased antibodies

### NURSING CONSIDERATIONS
#### Assessment
• Assess buccal cavity q8hr for dryness, sores or ulceration, white patches, oral pain, bleeding, dysphagia; obtain prescription for viscous lidocaine (Xylocaine)
• Assess symptoms indicating severe allergic reaction: rash, pruritus, urticaria, purpuric skin lesions, itching, flushing
• Assess tachypnea, ECG changes, dyspnea, edema, fatigue; identify dyspnea, crackles, unproductive cough, chest pain, tachypnea
• Monitor CBC, differential, platelet count weekly; withhold product if WBC is <3500/mm$^3$ or platelet count is <100,000/mm$^3$; notify prescriber of results if WBC <20,000/mm$^3$, platelets <150,000/mm$^3$; WBC, platelet nadirs occur on day 7
• Assess for increased uric acid levels, swelling, joint pain primarily in extremities; patient should be well hydrated to prevent urate deposits

Adverse effects: *italic* = common, **bold** = life-threatening

M

• Monitor renal function studies: BUN, creatinine, serum uric acid, urine CCr before and during therapy; check I&O ratio; report fall in urine output to <30 ml/hr
• Monitor temp (may indicate beginning of infection)
• Monitor liver function tests before and during therapy (bilirubin, AST, ALT, LDH) as needed or monthly; check for jaundice of skin and sclera, dark urine, clay-colored stools, itchy skin, abdominal pain, fever, diarrhea (hepatotoxicity)
• Assess for bleeding: hematuria, stool guaiac, bruising or petechiae, mucosa or orifices; check for inflammation of mucosa, breaks in skin
• Identify effects of alopecia on body image; discuss feelings about body changes
• Identify edema in feet, joint and stomach pain, shaking; prescriber should be notified
• Monitor methotrexate levels, adjust leucovorin dose based on the level

### Nursing diagnoses
• Body image, disturbed (adverse reactions)
• Infection, risk for (adverse reactions)
• Injury, risk for (adverse reactions)
• Knowledge, deficient (teaching)

### Implementation
• Avoid contact with skin, since product is very irritating; wash completely to remove
◆ Administer leucovorin calcium within 24 hr of giving this product to prevent tissue damage; check agency policy; continue until methotrexate level <$10^{-8}$ m
• Give fluids **IV** or PO before chemotherapy to hydrate patient
• Give antiemetic 30-60 min before giving product and prn to prevent vomiting; administer antibiotics for infection prophylaxis
• Give in AM so product can be eliminated before bedtime
• Provide liquid diet: carbonated beverages; gelatin may be added if patient is not nauseated or vomiting

**PO route**
• Give 1 hr before or 2 hr after meals to prevent vomiting
• Make sure product is taken weekly in RA, JRA

**IM route**
• Give deeply in large muscle mass

**IV route**
• Give **IV** after diluting 5 mg/2 ml of sterile water for inj; give through Y-tube or 3-way stopcock
• Give **IV** inf after diluting in 0.9% NaCl, D$_5$W, D$_5$/0.9% NaCl and give as prescribed

◆ Give sodium bicarbonate tabs or **IV** fluids to prevent precipitation of product at high doses, urine pH should be >7; may need to reduce dose if BUN is 20-30 mg/dl or creatinine is 1.2-2 mg/dl; stop product if BUN >30 mg/dl or creatitine is >2 mg/dl

*Syringe compatibilities:* Bleomycin, cisplatin, cyclophosphamide, doxapram, DOXOrubicin, fluorouracil, furosemide, heparin, leucovorin, mitomycin, vinBLAStine, vinCRIStine

*Syringe incompatibilities:* Droperidol, ranitidine

*Y-site compatibilities:* Allopurinol, amifostine, asparaginase, aztreonam, bleomycin, cefepime, ceftriaxone, cimetidine, cisplatin, cyclophosphamide, cytarabine, DAUNOrubicin, dexchlorpheniramine, diphenhydrAMINE, DOXOrubicin, etoposide, famotidine, filgrastim, fludarabine, fluorouracil, furosemide, gallium, ganciclovir, granisetron, heparin, hydromorphone, imipenem-cilastatin, leucovorin, lorazepam, melphalan, mesna, methylPREDNISolone, metoclopramide, mitomycin, morphine, ondansetron, oxacillin, paclitaxel, piperacillin/tazobactam, prochlorperazine, ranitidine, sargramostim, teniposide, thiotepa, vinBLAStine, vinCRIStine, vinorelbine

*Y-site incompatibilities:* Droperidol, idarubicin

*Additive compatibilities:* Cephalothin, cyclophosphamide, cytarabine, fluorouracil, hydrOXYzine, mercaptopurine, ondansetron, sodium bicarbonate, vinCRIStine

*Additive incompatibilities:* Bleomycin, prednisoLONE

*Solution compatibilities:* Amino acids, 4.25%/D$_{25}$, D$_5$W, sodium bicarbonate 0.05 mol/L, sodium chloride 0.9%

### Patient/family education
• Encourage patient to rinse mouth tid-qid with water, club soda; brush teeth bid-qid with soft brush or cotton-tipped applicators for stomatitis; use unwaxed dental floss
• Advise patient that contraceptive measures are recommended during therapy; product is teratogenic; contraception should be used for 3 mo (male) and 4-6 wk (female); to discontinue breastfeeding; toxicity to infant may occur
• Teach patient to avoid use of products containing aspirin or NSAIDs, razors, commercial mouthwash, since bleeding may occur; to report symptoms of bleeding (hematuria, tarry stools)
• Caution patient to report signs of anemia

(fatigue, headache, irritability, faintness, shortness of breath); seizures
• Advise patient to report any changes in breathing or coughing even several mo after treatment; to avoid crowds and persons with respiratory tract or other infections
• Advise patient to report stomatitis: any bleeding, white spots, ulcerations in mouth to prescriber; tell patient to examine mouth daily, report symptoms, use good oral hygiene
• Teach patient that hair may be lost during treatment; a wig or hairpiece may make patient feel better; new hair may be different in color, texture
• Caution patient not to have any vaccinations without the advice of the prescriber; serious reactions can occur
• Advise patient to use sunblock or protective clothing to prevent burns

## Evaluation
**Positive therapeutic outcome**
• Prevention of rapid division of malignant cells
• Decreased joint inflammation in RA

## methyldopa/ methyldopate (Rx)
(meth-ill-doe'pa)

Aldomet, Apo-methyldopa ✦,
Dopamet ✦, methyldopa/methyldopate,
Novo-medopa ✦, Nu-Medopa ✦
*Func. class.:* Antihypertensive
*Chem. class.:* Centrally acting α-adrenergic inhibitor

### Pregnancy category
B (PO)
C (IV)

### Do not confuse:
methyldopa/L-dopa (levodopa)

**Action:** Stimulates central $\alpha_2$-adrenergic receptors in the CNS, resulting in decreased sympathetic outflow from the brain with decreased peripheral resistance

**Therapeutic outcome:** Decreased B/P in hypertension

**Uses:** Hypertension, hypertensive crisis

### Dosage and routes
*Adult:* PO 250-500 mg bid or tid, then adjusted q2 days prn, 0.5-2 g/day in 2-4 divided doses (maintenance), max 3 g/day; **IV** 250-500 mg in 100 ml $D_5W$ q6hr, run over 30-60 min, not to exceed 1 g q6hr, switch to PO as soon as possible

*Geriatric:* PO 125 mg bid tid, increase q2 days as needed, max 3 g/day
*Child:* PO 10 mg/kg/day in 2-4 divided doses, max 65 mg/kg or 3 g/day, whichever is less; **IV** 20-40 mg/kg/day in 4 divided doses, max 65 mg/kg or 3 g, whichever is less

**Available forms:** Methyldopa: tabs 125, 250, 500 mg; oral susp 50 mg/ml; methyldopate: inj 50 mg/ml (250 mg/5 ml)

### Adverse effects
*CNS: Drowsiness, weakness, dizziness, sedation, headache,* depression, psychosis, paresthesias, parkinsonism, Bell's palsy, nightmares
*CV:* Bradycardia, **myocarditis,** orthostatic hypotension, angina, edema, weight gain, **CHF,** paradoxical pressor response (**IV** use)
*EENT:* Nasal congestion
*ENDO:* Breast enlargement, gynecomastia, breastfeeding, amenorrhea
*GI:* Nausea, vomiting, diarrhea, constipation, **hepatic dysfunction,** sore or "black" tongue, **pancreatitis,** colitis, flatulence
*GU:* Impotence, failure to ejaculate
*HEMA:* **Leukopenia, thrombocytopenia, hemolytic anemia, granulocytopenia,** positive Coombs' test
*INTEG:* Lupus-like syndrome, rash, **toxic epidural necrolysis**

**Contraindications:** Active hepatic disease, hypersensitivity

**Precautions:** Pregnancy **B** (PO), **C** (**IV**), eclampsia, severe cardiac disease, renal/hepatic disease, CHF, edema

### Pharmacokinetics
| | |
|---|---|
| **Absorption** | 50% (PO) |
| **Distribution** | Crosses placenta, blood-brain barrier |
| **Metabolism** | Liver, moderately |
| **Excretion** | Kidneys, unchanged (partially) |
| **Half-life** | 1½ hr |

### Pharmacodynamics
| | PO | IV |
|---|---|---|
| **Onset** | Unknown | Unknown |
| **Peak** | 2-4 hr | 2 hr |
| **Duration** | 12-24 hr | 10-16 hr |

### Interactions
*Individual drugs*
Alcohol: CNS depression
Haloperidol: increased psychosis
Iron: decreased methyldopa absorption
Levodopa: increased CNS toxicity, hypotension

M

Adverse effects: *italic* = common, **bold** = life-threatening

Lithium: increased lithium toxicity

TOLBUTamide: increased hypoglycemia

**Drug classifications**

Amphetamines, antidepressants (tricyclics), barbiturates, NSAIDs, phenothiazines: decreased antihypertensive effect

Analgesics, antidepressants, antihistamines, sedative/hypnotics: increased CNS depression

Antihypertensives, diuretics: increased hypotension

β-Adrenergic blockers: increased B/P

MAOIs: increased pressor effect

Sympathomimetic amines: increased pressor effect

**Drug/herb**

Aconite: increased toxicity, death

Astragalus, cola tree: increased or decreased antihypertensive effect

Barberry, betony, black catechu, black cohosh, bloodroot, broom, burdock, cat's claw, dandelion, goldenseal, hawthorn, Irish moss, Jamaican dogwood, kelp, khella, mistletoe, parsley: increased antihypertensive effect

Capsicum, Indian snakeroot: decreased effect

Coltsfoot, guarana, khat, licorice, yohimbe: decreased antihypertensive effect

**Drug/lab test**

Interference: urinary uric acid, serum creatinine, AST

False increase: urinary catecholamines

## NURSING CONSIDERATIONS
### Assessment

• Monitor blood tests: neutrophils, decreased platelets; direct Coombs' test before and after 6, 12 mo of therapy

• Monitor renal studies: protein, BUN, creatinine; watch for increased levels that may indicate nephrotic syndrome: polyuria, oliguria, frequency; report weight gain >5 lb

• Obtain baselines in renal, liver function tests before therapy begins; check potassium levels, although hyperkalemia rarely occurs

• Monitor B/P, pulse if the product is being used for hypertension; notify prescriber of changes

• Monitor edema in feet, legs daily; monitor I&O; check weight for decreasing output

• Assess for allergic reaction: rash, fever, pruritus, urticaria; product should be discontinued if antihistamines fail to help

• Monitor CNS symptoms, especially in the geriatric, depression, change in mental status

### Nursing diagnoses

• Cardiac output, decreased (uses)

• Injury, risk for (side effects)

• Knowledge, deficient (teaching)

• Noncompliance (teaching)

## Implementation
### PO route

• Give before meals

• Shake susp before using

• Store in airtight container at room temperature

### IV route

• Give by intermittent inf after diluting in 100 ml of 0.9% NaCl, $D_5W$, $D_5$/0.9% NaCl, 5% sodium bicarbonate, Ringer's; administer over 30-60 min

**Y-site compatibilities:** Esmolol, heparin, meperidine, morphine, theophylline

**Additive compatibilities:** Aminophylline, ascorbic acid, chloramphenicol, diphenhydrAMINE, heparin, magnesium sulfate, multivitamins, netilmicin, potassium chloride, promazine, sodium bicarbonate, succinylcholine, verapamil, vit B/C

**Additive incompatibilities:** Amphotericin B, barbiturates, methohexital, sulfonamides

**Solution compatibilities:** $D_5W$, $D_5$/0.9% NaCl, Ringer's, sodium bicarbonate 5%, 0.9% NaCl, amino acids 4.25%/$D_{25}$, Dextran$_6$/0.9% NaCl, Normosol R, Normosol M/$D_5W$

### Patient/family education

• Instruct patient not to discontinue product abruptly, or withdrawal symptoms may occur: anxiety, increased B/P, headache, insomnia, increased pulse, tremors, nausea, sweating

• Caution patient not to use OTC (cough, cold, or allergy) products unless directed by prescriber

• Teach patient to comply with dosage schedule even if feeling better; product controls symptoms, does not cure

• Caution patient to change position slowly, to rise slowly to sitting or standing position to minimize orthostatic hypotension, especially geriatric

• Teach patient about excessive perspiration, dehydration, vomiting, diarrhea, may lead to fall in B/P; consult prescriber if these occur

• Advise patient that product may cause dizziness, fainting; light-headedness may occur during 1st few days of therapy; that product may cause dry mouth; use hard candy, saliva product, or frequent rinsing of mouth

• Caution patient that compliance is necessary; not to skip or stop product unless directed by prescriber

• Teach patient that product may cause skin rash

• Teach patient to avoid hazardous activities, since product may cause drowsiness, dizziness

### Evaluation
**Positive therapeutic outcome**
- Decreased B/P

**Treatment of overdose:** Gastric evacuation, sympathomimetics, may be indicated if severe; hemodialysis

---

## methylergonovine (Rx)
(meth-ill-er-goe-noe'veen)
Methergine, methylergonovine
*Func. class.:* Oxytocic
*Chem. class.:* Ergot alkaloid

**Pregnancy category C**

**Action:** Stimulates uterine and vascular smooth muscle, causing contractions, decreased bleeding, arterial vasoconstriction

**Therapeutic outcome:** Absence of hemorrhage

**Uses:** Treatment of hemorrhage postpartum or after abortion, uterine contractions

### Dosage and routes
*Adult:* PO 200-400 mcg q6-12hr × 2-7 days
IM/**IV** 200 mcg q2-4hr for 1-5 doses

**Available forms:** Inj 200 mcg/ml; tabs 200 mcg

### Adverse effects
*CNS: Headache, dizziness,* **seizures**
*CV:* **Hypotension,** chest pain, palpitations, *hypertension,* **dysrhythmias; CVA (IV)**
*EENT:* Tinnitus
*GI: Nausea, vomiting*
*GU:* Cramping
*INTEG:* Sweating, rash, allergic reactions
*RESP: Dyspnea*

**Contraindications:** Pregnancy (4th stage of labor), hypersensitivity to ergot preparations, indication of labor, before delivery of placenta, hypertension, PID, respiratory disease, cardiac disease, peripheral vascular disease

**Precautions:** Pregnancy **C,** severe renal/hepatic disease, jaundice, diabetes mellitus, seizure disorders, sepsis, CAD

### Pharmacokinetics
| | |
|---|---|
| Absorption | Well absorbed (PO, IM) |
| Distribution | Unknown |
| Metabolism | Liver, possibly |
| Excretion | Unknown |
| Half-life | ½-2 hr |

### Pharmacodynamics
| | PO | IM | IV |
|---|---|---|---|
| Onset | 5-15 min | 5 min | Immediate |
| Peak | Unknown | Unknown | Unknown |
| Duration | 3 hr | 3 hr | Unknown |

### Interactions
*Individual drugs*
Smoking: increased vasoconstriction
*Drug classifications*
Vasopressors: increased vasoconstriction

### NURSING CONSIDERATIONS
**Assessment**
- Monitor B/P, pulse; watch for change that may indicate hemorrhage; check respiratory rate, rhythm, depth; notify prescriber of abnormalities
- Assess fundal tone, nonphasic contractions; check for relaxation or severe cramping
- Assess for ergotism or overdose: nausea, vomiting, weakness, muscular pain, insensitivity to cold, paresthesia of extremities; product should be decreased or infusion discontinued
- Before administering ergonovine, check calcium levels; if hypocalcemia is present, correction should be made to increase effectiveness of this product
- Monitor prolactin levels and for decreased breast milk production

**Nursing diagnoses**
- Injury, risk for (adverse reactions)
- Knowledge, deficient (teaching)
- Tissue perfusion, ineffective (uses)

**Implementation**
**PO route**
- PO is the preferred route
**IM route**
- Give inj deeply in large muscle mass
**IV route**
- Give by this route for severe, life-threatening hemorrhage
- Give directly undiluted or diluted with 5 ml of 0.9% NaCl given through Y-site or 3-way stopcock; give 0.2 mg/min; use clear, colorless sol
- Store up to 2 mo if unused
***Y-site compatibilities:*** Heparin, hydrocortisone sodium succinate, potassium chloride, vit B/C

**Patient/family education**
- Advise patient to stop smoking, since increased vasoconstriction will result
- Inform patient that abdominal cramps are a side effect of this medication

M

Adverse effects: *italic* = common, **bold** = life-threatening

• Instruct patient to notify prescriber if chest pain, nausea, vomiting, headache, muscle pain, weakness or cold, numb extremities occur

### Evaluation
**Positive therapeutic outcome**
• Prevention of hemorrhage

---

## methylphenidate (Rx)
(meth-ill-fen′i-date)
Concerta, Daytrana, Metadate CD, Methidate, Methylin, Methylin ER, PMS-Methylphenidate ✤, Riphenidate ✤, Ritalin, Ritalin SR, Ritalin LA
*Func. class.:* Cerebral stimulant
*Chem. class.:* Piperidine derivative

**Pregnancy category C**

**Controlled substance schedule II**

**Do not confuse:**
methylphenidate/methadone

**Action:** Increases release of norepinephrine and dopamine in cerebral cortex to reticular activating system; exact action not known

**Therapeutic outcome:** Increased alertness, decreased fatigue, ability to stay awake (narcolepsy), increased attention span, decreased hyperactivity (ADHD)

**Uses:** Attention deficit disorder with hyperactivity (ADHD), narcolepsy (except Concerta, Metadate CD, Ritalin LA), attention deficit disorder (ADD)

**Unlabeled uses:** Depression in the geriatric, cancer, poststroke, HIV, brain injury, improvement of pain control, sedation in patients receiving opiates

### Dosage and routes
*ADHD*
*Child >6 yr:* PO (immediate-release tab, chew tabs, oral sol) 5 mg before breakfast and lunch, increasing by 5-10 mg/wk, not to exceed 60 mg/day; EXT REL 20 mg daily-tid

*Attention deficit hyperactivity disorder, conversion from PO to transdermal*
*Child 6-12 yr:* Week 1, 12.5 cm$^2$ (10 mg); week 2, 18.75 cm$^2$ (15 mg); week 3, 25 cm$^2$ (20 mg); week 4, 37.5 cm$^2$ (30 mg)

*Narcolepsy*
*Adult:* PO 10 mg bid-tid, 30-45 min before meals; may increase up to 40-60 mg/day

*Major depression/poststroke depression*
*Adult and geriatric:* PO 2.5 mg q AM, increase q 3rd day by 2.5 mg to desired dose, max 20 mg/day

**Available forms:** Tabs 5, 10, 20 mg; ext rel tabs 10, 20 mg; ext rel tabs (Concerta) 18, 27, 36, 54 mg; chew tabs (Methylin) 2.5, 5, 10 mg; ext rel cap 10, 20, 30, 40 mg; oral sol 5 mg, 10 mg/ml; transdermal patch 12.5 cm$^2$ (10 mg), 18.75 cm$^2$ (15 mg), 25 cm$^2$ (20 mg), 37.5 cm$^2$ (30 mg)

### Adverse effects
*CNS: Hyperactivity, insomnia, restlessness, talkativeness,* dizziness, headache, akathisia, dyskinesia, masking or worsening of Gilles de la Tourette's syndrome, **seizures,** drowsiness, toxic psychosis
*CV: Palpitations, tachycardia,* B/P changes, angina, **dysrhythmias**
*ENDO:* Growth retardation
*GI:* Nausea, anorexia, dry mouth, weight loss, abdominal pain
*HEMA:* **Leukopenia,** anemia, **thrombocytopenic purpura**
*INTEG:* **Exfoliative dermatitis,** urticaria, rash, erythema multiforme
*MISC:* Fever, arthralgia, scalp hair loss

**Contraindications:** Hypersensitivity, anxiety, history of Gilles de la Tourette's syndrome, children <6 yr, glaucoma, anorexia nervosa, tartrazine dye hypersensitivity

**Precautions:** Pregnancy **C,** breastfeeding, hypertension, depression, seizures, product abuse

| Pharmacokinetics | |
|---|---|
| **Absorption** | Well absorbed (PO); delayed (ext rel) |
| **Distribution** | Widely distributed; crosses placenta |
| **Metabolism** | Liver |
| **Excretion** | Kidneys |
| **Half-life** | 1-3 hr |

| Pharmacodynamics | | |
|---|---|---|
| | PO | PO–EXT REL |
| **Onset** | ½-1 hr | 2 hr |
| **Peak** | 1-3 hr | 4 hr |
| **Duration** | 4-6 hr | 6-8 hr |

### Interactions
*Individual drugs*
Guanethidine: decreased effect of guanethidine

---

### Drug classifications
Anticonvulsants, antidepressants (tricyclics), selective serotonin reuptake inhibitors: increased effects
MAOIs (or within 14 days of MAOIs), vasopressors: hypertensive crisis
### Drug/herb
Cola nut, guarana, horsetail, yerba maté, yohimbe: increased CNS stimulation
Melatonin: synergistic effect
### Drug/food
Caffeine: increased stimulation

### NURSING CONSIDERATIONS
### Assessment
• Monitor VS, B/P, since this product may reverse antihypertensives; check patients with cardiac disease more often for increased B/P
• Perform CBC, urinalysis; for diabetic patients monitor blood glucose, urine glucose; insulin changes may be required, since eating will decrease
• Monitor height and weight q3 mo since growth rate in children may be decreased; appetite is suppressed, weight loss is common during the first few mo of treatment
• Monitor mental status: mood sensorium, affect, stimulation, insomnia; aggressiveness may occur; depression with crying spells may occur after product has worn off
• Assess for tolerance; should not be used for extended time except in ADHD; dosage should be discontinued gradually to prevent withdrawal symptoms
• Assess for narcoleptic symptoms before medication and after; ability to stay awake should increase significantly
• In children or adults with ADHD, monitor for improved organizational skills, attention span, attending to tasks, impulse control, socialization, and ability to get along better with others
◆ Assess for withdrawal symptoms: headache, nausea, vomiting, muscle pain, weakness; product tolerance will develop after long-term use; dosage should not be increased if tolerance develops
• Assess appetite, sleep, speech patterns

### Nursing diagnoses
• Coping, compromised family (uses)
• Coping, ineffective (uses)
• Knowledge, deficient (teaching)
• Thought processes, disturbed (uses, adverse reactions)

### Implementation
• Do not chew, crush time rel tabs; caps may be opened and beads sprinkled over spoonful of applesauce
• Give at least 6 hr before bedtime (regular release); at least 10 hr (ext rel) to avoid sleeplessness; titrate to patient's response; lowest dosage should be used to control symptoms
• Give gum, hard candy, frequent sips of water for dry mouth at beginning of treatment; these symptoms tend to lessen with time

### Patient/family education
• Teach patient to decrease caffeine consumption (coffee, tea, cola, chocolate); not to use guarana, cola nut, yerba maté, which may increase irritability and stimulation; to avoid OTC preparations unless approved by prescriber; to avoid alcohol ingestion; these may cause serious product interactions
• Advise patient to taper off product over several wk, or depression, increased sleeping, lethargy may occur
• Caution patient to avoid hazardous activities until stabilized on medication
• Instruct patient not to double doses if medication is missed; prescriber may suggest product holidays (ADHD) during the school year to assess progress and determine continued product necessity
• Instruct patient/family to notify prescriber if significant side effects occur: tremors, insomnia, palpitations, restlessness; product changes may be needed
• Inform patient that if dry mouth occurs to use frequent sips of water, sugarless gum, hard candy during beginning therapy; dry mouth lessens with continued treatment
• Encourage patient to get needed rest; patient will feel more tired at end of day; to take last dose at least 6 hr before bedtime to avoid insomnia
• Advise patient that shell of Concerta tab may appear in stools

### Evaluation
#### Positive therapeutic outcome
• Decreased hyperactivity in ADHD
• Improved attention span in ADHD
• Absence of sleeping during day in narcolepsy

### Treatment of overdose: Administer fluids, hemodialysis, peritoneal dialysis, antihypertensives for increased B/P

M

## *methylPREDNISolone (Rx)
(meth-ill-pred-niss'oh-lone)
A-Methapred, dep Medalone, Depoject, Depo-Medrol, Depopred, Depo-Predate, Duralone, Medralone, Medrol, Rep-Pred, Solu-Medrol
*Func. class.:* Corticosteroid, synthetic
*Chem. class.:* Glucocorticoid, immediate acting

**Pregnancy category C**

### Do not confuse:
methylPREDNISolone/medroxyPROGESTERone, predniSONE/methylTESTOSTERone

**Action:** Decreases inflammation by suppression of migration of polymorphonuclear leukocytes, fibroblasts; reverses increased capillary permeability and lysosomal stabilization; antipruritic, antiinflammatory (topical)

**Therapeutic outcome:** Decreased inflammation

**Uses:** Severe inflammation, shock, adrenal insufficiency, collagen disorders, management of acute spinal cord injury, multiple sclerosis

### Dosage and routes
*Adrenal insufficiency/ inflammation*
*Adult:* PO 2-60 mg in 4 divided doses; IM 10-80 mg (acetate); IM/**IV** 10-250 mg (succinate); intraarticular 4-30 mg (acetate); RECT 40 mg 3-7 × wk for ≥2 wk
*Child:* **IV** 0.5-1.7 mg/kg in 3-4 divided doses (succinate); RECT 0.5-1 mg/kg (15-30 mg/m²) daily or every other day × 1 wk or more

*Shock*
*Adult:* **IV** 100-250 mg q2-6hr or 30 mg/kg, then q4-6hr prn × 2-3 days (succinate)

*Multiple sclerosis*
*Adult:* PO 160 mg/day × 1 wk, then 64 mg every other day × 30 days

**Available forms:** Tabs 2, 4, 6, 8, 16, 24, 32 mg; inj 20, 40, 80 mg/ml acetate; inj 40, 125, 500, 1000, 2000 mg/vial succinate, dose pack 4 mg tabs; susp for inj 20, 40, 80 mg/ml; enema 40 mg

### Adverse effects
*CNS:* Depression, flushing, sweating, headache, mood changes
*CV:* Hypertension, **circulatory collapse, thrombophlebitis, embolism,** tachycardia
*EENT:* Fungal infections, increased intraocular pressure, blurred vision, cataracts
*GI:* Diarrhea, nausea, abdominal distention, **GI hemorrhage,** increased appetite, **pancreatitis**
*HEMA:* **Thrombocytopenia**
*INTEG:* Acne, poor wound healing, ecchymosis, petechiae
*MS:* Fractures, osteoporosis, weakness

**Contraindications:** Children <2 yr, hypersensitivity to corticosteroids, fungal infections, psychosis, idiopathic thrombocytopenia, acute glomerulonephritis, amebiasis, nonasthmatic bronchial disease, AIDS, TB

**Precautions:** Pregnancy **C**, breastfeeding, diabetes mellitus, glaucoma, osteoporosis, seizure disorders, ulcerative colitis, CHF, myasthenia gravis, renal disease, esophagitis, peptic ulcer

### Pharmacokinetics

| | |
|---|---|
| **Absorption** | Well absorbed (PO); systemic (topical) |
| **Distribution** | Crosses placenta |
| **Metabolism** | Liver, extensively |
| **Excretion** | Kidney |
| **Half-life** | 3-5 hr (plasma) 18-36 hr (tissue); adrenal suppression 3-4 days |

### Pharmacodynamics

| | PO | IM | IV | TOPICAL |
|---|---|---|---|---|
| **Onset** | Unknown | Unknown | Rapid | Min to hr |
| **Peak** | 2 hr | 4-8 days | Unknown | Hr to days |
| **Duration** | 1½ days | 1-4 wk | Unknown | Hr to days |

### Interactions
*Individual drugs*
Amphotericin B: increased side effects
Insulin: increased need for insulin
Phenytoin, rifampin, theophylline: decreased action; increased metabolism
Somatrem: decreased effect
*Drug classifications*
Contraceptives, oral: increased methylPREDNISolone action
CYP3A4 inducers (barbiturates, bosentan, carbamazepine, efavirenz, phenytoins, nevirapine, rifabutin, rifampin): decreased methylPREDNISolone effect
CYP3A4 inhibitors (aprepitant, antiretroviral protease inhibitors, clarithromycin, danazol, delavirdine, diltiazem, erythromycin, fluconazole, fluoxetine, fluvoxamine, imatinib, ketoconazole, mibefradil, nefazodone, telithromycin, voriconazole): increased adrenal suppression
Diuretics: increased side effects

Hypoglycemic agents: increased need for hypoglycemic agents

### Drug/herb
Aloe, buckthorn, cascara sagrada, Chinese rhubarb, senna: increased hypokalemia

Aloe, licorice, perilla: increased corticosteroid effect

### Drug/food
Grapefruit juice: increased methylPREDNISolone level; do not use concurrently

St. John's wort: avoid use

### Drug/lab test
Increased: cholesterol, sodium, blood glucose, uric acid, calcium, urine glucose

Decreased: calcium, potassium, $T_4$, $T_3$, thyroid radioactive iodine uptake test, urine 17-OHCS, 17-KS

False negative: skin allergy tests

## NURSING CONSIDERATIONS
### Assessment
• Monitor potassium, blood glucose, urine glucose while patient is on long-term therapy; hypokalemia and hyperglycemia

• Monitor weight daily; notify prescriber of weekly gain >5 lb

• Monitor B/P q4hr, pulse; notify prescriber if chest pain occurs

• Monitor I&O ratio; be alert for decreasing urinary output and increasing edema

• Monitor plasma cortisol levels during long-term therapy (normal level 138-635 nmol/L when drawn at 8 AM)

• Monitor adrenal function periodically for hypothalamic-pituitary-adrenal axis suppression

• Assess for infection: increased temp, WBC even after withdrawal of medication; product masks infection symptoms

• Assess for potassium depletion: paresthesias, fatigue, nausea, vomiting, depression, polyuria, dysrhythmias, weakness

• Assess for edema, hypertension, cardiac symptoms

• Assess mental status: affect, mood, behavioral changes, aggression

• Check temp; if fever develops, product should be discontinued

• Assess for systemic absorption: increased temp, inflammation, irritation (topical)

### Nursing diagnoses
• Infection, risk for (adverse reactions)
• Knowledge, deficient (teaching)
• Noncompliance (teaching)

## Implementation
### PO route
• Give with food or milk to decrease GI symptoms

### IM route
• Give IM inj deep in large muscle mass; rotate sites; avoid deltoid; use 21-G needle

• Give in one dose in AM to prevent adrenal suppression; avoid SUBCUT administration; may damage tissue

### Inhalation route
• Give inh with water to decrease possibility of fungal infections

• Give titrated dosage; use lowest effective dosage

• Clean aerosol topical daily with warm water; dry thoroughly

• Store in cool environment; do not puncture or incinerate container

### Topical route
• Cleanse area before applying product

• Apply only to affected areas; do not get in eyes

• Apply medication, then cover with occlusive dressing (only if prescribed); seal to normal skin; change q12hr; systemic absorption may occur

• Apply only to dermatoses; do not use on weeping, denuded, or infected area

• Apply treatment for a few days after area has cleared

• Store at room temperature

### IV route
• Give **IV**, use only sodium phosphate product; give >1 min; may be given by **IV** inf in compatible sol

• Give after shaking susp (parenteral)

• Give titrated dosage; use lowest effective dosage

*Syringe compatibilities:* Granisetron, metoclopramide

*Y-site compatibilities:* Acyclovir, amifostine, aztreonam, cefepime, cisplatin, cladribine, cyclophosphamide, cytarabine, DOPamine, DOXOrubicin, enalaprilat, famotidine, fludarabine, granisetron, heparin, inamrinone, melphalan, meperidine, methotrexate, metronidazole, midazolam, morphine, piperacillin/tazobactam, sodium bicarbonate, tacrolimus, teniposide, theophylline, thiotepa, vit B with C

*Y-site incompatibilities:* Ondansetron, paclitaxel, sargramostim, vinorelbine

*Additive compatibilities:* Chloramphenicol, cimetidine, clindamycin, DOPamine, granisetron, heparin, norepinephrine, penicillin G potassium, ranitidine, theophylline, verapamil

M

Adverse effects: *italic* = common, **bold** = life-threatening

### Patient/family education
• Teach patient that emergency ID as steroid user should be carried/worn
• Advise patient to notify prescriber if therapeutic response decreases; dosage adjustment may be needed
• Caution patient not to discontinue abruptly; adrenal crisis can result
• Caution patient to avoid OTC products: salicylates, alcohol in cough products, cold preparations unless directed by prescriber
• Teach patient all aspects of product usage including cushingoid symptoms
• Teach patient symptoms of adrenal insufficiency: nausea, anorexia, fatigue, dizziness, dyspnea, weakness, joint pain
• Inform patient that long-term therapy may be needed to clear infection (1-2 mo depending on type of infection)

**Nasal route**
• Advise patient to clear nasal passages if sneezing attack occurs; repeat dose
• Advise patient to continue using product even if mild nasal bleeding occurs; is usually transient
• Teach patient method of instillation after providing written instructions from manufacturer

**Topical route**
• Advise patient to avoid sunlight on affected area; burns may occur

### Evaluation
**Positive therapeutic outcome**
• Ease of respirations, decreased inflammation
• Absence of severe itching, patches on skin, flaking (top)

---

## metipranolol ophthalmic
*See Appendix D*

---

## metoclopramide (Rx)
(met-oh-kloe-pra′mide)
Apo-Metoclop , Emex , Maxeran , metoclopramide, Octamide, Reglan, Sensamide IV
*Func. class.:* Cholinergic, antiemetic
*Chem. class.:* Central dopamine receptor antagonist

**Pregnancy category** B

**Do not confuse:**
metoclopramide/metolazone, Reglan/Megace/Renagel

**Action:** Enhances response to acetylcholine of tissue in upper GI tract, which causes contraction of gastric muscle, relaxes pyloric, duodenal segments, increases peristalsis without stimulating secretions, blocks dopamine in chemoreceptor trigger zone of CNS

**Therapeutic outcome:** Decreased symptoms of delayed gastric emptying, decreased nausea, vomiting

**Uses:** Prevention of nausea, vomiting induced by chemotherapy, radiation; delayed gastric emptying, gastroesophageal reflux

**Unlabeled uses:** Hiccups, migraines, breastfeeding induction, lung cancer

### Dosage and routes
*Nausea/vomiting*
*Adult:* **IV** 1-2 mg/kg 30 min before administration of chemotherapy, then q2hr × 2 doses, then q3hr × 3 doses
*Child:* **IV** 0.1-0.2 mg/kg/dose

*Facilitation of small bowel intubation in radiologic exams*
*Adult and child >14 yr:* **IV** 10 mg over 1-2 min
*Child 6-14 yr:* **IV** 2.5-5 mg
*Child <6 yr:* **IV** 0.1 mg/kg

*Diabetic gastroparesis*
*Adult:* PO 10 mg 30 min before meals, at bedtime × 2-8 wk
*Geriatric:* PO 5 mg ½ hr before meals, at bedtime, increase to 10 mg if needed

*Gastroesophageal reflux*
*Adult:* PO 10-15 mg qid 30 min before meals
*Child:* PO 0.4-0.8 mg/kg/day divided in 4 doses

*Hiccups (unlabeled)*
*Adult:* PO/IM/**IV** 10 mg q6hr

*Lactation induction (unlabeled)*
*Adult:* PO 10 mg bid-tid, may increase to 20-45 mg/day in divided doses

*Non–small cell lung cancer (NSCLC) radiation sensitizer (unlabeled) (Sensamide IV)*
*Adult:* **IV** 2 mg/kg given 1 hr prior to radiation therapy 3 ×/wk

*Renal dose*
*Adult:* **IV** CCr <40 ml/min 50% of dose

**Available forms:** Tabs 5, 10 mg; syr 5 mg/5 ml; inj 5 mg/ml, conc sol 10 mg/ml

---

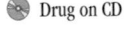

◆ Alert      ♣ Canada Only      🔊 Drug on CD      * "Tall Man" lettering (See Preface)

## Adverse effects
*CNS: Sedation, fatigue, restlessness, head-
ache, sleeplessness, dystonia,* dizziness,
drowsiness, **suicide ideation, seizures,** EPS
*CV:* Hypotension, **supraventricular tachycardia**
*GI:* Dry mouth, constipation, nausea, anorexia,
vomiting, diarrhea
*GU:* Decreased libido, prolactin secretion,
amenorrhea, galactorrhea
*HEMA:* **Neutropenia, leukopenia, agranulocytosis**
*INTEG:* Urticaria, rash

**Contraindications:** Hypersensitivity to
this product or procaine or procainamide,
seizure disorder, pheochromocytoma, breast
cancer (prolactin dependent), GI obstruction

**Precautions:** Pregnancy **B,** breastfeeding,
GI hemorrhage, CHF, Parkinson's disease,
tardive dyskinesia

### Pharmacokinetics

| | |
|---|---|
| **Absorption** | Well absorbed (PO) |
| **Distribution** | Widely distributed; crosses blood-brain barrier, placenta |
| **Metabolism** | Liver, minimally |
| **Excretion** | Kidneys, breast milk |
| **Half-life** | 4 hr |

### Pharmacodynamics

| | PO | IM | IV |
|---|---|---|---|
| **Onset** | ½-1 hr | 10-15 min | 1-3 min |
| **Peak** | Unknown | Unknown | Unknown |
| **Duration** | 1-2 hr | 1-2 hr | 1-2 hr |

## Interactions
### Individual drugs
Alcohol: increased sedation
Haloperidol: increased extrapyramidal reac-
tion
### Drug classifications
Anticholinergics, opiates: decreased action of
metoclopramide
CNS depressants: increased sedation
MAOIs: avoid use
Phenothiazines: increased extrapyramidal
reaction
### Drug/lab test
Increased: prolactin, aldosterone, thyrotropin

## NURSING CONSIDERATIONS
### Assessment
• Assess GI complaints: nausea, vomiting,
anorexia, constipation, abdominal distention
before and after administration
• Assess for EPS and tardive dyskinesia, more
likely to occur in geriatric patient: rigidity,

grimacing, shuffling gait, tremors, rhythmic
involuntary movements of tongue, mouth, jaw,
feet, hands; these side effects should be
reported to prescriber immediately; some
effects may be irreversible
• Assess mental status: depression, anxiety,
irritability during treatment

### Nursing diagnoses
• Injury, risk for (adverse reactions)
• Knowledge, deficient (teaching)

### Implementation
#### PO route
• Use gum, hard candy, frequent rinsing of
mouth for dryness of oral cavity
• Give ½-1 hr before meals for better absorption
#### IV route
• Give **IV** undiluted if dose is ≤10 mg; give
over 2 min
• Dilute more than 10 mg in 50 ml or more
$D_5W$, NaCl, Ringer's, LR and give over 15 min
or more
• Give diphenhydrAMINE **IV** for EPS
• Discard open ampules
***Syringe compatibilities:*** Aminophylline, ascorbic acid, atropine, benztropine,
bleomycin, butorphanol, chlorproMAZINE,
cisplatin, cyclophosphamide, cytarabine,
dexamethasone, dimenhyDRINATE, diphenhydrAMINE, DOXOrubicin, droperidol, fentanyl,
fluorouracil, heparin, hydrocortisone, hydrOXYzine, regular insulin, leucovorin, lidocaine, magnesium sulfate, meperidine, methotrimeprazine, methylPREDNISolone, midazolam,
mitomycin, morphine, pentazocine, perphenazine, prochlorperazine, promazine, promethazine, ranitidine, scopolamine, sufentanil,
vinBLAStine, vinCRIStine, vit B/C
***Syringe incompatibilities:*** Ampicillin,
calcium gluconate, cephalothin, chloramphenicol, furosemide, penicillin G potassium,
sodium bicarbonate
***Y-site compatibilities:*** Acyclovir,
aldesleukin, amifostine, aztreonam, bleomycin,
ciprofloxacin, cisplatin, cladribine, cyclophosphamide, cytarabine, diltiazem, DOXOrubicin,
droperidol, famotidine, filgrastim, fluconazole,
fludarabine, fluorouracil, foscarnet, gallium,
granisetron, heparin, idarubicin, leucovorin,
melphalan, meperidine, meropenem, methotrexate, mitomycin, morphine, ondansetron,
paclitaxel, piperacillin/tazobactam, propofol,
sargramostim, sufentanil, tacrolimus, teniposide, thiotepa, vinBLAStine, vinCRIStine,
vinorelbine, zidovudine
***Y-site incompatibilities:*** Furosemide

M

Adverse effects: *italic* = common, **bold** = life-threatening

**Additive compatibilities:** Clindamycin, meropenem, morphine, multivitamins, potassium acetate/chloride/phosphate, verapamil
**Additive incompatibilities:** Cisplatin, erythromycin, tetracycline

## Patient/family education

• Instruct patient to avoid driving, other hazardous activities until stabilized on this medication

• Advise patient to avoid alcohol and other CNS depressants that enhance sedating properties of this product

• Advise patient to notify prescriber if involuntary movements occur

## Evaluation

**Positive therapeutic outcome**

• Absence of nausea, vomiting, anorexia, fullness

---

## metolazone (Rx)

(me-tole'a-zone)
Zaroxolyn
*Func. class.:* Diuretic, antihypertensive
*Chem. class.:* Thiazide-like quinazoline derivative

**Pregnancy category B**

**Do not confuse:**
metolazone/methotrexate/metoclopramide

**Action:** Acts on the distal tubule and cortical thick ascending limb of the loop of Henle in the kidney, increasing excretion of sodium, water, chloride, magnesium, potassium, and bicarbonate

**Therapeutic outcome:** Decreased B/P, decreased edema in lung tissue and peripherally

**Uses:** Edema in CHF, nephrotic syndrome; may be used alone or as adjunct with antihypertensives for mild to moderate hypertension

## Dosage and routes
### Edema
**Adult:** PO 5-20 mg/day

### Hypertension
**Adult:** PO 2.5-5 mg/day

**Available forms:** Tabs 2.5, 5, 10 mg

## Adverse effects

**CNS:** Anxiety, depression, headache, *dizziness, fatigue, weakness*
**CV:** Orthostatic hypotension, palpitations, volume depletion, chest pain
**EENT:** Blurred vision

**ELECT:** *Hypokalemia,* hypercalcemia, hyponatremia
**GI:** *Nausea, vomiting, anorexia,* constipation, diarrhea, cramps, **pancreatitis,** GI irritation, dry mouth, jaundice
**GU:** *Frequency,* polyuria, **uremia,** glucosuria, nocturia, impotence
**HEMA: Aplastic anemia, hemolytic anemia, leukopenia, agranulocytosis, neutropenia**
**INTEG:** *Rash,* urticaria, purpura, photosensitivity, fever, dry skin
**META:** *Hyperglycemia,* increased creatinine, BUN

**Contraindications:** Hypersensitivity to thiazides or sulfonamides, anuria, hepatic coma

**Precautions:** Pregnancy **B**, breastfeeding, geriatric, hypokalemia, renal/hepatic disease, gout, COPD, lupus erythematosus, diabetes mellitus, hypotension

### Pharmacokinetics

| | |
|---|---|
| **Absorption** | GI tract (10%-20%) |
| **Distribution** | Crosses placenta |
| **Metabolism** | Urine, unchanged |
| **Excretion** | Breast milk |
| **Half-life** | 8 hr (extended); 14 hr (prompt) |

### Pharmacodynamics

| | |
|---|---|
| **Onset** | 1 hr |
| **Peak** | 2 hr |
| **Duration** | 12-24 hr |

## Interactions
### Individual drugs
Alcohol: increased hypotension (large amounts)
Amphotericin B, digoxin, mezlocillin, piperacillin: increased hypokalemia
Lithium: increased toxicity
### Drug classifications
Antihypertensives: increased antihypertensive effect
Barbiturates, nitrates, opioids: increased hypotension
Diuretics (loop): increased metolazone effect
Glucocorticoids, laxatives (stimulant): increased hypokalemia
NSAIDs, salicylates: decreased action of metolazone
### Drug/herb
Aconite: increased toxicity, death
Aloe, buckthorn, cascara sagrada, rhubarb, senna: increased hypokalemia

Astragalus, cola tree: increased or decreased antihypertensive effect

Barberry, betony, black catechu, black cohosh, bloodroot, broom, burdock, cat's claw, dandelion, goldenseal, Irish moss, Jamaican dogwood, kelp, khella, mistletoe, parsley: increased antihypertensive effect

Coltsfoot, guarana, khat, licorice: decreased antihypertensive effect

## NURSING CONSIDERATIONS
### Assessment

• Monitor blood glucose if patient is diabetic
• Check for rashes, temp elevation daily
• Monitor patients receiving cardiac glycosides for increased hypokalemia
• Monitor manifestations of hypokalemia; acidic urine, reduced urine, osmolality, nocturia; hypotension, broad T wave, U wave, ectopy, tachycardia, weak pulse; muscle weakness, altered LOC, drowsiness, apathy, lethargy, confusion, depression; anorexia, nausea, cramps, constipation, distention, paralytic ileus; hypoventilation, respiratory muscle weakness
• Monitor for manifestations of hypomagnesemia: agitation, muscle twitching, paresthesias, hyperactive reflexes, positive Babinski reflex, dysphagia, nystagmus seizures, tetany; nausea, vomiting, diarrhea, anorexia, abdominal distention; ectopy, tachycardia, broad, flat, or inverted T-waves, depressed ST segment, prolonged QT interval, decreased cardiac output, hypotension
• Monitor for manifestations of hyponatremia; increased B/P, cold, clammy skin, hypovolemia or hypervolemia; anorexia, nausea, vomiting, diarrhea, abdominal cramps; lethargy, increased ICP, confusion, headache, seizures, coma, fatigue, tremors, hyperreflexia
• Monitor for manifestations of hyperchloremia: weakness, lethargy, coma, deep rapid breathing
• Assess and record fluid volume status: I&O ratios; monitor weight, distended red veins, crackles in lung, color, quality and specific gravity of urine, skin turgor, adequacy of pulses, moist mucous membranes, bilateral lung sounds, peripheral pitting edema; dehydration symptoms of decreasing output, thirst, hypotension, dry mouth and mucous membranes should be reported
• Monitor electrolytes: potassium, sodium, calcium, magnesium; also include BUN, blood pH, ABGs, uric acid, CBC, blood glucose
• Assess B/P before and during therapy with patient lying, standing, and sitting as appropriate; orthostatic hypotension can occur rapidly

### Nursing diagnoses
• Fluid volume, deficient (adverse reactions)
• Fluid volume, excess (uses)
• Knowledge, deficient (teaching)
• Urinary elimination, impaired (adverse reactions)

### Implementation
• Give in AM to avoid interference with sleep
• Provide potassium replacement if potassium level is 3.0; product may be crushed if patient is unable to swallow
• Give with food; if nausea occurs, absorption may be increased; extended-release product is Zaroxolyn; prompt action product is Mykrox; the two formulations are not equivalent

### Patient/family education
• Teach patient to take the medication early in the day to prevent nocturia
• Instruct patient to take with food or milk if GI symptoms of nausea and anorexia occur
• Teach patient to maintain a weekly record of weight and notify prescriber of weight loss >5 lb
• Caution patient that this product causes a loss of potassium, so foods rich in potassium should be added to the diet; refer to a dietitian for assistance in planning
• Caution the patient to rise slowly from sitting or reclining positions, not to exercise in hot weather or stand for prolonged periods, since orthostatic hypotension will be enhanced; lie down if dizziness occurs
• Teach patient not to use alcohol or any OTC medications without prescriber's approval; serious product reactions may occur
• Emphasize the need to contact prescriber immediately if muscle cramps, weakness, nausea, dizziness, or numbness occurs
• Teach patient to take own B/P and pulse and record
• Advise patient to use sunscreen to prevent burns
• Teach patient to continue taking medication even if feeling better; this product controls symptoms but does not cure the condition
• Advise patient with hypertension to continue other medical regimen (exercise, weight loss, relaxation techniques, cessation of smoking)

### Evaluation
**Positive therapeutic outcome**
• Decreased edema
• Decreased B/P

### Treatment of overdose: Lavage if taken orally, monitor electrolytes; administer dextrose in saline; monitor hydration, CV, renal status

M

---

Adverse effects: *italic* = common, **bold** = life-threatening

## metoprolol (Rx)
(met-oh-proe'lole)
Betaloc ♥, Betaloc Durules ♥,
Lopresor ♥, Lopressor, Lopressor SR ♥,
Novometoprol ♥, Nu-Metop ♥,
Toprol XL
*Func. class.:* Antihypertensive, antianginal
*Chem. class.:* β₁-Adrenergic blocker

**Pregnancy category** C

### Do not confuse:
metoprolol/misoprostol

**Action:** Competitively blocks stimulation of β₁-adrenergic receptor within vascular smooth muscle; produces chronotropic, inotropic activity (decreases rate of SA node discharge, increases recovery time), slows conduction of AV node, decreases heart rate, which decreases $O_2$ consumption in myocardium; also decreases renin-aldosterone-angiotensin system at high doses, negative chronotropic effect

**Therapeutic outcome:** Decreased B/P, heart rate, AV conduction

**Uses:** Mild to moderate hypertension, acute MI to reduce cardiovascular mortality, angina pectoris, New York Heart Association class II, III heart failure

**Unlabeled uses:** Atrial ectopy, antipsychotic-induced akathisia, rapid heart rate control, unstable angina, variceal bleeding in portal hypertension, migraine prevention

### Dosage and routes
*Hypertension*
*Adult:* PO 50 mg bid, or 100 mg/day; may give 200-450 mg in divided doses; EXT REL TABS give daily
*Geriatric:* PO 25 mg/day initially, increase weekly as needed

*MI*
*Adult:* **IV** (early treatment) BOL 5 mg q2 min × 3 doses, then 50 mg PO 15 min after last dose and q6hr × 48 hr (late treatment) PO maintenance 100 mg bid for 3 mo

*Angina*
*Adult:* PO 100 mg/day as a single dose or in 2 divided doses, increase qwk as needed or 100 mg ext rel tab daily

*Migraine prevention (unlabeled)*
*Adult:* PO 50-100 mg bid-qid

**Available forms:** Tabs 50, 100 mg; inj 1 mg/ml; ext rel tabs (tartrate) 100 mg; ext rel tabs (succinate) (XL) 25, 50, 100, 200 mg

### Adverse effects
*CNS: Insomnia, dizziness,* mental changes, hallucinations, **depression,** anxiety, headaches, nightmares, confusion, fatigue
*CV:* **CHF,** *palpitations,* dysrhythmias, **cardiac arrest, AV block,** hypotension, **bradycardia, pulmonary/peripheral edema, chest pain**
*EENT:* Sore throat, dry burning eyes
*GI: Nausea, vomiting,* colitis, cramps, *diarrhea,* constipation, flatulence, dry mouth, *hiccups*
*GU:* Impotence
*HEMA:* **Agranulocytosis, eosinophilia, thrombocytopenic purpura**
*INTEG:* Rash, purpura, alopecia, dry skin, urticaria, pruritus
*RESP:* **Bronchospasm,** dyspnea, wheezing

**Contraindications:** Hypersensitivity to β-blockers, cardiogenic shock, heart block (2nd- and 3rd-degree), sinus bradycardia, bronchial asthma

**Precautions:** Pregnancy **C,** breastfeeding, geriatric, major surgery, diabetes mellitus, thyroid/renal/hepatic disease, COPD, CAD, nonallergic bronchospasm, CHF

### Pharmacokinetics
| | |
|---|---|
| **Absorption** | Well absorbed (PO); completely absorbed (**IV**) |
| **Distribution** | Crosses blood-brain barrier, placenta |
| **Metabolism** | Liver, extensively |
| **Excretion** | Kidneys, breast milk |
| **Half-life** | 3-4 hr |

### Pharmacodynamics
| | PO | IV |
|---|---|---|
| **Onset** | 15 min | Immediate |
| **Peak** | 2-4 hr | 20 min |
| **Duration** | 6-19 hr | 5-8 hr |

### Interactions
*Individual drugs*
Cimetidine: increased metoprolol level
DOBUTamine: decreased effect of DOBUTamine
DOPamine: decreased DOPamine
EpINEPHrine, hydrALAZINE, methyldopa prazosin, reserpine: increased hypotension, bradycardia
Indomethacin: decreased antihypertensive effect
Insulin: increased hypoglycemia
*Drug classifications*
Antidiabetics (oral): increased hypoglycemia
Amphetamines, calcium channel blockers,

histamine H$_2$ antagonists: increased hypotension, bradycardia

Barbiturates: decreased metoprolol level

Benzodiazepines: increased effect of benzodiazepines

MAOIs: do not use together

NSAIDs, salicylates: decreased antihypertensive effect

Sulfonylureas: increased hypoglycemic effect

Xanthines: decreased effects of xanthines

*Drug/herb*

Aconite: increased toxicity, death

Astragalus, cola tree: increased or decreased antihypertensive effect

Barberry, betony, black catechu, black cohosh, bloodroot, broom, burdock, cat's claw, dandelion, goldenseal, Irish moss, Jamaican dogwood, kelp, khella, mistletoe, parsley: increased antihypertensive effect

Coltsfoot, guarana, khat, licorice: decreased antihypertensive effect

*Drug/food*

Increased: absorption with food

*Drug/lab test*

Increased: BUN, potassium, ANA titer, serum lipoprotein, triglycerides, uric acid, alkaline phosphatase, LDH, AST, ALT

## NURSING CONSIDERATIONS
### Assessment

• Monitor B/P during beginning treatment, periodically thereafter; pulse q4hr; note rate, rhythm, quality; check apical/radial pulse before administration; notify prescriber of any significant changes (pulse <50 bpm)

• Check for baselines in renal, liver function tests before therapy begins and periodically thereafter

• Assess for edema in feet, legs daily; monitor I&O, daily weight; check for jugular vein distention, crackles bilaterally, dyspnea (CHF)

• Monitor skin turgor, dryness of mucous membranes for hydration status, especially geriatric

### Nursing diagnoses

• Cardiac output, decreased (uses)
• Injury, risk for (adverse reactions)
• Knowledge, deficient (teaching)
• Noncompliance (teaching)

### Implementation
#### PO route

• Do not break, crush, or chew ext rel tabs
• Give regular release tab before meals, at bedtime; tab may be crushed or swallowed whole; give with food to prevent GI upset; reduced dosage in renal dysfunction; take at same time each day

• Store protected from light, moisture; place in cool environment

#### IV route

• Give by direct **IV** 5 mg/2 min or more × 3 doses at 2 min intervals, start PO 15 min after last **IV** dose

*Y-site compatibilities:*

Alteplase, meperidine, morphine

### Patient/family education

• Teach patient not to discontinue product abruptly; taper over 2 wk; may cause precipitate angina if stopped abruptly

• Teach patient not to use OTC products containing α-adrenergic stimulants (such as nasal decongestants, cold preparations); to avoid alcohol, smoking and to limit sodium intake as prescribed

• Teach patient how to take pulse and B/P at home; advise when to notify prescriber

• Instruct patient to comply with weight control, dietary adjustments, modified exercise program

• Tell patient to carry/wear emergency ID to identify product being taken, allergies; tell patient product controls symptoms but does not cure

• Caution patient to avoid hazardous activities if dizziness, drowsiness is present, to avoid driving until product response is known

• Teach patient to report symptoms of CHF; difficult breathing, especially with exertion or when lying down, night cough, swelling of extremities or bradycardia, dizziness, confusion, depression, fever

• Teach patient to take product as prescribed, not to double doses or skip doses; take any missed doses as soon as remembered if at least 4 hr until next dose

### Evaluation
#### Positive therapeutic outcome

• Decreased B/P in hypertension (after 1-2 wk)
• Absence of dysrhythmias
• Decreased anginal pain

**Treatment of overdose:** Lavage, **IV** atropine for bradycardia, **IV** theophylline for bronchospasm, digoxin, O$_2$, diuretic for cardiac failure, hemodialysis, **IV** glucose for hyperglycemia, **IV** diazepam (or phenytoin) for seizures

M

## metronidazole (Rx)
(me-troe-ni′da-zole)
Apo-Metronidazole ♣, Flagyl, Flagyl ER, Flagyl IV, Flagyl IV RTU, Metronidazole, Novonidazole ♣, Protostat, Trikacide ♣
*Func. class.:* Trichomonacide, amebicide, antiinfective
*Chem. class.:* Nitroimidazole derivative

**Pregnancy category** B
(2nd, 3rd trimesters)

**Action:** Direct-acting amebicide/trichomonacide; binds, degrades DNA in organism

**Therapeutic outcome:** Trichomonacidal, amebicidal, bactericidal for the following susceptible organisms: *Bacteroides, Clostridium, Trichomonas vaginalis, Giardia lamblia, Entamoeba histolytica*

**Uses:** Intestinal amebiasis, amebic abscess, trichomoniasis, refractory trichomoniasis, bacterial anaerobic infections, giardiasis; septicemia, endocarditis, bone, joint, and lower respiratory tract infections

**Unlabeled uses:** Crohn's disease, antibiotic-associated diarrhea, rosacea

**Dosage and routes**
*Trichomoniasis*
*Adult:* PO 250 mg tid × 7 days or 2 g in single dose; do not repeat treatment for 4-6 wk
*Child:* PO 5 mg/kg/day divided in 3 doses × 7-10 days

*Refractory trichomoniasis*
*Adult:* PO 250 mg bid × 10 days

*Amebic hepatic abscess*
*Adult:* PO 500-750 mg tid × 5-10 days
*Child:* PO 35-50 mg/kg/day in 3 divided doses × 10 days

*Intestinal amebiasis*
*Adult:* PO 750 mg tid × 5-10 days
*Child:* PO 35-50 mg/kg/day in 3 divided doses × 10 days; then oral iodoquinol

*Anaerobic bacterial infections*
*Adult:* **IV** INF 15 mg/kg/over 1 hr, then 7.5 mg/kg **IV** or PO q6hr, max 4 g/day; first maintenance dose should be administered 6 hr after loading dose

*Giardiasis*
*Adult:* PO 250 mg tid × 5 days
*Child:* PO 5 mg/kg tid × 5 days

*Antibiotic-associated pseudomembranous colitis*
*Adult:* PO 250-500 mg 3-4 ×/day × 10-14 days

*Child:* PO 20 mg/kg/day (max 2 g) divided q6hr
*Bacterial vaginosis*
*Adult:* PO ext rel 750 mg/day × 7 days

**Available forms:** Tabs 250, 500 mg; ext rel tabs 750 mg; caps 375, 500 mg; inj 500 mg/100 ml; powder for inj 500 mg single dose

**Adverse effects**
***CNS:*** *Headache, dizziness,* confusion, irritability, restlessness, ataxia, depression, fatigue, drowsiness, insomnia, paresthesia, peripheral neuropathy, **seizures,** incoordination, depression, encephalopathy
***CV:*** Flat T-waves
***EENT:*** Blurred vision, sore throat, retinal edema, dry mouth, metallic taste, furry tongue, glossitis, stomatitis, photophobia
***GI:*** *Nausea, vomiting, diarrhea,* epigastric distress, *anorexia,* constipation, *abdominal cramps,* **pseudomembranous colitis**
***GU:*** Darkened urine, vaginal dryness, polyuria, **albuminuria,** dysuria, cystitis, decreased libido, **nephrotoxicity,** incontinence, dyspareunia, candidiasis
***HEMA:*** **Leukopenia, bone marrow depression, aplasia**
***INTEG:*** Rash, pruritus, urticaria, flushing

**Contraindications:** Pregnancy (1st trimester), breastfeeding, hypersensitivity to this product, renal/hepatic/GI disease, contracted visual or color fields, blood dyscrasias, CNS disorders

**Precautions:** Pregnancy **B** (2nd/3rd trimesters), candidal infections, heart failure, fungal infection, geriatric, dental disease, bone marrow suppression, hematologic disease

### Pharmacokinetics
| | |
|---|---|
| **Absorption** | 80% (PO) |
| **Distribution** | Widely distributed, crosses placenta |
| **Metabolism** | Liver |
| **Excretion** | Urine, unchanged; feces |
| **Half-life** | 6-11 hr |

### Pharmacodynamics
| | PO | IV |
|---|---|---|
| **Onset** | Rapid | Immediate |
| **Peak** | 1-2 hr | Infusion's end |
| **Duration** | Unknown | Unknown |

**Interactions**
*Individual drugs*
Alcohol: increased disulfiram-like reaction
Azathioprine, fluorouracil: increased leukopenia

 Alert     Canada Only    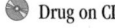 Drug on CD        * "Tall Man" lettering (See Preface)

Cimetidine, phenobarbital, phenytoin: decreased effect of metronidazole

Warfarin: increased action of warfarin

### Drug/herb
Acidophilus: do not use with antiinfectives; separate by several hours

### Drug/lab test
Altered: AST, ALT, LDH

## NURSING CONSIDERATIONS
### Assessment
• Assess patient for signs and symptoms of infection including characteristics of wounds, WBC >10,000/mm$^3$, vaginal secretions, fever; obtain baseline information and during treatment
• Obtain C&S before beginning product therapy to identify if correct treatment has been initiated
• Assess for allergic reactions: rash, urticaria, pruritus
• Identify urine output; if decreasing, notify prescriber (may indicate nephrotoxicity); also check for increased BUN, creatinine
• Assess bowel pattern daily; if severe diarrhea occurs, product should be discontinued
• Assess for overgrowth of infection: perineal itching, fever, malaise, redness, pain, swelling, drainage, rash, diarrhea, change in cough, sputum

### Nursing diagnoses
• Diarrhea (adverse reactions)
• Infection, risk for (uses)
• Injury, risk for (adverse reactions)
• Knowledge, deficient (teaching)
• Noncompliance (teaching)

### Implementation
**PO route**
• Give with or after a meal to avoid GI symptoms, metallic taste; crush tab if needed
• Store in light-resistant container; do not refrigerate

**Topical route**
• A thin coating should be applied to affected area after cleaning with soap and water and patting dry

**IV route**
• Give intermittent **IV** prediluted; for Flagyl **IV** dilute with 4.4 ml of sterile water or 0.9% NaCl; must be diluted further with 8 mg/ml or more 0.9% NaCl, D$_5$W, or LR; must neutralize with 5 mEq of NaCO$_3$/500 mg; CO$_2$ gas will be generated and may require venting; run over 1 hr or more; primary **IV** must be discontinued; may be given as cont inf; do not use aluminum products; **IV** may require venting

**Y-site compatibilities:** Acyclovir, allopurinol, amifostine, amiodarone, cefepime, cyclophosphamide, diltiazem, DOPamine, enalaprilat, esmolol, fluconazole, foscarnet, granisetron, heparin, hydromorphone, labetalol, lorazepam, magnesium sulfate, melphalan, meperidine, methylPREDNISolone, midazolam, morphine, perphenazine, piperacillin/tazobactam, sargramostim, tacrolimus, teniposide, theophylline, thiotepa, vinorelbine

**Additive compatibilities:** Amikacin, aminophylline, cefazolin, cefotaxime, ceftazidime, ceftizoxime, ceftriaxone, cefuroxime, chloramphenicol, ciprofloxacin, clindamycin, disopyramide, floxacillin, fluconazole, gentamicin, heparin, moxalactam, multielectrolyte concentrate, multivitamins, netilmicin, penicillin G potassium, tobramycin

### Patient/family education
• Teach patient to report sore throat, bruising, bleeding, joint pain; may indicate blood dyscrasias (rare)
• Advise patient to contact prescriber if vaginal itching, loose foul-smelling stools, furry tongue occur; may indicate superinfection
• Advise patient to notify physician of numbness or tingling of extremities
• Teach trichomoniasis patient that both partners need to be treated; condoms should be used during intercourse to prevent reinfection
• Advise patient of disulfiram-like reaction to alcohol ingestion; alcohol should not be used within 48 hr of this product
• Inform patient product has a metallic taste and urine may turn dark
• Advise patient to contact prescriber if pregnancy is suspected
• Advise patient to use sips of water, sugarless gum, candy for dry mouth

### Evaluation
**Positive therapeutic outcome**
• Decreased symptoms of infection

M

## metronidazole topical
*See Appendix D*

## mexiletine (Rx)
(mex-il'e-teen)
Mexitil
*Func. class.:* Antidysrhythmic (class IB)
*Chem. class.:* Lidocaine analog

### Pregnancy category C

**Action:** Increases electrical stimulation threshold of ventricle and His-Purkinje system, which stabilizes cardiac membrane and decreases automaticity

**Therapeutic outcome:** Decreased ventricular dysrhythmia

**Uses:** Life-threatening ventricular tachycardia; because of proarrhythmic effects, use with lesser dysrhythmias is not recommended

**Unlabeled uses:** Neuropathic pain

### Dosage and routes
*Adult:* PO 200-400 mg (loading dose), then 200 mg q8hr, then 200-400 mg q8hr

### Neuropathic pain (unlabeled)
*Adult:* PO 450-600 mg/day

**Available forms:** Caps 150, 200, 250 mg

### Adverse effects
*CNS:* Headache, dizziness, confusion, **seizures,** tremors, psychosis, nervousness, paresthesias, weakness, fatigue, coordination difficulties, change in sleep habits
*CV:* Hypotension, bradycardia, angina, PVCs, **heart block, cardiovascular collapse, arrest,** sinus node slowing, **left ventricular failure,** syncope, **cardiogenic shock, AV conduction disturbances, CHF, atrial dysrhythmias, palpitations, ventricular dysrhythmias, ventricular tachycardia, other ventricular arrhythmias in acute phase of MI**
*EENT:* Blurred vision, tinnitus
*GI:* Nausea, vomiting, anorexia, diarrhea, abdominal pain, **hepatitis,** dry mouth, peptic ulcer, altered taste, **GI bleeding,** constipation
*GU:* Urinary hesitancy, decreased libido
*HEMA:* **Thrombocytopenia, leukopenia, agranulocytosis**
*INTEG:* Rash, alopecia, dry skin
*MISC:* Edema, arthralgia, fever, systemic lupus erythematosus syndrome
*RESP:* Dyspnea

**Contraindications:** Hypersensitivity, cardiogenic shock, severe heart block (if no pacemaker)

**Precautions:** Pregnancy **C,** breastfeeding, children, hepatic disease, CHF, seizure disorders, hypotension

### Pharmacokinetics
| | |
|---|---|
| **Absorption** | Well absorbed |
| **Distribution** | Body tissues |
| **Metabolism** | Liver, extensively |
| **Excretion** | Kidneys, unchanged (10%) |
| **Half-life** | 12 hr |

### Pharmacodynamics
| | |
|---|---|
| **Onset** | ½-2 hr |
| **Peak** | 2-3 hr |
| **Duration** | 8-12 hr |

### Interactions
*Individual drugs*
Atropine, aluminum/magnesium hydroxide, phenobarbitol, phenytoin, rifampin: decreased mexiletine levels
Caffeine, theophylline: increased levels of each
Cimetidine: increased or decreased mexiletine effects
Metoclopramide: increased effects of mexiletine
*Drug classifications*
Acidifers (urinary), opiates: decreased mexiletine levels
Alkalinizers (urinary): increased mexiletine levels
Smoking: decreased mexiletine effect
*Drug/herb*
Aconite: increased toxicity, death
Aloe, broom, buckthorn (chronic use), cascara sagrada (chronic use), Chinese rhubarb, figwort, fumitory, goldenseal, kudzu, licorice: increased effect
Aloe, buckthorn, cascara sagrada, rhubarb, senna: increased hypokalemia, increased antidysrhythmic action
Coltsfoot: decreased effect
Horehound: increased serotonin effect
*Drug/lab test*
Increased: CPK

### NURSING CONSIDERATIONS
**Assessment**
• Assess for oxygenation or perfusion deficit: decreased B/P, chest pain, dizziness, loss of consciousness
• Assess respiratory status: auscultate lung fields for bibasilar crackles in patients with advanced CHF
• Assess for urinary retention: check for pain, abdominal absorption, palpate bladder; check males with benign prostatic hypertrophy; anticholinergic reaction may cause retention

- Monitor I&O ratio; electrolytes potassium, sodium, chloride; watch for decreasing urinary output, possible retention
- Monitor liver function tests: AST, ALT, bilirubin, alkaline phosphatase
- Monitor ECG periodically to determine product effectiveness; measure PR, QRS, QT intervals; check for PVCs, other dysrhythmias; assess B/P for hypo/hypertension, for rebound hypertension after 1-2 hr; for prolonged PR/QT intervals, QRS complex, if QT or QRS increase by 50% or more, withhold next dose, notify prescriber
- Monitor for dehydration and hypovolemia
- Monitor blood levels (therapeutic level 0.5-2 mcg/ml), notify prescriber of abnormal results
- Assess pulmonary toxicity: dyspnea, fatigue, cough, fever, chest pain; product should be discontinued
- Assess cardiac rate, respiration: rate, rhythm, character, chest pain, ventricular tachycardia, supraventricular tachycardia, fibrillation

## Nursing diagnoses
- Cardiac output, decreased (uses)
- Gas exchange, impaired (adverse reactions)
- Knowledge, deficient (teaching)

## Implementation
- Give with meals for GI upset

## Patient/family education
- Teach patient to report side effects immediately to prescriber; to take exactly as prescribed; if dose is missed, take when remembered if within 3-4 hr of next dose; do not double doses
- Caution patient to avoid temperature extremes; impairment of heat-regulating mechanism can occur
- Encourage patient to complete follow-up appointment with health care provider, including pulmonary function tests, chest x-ray
- Instruct patient that dry mouth may be relieved by frequent sips of water, hard candy, sugarless gum
- Caution patient to make position changes from lying to standing slowly to prevent orthostatic hypotension

## Evaluation
**Positive therapeutic outcome**
- Decreased B/P, dysrhythmias
- Decreased heart rate
- Normal sinus rhythm

**Treatment of overdose:** $O_2$, artificial ventilation, ECG monitoring, administer DOPamine for circulatory depression, administer diazepam or thiopental for seizures, isoproterenol

### micafungin (Rx)
(my-ca-fun′gin)
Mycamine
*Func. class.:* Antifungal, systemic
*Chem. class.:* Echinocandin

**Pregnancy category  C**

**Action:** Inhibits an essential component in fungal cell walls; causes direct damage to fungal cell wall

**Therapeutic outcome:** Prevention of *Candida* infection in HSTC; or decreased symptoms of candida infection, negative culture

**Uses:** Treatment of esophageal candidiasis; prophylaxis of *Candida* infections in patients undergoing hematopoietic stem cell transplantation (HSCT); susceptible *Candida* species: *C. albicans, C. glabrata, C. krusei, C. parapsilosis, C. tropicalis*

### Dosage and routes
*Esophageal candidiasis*
*Adult:* **IV** 150 mg/day, given over 1 hr
*Prophylaxis of* Candida *infections*
*Adult:* **IV** 50 mg/day, given over 1 hr

**Available forms:** Powder for injection 50 mg, in single-dose vials

### Adverse effects
*CNS:* **Convulsions,** dizziness, *headache, somnolence*
*CV:* Flushing, hypertension, phlebitis
*GI:* Abdominal pain, *nausea, anorexia, vomiting, diarrhea, increased AST, ALT, alkaline phosphatase, blood dehydrogenase, hyperbilirubinemia*
*HEMA:* **Neutropenia, thrombocytopenia, leukopenia, coagulopathy, anemia, hemolytic anemia**
*INTEG:* *Rash, pruritus, inj site pain*
*META:* Hypokalemia, hypocalcemia, hypomagnesemia
*MS:* *Rigors*

**Contraindications:** Hypersensitivity to this product or other echinocandins

**Precautions:** Pregnancy **C**, breastfeeding, children, geriatric, severe hepatic disease

M

## Pharmacokinetics

| | |
|---|---|
| **Absorption** | Unknown |
| **Distribution** | Protein binding 99% |
| **Metabolism** | Liver |
| **Excretion** | Feces, urine |
| **Half-life** | Terminal 14-20 hr |

## Pharmacodynamics
Unknown

## Interactions
### Individual drugs
Sirolimus, nifedipine: increased plasma concentrations; may need dosage reduction

## NURSING CONSIDERATIONS
### Assessment
• Assess for signs and symptoms of infection, clearing of cultures during treatment; obtain culture baseline and throughout; product may be started as soon as culture is taken (esophageal candidiasis); monitor cultures during HSCT, for prevention of *Candida* infections
• Monitor CBC (RBC, Hct, Hgb), differential, platelet count periodically; notify prescriber of results
• Monitor renal studies: BUN, urine CCr, electrolytes before and during therapy
• Monitor hepatic studies before and during treatment: bilirubin, AST, ALT, alkaline phosphatase, as needed
• Assess for bleeding: hematuria, heme-positive stools, bruising or petechiae, mucosa or orifices; blood dyscrasias can occur
• Assess for hypersensitivity: rash, pruritus, facial swelling; also for phlebitis
• Assess for hemolytic anemia
• Assess GI symptoms: frequency of stools, cramping; if severe diarrhea occurs, electrolytes may need to be given

### Nursing diagnoses
• Infection, risk for (uses)
• Injury, risk for (adverse reactions)
• Knowledge, deficient (teaching)

### Implementation
• Do not use if cloudy or precipitated; do not admix product
• Flush line before and after administration with 0.9% NaCl
**IV route**
• For *Candida* prevention, reconstitute with provided diluent 0.9% NaCl without bacteriostatic product; 50 mg vial/5 ml (10 mg/ml), swirl to dissolve, do not shake; further dilute with 100 ml 0.9% NaCl, only; run over 1 hr
• For *Candida* infection, reconstitute with provided diluent 50 mg/5 ml (10 mg/ml); further dilute 3 reconstituted vials in 100 ml of 0.9% NaCl, run over 1 hr
• Store at room temperature, away from light; do not freeze; discard unused solution

### Patient/family education
• Advise patient to notify prescriber if pregnancy is suspected or planned; use non-hormonal form of contraception while taking this product
• Teach patient to avoid breastfeeding while taking this product
• Teach patient to inform prescriber of renal or hepatic disease
• Teach patient to report bleeding, facial swelling, wheezing, difficulty breathing, itching, rash, hives, increasing warmth, flushing
• Instruct patient to report signs of infection: increased temp, sore throat, flulike symptoms
• Advise patient to notify prescriber of nausea, vomiting, diarrhea, jaundice, anorexia, clay-colored stools, dark urine; heptatotoxicity may occur

### Evaluation
**Positive therapeutic outcome**
• Prevention of *Candida* infection in HSTC; or decreased symptoms of *Candida* infection, negative culture

---

**miconazole** 🔵 **(Rx, OTC)**
(mi-kon′a-zole)
Femizole-M, Monistat, Monistat-Derm, Monistat 3, Monistat 7, Monistat Dual-Pak, M-Zole 7 Dual Pack, topical: Micatin, Micatin Liquid, miconazole nitrate
*Func. class.:* Antifungal
*Chem. class.:* Imidazole
**Pregnancy category C**

**Action:** Alters cell membranes, inhibits fungal enzymes, inhibits sterols so intracellular contents are lost, prevents biosynthesis of phospholipids/triglycerides

**Therapeutic outcome:** Fungistatic/fungicidal against *Aspergillus, Coccidioides, Cryptococcus, Candida, Dermatophytes, Histoplasma*

**Uses:** Coccidioidomycosis, candidiasis, cryptococcosis, paracoccidioidomycosis, chronic mucocutaneous candidiasis, fungal meningitis; **IV** used for severe infections only; (topical) tinea pedis, tinea cruris, tinea corporis, tinea versicolor, vaginal or vulva candidal infections

---

## Dosage and routes

*Adult:* **IV** INF 200-3600 mg/day; may be divided in 3 inf at 200-1200 mg/inf; may have to repeat course; IT 20 mg given simultaneously with **IV** for fungal meningitis q1-2 days

*Child:* **IV** 20-40 mg/kg/day, max 15 mg/kg/day

*Adult and child:* TOP Apply to affected area bid × 2-4 wk

*Adult:* INTRAVAGINAL 200 mg supp at bedtime × 3 days or 100 mg supp × 1 wk

**Available forms:** Inj 10 mg/ml; aerosol 2%; cream 2%; lotion 2%; powder 2%; spray 2%; vag cream 2%; vag supp 100, 200 mg

## Adverse effects

*CNS:* Drowsiness, headache, lethargy
*CV:* Tachycardia, **dysrhythmias** (rapid **IV**)
*GI:* Nausea, vomiting, anorexia, diarrhea, cramps
*GU:* Vulvovaginal burning, itching, hyponatremia, pelvic cramps (topical forms)
**HEMA: Decreased Hct, thrombocytopenia, hyperlipidemia**
*INTEG:* Pruritus, rash, fever, flushing, hives
*SYST:* Anaphylaxis

**Contraindications:** Hypersensitivity

**Precautions:** Pregnancy **C**, renal/hepatic disease

### Pharmacokinetics

| | |
|---|---|
| **Absorption** | Poorly absorbed (PO) |
| **Distribution** | Widely distributed (**IV**); bound to serum proteins (90%) |
| **Metabolism** | Liver, extensively |
| **Excretion** | Unknown |
| **Half-life** | Triphasic: 0.4, 2.1, 24 hr |

### Pharmacodynamics

| | IV | TOPICAL | VAG |
|---|---|---|---|
| **Onset** | Rapid | Unknown | Unknown |
| **Peak** | Infusion's end | Unknown | Unknown |
| **Duration** | Unknown | Unknown | Unknown |

## Interactions

*Individual drugs*

Amphotericin B: decreased effect of amphotericin B
Amphotericin B, isoniazid, rifampin: decreased effect of miconazole
Phenytoin: increased effect
Warfarin: increased anticoagulant effect

*Drug classifications*

Sulfonylureas: increased effect

*Drug/lab test*
False positive: urine glucose, urine protein

## NURSING CONSIDERATIONS
### Assessment

• Assess for signs and symptoms of infection: drainage, sore throat, urinary pain, hematuria, fever

• Obtain C&S before beginning treatment; therapy may be started after culture is taken; monitor signs of infection before and throughout treatment

• Monitor bowel pattern before and during treatment; diarrhea may occur

• Monitor cardiac system: B/P, pulse; watch for increasing pulse, cardiac dysrhythmias; product should be discontinued

• Monitor blood studies: WBC, RBC, Hgb, Hct, bleeding time; patients taking anticoagulants may need a decreased dosage; monitor liver and renal studies periodically for patients on long-term therapy

• Monitor I&O ratio; watch for decreasing urinary output, change in specific gravity; discontinue product to prevent renal damage; patients with renal disease may require lowered dose

• Monitor **IV** site for thrombophlebitis; site should be changed q48-72hr

• Monitor for allergies before initiation of treatment and reaction to each medication; highlight allergies on chart; check for allergic reaction: burning, stinging, swelling, redness (topical); observe for skin eruptions after administration of product to 1 wk after discontinuing product

### Nursing diagnoses

• Infection, risk for (uses)
• Injury, risk for (adverse reactions)
• Knowledge, deficient (teaching)
• Skin integrity, impaired (uses)

### Implementation

• Have adrenalin, suction, tracheostomy set, endotracheal intubation equipment available
**Topical route**
• Apply after cleansing area with soap and water before each application; use enough medication to cover lesions completely; dry well
• Store at room temperature in dry place
**Vaginal route**
• Administer 1 applicator full every night high into the vagina
• Store at room temperature in dry place
**IV route**
• Give 200 mg initially to prevent severe hypersensitive reaction

**M**

Adverse effects: *italic* = common, **bold** = life-threatening

- Give **IV** after diluting ≤1 g/10 ml of sterile water, $D_5W$, or 0.45% NaCl over 3-5 min
- Give by intermittent **IV** after diluting in 200 ml or more, $D_5W$ or 0.9% NaCl; give over 30-60 min
- Store at room temperature; reconstituted sol is stable for 24 hr refrigerated

*Y-site compatibilities:* Allopurinol, filgrastim, foscarnet, granisetron, melphalan, ondansetron, propofol, sargramostim, teniposide, thiotepa, vinorelbine

*Y-site incompatibilities:* Fludarabine

### Patient/family education
- Inform patient that culture may be performed after completed course of medication
- Advise patient to notify nurse of diarrhea, symptoms of candidal vaginitis

**Topical route**
- Teach patient to use medical asepsis (hand washing) before, after each application; to apply with glove to prevent further infection; to avoid contact with eyes; not to use occlusive dressings
- Caution patient to avoid use of OTC creams, ointments, lotions unless directed by prescriber
- Instruct patient to notify prescriber if no improvement in condition in 4 wk or if symptoms return in 2 mo; pregnancy or a serious medical condition may be the cause
- Teach patient to use for full prescribed treatment time, or reinfection may occur

**Vaginal route**
- Instruct patient in asepsis (hand washing) before, after each application
- Teach patient to apply with applicator only; to avoid use of any other vaginal product unless directed by prescriber; sanitary napkin may prevent soiling of undergarments; to abstain from sexual intercourse until treatment is completed; reinfection and irritation may occur
- Instruct patient to notify prescriber if symptoms persist

### Evaluation
**Positive therapeutic outcome**
- Decreasing oral candidiasis, fever, malaise, rash
- Negative C&S for infectious organism
- Decrease in size, number of lesions
- Decrease in itching or white discharge (vaginal)

**Treatment of overdose:** Withdraw product; maintain airway; administer epINEPHrine, aminophylline, $O_2$, **IV** corticosteroids for anaphylaxis

## miconazole topical
*See Appendix D*

## miconazole vaginal antifungal
*See Appendix D*

## midazolam (Rx)
(mid′ay-zoe-lam)
Versed
*Func. class.:* Sedative/hypnotic, antianxiety
*Chem. class.:* Benzodiazepine, short-acting

**Pregnancy category D**
**Controlled substance schedule IV**

**Do not confuse:**
Versed/Vepesid/Vistaril

**Action:** Depresses subcortical levels in CNS; may act on limbic system, reticular formation; may potentiate GABA by binding to specific benzodiazepine receptors

**Therapeutic outcome:** Sedation for anesthesia induction and procedures

**Uses:** Preoperative sedation, general anesthesia induction, sedation for diagnostic endoscopic procedures, intubation, anxiety

**Unlabeled uses:** Epileptic seizures, refractory status epilepticus

**Dosage and routes**
*Preoperative sedation*
*Adult and child ≥12 yr:* IM 0.07-0.08 mg/kg 30-60 min before general anesthesia
*Child 1-6 mo:* IM 0.1-0.15 mg/kg, may give up to 0.5 mg/kg if needed, max 10 mg
*Child 6 mo-5 yr:* PO 0.25-1 mg/kg, max 20 mg as a single dose
*Child 6 yr-11 yr:* PO/IM 0.25-0.5 mg/kg, max 20 mg as a single dose

*Induction of general anesthesia*
*Adult and child 12-16 yr:* IV (Unpremedicated patients) 150-350 mcg/kg over 30 sec, wait 2 min, follow with 20%-25% of initial dose if needed; (premedicated patients) 0.15-0.35 mg/kg over 20-30 sec, allow 2 min for effect
*Child 6-12 yr:* IV 0.025-0.05 mg/kg over 2-3 min; total dose up to 0.4 mg/kg if needed, max 10 mg
*Child 6 mo-5 yr:* IV 0.05-0.1 mg/kg over 2-3 min; total dose up to 0.6 mg/kg may be needed, max 6 mg

*Child <6 mo:* Titrate with small increments, adjust as needed

**Continuous infusion for intubation (critical care)**
*Adult:* **IV** 0.01-0.05 mg/kg over several min; repeat at 10-15 min intervals, until adequate sedation; then 0.02-0.10 mg/kg/hr maintenance, adjust as needed
*Child:* **IV** 0.05-0.2 mg/kg over 2-3 min then 0.06-0.12 mg/kg/hr by CONT INF; adjust as needed
*Neonates:* **IV** 0.03-0.06 mg/kg/hr titrate using lowest dose

**Available forms:** Inj 1, 5 mg/ml; syr 2 mg/ml

**Adverse effects**
*CNS:* Retrograde amnesia, euphoria, confusion, headache, anxiety, insomnia, slurred speech, paresthesia, tremors, weakness, chills
*CV:* Hypotension, PVCs, tachycardia, bigeminy, nodal rhythm, **cardiac arrest**
*EENT:* Blurred vision, nystagmus, diplopia, blocked ears, loss of balance
*GI: Nausea, vomiting,* increased salivation, hiccups
*INTEG:* Urticaria, pain, swelling at inj site, rash, pruritus
*RESP:* Coughing, **apnea, bronchospasm, laryngospasm,** dyspnea, **respiratory depression**

**Contraindications:** Pregnancy **D,** hypersensitivity to benzodiazepines, shock, coma, alcohol intoxication, acute angle-closure glaucoma, status asthmaticus

**Precautions:** Breastfeeding, neonates (contains benzyl alcohol), children, geriatric, COPD, CHF, chronic renal failure, chills, debilitated, hepatic disease

**Pharmacokinetics**

| Absorption | Well absorbed |
|---|---|
| Distribution | Crosses placenta, blood-brain barrier, protein binding 97% |
| Metabolism | Liver |
| Excretion | Kidneys, breast milk |
| Half-life | 1.8-6.4 hr |

**Pharmacodynamics**

| | PO | IM | IV |
|---|---|---|---|
| Onset | 20-30 min | 15 min | 3-5 min |
| Peak | Unknown | ½-1 hr | Unknown |
| Duration | Unknown | 2-3 hr | <2 hr |

**Interactions**
*Individual drugs*
Alcohol: increased respiratory depression
Cimetidine, erythromycin, ranitidine, theophylline: decreased midazolam metabolism
Fluvoxamine, indinavir, ritonavir, verapamil: increased respiratory depression
*Drug classifications*
Antifungals, azole, CYP3A4 inhibitors: increased levels of midalozam
Barbiturates, opiate analgesics, other CNS depressants: increased respiratory depression
CYP3A4 inducers, oral contraceptives: increased half-life of midazolam
Theophyllines: decreased effect of midazolam
*Drug/herb*
Black cohosh: increased hypotension
Catnip, chamomile, clary, cowslip, hops, kava, lavender, mistletoe, nettle, pokeweed, poppy, Queen Anne's lace, senega, skullcap, valerian: increased CNS depression
*Drug/food*
Grapefruit juice: increased midazolam effect

**NURSING CONSIDERATIONS**
**Assessment**
• Monitor B/P, pulse, respiration during **IV**; O₂ and emergency equipment should be nearby
• Monitor inj site for redness, pain, swelling
• Assess degree of amnesia in geriatric; may be increased
• Assess anterograde amnesia
• Assess vital signs for recovery period in obese patient, since half-life may be extended
• Assess for apnea, respiratory depression, which may be increased in the geriatric

**Nursing diagnoses**
• Knowledge, deficient (teaching)

**Implementation**
**PO route**
• Remove cap of press-in bottle adaptor and push adaptor into neck of bottle, close with cap, remove cap and insert tip of dispenser and insert into adaptor, turn upside-down and withdraw correct dose, place in mouth
**IM route**
• Give inj deep into large muscle mass
• Store at room temperature; protect from light
**IV route**
• Give **IV** undiluted or after diluting with D₅W or 0.9% NaCl to a conc of 0.25 mg/ml; give

M

over 2 min (conscious sedation) or over 30 sec (anesthesia induction)
• Ensure immediate availability of resuscitation equipment, $O_2$ to support airway; do not give by rapid bol

*Syringe compatibilities:* Alfentanil, atracurium, atropine, benzquinamide, buprenorphine, butorphanol, chlorproMAZINE, cimetidine, cisatracurium, diphenhyDRAMINE, droperidol, fentanyl, glycopyrrolate, hydromorphine, hydrOXYzine, ketamine, meperidine, metoclopramide, morphine, nalbuphine, promazine, promethazine, remifentanil, scopolamine, sufentanil, thiethylperazine, trimethobenzamide

*Syringe incompatibilities:* Dimenhydrinate, pentobarbital, perphenazine, prochlorperazine, ranitidine

*Y-site compatibilities:* Abciximab, alfentamil, amikacin, amiodarone, argatroban, atracurium, atropine, aztreonam, benzotropine, calcium gluconate, cefazolin, cefotaxime, cefoxitine, ceftriaxone, cimetidine, ciprofloxacin, cisplatin, clindamycin, clonidine, cyanocobalamin, cycloSPORINE, dactinomycin, digoxin, diltiazem, diphenhydramine, docetaxal, DOPamine, doxycycline, enalaprilat, epINEPHrine, erythromycin, esmolol, etomidate, etoposide, famotidine, fentanyl, fluconazole, folic acid, gatifloxacin, gemcitabine, gentamicin, glycopyrrolate, granisetron, heparin, hetastarch, hydromorphone, hydrOXYzine, inamrinone, isoproterenol, labetalol, lactated ringers, levofloxacin, lidocaine, linezolid, lorazepam, magnesium, mannitol, meperidine, methadone, methyldopa, methylPREDNISolone, metoclopromide, metomolol, metronidazole, milrinone, morphine, nalbuphine, naloxone, niCARdipine, nitroglycerin, nitroprusside, norepinephrine, ondansetron, oxacillin, oxytocin, paclitaxel, palonosetron, pancuronium, papaverin, phentolamine, phytonadione, piperacillin, potassium chloride, propanolol, protamine, pyridoxine, ranitidine, remifentanil, sodium nitroprusside, streptokinase, succinylcholine, sufentanil, teniposide, theophylline, thiotepa, ticarcillin, tobramycin, vancomycin, vasopressin, vecuronium, verapamil, voriconazole

*Y-site incompatibilities:* Foscarnet

## Patient/family education
• Inform patient that amnesia occurs; events may not be remembered
• Caution patient to avoid CNS depressants including alcohol for 24 hr after taking this product

## Evaluation
**Positive therapeutic outcome**
• Induction of sedation, amnesia

**Treatment of overdose:** $O_2$, flumazenil

---

**midodrine** (Rx)
(mye′doh-dreen)
ProAmatine
*Func. class.:* Proproduct
**Pregnancy category C**

**Do not confuse:**
ProAmatine/Protamine

**Action:** Activates α-adrenergic receptors of arteriolar, venous vasculature; increases vascular tone

**Therapeutic outcome:** Decreased feeling of faintness upon rising, absence of significant change in B/P

**Uses:** Orthostatic hypotension

**Dosage and routes**
*Adult:* PO 10 mg tid

**Renal dose**
*Adult:* PO 2.5 mg tid

**Available forms:** Tabs 2.5, 5 mg

**Adverse effects**
*CNS:* Drowsiness, restlessness, headache, paresthesia, pain, chills, confusion
*CV:* **Supine hypertension,** vasodilatation, flushing face
*EENT:* Dry mouth, blurred vision
*GI:* Nausea, anorexia
*GU:* Dysuria
*INTEG:* Pruritus, piloerection, rash

**Contraindications:** Hypersensitivity, severe organic heart disease, acute renal disease, urinary retention, pheochromocytoma, thyrotoxicosis, persistent/excessive supine hypertension

**Precautions:** Pregnancy C, breastfeeding, children, prostatic hypertrophy, hepatic function impairment, orthostatic diabetic patients, renal disease

| Pharmacokinetics | |
|---|---|
| **Absorption** | Bioavailability 90% |
| **Distribution** | Unknown |
| **Metabolism** | Unknown |
| **Excretion** | Urine 80%, active metabolite |
| **Half-life** | 3-4 hr |

| Pharmacodynamics | |
|---|---|
| Onset | Unknown |
| Peak | 1-2 hr |
| Duration | Unknown |

## Interactions
### Individual drugs:
Fludrocortisone: increased supine hypertension

Metformin: increased lactic acidosis

### Drug classifications
α-Adrenergic agonists: increased pressor effects

β-Adrenergic blockers, cardiac glycosides, psychotropics, tricyclics: increased bradycardia

## NURSING CONSIDERATIONS
### Assessment
• Monitor VS, B/P (standing, supine); notify prescriber if B/P supine is increased
• Observe for drowsiness, dizziness, LOC

### Nursing diagnoses
• Knowledge, deficient (teaching)

### Implementation
• Tablets may be swallowed whole, chewed, or allowed to dissolve
• Administer upon rising, at midday, and in late afternoon (no later than 6 PM)
• Avoid administering if patient is to be supine during day

### Patient/family education
• Advise patient to avoid hazardous activities; activities requiring alertness; dizziness may occur; instruct patient to request assistance with ambulation
• Advise patient to avoid alcohol, other depressants, OTC products

### Evaluation
**Positive therapeutic outcome**
• Decreased orthostatic hypotension

## mifepristone, RU-486 (Rx)
(mif-ee-press'tone)
Corlax, Mifeprex
*Func. class.:* Abortifacient
*Chem. class.:* Antiprogestational

### Pregnancy category C

**Action:** Stimulates uterine contractions, causing complete abortion

**Therapeutic outcome:** Termination of pregnancy

**Uses:** Abortion through 49 days gestation

**Unlabeled uses:** Postcoital contraception/contragestation, intrauterine fetal death, endometriosis, Cushing's syndrome, unresectable meningioma

## Dosage and routes
### Coadministration of mifepristone/misoprostol
• Day 1: PO single dose 600 mg mifepristone
• Day 3: 400 mcg misoprostol

**Available forms:** Tabs 200 mg

## Adverse effects
*CNS:* Dizziness, insomnia, anxiety, syncope, fainting, headache
*GI: Nausea, vomiting, diarrhea,* dyspepsia
*GU:* Uterine cramping, uterine hemorrhage, vaginitis, pelvic pain
*MISC:* Fatigue, back pain, fever, viral infections, chills, sinusitis

**Contraindications:** Hypersensitivity, severe renal/hepatic disease, PID, respiratory/cardiac disease, IUD, ectopic pregnancy, chronic adrenal failure, bleeding disorder, inherited porphyrias

**Precautions:** Pregnancy **C,** women >35 yr/smoking ≥10 cigarettes/day, asthma, anemia, jaundice, diabetes mellitus, seizure disorders, past uterine surgery

| Pharmacokinetics | |
|---|---|
| Absorption | Rapidly |
| Distribution | 98% protein binding, albumin, glycoprotein |
| Metabolism | Unknown |
| Excretion | Feces, urine |
| Half-life | Unknown |

| Pharmacodynamics | |
|---|---|
| Onset | Unknown |
| Peak | 90 min |
| Duration | Unknown |

## Interactions
### Individual drugs
Erythromycin, itraconazole, ketoconazole: decreased metabolism of each specific product
### Drug/herb
St. John's wort: decreased mifepristone action
### Drug/food
Grapefruit juice: decreased metabolism of mifepristone

## NURSING CONSIDERATIONS
### Assessment
• Monitor B/P, pulse; watch for change that may indicate hemorrhage

Adverse effects: *italic* = common, **bold** = life-threatening

- Monitor respiratory rate, rhythm, depth; notify prescriber of abnormalities
- Assess for length, duration of contraction; notify prescriber of contractions lasting over 1 min or absence of contractions
- Assess for incomplete abortion, pregnancy must be terminated by another method; product is teratogenic

### Nursing diagnoses
- Knowledge, deficient (teaching)
- Pain, acute (adverse reactions)

### Implementation
- Provide emotional support before and after abortion

### Patient/family education
- Advise patient to report increased blood loss, abdominal cramps, increased temp, foul-smelling lochia
- Teach patient some methods of comfort control and pain control
- Advise patient to continue with follow-up
- Advise patient that cramping and vaginal bleeding will occur

### Evaluation
**Positive therapeutic outcome**
- Expulsion of fetus

---

## miglitol (Rx)
(mig'le-tol)
Glyset
*Func. class.:* Oral hypoglycemic
*Chem. class.:* α-Glucosidase inhibitor

**Pregnancy category B**

**Action:** Delays the digestion/absorption of ingested carbohydrates, results in a smaller rise in blood glucose after meals; does not increase insulin production

**Therapeutic outcome:** Decreased blood glucose levels in diabetes mellitus

**Uses:** Type 2 diabetes mellitus

### Dosage and routes
*Initial dose*
*Adult:* PO 25 mg tid initially, with first bite of meal

*Maintenance dose*
*Adult:* PO may be increased to 50 mg tid; may increase to 100 mg tid if needed with dosage adjustment at 4-8 wk intervals

**Available forms:** Tabs 25, 50, 100 mg

### Adverse effects
***GI:*** *Abdominal pain, diarrhea, flatulence,* **hepatotoxicity**
***HEMA:*** Low iron
***INTEG:*** Rash

**Contraindications:** Hypersensitivity, diabetic ketoacidosis, cirrhosis, IBD, colonic ulceration, partial intestinal obstruction, chronic intestinal disease, ileus

**Precautions:** Pregnancy **B**, breastfeeding, children, renal/hepatic disease

| Pharmacokinetics | |
|---|---|
| **Absorption** | Unknown |
| **Distribution** | Unknown |
| **Metabolism** | Not metabolized |
| **Excretion** | Kidneys, unchanged product |
| **Half-life** | 2 hr |

| Pharmacodynamics | |
|---|---|
| **Onset** | Unknown |
| **Peak** | 2-3 hr |
| **Duration** | Unknown |

### Interactions
*Individual drugs*
Digoxin: decreased levels of digoxin
Propranolol: decreased levels of propranolol
Ranitidine: decreased levels of ranitidine
*Drug classifications*
Adsorbents (intestinal), enzymes (digestive): decreased miglitol levels; do not use together
*Drug/herb*
Broom, buchu, dandelion, juniper: decreased hypoglycemia
Chromium, fenugreek, ginseng: increased or decreased hypoglycemic effect
Karela: Improved glucose tolerance
*Drug/food*
Carbohydrates: increased diarrhea

### NURSING CONSIDERATIONS
**Assessment**
- Assess for hypo/hyperglycemia; even though this product does not cause hypoglycemia, if taking a sulfonylurea or insulin, hypoglycemia may be additive (rare)
- Monitor blood glucose levels, A1C, liver function tests; if hypoglycemia occurs with monotherapy, treat with glucose

**Nursing diagnoses**
- Knowledge, deficient (teaching)
- Noncompliance (teaching)
- Nutrition: less than body requirements, imbalanced (adverse reactions)

- Nutrition: more than body requirements, imbalanced (uses)

## Implementation
- Give tid with first bite of each meal
- Provide storage in airtight container in cool environment

## Patient/family education
- Teach patient the symptoms of hypo/hyperglycemia and what to do about each
- Instruct that medication must be taken as prescribed; explain consequences of discontinuing the medication abruptly; that during periods of stress, infection, surgery, insulin may be required
- Tell patient to avoid OTC medications unless approved by prescriber
- Teach patient that diabetes is a lifelong illness; product will not cure condition
- Instruct patient to carry/wear emergency ID as diabetic
- Teach patient that diet and exercise regimen must be followed
- Teach patient GI side effects and what to do about them

## Evaluation
**Positive therapeutic outcome**
- Decreased signs, symptoms of diabetes mellitus (polyuria, polydipsia, polyphagia, clear sensorium, absence of dizziness, stable gait)
- Improved blood glucose, A1c

---

## ⚠ HIGH ALERT

### milrinone (Rx)
(mill-re′none)
Primacor
*Func. class.:* Inotropic/vasodilator agent with phosphodiesterase activity
Chem. class.: Bipyridine derivative

**Pregnancy category C**

**Action:** Positive inotropic agent with vasodilator properties; increases contractility of cardiac muscle; reduces preload and afterload by direct relaxation of vascular smooth muscle; increases myocardial contractility

**Therapeutic outcome:** Increased inotropic effect resulting in increased cardiac output

**Uses:** Short-term management of advanced CHF that has not responded to other medication; can be used with digoxin

## Dosage and routes
*Adult:* **IV** BOL 50 mcg/kg given over 10 min; start INF of 0.375-0.75 mcg/kg/min; reduce dosage in renal impairment

**Available forms:** Inj 1 mg/ml; premixed inj 200 mcg/ml in D$_5$W

## Adverse effects
*CV:* Dysrhythmias, hypotension, chest pain
*GI:* Nausea, vomiting, anorexia, abdominal pain, **hepatotoxicity,** jaundice
*HEMA:* **Thrombocytopenia**
*MISC:* Headache, hypokalemia, tremor, injection site reactions

**Contraindications:** Hypersensitivity to this product, severe aortic disease, severe pulmonic valvular disease, acute MI

**Precautions:** Pregnancy **C**, breastfeeding, children, geriatric, renal/hepatic disease, atrial flutter/fibrillation

### Pharmacokinetics
| | |
|---|---|
| **Absorption** | Completely absorbed |
| **Distribution** | Unknown |
| **Metabolism** | Liver (50%) |
| **Excretion** | Kidney, unchanged (83%), metabolites (12%) |
| **Half-life** | 2.4 hr; increased in CHF |

### Pharmacodynamics
| | |
|---|---|
| **Onset** | 2-5 min |
| **Peak** | 10 min |
| **Duration** | Variable |

## NURSING CONSIDERATIONS
### Assessment
- Monitor manifestations of hypokalemia: acidic urine, reduced urine, osmolality, nocturia; hypotension, broad T-wave, U-wave, ectopy, tachycardia, weak pulse; muscle weakness, altered LOC, drowsiness, apathy, lethargy, confusion, depression; anorexia, nausea, cramps, constipation, distention, paralytic ileus; hypoventilation, respiratory muscle weakness
- Assess fluid volume status: complete I&O ratio and record; note weight, distended red veins, crackles in lung, color, quality, and specific gravity of urine, skin turgor, adequacy of pulses, moist mucous membranes, bilateral lung sounds, peripheral pitting edema; dehydration symptoms of decreasing output, thirst, hypotension, dry mouth and mucous membranes should be reported
◆ Monitor electrolytes: potassium, sodium, calcium, magnesium; also include BUN, blood pH, ABGs

Adverse effects: *italic* = common, **bold** = life-threatening

- Monitor B/P and pulse, ECG continuously during **IV**, ventricular dysrhythmia can occur, PCWP, CVP, index often during infusion; if B/P drops 30 mm Hg, stop infusion and call prescriber
- Monitor ALT, AST, bilirubin daily; if these are elevated, hepatoxicity is suspected
- Monitor platelets; if <150,000/mm³, product is usually discontinued and another product started
- Assess for extravasation: change site q48hr

### Nursing diagnoses
- Cardiac output, decreased (uses)
- Fluid volume, excess (uses)
- Knowledge, deficient (teaching)

### Implementation
**IV route**
- Give **IV** loading dose undiluted over 10 min
- Do not mix directly with glucose sol; chemical reaction occurs over 24 hr; precipitate forms if milrinone and furosemide come in contact
- Administer by direct **IV** into inf through Y-connector or directly into tubing; may give undiluted over 2-3 min
- Give by cont inf diluted with 0.9% NaCl to conc of 1-3 mg/ml, run at prescribed rate; give by infusion pump for doses other than bol
- Administer potassium supplements if ordered for potassium levels <3.0 mg/dl

**Syringe compatibilities:** Atropine, calcium chloride, digoxin, epINEPHrine, lidocaine, morphine, propranolol, sodium bicarbonate, verapamil

**Y-site compatibilities:** Digoxin, diltiazem, DOBUTamine, DOPamine, epINEPHrine, fentanyl, heparin, hydromorphone, labetalol, lorazepam, midazolam, morphine, niCARdipine, nitroglycerin, norepinephrine, propranolol, quinidine, ranitidine, thiopental, vecuronium

**Additive compatibilities:** Quinidine

### Patient/family education
- Teach patient reason for medication and expected results
- Instruct patient to make position changes slowly; orthostatic hypotension may occur
- Teach patient signs and symptoms of hypersensitivity reactions and hypokalemia

### Evaluation
**Positive therapeutic outcome**
- Increased cardiac output
- Decreased PCWP, adequate CVP
- Decreased dyspnea, fatigue, edema, ECG

**Treatment of overdose:** Discontinue product, support circulation

## minocycline (Rx)
(min-oh-sye'kleen)
Arestin, Dynacin, Minocin, Myrac, Vectrin
*Func. class.:* Antiinfective
*Chem. class.:* Tetracycline

**Pregnancy category D**

**Action:** Inhibits protein synthesis and phosphorylation in microorganisms by binding to 30S ribosomal subunits and reversibly binding to 50S ribosomal subunits; bacteriostatic

**Therapeutic outcome:** Bactericidal action against susceptible organisms, including *Neisseria meningitidis, Neisseria gonorrhoeae, Treponema pallidum, Chlamydia trachomatis, Ureaplasma urealyticum, Mycoplasma pneumoniae, Nocardia, Rickettsia*

**Uses:** Syphilis, chlamydial infection, gonorrhea, lymphogranuloma venereum, rickettsial infections, inflammatory acne, meningitis carriers, periodontitis, methicillin-resistant *Staphylococcus aureus* (MRSA) infections

**Unlabeled uses:** Rheumatoid arthritis

### Dosage and routes
*Adult:* PO/IV 200 mg, then 100 mg q12hr or 50 mg q6hr, max 400 mg/24 hr **IV**; subgingival insert into periodontal pocket
*Child >8 yr:* PO/IV 4 mg/kg then 4 mg/kg/day PO in divided doses q12hr

*Gonorrhea*
*Adult:* PO 200 mg, then 100 mg q12hr × 4 days or more

*C. trachomatis infection*
*Adult:* PO 100 mg bid × 7 days

*Syphilis*
*Adult:* PO 200 mg, then 100 mg q12hr × 10-15 days

*Uncomplicated gonococcal urethritis in men*
*Adult:* PO 100 mg q12hr × 5 days

*Rheumatoid arthritis (unlabeled)*
*Adult:* PO 100 mg bid for ≤48 wk

**Available forms:** Caps 50, 75, 100 mg; oral susp 50 mg/5 ml; powder for inj 100 mg; pellet filled caps 50, 100 mg; tabs 50, 75, 100 mg; ext rel tabs 45, 90, 135 mg

**Adverse effects**
*CNS: Dizziness,* fever, light-headedness, vertigo, seizures
*CV:* Pericarditis

**EENT:** Dysphagia, glossitis, decreased calcification, permanent discoloration of teeth, oral candidiasis

**GI:** *Nausea,* abdominal pain, *vomiting, diarrhea,* anorexia, enterocolitis, **hepatotoxicity,** flatulence, abdominal cramps, epigastric burning, stomatitis

**GU:** Increased BUN, polyuria, polydipsia, **renal failure, nephrotoxicity**

**HEMA:** **Eosinophilia, neutropenia, thrombocytopenia, hemolytic anemia,** pancytopenia

**INTEG:** *Rash, urticaria, photosensitivity, increased pigmentation,* **exfoliative dermatitis,** pruritus, blue-gray color of skin and mucous membranes

**SYST:** **Angioedema, Stevens-Johnson syndrome**

**Contraindications:** Pregnancy **D,** hypersensitivity to tetracyclines, children <8 yr

**Precautions:** Breastfeeding, hepatic disease

| Pharmacokinetics | |
|---|---|
| Absorption | Well absorbed (PO) |
| Distribution | Widely distributed (70%-75% protein bound); some distribution in CSF, crosses placenta |
| Metabolism | Liver, some |
| Excretion | Kidneys, unchanged (20%), bile, feces |
| Half-life | 11-17 hr |

| Pharmacodynamics | | |
|---|---|---|
| | PO | IV |
| Onset | Rapid | Rapid |
| Peak | 2-3 hr | Infusion's end |
| Duration | Unknown | Unknown |

## Interactions
### Individual drugs
Calcium: forms chelates, decreased absorption
Carbamazepine, phenytoin: decreased effect
Digoxin: increased effect
Insulin: increased effect
Kaolin/pectin, sodium bicarbonate, cimetidine, iron: decreased minocycline effect
Theophylline: increased effect
Warfarin: increased effect

### Drug classifications
Antacids, alkali products: decreased minocycline effect
Anticoagulants (oral): increased effect
Barbiturates, penicillins: decreased effect
Oral contraceptives: decreased effect of oral contraception

### Drug/herb
Acidophilus: do not use with antiinfectives; separate by several hours

### Drug/lab test
False negative: urine glucose with Clinistix, Tes-Tape

## NURSING CONSIDERATIONS
### Assessment
- Assess patient for previous sensitivity reaction
- Assess patient for signs and symptoms of infection including characteristics of wounds, sputum, urine, stool, WBC >10,000/mm$^3$, fever; obtain baseline information, before and during treatment
- Obtain C&S before beginning product therapy to identify if correct treatment has been initiated
- Assess for allergic reactions: rash, urticaria, pruritus
- Monitor blood studies: AST, ALT, CBC, Hct, bilirubin, alkaline phosphatase, amylase monthly if patient is on long-term therapy
- Assess bowel pattern daily; if severe diarrhea occurs, product should be discontinued
- Monitor for bleeding: ecchymosis, bleeding gums, hematuria, stool guaiac daily if on long-term therapy; blood dyscrasias may occur
- Assess for overgrowth of infection: perineal itching, fever, malaise, redness, pain, swelling, drainage, rash, diarrhea, change in cough, sputum; black; furry tongue

### Nursing diagnoses
- Diarrhea (adverse reactions)
- Infection, risk for (uses)
- Knowledge, deficient (teaching)
- Noncompliance (teaching)

### Implementation
#### PO route
- Give around the clock to maintain proper blood levels; give with food to increase absorption of product; do not give within 3 hr of other agents; product interactions may occur
- Give with 8 oz of water 1 hr before bedtime to prevent ulceration
- Shake liquid preparation well before giving; use calibrated device for proper dosing
- Do not give with iron, calcium, magnesium products, or antacids, which decrease absorption and form insoluble chelate

#### IV route
- Check for irritation, extravasation, phlebitis daily; change site q72hr
- For intermittent inf, dilute each 100 mg/10 ml of 0.9% NaCl, sterile water for inj; further

M

dilute in 500-1000 ml of 0.9% NaCl, D$_5$W, Ringer's, LR, D$_5$/LR; give over 6 hr

**Y-site compatibilities:** Cyclophosphamide, fludarabine, granisetron, heparin, hydrocortisone, magnesium sulfate, melphalan, perphenazine, potassium chloride, sargramostim, sodium succinate, vinorelbine, vit B/C

**Y-site incompatibilities:** Aztreonam, filgrastim, hydromorphone, meperidine, morphine, teniposide

### Patient/family education
• Teach patient to use sunscreen when outdoors to decrease photosensitivity reaction
• Teach patient to report sore throat, bruising, bleeding, joint pain; may indicate blood dyscrasias (rare)
• Advise patient to contact prescriber if vaginal itching, loose foul-smelling stools, furry tongue occur; may indicate superinfection; report itching, rash, pruritus, urticaria
• Instruct patient to take all medication prescribed for the length of time ordered; product must be taken around the clock to maintain blood levels; do not give medication to others; take with a full glass of water; may take with food; not to use outdated product, Fanconi's syndrome may occur
• Advise patient to use a form of contraception other than hormonal

### Evaluation
**Positive therapeutic outcome**
• Absence of signs/symptoms of infection (WBC <10,000/mm$^3$, temp WNL, absence of red, draining wounds)
• Reported improvement in symptoms of infection

---

**minoxidil** (Rx, OTC)
(mi-nox'i-dill)
Loniten, minoxidil, Rogaine (top)
*Func. class.:* Antihypertensive, hair growth stimulant
*Chem. class.:* Vasodilator, peripheral
**Pregnancy category** C

### Do not confuse:
minoxidil/Monopril, Loniten/Lotensin

**Action:** Directly relaxes arteriolar smooth muscle, causing vasodilatation; increased cutaneous blood flow; stimulation of hair follicles

**Therapeutic outcome:** Decreased B/P in hypertension; hair growth

**Uses:** Severe hypertension unresponsive to other therapy (use with diuretic); topically to treat alopecia

### Dosage and routes
**Severe hypertension**
**Adult:** PO 2.5-5 mg/day in 1-2 divided doses, max 100 mg/day; usual range 10-40 mg/day in single doses
**Geriatric:** PO 2.5 mg/day, may be increased gradually
**Child <12 yr:** PO Initial, 0.1-0.2 mg/kg/day; effective range, 0.25-1 mg/kg/day; max, 50 mg/day

**Alopecia**
**Adult:** TOP 1 ml bid rub into scalp daily, max 2 ml/day

**Available forms:** Tabs 2.5, 10 mg; topical 2% sol

### Adverse effects
*CNS:* Headache, fatigue
*CV: Severe rebound hypertension (on withdrawal in children),* tachycardia, angina, increased T-wave, **CHF, pulmonary edema, pericardial effusion,** edema, sodium retention, water retention
*GI:* Nausea, vomiting
*GU:* Breast tenderness
*HEMA:* Hct, Hgb, erythrocyte count may decrease initially
*INTEG:* Pruritus, **Stevens-Johnson syndrome,** rash, hirsutism

**Contraindications:** Acute MI, dissecting aortic aneurysm, hypersensitivity, pheochromocytoma

**Precautions:** Pregnancy **C**, breastfeeding, children, geriatric, renal disease, CAD, CHF, CVD

| Pharmacokinetics | |
|---|---|
| **Absorption** | Well absorbed (PO); minimally absorbed (topical) |
| **Distribution** | Widely distributed |
| **Metabolism** | Liver |
| **Excretion** | Kidneys, breast milk |
| **Half-life** | 4.2 hr |

| Pharmacodynamics | | |
|---|---|---|
| | PO | TOPICAL |
| **Onset** | ½ hr | 4 mo |
| **Peak** | 2-3 hr | Unknown |
| **Duration** | 75 hr | 4 mo |

---

 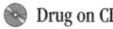

### Interactions
*Drug classifications*
Antihypertensives: increased orthostatic hypotension
NSAIDs, salicylates: decreased antihypertensive effect
*Drug/herb*
Hawthorn: increased antihypertensive effect
Yohimbe: decreased antihypertensive effect
*Drug/lab test*
Increased: renal function tests
Decreased: Hgb, Hct, RBC

### NURSING CONSIDERATIONS
**Assessment**
◆ Monitor closely, usually given with β-blocker to prevent tachycardia and increased myocardial workload, usually given with diuretic to prevent serious fluid accumulation, patient should be hospitalized during beginning treatment
• Monitor B/P, pulse, jugular venous distention periodically throughout treatment
• Monitor electrolytes, blood studies: potassium, sodium, chloride, carbon dioxide, CBC, serum glucose
◆ Monitor weight daily, I&O; assess edema in feet, legs daily; check skin turgor, dryness of mucous membranes for hydration status
• Assess for crackles, dyspnea, orthopnea, peripheral edema, fatigue, weight gain, jugular vein distention (CHF)
• Assess for signs of hyperglycemia: acetone breath, increased urinary output, severe thirst, lethargy, dizziness

**Nursing diagnoses**
• Cardiac output, decreased (adverse reactions)
• Injury, risk for (side effects)
• Knowledge, deficient (teaching)

**Implementation**
**PO route**
• Give with meals to decrease GI symptoms
• Give with β-blockers and/or diuretic for hypertension
• Store protected from light and heat
**Topical route**
• Administer 1 ml dose no matter how much balding has occurred; increasing dose does not speed hair growth
• Treatment must continue long term or new hair will be lost again

**Patient/family education**
**Topical route**
• Teach patient that new hair will be soft and hardly visible

• Caution patient not to use on other parts of the body; product is to be used on the scalp only
• Instruct patient that hair should be clean before applying medication; do not get on clothing
• Caution patient not to get medication near mucous membranes (mouth, nose, eyes) and to contact prescriber if burning, stinging, or rash occurs

**Evaluation**
**Positive therapeutic outcome**
• Decreased B/P in hypertension
• Hair growth (Top)

---

## mirtazapine (Rx)
(mer-ta′za-peen)
Remeron, Remeron Soltab
*Func. class.:* Antidepressant
*Chem. class.:* Tetracyclic

**Pregnancy category C**

**Action:** Blocks reuptake of norepinephrine, serotonin into nerve endings, increasing action of norepinephrine, serotonin in nerve cells; antagonist of central $\alpha_2$-receptors, blocks histamine receptors; has anticholinergic action

**Therapeutic outcome:** Decreased symptoms of depression after 2-3 wk

**Uses:** Depression, dysthymic disorder, bipolar disorder: depression, agitated depression

**Dosage and routes**
*Adult:* PO 15 mg/day at bedtime, maintenance to continue for 6 mo, titrate up to 45 mg/day; ORALLY DISINTEGRATING TABS open blister pack, place tab on tongue, allow to disintegrate, swallow
*Geriatric:* PO 7.5 mg nightly, increase by 7.5 mg q1-2 wk to desired dose, max 45 mg/day

**Available forms:** Tabs 15, 30, 45 mg; orally disintegrating tabs 15, 30, 45 mg

**Adverse effects**
*CNS: Dizziness, drowsiness,* confusion, headache, anxiety, tremors, stimulation, weakness, nightmares, EPS (geriatric), increased psychiatric symptoms, **seizures**
*CV: Orthostatic hypotension, ECG changes, tachycardia, hypertension,* palpitations
*EENT: Blurred vision,* tinnitus, mydriasis
*GI: Diarrhea, dry mouth,* nausea, vomiting, **paralytic ileus,** increased appetite; cramps, epigastric distress, **jaundice, hepatitis,**

M

stomatitis, constipation, increased cholesterol levels
*GU: Retention,* **acute renal failure**
*HEMA:* **Agranulocytosis, thrombocytopenia, eosinophilia, leukopenia**
*INTEG:* Rash, urticaria, sweating, pruritus, photosensitivity
*SYST:* Flulike symptoms

**Contraindications:** Hypersensitivity to tricyclics, recovery phase of MI, seizure disorders, prostatic hypertrophy

**Precautions:** Pregnancy **C**, geriatric, suicidal patients, severe depression, increased intraocular pressure, angle-closure glaucoma, urinary retention, cardiac/renal/hepatic disease, hypo/hyperthyroidism, electroshock therapy, elective surgery, suicidal ideation

### Pharmacokinetics

| | |
|---|---|
| **Absorption** | Slow, complete |
| **Distribution** | Widely distributed; crosses placenta |
| **Metabolism** | Liver, extensively |
| **Excretion** | Feces; breast milk |
| **Half-life** | 20-40 hr |

### Pharmacodynamics

| | |
|---|---|
| **Onset** | Unknown |
| **Peak** | 2 hr |
| **Duration** | Unknown |

### Interactions
*Individual drugs*
Alcohol: increased CNS depression
Clonidine: decreased effects
*Drug classifications*
Barbiturates, benzodiazepines, CNS depressants (other): increased effects
MAOIs: hypertensive episode, seizures, hyperpyretic crisis
Sympathomimetics, indirect acting (epHEDrine): decreased effects
*Drug/herb*
Belladonna, henbane: increased anticholinergic effect
Chamomile, hops, kava, skullcap, valerian: increased CNS depression
St. John's wort, SAM-e: serotonin syndrome
Scopolia: increased antidepressant effect
*Drug/lab test*
Increased: serum bilirubin, blood glucose, alkaline phosphatase
Decreased: VMA, 5-HIAA
False increase: urinary catecholamines

## NURSING CONSIDERATIONS
### Assessment
• Monitor B/P (with patient lying, standing), pulse q4hr during beginning treatment; if systolic B/P drops 20 mm Hg, hold product, notify prescriber; take VS q4hr in patients with CV disease
• Monitor blood studies: CBC, leukocytes, differential, cardiac enzymes if patient is receiving long-term therapy
• Monitor liver function tests: AST, ALT, bilirubin
• Check weight weekly, product may increase appetite
• Assess ECG for flattening of T-wave, bundle branch block, AV block, dysrhythmias in cardiac patients
• Assess for EPS primarily in geriatric: rigidity, dystonia, akathisia
• Assess mental status: mood, sensorium, affect, suicidal tendencies; assess increase in psychiatric symptoms: depression, panic
• Identify alcohol consumption; if alcohol is consumed, hold dose until AM

### Nursing diagnoses
• Coping, ineffective (uses)
• Injury, risk for (side effects)
• Knowledge, deficient (teaching)
• Noncompliance (teaching)

### Implementation
• Give with food or milk for GI symptoms; crush if patient is unable to swallow medication whole
• Give dose at bedtime if oversedation occurs during day; may take entire dose at bedtime; geriatric may not tolerate once/day dosing
• Store at room temperature; do not freeze
• Allow orally disintegrating tablets to dissolve on tongue; no water needed

### Patient/family education
• Inform patient that therapeutic effects may take 2-3 wk; take at bedtime
• Advise patient to use caution in driving and other activities requiring alertness because of drowsiness, dizziness, blurred vision; to avoid rising quickly from sitting to standing, especially geriatric
• Caution patient to avoid alcohol ingestion, other CNS depressants
• Teach patient to increase fluids, bulk in diet if constipation, urinary retention occur, especially geriatric
• Teach patient to use gum, hard sugarless candy, or frequent sips of water for dry mouth
• To report immediately urinary retention, worsening of depression, suicidal thoughts/behavior

mitomycin 643

## Evaluation
**Positive therapeutic outcome**
- Decrease in depression
- Absence of suicidal thoughts

**Treatment of overdose:** ECG monitoring, lavage, activated charcoal, administer anticonvulsant

---

## misoprostol (Rx)
(mye-soe-prost'ole)
Cytotec
*Func. class.:* Gastric mucosa protectant; antiulcer
*Chem. class.:* Prostaglandin $E_1$ analog
**Pregnancy category** X

**Do not confuse:**
misoprostol/metoprolol, Cytotec/Cytoxan

**Action:** Inhibits gastric acid secretion; may protect gastric mucosa; can increase bicarbonate, mucus production

**Therapeutic outcome:** Prevention of gastric ulcers

**Uses:** Prevention of NSAID-induced gastric ulcers

### Dosage and routes
*Adult:* PO 200 mcg qid with food for duration of NSAID therapy with last dose at bedtime; if 200 mcg is not tolerated, 100 mcg may be given

**Available forms:** Tabs 100, 200 mcg

### Adverse effects
*GI:* **Diarrhea,** nausea, vomiting, flatulence, constipation, dyspepsia, abdominal pain
*GU:* Spotting, cramps, hypermenorrhea, menstrual disorders

**Contraindications:** Pregnancy X, hypersensitivity to this product or prostaglandins

**Precautions:** Breastfeeding, children, geriatric, renal disease

### Pharmacokinetics
| Absorption | Well absorbed |
|---|---|
| Distribution | Unknown |
| Metabolism | Liver |
| Excretion | Kidneys |
| Half-life | ½-1 hr |

### Pharmacodynamics
| Onset | ½ hr |
|---|---|
| Peak | Unknown |
| Duration | 3 hr |

## Interactions
*Drug/food*
Decreased absorption with food

## NURSING CONSIDERATIONS
### Assessment
- Assess patient for GI symptoms: hematemesis, occult or frank blood in stools, also severe abdominal pain, cramping, severe diarrhea
- Obtain a negative pregnancy test in women of childbearing age before starting medication; miscarriages are common

### Nursing diagnoses
- Knowledge, deficient (teaching)
- Pain, chronic (uses)

### Implementation
- Give with meals for prolonged product effect; avoid use of magnesium antacids

### Patient/family education
- Advise patient to avoid black pepper, caffeine, alcohol, harsh spices, extremes in temperature of food, which may aggravate condition
- Caution patient to avoid OTC preparations: aspirin, cough, cold preparations; condition may worsen
- Teach patient that product must be continued for prescribed time to be effective and taken exactly as prescribed; doses are not to be doubled
- Instruct patient to report to prescriber diarrhea, black tarry stools, abdominal pain, cramping, menstrual disorders
- Caution patient to prevent pregnancy while taking this product; spontaneous abortion may occur

### Evaluation
**Positive therapeutic outcome**
- Prevention of ulcers

---

### ! HIGH ALERT
## mitomycin (Rx)
(mye-toe-mye'sin)
mitomycin, Mutamycin
*Func. class.:* Antineoplastic, antibiotic
**Pregnancy category** D

**Do not confuse:**
mitomycin/mithramycin/mitotane/mitoxantrone

**Action:** Inhibits DNA synthesis, primarily; derived from *Streptomyces caespitosus;* appears to cause cross-linking of DNA, a vesicant

Adverse effects: *italic* = common, **bold** = life-threatening

**Therapeutic outcome:** Prevention of rapidly growing malignant cells

**Uses:** Pancreas, stomach, colorectal, bladder cancer

**Unlabeled uses:** Palliative treatment of head, neck, colon, breast, biliary, cervical, lung malignancies

## Dosage and routes
*Adult:* **IV** 10-20 mg/m² q6-8 wk

**Available forms:** Inj 5, 20, 40 mg/vial

## Adverse effects
*CNS:* Fever, headache, confusion, drowsiness, syncope, fatigue
*EENT:* Blurred vision
*GI: Nausea, vomiting, anorexia, stomatitis,* **hepatotoxicity,** diarrhea
*GU:* Urinary retention, **renal failure,** edema
*HEMA:* **Thrombocytopenia, leukopenia, anemia**
*INTEG:* *Rash,* alopecia, **extravasation,** nail discoloration
*MISC:* **Hemolytic uremic syndrome, CHF**
*RESP:* **Fibrosis, pulmonary infiltrate,** dyspnea

**Contraindications:** Pregnancy **D** (1st trimester), breastfeeding, hypersensitivity, as a single agent, thrombocytopenia, coagulation disorders

**Precautions:** Renal disease, bone marrow depression

| Pharmacokinetics | |
|---|---|
| Absorption | Complete bioavailability |
| Distribution | Widely distributed; concentrates in tumor |
| Metabolism | Liver, extensively |
| Excretion | Kidneys, unchanged |
| Half-life | 1 hr |

| Pharmacodynamics |
|---|
| Unknown |

## Interactions
*Individual drugs*
Radiation: increased toxicity
*Drug classifications*
Anticoagulants, NSAIDs: increased bleeding risk
Antineoplastics: increased toxicity
*Drug/herb*
Black cohosh: avoid use

## NURSING CONSIDERATIONS
### Assessment
◆ Assess for fatal hemolytic uremic syndrome: hypertension, thrombocytopenia, microangiopathic hemolytic anemia, occurs during long-term therapy
• Assess buccal cavity q8hr for dryness, sores or ulceration, white patches, oral pain, bleeding, dysphagia; obtain prescription for viscous lidocaine (Xylocaine)
• Assess symptoms indicating severe allergic reaction: rash, pruritus, urticaria, purpuric skin lesions, itching, flushing
• Monitor CBC, differential, platelet count weekly; withhold product if WBC is <2000/mm³ or platelet count is <100,000/mm³ or granulocyte count is <1000/mm³, notify prescriber of results if WBC <20,000/mm³, platelets <150,000/mm³
• Monitor renal function tests: BUN, creatinine, serum uric acid, urine CCr before and during therapy; check I&O ratio; report fall in urine output to <30 ml/hr
◆ Assess for pulmonary fibrosis, bronchospasm, dyspnea, crackles, unproductive cough, chest pain, tachypnea, fatigue, increased pulse, pallor, lethargy
• Monitor temp q4hr (may indicate beginning of infection)
• Monitor liver function tests before and during therapy (bilirubin, AST, ALT, LDH) as needed or monthly; check for jaundiced skin and sclera, dark urine, clay-colored stools, itchy skin, abdominal pain, fever, diarrhea
• Assess for bleeding: hematuria, stool guaiac, bruising or petechiae, mucosa or orifices q8hr; inflammation of mucosa, breaks in skin
• Identify effects of alopecia on body image; discuss feelings about body changes
• Identify edema in feet, joint pain, stomach pain, shaking; check for inflammation of mucosa, breaks in skin

### Nursing diagnoses
• Body image, disturbed (adverse reactions)
• Infection, risk for (adverse reactions)
• Injury, risk for (adverse reactions)
• Knowledge, deficient (teaching)

### Implementation
#### IV route
• Avoid contact with skin, since medication is very irritating; wash completely to remove
• Give fluids **IV** or PO before chemotherapy to hydrate patient
• Provide antacid before oral agent; give product after evening meal, before bedtime; administer antiemetic 30-60 min before giving

product and prn to prevent vomiting; use antibiotics for prophylaxis of infection
• Give topical or systemic analgesics for pain
• Give in AM so product can be eliminated before bedtime
• Provide a liquid diet: carbonated beverages; gelatin may be added if patient is not nauseated or vomiting
• Product should be prepared by experienced personnel using proper precautions in a biologic cabinet using gown, gloves, mask
• Give by direct **IV** after diluting 5 mg/10, or 10 mg/40 ml sterile water for inj; shake, allow to stand, give through Y-tube or 3 way stopcock; give slow IV push or inf over 15-30 min through running D$_5$W, 0.9% NaCl **IV**; color of reconstituted sol is gray
• Apply ice compress for extravasation

*Syringe compatibilities:* Bleomycin, cisplatin, cyclophosphamide, DOXOrubicin, droperidol, fluorouracil, furosemide, heparin, leucovorin, methotrexate, metoclopramide, vinBLAStine, vinCRIStine

*Y-site compatibilities:* Allopurinol, amifostine, bleomycin, cisplatin, cyclophosphamide, DOXOrubicin, droperidol, fluorouracil, furosemide, granisetron, heparin, leucovorin, melphalan, methotrexate, metoclopramide, ondansetron, teniposide, thiotepa, vinBLAStine, vinCRIStine

*Y-site incompatibilities:* Sargramostim, vinorelbine

*Additive compatibilities:* Dexamethasone, hydrocortisone

*Additive incompatibilities:* Bleomycin

*Solution compatibilities:* LR, 0.3% NaCl, 0.5% NaCl

## Patient/family education
• Advise patient to get adequate fluids 2-3 L/day unless contraindicated
• Encourage patient to rinse mouth tid-qid with water, club soda, brush teeth bid-qid with soft brush or cotton-tipped applicators for stomatitis, use unwaxed dental floss
• Teach patient to avoid use of products containing aspirin or ibuprofen, razors, commercial mouthwash, since bleeding may occur; to report symptoms of bleeding (hematuria, tarry stools)
• Caution patient to report signs of anemia (fatigue, headache, irritability, faintness, shortness of breath)
• Advise patient to report any changes in breathing or coughing even several mo after treatment; to avoid crowds and persons with respiratory tract or other infections
• Inform patient that hair may be lost during

treatment; a wig or hairpiece may make patient feel better; new hair may be different in color, texture
• Advise patient not to have any vaccinations without the advice of the prescriber, serious reactions can occur
• Teach patient that contraception is needed during treatment and for several mo after completion of therapy
• Teach patient to report immediately urine retention, absence of urine, dyspnea, bleeding, jaundice

## Evaluation
**Positive therapeutic outcome**
• Prevention of rapid division of malignant cells

---

**⁄ HIGH ALERT**

**mitoxantrone** (Rx)
(mye-toe-zan'trone)
Novantrone
*Func. class.:* Antineoplastic-antibiotic, immunomodulator
*Chem. class.:* Synthetic anthraquinone

**Pregnancy category D**

**Action:** DNA reactive agent; cytocidal effect on both proliferating and nonproliferating cells, topoisomerase II inhibitor; a vesicant

**Therapeutic outcome:** Prevention of rapidly growing malignant cells

**Uses:** Acute myelogenous leukemia (adult), relapsed leukemia, breast cancer, multiple sclerosis; used with steroids to treat bone pain (advanced prostate cancer)

**Unlabeled uses:** Liver malignancies, non-Hodgkin's lymphoma, breast cancer, ALL

## Dosage and routes
*Acute nonlymphatic leukemia/ induction*
*Adult:* **IV** INF 12 mg/m$^2$/day on days 1-3, and 100 mg/m$^2$ cytosine arabinoside × 7 days as a CONT 24-hr INF

*Consolidation*
*Adult:* **IV** INF 12 mg/m$^2$ given as a short 5-15 min inf

*Advanced prostate cancer*
*Adult:* **IV** 12-14 mg/m$^2$ as a single dose or short INF

*Multiple sclerosis*
*Adult:* **IV** INF 12 mg/m$^2$ as a 5-15 min infusion q3 mo

M

Adverse effects: *italic* = common, **bold** = life-threatening

**Available forms:** Inj 2, 10, 12.5, 15 mg/ml

**Adverse effects**

*CNS:* Headache, **seizures**, fatigue
*CV:* **CHF, cardiomyopathy, dysrhythmias**
*EENT:* Conjunctivitis, blue-green sclera, blurred vision
*GI: Nausea, vomiting, diarrhea, anorexia, mucositis,* **hepatoxicity**
*GU:* Amenorrhea, menstrual disorders
*HEMA:* **Thrombocytopenia, leukopenia, myelosuppression, anemia, secondary leukemia**
*INTEG: Rash, necrosis at inj site,* alopecia, dermatitis, thrombophlebitis at inj site
*MISC:* Fever
*RESP:* Cough, dyspnea

**Contraindications:** Pregnancy **D**, hypersensitivity

**Precautions:** Breastfeeding, children, myelosuppression, cardiac/renal/hepatic disease, gout

| Pharmacokinetics | |
|---|---|
| Absorption | Completely absorbed |
| Distribution | Widely distributed, protein binding 78% |
| Metabolism | Liver |
| Excretion | Bile; kidneys, unchanged (<10%) |
| Half-life | 23-215 hr |

| Pharmacodynamics | |
|---|---|
| Unknown | |

**Interactions**
*Individual drugs*
Radiation: increased toxicity, bone marrow suppression
*Drug classifications*
Anticoagulants, NSAIDs: increased bleeding risk
Antineoplastics: increased toxicity, bone marrow suppression
Live virus vaccines: increased adverse reactions
*Drug/herb*
Black cohosh, dong quai: avoid use

**NURSING CONSIDERATIONS**
**Assessment**
• Multiple sclerosis: obtain baseline multigated angiogram, left ventricular ejection fraction (LVEF) if symptoms of CHF occur, repeat LVEF or if cumulative dose is >100 mg/m²; do not administer to patients who have received a lifetime dose of ≥140 mg/m² or if LVEF <50% or significant decrease in LVEF

• Do not administer in multiple sclerosis if neutrophils <1500/mm³
• Obtain pregnancy test in all women of childbearing age
◆ Monitor ECG; watch for ST-T wave changes, low QRS and T, possible dysrhythmias (sinus tachycardia, heart block, PVCs); also monitor ECHO, chest x-ray, RAI angiography to assess ejection fraction before and during treatment, product is cardiotoxic, may develop during treatment or months to years after treatment
• Assess buccal cavity q8hr for dryness, sores or ulceration, white patches, oral pain, bleeding, dysphagia; obtain prescription for viscous lidocaine (Xylocaine)
• Assess symptoms indicating severe allergic reaction: rash, pruritus, urticaria, purpuric skin lesions, itching, flushing
• Assess tachypnea, ECG changes, dyspnea, edema, fatigue
• Monitor CBC, differential, platelet count weekly; withhold product if WBC is <4000/mm³ or platelet count is <100,000/mm³, notify prescriber of results if WBC <20,000/mm³, platelets <150,000/mm³
• Assess for increased uric acid levels, swelling, joint pain primarily in extremities; patient should be well hydrated to prevent urate deposits
• Monitor renal function tests: BUN, creatinine, urine CCr before and during therapy; determine I&O ratio
• Monitor temp q4hr (may indicate beginning of infection)
• Monitor liver function tests before and during therapy (bilirubin, AST, ALT, LDH) as needed or monthly; dose reduction needed in hepatic disease; check for jaundiced skin and sclera, dark urine, clay-colored stools, itchy skin, abdominal pain, fever, diarrhea
• Assess for bleeding: hematuria, stool guaiac, bruising or petechiae, mucosa or orifices q8hr; check for inflammation of mucosa, breaks in skin
• Identify effects of alopecia on body image; discuss feelings about body changes
◆ Assess for MS: obtain MUGA, LVEF baselines; repeat LVEF if symptoms of CHF occur or if cumulative dose is >100 mg/m²; do not give to patients who have received a lifetime dose of ≥140 mg/m² or if LVEF <50% or significant LVEF
◆ Assess for secondary acute myelogenous leukemia (AML) that can develop after taking this product

### Nursing diagnoses
• Body image, disturbed (adverse reactions)
• Infection, risk for (adverse reactions)
• Injury, risk for (adverse reactions)
• Knowledge, deficient (teaching)

### Implementation
🔷 Do not mix with any other product
• Avoid contact with skin, since medication is very irritating; wash completely to remove
• Give fluids **IV** or PO before chemotherapy to hydrate patient
• Give antacid before oral agent; give product after evening meal, before bedtime; provide antiemetic 30-60 min before giving product and prn to prevent vomiting; administer antibiotics for prophylaxis of infection
• Give topical or systemic analgesics for pain
• Liquid diet: carbonated beverages; gelatin may be added if patient is not nauseated or vomiting
• Sol should be prepared by qualified personnel only under controlled conditions in a biologic cabinet using mask, gloves, gown
• Use Luer-Lok tubing to prevent leakage; do not let sol come in contact with skin; if contact occurs, wash well with soap and water
• Give by direct **IV** after diluting with 50 ml or more of 0.9% NaCl or D₅W; give over 3-5 min, running **IV** of D₅W or 0.9% NaCl
• Intermittent infusion may be diluted further in D₅W, 0.9% NaCl and run over 15-30 min; check for extravasation

*Y-site compatibilities:* Allopurinol, amifostine, cladribine, filgrastim, fludarabine, granisetron, melphalan, ondansetron, sargramostim, teniposide, thiotepa, vinorelbine
*Y-site incompatibilities:* Paclitaxel
*Additive compatibilities:* Cyclophosphamide, cytarabine, fluorouracil, hydrocortisone, potassium chloride
*Additive incompatibilities:* Heparin
*Solution compatibilities:* D₅/0.9 NaCl, D₅W, 0.9% NaCl

### Patient/family education
• Encourage patient to rinse mouth tid-qid with water, club soda, brush teeth bid-qid with soft brush or cotton-tipped applicators for stomatitis, use unwaxed dental floss
• Teach patient to avoid use of products containing aspirin or NSAIDs, razors, commercial mouthwash, since bleeding may occur; to report symptoms of bleeding (hematuria, tarry stools)
• Caution patient to report signs of anemia (fatigue, headache, irritability, faintness, shortness of breath)
• Inform patient that hair may be lost during

treatment; a wig or hairpiece may make patient feel better; new hair may be different in color, texture
• Caution patient not to have any vaccinations without the advice of the prescriber; serious reactions can occur
• Advise patient that contraception is needed during treatment and for several mo after completion of therapy
• Advise patient that sclera, urine may turn blue or green
• Advise patient to increase fluids to 2-3 L/day unless contraindicated
• Teach patient to avoid crowds, persons with infections
• Teach patient to report immediately bleeding, dyspnea, possible infections, seizure, jaundice

### Evaluation
**Positive therapeutic outcome**
• Prevention of rapid division of malignant cells

---

**moexipril** (Rx)
(moe-ex'i-pril)
Univasc
*Func. class.:* Antihypertensive
*Chem. class.:* Angiotensin-converting enzyme (ACE) inhibitor
**Pregnancy category  D**

M

---

**Action:** Selectively suppresses renin-angiotensin-aldosterone system; inhibits ACE; prevents conversion of angiotensin I to angiotensin II; results in dilatation of arterial, venous vessels

**Therapeutic outcome:** Decreased B/P in hypertension

**Uses:** Hypertension, alone or in combination with thiazide diuretics

### Dosage and routes
*Initial treatment*
*Adult:* PO 7.5 mg 1 hr before meals initially, may be increased or divided depending on B/P response

*Maintenance*
*Adult:* PO 7.5-30 mg/day in 1-2 divided doses 1 hr before meals

*Renal dose*
*Adult:* PO CCr <40 ml/min 3.75 mg/day titrate to desired dose, max 15 mg/day

**Available forms:** Tabs 7.5, 15 mg

---

Adverse effects: *italic* = common, **bold** = life-threatening

### Adverse effects

*CNS:* Fever, chills
*CV:* Hypotension, postural hypotension
*GI:* Loss of taste
*GU:* Impotence, dysuria, nocturia, proteinuria, nephrotic syndrome, acute reversible renal failure, polyuria, oliguria, frequency
*HEMA:* **Neutropenia**
*INTEG:* Rash
*META:* Hypokalemia
*RESP:* **Bronchospasm,** dyspnea, dry cough
*SYST:* **Angioedema, anaphylaxis**

**Contraindications:** Pregnancy **D**, breastfeeding, hypersensitivity, children, heart block, bilateral renal stenosis, history of angioedema

**Precautions:** Dialysis patients, hypovolemia, leukemia, scleroderma, lupus erythematosus, blood dyscrasias, CHF, diabetes mellitus, renal/thyroid disease, COPD, asthma, potassium-sparing diuretics

#### Pharmacokinetics

| | |
|---|---|
| **Absorption** | Unknown |
| **Distribution** | Unknown |
| **Metabolism** | Liver to metabolites |
| **Excretion** | Via kidneys, crosses placenta, excreted in breast milk |
| **Half-life** | Unknown |

#### Pharmacodynamics

Unknown

### Interactions
#### *Individual drugs*
Azathioprine: increased myelosuppression
CycloSPORINE: increased hyperkalemia
Digoxin, lithium: increased toxicity
#### *Drug classification*
Adrenergic blockers, antihypertensives, diuretics, ganglionic blockers, phenothiazines: increased hypotension
Diuretics (potassium-sparing), potassium supplements, sympathomimetics: do not use together
NSAIDs: decreased antihypertensive effect
#### *Drug/herb*
Hawthorn: increased antihypertensive effect
Yohimbe: decreased antihypertensive effect
#### *Drug/lab test*
False positive: urine acetone

### NURSING CONSIDERATIONS
#### Assessment
• Monitor blood studies: neutrophils, decreased platelets
• Monitor B/P

• Monitor renal function tests: protein, BUN, creatinine; watch for increased levels that may indicate nephrotic syndrome
• Monitor baselines in renal, liver function tests before therapy begins
• Monitor potassium levels, although hyperkalemia rarely occurs
• Assess edema in feet, legs daily
• Assess allergic reaction: rash, fever, pruritus, urticaria; product should be discontinued if antihistamines fail to help
• Assess for symptoms of CHF: edema, dyspnea, wet crackles, B/P
• Monitor for renal symptoms: polyuria, oliguria, frequency

#### Nursing diagnoses
• Knowledge, deficient (teaching)

#### Implementation
• Give PO 1 hr before meals
• Store in airtight container at 86° F or less

#### Patient/family education
• Instruct patient not to discontinue product abruptly
• Tell patient not to use OTC (cough, cold, allergy) products unless directed by prescriber
• Teach patient to comply with dosage schedule, even if feeling better
• Encourage patient to rise slowly to sitting or standing position to minimize orthostatic hypotension
• Teach patient to notify prescriber of mouth sores, sore throat, fever, swelling of hands or feet, irregular heartbeat, chest pain, signs of angioedema
• Tell patient that excessive perspiration, dehydration, vomiting, diarrhea may lead to fall in B/P; consult prescriber if this occurs
• Teach patient that dizziness, fainting, lightheadedness may occur during first few days of therapy
• Tell patient that skin rash or impaired perspiration may occur
• Teach patient how to take B/P

#### Evaluation
**Positive therapeutic outcome**
• Decreased B/P in hypertension

**Treatment of overdose:** 0.9% NaCl **IV** inf, hemodialysis

## montelukast (Rx)

(mon-teh-loo'kast)

Singulair

*Func. class.:* Bronchodilator

*Chem. class.:* Leukotriene antagonist, cysteinyl

**Pregnancy category** B

**Action:** Inhibits leukotriene (LTD$_4$) formation; leukotrienes exert their effects by increasing neutrophil, eosinophil migration; aggregation of neutrophils, monocytes; smooth muscle contraction, capillary permeability; these actions further lead to bronchoconstriction, inflammation, edema

**Therapeutic outcome:** Ability to breathe with ease

**Uses:** Chronic asthma

**Unlabeled uses:** Chronic urticaria

**Dosage and routes**

*Asthma*

*Adult and child ≥15 yr:* PO 10 mg/day PM

*Child 6-14 yr:* PO 5 mg chew tabs/day PM

*Child 2-5 yr:* PO chew tabs 4 mg/day

*Child 12-23 mo:* PO 1 packet of granules taken PM

*Exercise-induced bronchoconstriction*

*Adult and adolescent ≥15 yr:* PO 10 mg 2 hr prior to exercise; do not take another dose within 24 hr

**Available forms:** Tabs 10 mg; chewable tabs 4, 5 mg; oral granules 4 mg/packet

**Adverse effects**

*CNS:* Dizziness, fatigue, headache

*GI:* Abdominal pain, dyspepsia

*INTEG:* Rash

*MS:* Asthenia

*RESP:* Influenza, cough, nasal congestion

**Contraindications:** Hypersensitivity

**Precautions:** Pregnancy **B**, breastfeeding, children <6 yr, acute attacks of asthma, alcohol consumption, aspirin sensitivity

| Pharmacokinetics | |
|---|---|
| Absorption | Rapidly |
| Distribution | Protein binding 99% |
| Metabolism | Liver |
| Excretion | Bile |
| Half-life | 2.7-5.5 hr |

| Pharmacodynamics | |
|---|---|
| Onset | Unknown |
| Peak | 3-4 hr |
| Duration | Unknown |

**Interactions**

*Individual drugs*

Phenobarbital, rifampin: decreased montelukast levels

*Drug/herb*

Tea (green, black), guarana: increased stimulation

*Drug/lab test*

Increased: ALT, AST

**NURSING CONSIDERATIONS**

**Assessment**

◆ Assess adult patients carefully for symptoms of Churg-Strauss syndrome (rare), including eosinophilia, vasculitic rash, worsening pulmonary symptoms, cardiac complications and/or neuropathy

• Monitor CBC, blood chemistry during treatment

• Assess respiratory rate, rhythm, depth; auscultate lung fields bilaterally; notify prescriber of abnormalities

• Assess allergic reactions: rash, urticaria; product should be discontinued

**Nursing diagnoses**

• Activity intolerance (uses)

• Airway clearance, ineffective (uses)

• Knowledge, deficient (teaching)

**Implementation**

**PO route**

• Give PO in PM daily for all uses except exercise-induced bronchoconstriction; then take 2 hr prior to exercise

• Do not open packet until ready to use, mix whole dose, give within 15 min

• Granules may be given directly in mouth or mixed with a spoonful of soft food (carrots, applesauce, ice cream, rice)

**Patient/family education**

• Instruct patient to check OTC and current prescription medications for epHEDrine, which will increase stimulation; to avoid alcohol

• Advise patient to avoid hazardous activities; dizziness may occur

• Teach patient that product is not to be used for acute asthma attacks

• Advise patient to avoid NSAIDs if sensitive to aspirin

• Advise patient to continue to use inhaled β-agonists if exercise-induced asthma occurs

M

Adverse effects: *italic* = common, **bold** = life-threatening

### Evaluation
**Positive therapeutic outcome**
- Increased ease of breathing
- Decreased bronchospasm

---

**❗ HIGH ALERT**

## morphine (Rx)
(mor'feen)
Astramorph, Astramorph PF, Avinza,
Duramorph, Epimorph ✦, Infumorph,
Kadian, morphine sulfate, Morphitec ✦,
M.O.S. ✦, M.O.S.-S.R. ✦, MS Contin,
MSIR, OMS Concentrate, Oramorph SR,
RMS, Roxanol, Roxanol Rescudose,
Roxanol-T, Statex ✦
*Func. class.:* Opioid analgesic
*Chem. class.:* Alkaloid

**Pregnancy category** C

**Controlled substance schedule** II

**Do not confuse:**
morphine/hydromorphone, Roxanol/Roxicet

**Action:** Depresses pain impulse transmission at the spinal cord level by interacting with opioid receptors, produces CNS depression

**Therapeutic outcome:** Decreased pain

**Uses:** Moderate to severe pain; often given after or during an MI

### Dosage and routes
*Adult:* SUBCUT/IM 5-20 mg q4hr prn; PO 10-30 mg q4hr prn; EXT REL 15-30 mg q8-12hr; RECT 10-30 mg q4hr prn; **IV** 4-10 mg diluted in 4-5 ml of water for inj, over 5 min; SUS REL cap (Kadian), EXT REL cap (Avinza) give total daily dose q24hr; for those with no tolerance to opioids, 30 mg/day, may adjust by no more than 30 mg q4 days
*Child:* SUBCUT/**IV** 0.05-0.1 mg/kg, max 15 mg; PO 0.2-0.5 mg/kg q4-6hr (regular rel), q12hr (sus rel)

**Available forms:** Inj 0.5, 1, 2, 3, 4, 5, 8, 10, 15, 25, 50 mg/ml; sol tabs 10, 15, 30 mg; oral sol 10, 20 mg/5 ml, 20 mg/10 ml, 20 mg/ml; oral tabs 15, 30 mg; rect supp 5, 10, 20, 30 mg; ext rel tabs 15, 30, 60, 100, 200 mg; caps 15, 30 mg; syr 1, 5 mg/ml; cont rel cap pellets (Kadian) 20, 30, 50, 60, 100 mg; ext rel caps (Avinza) 30, 60, 90, 120 mg

### Adverse effects
***CNS:*** Drowsiness, dizziness, *confusion,* headache, *sedation,* euphoria, insomnia, **seizures**
***CV:*** Palpitations, **bradycardia**, change in B/P, **shock, cardiac arrest,** chest pain, hypertension, edema, **tachycardia**
***EENT:*** Tinnitus, blurred vision, miosis, diplopia
***GI:*** Nausea, vomiting, anorexia, *constipation,* cramps, biliary tract pressure
***GU:*** Urinary retention
***HEMA:*** **Thrombocytopenia**
***INTEG:*** Rash, urticaria, bruising, flushing, diaphoresis, pruritus
***RESP:*** **Respiratory depression, respiratory arrest, apnea**

**Contraindications:** Hypersensitivity, addiction (opioid), hemorrhage, bronchial asthma, increased ICP

**Precautions:** Pregnancy **C**, breastfeeding, children <18 yr, geriatric, addictive personality, acute MI, severe heart disease, respiratory depression, renal/hepatic disease, bowel impaction

| Pharmacokinetics | |
|---|---|
| **Absorption** | Variably absorbed (PO); well absorbed (IM, SUBCUT, RECT); completely absorbed (**IV**) |
| **Distribution** | Widely distributed; crosses placenta |
| **Metabolism** | Liver, extensively |
| **Excretion** | Kidneys |
| **Half-life** | 1½-2 hr |

### Interactions
*Individual drugs*
Alcohol: increased effects with other CNS depressants
Rifampin: decreased analgesic action
*Drug classifications*
Antipsychotics, opiates, sedative/hypnotics, skeletal muscle relaxants: increased effects with other CNS depressants
MAOIs: unpredictable reaction may occur, avoid use

| Pharmacodynamics | | | | | | | |
|---|---|---|---|---|---|---|---|
| | PO | PO–EXT REL | IM | SUBCUT | RECT | IV | IT |
| **Onset** | Variable | Unknown | 10-30 min | 20 min | Unknown | Rapid | Rapid |
| **Peak** | 1 hr | Unknown | ½-1 hr | 1-1½ hr | ½-1 hr | 20 min | Unknown |
| **Duration** | 4-5 hr | 8-12 hr | 3-7 hr | 4-5 hr | 4-5 hr | 4-5 hr | Ext |

---

### Drug/herb
Chamomile, hops, Jamaican dogwood, kava, lavender, mistletoe, nettle, pokeweed, poppy, senega, skullcap, St. John's wort, valerian: increased CNS depression
Corkwood: increased anticholinergic effect

### Drug/food
Cranberry juice (excessive amounts), oats: decreased morphine effect

### Drug/lab test
Increased: amylase

## NURSING CONSIDERATIONS
### Assessment
• Assess pain: location, type, character, intensity; give dose before pain becomes extreme
• Monitor I&O ratio; check for decreasing output; may indicate urinary retention; check for constipation; increase fluids, bulk in diet if needed or stool softeners may be prescribed
• Monitor CNS changes: dizziness, drowsiness, hallucinations, euphoria, LOC, pupil reactions
• Monitor allergic reactions: rash, urticaria
• Assess respiratory dysfunction: depression, character, rate, rhythm; notify prescriber if respirations are <10/min

### Nursing diagnoses
• Breathing pattern, ineffective (adverse reactions)
• Knowledge, deficient (teaching)
• Pain, acute (uses)
• Sensory perception, disturbed: visual, auditory (adverse reactions)

### Implementation
• Give with antiemetic if nausea, vomiting occur
• Administer when pain is beginning to return; determine dosage interval by patient response; continuous dosing of medication is more effective than giving prn
• Withdraw medication slowly after long-term use to prevent withdrawal symptoms
• Store in light-resistant container at room temperature
• Kadian is not bioequivalent to other controlled release forms

### PO route
• Swallow ext rel tabs whole; do not break, crush, or chew
◆ Kadian tabs may be opened and sprinkled on applesauce immediately before use; do not break, crush, chew, or dissolve pellets in Kadian cap, which may lead to an overdose; adjustments may need to be made when converting from another form of morphine
• May be given with food or milk to lessen GI upset; other forms may be crushed and mixed with food or fluids

**IM/SUBCUT route**
• Do not give if cloudy or a precipitate has formed

**IV route**
• Give direct **IV** by diluting with ≥5 ml of sterile water or 0.9% NaCl for inj; give 2.5-15 mg/4-5 min; rapid administration may lead to increased respiratory depression, death
• Give cont inf by adding to $D_5W$, $D_{10}W$, 0.9% NaCl, 0.45% NaCl, Ringer's, LR, any dextrose/saline sol, or any dextrose/Ringer's, 0.1-1 mg/ml
• Give by infusion pump to deliver correct dosage; titrate to provide adequate pain relief without serious sedation, respiratory depression, hypotension
• May be given by patient-controlled analgesia (PCA) pump in terminal illnesses; patient is able to control amount of morphine
• Administer epidurally with caution in the geriatric

*Syringe compatibilities:* Atropine, benzquinamide, bupivacaine, butorphanol, cimetidine, dimenhydRINATE, diphenhydrAMINE, droperidol, fentanyl, glycopyrrolate, hydrOXYzine, ketamine, metoclopramide, midazolam, milrinone, pentazocine, perphenazine, promazine, ranitidine, scopamine

*Syringe incompatibilities:* Meperidine, thiopental

*Y-site compatibilities:* Allopurinol, amifostine, amikacin, aminophylline, amiodarone, ampicillin, ampicillin/sulbactam, amsacrine, atenolol, atracurium, aztreonam, bumetanide, calcium chloride, cefamandole, cefazolin, cefmetazole, cefoperazone, cefotaxime, cefotetan, cefoxitin, ceftazidime, ceftizoxime, ceftriaxone, cefuroxime, cephalothin, cephapirin, chloramphenicol, cisplatin, cladribine, clindamycin, cyclophosphamide, cytarabine, dexamethasone, digoxin, diltiazem, dobutamine, DOPamine, doxycycline, enalaprilat, epINEPHrine, erythromycin, esmolol, etomidate, famotidine, fentanyl, filgrastim, fluconazole, fludarabine, foscarnet, gentamicin, granisetron, heparin, hydrocortisone, hydromorphone, IL-2, insulin (regular), kanamycin, labetalol, lidocaine, lorazepam, magnesium sulfate, melphalan, meropenem, methotrexate, methyldopate, methylPREDNISolone, metoclopramide, metoprolol, metronidazole, mezlocillin, midazolam, milrinone, moxalactam, nafcillin, niCARdipine, nitroglycerin, norepinephrine, ondansetron, oxacillin, oxytocin, paclitaxel, pancuronium, penicillin G potassium, piperacillin, piperacillin/tazobactam, potassium chloride, propofol, propranolol, ranitidine, sodium bicarbonate,

M

sodium nitroprusside, teniposide, thiotepa, ticarcillin, ticarcillin/clavulanate, tobramycin, trimethoprim/sulfamethoxazole, vancomycin, vecuronium, vinorelbine, vit B/C, warfarin, zidovudine

**Y-site incompatibilities:** Furosemide, minocycline, tetracycline

**Additive compatibilities:** Alteplase, atracurium, baclofen, bupivacaine, DOBUTamine, fluconazole, furosemide, meropenem, metoclopramide, ondansetron, succinylcholine, verapamil

**Additive incompatibilities:** Aminophylline

## Patient/family education

• Advise patient to report any symptoms of CNS changes, allergic reactions
• Caution patients to avoid CNS depressants (alcohol, sedative/hypnotics) for at least 24 hr after taking this product
• Discuss with patient that dizziness, drowsiness, and confusion are common; to avoid getting up without assistance
• Discuss in detail all aspects of the product and expected response

## Evaluation

**Positive therapeutic outcome**
• Decreased pain

**Treatment of overdose:** Naloxone (Narcan) 0.2-0.8 **IV**, O₂, **IV** fluids, vasopressors

---

## moxifloxacin (Rx)
(mox-i-floks′a-sin)
Avelox, Avelox IV
*Func. class.:* Antiinfective
*Chem. class.:* Fluoroquinolone

**Pregnancy category** C

**Action:** Interferes with conversion of intermediate DNA fragments into high molecular weight DNA in bacteria; DNA gyrase inhibitor

**Therapeutic outcome:** Bactericidal action against the following: *Staphylococcus aureus, Streptococcus pneumoniae, Haemophilus influenzae, Haemophilus parainfluenzae, Moraxella catarrhalis, Klebsiella pneumoniae, Mycoplasma pneumoniae, Chlamydia pneumoniae; Staphylococcus aureus, Streptococcus pyogenes, E. coli, Bacteroides fragilis, Streptococcus arginosus, Streptococcus constellatus, Enterococcus faecalis, Proteus mirabilis, Clostridium perfringens, Bacteroides thetalomicron, Peptostreptococcus, Enterobacter cloacae*

**Uses:** Acute bacterial sinusitis, acute bacterial exacerbation of chronic bronchitis, community-acquired pneumonia (mild to moderate), uncomplicated skin/skin structure infections, complicated intraabdominal infections including polymicrobial infections, complicated skin/skin structure infections

## Dosage and routes
*Acute bacterial sinusitis*
**Adult:** PO/**IV** 400 mg q24hr × 10 days

*Acute bacterial exacerbation of chronic bronchitis*
**Adult:** PO/**IV** 400 mg q24hr × 5 days

*Community-acquired pneumonia*
**Adult:** PO/**IV** 400 mg q24hr × 7-14 days

*Uncomplicated skin/skin structure infections*
**Adult:** PO/**IV** 400 mg q24hr × 7 days

*Complicated intraabdominal infections*
**Adult:** IV 400 mg/day × 5-14 days

*Complicated skin, skin structure infections*
**Adult:** PO/**IV** 400 mg/day × 7-21 days

**Available forms:** Tabs 400 mg; inj premix 400 mg

## Adverse effects
**CNS:** Headache, dizziness, fatigue, insomnia, depression, restlessness, **seizures,** confusion, **increased intracranial pressure**
**CV:** Prolonged QT interval, **dysrhythmias,** torsade de pointes, tachycardia
**EENT:** Blurred vision, tinnitus
**GI:** Nausea, increased ALT, AST, flatulence, heartburn, vomiting, diarrhea, oral candidiasis, dysphagia, **pseudomembranous colitis**
**INTEG:** Rash, pruritus, urticaria, photosensitivity, flushing, fever, chills
**MS:** Tremor, arthralgia, tendon rupture
**SYST:** **Anaphylaxis, Stevens-Johnson syndrome**

**Contraindications:** Hypersensitivity to quinolones

**Precautions:** Pregnancy **C**, breastfeeding, children, renal disease, epilepsy, uncorrected hypokalemia, prolonged QT interval, patients receiving class IA, III antidysrhythmics

| Pharmacokinetics | |
|---|---|
| **Absorption** | Well absorbed (75%) (PO) |
| **Distribution** | Widely distributed |
| **Metabolism** | Liver |
| **Excretion** | Kidneys |
| **Half-life** | Increased in renal disease |

---

## Pharmacodynamics

| | PO |
|---|---|
| **Onset** | Rapid |
| **Peak** | 1 hr |
| **Duration** | Unknown |

## Interactions
### Individual drugs
Aluminum hydroxide, calcium, didanosine, iron, sucralfate, zinc sulfate: decreased absorption of moxifloxacin

CycloSPORINE: increased cycloSPORINE effect

Probenecid: increased blood levels

Warfarin: increased warfarin effect

### Drug classifications
Antacids (magnesium), iron salts: decreased absorption of moxifloxacin

Antidysrhythmics IA, III: prolonged QT interval

### Drug/herb
Acidophilus: do not use with antiinfectives; separate by several hours

Cola tree: increased antiinfective effect

### Drug/food
Enteral feeding: decreased absorption of moxifloxacin

## NURSING CONSIDERATIONS
### Assessment
• Assess patient for previous sensitivity reaction

• Assess patient for signs and symptoms of infection including characteristics of wounds, sputum, urine, stool, WBC >10,000/mm³, fever; baseline and during treatment

• Obtain C&S before beginning product therapy to identify if correct treatment has been initiated

• Assess for allergic reactions and anaphylaxis: rash, urticaria, pruritus, chills, fever, joint pain; may occur a few days after therapy begins; epINEPHrine and resuscitation equipment should be available for anaphylactic reaction

• Assess for CNS symptoms: headache, dizziness, fatigue, insomnia, depression, **seizures**

• Identify urine output; if decreasing, notify prescriber (may indicate nephrotoxicity); also check for increased BUN, creatinine

• Monitor blood tests: AST, ALT, CBC, Hct, bilirubin, LDH, alkaline phosphatase, Coombs' test monthly if patient is on long-term therapy

• Monitor electrolytes: potassium, sodium chloride monthly if patient is on long-term therapy

• Assess bowel pattern daily; if severe diarrhea occurs, product should be discontinued

• Monitor for bleeding: ecchymosis, bleeding gums, hematuria, stool guaiac daily if on long-term therapy

• Assess for overgrowth of infection: perineal itching, fever, malaise, redness, pain, swelling, drainage, rash, diarrhea, change in cough, sputum

### Nursing diagnoses
• Diarrhea (side effects)
• Infection, risk for (uses)
• Injury, risk for (side effects)
• Knowledge, deficient (teaching)
• Noncompliance (teaching)

### Implementation
• Do not use theophylline with this product; may cause toxicity

**PO route**
• Give once a day for 5-10 days depending on condition

**IV route**
• Discontinue primary **IV** while administering moxifloxacin
• Do not give SUBCUT, IM

*Solution compatibilities:* 0.9% NaCl, $D_5$, $D_{10}$, LR, sterile water for inj

### Patient/family education
• Teach patient to report sore throat, bruising, bleeding, joint pain; may indicate blood dyscrasias (rare)

• Advise patient to contact prescriber if vaginal itching, loose foul-smelling stools, furry tongue occur; may indicate superinfection; report itching, rash, pruritus, urticaria

• Instruct patient to take all medication prescribed for the length of time ordered; do not give medication to others

• Advise patient to notify prescriber of diarrhea with blood or pus

• Advise patient to rinse mouth frequently, use sugarless candy or gum for dry mouth

• Advise patient to take as prescribed, not to double or miss doses

### Evaluation
#### Positive therapeutic outcome
• Absence of signs/symptoms of infection (WBC <10,000/mm³, temp WNL)
• Reported improvement in symptoms of infection

## moxifloxacin ophthalmic
*See Appendix D*

M

## multivitamins
### (PO, OTC, IV, Rx)
Adavite, Dayalets, LKV Drops, Multi-75, Multi-Day, One-A-Day, Optilets, Poly-Vi-Sol, Quintabs, Rulets, Sesame Street Vitamins, Tab-A-Vite, Therabid, Theragran, Unicaps, Vita-Bob, Vita-Kid, many other brands
*Func. class.:* Vitamins, multiple

**Pregnancy category A**

**Do not confuse:**
Theragran/Phenergan

**Action:** Needed for adequate metabolism

**Therapeutic outcome:** Prevention and treatment of vitamin deficiencies

**Uses:** Prevention and treatment of vitamin deficiencies

**Dosage and routes**
*Adult and child:* PO/**IV**—depends on brand

**Available forms:** Many forms available

**Adverse effects**
Rare at recommended dosage

**Precautions:** Pregnancy **A**

Pharmacokinetics

| | |
|---|---|
| **Absorption** | Well absorbed (PO) |
| **Distribution** | Widely distributed; crosses placenta |
| **Metabolism** | Widely metabolized |
| **Excretion** | Kidney, unchanged (water soluble) |
| **Half-life** | Unknown |

Pharmacodynamics
Unknown

### NURSING CONSIDERATIONS
**Assessment**
• Assess patient for vitamin deficiency; usually more than one vitamin deficiency is present

**Nursing diagnoses**
• Knowledge, deficient (teaching)
• Nutrition: less than body requirements, imbalanced (uses)

**Implementation**
**PO route**
• Liquid multivitamins can be diluted or dropped into patient's mouth using dropper provided with some brands
• Chew tabs should be chewed and not swallowed whole

**IV route**
• Give by cont inf only after diluting 5-10 ml (multivitamins)/500-1000 ml of $D_5W$, $D_{10}W$, $D_{20}W$, LR, $D_5$/LR, $D_5$/0.9% NaCl, 0.9% NaCl, 3% NaCl
• Do not use sol with crystals, precipitate, or color other than bright yellow
*Y-site compatibilities:* Acyclovir, ampicillin, cefazolin, cephalothin, cephapirin, diltiazem, erythromycin, fludarabine, gentamicin, tacrolimus, tetracycline
*Additive compatibilities:* Cefoxitin, isoproterenol, methyldopa, metoclopramide, metronidazole, netilmicin, norepinephrine, sodium bicarbonate, verapamil
*Additive incompatibilities:* Penicillin G, erythromycin, tetracycline, kanamycin, streptomycin, doxycycline, lincomycin should not be admixed

**Patient/family education**
• Advise patient that adequate nutrition must be maintained to prevent further deficiencies; to comply with treatment regimen
• Advise patient to avoid treating flavored multivitamins as candy; child may overdose
• Caution patient to store vitamins out of children's reach

**Evaluation**
**Positive therapeutic outcome**
• Check each individual vitamin for guidelines
• Absence of vitamin deficiencies

## mupirocin topical
*See Appendix D*

## muromonab-CD3 (Rx)
(mur-oe-mone'ab)
Orthoclone OKT3
*Func. class.:* Immunosuppressive
*Chem. class.:* Murine monoclonal antibody

**Pregnancy category C**

**Action:** Reverses graft rejection by blocking T-cell function

**Therapeutic outcome:** Prevention of graft rejection

**Uses:** Acute allograft rejection in renal, cardiac, hepatic transplant patients

**Dosage and routes**
*Adult:* **IV** BOL 5 mg/day × 10-14 days
*Child:* **IV** 100 mcg/kg/day × 10-14 day

 Alert　 Canada Only　 Drug on CD　　　* "Tall Man" lettering (See Preface)

### Cardiac/hepatic allograft rejection, steroid resistant

*Adult:* **IV** BOL 5 mg/day × 10-14 days; begin when it is known that rejection has not been reversed by steroids

**Available forms:** Inj 5 mg/5 ml

### Adverse effects

*CNS: Pyrexia, chills, tremors,* **aseptic meningitis,** fever
*CV: Chest pain*
*GI: Vomiting, nausea, diarrhea*
*MISC:* **Infection, cytokine release syndrome, anaphylaxis**
*RESP: Dyspnea, wheezing,* **pulmonary edema**

**Contraindications:** Hypersensitivity to murine origin, fluid overload

**Precautions:** Pregnancy **C,** children <2 yr, fever

| Pharmacokinetics | |
|---|---|
| **Absorption** | Completely absorbed |
| **Distribution** | Unknown |
| **Metabolism** | Unknown |
| **Excretion** | Unknown |
| **Half-life** | Unknown |

| Pharmacodynamics |
|---|
| Unknown |

### Interactions
*Individual drugs*
Azathioprine, cycloSPORINE: increased risk of infection
Indomethacin: increased CNS symptoms
*Drug classifications*
Corticosteroids: increased risk of infection
Immunosuppressants: increased immunosuppression
Live virus vaccines: decreased antibody response
*Drug/herb*
Astragalus, echinacea, melatonin: interference with immunosuppression
Ginseng, maitake, mistletoe, schisandra, St. John's wort, turmeric: decreased effect

### NURSING CONSIDERATIONS
**Assessment**
🔷 Assess for cytosine release syndrome (CRS): nausea, vomiting, chills, fever, joint pain, weakness, dizziness, diarrhea, tremors, abdominal pain; occurs 30-60 min after first dose; methylPREDNISolone sodium succinate may be prescribed to lessen this reaction
• Assess for hypersensitivity reaction, anaphylaxis: dyspnea, bronchospasm, urticaria, tachycardia, hypotension, angioedema; discontinue product; emergency equipment must be nearby
• Assess for headache, photophobia, fever, rigidity; indicate aseptic meningitis has developed
• Assess for sore throat, fever, chills, rash, dysuria, which may indicate infection; therapy may be discontinued
• Assess for fluid overload: edema, pulmonary edema, increasing weight
• Monitor blood studies: CBC with differential, platelets, BUN, creatinine, alkaline phosphatase, bilirubin during treatment monthly
• Monitor AST, ALT, BUN, creatinine, alkaline phosphatase, bilirubin
• Obtain human-mouse antibody; if titer is >1:1000, this product should not be used
• Monitor T-cells with CD3, CD4, CD8 antigen daily; report should be CD3 positive and T-cells <25/mm$^3$

### Nursing diagnoses
• Infection, risk for (uses)
• Knowledge, deficient (teaching)

### Implementation
• Give by direct **IV** undiluted; withdraw with a 0.2-0.22 low–protein binding μm filter; discard and use new needle for administration; give over 1 min
• Give for several days before transplant surgery

### Patient/family education
• Instruct patient to report fever, chills, sore throat, fatigue, since serious infections may occur; rash, rapid heartbeat
• Advise patient to use contraceptive measures during treatment and for 12 wk after ending therapy; product is mutagenic
• Advise patient to avoid crowds and persons with known infections to reduce risk of infection
• Advise patient to report symptoms of cytokine release syndrome, aseptic meningitis, give list of symptoms
• Instruct patient to avoid vaccinations during treatment

### Evaluation
**Positive therapeutic outcome**
• Absence of graft rejection

M

## mycophenolate (Rx)
(mie-koe-feen'oh-late)
CellCept, Myfortic
*Func. class.:* Immunosuppressant

**Pregnancy category** C

**Action:** Inhibits inflammatory responses that are mediated by the immune system; prolongs survival of allogenic transplants

**Therapeutic outcome:** Absence of graft rejection

**Uses:** Organ transplants to prevent rejection (renal); prophylaxis of rejection in allogenic cardiac, hepatic, renal transplants

**Unlabeled uses:** Refractory uveitis, 2nd-line therapy for Churg-Strauss syndrome, diffuse proliferative lupus nephritis (in combination), rheumatoid arthritis, psoriasis

### Dosage and routes
#### Renal transplant
*Adult:* PO/**IV** Give initial dose 72 hr before transplantation; 1 g bid given to renal transplant patients in combination with corticosteroids and cycloSPORINE; ER tab 720 mg bid on empty stomach
*Child:* PO-ER 400 mg/m$^2$ bid, max 720 mg bid

#### Renal dose
*Adult:* PO/**IV** GFR <25 ml/min, max 2 g/day

#### Cardiac transplant
*Adult:* PO/**IV** 1.5 g bid, **IV** can be started ≤24 hr after transplant, switch to PO when able

#### Hepatic transplant
*Adult:* PO/**IV** 1.5 g bid, give **IV** over ≥2 hr

**Available forms:** Caps 250 mg; tabs 500 mg; inj (powder) 500 mg/20 ml vial; powder for oral susp 200 mg/ml; ext rel tab (Myfortic) 180, 360 mg

### Adverse effects
*CNS:* Tremor, dizziness, insomnia, headache, fever
*CV:* Hypertension, chest pain
*GI:* Nausea, vomiting, stomatitis, diarrhea, constipation, **GI bleeding**
*GU:* UTI, hematuria, **renal tubular necrosis**
*HEMA:* Leukopenia, thrombocytopenia, anemia, pancytopenia
*INTEG:* Rash
*META:* Peripheral edema, hypercholesterolemia, hypophosphatemia, edema, hypo/hyperkalemia, hyperglycemia
*MS:* Arthralgia, muscle wasting

*RESP:* Dyspnea, respiratory infection, increased cough, pharyngitis, bronchitis, pneumonia
*SYST:* **Lymphoma, nonmelanoma skin carcinoma, sepsis**

**Contraindications:** Hypersensitivity to this product or mycophenolic acid

**Precautions:** Pregnancy C, breastfeeding, lymphomas, malignancies, neutropenia, renal disease

### Pharmacokinetics
| | |
|---|---|
| **Absorption** | Rapidly and completely absorbed |
| **Distribution** | Unknown |
| **Metabolism** | To active metabolite (MPA) |
| **Excretion** | Urine, feces |
| **Half-life** | Unknown |

### Pharmacodynamics
Unknown

### Interactions
#### Individual drugs
Acyclovir, ganciclovir: increased concentration of both products
Azathioprine: avoid use
Cholestyramine: decreased levels of mycophenolate
Phenytoin: increased effects; decreased protein binding of phenytoin
Probenecid: increased levels of mycophenolate
Theophylline: increased effects; decreased protein binding of theophylline
#### Drug classifications
Antacids: decreased levels of mycophenolate
Contraceptives (oral), live attenuated vaccines: decreased effects
Salicylates: increased levels of mycophenolate
#### Drug/herb
Astragalus, echinacea, melatonin: interferes with immunosuppression
#### Drug/food
Decreased absorption if taken with food

### NURSING CONSIDERATIONS
#### Assessment
- Monitor blood tests: CBC monthly during treatment
- Monitor liver function tests: alkaline phosphatase, AST, ALT, bilirubin
#### Nursing diagnoses
- Infection, risk for (uses)
- Knowledge, deficient (teaching)

 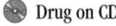

### Implementation
- Give 72 hr before transplantation; may be given in combination with corticosteroids and cycloSPORINE

**PO route**
- Do not crush, chew tabs; do not open caps; avoid inhalation or direct contact with skin, mucous membranes; tetragenic in animals
- Give alone for better absorption

**IV route**
- Do not give by rapid or bolus inj: reconstitute and dilute to 6 mg/ml with D$_5$, give over ≥2 hr
- Do not admix with mycophenolate **IV** in infusion catheter or with other **IV** product or infusion admixtures

### Patient/family education
- Teach patient to report fever, rash, severe diarrhea, chills, sore throat, fatigue, since serious infections may occur
- Instruct patient to avoid crowds to reduce risk of infection
- Advise patient that repeated lab tests are necessary
- Advise patient to limit exposure to sunlight/UV light
- Instruct patient to use contraception before, during, and 6 wk after therapy

### Evaluation
**Positive therapeutic outcome**
- Absence of graft rejection

---

### nabilone (Rx)
(nab′-ih-lohn)
Cesamet
*Func. class.:* Antiemetic
*Chem. class.:* Miscellaneous—cannabinoid

**Pregnancy category  C**

**Action:** Orally, active cannabinoid, chemically related to marijuana; may decrease nausea by action on cannabinoid receptors in the CNS

**Therapeutic outcome:** Decreased nausea and vomiting associated with chemotherapy

**Uses:** Prevention of nausea, vomiting associated with cancer chemotherapy, in those that have not responded to other treatment; not to be used on an as needed basis

### Dosage and routes
*Adult:* PO 1-2 mg bid; give initial dose 1-3 hrs prior to chemotherapy; start with lower dose and increase as needed; may give dose of 1-2 mg the night before chemotherapy; may give 2-3 times daily during chemotherapy cycle

**Available forms:** Caps 1 mg

### Adverse effects
*CNS: Headache, ataxia, drowsiness, dysphoria, euphoria, sleep disturbance, vertigo, asthenia, concentration difficulties, depression,* syncope, hallucinations
*CV:* Chest discomfort, **tachycardia,** orthostatic hypotension
*GI: Dry mouth,* nausea, *anorexia,* increased appetite
*INTEG:* Allergic reactions, rash, photosensitivity, pruritus
*MS:* Back, joint, muscle, neck pain

**Contraindications:** Hypersensitivity to this product or cannabinoids

**Precautions:** Pregnancy C, breastfeeding, depression, mental disorders, severe heptic/renal disease, hypertension, tachycardia, CV disorders

| Pharmacokinetics | |
|---|---|
| **Absorption** | Rapid 10-20% |
| **Distribution** | Unknown |
| **Metabolism** | Liver |
| **Excretion** | Biliary system in feces |
| **Half-life** | Terminal 2 hr |

| Pharmacodynamics | |
|---|---|
| **Onset** | Unknown |
| **Peak** | Unknown |
| **Duration** | Unpredictable, psychiatric symptoms may occur for up to 72 hr after treatment concludes |

### Interactions
*Individual drugs*
Disulfiram, possibly fluoxetine: hypomanic reaction
Naltrexone: increased action or nabilone
Theophylline: decreased metabolism of theophylline
*Drug classifications*
Anticholinergics (antihistamines, atropine, scopolamine): increased tachycardia, drowsiness
CNS depressants (alcohol, barbiturates, benzodiazepines, buspirone, lithium, muscle relaxants, opioids): increased drowsiness, CNS depression
Opioids: increased action of both products
Sympathomimetics (amphetamines, cocaine): increased hypertension, tachycardia, and possibly cardiotoxicity

---

Adverse effects: *italic* = common, **bold** = life-threatening

Tricyclic antidepressants: increased tachycardia, hypertension, drowsiness

## NURSING CONSIDERATIONS
### Assessment
- Assess for absence of nausea and vomiting during chemotherapy
- Assess for CNS symptoms: headache, depression, ataxia, drowsiness, dysphoria, euphoria, sleep disturbances, concentration difficulties
- Assess for CV symptoms, cardiac status: tachycardia, orthostatic hypotension, hypertension

### Nursing diagnoses
- Injury, risk for (uses, adverse reactions)
- Knowledge, deficient (teaching)
- Nutrition: less than body requirements, imbalanced (uses)

### Implementation
- Give PO, not to be used on an as needed basis
- Store capsules at room temperature, away from light and moisture

### Patient/family education
- Teach patient that mood, behavioral changes may occur while taking this product
- Advise patient to notify prescriber if pregnancy is suspected
- Advise patient to avoid breastfeeding while taking this product
- Instruct patient not to use alcohol or other CNS depressants unless approved by prescriber
- Instruct patient not to operate machinery or perform other hazardous activities while taking this product

### Evaluation
**Positive therapeutic outcome**
- Decreased nausea and vomiting associated with chemotherapy

---

## nabumetone (Rx)
(na-byoo'me-tone)
Relafen
*Func. class.:* Nonsteroidal antiinflammatory
*Chem. class.:* Acetic acid derivative

**Pregnancy category** C

**Action:** Inhibits prostaglandin synthesis by decreasing an enzyme needed for biosynthesis; analgesic, antiinflammatory

**Therapeutic outcome:** Decreased pain, swelling of joints

**Uses:** Osteoarthritis, rheumatoid arthritis, acute or chronic treatment

### Dosage and routes
*Adult:* PO 1 g as a single dose; may increase to 1.5-2 g/day if needed; may give daily or bid (as a divided dose)

**Available forms:** Tabs 500, 750 mg

### Adverse effects
*CNS:* Dizziness, headache, drowsiness, fatigue, tremors, confusion, insomnia, anxiety, depression, nervousness
*CV:* Tachycardia, peripheral edema, palpitations, **dysrhythmias, CHF, MI, stroke**
*GI:* Nausea, anorexia, vomiting, diarrhea, jaundice, cholestatic hepatitis, constipation, flatulence, cramps, dry mouth, peptic ulcer, gastritis, **ulceration, perforation,** bleeding
*GU:* **Nephrotoxicity, dysuria, hematuria, oliguria, azotemia,** cystitis
*HEMA:* **Blood dyscrasias**
*INTEG:* Purpura, rash, pruritus, sweating, photosensitivity
*RESP:* Dyspnea, pharyngitis, **bronchospasm**
*SYST:* **Anaphylaxis, angioneurotic edema**

**Contraindications:** Avoid in late pregnancy, hypersensitivity to this product or aspirin, iodides, NSAIDs, asthma, severe renal/hepatic disease, perioperative pain in CABG surgery

**Precautions:** Pregnancy **C**, breastfeeding, children, geriatric, bleeding disorders, GI/cardiac/renal disorders, hepatic dysfunction

### Pharmacokinetics
| | |
|---|---|
| **Absorption** | Well absorbed |
| **Distribution** | Unknown |
| **Metabolism** | Liver, extensively, to inactive metabolite |
| **Excretion** | Unknown |
| **Half-life** | 22-30 hr |

### Pharmacodynamics
| | |
|---|---|
| **Onset** | Unknown |
| **Peak** | 2½-4 hr |
| **Duration** | Unknown |

### Interactions
*Individual drugs*
Alcohol, potassium: increased GI reactions
Cefamandole, cefoperazone, cefotetan, clopidogrel, eptifibatide, plicamycin, ticlopidine, valproic acid: increased risk of bleeding
Radiation: increased risk of hematologic reactions

---

 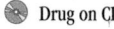

## Drug classifications

Anticoagulants, thrombolytics: increased risk of bleeding

Antihypertensives: decreased effect of antihypertensives

Antineoplastics: increased risk of hematologic reactions

Corticosteroids, NSAIDs, potassium supplements, salicylates: increased GI reactions

Diuretics: decreased effectiveness of diuretics

## Drug/herb

Arginine, gossypol: increased gastric irritation

Bearberry, bilberry: increased NSAIDs effect

Bogbean, chondroitin: increased bleeding risk

## Drug/lab test

Increased: bleeding time, K, BUN, AST, ALT, LDH, alkaline phosphatase, creatinine

Decreased: CCr, blood glucose, Hct, Hgb

## NURSING CONSIDERATIONS
### Assessment

• Assess for pain: frequency, characteristics, location, duration, intensity, relief of pain after medication; and for inflammation of joints, ROM

• Monitor blood counts during therapy; watch for decreasing platelets; if low, therapy may need to be discontinued, restarted after hematologic recovery; check for blood dyscrasias (thrombocytopenia): bruising, fatigue, bleeding, poor healing; monitor liver function tests: AST, ALT, alkaline phosphatase; LDH, blood glucose, WBC, CCr

• Assess for asthma, aspirin sensitivity, nasal polyps; increased hypersensitivity reactions

### Nursing diagnoses

• Injury, risk for (adverse reactions)
• Knowledge, deficient (teaching)
• Mobility, impaired physical (uses)
• Pain, acute (uses)
• Pain, chronic

### Implementation

• Administer tab to patient crushed or whole
• Give with food or milk to decrease gastric symptoms
• Patient should take with a full glass of water and sit upright

### Patient/family education

• Tell patient that product must be continued for prescribed time to be effective; to avoid aspirin, alcoholic beverages, NSAIDs, and OTC medications unless approved by prescriber

• Caution patient to report bleeding, bruising, fatigue, malaise, since blood dyscrasias do occur

• Instruct patient to use caution when driving; drowsiness, dizziness may occur

• Advise patient to use sunscreen, hat, and other protective clothing to prevent burns

• Advise patient to report dark stools, a change in urine pattern, increased weight, edema, increased pain in joints, fever, blood in urine, blurred vision, ringing or roaring in ears

### Evaluation
**Positive therapeutic outcome**

• Decreased pain
• Decreased inflammation
• Increased mobility

## nadolol (Rx)
(nay-doe′lole)
Corgard, Syn-Nadolol
*Func. class.:* Antihypertensive, antianginal
*Chem. class.:* β-Adrenergic receptor blocker

### Pregnancy category C

### Do not confuse:
Corgard/Cognex

**Action:** Competitively blocks stimulation of β-adrenergic receptor within vascular smooth muscle; produces chronotropic, inotropic activity (decreases rate of SA node discharge, increases recovery time), slows conduction of AV node, decreases heart rate, which decreases $O_2$ consumption in myocardium; also decreases renin-aldosterone-angiotensin system at high doses, inhibits $\beta_2$-receptors in bronchial system

**Therapeutic outcome:** Decreased B/P, heart rate

**Uses:** Chronic stable angina pectoris, mild to moderate hypertension

**Unlabeled uses:** Tachydysrhythmias, aggression, anxiety, tremors, esophageal varices (rebleeding only), prophylaxis of migraine headaches, hyperthyroidism adjunctive therapy

### Dosage and routes
*Adult:* PO 40 mg/day; increase by 40-80 mg q3-7 days; maintenance 40-240 mg/day for angina, 40-320 mg/day for hypertension
*Geriatric:* PO 20 mg/day, may increase by 20 mg until desired dose

### Renal dose
*Adult:* PO CCr 31-50 ml/min give q24-36hr; CCr 10-30 ml/min give q24-48hr; CCr <10 ml/min give q40-60hr

N

Adverse effects: *italic* = common, **bold** = life-threatening

**Available forms:** Tabs 20, 40, 80, 120, 160 mg

**Adverse effects**

***CNS:*** Depression, dizziness, fatigue, lethargy, paresthesia, headache, *weakness,* insomnia, memory loss, nightmares

***CV:*** **Bradycardia,** *hypotension,* **CHF,** palpitations, AV block, chest pain, peripheral ischemia, flushing, edema, vasodilatation, conduction disturbances

***EENT:*** Blurred vision, dry eyes, nasal congestion

***ENDO:*** Hyperglycemia, hypoglycemia

***GI:*** Nausea, vomiting, diarrhea, colitis, constipation, cramps, dry mouth, flatulence, hepatomegaly, **pancreatitis,** taste distortion

***GU: Impotence,*** decreased libido

***HEMA:*** **Agranulocytosis, thrombocytopenia**

***INTEG:*** Rash, pruritus, fever, alopecia

***RESP:*** Dyspnea, respiratory dysfunction, **bronchospasm,** cough, wheezing, pharyngitis, **laryngospasm, pulmonary edema**

**Contraindications:** Hypersensitivity to this product, cardiac failure, cardiogenic shock, 2nd- or 3rd-degree heart block, bronchospastic disease, sinus bradycardia, CHF, COPD

**Precautions:** Pregnancy **C,** breastfeeding, diabetes mellitus, renal disease, hyperthyroidism, peripheral vascular disease, myasthenia gravis, major surgery, nonallergic bronchospasm

| Pharmacokinetics | |
|---|---|
| **Absorption** | Variably absorbed |
| **Distribution** | Crosses placenta; minimal concentration in CNS, protein binding 30% |
| **Metabolism** | Unknown |
| **Excretion** | Kidneys, unchanged |
| **Half-life** | 10-24 hr; increased in renal disease |

| Pharmacodynamics | |
|---|---|
| **Onset** | Variable |
| **Peak** | 3-4 hr |
| **Duration** | 20-24 hr |

**Interactions**

*Individual drugs*

Clonidine, epINEPHrine: increased hypotension, bradycardia

Digoxin: increased bradycardia

Thyroid: decreased β-blocking effect

**Drug classifications**

Antihypertensives: increased hypotension

Ergots: peripheral ischemia

MAOIs: increased bradycardia; do not use together

NSAIDs: decreased antihypertensive effect

Phenothiazines: increased hypotensive effects

**Drug/herb**

Aconite: increased toxicity, death

Astragalus, cola tree: increased or decreased antihypertensive effect

Barberry, betony, black catechu, black cohosh, bloodroot, broom, burdock, cat's claw, dandelion, goldenseal, Irish moss, Jamaican dogwood, kelp, khella, mistletoe, parsley: increased antihypertensive effect

Coltsfoot, guarana, khat, licorice: decreased antihypertensive effect

**Drug/lab test**

Increased: serum potassium, serum uric acid, ALT, AST, alkaline phosphatase, LDH, blood glucose, cholesterol, ANA, triglycerides

**NURSING CONSIDERATIONS**

**Assessment**

• Monitor B/P at beginning of treatment, periodically thereafter; note rate, rhythm, quality of apical/radial pulse before administration; notify prescriber of any significant changes (pulse <55 bpm), orthostatic hypotension

• Check for baselines in renal, liver function tests before therapy begins

• Assess for edema in feet, legs daily; monitor I&O, daily weight; check for jugular vein distention and crackles bilaterally, dyspnea (CHF)

• Monitor skin turgor, dryness of mucous membranes for hydration status, especially geriatric

**Nursing diagnoses**

• Cardiac output, decreased (uses)

• Injury, risk for (adverse reactions)

• Knowledge, deficient (teaching)

• Noncompliance (teaching)

**Implementation**

• Given before meals, at bedtime; tab may be crushed or swallowed whole; give with food to prevent GI upset; give reduced dosage in renal dysfunction

• Store protected from light, moisture; place in cool environment

**Patient/family education**

• Teach patient not to discontinue product abruptly; taper over 2 wk; may cause precipitate angina, serious dysrhythmias if stopped abruptly

- Teach patient not to use OTC products containing α-adrenergic stimulants (such as nasal decongestants, cold preparations); to avoid alcohol, smoking and to limit sodium intake as prescribed
- Teach patient how to take pulse and B/P at home; to hold dose if pulse ≤50 bpm, systolic B/P <90 mm Hg; advise when to notify prescriber
- Instruct patient to comply with weight control, dietary adjustments, modified exercise program
- Advise patient to carry/wear emergency ID to identify product being taken, allergies; teach patient product controls symptoms but does not cure condition
- Caution patient to avoid hazardous activities if dizziness, drowsiness present; to rise slowly to prevent orthostatic hypotension
- Teach patient to report symptoms of CHF: difficult breathing, especially on exertion or when lying down, night cough, swelling of extremities or bradycardia, dizziness, confusion, depression, fever
- Teach patient to take product as prescribed, not to double doses, skip doses; take any missed doses as soon as remembered if at least 4 hr until next dose

### Evaluation
**Positive therapeutic outcome**
- Decreased B/P in hypertension

---

### nafarelin (Rx)
(naf-ah-rell′in)
Synarel
*Func. class.:* Gonadotropin
*Chem. class.:* Analog of gonadotropin-releasing hormone

**Pregnancy category X**

**Action:** Stimulates the release of LH and FSH, which increases ovarian steroid production; repeated dosing prevents stimulation of the pituitary gland

**Therapeutic outcome:** Decreased symptoms of endometriosis; resolution of central precocious puberty

**Uses:** Endometriosis, gonadotropin-dependent precocious puberty

### Dosage and routes
*Endometriosis*
**Adult:** NASAL 400 mcg/day as one spray (200 mcg) into one nostril in morning and 1 spray into other nostril in evening; start treatment between days 2 and 4 of menstrual cycle; may increase to 800 mcg/day (1 spray into each nostril twice a day); recommended duration of treatment is 6 mo

*Central precocious puberty*
**Child:** NASAL 2 sprays in each nostril AM and PM, may increase to 3 sprays after alternating nostril tid

**Available forms:** Nasal spray 2 mg/ml (200 mcg/spray)

### Adverse effects
*CNS:* Headache, flushing, depression, insomnia, emotional lability, hot flashes
*GU:* Decreased libido, vaginal dryness, breast tenderness, increased pubic hair, *impaired fertility, reduction in breast size,* impotence, irregular periods
*INTEG:* Acne
*META:* Decreased bone density, increased cholesterol, triglycerides
*MISC:* Body odor, seborrhea, rhinitis
*SENSITIVITY:* Shortness of breath, chest pain, urticaria, pruritus

**Contraindications:** Pregnancy **X;** breastfeeding; hypersensitivity to this product, GnRH, sorbitol; undiagnosed abnormal vaginal bleeding

**Precautions:** Children, polycystic ovary disease, bone mineral density loss

#### Pharmacokinetics

| | |
|---|---|
| **Absorption** | Well |
| **Distribution** | Unknown |
| **Metabolism** | Unknown |
| **Excretion** | 20%-40% feces, 3% urine, unchanged |
| **Half-life** | 3 hr |

#### Pharmacodynamics

| | |
|---|---|
| **Onset** | Up to 4 wk |
| **Peak** | 3-4 wk |
| **Duration** | Several months |

### Interactions
*Drug classifications*
Nasal decongestants (nasal sprays): decreased nafarelin absorbtion

### NURSING CONSIDERATIONS
#### Assessment
- Assess pain in endometriosis during treatment
- Assess endocrine studies, bone age, sex steroids, RHCG, GnRH, baseline q8 wk
- Assess for precocious puberty including secondary sex characteristics

- Assess test results: pituitary/hypothalamus dysfunction (decreased LH); postmenopausal (increased LH)

### Nursing diagnoses
- Knowledge, deficient (teaching)
- Pain, acute (uses)
- Sexual dysfunction (uses, adverse reactions)

### Implementation
- Repeated doses may be necessary to elevate pituitary gonadotropin reserve
- Tilt head back slightly, wait 30 sec between sprays; do not use decongestant until 2 hr later
- Store at room temperature; protect from light

### Patient/family education
- Teach patient to use nonhormonal contraception
- Teach patient about correct nasal use, 1 spray in right nostril AM, 1 in left nostril PM
- Teach patient that medication may cause hot flashes, decreased libido, vaginal dryness

### Evaluation
**Positive therapeutic outcome**
- Decreased symptoms of endometriosis; adequate resolution of central precocious puberty

---

### nafcillin (Rx)
(naf-sill'in)
Nafcillin sodium
*Func. class.:* Antiinfective—broad-spectrum
*Chem. class.:* Penicillinase-resistant penicillin

**Pregnancy category B**

**Action:** Interferes with cell wall replication of susceptible organisms; osmotically unstable cell wall swells, bursts from osmotic pressure

**Therapeutic outcome:** Bactericidal effects for gram-positive cocci *Staphylococcus aureus, Streptococcus viridans, Streptococcus pneumoniae* and infections caused by penicillinase-producing *Staphylococcus*

**Uses:** Infections caused by penicillinase-producing staphylococci, streptococci; respiratory tract, skin, skin structure, urinary tract, bone, joint infections, sinusitis, endocarditis, septicemia, meningitis

### Dosage and routes
*Adult:* **IV** 500-2000 mg q4hr
*Infant and child >1 mo:* **IV** 50-200 mg/kg/day in divided doses q4-6hr

*Neonate >7 days (weight >2 kg):*
**IV** 25 mg/kg q8hr
*Neonate ≤7 days (weight <2 kg):*
**IV** 25 mg/kg q12hr
*Meningitis*
*Adult:* **IV** 100-200 mg/kg/day divided q4-6hr, max 12 g/day
*Neonate >7 days (weight >2 kg):*
**IV** 50 mg/kg q6hr
*Neonate ≤7 days (weight <2 kg):*
**IV** 50 mg/kg q12hr

**Available forms:** Powder for inj 1, 2, 10 g

### Adverse effects
*CNS:* Lethargy, hallucinations, anxiety, depression, muscle twitching, **coma, seizures**
*GI: Nausea, vomiting, diarrhea,* increased AST, ALT, abdominal pain, glossitis, **pseudomembranous colitis**
*GU:* Oliguria, **proteinuria, hematuria,** vaginitis, moniliasis, **glomerulonephritis,** interstitial nephritis
*HEMA:* Anemia, increased bleeding time, **bone marrow depression, granulocytopenia**
*SYST:* **Anaphylaxis, serum sickness, Stevens-Johnson syndrome**

**Contraindications:** Hypersensitivity to penicillins

**Precautions:** Pregnancy **B**, breastfeeding, neonates, GI disease, asthma, hypersensitivity to cephalosporins

| Pharmacokinetics | |
| --- | --- |
| Absorption | Well absorbed (IM); erratic (PO) |
| Distribution | Widely distributed; crosses placenta |
| Metabolism | Not metabolized |
| Excretion | Kidneys, unchanged; breast milk |
| Half-life | 1 hr; increased in renal disease |

| Pharmacodynamics | | | |
| --- | --- | --- | --- |
| | PO | IM | IV |
| Onset | ½ hr | ½ hr | Immediate |
| Peak | 1-2 hr | 1-2 hr | Infusion end |
| Duration | Unknown | Unknown | Unknown |

### Interactions
*Individual drugs*
Probenecid: increased nafcillin levels
Heparin: decreased effect of heparin
*Drug classifications*
Anticoagulants (oral): decreased anticoagulant effects
Contraceptives (oral): decreased contraceptive effectiveness

---

 Alert     Canada Only     Drug on CD    * "Tall Man" lettering (See Preface)

*Drug/herb*
Acidophilus: do not use with antiinfectives; separate by several hours
Khat: decreased absorption
*Drug/food*
Food, carbonated drinks, citrus fruit juices: decreased absorption
*Drug/lab test*
False positive: urine glucose, urine protein

## NURSING CONSIDERATIONS
### Assessment
• Assess patient for previous sensitivity reaction to penicillins or other cephalosporins; cross-sensitivity between penicillins and cephalosporins is common
• Assess patient for signs and symptoms of infection including characteristics of wounds, sputum, urine, stool, WBC >10,000/mm³, earache, fever; obtain baseline information and during treatment
• Obtain C&S before beginning product therapy to identify if correct treatment has been initiated
• Assess for allergic reactions, anaphylaxis: rash, urticaria, pruritus, chills, fever, dyspnea, laryngeal edema, joint pain; angioedema may occur a few days after therapy begins; epI-NEPHrine, resuscitation equipment should be available for anaphylactic reaction
• Assess renal function tests: urinalysis, protein, blood, BUN, creatinine
◆ Identify urine output; if decreasing, notify prescriber (may indicate nephrotoxicity)
• Monitor blood studies: AST, ALT, CBC, Hct, bilirubin, LDH, alkaline phosphatase, Coombs' test monthly if patient is on long-term therapy
• Monitor electrolytes: potassium, sodium, chloride monthly if patient is on long-term therapy
• Assess bowel pattern daily; if severe diarrhea occurs, product should be discontinued; may indicate pseudomembranous colitis
• Monitor for bleeding: ecchymosis, bleeding gums, hematuria, stool guaiac daily if on long-term therapy
• Assess for overgrowth of infection: perineal itching, fever, malaise, redness, pain, swelling, drainage, rash, diarrhea, change in cough, sputum

### Nursing diagnoses
• Diarrhea (adverse reactions)
• Infection, risk for (uses)
• Injury, risk for (adverse reactions)
• Knowledge, deficient (teaching)
• Noncompliance (teaching)

### Implementation
#### PO route
• Give in even doses around the clock; if GI upset occurs, give with food; product must be given for 10-14 days to ensure organism death and prevent superinfection; store in airtight container.
• Shake susp; store in refrigerator for 2 wk, 1 wk at room temperature
#### IM route
• Reconstitute 500 mg/1.7-1.8 ml; 1 g/3.4 ml; 2 g/6.6-6.8 ml with sterile water or bacteriostatic water for a conc of 250 mg/ml; store unused portion in refrigerator for up to 7 days
• Give deep in large muscle mass
#### IV route
• Reconstitute 1 g/3.4 ml, 2 g/6.6-6.8 ml with sterile water or bacteriostatic water for a conc of 250 mg/ml; store unused portion in refrigerator for up to 7 days
• Give by direct **IV** by diluting reconstituted sol with 15-30 ml of sterile water or 0.9% NaCl; give over 5-10 min
• Give by intermittent inf by diluting to a conc of 2-40 mg/ml with 0.9% NaCl, D₅W, D₁₀W, D₅/0.9% NaCl, D₅/LR, LR, Ringer's; store in refrigerator for up to 96 hr or 24 hr room temperature; run over 30-60 min
*Syringe compatibilities:* Cimetidine, heparin
*Y-site compatibilities:* Acyclovir, atropine, cyclophosphamide, diazepam, enalaprilat, esmolol, famotidine, fentanyl, fluconazole, foscarnet, hydromorphone, magnesium sulfate, morphine, perphenazine, propofol, theophylline, zidovudine
*Y-site incompatibilities:* Droperidol, fentanyl/droperidol, labetalol, nalbuphine, pentazocine, regular insulin, verapamil
*Additive compatibilities:* Chloramphenicol, chlorothiazide, dexamethasone, diphenhydrAMINE, epHEDrine, heparin, hydrOXYzine, lidocaine, potassium chloride, prochlorperazine, sodium bicarbonate, sodium lactate
*Additive incompatibilities:* Ascorbic acid, aztreonam, bleomycin, cytarabine, gentamicin, hydrocortisone sodium succinate, methylPREDNISolone sodium succinate, promazine

### Patient/family education
• Teach patient to report sore throat, bruising, bleeding, joint pain; may indicate blood dyscrasias (rare)
• Advise patient to contact prescriber if vaginal itching, loose foul-smelling stools,

N

furry tongue occur; may indicate superinfection

- Instruct patient to take all medication prescribed for the length of time ordered
- Advise patient to notify prescriber of diarrhea with blood or pus, which may indicate pseudomembranous colitis
- Advise patient to carry/wear emergency ID if allergic to penicillins

### Evaluation
**Positive therapeutic outcome**
- Absence of signs/symptoms of infection (WBC <10,000/mm$^3$, temp WNL, absence of red, draining wounds, earache)
- Reported improvement in symptoms of infection

**Treatment of anaphylaxis:** Withdraw product, maintain airway, administer epINEPHrine, aminophylline, O$_2$, **IV** corticosteroids

---

### ! HIGH ALERT

### nalbuphine (Rx)
(nal'byoo-feen)
Nubain, nalbuphine HCl
*Func. class.:* Opioid analgesic
*Chem. class.:* Synthetic opioid agonist/antagonist

**Pregnancy category** C

**Action:** Inhibits ascending pain pathways in limbic system, thalamus, midbrain, hypothalamus by binding to opiate receptor sites, thus altering pain perception and response

**Therapeutic outcome:** Relief of pain

**Uses:** Moderate to severe pain

### Dosage and routes
*Analgesic*
**Adult:** SUBCUT/IM/**IV** 10 mg q3-6hr prn, not to exceed 160 mg/day

*Balanced anesthesia supplement*
**Adult: IV** 0.3-3 mg/kg given over 10-15 min; may give 0.25-0.5 mg/kg as needed (maintenance)

**Available forms:** Inj 10, 20 mg/ml

### Adverse effects
*CNS: Drowsiness, dizziness, confusion, headache, sedation, euphoria,* dysphoria (high doses), hallucinations, increased dreaming, tolerance, physical and psychologic dependency
*CV:* Palpitations, bradycardia, change in B/P, orthostatic hypotension, **cardiac arrest**

*EENT:* Tinnitus, blurred vision, miosis (high doses), diplopia
*GI: Nausea, vomiting, anorexia, constipation, cramps,* abdominal pain, dyspepsia, xerostomia, bitter taste
*GU:* Increased urinary output, dysuria, urinary retention, urgency
*INTEG: Rash,* urticaria, bruising, flushing, *diaphoresis,* pruritus
*RESP:* **Respiratory depression,** pulmonary edema

**Contraindications:** Hypersensitivity, addiction (opioid)

**Precautions:** Pregnancy C, breastfeeding, addictive personality, increased ICP, MI (acute), severe heart disease, respiratory depression, renal/hepatic disease, bowel impaction

### Pharmacokinetics
| | |
|---|---|
| **Absorption** | Well absorbed (SUBCUT, IM); completely absorbed (**IV**) |
| **Distribution** | Crosses placenta |
| **Metabolism** | Liver, extensively |
| **Excretion** | Feces, kidneys, unchanged (small amounts); breast milk |
| **Half-life** | 3-6 hr |

### Pharmacodynamics
| | IM | SUBCUT | IV |
|---|---|---|---|
| **Onset** | Up to 15 min | Up to 15 min | Rapid |
| **Peak** | 1 hr | Unknown | ½ hr |
| **Duration** | 3-6 hr | 3-6 hr | 3-6 hr |

### Interactions
*Individual drugs*
Alcohol: increased respiratory depression, hypotension, sedation
*Drug classifications*
Antipsychotics, CNS depressants, sedative/hypnotics, skeletal muscle relaxants: increased respiratory depression, hypotension
MAOIs: avoid use, results are unpredictable
Opiates: increased effects with other CNS depressants
*Drug/herb*
Chamomile, gotu kola, hops, Jamaican dogwood, kava, lavender, mistletoe, nettle, pokeweed, poppy, senega, skullcap, St. John's wort, valerian: increased CNS depression
Corkwood: increased anticholinergic effect
*Drug/lab test*
Increased: amylase

---

## NURSING CONSIDERATIONS
### Assessment
- Assess pain characteristics (location, intensity, type) before medication administration and after treatment
- Monitor VS after parenteral route; note muscle rigidity, product history, liver, kidney function tests; respiratory dysfunction: respiratory depression, character, rate, rhythm; notify prescriber if respirations are <10/min
- Monitor CNS changes: dizziness, drowsiness, hallucinations, euphoria, LOC, pupil reaction
- Monitor allergic reactions: rash, urticaria

### Nursing diagnoses
- Breathing pattern, ineffective (adverse reactions)
- Knowledge, deficient (teaching)
- Pain, acute (uses)
- Sensory perception, disturbed: visual, auditory (adverse reactions)

### Implementation
- Give by inj (IM, **IV**), only with resuscitative equipment available; give slowly to prevent rigidity
- Store in light-resistant area at room temperature
**IM route**
- Give inj deeply in large muscle mass; rotate inj sites
**IV route**
- Give direct **IV** undiluted 10 mg or less over 3-5 min or more
*Syringe compatibilities:* Atropine, cimetidine, diphenhydrAMINE, droperidol, glycopyrrolate, hydrOXYzine, lidocaine, midazolam, prochlorperazine, promethazine, ranitidine, scopolamine, trimethobenzamide
*Syringe incompatibilities:* Diazepam, pentobarbital
*Y-site compatibilities:* Amifostine, aztreonam, cefmetazole, cladribine, filgrastim, fludarabine, granisetron, melphalan, paclitaxel, propofol, teniposide, thiotepa, vinorelbine
*Y-site incompatibilities:* Nafcillin, sargramostim

### Patient/family education
- Instruct patient to report any symptoms of CNS changes, allergic reactions
- Caution patients to avoid CNS depressants: alcohol, sedative/hypnotics for at least 24 hr after taking this product
- Discuss with patient that dizziness, drowsiness, confusion are common; to avoid getting up without assistance
- Discuss in detail all aspects of the product: reason for taking product and expected results

- Instruct patient to change position slowly to prevent orthostatic hypotension
- Teach patient to turn, cough, deep breathe after surgery to prevent atelectasis

### Evaluation
**Positive therapeutic outcome**
- Relief of pain

**Treatment of overdose:** Naloxone (Narcan) 0.2-0.8 **IV**, $O_2$, **IV** fluids, vasopressors

## naloxone (Rx)
(nal-oks'one)
naloxone HCl, Narcan
*Func. class.:* Opioid antagonist, antidote
*Chem. class.:* Thebaine derivative
**Pregnancy category  C**

**Do not confuse:**
Narcan/Norcuron

**Action:** Competes with opioids at opioid receptor sites

**Therapeutic outcome:** Absence of opioid overdose

**Uses:** Respiratory depression induced by opioids, pentazocine, propoxyphene; refractory circulatory shock, asphyxia neonatorum, coma, hypotension

**Unlabeled uses:** IBS, opiate agonist dependence, opiate agonist-induced constipation, pruritus

**Dosage and routes**
*Opioid-induced respiratory depression*
*Adult:* **IV**/SUBCUT/IM 0.4-2 mg; repeat q2-3 min if needed, max 10 mg
*Child:* **IV**/SUBCUT/IM 0.01 mg/kg slowly followed by 0.1 mg/kg if needed or as an inf titrated to response

*Postoperative opioid-induced respiratory depression*
*Adult:* **IV** 0.1-0.2 mg q2-3 min prn
*Child:* **IV**/IM/SUBCUT 0.01 mg/kg q2-3 min prn

*Opioid overdose*
*Adult:* **IV**/SUBCUT/IM 0.4 mg (10 mcg/kg) (not opioid dependent) may repeat q2-3 min; 0.1-0.2 mg q2-3 min (opioid dependent)
*Child:* **IV**/SUBCUT/IM 10 mcg (0.01 mg/kg) q2-3 min

**Available forms:** Inj 0.02, 0.4 mg/ml

N

## Adverse effects

*CNS:* Drowsiness, nervousness

*CV:* Rapid pulse, **ventricular tachycardia, fibrillation,** increased systolic B/P (high doses), hypo/hypertension

*GI:* Nausea, vomiting, **hepatotoxicity**

*RESP:* Hyperpnea, pulmonary edema

**Contraindications:** Hypersensitivity

**Precautions:** Pregnancy **C**, breastfeeding, neonates, children, CV disease, opioid dependency, seizure disorder, drug dependency

### Pharmacokinetics

| | |
|---|---|
| **Absorption** | Well absorbed (SUBCUT, IM); completely absorbed (**IV**) |
| **Distribution** | Rapidly distributed; crosses placenta |
| **Metabolism** | Liver |
| **Excretion** | Kidneys |
| **Half-life** | 1 hr; up to 3 hr (neonates) |

### Pharmacodynamics

| | IV | IM/SUBCUT |
|---|---|---|
| **Onset** | 1 min | 2-5 min |
| **Peak** | Unknown | Unknown |
| **Duration** | 45 min | 45-60 min |

## Interactions
### Drug classifications
Analgesics (opioids): decreased effects of opioid analgesics
### Drug/lab test
Interference: urine VMA, 5-HIAA, urine glucose

## NURSING CONSIDERATIONS
### Assessment
• Assess for signs of opioid withdrawal in drug-dependent individuals: cramping, hypertension, anxiety, vomiting; may occur up to 2 hr after administration
• Monitor VS q3-5 min; ABGs including $Po_2$, $Pco_2$
• Assess cardiac status: tachycardia, hypertension; monitor ECG
• Assess for pain: duration, intensity, location before and after administration; may be used for respiratory depression
• Assess for respiratory dysfunction: respiratory depression, character, rate, rhythm; if respirations are <10/min, probably due to opioid overdose, administer naloxone; monitor LOC

### Nursing diagnoses
• Breathing pattern, ineffective (uses)
• Coping, ineffective (uses)
• Knowledge, deficient (teaching)
• Pain, acute (adverse reactions)

## Implementation
### IV route
• Give by direct **IV** undiluted; give 0.4 mg or less over 15 sec or titrate inf to response
• Give cont inf **IV** further diluted with 0.9% NaCl and $D_5$ and give as an inf
• Give only with resuscitative equipment, $O_2$ nearby
• Use only sol prepared within 24 hr
• Store at room temperature in darkness

*Syringe compatibilities:* Benzquinamide, heparin

*Y-site compatibilities:* Propofol

*Additive compatibilities:* Verapamil

### Patient/family education
• Explain reason for and expected results of medication when patient alert

### Evaluation
#### Positive therapeutic outcome
• Reversal of respiratory depression
• LOC: alert

---

## nandrolone (Rx)
(nan'droe-lone)
Deca-Durabolin, Hybolin Decanoate, Kabolin

*Func. class.:* Androgenic anabolic steroid, antianemic

*Chem. class.:* Halogenated testosterone derivative

**Pregnancy category X**

**Controlled substance schedule III**

**Action:** May stimulate bone marrow development, stimulates erythropoietin production

**Therapeutic outcome:** Increased Hgb, RBCs

**Uses:** Anemia associated with renal disease

### Dosage and routes
*Adult and child ≥14 yr:* IM (women) 50-100 mg q1-4 wk; (men) 100-200 mg q1-4 wk

*Child 2-13 yr:* IM 25-50 mg q3-4 wk

**Available forms:** Inj 50, 100, 200 mg/ml

### Adverse effects

*CNS:* Dizziness, headache, fatigue, tremors, paresthesias, flushing, sweating, anxiety, lability, insomnia, carpal tunnel syndrome, chills, depression

*CV:* Increased B/P, edema

*EENT:* Conjunctival edema, nasal congestion

*ENDO:* Abnormal GTT, *virilism (women, prepubescent boys)*

---

 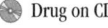

*GI:* Nausea, vomiting, constipation, weight gain, **cholestatic jaundice,** diarrhea
*GU:* **Hematuria,** amenorrhea, vaginitis, decreased libido, decreased breast size, clitoral hypertrophy, testicular atrophy, priapism, voice change
*INTEG:* Rash, acneiform lesions, oily hair/skin, flushing, sweating, acne vulgaris, alopecia, hirsutism
*MISC:* Hypercalcemia, chills, blood coagulation disorder, electrolyte imbalances
*MS:* Cramps, spasms

**Contraindications:** Pregnancy **X,** breastfeeding, males with cancer of breast, severe cardiac/renal/hepatic disease, hypersensitivity, abnormal genital bleeding, prostate

**Precautions:** Diabetes mellitus, CV disease, MI

| Pharmacokinetics | |
|---|---|
| **Absorption** | Well |
| **Distribution** | Unknown |
| **Metabolism** | Unknown |
| **Excretion** | Unknown |
| **Half-life** | Unknown |

| Pharmacodynamics | |
|---|---|
| **Onset** | Unknown |
| **Peak** | Up to 6 days |
| **Duration** | Unknown |

### Interactions
*Drug classifications*
Anticoagulants, NSAIDs, salicylates: increased bleeding risk
Hepatotoxics: increased hepatotoxicity
*Drug/lab test*
Increased: serum cholesterol, blood glucose, urine glucose
Decreased: serum calcium, serum potassium, $T_4$, $T_3$, thyroid $^{131}I$ uptake test, urine 17-OHCS, 17-KS

### NURSING CONSIDERATIONS
**Assessment**
• Assess for anemia symptoms: dyspnea, fatigue, weakness, pallor
• Monitor weight daily; notify prescriber if weekly weight gain is >5 lb
• Monitor B/P q4hr
• Monitor I/O ratio; be alert for decreasing urinary output, increasing edema
• Assess growth rate in children, since growth rate may be uneven (linear/bone growth) with extended use
• Monitor electrolytes: K, Na, Cl, Ca; cholesterol

• Monitor blood studies: CBC, Hct, Hgb, lipid panel
• Monitor liver function tests: ALT, AST, bilirubin
• Assess edema, hypertension, cardiac symptoms, jaundice
• Assess mental status: affect, mood, behavioral changes, aggression
• Assess signs of masculinization in female: increased libido, deepening of voice, decreased breast tissue, enlarged clitoris, menstrual irregularities; male: gynecomastia, impotence, testicular atrophy
• Assess hypercalcemia: lethargy, polyuria, polydipsia, nausea, vomiting, constipation, product may have to be decreased
• Assess for hypoglycemia in diabetics, since oral antidiabetic is increased

**Nursing diagnoses**
• Knowledge, deficient (teaching)

**Implementation**
• Give titrated dose; use lowest effective dose
• Inject deeply, use large muscle mass

**Patient/family education**
• Teach patient that product must be combined with complete health plan: diet, rest, exercise
• Teach patient to notify prescriber if therapeutic response decreases
• Teach patient not to discontinue abruptly
• Teach patient about changes in sex characteristics
• Teach patient that females should report menstrual irregularities
• Teach patient to increase calories, protein; decrease sodium if edema occurs

**Evaluation**
**Positive therapeutic outcome**
• Increased appetite, increased stamina

**naphazoline nasal**
*See Appendix D*

**naphazoline ophthalmic**
*See Appendix D*

N

Adverse effects: *italic* = common, **bold** = life-threatening

## naproxen (Rx, OTC)
(na-prox'en)
Apo-Naproxen ✤, EC-Naprosyn, Naprosyn, Naprosyn-E ✤, Naprosyn-SR ✤, Naxen ✤, Novo-Naprox ✤, Nu-Naprox ✤

## naproxen sodium (Rx, OTC)
Aleve, Anaprox, Anaprox DS, Apo-Napro-Na ✤, Midol Extended Relief, Naprelan, Novo-Naprox Sodium ✤, Novo-Naprox Sodium DS ✤, Synflex ✤, Synflex DS ✤
*Func. class.:* Nonsteroidal antiinflammatory, nonopioid analgesic
*Chem. class.:* Propionic acid derivative

**Pregnancy category**
B (1st trimester),
D (2nd/3rd trimesters)

**Action:** Inhibits prostaglandin synthesis by decreasing enzyme needed for biosynthesis; analgesic, antiinflammatory

**Therapeutic outcome:** Decreased pain, inflammation

**Uses:** Mild to moderate pain, osteoarthritis, rheumatoid arthritis, gouty arthritis, juvenile arthritis, primary dysmenorrhea

**Dosage and routes**
*Antiinflammatory/analgesic/antidysmenorrheal*
*Adult:* PO 250-500 mg bid, max 1.5 g/day; DEL REL TAB 375-500 mg bid
*Child >2 yr:* PO 5 mg/kg/day bid

*Antigout*
*Adult:* PO 750 mg, then 250 mg q8hr

*OTC use*
*Adult:* PO 200 mg q8-12hr or 400 mg, then 200 mg q12hr, max 600 mg/24 hr, taken no longer than 10 days

*Geriatric >65 yr:* PO max 200 mg q12hr

**Available forms:** Naproxen tabs: 250, 375, 500 mg; cont rel tabs (Naprelan) 375, 500 mg; del rel tabs (EC-Naprosyn, Naprosyn-E) 250✤, 375, 500 mg; oral susp 125 mg/5 ml; ext rel tabs (SR) 750 mg✤ naproxen sodium; tabs 250, 275, 375, 500 mg; supp (Naprosyn, Naxen) 500 mg✤

**Adverse effects**
*CNS:* Dizziness, drowsiness, fatigue, tremors, confusion, insomnia, anxiety, depression
*CV:* Tachycardia, peripheral edema, palpitations, **dysrhythmias, MI, stroke**
*EENT:* Tinnitus, hearing loss, blurred vision

*GI:* Nausea, anorexia, vomiting, diarrhea, jaundice, **cholestatic hepatitis,** constipation, flatulence, cramps, dry mouth, peptic ulcer, **GI ulceration, bleeding, perforation**
*GU:* **Nephrotoxicity: dysuria, hematuria,** oliguria, azotemia
*HEMA:* **Blood dyscrasias**
*INTEG:* Purpura, rash, pruritus, sweating
*SYST:* **Anaphylaxis**

**Contraindications:** Pregnancy **D** (2nd/3rd trimesters), hypersensitivity, asthma, severe renal/hepatic/ulcer disease, perioperative pain in CABG surgery

**Precautions:** Pregnancy **B** (1st trimester), breastfeeding, children <2 yr, geriatric, bleeding disorders, GI/cardiac disorders, hypersensitivity to other antiinflammatory agents, CCr <25 ml/min

### Pharmacokinetics
| | |
|---|---|
| **Absorption** | Completely absorbed |
| **Distribution** | Crosses placenta, 99% protein binding |
| **Metabolism** | Liver, extensively |
| **Excretion** | Breast milk |
| **Half-life** | 10-20 hr |

### Pharmacodynamics
| | |
|---|---|
| **Onset** | 1 hr |
| **Peak** | 2-4 hr |
| **Duration** | <7 hr |

**Interactions**
*Individual drugs*
Alcohol, aspirin: increased risk of GI side effects
Cefamandole, cefoperazone, cefotetan, clopidogrel, eptifibatide, plicamycin, ticlopidine, tirofiban, valproic acid: increased bleeding risk
Lithium: increased toxicity
Methotrexate: increased toxicity
Radiation: increased risk of hematologic toxicity
*Drug classifications*
ACE inhibitors: possible renal impairment
Anticoagulants, thrombolytics: increased risk of bleeding
Antihypertensives: decreased effect of antihypertensives
Antineoplastics: increased risk of hematologic toxicity
Corticosteroids, NSAIDs: increased risk of GI adverse reactions
Diuretics: decreased effectiveness of diuretics

*Drug/herb*

Anise, arnica, bogbean, chamomile, chondroitin, clove, dong quai, fenugreek, feverfew, garlic, ginger, ginkgo, ginseng *(Panax),* licorice: increased bleeding risk

Arginine, gossypol: increased gastric irritation

Bearberry, bilberry: increased NSAIDs effect

*Drug/lab test*

Increased: BUN, alkaline phosphatase

False: increased 5-HIAA, 17KS

## NURSING CONSIDERATIONS
### Assessment

• Monitor liver function, renal function, other blood tests: AST, ALT, bilirubin, creatinine, BUN, CBC, Hct, Hgb, protime, LDH, blood glucose, WBC, platelets; if patient is on long-term therapy

• Check I&O ratio; decreasing output may indicate renal failure (long-term therapy)

• Assess hepatotoxicity: dark urine, clay-colored stools, yellowing of the skin and sclera, itching, abdominal pain, fever, diarrhea if patient is on long-term therapy

• Assess for allergic reactions: rash, urticaria; if these occur, product may have to be discontinued

• Assess for ototoxicity: tinnitus, ringing, roaring in ears; audiometric testing needed before, after long-term therapy

• Assess for visual changes: blurring, halos; may indicate corneal, retinal damage

• Check for edema in feet, ankles, legs

• Identify prior product history; there are many product interactions

• Monitor pain: location, frequency, duration, characteristics, type, intensity before dose and 1 hour after; assess ROM before dose and after

• Assess for asthma, aspirin hypersensitivity, or nasal polyps, increased risk of hypersensitivity

### Nursing diagnoses

• Injury, risk for (adverse reactions)
• Knowledge, deficient (teaching)
• Mobility, impaired physical (uses)
• Pain, acute (uses)
• Pain, chronic

### Implementation

• Administer to patient crushed or whole

• Give OTC for 10 days or less unless approved by prescriber

• Give with food or milk to decrease gastric symptoms; give ½ hr before or 2 hr after meals for better absorption

• Patient should take with 8 oz of water and sit upright for 30 min after dose to prevent ulceration

### Patient/family education

• Teach patient to report any symptoms of renal/hepatic toxicity, visual changes, ototoxicity, allergic reactions, bleeding (long-term therapy)

• Caution patient not to exceed recommended dosage; acute poisoning may result; to take as prescribed, do not double dose

• Advise patient to use sunscreen to prevent photosensitivity reactions

• Teach patient to read label on other OTC products; many contain other antiinflammatories; caution patient to avoid alcohol ingestion; GI bleeding may occur

• Inform patient that the therapeutic response takes 2 wk (arthritis)

• Teach patient to report tinnitus, confusion, diarrhea, sweating, hyperventilation, blurred vision, fever, joint aches, black stools, flulike symptoms

### Evaluation
### Positive therapeutic outcome

• Decreased pain
• Decreased inflammation
• Increased mobility

---

## naratriptan (Rx)
(nair'ah-trip-tan)
Amerge
*Func. class.:* Migraine agent
*Chem. class.:* 5-HT₁-like receptor agonist

### Pregnancy category C

**Action:** Binds selectively to the vascular $5\text{-HT}_1$ receptor subtype, exerts antimigraine effect; causes vasoconstriction in cranial arteries

**Therapeutic outcome:** Decreased intensity and incidence of migraines

**Uses:** Acute treatment of migraine with or without aura

### Dosage and routes
*Adult:* PO 1 or 2.5 mg with fluids, if headache returns, repeat once after 4 hr, max 5 mg/24 hr

*Renal/hepatic dose*
Max 2.5 mg/24 hr

**Available forms:** Tabs 1, 2.5 mg

### Adverse effects
*CNS:* Dizziness, sedation, fatigue
*CV:* Increased B/P, palpitations, **tachydysrhythmias, PR, QT$_C$ prolongation, ST/T wave changes, PVCs, atrial flutter, fibrillation, coronary vasospasm**

N

**EENT:** EENT infections, photophobia
**GI:** *Nausea, vomiting*
**MISC:** Temp change sensations, tightness, pressure sensations
**MS:** *Weakness, neck stiffness,* myalgia

**Contraindications:** Angina pectoris, history of MI, documented silent ischemia, ischemic heart disease, concurrent ergotamine-containing preparations, uncontrolled hypertension, hypersensitivity, severe renal disease (CCr <15 ml/min), severe hepatic disease (Child-Pugh grade C), CV syndromes, hemiplegic or basilar migraines

**Precautions:** Pregnancy **C,** breastfeeding, children, postmenopausal women, men >40 yr, geriatric, risk factors for CAD, hypercholesterolemia, obesity, diabetes, impaired renal/hepatic function, peripheral vascular disease

### Pharmacokinetics

| | |
|---|---|
| **Absorption** | Unknown |
| **Distribution** | 28%-31% protein binding |
| **Metabolism** | Liver (metabolite) |
| **Excretion** | Urine/feces |
| **Half-life** | 6 hr |

### Pharmacodynamics

| | |
|---|---|
| **Onset** | Unknown |
| **Peak** | 2-3 hr |
| **Duration** | Unknown |

### Interactions
*Individual drugs*
Sibutramine: increased naratriptan effect
*Drug classifications*
5-HT agonists, ergot derivatives: increased vasospastic effect
MAOIs: increased risk of adverse reactions, do not use together
Selective serotonin release inhibitors (fluoxetine, fluvoxamine, paroxetine, sertraline): increased weakness, hyperreflexia, incoordination
*Drug/herb*
Butterbur: increased effect
SAM-e, St. John's wort: increased serotonin syndrome

### NURSING CONSIDERATIONS
**Assessment**
• Assess for stress level, activity, recreation, coping mechanisms
• Assess neurologic status: LOC, blurred vision, nausea, tics preceding headache

### Nursing diagnoses
• Knowledge, deficient (teaching)
• Noncompliance (teaching)
• Pain, acute (uses)

### Implementation
• Do not use product if another 5-HT agonist or an ergot preparation has been used in past 24 hr
• Give with fluids as soon as symptoms appear, may take another dose after 4 hr; do not take >5 mg in any 24-hr period
• Provide a quiet, calm environment with decreased stimulation for noise, bright light, excessive talking

### Patient/family education
• Teach patient to report pain, tightness in chest, neck, throat, or jaw; notify prescriber immediately if sudden, severe abdominal pain occurs
• Teach patient to use contraception while taking product, to notify prescriber if pregnancy is planned or suspected

### Evaluation
**Positive therapeutic outcome**
• Absence of migraine headaches

## natalizumab (Rx)
(na-ta-liz'u-mab)
Tysabri
*Func. class.:* Biological response modifier, immunoglobulins, monoclonal antibody

**Pregnancy category** C

**Action:** Action not clearly understood; biologic response modifying properties mediated through specific receptors on cells, may be secondary of blockade of the interaction by inflammatory cells on vascular endothelial cells

**Therapeutic outcome:** Decreased symptoms of multiple sclerosis

**Uses:** Ambulatory patients with relapsing-remitting multiple sclerosis who have not responded to other treatment

**Unlabeled uses:** Crohn's disease

**Dosage and routes**
*Adult:* **IV** INF 300 mg q 4 wks, give over 1 hr, observe during and for 1 hr after inf

**Available forms:** Single-use vial, 300 mg/100 ml 0.9% NaCl

**Adverse effects**
*CNS: Headache, fatigue,* rigors, syncope, tremors, *depression,* **PML (progressive**

**multifocal leukoencephalopathy), suicidal ideation**
*CV:* Chest discomfort, hyper/hypotension
*GI: Abdominal discomfort,* abnormal liver function tests, gastroenteritis
*GU:* Amenorrhea, *UTI, irregular menses,* vaginitis, urinary frequency
*INTEG: Rash,* dermatitis, pruritus
*MS: Arthralgia*
*RESP: Lower respiratory tract infection*
*SYST:* **Anaphylaxis, angioedema**

**Contraindications:** Hypersensitivity, immunocompromised individuals (HIV, AIDS, leukemia, lymphoma, transplants), PML, murine (mouse) protein allergy

**Precautions:** Pregnancy **C,** breastfeeding, geriatric, chronic progressive multiple sclerosis, depression, mental disorders, diabetes, TB, active infections

Pharmacokinetics

| | |
|---|---|
| **Absorption** | Unknown |
| **Distribution** | Unknown |
| **Metabolism** | Unknown |
| **Excretion** | Unknown |
| **Half-life** | Approximately 11 days |

Pharmacodynamics

Unknown

**Interactions**
*Drug classifications*
Do not use with vaccines
Immunosupressants, antineoplastics, immunomodulators: increased infection

**NURSING CONSIDERATIONS**
**Assessment**
• Monitor blood, renal, hepatic tests: CBC, differential, platelet counts, BUN, creatinine, ALT, urinalysis, for hypersensitivity reactions
• Assess CNS symptoms: headache, fatigue, depression, rigors, tremors
• Assess GI status: abdominal discomfort
• Assess mental status: depression, depersonalization, suicidal thoughts, insomnia
• Assess for multiple sclerosis symptoms; this product should only be used in patients who have not responded to other treatments
◆ Assess for anaphylaxis: shortness of breath, hives; swelling, tightness in throat, chest pain; usually within 2 hr of infusion
• Monitor PML using gadolinium-enhanced MRI scan of the brain, possibly CSF for JC viral DNA

**Nursing diagnoses**
• Injury, risk for (uses, adverse reactions)
• Knowledge, deficient (teaching)
• Mobility, impaired physical (uses)

**Implementation**
• Give acetaminophen for fever, headache
• Give only after being enrolled in the TOUCH Prescribing Program
**Intermittent IV inf**
• Use only clear, colorless solution, without particulates
• Withdraw 15 ml from the vial using aseptic technique: inject conc. into 100 ml 0.9% NaCl; do not use other diluents; mix completely; do not shake; infuse immediately or refrigerate for up to 8 hr; warm to room temperature before using; flush with 0.9% NaCl before and after infusion; do not admix or use in same line with other agents
• Withhold product at first sign of PML
• Store solution in refrigerator; do not freeze or shake; protect from light; use within 8 hr of preparation

**Patient/family education**
• Provide patient or family member with written, detailed information about the product
• Teach female patients they may experience irregular menses, amenorrhea
• Advise patient to use sunscreen to prevent photosensitivity
• Instruct patient to notify prescriber if pregnancy is suspected
• Instruct patient to avoid breastfeeding while taking this product
• Instruct patient to notify prescriber of possible infection: sore throat, cough, increased temp

**Evaluation**
**Positive therapeutic outcome**
• Decreased symptoms of multiple sclerosis

N

**natamycin ophthalmic**
*See Appendix D*

**nebivolol**
Bystolic
*See Appendix A, Selected New Drugs*

## nedocromil (Rx)
(ned-o-kroe'mil)
Tilade
*Func. class.:* Antiasthmatic
*Chem. class.:* Mast cell stabilizer
**Pregnancy category B**

**Action:** Stabilizes the membrane of the sensitized mast cell, preventing release of chemical mediators after an antigen-IgE interaction

**Therapeutic outcome:** Reduced symptoms of asthma

**Uses:** Severe perennial bronchial asthma, exercise-induced bronchospasm (prevention), prevention of acute bronchospasm induced by environmental pollutants, mastocytosis, not for treatment of acute asthma attacks

**Dosage and routes**
*Adult and child >12 yr:* 2 INH 2-4 ×/day at regular intervals to provide 14 g/day

**Available forms:** Inh cap 20 mg; inh aerosol spray 800 mcg/spray, 14.2-g container, neb sol 10 mg/ml; nasal sol 40 mg/ml; nasal insufflation 10 mg/cartridge

**Adverse effects**
*CNS:* Headache, dizziness, neuritis, dysphonia
*EENT:* Throat irritation, cough, nasal congestion, burning eyes, rhinitis
*GI:* Nausea, vomiting, anorexia, dry mouth, bitter taste
*MISC:* Anaphylaxis

**Contraindications:** Hypersensitivity to this product or lactose, status asthmaticus

**Precautions:** Pregnancy **B,** breastfeeding, children

| Pharmacokinetics | |
|---|---|
| **Absorption** | Poorly, 3% |
| **Distribution** | Unknown |
| **Metabolism** | Not usually metabolized |
| **Excretion** | Small amounts in bile, urine unchanged |
| **Half-life** | 80 min |

| Pharmacodynamics | |
|---|---|
| **Onset** | Unknown |
| **Peak** | 15 min |
| **Duration** | 4-6 hr |

**Interactions**
*Drug/lab test*
Increased: liver function tests

## NURSING CONSIDERATIONS
**Assessment**
- Assess pulmonary function testing baseline (asthma)
- Assess respiratory status: respiratory rate, rhythm, characteristics, cough, wheezing, dyspnea

**Nursing diagnoses**
- Airway clearance, ineffective (uses)
- Knowledge, deficient (teaching)

**Implementation**
- Give by inh only with spacer device if needed
- Encourage patient to gargle, sip water to decrease irritation in throat

**Patient/family education**
- Instruct patient to clear mucus before using
- Teach patient proper inhalation technique: exhale; using inhaler, inhale deeply with head tipped back to open airway; remove, hold breath, exhale; use Halermatic or Spinhaler with Intal caps
- Inform patient that therapeutic effect may take up to 4 wk
- Teach patient that product is preventive only, not restorative

**Evaluation**
**Positive therapeutic outcome**
- Decrease in asthmatic symptoms

## nelarabine (Rx)
(nella-ra'ben)
Arranon
*Func. class.:* Antineoplastic
*Chem. class.:* Purine analog
**Pregnancy category D**

**Action:** Leukemic blasts allow for incorporation into DNA, thus interfering with cell replication leading to cell death

**Therapeutic outcome:** Decreased growth of malignant cells

**Uses:** T-cell lymphoblastic leukemia, T-cell lymphoblastic lymphoma post relapse or treatment failure with at least two chemotherapeutic agents

**Dosage and routes**
*Adult:* IV 1500 mg/m$^2$ over 2 hr on days 1, 3, 5 repeated q 21 days
*Child:* IV 650 mg/m$^2$ over 1 hr/day × 5 days, repeated q 21 days

**Available forms:** Sol for inj 5 mg/ml (50 ml)

### Adverse effects
*CNS:* Dizziness, *fatigue,* insomnia, rigors, **seizures,** peripheral neuropathy, **paralysis,** confusion, headache
*CV:* Edema
*GI: Nausea, vomiting, anorexia, diarrhea, stomatitis, constipation*
*HEMA:* **Neutropenia,** leukopenia, **thrombocytopenia,** anemia
*META:* Decreased potassium, calcium, magnesium, albumin, bilirubin, AST, ALT, hyperuricemia; increased glucose
*MS:* Myalgia, arthralgia, back pain, weakness
*RESP:* **Pleural effusion,** cough, dyspnea, wheezing, epistaxis

**Contraindications:** Pregnancy **D,** hypersensitivity, severe neurotoxicity

**Precautions:** Breastfeeding, children, geriatric, renal/hepatic disease, seizure disorder

#### Pharmacokinetics

| | |
|---|---|
| **Absorption** | Unknown |
| **Distribution** | Unknown |
| **Metabolism** | Liver |
| **Excretion** | Kidneys |
| **Half-life** | 30 min-3hr |

#### Pharmacodynamics
Unknown

### Interactions
*Drug classifications*
Anticoagulants, NSAIDs: increased bleeding risk
Vaccinations (live virus): do not use

### NURSING CONSIDERATIONS
**Assessment**
• Monitor CBC (RBC, Hct, Hgb), differential platelet count weekly; withhold products if WBC is <4000/mm$^3$, platelet count is <75,000/mm$^3$, or RBC, Hct, Hgb low; notify prescriber of these results
• Monitor renal function tests: BUN, serum uric acid, urine CCr, electrolytes before and during therapy
• Monitor temp; fever may indicate beginning infection; no rectal temps
• Monitor liver function tests before and during therapy: bilirubin, ALT, AST, alkaline phosphatase as needed or monthly
• Assess for bleeding: hematuria, heme-positive stools, bruising or petechiae, mucosa or orifices
• Assess for neurotoxicity: somnolence, confusion, seizures, ataxia, paresthesias, hypoesthesia, coma, status epilepticus, craniospinal demyelination; contact prescriber immediately
• Assess for dyspnea, crackles, unproductive cough, chest pain, tachypnea, fatigue, increased pulse, pallor, lethargy, personality changes
• Assess buccal cavity q8hr for dryness, sores or ulceration, white patches, oral pain, bleeding, dysphagia
• Assess for GI symptoms: frequency of stools, cramping; if severe diarrhea occurs, fluid and electrolytes may need to be given

**Nursing diagnoses**
• Injury, risk for (uses, adverse reactions)

**Implementation**
• Provide **IV** hydration, and allopurinol in risk of hyperuricemia
• Use procedures for proper handling/ disposal of anticancer products
• Provide for rinsing of mouth tid-qid with water, club soda; brushing of teeth bid-tid with soft brush or cotton-tipped applicators for stomatitis; use unwaxed dental floss
• Store at room temperature

**Patient/family education**
• Advise patient to avoid foods with citric acid, hot or rough texture if stomatitis is present; OTC products
• Advise patient to use contraception while taking this product
• Advise patient to avoid using while breast-feeding
• Teach patient to report signs of infection: increased temp, sore throat, flulike symptoms
• Teach patient to report signs of anemia: fatigue, headache, faintness, shortness of breath, irritability
• Teach patient to report bleeding; to avoid use of razors, commercial mouthwash
• Advise patient that seizures may occur; do not operate machinery or drive until effects are known
• Advise patient not to receive vaccinations while taking this product

**Evaluation**
**Positive therapeutic outcome**
• Decreased spread of malignancy

**N**

## nelfinavir (Rx)
(nell-fin'a-ver)
Viracept
*Func. class.:* Antiretroviral
*Chem. class.:* HIV protease inhibitor

**Pregnancy category B**

**Action:** Inhibits HIV-1 protease

**Therapeutic outcome:** Prevents maturation of the infectious virus

**Uses:** HIV-1 in combination with other antiretrovirals

### Dosage and routes
*HIV Infection*
*Adult and child >13 yr:* PO 750 mg tid or 1250 mg bid
*Child 2-13 yr:* PO 20-30 mg/kg tid, max 2500 mg/day

*Prevention of HIV infection after exposure*
*Adult:* PO 750 mg tid with two other antiretroviral agents × 4 wk

**Available forms:** Tabs 250, 625 mg; oral powder 50 mg/g/scoop

### Adverse effects
*CNS:* Headache, asthenia, poor concentration, **seizures, suicidal ideation**
*CV:* Bleeding
*ENDO:* Hypoglycemia, hyperlipidemia
*GI:* Diarrhea, nausea, anorexia, dyspepsia, *flatulence,* **hepatitis, pancreatitis**
*HEMA:* Anemia, leukopenia, **thrombocytopenia, Hgb abnormalities**
*INTEG:* Rash, dermatitis
*MS:* Pain, arthralgia, myalgia, myopathy
*OTHER:* **Hypoglycemia,** redistribution/accumulation of body fat

**Contraindications:** Hypersensitivity to protease inhibitors

**Precautions:** Pregnancy **B**, breastfeeding, hemophilia, PKU, renal/hepatic disease, pancreatitis, diabetes

| Pharmacokinetics | |
|---|---|
| **Absorption** | Unknown |
| **Distribution** | 98% protein binding |
| **Metabolism** | Liver (minimal) |
| **Excretion** | Feces/urine |
| **Half-life** | 3½-5 hr |

| Pharmacodynamics | |
|---|---|
| **Onset** | Unknown |
| **Peak** | 2-4 hr |
| **Duration** | Unknown |

### Interactions
*Individual drugs*
Amiodarone, lovastatin, midazolam, pimozide, quinidine, simvastatin, triazolam: increased serious dysrhythmias
Atorvastatin, azithromycin, cycloSPORINE, indinavir, rifabutin, saquinavir, sildenafil, sirolimus, tacrolimus: increased effect
Carbamazepine, nevirapine, phenobarbital, phenytoin, rifamycin: decreased nelfinavir levels
Delavirdine: increased protease inhibitor levels
Didanosine, methadone, phenytoin: decreased effect
Indinavir, ketoconazole, ritonavir: increased nelfinavir levels
*Drug classifications*
Contraceptives (oral): decreased effect
Ergots: increased serious dysrhythmias
HIV protease inhibitors: increased protease inhibitor levels
*Drug/herb*
St. John's wort: decreased antiretroviral effect
*Drug/food*
Increased: absorption with food
*Drug/lab test*
Increased: AST, ALT, alkaline phosphatase, total bilirubin, CPK, LDH

### NURSING CONSIDERATIONS
**Assessment**
• Assess signs of infection, anemia
• Monitor liver function tests: ALT, AST
• Monitor C&S before product therapy; product may be taken as soon as culture is performed; repeat C&S after treatment; determine the presence of other STDs
• Assess bowel pattern before, during treatment; if severe abdominal pain with bleeding occurs, product should be discontinued; monitor hydration
• Assess skin eruptions, rash, urticaria, itching
• Assess allergies before treatment, reaction of each medication; place allergies on chart
• Monitor viral load, $CD_4$ cell counts baseline and throughout treatment

**Nursing diagnoses**
• Infection, risk for (uses)
• Knowledge, deficient (teaching)

**Implementation**
• Administer with food
• Oral powder can be mixed with fluids, do not mix with juice or acidic fluids, stable mixed for 6 hr

---

🔷 Alert    🍁 Canada Only    🔵 Drug on CD      * "Tall Man" lettering (See Preface)

### Patient/family education
• Advise patient to take with meal or snack; if dose is missed, take as soon as remembered up to 1 hr before next dose; do not double dose
• Advise patient to avoid taking with other medications, unless directed by prescriber
• Teach patient that product does not cure, but manages symptoms, does not prevent transmission of HIV to others
• Teach patient to use nonhormonal form of contraception while taking this product

### Evaluation
**Positive therapeutic outcome**
• Decreasing symptoms of HIV
• Improving viral load and CD4 cell counts

---

### neomycin topical
*See Appendix D*

---

### neostigmine (Rx)
(nee-oh-stig′meen)
neostigmine, Prostigmin
*Func. class.:* Cholinergic stimulant; anticholinesterase
*Chem. class.:* Quaternary compound

**Pregnancy category** C

**Action:** Inhibits destruction of acetylcholine, which increases concentration at sites where acetylcholine is released; this facilitates transmission of impulses across the myoneural junction

**Therapeutic outcome:** Increased strength in myasthenia gravis, reversal of nondepolarizing muscular blockers

**Uses:** Diagnosis/treatment of myasthenia gravis, nondepolarizing neuromuscular blocker antagonist, bladder distention, postoperative ileus

### Dosage and routes
*Myasthenia gravis diagnosis*
*Adult:* IM 0.02 mg/kg as a single dose
*Child:* IM 0.04 mg/kg as a single dose

*Myasthenia gravis treatment*
*Adult:* PO 15 mg q3-4hr, may increase to 375 mg/day; IM/**IV** 0.5-2 mg q1-3hr up to 10 mg/day
*Child:* PO 2 mg/kg/day q3-4hr; IM/**IV**/SUBCUT 0.01-0.04 mg/kg q2-4hr

*Nondepolarizing neuromuscular blocker antagonist*
*Adult:* **IV** 0.5-2 mg slowly; may repeat if needed, max 5 mg (give 0.6-1.2 mg atropine several min before this product)
*Infant and child:* **IV** 0.025-0.1 mg/kg/dose (give atropine several min before this product)

*Abdominal distention/postoperative ileus*
*Adult:* IM/SUBCUT 0.25-1 mg (1 : 4000) q4-6hr depending on condition × 2-3 days

*Urinary retention treatment*
*Adult:* IM/SUBCUT 0.25-1 mg (1 : 4000) q4-6hr depending on condition × 2-3 days

*Renal dose*
*Adult:* PO/IM/**IV** CCr 10-50 ml/min 50% of dose; CCr <10 ml/min 25% of dose

**Available forms:** Tabs 15 mg; inj 1 : 1000, 1 : 2000, 1 : 4000

**Adverse effects**
*CNS:* Dizziness, headache, sweating, weakness, **seizures,** incoordination, **paralysis,** drowsiness, LOC
*CV:* Tachycardia, **dysrhythmias,** bradycardia, hypotension, AV block, ECG changes, **cardiac arrest,** syncope
*EENT:* Miosis, blurred vision, lacrimation, visual changes
*GI: Nausea, diarrhea, vomiting, cramps,* increased peristalsis, salivary and gastric secretions
*GU:* Frequency, incontinence, urgency
*INTEG:* Rash, urticaria, flushing
*RESP:* **Respiratory depression, bronchospasm, constriction, laryngospasm, respiratory arrest, dyspnea**

**Contraindications:** Obstruction of intestine, renal system, bromide sensitivity, peritonitis, urinary tract obstruction, ileus

**Precautions:** Pregnancy **C,** breastfeeding, children, bradycardia, hypotension, seizure disorders, bronchial asthma, coronary occlusion, hyperthyroidism, dysrhythmias, peptic ulcer, megacolon, poor GI motility

| Pharmacokinetics | |
|---|---|
| **Absorption** | Poorly absorbed (PO), completely absorbed (**IV**) |
| **Distribution** | Unknown |
| **Metabolism** | Liver |
| **Excretion** | Kidneys |
| **Half-life** | 40-90 min |

N

### Pharmacodynamics

|  | PO | IM | IV |
|---|---|---|---|
| **Onset** | 45-75 min | 10-30 min | 4-8 min |
| **Peak** | Unknown | 30 min | 30 min |
| **Duration** | 2½-4 hr | 2½-4 hr | 2-4 hr |

### Interactions
*Individual drugs*
Atropine, disopyramide, haloperidol, quinidine: decreased neostigmine action
Decamethonium, succinylcholine: increased action of each specific product
Digoxin: increased bradycardia
*Drug classifications*
Aminoglycosides, anticholinergics, antidepressants, antihistamines, corticosteroids, local general anesthetics, phenothiazines: decreased neostigmine action
β-blockers, calcium channel blockers: increased bradycardia
*Drug/herb*
Pill bearing spurge: increased effect

### NURSING CONSIDERATIONS
Assessment
• Monitor VS, respiration during rest
◆ Monitor for bradycardia, hypotension, bronchospasm, headache, dizziness, seizures, respiratory depression; product should be discontinued if toxicity occurs

Nursing diagnoses
• Breathing pattern, ineffective (uses)
• Knowledge, deficient (teaching)

Implementation
**PO route**
• Give only after all other cholinergics have been discontinued
• Increased dosage as ordered may be needed if tolerance develops
• Give larger doses as ordered after exercise or fatigue
• Administer on empty stomach for better absorption
• Store at room temperature
**IV route**
• Give direct **IV** undiluted, through Y-tube or 3-way stopcock; give 0.5 mg or less over 1 min
• Give only with atropine sulfate available for cholinergic crisis
*Syringe compatibilities:* Glycopyrrolate, heparin, pentobarbital, thiopental
*Y-site compatibilities:* Heparin, hydrocortisone sodium succinate, potassium chloride, vit B/C
*Additive compatibilities:* Netilmicin

### Patient/family education
• Teach patient to carry/wear emergency ID specifying myasthenia gravis, products taken, prescriber's phone number

### Evaluation
**Positive therapeutic outcome**
• Increased muscle strength, hand grasp
• Improved gait
• Absence of labored breathing (if severe)

**Treatment of overdose:** Respiratory support, **IV** atropine 1-4 mg

---

### nepafenac ophthalmic
*See Appendix D*

---

### ! HIGH ALERT

### nesiritide (Rx)
(nes-eer'ih-tide)
Natrecor
*Func. class.:* Vasodilator
*Chem. class.:* Human B-type natriuretic peptide

**Pregnancy category** C

**Action:** Uses DNA technology; human B-type natriuretic peptide binds to the receptor in vascular smooth muscle and endothelial cells, leading to smooth muscle relaxation

**Therapeutic outcome:** Improvement in symptoms of CHF

**Uses:** Acutely decompensated CHF

**Dosage and routes**
*Adult:* BOL **IV** 2 mcg/kg, then CONT **IV** INF 0.01 mcg/kg/min

**Available forms:** Powder for inj, 1.5 mg single-use vial

**Adverse effects**
*CNS:* Headache, insomnia, dizziness, anxiety, confusion, paresthesia, tremor
*CV: Hypotension,* **tachycardia,** dysrhythmias, bradycardia, ventricular tachycardia, ventricular extrasystoles, **atrial fibrillation**
*GI:* Vomiting, nausea
*INTEG:* Rash, sweating, pruritus, inj site reaction
*MISC:* Back pain, abdominal pain
*RESP:* Increased cough, hemoptysis, **apnea**

**Contraindications:** Hypersensitivity, cardiogenic shock or B/P <90 mm Hg as primary therapy

---

 Alert       Canada Only       Drug on CD      * "Tall Man" lettering (See Preface)

**Precautions:** Pregnancy **C**, breastfeeding, children, mitral stenosis; significant valvular stenosis, restriction, or obstructive cardiomyopathy, or any condition that depends on venous return; renal disease, constrictive pericarditis

### Pharmacokinetics

| | |
|---|---|
| **Absorption** | Vascular smooth muscle and endothelial cells |
| **Distribution** | Unknown |
| **Metabolism** | Unknown |
| **Excretion** | Bound to cell surfaces, internalized, and proteolyzed; cleaved by endopeptidases on vascular lumenal surface; renal filtration |
| **Half-life** | 18 min |

### Pharmacodynamics

| | |
|---|---|
| **Onset** | 15 min |
| **Peak** | 1 hr |
| **Duration** | Unknown |

### Interactions
*Drug classifications*
ACE inhibitors: increased symptomatic hypotension

### NURSING CONSIDERATIONS
**Assessment**
• Assess PCWP, RAP, cardiac index, MPAP
• Assess B/P, pulse during treatment until stable

**Nursing diagnoses**
• Knowledge, deficient (teaching)
• Tissue perfusion, ineffective (uses)

**Implementation**
**IV route**
• Do not administer nesiritide through a central heparin-coated catheter; heparin should be administered through a separate catheter
• Prime **IV** fluid with inf of 25 ml before connecting to patient's vascular access port and before bolus dose or **IV** inf
• Reconstitute one 1.5 mg vial/5 ml of diluent from prefilled 250 ml plastic **IV** bag with diluent of choice (D₅, 0.9% NaCl, D₅/0.9% NaCl, D₅/0.2% NaCl); do not shake vial, roll gently; use only clear sol
• Withdraw all contents of reconstituted vial and add to the 250-ml plastic **IV** bag (6 mcg/ml); invert bag several times
• Use within 24 hr of reconstituting

**Patient/family education**
• Explain purpose of medication and expected results

### Evaluation
**Positive therapeutic outcome**
• Improvement in CHF with improved PCWP, RAP, MPAP

---

## nevirapine (Rx)
(ne-veer′a-peen)
Viramune
*Func. class.:* Antiretroviral
*Chem. class.:* Non-nucleoside reverse transcriptase inhibitor (NNRTI)
**Pregnancy category B**

**Do not confuse:**
nevirapine/nelfinavir, Viramune/Viracept

**Action:** Binds directly to reverse transcriptase and blocks RNA, DNA causing a disruption of the enzyme's site

**Therapeutic outcome:** Improvement of HIV-1 infection

**Uses:** HIV-1 in combination with other highly active antiretroviral treatments (HAART)

**Dosage and routes**
*Adult:* PO 200 mg/day × 2 wk, then 200 mg bid in combination
*Child ≥8 yr:* PO 4 mg/kg/day × 2 wk, then 4 mg/kg bid, max 200 mg bid
*Child 2 mo-8 yr:* PO 4 mg/kg/day × 2 wk, then 7 mg/kg bid

*Perinatal transmission prophylaxis*
*Females with no previous*
*antiretroviral therapy:* PO 200 mg as a single dose at onset of labor with zidovudine 2 mg/kg over 1 hr followed by zidovudine 1 mg/kg/hr until delivery
*Neonate:* PO Nevirapine 2 mg/kg as a single dose at age 48-72 hr and PO zidovudine 2 mg/kg q6hr for 6 wk

**Available forms:** Tabs 200 mg; oral susp 50 mg/5 ml

**Adverse effects**
*CNS: Paresthesia, headache, fever, peripheral neuropathy*
*GI: Diarrhea,* abdominal pain, *nausea, stomatitis,* hepatitis, **hepatotoxicity**
*HEMA:* **Neutropenia, anemia, thrombocytopenia**
*INTEG: Rash,* **toxic epidermal necrolysis**
*MISC:* **Stevens-Johnson syndrome**
*MS:* Pain, myalgia

**Contraindications:** Hypersensitivity

**Precautions:** Pregnancy **B**, breastfeeding, children, renal/hepatic disease

---

Adverse effects: *italic* = common, **bold** = life-threatening

### Pharmacokinetics

| | |
|---|---|
| **Absorption** | Rapid |
| **Distribution** | 60% bound to plasma proteins |
| **Metabolism** | Liver, by hepatic P450 enzyme system |
| **Excretion** | 91% urine |
| **Half-life** | 25-30 hr |

### Pharmacodynamics

| | |
|---|---|
| **Onset** | Unknown |
| **Peak** | 4 hr |
| **Duration** | Unknown |

### Interactions
#### *Individual drugs*
Cimetidine: increased nevirapine levels
Clonazepam, diazepam, warfarin: decreased nevirapine level
Itraconazole, ketoconazole: decreased effect of ketoconazole
Methadone: decreased effect of methadone
#### *Drug classifications*
Anticonvulsants, rifamycins: decreased nevirapine levels
Antiinfectives, macrolides: increased nevirapine levels
Oral contraceptives, protease inhibitors: decreased action
#### *Drug/herb*
St. John's wort: decreased nevirapine levels, do not use together
#### *Drug/lab test*
Increased: ALT, AST, GGT, bilirubin, Hgb
Decreased: neutrophil count

### NURSING CONSIDERATIONS
#### Assessment
- Assess signs of infection, anemia
- Assess liver, renal, blood tests: ALT, AST, viral load, CD4, glucose levels in diabetic patients; if liver function tests are elevated significantly, product should be withheld
- Assess C&S before product therapy; product may be taken as soon as culture is performed; repeat C&S after treatment; determine the presence of other sexually transmitted disease
- Assess bowel pattern before, during treatment; if severe abdominal pain with bleeding occurs, product should be discontinued; monitor hydration
- ◆ Assess skin eruptions; rash, urticaria, itching; if rash is severe or systemic symptoms occur, discontinue immediately
- Assess allergies before treatment, reaction to each medication

### Nursing diagnoses
- Diarrhea (side effects)
- Infection, risk for (uses)
- Knowledge, deficient (teaching)

### Implementation
- Give without regard to meals
- Give at equal intervals around the clock to maintain blood levels

### Patient/family education
- Instruct patient to report any right quadrant pain, jaundice, rash immediately
- Inform patient that product may be taken with food, antacids, didanosine
- Advise patient to take as prescribed; if dose is missed, take as soon as remembered up to 1 hr before next dose; do not double dose
- Advise patient that product must be taken in equal intervals around the clock to maintain blood levels for duration of therapy
- Advise patient that product is not a cure, controls symptoms of HIV
- Instruct patient to avoid OTC agents unless approved by prescriber
- Advise patient to use a nonhormonal form of contraception during treatment

### Evaluation
**Positive therapeutic outcome**
- Decreasing symptoms of HIV
- Improving viral load and CD4 cell counts

---

### niacin (Rx, OTC)
(nye′a-sin)
Edur-Acin, Nia-Bid, Niac, Niacels, Niacor, Niaspan, Nico-400, Nicobid, Nicolar, Nicotinex
### nicotinic acid (Rx, OTC)
(nick-oh-tin′ick)
Novo-Niacin ✿, Slo-Niacin, vitamin B
### niacinamide (Rx, OTC)
(nye-a-sin′a-mide)
### nicotinamide (Rx, OTC)
(nick-oh-tin′ah-mide)
*Func. class.:* Vitamin B₃
*Chem. class.:* Water-soluble vitamin, lipid-lowering product

**Pregnancy category** C

**Do not confuse:**
Nicobid/Nitro-Bid

**Action:** Needed for conversion of fats, protein, carbohydrates by oxidation-reduction; acts directly on vascular smooth muscle, causing vasodilatation; reduces LDL, VLDL,

---

total cholesterol, triglycerides, and lipoprotein A; increases HDL

**Therapeutic outcome:** Decreasing cholesterol and LDL levels, $B_3$ supplementation

**Uses:** Pellagra, hyperlipidemias (types IV, V), peripheral vascular disease, patients who present a risk for pancreatitis

### Dosage and routes
*Niacin deficiency*
*Adult:* PO 100-500 mg/day in divided doses; IM/SUBCUT 5-100 mg 5 or more times a day; **IV** 25-100 mg bid or tid
*Child:* PO Up to 300 mg/day in divided doses

*Adjunct in hyperlipidemia*
*Adult:* 250 mg after evening meal, may increase dose at 1-4 wk intervals to 1-2 g tid, max 6 g/day; EXT REL 500 mg at bedtime, ×4 wk, then 1000 mg at bedtime for wk 5-8, do not increase by more than 500 mg q4wk, max 2000 mg/day

*Pellagra*
*Adult:* PO 300-500 mg/day in divided doses
*Child:* PO 100-300 mg/day in divided doses

*Peripheral vascular disease*
*Adult:* PO 250-800 mg/day in divided doses

**Available forms:** Niacin: tabs 25, 50, 100, 250, 500, 1000 mg; time rel tabs 250, 500 mg; elixir 50 mg/5 ml; ext rel caps 250, 400 mg; sus rel tabs 500 mg; cont rel tabs 250, 500, 750 mg; sus rel cap 125, 500 mg; nicotinamide: tabs 100, 250, 500 mg

### Adverse effects
*CNS:* Paresthesias, headache, dizziness, anxiety
*CV:* Postural hypotension, vasovagal attacks, dysrhythmias, vasodilatation
*EENT:* Blurred vision, ptosis
*GI:* Nausea, vomiting, anorexia, *jaundice*, diarrhea, peptic ulcer, **hepatotoxicity**, dyspepsia
*GU:* Hyperuricemia, **glycosuria, hypoalbuminemia**
*INTEG:* Flushing, dry skin, rash, pruritus, itching, tingling

**Contraindications:** Breastfeeding, hypersensitivity, peptic ulcer, hepatic disease, hemorrhage, severe hypotension

**Precautions:** Pregnancy **C**, breastfeeding, glaucoma, CV disease, CAD, diabetes mellitus, gout, schizophrenia

### Pharmacokinetics

| | |
|---|---|
| **Absorption** | Well absorbed (PO) |
| **Distribution** | Widely distributed |
| **Metabolism** | Converted to niacinamide |
| **Excretion** | Urine, unchanged (30%); breast milk |
| **Half-life** | 45 min |

### Pharmacodynamics

| | PO | IV |
|---|---|---|
| **Onset** | Unknown | Unknown |
| **Peak** | 30-70 min | Unknown |
| **Duration** | Unknown | Unknown |

### Interactions
*Individual drugs*
Alcohol: increased flushing, pruritus, avoid use
*Drug classifications*
Ganglionic blockers: increased postural hypotension
HMG-CoA reductase inhibitors: increased myopathy, rhabdomyolysis
*Drug/lab test*
Increased: bilirubin, alkaline phosphatase, liver enzymes, LDH, uric acid, glucose
Decreased: cholesterol
False increase: urinary catecholamines
False positive: urine glucose

### NURSING CONSIDERATIONS
**Assessment**
• Assess for niacin deficiency (pellagra): nausea, vomiting, stomatitis, confusion, hallucinations before and throughout treatment
• Assess for symptoms of niacin deficiency: nausea, vomiting, anemia, poor memory, confusion, dermatitis
• Assess for lipid, triglyceride, cholesterol level, if using for hyperlipidemia
• Assess nutrition: fat, protein, carbohydrates, nutritional analysis should be completed by dietitian
• Monitor liver function tests: AST, ALT, bilirubin, uric acid, alkaline phosphatase; blood glucose before and during treatment; liver dysfunction: clay-colored stools, itching, dark urine, jaundice
• Monitor niacin levels during administration of this product
• Monitor cardiac status: rate, rhythm, quality; postural hypotension, dysrhythmias
• Monitor nutritional status: liver, yeast, legumes, organ meat, lean poultry; high-level niacin products should be included in the diet
• Assess for CNS symptoms: headache, paresthesias, blurred vision

N

Adverse effects: *italic* = common, **bold** = life-threatening

## Nursing diagnoses
• Knowledge, deficient (teaching)
• Noncompliance (teaching)
• Nutrition: less than body requirements, imbalanced (uses)

## Implementation
**PO route**
• Do not break, crush, or chew ext rel products
• Give with meals or milk for GI symptoms, and 81-325 mg of aspirin or NSAIDs ½ hr before dose to decrease flushing
**IV route**
• Give by direct **IV** after diluting to 2 mg/ml at a rate of ≤2 mg/min
• Give by inf by adding 500 ml of 0.9% NaCl at a rate of ≤2 mg/min
*Additive incompatibilities:* Acids (strong), alkalis, erythromycin, kanamycin, streptomycin
*Additive compatibilities:* TPN sol

## Patient/family education
• Advise patient that flushing and increase in feelings of warmth will occur several hr after taking product (PO); after 2 wk of therapy these side effects diminish
• Instruct patient to remain recumbent if postural hypotension occurs; to rise slowly from sitting or recumbent
• Caution patient to abstain from alcohol if product is prescribed for hyperlipidemia
• Caution patient to avoid sunlight if skin lesions are present
• Advise patient to report clay-colored stools, anorexia, jaundiced sclera, skin, dark urine; hepatotoxicity may occur

## Evaluation
**Positive therapeutic outcome**
• Decreased lipid levels
• Warm extremities
• Absence of numbness in extremities

---

## *niCARdipine (Rx)
(nye-card'i-peen)
Cardene, Cardene IV, Cardene SR
*Func. class.:* Calcium channel blocker, antianginal, antihypertensive
*Chem. class.:* Dihydropyridine
**Pregnancy category** C

## Do not confuse:
niCARdipine/NIFEdipine, Cardene/Cardizem, Cardene SR/Cardizem SR

**Action:** Inhibits calcium ion influx across cell membrane during cardiac depolarization, produces relaxation of coronary vascular smooth muscle and peripheral vascular smooth muscle, dilates coronary arteries, increases myocardial oxygen delivery in patients with vasospastic angina

**Therapeutic outcome:** Decreased angina pectoris, decreased B/P in hypertension

**Uses:** Chronic stable angina pectoris, hypertension

## Dosage and routes
*Hypertension*
*Adult:* PO 20 mg tid initially; may increase after 3 days (range 20-40 mg tid) or SUS REL 30 mg bid; may increase to 60 mg bid **IV** 5 mg/hr; may increase by 2.5 mg/hr q15 min, max 15 mg/hr

*Angina*
*Adult:* PO 20 mg tid, may be adjusted q3 days, may use 20-40 mg tid

*Renal dose*
*Adult:* PO 20 mg tid or SUS REL 30 mg bid

*Hepatic dose*
*Adult:* PO 20 mg bid

**Available forms:** Caps 20, 30 mg; sus rel caps 30, 45, 60 mg; inj 2.5 mg/ml

## Adverse effects
*CNS: Headache, dizziness,* anxiety, depression, confusion, paresthesia, somnolence, *flushing*
*CV:* Edema, bradycardia, hypotension, palpitations, **pulmonary edema,** chest pain, tachycardia, increased angina, **arrhythmias, CHF**
*GI:* Nausea, vomiting, gastric upset, constipation, **hepatitis,** abdominal cramps, dry mouth, sore throat
*GU:* Nocturia, polyuria, **acute renal failure**
*INTEG:* Rash, infusion site discomfort, **Stevens-Johnson syndrome**
*MISC:* Blurred vision, flushing, sweating, shortness of breath

**Contraindications:** Sick sinus syndrome, 2nd- or 3rd-degree heart block, hypersensitivity, advanced aortic stenosis

**Precautions:** Pregnancy **C,** breastfeeding, children, geriatric, CHF, hypotension, hepatic injury, renal disease

### Pharmacokinetics

| | |
|---|---|
| **Absorption** | Well absorbed (PO); bioavailability poor |
| **Distribution** | Unknown |
| **Metabolism** | Liver, extensively |
| **Excretion** | Kidneys 60%, feces 35% |
| **Half-life** | 2-5 hr |

---

 Alert     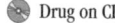 Canada Only     🐸 Drug on CD     * "Tall Man" lettering (See Preface)

| Pharmacodynamics | | |
|---|---|---|
| | PO | PO–SUS REL |
| **Onset** | ½ hr | Unknown |
| **Peak** | 1-2 hr | 2-6 hr |
| **Duration** | 8 hr | 10-12 hr |

### Interactions
*Individual drugs*

Alcohol: increased hypotension

Carbamazepine, cycloSPORINE, prazosin, propranolol, quinidine: increased risk of toxicity

Cimetidine: increased niCARdipine effects

Digoxin, quinidine, theophylline: increased effects

Rifampin: decreased antihypertensive effect

*Drug classifications*

Antihypertensives, neuromuscular blocking agents, nitrates: increased hypotension

NSAIDs: decreased antihypertensive effect

*Drug/herb*

Barberry, betel palm, burdock, goldenseal, khat, khella, lily of the valley, plantain: increased effect

Yohimbe: decreased effect

*Drug/food*

Grapefruit juice: increased hypotensive effect

### NURSING CONSIDERATIONS
**Assessment**

• Assess fluid volume status (I&O ratio) and record weight, color, quality and specific gravity of urine, skin turgor, adequacy of pulses, moist mucous membranes, bilateral lung sounds, peripheral pitting edema; dehydration symptoms of decreasing output, thirst, hypotension, dry mouth, and mucous membranes should be reported

• Monitor for CHF: weight gain, crackles, jugular venous distention, dyspnea

• Monitor B/P and pulse

• Assess anginal pain: intensity, location, duration, alleviating factors

• Monitor potassium, renal/liver function tests, periodically

**Nursing diagnoses**

• Cardiac output, decreased (uses)

• Knowledge, deficient (teaching)

**Implementation**

**PO route**

• Do not break, crush, chew, or open sus rel caps

• Give with or without regard to meals

• Store in airtight container at room temperature

**IV route**

• Dilute each 25 mg/240 ml of compatible sol (0.1 mg/ml), give slowly, stable for 24 hr at room temperature

*Solution compatibilities:* $D_5W$, $D_5$/0.45% NaCl, $D_5$/0.9% NaCl

*Y-site compatibilities:* Diltiazem, DOBUTamine, DOPamine, epINEPHrine, fentanyl, hydromorphone, labetalol, lorazepam, midazolam, milrinone, morphine, nitroglycerin, norepinephrine, ranitidine, vecuronium

**Patient/family education**

• Advise patient to avoid hazardous activities until stabilized on product and dizziness is no longer a problem

• Instruct patient to limit caffeine consumption; to avoid alcohol and OTC products unless directed by a prescriber

• Instruct patient to comply in all areas of medical regimen: diet, exercise, stress reduction, product therapy; to notify prescriber of irregular heart beat, shortness of breath, swelling of feet and hands, pronounced dizziness, constipation, nausea, hypotension

• Teach patient to use medication as directed even if feeling better; may be taken with other cardiovascular products (nitrates, β-blockers)

• Teach patient to take medication exactly as prescribed

• Advise patient to contact prescriber if anginal attacks continue or become worse

**Evaluation**

**Positive therapeutic outcome**

• Decreased angina attacks

• Decreased B/P

**Treatment of overdose:** Defibrillation, atropine for AV block, vasopressor for hypotension

### nicotinamide
*See niacin*

N

**nicotine** (OTC)
(nik′o-teen)
**nicotine chewing gum** (OTC)
Nicorette
**nicotine inhaler** (Rx)
Nicotrol Inhaler
**nicotine lozenge** (OTC)
Commit
**nicotine nasal spray** (Rx)
Nicotrol NS
**nicotine transdermal** (OTC)
Clear Nicoderm CQ, Habitrol, NicoDerm CQ, Nicotrol
*Func. class.:* Smoking deterrent
*Chem. class.:* Ganglionic cholinergic agonist

**Pregnancy category**
D (transdermal)
X (gum)

**Action:** Agonist at nicotinic receptors in the peripheral and central nervous systems; acts at sympathetic ganglia, on chemoreceptors of the aorta and carotid bodies; also affects adrenalin-releasing catecholamines

**Therapeutic outcome:** Decreased withdrawal effects when smoking cessation is attempted

**Uses:** Deter cigarette smoking

**Unlabeled uses:** Gilles de la Tourette's syndrome

**Dosage and routes**
*Habitrol, NicoDerm*
*Adult:* 21 mg/day × 4-8 wk; 14 mg/day × 2-4 wk; 7 mg/day × 2-4 wk

*Nicotine chewing gum*
*Adult:* If patient smokes <25 cigarettes/day, start with 2 mg gum; if >25 cigarettes/day, start with 4 mg gum; then 1 piece of gum q2-4hr × 2 wk, then 1 piece of gum q4-8hr × 2 wk, then discontinue; not to exceed 24/day

*Nicotine inhaler*
*Adult:* Inhale 6 cartridges/day for first 3-6 wk, max 16/day × 12 wk

*Nicotine lozenge*
*Adult:* If cigarette is desired >30 min after awakening, start with 1-2-mg lozenge; if <30 min after awakening, start with 4-mg lozenge; then 1 q1-2hr, max 20 lozenges/day or 5 lozenges/6 hr × 6 wk, then 1 lozenge q2-4hr × 2 wk, then 1 lozenge q4-8hr × 2 wk, then discontinue

*Nicotine nasal spray*
*Adult:* 1 spray in each nostril 1-2 ×/hr, max 5 ×/hr or 40 ×/day, max 3 mo

*Nicotrol*
*Adult:* 15 mg/day × 12 wk; 10 mg/day × 2 wk; 5 mg/day × 2 wk

*Nicotrol Inhaler*
*Adult:* Delivers 30% of what a smoker receives from an actual cigarette

*Gilles de la Tourette's Syndrome (unlabeled)*
*Adult and child:* Chewing gum 2 mg chewed × ½ hr bid × 1-6 mo; transdermal 7 or 10 mg patch daily × 2 days

**Available forms:** Gum: 2 mg/piece; nicotine transdermal system: (Habitrol, NicoDerm, Nicotine Transdermal System) 7, 14, 21 mg/day delivered; (NicoDerm) 5, 10, 15 mg/day; nicotine inhaler: 4 mg delivered; nasal spray: 0.5 mg of nicotine/actuation; lozenge: 2 mg, 4 mg

**Adverse effects**
*CNS:* Dizziness, vertigo, insomnia, headache, confusion, **seizures,** depression, euphoria, numbness, tinnitus, strange dreams
*CV:* **Dysrhythmias,** tachycardia, palpitations, edema, flushing, hypertension
*EENT:* Jaw ache, irritation in buccal cavity
*GI: Nausea, vomiting, anorexia, indigestion,* diarrhea, abdominal pain, constipation, eructation
*RESP:* Breathing difficulty, cough, hoarseness, sneezing, wheezing, bronchial spasm

**Contraindications:** Pregnancy **X** (gum), **D** (transdermal), hypersensitivity, immediate post-MI recovery period, severe angina pectoris

**Precautions:** Breastfeeding, vasospastic disease, dysrhythmias, diabetes mellitus, hyperthyroidism, pheochromocytoma, coronary disease, esophagitis, peptic ulcer, renal/hepatic disease

**Pharmacokinetics**

| | |
|---|---|
| **Absorption** | Slowly absorbed, buccal cavity |
| **Distribution** | Unknown |
| **Metabolism** | Liver; some by lungs, kidneys |
| **Excretion** | Kidneys, unchanged (20%); breast milk |
| **Half-life** | 1-2 hr |

**Pharmacodynamics**

| | |
|---|---|
| **Onset** | Rapid |
| **Peak** | ½ hr |
| **Duration** | Unknown |

 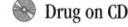

## Interactions
### Individual drugs
Acetaminophen, caffeine, furosemide, imipramine, oxazepam, pentazocine, propranolol: increased effects of each specific product with cessation of smoking

Glutethimide: decreased absorption

Insulin (SUBCUT): increased absorption

Propoxyphene: decreased propoxyphene metabolism

Theophylline: increased blood levels with cessation of smoking

### Drug/herb
Blue cohosh, lobelia: increased effect

Oats: decreased effect

## NURSING CONSIDERATIONS
### Assessment
• Assess for adverse reaction to gum: irritation of buccal cavity, dislike of taste, jaw ache

• Assess for withdrawal symptoms: headache, fatigue, drowsiness, restlessness, irritability, severe cravings for nicotine products before, during, and after treatment

• Obtain a nicotine assessment: brand of cigarettes, chewing tobacco, cigars, number of each used per day; what increases need or activities performed when each is used

• Gum should not be used if temporomandibular condition exists

• Assess for nicotine toxicity: GI symptoms (nausea, vomiting, diarrhea), cardiopulmonary symptoms (decreased B/P, dyspnea, change in pulse), weakness, abdominal cramping, headache, blurred vision, tinnitus; product should be discontinued

### Nursing diagnoses
• Coping, ineffective (uses)
• Knowledge, deficient (teaching)
• Noncompliance (teaching)

### Implementation
• Give only prescribed amount, or toxicity may occur

• Protect gum from light and heat

### Patient/family education
• Advise patient to begin product withdrawal after 3 mo use; do not exceed 6 mo

• Teach patient all aspects of product; give package insert to patient and explain; caution patient not to exceed prescribed dose

• Caution patient not to use during pregnancy; birth defects may occur

**Gum**
• Advise patient to chew gum slowly for 30 min to promote buccal absorption of the product; do not chew over 45 min

• Inform patient that gum will not stick to dentures, dental appliances

• Caution patient that gum is as toxic as cigarettes; it is to be used only to deter smoking

**Transdermal patch**
• Caution patient that patch is as toxic as cigarettes; to be used only to deter smoking

• Caution patient not to use during pregnancy; birth defects may occur

• Instruct patient to keep used and unused system out of reach of children and pets

• Instruct patient to apply once a day to a nonhairy, clean, dry area of skin on upper body or upper outer arm; to rotate sites to prevent skin irritation

• Instruct patient to stop smoking immediately when beginning patch treatment

• Teach patient to apply promptly after removing from protective pouch; system may lose strength

**Inhaler**
• Advise patient that puffing on mouthpiece delivers nicotine through the mouth lining

### Evaluation
**Positive therapeutic outcome**
• Decrease in urge to smoke
• Decreased need for gum after 3-6 mo

N

## *NIFEdipine (Rx)
(nye-fed′i-peen)
Adalat, Adalat CC, Apo-Nifed ✳, Novo-Nifedin ✳, Nu-Nifedin ✳, NIFEdipine, Procardia, Procardia XL
*Func. class.:* Calcium channel blocker, antianginal, antihypertensive
*Chem. class.:* Dihydropyridine
**Pregnancy category C**

**Do not confuse:**
NIFEdipine/niCARdipine

**Action:** Inhibits calcium ion influx across cell membrane during cardiac depolarization, produces relaxation of coronary vascular smooth muscle and peripheral vascular smooth muscle, dilates coronary vascular arteries, increases myocardial oxygen delivery in patients with vasospastic angina

**Therapeutic outcome:** Decreased angina pectoris, decreased B/P in hypertension

**Uses:** Chronic stable angina pectoris, vasospastic angina, hypertension

**Unlabeled uses:** Migraines, CHF, Raynaud's disease, anal fissures, preterm labor

## Dosage and routes
*Adult:* PO immediate release, 10 mg tid; increase in 10 mg increments q7-14 days, max 180 mg/24 hr or single dose of 30 mg; SUS REL, 30-60 mg/day; may increase q7-14 days; doses >120 mg not recommended
*Child:* PO 0.25-0.5 mg/kg/dose q4-6hr, max 1-2 mg/kg/day

**Available forms:** Caps 5 ♣, 10, 20 mg; ext rel tabs (CC, XL) 10 ♣, 20 ♣, 30, 60, 90 mg; tabs 10 mg ♣

## Adverse effects
*CNS: Headache,* fatigue, drowsiness, *dizziness,* anxiety, depression, weakness, insomnia, *light-headedness,* paresthesia, tinnitus, blurred vision, nervousness, tremor, flushing
*CV:* **Dysrhythmias,** edema, hypotension, palpitations, tachycardia
*GI: Nausea,* vomiting, diarrhea, gastric upset, constipation, increased liver function tests, dry mouth, flatulence, gingival hyperplasia, **hepatotoxicity**
*GU:* Nocturia, polyuria
*HEMA:* Bruising, bleeding, petechiae
*INTEG:* Rash, pruritus, *flushing,* hair loss
*MISC:* Sexual difficulties, cough, fever, chills
*SYST:* **Stevens-Johnson syndrome**

**Contraindications:** Hypersensitivity

**Precautions:** Pregnancy **C,** breastfeeding, children, CHF, hypotension, sick sinus syndrome, 2nd- or 3rd-degree heart block, hypotension less than 90 mm Hg systolic, hepatic injury, renal disease

### Pharmacokinetics

| | |
|---|---|
| **Absorption** | Well absorbed (PO) |
| **Distribution** | Unknown |
| **Metabolism** | Liver, extensively |
| **Excretion** | Unknown |
| **Half-life** | 2-5 hr |

### Pharmacodynamics

| | PO | PO–EXT REL |
|---|---|---|
| **Onset** | ½ hr | Unknown |
| **Peak** | Unknown | Unknown |
| **Duration** | 6-8 hr | 24 hr |

## Interactions
*Individual drugs*
Carbamazepine, cimetidine, cycloSPORINE, phenytoin, prazosin, ranitidine: increased risk of toxicity
Digoxin: increased digoxin levels
Quinidine: decreased effects
Smoking: decreased NIFEdipine level

*Drug classifications*
Antihypertensives, β-adrenergic blockers: increased effects
NSAIDs: decreased antihypertensive effect
*Drug/herb*
Barberry, betel palm, burdock, goldenseal, khat, khella, lily of the valley, plaintain: increased effect
Yohimbe: decreased effect
*Drug/food*
Grapefruit juice: increased NIFEdipine level
*Drug/lab test*
Positive: ANA titer, direct Coombs' test
Increased:
CPK, LDH, AST

## NURSING CONSIDERATIONS
### Assessment
• Assess anginal pain: location, intensity, duration, character, alleviating, aggravating factors
• Assess for bruising, petechiae, bleeding
• Monitor potassium, renal/liver function tests, periodically during treatment
• Assess fluid volume status (I&O ratio) and record weight, distended red veins, crackles in lung, color, quality and specific gravity of urine, skin turgor, adequacy of pulses, moist mucous membranes, bilateral lung sounds, peripheral pitting edema; dehydration symptoms of decreasing output, thirst, hypotension, dry mouth, and mucous membranes should be reported
• Monitor ALT, AST, bilirubin daily; if these are elevated, hepatotoxicity is suspected
• Monitor cardiac status: B/P, pulse, respirations, ECG

### Nursing diagnoses
• Cardiac output, decreased (uses)
• Knowledge, deficient (teaching)
• Pain, acute (uses)

### Implementation
**PO route**
• Give without regard to meals
• Store in airtight container at room temperature
**Sublingual route**
• Using a sterile needle puncture the cap and squeeze medication in buccal area (not an FDA-approved use)

### Patient/family education
• Advise patient to avoid hazardous activities until stabilized on product and dizziness is no longer a problem
• Instruct patient to limit caffeine consumption; to avoid alcohol and OTC products unless directed by prescriber

- Tell patient that ext rel tab has nonabsorbable shell, may appear in stools
- Instruct patient to comply in all areas of medical regimen: diet, exercise, stress reduction, product therapy; to notify prescriber of irregular heart beat, shortness of breath, swelling of feet and hands, pronounced dizziness, constipation, nausea, hypotension, severe rash
- Teach patient to use as directed even if feeling better; may be taken with other cardiovascular products (nitrates, β-blockers)
- Advise patient to increase fluid intake to prevent constipation
- Teach patient to check for gingival hyperplasia and report promptly
- Teach patient not to discontinue abruptly, gradually taper

### Evaluation
**Positive therapeutic outcome**
- Decreased angina attacks
- Decreased B/P

**Treatment of overdose:** Defibrillation, atropine for AV block, vasopressor for hypotension

## nilotinib
Tasigna
*See Appendix A, Selected New Drugs*

## nilutamide (Rx)
(nil-u'ta-mide)
Anandron ✤, Nilandron
*Func. class.:* Antineoplastic, hormone
*Chem. class.:* Antiandrogen

**Pregnancy category** C

**Action:** Interferes with testosterone uptake in the nucleus or testosterone activity in target tissues; arrests tumor growth in androgen-sensitive tissue, i.e., prostate gland, prostatic carcinoma is androgen-sensitive, so tumor growth is arrested

**Therapeutic outcome:** Decreased tumor size

**Uses:** Metastatic prostatic carcinoma, stage D2 in combination with surgical castration (only to be used by men)

### Dosage and routes
*Adult:* PO 300 mg/day × 30 days, then 150 mg/day

**Available forms:** Tabs 50, 100 ✤, 150 mg

### Adverse effects
*CNS:* Hot flashes, drowsiness, insomnia, dizziness, hyperthesia, depression
*CV:* **Heart failure,** hypertension
*EENT:* Delay in adaptation to dark
*GI:* Diarrhea, nausea, vomiting, elevated liver function tests, constipation, dyspepsia, **hepatotoxicity**
*GU:* Decreased libido, impotence, testicular atrophy, UTI, hematuria, nocturia, gynecomastia
*HEMA:* Anemia
*INTEG:* Rash, sweating, alopecia, dry skin
*MISC:* Edema
*RESP:* Dyspnea, URI, pneumonia, **interstitial pneumonitis**

**Contraindications:** Women, hypersensitivity, severe hepatic impairment, severe respiratory disease

**Precautions:** Pregnancy **C**

### Pharmacokinetics
| | |
|---|---|
| **Absorption** | Rapidly, completely |
| **Distribution** | Unknown |
| **Metabolism** | Unknown |
| **Excretion** | Urine, feces |
| **Half-life** | Unknown |

### Pharmacodynamics
Unknown

N

### Interactions
*Individual drugs*
Phenytoin, theophylline, vitamin K: increased toxicity

### NURSING CONSIDERATIONS
**Assessment**
- ◈ Monitor liver function tests: AST, ALT, alkaline phosphatase, which may be elevated; if elevated 3 × normal, discontinue product
- Monitor PSA, improvement in bone pain
- Monitor for CNS symptoms: drowsiness, insomnia, dizziness
- Monitor chest x-rays routinely, baseline pulmonary function tests, dyspnea, cough, may indicate interstitial pneumonitis, discontinue treatment if this condition is suspected
- Monitor for hyperglycemia, increased BUN, creatinine, alkaline phosphatase leukopenia

### Nursing diagnoses
- Infection, risk for (side effects)
- Knowledge, deficient (teaching)

### Implementation
- Administer without regard to meals
- Start therapy on day of or after surgery
- Store at room temperature

## Patient/family education
⚠ Advise patient to report side effects: decreased libido, impotence, breast enlargement, hot flashes, diarrhea, dyspnea, cough; symptoms of hepatotoxicity (dark urine, abdominal pain, clay-colored stools, jaundiced eyes, skin); notify prescriber immediately if shortness of breath occurs
• Advise patient to wear tinted lens to alleviate delay in adapting to the dark
• Advise patient that product is started on day of or day after surgical removal of testes
• Advise patient to avoid alcohol consumption

## Evaluation
**Positive therapeutic outcome**
• Decrease in prostatic tumor size, decrease in spread of cancer

**Treatment of overdose:** Induce vomiting, provide supportive care

---

## nimodipine (Rx)
(ni-moe′dip-een)
Nimotop
*Func. class.:* Calcium channel blocker
*Chem. class.:* Dihydropyridine

**Pregnancy category** C

**Action:** Unknown, may have greater effect on cerebral arteries

**Therapeutic outcome:** Prevention of vascular spasm (subarachnoid hemorrhage)

**Uses:** Prevention of cerebrovascular spasm in subarachnoid hemorrhage

## Dosage and routes
*Adult:* PO Begin therapy within 96 hr, 60 mg q4hr × 21 days

**Available forms:** Caps 30 mg

## Adverse effects
*CNS:* Headache, fatigue, drowsiness, dizziness, anxiety, depression, weakness, insomnia, confusion, paresthesia, somnolence
*CV:* Dysrhythmia, edema, CHF, bradycardia, hypotension, palpitations, **MI, pulmonary edema**
*GI:* Nausea, vomiting, diarrhea, gastric upset, constipation, **hepatitis,** abdominal cramps
*GU:* Nocturia, polyuria, **acute renal failure**
*INTEG:* Rash, pruritus, urticaria, photosensitivity, hair loss
*MISC:* Blurred vision, flushing, nasal congestion, sweating, shortness of breath, gynecomastia, hyperglycemia, sexual difficulties

**Contraindications:** Sick sinus syndrome, 2nd- or 3rd-degree heart block, hypotension less than 90 mm Hg systolic, hypersensitivity

**Precautions:** Pregnancy **C,** breastfeeding, children, geriatric, CHF, hypotension, hepatic injury, renal disease

### Pharmacokinetics
| | |
|---|---|
| **Absorption** | Well absorbed, bioavailability poor |
| **Distribution** | Crosses blood-brain barrier |
| **Metabolism** | Liver, extensively |
| **Excretion** | Kidneys |
| **Half-life** | 1-2 hr |

### Pharmacodynamics
| | |
|---|---|
| **Onset** | Unknown |
| **Peak** | 1 hr |
| **Duration** | Unknown |

## Interactions
*Individual drugs*
Alcohol: increased hypotension
Digoxin: increased digoxin levels, bradycardia
Phenobarbital, phenytoin: decreased effectiveness
Propranolol: increased toxicity
*Drug classifications*
Antihypertensives: increased hypotension
β-Adrenergic blockers: increased bradycardia
Nitrates: increased nitrates
*Drug/herb*
Barberry, betel palm, burdock, goldenseal, khat, khella, lily of the valley, plaintain: increased effect
Yohimbe: decreased effect

## NURSING CONSIDERATIONS
**Assessment**
• Assess fluid volume status (I&O ratio) and record weight; distended red veins; crackles in lung; color, quality, and specific gravity of urine; skin turgor; adequacy of pulses; moist mucous membranes; bilateral lung sounds; peripheral pitting edema; dehydration symptoms of decreasing output, thirst, hypotension, dry mouth and mucous membranes should be reported
• Monitor B/P and pulse; if B/P drops 30 mm Hg, call prescriber
• Monitor ALT, AST, bilirubin daily; if these are elevated, hepatotoxicity is suspected

**Nursing diagnoses**
• Injury, risk for (uses)
• Knowledge, deficient (teaching)

---

## Implementation
- May puncture cap and dilute in water and give through nasogastric tube; flush tube with 0.9% NaCl
- Store in airtight container at room temperature

## Evaluation
**Positive therapeutic outcome**
- Prevention of neurologic damage from subarachnoid hemorrhage

---

## nisoldipine (Rx)
(nye'sol-dye-peen)
Sular
*Func. class.:* Antihypertensive, calcium channel blocker
*Chem. class.:* Dihydropyridine
**Pregnancy category** C

**Action:** Inhibits calcium ion influx across cell membrane, resulting in dilation of peripheral arteries

**Therapeutic outcome:** Decreased B/P in hypertension

**Uses:** Essential hypertension, alone or with other antihypertensives

## Dosage and routes
*Adult:* PO 20 mg/day initially, may increase by 10 mg/wk, usual dose 20-40 mg/day, max 60 mg/day
*Geriatric/hepatic dose:* PO 10 mg/day, increase by 10 mg/wk

**Available forms:** Ext rel tabs 10, 20, 30, 40 mg

## Adverse effects
*CNS:* Headache, fatigue, drowsiness, dizziness, anxiety, depression, nervousness, insomnia, light-headedness, paresthesia, tinnitus, psychosis, somnolence, ataxia, confusion, malaise, migraine
*CV:* **Dysrhythmias,** edema, **CHF,** hypotension, palpitations, **MI, pulmonary edema,** tachycardia, syncope, AV block, angina, chest pain, ECG abnormalities
*GI:* Nausea, vomiting, diarrhea, gastric upset, constipation, elevated liver function tests, dry mouth, dyspepsia, dysphagia, flatulence
*GU:* Nocturia, hematuria, dysuria
*HEMA:* **Anemia, leukopenia,** petechiae
*INTEG:* Rash, pruritus
*MISC:* Sexual difficulties, gingival hyperplasia, chills, fever, gout, sweating, cough, nasal congestion, shortness of breath, wheezing, epistaxis, dyspnea

**Contraindications:** Hypersensitivity, sick sinus syndrome, 2nd- or 3rd-degree heart block, aortic stenosis

**Precautions:** Pregnancy **C,** breastfeeding, children, geriatric, CHF, hypotension <90 mm Hg systolic, hepatic injury, renal disease, acute MI, unstable angina, CAD

### Pharmacokinetics
| | |
|---|---|
| **Absorption** | Well absorbed |
| **Distribution** | Highly protein bound |
| **Metabolism** | Liver |
| **Excretion** | Kidneys |
| **Half-life** | Unknown |

### Pharmacodynamics
| | |
|---|---|
| **Onset** | Unknown |
| **Peak** | 6-12 hr |
| **Duration** | Unknown |

## Interactions
*Individual drugs*
Cimetidine, ranitidine: increased nisoldipine level
Digoxin: increased effects
*Drug classifications*
Antifungals (azole), CYP3A4 inhibitors: increased nisoldipine level
Antihypertensives: increased hypotension
β-Adrenergic blockers: increased effects
Hydantoins, CYP3A4 inducers: decreased nisoldipine effect
*Drug/herb*
Barberry, betel palm, burdock, goldenseal, khat, khella, lily of the valley, plaintain: increased effect
Yohimbe: decreased effect
*Drug/food*
Grapefruit juice: increased hypotension
High-fat foods: increased nisoldipine level

## NURSING CONSIDERATIONS
### Assessment
- Assess fluid volume status: I&O ratio and record; weight; skin turgor; adequacy of pulses; moist mucous membranes; bilateral lung sounds; peripheral pitting edema; dehydration symptoms of decreasing output, thirst, hypotension, dry mouth, and mucous membranes should be reported
- Monitor ALT, AST, bilirubin daily, if these are elevated and hepatotoxicity is suspected
- Monitor cardiac status: B/P, pulse, respiration, ECG

### Nursing diagnoses
- Cardiac output, decreased (uses)
- Knowledge, deficient (teaching)

Adverse effects: *italic* = common, **bold** = life-threatening

N

## Implementation
• Give once a day, with food to decrease GI symptoms, avoid high-fat foods, grapefruit

## Patient/family education
• Caution patient to avoid hazardous activities until stabilized on product and dizziness is no longer a problem
• Instruct patient to limit caffeine consumption; to avoid alcohol and OTC products unless directed by prescriber
• Urge patient to comply in all areas of medical regimen: diet, exercise, stress reduction, product therapy; to notify prescriber of irregular heart beat, shortness of breath, swelling of feet and hands, pronounced dizziness, constipation, nausea, hypotension
• Teach patient to use as directed even if feeling better; may be taken with other cardiovascular products (nitrates, β-blockers)
• Advise patient to rise slowly to prevent orthostatic hypotension
• Teach patient to report nausea, dizziness, edema, shortness of breath, palpitations

## Evaluation
**Positive therapeutic outcome**
• Decreased B/P

---

## nitazoxanide (Rx)
(nye-taz-ox′a-nide)
Alinia
*Func. class.:* Antiprotozoal

**Pregnancy category B**

**Action:** Interferes with DNA/RNA synthesis in protozoa

**Therapeutic outcome:** C&S negative for organism

**Uses:** Diarrhea caused by *Cryptosporidium parvum* or *Giardia lamblia*

## Dosage and routes
**Adult:** PO 500 mg q12hr × 3 days
**Child 4-11 yr:** **PO** 10 ml (200 mg) q12hr × 3 days
**Child 12-47 mo:** **PO** 5 ml (100 mg) q12hr × 3 days

**Available forms:** Powder for oral susp 100 mg/5 ml

## Adverse effects
*CNS:* Dizziness, fever, headache
*CV:* Hypotension
*GI:* Nausea, anorexia, flatulence, increased appetite, enlarged salivary glands, abdominal pain, diarrhea, vomiting

*HEMA:* Anemia, **leukopenia**, neutropenia
*INTEG:* Pruritus, sweating
*MISC:* Increased creatinine, pale yellow eye discoloration, rhinitis, discolored urine, infection, malaise

**Contraindications:** Hypersensitivity

**Precautions:** Pregnancy **B**, breastfeeding, children <1 yr or >11 yr, renal/hepatic disease, diabetes mellitus (contains sucrose), HIV, immunocompromised patients

### Pharmacokinetics
| | |
|---|---|
| **Absorption** | Unknown |
| **Distribution** | Metabolite protein binding >99% |
| **Metabolism** | Hydrolyzed to active metabolite, undergoes conjugation |
| **Excretion** | Urine, bile, feces |
| **Half-life** | Unknown |

### Pharmacodynamics
Unknown

## Interactions
*Drug classifications*
Other highly protein bound products (phenytoin, aspirin): competes for binding sites

## NURSING CONSIDERATIONS
### Assessment
• Assess for signs of infection
• Assess bowel pattern before, during treatment

### Nursing diagnoses
• Infection, risk for (uses)
• Knowledge, deficient (teaching)

### Implementation
**PO route**
• Give with food
• Shake oral susp before giving

### Patient/family education
• Advise to take with food; shake susp well before each dose

### Evaluation
**Positive therapeutic outcome**
• C&S negative for organism
• Decreased diarrhea

---

## nitisinone
Orfadin
*See Appendix A, Selected New Drugs*

---

## nitrofurantoin (Rx)
(nye-troe-fyoor'an-toyn)
Apo-Nitrofurantoin ✦, Furadantin,
Macrobid, Macrodantin, nitrofurantoin
*Func. class.:* Urinary tract antiinfective
*Chem. class.:* Synthetic nitrofuran derivative

**Pregnancy category** B

**Action:** Appears to inhibit bacterial enzymes

**Therapeutic outcome:** Resolution of infection

**Uses:** Urinary tract infections caused by *Escherichia coli, Klebsiella, Pseudomonas, Proteus vulgaris, Proteus morganii, Serratia, Citrobacter, Staphylococcus aureus, Staphylococcus epidermidis, Enterococcus, Salmonella, Shigella*

### Dosage and routes
*Active infections*
*Adult:* PO 50-100 mg qid after meals or 50-100 mg at bedtime for long-term treatment
*Child 1 mo:* PO 5-7 mg/kg/day in 4 divided doses; 1-3 mg/kg/day for long-term treatment; max 7 mg/day

*Chronic suppression*
*Adult:* PO 50-100 mg q PM
*Child:* PO 1 mg/kg/day q PM or 0.5-1 mg/kg q12hr if dose is not well tolerated

**Available forms:** Caps 25, 50, 100 mg; tabs 50, 100 mg; susp 25 mg/ml; macrocrystal caps (Macrodantin) 25, 50, 100 mg; cap (Macrobid) 100 mg (25 macrocrystals, 75 monohydrate)

### Adverse effects
*CNS: Dizziness, headache,* drowsiness, peripheral neuropathy, chills, confusion
*CV:* **Bundle branch block**
*GI: Nausea, vomiting, abdominal pain, diarrhea,* **cholestatic jaundice,** loss of appetite, **pseudomembranous colitis, hepatitis**
*HEMA:* **Anemia, agranulocytosis**
*INTEG:* Pruritus, rash, urticaria, **angioedema,** alopecia, tooth staining, exfoliative dermatitis
*SYST:* **Stevens-Johnson syndrome, superinfection**

**Contraindications:** Infants <1 mo, hypersensitivity, anuria, severe renal disease

**Precautions:** Pregnancy **B,** breastfeeding, geriatric, G6PD deficiency, CCr <60, GI disease, diabetes

### Pharmacokinetics
| | |
|---|---|
| **Absorption** | Readily |
| **Distribution** | Crosses placenta, excreted in breast milk |
| **Metabolism** | Liver, partially |
| **Excretion** | Kidneys, 30%-50% unchanged |
| **Half-life** | 20-60 min |

### Pharmacodynamics
| | |
|---|---|
| **Onset** | Unknown |
| **Peak** | 30 min |
| **Duration** | 6-12 hr |

### Interactions
*Individual products*
Magnesium trisilicate: decreased absorption
Norfloxacin: antagonist effect
Probenecid: increased nitrofurantoin levels
*Drug/herb*
Acidophilus: do not use with antiinfectives; separate by several hours
*Drug/lab test*
Increased: BUN, alkaline phosphatase, bilirubin, creatinine, blood glucose

### NURSING CONSIDERATIONS
**Assessment**
• Monitor blood count during chronic therapy
• Monitor I/O ratio: C&S before treatment, after completion; symptoms of UTI
• Assess CNS symptoms: insomnia, vertigo, headache, drowsiness, seizures
• Assess allergy: fever, flushing, rash, urticaria, pruritus

**Nursing diagnoses**
• Infection, risk for (uses)
• Knowledge, deficient (teaching)

**Implementation**
• Do not break, crush, chew, or open tabs, caps
• Give after clean-catch urine for C&S
• Give two daily doses if urine output is high or if patient has diabetes

**Patient/family education**
• Teach patient to take with food or milk; avoid alcohol
• Teach patient to protect susp from freezing and shake well before taking
• Teach patient that product may cause drowsiness; instruct client to seek aid in walking and other activities; advise patient not to drive or operate machinery while on medication
• Teach patient that diabetics should monitor blood glucose level

N

Adverse effects: *italic* = common, **bold** = life-threatening

- Teach patient that product may turn urine rust-yellow to brown

◆ Teach patient to notify prescriber of symptoms of pseudomembranous colitis: fever, diarrhea with mucous, pus, or blood

### Evaluation
**Positive therapeutic outcome**
- Decreased dysuria, fever; negative C&S

---

### nitrofurazone topical
*See Appendix D*

---

### nitroglycerin 🔘 (Rx)
(nye-troe-gli′ser-in)
**transmucosal tablets** (Rx)
Nitrogard, Nitrogard SR ✦
**extended release** (Rx)
Nitrocot, Nitroglyn E-R, Nitro-par, Nitro-Time, Nitrong
**extended release buccal tabs** (Rx)
Nitrogard, Nitrogard SR ✦
**intravenous** (Rx)
Nitro-Bid IV, Tridil
**spray** (Rx)
Nitrolingual Translingual Spray
**sublingual** (Rx)
Nitrostat, NitroQuick
**topical ointment** (Rx)
Nitro-Bid, Nitrol
**transdermal** (Rx)
Deponit, Minitran, Nitrek, Nitrocine, Nitrodisc, Nitro-Dur, Transderm-Nitro
*Func. class.:* Coronary vasodilator, antianginal
*Chem. class.:* Nitrate

**Pregnancy category** C

**Do not confuse:**
Nitro-Bid/Nicobid

**Action:** Decreases preload and afterload, which thus decreases left ventricular end-diastolic pressure and systemic vascular resistance; dilates coronary arteries and improves blood flow through coronary vasculature, dilates arterial, venous beds systemically

**Therapeutic outcome:** Prevention of anginal attack

**Uses:** Chronic stable angina pectoris, prophylaxis of angina pain, CHF associated with

acute MI, controlled hypotension in surgical procedures

### Dosage and routes
*Adult:* SL Dissolve tab under tongue when pain begins; may repeat q5 min until relief occurs; take no more than 3 tab/15 min; use 1 tab prophylactically 5-10 min before activities; SUS REL CAP q6-12hr on empty stomach; TOP 1-2 in q8hr; increase to 4 in q4hr as needed; **IV** 5 mcg/min, then increase by 5 mcg/min q3-5 min; if no response after 20 mcg/min, increase by 10-20 mcg/min until desired response; TRANSDERMAL apply a pad daily to a site free from hair; remove patch at bedtime to provide 10-12 hr nitrate-free interval to avoid tolerance; BUCCAL 1 mg q5hr
*Child:* **IV** Initial 0.25-0.5 mg/kg/min, titrate to patient response, usual dose 1-3 mg/kg/min

**Available forms:** Buccal tabs 1, 2, 3 mg; translingual aerosol 0.4 mg/m spray; sus rel caps 2.5, 6.5, 9, 13 mg; sus rel tabs 2.6, 6.5, 9 mg; SL tabs 0.3, 0.4, 0.6 mg; oint 2%; trans syst 0.1, 0.2, 0.3, 0.4, 0.6, 0.8 mg/hr; inj 25 mg/250 ml, 50 mg/250 ml, 100 mg/250 ml, 50 mg/500 ml, 100 mg/500 ml, 200 mg/500 ml

### Adverse effects
*CNS:* Headache, flushing, dizziness
*CV:* Postural hypotension, tachycardia, **collapse,** syncope, palpitations
*GI:* Nausea, vomiting
*INTEG:* Pallor, sweating, rash

**Contraindications:** Hypersensitivity to this product or nitrites, severe anemia, increased ICP, cerebral hemorrhage, angle-closure glaucoma

**Precautions:** Pregnancy C, breastfeeding, children, postural hypotension, severe renal/hepatic disease

| Pharmacokinetics | |
|---|---|
| **Absorption** | Well absorbed (PO, buccal, SL) |
| **Distribution** | Unknown |
| **Metabolism** | Liver, extensively |
| **Excretion** | Kidney |
| **Half-life** | 1-4 min |

### Interactions
*Individual drugs*
Alcohol: increased hypotension, CV collapse
Aspirin: increased nitrate level
Heparin: decreased effects (with IV nitroglycerin)
Sildenafil, tadalafil, vardenafil: increased hypotension

---

### Drug classifications
Antihypertensives, β-adrenergic blockers, calcium channel blockers, diuretics: increased hypotension

### Drug/lab test
Increased: urine catecholamine, urine VMA
False increase: cholesterol

## NURSING CONSIDERATIONS
### Assessment
- Monitor orthostatic B/P, pulse
- Assess pain: duration, time started, activity being performed, character; check for tolerance if taken over long period
- Monitor for headache, light-headedness, decreased B/P; may indicate a need for decreased dosage

### Nursing diagnoses
- Cardiac output, decreased (uses)
- Knowledge, deficient (teaching)
- Noncompliance (teaching)
- Poisoning, risk for (uses)
- Tissue perfusion, ineffective (uses)

### Implementation
**PO route**
- Swallow sus rel tabs whole; do not break, crush, or chew sus rel tabs
- Give 1 hr before or 2 hr after meals with 8 oz of water

**Transmucosal route**
- Tab should be placed between cheek and gum line
- Do not take anything PO when tab is in place

**Topical route**
- Apply ointment using dose-measuring papers supplied; apply to an area without hair; ointment should cover 2-3 in area; may apply an occlusive dressing as directed

**Transdermal route**
- Apply transdermal patches to area without hair; press hard to adhere; if patch becomes dislodged, apply a new one

**SL route**
- Keep tab in original container
- If 3 SL tab in 15 min do not relieve pain, consider diagnosis of MI
- SL tab should be held under tongue until dissolved (a few min); do not take anything by mouth when SL tab is in place

**IV route**
- Give **IV** diluted in amount specified D₅W, or 0.9% NaCl for inf; use glass inf bottles, non–polyvinyl chloride inf tubing; titrate to patient response; do not use filters

*Y-site compatibilities:* Amiodarone, amphotericin B cholesteryl, inamrinone, atracurium, cefmetazole, cisatracurium, diltiazem, DOBUTamine, DOPamine, epINEPHrine, esmolol, famotidine, fentanyl, fluconazole, furosemide, haloperidol, heparin, hydromorphone, regular insulin, labetalol, lidocaine, lorazepam, midazolam, milrinone, morphine, niCARDipine, nitroprusside, norepinephrine, pancuronium, ranitidine, remifentanil, streptokinase, tacrolimus, theophylline, vecuronium

*Y-site incompatibilities:* Alteplase
*Additive compatibilities:* Alteplase, aminophylline, DOBUTamine, DOPamine, enalaprilat, furosemide, lidocaine, verapamil
*Additive incompatibilities:* Manufacturer recommends that nitroglycerin not be admixed with other medications

### Patient/family education
- Instruct patient to avoid alcohol
- Advise patient that product may cause headache; tolerance usually develops; use nonopioid analgesic
- Teach patient that product may be taken before stressful activity, exercise, sexual activity
- Inform patient that SL tab may sting when product comes in contact with mucous membranes
- Caution patient to avoid hazardous activities if dizziness occurs
- Instruct patient to comply with complete medical regimen
- Advise patient to make position changes slowly to prevent fainting

### Evaluation
**Positive therapeutic outcome**
- Decreased, prevention of anginal pain

N

### Pharmacodynamics

|  | SUS REL | SL | TD | IV | TRANSMU-COSAL | AEROSOL | TOPICAL OINT |
|---|---|---|---|---|---|---|---|
| **Onset** | 20-45 min | 1-3 min | ½-1 hr | 1-2 min | 1-2 min | 2 min | ½-1 hr |
| **Peak** | Unknown | Unknown | Unknown | Unknown | Unknown | Unknown | Unknown |
| **Duration** | 3-8 hr | ½ hr | 12-24 hr | 3-5 min | 3-5 hr | ½-1 hr | 2-12 hr |

Adverse effects: *italic* = common, **bold** = life-threatening

## ! HIGH ALERT

### nitroprusside (Rx)
(nye-troe-pruss'ide)
Nitropress, Sodium nitroprusside
*Func. class.:* Antihypertensive, vasodilator

**Pregnancy category C**

**Action:** Directly relaxes arteriolar, venous smooth muscle, resulting in reduction in cardiac preload, afterload

**Therapeutic outcome:** Decreased B/P in hypertensive crisis, decreased preload, afterload

**Uses:** Hypertensive crisis, to decrease bleeding by creating hypotension during surgery, acute CHF

### Dosage and routes
*Adult and child:* IV INF 0.3-8 mcg/kg/min; max 10 mcg/kg/min

**Available forms:** Inj 50 mg

### Adverse effects
*CNS: Dizziness, headache,* agitation, twitching, decreased reflexes, restlessness
*CV:* Bradycardia, ECG changes, tachycardia, hypotension
*GI:* Nausea, vomiting, abdominal pain
*INTEG:* Pain, irritation at inj site, sweating
*MISC:* **Cyanide, thiocyanate toxicity,** flushing, hypothyroidism

**Contraindications:** Hypersensitivity, hypertension (compensatory) due to aortic coarctation or AV shunting, acute CHF associated with reduced peripheral vascular resistance

**Precautions:** Pregnancy **C**, breastfeeding, children, geriatric, fluid, electrolyte imbalances, renal/hepatic disease, hypothyroidism

### Pharmacokinetics
| | |
|---|---|
| **Absorption** | Complete bioavailability |
| **Distribution** | Not known |
| **Metabolism** | RBCs, tissues |
| **Excretion** | Kidneys |
| **Half-life** | 3 days; circulating half-life 2 min |

### Pharmacodynamics
| | |
|---|---|
| **Onset** | 1-2 min |
| **Peak** | Rapid |
| **Duration** | 1-10 min |

### Interactions
*Individual drugs*
Enflurane, halothane; severe hypotension

### Drug classifications
Circulatory depressants, ganglionic blockers, volatile liquid anesthetics: severe hypotension
*Drug/herb*
Aconite: increased toxicity, death
Astragalus, cola tree: increased or decreased antihypertensive effect
Barberry, betony, black catechu, black cohosh, bloodroot, broom, burdock, cat's claw, dandelion, goldenseal, Irish moss, Jamaican dogwood, kelp, khella, mistletoe, parsley: increased antihypertensive effect
Coltsfoot, guarana, khat, licorice: decreased antihypertensive effect

### NURSING CONSIDERATIONS
**Assessment**
• Monitor B/P q5 min × 2 hr, then q1hr × 2 hr; monitor pulse q4hr; monitor jugular venous distention q4hr; ECG should be monitored continuously; monitor PCWP; rebound hypertension may occur after nitroprusside is discontinued
• Monitor electrolytes, blood studies: potassium, sodium, chloride, $CO_2$, CBC, serum glucose, serum methemoglobin if pulmonary oxygen levels are decreased
• Check weight, I&O, edema in feet and legs daily; assess skin turgor, dryness of mucous membranes for hydration status
• Assess for signs of CHF: dyspnea, edema, wet crackles
◆ Monitor for increased lactate, cyanide, thiocyanate levels if on long-term treatment, thiocyanate level should be ≤1 millimole/L
• Monitor for decrease in bicarbonate, $P_{CO_2}$ and blood pH; acidosis may occur with this product

**Nursing diagnoses**
• Injury, risk for (adverse reactions)
• Knowledge, deficient (teaching)
• Tissue perfusion, ineffective (uses)

**Implementation**
• Give by cont inf after diluting 50 mg/2-3 ml of $D_5W$; further dilute in 250 ml of $D_5W$; use an infusion pump only; wrap bottle with aluminum foil to protect from light; observe for color change in inf; discard if highly discolored (blue, green, red); titrate to patient response; avoid extravasation
*Syringe compatibilities:* Heparin
*Y-site compatibilities:* Atracurium, diltiazem, DOBUTamine, DOPamine, enalaprilat, famotidine, inamrinone, lidocaine, nitroglycerin, pancuronium, tacrolimus, theophylline, vecuronium

---

 Alert     Canada Only    🔘 Drug on CD    * "Tall Man" lettering (See Preface)

*Additive incompatibilities:* Do not give with any other products

## Patient/family education
• Teach patient to report headache, dizziness, loss of hearing, blurred vision, dyspnea, faintness; may indicate adverse reactions

## Evaluation
**Positive therapeutic outcome**
• Decreased B/P in hypertension
• Absence of bleeding in surgery

**Treatment of overdose:** Administer amyl nitrate inh until 3% sodium nitrate sol can be prepared for **IV** administration, then inject sodium thiosulfate **IV**; correct drop in B/P with vasopressor

---

## nizatidine (Rx, OTC)
(ni-za'ti-deen)
Axid, Axid AR
*Func. class.:* H$_2$-Receptor antagonist
*Chem. class.:* Substituted thiazole
**Pregnancy category** B

**Action:** Blocks H$_2$ receptors thereby reducing gastric acid output

**Therapeutic outcome:** Healing of duodenal ulcers or gastric ulcers; prevention of duodenal ulcers; decreases symptoms of gastroesophageal reflux disease (GERD)

**Uses:** Benign gastric and duodenal ulceration, prevention of duodenal ulcer recurrence, symptomatic relief of gastroesophageal reflux, heartburn prevention

## Dosage and routes
*Prophylaxis of duodenal ulcer*
*Adult:* PO 150 mg/day at bedtime

*Gastric and duodenal ulcer disease*
*Adult:* PO 300 mg at night or 150 mg bid for 4-8 wk; maintenance 150 mg at night

*Gastroesophageal reflux*
*Adult:* PO 150 mg bid

*Heartburn prevention*
*Adult:* PO 75 mg before meals

*Renal dose*
*Adult:* PO CCr 20-50 ml/min give 150 mg/day; CCr <20 ml/min give 150 mg every other day

**Available forms:** Caps 150, 300 mg; tabs 75 mg

## Adverse effects
*CNS:* Headache, somnolence, confusion, abnormal dreams, dizziness
*CV:* **Dysrhythmias, cardiac arrest**
*ENDO:* Gynecomastia
*GI:* Elevated liver enzymes, hepatitis, jaundice, nausea
*HEMA:* **Thrombocytopenia, agranulocytosis, aplastic anemia**
*INTEG:* Pruritus, sweating, urticaria, **exfoliative dermatitis**
*META:* Hyperuricemia
*MS:* Myalgia
*RESP:* **Bronchospasm, laryngeal edema**

**Contraindications:** Hypersensitivity

**Precautions:** Pregnancy **B**, breastfeeding, renal/hepatic impairment (reduce dose in renal impairment)

### Pharmacokinetics
| | |
|---|---|
| **Absorption** | 70% |
| **Distribution** | Breast milk, crosses placenta |
| **Metabolism** | Liver, partially |
| **Excretion** | Kidney |
| **Half-life** | 1½ hr |

### Pharmacodynamics
| | |
|---|---|
| **Onset** | Variable |
| **Peak** | ½-3 hr |
| **Duration** | Unknown |

N

## NURSING CONSIDERATIONS
### Assessment
• Assess patient with ulcers or suspected ulcers: epigastric or abdominal pain, hematemesis, occult blood in stools, blood or gastric aspirate before and throughout treatment, monitor gastric pH (5 should be maintained)
◆ Monitor I&O ratio, BUN, creatinine, CBC with differential monthly; agranulocytosis may occur

### Nursing diagnoses
• Knowledge, deficient (teaching)
• Pain, chronic (uses)

### Implementation
• May be given with or without meals
• Give antacids 1 hr before or 1 hr after this product

### Patient/family education
• Caution patient that gynecomastia, impotence may occur and are reversible after treatment is discontinued

---

Adverse effects: *italic* = common, **bold** = life-threatening

- Advise patient to avoid driving, other hazardous activities until stabilized on this medication; drowsiness or dizziness may occur
- Caution patient to avoid black pepper, caffeine, alcohol, harsh spices, extremes in temperature of food; tell patient to avoid OTC preparations: aspirin, cough, cold preparations because condition may worsen
- Caution patient not to take OTC and ℞ forms concurrently
- Inform patient that smoking decreases the effectiveness of the product; that smoking cessation should be considered
- Instruct patient that product must be continued for prescribed time to be effective and taken exactly as prescribed; doses should not be doubled; a missed dose should be taken as soon as remembered up to 1 hr before next dose
- Advise patient to report bruising, fatigue, malaise; blood dyscrasias may occur
- Advise patient to report diarrhea, black tarry stools, sore throat, rash, dizziness, confusion, or delirium to prescriber immediately

## Evaluation
**Positive therapeutic outcome**
- Decreased pain in abdomen
- Healing of ulcers
- Absence of gastroesophageal reflux

---

## norfloxacin (Rx)
(nor-flox′a-sin)
Noroxin
*Func. class.:* Antiinfective—urinary
*Chem. class.:* Fluoroquinolone antibacterial

### Pregnancy category C

**Action:** Interferes with conversion intermediate DNA fragments into high-molecular weight DNA in bacteria

**Therapeutic outcome:** Bactericidal action against gram-positive *Staphylococcus epidermidis,* methicillin-resistant strains of *Staphylococcus aureus,* group D streptococci; gram-negative *Escherichia coli, Klebsiella pneumoniae, Enterobacter cloacae, Proteus mirabilis, Proteus vulgaris, Providencia rettgeri, Morganella morganii, Pseudomonas aeruginosa, Citrobacter freundii*

**Uses:** Adult UTIs (including complicated), uncomplicated gonorrhea, prostatitis, cystitis

### Dosage and routes
*Uncomplicated infections*
*Adult:* PO 400 mg bid × 3-10 days 1 hr before or 2 hr after meals

*Complicated infections*
*Adult:* PO 400 mg bid × 10-21 days; 400 mg/day × 7-10 days in impaired renal function

*Uncomplicated gonorrhea*
*Adult:* PO 800 mg as a single dose

*Prostatitis*
*Adult:* PO 400 mg bid × 4 wk

*Renal dose*
*Adult:* PO CCr ≤30 ml/min 400 mg/day

**Available forms:** Tabs 400 mg

### Adverse effects
*CNS: Headache, dizziness,* fatigue, somnolence, depression, insomnia
*CV:* QT prolongation
*EENT:* Visual disturbances
*GI: Nausea,* constipation, **hepatic necrosis,** increased ALT, AST, flatulence, heartburn, vomiting, diarrhea, dry mouth, **pseudomembranous colitis**
*HEMA:* **Agranulocytosis**
*INTEG:* Rash, photosensitivity
*SYST:* **Stevens-Johnson syndrome, angioedema**

**Contraindications:** Hypersensitivity to quinolones

**Precautions:** Pregnancy **C,** breastfeeding, children, renal disease, seizure disorders

| Pharmacokinetics | |
|---|---|
| **Absorption** | 30% (PO) |
| **Distribution** | Concentration in urinary system |
| **Metabolism** | Liver (minimal) |
| **Excretion** | Kidneys, unchanged (30%) |
| **Half-life** | 3-4 hr; increased in renal disease |

| Pharmacodynamics | |
|---|---|
| | PO |
| **Onset** | Unknown |
| **Peak** | 1 hr |
| **Duration** | Unknown |

### Interactions
*Individual drugs*
Caffeine, theophylline: possible increased levels, toxicity; do not use together
CycloSPORINE: increased serum concentrations
Nitrofurantoin: decreased effectiveness; monitor closely
Probenecid: increased norfloxacin level
Sucralfate: decreased absorption of norfloxacin, give 2 hr apart
Warfarin: increased anticoagulation

## Drug classifications
Antacids, iron salts: decreased absorption of norfloxacin; give 2 hr apart
Anticoagulants (oral): increased effect of anticoagulants
## Drug/herb
Acidophilus: do not use with antiinfectives; separate by several hours
## Drug/lab test
Increased: AST, ALT, BUN, creatinine, alkaline phosphatase

## NURSING CONSIDERATIONS
### Assessment
• Assess patient for previous sensitivity reaction
• Assess patient for signs and symptoms of infection including characteristics of urine, WBC >10,000/mm³, temp; obtain baseline information before and during treatment
• Obtain C&S before beginning product therapy to identify if correct treatment has been initiated
• Assess for allergic reactions: rash, urticaria, pruritus
• Monitor blood studies: AST, ALT, BUN, creatinine, alkaline phosphatase monthly if patient is on long-term therapy
• Assess bowel pattern daily; if severe diarrhea occurs, product should be discontinued
• Assess for overgrowth of infection: perineal itching, fever, malaise, redness, pain, swelling, drainage, rash, diarrhea, change in cough, sputum

### Nursing diagnoses
• Diarrhea (adverse reactions)
• Infection, risk for (uses)
• Injury, risk for (adverse reactions)
• Knowledge, deficient (teaching)
• Noncompliance (teaching)

### Implementation
• Give in equal intervals q12hr around the clock to maintain proper blood levels; give with food to increase absorption of product; do not give within 3 hr of other agents; product interactions may occur; give with 8 oz of water
• Do not give with iron, zinc products, or antacids, which decrease absorption

### Patient/family education
• Instruct patient to take all medication prescribed for the length of time ordered; product must be taken at same time of day to maintain blood levels; do not give medication to others; do not double doses; take any missed dose when remembered
• Advise patient to increase fluids to 2 L/day to prevent crystalluria
• Caution patient to avoid driving and other hazardous activities until response is known; dizziness may occur
• Instruct patient to use sunglasses to prevent photophobia
• Have patient use hard candy, frequent sips of water for dry mouth
• Teach patient correct instillation procedure (ophth)

### Evaluation
**Positive therapeutic outcome**
• Reported improvement in symptoms of infection
• Absence of red or itching eyes (ophth)

## norfloxacin ophthalmic
*See Appendix D*

## nortriptyline (Rx)
(nor-trip'ti-leen)
Aventyl, Pamelor
*Func. class.:* Antidepressant, tricyclic
*Chem. class.:* Dibenzocycloheptene, secondary amine
### Pregnancy category D

**N**

**Do not confuse:**
nortriptyline/amitriptyline

**Action:** Blocks reuptake of norepINEPHrine, serotonin into nerve endings, increasing action of norepINEPHrine, serotonin in nerve cells; has anticholinergic effects

**Therapeutic outcome:** Decreased symptoms of depression after 2-3 wk

**Uses:** Major depression

**Unlabeled uses:** Chronic pain management

### Dosage and routes
*Adult:* PO 25 mg tid or qid; may increase to 150 mg/day; may give daily dose at bedtime
*Geriatric:* PO 10-25 mg nightly, increase by 10-25 mg at weekly intervals to desired dose; usual maintenance 75 mg/day

**Available forms:** Caps 10, 25, 50, 75 mg; sol 10 mg/5 ml

### Adverse effects
*CNS: Dizziness, drowsiness,* confusion, headache, anxiety, tremors, stimulation, weakness, insomnia, nightmares, EPS

(geriatric), increased psychiatric symptoms, **seizures**

*CV: Orthostatic hypotension, ECG changes, tachycardia,* **hypertension,** palpitations, **dysrhythmias**

*EENT:* Blurred vision, tinnitus, mydriasis

*GI: Constipation, dry mouth,* nausea, vomiting, **paralytic ileus,** increased appetite, cramps, epigastric distress, jaundice, **hepatitis,** stomatitis

*GU: Retention,* **acute renal failure**

*HEMA:* **Agranulocytosis, thrombocytopenia, eosinophilia, leukopenia**

*INTEG:* Rash, urticaria, sweating, pruritus, photosensitivity

**Contraindications:** Pregnancy **D,** hypersensitivity to tricyclics, recovery phase of MI, seizure disorders, prostatic hypertrophy

**Precautions:** Breastfeeding, children, suicidal patients, severe depression, increased intraocular pressure, angle-closure glaucoma, urinary retention, cardiac/hepatic disease, hyperthyroidism, electroshock therapy, elective surgery, suicidal ideation

### Pharmacokinetics

| | |
|---|---|
| **Absorption** | Well absorbed |
| **Distribution** | Widely distributed; crosses placenta |
| **Metabolism** | Liver, extensively |
| **Excretion** | Kidneys, breast milk |
| **Half-life** | 18-28 hr; steady state 4-19 days |

### Pharmacodynamics

Unknown

### Interactions
#### Individual drugs
Alcohol: increased CNS depression
Clonidine, guanethidine: decreased effects
Smoking (heavy): decreased product effect

#### Drug classifications
Barbiturates, benzodiazepines, CNS depressants: increased effects
MAOIs: hypertensive episode, hyperpyretic crisis, seizures
Sympathomimetics (direct-acting), products increasing QT interval: increased effects
Sympathomimetics, indirect-acting: decreased effects

#### Drug/herb
Belladonna, corkwood, henbane, jimsonweed: increased anticholinergic effect
Hops, lavender: increased CNS effect
SAM-e, St. John's wort: serotonin syndrome
Scopolia: increased antidepressant action

#### Drug/lab test
Increased: serum bilirubin, blood glucose, alkaline phosphatase
Decreased: VMA, 5-HIAA
False increase: urinary catecholamines

## NURSING CONSIDERATIONS
### Assessment
• Monitor B/P (with patient lying, standing), pulse q4hr; if systolic B/P drops 20 mm Hg, hold product, notify prescriber; take VS q4hr of patients with CV disease
• Monitor blood studies: CBC, leukocytes, differential, cardiac enzymes if patient is receiving long-term therapy
• Monitor liver function tests: AST, ALT, bilirubin
• Check weight weekly; appetite may increase with product
• Assess ECG for flattening of T wave, bundle branch block, AV block, dysrhythmias in cardiac patients
• Assess for EPS primarily in geriatric: rigidity, dystonia, akathisia
• Assess mental status: mood, sensorium, affect, suicidal tendencies; increase in psychiatric symptoms: depression, panic
• Monitor urinary retention, constipation; constipation is more likely to occur in children or geriatric
 Assess for withdrawal symptoms: headache, nausea, vomiting, muscle pain, weakness; do not usually occur unless product was discontinued abruptly
• Identify alcohol consumption; if alcohol is consumed, hold dose until AM

### Nursing diagnoses
• Coping, ineffective (uses)
• Injury, risk for (adverse reactions)
• Knowledge, deficient (teaching)
• Noncompliance (teaching)

### Implementation
• Give with food or milk to decrease GI symptoms; mix conc with water, milk, fruit juice to disguise taste
• Give dose at bedtime if oversedation occurs during day; may take entire dose at bedtime; geriatric may not tolerate once/day dosing
• Store at room temperature; do not freeze

### Patient/family education
• Teach patient that therapeutic effects may take 2-3 wk
• Teach patient to use caution in driving and other activities requiring alertness because of drowsiness, dizziness, blurred vision; to avoid rising quickly from sitting to standing, especially geriatric

 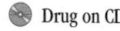

- Teach patient to avoid alcohol ingestion, other CNS depressants; teach patient not to discontinue medication quickly after long-term use; may cause nausea, headache, malaise
- Teach patient to wear sunscreen or large hat to avoid burns, because photosensitivity occurs
- Teach patient to increase fluids, bulk in diet if constipation, urinary retention occur, especially geriatric, worsening depression, suicidal thoughts/behavior
- Teach patient to take gum, hard sugarless candy, or frequent sips of water for dry mouth

## Evaluation
**Positive therapeutic outcome**
- Decrease in depression
- Absence of suicidal thoughts

**Treatment of overdose:** ECG monitoring, lavage, activated charcoal, administer anticonvulsant

## nystatin (Rx, OTC)
(nis′ta-tin)
Mycostatin, Nadostine ✦, Nilstat, nystatin, Nystex, Pastilles, PMS-Nystatin ✦; topical: Mycostatin, Nadostine ✦, Nyaderm ✦, Nystex vaginal
*Func. class.:* Antiinfective
*Chem. class.:* Antifungal

**Pregnancy category B**

**Action:** Interferes with fungal DNA replication; binds sterols in fungal cell membrane, which increases permeability, resulting in leaking of cell nutrients

**Therapeutic outcome:** Fungistatic/fungicidal against *Candida* organisms

**Uses:** *Candida* species causing oral, vaginal, intestinal infections; vaginal: cutaneous vulvovaginal candidiasis; topical: mucocutaneous fungal infections, infant eczema, pruritus ani and vulvae

## Dosage and routes
*Oral infection*
*Adult:* Susp 400,000-600,000 units qid, use ½ dose in each side of mouth, swish and swallow
*Infant:* 200,000 units qid (100,000 units in each side of mouth)
*Newborn and premature infant:* Susp 100,000 units qid
*Adult and child:* Troches 200,000-400,000 units qid × up to 2 wk

*GI infection*
*Adult:* PO 500,000-1,000,000 units tid

**Available forms:** Tabs 500,000 units; powder 50, 150, 500 million, 1, 2, 5 billion units; troches 200,000 units; susp 100,000 units/ml; oral caps 500,000, 1,000,000 units

**Adverse effects**
*GI:* Nausea, vomiting, anorexia, diarrhea, cramps
*INTEG:* Rash, urticaria (rare)

**Contraindication:** Hypersensitivity

**Precautions:** Pregnancy **B**

| Pharmacokinetics | |
|---|---|
| Absorption | Poorly absorbed |
| Distribution | Unknown |
| Metabolism | Not metabolized |
| Excretion | Feces, unchanged |
| Half-life | Unknown |

| Pharmacodynamics | |
|---|---|
| Onset | Rapid |
| Peak | Unknown |
| Duration | 6-12 hr |

## NURSING CONSIDERATIONS
### Assessment
- Assess for allergic reaction: rash, urticaria; product may have to be discontinued
- Assess for predisposing factors for candidal infection: antibiotic therapy, pregnancy, diabetes mellitus, sexual partner infection (vag infections), AIDS

### Nursing diagnoses
- Infection, risk for (uses)
- Knowledge, deficient (teaching)
- Skin integrity, impaired (uses)

### Implementation
**PO route**
- Give oral susp dose by placing ½ in each cheek, swish for several min, then swallow; shake susp before use
- Store oral susp in refrigerator, tab in airtight, light-resistant containers at room temperature
**Topical route**
- Administer by moistening lesions with a swab coated with cream or ointment; use enough medication to cover lesions completely; give after cleansing with soap, water before each application; dry well
**Vaginal route**
- Insert vag tab high into vagina with applicator provided; administer in gravid client 3-6

Adverse effects: *italic* = common, **bold** = life-threatening

wk before term to decrease candidiasis in the newborn
• Store at room temperature in dry place; protect from light, air, heat

### Patient/family education
• Instruct patient that long-term therapy may be needed to clear infection; to complete entire course of medication
• Teach patient proper hygiene: use no commercial mouthwashes for mouth infection
• Advise patient to avoid getting preparation on hands
• Instruct patient to wear light-day pad for vag preparations to avoid soiling clothing; to avoid sexual contact during treatment to minimize reinfection
• Instruct patient to notify prescriber if irritation occurs; product may have to be discontinued
• Inform patient that relief from itching may occur after 24-72 hr

**Topical route**
• Advise patient to discontinue use and notify prescriber if irritation occurs
• Teach patient to apply with glove to prevent further infection; product may stain
• Caution patient not to use occlusive dressings; to avoid use of OTC creams, ointments, lotions unless directed by prescriber

### Evaluation
**Positive therapeutic outcome**
• Culture negative for *Candida*
• Decrease in size, number of lesions
• Decreased itching, white patches on vulva (vaginal)

---

## nystatin topical
*See Appendix D*

---

## nystatin vaginal antifungal
*See Appendix D*

---

## octreotide (Rx)
(ok-tree′-o-tide)
Sandostatin, Sandostatin LAR Depot
*Func. class.:* Hormone, antidiarrheal
*Chem. class.:* Octapeptide

**Pregnancy category** B

**Action:** Action similar to somatostatin

**Therapeutic outcome:** Decreased diarrhea; decreased symptoms of acromegaly, carcinoid tumors, vasoactive intestinal peptide tumors (VIPomas)

**Uses:** Sandostatin: acromegaly, carcinoid tumors, VIPomas; LAR Depot: long-term maintenance of acromegaly, carcinoid tumors, VIPomas

**Unlabeled uses:** GI fistula, variceal bleeding, diarrheal conditions, pancreatic fistula, IBS, dumping syndrome

### Dosage and routes
*Acromegaly*
*Adult:* SUBCUT/**IV** 50-100 mcg bid-tid, adjust q2 wk based on growth hormone levels (Sandostatin) or IM 20 mg q4 wk × 3 mo, adjust by growth hormone levels (Sandostatin LAR)

*VIPomas*
*Adult:* SUBCUT/**IV** 0.2-0.3 mg/day in 2-4 doses for 2 wk, not to exceed 0.45 mg/day (Sandostatin) or IM 20 mg q2 wk × 2 mo, adjust dose (Sandostatin LAR)

*Carcinoid tumors*
*Adult:* SUBCUT/**IV** 0.1-0.6 mg/day in 2-4 doses for 2 wk, titrated to patient response (Sandostatin) or IM 20 mg q4 wk × 2 mo, adjust dose (Sandostatin LAR)

*GI fistula*
*Adult:* SUBCUT 50-200 mcg q8hr

*Irritable bowel syndrome (unlabeled)*
*Adult:* SUBCUT 100 mcg single dose to 125 mcg bid

*Antidiarrheal in AIDS patients*
*Adult:* SUBCUT/**IV** 100-1800 mcg/day

*Dumping syndrome (unlabeled)*
*Adult:* SUBCUT 50-150 mcg/day

*Variceal bleeding (unlabeled)*
*Adult:* **IV** 25-50 mcg/hr CONT **IV** INF for 18 hr-5 days

**Available forms:** Sandostatin: inj 0.05, 0.1, 0.2, 0.5, 1 mg/ml; LAR Depot: inj 10 mg, 20, 30 mg/5 ml

### Adverse effects
*CNS: Headache, dizziness, fatigue, weakness,* depression, anxiety, tremors, **seizures,** paranoia
*CV: Sinus bradycardia, conduction abnormalities,* **dysrhythmias,** chest pain, shortness of breath, thrombophlebitis, ischemia, **CHF,** hypertension, palpitations
*ENDO: Hypo/hyperglycemia, ketosis, hypothyroidism,* galactorrhea, diabetes insipidus
*GI: Diarrhea, nausea, abdominal pain, vomiting, flatulence, distension, constipa-*

---

*tion,* **hepatitis,** elevated liver function tests, **GI bleeding, pancreatitis**
*GU:* UTI, cholelithiasis
*HEMA:* Hematoma of inj site, bruise
*INTEG:* Rash, urticaria, pain, inflammation at inj site
*MS:* Joint and muscle pain

**Contraindications:** Hypersensitivity

**Precautions:** Pregnancy **B,** breastfeeding, children, geriatric, diabetes mellitus, hypothyroidism, renal disease

### Pharmacokinetics

| | |
|---|---|
| **Absorption** | Rapidly, completely |
| **Distribution** | Unknown |
| **Metabolism** | Little |
| **Excretion** | Urine, unchanged |
| **Half-life** | 1.7 hr |

### Pharmacodynamics

| | |
|---|---|
| **Onset** | Unknown |
| **Peak** | $\frac{1}{2}$ hr |
| **Duration** | 12 hr |

### Interactions
*Individual drugs*
CycloSPORINE: possible increased rejection
*Drug/food*
Decreased: absorption of dietary fat, vit $B_{12}$ levels
*Drug/lab test*
Decreased: $T_4$

### NURSING CONSIDERATIONS
**Assessment**
• Identify growth hormone antibodies, IGF-1, 1-4 hr intervals for 8-12 hr after dose in acromegaly; 5-HIAA, plasma serotonin, plasma substance P in carcinoid; VIP in VIPomas
• Fecal fat, serum carotene
• Monitor thyroid function tests: $T_3$, $T_4$, $T_7$, TSH to identify hypothyroidism
• Assess for allergic reaction: rash, itching, fever, nausea, wheezing
• Assess for cardiac status: bradycardia, conduction abnormalities, dysrhythmias; monitor ECG for QT prolongation, low voltage, axis shifts, early repolarization, R/S transition, early wave progression

**Nursing diagnoses**
• Body image, disturbed (uses)
• Knowledge, deficient (teaching)

**Implementation**
• Store unopened amps, vials in refrigerator; or room temperature for 2 wk, protect from light; do not use discolored or cloudy sol

**SUBCUT route**
• Rotate inj sites, use hip, thigh, abdomen
• Avoid using medication that is cold; allow to reach room temperature
**IM route**
• Reconstitute with diluent provided; give into gluteal muscle
**IV route**
• May use **IV** bolus if required; give over 3 min
• To use by intermittent infusion, dilute in 50-200 ml $D_5W$, 0.9% NaCl, give over 15-30 min
• In an emergency carcinoid crisis, give rapid bolus

**Patient/family education**
• Explain reason for medication and expected results
• Advise patient that routine follow-up is needed
• Instruct parents on procedure for medication preparation and inj use; request demonstration, return demonstration; provide written instructions
• Advise patient to change position slowly to prevent orthostatic hypotension

**Evaluation**
**Positive therapeutic outcome**
• Decreased symptoms of acromegaly, carcinoid, VIPoma
• Decreased diarrhea in AIDS

### ofloxacin (Rx)
(o-flox'a-sin)
Floxin
*Func. class.:* Antiinfective
*Chem. class.:* Fluoroquinolone
**Pregnancy category** C

**Action:** Interferes with conversion of intermediate DNA fragments into high molecular weight DNA in bacteria

**Therapeutic outcome:** Bactericidal action against gram-positive pathogens *Staphylococcus epidermidis,* methicillin-resistant strains of *Staphylococcus aureus, Streptococcus pyogenes, Streptococcus pneumoniae;* gram-negative pathogens *Escherichia coli, Klebsiella* species, *Enterobacter, Salmonella, Shigella, Proteus vulgaris, Proteus rettgeri, Providencia stuartii, Morganella morganii, Pseudomonas aeruginosa, Serratia, Haemophilus* species, *Acinetobacter, Neisseria gonorrhoeae, Neisseria meningitidis, Yersinia, Vibrio, Brucella, Campylobacter,* and

*Aeromonas* species; anaerobic pathogens *Bacteroides fragilis intermedius, Clostridium perfringens, Gardnerella vaginalis, Peptococcus niger, Peptostreptococcus* species; *Chlamydia pneumoniae, Chlamydia trachomatis, Legionella pneumoniae, Mycobacterium tuberculosis, Mycoplasma pneumoniae*

**Uses:** Treatment of lower respiratory tract infections (pneumonia, bronchitis), genitourinary infections (prostatitis, UTIs), skin and skin structure infections, conjunctivitis (ophth)

## Dosage and routes
### Lower respiratory tract infection/ skin and skin structure infections
*Adult:* PO/**IV** 400 mg q12hr × 10 days

### Cervicitis, urethritis
*Adult:* PO/**IV** 300 mg q12hr × 7 days

### Prostatitis
*Adult:* PO 300 mg q12hr × 6 wk

### Acute, uncomplicated gonorrhea
*Adult:* PO/**IV** 400 mg as a single dose

### Urinary tract infection
*Adult:* PO/**IV** 200-400 mg q12hr × 3-10 days

### Renal dose
*Adult:* PO CCr 20-50 ml/min give q24hr; CCr <20 ml/min give ½ of dose q24hr

**Available forms:** Tabs 200, 300, 400 mg; inj 20, 40 mg/ml; 200 mg/50 ml, 400 mg/100 ml

## Adverse effects
*CNS:* Dizziness, headache, fatigue, somnolence, depression, insomnia, lethargy, malaise, **seizures**
*CV:* **QT prolongation, dysrhythmias**
*EENT:* Visual disturbances
*GI:* Diarrhea, nausea, vomiting, anorexia, flatulence, heartburn, dry mouth, increased AST, ALT, abdominal pain, constipation, **pseudomembranous colitis**
*HEMA:* **Blood dyscrasias**
*INTEG:* Rash, pruritus
*SYST:* **Anaphylaxis, Stevens-Johnson syndrome, toxic epidermal necrosis**

**Contraindication:** Hypersensitivity to quinolones

**Precautions:** Pregnancy **C**, breastfeeding, children, geriatric, renal disease, seizure disorders, excessive sunlight

### Pharmacokinetics
| | |
|---|---|
| **Absorption** | Well absorbed (PO) |
| **Distribution** | Widely distributed |
| **Metabolism** | Unknown |
| **Excretion** | Kidneys, unchanged; breast milk |
| **Half-life** | 5-9 hr; increased in renal disease |

### Pharmacodynamics
| | PO | IV | OPHTH |
|---|---|---|---|
| **Onset** | Rapid | Rapid | Unknown |
| **Peak** | 1-2 hr | Inf end | Unknown |
| **Duration** | Unknown | Unknown | Unknown |

## Interactions
### Individual drugs
Sucralfate, zinc sulfate: decreased absorption of ofloxacin, separate by 2 hr
Theophylline: increased toxicity, do not use together
Warfarin: increased anticoagulation
### Drug classifications
Antacids with aluminum, iron salts, magnesium: decreased absorption of ofloxacin, separate by 2 hr
Antidiabetics: altered blood glucose levels
NSAIDs: increased CNS stimulation, seizures
### Drug/herb
Acidophilus: do not use with antiinfectives; separate by several hours
Cola nut: increased effect

## NURSING CONSIDERATIONS
### Assessment
• Assess patient for previous sensitivity reaction
• Assess patient for signs and symptoms of infection including characteristics of wounds, sputum, urine, stool, WBC >10,000/mm$^3$, fever; obtain baselines and monitor during treatment
• Obtain C&S before beginning product therapy to identify if correct treatment has been initiated
• Assess for allergic reactions: rash, urticaria, pruritus
• Monitor blood studies: AST, ALT, CBC, serum glucose monthly if patient is on long-term therapy
• Assess bowel pattern daily; if severe diarrhea occurs, product should be discontinued
• Assess for overgrowth of infection: perineal itching, fever, malaise, redness, pain, swelling, drainage, rash, diarrhea, change in cough, sputum
• Assess for CNS symptoms: seizures, vertigo, drowsiness, agitation, confusion, tremors

## Nursing diagnoses
- Diarrhea (adverse reactions)
- Infection, risk for (uses)
- Injury, risk for (adverse reactions)
- Knowledge, deficient (teaching)
- Noncompliance (teaching)

## Implementation
### PO route
- Give in equal intervals q12hr around the clock to maintain proper blood levels; do not give within 2 hr of other agents, since product interactions are possible: give with 8 oz of water
- Do not give with iron, aluminum, zinc products or antacids, which decrease absorption and form insoluble chelate

### IV route
- For intermittent inf, dilute to 4 mg/ml with $D_5W$, $D_5$/0.9% NaCl, 0.9% NaCl, $D_5$/LR, sodium bicarbonate, sodium lactate, $D_5$/Plasmalyte 56; give over 1 hr or more
- Store for 2 wk refrigerated or 6 mo frozen, after reconstitution

**Syringe compatibilities:** Cefotaxime
**Y-site compatibilities:** Ampicillin, cisatracurium, docetaxel, etoposide, gemcitabine, granisetron, linezolid, propofol, remifentanil, thiotepa
**Additive compatibilities:** Amoxicillin, ceftazidime, clindamycin, gentamicin, piperacillin, tobramycin, vancomycin

## Patient/family education
- Instruct patient to take all medication prescribed for the length of time ordered; product must be taken around the clock to maintain blood levels; do not give medication to others
- Teach patient to use sunscreen when outdoors to decrease phototoxicity
- Advise patient to increase fluids to 2 L/day to prevent crystalluria
- Caution patient to avoid driving and other hazardous activities until response is known; dizziness, confusion, drowsiness may occur

## Evaluation
### Positive therapeutic outcome
- Absence of signs/symptoms of infection
- Reported improvement in symptoms of infection
- Absence of red or itching eyes (ophth)

## ofloxacin ophthalmic
*See Appendix D*

---

## olanzapine (Rx)
(oh-lanz'a-peen)
Zydis, Zyprexa, Zyprexa Intramuscular
*Func. class.:* Antipsychotic/neuroleptic
*Chem. class.:* Thienobenzodiazepine

**Pregnancy category  C**

**Action:** Unknown; may mediate antipsychotic activity by both dopamine and serotonin type 2 ($5\text{-}HT_2$) antagonism; also, may antagonize muscarinic receptors, histaminic ($H_1$)- and $\alpha$-adrenergic receptors

**Therapeutic outcome:** Decreased psychotic symptoms

**Uses:** Schizophrenia, acute manic episodes in bipolar disorder

**Unlabeled uses:** Dementia related to Alzheimer's disease, OCD

### Dosage and routes
*Schizophrenia*
**Adult:** PO 5-10 mg/day initially, may increase dosage by 5 mg at 1 wk or more intervals; ORALLY DISINTEGRATING TABS open blister pack, place tab on tongue, let disintegrate, swallow, max 20 mg/day
**Geriatric:** PO 5 mg, may increase cautiously at 1 wk intervals, max 20 mg/day

*Bipolar mania*
**Adult:** PO 10-15 mg/day, may increase dose after 24 hr by 5 mg

*Agitation associated with schizophrenia, bipolar I mania*
**Adult:** IM 10 mg

**Available forms:** Tabs 2.5, 5, 7.5, 10, 15, 20 mg; orally disintegrating tabs 5, 10, 15, 20 mg; powder for injection 10 mg

### Adverse effects
***CNS:*** EPS (pseudoparkinsonism, akathisia, dystonia, tardive dyskinesia), **seizures,** headache, **neuroleptic malignant syndrome (rare),** somnolence, agitation, nervousness, hostility, dizziness, hypertonia, tremor, euphoria, confusion, *drowsiness,* fatigue, *abnormal gait, insomnia, fever*
***CV:*** Hypotension, tachycardia, chest pain, **heart failure, sudden death (geriatric, IM)**
***ENDO:*** Increased prolactin levels
***GI:*** Dry mouth, nausea, vomiting, anorexia, constipation, abdominal pain, weight gain, appetite, dyspepsia, jaundice, **hepatitis**
***GU:*** Urinary retention, urinary frequency, enuresis, impotence, amenorrhea, gynecomas-

---

Adverse effects: *italic* = common, **bold** = life-threatening

tia, breast engorgement, premenstrual syndrome

***HEMA:* Neutropenia**

***INTEG:*** Rash

***MISC:*** Peripheral edema, accidental injury, hypertonia

***MS:*** Joint pain, twitching

***RESP:*** *Cough, pharyngitis,* **fatal pneumonia (geriatric, IM)**

**Contraindications:** Hypersensitivity

**Precautions:** Pregnancy **C**, breastfeeding, geriatric, hypertension, cardiac/renal/hepatic disease, diabetes

### Pharmacokinetics

| | |
|---|---|
| **Absorption** | Well |
| **Distribution** | 93% plasma protein binding |
| **Metabolism** | Liver |
| **Excretion** | Kidneys |
| **Half-life** | Unknown |

### Pharmacodynamics

| | |
|---|---|
| **Onset** | Unknown |
| **Peak** | 6 hr |
| **Duration** | Unknown |

### Interactions
#### Individual drugs
Alcohol: increased sedation, hypotension

Bromocriptine, levodopa: decreased antiparkinson activity

Carbamazepine, omeprazole, rifampin: decreased levels of olanzapine

Diazepam: increased hypotension

Fluvoxamine: increased olanzapine levels

#### Drug classifications
Anesthetics (barbiturates), antidepressants, antihistamines, sedative/hypnotics, CNS depressants: increased sedation

Anticholinergics: increased anticholinergic effects

Antihypertensives: increased hypotension

Dopamine agonists: decreased antiparkinson activity

#### Drug/herb
Betel palm, kava: increased EPS

Cola tree, hops, nettle, nutmeg: increased action

#### Drug/lab test
Increased: liver function tests, prolactin, CPK

### NURSING CONSIDERATIONS
#### Assessment
• Assess mental status, orientation, mood, behavior, presence of hallucinations and type before initial administration and monthly

• Monitor swallowing of PO medication: check for hoarding or giving of medication to other patients

• Monitor I&O ratio; palpate bladder if low urinary output occurs, especially in geriatric

• Monitor bilirubin, CBC

• Monitor urinalysis; recommended before, during prolonged therapy

• Assess affect, orientation, LOC, reflexes, gait, coordination, sleep pattern disturbances

• Monitor B/P sitting, standing, lying; take pulse and respirations q4hr during initial treatment; establish baseline before starting treatment; report drops of 30 mm Hg; obtain baseline ECG

• Assess dizziness, faintness, palpitations, tachycardia on rising

• Assess for neuroleptic malignant syndrome: hyperpyrexia, muscle rigidity, increased CPK, altered mental status, for acute dystonia (check chewing, swallowing, eyes, pin rolling)

• EPS including akathisia (inability to sit still, no pattern to movements), tardive dyskinesia (bizarre movements of the jaw, mouth, tongue, extremities), pseudoparkinsonism (rigidity, tremors, pill rolling, shuffling gait)

• Monitor skin turgor daily

• Monitor constipation, urinary retention daily; increase bulk, $H_2O$ in diet

#### Nursing diagnoses
• Knowledge, deficient (teaching)

• Noncompliance (teaching)

• Thought processes, disturbed (uses)

#### Implementation
• Give antiparkinsonian agent for EPS

• Give decreased dose in geriatric

• Give PO with full glass of water, milk; or with food to decrease GI upset

• Provide decreased stimuli by dimming light, avoiding loud noises

• Provide supervised ambulation until stabilized on medication; do not involve in strenuous exercise program because fainting is possible; patients should not stand still for long periods

• Give increased fluids to prevent constipation

• Give sips of water, candy, gum for dry mouth

• Store in airtight, light-resistant container

• Give orally disintegrating tabs: open blister pack, place tab on tongue until dissolved, swallow; no water needed

#### Patient/family education
• Teach patient to use good oral hygiene; frequent rinsing of mouth, candy, ice chips, sugarless gum for dry mouth

• Advise patient to avoid hazardous activities until product response is determined

---

◆ Alert      ♣ Canada Only      💿 Drug on CD                    * "Tall Man" lettering (See Preface)

- Advise patient that orthostatic hypotension occurs often and to rise from sitting or lying position gradually
- Advise patient to avoid hot tubs, hot showers, tub baths, since hypotension may occur
- Advise patient to avoid abrupt withdrawal of this product, or EPS may result; product should be withdrawn slowly
- Advise patient to avoid OTC preparations (cough, hay fever, cold) unless approved by prescriber, since serious product interactions may occur; avoid use with alcohol, CNS depresssants, increased drowsiness may occur
- Advise patient that in hot weather, heat stroke may occur; take extra precautions to stay cool

### Evaluation
**Positive therapeutic outcome**
- Decrease in emotional excitement, hallucinations, delusions, paranoia, reorganization of patterns of thought, speech

**Treatment of overdose:** Lavage if orally ingested; provide airway; do not induce vomiting or use epINEPHrine

---

## olmesartan (Rx)
(ol-meh-sar′tan)
Benicar
*Func. class.:* Antihypertensive

**Pregnancy category**
C (1st trimester),
D (2nd/3rd trimesters)

**Action:** Blocks the vasoconstrictor and aldosterone-secreting effects of angiotensin II; selectively blocks the binding of angiotensin II to the $AT_1$ receptor found in tissues

**Therapeutic outcome:** Decreased B/P

**Uses:** Hypertension, alone or in combination with other antihypertensives

### Dosage and routes
*Adult:* **PO** Single agent 20 mg/day initially in patients who are not volume depleted; may be increased to 40 mg/day if needed after 2 wk

**Available forms:** Tabs 5, 20, 40 mg

### Adverse effects
*CNS: Dizziness,* fatigue, headache, insomnia
*CV:* Chest pain, peripheral edema, tachycardia
*EENT:* Sinusitis, rhinitis, pharyngitis
*GI: Diarrhea,* abdominal pain
*MS:* Arthralgia, pain
*RESP: Upper respiratory infection,* bronchitis
*SYST:* **Angioedema**

**Contraindications:** Pregnancy **D** (2nd/3rd trimesters), hypersensitivity

**Precautions:** Pregnancy **C** (1st trimester), breastfeeding, children, geriatric, hepatic disease

### Pharmacokinetics
| | |
|---|---|
| **Absorption** | Unknown |
| **Distribution** | Unknown |
| **Metabolism** | Unknown |
| **Excretion** | Urine, feces |
| **Half-life** | Unknown |

### Pharmacodynamics
Unknown

### Interactions
*Individual drugs*
Lithium: increased effect
*Drug classifications*
Antihypertensives (other), diuretics: increased antihypertensive effects
Potassium supplements, potassium-sparing diuretics: increased hyperkalemia
NSAIDs, salicylates: decreased antihypertensive effect
*Drug/herb*
Aconite: increased toxicity, death
Astragalus, cola tree: increased or decreased antihypertensive effect
Barberry, betony, black catechu, black cohosh, bloodroot, broom, burdock, cat's claw, dandelion, goldenseal, hawthorn, Irish moss, Jamaican dogwood, kelp, khella, mistletoe, parsley: increased antihypertensive effect
Coltsfoot, guarana, khat, licorice, yohimbe: decreased antihypertensive effect

### NURSING CONSIDERATIONS
**Assessment**
- Assess for pregnancy; this product can cause fetal death when given in pregnancy
- Assess response and adverse reactions, especially in renal disease
- Monitor B/P, pulse q4hr; note rate, rhythm, quality; electrolytes: K, Na, Cl; baselines in renal, liver function tests before therapy begins
- Assess skin turgor, dryness of mucous membranes for hydration status; for angioedema: facial swelling, dyspnea

**Nursing diagnoses**
- Cardiac output, decreased (uses)
- Knowledge, deficient (teaching)
- Noncompliance (teaching)
- Tissue perfusion, ineffective (uses)

## Implementation
- Give without regard to meals

## Patient/family education
- Advise to comply with dosage schedule, even if feeling better
- Advise patient to notify prescriber of mouth sores, fever, swelling of hands or feet, irregular heartbeat, chest pain
- Teach that excessive perspiration, dehydration, vomiting, diarrhea may lead to fall in B/P; to consult prescriber if these occur
- Teach that product may cause dizziness, fainting; light-headedness may occur
- Advise to rise slowly to sitting or standing position to minimize orthostatic hypotension
- Teach to notify prescriber immediately if pregnant; not to use during breastfeeding
- Advise to avoid all OTC medications, unless approved by prescriber
- Advise to inform all health care providers of medication use
- Advise to use proper technique for obtaining B/P and acceptable parameters

## Evaluation
**Positive therapeutic outcome**
- Decreased B/P

---

**olopatadine ophthalmic**
*See Appendix D*

---

**olsalazine** (Rx)
(ohl-sal'ah-zeen)
Dipetum ✤
*Func. class.:* Antiinflammatory
*Chem. class.:* Salicylate derivative

**Pregnancy category** C

**Action:** Bioconverted to 5-aminosalicylic acid, which decreases inflammation

**Therapeutic outcome:** Lessening of loose, diarrhea stools and cramping

**Uses:** Maintenance of remission of ulcerative colitis in patients intolerant to sulfasalazine

## Dosage and routes
*Adult:* PO 500 mg bid

**Available forms:** Caps 250 mg

## Adverse effects
*CNS:* Headache, hallucinations, depression, vertigo, fatigue, dizziness
*GI:* Nausea, vomiting, abdominal pain, **hepatitis**, diarrhea, bloating, **pancreatitis**

*HEMA:* **Leukopenia, neutropenia, thrombocytopenia, agranulocytosis, anemia**
*INTEG:* Rash, dermatitis, urticaria

**Contraindications:** Hypersensitivity to salicylates

**Precautions:** Pregnancy **C**, breastfeeding, children <14 yr, impaired renal/hepatic function, severe allergy, bronchial asthma

| Pharmacokinetics | |
|---|---|
| Absorption | Colon 99% converted to mesalamine |
| Distribution | Colon |
| Metabolism | Liver |
| Excretion | Feces |
| Half-life | 0.9 hr |

| Pharmacodynamics | |
|---|---|
| Onset | Unknown |
| Peak | 1 hr |
| Duration | 12 hr |

## Interactions
*Drug/lab test*
Increased: AST, ALT

## NURSING CONSIDERATIONS
### Assessment
🔷 Assess for blood dyscrasias: skin rash, fever, sore throat, bruising, bleeding, fatigue, joint pain (rare)
- Assess for allergic reaction: rash, dermatitis, urticaria, pruritus, dyspnea, bronchospasm

### Nursing diagnoses
- Diarrhea (uses)
- Knowledge, deficient (teaching)
- Pain, acute (uses)

### Implementation
- Give total daily dose evenly spaced to minimize GI intolerance, with food
- Store in tight, light-resistant container at room temperature

### Patient/family education
- Advise patient to take as prescribed, take missed dose as soon as remembered
- Inform patient not to operate machinery or drive until effects are known, may cause dizziness
- Advise patient to notify prescriber if symptoms do not improve or if allergic reaction or sore throat occurs

### Evaluation
**Positive therapeutic outcome**
- Absence of fever, mucus in stools

---

## omalizumab (Rx)
(oh-mah-lye-zoo'mab)
Xolair
*Func. class.:* Monoclonal antibody

**Pregnancy category B**

**Action:** Recombinant DNA-derived humanized IgG murine monoclonal antibody that selectively binds to IgE to limit the release of mediators in the allergic response

**Therapeutic outcome:** Ability to breathe more easily

**Uses:** Moderate to severe persistent asthma

**Unlabeled uses:** Seasonal allergic rhinitis, food allergy

**Dosage and routes**
*Adult:* SUBCUT 150-375 mg × 2-4 wk, divide inj into 2 sites, if dose is >150 mg; dose is adjusted based on IgE levels and significant changes in body weight

**Available forms:** Powder for inj, lyophilized 202.5 mg (150 mg/1.2 ml after reconstitution)

**Adverse effects**
*INTEG:* Pruritus, dermatitis, inj site reactions, rash
*MISC:* Earache, dizziness, fatigue, pain, **malignancies,** viral infections, **anaphylaxis, thrombocytopenia,** headache
*MS:* Arthralgia, fracture, leg, arm pain
*RESP:* Sinusitis, upper respiratory tract infections, pharyngitis

**Contraindications:** Hypersensitivity to this product or hamster protein

**Precautions:** Pregnancy **B**, breastfeeding, children <12 yr, acute attacks of asthma, lymphoma, nephrotic disease, bronchospasm, neoplastic disease, status asthmaticus

| Pharmacokinetics | |
|---|---|
| **Absorption** | Slow |
| **Distribution** | Unknown |
| **Metabolism** | Degradation by liver |
| **Excretion** | In bile |
| **Half-life** | 26 days |

| Pharmacodynamics | |
|---|---|
| **Onset** | Unknown |
| **Peak** | 7-8 days |
| **Duration** | Unknown |

**Interactions**
*Drug classifications*
Vaccines (live virus): avoid concurrent use

## NURSING CONSIDERATIONS
**Assess:**
• Monitor respiratory rate, rhythm, depth; auscultate lung fields bilaterally; notify prescriber of abnormalities; monitor pulmonary function tests
• Assess for allergic reactions: rash, urticaria; product should be discontinued

**Nursing diagnoses**
• Gas exchange, impaired (uses)
• Knowledge, deficient (teaching)

**Implementation**
**SUBCUT route**
• Given q2-4 wk; product is viscous; if >150 mg is given, divide into two sites; the inj may take 5-10 sec to administer
• Do not give more than 150 mg/inj site

**Patient/family education**
• Advise that improvement will not be immediate
• Teach not to stop taking or decrease current asthma medications unless instructed by prescriber

**Evaluation**
**Positive therapeutic outcome**
• Ability to breathe more easily

## omeprazole (Rx, OTC)
(oh-mep'ra-zole)
Losec ✦, Prilosec, Prilosec OTC, Zegerid
*Func. class.:* Antiulcer, proton pump inhibitor
*Chem. class.:* Benzimidazole

**Pregnancy category C**

**Do not confuse:**
Prilosec/Prinivil/predniSONE/Prozac

**Action:** Suppresses gastric secretion by inhibiting hydrogen/potassium ATPase enzyme system in the gastric parietal cell; characterized as a gastric acid pump inhibitor, since it blocks the final step of acid production

**Therapeutic outcome:** Absence of duodenal ulcers; decreased gastroesophageal reflux

**Uses:** Gastroesophageal reflux disease (GERD), severe erosive esophagitis, poorly responsive systemic GERD, pathologic hypersecretory conditions (Zollinger-Ellison syndrome, systemic mastocytosis, multiple endocrine adenomas); possibly effective for treatment of duodenal ulcers with or without antiinfectives for *Helicobacter pylori*

O

**Unlabeled uses:** GERD-related laryngitis, enhancing pancreatin

## Dosage and routes
### Active duodenal ulcers
*Adult:* PO 20 mg/day × 4-8 wk; associated with *H. pylori* 40 mg qᴀᴍ and clarithromycin 500 mg tid on days 1-14, then 20 mg/day days 15-28

### Severe erosive esophagitis/poorly responsive GERD
*Adult:* PO 20 mg/day × 4-8 wk

### Pathologic hypersecretory conditions
*Adult:* PO 60 mg/day; may increase to 120 mg tid; daily doses >80 mg should be divided

### Gastric ulcer
*Adult:* PO 40 mg/day × 4-8 wk
*Geriatric:* PO Max 20 mg/day

### Heartburn (OTC)
*Adult:* PO 1 delayed rel tab (20 mg) daily before ᴀᴍ meal with glass of water

### Laryngitis (unlabeled)
*Adult:* PO 20-40 mg nightly × 6-24 wk or 20 mg bid × 4-12 wk

**Available forms:** Delayed rel caps 10, 20, 40 mg, delayed rel tabs (Prilosec OTC) 20 mg

## Adverse effects
***CNS:*** *Headache, dizziness, asthenia*
***CV:*** Chest pain, angina, tachycardia, bradycardia, palpitations, peripheral edema, **heart failure**
***EENT:*** Tinnitus, taste perversion
***GI:*** *Diarrhea, abdominal pain, vomiting, nausea, constipation, flatulence, acid regurgitation,* abdominal swelling, anorexia, irritable colon, esophageal candidiasis, dry mouth, **hepatic failure**
***GU:*** UTI, frequency, increased creatinine, **proteinuria, hematuria,** testicular pain, glycosuria
***HEMA:*** **Pancytopenia, thrombocytopenia, neutropenia, leukocytosis,** anemia
***INTEG:*** Rash, dry skin, urticaria, pruritus, alopecia
***META:*** Hypoglycemia, increased hepatic enzymes, weight gain
***MISC:*** *Back pain,* fever, fatigue, malaise
***RESP:*** *Upper respiratory tract infections, cough,* epistaxis
***SYST:*** **Angioedema, exfoliative dermatitis, Stevens-Johnson syndrome, toxic epidermal necrolysis**

**Contraindications:** Hypersensitivity

**Precautions:** Pregnancy **C,** breastfeeding, children

### Pharmacokinetics
| | |
|---|---|
| **Absorption** | Rapidly absorbed |
| **Distribution** | Protein binding (95%); gastric parietal cells |
| **Metabolism** | Liver, extensively; by CYP450 enzyme system |
| **Excretion** | Kidneys, feces |
| **Half-life** | ½-1 hr; increased in the geriatric, hepatic disease |

### Pharmacodynamics
| | |
|---|---|
| **Onset** | 1 hr |
| **Peak** | ½-3½ hr |
| **Duration** | 3-4 days |

## Interactions
### Individual drugs
Calcium carbonate: decreased absorption of calcium carbonate
Cyanocobalamin: decreased absorption of cyanocobalamin
CycloSPORINE: increased cycloSPORINE levels
Diazepam: increased serum levels of diazepam
Digoxin: increased serum levels, delayed absorption of digoxin
Disulfiram: increased disulfiram levels
Flurazepam: increased flurazepam level
Iron salts: decreased absorption
Ketoconazole: decreased absorption of ketoconazole
Phenytoin: increased serum levels of phenytoin
Triazolam: increased triazolam level
Warfarin: increased bleeding tendencies
### Drug classifications
Iron products: decreased absorption of iron
### Drug/lab test
Increased: alkaline phosphatase, AST, ALT, bilirubin, gastrin

## NURSING CONSIDERATIONS
### Assessment
• Assess GI system: bowel sounds q8hr, abdomen for pain and swelling, anorexia
• Monitor hepatic enzymes: AST, ALT, increased alkaline phosphatase during treatment

### Nursing diagnoses
• Knowledge, deficient (teaching)
• Pain, chronic (uses)

### Implementation
• Swallow sus rel caps whole; do not break, crush, chew, or open
• Give before patient eats; may give with antacids

---

 Alert      Canada Only     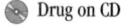 Drug on CD          * ''Tall Man'' lettering (See Preface)

## Patient/family education
• Advise patient to report severe diarrhea; product may have to be discontinued
• Caution patient to avoid driving and other hazardous activities until response to product is known
• Caution patient to avoid alcohol, salicylates, ibuprofen; may cause GI irritation

## Evaluation
**Positive therapeutic outcome**
• Absence of epigastric pain, swelling, fullness

---

## ondansetron (Rx)
(on-dan'sa-tron)
Zofran, Zofran ODT
*Func. class.:* Antiemetic
*Chem. class.:* 5-HT receptor antagonist

**Pregnancy category** B

**Do not confuse:**
Zofran/Zantac

**Action:** Prevents nausea, vomiting by blocking serotonin (5-HT) peripherally, centrally, and in the small intestine

**Therapeutic outcome:** Control of nausea, vomiting

**Uses:** Prevention of nausea, vomiting associated with cancer chemotherapy and prevention of postopertive nausea, vomiting

**Unlabeled uses:** Bulimia, pruritus (rectal use), alcoholism, hyperemesis gravidarum

## Dosage and routes
*Prevention of nausea/vomiting associated with cancer chemotherapy*
*Adult and child 4-18 yr:* **IV** 0.15 mg/kg infused over 15 min, 30 min before start of cancer chemotherapy; 0.15 mg/kg is given 4 hr and 8 hr after first dose or 32 mg as a single dose; dilute in 50 ml of $D_5$ or 0.9% NaCl before giving; RECT (unlabeled) 16 mg daily 2 hr before chemotherapy; PO 8 mg ½ hr prior to chemotherapy, repeat 8 hr later
*Child ≥4 yr:* PO 4 mg ½ hr prior to chemotherapy

*Prevention of nausea/vomiting of radiotherapy*
*Adult:* PO 8 mg tid, may repeat q8hr

*Prevention of postoperative nausea/vomiting*
*Adult:* **IV**/IM 4 mg undiluted over >30 sec prior to induction of anesthesia

*Child 2-12 yr:* **IV** 0.1 mg/kg (≤40 kg); 4 mg (≥40 kg) give ≥30 sec

*Hepatic dose*
*Adult:* PO/IM/**IV** max dose 8 mg daily

*Hyperemesis gravidarum (unlabeled)*
*Adult:* PO/**IV** 4-8 mg bid-tid

*Bulimia (unlabeled)*
*Adult:* PO 4 mg tid (base dose) prn during bingeing/purging

*Pruritus (unlabeled)*
*Adult:* PO 4 mg bid

*Alcoholism (unlabeled)*
*Adult:* PO 4 mcg/kg bid

**Available forms:** Inj 2 mg/ml, 32 mg/50 ml (premixed); tabs 4, 8 mg; oral sol 4 mg/5 ml; oral disintegrating tabs 4, 8 mg

## Adverse effects
*CNS: Headache,* dizziness, drowsiness, fatigue, EPS
*GI: Diarrhea, constipation, abdominal pain, dry mouth*
*MISC:* Rash, **bronchospasm** (rare), *musculoskeletal pain, wound problems, shivering, fever, hypoxia, urinary retention*

**Contraindications:** Hypersensitivity

**Precautions:** Pregnancy **B,** breastfeeding, children, geriatric, granisetron hypersensitivity

| Pharmacokinetics | |
|---|---|
| **Absorption** | Completely absorbed (**IV**) |
| **Distribution** | Unknown |
| **Metabolism** | Liver, extensively |
| **Excretion** | Kidneys |
| **Half-life** | 3.5-4.7 hr |

Pharmacodynamics
Unknown

## Interactions
*Individual drugs*
Rifampin: decreased ondansetron effect

## NURSING CONSIDERATIONS
**Assessment**
• Assess for absence of nausea, vomiting during chemotherapy
• Assess for hypersensitivity reaction: rash, bronchospasm
• Assess for EPS shuffling gait, tremors, grimacing, rigidity

## Nursing diagnoses
• Knowledge, deficient (teaching)
• Noncompliance (teaching)

## Implementation
### IV route
- Give **IV** after diluting a single dose in 50 ml of 0.9% NaCl or D$_5$W, 0.45% NaCl; give over 15 min
- Store at room temperature for 48 hr after dilution

*Y-site compatibilities:* Aldesleukin, amifostine, amikacin, aztreonam, bleomycin, carboplatin, carmustine, cefazolin, ceforanide, cefotazime, cefoxitin, ceftazidime, ceftizoxime, cefuroxime, chlorproMAZINE, cimetidine, cisatracurium, cisplatin, cladribine, clindamycin, cyclophosphamide, cytarabine, dacarbazine, dactinomycin, DAUNOrubicin, dexamethasone, diphenhydrAMINE, DOXOrubicin, DOXOrubicin liposome, doxycycline, droperidol, etoposide, famotidine, filgrastim, floxuridine, fluconazole, fludarabine, gentamicin, haloperidol, heparin, hydrocortisone, hydromorphone, hydrOXYzine, ifosfamide, imipenem/cilastatin, magnesium sulfate, mannitol, mechlorethamine, melphalan, meperidine, mesna, methotrexate, metoclopramide, miconazole, mitomycin, mitoxantrone, morphine, paclitaxel, pentostatin, potassium chloride, prochlorperazine, ranitidine, remifentanil, streptozocin, teniposide, thiotepa, ticarcillin, ticarcillin/clavulanate, vancomycin, vinBLAStine, vinCRIStine, vinorelbine, zidovudine

*Y-site incompatibilities:* Acyclovir, aminophylline, amphotericin B, ampicillin, ampicillin/sulbactam, cefoperazone, furosemide, ganciclovir, lorazepam, methylPREDNISolone, mezlocillin, piperacillin, sargramostim, sodium bicarbonate

*Additive compatibilities:* Cisplatin, cyclophosphamide, cytarabine, dacarbazine, dexamethasone, DOXOrubicin, etoposide, meperidine, methotrexate

*Solution compatibilities:* May also be diluted with D$_5$W, LR, D$_5$/0.9% NaCl, D$_5$/0.45% NaCl

## Patient/family education
- Instruct patient to report diarrhea, constipation, rash, changes in respirations, or discomfort at insertion site
- Teach patient reason for medication and expected results

## Evaluation
### Positive therapeutic outcome
- Absence of nausea, vomiting during cancer chemotherapy

---

## orlistat (Rx, OTC)
(or-li′-stat)
Alli, Xenical
*Chem. class.:* Weight control agent, lipase inhibitor

### Pregnancy category B

**Action:** Inhibits the absorption of dietary fat

**Therapeutic outcome:** Decrease in weight

**Uses:** Obesity management

### Dosage and routes
*Adult:* PO 60 mg (Alli)-120 mg (Xenical) tid with each main meal containing fat, max 360 mg/day

**Available forms:** Caps 60 mg (Alli), 120 mg (Xenical)

### Adverse effects
*CNS:* Insomnia, dizziness, headache, depression, anxiety, fatigue
*GI: Oily spotting, flatus with discharge, fecal urgency, fatty/oily stool, oily evacuation, fecal incontinence,* frequent defecation, nausea, vomiting, abdominal pain, infectious diarrhea, rectal pain, tooth disorder, hypovitaminosis
*GU:* UTI, vaginitis, menstrual irregularity
*INTEG:* Dry skin, rash
*MS:* Back pain, arthritis, myalgia, tendinitis
*RESP:* Influenza, upper, lower respiratory tract infection, EENT symptoms

**Contraindications:** Breastfeeding, hypersensitivity, chronic malabsorption syndrome, cholestasis

**Precautions:** Pregnancy **B,** children, hypothyroidism, other organic causes of obesity, anorexia nervosa, bulimia, nephrolithiasis, GI disease, diabetes, fat-soluble vitamin deficiency

### Pharmacokinetics
| | |
|---|---|
| **Absorption** | Minimal |
| **Distribution** | 99% protein binding |
| **Metabolism** | Unknown |
| **Excretion** | Feces |
| **Half-life** | 1-2 hr |

### Pharmacodynamics
| | |
|---|---|
| **Onset** | Unknown |
| **Peak** | 8 hr |
| **Duration** | Unknown |

---

## Interactions
### Individual drugs
Cyclosporine: decreased absorption
Pravastatin: increased lipid-lowering effect
Warfarin: increased effects of warfarin
### Drug classifications
Fat-soluble vitamins: decreased absorption

## NURSING CONSIDERATIONS
### Assessment
• Monitor weight weekly, diabetic patients may need reduction in oral hypoglycemics
• Assess for misuse in certain populations (anorexia nervosa, bulimia)

### Nursing diagnoses
• Knowledge, deficient (teaching)
• Noncompliance (teaching)

### Implementation
• Patient should be on a diet with 30% of calories from fat; omit dose of orlistat if a meal contains no fat

### Patient/family education
• Advise patient that 60 mg cap can be obtained OTC; 60 mg tid is the highest OTC dose
• Warn patient that safety and effectiveness beyond 2 yr have not been determined
• Instruct patient to read patient's information sheet, discuss unpleasant GI side effects
• Advise patient to avoid hazardous activities until stabilized on medication
• Instruct patient to take a multivitamin containing fat-soluble vitamins, take 2 hr before or after orlistat; psyllium taken with each dose or at bedtime may decrease GI symptoms
• Instruct patient/family to notify prescriber if significant side effects occur
• Advise prescriber if pregnancy is planned or suspected

### Evaluation
**Positive therapeutic outcome**
• Decreased weight

---

## oseltamivir (Rx)
(oh-sell-tam'ih-ver)
Tamiflu
*Func. class.:* Antiviral
*Chem. class.:* Neuramidase inhibitor
**Pregnancy category C**

**Action:** Inhibits influenza virus neuraminidase with possible alteration of virus particle aggregation and release

**Therapeutic outcome:** Decreased symptoms of influenza type A

**Uses:** Prevention/treatment of influenza type A or B

**Unlabeled uses:** Possibly effective for avian flu (H5N1)

## Dosage and routes
### Treatment
**Adult and child >40 kg:** PO 75 bid mg × 5 days, begin treatment within 2 days of onset of symptoms
**Child 23-40 kg and ≥1 yr:** PO 60 mg bid
**Child 15-23 kg and ≥1 yr:** PO 45 mg bid
**Child ≤15 kg and ≥1 yr:** PO 30 mg bid
### Renal dose
**Adult:** PO CCr 10-30 ml/min 75 mg/day × 5 days
### Prevention
**Adult and child ≥13 yr:** PO 75 mg/day × ≥7 days; begin treatment within 2 days of contact, max use 6 wk

**Available forms:** Caps 75 mg; powder for oral susp 12 mg/ml after reconstitution

## Adverse effects
*CNS:* Headache, fatigue, insomnia, dizziness, delirium, **self-injury (children)**
*GI: Nausea, vomiting,* diarrhea, abdominal pain
*INTEG:* **Toxic epidermal necrolysis, Stevens-Johnson syndrome, erythema multiforme**
*RESP:* Cough

**Contraindications:** Hypersensitivity

**Precautions:** Pregnancy **C**, geriatric, renal/hepatic disease

| Pharmacokinetics | |
|---|---|
| Absorption | Rapidly absorbed |
| Distribution | Protein binding is low |
| Metabolism | Converted to oseltamivir carboxylate |
| Excretion | Eliminated by conversion, urine 99% |
| Half-life | 1-3 hr |

| Pharmacodynamics | |
|---|---|
| Unknown | |

## NURSING CONSIDERATIONS
### Assessment
• Assess for symptoms of influenza A: increased temperature, malaise, aches and pains

### Nursing diagnoses
• Infection, risk for (uses)
• Knowledge, deficient (teaching)

Adverse effects: *italic* = common, **bold** = life-threatening

## Implementation
- Give within 2 days of symptoms of influenza; continue for 5 days
- Give at least 4 hr before bedtime to prevent insomnia
- Administer after meals for better absorption, to decrease GI symptoms: caps may be opened and mixed with food for easy swallowing
- Store in airtight, dry container

## Patient/family education
- Teach patient about aspects of product therapy: the need to report dyspnea, weight gain, dizziness, poor concentration, dysuria, behavioral changes
- Teach patient to avoid hazardous activities if dizziness occurs
- Advise patient to take missed dose as soon as remembered if within 2 hr of next dose

## Evaluation
**Positive therapeutic outcome**
- Absence of fever, malaise, cough, dyspnea in influenza A

## oxacillin (Rx)
(ox-a-sill′in)
Bactocill, oxacillin sodium
*Func. class.:* Broad-spectrum antiinfective
*Chem. class.:* Penicillinase-resistant penicillin

**Pregnancy category B**

**Action:** Interferes with cell wall replication of susceptible organisms; osmotically unstable cell wall swells, bursts from osmotic pressure

**Therapeutic outcome:** Bactericidal effects for gram-positive cocci *Staphylococcus aureus, Streptococcus pneumoniae,* infections caused by penicillinase-producing staphylococci

**Uses:** Infections caused by penicillinase-producing staphylococci, streptococci; respiratory tract, skin, skin structure, urinary tract, bone, joint infections, sinusitis, endocarditis, septicemia, meningitis

## Dosage and routes
*Adult:* IM/**IV** 2-12 g/day in divided doses q4-6hr
*Child:* IM/**IV** 50-100 mg/kg/day in divided doses q4-6hr

**Available forms:** Powder for inj 250, 500 mg, 1, 2, 4, 10 g

## Adverse effects
*CNS:* Lethargy, hallucinations, anxiety, depression, twitching, **coma, seizures**

*GI:* *Nausea, vomiting, diarrhea,* increased AST, ALT, abdominal pain, glossitis, colitis, **pseudomembranous colitis**
*GU:* **Oliguria, proteinuria, hematuria,** vaginitis, moniliasis, **glomerulonephritis**
*HEMA:* Anemia, increased bleeding time, **bone marrow depression, granulocytopenia**
*INTEG:* **Exfoliative dermatitis, Stevens-Johnson syndrome**
*SYST:* **Anaphylaxis, serum sickness**

**Contraindications:** Hypersensitivity to penicillins

**Precautions:** Pregnancy **B**, breastfeeding, neonates, hypersensitivity to cephalosporins, renal/hepatic/GI disease

### Pharmacokinetics
| | |
|---|---|
| **Absorption** | Rapid, incomplete (PO); well absorbed (IM); completely (**IV**) |
| **Distribution** | Widely distributed; crosses placenta |
| **Metabolism** | Liver |
| **Excretion** | Kidneys, unchanged (51%); breast milk |
| **Half-life** | 20-50 min; increased in severe hepatic disease |

### Pharmacodynamics
| | PO | IM | IV |
|---|---|---|---|
| **Onset** | Rapid | Rapid | Rapid |
| **Peak** | ½-1 hr | ½ hr | Inf end |
| **Duration** | Unknown | Unknown | Unknown |

## Interactions
*Individual drugs*
Chloramphenicol, colestipol, cholestyramine: decreased effectiveness of oxacillin
Probenecid: increased oxacillin levels
Rifampin: decreased oxacillin effect
*Drug classifications*
Contraceptives (oral): decreased contraceptive effectiveness
Erythromycins, tetracyclines: decreased antimicrobial effectiveness
*Drug/herb*
Acidophilus: do not use with antiinfectives; separate by several hours
Khat: decreased absorption, separate by ≥2 hr
*Drug/lab test*
False positive: urine glucose, urine protein

## NURSING CONSIDERATIONS
### Assessment
- Assess patient for previous sensitivity reaction to penicillins or other cephalosporins; cross-sensitivity between penicillins and cephalosporins is common

- Assess patient for signs and symptoms of infection including characteristics of wounds, sputum, urine, stool, WBC >10,000/mm$^3$, fever; obtain baseline information and during treatment
- Obtain C&S before beginning product therapy to identify if correct treatment has been initiated
- Assess for allergic reactions: rash, urticaria, pruritus, chills, fever, joint pain; angioedema may occur a few days after therapy begins; epINEPHrine, resuscitation equipment should be available for anaphylactic reaction
- ⬥ Assess urine output; if decreasing, notify prescriber (may indicate nephrotoxicity); also check for increased BUN, creatinine
- Monitor blood studies: AST, ALT, CBC, Hct, bilirubin, LDH, alkaline phosphatase, Coombs' test monthly if patient is on long-term therapy
- Monitor electrolytes: potassium, sodium, chloride monthly if patient is on long-term therapy
- Assess bowel pattern daily; if severe diarrhea occurs, product should be discontinued; may indicate pseudomembranous colitis
- Monitor for bleeding: ecchymosis, bleeding gums, hematuria, stool guaiac daily if on long-term therapy
- Assess for overgrowth of infection: perineal itching, fever, malaise, redness, pain, swelling, drainage, rash, diarrhea, change in cough, sputum

### Nursing diagnoses
- Diarrhea (adverse reactions)
- Infection, risk for (uses)
- Injury, risk for (adverse reactions)
- Knowledge, deficient (teaching)
- Noncompliance (teaching)

### Implementation
#### PO route
- Give in even doses around the clock; if GI upset occurs, give with food; product must be given for 10-14 days to ensure organism death and prevent superinfection; store in airtight container
- Shake susp; store in refrigerator for 2 wk, 1 wk at room temperature
#### IM route
- Reconstitute 250 mg/1.4 ml, 500 mg/2.7-2.8 ml, 1 g/5.7 ml, 2 g/11.4-11.5 ml, 4 g/21.8-23 ml of sterile water for a conc of 250 mg/1.5 ml; store unused portion in refrigerator for 1 wk or 3 days at room temperature
- Inject deeply in large muscle mass
#### IV route
- Reconstitute 250 mg/1.4 ml, 500 mg/2.7-2.8 ml, 1 g/5.7 ml, 2 g/11.4-11.5 ml, 4

g/21.8-23 ml of sterile water for a conc of 250 mg/1.5 ml; store unused portion in refrigerator for 1 week or 3 days at room temperature
- Give direct **IV** by diluting reconstituted sol with 250-500 mg/5 ml, 1 g/10 ml, 2 g/20 ml, 4 g/40 ml of sterile water or 0.9% NaCl, give over 10 min
- Give intermittent inf by diluting to a conc of 0.5-40 mg/ml with D$_5$W, 0.9% NaCl, D$_5$/0.9% NaCl, LR; give over 6 hr or less

*Y-site compatibilities:* Acyclovir, cyclophosphamide, diltiazem, famotidine, fluconazole, foscarnet, heparin, hydrocortisone, hydromorphone, labetalol, magnesium sulfate, meperidine, methotrexate, morphine, perphenazine, potassium chloride, tacrolimus, vit B with C, zidovudine

*Y-site incompatibilities:* Verapamil

*Additive compatibilities:* Cephapirin, chloramphenicol, DOPamine, potassium chloride, sodium bicarbonate

*Additive incompatibilities:* Cytarabine, tetracycline

### Patient/family education
- Teach patient to report sore throat, bruising, bleeding, joint pain; may indicate blood dyscrasias (rare)
- Advise patient to contact prescriber if vaginal itching, loose foul-smelling stools, furry tongue occur; may indicate superinfection
- Instruct patient to take all medication prescribed for the length of time ordered
- Advise patient to notify prescriber of diarrhea with blood or pus, which may indicate pseudomembranous colitis

### Evaluation
#### Positive therapeutic outcome
- Absence of signs/symptoms of infection (WBC <10,000/mm$^3$, temp WNL, absence of red, draining wounds)
- Reported improvement in symptoms of infection

**Treatment of anaphylaxis:** Withdraw product, maintain airway, administer epINEPHrine, aminophylline, O$_2$, **IV** corticosteroids

---

Adverse effects: *italic* = common, **bold** = life-threatening

## oxaliplatin (Rx)
(ox-al-i'plat-in)
Eloxitan
*Func. class.:* Antineoplastic
*Chem. class.:* 3rd generation platinum analog

### Pregnancy category D

**Action:** Forms cross links, inhibiting DNA replication and transcription, cell-cycle nonspecific

**Therapeutic outcome:** Decreased size of tumor, spread of malignancy

**Uses:** Metastatic carcinoma of the colon or rectum in combination with 5-FU/leucovorin

**Unlabeled uses:** Relapsed or refractory non-Hodgkin's lymphoma, advanced ovarian cancer

### Dosage and routes
Dosage protocols may vary
*Adult:* **IV** INF *Day 1:* oxaliplatin 85 mg/m$^2$ in 250-500 ml D$_5$W and leucovorin 200 mg/m$^2$ in D$_5$W, give both over 2 hr at the same time in separate bags using a Y-line, followed by 5-FU 400 mg/m$^2$ **IV** BOL over 2-4 min, then 5-FU 600 mg/m$^2$ **IV** INF in 500 ml D$_5$W as a 22-hr CONT INF; *Day 2:* leucovorin 200 mg/m$^2$ **IV** INF over 2 hr, then 5-FU 400 mg/m$^2$ **IV** BOL over 2-4 min, then 5-FU 600 mg/m$^2$ **IV** INF in 500 D$_5$W as a 22-hr CONT INF; repeat cycle q2 wk

**Available forms:** Powder for inj 50, 100 mg single-use vials

### Adverse effects
*CNS:* Peripheral neuropathy, fatigue, headache, dizziness, insomnia
*CV:* Cardiac abnormalities, thromboembolism
*EENT: Decreased visual acuity, tinnitus, hearing loss*
*GI: Severe nausea, vomiting, diarrhea, weight loss,* stomatitis, anorexia, gastroesophageal reflux, constipation, dyspepsia, mucositis, flatulence
*GU:* Hematuria, dysuria, creatinine
**HEMA: Thrombocytopenia, leukopenia, pancytopenia, neutropenia, anemia, hemolytic uremic syndrome**
*INTEG: Alopecia,* rash, flushing, extravasation, redness, swelling, pain at inj site
*META:* Hypokalemia
*RESP:* **Fibrosis,** dyspnea, cough, rhinitis, URI, pharyngitis
*SYST:* **Anaphylaxis, angioedema**

**Contraindications:** Pregnancy **D**, breastfeeding, hypersensitivity to this product or other platinum products; radiation therapy or chemotherapy within 1 mo, thrombocytopenia, smallpox vaccination

**Precautions:** Children, geriatric, pneumococcus vaccination, renal disease

### Pharmacokinetics
| | |
|---|---|
| **Absorption** | Unknown |
| **Distribution** | 15% of platinum in systemic circulation; 85% is either in tissues or being eliminated in urine |
| **Metabolism** | Liver |
| **Excretion** | Urine |
| **Half-life** | 40 days |

### Pharmacodynamics
Unknown

### Interactions
*Individual drugs*
Alcohol, aspirin: increased risk of bleeding
Radiation: increased myelosuppression
*Drug classifications*
Aminoglycosides, diuretics (loop): increased nephrotoxicity
Anticoagulants, NSAIDs: increased risk of bleeding
Live virus vaccines: decreased antibody response
Myelosuppressives: increased myelosuppression
Tannins: increased oxaliplatin
*Drug/lab test*
Increased: ALT, AST, bilirubin, creatinine
Decreased: potassium, neutrophils, WBC, platelets

### NURSING CONSIDERATIONS
Assessment
**For bone marrow depression**
• Monitor CBC, differential, platelet count weekly; withhold product if WBC is <4000 or platelet count is <100,000; notify prescriber of results
• Monitor renal function tests: BUN, creatinine, serum uric acid, urine CCr before, electrolytes during therapy; dose should not be given if BUN >19 mg/dl; creatinine <1.5 mg/dl; I&O ratio; report fall in urine output of <30 ml/hr
 Assess for anaphylaxis: wheezing, tachycardia, facial swelling, fainting; discontinue product and report to prescriber; resuscitation equipment should be nearby
• Monitor temp (may indicate beginning infection)

• Monitor liver function tests before, during therapy (bilirubin, AST, ALT, LDH) as needed or monthly

• Assess for bleeding: hematuria, guaiac, bruising or petechiae, mucosa or orifices q8hr; obtain prescription for viscous lidocaine (Xylocaine)

• Assess effects of alopecia on body image; discuss feelings about body changes

• Assess for jaundice of skin, sclera; dark urine; clay-colored stools; itchy skin; abdominal pain; fever; diarrhea

• Assess for edema in feet, joint pain, stomach pain, shaking

### Nursing diagnoses

• Infection, risk for (adverse reactions)
• Knowledge, deficient (teaching)
• Nutrition: less than body requirements, imbalanced (adverse reactions)

### Implementation

• Provide comprehensive oral hygiene
• Provide all medications PO, if possible, avoid IM inj when platelets <100,000/mm$^3$
• Increase fluid intake to 2-3 L/day to prevent urate deposits, calculi formation; elimination of product

**IV route**

• Do not reconstitute or dilute with sodium chloride or any chloride-containing solutions
• Do not use aluminum equipment during any preparation or administration, will degrade platinum; do not refrigerate unopened powder or solution
• Prepare in biologic cabinet using gown, gloves, mask; do not allow product to come in contact with skin, use soap and water if contact occurs
• Hydrate patient with 0.9% NaCl over 8-12 hr before treatment
• Have epINEPHrine, antihistamines, corticosteroids for hypersensitivity reaction
• Give antiemetic 30-60 min before giving product and prn
• Give diuretic (furosemide 40 mg **IV**) or mannitol after infusion
• Provide blankets, hat, gloves for cold prevention

### Patient/family education

• Advise to report signs of infection: increased temp, sore throat, flulike symptoms
• Advise to report signs of anemia: fatigue, headache, faintness, shortness of breath, irritability
• Advise to report bleeding; avoid use of razors, commercial mouthwash
• Advise to avoid aspirin, ibuprofen, NSAIDs, alcohol; may cause GI bleeding

• Advise to report any complaints or side effects to nurse or prescriber
• Advise to report any changes in breathing, coughing
• Advise that hair may be lost during treatment; a wig or hairpiece may make patient feel better; new hair may be different in color, texture
• Advise to report numbness, tingling in face or extremities, poor hearing or joint pain, swelling
• Advise not to receive vaccines during treatment
• Advise to use contraception during treatment and 4 mo after; this product may cause infertility
• Teach patient to avoid contact with cold (air, ice, liquid); causes acute dysesthesias

### Evaluation

**Positive therapeutic outcome**
• Decreased tumor size, spread of malignancy

---

## oxaprozin (Rx)
(ox-a-proe'zin)
Daypro, Daypro ALTA
*Func. class.:* Nonsteroidal antiinflammatory, antirheumatic
*Chem. class.:* Propionic acid derivative

### Pregnancy category C

**Do not confuse:**
Daypro/Diupres

**Action:** Inhibits prostaglandin synthesis by decreasing an enzyme needed for biosynthesis; analgesic, antiinflammatory

**Therapeutic outcome:** Decreased pain, inflammation

**Uses:** Acute and long-term management of osteoarthritis, rheumatoid arthritis, juvenile rheumatoid arthritis

### Dosage and routes
*Adult:* PO 600-1200 mg/day; max 1800 mg/day or 26 mg/kg, whichever is lower in divided doses
*Adult <50 kg:* PO 600 mg/day

*Juvenile rheumatoid arthritis*
*Child 6-16 yr:* PO 22-31 kg, 600 mg/dose; 32-54 kg, 900 mg/dose; ≥55 kg, 1200 mg/ dose

**Available forms:** Tabs 600 mg; tabs oxaprozin potassium 678 mg (equal to 600 mg oxaprozin); caps 600 mg

## Adverse effects

**CNS:** Dizziness, headache, drowsiness, fatigue, tremors, confusion, insomnia, anxiety, depression
**CV:** Tachycardia, peripheral edema, palpitations, dysrhythmias, **MI, stroke**
**EENT:** Tinnitus, hearing loss, blurred vision
**GI:** Nausea, *anorexia,* vomiting, *diarrhea,* jaundice, **cholestatic hepatitis,** constipation, flatulence, *cramps,* dry mouth, peptic ulcer, **GI bleeding,** perforation, ulceration
**GU: Nephrotoxicity: dysuria, hematuria, oliguria, azotemia**
**HEMA:** Increased bleeding time
**INTEG:** Purpura, rash, pruritus, sweating
**SYST: Anaphylaxis, angioneurotic edema, toxic epidermal necrolysis, Stevens-Johnson syndrome**

**Contraindications:** Hypersensitivity, asthma, patients in whom aspirin and iodides have induced symptoms of allergic reactions or asthma, perioperative pain in CABG surgery

**Precautions:** Pregnancy **C**, breastfeeding, children, geriatric, avoid in late pregnancy, bleeding/GI/cardiac disorders, CHF, hypersensitivity to other antiinflammatory agents, severe renal/hepatic disease

### Pharmacokinetics

| | |
|---|---|
| **Absorption** | Well absorbed |
| **Distribution** | Unknown |
| **Metabolism** | Liver, extensively |
| **Excretion** | Breast milk |
| **Half-life** | 40-50 hr |

### Pharmacodynamics

| | |
|---|---|
| **Onset** | Unknown |
| **Peak** | 2 hr |
| **Duration** | Unknown |

## Interactions
### Individual drugs
Alcohol: increased GI side effects
Aspirin: increased GI adverse reactions, toxicity
Cefamandole, cefoperazone, cefotetan, clopidogrel, eptifibatide, plicamycin, ticlopidine, tirofiban: increased bleeding risk
Cyclosporine, methotrexate: increased toxicity
Lithium: increased lithium levels, avoid concomitant use
Phenytoin: increased phenytoin level, avoid concomitant use
Radiation: increased risk of hematologic toxicity

### Drug classifications
Anticoagulants, thrombolytics: increased risk of bleeding
Antihypertensives: decreased effect of antihypertensives
Antineoplastics: increased risk of hematologic toxicity
Corticosteroids, NSAIDs: increased GI side effects
Diuretics: decreased effectiveness of diuretics
Potassium supplements: increased GI side effects

### Drug/herb
Anise, arnica, bogbean, chamomile, chondroitin, clove, dong quai, fenugreek, feverfew, garlic, ginger, ginkgo, ginseng *(Panax),* licorice: increased bleeding risk
Arginine, gossypol: increased gastric irritation
Bearberry, bilberry: increased NSAIDs effect

### Drug/lab test
Increased: BUN, alkaline phosphatase
False positive: increased 5-HIAA
False increase: 17-KS

## NURSING CONSIDERATIONS
### Assessment
• Assess for pain and ROM: intensity, location, duration
• Monitor blood studies: alkaline phosphatase, LDH, AST, ALT, and bleeding time (may be increased)
• Assess for asthma, aspirin hypersensitivity, nasal polyps; increased hypersensitivity reactions

### Nursing diagnoses
• Injury, risk for (adverse reactions)
• Knowledge, deficient (teaching)
• Mobility, impaired physical (uses)
• Pain, chronic (uses)

### Implementation
• Do not break, crush, or chew tabs
• Give with full glass of water to enhance absorption
• Give with food, antacids, milk to decrease gastric symptoms
• Sit upright for 30 min to prevent stomach irritation and ulceration

### Patient/family education
• Teach patient that product must be continued for prescribed time to be effective; to avoid aspirin, alcoholic beverages
• Instruct patient to use caution when driving; drowsiness, dizziness may occur
• Teach patient to take with a full glass of water to enhance absorption; patient should sit upright for 30 min to prevent stomach irritation and ulceration

 Alert      Canada Only      Drug on CD     * "Tall Man" lettering (See Preface)

- Instruct patient to use sunscreen and protective clothing to prevent burns
- Advise patient to report to prescriber severe abdominal pain, rash, itching, yellowing of skin or eyes, depression

### Evaluation
**Positive therapeutic outcome**
- Decreased pain
- Decreased inflammation
- Increased mobility

## oxazepam (Rx)
(ox-az′e-pam)
Apo-Oxazepam ✦, Novoxapam ✦, oxazepam, Serax
*Func. class.:* Sedative/hypnotic; antianxiety
*Chem. class.:* Benzodiazepine, short-acting

**Pregnancy category D**
**Controlled substance schedule IV**

**Action:** Depresses subcortical levels of CNS, including limbic system, reticular formation; potentiates GABA

**Therapeutic outcome:** Decreased anxiety, successful alcohol withdrawal, relaxation

**Uses:** Anxiety, alcohol withdrawal, insomnia

### Dosage and routes
*Anxiety*
*Adult:* PO 10-30 mg tid-qid, max 120 mg/day
*Geriatric:* PO 5 mg daily-bid initially, may increase, max 15 mg qid
*Alcohol withdrawal*
*Adult:* PO 15-30 mg tid-qid
**Available forms:** Caps 10, 15, 30 mg; tab 15 mg

### Adverse effects
*CNS: Dizziness, drowsiness,* confusion, headache, anxiety, tremors, fatigue, depression, insomnia, hallucinations, paradoxic excitement, transient amnesia
*CV: Orthostatic hypotension,* **ECG changes, tachycardia,** hypotension
*EENT: Blurred vision,* tinnitus, mydriasis
*GI:* Nausea, vomiting, anorexia
*HEMA:* Leukopenia
*INTEG:* Rash, dermatitis, itching
*SYST:* Dependence

**Contraindications:** Pregnancy **D**, breastfeeding, children <12 yr, hypersensitivity to benzodiazepines, angle-closure glaucoma, psychosis

**Precautions:** Geriatric, debilitated, renal/hepatic disease, depression, suicidal ideation

### Pharmacokinetics
| | |
|---|---|
| **Absorption** | Well absorbed |
| **Distribution** | Widely distributed; crosses placenta, blood-brain barrier |
| **Metabolism** | Liver |
| **Excretion** | Kidneys, breast milk |
| **Half-life** | 5-15 hr |

### Pharmacodynamics
| | |
|---|---|
| **Onset** | ½-1½ hr |
| **Peak** | Unknown |
| **Duration** | 6-12 hr |

### Interactions
*Individual drugs*
Alcohol: increased CNS depression
Disulfiram: increased oxazepam effects
Levodopa: decreased effects of levodopa
Phenytoin, theophylline, valproic acid: decreased oxazepam effects
*Drug classifications*
CNS depressants: increased oxazepam effects
Oral contraceptives: increased or decreased oxazepam effect
*Drug/herb*
Black cohosh: increased hypotension
Catnip, chamomile, clary, cowslip, hops, kava, lavender, mistletoe, nettle, pokeweed, poppy, Queen Anne's lace, senega, skullcap, valerian: increased CNS depression
*Drug/lab test*
Increased: AST, ALT, serum bilirubin
Decreased: radioactive iodine uptake
False increase: 17-OHCS

### NURSING CONSIDERATIONS
**Assessment**
- Assess mental status: mood, sensorium, anxiety, affect, sleeping pattern, drowsiness, dizziness, especially geriatric; physical dependency, withdrawal symptoms: anxiety, panic attacks, agitation, seizures, headache, nausea, vomiting, muscle pain, weakness; suicidal tendencies; indications of increasing tolerance and abuse
- Monitor B/P with patient lying, standing, pulse; if systolic B/P drops 20 mm Hg, hold product, notify prescriber
- Monitor blood tests: CBC during long-term therapy; blood dyscrasias have occurred rarely; decreased hematocrit, neutropenia may occur

- Monitor hepatic tests: AST, ALT, bilirubin, creatinine LDH, alkaline phosphatase if taking long term
- Monitor I&O; indicate renal dysfunction

### Nursing diagnoses
- Anxiety (uses)
- Injury, risk for (adverse reactions)
- Knowledge, deficient (teaching)

### Implementation
- Give with food or milk for GI symptoms; tab may be crushed if patient is unable to swallow medication whole

### Patient/family education
- Teach patient that product may be taken with food or fluids; tab may be crushed or swallowed whole
- Caution patient not to use for everyday stress or longer than 3 mo unless directed by prescriber; not to take more than prescribed amount; not to double doses or skip doses
- Advise patient to avoid OTC preparations unless approved by prescriber; alcohol and CNS depressants will increase CNS depression
- Caution patient to avoid driving and activities that require alertness, since drowsiness may occur; to avoid alcohol and other psychotropic medications; to rise slowly or fainting may occur, especially geriatric; that drowsiness may worsen at beginning of treatment
- Caution patient not to discontinue medication abruptly after long-term use; withdrawal symptoms include vomiting, cramping, tremors, seizures
- Advise patient to use sugarless gum, hard candy, frequent sips of water for dry mouth

### Evaluation
**Positive therapeutic outcome**
- Decreased anxiety, restlessness, sleeplessness (short-term treatment only)

### Treatment of overdose: Lavage, VS, supportive care

---

### oxcarbazepine (Rx)
(ox'kar-baz'uh-peen)
Trileptal
*Func. class.:* Anticonvulsant

**Pregnancy category C**

**Action:** May inhibit nerve impulses by limiting influx of sodium ions across cell membrane in motor cortex

**Therapeutic outcome:** Absence of seizures

**Uses:** Partial seizures

**Unlabeled uses:** Trigeminal neuralgia, atypical panic disorder, bipolar disorder

### Dosage and routes
*Seizures adjunctive therapy*
*Adult:* PO 300 mg bid, may be increased by 600 mg/day in divided doses bid; maintenance 1200 mg/day
*Child 4-16 yr:* PO 8-10 mg/kg/day divided bid, max 600 mg/day; dose is determined by weight

*Conversion to monotherapy in partial seizures*
*Adult:* PO 300 mg bid with reduction in other anticonvulsants, increase oxcarbazepine by 600 mg/day q1 wk over 2-4 wk; withdraw other anticonvulsants over 3-6 wk, max 2400 mg/day

*Initiation of monotherapy in partial seizures*
*Adult:* PO 300 mg bid, increase by 300 mg/day q3 days to 1200 mg divided bid

*Renal dose*
*Adult:* PO CCr <30 ml/min 150 mg bid and increase slowly

**Available forms:** Film-coated tabs 300 mg; oral susp 300 mg/5 ml

### Adverse effects
*CNS: Headache, dizziness, confusion, fatigue,* feeling abnormal, ataxia, abnormal gait, tremors, anxiety, agitation, **worsening of seizures**
*CV: Hypotension,* chest pain, edema
*EENT: Blurred vision, diplopia, nystagmus,* rhinitis, sinusitis
*GI: Nausea, constipation, diarrhea,* anorexia, vomiting, abdominal pain, gastritis, dry mouth, thirst, **rectal hemorrhage**
*GU: Frequency,* UTI, vaginitis
*INTEG:* Purpura, rash, acne
*RESP:* Rhinitis, URI
*SYST: Angioedema, anaphylaxis,* **Stevens-Johnson syndrome**

**Contraindications:** Hypersensitivity

**Precautions:** Pregnancy **C,** breastfeeding, children <4 yr, hypersensitivity to carbamazepine, renal disease, fluid restriction, hyponatremia

| Pharmacokinetics | |
|---|---|
| **Absorption** | Unknown |
| **Distribution** | Unknown |
| **Metabolism** | Liver |
| **Excretion** | Unknown |
| **Half-life** | Unknown |

---

| Pharmacodynamics | |
|---|---|
| **Onset** | Unknown |
| **Peak** | 4-6 hr |
| **Duration** | Unknown |

## Interactions
### Individual products
Alcohol: increased CNS depression
Carbamazepine: decreased carbamazepine level
Felodipine: decreased effects of felodipine
Phenobarbital, valproic acid, verapamil: decreased oxcarbazepine level
Phenytoin: decreased oxcarbazepine level
### Drug classifications
Contraceptives (oral): decreased oral contraceptive level
MAOIs: do not use concurrently
### Drug/herb
Ginkgo: increased anticonvulsant effect
Ginseng, santonica: decreased anticonvulsant effect

## NURSING CONSIDERATIONS
### Assessment
• Assess seizure activity including frequency, duration, and aura; provide seizure precautions
• Assess mental status including mood, sensorium, affect, behavioral changes; if mental status changes, notify prescriber
• Assess eye problems: ophthalmic examinations (slit lamp, funduscopy, tonometry) are needed before, during, after treatment
• Assess patient for hypersensitivity to carbamazepine
• Assess for serious reactions: angioedema, anaphylaxis, Stevens-Johnson syndrome
### Nursing diagnoses
• Injury, risk for (side effects)
• Knowledge, deficient (teaching)
### Implementation
• Store product at room temperature
• Provide assistance with ambulation during early part of treatment; dizziness may occur
• Give product with food, milk to decrease GI symptoms
### Patient/family education
• Caution patient to avoid driving, other activities that require alertness
• Advise patient not to discontinue medication quickly after long-term use
• Instruct patient to avoid use of alcohol while taking this medication
• Instruct patient to use alternate contraception if using hormonal method
• Advise patient to use hard candy or gum for dry mouth, rinse mouth frequently
• Advise patient to carry/wear emergency ID stating name, products taken, condition, prescriber's name and phone number
### Evaluation
**Positive therapeutic outcome**
• Decreased seizure activity
**Treatment of overdose:** Activated charcoal, give 0.9% NaCl (hypotensive state), atropine (bradycardia); use benzodiazepines, barbiturates for seizures

## oxybutynin (Rx)
(ox-i-byoo'ti-nin)
Ditropan, Ditropan XL, oxybutynin, Oxytrol Transdermal
*Func. class.:* Anticholinergic
*Chem. class.:* Synthetic tertiary amine
**Pregnancy category B**

**Do not confuse:**
Ditropan/diazepam

**Action:** Relaxes smooth muscles in urinary tract by inhibiting acetylcholine at postganglionic sites

**Therapeutic outcome:** Decreased symptoms of urgency, nocturia, incontinence

**Uses:** Antispasmodic for neurogenic bladder, overactive bladder

### Dosage and routes
*Adult:* PO 5 mg bid-tid, not to exceed 5 mg qid; EXT REL TABS 5 mg/day, may increase by 5 mg, max 30 mg/day; TRANSDERMAL apply one patch to abdomen, hip, buttock 2 ×/wk (q3-4 days)
*Geriatric:* PO 2.5-5 mg tid, increase by 2.5 mg q several days
*Child >6 yr:* PO 5 mg bid, not to exceed 5 mg tid; EXT REL 5 mg/day, max 20 mg/day
*Child 1-5 yr:* PO 0.2 mg/kg/dose 2-4 ×/day

**Available forms:** Syr 5 mg/5 ml; tabs 5 mg; ext rel tabs 5, 10, 15 mg; transdermal 3.9 mg/day

### Adverse effects
*CNS: Anxiety, restlessness, dizziness,* somnolence, insomnia, nervousness, **seizures,** headache, drowsiness, confusion
*CV: Palpitations, sinus tachycardia,* hypertension, peripheral edema
*EENT:* Blurred vision, increased intraocular tension, dry mouth, throat

Adverse effects: *italic* = common, **bold** = life-threatening

**GI:** *Nausea, vomiting, anorexia,* abdominal pain, constipation, *dyspepsia,* diarrhea, taste perversion, GERD

**GU:** Dysuria, impotence, retention, hesitancy

**Contraindications:** Hypersensitivity, GI obstruction, GU obstruction, glaucoma, severe colitis, myasthenia gravis, unstable CV

**Precautions:** Pregnancy **B**, breastfeeding, children <12 yr, geriatric, suspected glaucoma

### Pharmacokinetics

| | |
|---|---|
| **Absorption** | Rapidly absorbed |
| **Distribution** | Unknown |
| **Metabolism** | Liver |
| **Excretion** | Unknown |
| **Half-life** | Unknown |

### Pharmacodynamics

| | |
|---|---|
| **Onset** | ½-1 hr |
| **Peak** | 3-4 hr |
| **Duration** | 6-10 hr |

### Interactions
#### Individual drugs
Acetaminophen: decreased levels of acetaminophen

Amantadine: increased anticholinergic effects

Atenolol: increased levels of atenolol

Digoxin: increased levels of digoxin

Haloperidol: decreased levels of haloperidol

Levodopa: decreased levels of levodopa

Nitrofurantoin: increased levels of nitrofurantoin

#### Drug classifications
Antihistamines, other anticholinergics: increased anticholinergic effects

Phenothiazines: increased or decreased levels of phenothiazines

#### Drug/herb
Black catechu: increased constipation

Butterbur, jimsonweed, scopolia: increased anticholinergic action

Jamborandi tree, pill-bearing spurge: decreased anticholinergic effect

### NURSING CONSIDERATIONS
#### Assessment
• Assess for allergic reactions: rash, urticaria; if these occur, product should be discontinued
• Assess urinary patterns: distention, nocturia, frequency, urgency, incontinence; catheterization may be required to remove residual urine

#### Nursing diagnoses
• Knowledge, deficient (teaching)
• Pain, acute (uses)
• Urinary elimination, impaired (uses)

### Implementation
• Do not break, crush, or chew ext rel tabs
• May be given with meals or fluids or on an empty stomach

### Patient/family education
• Advise patient to avoid hazardous activities until response to product is known; dizziness, blurred vision may occur
• Caution patient to avoid OTC medication with alcohol or other CNS depressants
• Advise patient to prevent photophobia by wearing sunglasses
• Teach patient to use frequent rinsing of mouth, sips of water for dry mouth
• Teach patient to stay cool; avoid hot weather, strenuous activity since overheating may occur; product decreases perspiration
• Advise patient to report CNS effects: confusion, anxiety, anticholinergic effect in the geriatric

### Evaluation
**Positive therapeutic outcome**
• Absence of dysuria, frequency, nocturia, incontinence

---

### ⚠ HIGH ALERT

### oxycodone (Rx) ✓
(ox-i-koe'done)
Endocodone, M-oxy, OxyContin, OxyFast, Oxyl R, Roxicodone, Roxicodone SR, Supeudol ✦

### oxycodone/ acetaminophen (Rx) ✓
Endocet ✦, Oxycocet ✦, Percocet, Roxicet, Roxilox, Tylox

### oxycodone/aspirin (Rx)
Endodan ✦, Oxycodan ✦, Percodan, Percodan-Demi, Roxiprin

### oxycodone/ibuprofen (Rx)
Combunox
*Func. class.:* Opiate analgesic
*Chem. class.:* Semisynthetic derivative

**Pregnancy category B**
**Controlled substance schedule II**

**Do not confuse:**
Percodan/Decadron, Roxicet/Roxanol, Tylox/Trimox/Wymox/Xanax

**Action:** Inhibits ascending pain pathways in CNS, increases pain threshold, alters pain perception

**Therapeutic outcome:** Decreased pain

**Uses:** Moderate to severe pain

---

 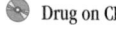

**Unlabeled uses:** Postherpetic neuralgia (cont rel)

## Dosage and routes
*Adult:* PO 10-30 mg q4hr (5 mg q6hr for Oxyl R, OxyFast); OxyFast conc sol is extremely concentrated, do not use interchangeably
*Child:* PO 0.05-0.15 mg/kg/dose up to 5 mg/dose q4-6hr; not recommended in children

**Available forms:** Oxycodone: cont rel tabs (OxyContin) 10, 20, 40, 80, 160 mg; immediate rel tabs 15, 30 mg; tabs 5 mg; immediate rel caps 5 mg; oral sol 5 mg/5 ml, 20 mg/ml; oxycodone with acetaminophen: tabs 5 mg/325 mg; caps 5 mg/500 mg; oral sol 5 mg/325 mg/5 ml; oxycodone with aspirin: 2.44, 4.88 mg/325 mg

## Adverse effects
*CNS: Drowsiness, dizziness, confusion, headache, sedation, euphoria,* fatigue, abnormal dreams, thoughts, hallucinations
*CV:* Palpitations, bradycardia, change in B/P
*EENT:* Tinnitus, blurred vision, miosis, diplopia
*GI: Nausea, vomiting, anorexia, constipation, cramps,* gastritis, dyspepsia, biliary spasms
*GU:* Increased urinary output, dysuria, urinary retention
*INTEG: Rash,* urticaria, bruising, flushing, diaphoresis, pruritus
***RESP: Respiratory depression***

**Contraindications:** Hypersensitivity, addiction (opiate)

**Precautions:** Pregnancy **B**, breastfeeding, children <18 yr, addictive personality, increased ICP, MI (acute), severe heart disease, respiratory depression, renal/hepatic disease, bowel impaction

### Pharmacokinetics

| | |
|---|---|
| Absorption | Well absorbed |
| Distribution | Widely distributed; crosses placenta, protein binding 45% |
| Metabolism | Liver, extensively |
| Excretion | Kidneys, breast milk |
| Half-life | 3-5 hr |

### Pharmacodynamics

| | PO | RECT |
|---|---|---|
| Onset | 15-30 min | Unknown |
| Peak | ½-1 hr | Unknown |
| Duration | 3-4 hr | 4-6 hr |

## Interactions
### Individual drugs
Alcohol: increased respiratory depression, hypotension, sedation
Cimetidine: increased toxicity
### Drug classifications
Antipsychotics, CNS depressants, opioids, sedative/hypnotics, skeletal muscle relaxants: increased respiratory depression, hypotension
MAOIs: increased toxicity
### Drug/herb
Corkwood: increased anticholinergic effect
Gotu kola, Jamaican dogwood, kava, lavender, mistletoe, nettle, pokeweed, poppy, senega, St. John's wort, valerian: increased sedative effect
### Drug/lab test
Increased: amylase, lipase

## NURSING CONSIDERATIONS
### Assessment
• Monitor VS after parenteral route; note muscle rigidity, product history, renal, liver function tests, respiratory dysfunction: respiratory depression, character, rate, rhythm; notify prescriber if respirations are <10/min
• Monitor CNS changes: dizziness, drowsiness, hallucinations, euphoria, LOC, pupil reaction
• Monitor allergic reactions: rash, urticaria

### Nursing diagnoses
• Breathing pattern, ineffective (adverse reactions)
• Injury, risk for (adverse reactions)
• Knowledge, deficient (teaching)
• Pain, acute (uses)
• Pain, chronic
• Sensory perception, disturbed: visual, auditory (adverse reactions)

### Implementation
• Give with antiemetic if nausea, vomiting occur
• Give when pain is beginning to return; determine dosage interval by patient response; continuous dosing of medication is more effective than when given prn
• Medication should be slowly withdrawn after long-term use to prevent withdrawal symptoms
• Store in light-resistant container at room temperature
**PO route**
• Do not break, crush, or chew cont rel tabs
• May be given with food or milk to lessen GI upset
• Use 80, 160 mg cont rel tabs only in opioid-tolerant patients

O

Adverse effects: *italic* = common, **bold** = life-threatening

**Rectal route**
• Store supp in the refrigerator; run under warm water before insertion

**Patient/family education**
• Advise patients to avoid CNS depressants: alcohol, sedative/hypnotics
• Discuss with patient that dizziness, drowsiness, and confusion are common; to avoid getting up without assistance
• Discuss in detail all aspects of the product, including purpose and what to expect
• Advise patient to make position changes slowly to lessen orthostatic hypotension
• Advise patient to avoid CNS depressants, alcohol
• Advise patient to avoid operating machinery, driving, if drowsiness occurs

**Evaluation**

**Positive therapeutic outcome**
• Decreased pain

**Treatment of overdose:** Naloxone 0.2-0.8 **IV**, O₂, **IV** fluids, vasopressors

---

**oxymetazoline nasal agent**
*See Appendix D*

---

**oxymetazoline ophthalmic**
*See Appendix D*

---

**❗ HIGH ALERT**

**oxymorphone** (Rx)
(ox-i-mor'fone)
Numorphan, Opana, Opana ER
*Func. class.:* Opiate analgesic
*Chem. class.:* Semisynthetic phenanthrene derivative

**Pregnancy category** B
**Controlled substance schedule** II

**Action:** Depresses pain impulse transmission at the spinal cord level by interacting with opioid receptors

**Therapeutic outcome:** Decreased pain

**Uses:** Moderate to severe pain

**Dosage and routes**
*Adult:* IM/SUBCUT 1-1.5 mg q4-6hr prn; **IV** 0.5 mg q4-6hr prn; RECT 5 mg q4-6hr prn; PO (immediate release only) 5-20 mg q4-6hr prn; PO-ER 5 mg q12hr in those requiring around the clock

*Labor analgesia*
*Adult:* IM 0.5-1 mg

**Available forms:** Inj 1, 1.5 mg/ml; supp 5 mg; ER tab 5, 10, 20, 40 mg; tabs 5, 10 mg

**Adverse effects**
***CNS:*** *Drowsiness, dizziness, confusion, headache, sedation, euphoria (geriatric)*, **seizures,** hallucinations, **increased ICP**
***CV:*** Palpitations, **bradycardia,** change in B/P, hypotension
***EENT:*** Tinnitus, blurred vision, miosis, diplopia
***GI:*** *Nausea, vomiting, anorexia, constipation, cramps*
***GU:*** Increased urinary output, dysuria, urinary retention
***INTEG:*** *Rash,* urticaria, bruising, flushing, diaphoresis, pruritus
***RESP:*** **Respiratory depression**

**Contraindications:** Hypersensitivity, addiction (opioid)

**Precautions:** Pregnancy **B** (short-term), breastfeeding, children <18 yr, addictive personality, increased ICP, MI (acute), severe heart disease, respiratory depression, renal/hepatic disease, bowel impaction

| Pharmacokinetics | |
|---|---|
| **Absorption** | Well absorbed (RECT, IM, SUBCUT); completely absorbed (**IV**) |
| **Distribution** | Widely distributed; crosses placenta |
| **Metabolism** | Liver, extensively |
| **Excretion** | Kidneys |
| **Half-life** | 2½-4 hr |

| Pharmacodynamics | | | |
|---|---|---|---|
| | IM/SUBCUT | IV | RECT |
| **Onset** | 15 min | 10 min | 30 min |
| **Peak** | 1-1½ hr | 15-30 min | Unknown |
| **Duration** | 3-6 hr | 3-4 hr | 3-6 hr |

**Interactions**
*Individual drugs*
Alcohol: increased respiratory depression, hypotension, sedation
*Drug classifications*
CNS depressants, opiates, antipsychotics, skeletal muscle relaxants, sedative/hypnotics: increased respiratory depression, hypotension
MAOIs: do not use 2 wk before oxymorphone; unpredictable effects
*Drug/herb*
Corkwood: increased anticholinergic effect
Gotu kola, Jamaican dogwood, kava, lavender,

mistletoe, nettle, pokeweed, poppy, senega, St. John's wort, valerian: increased sedative effect

*Drug/lab test*
Increased: amylase

## NURSING CONSIDERATIONS
### Assessment
• Monitor VS after parenteral route; note muscle rigidity, product history, liver, kidney function tests, respiratory dysfunction: respiratory depression, character, rate, rhythm; notify prescriber if respirations are <10/min
• Monitor CNS changes: dizziness, drowsiness, hallucinations, euphoria, LOC, pupil reaction
• Monitor allergic reactions: rash, urticaria

### Nursing diagnoses
• Breathing pattern, ineffective (adverse reactions)
• Injury, risk for (adverse reactions)
• Knowledge, deficient (teaching)
• Pain, acute (uses)
• Sensory perception, disturbed: visual, auditory (adverse reactions)

### Implementation
• Give 1 hr before or 2 hr after food (PO)
• Give with antiemetic if nausea, vomiting occur
• Give when pain is beginning to return; determine dosage interval by patient response; continuous dosing of medication is more effective than when given prn
• Medication should be slowly withdrawn after long-term use to prevent withdrawal symptoms
• Store in light-resistant container at room temperature
**Rectal route**
• Store in refrigerator
**IV route**
• Give by direct **IV** undiluted over 2-3 min
*Y-site compatibilities:* Glycopyrrolate, hydrOXYzine, ranitidine

### Patient/family education
• Advise patients to avoid CNS depressants: alcohol, sedative/hypnotics
• Discuss with patient that dizziness, drowsiness, and confusion are common; to avoid getting up without assistance
• Discuss in detail all aspects of the product, including purpose and what to expect
• Advise patient to make position changes slowly to lessen orthostatic hypotension
• Advise patient not to drive, operate machinery if drowsiness occurs
• Advise patient to avoid CNS depressants, alcohol

### Evaluation
**Positive therapeutic outcome**
• Decreased pain
**Treatment of overdose:** Naloxone (Narcan) 0.2-0.8 mg **IV**, O$_2$, **IV** fluids, vasopressors

---

## ! HIGH ALERT

## oxytocin (Rx)
(ox-i-toe'sin)
Pitocin
*Func. class.:* Oxytocic hormone
**Pregnancy category** N/A

**Action:** Acts directly on myofibrils, producing uterine contraction; stimulates breast milk letdown

**Therapeutic outcome:** Stimulation of labor, control of bleeding; stimulation of milk letdown

**Uses:** Stimulation, induction of labor; missed or incomplete abortion, postpartum bleeding, postpartum breast engorgement

### Dosage and routes
*Labor induction*
*Adult:* **IV** 1-2 milliunit/min, increase by 1-2 milliunit q15-60 min until regular contractions occur, then decrease dosage
*Postpartum hemorrhage*
*Adult:* **IV** 10-40 units in 1000 ml nonhydrating diluent infused at 20-40 mU/min
*Adult:* IM 10 units after placenta delivery
*Incomplete abortion*
*Adult:* **IV** INF 10 units/500 ml D$_5$W or 0.9% NaCl run at 20-40 mU/min; max 30 units/12 hr
*Fetal stress test*
*Adult:* **IV** 0.5 mU/min; increase q20 min until 3 contractions occur at 10 min
**Available forms:** Inj 10 units/ml
### Adverse effects
*CNS:* **Seizures, tetanic contractions**
*CV:* Hypo/hypertension, dysrhythmias, increased pulse, bradycardia, tachycardia, premature ventricular contractions
*FETUS:* Dysrhythmias, jaundice, hypoxia, **intracranial hemorrhage**
*GI:* Anorexia, nausea, vomiting, constipation
*GU:* **Abruptio placentae, decreased uterine blood flow**
*HEMA:* Increased hyperbilirubinemia
*INTEG:* Rash
*RESP:* **Asphyxia**
*SYST:* Water intoxication of mother

Adverse effects: *italic* = common, **bold** = life-threatening

**Contraindications:** Hypersensitivity, serum toxemia, cephalopelvic disproportion, fetal distress, hypertonic uterus, prolapsed umbilical cord, active genital herpes

**Precautions:** Cervical/uterine surgery, uterine sepsis, primipara >35 yr, 1st/2nd stage of labor

### Pharmacokinetics

| Absorption | Well absorbed (nasal); completely absorbed (**IV**) |
|---|---|
| Distribution | Widely distributed (extracellular fluid) |
| Metabolism | Liver, rapidly |
| Excretion | Kidneys |
| Half-life | 3-12 min |

### Pharmacodynamics

|  | NASAL | IV | IM |
|---|---|---|---|
| Onset | 5 min | Rapid | 3-7 min |
| Peak | Unknown | Unknown | Unknown |
| Duration | 20 min | 1 hr | 1 hr |

### Interactions
#### Drug classifications
Vasopressors: increased hypertension
#### Drug/herb
Ephedra: hypertension

### NURSING CONSIDERATIONS
#### Assessment
• Assess labor contractions: fetal heart tones, frequency, duration, intensity of contractions; if fetal heart tones increase or decrease significantly or if contractions are longer than 1 min, notify prescriber; turn patient on left side to increase oxygen to fetus
◆ Assess for water intoxication: confusion, anuria, drowsiness, headache; notify prescriber
• Watch for fetal distress, acceleration, deceleration, fetal presentation, pelvic dimensions
• Monitor B/P, pulse, respiratory rate, rhythm, depth
• Monitor I&O ratio
• Provide an environment conducive to letdown reflex

#### Nursing diagnoses
• Breastfeeding, ineffective (uses)
• Injury, risk for (uses)
• Knowledge, deficient (teaching)

#### Implementation
**IV route**
• Use an infusion pump; rotate sol for mixing; have magnesium sulfate available

• For labor induction administer after diluting 10 units/L of $D_5W$, 0.9% NaCl, 0.45% NaCl, LR, Ringer's for a conc of 10 units/ml; start at 1-2 units/min (0.1-0.2 ml); may increase by 1-2 units/min q15-30 min until labor begins
• For threatened abortion administer after diluting 10 units/500 ml of $D_5W$, $D_{10}W$, 0.9% NaCl, 0.45% NaCl, LR, Ringer's for a conc of 20 units/ml; give at 10-40 units/min
• For postpartum bleeding administer after diluting 10-40 units/L of $D_5W$, $D_{10}W$, 0.9% NaCl, 0.45% NaCl, LR, Ringer's for a conc of 10-40 units/ml; may titrate to response

**Y-site compatibilities:** Heparin, regular insulin, hydrocortisone, meperidine, morphine, potassium chloride, vit B/C, warfarin
**Additive compatibilities:** Chloramphenicol, metaraminol, netilmicin, sodium bicarbonate, thiopental, verapamil
**Additive incompatibilities:** Fibrinolysin, warfarin

#### Patient/family education
• Teach patient to report increased blood loss, abdominal cramps, increased temp or foul-smelling lochia
• Advise patient that contractions will be similar to menstrual cramps, gradually increasing in intensity

#### Evaluation
**Positive therapeutic outcome**
• Stimulation of milk letdown (nasal)
• Induction of labor
• Decreased postpartum bleeding

---

## paclitaxel (Rx)
(pa-kli-tax'el)
Onxol, Taxol
## paclitaxel protein-bound particles (Rx)
Abraxane
*Func. class.:* Antineoplastic—miscellaneous
*Chem. class.:* Natural diterpene, antimicrotubule

### Pregnancy category D

**Do not confuse:**
paclitaxel/paroxetine/Paxil, Taxol/Paxil/Taxotera

**Action:** Inhibits the reorganization of the microtubule network needed for interphase and mitotic cellular functions; also causes abnormal bundles of microtubules during cell cycle and multiple esters of microtubules during mitosis

**Therapeutic outcome:** Prevention of rapidly growing malignant cells

**Uses:** Taxol: metastatic carcinoma of the ovary unresponsive to other treatment, breast carcinoma; AIDS-related Kaposi's sarcoma (second line), non–small cell lung cancer (first line), adjuvant treatment for node-positive breast cancer; Onxol: failure of other treatment in breast cancer, advanced ovarian cancer, bladder cancer

**Unlabeled uses:** Advanced head, neck, small cell lung cancer; non-Hodgkin's lymphoma, adenocarcinoma of the upper GI tract, hormone-refractory prostate cancer

## Dosage and routes
### Paclitaxel
#### Ovarian carcinoma
**Adult: IV** INF 135 mg/m$^2$ given over 24 hr q3 wk, then cisplatin 75 mg/m$^2$ or 175 mg/m$^2$ over 3 hr q3 wk or 175 mg/m$^2$ over 3 hr

#### Advanced ovarian carcinoma
**Adult: IV** INF 175 mg/m$^2$ with cisplatin 75 mg/m$^2$ over 3 hr q3 wk

#### Breast carcinoma
**Adult: IV** INF 175 mg/m$^2$ over 3 hr q3 wk × 4 courses

#### AIDS-related Kaposi's sarcoma
**Adult: IV** INF 135 mg/m$^2$ over 3 hr q3 wk or 100 mg/m$^2$ over 3 hr q2 wk

#### 1st line non–small cell lung cancer
**Adult: IV** INF 135 mg/m$^2$/24 hr with cisplatin 75 mg/m$^2$ × 3 wk

### Paclitaxel protein-bound particles
**Adult: IV** 260 mg/m$^2$ q3wk

**Available forms:** Inj 30 mg/5-ml vial, 100 mg/16.7-ml vial, 150 mg/24-ml vial, 300 mg/5-ml vials; powder for inj, lyophilized 100 mg in single-use vials (Abraxane)

## Adverse effects
*CV: Bradycardia, hypotension, abnormal ECG*
*GI: Nausea, vomiting, diarrhea, mucositis; increased bilirubin, alkaline phosphatase, AST*
**HEMA: Neutropenia, leukopenia, thrombocytopenia, anemia,** bleeding, infections
*INTEG: Alopecia*
*MS: Arthralgia, myalgia*
*NEURO: Peripheral neuropathy*
*SYST: Hypersensitivity reactions,* **anaphylaxis, Stevens-Johnson syndrome, toxic epidermal necrolysis**

**Contraindications:** Pregnancy **D,** hypersensitivity to paclitaxel or other products with polyoxyethylated castor oil, neutropenia (neutrophils <1500/mm$^3$)

**Precautions:** Breastfeeding, children, CV/hepatic disease, CNS disorder

### Pharmacokinetics
| | |
|---|---|
| **Absorption** | Completely absorbed |
| **Distribution** | 89%-98% protein binding |
| **Metabolism** | Liver, extensively |
| **Excretion** | Unknown |
| **Half-life** | 5-17 hr |

### Pharmacodynamics
| | |
|---|---|
| **Onset** | Unknown |
| **Peak** | 1-2 wk |
| **Duration** | 3 wk |

## Interactions
### Individual drugs
CycloSPORINE, dexamethasone, diazepam, etoposide, quinidine, teniposide, testosterone, verapamil, vinCRIStine: decreased metabolism of paclitaxel
DOXOrubicin: increased levels of DOXOrubicin
Ketoconazole: increased toxicity, decreased metabolism; avoid concurrent use
Radiation: increased myelosuppression
### Drug classifications
Anticoagulants, NSAIDs: increased bleeding risk
Antineoplastics: increased myelosuppression
CYP2C8, CYP2C9 inducers: decreased paclitaxel level
Vaccines (live virus): decreased immune response

## NURSING CONSIDERATIONS
### Assessment
• Assess CNS changes: confusion, paresthesias, psychosis, tremors, seizures, neuropathies; product should be discontinued
• Check buccal cavity q8hr for dryness, sores or ulceration, white patches, oral pain, bleeding, dysphagia; obtain prescription for viscous lidocaine (Xylocaine) to use in mouth
• Assess symptoms indicating severe allergic reaction, anaphylaxis: rash, pruritus, urticaria, purpuric skin lesions, itching, flushing
• Monitor CBC, differential, platelet count weekly; withhold product if WBC is <1500/mm$^3$ or platelet count is <100,000/mm$^3$, notify prescriber of results
• Monitor renal function tests: BUN, creatinine, serum uric acid, urine CCr before and during therapy; check I&O ratio; report fall in urine output to <30 ml/hr

P

Adverse effects: *italic* = common, **bold** = life-threatening

- Monitor temp q4hr (may indicate beginning of infection)
- Monitor liver function tests before and during therapy (bilirubin, AST, ALT, LDH) as needed or monthly; check for jaundice of skin and sclera, dark urine, clay-colored stools, itchy skin, abdominal pain, fever, diarrhea
- Assess for bleeding: hematuria, stool guaiac, bruising or petechiae, mucosa or orifices q8hr; check for inflammation of mucosa, breaks in skin
- Assess effects of alopecia on body image; discuss feelings about body changes

## Nursing diagnoses
- Body image, disturbed (adverse reactions)
- Infection, risk for (adverse reactions)
- Injury, risk for (adverse reactions)
- Knowledge, deficient (teaching)

## Implementation
- Give fluids PO before chemotherapy to hydrate patient
- Give antacid before oral agent; give product after evening meal, before bedtime; provide antiemetic 30-60 min before giving product and prn to prevent vomiting; administer antibiotics for prophylaxis of infection
- Give topical or systemic analgesics for pain to lessen effects of stomatitis
- Give liquid diet: carbonated beverages; gelatin may be added if patient is not nauseated or vomiting

**IV route**
- Give after diluting in 0.9% NaCl, D$_5$, D$_5$ and 0.9% NaCl, D$_5$LR to a concentration of 0.3-1.2 mg/ml
- Use an in-line filter ≤0.22 mcg
- Give after premedicating with dexamethasone 20 mg PO 12 and 6 hr before paclitaxel, diphenhydrAMINE 50 mg **IV** ½-1 hr before paclitaxel and cimetidine 300 mg or ranitidine 50 mg **IV** ½-1 hr before paclitaxel
- Use only glass bottles, polypropylene, polyolefin bags and administration sets; do not use PVC infusion bags or sets
- Use gloves and cytotoxic handling precautions

**Abraxane**
- Reconstitute vial by injecting 20 ml of 0.9% NaCl
- Slowly inject the 20 ml of 0.9% NaCl over at least 1 min to direct the sol flow on wall of vial
- Do not inject 0.9% NaCl directly onto lyophilized cake (foaming will occur)
- Allow vial to sit for at least 5 min to ensure proper wetting of lyophilized cake
- Gently swirl or invert vial slowly for at least 2 min until completely dissolved

- Calculate dosing by: Dosing volume (ml) = total dose (mg) ÷ 5 (mg/ml)

**Y-site compatiblilities:** Acyclovir, amikacin, aminophylline, bleomycin, butorphanol, calcium chloride, carboplatin, cefepime, cefotetan, ceftazidime, ceftriaxone, cimetidine, cisplatin, cyclophosphamide, cytarabine, dacarbazine, dexamethasone, diphenhydrAMINE, DOXOrubicin, droperidol, etoposide, famotidine, floxuridine, fluconazole, fluorouracil, furosemide, ganciclovir, gentamicin, haloperidol, heparin, mannitol, meperidine, mesna, methotrexate, metoclopramide, morphine, nalbuphine, ondansetron, pentostatin, potassium chloride, prochlorperazine, propofol, ranitidine, sodium bicarbonate, vancomycin, vinBLAStine, vinCRIStine, zidovudine

## Patient/family education
- Inform patient that nonhormonal contraceptive measures are recommended during therapy and >4 mo after; teratogenic effects are possible
- Teach patient to avoid use of products containing aspirin or ibuprofen, razors, commercial mouthwash, since bleeding may occur; to report symptoms of bleeding (hematuria, tarry stools)
- Instruct patient to report signs of anemia (fatigue, headache, irritability, faintness, shortness of breath) and CNS reactions (confusion, psychosis, nightmares, seizures, severe headaches)
- Teach patient to rinse mouth tid-qid with water, club soda; brush teeth bid-qid with soft brush or cotton-tipped applicators for stomatitis; use unwaxed dental floss
- Inform patient that hair may be lost during treatment; a wig or hairpiece may make patient feel better; new hair may be different in color, texture
- Inform patient that receiving vaccinations during therapy may cause serious reactions

## Evaluation
**Positive therapeutic outcome**
- Prevention of rapid division of malignant cells

## paliperidone (Rx)

(pal-ee-per'i-done)

Invega

*Func. class.:* Antipsychotic

*Chem. class.:* Benzisoxazole derivative

**Pregnancy category C**

**Action:** Mediated through both dopamine type 2 ($D_2$) and serotonin type 2 (5-HT$_2$) antagonism

**Therapeutic outcome:** Decrease in emotional excitement, hallucinations, delusions, paranoia; reorganization of patterns of thought, speech

**Uses:** Schizophrenia

**Dosage and routes**

*Adult:* PO 6 mg/day

**Available forms:** Ext rel tabs 3, 6, 9 mg

**Adverse effects**

*CNS: EPS, pseudoparkinsonism, akathisia, dystonia, tardive dyskinesia; drowsiness, insomnia, agitation, anxiety, headache,* **seizures, neuroleptic malignant syndrome,** dizziness

*CV:* Orthostatic hypotension, **tachycardia, heart failure, QT prolongation**

*EENT:* Blurred vision

*GI: Nausea,* vomiting, *anorexia, constipation,* weight gain

**Contraindications:** Breastfeeding, seizure disorders, AV block, geriatric, QT prolongation, torsade de pointes, hypersensitivity to this product or risperidone

**Precautions:** Pregnancy **C**, children, renal/hepatic disease, obesity, Parkinson's disease

### Pharmacokinetics

| | |
|---|---|
| **Absorption** | Unknown |
| **Distribution** | Unknown |
| **Metabolism** | Unknown |
| **Excretion** | 80% urine, 11% feces |
| **Half-life** | Elimination 23 hr |

### Pharmacodynamics

| | |
|---|---|
| **Onset** | Unknown |
| **Peak** | 24 hr |
| **Duration** | Unknown |

**Interactions**

*Individual drugs*

Abarelix, alfuzosin, amoxapine, apomorphine, chloroquine, dasatinib, dolasetron, droperi-

dol, flecainide, pimozide, probucol: increased QT prolongation

Alcohol: increased sedation

Levodopa: decreased levodopa effect

Paliperidone: increased excretion

*Drug classifications*

Azole antifungals; β-blockers; class IA, III antidysrhythmics; halogenated anesthetics; some antipsychotics; some phenothiazines; tricyclics (high doses): increased QT prolongation

Other antipsychotics: increased EPS

Other CNS depressants: increased sedation

*Drug/herb*

Betel palm, kava: increased EPS

Cola tree, hops, nettle, nutmeg: increased action

Kava: increased CNS depression

*Drug/lab test*

Increased: prolactin levels

**NURSING CONSIDERATIONS**

**Assessment**

• Assess mental status before initial administration

• Monitor for swallowing of PO medication; check for hoarding or giving of medication to other patients

• Monitor I&O ratio; palpate bladder if urinary output is low

• Assess affect, orientation, LOC, reflexes, gait, coordination, sleep pattern disturbances

• Monitor B/P standing and lying; also pulse, respirations; take these q4hr during initial treatment; establish baseline before starting treatment; report drops of 30 mm Hg; watch for ECG changes

• Assess for dizziness, faintness, palpitations, tachycardia on rising

• Assess for EPS, including akathisia, tardive dyskinesia (bizarre movements of the jaw, mouth, tongue, extremities), pseudoparkinsonism (rigidity, tremors, pill rolling, shuffling gait)

⬥ Assess for serious reactions in the geriatric patient

⬥ Assess for neuroleptic malignant syndrome: hyperthermia, increased CPK, altered mental status, muscle rigidity

• Assess skin turgor daily

• Assess for constipation, urinary retention daily; if these occur, increase bulk and water in diet

**Nursing diagnoses**

• Knowledge, deficient (teaching)

• Noncompliance (teaching)

• Thought processes, disturbed (uses)

P

## Implementation

- Do not break, crush, or chew ext rel tabs
- Give without regard for food
- Give a reduced dose to the geriatric patient
- Give antiparkinsonian agent on order from prescriber; to be used for EPS
- Avoid use with CNS depressants
- Supervise ambulation until patient is stabilized on medication; do not involve in strenuous exercise program because fainting is possible; patient should not stand still for a long time
- Increase fluids to prevent constipation
- Provide sips of water, candy, gum for dry mouth
- Store in airtight, light-resistant container

## Patient/family education

- Advise patient that orthostatic hypotension may occur and to rise from sitting or lying position gradually
- Advise patient to avoid hot tubs, hot showers, tub baths; hypotension may occur
- Caution patient to avoid abrupt withdrawal of this product; EPS may result; product should be withdrawn slowly
- Teach patient to avoid OTC preparations (cough, hay fever, cold) unless approved by prescriber; serious product interactions may occur; avoid use of alcohol; increased drowsiness may occur
- Advise patient to avoid hazardous activities if drowsy or dizzy
- Teach patient compliance with product regimen
- Teach patient to report impaired vision, tremors, muscle twitching
- Caution patient that heat stroke may occur in hot weather; take extra precautions to stay cool
- Teach patient to use contraception, inform prescriber if pregnancy is planned or suspected

## Evaluation

**Positive therapeutic outcome**

- Decrease in emotional excitement, hallucinations, delusions, paranoia; reorganization of patterns of thought, speech

**Treatment of overdose:** Lavage if orally ingested; provide airway; *do not induce vomiting*

## palivizumab (Rx)

(pal-ih-viz'uh-mab)

Synagis

*Func. class.:* Monoclonal antibody

### Pregnancy category C

**Action:** A humanized monoclonal antibody that exhibits neutralizing and fusion-inhibitory activity against respiratory syncytial virus (RSV)

**Therapeutic outcome:** Absence of RSV

**Uses:** Prevention of serious lower respiratory tract disease caused by RSV in pediatric patients

### Dosage and routes

*Child:* IM 15 mg/kg, those patients who develop RSV should receive monthly doses during RSV season (November-April)

**Available forms:** Powder for reconstitution 50, 100 mg; solution 50 mg/0.5 ml, 100 mg/1 mg

### Adverse effects

*CNS:* Fever

*EENT:* Otitis media, rhinitis, pharyngitis

*GI:* Nausea, vomiting, diarrhea, increased AST

*INTEG:* Rash, inj site reaction

*RESP:* Upper respiratory tract infection, **apnea,** cough

*SYST:* **Anaphylaxis**

**Contraindications:** Hypersensitivity, adults, cyanotic congenital heart disease

**Precautions:** Pregnancy **C,** thrombocytopenia, coagulation disorders, established RSV, congenital heart disease, chronic lung disease, systemic allergic reactions

| Pharmacokinetics | |
|---|---|
| **Absorption** | Unknown |
| **Distribution** | Unknown |
| **Metabolism** | Unknown |
| **Excretion** | Unknown |
| **Half-life** | 20 days |

| Pharmacodynamics |
|---|
| Unknown |

## NURSING CONSIDERATIONS

### Assessment

- Assess for presence of RSV infection; product is given to prevent infection
- Assess for side effects and report if allergic reaction is evident

◆ Assess for anaphylaxis: difficulty breathing, product should be discontinued, have emergency equipment nearby

## Nursing diagnoses
• Infection, risk for (uses)
• Knowledge, deficient (teaching)

## Implementation
• Give IM only
• Give after adding 1 ml of sterile water for inj per 100 mg vial (add 0.6 ml sterile water for inj for 50 mg vial); gently swirl for 30 sec to avoid foaming, do not shake; let stand at room temperature for 20 min until sol clarifies; given within 6 hr of reconstitution

## Patient/family education
• Teach patient to report upper respiratory infections, earaches, rash, sore throat

## Evaluation
**Positive therapeutic outcome**
• Absence of RSV

## palonosetron (Rx)
(pa-lone-o'se-tron)
Aloxi
*Func. class.:* Antiemetic
*Chem. class.:* 5-HT$_3$ receptor antagonist
**Pregnancy category** B

**Action:** Prevents nausea, vomiting by blocking serotonin peripherally, centrally, and in the small intestine at the 5-HT$_3$ receptor

**Therapeutic outcome:** Decreased nausea, vomiting during chemotherapy

**Uses:** Prevention of nausea, vomiting associated with cancer chemotherapy

## Dosage and routes
*Adult:* **IV** 0.25 mg as a single dose over 30 sec, 30 min prior to chemotherapy, max 25 mg **IV** over q7 days

**Available forms:** Inj 0.25 mg/5 ml

## Adverse effects
*CNS: Headache, dizziness, drowsiness, fatigue, insomnia*
*GI: Diarrhea, constipation,* abdominal pain
*MISC:* Weakness, hyperkalemia, anxiety, rash, **bronchospasm** (rare), arthralgia, *fever, urinary retention*

**Contraindications:** Hypersensitivity

**Precautions:** Pregnancy **B**, breastfeeding, children, geriatric, prolongation of QT interval or other cardiac conduction intervals (patients with hypokalemia, hypomagnesemia, taking diuretics, with congenital QT syndrome, and taking antidysrhythmics or other products that may prolong QT interval and cumulative high-dose antithramycline therapy)

### Pharmacokinetics
| | |
|---|---|
| **Absorption** | Unknown |
| **Distribution** | 62% protein bound |
| **Metabolism** | Liver |
| **Excretion** | Unchanged product and metabolites excreted by kidney |
| **Half-life** | 40 hr |

### Pharmacodynamics
Unknown

## NURSING CONSIDERATIONS
### Assessment
• Monitor for absence of nausea, vomiting during chemotherapy
• Assess hypersensitivity reaction: rash, bronchospasm

### Nursing diagnoses
• Knowledge, deficient (teaching)

### Implementation
**IV route**
• Give as a single dose over 30 sec
• Do not mix with other products, flush **IV** line before and after administration
• Store at room temperature

### Patient/family education
• Teach to report diarrhea, constipation, rash, or changes in respirations or discomfort at insertion site

### Evaluation
**Positive therapeutic outcome**
• Absence of nausea, vomiting during cancer chemotherapy

## pamidronate (Rx)
(pam-i-drone'ate)
Aredia
*Func. class.:* Bone resorption inhibitor, electrolyte modifier
*Chem. class.:* Bisphosphonate
**Pregnancy category** D

**Do not confuse:**
Aredia/Adriamycin

**Action:** Inhibits bone resorption, apparently without inhibiting bone formation and mineralization; absorbs calcium phosphate crystals in bone and may directly block dissolution of hydroxyapatite crystals of bone

Adverse effects: *italic* = common, **bold** = life-threatening

**Therapeutic outcome:** Serum calcium at normal level

**Uses:** Moderate to severe Paget's disease associated with malignancy with or without bone metastases; osteolytic bone metastases in breast cancer patients, multiple myeloma

**Unlabeled uses:** Postmenopausal osteoporosis, hyperparathyroidism, reduction of bone pain in prostatic carcinoma, immobilization-related hypercalcemia

## Dosage and routes
*Hypercalcemia of malignancy*
*Adult:* **IV** INF 60-90 mg as a single dose in moderate hypercalcemia, 90 mg in severe hypercalcemia given over 24 hr; dose should be diluted in 1000 ml 0.45% NaCl, 0.9% NaCl, or D₅W; wait 7 days before 2nd course

*Osteolytic lesions from multiple myeloma*
*Adult:* **IV** 90 mg/500 ml of D₅W, 0.45% NaCl, or 0.9% NaCl given over 4 hr on a monthly basis

*Paget's disease*
*Adult:* **IV** 90-180 mg/treatment, may use 30 mg/day × 3 days

**Available forms:** Powder for inj 30, 90 mg/vial; inj 3, 6, 9 mg/ml

## Adverse effects
*CNS:* Fatigue, fever, psychosis
*CV:* Hypertension
*EENT:* Ocular pain, inflammation, vision impairment
*GI: Abdominal pain, anorexia, constipation, nausea, vomiting,* diarrhea, dyspepsia
*GU:* UTI, fluid overload, **renal failure**
*INTEG:* Redness, swelling, induration, pain on palpation at site of catheter insertion
*META:* Anemia, hypokalemia, hypomagnesemia, hypophosphatemia, hypocalcemia, hypothyroidism
*MS: Bone pain,* myalgia, **osteonecrosis of the jaw**
*RESP:* Coughing, dyspnea, URI
*SYST:* **Angioedema, anaphylaxis**

**Contraindications:** Pregnancy **D**, hypersensitivity to bisphosphonates

**Precautions:** Children, nursing mothers, renal dysfunction, poor dentition

| Pharmacokinetics | |
|---|---|
| **Absorption** | Rapidly cleared from circulation |
| **Distribution** | Mainly to bones, primarily in areas of high bone turnover |
| **Metabolism** | Unknown |
| **Excretion** | Kidneys, unchanged (50%) |
| **Half-life** | Biphasic 1½ hr; 27 hr; from bone to 300 days |

| Pharmacodynamics | |
|---|---|
| **Onset** | 1 day |
| **Peak** | 1 wk |
| **Duration** | Unknown |

## Interactions
*Individual drugs*
Calcium, vitamin D: decreased pamidronate effect
Digoxin: increased hypomagnesemia, hypokalemia

## NURSING CONSIDERATIONS
### Assessment
• Assess for hypocalcemia: Chvostek's, Trousseau's sign, paresthesia, twitching, laryngospasm
• Monitor manifestations of hypocalcemia: personality changes, anxiety, disturbances, depression, psychosis; nausea, vomiting, constipation, abdominal pain from muscle spasm; decreased contractility, decreased cardiac output, hypotension, lengthened ST segment, prolonged QT interval; scaling eczema, alopecia, hyperpigmentation; tetany, muscle twitching, cramping, grimacing, seizure, altered deep tendon reflexes, spasm
• Monitor manifestations of hypomagnesemia: agitation; muscle twitching, paresthesia, hyperactive reflexes, positive Babinski reflex, dysphagia, nystagmus, seizures, tetany; nausea, vomiting, diarrhea, anorexia, abdominal distention; ectopy, tachycardia, broad, flat, or inverted T waves, depressed ST segment, prolonged QT interval, decreased cardiac output, hypotension
• Monitor manifestations of hypokalemia: acidic urine, reduced urine osmolality, nocturia, polyuria, polydipsia; hypotension, broad T wave, U wave, ectopy, tachycardia, weak pulse; muscle weakness, altered LOC, drowsiness, apathy, lethargy, confusion, depression; anorexia, nausea, cramps, constipation, distention, paralytic ileus; hypoventilation, respiratory muscle weakness
• Assess fluid volume status: check I&O ratio and record, assess for distended red veins, crackles in lung, color, quality, and specific

gravity of urine, skin turgor, adequacy of pulses, moist mucous membranes, bilateral lung sounds, peripheral pitting edema
• Monitor electrolytes: phosphorus, potassium, sodium, calcium, magnesium; also include BUN, creatinine, CBC, platelets, hemoglobin
• Assess B/P before and during therapy
• Assess for pain: in joints or on exertion, duration and characteristics; analgesics may be ordered
• Assess for phlebitis at **IV** site: swelling, redness, pain, warmth

### Nursing diagnoses
• Fluid volume, excess (side effects)
• Injury, risk for (uses, adverse reactions)
• Knowledge, deficient (teaching)

### Implementation
• Give by **IV** inf after reconstituting by adding 10 ml of sterile water for inj to each vial, then adding to 1000 ml of sterile 0.45%, 0.9% NaCl, D$_5$W, run over 4 hr for hypercalcemia or 60 mg ≥4 hr, 90 mg/24 hr; dilute reconstituted sol in 500 ml of 0.9% NaCl, 0.45% NaCl, or D$_5$W, give over 4 hr (multiple myeloma, Paget's disease)
• Do not mix with calcium-containing infusion sol such as Ringer's sol
• Store inf sol for up to 24 hr at room temperature
• Reconstituted sol with sterile water may be stored under refrigeration for up to 24 hr

*Additive incompatibilities:*
Calcium products, sol

### Patient/family education
• Advise patient to report hypercalcemic relapse: nausea, vomiting, bone pain, thirst; unusual muscle twitching, muscle spasms, severe diarrhea, constipation, ocular symptoms
• Advise patient to continue with dietary recommendations, including calcium and vit D
• To obtain an analgesic from provider for bone pain
• That, if nausea/vomiting occur, small, frequent meals may help

### Evaluation
**Positive therapeutic outcome**
• Decreased calcium levels to normal

---

## pancrelipase (Rx)
(pan-kre-li´pase)
Cotazym, Cotazym-65B ♦, Cotazym E.C.S. 8, Cotazym E.C.S. 20, Cotazym Capsules, Cotazym-S, Creon, Ilozyme, Ku-Zyme HP, Lipram-PN16, Lipram-CR20, Lipram-UL12, Lipram-PN10, Pancrease Capsules, Pancrease MT 4, Pancrease MT 10, Pancrease MT 16, Protilase, Ultrase MT 12, Ultrase MT 20, Viokase, Zymase
*Func. class.:* Digestant
*Chem. class.:* Pancreatic enzyme (bovine/porcine)

**Pregnancy category  B**

**Action:** Pancreatic enzyme needed for breakdown of substances released from the pancreas

**Therapeutic outcome:** Increases protein, fat, carbohydrate digestion

**Uses:** Exocrine pancreatic secretion insufficiency, cystic fibrosis (digestive aid), steatorrhea, pancreatic enzyme deficiency

**Dosage and routes**
Many products listed above are not interchangeable
*Adult and child:* PO 1-3 cap/tab before or with meals, or 1 cap/tab with snack or 1-2 powder packets before meals

**Available forms:** Powder 16,800 units lipase/70,000 units protease and amylase; caps 8000 units lipase/30,000 units protease and amylase; delayed rel caps, 4000 units lipase/12,000 units protease and amylase, 4000 units lipase/25,000 units protease/20,000 units amylase, 5000 units lipase/20,000 units protease and amylase, 10,000 units lipase/30,000 units protease and amylase, 12,000 units lipase/24,000 units protease and amylase, 12,000 units lipase/39,000 units protease and amylase, 16,000 units lipase/48,000 units protease and amylase 20,000 units lipase/65,000 units protease and amylase, 24,000 units lipase/78,000 units protease and amylase

**Adverse effects**
*GI:* Anorexia, nausea, vomiting, diarrhea, cramping, bloating
*GU:* Hyperuricuria, hyperuricemia

**Contraindications:** Allergy to pork

**Precautions:** Pregnancy **B**, ileus, pancreatitis, Crohn's disease

P

## Pharmacokinetics
Unknown

## Pharmacodynamics
Unknown

## Interactions
*Individual drugs*
Acarbose, miglitol: decreased effects of each specific drug
Cimetidine, iron (oral): decreased absorption of pancrelipase
*Drug classifications*
Antacids: decreased absorption of pancreli- pase

## NURSING CONSIDERATIONS
### Assessment
• Monitor I&O ratio; watch for increasing urinary output
• Monitor fecal fat, nitrogen, pro-time, during treatment
• Monitor for polyuria, polydipsia, polyphagia (may indicate diabetes mellitus)
• Assess for allergy to pork; patient may also be sensitive to this product
• Assess for appropriate weight, height, development; there may be a developmental lag
• Check stools for steatorrhea, which signifies undigested fat content

### Nursing diagnoses
• Knowledge, deficient (teaching)
• Nutrition: less than body requirements, imbalanced (uses)

### Implementation
• Avoid inhaling powder
• Give tab with 8 oz of water and sitting up only; do not let tab sit in mouth; give with meals
• Give after antacid or cimetidine; decreased pH inactivates product
• Give powder mixed in prepared fruit for infants, children
• Administer low-fat diet to decrease GI symptoms
• Provide adequate hydration
• Store in airtight container at room tempera- ture

### Patient/family education
• Teach patient to take tab with 8 oz or more water, not to let tab sit in mouth; have patient take tab sitting up only
• Advise patient to notify prescriber of allergic reactions, abdominal pain, cramping, or hematuria

• Teach patient not to inhale powder, very irritating to mucous membranes, some powder may irritate skin

### Evaluation
**Positive therapeutic outcome**
• Absence of steatorrhea
• Improved digestion of carbohydrates, proteins, fat

---

## ⚠ HIGH ALERT

### pancuronium (Rx)
(pan-cure-oh'nee-yum)
pancuronium bromide, Pavulon
*Func. class.:* Neuromuscular blocker (nondepolarizing)
*Chem. class.:* Synthetic curariform

**Pregnancy category C**

**Action:** Inhibits transmission of nerve impulses by binding with cholinergic receptor sites, antagonizing action of acetylcholine; no analgesic response

**Therapeutic outcome:** Paralysis of all skeletal muscles

**Uses:** Facilitation of endotracheal intubation, skeletal muscle relaxation during mechanical ventilation, surgery, or general anesthesia

### Dosage and routes
*Adult/child/infant >1 mo:* **IV** 0.06-0.1 mg/kg initially or 0.05 mg/kg after initial dose of succinylcholine; maintenance 0.01 mg/kg 60-100 min after initial dose, then 0.01 mg/kg q25-60 min as needed
*Neonate <1 mo:* **IV** Test dose 0.02 mg/kg, then 0.03 mg/kg/dose initially, repeat 2× as needed at 5-10 min intervals; mainte- nance 0.03-0.09 mg/kg/dose q30 min-4 hr as needed

**Available forms:** Inj 1, 2 mg/ml

### Adverse effects
*CV:* Bradycardia, tachycardia, increased, decreased B/P, ventricular extrasystoles, edema, hypotension
*EENT:* Increased secretions
*INTEG:* Rash, flushing, pruritus, urticaria, sweating, salivation
*MS:* Weakness to prolonged skeletal muscle relaxation
***RESP:* Prolonged apnea, bronchospasm, cyanosis, respiratory depression,** dyspnea
*SYST:* **Anaphylaxis**

**Contraindications:** Hypersensitivity to bromide ion

---

**Precautions:** Pregnancy **C**, breastfeeding, children <2 yr, renal/hepatic/cardiac/neuromuscular/respiratory disease, electrolyte imbalances, dehydration, previous anaphylactic reactions (other neuromuscular blockers)

### Pharmacokinetics

| | |
|---|---|
| **Absorption** | Complete bioavailability |
| **Distribution** | Extracellular space; crosses placenta |
| **Metabolism** | Plasma |
| **Excretion** | Kidneys, unchanged |
| **Half-life** | 2 hr |

### Pharmacodynamics

| | |
|---|---|
| **Onset** | 3-5 min, dose dependent |
| **Peak** | 3-5 min |
| **Duration** | 35-40 min |

### Interactions
*Individual products*
Clindamycin, enflurane, isoflurane, lincomycin, lithium, quinidine: increased neuromuscular blockade
Theophylline: dysrhythmias
*Drug classifications*
Aminoglycosides, anesthetics (local), analgesics (opioid), polymyxin antiinfectives, thiazides: increased neuromuscular blockade
*Drug/lab test*
Decreased: cholinesterase

### NURSING CONSIDERATIONS
**Assessment**
• Monitor vital signs (B/P, pulse, respirations, airway) until fully recovered; note rate, depth, pattern of respirations, strength of hand grip; patient should be intubated before use
• Monitor for electrolyte imbalances (potassium, magnesium) before product is used; electrolyte imbalances may lead to increased action of this product
• Monitor for recovery: decreased paralysis of face, diaphragm, leg, arm, rest of body; residual weakness and respiratory problems may occur during recovery period
♦ Assess for hypersensitive reactions, anaphylaxis: rash, fever, respiratory distress, pruritus; product should be discontinued

**Nursing diagnoses**
• Breathing pattern, ineffective (uses)
• Communication, impaired verbal (adverse reactions)
• Fear (adverse reactions)
• Knowledge, deficient (teaching)

**Implementation**
• Use peripheral nerve stimulator (anesthesiologist) to determine neuromuscular blockade; deep tendon reflexes should be monitored during extended periods
• Give direct **IV** undiluted over 1-2 min, or diluted in D$_5$W or 0.9% NaCl and give as an inf at prescribed rate; titrate to patient response; should be administered only by qualified person, usually an anesthesiologist; do not administer IM
• Store in light-resistant area
• Give anticholinesterase to reverse neuromuscular blockade
*Syringe compatibilities:* Heparin
*Y-site compatibilities:* Aminophylline, cefazolin, cefuroxime, cimetidine, DOBUTamine, DOPamine, epINEPHrine, esmolol, fentanyl, fluconazole, gentamicin, heparin, hydrocortisone, isoproterenol, lorazepam, midazolam, morphine, nitroglycerin, nitroprusside, ranitidine, sulfamethoxazole/trimethoprim, vancomycin
*Y-site incompatibilities:* Diazepam
*Additive compatibilities:* Verapamil
*Additive incompatibilities:* Barbiturates

**Patient/family education**
• Provide reassurance if communication is difficult during recovery from neuromuscular blockade
• Provide explanation to patients regarding all procedures or treatments; patient will remain conscious if anesthesia is not given also

**Evaluation**
**Positive therapeutic outcome**
• Paralysis of jaw, eyelid, head, neck, rest of body as evaluated by peripheral nerve stimulator

**Treatment of overdose:** Edrophonium or neostigmine, atropine; monitor VS; may require mechanical ventilation

---

**panitumumab** (Rx)
(pan-i-tue′moo-mab)
Vectibix
*Func. class.:* Antineoplastic—miscellaneous
*Chem. class.:* Multikinase inhibitor, signal transduction inhibitor
**Pregnancy category** C

---

**Action:** Decreases growth and survival of cancer cells by competitive inhibition of EGF receptor

P

**Therapeutic outcome:** Decrease in colon carcinoma progression

**Uses:** EGFR expressing metastatic colorectal cancer

**Dosage and routes**
*Adult:* **IV** INF 6 mg/kg over 60 min every 2 wks

**Available forms:** Sol for inj 20 mg/ml

**Adverse effects**
*CNS:* Fatigue, ocular toxicity
*CV:* Peripheral edema
*GI: Nausea, diarrhea, vomiting,* anorexia, mouth ulceration, abdominal pain, constipation
*HEMA:* Thrombophlebitis
*INTEG: Rash,* pruritus, **exfoliative dermatitis,** skin fissure
*META:* Hypocalcemia, hypomagnesemia, antibody formation
*RESP:* **Bronchospasm, cough,** dyspnea, **hypoxia, pulmonary fibrosis,** pneumonitis, wheezing

**Contraindications:** Hypersensitivity

**Precautions:** Pregnancy **C,** breastfeeding, children, hepatic disease, acute bronchospasm, diarrhea, exfoliative dermatitis, hamster protein allergy, hypomagnesemia, hypotension, pulmonary fibrosis, sepsis

| Pharmacokinetics | |
|---|---|
| **Absorption** | 38%-49%, high-fat meal decreases absorption |
| **Distribution** | Protein binding 99.5% |
| **Metabolism** | Liver, oxidative metabolism by CYP3A4, glucuronidation by UGT1A9 |
| **Excretion** | Feces 77% |
| **Half-life** | Elimination 7.5 day |

| Pharmacodynamics | |
|---|---|
| **Onset** | Unknown |
| **Peak** | 3 hr |
| **Duration** | Unknown |

**NURSING CONSIDERATIONS**
**Assessment**
• Monitor serum electrolytes periodically
• Assess for signs of infection: increased temperature
• Assess for signs of infusion reactions: bronchospasm, fever, chills, hypotension
• Assess for signs of ocular toxicity

**Nursing diagnoses**
• Infection, risk for (uses)
• Knowledge, deficient (teaching)

• Nutrition: less than body requirements, imbalanced (adverse reactions)

**Implementation**
• Give in hospital or clinic setting with full resuscitation equipment
• Give only as IV infusion using controlled IV infusion pump; do not give IV push or bolus; use low-protein binding 0.2 or 0.22 micron in-line filter; flush line with 0.9% NaCl before and after administration
• Give over 60 min through a peripheral line or in-dwelling catheter; infuse doses of >1000 mg over 90 min
• Dilute in 100 ml of 0.9% NaCl; dilute doses >1000 mg in 150 ml of 0.9% NaCl; mix by inverting; do not exceed 10 mg/ml; use within 6 hr if stored at room temperature; can be stored between 2°-8° C for up to 24 hr
• Store unopened vials in refrigerator; do not shake; protect from direct sunlight; do not freeze

**Patient/family education**
◆ Instruct patient to report adverse reactions immediately: difficulty breathing, mouth sores, skin rash, ocular toxicity
• Teach patient reason for treatment, expected results, adverse reactions

**Evaluation**
**Positive therapeutic outcome**
• Decrease in colon carcinoma progression

**pantoprazole** (Rx)
(pan-toe-pray′zole)
Protonix, Protonix IV
*Func. class.:* Proton pump inhibitor
*Chem. class.:* Benzimidazole
**Pregnancy category C**

**Action:** Suppresses gastric secretion by inhibiting hydrogen/potassium ATPase enzyme system in gastric parietal cell; characterized as gastric acid pump inhibitor, since it blocks final step of acid production

**Therapeutic outcome:** Absence of epigastric fullness, pain, swelling

**Uses:** Gastroesophageal reflux disease (GERD), severe erosive esophagitis, maintenance, long-term pathological hypersecretory conditions including Zollinger-Ellison syndrome

**Dosage and routes**
*GERD*
*Adult:* PO 40 mg/day × 8 wk, may repeat course

### Erosive esophagitis
**Adult:** IV 40 mg/day × 7-10 days; PO 40 mg/day × 8 wk; may repeat PO course

### Pathologic hypersecretory conditions
**Adult:** IV 80 mg q12hr; max 240 mg/day

**Available forms:** Delayed rel tabs, 20, 40 mg; powder for inj, freeze dried 40 mg/vial

### Adverse effects
**CNS:** *Headache,* insomnia
**GI:** *Diarrhea, abdominal pain,* flatulence
**INTEG:** *Rash*
**META:** Hyperglycemia

**Contraindications:** Hypersensitivity

**Precautions:** Pregnancy **C,** breastfeeding, children

| Pharmacokinetics | |
|---|---|
| **Absorption** | Unknown |
| **Distribution** | Protein binding 97% |
| **Metabolism** | Unknown |
| **Excretion** | Urine-metabolites, feces, decreased rate in geriatric |
| **Half-life** | 1½ hr |

| Pharmacodynamics | |
|---|---|
| **Onset** | Unknown |
| **Peak** | 2.4 hr |
| **Duration** | >24 hr |

### Interactions
#### Individual drugs
Clarithromycin, diazepam, flurazepam, phenytoin, triazolam: increased levels of pantoprazole
Sucralfate: decreased absorption of pantoprazole
Warfarin: increased risk of bleeding

### NURSING CONSIDERATIONS
#### Assessment
• Assess GI system: bowel sounds q8hr, abdomen for pain, swelling, anorexia
• Monitor hepatic enzymes: AST, ALT, alkaline phosphatase during treatment

#### Nursing diagnoses
• Knowledge, deficient (teaching)

#### Implementation
• Swallow del rel tabs whole; do not break, crush, or chew
• May take with or without food
**IV route**
• May be given undiluted via rapid **IV** injection

### Patient/family education
• Advise patient to report severe diarrhea; product may have to be discontinued
• Advise patient with diabetes that hyperglycemia may occur
• Advise patient to avoid hazardous activities; dizziness may occur
• Advise patient to avoid alcohol, salicylates, ibuprofen; may cause GI irritation

### Evaluation
**Positive therapeutic outcome**
• Absence of epigastric pain, swelling, fullness

---

## paricalcitol (Rx)
(par-ih-cal'sih-tol)
Zemplar
*Func. class.:* Vitamin D analog
*Chem. class.:* Fat-soluble vitamin
**Pregnancy category C**

**Action:** Reduces parathyroid hormone (PTH) levels; suppresses PTH levels in patients with chronic renal failure with absence of hypercalcemia/hyperphosphatemia; serum $PO_4$, Ca, calcium-phosphate product (CaxP) may increase

**Therapeutic outcome:** Decreased symptoms of hyperparathyroidism

**Uses:** Hyperparathyroidism in chronic renal failure

### Dosage and routes
**Adult:** IV BOL 0.04-0.1 mcg/kg (2.8-7 mcg) no more than every other day during dialysis; may increase by 2-4 mcg q2-4 wk until target serum intact PTH (1.5-3 × nonuremic upper limit of normal) is achieved; PO 1 mcg/day or 2 mcg 3×/wk

**Available forms:** Inj 5 mcg/ml; caps 1, 2, 4 mcg

### Adverse effects
**CNS:** Light-headedness
**CV:** Palpitations
**GI:** Nausea, vomiting, anorexia, dry mouth
**MISC:** Pneumonia, edema, chills, fever, flu, **sepsis**

**Contraindications:** Hypersensitivity, hypercalcemia

**Precautions:** Pregnancy **C,** breastfeeding, children, geriatric, CV disease, renal calculi

P

| Pharmacokinetics | |
|---|---|
| **Excretion** | Crosses placenta, enters breast milk |

| Pharmacodynamics | |
|---|---|
| Unknown | |

## Interactions
### Individual products
Digitalis: increased toxicity

## NURSING CONSIDERATIONS
### Assessment
• Monitor Ca, $PO_4$, 2 ×/wk qwk during initial therapy; after dose is established measure calcium and phosphorus q mo

### Nursing diagnoses
• Knowledge, deficient (teaching)

### Implementation
• Give by **IV** bol only

### Patient/family education
• Advise patient to report weakness, lethargy, headache, anorexia, loss of weight
• Teach patient to report nausea, vomiting, palpitations

### Evaluation
**Positive therapeutic outcome**
• Decreased hypoparathyroidism in chronic renal disease

---

## paroxetine (Rx)
(par-ox′e-teen)
Paxeva, Paxil, Paxil CR
*Func. class.:* Antidepressant, selective serotonin reuptake inhibitor (SSRI)
*Chem. class.:* Phenylpiperidine derivative
**Pregnancy category  D**

### Do not confuse:
paroxetine/paclitaxel, Paxil/paclitaxel/Taxol

**Action:** Inhibits CNS neuron reuptake of serotonin but not of norepinephrine or DOPamine

**Therapeutic outcome:** Relief of depression

**Uses:** Major depressive disorder, obsessive-compulsive disorder, panic disorder, generalized anxiety disorder, posttraumatic stress disorder, premenstrual disorders, social anxiety disorder

**Unlabeled uses:** Diabetic neuropathy, headache, premature ejaculation, bipolar depression with lithium, fibromyalgia

## Dosage and routes
### Depression
*Adult:* PO 20 mg/day in AM; after 4 wk if no clinical improvement is noted, dosage may be increased by 10 mg/day weekly to desired response; not to exceed 60 mg/day; or CONTROLLED REL 25 mg/day, may increase by 12.5 mg/day weekly up to 62.5 mg/day
*Geriatric:* PO 10 mg/day, increase by 10 mg to desired dose, max 40 mg/day

### Obsessive-compulsive disorder
*Adult:* PO 40 mg/day in AM; start with 20 mg/day, increase 10 mg/day increments, max 60 mg/day

### Panic disorder
*Adult:* Start with 10 mg/day and increase in 10 mg/day increments to 40 mg/day, max 60 mg/day or CONTROLLED REL 12.5 mg/day max 75 mg/day

### Generalized anxiety disorder
*Adult:* PO 20 mg/day in AM, range 20-50 mg/day

### Posttraumatic stress disorder
*Adult:* PO 20 mg/day, range 20-60 mg/day

### Renal dose
*Adult:* PO CCr <30 ml/min 10 mg/day in AM, may increase by 10 mg/day q wk, max 50 mg/day or CONTROLLED REL 12.5 mg/day max 50 mg/day

### Premenstrual disorders
*Adult:* CONTROLLED REL 12.5 mg/day in AM

**Available forms:** Tabs 10, 20, 30, 40 mg; oral susp 10 mg/5 ml; controlled rel 12.5, 25, 37.5 mg

### Adverse effects
***CNS:*** *Headache, nervousness, insomnia, drowsiness, anxiety, tremor, dizziness, fatigue, sedation,* abnormal dreams, agitation, apathy, euphoria, hallucinations, delusions, psychosis, **seizures**
***CV:*** Vasodilatation, postural hypotension, palpitations
***EENT:*** Visual changes
***GI:*** *Nausea, diarrhea, constipation, dry mouth, anorexia,* dyspepsia, vomiting, taste changes, flatulence, decreased appetite, cramps
***GU:*** Dysmenorrhea, decreased libido, urinary frequency, UTI, amenorrhea, cystitis, impotence, *abnormal ejaculation* (male)
***INTEG:*** *Sweating,* rash
***MS:*** Pain, arthritis, myalgia, myopathy, myasthenia

---

**RESP:** Infection, pharyngitis, nasal congestion, sinus headache, sinusitis, cough, dyspnea, yawning
**SYST:** Asthenia, fever

**Contraindications:** Pregnancy **D**, hypersensitivity, patients taking MAOIs, alcohol use

**Precautions:** Breastfeeding, children, geriatric, seizure history, patients with history of mania, renal/hepatic disease, suicidal ideation

### Pharmacokinetics

| | |
|---|---|
| **Absorption** | Well absorbed |
| **Distribution** | Widely distributed; crosses blood-brain barrier, protein-binding 95% |
| **Metabolism** | Liver, mostly by CPY450 enzyme system |
| **Excretion** | Kidneys, unchanged (2%); breast milk |
| **Half-life** | 21 hr |

### Pharmacodynamics

| | |
|---|---|
| **Onset** | Unknown |
| **Peak** | 5.2 hr |
| **Duration** | Unknown |

### Interactions
*Individual drugs*
Cimetidine: increased paroxetine levels
Digoxin: decreased effect of digoxin
L-tryptophan: increased agitation
Phenobarbital: decreased paroxetine levels
Phenytoin: decreased effect of paroxetine
◆Pimozide: potentially fatal reactions
Theophylline: increased theophylline levels
◆Thioridazine: do not use with paroxetine; hypertensive crisis, seizures, potentially fatal reactions can occur
Warfarin: increased bleeding
*Drug classifications*
CYP2D6 inhibitors (aprepitant, delavirdine, imatinib, nefazodone): increased toxicity
Highly protein-bound products: increased side effects
◆MAOIs: hypertensive crisis, seizures; do not use together, potentially fatal reactions can occur
*Drug/herb*
Corkwood, jimsonweed: increased anticholinergic effect
Ephedra: hypertensive crisis
Hops, lavender: increased sedation
Kava, St. John's wort: avoid use
SAM-e, St. John's wort: possible serotonin syndrome
Yohimbe: increased CNS stimulation
*Drug/lab test*
Increased: serum bilirubin, blood glucose, alkaline phosphatase

Decreased: VMA, 5-HIAA
False increase: urinary catecholamines

### NURSING CONSIDERATIONS
**Assessment**
• Assess mental status: mood, sensorium, affect, suicidal tendencies; increase in psychiatric symptoms: depression, panic
• Assess for withdrawal symptoms: headache, nausea, vomiting, muscle pain, weakness; do not usually occur unless product was discontinued abruptly
• Monitor B/P (with patient lying, standing), pulse q4hr; if systolic B/P drops 20 mm Hg, hold product, notify prescriber; take VS q4hr in patients with CV disease
• Monitor blood studies: CBC, leukocytes, differential, cardiac enzymes if patient is receiving long-term therapy
• Monitor hepatic studies: AST, ALT, bilirubin
• Check weight weekly; appetite may increase with product
• Assess ECG for flattening of T wave, bundle branch block, AV block, dysrhythmias in cardiac patients
• Assess for EPS primarily in geriatric: rigidity, dystonia, akathisia
• Monitor urinary retention, constipation; constipation is more likely to occur in children or geriatric
• Identify alcohol consumption; if alcohol is consumed, hold dose until AM

**Nursing diagnoses**
• Coping, ineffective (uses)
• Injury, risk for (adverse reactions)
• Knowledge, deficient (teaching)
• Noncompliance (teaching)

**Implementation**
• Give with food or milk for GI symptoms; store at room temperature; do not freeze
• Give crushed if patient is unable to swallow whole, regular release only

**Patient/family education**
• Advise patient that therapeutic effects may take 1-4 wk
• Teach patient to use caution in driving and other activities requiring alertness because of drowsiness, dizziness, blurred vision; to avoid rising quickly from sitting to standing, especially geriatric
• Caution patient to avoid alcohol ingestion, other CNS depressants, and OTC medication unless prescribed
• Caution patient not to discontinue medication quickly after long-term use; may cause nausea, anxiety, headache, malaise; do not double doses if one is missed

P

• Advise patient to use gum, hard sugarless candy, or frequent sips of water for dry mouth; if dry mouth continues an artificial saliva product may be used

• Advise patient that depression may worsen, suicidal thoughts/behavior occur

### Evaluation
**Positive therapeutic outcome**
• Decrease in depression
• Absence of suicidal thoughts

**Treatment of overdose:** Activated charcoal, gastric lavage, maintain airway; for seizures give diazepam, symptomatic treatment

## pegaptanib (Rx)
(peg-ap′ta-nib)
Macugen
*Func. class:* Ophthalmic agent—miscellaneous

### Pregnancy category B

**Action:** Binds to vascular endothelial growth factor (VEGF), thereby inhibiting angiogenesis

**Therapeutic outcome:** Stabilization of vision in macular degeneration

**Uses:** Treatment of neovascular (wet) age-related macular degeneration. May be used alone or with photodynamic therapy (PDT).

### Dosage and routes
*Adult:* Intravitreal inj 0.3 mg injected q6 wk

**Available forms:** Inj 0.3 mg, single glass syringes

### Adverse effects
***EENT:*** *Anterior chamber inflammation, blurred vision, conjunctival hemorrhage, corneal edema, cataract, eye discharge, eye pain, increased intraocular pressure, punctate keratitis, reduced visual acuity, vitreous floaters, vitreous opacities, blepharitis, conjunctivitis, photophobia, retinal detachment, iatrogenic traumatic cataract*

**Contraindications:** Hypersensitivity, ocular or periocular infections

**Precautions:** Pregnancy **B**, inflammatory eye disease, ocular hypertension

### Pharmacokinetics
| | |
|---|---|
| **Absorption** | Unknown |
| **Distribution** | Unknown |
| **Metabolism** | Unknown |
| **Excretion** | Unknown |
| **Half-life** | 87-100 hr in vitreous humor of the monkey |

### Pharmacodynamics
| | |
|---|---|
| **Onset** | Unknown |
| **Peak** | Unknown |
| **Duration** | May remain fully active in the eye for 7-28 days |

## NURSING CONSIDERATIONS
### Assessment
• Test visual acuity periodically
• Assess treated eye for increased intraocular pressure, infection, endophthalmitis
• Monitor perfusion of the optic nerve head immediately after injection, tonometry ½ hr after inj, biomicroscopy 2-7 days after inj

### Nursing diagnoses
• Knowledge, deficient (teaching)
• Sensory perception, disturbed: visual (uses)

### Implementation
• Administer anesthesia and a broad-spectrum antiinfective prior to injection
• The inj should be done under aseptic conditions
• Remove all air bubbles prior to use
• Store at 36°-46° F, do not freeze or shake vigorously

### Patient/family education
• Instruct patient to report any inflammation, bleeding, eye discharge, opacities to prescriber.
• Instruct patient to continue with follow-up care during treatment

### Evaluation
**Positive therapeutic outcome**
• Macular degeneration stabilized

### ! HIGH ALERT

## pegaspargase (Rx)
(peg-as′per-gase)
Oncaspar, PEG-L-asparaginase
*Func. class.:* Antineoplastic
*Chem. class.:* *Escherichia coli* enzyme

### Pregnancy category C

**Action:** Indirectly inhibits protein synthesis in tumor cells; without amino acid, DNA, RNA synthesis is halted; asparagine, protein synthesis is halted; $G_1$ phase of cell cycle specific; a nonvesicant; a modified version of L-asparaginase

**Therapeutic outcome:** Prevention of rapidly growing malignant cells

**Uses:** Acute lymphocytic leukemia unresponsive to other agents in combination with other antineoplastics

## Dosage and routes
### In combination
### Adult and child with BSA ≥0.6 m²:
IV/IM 2500 international units/m² q14 days, run **IV** over 1-2 hr in 100 ml of NaCl or D₅ through a running **IV**; IM should be no more than 2 ml in one inj site
### Child with BSA <0.6 m²: IV/IM 82.5
international units/kg q14 days

**Available forms:** Inj 750 international units/ml in a phosphate-buffered saline sol

## Adverse effects
***CNS:*** Neuritis, dizziness, headache, **coma,** depression, fatigue, confusion, hallucinations, **seizures, intracranial bleeding**
***CV:*** Chest pain, **hypotension**
***ENDO:*** Hyperglycemia
***GI:*** *Nausea, vomiting, anorexia, cramps, stomatitis,* **hepatotoxicity, pancreatitis,** *diarrhea*
***GU:*** Urinary retention, **renal failure,** glycosuria, polyuria, azotemia, uric acid neuropathy
***HEMA:*** **Thrombocytopenia, leukopenia, myelosuppression, anemia, decreased clotting factors, pancytopenia, DIC**
***INTEG:*** *Rash,* urticaria, chills, fever
***RESP:*** **Fibrosis, pulmonary infiltrate, severe bronchospasm**
***SYST:*** **Anaphylaxis, hypersensitivity, angioedema**

**Contraindications:** Breastfeeding, infants, hypersensitivity, pancreatitis

**Precautions:** Pregnancy **C,** renal/hepatic/CNS disease

| Pharmacokinetics | |
|---|---|
| **Absorption** | Complete bioavailability |
| **Distribution** | Intravascular spaces |
| **Metabolism** | Unknown |
| **Excretion** | Reticuloendothelial system |
| **Half-life** | 5½ days |

| Pharmacodynamics | |
|---|---|
| **Onset** | Rapid |
| **Peak** | Unknown |
| **Duration** | 2 wk |

## Interactions
### Individual drugs
Aspirin, heparin, warfarin: coagulation factor imbalances
Methotrexate: decreased action of methotrexate
Radiation: do not use together
### Drug classifications
NSAIDs: coagulation factor imbalances

## NURSING CONSIDERATIONS
### Assessment
◆ Assess for signs and symptoms of pancreatitis (nausea, vomiting, severe abdominal pain), anaphylaxis (bronchospasm, dyspnea), cyanosis; monitor amylase, glucose
◆ Assess symptoms indicating severe allergic reaction: rash, pruritus, urticaria, purpuric skin lesions, itching, flushing; monitor for joint pain, bronchospasm, hypotension; epINEPHrine and crash carts should be nearby
• Monitor for frequency of stools, characteristics: cramping, acidosis; signs of dehydration: rapid respirations, poor skin turgor, decreased urine output, dry skin, restlessness, weakness
• Monitor CBC, differential, platelet count weekly; withhold product if WBC is <4000/mm³ or platelet count is <100,000/mm³; notify physician of results; also assess protime, PTT, and thrombin time, which may be increased
• Monitor renal function tests: BUN, creatinine, serum uric acid, urine CCr before and during therapy; check I&O ratio; report fall in urine output to <30 ml/hr; patient should be well hydrated with 2-3 L/day to prevent urate deposits
• Monitor temp q4hr (may indicate beginning of infection)
• Monitor liver function tests before and during therapy (bilirubin, AST, ALT, LDH) as needed or monthly; check for jaundice of skin and sclera, dark urine, clay-colored stools, itchy skin, abdominal pain, fever, diarrhea; also monitor cholesterol, alkaline phosphatase
• Assess for bleeding: hematuria, stool guaiac, bruising or petechiae, mucosa or orifices q8hr; check for inflammation of mucosa, breaks in skin
• Identify edema in feet, joint pain, stomach pain, shaking

### Nursing diagnoses
• Infection, risk for (adverse reactions)
• Injury, risk for (adverse reactions)
• Knowledge, deficient (teaching)

### Implementation
• Preparation by trained personnel is required in controlled environment
• Give fluids **IV** or PO before chemotherapy to hydrate patient
• Provide antiemetic 30-60 min before giving product and prn to prevent vomiting; administer antibiotics for prophylaxis of infection
• Provide a liquid diet: carbonated beverages; gelatin may be added if patient is not nauseated or vomiting

Adverse effects: *italic* = common, **bold** = life-threatening

## IM route

- Dilute 10,000 international units/2 ml of 0.9% NaCl with preservatives; give 2 ml or less per site

### Intradermal route

- After intradermal skin testing and desensitization, give 0.1 ml (2 international units) intradermally after reconstituting with 5 ml of sterile water or 0.9% NaCl for inj; then add 0.1 ml of reconstituted product to 9.9 ml of diluent (20 international units/ml); observe for 1 hr, check for wheal; desensitization may be required

### IV route

- For direct **IV** dilute 10,000 international units/5 ml of sterile water for inj or 0.9% NaCl without preservatives; give through 5-μm filter if fibers are present; do not use if sol cloudy or discolored, give over 30 min through Y-site of full-flowing **IV** of 0.9% NaCl or $D_5W$; run **IV** sol for at least 2 hr after direct administration
- Give **IV** inf using 21, 23, 25G needle; administer by slow **IV** inf via Y-tube or 3-way stopcock of flowing $D_5W$ or 0.9% NaCl inf over 30 min after diluting 10,000 international units/5 ml of sterile water or 0.9% NaCl (no preservatives) to 2000 international units/ml; filter may be necessary if fibers are present
- Provide allopurinol or sodium bicarbonate to reduce uric acid levels, alkalinization of urine

## Patient/family education

- Advise patient that contraceptive measures are recommended during therapy; product is teratogenic
- Teach patient to avoid use of products containing aspirin or NSAIDs, razors, commercial mouthwash, since bleeding may occur; to report symptoms of bleeding (hematuria, tarry stools)
- Teach patient to report signs of anemia (fatigue, headache, irritability, faintness, shortness of breath)
- Tell patient to avoid crowds and persons with respiratory tract infections to prevent patient infection
- Advise patient to avoid vaccinations, since serious reactions can occur
- Teach patient to report nausea, vomiting, bruising, bleeding, stomatitis, severe diarrhea, jaundice, chest pain, abdominal pain, trouble breathing, rash

## Evaluation

### Positive therapeutic outcome

- Prevention of rapid division of malignant cells

---

# pegfilgrastim (Rx)
(peg-fill-grass'stim)
Neulasta
*Func. class.:* Hematopoietic agent

## Pregnancy category C

**Action:** Stimulates proliferation and differentiation of neutrophils

**Therapeutic outcome:** Absence of infection

**Uses:** To decrease infection in patients receiving antineoplastics that are myelosuppressive; to increase WBC in patients with product-induced neutropenia

## Dosage and routes

*Adult:* SUBCUT 6 mg give once per chemotherapy cycle

**Available forms:** Sol for inj 10 mg/0.6 ml

## Adverse effects

*CNS:* Fever, fatigue, headache, dizziness, insomnia, peripheral edema
*GI: Nausea,* vomiting, diarrhea, mucositis, anorexia, constipation, dyspepsia, abdominal pain, stomatitis, **splenic rupture**
*HEMA:* **Leukocytosis, granulocytopenia, sickle cell crisis, hemoglobin S disease with crisis**
*INTEG:* Alopecia
*MISC:* Chest pain, hyperuricemia, **anaphylaxis, influenza-like syndrome**
*MS:* Skeletal pain
*RESP:* **Respiratory distress syndrome**

**Contraindications:** Hypersensitivity to proteins of *E. coli,* filgrastim

**Precautions:** Pregnancy **C**, breastfeeding, child <45 kg, adolescents, myeloid malignancies, sickle cell disease, leukocytosis, splenic rupture, allergic-type reactions, ARDS

### Pharmacokinetics

| Absorption | Unknown |
|---|---|
| Distribution | Unknown |
| Metabolism | Unknown |
| Excretion | Unknown |
| Half-life | 15-80 hr |

### Pharmacodynamics
Unknown

## Interactions
### Individual drug
Lithium: increased release of neutrophils

---

## Drug classifications

Cytotoxic chemotherapy agents: do not use this product concomitantly or 2 wk before or 24 hr after administration of cytotoxics

### Drug/lab test

Increased: uric acid, LDH, alkaline phosphatase

## NURSING CONSIDERATIONS
### Assessment

• Assess for allergic reactions, anaphylaxis: rash, urticaria; discontinue this product, have emergency equipment nearby
• Monitor blood studies: CBC, platelet count before treatment and twice weekly; neutrophil counts may be increased for 2 days after therapy
• Monitor B/P, respirations, pulse before and during therapy
• Assess for bone pain, give mild analgesics

### Nursing diagnoses

• Infection, risk for (uses)
• Knowledge, deficient (teaching)

### Implementation

• Give using single-use vials; after dose is withdrawn, do not reenter vial
• Do not use 6-mg fixed dose in infants, children, or others <45 kg
• Inspect sol for discoloration, particulates; if present, do not use
• Do not administer in the period 14 days before and 24 hr after cytotoxic chemotherapy
• Store in refrigerator; do not freeze; may store at room temperature up to 6 hr, avoid shaking, protect from light

### Patient/family education

• Teach the technique for self-administration: dose, side effects, disposal of containers and needles; provide instruction sheet

### Evaluation
**Positive therapeutic outcome**

• Absence of infection

## peginterferon alfa-2a (Rx)

(peg-in-ter-feer′on)

Pegasys

*Func. class.:* Immunomodulator

**Pregnancy category C**

**Action:** Stimulates genes to modulate many biologic effects, including inhibition of viral replication; inhibits ion cell proliferation, immunomodulation, stimulates effector proteins, decreases leukocyte, platelet counts

**Therapeutic outcome:** Undetectable viral load; decreasing signs, symptoms of chronic hepatitis C

**Uses:** Chronic hepatitis C infections in adults with compensated liver disease, chronic hepatitis B in adults with HBe AG–positive, HBe AG–negative

**Unlabeled uses:** Renal cell carcinoma, chronic myelogenous leukemia

### Dosage and routes

*Adult:* SUBCUT 180 mcg q wk × 48 wk; if poorly tolerated, reduce dose to 135 mcg q wk; in some cases reduction to 90 mcg may be needed

**Available forms:** Inj 180 mcg/ml

### Adverse effects

*CNS: Headache, insomnia, dizziness,* anxiety, hostility, lability, nervousness, depression, fatigue, poor concentration, pyrexia, **suicidal ideation, homicidal ideation,** relapse of drug addiction
*ENDO:* Hypothyroidism
*GI: Abdominal pain, nausea, diarrhea, anorexia, vomiting,* dry mouth, **fatal colitis, fatal pancreatitis**
*HEMA:* **Thrombocytopenia,** neutropenia, anemia, lymphopenia
*INTEG: Alopecia, pruritus, rash,* dermatitis
*MISC:* Blurred vision, inj site reaction, rigors
*MS: Back pain,* myalgia, arthralgia
*RESP:* Cough, dyspnea

**Contraindications:** Hypersensitivity to interferons, neonates, infants, autoimmune hepatitis, decompensated hepatic disease before use of this product

**Precautions:** Pregnancy C, breastfeeding, children <18 yr, geriatric, thyroid disorders, myelosuppression, cardiac/renal/hepatic disease, depression/suicide, preexisting ophthalmologic disorders, pancreatitis

P

| | |
|---|---|
| **Absorption** | Large variability |
| **Distribution** | Large variability |
| **Metabolism** | Large variability |
| **Excretion** | Large variability |
| **Half-life** | 15-80 hr |

Pharmacodynamics

Unknown

### Interactions
*Individual drugs*

Theophylline: use caution if giving together

*Adverse effects: italic = common, **bold** = life-threatening*

*Drug classifications*
Myelosuppressives: use caution if giving together
*Drug/lab test*
Increased: triglycerides, ALT, neutrophils, platelets
Abnormal: thyroid function test

## NURSING CONSIDERATIONS
### Assessment
• Monitor ALT, HCV viral load; patients who show no reduction in ALT, HCV are unlikely to show benefit of treatment after 6 mo
• Monitor platelet counts, heme concentration, ANC, serum creatinine concentration, albumin, bilirubin, TSH, $T_4$, AFP
• Assess for myelosuppression, hold dose if neutrophil count is $<500 \times 10^6$/L or if platelets are $<50 \times 10^9$/L
• Assess for hypersensitivity: discontinue immediately if hypersensitivity occurs

### Nursing diagnoses
• Infection, risk for (uses)
• Knowledge, deficient (teaching)

### Implementation
• Give in PM to reduce discomfort, sleep through side effects

### Patient/family education
• Provide patient or family member with written, detailed information about product
• Give instructions for home use if appropriate
• Advise to take in evening to reduce discomfort, sleep through some side effects

### Evaluation
**Positive therapeutic outcome**
• Decreased chronic hepatitis C signs/symptoms, undetectable viral load

---

**! HIGH ALERT**

### pemetrexed (Rx)
(pem-ah-trex'ed)
Alimta
*Func. class.:* Antineoplastic-antimetabolite
*Chem. class.:* Folic acid antagonist

**Pregnancy category D**

**Action:** Inhibits multiple enzymes that reduce folic acid, which is needed for cell replication

**Therapeutic outcome:** Decreased spread of mesothelioma, decreased tumor size

**Uses:** Malignant pleural mesothelioma in combination with cisplatin; non–small cell lung cancer as a single agent

### Dosage and routes
*Adult:* **IV** INF 500-600 mg/m² given over 10 min on day 1 of a 21-day cycle with cisplatin 75 mg/m² infused over 2 hr beginning ½ hr after end of pemetrexed infusion
Nadir ANC < 500/mm³ and platelets = 50,000/mm³ 75% of previous dose

**Available forms:** Inj, single-use vials, 500 mg

### Adverse effects
*CNS: Fatigue, fever, mood alteration, neuropathy*
*CV:* **Thrombosis/embolism,** *chest pain*
*GI:* **Nausea, vomiting, anorexia, diarrhea, ulcerative stomatitis, constipation, dysphagia, dehydration**
*GU:* **Renal failure,** *creatinine elevation*
*HEMA:* **Neutropenia, leukopenia, thrombocytopenia, myelosuppression, anemia**
*INTEG:* **Rash, desquamation**
*RESP: Dyspnea*
*SYST:* **Infection with/without neutropenia**

**Contraindications:** Pregnancy **D**, hypersensitivity, ANC <1500 cells/mm³, CCr < 45 ml/min, thrombocytopenia (<100,000/mm³), anemia

**Precautions:** Breastfeeding, children, renal/hepatic disease

| Pharmacokinetics | |
|---|---|
| **Absorption** | Unknown |
| **Distribution** | 81% protein binding |
| **Metabolism** | Not metabolized |
| **Excretion** | Excreted in urine (unchanged 70-90%) |
| | Not known if it is excreted in breast milk |
| **Half-life** | 3.5 hr |

| Pharmacodynamics |
|---|
| Unknown |

### Interactions
*Individual drugs*
Mannitol: do not use concurrently
*Drug classifications*
Anticoagulants, NSAIDs: increased bleeding risk
Nephrotoxic products (NSAIDs): decreased pemetrexed clearance

---

## NURSING CONSIDERATIONS
### Assessment

⬥ Monitor CBC, differential, platelet count, monitor for nadir and recovery; a new cycle should not begin if ANC < 1500 cells/mm$^3$, platelets are < 100,000 cells/mm$^3$, creatinine clearance < 45 ml/min
• Monitor renal tests: BUN, serum uric acid, urine CCr, electrolytes before, during therapy
• Monitor I&O ratio; report fall in urine output to <30 ml/hr
• Monitor temp q4hr; fever may indicate beginning infection; no rectal temps
• Assess bleeding time, coagulation time during treatment; bleeding: hematuria, guaiac, bruising or petechiae, mucosa or orifices q8hr
• Assess buccal cavity q8hr for dryness, sores, ulceration, white patches, oral pain, bleeding, dysphagia
⬥ Assess for symptoms indicating severe allergic reaction: rash, urticaria, itching, flushing

### Nursing diagnoses

• Body image, disturbed (adverse reactions)
• Infection, risk for (adverse reactions)
• Injury, risk for (adverse reactions)
• Knowledge, deficient (teaching)

### Implementation

• Administer vit B$_{12}$ and low-dose folic acid as a prophylactic measure to treat related hematologic, GI toxicity. At least 5 daily doses of folic acid must be taken in the 7 days preceding first dose
• Premedicate with a corticosteroid (dexamethasone) given PO bid the day before, day of, and day after administration of pemetrexed
**IV route**
• Use aseptic technique during reconstitution, dilution
• Reconstitute 500 mg vial/20 ml 0.9% NaCl injection (preservative free) = 25 mg/ml, swirl until dissolved, further dilute with 100 ml 0.9% NaCl injection (preservative free) give as **IV** infusion over 10 mg
• Use only 0.9% NaCl inj (preservative free) for reconstitution, dilution
• Follow strict medical asepsis and protective isolation if WBC levels are low
• Use a liquid diet: carbonated beverage, Jell-O; dry toast, crackers may be added when patient is not nauseated or vomiting
• Assist patient with rinsing of mouth tid-qid with water, club soda; brushing of teeth bid-tid with soft brush or cotton-tipped applicators for stomatitis; use unwaxed dental floss
• Store at 77° F, excursions permitted 59°-86° F, not light sensitive, discard unused portions

### Patient/family education

• Instruct patient to report any complaints, side effects to nurse or prescriber: black tarry stools, chills, fever, sore throat, bleeding, bruising, cough, shortness of breath, dark or bloody urine
• Instruct patient to avoid foods with citric acid, hot or rough texture if stomatitis is present
• Instruct patient to report stomatitis: any bleeding, white spots, ulcerations in mouth to prescriber; tell patient to examine mouth daily, report symptoms to nurse, use good oral hygiene
• Advise patient that contraceptive measures are recommended during therapy and for at least 8 wk following cessation of therapy, to discontinue breastfeeding; toxicity to infant may occur
• Advise patient to avoid alcohol, salicylates, live vaccines
• Advise patient to avoid use of razors, commercial mouthwash

### Evaluation
**Positive therapeutic outcome**
• Decreased spread of malignancy

### penciclovir topical
*See Appendix D*

## PENICILLINS

P

### penicillin G benzathine (Rx)
(pen-i-sill′in)
Bicillin L-A, Megacillin ✤, Permapen
### penicillin G (Rx)
Pfizerpen
### penicillin G procaine (Rx)
Ayercillin ✤, Wycillin
### penicillin V (Rx)
Apo-Pen-VK ✤, Beepen-VK, Nadopen-V ✤, Novopen-VK ✤, Pen-Vee K ✤, PVFK ✤, Veetids
*Func. class.:* Broad-spectrum antiinfective
*Chem. class.:* Natural penicillin
### Pregnancy category B

**Action:** Interferes with cell wall replication of susceptible organisms; osmotically unstable cell wall swells and bursts from osmotic pressure, resulting in cell death

Adverse effects: *italic* = common, **bold** = life-threatening

### Penicillin G benzathine

#### Pharmacokinetics

| | |
|---|---|
| **Absorption** | Delayed; prolonged product levels |
| **Distribution** | Widely distributed; crosses placenta |
| **Metabolism** | Liver, minimally |
| **Excretion** | Kidneys, unchanged; breast milk |
| **Half-life** | ½-1 hr |

#### Pharmacodynamics

| | |
|---|---|
| **Onset** | Slow |
| **Peak** | 12-24 hr |
| **Duration** | 1-4 wk |

### Penicillin G

#### Pharmacokinetics

| | |
|---|---|
| **Absorption** | Variably absorbed (PO); well absorbed (IM) |
| **Distribution** | Widely distributed; crosses placenta |
| **Metabolism** | Liver, minimally |
| **Excretion** | Kidneys, unchanged; breast milk |
| **Half-life** | ½-1 hr |

#### Pharmacodynamics

| | PO | IM | IV |
|---|---|---|---|
| **Onset** | Rapid | Rapid | Rapid |
| **Peak** | 1 hr | ¼-½ hr | Immediate |
| **Duration** | Unknown | Unknown | Unknown |

### Penicillin G procaine

#### Pharmacokinetics

| | |
|---|---|
| **Absorption** | Delayed; prolonged product levels |
| **Distribution** | Widely distributed; crosses placenta |
| **Metabolism** | Liver, minimally |
| **Excretion** | Kidneys, unchanged; breast milk |
| **Half-life** | ½-1 hr |

#### Pharmacodynamics

| | |
|---|---|
| **Onset** | Slow |
| **Peak** | 1-4 hr |
| **Duration** | 15 hr |

### Penicillin V

#### Pharmacokinetics

| | |
|---|---|
| **Absorption** | Widely absorbed |
| **Distribution** | Widely distributed; crosses placenta |
| **Metabolism** | Liver, minimally |
| **Excretion** | Kidneys, unchanged; breast milk |
| **Half-life** | ½-1 hr |

#### Pharmacodynamics

| | |
|---|---|
| **Onset** | Rapid |
| **Peak** | ½ hr |
| **Duration** | Unknown |

## Interactions
### Individual drugs
Aspirin, probenecid: increased penicillin levels
Aspirin: decreased renal excretion
Heparin: increased effect of heparin
Methotrexate: increased effect of methotrexate
Typhoid vaccine: decreased effect of toxoid vaccine

### Drug classifications
Anticoagulants (oral): increased anticoagulant effects
Contraceptives (oral): decreased contraceptive effectiveness
Tetracyclines: decreased antimicrobial effectiveness of penicillin

### Drug/herb
Acidophilus: do not use with antiinfectives; separate by several hours
Khat: decreased absorption of penicillin; separate doses by 2 hr or more

### Drug/lab test
False positive: urine glucose, urine protein

## NURSING CONSIDERATIONS
### Assessment
• Assess patient for previous sensitivity reaction to penicillins or cephalosporins; cross-sensitivity between penicillins and cephalosporins is common
• Assess patient for signs and symptoms of infection including characteristics of wounds, sputum, urine, stool, WBC >10,000/mm³, earache, fever; obtain baseline information and during treatment
• Obtain C&S before beginning product therapy to identify if correct treatment has been initiated
• Assess for allergic reactions: rash, urticaria, pruritus, chills, fever, joint pain; angioedema may occur a few days after therapy begins; epINEPHrine, resuscitation equipment should be available for anaphylactic reaction
◆ Identify urine output; if decreasing, notify prescriber (may indicate nephrotoxicity); also check for increased BUN, creatinine
• Monitor blood studies: AST, ALT, CBC, Hct, bilirubin, LDH, alkaline phosphatase, Coombs' test monthly if patient is on long-term therapy
• Monitor electrolytes: potassium, sodium, chloride monthly if patient is on long-term therapy
• Assess bowel pattern daily; if severe diarrhea occurs, product should be discontinued; may indicate pseudomembranous colitis
• Monitor for bleeding: ecchymosis, bleeding gums, hematuria, stool guaiac daily if on long-term therapy

**P**

Adverse effects: *italic* = common, **bold** = life-threatening

- Assess for overgrowth of infection: perineal itching, fever, malaise, redness, pain, swelling, drainage, rash, diarrhea, change in cough, sputum

## Nursing diagnoses
- Diarrhea (adverse reactions)
- Infection, risk for (uses)
- Injury, risk for (adverse reactions)
- Knowledge, deficient (teaching)
- Noncompliance (teaching)

## Implementation
### Penicillin G benzathine
**PO route**
- Give in even doses around the clock; if GI upset occurs, give with food, avoid acidic juices; carbonated beverages may decrease PO absorption; product must be given for 10-14 days to ensure organism death and prevent superinfection
- Shake susp

**IM route**
- Do not give **IV**
- Give inj deep in large muscle mass
- Reconstitute with 0.9% NaCl, sterile water for inj, D₅W; refrigerate unused portion

### Penicillin G
**IM route**
- Reconstitute with D₅W, 0.9% NaCl, sterile water for inj; shake well
- Give deep in large muscle mass; massage
- Do not use SUBCUT; may cause severe pain
- If injected near a nerve, loss of function and severe pain may occur

**IV route**
- Change **IV** sites q48hr to prevent pain and phlebitis
- Give by intermittent inf by diluting 3 million units or less/50 ml or more; dilute 3 million units or more/100 ml of D₅W, D₁₀W, 0.45% NaCl, 0.9% NaCl, LR, Ringer's, or any combination run over 1-2 hr (adult), 15-30 min (child)
- Give by cont inf by diluting and infusing over 24 hr

**Syringe compatibilities:** Heparin
**Syringe incompatibilities:** Metoclopramide
**Y-site compatibilities:** Acyclovir, amiodarone, cyclophosphamide, diltiazem, enalaprilat, esmolol, fluconazole, foscarnet, heparin, hydromorphone, labetalol, magnesium sulfate, meperidine, morphine, perphenazine, potassium chloride, tacrolimus, theophylline, verapamil, vit B/C
**Additive compatibilities:** Ascorbic acid, calcium chloride, calcium gluconate,

cephapirin, chloramphenicol, cimetidine, clindamycin, colistimethate, corticotropin, dimenhyDRINATE, diphenhydrAMINE, epHEDrine, erythromycin, furosemide, hydrocortisone, kanamycin, lidocaine, magnesium sulfate, methicillin, methylPREDNISolone, metronidazole, polymyxin B, prednisoLONE, potassium chloride, procaine, prochlorperazine, verapamil
**Additive incompatibilities:** Aminoglycosides, aminophylline, amphotericin B, chlorproMAZINE, DOPamine, floxacillin, hydrOXYzine, metaraminol, oxytetracycline, pentobarbital, prochlorperazine mesylate, promazine, tetracycline, thiopental

### Penicillin G procaine
- Do not give **IV**
- Give deeply in large muscle mass
- Reconstitute with 0.9% NaCl, sterile water for inj, D₅W; refrigerate unused portion
- Shake medication before administering
- IM route may include procaine reactions: fear of death, depression, seizures, anxiety, confusion, hallucinations

### Penicillin V
- Give in even doses around the clock; if GI upset occurs, give with food; product must be given for 10-14 days to ensure organism death and prevent superinfection; store in tight container
- Shake susp; store in refrigerator for 2 wk or for 1 wk at room temperature

## Patient/family education
- Teach patient to report sore throat, bruising, bleeding, joint pain; may indicate blood dyscrasias (rare)
- Advise patient to contact prescriber if vaginal itching, loose foul-smelling stools, furry tongue occur; may indicate superinfection
- Instruct patient to take all medication prescribed for the length of time ordered
- Advise patient to notify prescriber of diarrhea with blood or pus, which may indicate pseudomembranous colitis

## Evaluation
**Positive therapeutic outcome**
- Absence of signs/symptoms of infection (WBC <10,000/mm³, temp WNL, absence of red, draining wounds, earache)
- Reported improvement in symptoms of infection

**Treatment of anaphylaxis:** Withdraw product, maintain airway, administer epINEPHrine, aminophylline, O₂, **IV** corticosteroids

## pentamidine (Rx)
(pen-tam'i-deen)
Nebupent, Pentam 300, Pentacarinat �币,
Pneumopent ✚
*Func. class.:* Antiprotozoal
*Chem. class.:* Aromatic diamide derivative

**Pregnancy category C**

**Action:** Interferes with DNA/RNA synthesis in protozoa; has direct effect on islet cells in the pancreas

**Therapeutic outcome:** Protozoa death

**Uses:** Treatment/prevention of *Pneumocystis jiroveci* infections

**Unlabeled uses:** Leishmaniasis, African trypanosomiasis

### Dosage and routes
*Adult and child:* **IV**/IM 4 mg/kg/day × 2-3 wk; NEB 300 mg via specific nebulizer given q4 wk for prevention

**Available forms:** Inj; aerosol 300 mg/vial; sol for aerosol 60 mg/vial ✚

### Adverse effects
*CNS:* Disorientation, hallucinations, dizziness, confusion, drowsiness
*CV:* Hypotension, ventricular tachycardia, ECG abnormalities; **dysrhythmias**
*GI:* Nausea, vomiting, anorexia, increased AST, ALT, **acute pancreatitis**, metallic taste
*GU:* **Acute renal failure, increased serum creatinine, renal toxicity,** decreased urination
*HEMA:* Anemia, **leukopenia, thrombocytopenia**
*INTEG:* Sterile abscess, pain at inj site, pruritus, urticaria, rash
*META:* Hyperkalemia, hypocalcemia, *hypoglycemia,* fever
*MISC:* Fatigue, chills, night sweats, **anaphylaxis, Stevens-Johnson syndrome**
*RESP:* Cough, shortness of breath, **bronchospasm** (with aerosol), sore throat

**Contraindications:** Hypersensitivity

**Precautions:** Pregnancy **C**, breastfeeding, children, blood dyscrasias, cardiac/renal/hepatic disease, diabetes mellitus, hypocalcemia, hyper/hypotension, anemia

### Pharmacokinetics
| | |
|---|---|
| **Absorption** | Well absorbed (IM); minimally absorbed (inh); completely absorbed (**IV**) |
| **Distribution** | Widely distributed; does not appear in CSF |
| **Metabolism** | Not known |
| **Excretion** | Kidneys, unchanged (up to 30%) |
| **Half-life** | 6½-9½ hr; increased in renal disease |

### Pharmacodynamics
| | IM | IV | INH |
|---|---|---|---|
| **Onset** | Unknown | Unknown | Unknown |
| **Peak** | ½-1 hr | Inf end | Unknown |
| **Duration** | Unknown | Unknown | Unknown |

### Interactions
*Individual drugs*
Amphotericin B, cisplatin, vancomycin: increased nephrotoxicity
◆Erythromycin **IV:** fatal dysrhythmias
Radiation: bone marrow suppression
*Drug classifications*
Aminoglycosides NSAIDs: increased nephrotoxicity
Antineoplastics: increased bone marrow depression
Class IA, class III antidysrhythmics, phenothiazines: increased QT prolongation

### NURSING CONSIDERATIONS
**Assessment**
◆ Assess any patient with compromised renal system: product is excreted slowly in poor renal system function; toxicity may occur rapidly
• Assess patient for infection including increased temp, thick sputum, WBC >10,000/mm³; monitor these signs of infection throughout treatment; obtain C&S before beginning therapy; treatment may begin after culture is obtained
• Assess respiratory system including rate, rhythm, bilateral lung sounds, shortness of breath, wheezing, dyspnea
• Monitor ECG for cardiac dysrhythmias; ECG and pulse should be checked frequently during treatment, since cardiotoxicity can occur
• Assess for hypoglycemia including nausea, tremors, anxiety, chills, diaphoresis, headache, hunger, cold, pale skin; this side effect can last for several mo after treatment is completed
• Monitor for hyperglycemia including flushed, dry skin, acetone breath, thirst, anorexia, drowsiness, polyuria; this side effect can last for several mo after treatment is completed

P

*Adverse effects:* italic = common, **bold** = life-threatening

• Monitor renal function tests including BUN, urinalysis, creatinine; obtain at baseline and frequently during treatment; nephrotoxicity may occur; check I&O, report hematuria, oliguria
• Monitor blood studies including blood glucose, CBC, platelets; blood glucose fluctuations are common; anemia, leukopenia, thrombocytopenia can occur
• Monitor liver function studies including AST, ALT, alkaline phosphatase, bilirubin before beginning treatment and every 3 days during therapy
• Monitor calcium and magnesium before beginning treatment and every 3 days during therapy; hypocalcemia may occur

## Nursing diagnoses
• Infection, risk for (uses)
• Knowledge, deficient (teaching)

## Implementation
### IM route
• Reconstitute 300 mg/3 ml of sterile water for inj; give deep in large muscle mass by Z-track; IM is a painful route
• Do not mix in normal saline

### Inhalation route
• Dilute 300 mg/600 ml sterile water for inj; put reconstituted sol into nebulizer; do not use with other products or sol precipitate may occur; sol stable for 48 hr at room temperature; protect from light; administer over 30-45 min

### IV route
• For intermittent inf reconstitute 300 mg/3-5 ml of sterile water for inj, $D_5W$; withdraw dose and further dilute in 50-250 ml of $D_5W$; diluted sol is stable for 48 hr; discard unused sol; give over 1 hr or more

*Y-site compatibilities:* Zidovudine
*Y-site incompatibilities:* Foscarnet, fluconazole

## Patient/family education
• Teach patient to report sore throat, fever, fatigue; could indicate superinfection
• Advise patient not to drink alcohol or take aspirin, since gastric bleeding may occur
• Teach patient to make position changes slowly to prevent orthostatic hypotension
• Advise patient to maintain adequate fluid intake

## Evaluation
### Positive therapeutic outcome
• Decreased signs and symptoms of protozoan infections
• Decreased signs and symptoms of *P. jiroveci* pneumonia in HIV infections

---

## ! HIGH ALERT

# pentazocine (Rx)
(pen-taz'oh-seen)
Talwin, Talwin NX
*Func. class.:* Opiate analgesic
*Chem. class.:* Synthetic benzomorphan (agonist/antagonist)

**Pregnancy category** C
**Controlled substance schedule** IV

**Action:** Inhibits ascending pain pathways in limbic system, thalamus, midbrain, hypothalamus by binding to opiate receptor sites, altering pain perception and response

**Therapeutic outcome:** Relief of pain

**Uses:** Moderate to severe pain

## Dosage and routes
*Adult:* PO 50-100 mg q3-4hr prn, not to exceed 600 mg/day; IV/IM/SUBCUT 30 mg q3-4hr prn, not to exceed 360 mg/day

### Labor
*Adult:* IM 30-60 mg; IV 30 mg q2-3hr when contractions are regular

### Renal dose
*Adult:* CCr 10-50 ml/min reduce dose by 25%; CCr <10 ml/min reduce dose by 50%

**Available forms:** SUBCUT, IM, IV 30 mg/ml; tabs 50 mg

## Adverse effects
*CNS: Drowsiness, dizziness, confusion, headache, sedation, euphoria, hallucinations,* dreaming, insomnia, light-headedness
*CV:* Palpitations, bradycardia, change in B/P, tachycardia, increased B/P (high doses), hypotension, syncope, flushing
*EENT:* Tinnitus, blurred vision, miosis, diplopia
*GI: Nausea,* vomiting, anorexia, constipation, cramps, dry mouth
*GU:* Urinary retention, increased urinary output, dysuria
*INTEG: Rash,* urticaria, bruising, flushing, diaphoresis, pruritus, severe irritation at inj sites, **Stevens-Johnson syndrome**
*RESP:* **Respiratory depression**

**Contraindications:** Hypersensitivity, addiction (opioid)

**Precautions:** Pregnancy C, breastfeeding, child <18 yr, addictive personality, increased ICP, MI (acute), severe heart disease, respiratory depression, renal/hepatic disease, seizure disorder, head trauma, bowel impaction

---

## Pharmacokinetics

| | |
|---|---|
| **Absorption** | Well absorbed (PO, SUBCUT, IM); completely absorbed (**IV**) |
| **Distribution** | Widely distributed; crosses placenta |
| **Metabolism** | Liver, extensively |
| **Excretion** | Kidneys, small amounts (unchanged) |
| **Half-life** | 2-3 hr |

## Pharmacodynamics

| | PO | SUBCUT/IM | IV |
|---|---|---|---|
| **Onset** | 15-30 min | 15-30 min | Rapid |
| **Peak** | 1-3 hr | 1-2 hr | 15 min |
| **Duration** | 3 hr | 2-4 hr | 1 hr |

## Interactions
### Individual drugs
Alcohol: increased side effects
### Drug classifications
Antipsychotics, CNS depressants, sedative/ hypnotics, skeletal muscle relaxants: increased side effects

MAOIs: use cautiously; results are unpredictable

Opiates: decreased effects
### Drug/lab test
Increased: amylase

## NURSING CONSIDERATIONS
### Assessment
• Assess pain characteristics: location, intensity, type of pain before medication administration and after treatment
• Monitor VS after parenteral route; note muscle rigidity, product history, liver, kidney function tests, respiratory dysfunction: respiratory depression, character, rate, rhythm; notify prescriber if respirations are <10/min
• Monitor CNS changes: dizziness, drowsiness, hallucinations, euphoria, LOC, pupil reaction
• Monitor allergic reactions: rash, urticaria
• Assess for withdrawal symptoms in opiate-dependent patients

### Nursing diagnoses
• Breathing pattern, ineffective (adverse reactions)
• Knowledge, deficient (teaching)
• Pain, acute (uses)
• Sensory perception, disturbed: visual, auditory (adverse reactions)

### Implementation
• Give by inj (IM, **IV**), only when resuscitative equipment available; give slowly to prevent rigidity
• Store in light-resistant area at room temperature

### PO route
• Tabs made in the United States contain naloxone 0.5 mg to prevent abuse if the PO preparation is used **IV**
### IM/SUBCUT route
• Give IM inj deeply in large muscle mass; rotate inj sites; repeated SUBCUT inj may cause necrosis
### IV route
• Give by direct **IV** after diluting 5 mg/ml of sterile water for inj; give 5 mg or less over 1 min

*Syringe compatibilities:* Atropine, benzquinamide, butorphanol, chlorproMAZINE, cimetidine, dimenhyDRINATE, diphenhydrAMINE, droperidol, fentanyl, hydromorphone, hydrOXYzine, meperidine, metoclopramide, morphine, perphenazine, prochlorperazine, promazine, promethazine, propiomazine, ranitidine, scopolamine

*Syringe incompatibilities:* Glycopyrrolate, heparin, pentobarbital, other barbiturates

*Y-site compatibilities:* Heparin, hydrocortisone, potassium chloride, vit B/C

*Y-site incompatibilities:* Nafcillin

*Additive incompatibilities:* Aminophylline, amobarbital, pentobarbital, phenobarbital, secobarbital, sodium bicarbonate

### Patient/family education
• Teach patient to report any symptoms of CNS changes, allergic reactions
• Advise patients to avoid CNS depressants: alcohol, sedative/hypnotics for at least 24 hr after taking this product
• Discuss with patient that dizziness, drowsiness, and confusion are common; to avoid getting up without assistance
• Discuss in detail all aspects of the product
• Instruct patient to change position slowly to prevent orthostatic hypotension
• Teach patient to turn, cough, deep breathe after surgery to prevent atelectasis
• Advise patient to avoid CNS depressants, alcohol
• Teach patient to avoid operating machinery if drowsiness occurs

### Evaluation
#### Positive therapeutic outcome
• Relief of pain

**Treatment of overdose:** Naloxone (Narcan) 0.2-0.8 mg **IV**, O$_2$, **IV** fluids, vasopressors

P

## ⚠ HIGH ALERT

## pentobarbital (Rx)
(pen-toe-bar′bi-tal)
Nembutal, Novopentobarb ♣, Nova-Rectal ♣, pentobarbital sodium
*Func. class.:* Sedative/hypnotic barbiturate; anticonvulsant, anesthetic adjunct
*Chem. class.:* Barbitone, short acting

### Pregnancy category D

### Controlled substance schedule II (USA), schedule G (Canada)

### Do not confuse:
pentobarbital/phenobarbital

**Action:** Depresses activity in brain cells, primarily in reticular activating system in brain stem; also selectively depresses neurons in posterior hypothalamus, limbic structures; may decrease cerebral blood flow, ICP (**IV**) and cerebral edema; may potentiate GABA, an inhibitory neurotransmitter

**Therapeutic outcome:** Sedation, sleep

**Uses:** Insomnia, sedation, preoperative medication, increased ICP, dental anesthetic, status epilepticus

### Dosage and routes
#### Insomnia
*Adult:* PO 100-200 mg at bedtime; IM 150-200 mg at bedtime; **IV** 100 mg initially, then up to 500 mg; RECT 120-200 mg at bedtime
*Child:* IM 2-6 mg/kg, not to exceed 100 mg; PO 2-6 mg/kg/day in divided doses; PO preoperatively 2-6 mg/kg, max 100 mg/dose; **IV** 100 mg (hypnotic/anticonvulsant)

#### Status epilepticus
*Adult:* IM/**IV** 100 mg, then additional small doses at 1-min intervals

**Available forms:** Caps 50, 100 mg; elixir 20 mg/5 ml; rectal supp 30, 50, 120, 200 mg; inj 50 mg/ml

### Adverse effects
*CNS:* Lethargy, *drowsiness, hangover,* dizziness, paradoxic stimulation in geriatric and children, light-headedness, dependence, **CNS depression,** mental depression, slurred speech, agitation
*CV:* Hypotension, bradycardia
*GI:* Nausea, vomiting, diarrhea, constipation, hepatic injury
*HEMA:* **Agranulocytosis, thrombocytopenia, megaloblastic anemia** (long-term treatment)

*INTEG:* Rash, urticaria, pain, abscesses at inj site, **angioedema, thrombophlebitis**
*RESP:* **Respiratory depression, apnea, laryngospasm, bronchospasm**
*SYST:* **Stevens-Johnson syndrome**

**Contraindications:** Pregnancy **D**, hypersensitivity to barbiturates, respiratory depression, addiction to barbiturates, severe renal/hepatic impairment, porphyria, uncontrolled pain

**Precautions:** Breastfeeding, geriatric, anemia, renal/hepatic disease, hypertension, acute/chronic pain, suicidal ideation, depression, angioedema

### Pharmacokinetics
| | |
|---|---|
| **Absorption** | Well absorbed |
| **Distribution** | Widely distributed; crosses placenta, enters breast milk |
| **Metabolism** | Liver |
| **Excretion** | Kidneys, unchanged (minimally) |
| **Half-life** | 15-48 hr |

### Pharmacodynamics
| | PO | IM | IV | RECT |
|---|---|---|---|---|
| **Onset** | 15-30 min | 10-25 min | Immediate | Slow |
| **Peak** | 3-4 hr | Unknown | 1 min | Unknown |
| **Duration** | 4-6 hr | 1-4 hr | 15 min | 4-6 hr |

### Interactions
#### Individual drugs
Alcohol: increased CNS depression
CycloSPORINE, voriconazole: avoid concurrent use
Doxycycline: increased half-life
Griseofulvin, quinidine: decreased effectiveness
#### Drug classifications
Anticoagulants: decreased effectiveness
Antihistamines, CNS depressants, MAOIs, opiates, sedative/hypnotics: increased CNS depression
Corticosteroids: decreased effectiveness
#### Drug/herb
Eucalyptus, Jamaican dogwood, kava, lemon balm, nettle, pill-bearing spurge, poppy, quinine, senega, valerian: increased pentobarbital level
#### Drug/lab test
False increase: sulfobromophthalein

### NURSING CONSIDERATIONS
#### Assessment
• Assess mental status: mood, sensorium, affect, memory (long, short), especially geriatric; if using as a hypnotic, assess sleep

 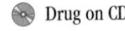

patterns during therapy; product suppresses REM sleep with dreaming; withdrawal insomnia may occur after short-term use; do not start using product again; insomnia will improve in 1-3 nights; may experience increased dreaming

• Monitor for respiratory dysfunction: respiratory depression, character, rate, rhythm (when using **IV**); hold product if respirations are <10/min or if pupils are dilated; also check VS q30 min after parenteral route for 2 hr

• Assess for blood dyscrasias: fever, sore throat, bruising, rash, jaundice, epistaxis (long-term treatment only)

• Assess seizure activity including type, location, duration, and character; provide seizure precaution

• Assess for pain in postoperative patients; pain threshold is lowered when patients are taking this medication

## Nursing diagnoses
• Injury, risk for (side effects)
• Knowledge, deficient (teaching)

## Implementation
• Administer only after removal of cigarettes, to prevent fires
• Reserve use until after trying conservative measures for insomnia

**PO route**
• Give 30 min before bedtime for expected sleeplessness
• May dilute elixir in juice, milk, or water if needed
• Give on empty stomach for best absorption

**IM route**
• Give deeply in muscle mass (gluteal) to minimize irritation to tissues; split inj >5 ml into 2 inj since irritation to tissues may occur; do not administer SUBCUT

**IV route**
• Use large vein to prevent extravasation; if extravasation occurs, use moist heat to the area and 5% procaine sol injected into area; give at 50 mg/1 min or more
• Give **IV** only with resuscitative equipment available (and only by qualified personnel)

*Syringe compatibilities:* Aminophylline, epHEDrine, hydromorphone, neostigmine, scopolamine, sodium bicarbonate, thiopental

*Syringe incompatibilities:* Benzquinamide, butorphanol, chlorproMAZINE, cimetidine, dimenhyDRINATE, diphenhydrAMINE, droperidol, fentanyl, glycopyrrolate, hydrOXYzine, meperidine, midazolam, nalbuphine, pentazocine, perphenazine, prochlorperazine, promazine, promethazine, ranitidine

*Y-site compatibilities:* Acyclovir, propofol, regular insulin

*Additive compatibilities:* Amikacin, aminophylline, calcium chloride, cephapirin, chloramphenicol, dimenhyDRINATE, erythromycin, lidocaine, thiopental, verapamil

*Additive incompatibilities:* Chlorpheniramine, codeine, epHEDrine, erythromycin gluceptate, hydrocortisone, hydrOXYzine, levorphanol, methadone, norepinephrine, pentazocine, penicillin G potassium, phenytoin, promazine, promethazine, regular insulin, sodium succinate, streptomycin, triflupromazine, vancomycin

## Patient/family education
• Teach patient to carry/wear emergency ID stating name, products taken, condition, prescriber's name, phone number
• Caution patient to avoid driving and other activities that require alertness
• Caution patient to avoid alcohol ingestion and CNS depressants; increased sedation may occur
• Teach patient not to discontinue medication quickly after long-term use; taper off over several wk

## Evaluation
**Positive therapeutic outcome**
• Improved sleeping patterns
• Decreased seizure activity
• Improved energy

**Treatment of overdose:** Lavage, activated charcoal, warming blanket, vital signs, hemodialysis

P

## ⚠ HIGH ALERT

### pentostatin (Rx)
(pen'toe-sta-tin)
Nipent
*Func. class.:* Antineoplastic, enzyme inhibitor
*Chem. class.: Streptomyces antibioticus* derivative

**Pregnancy category D**

**Action:** Inhibits the enzyme adenosine deaminase (ADA), which is able to block DNA synthesis and some RNA synthesis

**Therapeutic outcome:** Prevention of rapidly growing malignant cells

**Uses:** α-Interferon–refractory hairy cell leukemia, chronic lymphocytic leukemia

**Unlabeled uses:** Chronic lymphocytic leukemia, non-Hodgkin's lymphoma

Adverse effects: *italic* = common, **bold** = life-threatening

## Dosage and routes

*Adult:* **IV** 4 mg/m² every other wk; may be given **IV** BOL or diluted in a larger volume and given over 20-30 min

**Available forms:** Powder for inj 10 mg/vial

## Adverse effects

*CNS:* Headache, anxiety, confusion, depression, dizziness, insomnia, nervousness, paresthesia

*GI:* Nausea, vomiting, anorexia, diarrhea, constipation, flatulence, stomatitis, elevated liver function tests

*GU:* **Hematuria,** dysuria, increased BUN/creatinine, **acute renal failure**

*HEMA:* **Leukopenia, anemia, thrombocytopenia, ecchymosis, lymphadenopathy,** petechiae

*INTEG:* Rash, eczema, dry skin, pruritus, sweating, herpes simplex/zoster

*RESP:* Cough, upper respiratory tract infection, bronchitis, dyspnea, epistaxis, pneumonia, pharyngitis, rhinitis, sinusitis, **pulmonary edema**

*SYST:* Fever, infection, fatigue, pain, allergic reaction, chills, **death, sepsis,** chest pain, flulike symptoms

**Contraindications:** Pregnancy **D,** hypersensitivity to this product or mannitol

**Precautions:** Breastfeeding, children, renal/hepatic disease, bone marrow depression

| Pharmacokinetics | |
|---|---|
| **Absorption** | Completely absorbed |
| **Distribution** | Unknown; low protein binding |
| **Metabolism** | Unknown |
| **Excretion** | Kidneys |
| **Half-life** | 5-7 hr; increased in renal disease |

| Pharmacodynamics | |
|---|---|
| **Onset** | 4-5 mo |
| **Peak** | Unknown |
| **Duration** | 1½-34 mo |

## Interactions

### Individual drugs
Fludarabine: fatal pulmonary reaction
Vidarabine: increased adverse reactions

### Drug classifications
Anticoagulants, NSAIDs: increased bleeding risk

### Drug/lab test
Increased: uric acid

## NURSING CONSIDERATIONS
### Assessment
• Assess CNS changes: confusion, paresthesias, psychosis, tremors, seizures, neuropathies; product should be discontinued
• Assess for toxicity: facial flushing, epistaxis, increased pro-time, thrombocytopenia; product should be discontinued
• Assess acidosis, signs of dehydration: rapid respirations, poor skin turgor, decreased urine output, dry skin, restlessness, weakness
• Check buccal cavity q8hr for dryness, sores or ulceration, white patches, oral pain, bleeding, dysphagia; obtain prescription for viscous lidocaine (Xylocaine) to use in mouth
• Assess symptoms indicating severe allergic reaction: rash, pruritus, urticaria, purpuric skin lesions, itching, flushing
• Assess tachypnea, ECG changes, dyspnea, edema, fatigue; respiratory and CV reaction can be severe
• Monitor CBC, differential, platelet count weekly; withhold product if WBC is <2000/mm³ or platelet count is <100,000/mm³, notify prescriber of results
• Monitor renal function tests: BUN, creatinine, serum uric acid, urine CCr before and during therapy; I&O ratio; report fall in urine output to <30 ml/hr
• Monitor temp q4hr (may indicate beginning of infection)
• Monitor liver function tests before and during therapy (bilirubin, AST, ALT, LDH) as needed or monthly; check for jaundice of skin and sclera, dark urine, clay-colored stools, itchy skin, abdominal pain, fever, diarrhea
• Assess for bleeding: hematuria, stool guaiac, bruising or petechiae, mucosa or orifices q8hr; check for inflammation of mucosa, breaks in skin
• Assess effects of alopecia on body image; discuss feelings about body changes

### Nursing diagnoses
• Body image, disturbed (adverse reactions)
• Infection, risk for (adverse reactions)
• Injury, risk for (adverse reactions)
• Knowledge, deficient (teaching)

### Implementation
• Give fluids **IV** or PO before chemotherapy to hydrate patient
• Give antacid before oral agent, antiemetic 30-60 min before giving product and prn to prevent vomiting; allopurinol to prevent uric acid increases
• Give TOP or systemic analgesics for pain to lessen effects from stomatitis

• Give liquid diet: carbonated beverages; gelatin may be added if patient is not nauseated or vomiting
• Preparation should be done by personnel knowledgeable in preparing antineoplastics wearing gloves, gown, mask in biologic cabinet
• Give by direct **IV** by reconstituting 10 mg/5 ml of sterile water for inj (2 mg/ml); shake well
• Give over 5 min
• Give by intermittent inf after diluting 10 mg/25-50 ml of 0.9% NaCl, D$_5$W; give over 30 min
• Diluted sol should be used within 8 hr at room temperature

*Y-site compatibilities:* Fludarabine, melphalan, ondansetron, paclitaxel, sargramostim

*Solution compatibilities:* D$_5$W, 0.9% NaCl, LR

### Patient/family education

• Teach patient to avoid use of products containing aspirin or NSAIDs, razors, commercial mouthwash, since bleeding may occur; to report symptoms of bleeding (hematuria, tarry stools)
• Encourage patient to rinse mouth tid-qid with water, club soda; brush teeth bid-qid with soft brush or cotton-tipped applicators for stomatitis; use unwaxed dental floss
• Advise patient to report signs of anemia (fatigue, headache, irritability, faintness, shortness of breath); CNS reactions including confusion, psychosis, nightmares, seizures, severe headaches
• Inform patient that hair may be lost during treatment; a wig or hairpiece may make patient feel better; new hair may be different in color, texture
• Advise patient to use sunscreen and protective clothing to prevent photosensitive reactions

### Evaluation

**Positive therapeutic outcome**
• Prevention of rapid division of malignant cells
• Decreased bone marrow hairy cells

## pentoxifylline (Rx)

(pen-tox-if'i-lin)

Trental

*Func. class.:* Hemorheologic agent
*Chem. class.:* Dimethylxanthine derivative

### Pregnancy category C

**Action:** Decreases blood viscosity, stimulates prostacyclin formation, increases blood flow by increasing flexibility of RBCs; decreases RBC hyperaggregation; reduces platelet aggregation, decreases fibrinogen concentration

**Therapeutic outcome:** Decreased claudication and improved blood flow

**Uses:** Intermittent claudication related to chronic occlusive vascular disease, sickle cell anemia

**Unlabeled uses:** Diabetic neuropathies, sickle cell anemia

### Dosage and routes

*Adult:* PO 400 mg tid with meals, may decrease to bid if side effects occur, must be taken for ≥8 wk for maximal effect

**Available forms:** Cont rel tabs 400 mg; ext rel tabs 400 mg

### Adverse effects

*CNS: Headache,* anxiety, *tremors,* confusion, *dizziness*

*CV:* Angina, dysrhythmias, palpitations, hypotension, chest pain, dyspnea, edema

*EENT:* Blurred vision, earache, increased salivation, sore throat, conjunctivitis

*GI: Dyspepsia, nausea, vomiting,* anorexia, bloating, belching, constipation, cholecystitis, dry mouth, thirst, bad taste, flatulence

*INTEG:* Rash, pruritus, urticaria, brittle fingernails

*MISC:* Epistaxis, flulike symptoms, laryngitis, nasal congestion, **leukopenia,** malaise, weight changes

**Contraindications:** Hypersensitivity to this product or xanthines, retinal/cerebral hemorrhage, severe hepatic disease

**Precautions:** Pregnancy **C,** breastfeeding, children, angina pectoris, impaired renal function, recent surgery, peptic ulcer, cardiac/hepatic disease, bleeding disorders

P

## Pharmacokinetics

| | |
|---|---|
| **Absorption** | Well absorbed |
| **Distribution** | Unknown |
| **Metabolism** | Liver, degradation |
| **Excretion** | Kidneys |
| **Half-life** | ½-1 hr |

## Pharmacodynamics

| | |
|---|---|
| **Onset** | Unknown |
| **Peak** | 2-4 hr |
| **Duration** | Unknown |

## Interactions
### Individual drugs
Abciximab, eptifibatide, ticlopidine, tirofiban, warfarin: increased bleeding risk

Cimetidine, ciprofloxacin: increased pentoxifylline level

Theophylline: increased theophylline level

### Drug classifications
Antihypertensives, nitrates: increased hypotension

NSAIDs, salicylates, thrombolytics: increased bleeding risk

### Drug/herb
Anise, arnica, chamomile, clove, dong quai, fenugreek, feverfew, garlic, ginger, ginkgo, ginseng (Panax), licorice: increased bleeding risk

## NURSING CONSIDERATIONS
### Assessment
• Monitor B/P, respirations in patient taking antihypertensives
• Assess for intermittent claudication baseline and during treatment
• Monitor blood tests: PT, Hgb, Hct in patients at risk for hemorrhage

### Nursing diagnoses
• Activity intolerance (uses)
• Knowledge, deficient (teaching)
• Noncompliance (teaching)
• Pain, chronic (uses)

### Implementation
• Do not break, crush, or chew controlled rel or ext rel tab
• Give with meals to prevent GI upset

### Patient/family education
• Teach patient that therapeutic response may take 2-4 wk
• Instruct patient to observe feet for arterial insufficiency
• Instruct patient to use cotton socks, well-fitted shoes; not to go barefoot
• Advise patient to watch for bleeding, bruises, petechiae, epistaxis

## Evaluation
### Positive therapeutic outcome
• Decreased pain, cramping
• Increased ambulation

---

## perindopril (Rx)
(per-in-doe-pril)
Aceon
*Func. class.:* Antihypertensive
*Chem. class.:* Angiotensin-converting enzyme (ACE) inhibitor

**Pregnancy category  D**

**Action:** Selectively suppresses renin-angiotensin-aldosterone system; inhibits ACE; prevents conversion of angiotensin I to angiotensin II, resulting in dilatation of arterial and venous vessels

**Therapeutic outcome:** Decreased B/P in hypertension

**Uses:** Hypertension alone or in combination, stable artery disease

### Dosage and routes
#### Hypertension
*Adult:* PO 4 mg/day, may increase or decrease to desired response; range 4-8 mg/day may give in 2 divided doses or as a single dose, max 16 mg/day

#### Patients taking diuretics
Discontinue diuretic 2-3 days before perindopril, then resume diuretic if needed

#### Renal dose
*Adult:* PO CCr 16-29 ml/min, 2 mg every other day; CCr 30-59 ml/min 2 mg/day

#### Stable CAD
*Adult:* PO 4 mg/day × 2wk then increase as tolerated to 8 mg/day

**Available forms:** Tabs, scored 2, 4, 8 mg

### Adverse effects
*CNS: Insomnia, dizziness,* paresthesias, headache, fatigue, anxiety, depression
*CV: Hypotension,* chest pain, tachycardia, dysrhythmias, syncope
*EENT: Tinnitus,* visual changes, sore throat, double vision, dry burning eyes
*GI:* Nausea, vomiting, colitis, cramps, diarrhea, constipation, flatulence, dry mouth, loss of taste
*GU:* **Proteinuria, renal failure,** increased frequency of polyuria or oliguria
*HEMA:* **Agranulocytosis, neutropenia**

---

*INTEG:* Rash, purpura, alopecia, hyperhidrosis
*META:* Hyperkalemia
*RESP:* Dyspnea, dry cough, crackles
*SYST:* **Angioedema**

**Contraindications:** Pregnancy **D**, hypersensitivity, history of angioedema

**Precautions:** Breastfeeding, renal disease, hyperkalemia, hepatic failure, dehydration, bilateral renal artery stenosis, cough, angioedema, severe CHF

### Pharmacokinetics

| | |
|---|---|
| **Absorption** | Well absorbed |
| **Distribution** | Unknown |
| **Metabolism** | Liver |
| **Excretion** | Kidneys |
| **Half-life** | Unknown |

### Pharmacodynamics
Unknown

### Interactions
#### Individual drugs
Allopurinol: increased hypersensitivity
Lithium: increased serum levels
#### Drug classifications
Antihypertensives, diuretics: increased hypotension
Antihypertensives, neuromuscular blocking agents: increased effects
Diuretics (potassium-sparing), potassium supplements, salt substitutes: hyperkalemia
NSAIDs: decreased effects
NSAIDs, salicylates: decreased antihypertensive effect
#### Drug/herb
Aconite: increased toxicity, death
Astragalus, cola tree: increased or decreased antihypertensive effect
Barberry, betony, black catechu, black cohosh, bloodroot, broom, burdock, cat's claw, dandelion, goldenseal, hawthorn, Irish moss, Jamaican dogwood, kelp, khella, mistletoe, parsley: increased antihypertensive effect
Coltsfoot, guarana, khat, licorice, yohimbe: decreased antihypertensive effect
#### Drug/lab test
Interference: glucose/insulin tolerance tests

### NURSING CONSIDERATIONS
#### Assessment
• Monitor blood studies: neutrophils, decreased platelets
• Monitor B/P, orthostatic hypotension, syncope; if changes occur dosage change may be required
• Monitor renal studies: protein, BUN, creatinine; increased levels may indicate nephrotic syndrome and renal failure
• Monitor renal symptoms: polyuria, oliguria, frequency, dysuria
• Establish baselines in renal, liver function tests before therapy begins
• Check potassium levels throughout treatment, although hyperkalemia rarely occurs
• Check for edema in feet, legs daily
• Assess for allergic reactions: rash, fever, pruritus, urticaria; product should be discontinued if antihistamines fail to help

#### Nursing diagnoses
• Cardiac output, decreased (uses)
• Injury, risk for (adverse reactions)
• Knowledge, deficient (teaching)
• Noncompliance (teaching)

#### Implementation
• Store in airtight container at 86° F (30° C) or less
• Severe hypotension may occur after 1st dose of this medication; decreased hypotension may be prevented by reducing or discontinuing diuretic therapy 3 days before beginning perindopril therapy
• Give by **IV** inf of 0.9% NaCl (as ordered) to expand fluid volume if severe hypotension occurs

#### Patient/family education
• Advise patient not to discontinue product abruptly; advise patient to tell all persons associated with health care
• Teach patient not to use OTC products (cough, cold, allergy medications) unless directed by physician; serious side effects can occur; xanthines, such as coffee, tea, chocolate, cola can prevent action of product
• Instruct patient on the importance of complying with dosage schedule, even if feeling better; to continue with medical regimen to decrease B/P: exercise, cessation of smoking, decreasing stress, diet modifications
• Emphasize the need to rise slowly to sitting or standing position to minimize orthostatic hypotension; not to exercise in hot weather, which can cause increased hypotension
• Advise patient to notify prescriber of mouth sores, sore throat, fever, swelling of hands or feet, irregular heartbeat, chest pain, coughing, shortness of breath
• Caution patient to report excessive perspiration, dehydration, vomiting, diarrhea; may lead to fall in B/P

**P**

Adverse effects: *italic* = common, **bold** = life-threatening

- Caution patient that product may cause dizziness, fainting, light-headedness; may occur during 1st few days of therapy; to avoid activities that may be hazardous
- Teach patient how to take B/P, and normal readings for age-group

### Evaluation
**Positive therapeutic outcome**
- Decreased B/P in hypertension

**Treatment of overdose:** Lavage, **IV** atropine for bradycardia, **IV** theophylline for bronchospasm, digoxin, $O_2$; diuretic for cardiac failure, hemodialysis

---

## perphenazine (Rx)
(per-fen'a-zeen)
Apo-Perphenazine ✦, perphenazine, Phenazine ✦, PMS Perphenazine ✦, Trilafon
*Func. class.:* Antipsychotic/neuroleptic
*Chem. class.:* Phenothiazine piperidine

**Pregnancy category** C

**Action:** Depresses cerebral cortex, hypothalamus, limbic system, which control activity, aggression; blocks neurotransmission produced by dopamine at synapse; exhibits strong α-adrenergic, anticholinergic blocking action; as antiemetic inhibits medullary chemoreceptor trigger zone; mechanism for antipsychotic effects is unclear

**Therapeutic outcome:** Decreased signs and symptoms of psychosis; decreased nausea and vomiting

**Uses:** Psychotic disorders, schizophrenia, nausea, vomiting

### Dosage and routes
*Nausea/vomiting*
***Adult and child >12 yr:*** IM 5-10 mg prn, max 15 mg in ambulatory patients, 30 mg in hospitalized patients; PO 8-16 mg/day in divided doses, up to 24 mg; **IV** max 5 mg; give diluted or slow **IV** drip

*Psychiatric use in hospitalized patients*
***Adult:*** PO 8-16 mg bid-qid, gradually increased to desired dose, max 64 mg/day; IM 5 mg q6hr, max 30 mg/day
***Geriatric:*** PO 2-4 mg daily-bid, increase by 2-4 mg/wk to desired dose
***Child >12 yr:*** PO 6-12 mg in divided doses

*Nonhospitalized patients*
***Adult:*** PO 4-8 mg tid

**Available forms:** Tabs 2, 4, 8, 16 mg; oral conc 16 mg/5 ml; syr 2 mg/5 ml ✦

### Adverse effects
***CNS:*** *EPS (pseudoparkinsonism, akathisia, dystonia, tardive dyskinesia),* **neuroleptic malignant syndrome, seizures,** *headache,* dizziness
***CV:*** *Orthostatic hypotension (geriatric),* **cardiac arrest,** ECG changes, **tachycardia**
***EENT:*** Blurred vision, glaucoma
***GI:*** *Dry mouth, nausea, vomiting, anorexia, constipation,* diarrhea, jaundice, weight gain
***GU:*** Urinary retention, urinary frequency, enuresis, impotence, amenorrhea, gynecomastia
***HEMA:*** Anemia, **leukopenia, leukocytosis, agranulocytosis**
***INTEG:*** *Rash,* photosensitivity, dermatitis
***RESP:*** **Laryngospasm,** dyspnea, **respiratory depression**

**Contraindications:** Child <12 yr, hypersensitivity, blood dyscrasias, coma, brain damage, bone marrow depression

**Precautions:** Pregnancy C, breastfeeding, geriatric, seizure disorders, hypertension, renal/hepatic/cardiac disease, angle-closure glaucoma

### Pharmacokinetics

| | |
|---|---|
| **Absorption** | Variably absorbed (PO); well absorbed (IM) |
| **Distribution** | Widely distributed; high concentrations in CNS; crosses placenta; 91%-99% protein binding |
| **Metabolism** | Liver, extensively; GI mucosa |
| **Excretion** | Kidneys |
| **Half-life** | Unknown |

### Pharmacodynamics

| | PO | IM | IV |
|---|---|---|---|
| **Onset** | Erratic | 30-60 min | Rapid |
| **Peak** | 4-8 hr | 1-2 hr | Unknown |
| **Duration** | 6-12 hr | 6-12 hr | Unknown |

### Interactions
*Individual drugs*
Alcohol: increased effects of both products, oversedation
Aluminum hydroxide, magnesium hydroxide: decreased absorption
Epinephrine: increased toxicity
Levodopa: decreased antiparkinson activity
Lithium: increased risk of EPS
Ritonavir: increased perphenazine effect
Meperidine: increased hypotension

---

## Drug classifications

Anesthetics (barbiturates), CNS depressants, barbiturate anesthetics: increased sedation

Anticholinergics: increased anticholinergic effects

Anticoagulants (oral): decreased anticoagulant effect

β-Adrenergic blockers: increased effects of both products

Diuretics (thiazide): increased hypotension

## Drug/herb

Betel palm, kava: increased EPS

Cola tree, hops, nettle, nutmeg: increased action

Henbane: increased anticholinergic effect

## Drug/lab test

Increased: liver function tests, cardiac enzymes, cholesterol, blood glucose, prolactin, bilirubin, cholinesterase, iodine

Decreased: hormones (blood and urine)

False positive: pregnancy tests, PKU

False negative: urinary steroids, 17-OHCS

## NURSING CONSIDERATIONS
### Assessment

• Assess mental status: orientation, mood, behavior, presence and type of hallucinations before initial administration and monthly; this product should significantly reduce psychotic behavior

• Check for swallowing of PO medication; check for hoarding or giving medication to other patients

• Monitor I&O ratio; palpate bladder if low urinary output occurs, especially in geriatric; urinalysis recommended before, during prolonged therapy

• Monitor bilirubin, CBC, liver function tests monthly

• Assess affect, orientation, LOC, reflexes, gait, coordination, sleep pattern disturbances

• Monitor B/P with patient sitting, standing, and lying; take pulse and respirations q4hr during initial treatment; establish baseline before starting treatment; report drops of 30 mm Hg; obtain baseline ECG, with Q- and T-wave changes

• Check for dizziness, faintness, palpitations, tachycardia on rising; severe orthostatic hypotension is common

◆ Identify for neuroleptic malignant syndrome: hyperpyrexia, muscle rigidity, increased CPK, altered mental status; product should be discontinued

• Assess for EPS including akathisia (inability to sit still, no pattern to movements), tardive dyskinesia (bizarre movements of the jaw, mouth, tongue, extremities), pseudoparkin-

sonism (ragged tremors, pill rolling, shuffling gait); an antiparkinsonian product should be prescribed

• Assess for constipation, urinary retention daily; if these occur, increase bulk, water in diet

### Nursing diagnoses

• Coping, ineffective (uses)
• Knowledge, deficient (teaching)
• Noncompliance (teaching)
• Thought processes, disturbed (uses)

### Implementation
#### PO route

• Administer product in liquid form mixed in glass of juice or cola if hoarding is suspected; do not mix in caffeine drinks, tannics, pectins

• Administer decreased dose in geriatric, in whom metabolism is slowed

• Administer PO with full glass of water, milk; or give with food to decrease GI upset

• Give antacids 2 hr before or after taking this product

• Store in airtight, light-resistant container; oral sol in amber bottle

#### IM route

• Inject in deep muscle mass; do not give SUBCUT; do not administer sol with a precipitate

• Remain lying down after IM inj for at least 30 min

#### IV route

• Give by direct **IV** after diluting with 0.9% NaCl to a conc of 0.5 mg/1 ml; administer at 1 mg/min; may be further diluted and given as an inf

**Syringe compatibilities:** Atropine, benztropine, butorphanol, chlorproMAZINE, cimetidine, dimenhyDRINATE, diphenhydrA-MINE, droperidol, fentanyl, hydrOXYzine, meperidine, methotrimeprazine, metoclopramide, morphine, pentazocine, prochlorperazine, promethazine, ranitidine, scopolamine

**Syringe incompatibilities:** Midazolam, opium alkaloids, pentobarbital, thiethylperazine

**Y-site compatibilities:** Acyclovir, amikacin, ampicillin, azlocillin, cefamandole, cefazolin, cefotaxime, cefoxitin, cefuroxime, cephalothin, cephapirin, chloramphenicol, clindamycin, cotrimoxazole, doxycycline, erythromycin, famotidine, gentamicin, kanamycin, metronidazole, mezlocillin, minocycline, moxalactam, nafcillin, oxacillin, penicillin G potassium, piperacillin, sulfamethoxazole, tacrolimus, ticarcillin, ticarcillin/clavulanate, tobramycin, trimethoprim, vancomycin

P

Adverse effects: *italic* = common, **bold** = life-threatening

*Additive compatibilities:* Ascorbic acid, ethacrynate, netilmicin
*Additive incompatibilities:* Cefoperazone

## Patient/family education
• Teach patient to use good oral hygiene; frequent rinsing of mouth, sugarless gum for dry mouth
• Advise patient to avoid hazardous activities until product response is determined, dizziness, blurred vision may occur
• Inform patient that orthostatic hypotension occurs often and to rise from sitting or lying position gradually; to remain lying down after IM inj for at least 30 min; tell patient to avoid hot tubs, hot showers, tub baths, since hypotension may occur; teach patient that in hot weather heat stroke may occur; take extra precautions to stay cool
• Teach patient to avoid abrupt withdrawal of this product, or EPS may result; product should be withdrawn slowly
• Teach patient to avoid OTC preparations (cough, hay fever, cold) unless approved by prescriber, since serious product interactions may occur; avoid use with alcohol, CNS depressants; increased drowsiness may result
• Caution patient to use a sunscreen and sunglasses to prevent burns
• Teach patient about EPS and necessity of meticulous oral hygiene, since oral candidiasis may occur
• Instruct patient to take antacids 2 hr before or after taking this product
• Teach patient to report sore throat, malaise, fever, bleeding, mouth sores; if these occur, CBC should be performed and product discontinued
• Teach patient that urine may turn reddish brown

## Evaluation
**Positive therapeutic outcome**
• Decrease in emotional excitement, hallucinations, delusions, paranoia
• Reorganization of patterns of thought, speech

**Treatment of overdose:** Lavage if orally ingested; provide airway; *do not induce vomiting or use epINEPHrine*

## phenazopyridine (Rx, OTC)
(fen-az-o-peer'i-deen)
AZO-Standard, Baridium, Eridium, Geridium, Phenazo ✤, Phenazodine, phenazopyridine, Prodium, Pyridiate, Pyridium, Urodine, Urogesic
*Func. class.:* Nonopioid analgesic, urinary
*Chem. class.:* Azodye

### Pregnancy category B

**Action:** Exerts analgesic, anesthetic action on the urinary tract mucosa

**Uses:** Urinary tract irritation, infection (for symptoms only of pain, burning, itching) used with urinary antiinfectives

**Dosage and routes**
*Adult:* PO 200 mg tid × 2 days or less when used with antibacterial for UTI
*Child 6-12 yr:* PO 4 mg/kg tid × 2 days

**Renal dose**
*Adult:* PO CCr <50 ml/min do not use

**Available forms:** Tabs 95, 97.2, 100, 200 mg

**Adverse effects**
*CNS:* Headache, **aseptic meningitis**
*GI: Nausea, vomiting, diarrhea, heartburn,* anorexia, **hepatic toxicity**
*GU:* Renal toxicity, *orange-red urine*
*HEMA:* **Thrombocytopenia, agranulocytosis, leukopenia, neutropenia, hemolytic anemia, methemoglobinemia**
*INTEG:* Rash, pruritus, skin pigmentation
*SYST:* **Anaphylaxis**

**Contraindications:** Hypersensitivity, renal insufficiency

**Precautions:** Pregnancy **B**, breastfeeding, children <12 yr

| Pharmacokinetics | |
|---|---|
| Absorption | Well absorbed |
| Distribution | Unknown; crosses placenta |
| Metabolism | Unknown |
| Excretion | Kidneys, unchanged |
| Half-life | Unknown |

| Pharmacodynamics | |
|---|---|
| Onset | Unknown |
| Peak | 5-6 hr |
| Duration | 8 hr |

**Interactions**
*Drug/lab test*
Interference: urinalysis

 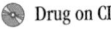

## NURSING CONSIDERATIONS
### Assessment

- Assess urinary status: burning, pain, itching, urgency, frequency, hematuria before, during, and after completion of product therapy
- Monitor liver function tests: AST, ALT, bilirubin if patient is on long-term therapy
♦ Assess for hepatotoxicity: dark urine, clay-colored stools, yellowing of skin and sclera, itching, abdominal pain, fever, diarrhea if patient is on long-term therapy
- Assess for allergic reactions: rash, urticaria; if these occur, product may have to be discontinued

### Nursing diagnoses

- Knowledge, deficient (teaching)
- Pain, acute (uses)
- Urinary elimination, impaired (uses)

### Implementation

- Give to patient crushed or whole; chew tab should be chewed
- Give with food or milk to decrease gastric symptoms

### Patient/family education

- Advise patient to report any symptoms of hepatotoxicity
- Caution patient not to exceed recommended dosage and to take with meals; to read label on other OTC products
- Teach patient not to discontinue after pain is relieved but continue to take concurrent prescribed antiinfective until finished
- Inform patient urine may turn red-orange, may stain clothing or contact lens

### Evaluation
**Positive therapeutic outcome**

- Decrease in pain, burning, itching when urinating

**Treatment of overdose:** Methylene blue 1-2 mg/kg **IV** or vit C 100-200 mg PO

---

### ! HIGH ALERT

### phenobarbital 😊 (Rx)
(fee-noe-bar'bit-tal)
Ancalixir ✤, Barbita, Luminal, phenobarbital sodium, Solfoton
*Func. class.:* Anticonvulsant, sedative/hypnotic
*Chem. class.:* Barbiturate

**Pregnancy category D**

**Controlled substance schedule IV**

**Do not confuse:**
phenobarbital/pentobarbital

**Action:** Depresses activity in brain cells primarily in reticular activating system in brain stem; also selectively depresses neurons in posterior hypothalamus, limbic structures; able to decrease seizure activity by inhibition of impulses in CNS; decreases motor activity

**Therapeutic outcome:** Sedation, anticonvulsant, improved energy

**Uses:** All forms of epilepsy, status epilepticus, febrile seizures in children, sedation, insomnia

**Unlabeled uses:** Hyperbilirubinemia, chronic cholestasis

### Dosage and routes
*Seizures*
*Adult:* PO 1-3 mg/kg/day in divided doses tid or total dose at bedtime
*Child 5-12 yr:* PO 3-6 mg/kg/day in 1-2 divided doses
*Child 1-5 yr:* PO 6-8 mg/kg/day in 1-2 divided doses
*Infant:* PO 5-6 mg/kg/day in 1-2 divided doses
*Neonate:* PO 3-4 mg/kg/day as a single dose

*Status epilepticus*
*Adult:* **IV** INF 10 mg/kg; run no faster than 50 mg/min; may give up to 30 mg/kg
*Child:* **IV** INF 5-10 mg/kg; may repeat q10-15 min up to 20 mg/kg; run no faster than 50 mg/min

*Insomnia*
*Adult:* PO/IM 100-200 mg
*Child:* PO/IM 3-5 mg/kg

*Sedation*
*Adult:* PO 30-120 mg/day in 2-3 divided doses
*Child:* PO 3-5 mg/kg/day in 3 divided doses

*Preoperative sedation*
*Adult:* IM 100-200 mg 1-1½ hr before surgery
*Child:* PO/IM/**IV** 1-3 mg/kg 1-1½ hr before surgery

**Available forms:** Caps 15 mg; elixir 20 mg/5 ml; tabs 8, 15, 30, 60, 100 mg; inj 30, 60, 65, 130 mg/ml

### Adverse effects
*CNS:* Paradoxic excitement (geriatric), drowsiness, lethargy, *hangover headache,* flushing, hallucinations, **coma**
*GI:* Nausea, vomiting, diarrhea, constipation
*HEMA:* **Agranulocytosis, megaloblastic anemia, thrombocytopenia, thrombophlebitis**

P

*INTEG:* Rash, urticaria, **Stevens-Johnson syndrome, angioedema,** local pain, swelling, necrosis, scaling eczema

**Contraindications:** Pregnancy **D,** breast-feeding, geriatric, hypersensitivity to barbiturates, porphyria, hepatic/respiratory disease, nephritis, hyperthyroidism, diabetes mellitus

**Precautions:** Anemia, renal disease

### Pharmacokinetics

| | |
|---|---|
| **Absorption** | Slow (70%-90%) (PO/IM/**IV**) |
| **Distribution** | Not known; crosses placenta |
| **Metabolism** | Liver (75%) |
| **Excretion** | Kidneys (25% unchanged) |
| **Half-life** | 2-6 days |

### Pharmacodynamics

| | PO | IM | IV |
|---|---|---|---|
| **Onset** | 30-60 min | 10-30 min | 5 min |
| **Peak** | Unknown | Unknown | 30 min |
| **Duration** | 6-8 hr | 4-6 hr | 4-6 hr |

### Interactions
*Individual drugs*
Alcohol: increased CNS depression
Chloramphenicol, disulfiram: increased effects
Doxycycline, quinidine, theophylline, metronidazole: decreased effectiveness
Furosemide: increased orthostatic hypotension
Valproic acid: increased sedation
*Drug classifications*
Anticoagulants, glucocorticoids: decreased effectiveness
CNS depressants: increased effects
Skeletal muscle relaxants (nondepolarizing), MAOIs, sulfonamides: increased effects
*Drug/herb*
Chamomile, eucalyptus, hops, Jamaican dogwood, kava, lemon balm, nettle, pill-bearing spurge, poppy, senega, skullcap, valerian: increased CNS depression
Quinine: increased phenobarbital levels
St. John's wort: decreased barbiturate effect

### NURSING CONSIDERATIONS
**Assessment**
• Assess mental status: mood, sensorium, affect, memory (long, short), especially geriatric; if using as a hypnotic, assess sleep patterns during therapy; product suppresses REM sleep with dreaming
• Withdrawal insomnia may occur after short-term use; do not start using product again; insomnia improves in 1-3 nights; may experience increased dreaming
• Assess respiratory dysfunction: respiratory depression, character, rate, rhythm when using

**IV**; hold product if respirations are <10/min or if pupils are dilated; also check VS q30 min after parenteral route for 2 hr
• Assess for barbiturate toxicity: hypotension, pulmonary constriction, cold, clammy skin, cyanosis of lips, CNS depression, nausea, vomiting, hallucinations, delirium, weakness, coma, pupillary constriction; mild symptoms occur in 8-12 hr without product
• Assess for pain in postoperative patients; pain threshold is lowered when patients are taking this medication
• Assess for blood dyscrasias: fever, sore throat, bruising, rash, jaundice, epistaxis (long-term treatment only)
• Assess seizure activity including type, location, duration, and character; provide seizure precaution

**Nursing diagnoses**
• Injury, risk for (adverse reactions)
• Knowledge, deficient (teaching)
• Sleep deprivation (uses)

**Implementation**
• Give medication after removal of cigarettes to prevent fires
• Give medication after trying conservative measures for insomnia
**PO route**
• Tab may be crushed and mixed with food if swallowing is difficult; also may be mixed with other fluids 30-60 min before bedtime for expected sleeplessness; on empty stomach for best absorption
**IM route**
• Give inj in deep muscle mass (gluteal) to minimize irritation to tissues
• Split inj of >5 ml into two, since irritation to tissues may occur
**IV, direct route**
• Use large vein to prevent extravasation; if extravasation occurs, use moist heat to the area and 5% procaine sol injected into area; give at 65 mg or less/min; titrate to patient response
*Syringe compatibilities:* Heparin
*Syringe incompatibilities:* Benzquinamide, ranitidine
*Y-site compatibilities:* Enalaprilat, meropenem, propofol, sufentanil
*Y-site incompatibilities:* Hydromorphone
*Additive compatibilities:* Amikacin, aminophylline, calcium chloride, calcium gluceptate, cephapirin, colistimethate, dimenhyDRINATE, meropenem, polymyxin B, sodium bicarbonate, thiopental, verapamil

 Alert     Canada Only    Drug on CD    * "Tall Man" lettering (See Preface)

**Additive incompatibilities:** Cephalothin, chlorproMAZINE, codeine, epHEDrine, hydrALAZINE, hydrocortisone sodium succinate, hydrOXYzine, insulin, levorphanol, meperidine, methadone, morphine, norepinephrine, pentazocine, procaine, prochlorazine mesylate, promazine, promethazine, streptomycin, vancomycin

**Solution compatibilities:** $D_5W$, $D_{10}W$, 0.45% NaCl, 0.9% NaCl, Ringer's, dextrose/saline combinations, dextrose/Ringer's, dextrose/LR combinations, sodium lactate

## Patient/family education

• Teach patient that hangover is common
• Instruct patient that product is indicated only for short-term treatment of insomnia and is probably ineffective after 2 wk
• Inform patient that physical dependency may result when used for extended time (45-90 days depending on dosage)
• Teach patient to avoid driving and other activities requiring alertness
• Caution patient to avoid alcohol ingestion and CNS depressants; serious CNS depression may result
• Instruct patient not to discontinue medication quickly after long-term use; may cause seizures; product should be tapered over 1 wk; take exactly as prescribed
• Emphasize the need to tell all prescribers that a barbiturate is being taken
• Teach the patient to make position changes slowly; orthostatic hypotension may occur
• Teach patient that response may take 4 days to 2 wk
• Instruct patient to notify prescriber immediately if bruising, bleeding occur, which may indicate blood dyscrasias

## Evaluation

**Positive therapeutic outcome**
• Improved sleeping patterns
• Decreased seizure activity
• Sedative preoperatively

**Treatment of overdose:** Lavage, activated charcoal, warming blanket, VS, hemodialysis, alkalinize urine, give **IV** volume expanders, **IV** fluids

## phentolamine (Rx)
(fen-tole'a-meen)
Regitine, Rogitine ♣
*Func. class.:* Antihypertensive
*Chem. class.:* α-Adrenergic blocker

**Pregnancy category C**

**Action:** α-Adrenergic blocker, binds to α-adrenergic receptors, dilating peripheral blood vessels, lowering peripheral resistance, lowering blood pressure

**Therapeutic outcome:** Decreased B/P, reversal of vasoconstriction (dermal necrosis)

**Uses:** Hypertension, pheochromocytoma, prevention, treatment of dermal necrosis after extravasation of norepinephrine or DOPamine

**Unlabeled uses:** Impotence, hypertensive crisis due to MAOIs

## Dosage and routes
*Treatment of hypertensive episodes in pheochromocytoma*
**Adult: IV**/IM 5 mg; repeat if necessary
**Child: IV**/IM 0.05-0.1 mg/kg; repeat if necessary, max 5 mg

*Diagnosis of pheochromocytoma*
**Adult: IV** 2.5 mg; if negative, repeat with 5 mg **IV**
**Child: IV** 0.05 mg/kg; if negative, repeat with 0.1 mg/kg **IV**

*Treatment of necrosis*
**Adult:** 5-10 mg/10 ml NS injected into area of extravasation within 12 hr
**Child:** 0.1-0.2 mg/kg; max 5 mg

*Prevention of dermal necrosis*
**Adult: IV** 10 mg/L of norepinephrine-containing sol
**Child: IV** 0.1-0.2 mg/kg, max 5 mg

**Available forms:** Inj 5 mg/ml

**Adverse effects**
*CNS: Dizziness,* flushing, weakness, **cerebrovascular spasm**
*CV: Hypotension,* **tachycardia,** *angina,* **dysrhythmias, MI**
*EENT:* Nasal congestion
*GI: Dry mouth, nausea, vomiting, diarrhea, abdominal pain*

**Contraindications:** Hypersensitivity, MI, coronary insufficiency, angina

**Precautions:** Pregnancy **C,** breastfeeding, dysrhythmia

P

## Pharmacokinetics

| Absorption | Well absorbed (IM); completely absorbed (**IV**) |
|---|---|
| Distribution | Unknown |
| Metabolism | Unknown |
| Excretion | Kidneys, unchanged (10%) |
| Half-life | Unknown |

## Pharmacodynamics

| | IM | IV |
|---|---|---|
| Onset | Unknown | Rapid |
| Peak | 20 min | 2 min |
| Duration | ½-1 hr | ½ hr |

## Interactions
### Individual drugs
EpINEPHrine: increased effects of epINEPHrine
### Drug classifications
Antihypertensives: increased effects of antihypertensives
### Drug/herb
Aconite: increased toxicity, death

Astragalus, cola tree: increased or decreased antihypertensive effect

Barberry, betony, black catechu, black cohosh, bloodroot, broom, burdock, cat's claw, dandelion, goldenseal, hawthorn, Irish moss, Jamaican dogwood, kelp, khella, mistletoe, parsley: increased antihypertensive effect

Coltsfoot, guarana, khat, licorice, yohimbe: decreased antihypertensive effect

## NURSING CONSIDERATIONS
### Assessment
• Monitor B/P, orthostatic hypotension, syncope, pulse and ECG until stable

### Nursing diagnoses
• Cardiac output, decreased (uses)
• Injury, risk for (adverse reactions)
• Knowledge, deficient (teaching)
• Noncompliance (teaching)

### Implementation
• Give with vasopressor nearby
**IV route**
• Give by direct **IV** after diluting 5 mg/1 ml of sterile water for inj or 0.9% NaCl; give 5 mg or less/min
• Give by cont inf by further diluting 5-10 mg/500 ml of D₅W, titrate to patient response
• Add 10 mg/L to norepINEPHrine in **IV** sol for prevention of dermal necrosis
*Syringe compatibilities:* Papaverine
*Y-site compatibilities:* Amiodarone
*Additive compatibilities:* DOBUTamine, verapamil

### Patient/family education
• Caution patient not to discontinue product abruptly
• Teach patient not to use OTC products (cough, cold, allergy) unless directed by prescriber
• Teach patient the importance of complying with dosage schedule, even if feeling better
• Emphasize the need to rise slowly to sitting or standing position to minimize orthostatic hypotension
• Teach patient to notify prescriber of mouth sores, sore throat, fever, swelling of hands or feet, irregular heartbeat, chest pain
• Caution patient to report excessive perspiration, dehydration, vomiting, diarrhea; may lead to fall in B/P
• Caution patient that product may cause dizziness, fainting, light-headedness; may occur during 1st few days of therapy
• Teach patient how to take B/P, and normal readings for age-group

### Evaluation
**Positive therapeutic outcome**
• Decreased B/P in hypertension
• Resolution of impotence
• Prevention of dermal necrosis

**Treatment of overdose:** Administer norepinephrine; discontinue product

---

## phenylephrine (Rx)
(fen-ill-ef′rin)
Neo-Synephrine
*Func. class.:* Adrenergic, direct acting
*Chem. class.:* Direct sympathomimetic amine (α-agonist)
### Pregnancy category C

**Action:** Powerful and selective receptor agonist causing contraction of blood vessels, vasoconstriction of eye arterioles; decreases eye engorgement by stimulation of α-adrenergic receptors

**Therapeutic outcome:** Increased B/P, decreased nasal congestion, decreased eye irritation

**Uses:** Hypotension, paroxysmal supraventricular tachycardia, shock, B/P maintenance during spinal anesthesia, topical ocular vasoconstrictor in uveitis, open-angle glaucoma, preoperatively, diagnostic procedures, refraction without cycloplegia, nasal congestion

## Dosage and routes
### Hypotension
*Adult:* SUBCUT/IM 2-5 mg; may repeat q10-15 min if needed, do not exceed initial dose; **IV** 0.1-0.5 mg; may repeat q10-15 min if needed, do not exceed initial dose
*Child:* IM/SUBCUT 0.1 mg/kg/dose q1-2hr prn

### Supraventricular tachycardia
*Adult:* **IV** BOL 0.5-1 mg given rapidly, not to exceed prior dose by >0.1 mg; total dose ≤1 mg

### Shock
*Adult:* **IV** INF 10 mg/500 ml of D₅W given 100-180 mcg/min (if 20 gtt/ml device is used), then maintenance of 40-60 mcg/min (if 20 gtt/ml device is used); use infusion pump
*Child:* **IV** BOL 5-20 mcg/kg/dose q10-15 min; **IV** INF 0.1-0.5 mg/kg/min

**Available forms:** Inj 1% (10 mg/ml)

## Adverse effects
*CNS: Headache, dizziness, anxiety, tremor, insomnia*
*CV:* Reflex bradycardia, **dysrhythmias,** *hypertension,* **tachycardia,** palpitations, ectopic beats, angina
*GI: Nausea, vomiting*
*INTEG:* Necrosis, tissue sloughing with extravasation, **gangrene**
*MISC:* **Anaphylaxis**

**Contraindications:** Hypersensitivity, angle-closure glaucoma, ventricular fibrillation, tachydysrhythmias, pheochromocytoma, severe hypertension

**Precautions:** Pregnancy **C,** breastfeeding, geriatric, hyperthyroidism, severe arteriosclerosis, arterial embolism, peripheral vascular disease, bradycardia, myocardial disease, partial heart block

### Pharmacokinetics

| | |
|---|---|
| Absorption | Well absorbed (IM); completely absorbed (**IV**); minimally absorbed (nasal, ophth) |
| Distribution | Unknown |
| Metabolism | Liver |
| Excretion | Unknown |
| Half-life | Unknown |

### Pharmacodynamics

| | SUBCUT/IM | IV |
|---|---|---|
| Onset | 15 min | Rapid |
| Peak | Unknown | Unknown |
| Duration | 45-60 min | 20-30 min |

## Interactions
### Individual drugs
Bretylium, digoxin: increased dysrhythmias
### Drug classifications
α-Blockers: decreased phenylephrine action
Antidepressants (tricyclics), β-adrenergic blockers, H₁ antihistamines: increased pressor effect
General anesthetics: increased dysrhythmias
MAOIs: do not use within 2 wk, hypertensive crisis may result
Oxytocics: increased B/P

## NURSING CONSIDERATIONS
### Assessment
• Monitor I&O ratio; notify prescriber if output <30 ml/hr
• Monitor ECG during administration continuously; if B/P increases, product is decreased
• Monitor B/P and pulse q5 min after parenteral route; CVP or PWP during inf if possible
• Assess for paresthesias and coldness of extremities; peripheral blood flow may decrease

### Nursing diagnoses
• Cardiac output, decreased (uses)
• Knowledge, deficient (teaching)
• Tissue perfusion, ineffective (uses)

### Implementation
#### IV route
• Give plasma expanders for hypovolemia
• Give **IV** after diluting 1 mg/9 ml of sterile water for inj; give dose over 30-60 sec; may be diluted 10 mg/500 ml of D₅W or 0.9% NaCl; titrate to patient response; low normal B/P; check for extravasation; check site for infiltration; use infusion pump
• Store reconstituted sol in refrigerator for no longer than 24 hr
• Do not use discolored sol
*Y-site compatibilities:* Famotidine, haloperidol, inamrinone, zidovudine
*Additive compatibilities:* Chloramphenicol, DOBUTamine, lidocaine, potassium chloride, sodium bicarbonate

### Patient/family education
• Inform patient of reason for product administration and expected result
• Advise patient to report pain at inf site immediately
• Instruct patient to report change in vision, blurring, loss of sight; breathing trouble, sweating, flushing

### Evaluation
**Positive therapeutic outcome**
• Increased B/P with stabilization

Adverse effects: *italic* = common, **bold** = life-threatening

## phenylephrine nasal agent
*See Appendix D*

## phenylephrine ophthalmic
*See Appendix D*

## phenytoin 🐾 (Rx)
(fen'i-toyn)
Dilantin, Dilantin Infatab, Phenytex
*Func. class.:* Anticonvulsant/antidysrhythmic
(class IB)
*Chem. class.:* Hydantoin

**Pregnancy category** D

**Action:** Inhibits spread of seizure activity in motor cortex by altering ion transport; increases AV conduction to decrease dysrhythmias

**Therapeutic outcome:** Decreased seizures, absence of dysrhythmias

**Uses:** Generalized tonic-clonic seizures, status epilepticus, nonepileptic seizures associated with Reye's syndrome or after head trauma, migraines, trigeminal neuralgia, Bell's palsy, ventricular dysrhythmias uncontrolled by antidysrhythmics

### Dosage and routes
#### Seizures
*Adult:* PO 1 g or 20 mg/kg (ext rel) in 3-4 divided doses given q2hr or 400 mg, then 300 mg q2hr × 2 doses, maintenance 300-400 mg/day; max 600 mg/day; **IV** 15-20 mg/kg, max 25-50 mg/min then 100 mg q6-8hr
*Child:* PO 5 mg/kg/day in 2-3 divided doses, maintenance 4-8 mg/kg/day in 2-3 divided doses, max 300 mg/day; **IV** 15-20 mg/kg at 1-3 mg/kg/min

#### Status epilepticus
*Adult:* **IV** 15-20 mg/kg, max 25-50 mg/min; may give 100 mg q6-8hr thereafter
*Child:* **IV** 15-20 mg/kg, max in divided doses 1-3 mg/kg/min

#### Neuritic pain
*Adult:* PO 200-600 mg/day in divided doses

#### Ventricular dysrhythmias
*Adult:* PO Loading dose 1 g divided over 24 hr, then 500 mg/day × 2 days; **IV** 250 mg given over 5 min until dysrhythmias subside or 1 g is given, or 100 mg q15 min until dysrhythmias subside or 1 g is given

*Child:* PO 3-8 mg/kg or 250 mg/m$^2$/day as single dose or divided in 2 doses; **IV** 3-8 mg/kg given over several min, or 250 mg/m$^2$/day as single dose or divided in 2 doses

#### Renal dose
*Adult:* Do not use loading dose CCr <10 ml/min or hepatic failure

**Available forms:** Susp 30, 125 mg/5 ml; chew tabs 50 mg; inj 50 mg/ml; ext rel caps 30, 100 mg; prompt rel caps 30, 100 mg

### Adverse effects
*CNS:* Drowsiness, dizziness, insomnia, paresthesias, depression, suicidal tendencies, aggression, headache, confusion, slurred speech, peripheral neuropathy
*CV:* Hypotension, **ventricular fibrillation**
*EENT:* Nystagmus, diplopia, blurred vision
*ENDO:* Diabetes insipidus
*GI:* Nausea, vomiting, constipation, anorexia, weight loss, **hepatitis,** jaundice, gingival hyperplasia
*GU:* **Nephritis,** urine discoloration
*HEMA:* **Agranulocytosis, leukopenia, aplastic anemia, thrombocytopenia, megaloblastic anemia**
*INTEG:* Rash, **lupus erythematosus, Stevens-Johnson syndrome,** hirsutism, **toxic epidermal necrolysis**
*SYST:* Hypocalcemia

**Contraindications:** Pregnancy **D**, hypersensitivity, psychiatric condition, bradycardia, SA and AV block, Stokes-Adams syndrome, hepatic failure, acute intermittent porphyria

**Precautions:** Geriatric, allergies, renal/hepatic disease, petit mal seizures, hypotension, myocardial insufficiency

### Pharmacokinetics
| | |
|---|---|
| Absorption | Slowly absorbed from GI tract; erratic (IM) |
| Distribution | Crosses placenta, 90%-95% protein binding |
| Metabolism | Liver, extensively |
| Excretion | Kidneys, minimally; enters breast milk |
| Half-life | 7-42 hr, dose dependent |

### Pharmacodynamics
| | PO | PO–EXT REL | IM | IV |
|---|---|---|---|---|
| Onset | 2-24 hr | 2-24 hr | Erratic | 1-2 hr |
| Peak | 1½-3 hr | 4-12 hr | Erratic | Unknown |
| Duration | 6-12 hr | 12-36 hr | 12-24 hr | 12-24 hr |

## Interactions
### Individual drugs
Alcohol (chronic use), carbamazepine, diazoxide, folic acid, rifampin: decreased effects of phenytoin

Chloramphenicol, cimetidine, cycloSERINE, diazepam, valproate: increased phenytoin effect

### Drug classifications
Antacids, barbiturates: decreased effect of phenytoin

Antidepressants (tricyclics), benzodiazepines, salicylates: increased phenytoin level

### Drug/herb
Aloe, buckthorn, cascara sagrada, senna: increased hypokalemia, antidysrhythmic action

Ginkgo: increased effect

Ginseng, santonica, valerian: decreased anticonvulsant effect

### Drug/lab test
Increased: glucose, alkaline phosphatase, BSP

Decreased: dexamethasone, metyrapone test serum, urinary steroids

## NURSING CONSIDERATIONS
### Assessment
- Assess product level: toxic level 30-50 mcg/ml; therapeutic level 7.5-20 mcg/ml, wait ≥1 wk to determine level
- Assess mental status: mood, sensorium, affect, memory (long, short), especially geriatric
- Assess for beginning rash that may lead to Stevens-Johnson syndrome or toxic epidermal necrolysis; phenytoin should not be used again
- Assess for blood dyscrasias: fever, sore throat, bruising, rash, jaundice, epistaxis (long-term treatment only)
- Assess seizure activity including type, location, duration, and character; provide seizure precaution
- Assess renal studies: urinalysis, BUN, urine creatinine
- Monitor blood studies: RBC, Hct, Hgb, reticulocyte counts weekly for 4 wk then monthly; also check thyroid function tests, serum calcium
- Monitor liver function tests: ALT, AST, bilirubin, creatinine; for renal failure
- Assess for signs of physical withdrawal if medication suddenly discontinued
- Assess eye problems: need for ophth exam before, during, after treatment (slit lamp, funduscopy, tonometry)
- Assess allergic reaction: red raised rash, increased temp, lymphadenopathy; if this occurs, product should be discontinued,

usually occurs 3-12 wk after start of treatment; may also cause hepatotoxicity, rhabdomyolysis
- Monitor for toxicity: bone marrow depression, nausea, vomiting, ataxia, diplopia, CV collapse, slurred speech, confusion

### Nursing diagnoses
- Injury, risk for (uses, adverse reactions)
- Knowledge, deficient (teaching)
- Noncompliance (teaching)

### Implementation
#### PO route
- Give with meals to decrease GI upset
- Chew tab can be crushed or chewed; cap can be opened and mixed with foods or fluids; cap and tab are not interchangeable, only ext rel cap are to be used for once a day dosing
- Do not take antacids or antidiarrheals within 2-3 hr of taking phenytoin
- Give by gastric/NG tube: dilute susp before administration, flush tube with 20 ml of $H_2O$ after dose
- Shake oral susp well; use measuring device for correct dose
- Allow 7-10 days between dosage changes
#### IV route
- Administer by direct **IV** after diluting with special diluent provided (1 ml/50 mg, 2.2 ml/100 mg, 5.2 ml/250 mg); shake; give through Y-tube or 3-way stopcock; inject slowly <50 mg/min
- Give intermittent **IV** after diluting to a conc of 1-10 mg/ml
- Clear **IV** tubing first with 0.9% NaCl sol; use in-line filter; discard sol 4 hr after preparation; inject into large veins to prevent purple glove syndrome

**Additive compatibilities:** Bleomycin, verapamil

**Y-site compatibilities:** Esmolol, famotidine, fluconazole, foscarnet, tacrolimus

**Y-site incompatibilities:** Enalaprilat, potassium chloride, vit B/C

### Patient/family education
- Teach patient to carry/wear emergency ID stating name, products taken, condition, prescriber's name and phone number
- Advise patient to avoid driving and other activities that require alertness until product response is known; dizziness, drowsiness can occur
- Advise patient to avoid alcohol ingestion and CNS depressants unless approved by prescriber; increased sedation may occur
- Teach patient not to discontinue medication quickly after long-term use; taper off over several wk

P

Adverse effects: *italic* = common, **bold** = life-threatening

- Advise patient that urine may turn pink, red, or brown
- Caution patient to avoid antacids or antidiarrheals within 2-3 hr of taking phenytoin
- Instruct patient in proper oral hygiene to prevent gingival hyperplasia; to visit dentist routinely

### Evaluation
**Positive therapeutic outcome**
- Decreased seizure activity
- Decreased dysrhythmias
- Relief of pain

## physostigmine ophthalmic
*See Appendix D*

## phytonadione (vit K₁) (Rx)
(fye-toe-na-dye'one)
AquaMEPHYTON, Mephyton
*Func. class.:* Vitamin K₁, fat-soluble vitamin
**Pregnancy category** C

**Action:** Needed for adequate blood clotting (factors II, VII, IX, X)

**Therapeutic outcome:** Prevention of bleeding

**Uses:** Vitamin K malabsorption, hypoprothrombinemia, prevention of hypoprothrombinemia caused by oral anticoagulants, prevention of hemorrhagic disease of the newborn

### Dosage and routes
*Hypoprothrombinemia caused by vitamin K malabsorption*
*Adult:* PO/IM 2.5-25 mg; may repeat or increase to 50 mg
*Child:* PO/IM 5-10 mg
*Infant:* PO/IM 2 mg

*Prevention of hemorrhagic disease of the newborn*
*Neonate:* IM 0.5-1 mg within 1 hr after birth; repeat in 2-3 wk if required

*Hypoprothrombinemia caused by oral anticoagulants*
*Adult and child:* PO/SUBCUT/IM 1-10 mg, may repeat 12-48 hr after PO dose or 6-8 hr after SUBCUT/IM dose, based on protime

**Available forms:** Tabs 5 mg; inj 2 mg/ml; aqueous colloidal (IM, **IV**); inj aqueous dispersion 10 mg/ml (IM)

### Adverse effects
*CNS:* Headache, **brain damage** (large doses)
*GI:* Nausea, decreased liver function tests

*HEMA:* Hemolytic anemia, hemoglobinuria, hyperbilirubinemia
*INTEG:* Rash, urticaria
*RESP:* **Bronchospasm**, dyspnea, chest constriction, **respiratory arrest**

**Contraindications:** Hypersensitivity, severe hepatic disease, last few wk of pregnancy
**Precautions:** Pregnancy C, neonates

### Pharmacokinetics
| | |
|---|---|
| **Absorption** | Well absorbed (PO, IM, SUBCUT) |
| **Distribution** | Crosses placenta |
| **Metabolism** | Liver, rapidly |
| **Excretion** | Breast milk |
| **Half-life** | Unknown |

### Pharmacodynamics
| | PO | SUBCUT/IM |
|---|---|---|
| **Onset** | 6-12 hr | 1-2 hr |
| **Peak** | Unknown | 6 hr |
| **Duration** | Unknown | 14 hr |

### Interactions
*Individual drugs*
Cholestyramine, mineral oil: decreased action of phytonadione
*Drug classifications*
Oral anticoagulants: decreased anticoagulant effect
*Drug/food*
Olestra: decreased vit K levels

### NURSING CONSIDERATIONS
**Assessment**
- Monitor protime during treatment (2-sec deviation from control time, bleeding time, and clotting time); monitor for bleeding, pulse, and B/P
- Assess nutritional status: liver (beef), spinach, tomatoes, coffee, asparagus, broccoli, cabbage, lettuce, greens
- Assess for bleeding or bruising: hematuria, black tarry stools, hematemesis

**Nursing diagnoses**
- Knowledge, deficient (teaching)
- Nutrition: less than body requirements, imbalanced (uses)
- Tissue perfusion, ineffective (uses)

**Implementation**
**IV route**
- Give **IV** after diluting with D₅ NS 10 ml or more; give 1 mg/min or more
- Give **IV** only when other routes not possible (deaths have occurred)
- Store in airtight, light-resistant container
*Syringe compatibilities:* Doxapram

*Y-site compatibilities:* Ampicillin, epINEPHrine, famotidine, heparin, hydrocortisone, potassium chloride, tolazoline, vit B/C
*Additive compatibilities:* Amikacin, calcium gluceptate, cephapirin, chloramphenicol, cimetidine, netilmicin, sodium bicarbonate

### Patient/family education

• Teach patient not to take other supplements, unless directed by prescriber; to take this medication as directed
• Teach patient necessary foods high in vit K to be included in diet
• Advise patient to avoid IM inj, hard toothbrush, flossing; use electric razor until treatment is terminated
• Instruct patient to report symptoms of bleeding: bruising, nosebleeds, blood in urine, heavy menstruation, black tarry stools
• Caution patient not to use OTC medications unless approved by prescriber
• Stress the need for periodic lab tests to monitor coagulation levels
• Stress the need for patient to carry/wear emergency ID with condition, treatment, and medications taken

### Evaluation

**Positive therapeutic outcome**
• Decreased bleeding tendencies
• Decreased protime
• Decreased clotting time

---

### pilocarpine ophthalmic
*See Appendix D*

---

### pimecrolimus topical
*See Appendix D*

---

### pindolol (Rx)
(pin′doe-lole)
Novo-Pindol ✤, Syn-Pindol ✤, Visken
*Func. class.:* Antihypertensive
*Chem. class.:* Nonselective β-blocker

**Pregnancy category B**

**Do not confuse:**
pindolol/Parlodel/Plendil

**Action:** Competitively blocks stimulation of β-adrenergic receptor within vascular smooth muscle; produces chronotropic, inotropic activity (decreases rate of SA node discharge, increases recovery time), slows conduction of AV node, decreases heart rate, which de-

creases $O_2$ consumption in myocardium; also decreases renin-aldosterone-angiotensin system and at high doses inhibits $\beta_2$ receptors in bronchial system

**Therapeutic outcome:** Decreased B/P in hypertension, heart rate

**Uses:** Mild to moderate hypertension

### Dosage and routes

*Adult:* PO 5 mg bid; usual dose 15 mg/day (5 mg tid); may increase by 10 mg/day q3-4 wk to a max of 60 mg/day
*Geriatric:* PO 5 mg/day increase by 5 mg q3-4 wk

**Available forms:** Tabs 5, 10 mg

### Adverse effects

*CNS: Insomnia, dizziness,* hallucinations, anxiety, fatigue, headache, depression
*CV:* Hypotension, bradycardia, **CHF,** edema, chest pain, palpitations, claudication, tachycardia, **AV block, pulmonary edema, bradycardia, dysrhythmias**
*EENT: Visual changes,* sore throat, *double vision,* dry burning eyes, nasal stuffiness
*GI: Nausea,* vomiting, **ischemic colitis,** diarrhea, *abdominal pain,* **mesenteric arterial thrombosis,** flatulence, constipation
*GU:* Impotence, urinary frequency
*HEMA:* **Agranulocytosis, thrombocytopenia, purpura**
*INTEG:* Rash, alopecia, pruritus, fever
*MISC: Joint pain, muscle pain*
*RESP:* **Bronchospasm,** *dyspnea,* cough, crackles

**Contraindications:** Hypersensitivity to β-blockers, cardiogenic shock, 2nd- or 3rd-degree heart block, sinus bradycardia, CHF, cardiac failure, bronchial asthma, severe COPD

**Precautions:** Pregnancy **B,** breastfeeding, major surgery, diabetes mellitus, renal/hepatic disease, thyroid disease, COPD, well-compensated heart failure, CAD, nonallergic bronchospasm, peripheral vascular disease

**P**

### Pharmacokinetics

| | |
|---|---|
| **Absorption** | Well absorbed |
| **Distribution** | Crosses placenta; some penetration in CNS, protein binding 40% |
| **Metabolism** | Liver, moderately (60%-65%) |
| **Excretion** | Kidneys, unchanged (30%-45%) |
| **Half-life** | 3-4 hr |

### Pharmacodynamics

| | |
|---|---|
| **Onset** | Unknown |
| **Peak** | 2-4 hr |
| **Duration** | 8-24 hr |

Adverse effects: *italic* = common, **bold** = life-threatening

## Interactions
### Individual drugs
Hydralazine, methyldopa, prazosin, reserpine: increased hypotension, bradycardia

Insulin: may alter hypoglycemic effect

Thyroid: decreased effect of β-blockers

### Drug classifications
Anticholinergics: increased hypotension, bradycardia

β2-Adrenergic agonists: increased effect of β-blockers

Calcium channel blockers: increased effects of calcium channel blockers

NSAIDs, sympathomimetics: decreased antihypertensive effect

Oral hypoglycemics: may alter hypoglycemic effect

Theophyllines, β2-agonists: decreased bronchodilatation

### Drug/herb
Aconite: increased toxicity, death

Astragalus, cola tree: increased or decreased antihypertensive effect

Barberry, betony, black catechu, black cohosh, bloodroot, broom, burdock, cat's claw, dandelion, goldenseal, Irish moss, Jamaican dogwood, kelp, khella, mistletoe, parsley: increased antihypertensive effect

Coltsfoot, guarana, khat, licorice: decreased antihypertensive effect

### Drug/lab test
Increased: renal/liver function tests

Interference: glucose, insulin tolerance test

## NURSING CONSIDERATIONS
### Assessment
• Monitor B/P during beginning treatment, periodically thereafter; pulse q4hr; note rate, rhythm, quality: apical/radial pulse before administration; notify prescriber of any significant changes (pulse <50 bpm)

• Obtain baselines in renal, liver function tests before therapy begins

• Assess for edema in feet, legs daily; monitor I&O, daily weight; check for jugular vein distention, crackles bilaterally, dyspnea (CHF)

• Monitor skin turgor, dryness of mucous membranes for hydration status, especially geriatric

### Nursing diagnoses
• Cardiac output, decreased (uses)
• Injury, risk for (adverse reactions)
• Knowledge, deficient (teaching)
• Noncompliance (teaching)

## Implementation
• Give before meals, at bedtime; tab may be crushed or swallowed whole; give with food to prevent GI upset

• Store protected from light, moisture; place in cool environment

### Patient/family education
◆ Teach patient not to discontinue product abruptly; taper over 2 wk; may cause precipitate angina if stopped abruptly

• Teach patient not to use OTC products containing α-adrenergic stimulants (such as nasal decongestants, cold preparations); to avoid alcohol, smoking, and to limit sodium intake as prescribed

• Teach patient how to take pulse and B/P at home; advise when to notify prescriber

• Instruct patient to comply with weight control, dietary adjustments, modified exercise program

• Tell patient to carry/wear emergency ID to identify product being taken, allergies; tell patient product controls symptoms but does not cure

• Caution patient to avoid hazardous activities if dizziness, drowsiness present

• Teach patient to report symptoms of CHF: difficult breathing, especially on exertion or when lying down, night cough, swelling of extremities or bradycardia, dizziness, confusion, depression, fever

• Teach patient to take product as prescribed, not to double doses, skip doses; take any missed doses as soon as remembered if at least 4 hr until next dose; to take with or immediately after meals if GI symptoms occur

### Evaluation
**Positive therapeutic outcome**
• Decreased B/P in hypertension (after 1-2 wk)

**Treatment of overdose:** Lavage, **IV** atropine for bradycardia, **IV** theophylline for bronchospasm, digoxin, O2, diuretic for cardiac failure, hemodialysis, **IV** glucose for hyperglycemia, **IV** diazepam (or phenytoin) for seizures

## pioglitazone (Rx)
(pie-oh-glye′ta-zone)

Actos

*Func. class.:* Antidiabetic, oral
*Chem. class.:* Thiazolidinedione

**Pregnancy category C**

**Action:** Specifically targets insulin resistance, an insulin sensitizer; regulates the transcription of a number of insulin responsive genes

**Therapeutic outcome:** Decreased symptoms of diabetes mellitus

**Uses:** Type 2 diabetes mellitus

### Dosage and routes
*Monotherapy*
*Adult:* PO 15-30 mg/day, may increase to 45 mg/day

*Combination therapy*
*Adult:* PO 15-30 mg/day with a sulfonylurea, metformin, or insulin; decrease sulfonylurea dose if hypoglycemia occurs; decrease insulin dose by 10%-25% if hypoglycemia occurs or if plasma glucose is <100 mg/dl, max 45 mg/day

*Hepatic dose*
Do not use in active liver disease or if ALT >2.5 × ULN

**Available forms:** Tabs 15, 30, 45 mg

### Adverse effects
*CNS: Headache*
*ENDO: Aggravated diabetes mellitus*
*MISC: Myalgia, sinusitis, upper respiratory tract infection, pharyngitis,* **hepatotoxicity,** edema, weight gain, anemia, macular edema
*MS: Fractures (females), myalgia*

**Contraindications:** Breastfeeding, children, hypersensitivity to thiazolidinediones, diabetic ketoacidosis, CHF

**Precautions:** Pregnancy C, geriatric, thyroid/renal/hepatic disease, edema, CHF

### Pharmacokinetics

| | |
|---|---|
| **Absorption** | Unknown |
| **Distribution** | Unknown |
| **Metabolism** | Unknown |
| **Excretion** | Kidneys |
| **Half-life** | 3-7 hr, terminal 16-24 hr |

### Pharmacodynamics

| | |
|---|---|
| **Onset** | Unknown |
| **Peak** | 6-12 wk |
| **Duration** | Unknown |

### Interactions
*Individual drugs*
Fluconazole, itraconazole, ketoconazole, miconazole, voriconazole: decreased pioglitazone effect
Gatifloxacin: poor glucose control
*Drug classifications*
CYP2C8 inducers: decreased pioglitazone effect
Oral contraceptives: decreased effect, use an alternative contraceptive method
*Drug/herb*
Alfalfa, aloe, basil, bay, bilberry, bitter melon, black catechu, buchu, burdock, coriander, dandelion, eyebright (po), fenugreek, garlic, ginseng, glucomannan, glucosamine, goat's rue, gymnema, horehound, horse chestnut, jambul, myrrh, myrtle: increased antidiabetic effect
Bee pollen, blue cohosh, broom, chromium, elecampane, eucalyptus, gotu kola: decreased antidiabetic effect
Chromium, coenzyme Q10, fenugreek: increased hypoglycemia
Glucosamine: decreased blood glucose control

### NURSING CONSIDERATIONS
**Assessment**
• Assess for hypoglycemic reactions (sweating, weakness, dizziness, anxiety, tremors, hunger), hyperglycemic reactions soon after meals (rare)
• Check liver function tests periodically; AST, LDH, FBS, glycosylated Hgb, plasma lipids, lipoproteins, B/P, body weight during treatment

**Nursing diagnoses**
• Knowledge, deficient (teaching)
• Nutrition: more than body requirements, imbalanced (uses)

**Implementation**
• Convert from other oral hypoglycemic agents; change may be made with gradual dosage change; monitor serum glucose during conversion
• Give once a day; give with meals to decrease GI upset
• Give tabs crushed and mixed with meal or fluids for patients with difficulty swallowing
• Store in airtight container in cool environment

**Patient/family education**
• Teach patient to self-monitor using a blood glucose meter
• Teach patient symptoms of hypo/hyperglycemia, what to do about each (rare)

P

- Advise patient that product must be continued on daily basis; explain consequence of discontinuing product abruptly
- Advise patient to avoid OTC medications or herbal preparations unless approved by prescriber; to report weight gain, edema
- Advise patient that diabetes is life-long illness; that this product is not a cure, only controls symptoms
- Instruct patient to notify prescriber if oral contraceptives are used
- Teach patient not to use if breastfeeding

### Evaluation
**Positive therapeutic outcome**
- Decrease in polyuria, polydipsia, polyphagia; clear sensorium; absence of dizziness; stable gait; blood glucose, A1c improvement

---

## piperacillin (Rx)
(pi-per'a-sill-in)
Pipracil
*Func. class.:* Broad-spectrum antiinfective
*Chem. class.:* Extended-spectrum penicillin
**Pregnancy category B**

**Action:** Interferes with cell wall replication of susceptible organisms; osmotically unstable cell wall swells and bursts from osmotic pressure

**Therapeutic outcome:** Bactericidal effects for gram-positive cocci *Staphylococcus aureus, Streptococcus pyogenes, Streptococcus viridans, Streptococcus faecalis, Streptococcus bovis, Streptococcus pneumoniae;* gram-negative cocci *Neisseria gonorrhoeae, Neisseria meningitidis;* gram-positive bacilli *Acinetobacter, Clostridium perfringens, Clostridium tetani;* gram-negative bacilli *Bacteroides, Fusobacterium nucleatum, Escherichia coli, Klebsiella, Proteus mirabilis, Proteus vulgaris, Proteus rettgeri, Morganella morganii, Enterobacter, Citrobacter, Pseudomonas aeruginosa, Serratia, Peptococcus, Peptostreptococcus, Eubacterium*

**Uses:** Respiratory tract, skin, skin structure, urinary tract, bone, and joint infections; gonorrhea, pneumonia, endocarditis, septicemia, meningitis, sinusitis; infections caused by penicillinase-producing staphylococci, streptococci; may be combined with an aminoglycoside for *Pseudomonas* infection

### Dosage and routes
*Urinary tract infections*
*Adult:* **IV** 8-16 g/day (125-200 mg/kg/day) in divided doses q6-8hr
*Serious systemic infections*
*Adult and child >12 yr:* IM/**IV** 2-4 g q4-6hr (2 g/site IM)
*Child <12 yr:* IM/**IV** 200-300 mg/kg/day in divided doses q4-6hr
*Neonate <36 wk:* **IV** 75 mg/kg q12hr in the 1st wk of life, then q8hr in 2nd wk
*Full-term infant:* **IV** 75 mg/kg q8hr in 1st wk of life, then q6hr thereafter

*Prophylaxis of surgical infections*
*Adult:* **IV** 2 g 30-60 min before procedure; may be repeated during or after surgery

*Renal dose*
*Adult:* **IV** CCr 20-40 ml/min give q8hr, CCr <20 ml/min give q12hr

**Available forms:** Powder for inj 2, 3, 4, 40 g

### Adverse effects
*CNS:* Lethargy, hallucinations, anxiety, depression, twitching, **coma, seizures**
*GI:* Nausea, vomiting, diarrhea, increased AST, ALT, abdominal pain, glossitis, colitis, **pseudomembranous colitis**
*GU:* Oliguria, proteinuria, hematuria, vaginitis, moniliasis, **glomerulonephritis**
*HEMA:* Anemia, increased bleeding time, **bone marrow depression, thrombocytopenia**
*META:* Hypokalemia, hypernatremia
*SYST:* Serum sickness, anaphylaxis, Stevens-Johnson syndrome, exfoliative dermatitis

**Contraindications:** Neonates, hypersensitivity to penicillins

**Precautions:** Pregnancy **B**, breastfeeding, hypersensitivity to cephalosporins, CHF, renal/GI disease, seizures

| Pharmacokinetics | |
|---|---|
| Absorption | Well absorbed (80%) |
| Distribution | Widely distributed; crosses placenta |
| Metabolism | Not metabolized |
| Excretion | Kidneys, unchanged (90%); bile (10%); breast milk |
| Half-life | 0.7-1.3 hr |

| Pharmacodynamics | IM | IV |
|---|---|---|
| Onset | Rapid | Rapid |
| Peak | 30-50 min | Inf end |
| Duration | Unknown | Unknown |

### Interactions
*Individual drugs*
Aspirin, probenecid: increased piperacillin levels
Methotrexate: increased levels of methotrexate
*Drug classifications*
Aminoglycosides: decreased antimicrobial effect of piperacillin
Contraceptives (oral): decreased contraceptive effectiveness
Neuromuscular blockers: increased levels of neuromuscular blockers
Tetracyclines: decreased antimicrobial effectiveness (with high concentrations of piperacillin)
*Drug/herb*
Acidophilus: do not use with antiinfectives; separate by several hours
Khat: decreased absorption
*Drug/lab test*
False positive: urine glucose, urine protein, Coombs' test

### NURSING CONSIDERATIONS
**Assessment**
- Assess patient for previous sensitivity reaction to penicillins or other cephalosporins; cross-sensitivity between penicillins and cephalosporins is common
- Assess patient for signs and symptoms of infection including characteristics of wounds, sputum, urine, stool, WBC >10,000/mm³, fever; obtain baseline information and during treatment
- Obtain C&S before beginning product therapy to identify if correct treatment has been initiated
- Assess for allergic reactions: rash, urticaria, pruritus, chills, fever, joint pain; angioedema may occur a few days after therapy begins; epINEPHrine, resuscitation equipment should be available for anaphylactic reaction
- ◆ Identify urine output; if decreasing, notify prescriber (may indicate nephrotoxicity); also check for increased BUN, creatinine
- Monitor blood studies: AST, ALT, CBC, Hct, bilirubin, LDH, alkaline phosphatase, Coombs' test monthly if patient is on long-term therapy
- Monitor electrolytes: potassium, sodium, chloride monthly if patient is on long-term therapy
- Assess bowel pattern daily; if severe diarrhea occurs, product should be discontinued; may indicate pseudomembranous colitis
- Monitor for bleeding: ecchymosis, bleeding gums, hematuria, stool guaiac daily if on long-term therapy
- Assess for overgrowth of infection: perineal itching, fever, malaise, redness, pain, swelling, drainage, rash, diarrhea, change in cough, sputum

**Nursing diagnoses**
- Diarrhea (adverse reactions)
- Infection, risk for (uses)
- Injury, risk for (adverse reactions)
- Knowledge, deficient (teaching)
- Noncompliance (teaching)

**Implementation**
**IM route**
- Reconstitute 2 g/4 ml, 3 g/6 ml, 4 g/7.8 ml with sterile water, 0.9% NaCl, bacteriostatic water, 0.5% or 1% lidocaine without epINEPHrine
- Inject deep in large muscle mass, massage; split inj >2 g into 2 inj
**IV route**
- Reconstitute with 5 ml or more 0.9% NaCl, bacteriostatic water; shake sol to dissolve
- Change **IV** sites q48hr to prevent phlebitis and pain
- Give direct **IV** over 3-5 min
- Give by intermittent inf by diluting in 50 ml or more D₅W, 0.9% NaCl, D₅/0.9% NaCl, LR, give over 20-30 min by Y-site; discontinue primary inf during intermittent inf
*Syringe compatibilities:* Heparin
*Y-site compatibilities:* Acyclovir, aldesleukin, allopurinol, amifostine, aztreonam, ciprofloxacin, cyclophosphamide, diltiazem, enalaprilat, esmolol, famotidine, fludarabine, foscarnet, heparin, hydromorphone, IL-2, labetalol, lorazepam, magnesium sulfate, melphalan, meperidine, midazolam, morphine, perphenazine, propofol, ranitidine, tacrolimus, teniposide, theophylline, thiotepa, verapamil, zidovudine
*Y-site incompatibilities:* Ondansetron, fluconazole, sargramostim, vinorelbine
*Additive compatibilities:* Ciprofloxacin, clindamycin, fluconazole, hydrocortisone sodium succinate, ofloxacin, potassium chloride, verapamil
*Additive incompatibilities:* Aminoglycosides

**Patient/family education**
- Teach patient to report sore throat, bruising, bleeding, joint pain; may indicate blood dyscrasias (rare)
- Advise patient to contact prescriber if vaginal itching, loose foul-smelling stools, furry tongue occur; may indicate superinfection
- Advise patient to notify prescriber of diarrhea with blood or pus, which may indicate pseudomembranous colitis

Adverse effects: *italic* = common, **bold** = life-threatening

## Evaluation
**Positive therapeutic outcome**
- Absence of signs/symptoms of infection (WBC <10,000/mm$^3$, temp WNL, absence of red, draining wounds)
- Reported improvement in symptoms of infection

**Treatment of anaphylaxis:** Withdraw product, maintain airway, administer epINEPHrine, aminophylline, O$_2$, **IV** corticosteroids

## piperacillin/tazobactam (Rx)
Zosyn
*Func. class.:* Broad-spectrum antiinfective
*Chem. class.:* Extended-spectrum penicillin

**Pregnancy category B**

**Action:** Interferes with cell wall replication of susceptible organisms; osmotically unstable cell wall swells and bursts from osmotic pressure; tazobactam is a β-lactamase inhibitor, protects piperacillin from enzymatic degradation

**Therapeutic outcome:** Bactericidal effects for piperacillin-resistant β-lactamase, *Escherichia coli, Staphylococcus aureus, Bacteroides fragilis, Bacteroides ovatus, Bacteroides thetaiotaomicron, Bacteroides vulgatus, Haemophilus influenzae*

**Uses:** Moderate to severe infections: piperacillin-resistant, β-lactamase strains causing infections in respiratory tract, skin, skin structure, urinary tract, bone, and joint; gonorrhea, pneumonia, infections from penicillinase-producing staphylococci, streptococci

### Dosage and routes
*Nosocomial pneumonia*
*Adult:* **IV** 3.375 g q6-8hr with an aminoglycoside × 1-2 wk; continue aminoglycoside only if *Pseudomonas aeruginosa* is isolated

*Other infections*
*Adult:* **IV** INF 6-12 g/day, given 2.25 g q8hr to 3.375 g q6hr over 30 min × 7-10 days

*Renal dose*
*Adult:* **IV** CCr 20-40 ml/min 2.25 g q6hr; CCr <20 ml/min 2.25 g q8hr

**Available forms:** Powder for inj 2 g piperacillin/0.25 g tazobactam; 3 g piperacillin/0.375 g tazobactam, 4 g piperacillin/0.5 g tazobactam, 36 g piperacillin/4.5 g tazobactam

## Adverse effects
*CNS:* Headache, insomnia, dizziness, fever, lethargy, hallucinations, anxiety, depression, twitching, **seizures**
*GI: Nausea, vomiting, diarrhea,* increased AST, ALT, abdominal pain, glossitis, constipation, **pseudomembranous colitis**
*GU:* **Oliguria, proteinuria, hematuria,** *vaginitis, moniliasis,* **glomerulonephritis, renal failure**
*HEMA:* Anemia, increased bleeding time, **bone marrow depression, agranulocytosis**
*INTEG:* Rash, pruritus, **exfoliative dermatitis**
*META:* Hypokalemia, hypernatremia
*SYST:* **Serum sickness, anaphylaxis**

**Contraindications:** Hypersensitivity to penicillins; neonates, carbapenem allergy

**Precautions:** Pregnancy **B**, breastfeeding, CHF, seizures, hypersensitivity to cephalosporins, renal insufficiency in children, GI disease, electrolyte imbalances

### Pharmacokinetics
| | |
|---|---|
| **Absorption** | Well absorbed (80%) |
| **Distribution** | Widely distributed; crosses placenta |
| **Metabolism** | Not metabolized |
| **Excretion** | Kidneys, unchanged (90%); bile (10%); breast milk |
| **Half-life** | 0.7-1.3 hr |

### Pharmacodynamics
| | |
|---|---|
| **Onset** | Rapid |
| **Peak** | Inf end |
| **Duration** | Unknown |

### Interactions
*Individual drugs*
Aspirin, probenecid: increased piperacillin levels
Methotrexate: increased effect of methotrexate
*Drug classifications*
Aminoglycosides (**IV**): decreased piperacillin effect
Anticoagulants (oral): increased anticoagulant effects
Contraceptives (oral): decreased contraceptive effectiveness
Neuromuscular blockers: increased effects
Tetracyclines: decreased antimicrobial effectiveness of piperacillin
*Drug/herb*
Acidophilus: do not use with antiinfectives; separate by several hours
Khat: decreased absorption

## *Drug/lab test*
Increased: platelet count, eosinophilia, neutropenia, leucopenia, serum creatinine, PTT, AST, ALT, alkaline phosphatase, bilirubin, BUN, electrolytes

Decreased: Hct, Hgb, electrolytes

False positive: urine glucose, urine protein, Coombs' test

## NURSING CONSIDERATIONS
### Assessment
• Assess patient for previous sensitivity reaction to penicillins or other cephalosporins, cross-sensitivity between penicillins and cephalosporins is common

• Assess patient for signs and symptoms of infection including characteristics of wounds, sputm, urine, stool, WBC >10,000/mm$^3$, fever; obtain baseline information and during treatment

• Obtain C&S before beginning product therapy to identify if correct treatment has been initiated

• Assess for allergic reactions: rash, urticaria, pruritus, chills, fever, joint pain; angioedema may occur a few days after therapy begins; epINEPHrine, resuscitation equipment should be available for anaphylactic reaction

⏺ Identify urine output; if decreasing, notify prescriber (may indicate nephrotoxicity); also check for increased BUN, creatinine

• Monitor blood studies: AST, ALT, CBC, Hct, bilirubin, LDH, alkaline phosphatase, Coombs' test monthly if patient is on long-term therapy

• Monitor electrolytes: potassium, sodium, chloride monthly if patient is on long-term therapy

• Assess bowel pattern daily; if severe diarrhea occurs, product should be discontinued; may indicate pseudomembranous colitis

• Monitor for bleeding: ecchymosis, bleeding gums, hematuria, stool guaiac daily if on long-term therapy

• Assess for overgrowth of infection: perineal itching, fever, malaise, redness, pain, swelling, drainage, rash, diarrhea, change in cough, sputum

### Nursing diagnoses
• Diarrhea (adverse reactions)
• Infection, risk for (uses)
• Injury, risk for (adverse reactions)
• Knowledge, deficient (teaching)
• Noncompliance (teaching)

### Implementation
• Reconstitute with 5 ml or more 0.9% NaCl, bacteriostatic water; shake sol to dissolve

• Give by intermittent inf by diluting in 50 ml or more D$_5$W, 0.9% NaCl, D$_5$/0.9% NaCl, LR; give over 20-30 min by Y-site; discontinue primary inf during intermittent inf

• Change **IV** sites q48hr to prevent phlebitis and pain

• Give direct **IV** over 3-5 min

*Y-site compatibilities:* Aminophylline, aztreonam, bleomycin, bumetanide, buprenorphine, butorphanol, calcium gluconate, carboplatin, carmustine, cefepime, cimetidine, clindamycin, cyclophosphamide, cytarabine, dexamethasone, diphenhydrAMINE, DOPamine, enalaprilat, etoposide, floxuridine, fluconazole, fludarabine, fluorouracil, furosemide, gallium, granisetron, heparin, hydrocortisone, hydromorphone, ifosfamide, leucovorin, lorazepam, magnesium sulfate, mannitol, meperidine, mesna, methotrexate, methylPREDNISolone, metoclopramide, metronidazole, morphine, ondansetron, plicomycin, potassium chloride, ranitidine, sargramostim, sodium bicarbonate, thiotepa, trimethoprim/sulfamethoxazole, vinBLAStine, vinCRIStine, zidovudine

*Y-site incompatibilities:* Fluconazole, ondansetron, sargramostim, vinorelbine

### Patient/family education
• Teach patient to report sore throat, bruising, bleeding, joint pain; may indicate blood dyscrasias (rare)

• Advise patient to contact prescriber if vaginal itching, loose foul-smelling stools, furry tongue occur; may indicate superinfection

• Advise patient to notify prescriber of diarrhea with blood or pus, which may indicate pseudomembranous colitis

### Evaluation
**Positive therapeutic outcome**
• Absence of signs/symptoms of infection (WBC <10,000/mm$^3$, temp WNL, absence of red, draining wounds)

• Reported improvement in symptoms of infection

**Treatment of anaphylaxis:** Withdraw product, maintain airway, administer epINEPHrine, aminophylline, O$_2$, **IV** corticosteroids

P

## pirbuterol (Rx)
(peer-byoo'ter-ole)
Maxair
*Func. class.:* Bronchodilator
*Chem. class.:* β-Adrenergic agonist

**Pregnancy category C**

**Action:** Relaxes bronchial smooth muscle by direct action on $\beta_2$-adrenergic receptors, with increased levels of cAMP and increased bronchodilatation, diuresis, and cardiac and CNS stimulation

**Therapeutic outcome:** Bronchodilatation with ease of breathing

**Uses:** Reversible bronchospasm (prevention, treatment), including asthma, may be given with theophylline or steroids

### Dosage and routes
***Adult and child >12 yr:*** INH 1-2 (0.4 mg) q4-6hr; max 12 inh/day

**Available forms:** Aerosol delivers 0.2 mg pirbuterol/actuation

### Adverse effects
*CNS:* Tremors, anxiety, insomnia, headache, dizziness, stimulation, restlessness, hallucinations, drowsiness, irritability
*CV:* Palpitations, tachycardia, hypo/hypertension, angina, **dysrhythmias**
*EENT:* Dry nose and mouth, irritation of nose, throat
*GI:* Gastritis, nausea, vomiting, anorexia
*MS:* Muscle cramps
*RESP:* **Paradoxical bronchospasm**, dyspnea, coughing

**Contraindications:** Hypersensitivity to sympathomimetics, tachycardia

**Precautions:** Pregnancy **C**, breastfeeding, cardiac disorders, hyperthyroidism, hypertension, diabetes mellitus, prostatic hypertrophy

### Pharmacokinetics

| | |
|---|---|
| **Absorption** | Minimally absorbed |
| **Distribution** | Unknown |
| **Metabolism** | Liver |
| **Excretion** | Unknown |
| **Half-life** | 2 hr |

### Pharmacodynamics

| | |
|---|---|
| **Onset** | 5-15 min |
| **Peak** | 1-1½ hr |
| **Duration** | 5 hr |

### Interactions
***Individual drugs***
Levothyroxine: increased pirbuterol action
***Drug classifications***
Antidepressants (tricyclics), antihistamines: increased pirbuterol action
β-Adrenergic blockers: block therapeutic effect
Bronchodilators, aerosol: increased action of bronchodilator
MAOIs: increased chance of hypertensive crisis
***Drug/herb***
Cola nut, guarana, yerba maté: increased action of both
Green tea (large amounts), guarana: increased effect

## NURSING CONSIDERATIONS
### Assessment
• Monitor respiratory function: vital capacity, FEV, ABGs, lung sounds, heart rate, rhythm (baseline)
• Monitor for evidence of allergic reactions, paradoxic bronchospasm (can occur rapidly); withhold dose and notify prescriber

### Nursing diagnoses
• Airway clearance, ineffective (uses)
• Gas exchange, impaired (uses)
• Knowledge, deficient (teaching)

### Implementation
• Give after shaking; have patient exhale, place mouthpiece in mouth, inhale slowly, hold breath, remove, exhale slowly; allow at least 1 min between inhalations
• Give this medication before other medications and allow at least 1 min between each to prevent overstimulation
• Store in light-resistant container; do not expose to temperature over 86° F (30° C)

### Patient/family education
• Advise patient not to use OTC medications; extra stimulation may occur; to use this medication before other medications and allow at least 1 min between each to prevent overstimulation
• Teach patient use of inhaler; to avoid getting aerosol in eyes; blurring may result; to wash inhaler in warm water and dry daily; to avoid smoking, smoke-filled rooms, persons with respiratory tract infections; review package insert with patient
• Teach patient that paradoxic bronchospasm may occur and to stop product immediately and notify prescriber; to limit caffeine products such as chocolate, coffee, tea, and colas

- Instruct patient on administration of dose; not to use more than prescribed; serious side effects may occur

### Evaluation
#### Positive therapeutic outcome
- Absence of dyspnea, wheezing after 1 hr
- Improved airway exchange
- Improved ABGs

**Treatment of overdose:** Administer a β₂-adrenergic blocker

---

### piroxicam (Rx)
(peer-ox'i-kam)
Apo-Piroxicam ✦, Feldene, Novopirocam ✦, PMS-Piroxicam ✦
*Func. class.:* Nonsteroidal antiinflammatory
*Chem. class.:* Oxicam derivative

#### Pregnancy category B

**Action:** Inhibits prostaglandin synthesis by decreasing an enzyme needed for biosynthesis; analgesic, antiinflammatory

**Therapeutic outcome:** Decreased pain, inflammation

**Uses:** Mild to moderate pain, osteoarthritis, rheumatoid arthritis

### Dosage and routes
*Adult:* PO 20 mg/day or 10 mg bid

**Available forms:** Caps 10, 20 mg

### Adverse effects
*CNS:* Dizziness, *drowsiness,* fatigue, tremors, confusion, insomnia, anxiety, depression, *headache*
*CV:* Tachycardia, peripheral edema, palpitations, **dysrhythmias,** hypertension, **MI, stroke**
*EENT:* Tinnitus, hearing loss, blurred vision
*GI:* Nausea, anorexia, vomiting, diarrhea, jaundice, **cholestatic hepatitis,** constipation, flatulence, cramps, dry mouth, peptic ulcer, **bleeding, ulceration, perforation**
*GU:* Nephrotoxicity: dysuria, **hematuria, oliguria, azotemia**
*HEMA:* Blood dyscrasias
*INTEG:* Purpura, rash, pruritus, sweating, photosensitivity
*SYST:* Anaphylaxis

**Contraindications:** Hypersensitivity, asthma, severe renal/hepatic/ulcer/cardiac disease, perioperative pain in CABG surgery

**Precautions:** Pregnancy **B**, breastfeeding, children, bleeding disorders, GI/cardiac

disorders, hypersensitivity to other antiinflammatory agents, CHF, avoid in late pregnancy

#### Pharmacokinetics
| | |
|---|---|
| **Absorption** | Well absorbed |
| **Distribution** | Unknown |
| **Metabolism** | Liver, extensively |
| **Excretion** | Kidneys, minimal; breast milk |
| **Half-life** | 50 hr |

#### Pharmacodynamics
| | |
|---|---|
| **Onset** | 1 hr |
| **Peak** | 3-5 hr |
| **Duration** | 48-72 hr |

### Interactions
#### Individual drugs
Alcohol, aspirin, cycloSPORINE, lithium, methotrexate: increased toxicity
#### Drug classifications
Anticoagulants (oral), corticosteroids: increased toxicity
Antidiabetics (oral): hypoglycemia
Antihypertensives: decreased effect of antihypertensives
Diuretics: decreased effectiveness of diuretics
#### Drug/herb
Arginine, gossypol: increased gastric irritation
Bearberry, bilberry: increased NSAIDs effect
Bogbean, chondroitin: increased bleeding risk

### NURSING CONSIDERATIONS
#### Assessment
- Monitor blood counts during therapy; watch for decreasing platelets; if low, therapy may need to be discontinued, restarted after hematologic recovery; check for blood dyscrasia (thrombocytopenia): bruising, fatigue, bleeding, poor healing
- Assess for pain: location, duration, ROM, before and 1-2 hr after administration
- Assess for aspirin sensitivity, asthma, nasal polyps; these may develop into allergic reactions

#### Nursing diagnoses
- Injury, risk for (adverse reactions)
- Knowledge, deficient (teaching)
- Mobility, impaired physical (uses)
- Pain, chronic (uses)

#### Implementation
- Swallow caps whole; do not break, crush, or chew
- Give with food or milk to decrease gastric symptoms, water to enhance absorption

**P**

## Patient/family education
- Teach patient that product must be continued for prescribed time to be effective; to avoid aspirin, alcoholic beverages, and other OTC medications unless approved by prescriber
- Caution patient to report bleeding, bruising, fatigue, malaise, since blood dyscrasias do occur
- Instruct patient to use caution when driving; drowsiness, dizziness may occur
- Teach patient to take with a full glass of water to enhance absorption

## Evaluation
**Positive therapeutic outcome**
- Decreased pain
- Decreased inflammation
- Increased mobility

---

## plasma protein fraction (Rx)
Plasmanate, Plasma Plex, Plasmatein, Protenate
*Func. class.:* Blood derivative
*Chem. class.:* Human plasma in sodium chloride

**Pregnancy category** C

---

**Action:** Exerts similar oncotic pressure as human plasma, expands blood volume, shifts water from extravascular space to intravascular space

**Therapeutic outcome:** Shift of fluid from extravascular into intravascular space

**Uses:** Hypovolemic shock, hypoproteinemia, ARDS, preoperative cardiopulmonary bypass, acute liver failure, nephrotic syndrome, cardiogenic shock

## Dosage and routes
*Hypovolemia*
**Adult:** **IV** INF 250-500 ml (12.5-25 g of protein), max 10 ml/min
**Child:** **IV** INF 22-33 ml/kg at 5-10 ml/min

*Hypoproteinemia*
**Adult:** **IV** INF 1000-1500 ml/day, max 8 ml/min

**Available forms:** Inj 5%

## Adverse effects
*CNS:* Fever, chills, headache, paresthesias, flushing
*CV:* **Fluid overload,** hypotension, erratic pulse
*GI:* Nausea, vomiting, increased salivation
*INTEG:* Rash, urticaria, cyanosis

*RESP:* Altered respirations, dyspnea, **pulmonary edema**

**Contraindications:** Hypersensitivity, CHF, severe anemia, renal insufficiency, hyponatremia, cardiopulmonary bypass

**Precautions:** Pregnancy **C**, decreased salt intake, decreased cardiac reserve, lack of albumin deficiency, hepatic disease

### Pharmacokinetics
| | |
|---|---|
| **Absorption** | Completely absorbed |
| **Distribution** | Intravascular space |
| **Metabolism** | Unknown |
| **Excretion** | Unknown |
| **Half-life** | Unknown |

### Pharmacodynamics
| | |
|---|---|
| **Onset** | 15-30 min |
| **Peak** | Unknown |
| **Duration** | Unknown |

## Interactions
*Drug/lab test*
False increase: alkaline phosphatase

## NURSING CONSIDERATIONS
### Assessment
- Monitor blood studies: Hct, Hgb; electrolytes, serum protein, if serum protein declines, dyspnea, hypoxemia can result
- Monitor B/P (decreased), pulse (erratic), respiration during inf; CVP, jugular vein distention, PWP (increases if overload occurs); shortness of breath, anxiety, insomnia, expiratory crackles, frothy blood-tinged cough, cyanosis indicate pulmonary overload
- Monitor I&O ratio; urinary output may decrease
- Assess for allergy: fever, rash, itching, chills, flushing, urticaria, nausea, vomiting, or hypotension requires discontinuation of inf; use new lot if therapy reinstituted, premedicate with diphenhydrAMINE

### Nursing diagnoses
- Cardiac output, decreased (uses)
- Fluid volume, deficient (uses)
- Fluid volume, excess (adverse reactions)

### Implementation
- Give by **IV**; no dilution required; use infusion pump, large-gauge needle (≥20G); discard unused portion; infuse slowly to prevent hypotension; give within 4 hr of opening
- Provide adequate hydration before administration
- Do not use sol that has been frozen
- Adjust rate to changes in B/P

---

- When storing, check type of albumin, date; may have to refrigerate

**Additive compatibilities:**
Carbohydrate and electrolyte sol, whole blood, packed RBCs, chloramphenicol, tetracycline

**Additive incompatibilities:**
Protein hydrolysate sol, amino acids sol, alcohol, norepinephrine

### Patient/family education
- Explain reason for and expected result of medication

### Evaluation
**Positive therapeutic outcome**
- Increased B/P
- Decreased edema
- Increased serum albumin

---

## porfirmer (Rx)
(pour'fur-meer)
Photofrin
*Func. class.:* Antineoplastic—miscellaneous
*Chem. class.:* Photosensitizing agent, hematoporphyrin derivative

**Pregnancy category** C

**Action:** Used in photodynamic treatment (PDT) of tumors; antitumor and cytotoxic actions are light and $O_2$ dependent; used with 630-nm laser light

**Therapeutic outcome:** Prevention of growth of tumor

**Uses:** Esophageal cancer (completely obstructing), endobronchial non–small-cell lung cancer, Barrett's esophagus

### Dosage and routes
Refer to Optiguide for complete instructions
*Adult:* **IV** 2 mg/kg over 3-5 min, then illumination with laser light 40-50 hr after inj; a second laser light application may be given 96-120 hr after inj; may repeat q30 days × 3

*Endobronchial cancer*
*Adult:* 200 joules/cm of tumor length

**Available forms:** Cake/powder for inj 75 mg

### Adverse effects
*CNS: Anxiety, confusion, insomnia*
*CV: Hypo/hypertension,* **atrial fibrillation, cardiac failure,** *tachycardia,* chest pain
*GI: Abdominal pain, constipation, diarrhea, dyspepsia, dysphagia, eructation, esophageal edema/bleeding, hematemesis, melena, nausea, vomiting, anorexia*

*MISC:* Dehydration, weight decrease, anemia, photosensitivity reaction, UTI, moniliasis
*RESP:* **Pleural effusion,** pneumonia, dyspnea, respiratory insufficiency, **tracheoesophageal fistula,** stricture/ulceration

**Contraindications:** Porphyria, porphyrin allergy (porfirmer); tracheoesophageal, bronchoesophageal fistula; major blood vessels with eroding tumors (PDT)

**Precautions:** Pregnancy **C,** breastfeeding, children, geriatric

### Pharmacokinetics
| | |
|---|---|
| **Absorption** | Unknown |
| **Distribution** | In tissues |
| **Metabolism** | Unknown |
| **Excretion** | Cleared by biliary excretion |
| **Half-life** | 250 hr |

### Pharmacodynamics
| | |
|---|---|
| **Onset** | Unknown |
| **Peak** | 5-10 hr |
| **Duration** | Unknown |

### Interactions
*Drug classifications*
Anticoagulants, NSAIDS, platelet inhibitors, thrombolytics: decreased porfirmer effect
Phenothiazines, sulfonamides, sulfonylureas, tetracyclines, thiazides: increased photosensitivity

### NURSING CONSIDERATIONS
**Assessment**
- Assess for ocular sensitivity; sensitivity to sun, bright lights, car headlights; patients should wear dark sunglasses with an average white light transmittance of <4%
- Assess for chest pain: may be so severe as to necessitate opiate analgesics
- Assess for extravasation at inj site: take care to protect from light

**Nursing diagnoses**
- Infection, risk for (adverse reactions)
- Knowledge, deficient (teaching)

**Implementation**
- Give as a single slow **IV** inj over 3-5 min at 2 mg/kg; reconstitute each vial with 31.8 ml of $D_5$ or 0.9% NaCl (2.5 mg/ml), shake well, do not mix with other products or sol, protect from light, and use immediately
- Laser light is initiated 630-nm wavelength laser light
- Wipe spills with damp cloth, avoid skin/eye contact, use rubber gloves, eye protection;

P

Adverse effects: *italic* = common, **bold** = life-threatening

dispose of material in polyethylene bag according to policy

### Patient/family education
• Advise patient to report chest pain, eye sensitivity
• Advise patient to wear sunglasses; avoid exposure to sunlight or bright light for 30 days

### Evaluation
**Positive therapeutic outcome**
• Reducing number and spread of malignant cells

---

## posaconazole (Rx)
(poe'sa-kon'a-zole)
Noxafil
*Func. class.:* Antifungal, systemic
*Chem. class.:* Triazole derivative

**Pregnancy category** C

**Action:** Inhibits a portion of cell wall synthesis; alters cell membranes and inhibits several fungal enzymes

**Therapeutic outcome:** Decreased fever, malaise, rash, negative C&S for infecting organism

**Uses:** Prevention of aspergillus, candida infection, oropharyngeal candidiasis in the immunocompromised

### Dosage and routes
*Adult:* PO 800 mg/day in 2-4 divided doses
*Child:* PO 100 mg tid

**Available forms:** Oral susp 200 mg/5 ml

### Adverse effects
*CNS: Headache, dizziness,* insomnia, fever, rigors, weakness, anxiety
*CV:* Hypo/hypertension, tachycardia, anemia
*GI: Nausea, vomiting, anorexia, diarrhea,* cramps, abdominal pain, flatulence, **GI bleeding, hepatotoxicity**
*GU:* Gynecomastia, impotence, decreased libido
*INTEG: Pruritus,* fever, *rash,* **toxic epidermal necrolysis**
*MISC: Edema, fatigue,* malaise, hypokalemia, tinnitus, **rhabdomyolysis**

**Contraindications:** Hypersensitivity to this product or other systemic antifungal or azoles, fungal meningitis, onchomycosis or dermatomycosis in cardiac dysfunction

**Precautions:** Pregnancy **C**, breastfeeding, children, hepatic/cardiac disease

### Pharmacokinetics
| | |
|---|---|
| **Absorption** | Well, enhanced by food |
| **Distribution** | Protein binding 98-99% |
| **Metabolism** | Liver |
| **Excretion** | Feces, 77% unchanged |
| **Half-life** | 19-35 hr |

### Pharmacodynamics
| | |
|---|---|
| **Onset** | Unknown |
| **Peak** | 4-11 hr |
| **Duration** | Unknown |

### Interactions
*Individual drugs*
🔷 BusPIRone, busulfan, clarithromycin, cycloSPORINE, diazepam, digoxin, felodipine, indinavir, isradipine, niCARdipine, niFEDipine, nimodipine, phenytoin, quinidine, ritonavir, saquinavir, tacrolimus, warfarin: increased levels, toxicity
Didanosine: decreased posaconazole action
🔷 Dofetilide, pimozide, quinidine: life-threatening reactions
Midazolam (oral), triazolam: increased sedation
Quinidine: increased tinnitus, hearing loss
*Drug classifications*
Antacids, H$_2$-receptor antagonists, rifamycins: decreased posaconazole action
Calcium channel blockers: Increased edema
🔷 Ergots: life-threatening reactions
Other hepatotoxic products: increased hepatotoxicity
Oral contraceptives: decreased effect, use other contraceptives
Oral hypoglycemics: increased severe hypoglycemia
*Drug/herb*
Gossypol: nephrotoxicity
*Drug/food*
Food: increased absorption

### NURSING CONSIDERATIONS
Assessment
• Assess for type of infection; may begin treatment prior to obtaining results
• Assess for infection: temp, WBC, sputum, baseline and periodically
• Monitor I&O ratio, potassium levels
• Monitor liver function tests (ALT, AST, bilirubin) if on long-term therapy
• Assess for allergic reaction: rash, photosensitivity, uricaria, dermatitis
🔷 Assess for hepatotoxicity: nausea, vomiting, jaundice, clay-colored stools, fatigue

---

### Nursing diagnoses
- Infection, risk for (uses)
- Knowledge, deficient (teaching)

### Implementation
- Give after shaking well; use calibrated measuring device; take only with a full meal or liquid nutritional supplements such as Ensure; rinse measuring device after each use
- Store in a tight container in refrigerator; do not freeze

### Patient/family education
- Teach patient that long-term therapy may be needed to clear infection (1 wk-6 mo depending on infection)
- Advise patient to avoid hazardous activities if dizziness occurs
- Advise patient to take 2 hr before administration of other products that increase gastric pH (antacids, $H_2$-blockers, omeprazole, sucralfate, anticholinergics); to notify health care provider of all medications taken
- Teach the patient the importance of compliance with product regimen; to use alternative method of contraceptive
- Teach patient to notify prescriber of GI symptoms, signs of hepatic dysfunction (fatigue, nausea, anorexia, vomiting, dark urine, pale stools)

### Evaluation
**Positive therapeutic outcome**
- Decreased fever, malaise, rash, negative C&S for infecting organism

## potassium acetate/ potassium bicarbonate (Rx, OTC)
K+Care ET, K-Electrolyte, K-Ide, Klor-Con EF, K-Lyte, K-Vescent

## potassium bicarbonate/ potassium chloride (Rx, OTC)
Klorvess, Klorvess Effervescent Granules, K-Lyte/Cl, Neo-K ✦

## potassium bicarbonate/ potassium citrate (Rx, OTC)
Effer-K, K-Lyte DS

## potassium chloride (Rx, OTC)
Apo-K ✦, Cena-K, Gen-K, K+care, K+10, Kalium Durules ✦, Kaochlor, Kaochlor S-F, Kaon-Cl, Kay Ciel, KCl, K-Dur, K-Lease, K-Long ✦, K-Lor, Klor-Con, Klorvess, Klotrix, K-Lyte/Cl powder, K-med, K-Norm, K-Sol, K-Tab, Micro-K, Micro-LS, Potasalan, Roychlor, Rum-K, Slow-K, Ten-K

## potassium chloride/ potassium bicarbonate/ potassium citrate (Rx, OTC)
Kaochlor Eff

## potassium gluconate (Rx, OTC)
Kaon, Kaylixir, K-G Elixir, Potassium-Rougier ✦

## potassium gluconate/ potassium chloride (Rx, OTC)
Kolyum

## potassium gluconate/ potassium citrate (Rx, OTC)
Twin-K

*Func. class.:* Electrolyte, mineral replacement
*Chem. class.:* Potassium

**Pregnancy category C**

**Action:** Needed for adequate transmission of nerve impulses and cardiac contraction, renal function, intracellular ion maintenance

**Therapeutic outcome:** Potassium level 3.0-5.0 mg/dl

**Uses:** Prevention and treatment of hypokalemia

### Dosage and routes
*Potassium bicarbonate*
*Adult:* PO Dissolve 25-50 mEq in water daily-qid

Adverse effects: *italic* = common, **bold** = life-threatening

*Hypokalemia (prevention)*
**Adult and child:** PO 20 mEq/day in 2-4 divided doses

*Potassium acetate—hypokalemia*
**Adult and child:** PO 40-100 mEq/day in divided doses × 2-4 days

*Potassium chloride*
**Adult:** PO 40-100 mEq in divided doses tid-qid; **IV** 20 mEq/hr when diluted as 40 mEq/1000 ml, max 150 mEq/day
**Child:** PO 2-4 mEq/kg/day

*Potassium gluconate*
**Adult:** PO 40-100 mEq in divided doses tid-qid

*Potassium phosphate*
**Adult:** **IV** 1 mEq/hr in sol of 60 mEq/L, max 150 mEq/day; PO 40-100 mEq/day in divided doses
**Child:** **IV** Max rate of infusion 1 mEq/kg/min

**Available forms:** Tabs for sol 6.5, 25 mEq; ext rel caps 8, 10 mEq; powder for sol 3.3, 5, 6.7, 10, 13.3 mEq/5 ml; tabs 2, 4, 5, 13.4 mEq; ext rel tabs 6.7, 8, 10 mEq; elixir 6.7 mEq/5 ml; oral sol 2.375 mEq/5 ml; inj for prep of **IV** 1.5, 2, 2.4, 3, 3.2, 4.4, 4.7 mEq

**Adverse effects**
***CNS:*** Confusion
***CV:*** Bradycardia, *cardiac depression,* **dysrhythmias, arrest, peaking T waves, lowered R and depressed RST, prolonged PR interval, widened QRS complex**
***GI:*** *Nausea, vomiting, cramps,* pain, *diarrhea,* ulceration of small bowel
***GU:*** Oliguria
***INTEG:*** Cold extremities, rash

**Contraindications:** Renal disease (severe), severe hemolytic disease, Addison's disease, hyperkalemia, acute dehydration, extensive tissue breakdown

**Precautions:** Pregnancy C, cardiac disease, potassium-sparing diuretic therapy, systemic acidosis

| Pharmacokinetics | |
|---|---|
| **Absorption** | Unknown |
| **Distribution** | Unknown |
| **Metabolism** | Unknown |
| **Excretion** | Kidneys, feces |
| **Half-life** | Unknown |

| Pharmacodynamics | | |
|---|---|---|
| | PO | IV |
| **Onset** | 30 min | Immediate |
| **Peak** | Unknown | Unknown |
| **Duration** | Unknown | Unknown |

**Interactions**
*Drug classifications*
Angiotensin-converting enzyme inhibitors, calcium, diuretics (potassium-sparing), magnesium, potassium phosphate, **IV**, other potassium products: increased hyperkalemia
*Drug/food*
Licorice: avoid large amounts

**NURSING CONSIDERATIONS**
**Assessment**
• Assess ECG for peaking T waves, lowered R, depressed RST, prolonged PR interval, widening QRS complex, hyperkalemia; product should be reduced or discontinued
• Monitor potassium level during treatment (3.5-5.0 mg/dl is normal level)
• Monitor I&O ratio; watch for decreased urinary output; notify prescriber immediately; check urinary pH in patients receiving the product as a urinary acidifier
• Assess cardiac status: rate, rhythm, CVP, PWP, PAWP if being monitored directly

**Nursing diagnoses**
• Knowledge, deficient (teaching)
• Nutrition: less than body requirements, imbalanced (uses)

**Implementation**
**PO route**
• Do not break, crush, or chew ext rel tabs/caps or enteric-coated products
• Give with meal or after meal; take cap with full glass of liquid; dissolve effervescent tab, powder in 8 oz of cold water or juice; do not give IM, SUBCUT
• Store at room temperature
**IV route**
• Give through large-bore needle to decrease vein inflammation; check for extravasation; administer in large vein, avoiding scalp vein in child
• After diluting in large volume of **IV** sol give as an **IV** inf slowly to prevent toxicity; never give **IV** bol or IM
*Potassium acetate*
***Additive compatibilities:*** Metoclopramide
*Potassium chloride*
***Y-site compatibilities:*** Acyclovir, aldesleukin, allopurinol, amifostine, aminophylline, amiodarone, ampicillin, ininamrinone, atropine, aztreonam, betamethasone, calcium gluconate, cefmetazole, cephalothin, cephapirin, chlordiazepoxide, chlorproMAZINE, ciprofloxacin, cladribine, cyanocobalamin, dexamethasone, digoxin, diltiazem, diphenhydrAMINE, DOBUTamine, DOPamine, droperi-

 Alert     ♣ Canada Only      Drug on CD     * "Tall Man" lettering (See Preface)

dol, edrophonium, enalaprilat, epINEPHrine, esmolol, estrogens, ethacrynate, famotidine, fentanyl, filgrastim, fludarabine, fluorouracil, furosemide, gallium, granisetron, heparin, hydrALAZINE, idarubicin, indomethacin, insulin, regular, isoproterenol, kanamycin, labetalol, lidocaine, lorazepam, magnesium sulfate, melphalan, meperidine, methicillin, methoxamine, methylergonovine, midazolam, minocycline, morphine, neostigmine, norepinephrine, ondansetron, oxacillin, oxytocin, paclitaxel, penicillin G potassium, pentazocine, phytonadione, piperacillin/tazobactam, predniSOLONE, procainamide, prochlorperazine, propofol, propranolol, pyridostigmine, sargramostim, scopolamine, sodium bicarbonate, succinylcholine, tacrolimus, teniposide, theophylline, thiotepa, trimethaphan, trimethobenzamide, vinorelbine, zidovudine

*Additive compatibilities:* Aminophylline, amiodarone, atracurium, bretylium, calcium chloride, cefepime, cephalothin, cephapirin, chloramphenicol, cimetidine, ciprofloxacin, clindamycin, cloxacillin, corticotropin, cytarabine, dimenhyDRINATE, DOPamine, enalaprilat, erythromycin, floxacillin, fluconazole, furosemide, heparin, hydrocortisone, isoproterenol, lidocaine, metaraminol, methicillin, methyldopate, metoclopramide, mitoxantrone, nafcillin, netilmicin, norepinephrine, oxacillin, penicillin G potassium or sodium, phenylephrine, piperacillin, ranitidine, sodium bicarbonate, thiopental, vancomycin, verapamil, vit B/C

*Potassium chloride*
*Y-site compatibilities:* Aldesleukin, amifostine, granisetron, lorazepam, midazolam, thiotepa

**Patient/family education**
• Teach patient to eat foods rich in potassium after medication is discontinued
• Advise patient to avoid OTC products: antacids, salt substitutes, analgesics, vit preparations, unless specifically directed by prescriber; avoid licorice in large amounts, may cause hypokalemia, sodium retention
• Advise patient to report hyperkalemia symptoms or continued hypokalemia symptoms
• Tell patient to take cap with full glass of liquid; to dissolve powder or tab completely in at least 120 ml of water or juice; not to crush, chew caps or tabs
• Emphasize importance of regular follow-up and periodic potassium levels

**Evaluation**
**Positive therapeutic outcome**
• Absence of fatigue, muscle weakness, and decreased thirst and urinary output, cardiac changes
• Potassium level normal

**pramipexole** (Rx)
(pra-mi-pex'ol)
Mirapex
*Func. class.:* Antiparkinsonian agent
*Chem. class.:* Dopamine receptor agonist, nonergot
**Pregnancy category C**

**Action:** Selective agonist for $D_2$ receptors (presynaptic/postsynaptic sites); binding at $D_3$ receptor contributes to antiparkinson effects

**Therapeutic outcome:** Decreased symptoms of Parkinson's disease (involuntary movements)

**Uses:** Parkinsonism, restless leg syndrome

**Dosage and routes**
*Initial treatment*
*Adult:* PO From a starting dose of 0.375 mg/day given in 3 divided doses; increase gradually by 0.125 mg/dose at 5-7-day intervals until total daily dose of 4.5 mg is reached
*Maintenance treatment*
*Adult:* PO 1.5-4.5 mg/day in 3 divided doses
*Renal dose*
*Adult:* PO CCr 35-59 ml/min 0.125 mg bid, may increase q5-7 days to 1.5 mg bid; CCr 15-34 ml/min 0.125 mg/day, may increase q5-7 days to 1.5 mg/day
*Restless leg syndrome*
*Adult:* PO 0.125-0.375 mg 2-3 hr before bedtime, increase gradually

**Available forms:** Tabs 0.125, 0.25, 1, 1.5 mg

**Adverse effects**
*CNS: Agitation, insomnia,* psychosis, hallucinations, depression, dizziness, headache, confusion, amnesia, dream disorder, asthenia
*CV: Orthostatic hypotension,* edema, syncope, tachycardia
*EENT:* Blurred vision
*GI: Nausea, anorexia,* constipation, dysphagia, dry mouth
*GU:* Impotence, urinary frequency
*HEMA:* **Hemolytic anemia, leukopenia, agranulocytosis**

**Contraindications:** Hypersensitivity

Adverse effects: *italic* = common, **bold** = life-threatening

**Precautions:** Pregnancy **C**, renal/cardiac disease, MI with dysrhythmias, affective disorders, psychosis, preexisting dyskinesias

### Pharmacokinetics

| | |
|---|---|
| **Absorption** | Well absorbed |
| **Distribution** | Widely distributed |
| **Metabolism** | Liver, minimally |
| **Excretion** | Kidneys, unchanged |
| **Half-life** | 8 hr; 12 hr in geriatric |

### Pharmacodynamics

| | |
|---|---|
| **Onset** | Unknown |
| **Peak** | 2 hr |
| **Duration** | Unknown |

### Interactions
*Individual drugs*

Cimetidine, diltiazem, levodopa, quinidine, ranitidine, triamterine, verapamil: increased pramipexole levels
Metoclopramide: decreased pramipexole levels
*Drug classifications*

Butyrophenones, DOPamine agonists, phenothiazines: decreased pramipexole effect
*Drug/herb*

Chaste tree fruit, kava: decreased pramipexole effect

### NURSING CONSIDERATIONS
**Assessment**

• Monitor B/P, ECG, respiration during initial treatment; hypo/hypertension should be reported
• Assess mental status: affect, mood, behavioral changes, depression; complete suicide assessment
• Monitor renal function tests
• Assess for involuntary movements in parkinsonism: akinesia, tremors, staggering gait, muscle rigidity, drooling; these symptoms should improve with therapy
🔷 Assess for sleep attacks: may fall asleep during activities, without warning; may need to discontinue medication

**Nursing diagnoses**

• Injury, risk for (uses)
• Knowledge, deficient (teaching)
• Mobility, impaired physical (uses)
• Noncompliance (teaching)

**Implementation**

• Adjust dosage to patient response
• Give with meals to decrease GI upset

### Patient/family education

• Advise patient that therapeutic effects may take several wk to a few mo
• Caution patient to change positions slowly to prevent orthostatic hypotension
• Instruct patient to use product exactly as prescribed; if product is discontinued abruptly, parkinsonian crisis may occur; if treatment is to be discontinued, taper over 1 wk; avoid alcohol, OTC sleeping products
• Advise patient to notify prescriber if pregnancy is planned or suspected

### Evaluation
**Positive therapeutic outcome**

• Decreased akathisia, other involuntary movements
• Improved mood

---

### pramlintide (Rx)
(pram′lin-tide)
Symlin
*Func. class.:* Antidiabetic
*Chem. class.:* Synthetic human amylin analog

**Pregnancy category C**

**Action:** Modulates and slows stomach emptying, prevents postprandial rise in plasma glucagon, decreases appetite, leads to decreased caloric intake and weight loss

**Therapeutic outcome:** Decreased polyuria, polydipsia, polyphagia; improved A1c

**Uses:** As an adjunct to insulin therapy with uncontrolled type 1 or type 2 diabetes

### Dosage and routes
*Type 1 diabetes*

**Adult:** SUBCUT Prior to each meal (≥30 g CHO), titrate up to 15 mcg to target dose of 60 mg/dose, each dose titration should occur after no nausea for 3 days

*Type 2 diabetes*

**Adult:** SUBCUT 60 mcg prior to each meal (≥30 g CHO), titrate up to 120 mcg SUBCUT with each meal after no nausea for 3-7 days

**Available forms:** Inj 5 ml vials (0.6 mg/ml)

### Adverse effects

*CNS:* Headache, fatigue, dizziness
*GI:* Nausea, vomiting, anorexia, abdominal pain
*INTEG:* Inj site reactions
*META:* Hypoglycemia (while used with insulin)
*MS:* Arthralgia

---

 Alert     Canada Only     Drug on CD    \* "Tall Man" lettering (See Preface)

*RESP: Cough,* pharyngitis
*SYST: Systemic allergy*

**Contraindications:** Hypersensitivity to this product or metacresol, gastroparesis

**Precautions:** Pregnancy **C**, breastfeeding, frequent hypoglycemia

### Pharmacokinetics

| | |
|---|---|
| **Absorption** | 30%-40% |
| **Distribution** | Extensively bound to blood cells or albumin |
| **Metabolism** | Kidneys |
| **Excretion** | Unknown |
| **Half-life** | 48 min |

### Pharmacodynamics

Unknown

### Interactions
*Individual drugs*

Acetaminophen: may increase effect of acetaminophen

Alcohol, disopyramide: increased hypoglycemia

Dextrothyroxine, niacin, triamterene: decreased hypoglycemia

Diphenoxylate, loperamide, octreotide: increased pramlintide action

Erythromycin, metoclopramide: do not use
*Drug classifications*

ACE inhibitors, anabolic steroids, androgens, corticosteroids, fibric acid derivatives: increased hypoglycemia

α-Glucosidase inhibitors, antimuscarinics, opiate agonist, tricyclics: increased pramlintide action

Estrogens, MAOIs, oral contraceptives, progestins, thiazide diuretics: decreased hypoglycemia

Phenothiazines: increased hyperglycemia

### NURSING CONSIDERATIONS
**Assessment**

• Monitor fasting blood glucose, 2 hr PP (80-150 mg/dl, normal fasting level; 70-130 mg/dl, normal 2 hr level); A1c may also be drawn to identify treatment effectiveness; also monitor weight, appetite

• Assess for hypoglycemic reaction (sweating, weakness, dizziness, chills, confusion, headache, nausea, rapid weak pulse, fatigue, tachycardia, memory lapses, slurred speech, staggering gait, anxiety, tremors, hunger)

• Assess for hyperglycemia: acetone breath, polyuria, fatigue, polydipsia, flushed, dry skin, lethargy

**Nursing diagnoses**

• Injury, risk for (uses)
• Knowledge, deficient (teaching)
• Noncompliance (teaching)

**Implementation**

• Pre-meal insulin should be decreased by 50% when starting and adjusted to therapeutic dose to prevent hypoglycemia

**SUBCUT route**

• Give immediately before mealtime or if 30 g of carbohydrates will be consumed
• Do not use if a meal is skipped
• Do not use if discolored; do not give in arm; absorption is variable
• Store at room temperature, keep away from heat and sunlight; refrigerate all other supply

*Syringe compatibilities:* Do not mix with insulin, give separately

**Patient/family education**

• Advise patient that product does not cure diabetes but controls symptoms
• Advise patient to carry emergency ID as diabetic
• Teach patient to recognize hypoglycemia reaction: headache, fatigue, weakness
• Teach patient the dosage, route, mixing instructions, if any diet restrictions, disease process
• Advise patient to carry a glucose source (candy or lump sugar) to treat hypoglycemia
• Teach patient symptoms of ketoacidosis: nausea, thirst, polyuria, dry mouth, decreased B/P, dry, flushed skin, acetone breath, drowsiness, Kussmaul respirations
• Advise patient that a plan is necessary for diet, exercise; all food on diet should be eaten; exercise routine should not vary
• Teach patient about blood glucose testing; make sure patient is able to determine glucose level
• Advise patient to avoid OTC products unless directed by prescriber, alcohol
• Advise patient not to operate machinery or drive until effect is known

**Evaluation**
**Positive therapeutic outcome**

• Decrease in polyuria, polydipsia, polyphagia, clear sensorium; improved A1c, blood glucose; absence of dizziness; stable gait

**Treatment of overdose:** Glucose 25 g **IV**, via dextrose 50% sol, 50 ml or glucagon 1 mg SUBCUT

P

## pramoxine topical
*See Appendix D*

## pravastatin (Rx)
(pra'va-sta-tin)
Pravachol
*Func. class.:* Antilipidemic

### Pregnancy category X

**Do not confuse:**
Pravachol/Prevacid

**Action:** Inhibits biosynthesis of VLDL, LDL, which are responsible for cholesterol development, by inhibiting the enzyme HMG-CoA reductase

**Therapeutic outcome:** Decreasing cholesterol levels and LDL, increased HDL

**Uses:** As an adjunct in primary hypercholesterolemia types IIa, IIb, III, IV, artherosclerosis, to reduce the risk of recurrent MI

### Dosage and routes
*Adult:* PO 40-80 mg/day at bedtime (range 20-80 mg/day)
*Adolescent 14-18 yr:* PO 40 mg/day
*Child 8-13 yr:* PO 20 mg/day
*Geriatric/renal/hepatic dose:* PO 10 mg/day, initially

**Available forms:** Tabs 10, 20, 40, 80 mg

### Adverse effects
*CNS:* Headache, dizziness, fatigue
*CV:* Chest pain
*EENT:* Lens opacities
*GI:* Nausea, constipation, diarrhea, flatus, abdominal pain, heartburn, **liver dysfunction, pancreatitis, hepatitis**
*INTEG:* Rash, pruritus, photosensitivity
*MS:* Muscle cramps, myalgia, **myositis, rhabdomyolysis**
*RESP:* Common cold, rhinitis, cough

**Contraindications:** Pregnancy **X**, breastfeeding, hypersensitivity, active liver disease

**Precautions:** Past liver disease, alcoholism, severe acute infections, trauma, severe metabolic disorders, electrolyte imbalances

### Pharmacokinetics

| | |
|---|---|
| **Absorption** | Poorly absorbed, erratic |
| **Distribution** | Protein binding 80% |
| **Metabolism** | Liver, extensively |
| **Excretion** | Feces (70%-75%); kidneys, unchanged (20%); breast milk (minimal) |
| **Half-life** | 2 hr |

### Pharmacodynamics

| | |
|---|---|
| **Onset** | Unknown |
| **Peak** | 1-1½ hr |
| **Duration** | Unknown |

### Interactions
*Individual drugs*
Clarithromycin, clofibrate, cycloSPORINE, erythromycin, gemfibrozil, itraconazole, niacin: increased risk for myopathy
Digoxin: increased effects of digoxin
Warfarin: increased bleeding
*Drug classifications*
Bile acid sequestrants: decreased pravastat in bioavailability
Protease inhibitors: increased risk of myopathy
*Drug/herb*
Glucomannan: increased effect
Gotu kola, oat bran, St. John's wort: decreased effect
*Drug/lab test*
Increased: CPK, liver function tests
Altered: thyroid function tests

### NURSING CONSIDERATIONS
**Assessment**
• Assess nutrition: fat, protein, carbohydrates; nutritional analysis should be completed by dietitian before treatment
• Monitor triglycerides, esterol, cholesterol at baseline and throughout treatment; LDL and HDL should be watched closely; if increased, product should be discontinued
◆ Assess for muscle tenderness, pain, obtain CPK; rhabdomyolysis may occur, therapy should be discontinued
• Monitor ophthal status yearly

**Nursing diagnoses**
• Knowledge, deficient (teaching)
• Noncompliance (teaching)

**Implementation**
• Give at bedtime only; give 1 hr before or 2 hr after bile acid sequestrants
• Store in cool environment in airtight, light-resistant container

**Patient/family education**
• Inform patient that compliance is needed for positive results to occur; not to double doses or skip doses
• Teach patient that risk factors should be decreased: high-fat diet, smoking, alcohol consumption, absence of exercise
• Advise patient to notify prescriber of weakness, tenderness, or limited mobility

- Explain to patient that contraception is necessary, since product produces teratogenic effects
- Advise patient to use sunscreen, protective clothing to prevent burns

### Evaluation
**Positive therapeutic outcome**
- Decreased cholesterol, serum triglyceride levels and improved ratio with HDL

---

## prazosin (Rx)
(pra'zoe-sin)
Minipress, prazosin
*Func. class.:* Antihypertensive
*Chem. class.:* α₁-Adrenergic blocker

**Pregnancy category C**

**Action:** Blocks α-mediated vasoconstriction of adrenergic receptors, inducing peripheral vasodilatation

**Therapeutic outcome:** Decreased B/P in hypertension; decreased cardiac preload, afterload

**Uses:** Hypertension, refractory CHF, Raynaud's vasospasm

**Unlabeled uses:** Benign prostatic hypertrophy to decreased urine outflow obstruction

### Dosage and routes
*Hypertension*
*Adult:* PO 1 mg bid or tid, increasing to 20 mg/day in divided doses if required, usual range 6-15 mg/day, not to exceed 1 mg initially; max 20-40 mg/day
*Child:* PO 5 mcg/kg q6hr; max 400 mcg/kg/day

*Benign prostatic hyperplasia*
*Adult:* PO 1-9 mg/day

**Available forms:** Caps 1, 2, 5 mg

### Adverse effects
*CNS: Dizziness, headache, drowsiness,* anxiety, depression, vertigo, weakness, fatigue
*CV: Palpitations, orthostatic hypotension,* tachycardia, edema, rebound hypertension
*EENT:* Blurred vision, epistaxis, tinnitus, dry mouth, red sclera
*GI: Nausea,* vomiting, diarrhea, constipation, abdominal pain
*GU:* Urinary frequency, incontinence, impotence, priapism, water and sodium retention

**Contraindications:** Hypersensitivity

**Precautions:** Pregnancy **C**, breastfeeding, children, hepatic disease, prostate cancer

### Pharmacokinetics
| | |
|---|---|
| **Absorption** | 60% |
| **Distribution** | Widely distributed |
| **Metabolism** | Liver, extensively; protein binding 97% |
| **Excretion** | Kidneys, unchanged (10%); bile (90%) |
| **Half-life** | 2-3 hr |

### Pharmacodynamics
| | |
|---|---|
| **Onset** | 2 hr |
| **Peak** | 1-3 hr |
| **Duration** | 6-12 hr |

### Interactions
*Individual drugs*
Alcohol, nitroglycerin, verapamil: increased hypotension
Clonidine: decreased antihypertensive effect
*Drug classifications*
Antihypertensives, β-adrenergic blockers: increased hypotension
NSAIDs: decreased antihypertensive effect
*Drug/herb*
Aconite: increased toxicity, death
Astragalus, cola tree: increased or decreased antihypertensive effect
Barberry, betony, black catechu, black cohosh, bloodroot, broom, burdock, cat's claw, dandelion, goldenseal, hawthorn, Irish moss, Jamaican dogwood, kelp, khella, mistletoe, parsley: increased antihypertensive effect
Coltsoot, guarana, khat, licorice, yohimbe: decreased antihypertensive effect
*Drug/lab test*
Increased: urinary norepinephrine, VMA

### NURSING CONSIDERATIONS
**Assessment**
- Monitor B/P, orthostatic hypotension, syncope; check for edema in feet, legs daily; monitor I&O, weight daily; notify prescriber of changes
- Assess for allergic reactions: rash, fever, pruritus, urticaria; product should be discontinued if antihistamines fail to help
- Assess for orthostatic hypotension; tell patient to rise slowly from sitting or lying position

**Nursing diagnoses**
- Cardiac output, decreased (uses)
- Injury, risk for (adverse reactions)
- Knowledge, deficient (teaching)
- Noncompliance (teaching)

**Implementation**
- Severe hypotension may occur after first dose of this medication; hypotension may be prevented by reducing or discontinuing

Adverse effects: *italic* = common, **bold** = life-threatening

diuretic therapy 3 days before beginning prazosin therapy
• Give same time each day
• Store in airtight container at 86° F (30° C) or less

### Patient/family education
• Instruct patient not to discontinue product abruptly; stress the importance of complying with dosage schedule, even if feeling better; if dose is missed, take as soon as remembered; take at same time each day
• Advise patient not to use OTC products (cough, cold, allergy) unless directed by prescriber; also to avoid large amounts of caffeine
• Emphasize the need to rise slowly to sitting or standing position to minimize orthostatic hypotension
• Teach patient to notify prescriber of mouth sores, sore throat, fever, swelling of hands or feet, irregular heartbeat, chest pain
• Caution patient to report excessive perspiration, dehydration, vomiting, diarrhea; may lead to fall in B/P
• Caution patient that product may cause dizziness, fainting, light-headedness; may occur during 1st few days of therapy; to avoid hazardous activities
• Teach patient how to take B/P and normal readings for age-group; instruct to take B/P q7 days

### Evaluation
**Positive therapeutic outcome**
• Decreased B/P in hypertension

**Treatment of overdose:** Administer volume expanders or vasopressors, discontinue product, place patient in supine position

---

**\*prednisoLONE** (Rx)
(pred-niss'oh-lone)
Articulose-50, Delta-Cortef, prednisoLONE, Prelone, Key-Pred 25, Key-Pred 50, Predaject-50, Predalone 50, Predcor-25, Predcor-50, Prednisolone Acetate, Orapred, Hydeltrasol, Key-Pred-SP, Pediapred, Hydeltra-T.B.A., Predalone-T.B.A., Prednisol TBA
*Func. class.:* Corticosteroid, synthetic
*Chem. class.:* Intermediate-acting glucocorticoid

**Pregnancy category  C**

**Do not confuse:**
prednisoLONE/predniSONE

**Action:** Decreases inflammation by suppressing migration of polymorphonuclear leukocytes, fibroblasts; reversal to increase capillary permeability and lysosomal stabilization, minimal mineralocorticoid

**Therapeutic outcome:** Decreased inflammation, decreased adrenal insufficiency

**Uses:** Severe inflammation, immunosuppression, neoplasms

### Dosage and routes
*Adult:* PO 2.5-15 mg bid-qid

### Asthma/antiinflammatory
*Child:* PO 1 mg/kg q6hr × 2 days, then 1-2 mg/kg, max 60 mg/day

**Available forms:** PrednisoLONE: tabs 5 mg, syr 5 mg/5 ml, 15 mg/5 ml; prednisoLONE phosphate: oral liquid 5 mg/5 ml; tabs 1, 2.5, 5, 10, 20, 50 mg, oral sol 5 mg/ml, 5 mg/5 ml, syr 5 mg/5 ml; oral dissolving tab 10, 15, 30 mg

### Adverse effects
*CNS: Depression,* flushing, sweating, headache, mood changes
*CV: Hypertension,* **circulatory collapse, thrombophlebitis, embolism,** tachycardia
*EENT:* Fungal infections, increased intraocular pressure, blurred vision
*GI: Diarrhea, nausea, abdominal distention,* **GI hemorrhage,** increased appetite, **pancreatitis**
*HEMA:* **Thrombocytopenia**
*INTEG:* Acne, poor wound healing, ecchymosis, petechiae
*MS:* Fractures, osteoporosis, weakness, arthralgia, myopathy, tendon rupture

**Contraindications:** Child <2 yr, psychosis, hypersensitivity, idiopathic thrombocytopenia, acute glomerulonephritis, amebiasis, fungal infections, nonasthmatic bronchial disease, measles, varicella, Cushing's syndrome

**Precautions:** Pregnancy **C,** breastfeeding, children, diabetes mellitus, glaucoma, osteoporosis, seizure disorders, ulcerative colitis, CHF, myasthenia gravis

| Pharmacokinetics | |
| --- | --- |
| **Absorption** | Well absorbed (PO, IM), completely absorbed (**IV**) |
| **Distribution** | Widely distributed, crosses placenta |
| **Metabolism** | Liver, extensively |
| **Excretion** | Kidney, breast milk |
| **Half-life** | 2-4 hr |

---

## Pharmacodynamics

|  | PO | IM (phosphate) | IV | IA/IL |
|---|---|---|---|---|
| **Onset** | 1 hr | Rapid | Rapid | Slow |
| **Peak** | 2 hr | 1 hr | Unknown | Unknown |
| **Duration** | 1½ days | Unknown | Unknown | Up to 1 mo |

## Interactions
### Individual drugs
Alcohol, amphotericin B, cycloSPORINE, digoxin, indomethacin: increased side effects

Ambenonium, isoniazid, neostigmine, somatrem: decreased effects of each specific product

Cholestyramine, colestipol, epHEDrine, phenytoin, rifampin, theophylline: decreased action of prednisoLONE

Indomethacin, ketoconazole: increased action of prednisoLONE
### Drug classifications
Antibiotics (macrolide), contraceptives (oral), estrogens, salicylates: increased action of prednisoLONE

Anticholinesterases, anticoagulants, anticonvulsants, antidiabetics, salicylates, toxoids, vaccines: decreased effects of each specific product

Barbiturates: decreased action of prednisoLONE

Diuretics, salicylates: increased side effects
### Drug/herb
Aloe, buckthorn, cascara sagrada, Chinese rhubarb, senna: increased hypokalemia

Aloe, licorice, perilla: increased effect
### Drug/lab test
Increased: cholesterol, sodium, blood glucose, uric acid, calcium, urine glucose

Decreased: calcium, potassium, $T_4$, $T_3$, thyroid $^{131}I$ uptake test, urine 17-OHCS, 17-KS

False negative: skin allergy tests

## NURSING CONSIDERATIONS
### Assessment
• Monitor potassium, blood glucose, urine glucose while patient is on long-term therapy; hypokalemia and hyperglycemia may occur

• Monitor weight daily; notify prescriber of weekly gain >5 lb; monitor I&O ratio; be alert for decreasing urinary output and increasing edema

• Monitor B/P q4hr, pulse; notify prescriber if chest pain occurs

• Monitor plasma cortisol levels during long-term therapy (normal level; 138-635 nmol/L [SI units] when measured at 8 AM)

• Assess adrenal function periodically for hypothalamic-pituitary-adrenal axis suppression

• Assess infection: increased temp, WBC even after withdrawal of medication; product masks infection symptoms

• Assess for potassium depletion: paresthesias, fatigue, nausea, vomiting, depression, polyuria, dysrhythmias, weakness, edema, hypertension, cardiac symptoms

• Assess mental status: affect, mood, behavioral changes, aggression

• Monitor temp; if fever develops, product should be discontinued

• Assess for systemic absorption: increased temp, inflammation, irritation (topical)
### Nursing diagnoses
• Infection, risk for (adverse reactions)
• Knowledge, deficient (teaching)
• Noncompliance (teaching)
### Implementation
• Oral sol: use calibrated measuring devices
• Orally disintegrating tabs: place on tongue, allow to dissolve, swallow; or swallow whole; do not cut, split
### Patient/family education
• Advise patient to carry/wear emergency ID as steroid user

• Advise patient to notify prescriber if therapeutic response decreases; dosage adjustment may be needed

• Caution patient not to discontinue abruptly; adrenal crisis can result; take exactly as prescribed

• Caution patient to avoid OTC products: salicylates, cough products with alcohol, cold preparations unless directed by prescriber

• Teach patient all aspects of product usage including cushingoid symptoms

• Teach patient symptoms of adrenal insufficiency: nausea, anorexia, fatigue, dizziness, dyspnea, weakness, joint pain

• Advise patient that long-term therapy may be needed to clear infection (1-2 mo depending on type of infection)
### Evaluation
**Positive therapeutic outcome**
• Decreased inflammation

## *prednisoLONE ophthalmic
*See Appendix D*

Adverse effects: *italic* = common, **bold** = life-threatening

## *predniSONE  (Rx)

(pred'ni-sone)

Apo-Prednisone ✤, Deltasone, Liquid Pred, Meticorten, Orasone, Panasol-S, Prednicen-M, predniSONE, Sterapred, Winpred

*Func. class.:* Corticosteroid
*Chem. class.:* Intermediate-acting glucocorticoid

### Pregnancy category C

### Do not confuse:
predniSONE/methylPREDNISolone/prednisoLONE/Prilosec

**Action:** Decreases inflammation by suppressing migration of polymorphonuclear leukocytes, fibroblasts; reversal to increase capillary permeability and lysosomal stabilization, minimal mineralocorticoid activity

**Therapeutic outcome:** Decreased inflammation, decreased adrenal insufficiency

**Uses:** Severe inflammation, immunosuppression, neoplasms, multiple sclerosis, collagen disorders, dermatologic disorders

### Dosage and routes
*Adult:* PO 5-60 mg/day or divided bid-qid
*Child:* PO 0.05-2 mg/kg/day divided 1-4 ×/day

*Nephrosis*
*Child:* PO 2 mg/kg/day in divided doses, max 28 days, then 1-1.5 mg/kg/day every other day × 4 wk

*Multiple sclerosis*
*Adult:* PO 200 mg/day × 1 wk, then 80 mg every other day × 1 mo

**Available forms:** Tabs 1, 2.5, 5, 10, 20, 50 mg; oral sol 5 mg/5 ml; syr 5 mg/5 ml

### Adverse effects
*CNS:* Depression, flushing, sweating, headache, mood changes
*CV:* Hypertension, **circulatory collapse, thrombophlebitis, embolism,** tachycardia
*EENT:* Fungal infections, increased intraocular pressure, blurred vision
*GI:* Diarrhea, nausea, abdominal distention, **GI hemorrhage,** increased appetite, **pancreatitis**
*HEMA:* **Thrombocytopenia**
*INTEG:* Acne, poor wound healing, ecchymosis, petechiae
*META:* Hyperglycemia
*MS:* Fractures, osteoporosis, weakness

**Contraindications:** Psychosis, hypersensitivity, idiopathic thrombocytopenia, acute glomerulonephritis, amebiasis, fungal infec-

tions, nonasthmatic bronchial disease, child <2 yr, AIDS, TB

**Precautions:** Pregnancy **C,** diabetes mellitus, glaucoma, osteoporosis, seizure disorders, ulcerative colitis, CHF, myasthenia gravis, renal disease, esophagitis, peptic ulcer, cataracts, coagulopathy

### Pharmacokinetics

| | |
|---|---|
| **Absorption** | Well absorbed |
| **Distribution** | Widely distributed, crosses placenta |
| **Metabolism** | Liver, extensively |
| **Excretion** | Kidney, breast milk |
| **Half-life** | 3-4 hr |

### Pharmacodynamics

| | |
|---|---|
| **Onset** | Unknown |
| **Peak** | 1-2 hr |
| **Duration** | 1½ days |

### Interactions
*Individual drugs*
Alcohol, amphotericin B, cycloSPORINE, digoxin: increased side effects
Ambenonium, isoniazid, neostigmine, sometrem: decreased effects of each specific product
Cholestyramine, colestipol, epHEDrine, phenytoin, rifampin, theophylline: decreased action of predniSONE
Indomethacin: increased side effects, increased action of predniSONE
Ketoconazole: increased action of predniSONE
*Drug classifications*
Anticholinesterases, anticoagulants, anticonvulsants, antidiabetics, toxoids, vaccines: decreased effects of each specific product
Antiinfectives (macrolide), contraceptives (oral), estrogens: increased action of predniSONE
Barbiturates: decreased action of predniSONE
Diuretics: increased side effects
Salicylates: increased side effects, action of predniSONE, decreased effects of salicylates
*Drug/herb*
Aloe, buckthorn, Chinese rhubarb, senna: increased hypokalemia
Aloe, licorice, perilla: increased effect
Ephedra (Ma huang): decreased predniSONE effect
*Drug/lab test*
Increased: cholesterol, sodium, blood glucose, uric acid, calcium, urine glucose
Decreased: calcium, potassium, $T_4$, $T_3$, thyroid [131]I uptake test, urine 17-OHCS, 17-KS, PBI
False negative: skin allergy tests

---

 Alert     ✤ Canada Only      Drug on CD     * "Tall Man" lettering (See Preface)

## NURSING CONSIDERATIONS
### Assessment
• Monitor potassium, blood glucose, urine glucose while on long-term therapy; hypokalemia and hyperglycemia may occur
• Monitor weight daily; notify prescriber of weekly gain >5 lb; monitor I&O ratio; be alert for decreasing urinary output and increasing edema
• Monitor B/P q4hr, pulse; notify prescriber if chest pain occurs
• Monitor plasma cortisol levels during long-term therapy (normal level 138-635 nmol/L when measured at 8 AM)
• Assess adrenal function periodically for hypothalamic-pituitary-adrenal axis suppression
• Assess infection: increased temp, WBC even after withdrawal of medication; product masks infection symptoms
• Assess for potassium depletion: paresthesias, fatigue, nausea, vomiting, depression, polyuria, dysrhythmias, weakness, edema, hypertension, cardiac symptoms
• Assess mental status: affect, mood, behavioral changes, aggression
• Monitor temp; if fever develops, product should be discontinued
• Assess for systemic absorption: increased temp, inflammation, irritation (topical)

### Nursing diagnoses
• Infection, risk for (adverse reactions)
• Knowledge, deficient (teaching)
• Noncompliance (teaching)

### Implementation
• Give with food or milk to decrease GI symptoms; use measuring device for liquid route
• For long-term use, alternative product therapy is recommended, to decrease adverse reactions

### Patient/family education
• Advise patient that emergency ID as steroid user should be carried or worn
• Advise patient to notify prescriber if therapeutic response decreases; dosage adjustment may be needed
• Caution patient not to discontinue abruptly; adrenal crisis can result
• Caution patient to avoid OTC products: salicylates, cough products with alcohol, cold preparations unless directed by prescriber
• Teach patient all aspects of product usage including cushingoid symptoms
• Teach patient symptoms of adrenal insufficiency: nausea, anorexia, fatigue, dizziness, dyspnea, weakness, joint pain

• Advise patient that long-term therapy may be needed to clear infection (1-2 mo depending on type of infection)

### Evaluation
**Positive therapeutic outcome**
• Decreased inflammation

## pregabalin (Rx)
(pre-gab'a-lin)
Lyrica
*Func. class.:* Anticonvulsant

**Pregnancy category** C

**Controlled substance schedule** V

**Action:** Binds to high-voltage–gated calcium channels in CNS tissues; this may lead to anticonvulsant action, similar to the inhibitory neurotransmitter GABA, anxiolytic, analgesics, and antiepileptic properties

**Therapeutic outcome:** Decreased seizure activity, decreased neuropathic pain

**Uses:** Neuropathic pain associated with diabetic peripheral neuropathy, partial onset seizures, postherpetic neuralgia, fibromyalgia

**Unlabeled uses:** Generalized anxiety disorder (GAD), moderate pain, social anxiety disorder

### Dosage and routes
*Diabetic peripheral neuropathic pain*
*Adult:* PO 50 mg tid, may increase to 300 mg/day (max) within 1 wk, adjust in renal disease

*Partial onset seizures*
*Adult:* PO 75 mg bid or 50 mg tid; may increase to 600 mg/day (max)

*Postherpetic neuralgia*
*Adult:* PO 75-150 mg bid or 50-100 mg tid in patient with CCr ≥60 ml/min, initially give 75 mg bid or 50 mg tid and may increase to 600 mg/day (max) within 1 wk

**Available forms:** Caps 25, 50, 75, 100, 150, 200, 225, 300 mg

### Adverse effects
*CNS:* Dizziness, fatigue, confusion, euphoria, incoordination, nervousness, neuropathy, tremor, vertigo, somnolence, ataxia, amnesia, abnormal thinking
*EENT:* Dry mouth, blurred vision, nystagmus, amblyopia
*GI:* Constipation, flatulence, abdominal pain, weight gain
*HEMA:* Ecchymosis

Adverse effects: *italic* = common, **bold** = life-threatening

***MS:*** Back pain
***OTHER:*** Pruritus, impotence, peripheral edema
***RESP:*** Dyspnea

**Contraindications:** Hypersensitivity, abrupt discontinuation

**Precautions:** Pregnancy **C,** breastfeeding, children <12 yr, geriatric, renal disease, PR interval prolongation, creatine kinase elevations, CHF (class III, IV), decreased platelets, drug abuse, dependence, glaucoma, myopathy

| Pharmacokinetics | |
|---|---|
| **Absorption** | Well, decreased by food |
| **Distribution** | Not bound to plasma proteins |
| **Metabolism** | Negligible |
| **Excretion** | 90% unchanged, urine |
| **Half-life** | 6 hr |

| Pharmacodynamics | |
|---|---|
| **Onset** | Unknown |
| **Peak** | 1.5 hr |
| **Duration** | Unknown |

**Interactions**
***Drug classifications***
Anxiolytics, barbiturates, general anesthetics, hypnotics, opiate agonists, phenothiazines, sedating H$_1$ blockers, sedatives, thiazolidinediones, tricyclics: increased CNS depression
Thiazolidinediones: increased weight gain/fluid retention; avoid use if possible

**NURSING CONSIDERATIONS**
**Assessment**
• Assess for seizures: aura, location, duration, activity at onset
• Assess for pain: location, duration, characteristics if using for diabetic neuropathy
• Monitor renal function tests: urinalysis, BUN, urine creatinine q3 mo, creatine kinase; if markedly increased, discontinue
• Assess mental status: mood, sensorium, affect, behavioral changes; if mental status changes, notify prescriber

**Nursing diagnoses**
• Knowledge, deficient (teaching)
• Pain, chronic  (uses)

**Implementation**
• Do not crush or chew caps; caps may be opened and contents put in applesauce or dissolved in juice
• Give without regard to meals
• Gradually withdraw over 7 days; abrupt withdrawal may precipitate seizures

• Store at room temperature away from heat and light
• Give hard candy, frequent rinsing of mouth, gum for dry mouth
• Provide assistance with ambulation during early part of treatment; dizziness occurs
• Provide seizure precautions: padded side rails; move objects that may harm patient
• Provide increased fluids, bulk in diet for constipation

**Patient/family education**
• Advise patient to carry emergency ID stating patient's name, products taken, condition, prescriber's name and phone number
• Advise patient to avoid driving, other activities that require alertness: dizziness, drowsiness may occur
• Teach patient not to discontinue medication quickly after long-term use, taper over ≥1 wk; withdrawal-precipitated seizures may occur, not to double doses if dose is missed, take if 2 hr or more before next dose
• Teach patient to notify prescriber if pregnancy planned or suspected; avoid breastfeeding
• Teach patient to report muscle pain, tenderness, weakness, when accompanied by fever, malaise
• Advise patient to avoid alcohol

**Evaluation**
**Positive therapeutic outcome**
• Decreased seizure activity; decrease in neuropathic pain

**Treatment of overdose:** Lavage, VS, hemodialysis

**primidone** (Rx)
(pri′mi-done)
Apo-Primidone ✖, Mysoline, PMS-Primidone ✖, primidone, Sertan ✖
*Func. class.:* Anticonvulsant
*Chem. class.:* Barbiturate derivative
**Pregnancy category D**

**Action:** Raises seizure threshold by conversion of product to phenobarbital; decreases neuron firing

**Therapeutic outcome:** Reduction in seizure activity

**Uses:** Generalized tonic-clonic (grand mal), complex-partial, psychomotor seizures, essential tremors

 Alert     Canada Only     Drug on CD        * "Tall Man" lettering (See Preface)

### Dosage and routes
*Adult and child >8 yr:* PO 100-125 mg at bedtime on days 1, 2, 3; then 100-125 mg bid on days 4, 5, 6; then 100-125 mg tid on days 7, 8, 9; then maintenance 250 mg tid-qid, max 2 g/day in divided doses
*Child <8 yr:* PO 50 mg at bedtime on days 1, 2, 3; then 50 mg bid on days 4, 5, 6; then 100 mg bid on days 7, 8, 9; maintenance 125-250 mg tid or 10-25 mg/kg/day in divided doses

**Available forms:** Tabs 50, 250 mg; susp 250 mg/5 ml ✽; chew tabs 125 mg ✽

### Adverse effects
*CNS: Stimulation, drowsiness,* irritability, fatigue, emotional disturbances, mood changes, paranoia, psychosis, ataxia, *vertigo*
*EENT:* Diplopia, nystagmus, edema of eyelids
*GI: Nausea, vomiting, anorexia,* **hepatitis**
*GU:* Impotence
*HEMA:* **Thrombocytopenia, leukopenia, neutropenia, eosinophilia, megaloblastic anemia,** decreased serum folate level, lymphadenopathy
*INTEG:* Rash, edema, alopecia, lupus-like syndrome

**Contraindications:** Pregnancy **D,** hypersensitivity, porphyria, hepatic encephalopathy

**Precautions:** COPD, renal/hepatic disease, hyperactive children

#### Pharmacokinetics

| | |
|---|---|
| **Absorption** | 60%-80% |
| **Distribution** | Widely distributed, crosses placenta |
| **Metabolism** | Liver, converted to phenobarbital + PEMA |
| **Excretion** | Kidneys, breast milk |
| **Half-life** | 3-12 hr |

#### Pharmacodynamics

| | |
|---|---|
| **Onset** | Unknown |
| **Peak** | 4 hr |
| **Duration** | Unknown |

### Interactions
*Individual drugs*
Acebutolol, metoprolol, propranolol: decreased effectiveness
Acetazolamide, carbamazepine: decreased primidone levels
Alcohol, heparin, isoniazid, nicotinamide, phenobarbital, phenytoin: increased primidone levels

*Drug classifications*
Antidepressants (tricyclic), oral contraceptives, phenothiazines: decreased effectiveness
CNS depressants, hydantoins: increased primidone levels
CYP3A4 inducers (barbiturates, carbamazepine, efavirenz, phenytoins, nevirapine): decreased primidone effect
CYP3A4 inhibitors (aprepitant, antiretroviral protease inhibitors, delavirdine, fluconazole, imatinib, voriconazole): increased toxicity
Succinimides: decreased primidone levels

*Drug/herb*
Ginkgo: increased effect
Ginseng, santonica: decreased effect
St. John's wort: avoid use

### NURSING CONSIDERATIONS
**Assessment**
• Assess mental status: mood, sensorium, affect, memory (long, short), especially geriatric
• Assess for blood dyscrasias: fever, sore throat, bruising, rash, jaundice, epistaxis (long-term treatment only)
• Assess seizure activity including type, location, duration, and character; provide seizure precaution
• Assess renal function tests: urinalysis, BUN, urine creatinine
• Monitor blood studies: RBC, Hct, Hgb, reticulocyte counts weekly for 4 wk then monthly
• Monitor liver function tests: ALT, AST, bilirubin, creatinine
• Monitor product levels during initial treatment: therapeutic level 5-15 mcg/ml
• Assess for signs of physical withdrawal if medication is suddenly discontinued
• Assess eye problems: need for ophthal exam before, during, after treatment (slit lamp, funduscopy, tonometry)
• Assess allergic reaction: red raised rash; if this occurs, product should be discontinued
• Monitor for toxicity: bone marrow depression, nausea, vomiting, ataxia, diplopia, CV collapse

**Nursing diagnoses**
• Injury, risk for (side effects)
• Knowledge, deficient (teaching)

**Implementation**
• May give with food to decrease gastric irritation
• May crush tab and mix with food or fluid

**P**

### Patient/family education
- Teach patient to carry/wear emergency ID stating name, products taken, condition, prescriber's name, phone number
- Advise patient to avoid driving and other activities that require alertness
- Caution patient to avoid alcohol and CNS depressants; increased sedation may occur
- Teach patient not to discontinue medication quickly after long-term use; taper off over several wk

### Evaluation
**Positive therapeutic outcome**
- Decreased seizure activity

---

### probenecid (Rx)
(proe-ben′e-sid)
Benemid, Benuryl ✤, probenecid
*Func. class.:* Uricosuric; antigout
*Chem. class.:* Sulfonamide derivative

**Pregnancy category B**

**Action:** Inhibits tubular reabsorption of urates, with increased excretion of uric acids

**Therapeutic outcome:** Decreased uric acid levels

**Uses:** Hyperuricemia in gout, gouty arthritis; adjunct to cephalosporin, cidofovir, or penicillin treatment (gonorrhea)

### Dosage and routes
*Gonorrhea*
*Adult:* PO 1 g with 3.5 g of ampicillin or 1 g 30 min before 4.8 million units of aqueous penicillin G procaine injected into 2 sites IM

*Gout/gouty arthritis*
*Adult:* PO 250 mg bid for 1 wk, then 500 mg bid, not to exceed 2 g/day; maintenance 500 mg/day × 6 mo

*Adjunct in penicillin/cephalosporin treatment*
*Adult and child >50 kg:* PO 500 mg qid
*Child <50 kg:* PO 25 mg/kg, then 40 mg/kg in divided doses qid

*Minimize toxicity in cidofovir therapy*
*Adult:* PO 2 g 3 hr prior to cidofovir dose, followed by 1 g at 2 and 8 hr after end of cidofovir infusion

*Renal dose*
*Adult:* PO CCr <50 ml/min avoid use

**Available forms:** Tabs 0.5 g

### Adverse effects
***CNS:*** Drowsiness, headache
***CV:*** Bradycardia
***GI:*** *Gastric irritation, nausea, vomiting, anorexia,* **hepatic necrosis**
***GU:*** Glycosuria, thirst, frequency, **nephrotic syndrome**
***INTEG:*** Rash, dermatitis, pruritus, fever
***META:*** *Acidosis, hypokalemia, hyperchloremia,* hyperglycemia
***RESP:*** **Apnea,** irregular respirations

**Contraindications:** Hypersensitivity, severe renal/hepatic disease, CCr <50 mg/min, history of uric acid calculus

**Precautions:** Pregnancy **B**, children <2 yr, sulfonamide hypersensitivity

#### Pharmacokinetics

| | |
|---|---|
| **Absorption** | Well absorbed |
| **Distribution** | Crosses placenta |
| **Metabolism** | Liver |
| **Excretion** | Kidneys |
| **Half-life** | 5-8 hr |

#### Pharmacodynamics

| | |
|---|---|
| **Onset** | ½ hr |
| **Peak** | 2-4 hr |
| **Duration** | 8 hr |

### Interactions
*Individual drugs*
Acyclovir, allopurinol, dyphylline, zidovudine: increased effect
Clofibrate, dapsone, indomethacin, methotrexate, naproxen, rifampin: increased toxicity
*Drug classifications*
Barbiturates, benzodiazepines: increased effect
Salicylates: decreased action of probenecid
Sulfa products: increased toxicity
*Drug/lab test*
Increased: BSP/urinary PSP, theophylline levels
False positive: urine glucose with copper sulfate test (Clinitest)

### NURSING CONSIDERATIONS
#### Assessment
- Monitor I&O ratio; observe for decrease in urinary output; increase fluids to 2-3 L/day; urine may be alkalized with sodium bicarbonate acetaZOLAMIDE
- Assess mobility, joint pain, and swelling in the joints
- Monitor CBC, urine pH, uric acid and BUN, creatinine before and periodically during treatment

---

## Nursing diagnoses
- Knowledge, deficient (teaching)
- Mobility, impaired physical (uses)
- Pain, chronic (uses)

## Implementation
- Give with food or antacid to decrease GI upset
- Reduce dosage gradually if uric acid levels are normal after 6 mo

## Patient/family education
- Advise patient to increase fluids to 2-3 L/day, avoid caffeine, alcohol
- Caution patient to avoid salicylates; probenecid levels will be decreased
- Advise patient to report any pain, redness, or hard area, usually in legs
- Instruct patient on importance of complying with medical regimen including weight loss program, diet restrictions, and alcohol intake

## Evaluation
**Positive therapeutic outcome**
- Decreased pain in joints
- Normal serum uric acid levels
- Increased duration of antiinfectives

---

## procainamide 🔹 (Rx)
(proe'kane-ah-mide)
Promine, procainamide, Procanbid, Pronestyl, Pronestyl-SR
*Func. class.:* Antidysrhythmic (class IA)
*Chem. class.:* procaine HCl amide analog

**Pregnancy category C**

**Action:** Depresses excitability of cardiac muscle to electrical stimulation and slows conduction in atrium, bundle of His, and ventricle increases refractory period

**Therapeutic outcome:** Prevention of dysrhythmias

**Uses:** Life-threatening ventricular dysrhythmias

## Dosage and routes
### Atrial fibrillation/PAT
*Adult:* PO 1-1.25 g; may give another 750 mg if needed; if no response, 500 mg-1g q2hr until desired response; maintenance 50 mg/kg in divided doses q6hr

### Ventricular tachycardia
*Adult:* PO 1 g; maintenance 50 mg/kg/day given in 3-hr intervals; SUS REL TAB 500 mg-1.25 g q6hr

### Other dysrhythmias
*Adult:* IV BOL 100 mg q5 min, given 25-50 mg/min, max 500 mg; or 17 mg/kg total, then IV INF 2-6 mg/min

### Renal dose
*Adult:* IV CCr 10-50 ml/min give q6-12hr; CCr <10 ml/min give q8-24hr

**Available forms:** Caps 250, 375, 500 mg; tabs 250, 375, 500 mg; sus rel tabs 500, 750, 1000 mg; inj IV 100, 500 mg/ml

## Adverse effects
*CNS: Headache, dizziness,* confusion, psychosis, restlessness, irritability, weakness
*CV: Hypotension,* **heart block, cardiovascular collapse, arrest**
*GI:* Nausea, vomiting, anorexia, diarrhea, hepatomegaly, pain, bitter taste
*HEMA:* Systemic lupus erythematosus syndrome, **agranulocytosis, thrombocytopenia, neutropenia, hemolytic anemia**
*INTEG:* Rash, urticaria, edema, swelling (rare), pruritus, flushing

**Contraindications:** Hypersensitivity, severe heart block, lupus erythromatosis, torsades de pointes

**Precautions:** Pregnancy C, breastfeeding, children, renal/hepatic disease, CHF, respiratory depression, cytopenia, bone marrow failure, dysrhythmia associated with digoxin toxicity, myasthenia gravis, digoxin toxicity

### Pharmacokinetics
| | |
|---|---|
| **Absorption** | Well absorbed |
| **Distribution** | Rapidly distributed |
| **Metabolism** | Liver |
| **Excretion** | Kidneys, unchanged (50%-70%) |
| **Half-life** | 2½-4½ hr; increased in renal disease |

### Pharmacodynamics
| | PO | PO–EXT REL | IV |
|---|---|---|---|
| **Onset** | ½ hr | Unknown | Rapid |
| **Peak** | 1-1½ hr | Unknown | ½-1 hr |
| **Duration** | 3 hr | Up to 8 hr | 3-4 hr |

## Interactions
### Individual drugs
Cimetidine, quinidine, ranitidine, trimethoprim: increased procainamide effect
Thioridazine: increased toxicity
### Drug classifications
Antidysrhythmics, quinolones: increased toxicity
β-Adrenergic blockers: increased procainamide effects

Neuromuscular blockers: increased neuromuscular blocking effect

### Drug/herb
Aconite: increased toxicity, death
Aloe, broom, buckthorn (chronic use), cascara sagrada (chronic use), Chinese rhubarb, figwort, fumitory, goldenseal, kudzu, licorice: increased effect
Coltsfoot: decreased effect
Horehound: increased serotonin effect

### Drug/lab test
Increased: ALT, AST, alkaline phosphatase, LDH, bilirubin

## NURSING CONSIDERATIONS
### Assessment
- Assess for oxygenation or perfusion deficit: decreased B/P, chest pain, dizziness, loss of consciousness
- Assess respiratory status: auscultate lung fields for bibasilar crackles in patients with advanced CHF
- Monitor I&O ratio; electrolytes: potassium, sodium, chloride; watch for decreasing urinary output, possible retention
- Monitor liver function tests: AST, ALT, bilirubin, alkaline phosphatase
- Monitor ECG continuously to determine product effectiveness; measure PR, QRS, QT intervals; check for PVCs, other dysrhythmias; check B/P continuously for hypo/hypertension; for rebound hypertension after 1-2 hr; prolonged PR/QT intervals, QRS complex; if QT or QRS increases by 50% or more, withhold next dose, notify prescriber
- Monitor ANA titer; during long-term treatment, watch for lupuslike symptoms
- Monitor for dehydration or hypovolemia
- Monitor for CNS symptoms: confusion, seizures, psychosis, numbness, depression, involuntary movements; if these occur, product should be discontinued
- Monitor blood levels (therapeutic level 3-10 mcg/ml), ANA titer or *N*-acetylprocainamide levels 10-20 mcg/ml; notify prescriber of abnormal results; assess for toxicity: confusion, drowsiness, nausea, vomiting, tachydysrhythmias, oliguria
- Assess cardiac rate, respiration: rate, rhythm, character, chest pain, ventricular tachycardia, supraventricular tachycardia or fibrillation

### Nursing diagnoses
- Cardiac output, decreased (uses)
- Gas exchange, impaired (adverse reactions)
- Knowledge, deficient (teaching)

### Implementation
**PO route**
- Do not break, crush, or chew sus rel tab
- Give on an empty stomach with a full glass of water
- May be given with meals if GI irritation occurs; absorption will be decreased
- Tab may be crushed and mixed with fluid or foods for patients with swallowing difficulties

**IV route**
- Give by direct **IV** after diluting 100 mg/10 ml of $D_5W$ or sterile water for inj; give 50 mg/min or less
- Give by intermittent inf after diluting to a conc of 2-4 mg/ml, 200 mg up to 1 g/50-500 ml of $D_5W$; give over 30 min (2-6 mg/min maintenance); use infusion pump for correct dosage
- Do not use if sol is dark or if precipitate is present

**Y-site compatibilities:** Amiodarone, famotidine, heparin, hydrocortisone, potassium chloride, ranitidine, vit B/C

**Y-site incompatibilities:** Milrinone

**Additive compatibilities:** Amiodarone, DOBUTamine, flumazenil, lidocaine, netilmicin, verapamil

**Additive incompatibilities:** Esmolol, ethacrynate, milrinone

**Solution compatibilities:** $D_5W$, $D_5$/0.9% NaCl, 0.45% NaCl, 0.9% NaCl, water for inj

### Patient/family education
- Advise patient to report side effects immediately to prescriber; to take exactly as prescribed; if dose is missed take when remembered if within 3-4 hr of next dose, do not double doses
- Caution patient that dark glasses may be needed for photophobia; to use sunscreen or stay out of sun to prevent burns; avoid temperature extremes; impairment of heat-regulating mechanism can occur
- Advise patient to complete follow-up appointment with prescriber including pulmonary function tests, chest x-ray
- Instruct patient that dry mouth may be relieved by frequent sips of water, hard candy, sugarless gum
- Caution patient to make position changes from lying to standing slowly to prevent orthostatic hypotension
- Advise prescriber immediately if lupuslike symptoms appear (joint pain, butterfly rash, fever, chills, dyspnea), or leukopenia (sore mouth, gums, throat) or thrombocytopenia (bleeding, bruising)

- Teach patient how to take pulse and when to report to prescriber

### Evaluation
**Positive therapeutic outcome**
- Decreased PVCs, ventricular tachycardia

**Treatment of overdose:** $O_2$, artificial ventilation, ECG, administer DOPamine for circulatory depression, diazepam or thiopental for seizures, isoproterenol

---

## procarbazine (Rx)
(proe-kar'ba-zeen)
Matulane, Natulan ✤
*Func. class.:* Antineoplastic, alkylating agent
*Chem. class.:* Hydrazine derivative

**Pregnancy category D**

**Action:** Inhibits DNA, RNA, protein synthesis, cell cycle S phase specific; has multiple sites of action; a nonvesicant

**Therapeutic outcome:** Prevention of rapidly growing malignant cells

**Uses:** Lymphoma, Hodgkin's disease, cancers resistant to other therapy

**Unlabeled uses:** Brain, lung malignancies, other lymphomas, multiple myeloma, malignant melanoma, polycythemia vera

### Dosage and routes
*Adult:* PO 2-4 mg/kg/day for first wk; maintain dosage of 4-6 mg/kg/day until platelets and WBC fall; after recovery, 1-2 mg/kg/day
*Child:* PO 50 mg/m$^2$/day for 7 days, then 100 mg/m$^2$ until desired response, leukopenia, or thrombocytopenia occurs; 50 mg/day is maintenance after bone marrow recovery

**Available forms:** Caps 50 mg

### Adverse effects
*CNS:* Headache, dizziness, **seizures,** insomnia, hallucinations, confusion, **coma,** pain, chills, fever, sweating, paresthesias
*EENT:* Retinal hemorrhage, nystagmus, photophobia, diplopia, dry eyes
*GI: Nausea, vomiting,* anorexia, diarrhea, constipation, dry mouth, stomatitis
*GU:* Azoospermia, cessation of menses
*HEMA:* **Thrombocytopenia, anemia, leukopenia, myelosuppression, bleeding tendencies,** purpura, petechiae, epistaxis
*INTEG: Rash,* pruritus, dermatitis, alopecia, herpes, hyperpigmentation
*MS:* Arthralgias, myalgias
*RESP:* Cough, pneumonitis

**Contraindications:** Pregnancy **D**, breast-feeding, hypersensitivity, thrombocytopenia, bone marrow depression

**Precautions:** Cardiac/renal/hepatic disease, radiation therapy, seizure disorder, anemia

### Pharmacokinetics
| | |
|---|---|
| **Absorption** | Well absorbed |
| **Distribution** | Widely distributed, crosses blood-brain barrier |
| **Metabolism** | Liver |
| **Excretion** | Kidneys |
| **Half-life** | 1 hr |

### Pharmacodynamics
Unknown

### Interactions
*Individual drugs*
Alcohol: increased CNS depression, disulfiram-like reaction
Caffeine, guanethidine, levodopa, methyldopa, reserpine: increased hypertension
Insulin: increased hypoglycemia
Meperidine: hypotension; do not use together
*Drug classifications*
Anticoagulants, NSAIDs, platelet inhibitors, thrombolytics: increased bleeding risk
Antidepressants, local anesthetics: increased hypertensive crisis
Antidepressants (tricyclics), MAOIs: disulfiram-like reaction
Antihistamines, barbiturates, hypotensive agents, opiates, phenothiazines: increased CNS depression
Hypoglycemics (oral): increased hypoglycemia
Selective serotonin reuptake inhibitors: confusion, seizures, hypertension
Sympathomimetics: disulfiram-like reaction, life-threatening hypertensive crisis
*Drug/food*
Tyramine-foods: increased disulfiram-like reaction, hypertensive crisis

### NURSING CONSIDERATIONS
**Assessment**
- Monitor CBC, differential, platelet count weekly; withhold product if WBC is <4000/mm$^3$ or platelet count is <75,000/mm$^3$; notify prescriber of results if WBC <20,000/mm$^3$, platelets <150,000/mm$^3$
- Monitor pulmonary function tests, chest x-ray films before, during therapy; chest film should be obtained q2 wk during treatment; check for dyspnea, crackles, unproductive cough, chest pain, tachypnea

Adverse effects: *italic* = common, **bold** = life-threatening

• Monitor renal function tests: BUN, serum uric acid, urine CCr before, during therapy; I&O ratio; report fall in urine output of 30 ml/hr; check for decreased hyperuricemia
• Monitor for cold, fever, sore throat (may indicate beginning of infection); identify edema in feet, joint and stomach pain, shaking; prescriber should be notified
• Assess for bleeding: hematuria, guaiac, bruising or petechiae, mucosa or orifices, no rectal temp
• Assess for tyramine-containing foods in the diet; hypertensive crisis can occur

### Nursing diagnoses
• Body image, disturbed (adverse reactions)
• Infection, risk for (adverse reactions)
• Injury, risk for (adverse reactions)
• Knowledge, deficient (teaching)

### Implementation
• Give with foods, fluids for GI upset; open cap and give with food/fluids for swallowing difficulty; administer as directed

### Patient/family education
• Teach patient to avoid use of products containing aspirin or NSAIDs, razors, commercial mouthwash, since bleeding may occur; to report symptoms of bleeding (hematuria, tarry stools)
• Caution patient to report signs of anemia (fatigue, headache, irritability, faintness, shortness of breath)
• Advise patient to report any changes in breathing or coughing even several mo after treatment; to avoid crowds and persons with respiratory tract or other infections
• Inform patient hair loss is common; discuss the use of wigs or hairpieces
• Caution patient not to have any vaccinations without the advice of the prescriber; serious reactions can occur
• Advise patient that contraception is needed during treatment and for several mo after the completion of therapy; avoid breastfeeding
• To avoid sunlight, or UV exposure, wear sunscreen or protective clothing

### Evaluation
**Positive therapeutic outcome**
• Absence of swelling at night
• Increased appetite, increased weight
• Decreasing malignancy

## prochlorperazine (Rx)
(proe-klor-pair′a-zeen)
Chlorpazine, Compa-Z, Compazine, Contranzine, Provazin ✤, Stemetil ✤, Ultrazine
*Func. class.:* Antiemetic/antipsychotic
*Chem. class.:* Phenothiazine, piperazine derivative

### Pregnancy category C

**Do not confuse:**
prochlorperazine/chlorproMAZINE,
Compazine/Coumadin

**Action:** Depresses cerebral cortex, hypothalamus, limbic system, which control activity aggression; blocks neurotransmission produced by DOPamine at synapse; exhibits a strong α-adrenergic, anticholinergic blocking action; mechanism for antipsychotic effects is unclear; acts centrally by blocking chemoreceptor trigger zone, which in turn acts on vomiting center

**Therapeutic outcome:** Decreased nausea, vomiting, decreased signs and symptoms of psychosis

**Uses:** Nausea, vomiting, psychosis

### Dosage and routes
*Postoperative nausea/vomiting*
**Adult:** IM 5-10 mg 1-2 hr before anesthesia; may repeat in 30 min; **IV** 5-10 mg 15-30 min before anesthesia; **IV** INF 20 mg/L D₅W or 0.9% NaCl 15-30 min before anesthesia, max 40 mg/day

*Severe nausea/vomiting*
**Adult:** PO 5-10 mg tid-qid; SUS REL 15 mg/day in ᴀᴍ or 10 mg q12hr; RECT 25 mg/bid; IM 5-10 mg; may repeat q4hr, max 40 mg/day
**Child 18-39 kg:** PO 2.5 mg tid or 5 mg bid; max 15 mg/day; IM 0.132 mg/kg
**Child 14-17 kg:** PO/RECT 2.5 mg bid-tid, max 10 mg/day; IM 0.132 mg/kg
**Child 9-13 kg:** PO/RECT 2.5 mg daily-bid, max 7.5 mg/day; IM 0.132 mg/kg

*Antipsychotic*
**Adult and child ≥12 yr:** PO 5-10 mg tid-qid; may increase q2-3 day, max 150 mg/day; IM 10-20 mg q2-4hr up to 4 doses, then 10-20 mg q4-6hr, max 200 mg/day; RECT 10 mg tid-qid may increase by 5-10 mg q2-3 days as needed
**Child 2-12 yr:** PO 2.5 mg bid-tid; IM 0.132 mg/kg

*Antianxiety*
**Adult and child ≥12 yr:** PO 5 mg
tid-qid, max 20 mg/day or >12 wk; IM 5-10
mg q3-4hr, max 40 mg/day; **IV** 2.5-10 mg;
max 40 mg/day
**Child 2-12 yr:** IM 132 mcg/kg

**Available forms:** Syr 5 mg/ml; inj 5
mg/ml; tabs 5, 10, 25 mg; sus rel caps 10, 15
mg; supp 2.5, 5, 25 mg

**Adverse effects**
*CNS:* Tardive dyskinesia, *euphoria,* **depression, EPS,** restlessness, tremor, dizziness,
**neuroleptic malignant syndrome,** drowsiness, headache
*CV:* **Circulatory failure, tachycardia**
*EENT:* Blurred vision
*GI:* Nausea, vomiting, anorexia, dry mouth,
diarrhea, constipation, weight loss, metallic
taste, cramps
*HEMA:* **Agranulocytosis**
*MISC:* Impotence
*RESP:* **Respiratory depression**

**Contraindications:** Hypersensitivity to
phenothiazines, bone marrow depression

**Precautions:** Pregnancy **C,** breastfeeding,
children <2 yr, geriatric, coma, seizure,
encephalopathy, angle-closure glaucoma

### Pharmacokinetics
| | |
|---|---|
| **Absorption** | Variably absorbed (PO); well absorbed (IM) |
| **Distribution** | Widely distributed, high concentration in CNS, crosses placenta |
| **Metabolism** | Liver, extensively; GI mucosa |
| **Excretion** | Kidneys, breast milk |
| **Half-life** | Unknown |

### Pharmacodynamics
| | PO | PO-SUS REL | RECT | IM | IV |
|---|---|---|---|---|---|
| **Onset** | ½ hr | ½ hr | 1 hr | 10-20 min | 4-5 min |
| **Peak** | Unkn | Unkn | Unkn | Unkn | Unkn |
| **Duration** | 3-4 hr | 10-12 hr | 3-4 hr | 3-4 hr | 3-4 hr |

**Interactions**
*Drug classifications*
Antacids, barbiturates: decreased prochlorperazine effect
Anticholinergics, antidepressants, antiparkinson products: increased anticholinergic effects
*Drug/herb*
Betel palm, kava: increased EPS
Chamomile, cola nut, hops, kava, nettle,
nutmeg, skullcap, valerian: increased CNS
depression
Henbane, jimsonweed, scopolia: increased
anticholinergic effect
*Drug/lab test*
Increased: liver function tests, cardiac enzymes, cholesterol, blood glucose, prolactin,
bilirubin, PBI, $^{131}$I, alkaline phosphatase,
leukocytes, granulocytes, platelets
Decreased: hormones (blood and urine)
False positive: pregnancy tests, urine bilirubin
False negative: urinary steroids, 17-OHCS,
pregnancy tests

## NURSING CONSIDERATIONS
### Assessment
• Assess mental status: orientation, mood,
behavior, presence and type of hallucinations
before initial administration and monthly; this
product should significantly reduce psychotic
behavior
• Check for swallowing of PO medication;
check for hoarding or giving of medication to
other patients
• Monitor I&O ratio; palpate bladder if low
urinary output occurs, especially in geriatric;
urinalysis recommended before, during
prolonged therapy
⚑ Monitor bilirubin, CBC, liver function tests
monthly; blood dyscrasias, hepatotoxicity may
occur
• Assess affect, orientation, LOC, reflexes, gait,
coordination, sleep pattern disturbances
• Monitor B/P with patient sitting, standing,
and lying; take pulse and respirations q4hr
during initial treatment; establish baseline
before starting treatment; report drops of 30
mm Hg; obtain baseline ECG, Q-wave and
T-wave changes
• Check for dizziness, faintness, palpitations,
tachycardia on rising; severe orthostatic
hypotension is common
⚑ Identify neuroleptic malignant syndrome:
hyperpyrexia, muscle rigidity, increased CPK,
altered mental status, seizures, fever, tachycardia, dyspnea, fatigue, loss of bladder control;
notify prescriber immediately; product should
be discontinued
• Assess for EPS including akathisia (inability
to sit still, no pattern to movements), tardive
dyskinesia (bizarre movements of the jaw,
mouth, tongue, extremities), pseudoparkinsonism (ragged tremors, pill rolling, shuffling
gait); an antiparkinsonism product should be
prescribed
• Assess for constipation, urinary retention
daily; if these occur, increase bulk, water in
diet

P

## Nursing diagnoses
- Coping, ineffective (uses)
- Knowledge, deficient (teaching)
- Noncompliance (teaching)
- Thought processes, disturbed (uses)

## Implementation
**PO route**
- Do not break, crush, or chew sus rel caps
- Give product in liquid form mixed in glass of juice or cola if hoarding is suspected; do not mix in caffeine drinks, tannics, pectins
- Give decreased dosage in geriatric since metabolism is slowed
- Give PO with full glass of water, milk; or give with food to decrease GI upset
- Give antacids 2 hr before or after taking this product
- Store in airtight, light-resistant container; oral sol in amber bottle

**IM route**
- Inject slowly in deep muscle mass; do not give SUBCUT; aspirate to avoid **IV** administration; do not administer sol with a precipitate; have patient lie down afterward for at least 30 min

**IV route**
- Give by direct **IV** after diluting **IV** using 0.9% NaCl to 1 mg/1 ml; administer at 1 mg/min or less
- Administer by intermittent inf after diluting 20 mg/L or less LR, Ringer's, dextrose, saline, or any combination

*Syringe compatibilities:* Atropine, butorphanol, chlorproMAZINE, cimetidine, diamorphine, diphenhydrAMINE, droperidol, fentanyl, glycopyrrolate, hydrOXYzine, meperidine, metoclopramide, nalbuphine, pentazocine, perphenazine, promazine, promethazine, ranitidine, scopolamine, sufentanil

*Syringe incompatibilities:* Dimenhy-DRINATE, midazolam, pentobarbital, thiopental

*Y-site compatibilities:* Amsacrine, calcium gluconate, cisplatin, cladribine, cyclophosphamide, cytarabine, DOXOrubicin, fluconazole, granisetron, heparin, hydrocortisone, melphalan, methotrexate, ondansetron, paclitaxel, potassium chloride, propofol, sargramostim, sufentanil, teniposide, thiotepa, vinorelbine, vit B/C

*Y-site incompatibilities:* Foscarnet
*Additive compatibilities:* Amikacin, ascorbic acid, dexamethasone, dimenhy-DRINATE, erythromycin, ethacrynate, lidocaine, nafcillin, netilmicin, sodium bicarbonate, vit B/C

*Additive incompatibilities:* Aminophylline, amphotericin B, ampicillin, calcium gluceptate, cefoperazone, cephalothin, chloramphenicol, chlorothiazide, floxacillin, furosemide, hydrocortisone sodium succinate, methohexital sodium, penicillin G sodium, phenobarbital, thiopental

## Patient/family education
- Teach patient to use good oral hygiene; frequent rinsing of mouth, sugarless gum for dry mouth since oral candidiasis may occur
- Caution patient to avoid hazardous activities until product response is determined; dizziness, blurred vision may occur
- Inform patient that orthostatic hypotension occurs often and to rise from sitting or lying position gradually; to remain lying down after IM inj for at least 30 min; tell patient to avoid hot tubs, hot showers, tub baths, since hypotension may occur; tell patient that in hot weather heat stroke may occur; take extra precautions to stay cool
- Advise patient to avoid abrupt withdrawal of this product, or EPS may result; product should be withdrawn slowly
- Teach patient to avoid OTC preparations (cough, hay fever, cold) unless approved by prescriber, since serious product interactions may occur; avoid use with alcohol, CNS depressants; increased drowsiness may occur; avoid activities requiring mental alertness
- Instruct patient to avoid sun or use sunscreen, sunglasses and protective clothing to prevent burns
- Advise patient to take antacids 2 hr before or after taking this product
- Advise patient to report sore throat, malaise, fever, bleeding, mouth sores; if these occur, CBC should be done and product discontinued
- Teach patient not to double or skip doses
- Teach patient urine may turn pink to reddish brown
- Instruct patient to report dark urine, clay-colored stools, bleeding, bruising, rash, blurred vision
- Advise patient that suppositories may contain coconut/palm oil

## Evaluation
**Positive therapeutic outcome**
- Relief of nausea and vomiting
- Decrease in emotional excitement, hallucinations, delusions, paranoia
- Reorganization of patterns of thought, speech

**Treatment of overdose:** Lavage if orally ingested; provide airway; *do not induce vomiting or use epINEPHrine*

---

**progesterone** 🚫 (Rx)
(proe-jess′ter-one)
Crinone, Endometrin, Prochieve, progesterone, Prometrium
*Func. class.:* Progestogen
*Chem. class.:* Progesterone derivative
**Pregnancy category D**

**Action:** Inhibits secretion of pituitary gonadotropins, which prevents follicular maturation, ovulation; stimulates growth of mammary tissue; antineoplastic action against endometrial cancer

**Therapeutic outcome:** Decreased abnormal uterine bleeding, absence of amenorrhea

**Uses:** Contraception, amenorrhea, premenstrual syndrome, abnormal uterine bleeding, endometrial hyperplasia prevention, assisted reproductive technology (ART) gel

**Unlabeled uses:** Corpus luteum insufficiency

**Dosage and routes**
*Infertility*
*Adult:* VAG 90 mg/day

*Amenorrhea/uterine bleeding*
*Adult:* IM 5-10 mg/day × 6-8 doses

*Endometrial hyperplasia prevention*
*Adult:* PO 200 mg/day × 12 days

*ART*
*Adult:* GEL 90 mg (8%) vaginally daily, for supplementation; 90 mg (8%) vaginally bid for replacement; if pregnancy occurs, continue × 10-12 wk

*Corpus luteum insufficiency (unlabeled)*
*Adult:* VAG insert 100 mg bid-tid starting at oocyte retrieval and continuing up to 10-12 wk gestation

**Available forms:** Caps 100, 200 mg; inj 50 mg/ml; powder micronized; vag gel 4%, 8%; vag insert 100 mg; supp 25, 100, 200, 500 mg

**Adverse effects**
*CNS:* Dizziness, headache, migraines, depression, fatigue, mood swings, dementia

*CV:* Hypotension, **thrombophlebitis,** edema, **thromboembolism, stroke, pulmonary embolism, MI**
*EENT:* Diplopia, retinal thrombosis
*GI: Nausea,* vomiting, anorexia, cramps, increased weight, **cholestatic jaundice,** constipation
*GU:* Amenorrhea, cervical erosion, breakthrough bleeding, dysmenorrhea, vaginal candidiasis, breast changes, *gynecomastia, testicular atrophy, impotence,* endometriosis, **spontaneous abortion,** breast pain, ectopic pregnancy
*INTEG:* Rash, urticaria, acne, hirsutism, alopecia, oily skin, seborrhea, purpura, melasma
*META:* Hyperglycemia
*SYST:* **Angioedema, anaphylaxis**

**Contraindications:** Pregnancy **D**, breast cancer, thromboembolic disorders, reproductive cancer, genital bleeding (abnormal, undiagnosed), cerebral hemorrhage, ectopic pregnancy, PID, STDs, hypersensitivity to this product or peanut oil

**Precautions:** Breastfeeding, hypertension, asthma, blood dyscrasias, gallbladder disease, CHF, diabetes mellitus, bone disease, depression, migraine headache, seizure disorders, renal/hepatic disease, family history of breast or reproductive tract cancer

| Pharmacokinetics | |
|---|---|
| **Absorption** | Unknown |
| **Distribution** | Unknown |
| **Metabolism** | Unknown |
| **Excretion** | Breast milk |
| **Half-life** | Unknown |

| Pharmacodynamics | | | |
|---|---|---|---|
| | IM | RECT | VAG |
| **Onset** | Unknown | Unknown | Unknown |
| **Peak** | Unknown | Unknown | Unknown |
| **Duration** | 24 hr | 24 hr | 24 hr |

**Interactions**
*Drug classifications*
Barbiturates, phenytoins: decreased progesterone effect
*Drug/herb*
Alfalfa: increased hormonal effect
*Drug/lab test*
Increased: alkaline phosphatase, nitrogen (urine), pregnanediol, amino acids, factors VII, VIII, IX, X
Decreased: GTT, HDL

P

## NURSING CONSIDERATIONS
### Assessment
- Monitor B/P at beginning of treatment and periodically; check weight daily; notify prescriber of weekly weight gain >5 lb
- Monitor I&O ratio: be alert for decreasing urinary output, increasing edema, hypertension
- Assess liver function tests: ALT, AST, bilirubin periodically during long-term therapy
- Assess edema, hypertension, cardiac symptoms, jaundice
- Assess mental status: affect, mood, behavioral changes, depression
- Assess for hypercalcemia
- Assess cervical cytology

### Nursing diagnoses
- Injury, risk for (adverse reactions)
- Knowledge, deficient (teaching)
- Sexual dysfunction (uses)
- Tissue perfusion, ineffective (adverse reactions)

### Implementation
- Wait at least 6 hr after any vaginal treatment before using vaginal gel
- Start progesterone 14 days after estrogen dose, if given concomitantly

**IM route**
- Store in dark area
- Give titrated dose; use lowest effective dosage; give oil sol deep in large muscle mass; rotate sites; use after warming to dissolve crystals

### Patient/family education
- Teach patient to report breast lumps, vaginal bleeding, edema, jaundice, dark urine, clay-colored stools, dyspnea, headache, blurred vision, abdominal pain, numbness or stiffness in legs, chest pain
- Teach patient to report suspected pregnancy

### Evaluation
**Positive therapeutic outcome**
- Decreased abnormal uterine bleeding
- Absence of amenorrhea
- Prevented pregnancy

---

**promethazine** (Rx)
(proe-meth′a-zeen)
Histanil ✦, Phenadoz, Phenergan, promethazine HCl
*Func. class.:* Antihistamine, H$_1$-receptor antagonist; antiemetic; sedative/hypnotic
*Chem. class.:* Phenothiazine derivative

**Pregnancy category** C

**Do not confuse:**
Phenergan/Theragran

**Action:** Acts on blood vessels, GI, respiratory system by competing with histamine for H$_1$-receptor site; decreases allergic response by blocking histamine; also acts on chemoreceptor trigger zone to decrease vomiting; increases CNS stimulation, has anticholinergic response

**Therapeutic outcome:** Absence of allergy symptoms and rhinitis, absence of nausea/vomiting, sedation

**Uses:** Motion sickness, rhinitis, allergy symptoms, sedation, nausea, preoperative and postoperative sedation

**Dosage and routes**
*Nausea*
*Adult:* PO/IM/**IV**/RECT 12.5-25 mg; may repeat 12.5-25 mg q4-6hr prn
*Child >2 yr:* PO/IM/**IV**/RECT 0.25-0.5 mg/kg q4-6hr prn

*Motion sickness*
*Adult:* PO 25 mg bid; give 30-60 min before departure and q8-12hr prn
*Child >2 yr:* PO/IM/RECT 12.5-25 mg bid; give 30-60 min before departure and q8-12hr prn

*Allergy/rhinitis*
*Adult:* PO 12.5 mg qid, or 25 mg at bedtime
*Child >2 yr:* PO 6.25-12.5 mg tid or 25 mg at bedtime

*Sedation*
*Adult:* PO/IM/**IV**/RECT 25-50 mg at bedtime
*Child >2 yr:* PO/IM/RECT 12.5-25 mg at bedtime

*Sedation (preoperative/ postoperative)*
*Adult:* PO/IM/**IV** 25-50 mg
*Child >2 yr:* PO/IM/**IV** 0.5-1.1 mg/kg

**Available forms:** Tabs 12.5, 25, 50 mg; supp 12.5, 25 mg; inj 25, 50 mg/ml; syr 6.25 mg/5 ml

**Adverse effects**
*CNS: Dizziness, drowsiness,* poor coordination, fatigue, anxiety, euphoria, confusion,

---

paresthesia, neuritis, EPS, **neuroleptic malignant syndrome**
*CV:* Hyper/hypotension, palpitations, tachycardia
*EENT:* Blurred vision, dilated pupils, tinnitus, nasal stuffiness, dry nose, throat, mouth, photosensitivity
*GI: Constipation,* dry mouth, nausea, vomiting, anorexia, diarrhea
*GU: Retention,* dysuria, frequency
*HEMA:* **Thrombocytopenia, agranulocytosis, hemolytic anemia**
*INTEG:* Rash, urticaria, photosensitivity
*RESP:* Increased thick secretions, wheezing, chest tightness, **apnea in pediatric patients**

**Contraindications:** Hypersensitivity to $H_1$-receptor antagonist, sulfite allergy, child <2 yr, acute asthma attack, lower respiratory tract disease

**Precautions:** Pregnancy **C**, increased intraocular pressure, renal/cardiac disease, hypertension, bronchial asthma, seizure disorder, stenosed peptic ulcers, hyperthyroidism, prostatic hypertrophy, bladder neck obstruction

### Pharmacokinetics

| | |
|---|---|
| **Absorption** | Well absorbed (PO, IM); erratically absorbed (RECT) |
| **Distribution** | Widely distributed; crosses the blood-brain barrier, placenta |
| **Metabolism** | Liver |
| **Excretion** | Kidneys, breast milk |
| **Half-life** | Unknown |

### Pharmacodynamics

| | PO/IM/RECT | IV |
|---|---|---|
| **Onset** | 20 min | 3-5 min |
| **Peak** | Unknown | Unknown |
| **Duration** | 4-12 hr | 4-6 hr |

### Interactions
*Individual drugs*
Alcohol: increased CNS depression
Heparin: decreased oral anticoagulants effect
*Drug classifications*
Anticoagulants, oral: decreased anticoagulant effect
Antidepressants (tricyclics), barbiturates, CNS depressants, opiates, sedative/hypnotics: increased CNS depression
Heparin: decreased oral anticoagulant effect
MAOIs: increased promethazine effect
*Drug/herb*
Henbane, jimsonweed, scopolia: increased anticholinergic effect

*Drug/lab test*
False-negative: skin allergy tests (discontinue antihistamines 3 days before testing)
False-positive: urine pregnancy test

## NURSING CONSIDERATIONS
### Assessment
• Assess respiratory status: rate, rhythm, increase in bronchial secretions, wheezing, chest tightness; provide fluids to 2 L/day to decrease secretion thickness
• Monitor I&O ratio: be alert for urinary retention, frequency, dysuria, especially geriatric; product should be discontinued if these occur
• Monitor CBC during long-term therapy; blood dyscrasias may occur but are rare
• Monitor cardiac status: VS, palpitations, increased pulse, hypo/hypertension

### Nursing diagnoses
• Airway clearance, ineffective (uses)
• Injury, risk for (adverse reactions)
• Knowledge, deficient (teaching)
• Noncompliance (teaching, overuse)

### Implementation
**PO route**
• Give 1 hr before or 2 hr after meals to facilitate absorption
• Give with meals to decrease GI upset
• Store in airtight, light-resistant container
**IM route**
• Give IM inj in large muscle mass; aspirate to avoid **IV** administration; do not give SUBCUT; necrosis may occur
**IV route**
• Do not use if precipitate is present
• Rapid administration may cause transient decrease in B/P
• Give **IV** directly; give 25 mg or less over 1 min; rapid drop in B/P may occur with rapid administration
*Syringe compatibilities:* Atropine, butorphanol, chlorproMAZINE, cimetidine, diphenhydrAMINE, droperidol, fentanyl, glycopyrrolate, hydromorphone, hydrOXYzine, meperidine, metoclopramide, midazolam, pentazocine, perphenazine, prochlorperazine, promazine, ranitidine, scopolamine
*Syringe incompatibilities:* DimenhyDRINATE, heparin, pentobarbital, thiopental
*Y-site compatibilities:* Amifostine, amsacrine, aztreonam, ciprofloxacin, cisplatin, cladribine, cyclophosphamide, cytarabine, DOXOrubicin, filgrastim, fluconazole, fludarabine, granisetron, melphalan, ondansetron, sargramostim, teniposide, thiotepa, vinorelbine

**P**

**Y-site incompatibilities:** Cefoperazone, foscarnet, heparin

**Additive compatibilities:** Amikacin, ascorbic acid, chloroquine, hydromorphone, netilmicin, vit B/C

**Additive incompatibilities:** Aminophylline, carbenicillin, chloramphenicol, chlorothiazide, floxacillin, furosemide, heparin, hydrocortisone sodium succinate, methicillin, methohexital, penicillin G, pentobarbital, phenobarbital, thiopental

### Patient/family education
• Inform patient that a false-negative result may occur with skin testing; these procedures should not be scheduled until 3 days after discontinuing use
• Advise patient to take 30 min before departure to prevent motion sickness
• Caution patient to avoid hazardous activities, activities requiring alertness, since dizziness may occur; instruct patient to request assistance with ambulation
• Advise patient to avoid alcohol, other depressants; serious CNS depression may occur
• Teach patient all aspects of product use; to notify prescriber if confusion, sedation, hypotension, jaundice, fever occur; to avoid driving and other hazardous activity if drowsiness occurs
• Advise patient to take 1 hr before or 2 hr after meals to facilitate absorption
• Caution patient not to exceed recommended dosage; dysrhythmias may occur
• Inform patient hard candy, gum, frequent rinsing of mouth may be used for dryness

### Evaluation
**Positive therapeutic outcome**
• Absence of motion sickness
• Absence of nausea, vomiting

---

## propafenone (Rx)
(pro-faff'e-nown)
Rythmol
*Func. class.:* Antidysrhythmic (Class IC)

**Pregnancy category C**

**Action:** Slows conduction velocity; reduces membrane responsiveness; inhibits automaticity; increases ratio of effective refractory period to action potential duration; β-blocking activity

**Uses:** Life-threatening dysrhythmias, sustained ventricular tachycardia

**Unlabeled uses:** Atrial fibrillation (single dose)

### Dosage and routes
*Adult:* PO 150 mg q8hr; allow a 3-4 day interval before increasing dose, max 900 mg/day

*Atrial fibrillation (unlabeled)*
*Adult:* PO 450 or 600 mg as a single dose

**Available forms:** Tabs 150, 225, 300 mg

### Adverse effects
*CNS:* Headache, dizziness, abnormal dreams, syncope, confusion, **seizures**
*CV:* **Supraventricular dysrhythmia, ventricular dysrhythmia, bradycardia**, prodysrhythmia, palpitations, AV block, intraventricular conduction delay, AV dissociation, hypotension, chest pain
*EENT:* Blurred vision, altered taste, tinnitus
*GI: Nausea, vomiting,* constipation, dyspepsia, cholestasis, abnormal hepatic studies, dry mouth
*HEMA:* **Leukopenia, agranulocytosis, granulocytopenia, thrombocytopenia,** anemia, bruising
*INTEG:* Rash
*RESP:* Dyspnea

**Contraindications:** 2nd-, 3rd-degree AV block, right bundle branch block, cardiogenic shock, hypersensitivity, bradycardia, uncontrolled CHF, sick sinus syndrome, marked hypotension, bronchospastic disorders

**Precautions:** Pregnancy **C,** breastfeeding, children, geriatric, CHF, hypo/hyperkalemia, recent MI, nonallergic bronchospasm, renal/hepatic disease

| Pharmacokinetics | |
|---|---|
| Absorption | Well |
| Distribution | Widely, crosses placenta |
| Metabolism | Rapid, liver, CYP1A2, CYP2D6, CYP3A4 |
| Excretion | Kidneys |
| Half-life | 2-32 hr |

| Pharmacodynamics (antiarrhythmic) | |
|---|---|
| Onset | Hours-several days |
| Peak | 4-5 days |
| Duration | Several hr |

### Interactions
*Individual products*
Cimetidine, quinidine, rifampin: decreased propafenone effect

CycloSPORINE, digoxin: increased serum levels

Metropolol, propranolol: increased β-blocker effect

Warfarin: increased anticoagulation

### Drug classifications

Local anesthetics: increased CNS effects

### Drug/herb

Aconite: increased toxicity, death

Aloe, broom, buckthorn (chronic use), cascara sagrada (chronic use), Chinese rhubarb, figwort, fumitory, goldenseal, kudzu, licorice: increased effect

Aloe, buckthorn, cascara sagrada, senna pod/leaf: hypokalemia, increased antidysrhythmic action

Coltsfoot: decreased effect

Horehound: increased serotonin effect

### Drug/lab test

Increased: CPK

## NURSING CONSIDERATIONS
### Assessment

• Monitor GI status: bowel pattern, number of stools

◆ Assess cardiac status: rate, rhythm, quality; ECG or Holter monitor prior to and during therapy; watch for PR, QT prolongation

• Monitor chest x-ray film, pulmonary function test during treatment

• Monitor I/O ratio; check for decreasing output; daily weight

• Monitor B/P for fluctuations

• Assess lung fields; bilateral crackles, dyspnea, peripheral edema, weight gain, jugular venous distention may occur in CHF patient

◆ Assess toxicity: fine tremors, dizziness, hypotension, drowsiness, abnormal heart rate

### Nursing diagnoses

• Cardiac output, decreased (uses)

• Knowledge, deficient (teaching)

### Implementation

• Begin treatment in hospital

• Remove other antiarrhythmics before starting propafenone

• Adjust dosage q3-4 days, no sooner

### Patient/family education

• Advise patient to avoid hazardous activities until response is known

• Advise patient to report fever, chills, sore throat, bleeding, shortness of breath, chest pain, palpitations, blurred vision

• Advise patient to take medication with food

• Advise patient to carry emergency ID identifying medication and prescriber

### Evaluation
#### Positive therapeutic outcome

• Absence of dysrhythmias

**Treatment of overdose:** $O_2$, artificial ventilation, defibrillation ECG; administer DOPamine for circulatory depression, diazepam or thiopental for seizures, isoproterenol

## propantheline (Rx)
(proe-pan'the-leen)
Pro-Banthine, Propanthel ✦
*Func. class.:* GI anticholinergic; antiulcer agent
*Chem. class.:* Synthetic quaternary ammonium compound

**Pregnancy category** C

**Action:** Inhibits muscarinic actions of acetylcholine at postganglionic parasympathetic neuroeffector sites

**Therapeutic outcome:** Absence of peptic ulcer disease symptoms

**Uses:** Treatment of peptic ulcer disease, irritable bowel syndrome, duodenography, urinary incontinence

**Dosage and routes**
*Adult:* PO 15 mg tid before meals, 30 mg at bedtime
*Geriatric/small patients:* PO 7.5 mg tid before meals
*Child:* 0.375 mg/kg (10 mg/m$^2$) qid

**Available forms:** Tabs 7.5, 15 mg

**Adverse effects**
*CNS: Confusion, stimulation in geriatric,* headache, insomnia, dizziness, drowsiness, anxiety, weakness, hallucinations
*CV:* Palpitations, tachycardia, orthostatic hypotension (geriatric)
*EENT: Blurred vision,* photophobia, mydriasis, cycloplegia, increased ocular tension
*GI: Dry mouth, constipation,* **paralytic ileus,** heartburn, nausea, vomiting, dysphagia, absence of taste
*GU:* Hesitancy, retention, impotence
*INTEG:* Urticaria, rash, pruritus, anhidrosis, fever, allergic reactions

**Contraindications:** Hypersensitivity to anticholinergics, angle-closure glaucoma, GI obstruction, myasthenia gravis, paralytic ileus, GI atony, toxic megacolon, urinary tract obstruction

**Precautions:** Pregnancy C, geriatric, hyperthyroidism, CAD, dysrhythmias, CHF, ulcerative colitis, hypertension, hiatal hernia, renal/hepatic disease, urinary retention, prostatic hypertrophy

P

## Pharmacokinetics

| | |
|---|---|
| **Absorption** | Moderately absorbed |
| **Distribution** | Unknown |
| **Metabolism** | Unknown |
| **Excretion** | Unknown |
| **Half-life** | Unknown |

## Pharmacodynamics

| | |
|---|---|
| **Onset** | ½ hr |
| **Peak** | 2-6 hr |
| **Duration** | 4-6 hr |

## Interactions
### Individual products
Disopyramide, procainamide, quinidine: increased anticholinergic effect
### Drug classifications
Antidepressants (tricyclics), H$_1$-antihistamines, belladonna alkaloids, MAOIs, opioids, phenothiazenes: increased anticholinergic effect
### Drug/herb
Henbane, jimsonweed, scopolia: increased anticholinergic effect

## NURSING CONSIDERATIONS
### Assessment
• Assess for the pain of peptic ulcer disease before, during, and after treatment

### Nursing diagnoses
• Constipation (adverse reactions)
• Knowledge, deficient (teaching)
• Pain, chronic (uses)
• Thought processes, disturbed (adverse reactions)

### Implementation
• Give 30 min before meals and at bedtime; do not give with antacids; separate by at least 1 hr

### Patient/family education
• Teach patient to report blurred vision, chest pain, allergic reactions
• Advise patient not to perform strenuous activity in high temperatures; heat stroke may result due to decreased perspiration
• Instruct patient to take as prescribed; not to skip doses
• Instruct patient to report change in vision; blurring or loss of sight; product should be discontinued
• Advise patient not to operate machinery or drive if dizziness occurs
• Caution patient not to take OTC products without approval of prescriber

### Evaluation
**Positive therapeutic outcome**
• Decreased pain in peptic ulcer disease

## proparacaine ophthalmic
*See Appendix D*

## ❕ HIGH ALERT

## propofol (Rx)
(pro′poh-fole)
Diprivan, Disoprofol
*Func. class.:* General anesthetic
**Pregnancy category B**

**Action:** Produces dose-dependent CNS depression by activation of GABA receptor

**Therapeutic outcome:** Induction of anesthesia

**Uses:** Induction or maintenance of anesthesia as part of balanced anesthetic technique; sedation in mechanically ventilated patients

### Dosage and routes
#### Induction
*Adult:* **IV** 2-2.5 mg/kg, approximately 40 mg q10 sec until induction onset
*Child 3-16 yr:* **IV** 2.5-3.5 mg/kg over 20-30 sec
*Geriatric:* **IV** 1-1.5 mg/kg, approximately 20 mg q10 sec until induction onset

#### Maintenance
*Adult:* **IV** 0.1-0.2 mg/kg/min (6-12 mg/kg/hr)
*Child ≥3 yr:* **IV** 0.125-0.3 mg/kg/min (7.5-18 mg/kg/hr)
*Geriatric:* **IV** 0.05-0.1 mg/kg/min (3-6 mg/kg/hr)

#### ICU sedation
*Adult:* **IV** 5 mcg/kg/min over 5 min; may increase by 5-10 mcg/kg/min over 5-10 min until desired response

**Available forms:** Inj 10 mg/ml in 20 ml ampule, 50 ml and 100 ml vials

### Adverse effects
*CNS:* Involuntary movement, headache, jerking, fever, dizziness, shivering, tremor, confusion, somnolence, paresthesia, agitation, abnormal dreams, euphoria, fatigue, **increased ICP, impaired cerebral flow, seizures**
*CV:* Bradycardia, hypotension, hypertension, PVC, PAC, tachycardia, abnormal ECG, ST segment depression, **asystole**

**EENT:** Blurred vision, tinnitus, eye pain, strange taste, diplopia
**GI:** *Nausea, vomiting, abdominal cramping,* dry mouth, swallowing, hypersalivation, **pancreatitis**
**GU:** Urine retention, green urine, cloudy urine, oliguria
**INTEG:** *Flushing, phlebitis, hives, burning/ stinging at inj site,* rash, pain of extremities
**MS:** Myalgia
**RESP:** *Apnea, cough, hiccups,* dyspnea, hypoventilation, sneezing, wheezing, tachypnea, hypoxia, respiratory acidosis

**Contraindications:** Hypersensitivity to product or soybean oil, egg

**Precautions:** Pregnancy **B**, breastfeeding, children, geriatric, respiratory depression, severe respiratory disorders, cardiac dysrhythmias, labor and delivery, renal disease, hyperlipidemia

Pharmacokinetics

| | |
|---|---|
| **Absorption** | Completely |
| **Distribution** | Rapid |
| **Metabolism** | Liver, conjugation to active metabolites; 95%-99% protein binding |
| **Excretion** | Urine |
| **Half-life** | 3-12 hr |

Pharmacodynamics

| | |
|---|---|
| **Onset** | 15-30 sec |
| **Peak** | Unknown |
| **Duration** | Unknown |

**Interactions**
*Individual drugs*
Alcohol: increased CNS depression

*Drug classifications*
Antipsychotics, CNS depressants (sedative/ hypnotics, opioid analgesics), inhalational anesthetics, skeletal muscle relaxants: increased CNS depression
MAOIs: do not use within 10 days

*Drug/herb*
St. John's wort: increased propofol effect

**NURSING CONSIDERATIONS**
**Assessment**
• Assess inj site: phlebitis, burning, stinging
• Monitor ECG for changes: PVC, PAC, ST segment changes; monitor VS
• Assess CNS changes: movement, jerking, tremors, dizziness, LOC, pupil reaction
• Assess allergic reactions: hives

◆ Assess respiratory dysfunction: respiratory depression, character, rate, rhythm; notify prescriber if respirations are <10/min

**Nursing diagnoses**
• Breathing pattern, ineffective (adverse reactions)
• Injury, risk for (adverse reactions)
• Knowledge, deficient (teaching)

**Implementation**
• Shake well before use; if diluted, use only D₅W to not less than 2 mg/ml; give over 3-5 min, titrate to needed level of sedation; use only glass containers when mixing, not stable in plastic
• May be given by cont inf; give by infusion pump
• Give only with resuscitative equipment available
• Give only by qualified persons trained in anesthesia
• Store in light-resistant area at room temperature; use within 6 hr of opening
• If transferred from original container to another container, complete infusion within 12 hr

*Y-site compatibilities:* Acyclovir, alfentanil, aminophylline, ampicillin, aztreonam, bumetanide, buprenorphine, butorphanol, calcium gluconate, carboplatin, cefazolin, cefoperazone, cefotaxime, cefotetan, cefoxitin, ceftizoxime, ceftriaxone, cefuroxime, chlorproMAZINE, cimetidine, cisplatin, clindamycin, cyclophosphamide, cycloSPORINE, cytarabine, dexamethasone, diphenhydrAMINE, DOBUTamine, DOPamine, doxycycline, droperidol, enalaprilat, epHEDrine, epINEPHrine, esmolol, famotidine, fentanyl, fluconazole, fluorouracil, furosemide, ganciclovir, glycopyrrolate, granisetron, haloperidol, heparin, hydrocortisone, hydromorphone, hydrOXYzine, ifosfamide, imipenem/cilastatin, inamrinone, insulin (regular), isoproterenol, ketamine, labetalol, levorphanol, lidocaine, lorazepam, magnesium sulfate, mannitol, meperidine, mezlocillin, miconazole, morphine, nafcillin, nalbuphine, naloxone, nitroglycerin, norepinephrine, ofloxacin, paclitaxel, pentobarbital, phenobarbital, piperacillin, potassium chloride, prochlorperazine, propranolol, ranitidine, scopolamine, sodium bicarbonate, sodium nitroprusside, succinylcholine, sufentanil, thiopental, ticarcillin, ticarcillin/clavulanate, vecuronium, verapamil
*Solution compatibilities:* (Is given together via Y-site) D₅W, D₅LR, LR, D₅/0.45% NaCl, D₅/0.2% NaCl

**P**

### Patient/family education
• Teach patient that this medication will cause dizziness, drowsiness, sedation

### Evaluation
**Positive therapeutic outcome**
• Induction of anesthesia

**Treatment of overdose:** Discontinue product; administer vasopressor agents or anticholinergics, artificial ventilation

---

**⚠ HIGH ALERT**

## propoxyphene (Rx)
(proe-pox′i-feen)
Darvon, Darvon-N, Dolene, Novapropoxyn ✦
*Func. class.:* Opiate analgesics
*Chem. class.:* Synthetic opiate

**Pregnancy category** C

**Controlled substance schedule** IV

**Action:** Depresses pain impulse transmission at the spinal cord level by interacting with opioid receptors

**Therapeutic outcome:** Decreased pain

**Uses:** Mild to moderate pain

### Dosage and routes
*Adult:* PO (HCl) 65 mg q4hr prn, max 390 mg/day
*Adult:* PO (napsylate) 100 mg q4hr prn, max 600 mg/day

**Available forms:** Propoxyphene HCl: caps 32, 65 mg; propoxyphene napsylate: tabs 100 mg; oral susp 50 mg/5 ml

### Adverse effects
***CNS:*** *Drowsiness, dizziness, confusion,* **increased ICP,** *headache, sedation,* euphoria, **seizures, hyperthermia (geriatric)**
***CV:*** Palpitations, bradycardia, change in B/P, **dysrhythmias**
***EENT:*** Tinnitus, blurred vision, miosis, diplopia
***GI:*** *Nausea, vomiting, anorexia, constipation, cramps,* abdominal pain, jaundice
***GU:*** Urinary retention, dysuria
***INTEG:*** *Rash,* urticaria, bruising, flushing, diaphoresis, pruritus
***RESP:*** **Respiratory depression, pulmonary edema**

**Contraindications:** Hypersensitivity to acetylsalicylic acid products (some preparations), addiction (opioid)

**Precautions:** Pregnancy **C**, breastfeeding, children <18 yr, geriatric, addictive personality, increased ICP, MI (acute), severe heart disease, respiratory depression, renal/hepatic disease

### Pharmacokinetics
| | |
|---|---|
| **Absorption** | Well absorbed |
| **Distribution** | Widely distributed, crosses placenta |
| **Metabolism** | Liver, extensively |
| **Excretion** | Kidneys, breast milk |
| **Half-life** | 6-12 hr |

### Pharmacodynamics
| | |
|---|---|
| **Onset** | ½-1 hr |
| **Peak** | 2-3 hr |
| **Duration** | 4-6 hr |

### Interactions
*Individual drugs*
Alcohol: possible fatal reactions
Nalbuphine, pentazocine: decreased analgesia
*Drug classifications*
Antipsychotics, CNS depressants, opioids, sedative/hypnotics, skeletal muscle relaxants: increased effects
MAOIs: possible fatal reactions
*Drug/herb*
Chamomile, hops, kava, Jamaican dogwood, lavender, mistletoe, nettle, pokeweed, poppy, senega, skullcap, valerian: increased CNS depression
Corkwood: increased anticholinergic effects
*Drug/lab test*
Increased: amylase
False positive: methadone test

### NURSING CONSIDERATIONS
#### Assessment
• Assess pain: location, duration, intensity before and 1 hr after administration
• Monitor CNS changes: dizziness, drowsiness, euphoria, LOC, pupil reaction
• Monitor allergic reactions: rash, urticaria

#### Nursing diagnoses
• Breathing pattern, ineffective (adverse reactions)
• Injury, risk for (adverse reactions)
• Knowledge, deficient (teaching)
• Pain, acute (uses)
• Sensory perception, disturbed: visual, auditory (adverse reactions)

#### Implementation
• Give with antiemetic if nausea, vomiting occur
• Give when pain is beginning to return; determine dosage interval by patient response;

---

continuous dosing of medication is more effective than when given prn
- Withdraw medication slowly after long-term use to prevent withdrawal symptoms
- Store in light-resistant container at room temperature
- May be given with food or milk to lessen GI upset

### Patient/family education
- Teach patient to avoid CNS depressants: alcohol, sedative/hypnotics for at least 24 hr after taking this product
- Discuss with patient that dizziness, drowsiness, and confusion are common; to avoid getting up without assistance
- Discuss in detail all aspects of the product, including purpose and what to expect after anesthesia
- Advise patient to make position changes slowly to lessen orthostatic hypotension

### Evaluation
**Positive therapeutic outcome**
- Decreased pain

### Treatment of overdose: Naloxone
0.2-0.8 mg **IV**, O₂, **IV** fluids, vasopressors

---

### propranolol  (Rx)
(proe-pran′oh-lole)
Apo-Propranolol ✦, Betaclinron E-R ✦, Detensol ✦, Inderal, Inderal LA, InnoPran XL, NovoPranol ✦, PMS-Propranol, propranolol HCl
*Func. class.:* Antihypertensive, antianginal, antidysrhythmic (class III)
*Chem. class.:* β-Adrenergic blocker

### Pregnancy category C

### Do not confuse:
Inderal/Toradol, Inderal LA/IMDUR

**Action:** Competitively blocks stimulation of β-adrenergic receptor within vascular smooth muscle; produces chronotropic, inotropic activity (decreases rate of SA node discharge, increases recovery time), slows conduction of AV node, decreased heart rate, which decreases O₂ consumption in myocardium; also suppresses renin-aldosterone-angiotensin system at high doses, inhibits β₂-receptors in bronchial system (high doses)

**Therapeutic outcome:** Decreased B/P, heart rate

**Uses:** Chronic stable angina pectoris, hypertension, supraventricular dysrhythmias, migraine prophylaxis, pheochromocytoma,

cyanotic spells related to hypertrophic subaortic stenosis

**Unlabeled uses:** Parkinson's tremor, prevention of variceal bleeding caused by portal hypertension, akathisia induced by antipsychotics

### Dosage and routes
*Dysrhythmias*
*Adult:* PO 10-30 mg tid-qid; **IV** BOL 0.5-3 mg given 1 mg/min; may repeat in 2 min; may repeat q4hr thereafter
*Child:* PO 1 mg/kg/day divided in 2 doses, **IV** 0.01-0.1 mg/kg over 5 min

*Hypertension*
*Adult:* PO 40 mg bid or 80 mg/day (sus rel) initially; usual dosage 120-240 mg/day bid-tid or 120-160 mg/day (sus rel)
*Child:* PO 0.5-1 mg/kg/day divided q6-12hr

*Angina*
*Adult:* PO 80-320 mg in divided doses bid-qid or 80 mg/day (sus rel); usual dosage 160 mg/day (sus rel)

*MI prophylaxis*
*Adult:* PO 180-240 mg/day tid-qid starting 5 days to 3 wk after MI

*Pheochromocytoma*
*Adult:* PO 60 mg/day × 3 days preoperatively in divided doses or 30 mg/day in divided doses (inoperable tumor)

*Migraine*
*Adult:* PO 80 mg (sus rel) or in divided doses; may increase to 160-240 mg/day in divided doses
*Child:* PO 0.6-1.5 mg/kg/day divided q8hr

*Essential tremor*
*Adult:* PO 40 mg bid; usual dosage 120 mg/day

**Available forms:** Sus rel caps 60, 80, 120, 160 mg; tabs 10, 20, 40, 60, 80, 90 mg; inj 1 mg/ml; oral sol 4 mg, 8 mg/ml; conc oral sol 80 mg/ml

### Adverse effects
*CNS:* Depression, hallucinations, dizziness, *fatigue*, lethargy, paresthesia, bizarre dreams, disorientation
*CV:* **Bradycardia**, *hypotension*, **CHF,** palpitations, AV block, peripheral vascular insufficiency, vasodilatation, **pulmonary edema,** **dysrhythmias,** cold extremities
*EENT:* Sore throat, **laryngospasm,** blurred vision, dry eyes
*GI:* Nausea, vomiting, diarrhea, colitis, constipation, cramps, dry mouth, hepatomegaly, gastric pain, acute pancreatitis

**P**

Adverse effects: *italic* = common, **bold** = life-threatening

*GU:* Impotence, decreased libido, UTIs
**HEMA: Agranulocytosis, thrombocytopenia**
*INTEG:* Rash, pruritus, fever
*META:* Hyperglycemia, hypoglycemia
*MISC:* Facial swelling, weight change, Raynaud's phenomenon
*MS:* Joint pain, arthralgia, muscle cramps, pain
*RESP:* Dyspnea, respiratory dysfunction, **bronchospasm,** cough

**Contraindications:** Hypersensitivity to this product, cardiac failure, cardiogenic shock, 2nd- or 3rd-degree heart block, bronchospastic disease, sinus bradycardia, CHF, bronchospasm

**Precautions:** Pregnancy **C,** breastfeeding, children, diabetes mellitus, renal/hepatic disease, hyperthyroidism, COPD, myasthenia gravis, peripheral vascular disease, hypotension, CHF

### Pharmacokinetics

| | |
|---|---|
| Absorption | Well absorbed (PO); slowly absorbed (ext rel); completely absorbed (**IV**) |
| Distribution | Widely distributed, crosses blood-brain barrier, protein binding 90% |
| Metabolism | Liver, extensively |
| Excretion | Kidneys |
| Half-life | 3-5 hr; ext rel 8-11 hr |

### Pharmacodynamics

| | PO | PO–EXT REL | IV |
|---|---|---|---|
| Onset | ½ hr | Unknown | Rapid |
| Peak | 1-1½ hr | 6 hr | 1 min |
| Duration | 6-12 hr | 24 hr | 4-6 hr |

### Interactions
*Individual drugs*
Cimetidine: increased β-blocking effect
Disopyramide: increased negative inotropic effects
Haloperidol, prazosin, quinidine: increased hypotension
Smoking: decreased propranolol levels
*Drug classifications*
Barbiturates: decreased β-blocking effect
Calcium channel blockers, neuromuscular blockers: increased effects
*Drug/herb*
Aconite: increased toxicity, death
Astragalus, cola tree: increased or decreased antihypertensive effect
Barberry, betony, black catechu, black cohosh, bloodroot, broom, burdock, cat's claw, dandelion, goldenseal, Irish moss, Jamaican

dogwood, kelp, khella, mistletoe, parsley: increased antihypertensive effect
Coltsfoot, guarana, khat, licorice: decreased antihypertensive effect
*Drug/lab test*
Increased: serum potassium, serum uric acid, AST, ALT, alkaline phosphatase, LDH
Decreased: blood glucose
Interference: glaucoma testing

## NURSING CONSIDERATIONS
### Assessment
• Monitor B/P during beginning treatment, periodically thereafter; pulse q4hr; note rate, rhythm, quality; check apical/radial pulse before administration; notify prescriber of any significant changes (pulse <50 bpm or systolic B/P <90 mmHg)
• Check for baselines in renal, liver function tests before therapy begins and periodically thereafter
• Assess for edema in feet, legs daily; monitor I&O, weight daily; check for jugular vein distention, crackles bilaterally; dyspnea (CHF)
• Monitor skin turgor, dryness of mucous membranes for hydration status, especially geriatric
• Assess for headache, light-headedness, decreased B/P; may indicate need for decreased dose; may aggravate symptoms of arterial insufficiency

### Nursing diagnoses
• Cardiac output, decreased (uses)
• Injury, risk for (adverse reactions)
• Knowledge, deficient (teaching)
• Noncompliance (teaching)

### Implementation
**PO route**
• Do not break, crush, or chew sus rel cap
• Given before meals, at bedtime, tab may be crushed or swallowed whole; give with food to prevent GI upset; reduce dosage in renal dysfunction
• May mix oral sol with liquid or semisolid food, rinse container to get entire dose
• Store protected from light, moisture; placed in cool environment
**IV route**
• Give by direct **IV** undiluted or diluted 1 mg/10 ml of D₅W for inj; administer over 1 min or more
• Give by intermittent inf after diluting in 50 ml of D₅W, 0.9% NaCl, D₅/0.45% NaCl, D₅/0.9% NaCl, LR; administer over 15 min

---

## Y-site compatibilities:
Heparin, hydrocortisone, inamrinone, meperidine, milrinone, morphine, potassium chloride, tacrolimus, vit B/C

**Y-site incompatibilities:** Diazoxide

**Additive compatibilities:** DOBUTamine, verapamil

**Solution compatibilities:** 0.9% NaCl, 0.45% NaCl, Ringer's, D$_5$W, D$_5$/0.9% NaCl, D$_5$/0.45% NaCl

## Patient/family education

• Teach patient not to discontinue product abruptly, taper over 2 wk; may cause precipitate angina, MI if stopped abruptly

• Teach patient not to use OTC products containing α-adrenergic stimulants (such as nasal decongestants, cold preparations); to avoid alcohol, smoking and to limit sodium intake as prescribed

• Teach patient how to take pulse and B/P at home; advise when to notify prescriber

• Instruct patient to comply with weight control, dietary adjustments, modified exercise program

• Instruct patient to carry/wear emergency ID to identify product being taken, allergies; tell patient product controls symptoms but does not cure

• Caution patient to avoid hazardous activities if dizziness, drowsiness is present

• Teach patient to report symptoms of CHF: difficult breathing, especially on exertion or when lying down, night cough, swelling of extremities or bradycardia, dizziness, confusion, depression, fever

• Teach patient to take product as prescribed, not to double doses, skip doses; take any missed doses as soon as remembered if at least 8 hr until next dose

• Advise patient that sensitivity to cold may occur

• Teach patient to monitor blood glucose, may mask symptoms of hypoglycemia

• Teach patient how to take pulse, B/P; withhold if <50 bpm or systolic B/P <90 mmHg

## Evaluation
**Positive therapeutic outcome**

• Decreased B/P in hypertension (after 1-2 wk)

• Decreased tremors

• Absence of dysrhythmias

• Decreased migraine headaches

**Treatment of overdose:** Lavage, **IV** atropine for bradycardia, **IV** theophylline for bronchospasm, digoxin, O$_2$, diuretic for cardiac failure, hemodialysis, **IV** glucose for hyperglycemia, **IV** diazepam (or phenytoin) for seizures

---

### propylhexadrine nasal
*See Appendix D*

---

### propylthiouracil (Rx)
(proe-pill-thye-oh-yoor'a-sill)
propylthiouracil, Propyl-Thyracil ✦, PTU
*Func. class.:* Thyroid hormone antagonist (antithyroid)
*Chem. class.:* Thioamide

### Pregnancy category D

**Action:** Blocks synthesis peripherally of T$_3$, T$_4$, inhibits organification of iodine

**Therapeutic outcome:** Decreased T$_3$, T$_4$ levels, hyperthyroid symptoms

**Uses:** Preparation for thyroidectomy, thyrotoxic crisis, hyperthyroidism, thyroid storm

### Dosage and routes
*Thyrotoxic crisis*
**Adult and child:** PO same as hyperthyroidism with iodine and propranolol

*Preparation for thyroidectomy*
**Adult:** PO 600-1200 mg/day
**Child:** PO 10 mg/kg/day in divided doses

*Hyperthyroidism*
**Adult:** PO 100 mg tid increasing to 300 mg q8hr if condition is severe; continue to euthyroid state, then 100 mg daily-tid
**Child >10 yr:** PO 100 mg tid; continue to euthyroid state, then 25 mg tid to 100 mg bid
**Child 6-10 yr:** PO 50-150 mg in divided doses q8hr
**Neonate:** PO 10 mg/kg/day in divided doses

**Available forms:** Tabs 50, 100 mg

### Adverse effects
*CNS: Drowsiness, headache, vertigo, fever,* paresthesias, neuritis
*GI: Nausea, diarrhea, vomiting, jaundice, hepatitis,* loss of taste
*GU:* **Nephritis**
*HEMA:* **Agranulocytosis, leukopenia, thrombocytopenia, hypothrombinemia, lymphadenopathy,** bleeding, vasculitis, periarteritis
*INTEG: Rash, urticaria, pruritus, alopecia, hyperpigmentation,* lupus-like syndrome
*MS: Myalgia, arthralgia, nocturnal muscle cramps, osteoporosis*

**P**

---

Adverse effects: *italic* = common, **bold** = life-threatening

**Contraindications:** Pregnancy **D**, breast-feeding, hypersensitivity

**Precautions:** Infection, bone marrow depression, hepatic disease

### Pharmacokinetics

| | |
|---|---|
| **Absorption** | Rapidly absorbed |
| **Distribution** | Crosses placenta, concentration in thyroid gland |
| **Metabolism** | Liver |
| **Excretion** | Urine, bile, breast milk |
| **Half-life** | 1-2 hr |

### Pharmacodynamics

| | |
|---|---|
| **Onset** | 30-40 min |
| **Peak** | Unknown |
| **Duration** | 2-4 hr |

## Interactions
### Individual drugs
Heparin: increased anticoagulant effect
Lithium: increased antithyroid effect
Potassium/sodium iodide: increased effects
Radiation: increased bone marrow depression
### Drug classifications
Anticoagulants (oral): increased anticoagulant effect
Antineoplastics: increased bone marrow depression
Phenothiazines: increased agranulocytosis
### Drug/lab test
Increased: pro-time, AST, ALT, alkaline phosphatase

## NURSING CONSIDERATIONS
### Assessment
• Monitor pulse, B/P, temp; I&O ratio; check for edema (puffy hands, feet, periorbits); indicates hypothyroidism
• Check weight daily with same clothing, scale, time of day
• Monitor $T_3$, $T_4$, which are increased; check serum TSH, which is decreased; assess free thyroxine index, which is increased if dosage is too low; discontinue product 3-4 wk before radioactive iodine uptake test
• Monitor blood tests: CBC for blood dyscrasias (leukopenia, thrombocytopenia, agranulocytosis); liver function tests
◆ Assess overdose (peripheral edema, heat intolerance, diaphoresis, palpitations, dysrhythmias, severe tachycardia, increased temp, delirium, CNS irritability); product should be discontinued
• Assess for hypersensitivity (rash, enlarged cervical lymph nodes); product may have to be discontinued

• Assess for hypoprothrombinemia (bleeding, petechiae, ecchymosis)
• Monitor clinical response: after 3 wk should include increased weight, decreased pulse, decreased $T_4$
• Assess for bone marrow depression: sore throat, fever, fatigue

### Nursing diagnoses
• Knowledge, deficient (teaching)
• Noncompliance (teaching)

### Implementation
• Give with meals to decrease GI upset
• Give at same time each day to maintain product level
• Give lowest dosage that relieves symptoms
• Store in light-resistant container
• Increase fluids to 3-4 L/day, unless contraindicated

### Patient/family education
• Advise patient to abstain from breastfeeding after delivery; product appears in breast milk
• Teach patient to take pulse daily and to keep graph of weight, pulse, mood
• Advise patient to report redness, swelling, sore throat, mouth lesions, which indicate blood dyscrasias
• Caution patient to avoid OTC products that contain iodine; that seafood, other iodine-containing foods may be restricted by prescriber
• Caution patient not to discontinue this medication abruptly; thyroid crisis may occur; stress patient compliance
• Teach patient that response may take several mo if thyroid is large
• Teach patient symptoms/signs of overdose: periorbital edema, cold intolerance, mental depression; notify prescriber at once
• Teach patient symptoms of inadequate dose: tachycardia, diarrhea, fever, irritability; prescriber should be notified to adjust dosage
• Teach patient to take medication exactly as prescribed, not to skip or double doses; missed doses should be taken when remembered up to 1 hr before next dose
• Instruct patient to carry/wear emergency identification indicating medication taken and condition being treated

### Evaluation
**Positive therapeutic outcome**
• Weight gain
• Decreased pulse
• Decreased $T_4$
• Decreased B/P

## protamine (Rx)

(proe'ta-meen)
*Func. class.:* Heparin antagonist
*Chem. class.:* Low-molecular-weight protein

**Pregnancy category  C**

**Action:** Binds heparin, making it ineffective

**Therapeutic outcome:** Prevention of heparin overdose

**Uses:** Heparin overdose; neutralizes heparin in procedures, hemorrhage

### Dosage and routes

*Adult and child:* **IV** 1 mg of protamine/100 units of heparin given or 100 anti-XA units of LMWH; administer slowly over 1-3 min; not to exceed 50 mg/10 min

**Available forms:** Inj 10 mg/ml

### Adverse effects

*CNS:* Lassitude, flushing
*CV:* Hypotension, bradycardia, **circulatory collapse,** capillary leak
*GI:* Nausea, vomiting, anorexia
*HEMA:* Bleeding
*INTEG:* Rash, dermatitis, urticaria
*RESP:* Dyspnea, **pulmonary edema, severe respiratory distress, bronchospasm**
*SYST:* **Anaphylaxis, angioedema**

**Contraindication:** Hypersensitivity

**Precautions:** Pregnancy **C,** breastfeeding, children, allergy to salmon, diabetes mellitus, infertile/vasectomized men, previous exposure to protamine, heparin rebound or bleeding

### Pharmacokinetics

| Absorption | Completely absorbed |
|---|---|
| Distribution | Unknown |
| Metabolism | Unknown |
| Excretion | Unknown |
| Half-life | Unknown |

### Pharmacodynamics

| Onset | 5 min |
|---|---|
| Peak | Unknown |
| Duration | 2 hr |

## NURSING CONSIDERATIONS

### Assessment

• Monitor blood studies (Hct, platelets, occult blood stools) q3 mo
• Monitor coagulation tests (APTT, ACT) 15 min after dose, then in several hr
• Monitor VS, B/P, pulse q30 min, plus 3 hr after dose
◆ Assess for hypersensitivity: skin rash, urti-caria, dermatitis, cough, wheezing, have emergency equipment nearby; men who have had a vasectomy may be more prone to hypersensitivity
◆ Assess for allergy to salmon; use with caution in these patients

### Nursing diagnoses

• Injury, risk for (uses)
• Knowledge, deficient (teaching)
• Tissue perfusion, ineffective (uses)

### Implementation

• Give by direct **IV** after diluting 50 mg/5 ml of sterile bacteriostatic water for inj; shake; give 20 mg or less over 1-3 min
• Give by intermittent inf after further diluting with equal volume of NaCl or $D_5W$ and run over 2-3 hr; titrate to APTT, ACT; use infusion pump
• Too rapid infusion leads to hypotension, anaphylactoid reactions
• Store at 36-46° F (2-8° C)

*Additive compatibilities:*
Cimetidine, ranitidine, verapamil

*Additive incompatibilities:*
Penicillins, cephalosporins

### Patient/family education

• Explain reason for medication and expected results
• Caution patient to avoid contact activities that may result in bleeding

### Evaluation

**Positive therapeutic outcome**
• Reversal of heparin overdose

## pseudoephedrine (OTC)

(soo-doe-e-fed'rin)
Afrin, Allermed, Canafed, Cenafed, Children's Congestion Relief, Children's Silfedrine, Congestion Relief, Decofed Syrup, DeFed-60, Dorcol Children's Decongestant, Drixoral Non-Drowsy Formula, Dynafed, Efidac/24, Eltor ✦, Genaphed, Halofed, Mini Thin Pseudo, pseudoepHEDrine HCl, Pseudo, Pseudogest, Seudotabs, Sinustop Pro, Sudafed, Sudafed 12 hour, Sudex, Triaminic AM Decongestant Formula
*Func. class.:* Adrenergic
*Chem. class.:* Substituted phenylethylamine

**Pregnancy category  C**

**Action:** Primary activity through α-adrenergic effects on respiratory mucosal membranes reducing congestion, hyperemia,

Adverse effects: *italic* = common, **bold** = life-threatening

edema; minimal bronchodilatation secondary to β-adrenergic effects

**Therapeutic outcome:** Decreased nasal congestion, swelling

**Uses:** Nasal decongestant, otitis media adjustment, adjunct with antihistamines

### Dosage and routes
*Adult and child >12 yr:* PO 60 mg q6hr; EXT REL 120 mg q12hr or 240 mg q24hr
*Geriatric:* PO 30-60 mg q6hr prn
*Child 6-12 yr:* PO 30 mg q6hr, max 120 mg/day
*Child 2-6 yr:* PO 15 mg q6hr, max 60 mg/day

**Available forms:** Ext rel caps 120, 240 mg; oral sol 15 mg, 30 mg/5 ml; drops 7.5 mg/0.8 ml; tabs 30, 60 mg; caps 60 mg; ext rel tabs 120, 240 mg

### Adverse effects
*CNS: Tremors, anxiety,* stimulation, insomnia, headache, dizziness, hallucinations, **seizures** (geriatric)
*CV:* Palpitations, tachycardia, hypertension, chest pain, **dysrhythmias, CV collapse**
*EENT:* Dry nose, irritation of nose and throat
*GI: Anorexia, nausea, vomiting,* dry mouth
*GU:* Dysuria

**Contraindications:** Hypersensitivity to sympathomimetics, angle-closure glaucoma

**Precautions:** Pregnancy **C,** breastfeeding, cardiac disorders, hyperthyroidism, diabetes mellitus, prostatic hypertrophy, hypertension

#### Pharmacokinetics
| | |
|---|---|
| **Absorption** | Well absorbed |
| **Distribution** | Enters CSF, crosses placenta |
| **Metabolism** | Liver, partially |
| **Excretion** | Kidneys, unchanged (75%); breast milk |
| **Half-life** | 7 hr |

#### Pharmacodynamics
| | PO | PO–EXT REL |
|---|---|---|
| **Onset** | 15-30 min | 1 hr |
| **Peak** | Unknown | Unknown |
| **Duration** | 4-6 hr | 12 hr |

### Interactions
*Individual products*
Methyldopa: decreased effect of pseudo-ephedrine
*Drug classifications*
Antidepressants (tricyclics), MAOIs: hypertensive crisis, do not use together

Rauwolfia alkaloids, urinary acidifiers: decreased effect of pseudoephedrine
Urinary alkalizers: increased effect of pseudoephedrine

### NURSING CONSIDERATIONS
#### Assessment
• Assess for CNS side effects in the geriatric: excitation, seizures, hallucinations
• Monitor for nasal congestion; auscultate lung sounds; check for tenacious bronchial secretions; children with otitis media should be assessed for eustachian tube congestion
• Monitor B/P and pulse throughout treatment

#### Nursing diagnoses
• Airway clearance, ineffective (uses)
• Knowledge, deficient (teaching)

#### Implementation
• Swallow tab and ext rel cap whole; do not break, crush, or chew
• Give several hr before bedtime if insomnia occurs
• Store at room temperature

#### Patient/family education
• Teach patient reason for product administration and expected results
• Instruct patient not to use continuously, or more than recommended dose; rebound congestion may occur
• Advise patient to check with prescriber before using other products, as product interactions may occur
• Advise patient to avoid taking near bedtime; stimulation can occur
• Caution patient not to use if stimulation, restlessness, tremors occur
• Notify parents of possible excessive agitation in children
◆ Advise patient to notify prescriber of anxiety, slow or fast heart rate, dyspnea, seizures

#### Evaluation
**Positive therapeutic outcome**
• Decreased nasal congestion

### pseudoephedrine nasal agent
*See Appendix D*

## psyllium (OTC)
(sill'i-um)

Fiberall, Fiberall Natural Flavor and Orange Flavor, Genifiber, Hydrocil Instant, Karacil ♣, Konsyl, Konsyl Orange, Maalox Daily Fiber Therapy, Metamucil, Metamucil Lemon Lime, Metamucil Orange Flavor, Metamucil Sugar Free, Metamucil Sugar Free Orange Flavor, Modane Bulk, Mylanta Natural Fiber Supplement, Natural Fiber Laxative, Natural Fiber Laxative Sugar Free, Natural Vegetable Reguloid, Prodiem Plain ♣, Reguloid Natural, Reguloid Orange, Reguloid Sugar Free Orange, Reguloid Sugar Free Regular, Restore, Restore Sugar Free, Serutan, Syllact

*Func. class.:* Laxative, bulk-forming
*Chem. class.:* Psyllium colloid

### Pregnancy category C

**Action:** Promotes peristalsis by combining with water in the intestine to form a gel-like substance that is easily evacuated

**Therapeutic outcome:** Decreased constipation, decreased diarrhea in colitis

**Uses:** Chronic constipation, ulcerative colitis, irritable bowel syndrome

### Dosage and routes
*Adult:* PO 1-2 tsp in 8 oz of water bid or tid, then 8 oz of water or 1 premeasured packet in 8 oz of water bid or tid, then 8 oz of water
*Child >6 yr:* 1 tsp in 4 oz of water at bedtime

**Available forms:** Chew pieces 1.7, 3.4 g/piece; powder effervescent 3.4, 3.7 g/packet; powder 3.3, 3.4, 3.5, 4.94 g/tsp; wafers 3.4 g/wafer

### Adverse effects
*GI: Nausea, vomiting, anorexia, diarrhea,* cramps, intestinal/esophageal blockage

**Contraindications:** Hypersensitivity, intestinal obstruction, abdominal pain, nausea/vomiting, fecal impaction

**Precautions:** Pregnancy **C**

### Pharmacokinetics

| | |
|---|---|
| **Absorption** | None |
| **Distribution** | None |
| **Metabolism** | Unknown |
| **Excretion** | Feces |
| **Half-life** | Unknown |

### Pharmacodynamics

| | |
|---|---|
| **Onset** | 12-24 hr |
| **Peak** | 2-4 days |
| **Duration** | Unknown |

### Interactions
*Drug classifications*
Cardiac glycosides, oral anticoagulants, salicylates: decreased absorption of each specific product
*Drug/herb*
Flax, senna: increased laxative

### NURSING CONSIDERATIONS
#### Assessment
• Monitor blood, urine electrolytes if used often by patient; check I&O ratio to identify fluid loss
• Assess for cramping, rectal bleeding, nausea, vomiting; if these symptoms occur, product should be discontinued; identify cause of constipation; identify whether fluids, bulk, or exercise is missing from lifestyle
• Assess stool for color, consistency, amount, presence of flatulence

#### Nursing diagnoses
• Constipation (uses)
• Knowledge, deficient (teaching)
• Noncompliance (teaching)

#### Implementation
• Give alone for better absorption; give after mixing with water immediately before use; administer with 8 oz of water or juice followed by another 8 oz of fluid
• Administer in AM or PM (oral dose)
• Shake susp well

#### Patient/family education
• Discuss with patient that adequate fluid consumption is necessary
• Teach patient that normal bowel movements do not always occur daily
• Caution patient not to use in presence of abdominal pain, nausea, vomiting; tell patient to notify prescriber if constipation is unrelieved or if symptoms of electrolyte imbalance occur (muscle cramps, pain, weakness, dizziness, excessive thirst)
• Teach patient not to use laxatives for long-term therapy; bowel tone will be lost and will decrease
• Teach patient not to take at bedtime as a laxative; may interfere with sleep; also problems with lipid pneumonia
• Teach patient not to use with food or vitamin preparations; delays digestion and absorption of fat-soluble vitamins

**P**

## Evaluation
**Positive therapeutic outcome**
• Decreased constipation in 12-24 hr

---

## pyrazinamide (Rx)
(peer-a-zin'a-mide)
PMS Pyrazinamide ✤, pyrazinamide,
Tebrazid ✤
*Func. class.:* Antitubercular agent
*Chem. class.:* Pyrazinoic acid amine/
nicoturimide analog

**Pregnancy category** C

**Action:** Bactericidal interference with lipid;
nucleic acid biosynthesis is possible

**Therapeutic outcome:** Bactericidal for
*Mycobacterium* species

**Uses:** Tuberculosis, as an adjunct when other
products are not feasible

**Dosage and routes**
*HIV negative*
*Adult:* PO 15-30 mg/kg/day, max 2 g/day
*Child:* PO 7.5-15 mg/kg bid or 15-30 mg/kg/
day, max 2 g

*HIV positive*
*Adult:* PO 15-30 mg/kg/day, max 2 g × 2 mo
used with a rifamycin
*Child:* PO 20-40 mg/kg/day, max 2 g/day × 2
mo given with a rifamycin

*Renal dose*
*Adult:* PO CCr 10-50 ml/min, give dose
q48-72hr; CCr <10 ml/min give dose q72hr

**Available forms:** Tabs 500 mg

**Adverse effects**
*CNS:* Headache
*GI:* **Hepatotoxicity,** abnormal liver function
tests, peptic ulcer, nausea, vomiting, anorexia,
cramps, diarrhea
*GU:* Urinary difficulty, increased uric acid
***HEMA:* Hemolytic anemia**
*INTEG:* Photosensitivity, urticaria

**Contraindications:** Hypersensitivity,
severe hepatic damage, acute gout

**Precautions:** Pregnancy C, child <13 yr,
renal failure, diabetes, porphyria, chronic gout

### Pharmacokinetics
| | |
|---|---|
| **Absorption** | Well absorbed |
| **Distribution** | Widely distributed |
| **Metabolism** | Liver, extensively |
| **Excretion** | Kidneys, breast milk |
| **Half-life** | 9-10 hr |

### Pharmacodynamics
| | |
|---|---|
| **Onset** | Unknown |
| **Peak** | 2 hr |
| **Duration** | 9½ hr; metabolites 12 hr |

## Interactions
*Drug/lab test*
Decreased: 17-KS

## NURSING CONSIDERATIONS
### Assessment
• C&S studies should be done before treatment begins, and periodically during treatment
• Monitor serum uric acid, which may be
elevated and cause gout symptoms
• Monitor liver function tests weekly: ALT, AST,
bilirubin; hepatic status: decreased appetite,
jaundice, dark urine, fatigue
• Monitor renal status before treatment and
monthly thereafter: BUN, creatinine, output,
specific gravity, urinalysis, uric acid
• Monitor mental status often: affect, mood,
behavioral changes; psychosis may occur

### Nursing diagnoses
• Diarrhea (adverse reactions)
• Infection, risk for (uses)
• Injury, risk for (adverse reactions)
• Knowledge, deficient (teaching)
• Noncompliance (teaching)

### Implementation
• Give with meals to decrease GI symptoms
• Give antiemetic if vomiting occurs
• May be given with other antitubercular
products

### Patient/family education
• Instruct patient that compliance with dosage
schedule, duration is necessary; that scheduled
appointments must be kept or relapse may
occur
• Advise diabetic patient to use blood glucose
monitor to obtain correct result
• Advise patient to report weakness, fatigue,
loss of appetite, nausea, vomiting, yellowing of
skin or eyes, tingling/numbness of hands/feet

### Evaluation
**Positive therapeutic outcome**
• Decreased symptoms of TB
• Sputum culture negative × 3

---

## pyridostigmine (Rx)

(peer-id-oh-stig′meen)

Mestinon, Mestinon SR, Mestinon Timespan, Regonol

*Func. class.:* Cholinergic, anticholinesterase

*Chem. class.:* Tertiary amine carbamate

**Pregnancy category** C

**Action:** Inhibits destruction of acetylcholine, which increases concentration at sites where acetylcholine is released; this facilitates transmission of impulses across myoneural junction

**Therapeutic outcome:** Decreased action of nondepolarizing muscle relaxant; increased muscle strength in myasthenia gravis

**Uses:** Nondepolarizing muscle relaxant antagonist, myasthenia gravis

### Dosage and routes
*Myasthenia gravis*
*Adult:* PO 600 mg/day in 5-6 divided doses, max 1.5 g/day; IM/**IV** 2 mg or 1/30 of PO dose; SUS REL 180-540 mg/day or bid at intervals of at least 6 hr
*Child:* PO 7 mg/kg/day in 5-6 divided doses; IM/**IV** 0.05-0.15 mg/kg/dose

*Nondepolarizing neuromuscular blocker antagonist*
*Adult:* 0.6-1.2 mg **IV** atropine, then 0.1-0.25 mg/kg/dose
*Child:* **IV** 0.1-0.25 mg/kg/dose

**Available forms:** Tabs 60 mg; ext rel tabs 180 mg; syr 60 mg/5 ml; inj 5 mg/ml

### Adverse effects
*CNS:* Dizziness, headache, sweating, weakness, **seizures,** uncoordination, paralysis, drowsiness, LOC
*CV:* Tachycardia, dysrhythmias, bradycardia, AV block, hypotension, ECG changes, **cardiac arrest,** syncope
*EENT:* Miosis, blurred vision, lacrimation, visual changes
*GI: Nausea, diarrhea, vomiting, cramps, increased salivary and gastric secretions, peristalsis*
*GU:* Frequency, incontinence, urgency
*INTEG:* Rash, urticaria, flushing
*RESP:* **Respiratory depression, bronchospasm, constriction, laryngospasm, respiratory arrest**

**Contraindications:** Bradycardia, hypotension, obstruction of intestine, renal system, bromide sensitivity

**Precautions:** Pregnancy **C,** seizure disorders, bronchial asthma, coronary occlusion, hyperthyroidism, dysrhythmias, peptic ulcer, megacolon, poor GI motility

### Pharmacokinetics
| | |
|---|---|
| **Absorption** | Poorly absorbed (PO) |
| **Distribution** | Widely distributed, crosses placenta |
| **Metabolism** | Liver, plasma cholinesterase |
| **Excretion** | Kidneys |
| **Half-life** | 2 hr (**IV**); 4 hr (PO) |

### Pharmacodynamics
| | PO | PO–EXT REL | IM/IV |
|---|---|---|---|
| **Onset** | 20-30 min | ½-1 hr | 2-15 min |
| **Peak** | Unknown | Unknown | Unknown |
| **Duration** | 3-6 hr | 3-6 hr | 2-4 hr |

### Interactions
*Individual drugs*
Atropine, gallamine, metocurine, pancuronium, tubocurarine: decreased action
Decamethonium, succinylcholine: increased action of pyridostigmine
Magnesium, mecamylamine, polymyxin, procainamide, quinidine: decreased action of pyridostigmine
*Drug classifications*
Aminoglycosides, anesthetics, antidysrhythmics, corticosteroids, quinolones: decreased action of pyridostigmine
*Drug/herb*
Jaborandi tree, pill-bearing spurge: increased effect

### NURSING CONSIDERATIONS
#### Assessment
• Monitor VS, respiration; increased B/P during test and at baseline
• Monitor diabetic patient carefully, since this product lowers blood glucose

#### Nursing diagnoses
• Breathing pattern, ineffective (uses)
• Knowledge, deficient (teaching)

#### Implementation
**PO route**
• Give only after all other cholinergics have been discontinued
• Give increased doses as ordered if tolerance occurs
• Give larger doses as ordered after exercise or fatigue
• Give on empty stomach for better absorption
• Store at room temperature
**IV route**
• Give **IV** undiluted, give through Y-tube or 3-way stopcock; give 0.5 mg or less/min

P

- Give only when atropine sulfate available for cholinergic crisis

*Syringe compatibilities:* Glycopyrrolate

*Y-site compatibilities:* Heparin, hydrocortisone, potassium chloride, vit B/C

**Patient/family education**

- Advise patient to carry/wear emergency ID specifying myasthenia gravis, products taken

**Evaluation**

**Positive therapeutic outcome**

- Increased muscle strength, hand grasp
- Improved gait
- Absence of labored breathing (if severe)

**Treatment of overdose:** Discontinue product, atropine 1-4 mg **IV**

---

**pyridoxine (vitamin B$_6$)**
**(OTC, Rx)**
(peer-i-dox'een)
Beesix, Doxine, Nestrex, pyridoxine HCl, Pyri, Rodex, Vitabee 6, Vitamin B$_6$
*Func. class.:* Vitamin B$_6$, water soluble

**Pregnancy category   A**

**Action:** Needed for fat, protein, carbohydrate metabolism; enhances glycogen release from liver and muscle tissue; needed as coenzyme for metabolic transformations of a variety of amino acids

**Therapeutic outcome:** Absence of vit B$_6$ deficiency

**Uses:** Vitamin B$_6$ deficiency associated with the following: inborn errors of metabolism, seizures, cycloSERINE, hydrALAZINE penicillamine, isoniazid therapy, oral contraceptives, alcoholism, polyneuritis

**Unlabeled uses:** Palmar-plantar erythrodysesthesia syndrome

**Dosage and routes**
*RDA*
*Adult:* PO (male) 1.7-2 mg; (female) 1.4-1.6 mg
*Adult and child >11 yr:* PO (male) 2.2 mg; (female) 2.0 mg
*Child 7-10 yr:* PO 1.8 mg
*Child 4-6 yr:* PO 1.3 mg
*Child 1-3 yr:* PO 0.9 mg
*Infant 6-12 mo:* PO 0.6 mg

*Vitamin B$_6$ deficiency*
*Adult:* PO/IM/**IV** 5-25 mg/day × 3 wk
*Child:* PO/IM/**IV** 10 mg until desired response

*Deficiency caused by isoniazid, cycloSERINE, hydrALAZINE, penicillamine*
*Adult:* PO 6-100 mg/day
*Child:* PO 5-25 mg/day

*Prevention of deficiency caused by isoniazid, cycloSERINE, hydrALAZINE, penicillamine*
*Adult:* PO 6-50 mg/day
*Child:* PO 0.5-1.5 mg/day
*Infant:* PO 0.1-0.5 mg/day

*Palmar-plantar erythrodysesthesia syndrome (unlabeled)*
*Adult:* PO 50-150 mg/day

**Available forms:** Tabs 10, 25, 50, 100 mg; ext rel tabs 100 mg; inj 100 mg/ml; ext rel caps 150 mg

**Adverse effects**
*CNS:* Paresthesia, flushing, warmth, lethargy (rare with normal renal function)
*INTEG:* Pain at inj site

**Contraindication:** Hypersensitivity

**Precautions:** Pregnancy **A**, breastfeeding, children, Parkinson's disease, patients taking levodopa should avoid supplemental vitamins with >5 mg pyridoxine

| Pharmacokinetics | |
|---|---|
| Absorption | Well absorbed (PO) |
| Distribution | Stored in liver, muscle, brain; crosses placenta |
| Metabolism | Unknown |
| Excretion | Kidneys, unchanged (not used) |
| Half-life | Unknown |

| Pharmacodynamics |
|---|
| Unknown |

**Interactions**
*Individual drugs*
Chloramphenicol, cycloSERINE, hydrALAZINE, isoniazid, penicillamine: decreased effects of pyridoxine
Levodopa: decreased effects of levodopa
*Drug classifications*
Contraceptives (oral), immunosuppressants: decreased effects of pyridoxine

**NURSING CONSIDERATIONS**
**Assessment**

- Monitor pyridoxine levels throughout treatment
- Assess nutritional status: yeast, liver, legumes, bananas, green vegetables, whole grains

---

• Assess for pyridoxine ($B_6$) deficiency: nausea, vomiting, dermatitis, cheilosis, seizures, irritability, dermatitis before and during treatment
• Assess neurologic status: paresthesia, lethargy
• Monitor blood tests: Hct, Hgb

## Nursing diagnoses
• Knowledge, deficient (teaching)
• Noncompliance (teaching, overuse)
• Nutrition: less than body requirements, imbalanced (uses)

## Implementation
**PO route**
• Swallow ext rel cap and ext rel tabs whole; do not break, crush, or chew
**IM route**
• Rotate sites to avoid pain; burning or stinging at site may occur; give by Z-track to minimize pain
• Store in airtight, light-resistant container
**IV route**
• Give **IV** undiluted or added to most **IV** sol; give 50 mg or less/1 min if undiluted
*Syringe compatibilities:*
Doxapram
*Additive incompatibilities:*
Erythromycin, iron salts, kanamycin, riboflavin, streptomycin

## Patient/family education
• Teach patient to avoid other vitamin supplements unless directed by prescriber
• Advise patient to increase meat, bananas, potatoes, lima beans, whole grain cereals in diet which are high in vit $B_6$
• Caution patient not to increase dosage, since serious reactions may occur

## Evaluation
**Positive therapeutic outcome**
• Absence of nausea, vomiting, anorexia, skin lesions, glossitis, stomatitis, edema, seizures, restlessness, paresthesia

---

## pyrimethamine (Rx)
(peer-i-meth'a-meen)
Daraprim, Fansidar (with sulfadoxine)
*Func. class.:* Antimalarial, antiprotozoal
*Chem. class.:* Folic acid antagonist
**Pregnancy category** C

**Action:** Inhibits folic acid metabolism in parasite; prevents transmission by stopping growth of fertilized gametes

**Therapeutic outcome:** Prevention of malaria

**Uses:** Malaria prophylaxis, antiprotozoal action against *Plasmodium vivax*

**Unlabeled uses:** *Pneumocystis jiroveci* pneumonia as an adjunct

## Dosage and routes
*Prophylaxis of malaria*
*Adult and child >10 yr:* PO 25 mg qwk
*Child 4-10 yr:* PO 12.5 mg qwk
*Child <4 yr:* PO 6.25 mg qwk

*Toxoplasmosis*
*Adult:* PO 100 mg, then 25 mg/day × 4-5 wk, with 1 g sulfADIAZINE q6hr
*Child:* PO 1 mg/kg/day in 2 divided doses or 2 mg/kg/day × 3 days, then 1 mg/kg/day or divided twice daily × 4 wk, max 25 mg/day

*Toxoplasmosis in AIDS patients*
*Adult:* PO 100-200 mg/day × 1-2 days, then 50-100 mg/day × 3-6 wk, then 25-50 mg/day for life (given with clindamycin or sulfADIAZINE)

**Available forms:** Tabs 25 mg; combo tabs 500 mg sulfadoxine/25 mg pyrimethamine

## Adverse effects
*CNS:* Stimulation, irritability, **seizures,** tremors, ataxia, fatigue
*CV:* Dysrhythmias
*GI: Nausea, vomiting, cramps, anorexia, diarrhea, atrophic glossitis, gastritis*
*HEMA:* **Thrombocytopenia, leukopenia, pancytopenia, megaloblastic anemia,** decreased folic acid, **agranulocytosis**
*INTEG:* Skin eruptions, photosensitivity
*RESP:* **Respiratory failure**

**Contraindications:** Hypersensitivity, chloroquine-resistant malaria, megaloblastic anemia caused by folate deficiency

**Precautions:** Pregnancy **C**, breastfeeding, blood dyscrasias, seizure disorder, glucose-6-phosphate dehydrogenase disease, renal/hepatic disease

P

### Pharmacokinetics
| | |
|---|---|
| **Absorption** | Well absorbed |
| **Distribution** | Widely; crosses placenta |
| **Metabolism** | Liver, extensively |
| **Excretion** | Kidneys, unchanged (30%); breast milk |
| **Half-life** | 4 days |

### Pharmacodynamics
| | |
|---|---|
| **Onset** | Unknown |
| **Peak** | 2 hr |
| **Duration** | Unknown |

Adverse effects: *italic* = common, **bold** = life-threatening

## Interactions
### Individual drugs
Folic acid: increased synergistic action
Radiation: increased bone marrow suppression
### Drug classifications
Bone marrow depressants: increased bone marrow suppression

## NURSING CONSIDERATIONS
### Assessment
• C&S studies should be done before treatment begins and periodically during treatment
• Monitor serum uric acid, which may be elevated and cause gout symptoms
• Monitor liver function tests weekly: ALT, AST, bilirubin; hepatic status: decreased appetite, jaundice, dark urine, fatigue
• Monitor renal status before therapy and monthly thereafter: BUN, creatinine, output, specific gravity, urinalysis
• Monitor mental status often: affect, mood, behavioral changes; psychosis may occur

### Nursing diagnoses
• Diarrhea (adverse reactions)
• Infection, risk for (uses)
• Injury, risk for (adverse reactions)
• Knowledge, deficient (teaching)
• Noncompliance (teaching)

### Implementation
• Give with meals to decrease GI symptoms
• Give antiemetic if vomiting occurs

### Patient/family education
• Instruct patient that compliance with dosage schedule, duration is necessary; that scheduled appointments must be kept or relapse may occur
• Advise diabetic patient to use blood glucose monitor to obtain correct result
• Advise patient to report weakness, fatigue, loss of appetite, nausea, vomiting, yellowing of skin or eyes, sore throat, glossitis

### Evaluation
**Positive therapeutic outcome**
• Decreased symptoms of toxoplasmosis
• Decreased symptoms of *Pneumocystis jiroveci* pneumonia

## quetiapine (Rx)
(kwe-tie′a-peen)
Seroquel, Seroquel XR
*Func. class.:* Antipsychotic
*Chem. class.:* Dibenzodiazepine

### Pregnancy category C

**Action:** Functions as an antagonist at multiple neurotransmitter receptors in the brain including $5\text{-}HT_{1A}$, $5\text{-}HT_2$, dopamine $D_1$, $D_2$, $H_1$, adrenergic $\alpha_1$, $\alpha_2$ receptors

**Therapeutic outcome:** Decreased hallucination and disorganized thought

**Uses:** Bipolar disorder, depression, mania, schizophrenia

### Dosage and routes
#### Bipolar disorder
*Adult:* PO At bedtime 50 mg on day 1, 100 mg on day 2, 200 mg on day 3, 300 mg on day 4

#### Psychotic disorders
*Adult:* PO 25 mg bid, titrate upward; (XR) 300 mg/day in PM

**Available forms:** Tabs 25, 50, 100, 200, 300 mg; ext rel tab 200, 300, 400 mg

### Adverse effects
*CNS:* EPS, pseudoparkinsonism, akathisia, dystonia, tardive dyskinesia, drowsiness, insomnia, agitation, anxiety, *headache,* seizures, **neuroleptic malignant syndrome,** dizziness
*CV:* Orthostatic hypotension, **tachycardia,** QT prolongation
*GI:* Nausea, anorexia, constipation, abdominal pain, dry mouth
*INTEG:* Rash
*MISC:* Asthenia, back pain, fever, ear pain
*RESP:* Rhinitis

**Contraindications:** Hypersensitivity, torsade de pointes

**Precautions:** Pregnancy **C**, breastfeeding, children, geriatric, suicide, long-term use, seizures, dementia, hepatic disease, breast cancer, QT prolongation, CV disease, Parkinson's

### Pharmacokinetics

| | |
|---|---|
| **Absorption** | Rapidly |
| **Distribution** | Widely |
| **Metabolism** | Liver, extensively; inhibits P450 CYP3A4 enzyme system; 83% protein binding |
| **Excretion** | Urine, feces |
| **Half-life** | ≥6 hr |

| Pharmacodynamics | |
| --- | --- |
| **Onset** | Unknown |
| **Peak** | 1.5 hr |
| **Duration** | Up to 12 hr |

## Interactions
### Individual drugs
Alcohol: increased CNS depression
Carbamazepine, phenytoin, rifampin, thioridazine: increased quetiapine clearance
Cimetidine: decreased quetiapine clearance
Erythromycin: increased effects of erythromycin
Fluconazole, itraconazole, ketoconazole: increased action of quetiapine
Levodopa: decreased effect of levodopa
Lorazepam: decreased effect of lorazepam

### Drug classifications
Analgesics (opioid), antihistamines, sedative/hypnotics: increased CNS depression
Barbiturates, glucocorticoids: increased clearance of quetiapine
DOPamine agonists: decreased effects of DOPamine agonists

### Drug/herb
Cola tree, hops, nettle, nutmeg: increased action
Betel palm, kava: increased EPS

## NURSING CONSIDERATIONS
### Assessment
• Assess CV status: QT prolongation, tachycardia
• Assess mental status: orientation, mood, AIMS assessment, presence and type of hallucinations before initial administration and monthly; this product should significantly reduce psychotic behavior
• Check that patient swallows all PO medication; check for hoarding or giving of medication to other patients
• Obtain baselines in blood glucose, liver function tests, neurologic status, ophthalmologic exam, cholesterol profile, weight
• Assess affect, orientation, LOC, reflexes, gait, coordination, sleep pattern disturbances
• Monitor B/P with patient in sitting, standing, and lying positions; take pulse and respirations q4hr during initial treatment; establish baseline before starting treatment; report drops of 30 mm Hg; obtain baseline ECG and monitor Q- and T-wave changes
• Check for dizziness, faintness, palpitations, tachycardia on rising; severe orthostatic hypotension is common
◆ Identify for neuroleptic malignant syndrome: hyperpyrexia, muscle rigidity, increased CPK, altered mental status, seizures, tachycardia, diaphoresis, hyper/hypotension, fatigue; product should be discontinued and prescriber notified immediately
• Assess for EPS including akathisia (inability to sit still, no pattern to movements), tardive dyskinesia (bizarre movements of the jaw, mouth, tongue, extremities), pseudoparkinsonism (rigidity, tremors, pill rolling, shuffling gait); an antiparkinson product should be prescribed

### Nursing diagnoses
• Coping, ineffective (uses)
• Knowledge, deficient (teaching)
• Noncompliance (teaching)
• Thought processes, disturbed (uses)

### Implementation
• PO with full glass of water, milk; or give with food to decrease GI upset
• Store in airtight, light-resistant container

### Patient/family education
• Teach patient to use good oral hygiene; frequent rinsing of mouth, sugarless gum for dry mouth
• Caution patient to avoid hazardous activities until product response is determined; dizziness, blurred vision may occur
• Inform patient that orthostatic hypotension occurs often; patient should rise from sitting or lying position gradually; avoid hot tubs, hot showers, and tub baths because hypotension may occur
• Inform patient that heat stroke may occur in hot weather, and to take extra precautions to stay cool
• Advise patient to avoid abrupt withdrawal of this product or EPS may result; product should be withdrawn slowly
• Teach patient to avoid OTC preparations (cough, hayfever, cold) unless approved by prescriber; serious product interactions may occur; avoid use with alcohol, CNS depressants because increased drowsiness may occur

### Evaluation
**Positive therapeutic outcome**
• Decrease in emotional excitement, hallucinations, delusions, paranoia
• Reorganization of patterns of thought, speech

**Treatment of overdose:** Lavage, provide airway

Q

## quinapril (Rx)
(kwin'a-pril)

Accupril

*Func. class.:* Antihypertensive
*Chem. class.:* Angiotensin-converting enzyme (ACE) inhibitor

**Pregnancy category D**

**Action:** Selectively suppresses renin-angiotensin-aldosterone system; inhibits ACE, prevents conversion of angiotensin I to angiotensin II; results in dilation of arterial, venous vessels

**Therapeutic outcome:** Decreased B/P in hypertension

**Uses:** Hypertension, alone or in combination with thiazide diuretics, systolic CHF

### Dosage and routes
**Hypertension (monotherapy)**
*Adult:* PO 10-20 mg/day initially, then 20-80 mg/day divided bid or daily
*Geriatric:* PO 10 mg/day, titrate to desired response

**Congestive heart failure**
*Adult:* PO 5 mg bid, may increase qwk unitl 20-40 mg/day in 2 divided doses

**Renal dose**
*Adult:* PO CCr 30-60 ml/min 5 mg/day initially; CCr <30 ml/min 2.5 mg/day initially

**Available forms:** Tabs 5, 10, 20, 40 mg

### Adverse effects
*CNS:* Headache, dizziness, fatigue, somnolence, depression, malaise, nervousness, vertigo
*CV:* Hypotension, postural hypotension, syncope, palpitations, angina pectoris, **MI, tachycardia,** vasodilation, chest pain
*GI:* Nausea, diarrhea, constipation, vomiting, gastritis, GI hemorrhage, dry mouth
*GU:* Increased BUN, creatinine, decreased libido, impotence
*HEMA:* **Thrombocytopenia, agranulocytosis**
*INTEG:* **Angioedema,** rash, sweating, photosensitivity, pruritus
*META:* Hyperkalemia
*MISC:* Back pain, amblyopia
*MS:* Myalgia
*RESP:* Cough, pharyngitis, dyspnea

**Contraindications:** Pregnancy **D,** children, hypersensitivity to ACE inhibitors, angioedema

**Precautions:** Breastfeeding, geriatric, impaired renal/liver function, dialysis patients, hypovolemia, blood dyscrasias, COPD, asthma, bilateral renal stenosis, cough

### Pharmacokinetics
| | |
|---|---|
| **Absorption** | Well absorbed |
| **Distribution** | Unknown, crosses placenta |
| **Metabolism** | Unknown |
| **Excretion** | Urine (60%), feces (37%) |
| **Half-life** | 2 hr |

### Pharmacodynamics
| | |
|---|---|
| **Onset** | ½-1 hr |
| **Peak** | 2-6 hr |
| **Duration** | 12-24 hr |

### Interactions
*Individual drugs*
Alcohol: increased hypotension (large amounts)
Digoxin, lithium: increased toxicity
Hydralazine, prazosin: use caution
Indomethacin: decreased antihypertensive effect of quinapril
Tetracycline: decreased absorption of tetracycline
*Drug classifications*
Adrenergic blockers, antihypertensives, diuretics, ganglionic blockers, nitrates, phenothiazines: increased hypotension
Diuretics (potassium sparing), potassium supplements, sympathomimetics, combine vasodilators: use caution
*Drug/herb*
Aconite: increased toxicity, death
Astragalus, cola tree: increased or decreased antihypertensive effect
Barberry, betony, black catechu, black cohosh, bloodroot, broom, burdock, cat's claw, dandelion, goldenseal, Irish moss, Jamaican dogwood, kelp, khella, mistletoe, parsley: increased antihypertensive effect
Coltsfoot, guarana, khat, licorice, yohimbe: decreased antihypertensive effect
*Drug/lab test*
False positive: urine acetone, ANA titer

### NURSING CONSIDERATIONS
**Assessment**
- Monitor blood studies: neutrophils, decreased platelets; WBC with differential baseline and periodically q3 mo; if neutrophils <1000/mm$^3$ discontinue treatment
- Monitor B/P, check for orthostatic hypotension, syncope; if changes occur, dosage change may be required

• Monitor renal function tests (protein, BUN, creatinine); and periodically liver function tests, uric acid, also glucose may be elevated; watch for increased levels that may indicate nephrotic syndrome and renal failure; monitor renal symptoms: polyuria, oliguria, frequency, dysuria

• Check potassium levels throughout treatment, although hyperkalemia rarely occurs

• Check for edema in feet, legs daily, weight daily in CHF

• Assess for allergic reactions: rash, fever, pruritus, urticaria; product should be discontinued if antihistamines fail to help

## Nursing diagnoses

• Cardiac output, decreased (uses)
• Injury, risk for (adverse reactions)
• Knowledge, deficient (teaching)
• Noncompliance (teaching)

## Implementation

• Tabs may be crushed if necessary
• Store in airtight container at 86° F (30° C) or less
• Severe hypotension may occur after 1st dose of this medication; may be prevented by reducing or discontinuing diuretic therapy 3 days before beginning quinapril therapy

## Patient/family education

• Advise patient not to discontinue product abruptly; advise patient to tell all persons associated with care

• Teach patient not to use OTC products (cough, cold, allergy) unless directed by physician; serious side effects can occur

• Inform patient that xanthines such as coffee, tea, chocolate, cola can prevent action of product

• Caution patient on the importance of complying with dosage schedule, even if feeling better; to continue with medical regimen to decrease B/P: exercise, cessation of smoking, decreasing stress, diet modifications

• Emphasize the need to rise slowly to sitting or standing position to minimize orthostatic hypotension; not to exercise in hot weather or increased hypotension can occur

• Teach patient to notify prescriber of mouth sores, sore throat, fever, swelling of hands or feet, irregular heartbeat, chest pain, coughing, shortness of breath

• Caution patient to report excessive perspiration, dehydration, vomiting, diarrhea; may lead to fall in B/P

• Caution patient that product may cause dizziness, fainting, light-headedness; may occur during 1st few days of therapy; to avoid activities that may be hazardous

• Teach patient how to take B/P, and normal readings for age-group

## Evaluation

### Positive therapeutic outcome
• Decreased B/P in hypertension

**Treatment of overdose:** 0.9% NaCl **IV** inf, hemodialysis

## quinidine (Rx)
(kwin'i-deen)
## quinidine gluconate (Rx)
Quinaglute Dura-Tabs, Quinalan, Quinate ✦
## quinidine polygalacturonate (Rx)
Cardioquin
## quinidine sulfate (Rx)
Apo-Quinidine ✦, Cin-Quin, Novoquinidine ✦, Quinidex Extentabs, Quinora
*Func. class.:* Antidysrhythmic (class IA)
*Chem. class.:* Quinine dextro isomer

### Pregnancy category  C

**Action:** Prolongs action potential duration and effective refractory period, thus decreasing myocardial excitability; anticholinergic properties

**Therapeutic outcome:** Treatment of dysrhythmias

**Uses:** Premature ventricular contractions (PVCs), atrial fibrillation, flutter; paroxysmal atrial tachycardia, ventricular tachycardia, malaria/**IV** quinidine gluconate

## Dosage and routes
### Quinidine sulfate
### Atrial fibrillation/flutter
*Adult:* PO 200 mg q2-3hr × 5-8 doses; may increase daily until sinus rhythm is restored; max 4 g/day given only after digitalization, maintenance 200-300 mg tid-qid or 300-600 mg q8-12hr (sus rel)

### Paroxysmal supraventricular tachycardia
*Adult:* PO 400-600 mg q2-3hr, then 200-300 mg q6-8hr or 300-600 mg q8-12hr (sus rel)

### Premature atrial/ventricular contraction
*Adult:* PO 200-300 mg q6-8hr or 300-600 mg (sus rel) q8-12hr, not to exceed 4 g/day
*Child:* PO 30 mg/kg/day or 900 mg/m$^2$/day in 5 divided doses

Q

Adverse effects: *italic* = common, **bold** = life-threatening

*Quinidine gluconate*
**Adult:** PO 324-660 mg q6-12hr (sus rel);
IM 600 mg, then 400 mg q2hr; **IV** give 16
mg/min

**Available forms:** Gluconate: sus rel tabs
324, 330 mg; inj gluconate 80 mg/ml; sulfate:
tabs 200, 300 mg; sus rel tabs 300 mg;
polygalacturonase: tabs 275 mg

### Adverse effects
**CNS:** *Headache, dizziness,* involuntary
movement, confusion, psychosis, restlessness,
irritability, syncope, excitement, depression,
ataxia
**CV: Hypotension,** *bradycardia, PVCs,* **heart
block, cardiovascular collapse, arrest,
torsade de pointes,** widening QRS complex,
**ventricular tachycardia**
**EENT:** Cinchonism: tinnitus, blurred vision,
hearing loss, mydriasis, disturbed color vision
**GI:** Nausea, vomiting, anorexia, *diarrhea,*
**hepatotoxicity,** abdominal pain
**HEMA: Thrombocytopenia, hemolytic
anemia, agranulocytosis,** hypoprothrombinemia
**INTEG:** Rash, urticaria, **angioedema,** swelling, photosensitivity, flushing with severe
pruritus
**RESP:** Dyspnea, **respiratory depression**

**Contraindications:** Hypersensitivity or
idiosyncratic response, digoxin toxicity, history
of long QT syndrome, product-induced torsades de pointes, blood dyscrasias, severe
heart block, myasthenia gravis

**Precautions:** Pregnancy **C,** breastfeeding,
children, geriatric, renal/hepatic disease,
potassium imbalance, CHF, respiratory depression

### Pharmacokinetics

| | |
|---|---|
| **Absorption** | Well absorbed (PO, IM), slowly absorbed (sus rel) |
| **Distribution** | Widely distributed, crosses placenta, protein binding (80%-90%) |
| **Metabolism** | Liver |
| **Excretion** | Kidney unchanged, 10%-50% breast milk |
| **Half-life** | 6-8 hr |

### Interactions
*Individual drugs*
Amiodarone, cimetidine, NIFEdipine: in-
creased quinidine level
Digoxin: increased digoxin level
NIFEdipine, sodium bicarbonate, verapamil:
increased quinidine effect
Phenytoin, rifampin, sucralfate: decreased
effects of quinidine
Propranolol: increased effect of propranolol
Reserpine: increased cardiac depression
Warfarin: increased levels of warfarin
*Drug classifications*
Antacids, carbonic anhydrase inhibitors,
diuretics (thiazide), hydroxide suspensions:
increased effects of quinidine
Anticholinergic blockers: increased vagolytic
effects
Anticoagulants (oral): increased levels of
anticoagulant
Antidepressants (tricyclics): increased effect of
antidepressant
Antidysrhythmics: increased cardiac depres-
sion
Barbiturates, cholinergics: decreased effects of
quinidine
Neuromuscular blockers: increased neuro-
muscular blocking
Phenothiazines: increased cardiac depression
*Drug/herb*
Aconite: increased toxicity, death
Aloe, broom, buckthorn (chronic use),
cascara sagrada (chronic use), Chinese
rhubarb, figwort, fumitory, goldenseal,
kudzu, licorice: increased effect
Aloe, buckthorn, cascara sagrada, senna:
increased hypokalemia, increased antidys-
rhythmic action
Coltsfoot: decreased effect
Horehound: increased serotonin effect
*Drug/food*
Grapefruit juice: decreased absorption, de-
creased metabolism
*Drug/lab test*
Increased: CPK
Interference: triamterene therapy interferes
with quinidine test levels

### Pharmacodynamics

| | PO (SULFATE) | PO-SUS REL | PO (GLUCONATE) | IM | IV |
|---|---|---|---|---|---|
| **Onset** | ½ hr | Unknown | Unknown | ½ hr | 5 min |
| **Peak** | 1-1½ hr | 4 hr | 4 hr | ½-1½ hr | Unknown |
| **Duration** | 6-8 hr | 8-12 hr | 6-8 hr | 6-8 hr | 6-8 hr |

## NURSING CONSIDERATIONS
### Assessment
• Monitor ECG continuously to determine product effectiveness, measure PR, QRS, QT intervals, check for PVCs, other dysrhythmias; monitor B/P continuously for hypo/hypertension; for rebound hypertension after 1-2 hr; check for dehydration or hypovolemia
• Monitor blood levels (therapeutic level 2-7 mcg/ml)
• Monitor I&O ratio, electrolytes (potassium, sodium, chloride); check weight daily; check for signs of CHF or pulmonary toxicity: dyspnea, fatigue, cough, fever, chest pain; if these occur, product should be discontinued
• Monitor liver function tests: AST, ALT, bilirubin, alkaline phosphatase
• Assess for CNS symptoms: confusion, psychosis, numbness, depression, involuntary movements; if these occur, product should be discontinued
• Monitor cardiac rate, respiration: rate, rhythm, character, chest pain; watch for ventricular tachycardia, supraventricular tachycardia, or fibrillation that indicates toxicity

### Nursing diagnoses
• Cardiac output, decreased (uses)
• Gas exchange, impaired (adverse reactions)
• Knowledge, deficient (teaching)

### Implementation
**PO route**
• Do not break, crush, or chew sus rel tab
• Give on an empty stomach with a full glass of water
• May be given with meals if GI irritation occurs, absorption will be decreased
• Sus rel forms not interchangeable
• Tab may be crushed and mixed with fluid or foods for patients with swallowing difficulties
**IV route**
• Give by intermittent inf after diluting 800 mg/50 ml of D₅W; gluconate: (16 mg/ml) give at 1 ml/min or less using an infusion pump for correct dose
• Do not use colored sol or sol with precipitate
• Diluted quinidine is stable for 24 hr at room temperature
*Y-site compatibilities:* Diazepam, milrinone
*Y-site incompatibilities:* Furosemide
*Additive compatibilities:* Bretylium, cimetidine, milrinone, ranitidine, verapamil
*Additive incompatibilities:* Amiodarone

### Patient/family education
• Instruct patient to report adverse effects immediately to prescriber
• Caution patient that sunglasses may be needed for photophobia; to use sunscreen, protective clothing, or stay out of sun to prevent burns
• Instruct patient to complete follow-up appointments with health care provider including pulmonary function tests, chest x-ray, ophth and otoscopic exams

### Evaluation
**Positive therapeutic outcome**
• Resolution of dysrhythmias

## quinine (OTC, Rx)
(kwye′nine)
*Func. class.:* Antimalarial
*Chem. class.:* Cinchona tree alkaloid
**Pregnancy category  X**

**Action:** Inhibits parasite replications, transcription of DNA to RNA by forming complexes with DNA of parasite

**Therapeutic outcome:** Reduction/death of *Plasmodium falciparum*; decreased leg cramps

**Uses:** *P. falciparum*, malaria

### Dosage and routes
*Malaria*
*Adult:* PO 650 mg q8hr × 10 days, given with pyrimethamine 25 mg q12hr × 3 days, with sulfADIAZINE 500 mg qid × 5 days
*Child:* PO 25 mg/kg/day divided q8hr for 3-7 days in conjunction with another agent

**Available forms:** Caps 200, 300, 325 mg; tabs 260, 325 mg

### Adverse effects
*CNS:* Headache, stimulation, fatigue, irritability, **seizures**, bad dreams, dizziness, fever, confusion, anxiety
*CV:* Angina, dysrhythmias, tachycardia, hypotension, **acute circulatory failure**
*EENT: Blurred vision, corneal changes, retinal changes, difficulty focusing,* tinnitus, vertigo, deafness, photophobia, diplopia, night blindness
*ENDO:* Hypoglycemia
*GI: Nausea, vomiting, anorexia,* diarrhea, epigastric pain
*GU:* Renal tubular damage, **anuria**
*HEMA:* **Thrombocytopenia, purpura, hypothrombinemia, hemolysis**

Q

Adverse effects: *italic* = common, **bold** = life-threatening

*INTEG:* Pruritus, pigmentary changes, skin eruptions, lichen planus–like eruptions, flushing, facial edema, sweating
*MISC:* **Hemolytic uremic syndrome**
*RESP:* Dyspnea

**Contraindications:** Pregnancy **X**, breast-feeding, hypersensitivity, G6PD deficiency, retinal field changes, myasthenia gravis

**Precautions:** Blood dyscrasias, severe GI/hepatic disease, neurologic disease, psoriasis, cardiac dysrhythmias, tinnitus, hypoglycemia, nocturnal leg cramps

### Pharmacokinetics

| | |
|---|---|
| **Absorption** | Rapidly, 80% |
| **Distribution** | Crosses placenta, excreted breast milk, protein binding >90% in malaria |
| **Metabolism** | Liver, extensively 80% |
| **Excretion** | Urine, 20% unchanged |
| **Half-life** | 11 hr, increases in malaria |

### Pharmacodynamics

| | |
|---|---|
| **Onset** | Unknown |
| **Peak** | 3½-6 hr |
| **Duration** | 8 hr |

### Interactions
*Individual products*
Acetazolamide, NaHCO$_3$: increased toxicity
Digoxin: increased levels
Rifampin: increased treatment failure
Warfarin: increased bleeding risk
*Drug classifications*
Antacids: decreased absorption of quinine
Anticoagulants: increased levels of anticoagulants
Neuromuscular blockers: increased effect of neuromuscular blockers
*Drug/lab test*
Increased: 17-KS

### NURSING CONSIDERATIONS
**Assessment**
• Monitor B/P, pulse; watch for hypotension, tachycardia
• Assess liver studies qwk: ALT, AST, bilirubin
• Assess blood tests, CBC, since blood dyscrasias occur
• Assess for cinchonism: nausea, blurred vision, tinnitus, headache, difficulty focusing; quinidine levels >10 mcg/ml
• Assess for symptoms of malaria and improvement
• Assess frequency/duration of nocturnal leg cramps

**Nursing diagnoses**
• Infection, risk for (uses)
• Knowledge, deficient (teaching)
• Noncompliance (teaching)

**Implementation**
• Give before or after meals at same time each day to maintain level
• Store in airtight, light-resistant container

**Patient/family education**
• Advise patient to avoid OTC preparations: cold preparations, tonic water
• Advise patient to take only as prescribed
• Teach patient visual changes may occur, to avoid driving or hazardous activities until response is known
• Teach patient to stop product and call prescriber if difficulty breathing, ringing in the ears, or allergic reaction occurs
• Teach patient to use insect repellant, protective clothing if in area with mosquitoes

**Evaluation**
**Positive therapeutic outcome**
• Decreased symptoms of malaria

---

### rabeprazole (Rx)
(rab-ee-pray′zole)
Aciphex
*Func. class.:* Proton pump inhibitor
*Chem. class.:* Benzimidazole
**Pregnancy category** C

**Action:** Suppresses gastric secretion by inhibiting hydrogen/potassium ATPase enzyme system in the gastric parietal cell; characterized as a gastric acid pump inhibitor, since it blocks the final step of acid production

**Therapeutic outcome:** Absence of duodenal ulcers; decreased gastroesophageal reflux

**Uses:** Gastroesophageal reflux disease (GERD), severe erosive esophagitis, poorly responsive systemic GERD, pathologic hypersecretory conditions (Zollinger-Ellison syndrome, systemic mastocytosis, multiple endocrine adenomas); possibly effective for treatment of duodenal ulcers with or without antiinfectives for *Helicobacter pylori;* daytime, nighttime heartburn

**Dosage and routes**
*Healing of duodenal ulcers*
*Adult:* PO 20 mg/day × ≤4 wk, to be taken after breakfast

*Erosive esophagitis/GERD*
*Adult:* PO 20 mg/day × 4-8 wk

*Pathologic hypersecretory conditions*
*Adult:* PO 60 mg/day; may increase to 120 mg in 2 divided doses

**Available forms:** Delayed rel tabs, 20 mg

**Adverse effects**
*CNS: Headache, dizziness, asthenia*
*CV:* Chest pain, angina, tachycardia, bradycardia, palpitations, peripheral edema
*EENT:* Tinnitus, taste perversion
*GI: Diarrhea, abdominal pain, vomiting, nausea, constipation, flatulence, acid regurgitation,* abdominal swelling, anorexia, irritable colon, esophageal candidiasis, dry mouth
*GU:* UTI, frequency, increased creatinine, **proteinuria, hematuria,** testicular pain, glycosuria
*HEMA:* **Pancytopenia, thrombocytopenia, neutropenia, leukocytosis,** anemia
*INTEG:* Rash, dry skin, urticaria, pruritus, alopecia
*META:* Hypoglycemia, increased hepatic enzymes, weight gain
*MISC: Back pain,* fever, fatigue, malaise
*RESP: Upper respiratory tract infections, cough,* epistaxis

**Contraindications:** Hypersensitivity

**Precautions:** Pregnancy **C,** breastfeeding, children

| Pharmacokinetics | |
|---|---|
| **Absorption** | Unknown |
| **Distribution** | Unknown |
| **Metabolism** | Liver, extensively |
| **Excretion** | Kidneys, feces |
| **Half-life** | Unknown |

| Pharmacodynamics |
|---|
| Unknown |

**Interactions**
*Individual drugs*
Calcium carbonate, sucralfate, vitamin $B_{12}$: decreased rabeprazole levels
Clarithromycin, phenytoin: increased levels of rabeprazole
*Drug classifications*
Benzodiazepines: increased levels of rabeprazole

**NURSING CONSIDERATIONS**
**Assessment**
• Assess GI system: bowel sounds q8hr, abdomen for pain and swelling, anorexia
• Monitor hepatic enzymes: AST, ALT, increased alkaline phosphatase during treatment

**Nursing diagnoses**
• Knowledge, deficient (teaching)
• Pain, chronic (uses)

**Implementation**
• Do not break, crush, or chew delayed rel tab
• Give after breakfast daily

**Patient/family education**
• Advise patient to report severe diarrhea; product may have to be discontinued
• Caution patient to avoid driving and other hazardous activities until response to product is known
• Caution patient to avoid alcohol, salicylates, NSAIDs; may cause GI irritation
• Advise patient to wear sunscreen, protective clothing to prevent burns

**Evaluation**
**Positive therapeutic outcome**
• Absence of epigastric pain, swelling, fullness

**raloxifene (Rx)**
(ral-ox'ih-feen)
Evista
*Func. class.:* Hormone modifier, selective estrogen receptor modulator (SERM)
*Chem. class.:* Benzothiophene
**Pregnancy category X**

**Action:** Reduces resorption of bone and decreases bone turnover; mediated through estrogen receptor binding

**Therapeutic outcome:** Absence, or decrease of osteoporosis in postmenopausal women

**Uses:** Prevention, treatment of osteoporosis in postmenopausal women

**Dosage and routes**
*Hormone replacement*
*Adult:* PO 60 mg/day, max 60 mg/day

**Available forms:** Tabs 60 mg

**Adverse effects**
*CNS:* Insomnia, migraines, depression, fever, CVA
*CV:* Hot flashes, chest pain
*GI:* **Nausea,** vomiting, diarrhea, anorexia, cramps, dyspepsia

R

Adverse effects: *italic* = common, **bold** = life-threatening

***GU:*** Vaginitis, UTI, leukorrhea, *hot flashes,* cystitis
***INTEG:*** Rash, sweating
***META:*** Weight gain, peripheral edema
***MS:*** Arthralgia, myalgia, *leg cramps,* arthritis
***RESP:*** Sinusitis, pharyngitis, increased cough, pneumonia, laryngitis, rhinitis, bronchitis, **pulmonary embolism**

**Contraindications:** Pregnancy **X,** breast-feeding, hypersensitivity, women with active or history of venous thromboembolic events

**Precautions:** Venous thromboembolic events, hepatic/CV disease, cervical/uterine cancer, elevated triglycerides, pulmonary embolism

### Pharmacokinetics

| | |
|---|---|
| **Absorption** | Unknown |
| **Distribution** | Highly protein bound |
| **Metabolism** | Unknown |
| **Excretion** | Feces, breast milk |
| **Half-life** | 28-32 hr (elimination) |

### Pharmacodynamics

Unknown

### Interactions
*Individual drugs*
Ampicillin, cholestyramine: decreased action of raloxifene
*Drug classifications*
Anticoagulants: decreased action of anticoagulants
Highly protein-bound products: administer cautiously
*Drug/lab test*
Increased: apolipoprotein, corticosteroid-binding globulin, thyroxine-binding globulin (TBG)
Decreased: lipoprotein, fibrinogen, LDL cholesterol, total cholesterol, calcium, total protein, albumin, platelets

### NURSING CONSIDERATIONS
**Assessment**
• Obtain bone density test baseline and periodically throughout treatment; bone-specific alkaline phosphatase; osteocalcin, collagen breakdown
• Monitor weight daily, notify prescriber of weekly weight gain >5 lb
• Monitor B/P q4hr, watch for increase caused by $H_2O$ and sodium retention
• Monitor liver function tests: AST, ALT, bilirubin, alkaline phosphatase
• Monitor I&O ratio; decreasing urinary output, increasing edema

**Nursing diagnoses**
• Knowledge, deficient (teaching)
• Mobility, impaired physical (uses)

**Implementation**
• Administer without regard to meals
• Add calcium supplement, vit D if lacking

**Patient/family education**
• Teach patient to weigh weekly, report gain >5 lb
• Teach patients to discontinue product 72 hr before prolonged bedrest
• Advise patient to avoid maintaining one position for long periods
• Advise patient to take calcium supplements, vit D if intake is inadequate
• Advise patient to increase exercise using weights
• Advise patient to stop smoking and to decrease alcohol consumption
• Inform patient that this product does not help control hot flashes
• Teach patient to report fever, acute migraine, insomnia, emotional distress; UTI or vaginal burning/itching; swelling, warmth, or pain in calves

**Evaluation**
**Positive therapeutic outcome**
• Prevention, treatment of osteoporosis

## raltegravir (Rx)
(ral-teg'ra-vir)
Isentress
*Func. class.:* Antiretroviral
*Chem. class.:* HIV integrase strand transfer inhibitor (ISTIs)
### Pregnancy category C

**Action:** Inhibits catalytic activity of HIV integrase, which is an HIV-encoded enzyme needed for replication

**Therapeutic outcome:** Improvement in CD4, T-cell counts

**Uses:** HIV in combination with other antiretrovirals

**Dosage and routes**
*Adult and adolescent ≥16 yr:* PO 400 mg bid, max 800 mg/day with or without food

**Available forms:** Tabs 400 mg

**Adverse effects**
***CNS:*** Fatigue, fever, dizziness, *headache*
***CV:*** **MI**
***GI:*** Nausea, vomiting, diarrhea, abdominal pain, asthenia, gastritis, **hepatitis**

 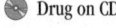

*GU:* **Oliguria, proteinuria, hematuria, glomerulonephritis, acute renal failure, renal tubular necrosis**
*HEMA:* **Anemia, neutropenia**
*INTEG:* Rash, urticaria, pruritus, pain or phlebitis at IV site, unusual sweating, alopecia
*META:* Hyperamylasia, hyperglycemia
*MS:* Myopathy, **rhabdomyolysis**

**Contraindications:** Hypersensitivity, breastfeeding

**Precautions:** Pregnancy **C**, children, geriatric, hepatic disease, immune reconstitution syndrome, hepatitis, antimicrobial resistance, lactase deficiency

Pharmacokinetics

| | |
|---|---|
| **Absorption** | Max 3 hr if taken on empty stomach |
| **Distribution** | Unknown |
| **Metabolism** | Unknown |
| **Excretion** | 51% feces, 32% urine |
| **Half-life** | Terminal 9 hr |

Pharmacodynamics
Unknown

**Interactions**
*Individual drugs*
Rifampin: decreased raltegravir levels
*Drug classifications*
Fibric acid derivatives, HMG-CoA reductase inhibitors: increased rhabdomyolysis, myopathy, elevated CPK

**NURSING CONSIDERATIONS**
**Assessment**
• Assess for signs of infection, anemia
• Monitor blood tests: CD4, T-cell count, plasma HIV RNA
• Assess skin eruptions: rash, urticaria, itching
• Assess for allergies before treatment, reaction of each medication; place allergies on chart in bright red letters

**Nursing diagnoses**
• Infection, risk for (uses)
• Knowledge, deficient (teaching)
• Noncompliance (teaching)

**Implementation**
• Do not break, crush, or chew tabs
• May give without regard to meals, with 8 oz of water
• Store at room temperature

**Patient/family education**
• Teach patient to take as prescribed; if dose is missed, take as soon as remembered up to 1 hr before next dose; do not double dose
• Teach patient that sexual partners need to be told that patient has HIV
• Advise patient that product does not cure infection, just controls symptoms and does not prevent infecting others
◆ Teach patient to report sore throat, fever, fatigue (may indicate superinfection)
• Advise patient that product must be taken in equal intervals around the clock to maintain blood levels for duration of therapy

**Evaluation**
**Positive therapeutic outcome**
• Improvement in CD4, T-cell counts

## ramelteon (Rx)
(rah-mel′tee-on)
Rozerem
*Func. class.:* Sedative/hypnotic, antianxiety
*Chem. class.:* Melatonin receptor agonist

**Pregnancy category C**

**Action:** Binds selectively to melatonin receptors ($MT_1$, $MT_2$); thought to be involved in circadian rhythm and the normal sleep/wake cycle

**Therapeutic outcome:** Ability to fall asleep easily and decrease early-morning awakenings

**Uses:** Insomnia

**Dosage and routes**
*Adult:* PO 8 mg at bedtime

*Hepatic dose*
Do not use in severe hepatic disease; use with caution in mild to moderate hepatic disease

**Available forms:** Tabs 8 mg

**Adverse effects**
*CNS:* Dizziness, somnolence, fatigue, headache, insomnia, depression
*GI:* Nausea, diarrhea, dysgeusia, vomiting
*MISC:* Myalgia, arthralgia, decreased blood cortisol, influenza, upper respiratory tract infection

**Contraindications:** Breastfeeding, infants, children, hypersensitivity, alcohol intoxication, hepatic encephalopathy

**Precautions:** Pregnancy **C**, hepatic disease, alcoholism, COPD, seizure disorder, sleep apnea, suicidal ideation, angioedema, depression, sleep-related behavior (sleepwalking)

R

## Pharmacokinetics

| | |
|---|---|
| **Absorption** | Rapidly |
| **Distribution** | Protein binding 82% |
| **Metabolism** | Rapid first pass metabolism, liver |
| **Excretion** | 84% urine, 4% feces |
| **Half-life** | 2-5 hr |

## Pharmacodynamics

| | |
|---|---|
| **Onset** | Unknown |
| **Peak** | 0.75 hr |
| **Duration** | Unknown |

## Interactions
### Individual drugs
Alcohol, ciprofloxacin, fluconazole, fluvox-amine, ketoconazole: increased ramelteon effect

Rifampin: decreased effect of ramelteon
### Drug classifications
Antiretroviral protease inhibitors: possible toxicity

Anxiolytics, azole antifungals, barbiturates, CYP1A2 inhibitors, hypnotics, sedatives: increased ramelteon effect
### Drug/herb
Do not use with melatonin

Catnip, chamomile, clary, cowslip, hops, kava, lavender, mistletoe, nettle, pokeweed, poppy, Queen Anne's lace, senega, skullcap, valerian: increased CNS depression
### Drug/food
High-fat/heavy meal: prolonged absorption, sleep onset reduced

## NURSING CONSIDERATIONS
### Assessment
• Assess mental status: mood, sensorium, affect, memory (long, short)
• Assess type of sleep problem: falling asleep, staying asleep

### Nursing diagnoses
• Injury, risk for (adverse reactions)
• Knowledge, deficient (teaching)
• Sleep deprivation (uses)

### Implementation
• Give after removal of cigarettes to prevent fires
• Give after trying conservative measures for insomnia
• Give within 30 min of bedtime for sleeplessness
• Give on empty stomach for fast onset
• Provide assistance with ambulation after receiving dose
• Provide safety measure: nightlight, call bell within easy reach

• Check to see if PO medication has been swallowed
• Store in tight container in cool environment

### Patient/family education
• Advise patient to avoid driving or other activities requiring alertness until product is stabilized
• Advise patient to avoid alcohol ingestion or CNS depressants
• Teach patient alternative measures to improve sleep: reading, exercise several hr before bedtime, warm bath, warm milk, TV, self-hypnosis, deep breathing
• Advise patient to take immediately before going to bed
• Advise patient not to ingest a high-fat/heavy meal before taking
• Teach patient to report cessation of menses, galactorrhea (women), decreased libido, infertility; worsening of insomnia, or behavioral changes

### Evaluation
**Positive therapeutic outcome**
• Ability to sleep at night, decreased amount of early-morning awakening

## ramipril (Rx)
(ra-mi′pril)
Altace
*Func. class.:* Antihypertensive
*Chem. class.:* Angiotensin-converting enzyme (ACE) inhibitor

### Pregnancy category D

**Do not confuse:**
ramipril/enalapril, Altace/alteplase/Artane

**Action:** Selectively suppresses renin-angiotensin-aldosterone system; inhibits ACE; prevents conversion of angiotensin I to angiotensin II; results in dilation of arterial, venous vessels

**Therapeutic outcome:** Decreased B/P in hypertension

**Uses:** Hypertension, alone or in combination with thiazide diuretics; CHF (after MI), reduction in risk of MI, stroke, death from CV disorders

### Dosage and routes
#### Hypertension
*Adult:* PO 2.5 mg/day initially, then 2.5-20 mg/day divided bid or daily

#### Renal impairment
*Adult:* 1.25 mg/day with CCr <40 ml/min/ 1.73 m², increase as needed to max 5 mg/day

**CHF/Post MI**
*Adult:* PO 1.25-2.5 mg bid, may increase to 5 mg bid

**Reduction in risk of MI, stroke, death**
*Adult:* PO 2.5 mg/day × 7 days, then 5 mg/day × 21 days, then may increase to 10 mg/day

**Renal dose**
*Adult:* PO CCr <40 ml/min 1.73 m² 50% of dose

**Available forms:** Caps 1.25, 2.5, 5, 10 mg

## Adverse effects

*CNS: Headache, dizziness,* anxiety, insomnia, paresthesia, fatigue, depression, malaise, vertigo, **seizures**
*CV: Hypotension,* chest pain, palpitations, angina, syncope, **dysrhythmia**
*EENT:* Hearing loss
*GI:* Nausea, constipation, vomiting, dyspepsia, dysphagia, anorexia, diarrhea, abdominal pain
*GU:* **Proteinuria,** increased BUN, creatinine, impotence
*HEMA:* Decreased Hct, Hgb, **eosinophilia, leukopenia**
*INTEG:* Rash, sweating, photosensitivity, pruritus
*META:* Hyperkalemia
*MISC:* **Angioedema**
*MS:* Arthralgia, arthritis, myalgia
*RESP:* Cough, dyspnea

**Contraindications:** Pregnancy **D,** breast-feeding, children, hypersensitivity to ACE inhibitors, history of angioedema

**Precautions:** Impaired renal/liver function, dialysis patients, hypovolemia, blood dyscrasias, COPD, CHF, asthma, geriatric, renal artery stenosis, cough

### Pharmacokinetics

| | |
|---|---|
| **Absorption** | Well absorbed |
| **Distribution** | Not known, crosses placenta |
| **Metabolism** | Liver, extensively; protein binding 73% |
| **Excretion** | Urine |
| **Half-life** | Ramipril (5 hr), ramiprilat (24 hr) |

### Pharmacodynamics

| | |
|---|---|
| **Onset** | ½-1 hr |
| **Peak** | 6-8 hr |
| **Duration** | 24-72 hr |

## Interactions

### Individual drugs
Alcohol: increased hypotension (large amounts)
Digoxin, lithium: increased serum levels
Hydralazine, prazocin: increased toxicity
Indomethacin: decreased antihypertensive effect

### Drug classifications
Adrenergic blockers, antihypertensives, diuretics, ganglionic blockers, nitrates: increased hypotension
Antacids: decreased absorption
Diuretics (potassium sparing), potassium supplements, sympathomimetics, vasodilators: increased toxicity
NSAIDs, salicylates: decreased antihypertensive effect

### Drug/herb
Aconite: increased toxicity, death
Astragalus, cola tree: increased or decreased antihypertensive effect
Barberry, betony, black catechu, black cohosh, bloodroot, broom, burdock, cat's claw, dandelion, goldenseal, hawthorn, Irish moss, Jamaican dogwood, kelp, khella, mistletoe, parsley: increased antihypertensive effect
Coltsfoot, guarana, khat, licorice, yohimbe: decreased antihypertensive effect

### Drug/lab test
False positive: urine acetone, ANA titer

## NURSING CONSIDERATIONS
### Assessment
• Monitor blood tests: neutrophils, decreased platelets; WBC with differential baseline and periodically q3 mo, if neutrophils <1000/mm³, discontinue treatment
• Monitor B/P, check for orthostatic hypotension, syncope; if changes occur, dosage may need to be changed
• Monitor renal function tests: protein, BUN, creatinine; watch for increased levels that may indicate nephrotic syndrome and renal failure; monitor renal symptoms: polyuria, oliguria, frequency, dysuria
• Establish baselines in renal, liver function tests before therapy begins and monitor periodically; liver function tests, uric acid, and glucose may be increased
• Check potassium levels throughout treatment, although hyperkalemia rarely occurs
• Check for edema in feet, legs daily, weight daily in CHF
• Assess for allergic reactions: rash, fever, pruritus, urticaria; product should be discontinued if antihistamines fail to help

R

Adverse effects: *italic* = common, **bold** = life-threatening

## Nursing diagnoses
- Cardiac output, decreased (uses)
- Injury, risk for (side effects)
- Knowledge, deficient (teaching)
- Noncompliance (teaching)

## Implementation
- Caps can be opened and added to food
- Store in airtight container at 86° F (30° C) or less
- Severe hypotension may occur after 1st dose of this medication; decreased hypotension may be prevented by reducing or discontinuing diuretic therapy 3 days before beginning benazepril therapy
- Give **IV** inf of 0.9% NaCl (as ordered) to expand fluid volume if severe hypotension occurs

## Patient/family education
- Caution patient not to discontinue product abruptly; advise patient to tell all persons associated with care
- Teach patient not to use OTC products (cough, cold, allergy) unless directed by physician; serious side effects can occur; xanthines such as coffee, tea, chocolate, cola can prevent action of product
- Instruct patient on the importance of complying with dosage schedule, even if feeling better; to continue with medical regimen to decrease B/P: exercise, cessation of smoking, decreasing stress, diet modifications
- Emphasize the need to rise slowly to sitting or standing position to minimize orthostatic hypotension; not to exercise in hot weather because increased hypotension can occur
- Teach patient to notify prescriber of mouth sores, sore throat, fever, swelling of hands or feet, irregular heartbeat, chest pain, coughing, shortness of breath
- Caution patient to report excessive perspiration, dehydration, vomiting, diarrhea; may lead to fall in B/P
- Caution patient that product may cause dizziness, fainting, light-headedness; may occur during 1st few days of therapy; to avoid activities that may be hazardous
- Teach patient how to take B/P, and normal readings for age-group

## Evaluation
**Positive therapeutic outcome**
- Decreased B/P in hypertension

**Treatment of overdose:** 0.9% NaCl **IV** inf, hemodialysis

## ranibizumab (Rx)
(ran-ih-biz'oo-mab)
Lucentis
*Func. class.:* Ophthalmic
*Chem. class.:* Selective vascular endothelial growth factor antagonist

### Pregnancy category C

**Action:** Binds to receptor-binding site of active forms of vascular endothelial growth factor A (VEGF-A) that causes angiogenesis and cell proliferation

**Therapeutic outcome:** Prevention of increasing neovascular macular degeneration

**Uses:** Macular degeneration (neovascular) (wet)

### Dosage and routes
*Adult:* INTRAVITREAL 0.5 mg (0.05 ml) qmo

**Available forms:** Sol for inj 0.5 mg/0.05 ml

### Adverse effects
*CNS:* Dizziness, headache
*EENT:* Blepharitis, cataract, conjunctival hemorrhage/hyperemia, detachment of the retinal pigment epithelium, dry/irritation/pain in the eye, visual impairment, vitreous floaters, ocular infection
*GI:* Constipation, nausea
*MISC:* Hypertension, UTI, thromboembolism
*RESP:* Bronchitis, cough, sinusitis, URI

**Contraindications:** Hypersensitivity, ocular infections

**Precautions:** Pregnancy **C**, breastfeeding, children, retinal detachment, increased intraocular pressure

### Pharmacokinetics
| | |
|---|---|
| Absorption | Minimal |
| Distribution | None |
| Metabolism | None |
| Excretion | None |
| Half-life | Elimination 9 days |

### Pharmacodynamics
Unknown

### Interactions
*Individual drugs*
Verteporfin photodynamic therapy (PDT): increased severe inflammation

## NURSING CONSIDERATIONS
### Assessment
• Assess for eye changes: redness, sensitivity to light, vision change, intraocular pressure change; report to ophthalmologist immediately

### Nursing diagnoses
• Knowledge, deficient (teaching)

### Implementation
• Given by ophthalmologist via intravitreal injection
• Store in refrigerator; do not freeze
• Protect from light

### Patient/family education
• Teach patient that if eye becomes red, sensitive to light, painful or if there is a change in vision, seek immediate care from ophthalmologist
• Teach patient reason for treatment, expected results

### Evaluation
**Positive therapeutic outcome**
• Prevention of increasing neovascular macular degeneration

---

## ranitidine (Rx)
(ra-nit'i-deen)
Apo-Ranitidine ✦, Equaline, Gen-Ranitidine ✦, Leader Ranitidine, Novo-Ranidine ✦, Nu-Ranit ✦, PMS-Ranitidine ✦, Wal-Zan, Zantac, Zantac-C ✦, Zantac EFFER-dose, Zantac GELdose
### ranitidine bismuth citrate
Tritec
*Func. class.:* H$_2$ histamine receptor antagonist

**Pregnancy category B**

**Do not confuse:**
ranitidine/amantadine, Zantac/Xanax/Zofran

**Action:** Inhibits histamine at H$_2$ receptor site in the gastric parietal cells, which inhibits gastric acid secretion

**Therapeutic outcome:** Healing of duodenal ulcers or gastric ulcers; prevention of duodenal ulcers; decreases symptoms of gastroesophageal reflux disease (GERD), Zollinger-Ellison syndrome, or heartburn

**Uses:** Short-term treatment of duodenal and gastric ulcers and maintenance; management of GERD, Zollinger-Ellison syndrome, active duodenal ulcers with *Helicobacter pylori* in combination with clarithromycin, hypersecretory conditions, stress ulcers, erosive esopha-gitis (maintenance), systemic mastocytosis, multiple endocrine adenoma syndrome, heartburn

**Unlabeled uses:** Prevention of aspiration pneumonitis, stress ulcers, upper GI bleeding

### Dosage and routes
*Ranitidine*
*Renal dose*
*Adult:* CCr <50 ml/min PO q24hr; IM/**IV** q18-24hr

*Erosive esophagitis*
*Adult:* PO 150 mg qid for up to 12 wk
*Child ≥1 mo:* PO 5-10 mg/kg/day in 2-3 divided doses

*Duodenal ulcer*
*Adult:* PO 150 mg bid, maintenance 150 mg at bedtime

*Zollinger-Ellison syndrome*
*Adult:* PO 150 mg bid, may increase if needed

*Gastric ulcer*
*Adult:* PO 150 mg bid × 6 wk, then 150 mg at bedtime

*GERD*
*Adult:* PO 150 mg bid

*Ranitidine bismuth citrate*
*Adult:* PO 400 mg bid × 4 wk with clarithro-mycin 500 mg tid × first 2 wk

**Available forms:** Ranitidine: tabs 75, 150, 300 mg; caps 150, 300 mg; syr 15 mg/ml; sol for inj 25 mg/ml; effervescent tabs 25 mg; ranitidine bismuth citrate: tabs 400 mg

### Adverse effects
*CNS:* Headache, sleeplessness, dizziness, confusion, agitation, depression; hallucination (geriatric)
*CV:* Tachycardia, bradycardia, premature ventricular contractions
*EENT:* Blurred vision, increased ocular pressure
*GI:* Constipation, abdominal pain, diarrhea, nausea, vomiting, **hepatotoxicity**
*GU:* Impotence, gynecomastia
*INTEG:* Urticaria, rash, fever
*SYST:* Anaphylaxis **(rare)**

**Contraindications:** Hypersensitivity

**Precautions:** Pregnancy **B,** breastfeeding, child <12 yr, renal/hepatic disease

R

---

Adverse effects: *italic* = common, **bold** = life-threatening

## Pharmacokinetics

| | |
|---|---|
| **Absorption** | Well absorbed (PO, IM), completely absorbed (**IV**) |
| **Distribution** | Widely distributed, crosses placenta |
| **Metabolism** | Liver (30%) |
| **Excretion** | Kidneys unchanged (70%) |
| **Half-life** | 2-3 hr, increased renal disease |

## Pharmacodynamics

| | PO | IM/IV |
|---|---|---|
| **Onset** | Unknown | Unknown |
| **Peak** | 2-3 hr | 15 min |
| **Duration** | 8-12 hr | 8-12 hr |

## Interactions
### Individual drugs
Diazepam, metoclopramide: decreased absorption of ranitidine
Ketoconazole: decreased effect of ketoconazole
Procainamide: increased absorption, toxicity
### Drug classifications
Anticholinergics, antacids: decreased ranitidine absorption
Anticoagulants, sulfonylureas: increased absorption, toxicity
Benzodiazepines: increased effects of benzodiazepines
Calcium channel blockers: increased effect of calcium channel blockers
Cephalosporins: decreased effects of cephalosporins
Iron salts: decreased effects of iron salts
### Drug/lab test
Increased: alkaline phosphatase, AST, creatinine, LDH, ALT, bilirubin
False positive: urine protein

## NURSING CONSIDERATIONS
### Assessment
• Assess patient with ulcers or suspected ulcers: epigastric or abdominal pain, hematemesis, occult blood in stools, blood in gastric aspirate before and throughout treatment, monitor gastric pH (5 should be maintained)
• Monitor I&O ratio, BUN, creatinine, CBC with differential monthly

### Nursing diagnoses
• Knowledge, deficient (teaching)
• Pain, chronic (uses)

### Implementation
#### PO route
• May be given with or without meals
• Give antacids 1 hr before or 1 hr after this product

#### IV, direct route
• Give by direct **IV** after diluting 50 mg/20 ml of 0.9% $D_5W$, NaCl over 5 min or more
#### Intermittent IV inf route
• Give by intermittent inf over 15 min after diluting 50 mg/100 ml of $D_5W$, 0.9% NaCl
#### Continuous inf route
• Give by continuous inf for a concentration 150 mg/250 ml, give 6.25 mg/hr
• Give Zollinger-Ellison patients up to a conc of 2.5 mg/ml at 1 mg/kg/hr initially
*Syringe compatibilities:* Atropine, cyclizine, dexamethasone, dimenhyDRINATE, diphenhydrAMINE, DOBUTamine, DOPamine, fentanyl, glycopyrrolate, hydromorphone, meperidine, metoclopramide, morphine, nalbuphine, oxymorphone, pentazocine, perphenazine, prochlorperazine, promethazine, scopolamine
*Syringe incompatibilities:* Hydroxyzine, methotrimeprazine, midazolam, pentobarbital, phenobarbital
*Y-site compatibilities:* Acyclovir, aldesleukin, allopurinol, amifostine, aminophylline, atracurium, aztreonam, bretylium, DOBUTamine, DOPamine, DOXOrubicin, enalaprilat, epINEPHrine, esmolol, fentanyl, filgrastim, fluconazole, fludarabine, foscarnet, furosemide, gallium, granisetron, heparin, hydromorphone, idarubicin, labetalol, lorazepam, melphalan, meperidine, methotrexate, midazolam, milrinone, morphine, niCARdipine, nitroglycerin, norepinephrine, ondansetron, paclitaxel, pancuronium, piperacillin, piperacillin/tazobactam, procainamide, propofol, sargramostim, vecuronium, zidovudine
*Additive compatibilities:* Acetazolamide, amikacin, aminophylline, chloramphenicol, chlorothiazide, ciprofloxacin, colistimethate, dexamethasone, digoxin, DOBUTamine, DOPamine, doxycycline, furosemide, gentamicin, heparin, lidocaine, penicillin G sodium, potassium chloride, ticarcillin, tobramycin, vancomycin
*Additive incompatibilities:* Amphotericin B, clindamycin

### Patient/family education
• Caution patient that gynecomastia, impotence may occur and are reversible after treatment is discontinued
• Advise patient to avoid driving, other hazardous activities until stabilized on this medication; drowsiness or dizziness may occur
• Inform patient that smoking decreases the effectiveness of the product; that smoking cessation should be considered

- Instruct patient that product must be continued for prescribed time to be effective and taken exactly as prescribed; doses should not be doubled; a missed dose should be taken when remembered up to 1 hr before next dose
- Advise patient to report bruising, fatigue, malaise; blood dyscrasias may occur
- Inform patient to report diarrhea, black tarry stools, sore throat, rash, dizziness, confusion, rash, or delirium to prescriber immediately

### Evaluation
**Positive therapeutic outcome**
- Decreased pain in abdomen, heartburn
- Healing of ulcers
- Absence of gastroesophageal reflux

---

## ranolazine (Rx)
(ruh-no'luh-zeen)
Ranexa
*Func. class:* Antianginal
**Pregnancy category** C

**Action:** Antiaginal, antiischemic; unknown, may work by inhibiting portal fatty-acid oxidation

**Therapeutic outcome:** Decreased anginal pain and number of episodes

**Uses:** Chronic stable angina pectoris; use in those that have not responded to other treatment options; should be used in combination with other antianginals such as amlodipine, beta blockers, or nitrates

### Dosage and routes
*Adult:* PO 500 mg bid and increased to 1000 mg bid based on response; max 1000 mg bid

**Available forms:** Ext rel tabs 500 mg

### Adverse effects
*CNS:* Headache, dizziness
*CV:* Palpitations, **QT prolongation**
*GI:* Nausea, vomiting, constipation, dry mouth
*MISC:* Peripheral edema
*RESP:* Dyspnea

**Contraindications:** Preexisting QT prolongation, hepatic disease (Child-Pugh class A, B, C), hypersensitivity, hypokalemia, renal failure, torsade de pointes, ventricular dysrhythmia, ventricular tachycardia

**Precautions:** Pregnancy C, breastfeeding, children, geriatric, renal disease, hypotension

### Pharmacokinetics
| | |
|---|---|
| **Absorption** | Varied |
| **Distribution** | Protein binding 62% |
| **Metabolism** | By CYP3A, CYP2D6 (lesser) |
| **Excretion** | Urine 75%, feces 25% |
| **Half-life** | 7 hr |

### Pharmacodynamics
| | |
|---|---|
| **Onset** | Unknown |
| **Peak** | 2-5 hr |
| **Duration** | Unknown |

### Interactions
*Individual drugs*
Arsenic trioxide, chloroquine, droperidol, grepafloxacin, halofantrine, haloperidol, levomethadyl, methadone, pentamidine, chlorpromazine, mesoridazine, thioridazine, pimozide, probucol, sparfloxacin: increased QT prolongation and torsade de pointes
Digoxin, simvastatin: increased action of digoxin, simvastatin
Diltiazem, ketoconazole, dofetilide, paroxetine, quinidine, sotalol, thioridazine, verapamil, ziprasidone: increased ranolazine action
*Drug classifications*
Anti-retroviral protease inhibitors: increased ranolazine absorption, toxicity
Class IA/III antidysrhythmics: increased QT prolongation and torsade de pointes
CYP3A4 inhibitors (ketoconazole, fluconazole, itraconazole, IV miconazole, voriconazole, diltiazem, verapamil): increased ranzolazine action and QT prolongation; do not use concurrently
Macrolide antibiotics, protease inhibitors: increased ranolazine action
Macrolides (clarithromycin, erythromycin, troleandomycin): increased QTc interval
*Drug/food*
Do not use with grapefruit or grapefruit juice

R

### NURSING CONSIDERATIONS
### Assessment
- Assess cardiac status: B/P, pulse, respiration, ECG; watch for prolongation of QT

### Nursing diagnoses
- Knowledge, deficient (teaching)
- Pain, acute (uses)
- Tissue perfusion, ineffective (uses)

### Implementation
- Do not break, crush, or chew tabs; to take products as prescribed; do not double or skip dose
- Give bid, without regard to meals

Adverse effects: *italic* = common, **bold** = life-threatening

### Patient/family education
• Teach patient to avoid hazardous activities until stabilized on product, dizziness is no longer a problem
• Advise patient to avoid OTC drugs, grapefruit juice, drugs prolonging QTc (quinidine, dofetilide, sotalol, erythromycin, thioridazine, ziprasidone or protease inhibitors, diltiazem, ketoconazole, macrolide antibiotics, verapamil) unless directed by prescriber
• Advise patient to comply in all areas of medical regimen
• Teach patient to notify prescriber of palpitations, fainting
• Teach patient to notify all health care providers of this product use

### Evaluation
**Positive therapeutic outcome**
• Decreased anginal pain and number of episodes

---

**rasagiline** (Rx)
(ra-sa'-ji-leen)
Azilect
*Func. class.:* Antiparkinson agent
*Chem. class.:* MAOI

**Pregnancy category C**

**Action:** Inhibits MAOI type B; may increase dopamine levels

**Therapeutic outcome:** Improved symptoms in those with Parkinson's disease

**Uses:** Idiopathic Parkinson's disease monotherapy or with levodopa

### Dosage and routes
*Monotherapy*
*Adult:* PO 1 mg/day

*Adjunctive therapy*
*Adult:* PO 0.5 mg/day, may be increased to 1 mg/day; change of levodopa dose in adjunct therapy; reduced levodopa dose may be needed

*Hepatic dose*
*Adult:* PO 0.5 mg in mild hepatic disease

*Concomitant ciprofloxacin, other CYP1A2 inhibitors*
*Adult:* PO 0.5 mg; plasma concentrations of rasagiline may double

**Available forms:** Tabs 0.5, 1 mg

### Adverse effects
*CNS:* Drowsiness, hallucinations, depression, headache, malaise, paresthesia, vertigo, syncope

*CV:* Angina, **hypertensive crisis** (ingestion of tyramine products), orthostatic hypotension
*GI: Nausea,* diarrhea, dry mouth, dyspepsia
*GU:* Impotence, decreased libido
*MISC:* Conjunctivitis, fever, flu syndrome, neck pain, allergic reaction, alopecia
*MS:* Arthralgia, arthritis, dyskinesia, falls
*RESP:* Rhinitis

**Contraindications:** Breastfeeding, hypersensitivity to this product or MAOIs, pheochromocytoma

**Precautions:** Pregnancy **C**, children, psychiatric disorders, severe hepatic disorders

| Pharmacokinetics | |
|---|---|
| Absorption | Well |
| Distribution | Protein binding >88-94% |
| Metabolism | Liver, CYP1A2 |
| Excretion | Kidneys |
| Half-life | Unknown |

| Pharmacodynamics |
|---|
| Unknown |

### Interactions
*Individual drugs*
Ciprofloxacin: increased levels of rasagiline up to 2-fold
◆ Meperidine: do not give; serious reaction including coma and death may occur
*Drug classifications*
◆ Analgesics, sympathomimetics: do not give; serious reaction including coma and death may occur
◆ Antidepressants (tricyclics, selective serotonin reuptake inhibitors, SNRIs, mirtazapine, cyclobenzaprine): increased severe CNS toxicity
CYP1A2 inhibitors (atazanavir, mexiletine, taurine): increased levels of rasagiline up to twofold
◆ MAOIs: increased hypertensive crisis
*Drug/herb*
◆ St. John's wort: do not give

### NURSING CONSIDERATIONS
**Assessment**
• Assess for Parkinson's symptoms: tremor, ataxia, muscle weakness and rigidity; baseline and periodically
• Assess mental status: hallucinations, confusion, notify prescriber
• Assess for hypertensive crisis: severe headache, blurred vision, seizures, chest pain, difficulty thinking, nausea/vomiting, signs of stroke; any unexplained severe headache should be considered to be hypertensive crisis

---

- Assess for increased dyskinesia and postural hypotension if used in combination with levodopa
- Assess for melanomas frequently, perform periodic skin exams by a dermatologist
- Monitor cardiac status: B/P, ECG; periodically during beginning treatment

## Nursing diagnoses
- Injury, risk for (uses, adverse reactions)
- Knowledge, deficient (teaching)
- Mobility, impaired physical (uses)

## Implementation
- Give with meals to prevent nausea; continuing therapy usually reduces or eliminates nausea
- Give reduced dose of carbidopa/levodopa, cautiously

## Patient/family education
- Advise patient to change positions slowly to prevent orthostatic hypotension
- Instruct patient to avoid hazardous activities until stabilized; dizziness can occur
- Advise patient to rinse mouth frequently, use sugarless gum to alleviate dry mouth
- Teach patient to take as prescribed, not to miss dose or double doses; take missed dose as soon as remembered, if several hours before next dose
- Teach patient to prevent hypertensive crisis by avoiding tyramine foods
- Teach patient to report signs of hypertensive crisis

## Evaluation
**Positive therapeutic outcome**
- Improved symptoms in those with Parkinson's disease (decreasing tremors, ataxia, muscle weakness/rigidity)

---

## rasburicase (Rx)
(rass-burr'i-case)
Elitek
*Func. class.:* Enzyme
*Chem.class.:* Recombinant urate-oxidase enzyme

### Pregnancy category C

**Action:** Catalyzes enzymatic oxidation of uric acid into an inactive and a soluble metabolite

**Therapeutic outcome:** Uric acid levels are decreased

**Uses:** To reduce uric acid levels in children with leukemia, lymphoma, solid tumor malignancies who are receiving chemotherapy

## Dosage and routes
*Adult:* **IV** INF 0.2 mg/kg as a single daily dose given as **IV** INF over ½ hr × 5 days
*Adolescent/child/infant:* **IV** INF 0.15-0.2 mg/kg/day q1-7 days

**Available forms:** Powder for inj 1.5 mg/vial

## Adverse effects
*CNS:* Headache
*CV:* Chest pain, hypotension
*GI: Nausea, vomiting, anorexia, diarrhea, abdominal pain, constipation, dyspepsia,* mucositis
*HEMA:* **Neutropenia with fever**
*INTEG:* Rash
*MISC:* Edema
*RESP:* **Bronchospasm,** wheezing, dyspnea
*SYST:* **Anaphylaxis, hemolysis, methemoglobinemia, sepsis**

**Contraindications:** Hypersensitivity, G6PD deficiency, hemolytic reactions, or methemoglobinemia reactions to this product

**Precautions:** Pregnancy **C**, breastfeeding, children <2 yr, acute bronchospasm, anemia

| Pharmacokinetics | |
|---|---|
| **Absorption** | Unknown |
| **Distribution** | Unknown |
| **Metabolism** | Unknown |
| **Excretion** | Unknown |
| **Half-life** | Elimination 16-21 hr |

| Pharmacodynamics |
|---|
| Unknown |

## Interactions
*Individual drugs*
Allopurinol: increased toxicity

## NURSING CONSIDERATIONS
### Assessment
- Monitor renal function tests: BUN, serum uric acid, urine CCr, electrolytes before and during therapy
- Monitor temp q4hr; fever may indicate beginning infection; no rectal temps
- Assess for anaphylaxis, have emergency equipment nearby
- Assess for G6PD deficiency, hemolytic reactions, methemoglobinemia; these patients should not be given this agent
- Assess for toxicity: severe diarrhea, nausea, vomiting
- Assess GI symptoms: frequency of stools, cramping; if severe diarrhea occurs, fluid and electrolytes may need to be given

R

Adverse effects: *italic* = common, **bold** = life-threatening

**Nursing diagnoses**
- Injury, risk for (adverse reactions, uses)
- Knowledge, deficient (teaching)

**Implementation**
- Give antiemetic 30-60 min before giving product and prn
- Infuse over 30 min; do not filter

**Patient/family education**
- Advise of reason for therapy, expected results

**Evaluation**
**Positive therapeutic outcome**
- Decreased uric acid levels

---

**⚠ HIGH ALERT**

**remifentanil** (Rx)
(re-me-fin′ta-nill)
Ultiva
*Func. class.:* Opiate agonist analgesic
*Chem. class.:* μ-Opioid agonist

**Pregnancy category** C

**Controlled substance schedule** II

**Action:** Inhibits ascending pain pathways in limbic system, thalamus, midbrain, hypothalamus

**Therapeutic outcome:** Maintenance of anesthesia

**Uses:** In combination with other products in general anesthesia to provide analgesia

**Dosage and routes**
*Adult:* Induction **IV** 0.5-1 mcg/kg/min with a hypnotic or volatile agent; maintenance with isoflurane (0.4-1.5 MAC) or propofol (100-200 mcg/kg/min); CONT INF 0.25-0.4 mcg/kg/min

**Available forms:** Powder for inj, lyophilized 1 mg/ml after reconstitution

**Adverse effects**
*CNS:* Drowsiness, *dizziness,* confusion, *headache,* sedation, euphoria, delirium, agitation, anxiety
*CV:* Palpitations, **bradycardia,** change in B/P; facial flushing, syncope, **asystole**
*EENT:* Tinnitus, blurred vision, miosis, diplopia
*GI:* Nausea, vomiting, anorexia, constipation, cramps, dry mouth
*GU:* Urinary retention, dysuria
*INTEG:* Rash, urticaria, bruising, flushing, diaphoresis, pruritus
*MS:* Rigidity
*RESP:* **Respiratory depression, apnea**

**Contraindications:** Child <12 yr, hypersensitivity

**Precautions:** Pregnancy **C,** breastfeeding, geriatric, increased ICP, acute MI, severe heart disease, GI/renal/hepatic disease, asthma, respiratory conditions, seizure disorders, bradyarrhythmias

| Pharmacokinetics | |
|---|---|
| **Absorption** | Complete |
| **Distribution** | 70% protein binding |
| **Metabolism** | Unknown |
| **Excretion** | Unknown |
| **Half-life** | Terminal 3-10 min |

| Pharmacodynamics | |
|---|---|
| **Onset** | Immediate |
| **Peak** | Unknown |
| **Duration** | Unknown |

**Interactions**
*Individual drugs*
Alcohol: increased respiratory depression, hypotension, profound sedation
*Drug classifications*
Antihistamines, CNS depressants, phenothiazines, sedative/hypnotics: increased respiratory depression, hypotension, profound sedation
*Drug/herb*
Kava: increased CNS depression

**NURSING CONSIDERATIONS**
**Assessment**
- Monitor I&O ratio, check for decreasing output; may indicate urinary retention, especially in geriatric
- Assess CNS changes: dizziness, drowsiness, hallucinations, euphoria, LOC pupil reaction
- Assess allergic reactions: rash, urticaria
- Assess respiratory dysfunction: respiratory depression, character, rate, rhythm; notify prescriber if respirations are <12/min; CV status, bradycardia, syncope
- Monitor GI status: nausea, vomiting, anorexia, constipation
- Use pain scoring to determine pain perception

**Nursing diagnoses**
- Knowledge, deficient (teaching)

**Implementation**
- Add 1 ml diluent per mg remifentanil
- Interruption of infusion results in rapid reversal (no residual opioid effect within 5-10 min)

---

- Store in light-resistant area at room temperature

**Y-site compatibilities:** Acyclovir, alfentanil, amikacin, aminophylline, ampicillin, ampicillin/sulbactam, aztreonam, bretylium, bumetanide, buprenorphine, butorphanol, calcium gluconate, cefazolin, cefepime, cefotaxime, cefotetan, cefoxitin, ceftazidime, ceftizoxime, ceftriaxone, cefuroxime, cimetidine, ciprofloxacin, cisatracurium, cisplatin, clindamycin, dactinomycin, dexamethasone, digoxin, diltiazem, diphenhydrAMINE, DOBUTamine, docetaxel, DOPamine, doxacurium, doxycycline, droperidol, enalaprilat, epINEPHrine, esmolol, etoposide, famotidine, fentanyl, fluconazole, furosemide, ganciclovir, gatifloxacin, gemcitabine, gentamicin, granisetron, haloperidol, heparin, hetastarch, hydrocortisone sodium succinate, hydromorphone, hydrOXYzine, imipenem/cilastatin, inamrinone, isoproterenol, ketorolac, levofloxacin, lidocaine, lorazepam, magnesium sulfate, mannitol, meperidine, methlyprednisoLONE sodium succinate, metoclopramide, metronidazole, mezlocillin, midazolam, minocycline, morphine, nalbuphine, netilmicin, nitroglycerin, norepinephrine, ofloxacin, ondansetron, paclitaxel, palonsetron, phenylephrine, pipericillin, potassium chloride, procainamide, prochlorperazine, promethazine, ranitidine, sulfamethoxazole/trimethroprim, sulfentanil, teniposide, theophylline, thiopental, thiotepa, ticarcillin, ticarcillin/clavulate, tobramycin, vancomycin, voriconazole, zidovudine

**Solution compatibilities:** $D_5$, 0.45% NaCl, LR, $D_5$LR, 0.9% NaCl

## Patient/family education
- Advise patient to call for assistance when ambulating or smoking; drowsiness, dizziness may occur
- Advise patient to make position changes slowly to prevent orthostatic hypotension

## Evaluation
**Positive therapeutic outcome**
- Maintenance of anesthesia

## repaglinide (Rx)
(re-pag'lih-nide)
Gluco Norm ✤, Prandin
*Func. class.:* Antidiabetic
*Chem. class.:* Meglitinides

**Pregnancy category  C**

**Action:** Causes functioning β-cells in pancreas to release insulin, leading to drop in blood glucose levels; closes ATP-dependent potassium channels in the β-cell membrane; this leads to opening of calcium channels; increased calcium influx induces insulin secretion

**Therapeutic outcome:** Blood glucose controlled

**Uses:** Type 2 diabetes mellitus

## Dosage and routes
*Adult:* PO 1-2 mg with each meal, max 16 mg/day, adjust at weekly intervals; oral hypoglycemic naive patients or those with A1c <8% should start with 0.5 mg with each meal

**Renal/hepatic dose**
*Adult:* PO 0.5 mg/day; titrate upward cautiously

**Available forms:** Tabs 0.5, 1, 2 mg

## Adverse effects
*CNS: Headache, weakness,* paresthesia
*ENDO:* **Hypoglycemia**
*GI:* Nausea, vomiting, diarrhea, constipation, dyspepsia
*INTEG:* Rash, allergic reactions
*MISC:* Chest pain, UTI, allergy
*MS:* Back pains, arthralgia
*RESP:* URI, sinusitis, rhinitis, bronchitis

**Contraindications:** Hypersensitivity to meglitinides, diabetic ketoacidosis, type 1 diabetes

**Precautions:** Pregnancy **C,** breastfeeding, children, geriatric, cardiac disease, severe renal/hepatic disease, thyroid disease, severe hypoglycemic reactions

| Pharmacokinetics | |
|---|---|
| **Absorption** | Complete |
| **Distribution** | 98% protein binding, crosses placenta |
| **Metabolism** | Liver |
| **Excretion** | Urine/feces |
| **Half-life** | 1 hr |

| Pharmacodynamics | |
|---|---|
| **Onset** | 30 min |
| **Peak** | 1-1½ hr |
| **Duration** | <4 hr |

## Interactions
*Individual drugs*
Carbamazepine, rifampin: increased repaglinide metabolism
Chloramphenicol, fenofibrate, gemfibrozil, probenecid, simvastatin: increased effect of repaglinide

R

Adverse effects: *italic* = common, **bold** = life-threatening

Erythromycin, ketoconazole, miconazole: decreased repaglinide metabolism

Isoniazid, phenobarbital, phenytoin, rifampin: decreased action of repaglinide

Levonorgestrel/ethinyl estradol: increase in both

*Drug classifications*

Antifungals, macrolides, CYP450 inhibitors: decreased repaglinide metabolism

CYP450 inducers, barbiturates: increased repaglinide metabolism

β-Adrenergic blockers, coumarins, MAOIs, NSAIDs, salicylates, sulfonamides: increased repaglinide effect

Calcium channel blockers, contraceptives (oral), corticosteroids, diuretics (thiazide), estrogens, phenothiazines, sympathomimetics, thyroid preparations: decreased repaglinide effect

*Drug/herb*

Alfalfa, aloe, basil, bay, bilberry, bitter melon, black catechu, buchu, burdock, coriander, dandelion, eyebright (po), fenugreek, garlic, ginseng, glucomannan, glucosamine, goat's rue, gymnema, horehound, horse chestnut, jambul, myrrh, myrtle: increased antidiabetic effect

Bee pollen, blue cohosh, broom, chromium, elecampane, eucalyptus, gotu kola: decreased antidiabetic effect

Broom, buchu, dandelion, juniper: decreased hypoglycemia

Chromium, fenugreek, ginseng: increased or decreased hypoglycemia

Karela: decreased glucose tolerance

*Drug/food*

Decreased: repaglinide level, give before meals

**NURSING CONSIDERATIONS**
**Assessment**

⬧ Assess for hypoglycemic or hyperglycemic reaction, which can occur soon after meals; dizziness, weakness, headache, tremor, anxiety, tachycardia, hunger, sweating, abdominal pain

• Monitor A1c, fasting, postprandial glucose during treatment

**Nursing diagnoses**

• Knowledge, deficient (teaching)

• Noncompliance (teaching)

• Nutrition: more than body requirements, imbalanced (uses)

**Implementation**

• 15 min before meals: 2, 3, or 4 ×/day preprandially

• Skip dose if meal is skipped; add dose if meal is added

• Store in airtight container in cool environment

**Patient/family education**

• Teach patient technique of blood glucose monitoring using blood glucose meter

• Teach patient the symptoms of hypoglycemia and hyperglycemia; what to do about each

• Teach patient that product must be continued on daily basis; explain consequence of discontinuing product abruptly

• Advise patient to avoid OTC medications unless ordered by prescriber

• Advise patient that diabetes is a lifelong illness; product will not cure disease

• Advise patient to eat all food included in diet plan to prevent hypoglycemia; to have glucagon emergency kit available

• Instruct patient to carry/wear emergency ID for emergency purposes

**Evaluation**
**Positive therapeutic outcome**

• Decrease in polyuria, polydipsia, polyphagia, clear sensorium; absence of dizziness; stable gait; blood glucose; A1c improvement

**Treatment of overdose:** Glucose 25 g **IV** via D$_{50}$ sol, 50 ml or 1

---

**retapamulin topical**
*See Appendix D*

---

**retinoic acid**
*See tretinoin*

---

**Rh$_o$ (D) immune globulin, standard dose IM**
BayRho (HyperRHO SD), Rho Gam Ultra Filtered Plus Solution for Injection

**Rh$_o$ (D) immune globulin microdose IM**
MICRhoGAM Ultra Filtered Plus Solution for Injection

**Rh$_o$ (D) immune globulin IV**
Rhophylac Pre-Filled Syringes, WinRho SDF
*Func. class.:* Immune globulins

**Pregnancy category C**

**Action:** Suppresses immunenonsensitized Rh$_o$ (D or D$^u$)-negative patients who are exposed to Rh$_o$ (D or D$^u$)-positive blood

**Therapeutic outcome:** Absence of Rh factor and transfusion error

**Uses:** Prevention of isoimmunization in Rh-negative women exposed to Rh-positive blood given after abortions, miscarriages,

---

⬧ Alert     ♣ Canada Only     🌐 Drug on CD     * "Tall Man" lettering (See Preface)

amniocentesis, chronic idiopathic thrombocytopenic purpura (Rhophylac)

## Dosage and routes
### To reduce risk of Rh isoimmunization antepartum/suppression of Rh isoimmunization postpartum following delivery of full-term infant
**Adult and adolescent ≥16 yr:** IM (BayRho-D [HyperRHO SD] [full dose only]) 300 mcg (1500 international units) at 28 wk gestation, repeat within 72 hr of delivery of confirmed Rho(D)-positive infant; a dose is not needed after delivery, if delivery is within 3 wk of last dose and no fetal maternal hemorrhage of >15 ml of RBC; IM (RhoGam only) 300 mcg (1500 international units) at 26-28 wk gestation, repeat within 72 hr even if status of Rho is unknown or if 72 hr have passed; IM/**IV** (WinRho SDF only) 300 mcg (1500 international units) at 28 wk gestation; if given earlier in pregnancy, give at 12-wk intervals during pregnancy, a 120 mcg (600 international units) dose; IM/**IV** should be given as soon as possible and preferably with 72 hr of delivery of a confirmed Rho(D)-positive infant and even if status is unknown, give up to 28 days after delivery

### Known or suspected massive fetomaternal hemorrhage (>15 ml of fetal RBC or >30 ml of fetal whole blood)
**Adult and adolescent ≥16 yr:** IM (BayRho-D [HyperRHO SD] [full dose only]) 300 mcg (1500 international units) per every 15 ml of fetal blood cells or 30 ml of whole blood, multiple syringes may be injected IM at the same time in different sites, give within 72 hr of exposure, repeat dose within 72 hr of delivery; IM (RhoGAM only) 300 mcg (1500 international units) for every 15 ml of fetal blood cells or 30 ml of whole blood, give total dose within 72 hr of exposure; IM/**IV** (WinRho SDF only) if large fetomaternal hemorrhage is suspected, give **IV** 9 mcg (45 international units) or IM 12 mcg (60 international units) for every ml of fetal whole blood, give **IV** 600 mcg (3000 international units) q8hr or IM 1200 mcg (6000 international units) q12hr until total dose is given, total dose should be given within 72 hr of exposure

### Threatened abortion at any stage of pregnancy
**Adult and adolescent ≥16 yr:** IM (BayRho-D [HyperRHO SD] [full dose only]) 300 mcg (1500 international units) as soon as possible; if given 13-18 wk gestation, give another 300 mcg (1500 international units) at 26-28 wk gestation; repeat dose within 72 hr of delivery; IM (RhoGam only) 300 mcg (1500 international units) as soon as possible and within 72 hr; IM/**IV** (Rhophylac only) 300 mcg (1500 international units) as soon as possible and within 72 hr; IM/**IV** (WinRho SDF only) 300 mcg (1500 international units) as soon as possible and within 72 hr, repeat dose at 12-wk intervals during pregnancy and 120 mcg (600 international units) as soon as possible after delivery and within 72 hr

### Following spontaneous abortion, induced termination of pregnancy or ectopic pregnancy that occurs ≤12 wk gestation
**Adult and adolescent ≥16 yr:** IM (BayRho-D Minidose, HYperRHO Minidose, MICRORhoGAM only) 50 mcg (250 international units) as soon as possible, give within 3 hr of spontaneous or surgical removal, if possible within 72 hr

### Following spontaneous abortion, induced termination or pregnancy, or ruptured tubal pregnancy that occur ≥13 wk
**Adult and adolescent ≥16 yr:** IM (BayRho-D full dose [HyperRHO SD full dose] RhoGAM only) 300 mcg (1500 international units) as soon as possible and within 72 hr of event

### Following spontaneous abortion, induced termination of pregnancy, aminocentesis, chorionic villus sampling, abdominal trauma, ruptured tubal pregnancy, or percutaneous umbilical cord sampling up to 34 wk gestation
**Adult and adolescent ≥16 wk:** IM/**IV** (WinRho SDF only) 300 mcg (1500 international units) within 72 hr, repeat at 12-wk intervals during pregnancy, give 120 mcg (600 international units) as soon as possible and preferably within 72 hr of delivery

**Available forms:** BayRho-D solution for injection 300 mcg/ml (HyperRHO SD solution for injection); MICRhoGAM Ultra Filtered Plus Solution for injection 50 mcg/ml; RhoGam Ultra Filtered Plus Solution for injection 50 mcg; Rhophylac Pre-Filled Syringes Solution for injection 300 mcg/2 ml; WinRho SDF Liquid for injection; WinRho powder for injection

R

**Adverse effects**
*CNS:* Lethargy
*INTEG:* Irritation at inj site, fever
*MS:* Myalgia

**Contraindications:** Previous immunization with this product, $Rh_o$ (O)-positive/$D^u$-positive patient

**Precautions:** Pregnancy **C**

### Pharmacokinetics

| | |
|---|---|
| **Absorption** | Well absorbed |
| **Distribution** | Unknown |
| **Metabolism** | Unknown |
| **Excretion** | Unknown |
| **Half-life** | Unknown |

### Pharmacodynamics

| | |
|---|---|
| **Onset** | Rapid |
| **Peak** | Unknown |
| **Duration** | Unknown |

### Interactions
*Drug classifications*
Live virus vaccines (measles, mumps, rubella): decreased antibody response to vaccine

### NURSING CONSIDERATIONS
**Assessment**
◆ Assess for allergies, reactions to immunizations; previous immunization with this product
• Obtain type and cross-match of mother's blood and of neonate's cord blood; neonate must be $Rh_o$(D)-positive, mother must be $Rh_o$(D)-negative and ($D^u$)-negative, medication should be given if there is a doubt
◆ Assess for intravascular hemolysis: back pain, chills, hemoglobinuria, renal insufficiency, idiopathic thrombocytopenic purpura

**Nursing diagnoses**
• Knowledge, deficient (teaching)

**Implementation**
• BayRho-D is being changed to HyperRHO SD
• BayRho-D (HyperRHO SD), MICRhoGAM, RhoGAM are given by IM only; do not give **IV**
• WinRhoSDF and Rhophylac can be given IM or **IV**
• Inspect for particulate matter; do not use if particulate matter is present
• Reconstitute/dilution: no reconstitution or dilution is needed for BayRho-D (HyperRHO SD), Rhophylac, MICRoGAM, RhoGAM, or the liquid formulation of WinRho SDF
• WinRho SDF powder for **IV** use: if giving **IV**, reconstitute 600 international units or 1500 international units immediately before

use with 2.5 ml of sterile diluent; reconstitute 5000 international units with 8.5 ml sterile diluent; add diluent to vial slowly down the wall of the vial; gently swirl until powder is dissolved; do not shake
• Win Rho SDF powder for IM use: **IV** giving IM, reconstitute 600 international units or 1500 international units immediately before use with 1.25 ml of sterile diluent; 5000 international units with 8.5 ml of sterile diluent; add diluent to the vial slowly down the wall of the vial; gently swirl until powder is dissolved; do not shake
**IM route**
• Use aseptic technique, observe for 20 min after administration
• Bring Rhophylac to room temperature before using
• Inject into the deltoid muscle of upper arm or anterolateral portion of the upper thigh; do not inject into gluteal muscle
• If dose calculated will need multiple vials or syringes, use different site at the same time
**IV route**
• Use aseptic technique
• WinRhoSDF: remove entire contents of vial to obtain calculated dose; if partial vial contents are required for dosage calculation, withdraw the entire vial contents to ensure correct calculation; infuse correct calculated dose over 3-5 min; do not infuse with other fluids or products
• Rhophylac: bring to room temperature; infuse by slow **IV**; observe for 20 min

**Patient/family education**
• Teach patient how product works; that product must be given after subsequent deliveries if subsequent babies are Rh-positive

**Evaluation**
**Positive therapeutic outcome**
• Prevention of $Rh_o$(D) sensitization in transfusion error
• Prevention of erythroblastosis fetalis in subsequent $Rh_o$(D)-positive neonates

---

**ribavarin** (Rx)
(rye-ba-vye′rin)
Virazole
*Func. class.:* Synthetic antiviral
*Chem. class.:* Tricyclic amine
**Pregnancy category X**

**Action:** Prevents replication of DNA and RNA synthesis

**Therapeutic outcome:** Resolution of severe lower respiratory tract infections

---

**Uses:** Severe lower respiratory tract infections in infants and children

**Unlabeled uses:** Influenza A or B (early)

**Dosage and routes**
*Infant and young child:* INH 20 mg/ml × 12-18 hr/day × 3-7 days

**Available forms:** Powder for reconstitution for aerosol 6 g/vial

**Adverse effects**
*CNS:* Dizziness, faintness
*CV:* Hypotension, cardiac arrest
*EENT:* Eye irritation, conjunctivitis, blurred vision, photosensitivity
*INTEG:* Rash

**Contraindications:** Pregnancy **X**, breastfeeding, children <1 yr, hypersensitivity

**Precautions:** Epilepsy, renal/hepatic disease

| Pharmacokinetics | |
|---|---|
| **Absorption** | Inh (systemic) |
| **Distribution** | To respiratory tract |
| **Metabolism** | Liver |
| **Excretion** | Respiratory tract |
| **Half-life** | 9½ hr |

| Pharmacodynamics | |
|---|---|
| **Onset** | Unknown |
| **Peak** | Inh end |
| **Duration** | Unknown |

**Interactions**
*Individual products*
Zidovudine: decreased antiviral action, increased toxicity
*Drug classification*
Cardiac glycosides: increased toxicity

**NURSING CONSIDERATIONS**
**Assessment**
• Assess allergies before initiation of treatment, reaction of each medication; list allergies on chart in bright red letters
• Monitor respiratory status: rate, character, wheezing, tightness in chest
• Obtain C&S test results before starting treatment

**Nursing diagnoses**
• Gas exchange, impaired (uses)
• Infection, risk for (uses)
• Knowledge, deficient (teaching)

**Implementation**
• Give by the Viratek small particle aerosol generator (SPAG-2), do not use other inhalation equipment

• May be given by an oxygen hood for infants, or a face mask may be attached to the SPAG-2
• Reconstitute 6 g of sterile water for inj or inh, place sol in the Erlenmeyer flask and dilute further to 20 mg/ml

**Patient/family education**
• Teach patient and parents aspects of product therapy

**Evaluation**
**Positive therapeutic outcome**
• Absence of respiratory syncytial virus

## riboflavin (vitamin B$_2$) (OTC)
(rye′boo-flay-vin)
*Func. class.:* Vitamin B$_2$, water soluble

**Pregnancy category  A**

**Action:** Needed for respiratory reactions (catalyzes proteins) and for normal vision

**Therapeutic outcome:** Prevention or treatment of riboflavin deficiency

**Uses:** Vitamin B$_2$ deficiency or polyneuritis; cheilosis adjunct with thiamine

**Dosage and routes**
*Deficiency*
*Adult and child >12 yr:* PO 5-25 mg/day
*Child <12 yr:* PO 2-10 mg/day, then 0.6 mg/1000 cal ingested

*RDA*
*Adult:* PO (Males) 1.4-1.8 mg; (females) 1.2-1.3 mg

**Available forms:** Tabs 5, 10, 25, 50, 100, 250 mg

**Adverse effects**
*GU:* Yellow discoloration of urine (large doses)

**Precautions:** Pregnancy **A**

| Pharmacokinetics | |
|---|---|
| **Absorption** | Well absorbed (by active transport) |
| **Distribution** | 60% protein bound, widely distributed, crosses placenta |
| **Metabolism** | Unknown |
| **Excretion** | Kidneys (unchanged), excess amounts |
| **Half-life** | 1-1½ hr |

| Pharmacodynamics | |
|---|---|
| Unknown | |

**R**

## Interactions
### Individual drugs
Alcohol, probenecid: increased riboflavin need
Tetracycline: decreased action of tetracycline
### Drug classifications
Antidepressants (tricyclics), phenothiazines: increased riboflavin need
### Drug/lab test
False increase: urinary catecholamines

## NURSING CONSIDERATIONS
### Assessment
• Assess patient's nutritional status: liver, eggs, dairy products, yeast, whole grain, green vegetables
• Assess for vit $B_2$ deficiency: photophobia, cheilosis, stomatitis, ocular swelling

### Nursing diagnoses
• Knowledge, deficient (teaching)
• Nutrition: less than body requirements, imbalanced (uses)

### Implementation
• Give with food for better absorption
• Store in airtight, light-resistant container

### Patient/family education
• Inform patient that urine may turn bright yellow
• Instruct patient about addition of needed foods that are rich in riboflavin

### Evaluation
**Positive therapeutic outcome**
• Absence of headache, GI problems, cheilosis, skin lesions, depression, burning, itchy eyes, anemia

## rifabutin (Rx)
(riff'a-byoo-tin)
Mycobutin
*Func. class.:* Antimycobacterial
*Chem. class.:* Rifamycin S derivative

**Pregnancy category B**

### Do not confuse:
rifabutin/rifampin

**Action:** Inhibits DNA-dependent RNA polymerase in susceptible strains

**Therapeutic outcome:** Antimycobacterial death of *Escherichia coli, Bacillus subtilis,* and *Mycobacterium avium*

**Uses:** Prevention of *M. avium* complex (MAC) in patients with advanced HIV infection

**Unlabeled uses:** *Helicobacter pylori* that has not responded to other treatment

## Dosage and routes
*Adult:* PO 300 mg/day (may take as 150 mg bid)
### Renal dose
*Adult:* PO CCr <30 ml/min reduce dose by 50%

**Available forms:** Caps 150 mg

## Adverse effects
*CNS:* Headache, fatigue, anxiety, confusion, insomnia
*GI: Nausea, vomiting, anorexia, diarrhea,* heartburn, **hepatitis,** discolored saliva
*GU:* Hematuria, discolored urine
*HEMA:* **Hemolytic anemia, eosinophilia, thrombocytopenia, leukopenia**
*INTEG:* Rash
*MISC:* Flulike syndrome, shortness of breath, chest pressure
*MS:* Asthenia, arthralgia, myalgia

**Contraindications:** Hypersensitivity, active TB, WBC <1000/mm$^3$, platelets <50,000/mm$^3$

**Precautions:** Pregnancy **B**, breastfeeding, children, hepatic disease, blood dyscrasias

### Pharmacokinetics
| | |
|---|---|
| **Absorption** | Well absorbed |
| **Distribution** | Widely distributed |
| **Metabolism** | Liver |
| **Excretion** | Kidney |
| **Half-life** | 45 hr |

### Pharmacodynamics
| | |
|---|---|
| **Onset** | Unknown |
| **Peak** | 2-3 hr |
| **Duration** | Unknown |

## Interactions
### Individual drugs
Amprenavir, busPIRone, clofibrate, cycloSPORINE, dapsone, delavirdine, digoxin, disopyramide, doxycycline, efavirenz, fluconazole, indinavir, ketoconazole, losartan, nelfinavir, nevirapine, phenytoin, quinidine, saquinavir, theophylline, tocainide, verapamil, zidovudine, zolpidem: decreased action of each specific product
Ritonavir: increased rifabutin level
### Drug classifications
Analgesics (opioid), anticoagulants, antidepressants (tricyclics), barbiturates, β-blockers, contraceptives (oral), corticosteroids, estrogens, sulfonylureas: decreased action of each specific product

*Drug/food*
High-fat foods: decreased absorption
*Drug/lab test*
Interference: folate level, vit B$_{12}$, BSP, gallbladder tests

## NURSING CONSIDERATIONS
### Assessment
• Assess for active TB: chest x-ray, sputum culture, blood culture, biopsy of lymph nodes, obtain PPD test; product should be given only for MAC and never for TB
• Monitor CBC for neutropenia, thrombocytopenia, eosinophilia

### Nursing diagnoses
• Diarrhea (adverse reaction)
• Infection, risk for (uses)
• Injury, risk for (adverse reaction)
• Knowledge, deficient (teaching)
• Noncompliance (teaching)

### Implementation
• Give with meals to decrease GI symptoms; better to take on empty stomach 1 hr before or 2 hr after meals; high-fat food slows absorption
• Give antiemetic if vomiting occurs

### Patient/family education
• Caution patient that compliance with dosage schedule and duration is necessary
• Instruct patient that scheduled appointments must be kept or relapse may occur
• Instruct patient to notify prescriber if hepatitis, neutropenia, or thrombocytopenia occurs: sore throat, fever, bleeding, bruising, yellow sclera, anorexia, nausea, vomiting, fatigue, weakness; myositis: muscle or bone pain
• Advise patient that urine, feces, saliva, sputum, sweat, tears may be colored red-orange; soft contact lens may become permanently stained
• Caution patients using oral contraceptives to use a nonhormonal method of birth control because rifabutin may decrease efficiency of oral contraceptives

### Evaluation
**Positive therapeutic outcome**
• Decreased symptoms of *M. avium* in patients with HIV

---

**rifampin** (Rx)
(rif´am-pin)
Rifadin, Rimactane, Rofact ✦
*Func. class.:* Antitubercular
*Chem. class.:* Rifamycin B derivative

**Pregnancy category  C**

**Do not confuse:**
rifampin/rifabutin

**Action:** Inhibits DNA-dependent polymerase, decreases replication

**Therapeutic outcome:** Bactericidal against the following organisms: mycobacteria, *Staphylococcus aureus, Haemophilus influenzae, Neisseria meningitidis, Legionella pneumophila*

**Uses:** Pulmonary TB, meningococcal carriers (prevention)

**Dosage and routes**
*Tuberculosis*
*Adult:* PO/**IV** max 600 mg/day as single dose 1 hr before or 2 hr after meals, or 10 mg/kg/day 2-3 ×/wk
*Child >5 yr:* PO/**IV** 10-20 mg/kg/day as single dose 1 hr before or 2 hr after meals, max 600 mg/day, with other antitubercular products

*6-mo regimen:* 2-mo treatment of isoniazid, rifampin, pyrazinamide, and possibly streptomycin or ethambutol; then rifampin and isoniazid × 4 mo

*9-mo regimen:* Rifampin and isoniazid supplemented with pyrazinamide, or streptomycin or ethambutol

*Meningococcal carriers*
*Adult:* PO/**IV** 600 mg bid × 2 days
*Child >5 yr:* PO/**IV** 10-20 mg/kg bid × 2 days, max 600 mg/dose
*Infant 3 mo-1 yr:* PO 5 mg/kg bid for 2 days

*Prevention of* H. influenzae *type B infection*
*Adult:* PO 600 mg/day × 4 days
*Child:* PO 20 mg/kg/day × 4 days

**Available forms:** Caps 150, 300 mg; powder for inj 600 mg/vial

**Adverse effects**
*CNS:* Headache, fatigue, anxiety, drowsiness, confusion
*EENT:* Visual disturbances

*GI:* *Nausea, vomiting, anorexia, diarrhea,* **pseudomembranous colitis,** *heartburn,* sore mouth and tongue, **pancreatitis,** elevated liver function tests
*GU:* **Hematuria, acute renal failure, hemoglobinuria**
*HEMA:* **Hemolytic anemia, eosinophilia, thrombocytopenia, leukopenia**
*INTEG:* Rash, pruritus, urticaria
*MISC:* Flulike syndrome, menstrual disturbances, edema, shortness of breath
*MS:* Ataxia, weakness

**Contraindications:** Hypersensitivity

**Precautions:** Pregnancy **C,** breastfeeding, children <5 yr, hepatic disease, blood dyscrasias

| Pharmacokinetics | |
|---|---|
| **Absorption** | Well absorbed (PO), completely absorbed (**IV**) |
| **Distribution** | Widely distributed, crosses placenta |
| **Metabolism** | Liver—extensively |
| **Excretion** | Feces |
| **Half-life** | 3 hr |

| Pharmacodynamics | | |
|---|---|---|
| | PO | IV |
| **Onset** | Rapid | Rapid |
| **Peak** | 2-3 hr | Inf end |
| **Duration** | Unknown | Unknown |

## Interactions
### Individual drugs
Acetaminophen, alcohol, chloramphenicol, clofibrate, cycloSPORINE, dapsone, digoxin, diltiazem, doxycycline, haloperidol, NIFEdipine, phenytoin, theophylline, verapamil, zidovudine: decreased effect of specific product
Imidazole: decreased antifungal action
Isoniazid: increased hepatotoxicity
Lithium: increased lithium toxicity
Sodium lactate: products are incompatible
### Drug classifications
Anticoagulants: decreased action of anticoagulants
Antidiabetics: decreased action of antidiabetics
Barbiturates: decreased action of barbiturates
Benzodiazepines: decreased action of benzodiazepines
β-blockers: decreased action of β-blockers
Contraceptives (oral), glucocorticoids: decreased effect
Fluroquinolones: decreased action of fluoroquinolones

Hormones: decreased action of hormones
Imidazole antifungals: decreased antifungal action
Sulfonamides: decreased action of sulfonamides
Protease inhibitors: decreased action of protease inhibitors
### Drug/lab test
Interference: folate level, vit $B_{12}$ gallbladder studies, dexamethasone suppression test
False positive: direct Coombs' test

## NURSING CONSIDERATIONS
### Assessment
- Monitor liver function tests qmo: ALT, AST, bilirubin
- Monitor renal status: before, qmo: BUN, creatinine, output, specific gravity, urinalysis
- Monitor mental status: affect, mood, behavioral changes; psychosis may occur
- Monitor hepatic status: decreased appetite, jaundice, dark urine, fatigue
- Assess for infection: sputum culture, lung sounds
- C&S should be performed before beginning treatment, during, and after therapy is completed

### Nursing diagnoses
- Diarrhea (adverse reactions)
- Infection, risk for (uses)
- Injury, risk for (adverse reactions)
- Knowledge, deficient (teaching)
- Noncompliance (teaching)

### Implementation
- Administer with meals to decrease GI symptoms; better to take on empty stomach 1 hr before or 2 hr after meals, with full glass of water

**Intermittent IV route**
- Give by intermittent inf after reconstituting 600 mg/10 ml of sterile water for inj, agitate gently; dilute further in 100 or 500 ml of 0.9% NaCl or $D_5W$; give 100 ml/30 min or 500 ml/3 hr
- Do not mix with other products or sols

### Patient/family education
- Instruct patient that compliance with dosage schedule, duration is necessary
- Instruct patient that scheduled appointments must be kept or relapse may occur
- Instruct patient to notify prescriber if hepatitis, neutropenia, or thrombocytopenia occurs: sore throat, fever, bleeding, bruising, yellow sclera, anorexia, nausea, vomiting, fatigue, weakness

• Advise patient that urine, feces, saliva, sputum, sweat, tears may be colored red-orange; soft contact lens may be permanently stained

• Caution patients using oral contraceptives to use a nonhormonal method of birth control because rifabutin may decrease the efficiency of oral contraceptives

• Advise patient to avoid alcohol, hepatotoxicity may occur

### Evaluation
**Positive therapeutic outcome**
• Decreased symptoms of TB

---

## rifapentine (Rx)
(riff'ah-pen-teen)
Priftin
*Func. class.:* Antitubercular
*Chem. class.:* Rifamycin derivative

**Pregnancy category C**

**Action:** Inhibits DNA-dependent polymerase, decreases tubercule bacilli replication

**Therapeutic outcome:** Resolution of pulmonary TB

**Uses:** Pulmonary TB; must be used with at least one other antitubercular product

### Dosage and routes
*Intensive phase*
**Adult:** PO 600 mg (4 150-mg tabs 2 ×/wk), with an interval of 72 hr between doses × 2 mo; must be given with at least one other antitubercular product

*Continuation phase*
**Adult:** 600 mg qwk × 4 mo in combination with isoniazid or other appropriate antitubercular product

**Available forms:** Tabs 150 mg

### Adverse effects
***CNS:*** Headache, fatigue, anxiety, dizziness
***EENT:*** Visual disturbances
***GI:*** *Nausea, vomiting, anorexia, diarrhea,* bilirubinemia, hepatitis, increased ALT, AST, *heartburn,* **pancreatitis**
***GU:*** **Hematuria,** pyuria, proteinuria, urinary casts, urine discoloration
***HEMA:*** **Thrombocytopenia, leukopenia, neutropenia, lymphopenia,** anemia, **leukocytosis,** purpura, hematoma
***INTEG:*** Rash, pruritus, urticaria, acne
***MISC:*** Edema, aggressive reaction, increased B/P
***MS:*** Gout, arthrosis

**Contraindications:** Hypersensitivity to rifamycins, porphyria

**Precautions:** Pregnancy **C,** breastfeeding, children <12 yr, geriatric, hepatic disease, blood dyscrasias

Pharmacokinetics
Unknown

Pharmacodynamics
Unknown

### Interactions
*Individual drugs*
Amitriptyline, chloramphenicol, clarithromycin, clofibrate, cycloSPORINE, dapsone, delaviridine, diazepam, digoxin, diltiazem, disopyramide, doxycycline, fentanyl, fluconazole, haloperidol, indinavir, itraconazole, ketoconazole, methadone, mexiletine, nelfinavir, NIFEdipine, nortriptyline, phenytoin, quinidine, quinine, ritonavir, saquinavir, sildenafil, tacrolimus, theophylline, tocainide, verapamil, warfarin, zidovudine: decreased action of each specific product

*Drug classifications*
Anticoagulants, antidiabetics, barbiturates, β-adrenergic blockers, corticosteroids, fluoroquinolones, oral contraceptives, phenothiazines, progestins, thyroid preparations: decreased action of each product class
Protease inhibitors: use extreme caution

*Drug/food*
Food: increased absorption with food

*Drug/lab test*
Interference: folate level, vit $B_{12}$

### NURSING CONSIDERATIONS
**Assessment**
• Obtain baselines in CBC, AST, ALT, bilirubin, platelets
• Assess for infection: sputum culture, lung sounds
• Assess signs of anemia: Hct, Hgb, fatigue
• Monitor liver function tests qmo: ALT, AST, bilirubin
• Monitor renal status qmo: BUN, creatinine, output, specific gravity, urinalysis
• Assess hepatic status: decreased appetite, jaundice, dark urine, fatigue

**Nursing diagnoses**
• Diarrhea (side effects)
• Infection, risk for (uses)
• Knowledge, deficient (teaching)
• Noncompliance (teaching)

R

## Implementation
- May be given with food for GI upset
- Give antiemetic if vomiting occurs
- Administer after C&S is completed; qmo to detect resistance

## Patient/family education
- Advise patient that compliance with dosage schedule, duration is necessary
- Instruct patient that scheduled appointments must be kept; relapse may occur
- Teach patient that urine, feces, saliva, sputum, sweat, tears may be colored red-orange; soft contact lenses, dentures may be permanently stained
- Teach patient to use alternative method of contraception; oral contraceptive action may be decreased
- Teach patient to report flulike symptoms: excessive fatigue, anorexia, vomiting, sore throat; unusual bleeding, jaundice of skin, eyes

## Evaluation
**Positive therapeutic outcome**
- Decreased symptoms of TB
- Negative culture

---

## rifaximin (Rx)
(rif-ax′i-min)
Xifaxan
*Func. class:* Misc. antiinfective
*Chem. class:* Analog of rifampin
**Pregnancy category C**

**Action:** Binds to bacterial DNA dependent RNA polymerase, thereby inhibiting bacterial RNA synthesis.

**Therapeutic outcome:** Bacterial action against *E. coli*

**Uses:** Traveler's diarrhea in those ≥12 yr old, caused by *E. coli*

## Dosage and routes
***Adult and child ≥12 yr:*** PO 200 mg tid × 3 days without regard to meals

**Available forms:** Tabs 200 mg

## Adverse effects
***CNS:*** Abnormal dreams, dizziness, insomnia
***GI:*** *Abdominal pain, constipation, defecation urgency, flatulence, nausea, rectal tenesmus,* vomiting
***MISC:*** *Headache, pyrexia*

**Contraindications:** Hypersensitivity, diarrhea with fever, blood in stool

**Precautions:** Pregnancy **C**, breastfeeding, children

### Pharmacokinetics
| | |
|---|---|
| **Absorption** | Unknown |
| **Distribution** | Unknown |
| **Metabolism** | Induces P450 3A4 (CYP3A4) |
| **Excretion** | Feces |
| **Half-life** | 6 hr |

### Pharmacodynamics
Unknown

## Interactions
*Drug/herb*
Acidophilus: do not use with antiinfectives; separate by several hours

## NURSING CONSIDERATIONS
### Assessment
- Assess for GI symptoms: amount and character of diarrhea, abdominal pain, nausea, vomiting
 Assess for overgrowth of infection and pseudomembranous colitis

### Nursing diagnoses
- Infection, risk for (uses)
- Knowledge, deficient (teaching)
- Noncompliance (teaching)

### Implementation
- May be administered without regard to food

### Patient/family education
- Instruct patient to discontinue rifaximin and notify prescriber if diarrhea persists for more than 24-48 hr, if diarrhea worsens, or if blood is in stools and fever is present

### Evaluation
**Positive therapeutic outcome**
- Absence of infection

---

## riluzole (Rx)
(ri-loo′zole)
Rilutek
*Func. class.:* Amyotropic lateral sclerosis (ALS) agent
*Chem. class.:* Benzathiazole
**Pregnancy category C**

**Action:** Unknown; may act by inhibiting glutamate, interfering with binding of amino acid receptors, inactivation of voltage-dependent sodium channels

**Therapeutic outcome:** Decreased symptoms of ALS

---

 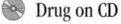

Uses: ALS

## Dosage and routes
*Adult:* PO 50 mg q12hr; take 1 hr before or 2 hr after meals

**Available forms:** Tabs 50 mg

## Adverse effects
*CNS:* Hypertonia, depression, dizziness, insomnia, somnolence, vertigo, paresthesia
*CV:* Hypertension, tachycardia, phlebitis, palpitation, postural hypertension
*GI:* Nausea, vomiting, dyspepsia, anorexia, diarrhea, flatulence, stomatitis, dry mouth, increased liver function tests, jaundice, abdominal pain
*GU:* UTI, dysuria
***HEMA:* Neutropenia**
*INTEG:* Pruritus, eczema, alopecia, **exfoliative dermatitis**
*MS:* Arthralgia
*RESP:* Decreased lung function; rhinitis, increased cough, pneumonia

**Contraindications:** Hypersensitivity

**Precautions:** Pregnancy **C**, breastfeeding, children, geriatric, neutropenia, renal/hepatic disease, cigarette smoking, febrile illness, pneumonia

### Pharmacokinetics
| | |
|---|---|
| **Absorption** | Well |
| **Distribution** | Unknown |
| **Metabolism** | Extensively—live |
| **Excretion** | Urine, feces |
| **Half-life** | Unknown |

### Pharmacodynamics
Unknown

## Interactions
*Individual drugs*
Allopurinol, leflunomide, methotrexate, methyldopa, sulfasalazine, tacrine: increased hepatic injury
Amitriptyline, caffeine, theophylline: decreased elimination of riluzole
Carbamazepine: increased liver function tests
Cigarette smoke, omeprazole, rifampin: increased elimination of riluzole
*Drug classifications*
Barbiturates: increased liver function tests
Quinolones: decreased elimination of riluzole
*Drug/food*
Charcoal-broiled foods: increased elimination of riluzole
High-fat meal: decreased absorption

## NURSING CONSIDERATIONS
### Assessment
• Assess for clinical improvement
• Monitor liver function tests: AST, ALT, bilirubin, GGT, baseline and qmo × 3 mo, then q3 mo
• Assess for neutropenia (neutrophils <500/mm$^3$)

### Nursing diagnoses
• Knowledge, deficient (teaching)
• Mobility, impaired physical (uses)

### Implementation
• Give 1 hr before or 2 hr after meals; a high-fat meal decreases absorption

### Patient/family education
• Advise to report febrile illness, may indicate neutropenia; cardiac/respiratory changes
• Teach reason for product and expected results

### Evaluation
**Positive therapeutic outcome**
• Decreasing symptoms of ALS

---

## rimantadine (Rx)
(ri-man'ti-deen)
Flumadine
*Func. class.:* Synthetic antiviral
*Chem. class.:* Tricyclic amine
**Pregnancy category C**

**Do not confuse:**
rimantadine/amantadine/ranitidine

**Action:** Prevents uncoating of nucleic acid in viral cell, preventing penetration of virus to host; causes release of dopamine from neurons

**Therapeutic outcome:** Prevention of influenza type A

**Uses:** Prophylaxis or treatment of influenza type A

## Dosage and routes
*Renal/hepatic dose*
Reduce as needed

*Influenza type A prophylaxis*
*Adult and child 1-10 yr:* PO 100 mg bid; in renal/hepatic disease, lower dose to 100 mg/day
*Child 1-10 yr:* PO 5 mg/kg/day, max 150 mg

R

Adverse effects: *italic* = common, **bold** = life-threatening

## Treatment

**Adult:** PO 100 mg bid; in renal/hepatic disease, lower dose to 100 mg/day; start treatment at onset of symptoms, continue for at least 1 wk

**Geriatric:** PO 100 mg/day × 5-7 days

**Available forms:** Tabs 100 mg; syr 50 mg/5 ml

## Adverse effects

*CNS:* *Headache, dizziness,* fatigue, depression, hallucinations, tremors, **seizures,** insomnia, poor concentration, asthenia, gait abnormalities, anxiety, confusion
*CV:* Pallor, palpitations, edema
*EENT:* Tinnitus, taste abnormality, eye pain
*GI:* *Nausea, vomiting,* constipation, *dry mouth, anorexia, abdominal pain, diarrhea,* dyspepsia
*INTEG:* Rash

**Contraindications:** Hypersensitivity to products of adamantine class (this product, amantadine)

**Precautions:** Pregnancy **C**, breastfeeding, children <1 yr, epilepsy, renal/hepatic disease

### Pharmacokinetics

| | |
|---|---|
| **Absorption** | Minimally absorbed (PO) |
| **Distribution** | Widely distributed, crosses placenta, CSF concentration 50% plasma |
| **Metabolism** | Liver |
| **Excretion** | 95% unchanged—kidneys |
| **Half-life** | 13-65 hr, increased in renal disease |

### Pharmacodynamics

| | PO |
|---|---|
| **Onset** | Unknown |
| **Peak** | 1½-2½ |
| **Duration** | Unknown |

## Interactions
### Individual drugs

Acetaminophen, aspirin, intranasal influenza vaccine: decreased peak concentration of rimantadine
Cimetidine: increased rimantidine concentration

## NURSING CONSIDERATIONS
### Assessment

• Assess for seizures; if seizures occur, product should be discontinued
• Assess allergies before initiation of treatment, patient's reaction to each medication; list allergies on chart

• Monitor respiratory status: rate, character, wheezing, tightness in chest

### Nursing diagnoses

• Infection, risk for (uses)
• Knowledge, deficient (teaching)

### Implementation

• Give before exposure to influenza; continue for 10 days after contact
• Give at least 4 hr before bedtime to prevent insomnia
• Administer after meals for better absorption, to decrease GI symptoms; cap may be opened and mixed with food for easy swallowing
• Give in divided doses to prevent CNS disturbances: headache, dizziness, fatigue, drowsiness
• Store in airtight, dry container

### Patient/family education

• Instruct patient about aspects of product therapy: need to report dyspnea, dizziness, poor concentration, behavioral changes
• Advise patient to avoid hazardous activities if dizziness occurs
• Caution patient to consult prescriber before taking OTC medications, alcohol; serious product interactions may result

### Evaluation
**Positive therapeutic outcome**

• Absence of fever, malaise, cough, dyspnea

---

### rimexolone ophthalmic
*See Appendix D*

---

### risedronate (Rx)
(rih-sed'roh-nate)
Actonel
*Func. class:* Bone resorption inhibitor
*Chem. class.:* Bisphosphonate

**Pregnancy category C**

**Action:** Inhibits bone resorption; absorbs calcium phosphate crystal in bone and may directly block dissolution of hydroxyapatite crystals of bone

**Therapeutic outcome:** Increased bone mass, activity without fractures

**Uses:** Paget's disease; prevention, treatment of osteoporosis in postmenopausal women; glucocorticoid-induced osteoporosis; osteoporosis in men

---

## Dosage and routes
### Paget's disease
*Adult:* PO 30 mg/day × 2 mo; give calcium and vit D if dietary intake is lacking; if relapse occurs, retreatment is advised

### Postmenopausal osteoporosis/glucocorticoid-induced osteoporosis
*Adult:* PO 35 mg qwk (postmenopausal osteoporosis) or 5 mg/day

### Osteoporosis in men
*Adult:* PO 35 mg q wk

**Available forms:** Tabs 5, 30, 35 mg

### Adverse effects
*CNS:* Dizziness, headache, depression
*CV:* Chest pain, hypertension
*GI:* *Abdominal pain, anorexia,* diarrhea, *nausea,* constipation
*MS:* *Bone pain,* arthralgia, osteonecrosis of the jaw
*MISC:* Rash, UTI, pharyngitis, hypocalcemia, hypophosphatemia, increased PTH

**Contraindications:** Hypersensitivity to bisphosphonates, inability to stand or sit upright for ≥30 min

**Precautions:** Pregnancy **C**, breastfeeding, children, renal disease, active upper GI disorders

### Pharmacokinetics
| | |
|---|---|
| **Absorption** | Unknown |
| **Distribution** | To bones |
| **Metabolism** | Unknown |
| **Excretion** | Kidneys |
| **Half-life** | Unknown |

### Pharmacodynamics
Unknown

### Interactions
#### Drug classifications
Antacids, calcium, iron, magnesium salts: decreased absorption of risedronate
NSAIDs, salicylates: increased GI irritation
#### Drug/food
Food: decreased bioavailability; take ½ hr before food or drinks other than water
#### Drug/lab test
Increased: bone imaging agents

### NURSING CONSIDERATIONS
#### Assessment
• Assess for symptoms of Paget's disease: headache, bone pain, increased head circumference

• Monitor phosphate, alkaline phosphatase, calcium; creatinine, BUN (renal disease)
• Assess for hypercalcemia: paresthesia, twitching, laryngospasm, Chvostek's/Trousseau's signs

#### Nursing diagnoses
• Knowledge, deficient (teaching)
• Mobility, impaired physical (uses)
• Nutrition: less than body requirements, imbalanced (uses)

#### Implementation
• Give PO for 2 mo to be effective in Paget's disease
• Give with a full glass of water; patient should be in upright position
• Administer supplemental calcium and vit D in Paget's disease
• Give daily ≥30 min before meals
• Store in cool environment, out of direct sunlight

#### Patient/family education
• Advise patient to sit upright for ½ hr after dose to prevent irritation
• Instruct patient to comply with dietary restrictions
• Advise patient to notify prescriber if pregnancy is planned or suspected

#### Evaluation
**Positive therapeutic outcome**
• Increased bone mass, absence of fractures

## risperidone (Rx)
(res-pare'a-done)
Risperdal, Risperdal M-TAB
*Func. class:* Antipsychotic
*Chem. class.:* Benzisoxazole derivative
**Pregnancy category C**

R

**Do not confuse:**
Risperdal/reserpine

**Action:** Unknown; may be mediated through both dopamine type 2 ($D_2$) and serotonin type 2 (5-$HT_2$) antagonism

**Therapeutic outcome:** Decreased hallucinations and disorganized thought

**Uses:** Psychotic disorders, irritability associated with autism

### Dosage and routes
*Adult:* PO 1 mg bid, with incremental increases of 1 mg bid on days 2 and 3 to a dose of 3 mg bid by day 3, then do not increase dose for at least 1 wk; IM 25 mg q2 wk, may increase to max 50 mg q2 wk

Adverse effects: *italic* = common, **bold** = life-threatening

*Geriatric:* PO 0.5 mg daily-bid increase by 1 mg qwk

*Hepatic dose/renal dose*
*Adult:* PO 0.5 mg, increase by 0.5 mg bid, then increase to 1.5 mg bid

**Available forms:** Tabs 0.25, 0.5, 1, 2, 3, 4 mg; oral sol 1 mg/ml; orally disintegrating tabs 0.5, 1, 2, 3, 4 mg; oral sol 1 mg/ml (30 ml); long-acting inj kit (Risperdal Consta) 12.5, 25, 37.5, 50 mg

**Adverse effects**
*CNS: EPS (pseudoparkinsonism, akathisia, dystonia, tardive dyskinesia), drowsiness, insomnia, agitation, anxiety, headache,* **neuroleptic malignant syndrome,** dizziness, **seizures**
*CV:* Orthostatic hypotension, **tachycardia, heart failure, sudden death (geriatric)**
*EENT:* Blurred vision
*GI: Nausea,* vomiting, *anorexia, constipation,* jaundice, weight gain
*GU:* Hyperprolactinemia, gynecomastia
*MISC:* **Renal artery disease**
*RESP:* Rhinitis, **fatal pneumonia (geriatric)**

**Contraindications:** Breastfeeding, hypersensitivity, seizure disorders

**Precautions:** Pregnancy **C,** children, geriatric, renal/hepatic disease, breast cancer, Parkinson's disease, dementia with Lewy bodies

| Pharmacokinetics | |
| --- | --- |
| **Absorption** | Unknown |
| **Distribution** | Unknown |
| **Metabolism** | Liver, extensively |
| **Excretion** | Urine 90% |
| **Half-life** | 3-24 hr |

| Pharmacodynamics | |
| --- | --- |
| **Onset** | Unknown |
| **Peak** | 1-2 hr |
| **Duration** | Up to 12 hr |

**Interactions**
*Individual drugs*
Alcohol: increased sedation
◆Bepridil, chloroquine, clarithromycin, droperidol, erythromycin, grepafloxacin, halofantrine, haloperidol, methadone, pentamidine, probucol, sparfloxacin: increased QT prolongation
Carbamazepine: increased risperidone excretion

◆Furosemide: possible death in dementia-related psychosis
Levodopa: decreased levodopa effect
*Drug classifications*
Antipsychotics: increased EPS
◆β-agonists, class IA/III antidysrhythmics, local anesthetics, some phenothiazines, tricyclics: increased QT prolongation
CNS depressants: increased sedation
CYP2D6 inducers (carbamazepine, barbiturates, phenytoin, rifampin): decreased risperidone action
CYP2D6 inhibitors (selective serotonin reuptake inhibitors): increased EPS
*Drug/herb*
Betel palm, kava: increased EPS
Cola tree, hops, nettle, nutmeg: increased action
Kava: increased CNS depression
*Drug/lab test*
Increased: prolactin levels

**NURSING CONSIDERATIONS**
**Assessment**
• Assess mental status: orientation, mood, behavior, presence and type of hallucinations before initial administration and monthly; this product should significantly reduce psychotic behavior
• Check that patient swallows all PO medication; check for hoarding or giving of medication to other patients
• Monitor I&O ratio, palpate bladder if low urinary output occurs, especially in geriatric; urinalysis recommended before, during prolonged therapy
• Monitor bilirubin, CBC, liver function tests monthly
• Assess affect, orientation, LOC, reflexes, gait, coordination, sleep pattern disturbances
• Monitor B/P with patient in sitting, standing, and lying positions; take pulse and respirations q4hr during initial treatment; establish baseline before starting treatment; report drops of 30 mm Hg; obtain baseline ECG and monitor Q- and T-wave changes
• Check for dizziness, faintness, palpitations, tachycardia on rising; severe orthostatic hypotension is common
◆ Identify for neuroleptic malignant syndrome: hyperpyrexia, muscle rigidity, increased CPK, altered mental status; product should be discontinued
• Assess for EPS including akathisia (inability to sit still, no pattern to movements), tardive dyskinesia (bizarre movements of the jaw, mouth, tongue, extremities), pseudoparkinsonism (rigidity, tremors, pill rolling, shuffling

gait); an antiparkinsonian product should be prescribed
• Assess for constipation, urinary retention daily; if these occur, increase bulk, water in diet

### Nursing diagnoses
• Coping, ineffective (uses)
• Knowledge, deficient (teaching)
• Noncompliance (teaching)
• Thought processes, disturbed (uses)

### Implementation
**PO route**
• Give with full glass of water, milk; or give with food to decrease GI upset
• Do not open blister pack or orally disintegrating tabs until ready to use; tear one of the four units apart at perforation; bend corner where indicated; peel back foil; do not push tab through foil; remove from pack and place on tongue; tab disintegrates in seconds and can be swallowed with or without liquids
• Store in airtight, light-resistant container
**IM route**
• Only use provided diluent and needle; do not substitute
• Do not give **IV**
• Inject deeply in large muscle mass
• Store unopened vials in refrigerator; protect from light; do not freeze
• Patient should lie down 30 min after IM inj

### Patient/family education
• Teach patient to use good oral hygiene; frequent rinsing of mouth, sugarless gum for dry mouth
• Caution patient to avoid hazardous activities until product response is determined; dizziness, blurred vision may occur
• Inform patient that orthostatic hypotension occurs often; patient should rise from sitting or lying position gradually and remain lying down for at least 30 min after IM inj
• Instruct patient to avoid hot tubs, hot showers, tub baths; hypotension may occur
• Inform patient that heat stroke may occur in hot weather, and to take extra precautions to stay cool
• Advise patient to avoid abrupt withdrawal of this product, or EPS may result; product should be withdrawn slowly
• Teach patient to avoid OTC preparations (cough, hay fever, cold) unless approved by prescriber; serious product interactions may occur; avoid use with alcohol, CNS depressants because increased drowsiness may occur
• Advise patient to use contraception, to inform prescriber if pregnancy is planned or suspected

### Evaluation
**Positive therapeutic outcome**
• Decrease in emotional excitement, hallucinations, delusions, paranoia
• Reorganization of patterns of thought, speech

**Treatment of overdose:** Lavage, provide airway

### ritonavir (Rx)
(ri-toe′na-veer)
Norvir
*Func. class.:* Antiretroviral
*Chem. class.:* Protease inhibitor
**Pregnancy category B**

**Do not confuse:**
ritonavir/retrovir

**Action:** Inhibits HIV-1 protease and prevents maturation of the infectious virus

**Therapeutic outcome:** Improvement of HIV-1 infection

**Uses:** HIV-1 in combination with other antiretrovirals

### Dosage and routes
*Adult:* PO 600 mg bid; if nausea occurs, begin dose at ½ and gradually increase
*Child 2-16 yr:* PO 400 mg/m$^2$ bid up to 1200 mg/day

**Available forms:** Caps 100 mg; oral sol 80 mg/ml

### Adverse effects
*CNS:* Paresthesia, headache, **seizures**, dizziness, insomnia, headache, fever
*GI: Diarrhea,* buccal mucosa ulceration, abdominal pain, *nausea,* taste perversion, dry mouth, vomiting, anorexia
*INTEG:* Rash
*MISC:* Asthenia, **angioedema, anaphylaxis, Stevens-Johnson syndrome,** increased lipids, lipodystrophy
*MS:* Pain

**Contraindications:** Hypersensitivity

**Precautions:** Pregnancy **B**, breastfeeding, children, liver disease, pancreatitis, diabetes, hemophilia

| Pharmacokinetics | |
|---|---|
| Absorption | Well |
| Distribution | Unknown |
| Metabolism | 98% protein binding, liver |
| Excretion | Unknown |
| Half-life | 3-5 hr |

Adverse effects: *italic* = common, **bold** = life-threatening

| Pharmacodynamics | |
|---|---|
| **Onset** | Unknown |
| **Peak** | 2-4 hr |
| **Duration** | Unknown |

## Interactions
### Individual drugs
Amiodarone, bepridil, buPROPion, clozapine, desipramine, dihydroergotamine, encainide, ergotamine, flecainide, meperedine, midazolam, pimozide, piroxicam, propafenone, propoxyphene, quinidine, saquinavir, terfenadine, triazolam, zolpidem: toxicity, do not use together

Atovaquone: decreased levels of atovaquone

Clarithromycin: increased level of both products

ddI: increased levels of ritonavir

Fluconazole: increased ritonavir level

Divalproex: decreased levels of divalproex

Ethinyl estradiol: decreased levels of ethinyl estradiol

Lamotrigine: decreased levels of lamotrigine

Nevirapine, phenytoin: decreased ritonavir levels

Phenytoin: decreased levels of phenytoin

Sulfamethoxazole: decreased levels of sulfamethoxazole

Theophylline: decreased levels of theophylline

Zidovudine: decreased levels of zidovudine

### Drug classifications
Anticoagulants: decreased levels of anticoagulants

Azole antifungals, benzodiazepines, HMG-CoA reductase inhibitors, interleukins: toxicity, do not use together

Barbiturates, rifamycins: decreased ritonavir level

### Drug/herb
St. John's wort: decreased ritonavir levels, avoid concurrent use

### Drug/lab test
Increased: ALT, GGT, AST, CPK, cholesterol, triglycerides, uric acid

Decreased: Hct, RBC, Hgb, neutrophils, WBC

## NURSING CONSIDERATIONS
### Assessment
- Assess signs of infection, anemia
- Monitor viral load and CD4 baseline and throughout therapy
- Assess liver function tests: ALT, AST
- Monitor C&S before product therapy; product may be taken as soon as culture is done; repeat C&S after treatment; determine the presence of other STDs
- Assess bowel pattern before, during treatment; if severe abdominal pain with bleeding occurs, product should be discontinued; monitor hydration
- Assess skin eruptions, rash
- Assess allergies before treatment, reaction to each medication; place allergies on chart

### Nursing diagnoses
- Infection, risk for (uses)
- Knowledge, deficient (teaching)

### Implementation
- Administer with food at equal intervals around the clock
- Mix oral powder with high-calorie drink
- Store caps in refrigerator

### Patient/family education
- Teach patient to take as prescribed; if dose is missed, take as soon as remembered up to 1 hr before next dose; do not double dose
- Teach patient that product must be taken in equal intervals around the clock to maintain blood levels for duration of therapy
- Teach patient that product is not a cure for HIV; opportunistic infections may continue to be acquired, and others may continue to contract HIV from the patient
- Advise patient not to use St. John's wort, that it decreases this product's effect
- Inform that redistribution of body fat or accumulation of body fat may occur

### Evaluation
**Positive therapeutic outcome**
- Decreasing symptoms of HIV
- Improving viral load and CD4 cell counts

## rituximab (Rx)
(rih-tuks'ih-mab)
Rituxan
*Func. class.:* Antineoplastic—miscellaneous; DMARDs
*Chem. class.:* Murine/human monoclonal antibody

### Pregnancy category C

**Action:** Directed against the CD20 antigen that is found on malignant B lymphocytes; CD20 regulates a portion of cell cycle initiation/differentiation

**Therapeutic outcome:** Decreased tumor size, prevention of spread of cancer

**Uses:** Non-Hodgkin's lymphoma (CD20 positive, B-cell), bulky disease (tumors >10 cm)

### Dosage and routes
*Adult:* **IV** INF 375 mg/m$^2$ qwk × 4 doses; give at 50 mg/hr for 1st inf; if hypersensitivity

does not occur, increase rate by 50 mg/hr q½hr, max 400 mg/hr; slow/interrupt INF if hypersensitivity occurs; other inf can be given at 100 mg/hr and increased by 100 mg/hr, max 400 mg/hr

**Available forms:** Inj 10 mg/ml

## Adverse effects

*CNS:* **Life-threatening brain infection**
*CV:* **Cardiac dysrhythmias, heart failure, MI, superventricular tachycardia, hypertension**
*GI: Nausea, vomiting, anorexia,* **GI obstruction/perforation**
*GU:* **Renal failure**
*HEMA:* **Leukopenia, neutropenia, thrombocytopenia**
*INTEG: Irritation at inj site, rash,* **fatal mucocutaneous infections (rare)**
*MISC:* Fever, chills, asthenia, headache, **angioedema,** hypotension, myalgia, bronchospasm, ARDs
*SYST:* **Stevens-Johnson syndrome, exfoliative dermatitis, toxic epidermal necrolysis, tumor lysis syndrome**

**Contraindications:** Hypersensitivity, murine proteins

**Precautions:** Pregnancy **C,** breastfeeding, children, geriatric, cardiac/renal/pulmonary conditions

### Pharmacokinetics

| | |
|---|---|
| **Absorption** | Unknown |
| **Distribution** | Unknown |
| **Metabolism** | Unknown |
| **Excretion** | Unknown |
| **Half-life** | 31-152 hr |

### Pharmacodynamics

Unknown

## Interactions
*Drug classifications*
Anticoagulants, NSAIDs: increased bleeding risk

## NURSING CONSIDERATIONS
### Assessment
◆ Assess for signs of fatal infusion reaction: hypoxia, pulmonary infiltrates, ARDS, MI, ventricular fibrillation, cardiogenic shock; most fatal infusion reactions occur with first INF, discontinue product
◆ Assess for signs of severe mucocutaneous reactions: Stevens-Johnson syndrome, lichenoid dermatitis, toxic epidermal lysis; signs occur 1-13 wk after product was given

◆ Assess for tumor lysis syndrome: acute renal failure requiring hemodialysis, hyperkalemia, hypocalcemia, hyperuricemia, hyperphosphatasemia
• Monitor CBC, differential, platelet count weekly; withhold product if WBC is <3500/mm$^3$, or platelet count <100,000/mm$^3$; notify prescriber of these results; product should be discontinued
• Assess GI symptoms: frequency of stools
• Assess signs of dehydration: rapid respirations, poor skin turgor, decreased urine output, dry skin, restlessness, weakness

### Nursing diagnoses
• Injury, risk for (side effects)
• Knowledge, deficient (teaching)

### Implementation
**IV route**
• Hold antihypertensive 2 hr prior to administration
• Administer after diluting to a final conc of 1-4 mg/ml; use 0.9% NaCl, D$_5$W, gently invert bag to mix; do not mix with other products
• Increase fluid intake to 2-3 L/day to prevent dehydration, unless contraindicated
• Provide nutritious diet with iron, vitamin supplement, low fiber, few dairy products
• Store vials at 36°-40° F, protect vials from direct sunlight, inf sol is stable at 36°-46° F × 24 hr and room temperature for another 12 hr

### Patient/family education
• Teach patient to report adverse reactions
• Advise to avoid OTC products

### Evaluation
**Positive therapeutic outcome**
• Prevention of increasing cancer progression

## rivastigmine (Rx)   R
(riv-as-tig′mine)
Exelon, Exelon Patch
*Func. class.:* Anti-Alzheimer's agent
*Chem. class.:* Cholinesterase inhibitor
**Pregnancy category B**

**Action:** May enhance cholinergic functioning by increasing acetylcholine

**Therapeutic outcome:** Decreased signs and symptoms of Alzheimer's dementia

**Uses:** Mild-moderate Alzheimer's dementia, dementia associated with Parkinson's disease

### Dosage and routes
*Adult:* PO 1.5 mg bid for 2 wk or more, may increase to 3 mg bid after 2 wk or more; may increase to 4.5 mg bid and thereafter 6 mg

Adverse effects: *italic* = common, **bold** = life-threatening

bid, max 12 mg/day; TRANSDERMAL apply 4.6 mg/24 hr after 4 wk or more, may increase to 9.6 mg/24 hr

**Available forms:** Caps 1.5, 3, 4.5, 6 mg; sol 2 mg/ml; transdermal patch 4.6, 9.6 mg/24 hr

### Adverse effects

***CNS:*** *Tremors, confusion, insomnia,* psychosis, hallucination, depression, dizziness, headache, anxiety, somnolence, fatigue, syncope, EPS, exacerbation of Parkinson's disease

***GI:*** *Nausea, vomiting, anorexia, abdominal distress, flatulence,* diarrhea, constipation, dyspepsia

***MISC:*** UTI, asthenia, increased sweating, hypertension, influenza-like syncope, weight change

**Contraindications:** Hypersensitivity to this product, other carbamates; angle-closure glaucoma, undiagnosed skin lesions

**Precautions:** Pregnancy **B**, breastfeeding, children, renal/hepatic/respiratory disease, seizure disorder, asthma, urinary obstruction, peptic ulcer

### Pharmacokinetics

| | |
|---|---|
| **Absorption** | Rapidly, completely |
| **Distribution** | Not known |
| **Metabolism** | To decarbamylated metabolite |
| **Excretion** | Kidney—metabolites, clearance lowered in geriatric, hepatic disease, increased nicotine use |
| **Half-life** | 1½ hr |

### Pharmacodynamics

Unknown

### Interactions
***Individual drugs***

Nicotine: increased metabolism, decreased blood level of rivastigmine

***Drug classifications***

Cholinesterase inhibitors: increased synergistic effect

***Drug/herb***

Pill-bearing spurge: increased effect

### NURSING CONSIDERATIONS
**Assessment**

• Monitor liver function tests: AST, ALT, alkaline phosphatase, LDH, bilirubin, CBC
• Assess for severe GI effects: nausea, vomiting, anorexia, weight loss
• Monitor B/P, respiration during initial treatment; hypo/hypertension should be reported
• Assess mental status: affect, mood, behavioral changes, depression; complete suicide assessment

### Nursing diagnoses
• Knowledge, deficient (teaching)

### Implementation
• Give with meals; take with AM and PM meal even though absorption may be decreased
• Provide assistance with ambulation during beginning therapy
• Discontinue treatment for several doses and restart at same or next lower dosage level if adverse reactions cause intolerance
• If treatment is interrupted for longer than several days treatment should be initiated with the lowest daily dose and titrated as indicated above

**Transdermal route**
• Apply to clean, hairless, dry skin; not in an area that clothing will rub; rotate sites daily; remove liner; apply firmly; may be used during water activities; avoid saunas

### Patient/family education
• Teach patient procedure for giving oral sol; use instruction sheet provided
• Teach patient to notify prescriber of severe GI effects
• Teach patient that product may cause dizziness, anorexia, weight loss

### Evaluation
**Positive therapeutic outcome**
• Increased coherence, decreased symptoms of Alzheimer's disease

---

## rizatriptan (Rx)
(rye-zah-trip′tan)
Maxalt, Maxalt-MLT
*Func. class.:* Migraine agent
*Chem. class.:* 5-HT₁-like receptor agonist

**Pregnancy category C**

**Action:** Binds selectively to the vascular serotonin type 1 (5-HT₁) receptor, exerts antimigraine effect; causes vasoconstriction in cranial arteries

**Therapeutic outcome:** After treatment, relief of migraine

**Uses:** Acute treatment of migraine

### Dosage and routes
***Adult:*** **PO** 5-10 mg single dose, redosing separate by 2 hr or more; max 30 mg/24 hr,

use 5 mg in patient on propanolol; max 15 mg/24 hr

**Available forms:** Tabs (Maxalt) 5, 10 mg; orally disintegrating tabs (Maxalt-MLT) 2.5, 5, 10 mg

**Adverse effects**

*CNS: Dizziness,* drowsiness, *headache, fatigue,* warm/cold sensation, flushing
*CV:* **MI, ventricular fibrillation, ventricular tachycardia, coronary artery vasospasm**
*ENDO:* Hot flashes, mild increase in growth hormone
*GI: Nausea,* dry mouth, diarrhea, abdominal pain
*RESP:* Chest tightness, pressure, dyspnea

**Contraindications:** Angina pectoris, history of MI, documented silent ischemia, Prinzmetal's angina, ischemic heart disease, concurrent ergotamine-containing preparations, uncontrolled hypertension, hypersensitivity, basilar or hemiplegic migraine

**Precautions:** Pregnancy **C**, breastfeeding, children, postmenopausal women, men >40 yr, geriatric, risk factors for CAD, hypercholesterolemia, obesity, diabetes, impaired renal/hepatic function

| Pharmacokinetics | |
|---|---|
| **Absorption** | Unknown |
| **Distribution** | Unknown |
| **Metabolism** | Liver (metabolite) |
| **Excretion** | Urine/feces |
| **Half-life** | 2-3 hr |

| Pharmacodynamics | |
|---|---|
| **Onset** | 10 min-2 hr |
| **Peak** | Unknown |
| **Duration** | Unknown |

**Interactions**
*Individual drugs*
Cimetidine, isocarboxazide, pargyline, phenelzine, propranolol, trancyclomine: increased rizatriptan action
Ergot: increased vasospastic effects
Sibutramine: increased levels of sibutramine
*Drug classifications*
Contraceptives (oral), MAOIs, MAOIs (nonselective types A and B): increased rizatriptan action
Ergot derivatives, 5-HT$_1$ receptor agonists: increased vasospastic effects
Selective serotonin reuptake inhibitors: increased weakness, hyperreflexia, incoordination

*Drug/herb*
SAM-e, St. John's wort: serotonin syndrome
Butterbur, feverfew: increased effect

**NURSING CONSIDERATIONS**
**Assessment**
• Assess for stress level, activity, recreation, coping mechanisms
• Assess neurologic status: LOC, blurring vision, nausea, vomiting, tingling in extremities preceding headache
• Monitor for ingestion of tyramine-containing foods (pickled products, beer, wine, aged cheese), food additives, preservatives, colorings, artificial sweeteners, chocolate, caffeine, which may precipitate these types of headaches

**Nursing diagnoses**
• Knowledge, deficient (teaching)
• Pain, acute (uses)

**Implementation**
• Provide quiet, calm environment with decreased stimulation for noise, bright light, excessive talking
• Do not open blister pack until ready to use
• Put orally disintegrating tab on tongue to dissolve; swallow with saliva

**Patient/family education**
• Teach patient use of orally disintegrating tab: instruct patient not to open blister until use, to peel blister open with dry hands, to place tab on tongue, where it will dissolve, and to swallow with saliva (contains phenylalanine)
• Advise patient to report any side effects to prescriber
• Advise patient to use alternate contraception while taking product if oral contraceptives are being used

**Evaluation**
**Positive therapeutic outcome**
• Decrease in frequency, severity of headache

**ropinirole** (Rx)
(roe-pin'e-role)
Requip
*Func. class.:* Antiparkinsonian agent
*Chem. class.:* Dopamine-receptor agonist, nonergot

**Pregnancy category** C

**Action:** Selective agonist for dopamine D$_2$ receptors (presynaptic/postsynaptic sites); binding at D$_3$ receptor contributes to antiparkinson effects

**Therapeutic outcome:** Decreased symptoms of Parkinson's disease (involuntary movements)

**Uses:** Parkinsonism, restless leg syndrome

## Dosage and routes
*Adult:* PO 0.25 mg tid, titrate weekly to max of 24 mg/day

### Restless leg syndrome
*Adult:* PO 0.25 mg at bedtime, may increase until symptoms resolve

**Available forms:** Tabs 0.25, 0.5, 1, 2, 3, 4, 5 mg

## Adverse effects
*CNS:* Dystonia, *agitation, insomnia,* dizziness, psychosis, hallucinations, depression, somnolence, **sleep attacks**
*CV: Orthostatic hypotension,* hypotension, syncope, palpitations, **tachycardia,** hypertension
*EENT:* Blurred vision
*GI: Nausea, vomiting, anorexia, dry mouth,* constipation, dyspepsia, flatulence
*GU:* Impotence, urinary frequency
*HEMA:* **Hemolytic anemia, leukopenia, agranulocytosis**
*INTEG:* Rash, sweating
*RESP:* Pharyngitis, rhinitis, sinusitis, bronchitis, dyspnea

**Contraindications:** Hypersensitivity

**Precautions:** Pregnancy **C,** cardiac/renal/hepatic disease, dysrhythmias, affective disorders, psychosis

| Pharmacokinetics | |
|---|---|
| **Absorption** | Well absorbed |
| **Distribution** | Widely distributed |
| **Metabolism** | Liver, extensively by the liver by CYP450 CYP1A2 enzyme system |
| **Excretion** | Kidneys |
| **Half-life** | 6 hr |

| Pharmacodynamics | |
|---|---|
| Unknown | |

## Interactions
### Individual drugs
Cimetidine, ciprofloxacin, digoxin, diltiazem, enoxacin, erythromycin, fluvoxamine, levodopa, mexiletine, norfloxacin, tacrine, theophylline: increased effect of ropinirole
Metoclopramide: decreased ropinirole effect
### Drug classifications
Butyrophenones, phenothiazines, thioxanthenes: decreased ropinirole effect

### Drug/herb
Chaste tree fruit, kava: decreased ropinirole action

## NURSING CONSIDERATIONS
### Assessment
• Monitor B/P, respiration during initial treatment; hypotension or hypertension should be reported
• Assess mental status: affect, mood, behavioral changes, depression; complete suicide assessment
• Assess for involuntary movements in parkinsonism: akinesia, tremors, staggering gait, muscle rigidity, drooling; these symptoms should improve with therapy
 Assess for sleep attacks, drowsiness, falling asleep without warning even during hazardous activities

### Nursing diagnoses
• Injury, risk for (uses)
• Knowledge, deficient (teaching)
• Mobility, impaired physical (uses)
• Noncompliance (teaching)

### Implementation
• Give product until NPO before surgery
• Adjust dosage to patient response
• Give with meals to decrease GI upset

### Patient/family education
• Advise patient that therapeutic effects may take several wk to a few mo
• Caution patient to change positions slowly to prevent orthostatic hypotension
• Instruct patient to use product exactly as prescribed; if product is discontinued abruptly, parkinsonian crisis may occur

### Evaluation
**Positive therapeutic outcome**
• Decreased akathisia, other involuntary movements
• Increased mood

## ropivacaine (Rx)
(roe-pi'va-kane)
Naropin
*Func. class.:* Local anesthetic
*Chem. class.:* Amide
**Pregnancy category B**

**Action:** Competes with calcium for sites in nerve membrane that control sodium transport across cell membrane; decreases rise of depolarization phase of action potential

**Therapeutic outcome:** Maintenance of local anesthesia

 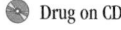

**Uses:** Peripheral nerve block, caudal anesthesia, central neural block, vaginal, epidural, spinal block

## Dosage and routes
*Lumbar epidural block for C-section*
*Adult:* 20-30 ml of 0.5% sol, or 15-20 ml of 0.75% sol

*Thoracic epidural*
*Adult:* 5-15 ml of 0.5%-0.75% sol

*Major nerve block*
*Adult:* 35-50 ml of 0.5% sol or 10-40 ml of 0.75% sol

*Labor pain epidural*
*Adult:* 10-20 ml of 0.2% sol, then 6-14 ml/hr

*Postoperative (lumbar/thoracic epidural)*
*Adult:* 6-14 ml/hr of 0.2% sol

*Infiltration/minor nerve block*
*Adult:* 1-100 ml of 0.2% sol or 1-40 ml of 0.5% sol

**Available forms:** Inj 2, 5, 7.5 mg/ml

## Adverse effects
*CNS:* Anxiety, restlessness, **seizures, loss of consciousness,** drowsiness, disorientation, tremors, shivering, paresthesia
*CV:* **Myocardial depression, cardiac arrest, dysrhythmias,** bradycardia, hypo/hypertension, **fetal bradycardia**
*EENT:* Blurred vision, tinnitus, pupil constriction
*ENDO:* Hypokalemia
*GI:* Nausea, vomiting
*GU:* Urinary retention
*INTEG:* Rash, urticaria, allergic reactions, edema, burning, skin discoloration at injection site, tissue necrosis
*RESP:* **Status asthmaticus, respiratory arrest, anaphylaxis**

**Contraindications:** Children <12 yr, geriatric, hypersensitivity to amide local anesthetics, severe liver disease, severe hypotension, complete heart block

**Precautions:** Pregnancy **B**, severe product allergies, hyperthyroidism, CV, hepatic/neurologic disease

### Pharmacokinetics
| | |
|---|---|
| Absorption | Complete |
| Distribution | Unknown |
| Metabolism | Liver |
| Excretion | Kidneys |
| Half-life | Unknown |

### Pharmacodynamics
| | |
|---|---|
| Onset | 2-8 min |
| Peak | Unknown |
| Duration | 3 hr, varies with inj site |

## Interactions
*Individual drugs*
Amiodarone, cimetidine, ciprofloxacin, fluvoxamine, imipramine, theophylline: increased effect
Chloroprocaine: decreased action of ropivacaine
Enflurane, epINEPHrine, halothane: increased dysrhythmias
*Drug classifications*
Antidepressants (tricyclics), MAOIs, phenothiazines: increased hypertension
Azole antifungals: increased effect

## NURSING CONSIDERATIONS
### Assessment
- Assess B/P, pulse, respiration during treatment
- Assess fetal heart tones during labor
- Assess allergic reactions: rash, urticaria, itching
- Assess cardiac status: ECG for dysrhythmias, pulse, B/P during anesthesia

### Nursing diagnoses
- Knowledge, deficient (teaching)

### Implementation
- Give only with resuscitative equipment nearby
- Give only products without preservatives for epidural or caudal anesthesia
- Use new sol; discard unused portions

### Evaluation
**Positive therapeutic outcome**
- Anesthesia necessary for procedure

**Treatment of overdose:** Airway, O₂, vasopressor, **IV** fluids, anticonvulsants for seizures

## rosiglitazone (Rx)
(roes-i-glye′ta-zone)
Avandia
*Func. class.:* Antidiabetic, oral
*Chem. class.:* Thiazolidinedione
**Pregnancy category** C

**Action:** Improves insulin resistance by hepatic glucose metabolism, insulin receptor kinase activity, insulin receptor phosphorylation

Adverse effects: *italic* = common, **bold** = life-threatening

**Therapeutic outcome:** Decreased symptoms of diabetes mellitus

**Uses:** Stable type 2 diabetes mellitus alone or in combination with sulfonylureas, metformin, or insulin

**Unlabeled uses:** Increased ovulation frequency in those with polycystic ovary syndrome; reduced in-stent restenosis in those with diabetes

### Dosage and routes
*Monotherapy*
*Adult:* PO 4 mg/day or in 2 divided doses, may increase to 8 mg/day or in 2 divided doses after 12 wk; may be added to metformin, sulfonylureas at the adult dose

**Available forms:** Tabs 2, 4, 8 mg

### Adverse effects
*CNS:* Fatigue, *headache*
*CV:* **Heart failure, CHF, MI**
*ENDO:* Hyper/hypoglycemia
*GI:* Weight gain, **hepatotoxicity**
*MISC:* Accidental injury, upper respiratory tract infection, sinusitis, anemia, back pain, diarrhea, edema, **CV risk**
*SYST:* **Anaphylaxis, Stevens-Johnson syndrome**

**Contraindications:** Breastfeeding, children, hypersensitivity to thiazolidinediones, diabetic ketoacidosis, jaundice, CAD

**Precautions:** Pregnancy **C**, geriatric, thyroid/renal/hepatic disease, heart failure, MI

| Pharmacokinetics | |
|---|---|
| **Absorption** | Unknown |
| **Distribution** | Protein binding 99.8% |
| **Metabolism** | Unknown |
| **Excretion** | Urine, feces, breast milk |
| **Half-life** | Elimination 3-4 hr |

| Pharmacodynamics | |
|---|---|
| **Onset** | Unknown |
| **Peak** | 6-12 wk |
| **Duration** | Unknown |

### Interactions
*Drug classification*
CYP2CS inducers/inhibitors: may increase/ decrease effect
*Drug/herb*
Alfalfa, aloe, basil, bay, bilberry, bitter melon, black catechu, buchu, burdock, coriander, dandelion, eyebright (po), fenugreek, garlic, ginseng, glucomannan, glucosamine, goat's rue, gymnema, horehound, horse chestnut, jambul, myrrh, myrtle: increased antidiabetic effect

Bee pollen, blue cohosh, broom, chromium, elecampane, eucalyptus, gotu kola: decreased antidiabetic effect

Chromium, coenzyme Q10, fenugreek: hypoglycemia

Glucosamine: decreased glucose control

### NURSING CONSIDERATIONS
**Assessment**
◆ Assess for CV status; those with CV disease should be monitored carefully
• Assess for hypoglycemic reactions (sweating, weakness, dizziness, anxiety, tremors, hunger), hyperglycemic reactions soon after meals
• Assess for systemic reactions: anaphylaxis, Stevens-Johnson syndrome
• Check liver function tests periodically; AST, FBS, ALT (if ALT >2.5 × ULN, do not use), HbA$_{2c}$, plasma lipids, lipoproteins, B/P, body weight during treatment

**Nursing diagnoses**
• Knowledge, deficient (teaching)
• Nutrition: more than body requirements, imbalanced (uses)

**Implementation**
• Convert from other oral hypoglycemic agents if needed; change may be made without gradual dosage change; monitor serum or urine glucose and ketones tid during conversion
• Give tabs crushed and mixed with meal or fluids for patients with difficulty swallowing
• Store in airtight container in cool environment

**Patient/family education**
• Teach patient to monitor capillary blood glucose test, that periodic liver function tests are mandatory; to report edema, weight gain
• Teach patient symptoms of hypo/ hyperglycemia, what to do about each
• Advise patient that product must be continued on daily basis; explain consequence of discontinuing product abruptly
• Advise patient to avoid OTC medications or herbal preparations unless approved by prescriber
• Advise patient that diabetes is lifelong illness; that this product is not a cure, only controls symptoms
• Advise patient that all food included in diet plan must be eaten to prevent hypoglycemia
• Advise patient to carry/wear emergency ID and glucagon emergency kit for emergencies

- Instruct patient to notify prescriber if oral contraceptives are used
- Teach patient not to use if breastfeeding, may be secreted in breast milk

## Evaluation
**Positive therapeutic outcome**
- Decrease in polyuria, polydipsia, polyphagia; clear sensorium; absence of dizziness; stable gait; blood glucose, A1c improvement

## rosuvastatin (Rx)
(roe-soo'va-sta-tin)
Crestor
*Func. class.:* Antilipemic
*Chem. class.:* HMG-CoA reductase inhibitor

**Pregnancy category X**

**Action:** Inhibits HMG-CoA reductase enzyme, which reduces cholesterol synthesis

**Therapeutic outcome:** Decreasing cholesterol levels

**Uses:** As an adjunct in primary hypercholesterolemia (types IIa, IIb), mixed dyslipidemia elevated serum triglycerides, homozygous familial hypercholesterolemia (FH), slowing of atherosclerosis

## Dosage and routes
Patient should first be placed on a cholesterol-lowering diet

*Hypercholesterolemia*
*Adult:* PO 5-40 mg/day; initial dose 10 mg/day, reanalyze lipid levels at 2-4 wk and adjust dosage accordingly

*Homozygous FH*
*Adult:* PO 20 mg/day, max 40 mg

*Dose in patients taking cycloSPORINE*
*Adult:* 5 mg/day

*Dose when taken with gemfibrozil*
*Adult:* 10 mg/day

*Asian patients/predisposition for myopathy*
*Adult:* PO 5 mg/day

*Atherosclerosis slowing*
*Adult:* PO 10 mg/day (for those not taking cycloSPORINE or gemfibrozil)

*Renal dose*
*Adult:* PO CCr <30 ml/min 5 mg daily; max 10 mg daily

**Available forms:** Tabs 5, 10, 20, 40 mg

## Adverse effects
*CNS: Headache, dizziness,* insomnia, paresthesia
*GI: Nausea, constipation, abdominal pain, flatus, diarrhea, dyspepsia, heartburn,* **kidney failure, liver dysfunction,** vomiting
*HEMA:* **Thrombocytopenia, hemolytic anemia,** leukopenia
*INTEG: Rash, pruritus,* photosensitivity
*MS: Asthenia, muscle cramps, arthritis, arthralgia, myalgia,* **myositis, rhabdomyolysis,** leg, shoulder or localized pain
*RESP:* Rhinitis, sinusitis, *pharyngitis,* bronchitis, increased cough

**Contraindications:** Pregnancy **X,** breastfeeding, hypersensitivity, active liver disease

**Precautions:** Children, geriatric, past liver disease, alcoholism, severe acute infections, trauma, hypotension, uncontrolled seizure disorders, severe metabolic disorders, electrolyte imbalances, severe renal impairment, hypothyroidism

### Pharmacokinetics
| | |
|---|---|
| **Absorption** | Unknown |
| **Distribution** | 88% protein bound, crosses placenta |
| **Metabolism** | Minimal liver metabolism (about 10%) |
| **Excretion** | Primarily in feces (90%) |
| **Half-life** | 19 hr |

### Pharmacodynamics
| | |
|---|---|
| **Onset** | Unknown |
| **Peak** | 3-5 hr |
| **Duration** | Unknown |

## Interactions
*Individual drugs*
Clofibrate, cycloSPORINE, gemfibrozil, niacin: increased myalgia, myositis
Warfarin: increased bleeding
*Drug classifications*
Antifungals (azole): increased myalgia, myositis
Bile acid sequestrants: increased effects
*Drug/herb*
St. John's wort: decreased rosuvastatin effect
*Drug/food*
Grapefruit juice: possible toxicity
*Drug/lab test*
Increased: CPK, liver function tests

## NURSING CONSIDERATIONS
### Assessment
- Assess diet: obtain diet history including fat, cholesterol in diet

R

## Nursing diagnoses
- Injury, risk for (uses)
- Knowledge, deficient (teaching)
- Mobility, impaired physical (uses)

## Implementation
- Apply patch at same time each day; remove old patch before applying new patch

## Patient/family education
- Instruct patient to change positions slowly to prevent orthostatic hypotension
- Advise patient to avoid hazardous activities until stabilized; dizziness can occur
- Teach patient to take as prescribed, not to miss dose or double doses

## Evaluation
**Positive therapeutic outcome**
- Improved symptoms in those with Parkinson's disease

## salicylic acid topical
*See Appendix D*

## salmeterol (Rx)
(sal-met'er-ole)
Serevent
*Func. class.:* Adrenergic β₂ agonist, bronchodilator

**Pregnancy category C**

**Action:** Causes bronchodilatation by action on β₂ (pulmonary) receptors by increasing levels of cAMP, which relaxes smooth muscle; with very little effect on heart rate, maintains improvement in FEV from 3 to 12 hr; prevents nocturnal asthma symptoms

**Therapeutic outcome:** Ease of breathing

**Uses:** Prevention of exercise-induced asthma, bronchospasm, COPD

## Dosage and routes
*Adult:* INH 50 mcg (one inhalation as dry powder); exercise-induced bronchospasm: 50 mcg (2 inh) ½-1 hr prior to exercise
*Child 4-12 yr:* INH 50 mcg as dry powder bid; exercise-induced bronchospasm 50 mcg as dry powder ½-1 hr prior to exercise

**Available forms:** Inhalation powder 50 mcg/blister

## Adverse effects
*CNS: Tremors, anxiety,* insomnia, headache, dizziness, stimulation, restlessness, hallucinations, flushing, irritability

*CV:* Palpitations, **tachycardia**, angina, hypo/hypertension, **dysrhythmias**
*EENT:* Dry nose, irritation of nose and throat
*GI:* Heartburn, nausea, vomiting
*MS:* Muscle cramps
*RESP:* **Bronchospasm**

**Contraindications:** Hypersensitivity to sympathomimetics, tachydysrhythmias, severe cardiac disease

**Precautions:** Pregnancy **C**, breastfeeding, cardiac disorders, hyperthyroidism, diabetes mellitus, hypertension, prostatic hypertrophy, angle-closure glaucoma, seizures, acute asthma, as a substitute for corticosteroids

### Pharmacokinetics
Unknown

### Pharmacodynamics
| | |
|---|---|
| **Onset** | 5-15 min |
| **Peak** | 4 hr |
| **Duration** | 12 hr |

## Interactions
*Drug classifications*
Antidepressants (tricyclics): increased salmeterol action
β-Adrenergic blockers: block therapeutic effect
Bronchodilators, aerosol: increased action of bronchodilator
MAOIs: increased action of salmeterol
*Drug/herb*
Betel palm, butterbur, coffee, cola nut, figwort, fumitory, guarana, hawthorn, lily of the valley, motherwort, plantain, tea (black, green), yerba maté: increased stimulation

## NURSING CONSIDERATIONS
### Assessment
- Monitor respiratory function tests: vital capacity, FEV, ABGs, lung sounds, heart rate, rhythm (baseline)

### Nursing diagnoses
- Airway clearance, ineffective (uses)
- Gas exchange, impaired (uses)
- Knowledge, deficient (teaching)

### Implementation
- Shake aerosol container, ask patient to exhale, then place mouthpiece in mouth, inhale slowly, hold breath, remove, exhale slowly; allow at least 1 min between inhalations
- Use this medication before other medications and allow at least 1 min between each
- Use spacing device for pediatric/geriatric patients
- Store in light-resistant container, do not expose to temperatures over 86° F (30° C)

S

## Patient/family education

• Caution patient not to use OTC medications because extra stimulation may occur
• Instruct patient to use this medication before other medications and to allow at least 1 min between each, to prevent overstimulation
• Teach patient how to use inhaler; to avoid getting aerosol in eyes; blurring may result; to wash inhaler in warm water daily and dry; to avoid smoking, smoke-filled rooms, and persons with respiratory infections; review package insert with patient
• Instruct patient on administration of dose, not to use more than prescribed; serious side effects may occur

## Evaluation

**Positive therapeutic outcome**
• Absence of dyspnea, wheezing
• Improved airway exchange
• Improved ABGs

**Treatment of overdose:** Administer a $\beta_2$-adrenergic blocker

---

## salsalate (Rx)

(sal-sa'late)
Amigesic, Anaflex, Disalcid, Marthritic, Mono-Gesic, Salflex, Salgesic, Salsalate, Salsitab
*Func. class.:* Nonopioid analgesic; nonsteroidal antiinflammatory agent
*Chem. class.:* Salicylate

**Pregnancy category C**

---

**Action:** Blocks formation of peripheral prostaglandins, which cause pain and inflammation; antipyretic action results from inhibition of hypothalamic heat-regulating center; does not inhibit platelet aggregation

**Therapeutic outcome:** Decreased pain, inflammation

**Uses:** Mild to moderate pain or fever, including arthritis, juvenile rheumatoid arthritis

## Dosage and routes
*Adult:* PO 3 g/day in divided doses

**Available forms:** Caps 500 mg; tabs 500, 750 mg

## Adverse effects
*CNS:* Stimulation, drowsiness, dizziness, confusion, **seizures**, headache, flushing, hallucinations, coma
*CV:* Rapid pulse, **pulmonary edema**
*EENT:* Tinnitus, hearing loss

*ENDO:* Hypoglycemia, hyponatremia, hypokalemia, alteration in acid-base balance
*GI: Nausea, vomiting, GI bleeding, diarrhea, heartburn,* anorexia, **hepatotoxicity**
*HEMA:* **Thrombocytopenia, agranulocytosis, leukopenia, neutropenia, hemolytic anemia,** increased protime
*INTEG:* Rash, urticaria, bruising
*RESP:* Wheezing, hyperpnea

**Contraindications:** Children <3 yr, hypersensitivity to salicylates, NSAIDs, GI bleeding, bleeding disorders, vit K deficiency

**Precautions:** Pregnancy **C** (1st trimester), breastfeeding, geriatric, anemia, renal/hepatic disease, Hodgkin's disease

### Pharmacokinetics

| | |
|---|---|
| **Absorption** | Absorbed in small intestine, full benefit 3-4 days |
| **Distribution** | Rapidly and widely distributed, crosses placenta |
| **Metabolism** | Not metabolized |
| **Excretion** | Unchanged—kidneys |
| **Half-life** | 2-3 hr (low doses), 15-30 hr (high doses) |

### Pharmacodynamics

| | |
|---|---|
| **Onset** | 30 min |
| **Peak** | 1-3 hr |
| **Duration** | 3-6 hr |

## Interactions
### Individual drugs
Alcohol, heparin, warfarin: increased bleeding
Insulin, methotrexate, phenytoin, probenecid: increased effects
*p*-Aminobenzoic acid: increased toxic effects
Spironolactone, sulfinpyrazone: decreased effects
### Drug classifications
Antacids, steroids, urinary alkalizers: decreased effects of salsalate
Anticoagulants, penicillins: increased effects
Salicylates: decreased blood glucose levels
Diuretics (loop), sulfonylamides: decreased effects
NSAIDs, platelet inhibitors, thrombolytics: increased bleeding risk
### Drug/herb
Feverfew: decreased effect of this herb
### Drug/food
Foods causing acidic urine may increase level
### Drug/lab test
Increased: coagulation studies, liver function tests, serum uric acid, amylase, $CO_2$, urinary protein

---

Decreased: serum potassium, cholesterol, blood glucose

Interference: urine catecholamines, pH, pregnancy test

## NURSING CONSIDERATIONS
### Assessment

- Monitor liver function tests: AST, ALT, bilirubin, creatinine if patient is on long-term therapy
- Monitor renal function tests: BUN, urine creatinine if patient is on long-term therapy
- Monitor blood tests: CBC, Hct, Hgb, Protime, stool guaiac, serum salicylate if patient is on long-term therapy
- Check I&O ratio; decreasing output may indicate renal failure if patient is on long-term therapy
- Assess hepatotoxicity: dark urine, clay-colored stools, yellowing of the skin and sclera, itching, abdominal pain, fever, diarrhea if patient is on long-term therapy
- Assess for allergic reactions: rash, urticaria; if these occur, product may have to be discontinued; assess for asthma, aspirin sensitivity, nasal polyps, may develop hypersensitivity
- Assess for ototoxicity: tinnitus, ringing, roaring in ears; audiometric testing needed before, after long-term therapy
- Assess for visual changes
- Check edema in feet, ankles, legs
- Identify prior product history; many product interactions are possible
- Monitor pain: location, duration, type, intensity, prior to dose and 1 hr after
- Monitor musculoskeletal status: ROM before dose
- Identify fever, length of time, and related symptoms

### Nursing diagnoses
- Injury, risk for (side effects)
- Knowledge, deficient (teaching)
- Mobility, impaired physical (uses)
- Pain, chronic (uses)

### Implementation
- Give with 8 oz of water and sit upright ½ hr after dose; with food or milk to decrease gastric symptoms
- Give antacids 1-2 hr after enteric products

### Patient/family education
- Advise patient to report any symptoms of renal/hepatic toxicity, visual changes, ototoxicity, allergic reactions, bleeding (long-term therapy)
- Instruct patient to take with 8 oz of water and sit upright for ½ hr after dose

- Caution patient not to exceed recommended dosage; acute poisoning may result
- Advise patient to read label on other OTC products; many contain aspirin
- Inform patient that the therapeutic response takes 2 wk (arthritis)
- Teach patient to report tinnitus, confusion, diarrhea, sweating, hyperventilation
- Caution patient to avoid alcohol ingestion; GI bleeding may occur
- Inform patient that patients who have allergies may develop allergic reactions

### Evaluation
**Positive therapeutic outcome**
- Decreased pain
- Decreased inflammation

**Treatment of overdose:** Lavage, activated charcoal, monitor electrolytes, VS

---

### saquinavir (Rx)
(sa-quen′a-ver)
Invirase
*Func. class.:* Antiretroviral
*Chem. class.:* Protease inhibitor
**Pregnancy category B**

**Action:** Inhibits HIV-1 protease

**Therapeutic outcome:** Prevents maturation of the infectious virus

**Uses:** HIV-1 in combination with other antiretrovirals

### Dosage and routes
*Adult:* PO 1000 mg bid with 100 mg ritonavir

**Available forms:** Caps 200, 500 mg

### Adverse effects
*CNS: Paresthesia*, headache
*GI: Diarrhea*, buccal mucosa ulceration, *abdominal pain, nausea*, vomiting
*INTEG: Rash*
*MISC:* Asthenia, *hyperglycemia*
*MS:* Pain

**Contraindications:** Hypersensitivity

**Precautions:** Pregnancy **B**, breastfeeding, children, hepatic, diabetes, pancreatitis

| Pharmacokinetics | |
|---|---|
| **Absorption** | Increased with food |
| **Distribution** | Protein-binding 98% |
| **Metabolism** | Extensively |
| **Excretion** | Unknown |
| **Half-life** | Terminal 12 hr |

S

## Interactions
### Individual drugs
Clarithromycin, delavirdine, indinavir, ketoconazole, nelfinavir, ritonavir: increased saquinavir level

Carbamazepine, dexamethasone, nevirapine, phenobarbital, phenytoin, rifamycins: decreased saquinavir levels

Clindamycin, dapsone, quinidine: increased toxicity

Midazolam, triazolam: increased toxicity, increased CNS depression; do not use concurrently

### Drug classifications
Calcium channel blockers: increased toxicity

Ergots: toxicity, increased vasoconstriction; do not use together

HMG-CoA reductase inhibitors: avoid use with saquinavir

### Drug/herb
Garlic, St. John's wort: decreased saquinavir level, avoid concurrent use

### Drug/food
Increased: bioavailability after high-fat meal
Grapefruit juice: increased saquinivir level

### Drug/lab test
Interference: CPK, glucose (low)

## NURSING CONSIDERATIONS
### Assessment
- Assess signs of infection, anemia
- Monitor liver function tests: ALT, AST
- Monitor C&S before product therapy; product may be taken as soon as culture is done; repeat C&S after treatment; determine the presence of other STDs
- Assess bowel pattern before, during treatment; if severe abdominal pain with bleeding occurs, product should be discontinued; monitor hydration
- Assess skin eruptions, rash, urticaria, itching
- Assess allergies before treatment, reaction of each medication; place allergies on chart

### Nursing diagnoses
- Infection, risk for (uses)
- Knowledge, deficient (teaching)

### Implementation
- Give in equal intervals around the clock for duration of therapy

### Patient/family education
- Advise patient to take as prescribed within 2 hr of a full meal; if dose is missed, take as soon as remembered up to 1 hr before next dose; do not double dose
- Advise patient that product must be taken in equal intervals around the clock to maintain blood levels for duration of therapy; that product is not a cure

### Evaluation
**Positive therapeutic outcome**
- Decreasing symptoms of HIV
- Improving viral load and CD4 cell counts

---

## sargramostim (Rx)
(sar-gram'oh-stim)
Leukine, rhu GM-CSF
*Func. class.:* Biologic modifier: cytokine
*Chem. class.:* Granulocyte/macrophage colony stimulating factor (GM-CSF)

### Pregnancy category C

**Do not confuse:**
Leukine/leucovorin/Leukeran

**Action:** Stimulates proliferation and differentiation of hematopoietic progenitor cells (granulocyte, macrophage)

**Uses:** Acceleration of myeloid recovery in patients with non-Hodgkin's lymphoma, acute lymphoblastic leukemia, autologous bone marrow transplantation in Hodgkin's disease; bone marrow transplantation failure or engraftment delay; mobilization and transplant of peripheral blood progenitor cells (PBPCs)

**Unlabeled uses:** Aplastic anemia, Crohn's disease, ganciclovir- or zidovudine-induced neutropenia

### Dosage and routes
#### Myeloid reconstitution after autologous bone marrow transplantation
*Adult:* **IV** 250 mcg/m$^2$/day × 3 wk; give over 2 hr, 2-4 hr after autologous bone marrow inf, and not less than 24 hr after last dose of antineoplastics and 12 hr after last dose of radiotherapy, bone marrow transplantation failure, or engraftment delay

#### Acceleration of myeloid recovery
*Adult:* **IV** 250 mcg/m$^2$/day × 14 days; give over 2 hr; may repeat in 7 days, may repeat 500 mcg/m$^2$/day × 14 days after another 7 days if no improvement

#### Mobilization of PBPCs
*Adult:* **IV**/SUBCUT 250 mcg/m$^2$/day during collection of PBPCs

*After PBPC transplantation*
*Adult:* **IV**/SUBCUT 250 mcg/m$^2$/day until
ANC >1500/mm$^3$ × 3 days

**Available forms:** Powder for inj lyophilized 250, 500 mcg

**Adverse effects**
*CNS:* Fever, malaise, CNS disorder, weakness, chills, dizziness, syncope
*CV:* **Transient supraventricular tachycardia,** peripheral edema, **pericardial effusion,** hypotension, tachycardia
*GI:* Nausea, vomiting, diarrhea, anorexia, **GI hemorrhage,** stomatitis, **liver damage**
*GU:* Urinary tract disorder, abnormal kidney function
*HEMA:* **Blood dyscrasias, hemorrhage**
*INTEG:* Alopecia, rash, peripheral edema
*MS:* Bone pain, myalgia
*RESP:* Dyspnea

**Contraindications:** Hypersensitivity to GM-CSF, benzyl alcohol, yeast products; excessive leukemic myeloid blast in the bone marrow or peripheral blood, neonates

**Precautions:** Pregnancy **C,** breastfeeding, children, renal/hepatic/lung/cardiac disease, pleural/pericardial effusions, peripheral edema, leukocytosis

| Pharmacokinetics | |
|---|---|
| **Absorption** | Completely absorbed |
| **Distribution** | Unknown |
| **Metabolism** | Unknown |
| **Excretion** | Unknown |
| **Half-life** | 2 hr |

| Pharmacodynamics | |
|---|---|
| **Onset** | Rapid |
| **Peak** | 2 hr |
| **Duration** | Unknown |

**Interactions**
*Individual drugs*
Lithium: increased myeloproliferation
*Drug classifications*
Antineoplastics: do not use together
Corticosteroids: increased myeloproliferation

**NURSING CONSIDERATIONS**
**Assessment**
• Monitor blood studies: CBC, differential count before treatment and twice weekly; leukocytosis may occur (WBC >50,000 cells/mm$^3$, ANC >20,000 cells/mm$^3$), platelets; if ANC >20,000/mm$^3$ or 10,000/mm$^3$ after nadir has occurred, or platelets >500,000/mm$^3$ reduce dose by ½ or discontinue; if blast cells occur, discontinue

• Monitor renal, liver function tests before treatment: BUN, creatinine, urinalysis; AST, ALT, alkaline phosphatase; monitoring is needed twice a week in renal/hepatic disease
• Assess for hypersensitivity reactions/rashes, and local inj site reactions; usually transient
• Assess for increased fluid retention in cardiac disease, body weight hydration status
• Assess for myalgia, arthralgia in legs, feet; use analgesics

**Nursing diagnoses**
• Infection, risk for (uses)
• Knowledge, deficient (teaching)

**Implementation**
• Reconstitute with 1 ml of sterile water for inj without preservative; do not reenter vial; discard unused portion; direct reconstitution sol at side of vial; rotate contents; do not shake
**SUBCUT route**
• Use reconstituted sol
**IV route**
• Give by intermittent inf after diluting in 0.9% NaCl inj to prepare **IV** inf; if final conc is <10 mcg/ml, add human albumin to make a final conc of 0.1% to the NaCl before adding sargramostim to prevent absorption; for a final conc of 0.1% albumin, add 1 mg of human albumin/1 ml of 0.9% NaCl inj; run over 2 hr (bone marrow transplant or failure of graft); over 4 hr (chemotherapy for acute myeloid leukemia); over 24 hr as cont inf (PBPCs); give within 6 hr after reconstitution
• Store in refrigerator; do not freeze

*Y-site compatibilities:* Amikacin, aminophylline, aztreonam, bleomycin, butorphanol, calcium gluconate, carboplatin, carmustine, cefazolin, cefepime, cefotaxime, cefotetan, ceftizoxime, ceftriaxone, cefuroxime, cimetidine, cisplatin, clindamycin, cyclophosphamide, cycloSPORINE, cytarabine, dacarbazine, dactinomycin, dexamethasone, diphenhydrAMINE, DOPamine, DOXOrubicin, doxycycline, droperidol, etoposide, famotidine, fentanyl, floxuridine, fluconazole, fluorouracil, furosemide, gentamicin, granisetron, heparin, idarubicin, ifosfamide, immune globulin, magnesium sulfate, mannitol, mechlorethamine, meperidine, mesna, methotrexate, metoclopramide, metronidazole, mezlocillin, miconazole, minocycline, mitoxantrone, netilmicin, pentostatin, piperacillin/tazobactam, potassium chloride, prochlorperazine, promethazine, ranitidine, teniposide, ticarcillin, ticarcillin/clavulanate, trimethoprim/sulfamethoxazole, vinBLAStine, vinCRIStine, zidovudine

**S**

*Y-site incompatibilities:* Acyclovir, ampicillin, ampicillin/sulbactam, cefonicid, cefoperazine, ceftazidime, chlorproMAZINE, ganciclovir, haloperidol, hydrocortisone, hydromorphone, hydrOXYzine, idarubicin, imipenem/cilastatin, lorazepam, methylPRED-NISolone sodium succinate, mitomycin, morphine, nalbuphine, ondansetron, piperacillin, sodium bicarbonate, tobramycin

### Patient/family education
• Teach patient reason for medication and expected results
• Advise patient to notify nurse or prescriber of side effects

### Evaluation
**Positive therapeutic outcome**
• WBC and differential recovery
• Absence of infection

---

## scopolamine (Rx)
(skoe-pol'a-meen)
Scopolamine Hydrobromide, Transderm-Scop, Transderm-V
*Func. class.:* Antiemetic, anticholinergic, mydriatic
*Chem. class.:* Belladonna alkaloid

**Pregnancy category** C

---

**Action:** Inhibits acetylcholine at receptor sites in autonomic nervous system, which controls secretions, free acids in stomach; blocks central muscarinic receptors, which decreases involuntary movements; blocks response of iris sphincter muscle, muscle of accommodation of ciliary body to cholinergic stimulation, resulting in dilatation, paralysis of accommodation

**Therapeutic outcome:** Absence of vomiting, secretions (preoperatively), involuntary movements

**Uses:** Reduction of secretions before surgery, calm delirium, uveitis, iritis, cycloplegia, mydriasis; prevention of motion sickness, Parkinson's symptoms

**Unlabeled uses:** Drooling (TD)

### Dosage and routes
*Ophthalmic route*
**Adult:** Instill 1-2 gtt before refraction or 1-2 gtt daily-tid for iritis or uveitis
**Child:** Instill 1 gtt bid × 2 days before refraction

*Prevention of motion sickness*
**Adult:** TRANSDERMAL 1 patch placed behind ear 4-5 hr before travel, reapply q3 days; alternate ears; not recommended for children

*Parkinson's symptoms*
**Adult:** IM/SUBCUT/**IV** 0.3-0.6 mg tid-qid diluted using dilution provided

*Preoperatively*
**Adult:** SUBCUT 0.3-0.5 mg; may repeat q4-6hr

*Nausea and vomiting*
**Child:** SUBCUT 0.006 mg/kg or 0.2 mg/m$^2$; max 0.3 mg/dose

*Drooling (unlabeled)*
**Adult:** TRANSDERMAL 1.5 mg patch q3 days

**Available forms:** Patch 0.5, 1 mg delivered in 72 hr; inj 0.3, 0.4, 0.86, 1 mg/ml

### Adverse effects
***CNS:*** Confusion, drowsiness, disorientation, anxiety, restlessness, irritability, delusions, hallucinations, sedation, depression, incoherence, dizziness, excitement, delirium, flushing, weakness; transdermal: memory disturbances
***CV:*** Palpitations, **tachycardia,** postural hypotension, paradoxical bradycardia
***EENT TD:*** Blurred vision, photophobia, dilated pupils, difficulty swallowing, mydriasis, cycloplegia, altered depth perception, *dry mouth,* dry, itchy red eyes, acute glaucoma
***GI:*** *Dryness of mouth, constipation,* nausea, vomiting, abdominal distress, **paralytic ileus**
***GU:*** Hesitancy, retention, difficult urination (patch)
***INTEG:*** Rash, erythema (patch), urticaria, dry skin
***MISC:*** Suppression of breastfeeding, nasal congestion, decreased sweating

**Contraindications:** Hypersensitivity, angle-closure glaucoma, myasthenia gravis, GI/GU obstruction, hypersensitivity to belladonna, barbiturates

**Precautions:** Pregnancy **C,** breastfeeding, children, geriatric, prostatic hypertrophy, CHF, hypertension, dysrhythmias, gastric ulcer, renal/hepatic disease, hiatal hernia, GERD, ulcerative colitis, hyperthyroidism; transdermal: pyloric urinary; bladder neck, intestinal obstruction; renal/hepatic disease

| Pharmacokinetics | |
|---|---|
| Absorption | Well absorbed (IM, SUBCUT, TRANSDERMAL) |
| Distribution | Crosses placenta, blood-brain barrier |
| Metabolism | Liver |
| Excretion | Unknown |
| Half-life | 8 hr |

## Pharmacodynamics

|  | SUBCUT/IM | IV | TRANS-DERMAL | OPHTH |
|---|---|---|---|---|
| **Onset** | 30-45 min | 10-15 min | 4-5 hr | Unknown |
| **Peak** | 1 hr | 1 hr | Unknown | 20-30 min |
| **Duration** | 6 hr | 4 hr | 72 hr | 3-7 days |

## Interactions
### Individual drugs
Alcohol: increased anticholinergic effect
### Drug classifications
Antidepressants (tricyclics), antihistamines, opioids, phenothiazines: increased anticholinergic effect
### Drug/herb
Henbane, jimsonweed, scopolia: increased anticholinergic effects

## NURSING CONSIDERATIONS
### Assessment
• Assess for eye pain; discontinue use (opticue)
• Monitor I&O ratio; retention commonly causes decreased urinary output
• Assess for parkinsonism, EPS: shuffling gait, muscle rigidity, involuntary movements
• Assess for urinary hesitancy, retention; palpate bladder if retention occurs
• Assess for constipation; increase fluids, bulk, exercise if this occurs
• Assess for tolerance over long-term therapy; dose may have to be increased or changed
• Assess mental status: affect, mood, CNS depression, worsening of mental symptoms during early therapy

### Nursing diagnoses
• Fluid volume, deficient (uses)
• Knowledge, deficient (teaching)

### Implementation
**IM/SUBCUT/IV route**
• Administer parenteral dose with patient recumbent to prevent postural hypotension
**Transdermal route**
• Instruct patient to wash, dry hands before and after applying to surface behind ear; to change patch q72hr; to apply at least 4 hr before traveling
**Ophthalmic route**
• Apply pressure on lacrimal sac for 1 min; do not touch dropper to eye
• Wait 5 min to use other drops; blink more than usual

**IV route**
• Give by direct **IV** after diluting with sterile water; give slowly
*Syringe compatibilities:* Atropine, benzquinamide, butorphanol, chlorproMAZINE, cimetidine, dimenhyDRINATE, diphenhydrAMINE, droperidol, fentanyl, glycopyrrolate, hydromorphone, hydrOXYzine, meperidine, metoclopramide, midazolam, morphine, nalbuphine, pentazocine, pentobarbital, perphenazine, prochlorperazine, promazine, promethazine, ranitidine, sufentanil, thiopental
*Y-site compatibilities:* Heparin, hydrocortisone, potassium chloride, propofol, sufentanil, vit B/C
*Additive compatibilities:* Floxacillin, furosemide, meperidine, succinylcholine

### Patient/family education
• Tell patient to avoid hazardous activities, activities requiring alertness; dizziness may occur
• Advise patient to discontinue use if blurred vision, severe dizziness, drowsiness occurs; another type of antiemetic may be used or the patch rotated to the other ear
• Instruct patient to read labels of all OTC medications; if any scopolamine is found in product, avoid use
• Advise patient to keep medication out of children's reach
• Caution patient to report change in vision, blurring or loss of sight, trouble breathing, inhibition of sweating, flushing
• Teach patient method of ophthalmic instillation
• Inform patient that blurred vision will decrease with repeated use of ophthalmic product
• Caution patient not to discontinue this product abruptly; to taper off over 1 wk

### Evaluation
**Positive therapeutic outcome**
• Decrease in inflammation, cycloplegic refraction
• Decreased secretions
• Absence of motion sickness

### scopolamine ophthalmic
*See Appendix D*

S

## selegiline (Rx)
(se-le'ji-leen)
Carbex, Eldepryl, Emsam, Novo-
Selegiline ✦, Zelapar
*Func. class.:* Antiparkinson agent
*Chem. class.:* MAOI, type B

**Pregnancy category** C

### Do not confuse:
Eldepryl/enalapril

**Action:** Increased dopaminergic activity by inhibition of MAO type B activity; not fully understood

**Therapeutic outcome:** Decreased symptoms of Parkinson's disease

**Uses:** Adjunct management of Parkinson's disease in patients being treated with levodopa/carbidopa who have responded poorly to therapy

**Unlabeled use:** Alzheimer's disease, depression

### Dosage and routes
*Adult:* PO 10 mg/day in divided doses, 5 mg at breakfast and lunch with levodopa/carbidopa; after 2-3 days begin to reduce the dose of levodopa/carbidopa 10%-30%; oral disintegrating tab 2.5 mg (2 tabs) initially, then 1.25 (1 tab) dissolved on tongue daily before breakfast × 6 wk or more; max 2.5 mg/day; TRANSDERMAL 6 mg/24 hr initially, increase by 3 mg/24 hr at ≥2 wk, up to 12 mg/24 hr if needed

### Alzheimer's disease (unlabeled)
*Adult:* PO 5 mg bid AM, PM

**Available forms:** Tabs 5 mg, caps 5 mg; oral disintegrating tabs 1.25 mg; transdermal 6 mg/24 hr (20 mg/20 cm²), 9 mg/24 hr (30 mg/30 cm²), 12 mg/24 hr (40 mg/40 cm²)

### Adverse effects
*CNS:* Increased tremors, chorea, restlessness, blepharospasm, increased bradykinesia, grimacing, tardive dyskinesia, dystonic symptoms, involuntary movements, increased apraxia, hallucinations, dizziness, mood changes, nightmares, delusions, lethargy, apathy, overstimulation, sleep disturbances, headache, migraine, numbness, muscle cramps, confusion, anxiety, tiredness, vertigo, personality change, back/leg pain, **suicide in children/adolescents**
*CV:* Orthostatic hypotension, hypertension, **dysrhythmia**, palpitations; angina pectoris, hypotension, tachycardia, edema, sinus bradycardia, syncope, **hypertensive crisis**

*EENT:* Diplopia, dry mouth, blurred vision, tinnitus
*GI:* *Nausea,* vomiting, constipation, weight loss, anorexia, diarrhea, heartburn, rectal bleeding, poor appetite, dysphagia, xerostomia
*GU:* Slow urination, nocturia, prostatic hypertrophy, hesitation, retention, frequency, sexual dysfunction
*INTEG:* Increased sweating, alopecia, hematoma, rash, photosensitivity, facial hair
*RESP:* Asthma, shortness of breath

**Contraindications:** Children/adolescents, hypersensitivity

**Precautions:** Pregnancy C, breastfeeding

| Pharmacokinetics | |
|---|---|
| Absorption | Well absorbed |
| Distribution | Widely distributed |
| Metabolism | Rapidly, liver |
| Excretion | Metabolites-N-desmethyldeprenyl, amphetamine, methamphetamine |
| Half-life | 9 min |

| Pharmacodynamics | |
|---|---|
| Onset | Unknown |
| Peak | ½-2 hr |
| Duration | Unknown |

### Interactions
*Individual drugs*
Dextromethorphan: increased unusual behavior, psychosis
Fluoxetine, fluvoxamine, paroxetine, sertraline: increased serotonin syndrome (confusion, seizures, fever, hypertension, agitation) discontinue 5 wk before selegiline
Levodopa/carbidopa: increased side effects
◆Meperidine: do not use, fatal reaction
*Drug classifications*
◆Antidepressants (tricyclics), opioids: do not use, fatal reaction
Antihypertensives: increased hypotension
*Drug/herb*
Chaste tree fruit, kava: decreased selegiline action
*Drug/lab test*
Decreased: VMA
False positive: urine ketones, urine glucose
False negative: urine glucose (glucose oxidase)
False increase: uric acid, urine protein

### NURSING CONSIDERATIONS
Assessment
• Monitor B/P, respiration throughout treatment
• Assess mental status: affect, mood, behav-

ioral changes, depression; perform suicide assessment
• Assess for decreased Parkinson's symptoms: rigidity, unsteady gait, weakness, tremors; these should decrease in severity

### Nursing diagnoses
• Knowledge, deficient (teaching)
• Mobility, impaired physical (uses)

### Implementation
• Adjust dosage to patient response
• Give with meals; limit protein taken with product
• Give at doses <10 mg/day because of risks associated with nonselective inhibition of MAO

### Patient/family education
• Caution patient to change positions slowly to prevent orthostatic hypotension
• Advise patient to report side effects: twitching, eye spasms; may indicate overdose
• Caution patient to use product exactly as prescribed; if product is discontinued abruptly, parkinsonian crisis may occur
• Instruct patient to avoid foods high in tyramine: cheese, pickled products, wine, beer, large amounts of caffeine
• Instruct patient not to exceed recommended dose of 10 mg; might precipitate a hypertensive crisis; report severe headache or other unusual symptoms

### Evaluation
**Positive therapeutic outcome**
• Decreased symptoms of Parkinson's disease

**Treatment of overdose: IV** fluids for hypertension, **IV** dilute pressure agent for B/P titration

---

### selenium topical
*See Appendix D*

---

### senna, sennosides (OTC)
(sin'na)
Black Draught, Dr. Caldwell Dosalax, Ex-Lax Gentle, Fletcher's Castoria, Gentlax, Senexon, Senna-Gen, Senokot, Senokotxtra, Senolax
*Func. class.:* Laxative-stimulant
*Chem. class.:* Anthraquinone

**Pregnancy category C**

**Action:** Stimulates peristalsis by action on Auerbach's plexus; softens feces by increasing water and electrolytes in large intestine

**Therapeutic outcome:** Decreased constipation

**Uses:** Acute constipation; bowel preparation for surgery or exam

### Dosage and routes
*Adult:* PO (Senokot) 1-8 tabs/day or ½ to 4 tsp of granules added to water or juice; RECT supp 1-2 at bedtime; syr 1-4 tsp at bedtime (1 tsp = 4 ml), 7.5-15 ml; (Black Draught) ¾ oz dissolved in 2.5 oz of liquid given between 2-4 PM the day before procedure (X-Prep)
*Child >27 kg:* PO ½ adult dose; do not use Black Draught for children
*Child 1 mo-1 yr:* Syr 1.25-2.5 ml (Senokot) at bedtime

**Available forms:** Tabs 6, 8.6, 15, 25 mg; granules 15, 20 mg/5 ml; syrup 8.8 mg/5 ml; liquid 33.3 mg/ml

### Adverse effects
*GI: Nausea, vomiting, anorexia, abdominal cramps,* diarrhea, flatulence
*GU:* Pink-red or brown-black discoloration of urine
*META:* Hypocalcemia, enteropathy, alkalosis, hypokalemia, **tetany**

**Contraindications:** Breastfeeding, hypersensitivity, GI bleeding, intestinal obstruction, CHF, abdominal pain, nausea/vomiting, appendicitis, acute surgical abdomen

**Precautions:** Pregnancy **C**

#### Pharmacokinetics
| | |
|---|---|
| **Absorption** | Minimally absorbed (PO) |
| **Distribution** | Unknown |
| **Metabolism** | Not metabolized |
| **Excretion** | Kidneys, feces |
| **Half-life** | Unknown |

#### Pharmacodynamics
| | PO | RECT |
|---|---|---|
| **Onset** | 6-24 hr | Unknown |
| **Peak** | Unknown | Unknown |
| **Duration** | 3-4 days | Unknown |

### Interactions
*Individual drugs*
Disulfiram: do not use together
*Drug/herb*
Flax, senna: increased laxative effect

### NURSING CONSIDERATIONS
#### Assessment
• Monitor blood, urine electrolytes if used often by patient; check I&O ratio to identify fluid loss

Adverse effects: *italic* = common, **bold** = life-threatening

- Assess cramping, rectal bleeding, nausea, vomiting; if these symptoms occur, product should be discontinued; identify cause of constipation; identify whether fluids, bulk, or exercise is missing from lifestyle
- Assess for magnesium toxicity: thirst, confusion, decrease in reflexes
- Monitor blood ammonia level (30-70 mg/100 ml); monitor for clearing of confusion, lethargy, restlessness, irritability (hepatic encephalopathy)

### Nursing diagnoses
- Constipation (uses)
- Diarrhea (side effects)
- Knowledge, deficient (teaching)
- Noncompliance (teaching)

### Implementation
**PO route**
- Administer on empty stomach for more rapid results
- Give with a full glass of water in AM or PM (oral dose); evacuation occurs 6-12 hr later
- Dissolve granules in water or juice before administration
- Shake oral sol before giving

### Patient/family education
- Discuss with patient that adequate fluid consumption is necessary
- Inform patient that normal bowel movements do not always occur daily
- Teach patient not to use in presence of abdominal pain, nausea, vomiting; tell patient to notify prescriber if constipation is unrelieved or if symptoms of electrolyte imbalance occur: muscle cramps, pain, weakness, dizziness, excessive thirst

### Evaluation
**Positive therapeutic outcome**
- Decreased constipation in 8-10 hr

---

### sertraline (Rx)
(ser'tra-leen)
Zoloft
*Func. class.:* Antidepressant
*Chem. class.:* Selective serotonin reuptake inhibitor (SSRI)

**Pregnancy category** C

**Do not confuse:**
Zoloft/Zocor

**Action:** Inhibits serotonin reuptake in CNS, thus increasing action of serotonin; does not affect dopamine, norepinephrine

**Therapeutic outcome:** Relief of depression, obsessive-compulsive disorder (OCD), posttraumatic stress disorder (PTSD), panic disorder

**Uses:** Major depression, OCD, PTSD, social anxiety disorder, panic disorder, premenstrual dysphoric disorder (PMDD)

**Unlabeled uses:** Extended interval dosing

### Dosage and routes
*Adult:* PO 50 mg/day; may increase to a maximum of 200 mg/day, do not change dose at intervals of <1 wk; administer daily in AM or PM
*Geriatric:* PO 25 mg/day, increase by 25 mg q3 days to desired dose
*Child 6-12 yr:* PO 25 mg/day
*Child 13-17 yr:* PO 50 mg/day

*Premenstrual disorders*
*Adult:* PO 50-150 mg nightly

**Available forms:** Tabs 25, 50, 100 mg; oral conc 20 mg/ml

### Adverse effects
*CNS: Insomnia, agitation, somnolence, dizziness, headache, tremor, fatigue,* paresthesia, twitching, confusion, ataxia, fever, gait abnormality (geriatric), **seizures**
*CV:* Palpitations, chest pain
*EENT:* Vision abnormalities, yawning
*ENDO:* Syndrome of inappropriate antidiuretic hormone (geriatric)
*GI: Diarrhea, nausea, constipation, anorexia, dry mouth,* dyspepsia, *vomiting, flatulence*
*GU: Male sexual dysfunction,* micturition disorder
*INTEG:* Increased sweating, rash, hot flashes
*MISC:* Hyponatremia

**Contraindications:** Hypersensitivity to this product or selective serotonin reuptake inhibitors

**Precautions:** Pregnancy **C**, breastfeeding, geriatric, renal/hepatic disease, epilepsy, recent MI, latex sensitivity (dropper of oral conc), suicidal ideation

### Pharmacokinetics

| | |
|---|---|
| **Absorption** | Well absorbed |
| **Distribution** | Unknown, steady state 1 wk |
| **Metabolism** | Liver, extensively |
| **Excretion** | Feces (14%) |
| **Half-life** | 26 hr |

---

## Pharmacodynamics

| | |
|---|---|
| **Onset** | Unknown |
| **Peak** | 4.5-8.4 hr |
| **Duration** | Unknown |

## Interactions
### Individual drugs
Cimetidine, warfarin: increased sertraline effect

Diazepam: increased diazepam effect

Disulfiram: disulfiram reaction with oral conc due to alcohol content

Lithium: altered lithium levels

Pimozide: sertraline is contraindicated with pimozide

Sumatriptan: increased sumatriptan effects

TOLBUTamide: increased effect of TOLBUTamide

Warfarin: increased warfarin effect

### Drug classifications
Antidepressants (tricyclics), benzodiazepines: increased effect

Highly protein-bound products: increased sertraline levels

◆ MAOIs: fatal reactions

### Drug/herb
Corkwood, jimsonweed: increased anticholinergic effect

Ephedra: hypertensive crisis

Hops, lavender: increased CNS effect

SAM-e, St. John's wort: increased effect of selective serotonin reuptake inhibitors, serotonin syndrome; do not use together

### Drug/lab test
Increased: AST, ALT

## NURSING CONSIDERATIONS
### Assessment
• Assess mental status: mood, sensorium, affect, suicidal tendencies; increase in psychiatric symptoms: depression, panic

• Identify alcohol consumption; if alcohol is consumed, hold dose until AM

### Nursing diagnoses
• Coping, ineffective (uses)
• Injury, risk for (adverse reactions)
• Knowledge, deficient (teaching)
• Noncompliance (teaching)

### Implementation
• Administer dosage at bedtime if oversedation occurs during day; may take entire dose at bedtime; may crush

• Store at room temperature; do not freeze

### Patient/family education
• Teach patient that therapeutic effects may take 1 wk or longer

• Instruct patient to use caution in driving or other activities requiring alertness because of drowsiness, dizziness, blurred vision; to avoid rising quickly from sitting to standing, especially geriatric

• Advise patient to avoid alcohol ingestion, other CNS depressants

◆ Teach patient not to discontinue medication quickly after long-term use: may cause nausea, headache, malaise

• Caution patient to wear sunscreen or large hat because photosensitivity can occur

• Teach patient to increase fluids, bulk in diet if constipation, urinary retention occur, especially geriatric

• Instruct patient to take gum, hard sugarless candy, or frequent sips of water for dry mouth

• Teach patient that suicidal thoughts/behavior may occur (children/adolescents)

### Evaluation
#### Positive therapeutic outcome
• Decrease in depression, OCD
• Absence of suicidal thoughts

**Treatment of overdose:** ECG monitoring, induce emesis, lavage, activated charcoal, administer anticonvulsant

## sildenafil (Rx)
(sil-den'a-fill)
Revatio, Viagra
*Func. class.:* Erectile agent
*Chem. class.:* Selective inhibitor of cGMP-PDE5

### Pregnancy category B

**Action:** Enhances the effect of nitric oxide (NO) by inhibiting phosphodiesterase type 5 (PDE5), which is necessary for degrading cGMP in the corpus cavernosum

**Therapeutic outcome:** Ability to achieve and maintain erection

**Uses:** Treatment of erectile dysfunction, pulmonary hypertension

**Unlabeled uses:** Sexual dysfunction (women)

### Dosage and routes
#### Erectile dysfunction (Viagra only)
*Adult:* PO 50 mg 1 hr before sexual activity or may be taken ½-4 hr before sexual activity; may be increased to 100 mg or decreased to 25 mg; max once/day

#### Renal/hepatic dose
*Adult:* PO 25 mg, take 1 hr before sexual activity, do not use more than 1 ×/day

Adverse effects: *italic* = common, **bold** = life-threatening

***Pulmonary hypertension (Revatio only)***
*Adult:* PO 20 mg tid, take 4-6 hr apart

**Available forms:** Tabs 20, 25, 50, 100 mg

**Adverse effects**
*CNS: Headache, flushing, dizziness*
*CV:* **MI, sudden death, CV collapse**
*MISC: Dyspepsia, nasal congestion, UTI, abnormal vision, diarrhea, rash,* **NAION (nonarteritic ischemic optic neuropathy),** hearing loss

**Contraindications:** Hypersensitivity to this product or nitrates

**Precautions:** Pregnancy **B,** anatomical penile deformities, sickle cell anemia, leukemia, multiple myeloma, retinitis pigmentosa, bleeding disorders, active peptic ulceration, CV/renal/hepatic disease, multidrug antihypertensive regimens

| Pharmacokinetics | |
| --- | --- |
| **Absorption** | Rapidly, bioavailability (40%) |
| **Distribution** | Unknown |
| **Metabolism** | Liver (active metabolites) |
| **Excretion** | Feces, urine |
| **Half-life** | 4 hr |

| Pharmacodynamics | |
| --- | --- |
| **Onset** | Unknown |
| **Peak** | ½-1½ hr |
| **Duration** | Unknown |

**Interactions**
*Individual drugs*
Alcohol, amlodipine: decreased B/P
Bosentan, cimetidine, erythromycin, itraconazole, ketoconazole: increased sildenafil levels
Rifampin: decreased sildenafil levels
*Drug classifications*
Antacids, barbiturates: decreased sildenafil levels
Antiretroviral protease inhibitors: increased sildenafil levels
α-Blockers, angiotensin II receptor blockers: decreased B/P
⬧ Nitrates: fatal reaction, do not use together

**NURSING CONSIDERATIONS**
**Assessment**
• Identify organic nitrates that should not be used with this product
• Assess for any severe loss of vision while taking this or any similar products; these products should not be used if vision loss has occurred

**Nursing diagnoses**
• Knowledge, deficient (teaching)
• Noncompliance (teaching)

**Implementation**
• Give approximately 1 hr before sexual activity, do not use more than once a day
• Tab may be split

**Patient/family education**
• Teach patient that product does not protect against STDs, including HIV
• Teach patient that product absorption is reduced with a high-fat meal
• Teach patient that product should not be used with nitrates in any form
• Teach patient that tab may be split
• Teach patient to notify prescriber immediately and stop taking product if vision loss occurs

**Evaluation**
**Positive therapeutic outcome**
• Ability to achieve and maintain an erection

**silver nitrate 1% ophthalmic**
*See Appendix D*

**silver nitrate sulfacetamide sodium ophthalmic**
*See Appendix D*

**\*silver sulfADIAZINE topical**
*See Appendix D*

## simethicone (Rx, OTC)
(si-meth'i-kone)

Extra Strength Gas-X, Extra Strength Maalox Anti-Gas, Extra Strength Maalox GRF Gas Relief Formula ✦, Flatulex, Gas Relief, Gas-X, Genasyme, Maalox Anti-Gas, Maalox GRF Gas Relief Formula ✦, Maximum Strength Gas Relief, Maximum Strength Mylanta Gas Relief, Maximum Strength Phazyme, Mylanta Gas, Mylicon, Ovol ✦, Phazyme, Phazyme-95, Phazyme-125

*Func. class.:* Antiflatulent

**Pregnancy category C**

**Do not confuse:**
Mylicon/Mylanta Gas

**Action:** Disperses, prevents gas pockets in GI system; lowers surface tension of gas bubbles

**Therapeutic outcome:** Belching or flatus

**Uses:** Flatulence

**Unlabeled uses:** Dyspepsia

**Dosage and routes**
*Adult and child >12 yr:* PO 40-360 mg after meals, at bedtime, max 500 mg/day
*Child 2-12 yr:* PO 40 mg after meals and at bedtime, max 240 mg/day
*Child <2 yr:* PO 20 mg qid

**Available forms:** Chew tabs 40, 80, 125, 150, 166 mg; tabs 60, 80, 95, 125 mg; drops 40 mg/0.6 ml, 40 mg/ml, 95 mg/1.425 ml; caps 95, 125, 166 mg; caps, soft gel 125 mg

**Adverse effects**
*GI:* Belching, rectal flatus, diarrhea

**Contraindications:** Hypersensitivity, GI obstruction/perforation

**Precautions:** Pregnancy C, abdominal pain, fistula, hiatal hernia

| Pharmacokinetics | |
|---|---|
| Absorption | None |
| Distribution | None |
| Metabolism | None |
| Excretion | None |
| Half-life | Unknown |

| Pharmacodynamics | |
|---|---|
| Onset | Rapid |
| Peak | Unknown |
| Duration | 3 hr |

## NURSING CONSIDERATIONS
**Assessment**
• Identify the reason for excess gas production: decreased bowel sounds, recent surgery, other GI conditions

**Nursing diagnoses**
• Knowledge, deficient (teaching)
• Pain, acute (uses)

**Implementation**
• Give after meals and at bedtime
• Shake susp well before administration
• Chew tab should be chewed and not swallowed whole

**Patient/family education**
• Caution patient that tab must be chewed; to shake susp well before pouring

**Evaluation**
**Positive therapeutic outcome**
• Absence of flatulence

## simvastatin (Rx)
(sim-va-stat'in)
Zocor
*Func. class.:* Antilipidemic
*Chem. class.:* HMG-CoA reductase inhibitor

**Pregnancy category X**

**Do not confuse:**
Zocor/Cozaar/Zoloft

**Action:** Inhibits HMG-CoA reductase enzyme, which reduces cholesterol synthesis; this enzyme is needed for cholesterol production

**Therapeutic outcome:** Decreasing cholesterol levels and LDLs, increased HDLs

**Uses:** As an adjunct in primary hypercholesterolemia (types IIa, IIb), mixed hyperlipidemia, CAD, isolated hypertriglyceridemia (Frederickson type IV) and type III hyperlipoproteinemia

**Dosage and routes**
*Adult:* PO 20 mg/day in PM initially, usual range 5-40 mg/day daily in PM, not to exceed 80 mg/day; dosage adjustments may be made at 4-wk intervals or more; those taking verapamil, max 20 mg/day

*Geriatric/renal dose/those taking cycloSPORINE:* PO 5 mg/day, initially

*Cardiac/renal transplantation*
*Adult:* PO 5 mg/day, max 10 mg/day

*With amiodarone or verapamil*
*Adult:* PO Max 20 mg/day

**S**

**With fibrates or niacin**
*Adult:* PO max 10 mg/day

**Available forms:** Tabs 5, 10, 20, 40, 80 mg

**Adverse effects**
*CNS:* Headache
*EENT:* Lens opacities
*GI:* Nausea, constipation, diarrhea, dyspepsia, flatus, abdominal pain, **liver dysfunction, pancreatitis**
*INTEG:* Rash, pruritus, photosensitivity
*MS:* Muscle cramps, myalgia, **myositis, rhabdomyolysis**
*RESP:* Upper respiratory tract infection

**Contraindications:** Pregnancy **X**, breastfeeding, hypersensitivity, active liver disease

**Precautions:** Past liver disease, alcoholism, severe acute infections, trauma, severe metabolic disorders, electrolyte imbalances

| Pharmacokinetics | |
|---|---|
| **Absorption** | 85% |
| **Distribution** | Unknown |
| **Metabolism** | Liver—extensively |
| **Excretion** | 70% feces, 20% kidneys |
| **Half-life** | 3 hr |

| Pharmacodynamics |
|---|
| Unknown |

**Interactions**
*Individual drugs*
Clarithromycin, clofibrate, cycloSPORINE, erythromycin, gemfibrozil, itraconazole, ketoconazole, niacin: increased myalgia, myositis
Digoxin: increased digoxin levels
Warfarin: increased risk of bleeding
*Drug classifications*
Protease inhibitors: increased myalgia, myositis
*Drug/herb*
Glucomannan: increased effect
Gotu kola: decreased effect
*Drug/lab test*
Increased: CPK, liver function tests

**NURSING CONSIDERATIONS**
**Assessment**
• Assess nutrition: fat, protein, carbohydrates; nutritional analysis should be completed by dietitian before treatment is initiated
◆ Assess for rhabdomyolysis: muscle tenderness, increased CPK levels; therapy should be discontinued

• Monitor bowel pattern daily; diarrhea may be a problem
• Monitor triglycerides, cholesterol baseline and throughout treatment; LDL, HDL, triglycerides and cholesterol at 6-8 wk and q6 mo should be watched closely; if increased, product should be discontinued

**Nursing diagnoses**
• Diarrhea (adverse reactions)
• Knowledge, deficient (teaching)
• Noncompliance (teaching)

**Implementation**
• Give 30 min before AM and PM meals

**Patient/family education**
• Inform patient that compliance is needed for positive results to occur; not to double doses
• Advise patient to lower risk factors: high-fat diet, smoking, alcohol consumption, absence of exercise
• Advise patient to notify health care prescriber if the GI symptoms of diarrhea, abdominal or epigastric pain, nausea, vomiting occur; or if chills, fever, sore throat occur

**Evaluation**
**Positive therapeutic outcome**
• Decreased cholesterol levels, serum triglycerides and improved ratio with HDLs

**sirolimus (Rx)**
(seer-roe′-li-mus)
Rapamune
*Func. class.:* Immunosuppressant
*Chem. class.:* Macrolide
**Pregnancy category** C

**Action:** Produces immunosuppression by inhibiting T-lymphocyte activation and proliferation

**Therapeutic outcome:** Prevention of rejection in organ transplant

**Uses:** Organ transplants: to prevent rejection, recommended use is with cycloSPORINE and corticosteroids

**Dosage and routes**
*Adult:* PO 2 mg daily with 6 mg loading dose, may use 5 mg/day with a 15 mg loading dose
*Child >13 yr <40 kg (88 lb):* PO 1 mg/m²/day, 3 mg/m²/loading dose

**Hepatic dose**
*Adult and child ≥13 yr <40 kg:* PO reduce by 33% in maintenance dose

**Available forms:** Oral sol 1 mg/ml

**Adverse effects**

*CNS: Tremors, headache, insomnia,* paresthesia, chills, fever

*CV:* Hypo/hypertension, **atrial fibrillation, CHF,** palpitations, **tachycardia**

*EENT:* Blurred vision, photophobia

*GI:* Nausea, vomiting, diarrhea, constipation

*GU:* UTI, **albuminuria, hematuria, proteinuria, renal failure,** nephrotic syndrome

*HEMA:* Anemia, **thrombocytopenia purpura, leukopenia**

*INTEG: Rash, acne,* photosensitivity

*META:* Increased creatinine, edema, hypercholesterolemia, *hyperlipemia,* hypophosphatemia, weight gain, hyperglycemia, hypo/hyperkalemia, hyperuricemia, hypomagnesemia

*RESP:* **Pleural effusion, atelectasis,** *dyspnea*

*SYST:* **Lymphoma,** exfoliative dermatitis

**Contraindications:** Breastfeeding, hypersensitivity to this product or to components of the product

**Precautions:** Pregnancy **C,** children <13 yr, severe renal/hepatic disease, diabetes mellitus, hyperkalemia, hyperuricemia, lymphomas, hypertension, infection, other malignancies

| Pharmacokinetics | |
|---|---|
| Absorption | Rapidly absorbed |
| Distribution | 92% protein binding |
| Metabolism | Liver; extensively by CYP3A4 enzyme system |
| Excretion | Unknown |
| Half-life | Unknown |

| Pharmacodynamics | |
|---|---|
| Onset | Unknown |
| Peak | 1 hr single dose, 2 hr multiple dosing |
| Duration | Unknown |

**Interactions**

*Individual drugs*

Bromocriptine, cimetidine, cycloSPORINE, danazol, erythromycin, metoclopramide: increased blood level

Carbamazepine, phenobarbital, phenytoin, rifamycin, rifapentine: decreased blood levels

*Drug classifications*

ACE inhibitors, angiotensin II receptor antagonists, cephalosporins, iodine-containing radiopaque contrast media, neuromuscular blockers, NSAIDs, penicillins, salicylates, thrombolytics: increased angioedema

Antifungal agents, calcium channel blockers, HIV protease inhibitors: increased blood levels

Live virus vaccines: decreased effect of vaccines

*Drug/herb*

Astragalus, echinacea, melatonin: decreased immunosuppression

Ginseng, maitake, mistletoe: increased effect

St. John's wort: decreased sirolimus effect

*Drug/food*

Food: alters bioavailability, use consistently with or without food

Grapefruit juice: do not use with grapefruit juice

**NURSING CONSIDERATIONS**

**Assessment**

• Monitor blood studies: Hgb, WBC, platelets monthly during treatment; if leukocytes are <3000/mm$^3$, or platelets <100,000/mm$^3$, product should be discontinued or reduced; decreased Hgb level may indicate bone marrow suppression

• Monitor blood levels in those who may have altered metabolism, trough levels ≥15 ng/ml are associated with increased adverse reactions

• Monitor lipid profile: cholesterol, triglycerides; a lipid-lowering agent may be needed

• Assess for infection and development of lymphoma

• Monitor liver function tests: alkaline phosphatase, AST, ALT, amylase, bilirubin, and for hepatotoxicity: dark urine, jaundice, itching, light-colored stools; product should be discontinued

**Nursing diagnoses**

• Infection, risk for (uses)

• Knowledge, deficient (teaching)

**Implementation**

• Administer prophylaxis for *Pneumocystis jiroveci* pneumonia for 1 yr after transplantation; prophylaxis for cytomegalovirus (CMV) is recommended for 90 days after transplantation in those at increased risk for CMV

• Use amber oral dose syringe and withdraw amount of oral sol needed from the bottle, empty correct dose into plastic/glass container holding 60 ml of water/orange juice, stir vigorously and have patient drink at once, refill container with additional 120 ml of water/orange juice, stir vigorously, and have patient drink at once; if using a pouch squeeze entire

**S**

contents into container and follow preceding directions
• Give all medications PO if possible; avoid IM inj because bleeding may occur
• Give for 3 days before transplant surgery; patients should be placed in protective isolation
• Store protected from light; refrigerate; stable for 24 months

### Patient/family education
• Instruct patient to report fever, rash, severe diarrhea, chills, sore throat, fatigue because serious infections may occur; clay-colored stools, cramping may indicate hepatotoxicity
• Caution patient to avoid crowds or persons with known infections to reduce risk of infection
• Teach patient to use contraception before, during, and 12 wk after product has been discontinued, avoid breastfeeding
• Teach patient to use sunscreen, protective clothing to prevent burns

### Evaluation
**Positive therapeutic outcome**
• Absence of graft rejection

---

### sitagliptin (Rx)
(sit-a-glip′tin)
Januvia
*Func. class.:* Antidiabetic, oral
*Chem. class.:* Dipeptidyl-peptidase-4 inhibitor (DPP-4 inhibitor)

**Pregnancy category** C

**Action:** Slows the inactivation of incretin hormones; improves glucose homeostasis, improves glucose-dependent insulin synthesis, lowers glucagon secretions and slows gastric emptying time

**Therapeutic outcome:** Decrease in polyuria, polydipsia, polyphagia; clear sensorium; absence of dizziness; stable gait, blood glucose at normal level

**Uses:** Type 2 diabetes mellitus as monotherapy or in combination with other antidiabetic agents

### Dosage and routes
*Adult:* PO 100 mg/day; may use with other antidiabetic agents (metformin, pioglitazone, rosiglitazone)

**Available forms:** Tabs 25, 50, 100 mg

### Adverse effects
*CNS: Headache*
*ENDO:* Hypoglycemia
*GI: Nausea, vomiting,* abdominal pain

**Contraindications:** Hypersensitivity, diabetic ketoacidosis (DKA)

**Precautions:** Pregnancy **C**, geriatric, hypersensitivity, GI obstruction, thyroid disease, surgery, renal/hepatic disease, trauma

| Pharmacokinetics | |
|---|---|
| **Absorption** | Rapidly |
| **Distribution** | Unknown |
| **Metabolism** | Unknown |
| **Excretion** | Kidneys, 79% unchanged |
| **Half-life** | Terminal 12.4 hr |

| Pharmacodynamics | |
|---|---|
| **Onset** | Unknown |
| **Peak** | 1-4 hr |
| **Duration** | Unknown |

### Interactions
*Individual drugs*
Cimetidine, fluoxetine: increased hypoglycemia
Cimetidine, disopyramide: increased sitagliptan level
Digoxin: increased levels of digoxin
Aripiprazole, clozapine, olanzapine, quetiapine, risperidone, ziprasidone, phenytoin, fosphenytoin: decreased antidiabetic effect
*Drug classifications*
Androgens, insulins, β-blockers, corticosteroids, salicylates, MAOIs, fibric acid derivatives: increased hypoglycemia
Thiazide diuretics, ACE inhibitors, protease inhibitors, sympathomimetics, phenothiazines, estrogens, progestins, oral contraceptives: decreased antidiabetic effect
*Drug/herb*
Alfalfa, aloe, basil, bay, bilberry, bitter melon, black catechu, buchu, burdock, coriander, dandelion, eyebright (po), fenugreek, garlic, ginseng, glucomannan, glucosamine, goat's rue, gymnema, horehound, horse chestnut, jambul, myrrh, myrtle: increased antidiabetic effect
Bee pollen, blue cohosh, broom, chromium, elecampane, eucalyptus, gotu kola: decreased antidiabetic effect
Chromium, coenzyme Q-10, fenugreek: increased hypoglycemia
Glucosamine: increased hyperglycemia

## NURSING CONSIDERATIONS
### Assessment
- Assess for hypoglycemic reactions (sweating, weakness, dizziness, anxiety, tremors, hunger), hyperglycemic reactions soon after meals
- Monitor CBC (baseline, q3 mo) during treatment; check liver function tests periodically, AST, LDH, renal studies: BUN, creatinine during treatment; glycosylated hemoglobin A1c
- Monitor blood glucose (BG) as needed

### Nursing diagnoses
- Knowledge, deficient (teaching)
- Noncompliance (teaching)
- Nutrition: more than body requirements, imbalanced (uses)

### Implementation
- May be taken with or without food
- Give 100 mg daily
- Conversion from other antidiabetic agents; change may be made with gradual dosage change
- Store in tight container in cool environment

### Patient/family education
- Teach patient to use regular self-monitoring of blood glucose using blood glucose meter
- Teach patient the symptoms of hypo/hyperglycemia; what to do about each
- Teach patient that product must be continued on daily basis; explain consequence of discontinuing product abruptly
- Advise patient to avoid OTC medications, alcohol, digoxin, exenatide, insulins, nateglinide, repaglinide and other products that lower blood sugar, unless approved by prescriber
- Teach patient that diabetes is a lifelong illness; that this product is not a cure, only controls symptoms
- Teach patient that all food included in diet plan must be eaten to prevent hypo/hyperglycemia
- Teach patient to carry emergency ID

### Evaluation
**Positive therapeutic outcome**
- Decrease in polyuria, polydipsia, polyphagia; clear sensorium; absence of dizziness; stable gait, blood glucose at normal level

---

### sodium bicarbonate (Rx, OTC)
baking soda, Bellans, Brosch-Neut, Citrocarbonate, Neut, Sellymin ✤, Soda Mint
*Func. class.:* Alkalinizer; antacid
**Pregnancy category** C

**Action:** Orally neutralizes gastric acid, which forms water, NaCl, $CO_2$; increases plasma bicarbonate, which buffers $H^+$ ion concentration; reverses acidosis **IV**

**Therapeutic outcome:** Correction of acidosis, gastric acid neutralization

**Uses:** Acidosis (metabolic), cardiac arrest, alkalinization (systemic/urinary); antacid (PO); salicylate poisoning

### Dosage and routes
*Acidosis, metabolic*
*Adult and child:* IV INF 2-5 mEq/kg over 4-8 hr depending on $CO_2$, pH

*Cardiac arrest*
*Adult and child:* IV BOL 1 mEq/kg of 7.5% or 8.4% sol, then 0.5 mEq/kg q5-10 min, then doses based on ABGs
*Infant:* IV INF not to exceed 8 mEq/kg/day based on ABGs (4.2% sol)

*Alkalinization of urine*
*Adult:* PO 325 mg-2 g qid or 48 mEq/kg (4 g), then 12-24 mEq q4hr
*Child:* PO 12-120 mg/kg/day (1-10 mEq/kg)

*Antacid*
*Adult:* PO 300 mg-2 g chewed, taken with water daily-qid

**Available forms:** Tabs 300, 325, 600, 650 mg; inj 4.2%, 5%, 7.5%, 8.4%

### Adverse effects
*CNS:* Irritability, headache, confusion, stimulation, tremors, *twitching, hyperreflexia,* **tetany,** weakness, **seizures** caused by alkalosis
*CV:* Irregular pulse, **cardiac arrest,** water retention, edema, weight gain
*GI:* Flatulence, *belching, distention,* **paralytic ileus,** acid rebound, nausea
*GU:* Calculi
*META:* Alkalosis
*MS:* Muscular twitching, tetany, irritability
*RESP:* Shallow, slow respirations, cyanosis, **apnea**

**Contraindications:** Hypertension, peptic ulcer, hypocalcemia

**Precautions:** Pregnancy **C,** CHF, cirrhosis, toxemia, renal disease

**S**

---

Adverse effects: *italic* = common, **bold** = life-threatening

### Pharmacokinetics

| | |
|---|---|
| **Absorption** | Unknown |
| **Distribution** | Widely distributed—extracellular fluids |
| **Metabolism** | Unknown |
| **Excretion** | Kidneys |
| **Half-life** | Unknown |

### Pharmacodynamics

| | PO | IV |
|---|---|---|
| **Onset** | 2 min | Rapid |
| **Peak** | ½ hr | Rapid |
| **Duration** | 1-3 hr | Unknown |

## Interactions
### Individual drugs
Chlorpropamide, lithium: decreased effect of each specific product

Flecainide, mecamylamine, pseudoephedrine, quinidine, quinine: increased effects of each specific product

### Drug classifications
Amphetamines, anorexiants: increased effects

Barbiturates: decreased effects of barbiturates

Benzodiazepines: decreased effects

Corticosteroids: increased sodium; decreased potassium

Salicylates: decreased effect of salicylates

### Drug/herb
Oak bark: decreased action of sodium bicarbonate

### Drug/lab test
Increased: urinary urobilinogen

False positive: urinary protein, blood lactate

## NURSING CONSIDERATIONS
### Assessment
• Assess respiratory and pulse rate, rhythm, depth, lung sounds; notify prescriber of abnormalities

• Assess for $CO_2$ in GI tract; may lead to perforation if ulcer is severe

• Monitor fluid balance (I&O ratio, weight daily, edema); notify prescriber of fluid overload

• Monitor electrolytes, blood pH, $PO_2$, $HCO_3$, during beginning treatment; ABGs frequently during emergencies

• Monitor urine pH, urinary output, during beginning treatment

• Monitor extravasation with **IV** administration (tissue sloughing, ulceration, and necrosis)

• Assess for alkalosis: irritability, confusion, twitching, hyperreflexia, stimulation, slow respirations, cyanosis, irregular pulse

• Monitor manifestations of hypokalemia: *RENAL:* acidic urine, reduced urine osmolality, nocturia, polyuria, polydipsia; *CV:* hypotension, broad T wave, U wave, ectopy, tachycardia, weak pulse; *NEURO:* muscle weakness, altered LOC, drowsiness, apathy, lethargy, confusion, depression; *GI:* anorexia, nausea, cramps, constipation, distention, paralytic ileus; *RESP:* hypoventilation, respiratory muscle weakness

• Monitor for manifestations of hyponatremia: *CV:* increased B/P, cold, clammy skin, hypo/hypervolemia; *GI:* anorexia, nausea, vomiting, diarrhea, abdominal cramps; *NEURO:* lethargy, increased ICP, confusion, headache, seizures, coma, fatigue, tremors, hyperreflexia

• Assess for milk-alkali syndrome: confusion, headache, nausea, vomiting, anorexia, urinary stones, hypercalcemia

### Nursing diagnoses
• Fluid volume, excess (adverse reactions)

• Gas exchange, impaired (uses)

• Knowledge, deficient (teaching)

### Implementation
#### PO route
• Antacid tab must be chewed and taken with 8 oz of water

• Dissolve effervescent tab in water

• May be used to neutralize gastric acid in peptic ulcer disease, given 1 and 3 hr after meals and at bedtime

#### IV route
• Give **IV** bol in cardiac arrest, may be repeated q10 min

• Give by intermittent or cont inf in prepared sol or diluted in an equal amount of any dextrose/saline combination; administer 2-5 mEq/kg over 4-8 hr, not to exceed 50 mEq/hr; slower rate in children

*Syringe compatibilities:* Milrinone, pentobarbital

*Syringe incompatibilities:* Glycopyrrolate, metoclopramide, thiopental

*Y-site compatibilities:* Acyclovir, amifostine, asparaginase, aztreonam, cefepime, cefmetazole, ceftriaxone, cladribine, cyclophosphamide, cytarabine, DAUNOrubicin, dexamethasone, dexchlorpheniramine, DOXOrubicin, etoposide, famotidine, filgrastim, fludarabine, gallium, granisetron, heparin, ifosfamide, indomethacin, insulin, melphalan, mesna, methylPREDNISolone, morphine, paclitaxel, piperacillin/tazobactam, potassium chloride, propofol, tacrolimus, teniposide, thiotepa, tolazoline, vancomycin, vit B/C

*Y-site incompatibilities:* Calcium chloride, idarubicin, imanrinone, sargramostim, verapamil, vinorelbine

*Additive compatibilities:* Amikacin, aminophylline, amobarbital, amphotericin B, atropine, bretylium, calcium gluceptate, cefoxitin, ceftazidime, cephalothin, cephapirin, chloramphenicol, chlorothiazide, cimetidine, clindamycin, cytarabine, droperidol/fentanyl, ergonovine, erythromycin, esmolol, floxacillin, furosemide, heparin, hyaluronidase, hydrocortisone, kanamycin, lidocaine, mannitol, metaraminol, methotrexate, methyldopate, multivitamins, nafcillin, nalmefene, netilmicin, nizatidine, ofloxacin, oxacillin, oxytocin, phenobarbital, phenylephrine, phenytoin, phytonadione, potassium chloride, prochlorperazine, thiopental, verapamil

*Additive incompatibilities:* Amoxicillin, ascorbic acid, carboplatin, carmustine, cefotaxime, cisplatin, codeine, DOBUTamine, epINEPHrine, hydromorphone, imipenem/cilastatin, insulin, isoproterenol, labetalol, levorphanol, magnesium sulfate, methadone, morphine, norepinephrine, pentazocine, pentobarbital, procaine, secobarbital, streptomycin, succinylcholine, tetracycline, vit B/C

## Patient/family education
• Instruct patient to chew antacid tab and drink 8 oz of water; not to take antacid with milk because milk-alkali syndrome may result; not to use antacid for more than 2 wk
• Advise patient to notify prescriber if indigestion is accompanied by chest pain; dyspnea; diarrhea; dark, tarry stools; coffee grounds–looking vomit; swelling of feet/ankles
• Teach patient about sodium-restricted diet; to avoid use of baking soda for indigestion

## Evaluation
**Positive therapeutic outcome**
• ABGs, electrolytes, blood pH, $HCO_3$ normal levels
• Decreased gastric pain

---

## sodium biphosphate/ sodium phosphate (OTC)
Fleet Enema, Phospho-soda
*Func. class.:* Laxative, saline
**Pregnancy category C**

**Action:** Increases water absorption in the small intestine by osmotic action; laxative effect occurs by increased peristalsis and water retention

**Therapeutic outcome:** Absence of constipation

**Uses:** Constipation, bowel or rectal preparation for surgery, examination

## Dosage and routes
*Adult:* PO 20-30 ml (Phospho-soda)
*Child:* PO 5-15 ml (Phospho-soda)
*Adult and child >12 yr:* RECT enema (118 ml)
*Child 2-12 yr:* RECT ½ enema (59 ml)

**Available forms:** Enema 7 g/phosphate and 19 g/biphosphate/118 ml; oral sol 18 g phosphate/48 g biphosphate/100 ml

## Adverse effects
*CV:* **Dysrhythmias, cardiac arrest,** hypotension, widening QRS complex
*GI:* *Nausea, cramps,* diarrhea
*META:* Electrolyte, fluid imbalances

**Contraindications:** Hypersensitivity, rectal fissures, abdominal pain, nausea/vomiting, appendicitis, acute surgical abdomen, ulcerated hemorrhoids, Na-restricted diets, renal failure, hyperphosphatemia, hypocalcemia, hypokalemia, hypernatremia, Addison's disease, CHF, ascites, bowel perforation; megacolon, imperforate anus

**Precautions:** Pregnancy **C**

### Pharmacokinetics
| | |
|---|---|
| Absorption | Up to 20% (rec) |
| Distribution | Unknown |
| Metabolism | Unknown |
| Excretion | Kidneys |
| Half-life | Unknown |

### Pharmacodynamics
| | PO | RECT |
|---|---|---|
| Onset | ½-3 hr | 5 min |
| Peak | Unknown | Unknown |
| Duration | Unknown | Unknown |

---

## NURSING CONSIDERATIONS
### Assessment
• Assess stools: color, amount, consistency
• Assess for bowel pattern, bowel sounds (frequency, intensity), flatulence, distention, increased temp, dietary patterns (fluid, bulk), exercise
• Assess for cramping, rectal bleeding, nausea, vomiting; if these symptoms occur, product should be discontinued

### Nursing diagnoses
• Constipation (uses)
• Knowledge, deficient (teaching)

### Implementation
**PO route**
• Give on empty stomach
• Mix oral sol in cold water

Adverse effects: *italic* = common, **bold** = life-threatening

- Take alone for better absorption; do not take within 1 hr of other products

**Patient/family education**
- Advise patient not to use laxatives or enema for long-term therapy; bowel tone will be lost
- Teach patient that normal bowel movements do not always occur daily
- Caution patient not to use in presence of abdominal pain, nausea, vomiting
- Caution patient to notify prescriber if constipation is unrelieved or if symptoms of electrolyte imbalance occur: muscle cramps, pain, weakness, dizziness, excessive thirst
- Instruct patient to maintain adequate fluid consumption to help prevent constipation

**Evaluation**
**Positive therapeutic outcome**
- Decrease in constipation

---

**sodium polystyrene sulfonate** (Rx)
(po-lee-stye'reen)
Kayexalate, K-Exit ♣, Kionex, PMS Sodium Polystyrene Sulfonate ♣, SPS
*Func. class.:* Potassium-removing resin
*Chem. class.:* Cation exchange resin

**Pregnancy category** C

**Action:** Removes potassium by exchanging sodium for potassium in body; occurs primarily in large intestine

**Therapeutic outcome:** Potassium levels within accepted range

**Uses:** Hyperkalemia in conjunction with other measures

**Dosage and routes**
*Adult:* PO 15 g daily-qid; RECT enema 30-50 g/100 ml of sorbitol warmed to body temp q6hr
*Child:* PO/RECT 1 mEq of K exchanged/g of resin, approximate dose 1 g/kg q6hr

**Available forms:** Susp, 15 g polystyrene sulfonate, 21.5 ml sorbitol, 15 g (65 mEq) sodium/60 ml; powder 15 g/4 level tsp

**Adverse effects**
*GI: Constipation,* anorexia, nausea, vomiting, diarrhea (sorbitol), *fecal impaction,* gastric irritation
*META:* Hypocalcemia, hypokalemia, hypomagnesemia, sodium retention

**Contraindications:** Hypersensitivity to saccharin or parabens that may be in some products; ileus

**Precautions:** Pregnancy C, geriatric, renal failure, CHF, severe edema, severe hypertension, sodium restriction, constipation

**Pharmacokinetics**
| | |
|---|---|
| Absorption | None |
| Distribution | None |
| Metabolism | None |
| Excretion | Feces |
| Half-life | Unknown |

**Pharmacodynamics**
| | PO | RECT |
|---|---|---|
| Onset | 2-12 hr | 2-12 hr |
| Peak | Unknown | Unknown |
| Duration | 6-24 hr | 4-6 hr |

**Interactions**
*Drug classifications*
Antacids (calcium or magnesium), laxatives: decreased effect of sodium polystyrene
Diuretics (loop): increased hypokalemia

**NURSING CONSIDERATIONS**
**Assessment**
- Assess bowel function daily: amount of stool, color, characteristics
- Assess for hypotension: confusion, irritability, muscular pain, weakness
- Monitor for manifestations of hypokalemia: *RENAL:* acidic urine, reduced urine osmolality, nocturia, polyuria, polydipsia; *CV:* hypotension, broad T wave, U wave, ectopy, tachycardia, weak pulse; *NEURO:* muscle weakness, altered LOC, drowsiness, apathy, lethargy, confusion, depression; *GI:* anorexia, nausea, cramps, constipation, distention, paralytic ileus; *RESP:* hypoventilation, respiratory muscle weakness
- Monitor for manifestations of hyperkalemia: confusion, dyspnea, weakness, dysrhythmias
- Monitor for manifestations of hypocalcemia: *CNS:* personality changes, anxiety, disturbances, depression, psychosis, nausea, vomiting, *GI:* constipation, abdominal pain from muscle spasm; *CV:* decreased contractility, decreased cardiac output, hypotension, lengthened ST segment, prolonged QT interval; *INTEG:* scaling eczema, alopecia, hyperpigmentation; *NEURO:* tetany, muscle twitching, cramping grimacing, seizure, altered deep tendon reflexes, spasm
- Monitor for manifestations of hypomagnesemia; *CNS:* agitation; *NEURO:* muscle twitching, paresthesias, hyperactive reflexes, positive Babinski reflex, dysphagia, nystagmus, seizures, tetany; *GI:* nausea, vomiting, diarrhea, anorexia, abdominal

distention; *CV:* ectopy; tachycardia, broad, flat, or inverted T waves; depressed ST segment; prolonged QT interval; decreased cardiac output; hypotension
• Monitor electrolytes: potassium, sodium, calcium, magnesium; I&O ratio, weight daily
• Monitor ECG for spiked T waves, depressed ST segments, prolonged QT interval and widening QRS complex

### Nursing diagnoses
• Constipation (adverse reactions)
• Diarrhea (adverse reactions)
• Knowledge, deficient (teaching)

### Implementation
**PO route**
• Give oral dose as susp mixed with $H_2O$ or syr (20-100 ml)
• Give mild laxative as ordered to prevent constipation and fecal impaction; sorbitol as ordered to prevent constipation

**Rectal route**
• Give by retention enema after mixing with warm water; introduce by gravity, continue stirring, flush with 100 ml of fluid, clamp, and leave in place for at least ½-1 hr
• Complete irrigation of colon after enema with 1-2 qt of nonsodium sol, drain
• Store freshly prepared sol for 24 hr at room temperature

### Patient/family education
• Explain reason for medication and expected results

### Evaluation
**Positive therapeutic outcome**
• Potassium level 3.5-5 mg/dl

---

## solifenacin (Rx)
(sol-i-fen′a-sin)
VESIcare
*Func. class.:* Overactive bladder product, anticholinergic
*Chem. class.:* Muscarinic receptor antagonist

### Pregnancy category  C

**Action:** Relaxes smooth muscles in urinary tract by inhibiting acetylcholine at postganglionic sites

**Therapeutic outcome:** Decreased dysuria, frequency, nocturia, incontinence

**Uses:** Overactive bladder (urinary frequency, urgency, incontinence)

### Dosage and routes
*Adult:* PO 5 mg/day, max 10 mg/day

### Renal/hepatic dose
*Adult:* PO CCr <30 ml/min 5 mg/day

**Available forms:** Tabs 5, 10 mg

### Adverse effects
*CNS:* Anxiety, paresthesia, fatigue, *dizziness,* headache
*CV:* Chest pain, hypertension, **QTc prolongation, edema**
*EENT: Vision abnormalities, xerophthalmia,* nasal dryness
*GI: Nausea, vomiting, anorexia,* abdominal pain, *constipation,* dry mouth, dyspepsia
*GU:* Dysuria, urinary retention, frequency, UTI
*INTEG:* Rash, pruritus
*RESP:* Bronchitis, cough, pharyngitis, URI

**Contraindications:** Hypersensitivity, uncontrolled angle-closure glaucoma, urinary retention, gastric retention

**Precautions:** Pregnancy **C**, breastfeeding, children, renal/hepatic disease, controlled angle-closure glaucoma, bladder outflow obstruction, GI obstruction, decreased GI motility, history of QT prolongation

### Pharmacokinetics
| | |
|---|---|
| **Absorption** | Rapid |
| **Distribution** | 98% highly protein bound |
| **Metabolism** | Extensively metabolized by CYP3A4 |
| **Excretion** | Excreted in urine/feces |
| **Half-life** | Terminal half-life 45-68 hr |

### Pharmacodynamics
Unknown

### Interactions
*Drug classifications*
CYP3A4 inducers (carbamazepine, nevirapine, phenobarbitol, phenytoin): decreased effects of solifenacin
CYP3A4 inhibitors (clarithromycin, diclofenac, doxycycline, erythromycin, isoniazid, ketoconazole, nefazodone, propofol, protease inhibitors, verapamil): increased action of solifenacin, with max dose 5 mg
*Drug/herb*
Henbane, jimsonweed, scopolia: increased effects
St. John's wort: decreased effects
*Drug/food*
Grapefruit juice: increased effect

### NURSING CONSIDERATIONS
### Assessment
• Assess urinary patterns: distention, nocturia, frequency, urgency, incontinence

---

Adverse effects: *italic* = common, **bold** = life-threatening

- Assess for allergic reactions: rash; if this occurs, product should be discontinued

### Nursing diagnoses
- Knowledge, deficient (teaching)
- Urinary elimination, impaired (uses)

### Patient/family education
- Caution patient to avoid hazardous activities; dizziness may occur
- Advise patient that constipation, blurred vision may occur
- Instruct patient to call prescriber if severe abdominal pain or constipation lasts for 3 or more days
- Advise patient that heat prostration may occur if used in a hot environment

### Evaluation
**Positive therapeutic outcome**
- Urinary status: dysuria, frequency, nocturia, incontinence

---

### somatropin (Rx)
(soe-ma-troe′pin)
Genotropin, Genotropin-MinQuick, Humatrope, Norditropin, Nutropin, Nutropin AQ, Nutropin Depot, Omnitrope, Saizen, Serostim, Tev-Tropin
*Func. class.:* Pituitary hormone
*Chem. class.:* Growth hormone

**Pregnancy category** C

**Action:** Stimulates growth; similar to natural growth hormone—both preparations are developed by recombinant DNA technique

**Therapeutic outcome:** Increase in height as a result of skeletal growth in pituitary growth hormone deficiency

**Uses:** Pituitary growth hormone deficiency (hypopituitary dwarfism), children with human growth hormone deficiency, AIDS wasting syndrome, cachexia, adults with somatropin deficiency syndrome (SDS), short stature in Noonan syndrome, SHOX deficiencies

### Dosage and routes
*Genotropin*
*Child:* SUBCUT 0.16-0.24 mg/kg/wk, divided into 6 or 7 inj, give in abdomen, thigh, buttocks
*Adult:* SUBCUT 0.4-0.8 mg/kg/wk divided in 6-7 daily doses

*Humatrope*
*Child:* SUBCUT/IM 0.18 mg/kg divided into equal doses either on 3 alternate days or 6 ×/wk, max wk dose is 0.3 mg/kg

*Adult:* IM 0.018 units/kg/day, max 0.0375 units/kg/day

*Growth hormone deficiency Nutropin/Nutropin AQ*
*Child:* SUBCUT 0.3 mg/kg/wk

*Serostim*
*Adult:* SUBCUT at bedtime >55 kg 6 mg, 45-55 kg 5 mg, 35-45 kg 4 mg

*Norditropin*
*Child:* SUBCUT 0.024-0.034 mg/kg 6-7 ×/wk

*Replacement of GH in GH deficiency*
*Adult:* SUBCUT (Saizen) 0.005 mg/kg/day; may increase after 4 wk to max 0.01 mg/kg/day

**Available forms:** Powder for inj (lyophilized) 1.5 mg (4 international units/ml), 4 mg (12 international units/vial), 5 mg (13 international units/vial), 5 mg (15 international units/vial), rDNA origin, 5.8 mg (15 international units/ml), 6 mg (18 international units/ml), 8 mg (24 international units/vial), 10 mg (26 international units/vial), inj 10 mg (30 international units/vial); 5, 10, 15 mg/1.5 ml

### Adverse effects
*CNS:* Headache, **growth of intracranial tumor,** fever, aggressive behavior
*ENDO: Hyperglycemia, ketosis, hypothyroidism*
*GI:* Nausea, vomiting
*GU: Hypercalciuria*
*INTEG:* Rash, urticaria, pain, inflammation at inj site
*MS:* Tissue swelling, joint and muscle pain
*SYST: Antibodies to growth hormone*

**Contraindications:** Hypersensitivity to benzyl alcohol, closed epiphyses, intracranial lesions, acute respiratory failure, Prader-Willi syndrome

**Precautions:** Pregnancy C, breastfeeding, newborns, geriatric, diabetes mellitus, hypothyroidism, intracranial lesions, prolonged treatment in adults, scoliosis

| Pharmacokinetics | |
|---|---|
| **Absorption** | Well absorbed (SUBCUT/IM) |
| **Distribution** | Unknown |
| **Metabolism** | Unknown |
| **Excretion** | Unknown |
| **Half-life** | 15-60 min |

### Pharmacodynamics

|  | IM/SUBCUT (GROWTH) |
|---|---|
| **Onset** | Unknown |
| **Peak** | Unknown |
| **Duration** | 7 days |

## Interactions
### Drug classifications
Androgens, thyroid hormones: increased epiphyseal closure
Glucocorticosteroids: decreased growth

## NURSING CONSIDERATIONS
### Assessment
- Identify growth hormone antibodies if patient fails to respond to therapy
- Monitor thyroid function tests: $T_3$, $T_4$, $T_7$, TSH to identify hypothyroidism
- Assess for allergic reaction: rash, itching, fever, nausea, wheezing
- Assess for hypercalciuria: urinary stones; groin, flank pain; nausea, vomiting, frequency, hematuria, chills
- Monitor growth rate of child at intervals during treatment

### Nursing diagnoses
- Body image, disturbed (uses)
- Knowledge, deficient (teaching)

### Implementation
- Store in refrigerator for <1 mo; if reconstituted, <1 wk; do not use discolored or cloudy sol

**IM route**
- Norditropin: After reconstituting 4-8 mg/2 ml diluent
- Humetrope: 5 mg/1.5-5 ml dilute, do not shake
- Nutropin/Nutropin AQ: Reconstitute 5 mg/1-5 ml or 10 mg/1-10 ml of bacteriostatic water for inj (benzyl alcohol preserved)

### Patient/family education
- Explain reason for medication and expected results; that treatment may continue for yr
- Advise patient that routine follow-up is needed to monitor growth rate
- Instruct parents on procedure for medication preparation and inj use; request demonstration, return demonstration; provide written instructions
- Teach patient to maintain growth record, report knee, hip pain or limping
- Advise patient treatment is very expensive

### Evaluation
**Positive therapeutic outcome**
- Growth in children until epiphyseal plates close

## sorafenib (Rx)
(sore-ah-fen'ib)
Nexavar
*Func. class.:* Antineoplastic—miscellaneous
*Chem. class.:* Multikinase inhibitor, signal transduction inhibitor
### Pregnancy category D

**Action:** Multikinase inhibitor that decreases tumor cell proliferation

**Therapeutic outcome:** Prevent spread of malignancy

**Uses:** Advanced/metastatic murine renal cell carcinoma

### Dosage and routes
*Adult:* PO 400 mg bid without food, continue until no longer benefiting or until unacceptable toxicity occurs

**Available forms:** Tabs 200 mg

### Adverse effects
*CNS:* Fatigue, weight loss, headache
*CV:* **Hypertension, cardiac ischemia, infarction, hypertensive crisis**
*GI:* *Nausea, diarrhea, vomiting,* anorexia, **pancreatitis,** mouth ulceration, abdominal pain, constipation, **GI perforation**
*HEMA:* **Hemorrhage, leukopenia, lymphopenia, anemia, neutropenia, thrombocytopenia, pancytopenia**
*INTEG:* *Rash,* pruritus, *dry skin,* erythema, hand-foot syndrome, **exfoliative dermatitis,** acne, flushing, alopecia
*META:* *Hypophosphatemia*
*MS:* *Arthralgia, myalgia*
*RESP:* *Hoarseness*

**Contraindications:** Pregnancy **D,** hypersensitivity

**Precautions:** Breastfeeding, children, geriatric, cardiac/renal/hepatic disease

S

### Pharmacokinetics

| | |
|---|---|
| **Absorption** | 38%-49%, high fat meal decreases bioavailability |
| **Distribution** | Protein binding 99.5% |
| **Metabolism** | Liver, oxidative metabolism by CYP3A4, glucuronidation by UGT1A9 |
| **Excretion** | 77% feces |
| **Half-life** | Elimination 25-48 hr |

### Pharmacodynamics

| | |
|---|---|
| **Onset** | Unknown |
| **Peak** | 3 hr |
| **Duration** | Unknown |

Adverse effects: *italic* = common, **bold** = life-threatening

## Interactions
### Drug classifications
Anticoagulants, NSAIDs, platelet inhibitors, thrombolytics: increased bleeding risk

CYP3A4 inducers (barbiturates, bosentan, carbamazepine, efavirenz, nevirapine, phenytoins, rifabutin, rifampin): may decrease sorafenib effect

UGT1A1 drugs (irinotecan, DOXOrubicin, morphine, naltrexone, estradiol, buprenorphine): increased effect of sorafenib

### Drug/lab test
Increased: lipase, amylase

## NURSING CONSIDERATIONS
### Assessment
• Assess for skin toxicities: Grade 1, continue therapy, topical treatment for relief; grade 2 (1st episode), continue therapy, if no improvement after 7 days, delay treatment until resolved to grade ≤1, resume dose by one dose level; grade 2 (2nd or 3rd episode), delay treatment until resolved to grade ≤1, resume dose by one dose level; grade 2 (4th episode), discontinue therapy; grade 3 (1st or 2nd episode), delay treatment until resolved to grade ≤1, resume dose by one dose level; grade 3 (3rd episode), discontinue therapy.

### Nursing diagnoses
• Injury, risk for (uses, adverse reactions)

### Implementation
• Swallow tab whole; do not break, crush, or chew
• Give on empty stomach 1 hr before or 2 hr after meal
• Store at room temp, in dry place

### Patient/family education
◆ Teach patient to report adverse reactions immediately
• Teach patient the reason for treatment, expected results
• Advise patient to use contraception during treatment, birth defects may occur; avoid breastfeeding
• Advise patient not to double dose if missed
• Advise patient to avoid OTC products without approval of prescriber

### Evaluation
**Positive therapeutic outcome**
• Decrease in renal cell carcinoma stabilization

---

## sotalol (Rx)
(soe-ta'lole)
Betapace, Betapace AF, Sotacar ✦
*Func. class.:* Antidysrhythmic, group III
*Chem. class.:* Nonselective β-blocker

**Pregnancy category B**

**Action:** Competitively blocks stimulation of β-adrenergic receptor within vascular smooth muscle; produces chronotropic, inotropic activity (decreases rate of SA node discharge, increases recovery time), slows conduction of AV node, decreases heart rate, which decreases $O_2$ consumption in myocardium; also decreases renin-aldosterone-angiotensin system at high doses, inhibits $β_2$ receptors in bronchial system (high doses)

**Therapeutic outcome:** Decreased B/P, heart rate, AV conduction

**Uses:** Life-threatening ventricular dysrhythmias; Betapace AF: to maintain sinus rhythm in symptomatic atrial fibrillation/flutter

**Dosage and routes**
*Adult:* PO Initial 80 mg bid, may increase to total of 240-320 mg/day

**Renal dose**
*Adult:* PO CCr 30-60 ml/min q24hr; CCr 10-29 ml/min q36-48hr; CCr <10 ml/min individualize dose

**Betapace AF**
*Adult:* PO Initial 80 mg bid, titrate upward to 120 mg bid during initial hospitalization

**Renal dose (Betapace AF)**
CCr >60 ml/min q12hr; CCr 40-60 ml/min q24hr; CCr <40 ml/min do not use

**Available forms:** Tabs 80, 120, 160, 240 mg; (Betapace AF) 80, 120, 160 mg

**Adverse effects**
*CNS:* Dizziness, mental changes, drowsiness, fatigue, headache, catatonia, depression, anxiety, nightmares, paresthesia, lethargy, insomnia, decreased concentration
*CV:* Orthostatic hypotension, bradycardia, **CHF**, chest pain, **ventricular dysrhythmias,** AV block, peripheral vascular insufficiency, palpitations, **prodysrhythmia, torsades de pointes; Betapace AF: life-threatening ventricular dysrhythmias**
*EENT:* Tinnitus, visual changes, sore throat, double vision, dry, burning eyes
*GI:* Nausea, vomiting, diarrhea, dry mouth, flatulence, constipation, anorexia
*GU:* Impotence, dysuria, ejaculatory failure, urinary retention

---

*HEMA:* **Agranulocytosis, thrombocytopenic purpura (rare), thrombocytopenia, leukopenia**

*INTEG:* Rash, alopecia, urticaria, pruritus, fever

*MISC:* Facial swelling, decreased exercise tolerance, weight change, Raynaud's disease

*MS:* Joint pain, arthralgia, muscle cramps, pain

*RESP:* **Bronchospasm,** dyspnea, wheezing, nasal stuffiness, pharyngitis

**Contraindications:** Hypersensitivity to β-blockers, cardiogenic shock, heart block (2nd or 3rd degree), sinus bradycardia, CHF, bronchial asthma, congenital or acquired long QT syndrome, CCr <40 ml/min

**Precautions:** Pregnancy **B**, breastfeeding, major surgery, diabetes mellitus, renal/thyroid disease, COPD, well-compensated heart failure, CAD, nonallergic bronchospasm, electrolyte disturbances, bradycardia, cardiac dysrhythmias, peripheral vascular disease

| Pharmacokinetics | |
|---|---|
| **Absorption** | Variable (30%) |
| **Distribution** | Crosses placenta, minimal penetration in CNS |
| **Metabolism** | Liver, protein binding 0% |
| **Excretion** | 70% unchanged—kidneys |
| **Half-life** | 10-24 hr, increased in renal disease |

| Pharmacodynamics | |
|---|---|
| **Onset** | Several hr |
| **Peak** | Unknown |
| **Duration** | Unknown |

**Interactions**
*Individual drugs*
Insulin: increased hypoglycemia
Lidocaine: increased effects of lidocaine
Nitroglycerin: increased hypotension
Theophylline: decreased bronchodilating effects of theophylline
*Drug classifications*
Antihypertensives, diuretics: increased hypotension
β$_2$-Agonists: decreased bronchodilating effects
Sulfonylureas: decreased hypoglycemic effects
Sympathomimetics: decreased β-blocker effects
*Drug/herb*
Aconite: increased toxicity, death
Aloe, broom, buckthorn, cascara sagrada, Chinese rhubarb, figwort, fumitory, goldenseal, kudzu, licorice: increased effect

Coltsfoot: decreased effect
Horehound: increased serotonin effect
*Drug/lab test*
False: increased urinary catecholamines
Interference: glucose, insulin tolerance tests

**NURSING CONSIDERATIONS**
**Assessment**
• Monitor B/P during beginning treatment, periodically thereafter; pulse q4hr; note rate, rhythm, quality: apical/radial pulse before administration; notify prescriber of any significant changes (pulse <50 bpm); monitor ECG continuously (Betapace AF); use QT interval to determine patient eligibility; baseline QT must be ≤450 msec
• Check for baselines in renal function tests, before therapy begins
• Assess for edema in feet, legs daily, monitor I&O ratio, daily weight; check for jugular vein distention, crackles, bilaterally, dyspnea (CHF)
• Monitor skin turgor, dryness of mucous membranes for hydration status, especially in geriatric

**Nursing diagnoses**
• Cardiac output, decreased (uses)
• Injury, risk for (adverse reactions)
• Knowledge, deficient (teaching)
• Noncompliance (teaching)

**Implementation**
• Given before meals, at bedtime, tab may be crushed or swallowed whole; give with food to prevent GI upset; reduce dosage in renal dysfunction
• Betapace and Betapace AF are not interchangeable
• Store protected from light, moisture; place in cool environment

**Patient/family education**
• Teach patient not to discontinue product abruptly, taper over 2 wk; may cause precipitate angina if stopped abruptly
• Teach patient not to use OTC products containing α-adrenergic stimulants (such as nasal decongestants, cold preparations); to avoid alcohol and smoking and to limit sodium intake as prescribed
• Teach patient how to take pulse and B/P at home, advise when to notify prescriber
• Instruct patient to comply with weight control, dietary adjustments, modified exercise program
• Caution patient to carry/wear emergency ID to identify product being taken, allergies
• Inform patient that product controls symptoms but does not cure

S

Adverse effects: *italic* = common, **bold** = life-threatening

- Caution patient to avoid hazardous activities if dizziness, drowsiness is present
- Teach patient to report symptoms of CHF: difficulty breathing, especially on exertion or when lying down; night cough; swelling of extremities; bradycardia; dizziness; confusion; depression; fever
- Teach patient to take product as prescribed, not to double or skip doses; take any missed doses as soon as remembered if at least 4 hr until next dose

### Evaluation
**Positive therapeutic outcome**
- Absence of dysrhythmias

**Treatment of overdose:** Lavage; **IV** atropine for bradycardia; **IV** theophylline for bronchospasm; digoxin, O₂, diuretic for cardiac failure; hemodialysis; **IV** glucose for hyperglycemia; **IV** diazepam (or phenytoin) for seizures

---

### spironolactone (Rx)
(speer'on-oh-lak'tone)
Aldactone, Novospiroton ✦
*Func. class:* Potassium-sparing diuretic
*Chem. class.:* Aldosterone antagonist

**Pregnancy category  D**

---

**Action:** Competes with aldosterone at receptor sites in the distal tubule in the renal system, resulting in excretion of sodium, chloride, water, bicarbonate, and calcium; potassium, phosphate, and hydrogen are retained

**Therapeutic outcome:** Diuretic and antihypertensive effect while retaining potassium; lowered aldosterone levels

**Uses:** Edema of CHF, hypertension, diuretic-induced hypokalemia, primary hyperaldosteronism (diagnosis, short-term treatment, long-term treatment), edema of nephrotic syndrome, cirrhosis of the liver with ascites

**Unlabeled uses:** CHF, hirsutism in women

### Dosage and routes
*Edema/hypertension*
*Adult:* PO 25-200 mg/day in 1-2 divided doses

*CHF*
*Adult:* PO 12.5-25 mg/day, max 50 mg/day

*Edema*
*Child:* PO 3.3 mg/kg/day in single or divided doses

*Hypertension*
*Child:* PO 1-2 mg/kg in divided doses

*Hypokalemia*
*Adult:* PO 25-100 mg/day; if PO, potassium supplements must not be used

*Primary hyperaldosteronism diagnosis*
*Adult:* PO 400 mg/day × 4 days or 4 wk depending on the test, then 100-400 mg/day maintenance

*Renal dose*
*Adult:* PO CCr 10-50 ml/min; give dose q12-24hr; CCr <10 ml/min, avoid use

*Polycystic ovary syndrome/hirsutism in women (unlabeled)*
*Adult:* PO 50-200 mg in 1-2 divided doses

**Available forms:** Tabs 25, 50, 100 mg

### Adverse effects
*CNS:* Headache, confusion, drowsiness, lethargy, ataxia
*ELECT:* Hyperchloremic metabolic acidosis, **hyperkalemia,** hyponatremia
*ENDO:* Impotence, gynecomastia, irregular menses, amenorrhea, postmenopausal bleeding, hirsutism, deepening voice, breast pain
*GI:* Diarrhea, cramps, bleeding, gastritis, vomiting, anorexia, nausea, **hepatocellular toxicity**
*HEMA:* **Agranulocytosis**
*INTEG:* Rash, pruritus, urticaria

**Contraindications:** Pregnancy **D**, hypersensitivity, anuria, severe renal disease, hyperkalemia

**Precautions:** Breastfeeding, dehydration, renal/hepatic disease, electrolyte imbalances, metabolic acidosis, gynecomastia

| Pharmacokinetics | |
|---|---|
| Absorption | GI tract; well absorbed |
| Distribution | Crosses placenta |
| Metabolism | Liver to canrenone (active metabolite) |
| Excretion | Renal; breast milk |
| Half-life | 12-24 hr (canrenone) |

| Pharmacodynamics | |
|---|---|
| Onset | 24-48 hr |
| Peak | 48-72 hr |
| Duration | Unknown |

---

## Interactions
### Individual drugs
Aspirin: decreased action of spironolactone

Cholestyramine: increased hyperchloremic acidosis in cirrhosis

Digoxin: increased digoxin action

Lithium: increased action, toxicity

### Drug classifications
ACE inhibitors, diuretics (potassium-sparing), potassium products, salt substitute: increased hyperkalemia

Anticoagulants: decreased effects of anticoagulants

Antihypertensives: increased action

NSAIDs: decreased effect of spironolactone

### Drug/herb
Arginine: fatal hypokalemia

Bearberry, gossypol: hypokalemia

Cucumber, dandelion, horsetail, licorice nettle, pumpkin, Queen Anne's lace: increased effect

Khella: increased hypotension

St. John's wort: severe photosensitivity

### Drug/lab test
Interference: 17-OHCS, 17-KS, radioimmunoassay, digoxin assay

## NURSING CONSIDERATIONS
### Assessment
• Monitor for manifestations of hyperkalemia: *MS:* fatigue, muscle weakness; *CV:* arrhythmias, hypotension, *NEURO:* paresthesias, confusion, *RESP:* dyspnea

• Monitor for manifestations of hyponatremia: *CV:* increased B/P, cold, clammy skin, hypo- or hypervolemia; *GI:* anorexia, nausea, vomiting, diarrhea, abdominal cramps; *NEURO:* lethargy, increased ICP, confusion, headache, seizures, coma, fatigue, tremors, hyperreflexia

• Monitor for manifestations of hyperchloremia: *NEURO:* weakness, lethargy, coma; *RESP:* deep rapid breathing

• Assess fluid volume status: I&O ratios and record, count or weigh diapers as appropriate, weight, distended red veins, crackles in lung, color, quality, and specific gravity of urine, skin turgor, adequacy of pulses, moist mucous membranes, bilateral lung sounds, peripheral pitting edema; dehydration symptoms of decreasing output, thirst, hypotension, dry mouth and mucous membranes should be reported

• Monitor electrolytes: potassium, sodium, calcium, magnesium; also include BUN, ABGs, uric acid, CBC, blood glucose

### Nursing diagnoses
• Fluid volume, deficient (adverse reactions)
• Fluid volume, excess (uses)
• Knowledge, deficient (teaching)
• Urinary elimination, impaired (adverse reactions)

### Implementation
• Give in AM to avoid interference with sleep
• With food, if nausea occurs, absorption may be increased; take at same time each day

### Patient/family education
• Teach patient to take medication early in day to prevent nocturia

• Instruct patient to take with food or milk if GI symptoms of nausea and anorexia occur

• Teach patient to maintain a record of weight on a weekly basis and notify prescriber of weight loss of >5 lb

• Caution patient that this product causes an increase in potassium levels, that foods high in potassium should be avoided; refer to dietitian for assistance planning

• Teach patient not to use alcohol, or any OTC medications without prescriber's approval; serious product reactions may occur

• Emphasize the need to contact prescriber immediately if muscle cramps, weakness, nausea, dizziness, or numbness occurs

• Teach patient to take own B/P and pulse and record

• Advise patient that dizziness and confusion may occur; avoid driving or other hazardous activities if alertness is decreased

• Teach patient to continue taking medication even if feeling better; this product controls symptoms but does not cure the condition

• Advise patient with hypertension to continue other treatment (exercise, weight loss, relaxation techniques, cessation of smoking)

### Evaluation
**Positive therapeutic outcome**
• Prevention of hypokalemia (diuretic use)
• Decreased edema
• Decreased B/P
• Decreased aldosterone levels
• Increased diuresis

### Treatment of overdose:
• Lavage if taken orally, monitor electrolytes
• Administer sodium bicarbonate
• Monitor hydration, CV, renal status

S

## stavudine (Rx)

(sta'vu-deen)

d4T, Zerit

*Func. class.:* Antiretroviral

*Chem. class.:* Nucleoside reverse transcriptase inhibitor

### Pregnancy category C

**Action:** Prevents replication of HIV-1 by the inhibition of the enzyme reverse transcriptase, causes DNA chain termination

**Therapeutic outcome:** Decreasing diarrhea, fatigue, night sweats; increased body weight

**Uses:** Treatment of HIV-1; used in combination with other antiretrovirals

### Dosage and routes

*Adult >60 kg:* PO 40 mg q12hr

*Adult <60 kg:* 30 mg q12hr

*Child <30 kg:* PO 1 mg/kg q12hr

*Child ≥30 kg ≤60 kg:* PO 30 mg q12hr

*Child >60 kg:* PO 40 mg q12hr

### Renal dose

*Adult >60 kg:* CCr 26-50 ml/min 20 mg q12hr; CCr 10-25 ml/min 20 mg q24hr

*Adult <60 kg:* CCr 26-50 ml/min 15 mg q12hr; CCr 10-25 ml/min 15 mg q24hr

**Available forms:** Caps 15, 20, 30, 40 mg; oral powder for sol 1 mg/ml

### Adverse effects

*CNS: Peripheral neuropathy,* insomnia, anxiety, neuropathy, depression, dizziness, confusion, headache, chills/fever, malaise

*CV:* Chest pain, vasodilatation, hypertension

*EENT:* Conjunctivitis, abnormal vision

*GI:* **Hepatotoxicity,** diarrhea, nausea, vomiting, anorexia, dyspepsia, constipation, stomatitis, **pancreatitis**

*HEMA:* **Bone marrow suppression**

*INTEG:* Rash, sweating, pruritus, benign neoplasms

*MISC:* **Lactic acidosis,** asthenia, lipodystrophy

*MS:* Myalgia, arthralgia

*RESP:* Dyspnea, pneumonia, asthma

**Contraindications:** Hypersensitivity to this product or zidovudine, didanosine, zalcitabine; severe peripheral neuropathy, lactic acidosis

**Precautions:** Pregnancy **C,** breastfeeding, advanced HIV infections, bone marrow suppression, renal/hepatic disease, peripheral neuropathy, osteoporosis, pancreatitis

### Pharmacokinetics

| | |
|---|---|
| **Absorption** | Rapidly absorbed, 82% bioavailability |
| **Distribution** | Cerebrospinal fluid |
| **Metabolism** | Unknown |
| **Excretion** | Kidneys, breast milk |
| **Half-life** | Elimination: 1-1.6 hr, intracellular: 3-3.5 hr |

### Pharmacodynamics

| | |
|---|---|
| **Onset** | Unknown |
| **Peak** | 1 hr |
| **Duration** | Unknown |

### Interactions

#### Individual drugs

Chloramphenicol, cisplatin, dapsone, didanosine, ethambutol, hydrALAZINE, lithium, phenytoin, vinCRIStine, zalcitabine: increased peripheral neuropathy

Methadose: decreased stavudine effect

Probenecid: increased stavudine levels

#### Drug classifications

Myelosuppressants: increased myelosuppression

### NURSING CONSIDERATIONS

#### Assessment

 Assess for lactic acidosis and severe hepatomegaly with steatosis; death may result

• Monitor viral load and CD4 counts baseline and throughout treatment

• Monitor for peripheral neuropathy: tingling, pain in extremities; if these occur, discontinue product

• Monitor for pancreatitis: severe upper abdominal pain, nausea, vomiting throughout treatment; if these occur, discontinue product

• Monitor blood tests: WBC, differential, RBC, Hct, Hgb, platelets

• Monitor renal function tests: urinalysis, protein, blood

• Obtain C&S before product therapy; product may be taken as soon as culture is performed; repeat C&S after therapy

• Monitor bowel pattern before, during treatment

• Monitor fluid overload; product requires large volume to stay in sol

• Assess for weakness, tremors, confusion, dizziness, psychosis; if these occur, product may have to be decreased or discontinued

#### Nursing diagnoses

• Infection, risk for (uses)

• Knowledge, deficient (teaching)

---

## Implementation

• Give with or without meals; absorption does not appear to be lowered when taken with food
• Give product q4hr around the clock, even during night

## Patient/family education

• Teach patient signs of peripheral neuropathy: burning, weakness, pain, pricking feeling in the extremities
• Caution patient that this product should not be given with antineoplastics
• Inform patient that GI complaints and insomnia resolve after 3-4 wk of treatment
• Inform patient that product is not a cure for AIDS, but will control symptoms
• Advise patient to call prescriber if sore throat, swollen lymph nodes, malaise, fever occur; may indicate presence of other infections
• Caution patient that even with product administration, virus is still infective and may be passed on to others
• Caution patient that follow-up visits must be continued because serious toxicity may occur; blood counts must be done q2 wk
• Teach patient that product must be taken q4hr around the clock even during night
• Caution patient that serious product interactions with other medications may occur, check with prescriber first if taking chloramphenicol, dapsone, cisplatin, didanosine, ethambutol, lithium, antifungals
• Inform patient that other products may be necessary to prevent other infections
• Inform patient that product may cause fainting or dizziness

## Evaluation

**Positive therapeutic outcome**

• Decreased symptoms of HIV infection

---

### ❗ HIGH ALERT

### streptokinase 😊 (Rx)
(strep-toe-kye′nase)
Streptase
*Func. class.:* Thrombolytic enzyme
*Chem. class.:* β-Hemolytic *Streptococcus* filtrate (purified)

### Pregnancy category C

**Action:** Activates conversion of plasminogen to plasmin (fibrinolysin): plasmin breaks down clots (fibrin), fibrinogen, factors V, VII; occlusion of venous access lines

**Therapeutic outcome:** Lysis of emboli, or thrombosis in various parts of the body

**Uses:** Deep vein thrombosis (DVT), pulmonary embolism, arterial thrombosis, arterial embolism, lysis of coronary artery thrombi after MI, acute evolving transmural MI

**Unlabeled uses:** Arteriovenous cannula occlusion

## Dosage and routes
*Lysis of coronary artery thrombi*
*Adult:* IC 20,000 international units, then 2000 international units/min over 1 hr as **IV** INF

*Thrombosis/embolism/DVT/ pulmonary embolism*
*Adult:* **IV** INF 250,000 international units over ½ hr, then 100,000 international units/hr for 72 hr for DVT; 100,000 international units/hr over 24-72 hr for pulmonary embolism; 100,000 international units/hr × 24-72 hr for arterial thrombosis or embolism

*Acute evolving transmural MI*
*Adult:* **IV** INF 1,500,000 international units diluted to a volume of 45 ml; give within 1 hr; intracoronary inf 20,000 international units by bol, then 2000 international units/min × 1 hr, total dose 140,000 international units

*Arteriovenous cannula occlusion (unlabeled)*
*Adult:* **IV** INF 10,000 international units/3 ml sol into occluded limb of cannula; clamp for 1 hr distally; aspirate contents; flush with NaCl sol and reconnect (serious reactions have been reported)

**Available forms:** Powder for inj, lyophilized 250,000, 600,000, 750,000, 1,500,000 international units/vial

## Adverse effects
*CNS:* Headache, fever
*CV:* **Dysrhythmias**, hypotension, noncardiogenic pulmonary edema, **pulmonary embolism**
*EENT:* Periorbital edema
*GI:* Nausea
*HEMA:* Decreased Hct, **bleeding**
*INTEG:* Rash, urticaria, phlebitis at infusion site, itching, flushing
*MS:* Low back pain
*RESP:* Altered respirations, shortness of breath, **bronchospasm**
*SYST:* GI, GU, **intracranial retroperitoneal bleeding, surface bleeding, anaphylaxis**

**S**

---

**Contraindications:** Breastfeeding, children, hypersensitivity, active internal bleeding, intraspinal surgery, CNS neoplasms, uncontrolled severe hypertension, recent CVA, intracranial, intrapleural surgery

**Precautions:** Pregnancy **C**, arterial emboli from left side of heart, ulcerative colitis, enteritis, severe renal disease, hepatic disease, hypocoagulation, COPD, subacute bacterial endocarditis, rheumatic valvular disease, cerebral embolism/thrombosis/hemorrhage, intraarterial diagnostic procedure or surgery (10 days), recent major surgery

### Pharmacokinetics

| | |
|---|---|
| **Absorption** | Completely absorbed |
| **Distribution** | Unknown |
| **Metabolism** | >80%—liver, rapidly cleared by reticuloendothelial system |
| **Excretion** | Kidneys |
| **Half-life** | 35 min |

### Pharmacodynamics

| | |
|---|---|
| **Onset** | Immediate |
| **Peak** | Rapid |
| **Duration** | <12 hr |

### Interactions
*Individual drugs*
Abciximab, aspirin, clopidogrel, dipyridamole, eptifibatide, indomethacin, phenylbutazone, plicamycin, ticlopidine, tirofiban, valproic acid: increased bleeding risk
*Drug classifications*
Anticoagulants (oral), cephalosporins (some), glycoprotein IIb/IIIa inhibitors, NSAIDs: increased bleeding risk
*Drug/lab test*
Increased: pro-time, APTT, TT
Decreased: plasminogen, fibrinogen

### NURSING CONSIDERATIONS
**Assessment**
• Monitor VS, B/P, pulse, respirations (including peripheral), neurologic signs, temp at least q4hr; temp >104° F (40° C) indicates internal bleeding; monitor rhythm closely; ventricular dysrhythmias may occur with hyperfusion; monitor heart, breath sounds, neurologic status, peripheral pulses
🔴 Assess for bleeding during first hr of treatment: hematuria, hematemesis, bleeding from mucous membranes, epistaxis, ecchymosis; guaiac, all body fluids, stools; may require transfusion (rare); blood studies (Hct, platelets, PTT, pro-time, TT, APTT) before starting therapy; pro-time or APTT must be less

than 2 × control before starting therapy; TT or protime q3-4hr during treatment
• Assess allergy: fever, rash, itching, chills; mild reaction may be treated with antihistamines; report to prescriber
• Monitor ECG on monitor, watch for segment changes, changes in rhythm; sinus bradycardia, ventricular tachycardia, accelerated idioventricular rhythm may occur as a result of reperfusion (coronary thrombosis); cardiac enzymes, radionuclide myocardial scanning/coronary angiography
• Monitor ABGs, respiratory rate (depth, characteristics), pulse, B/P, hemodynamics (pulmonary embolism)
• Monitor peripheral pulses, assess Homan's sign, check for redness, swelling qhr; notify prescriber of changes; B/P should not be taken in extremities (deep vein thrombosis)
• Check catheter for ability to aspirate blood from port; patient must exhale and hold breath when inserting and removing syringe to prevent air embolism (catheter/cannula occlusion)
• Assess for Guillain-Barré syndrome that may occur after treatment with this product
• Assess for respiratory depression

**Nursing diagnoses**
• Gas exchange, impaired (uses)
• Injury, risk for (adverse reactions)
• Knowledge, deficient (teaching)
• Tissue perfusion, ineffective (uses)

**Implementation**
• Give after reconstituting with provided diluent; add appropriate amount of sterile water for inj (no preservatives) 20-mg vial/20 ml or 50-mg vial/50 ml to make 1 mg/ml, mix by slow inversion or dilute with NaCl, $D_5W$ to a concentration of 0.5 mg/ml; further dilution, 1.5-<0.5 mg/ml may result in precipitation of product; use 18G needle; flush line with NaCl after administration; reconstituted **IV** sol within 8 hr; within 6 hr of coronary occlusion for best results
• Give **IV** loading dose over 30 min to avoid hypotension
• Give **IV** over 1 hr after dilution with 4-5 g/250 ml of 0.9% NaCl, $D_5W$, LR; may give by cont inf after loading dose(s) of 1 g/hr diluted in 50-100 ml of compatible sol; use infusion pump; do not give by direct **IV**
• Give heparin therapy after thrombolytic therapy is discontinued, TT, ACT, or APTT less than 2 × control (about 3-4 hr); **IV** heparin with loading dose is recommended after

discontinuing streptokinase to prevent redevelopment of thrombis
- Avoid invasive procedures, injection, taking temp via rectal route
- Apply pressure for 30 sec to minor bleeding sites; 30 min to sites of atrial puncture, followed by pressure dressing; inform prescriber if this does not attain hemostasis; apply pressure dressing
- Store powder at room temperature or refrigerate; protect from excessive light

*Y-site compatibilities:* Dobutamine, DOPamine, heparin, lidocaine, nitroglycerin
*Additive incompatibilities:* Do not mix with other medications

### Patient/family education
- Teach patient reason for medication, signs and symptoms of bleeding, allergic reactions, when to notify prescriber
- Explain that patient is to continue bed rest to avoid injury

### Evaluation
**Positive therapeutic outcome**
- Lysis of thrombi or emboli

---

## streptomycin (Rx)
(strep-toe-mye′sin)
*Func. class.:* Antiinfective, antituberculosis
*Chem. class.:* Aminoglycoside
**Pregnancy category  D**

**Action:** Interferes with protein synthesis in bacterial cell by binding to ribosomal subunit, causing inaccurate peptide sequence to form in protein chain, resulting in bacterial death

**Therapeutic outcome:** Bactericidal effects for the following organisms: sensitive strains of *Mycobacterium tuberculosis,* nontuberculous infections caused by sensitive strains of *Yersinia pestis, Brucella, Haemophilus influenzae, Klebsiella pneumoniae, Escherichia coli, Enterobacter aerogenes, Streptococcus viridans, Francisella tularensis, Proteus*

**Uses:** Active TB; used in combination for streptococcal and enterococcal infections; endocarditis, tularemia, plague

### Dosage and routes
*Tuberculosis*
*Adult:* IM 15 mg/kg (max 1 g) daily × 2-3 mo, then 1 g 2-3 ×/wk given with other antitubercular products

*Child:* IM 20-40 mg/kg/day in divided doses given with other antituberculosis products; max 15 mg/kg/day

*Streptococcal endocarditis*
*Adult:* IM 1 g q12hr × 1 wk with penicillin, then 500 mg bid × 1 wk

*Enterococcal endocarditis*
*Adult:* IM 1 g q12hr × 2 wk, then 500 mg q12hr × 4 wk with penicillin, max 15 mg/kg/day

**Available forms:** Inj 500 mg ♣, 1 g/ml

### Adverse effects
*CNS:* Confusion, dizziness, depression, numbness, tremors, **seizures,** muscle twitching, **neurotoxicity**
*CV:* Hypotension, myocarditis, palpitations
*EENT: Ototoxicity,* tinnitus, deafness, visual disturbances
*GI: Nausea, vomiting, anorexia,* increased ALT, AST, bilirubin, hepatomegaly, **hepatic necrosis,** splenomegaly
*GU:* **Oliguria, hematuria, renal damage, azotemia, renal failure, nephrotoxicity**
*HEMA:* **Agranulocytosis, thrombocytopenia, leukopenia, eosinophilia, anemia**
*INTEG: Rash,* burning, urticaria, dermatitis, alopecia

**Contraindications:** Pregnancy **D,** severe renal disease, hypersensitivity

**Precautions:** Breastfeeding, geriatric, neonates, mild renal disease, myasthenia gravis, hearing deficits, Parkinson's disease, hepatic disease

### Pharmacokinetics
| | |
|---|---|
| **Absorption** | Well absorbed |
| **Distribution** | Widely distributed in extracellular fluids, poorly distributed in CSF; crosses placenta |
| **Metabolism** | Minimal—liver |
| **Excretion** | Mostly unchanged (>90%) kidneys |
| **Half-life** | 2-2½ hr, increase in renal disease |

### Pharmacodynamics
| | |
|---|---|
| **Onset** | Rapid |
| **Peak** | 1-2 hr |
| **Duration** | Unknown |

### Interactions
*Individual drugs*
Amphotericin B, cidofovir, cisplatin, ethacrynic acid, furosemide, mannitol, methoxyflurane, polymyxin, vancomycin: increased ototoxicity, neurotoxicity, nephrotoxicity

S

Succinylcholine, warfarin: increased effects of streptomycin

*Drug classifications*

Aminoglycosides, cephalosporins: increased ototoxicity, neurotoxicity, nephrotoxicity

Nondepolarizing neuromuscular blockers, NSAIDs: increased effects of streptomycin

*Drug/herb*

Acidophilus: do not use with antiinfectives; separate by several hours

Lysine (large amounts): increased toxicity

## NURSING CONSIDERATIONS
### Assessment
- Assess patient for previous sensitivity reaction
- Assess patient for signs and symptoms of infection including characteristics of sputum, urine, stool WBC >10,000/mm³, temp
- Obtain baseline information before and during treatment
- Complete C&S testing before and after product therapy to identify if correct treatment has been initiated
- Assess for allergic reactions: rash, urticaria, pruritus, chills, fever, joint pain; angioedema may occur a few days after therapy begins; epINEPHrine, resuscitation equipment should be available for anaphylactic reaction
- Identify urine output; if decreasing, notify prescriber (may indicate nephrotoxicity); also increased BUN, creatinine, urine CCr <80 ml/min
- Monitor blood tests: AST, ALT, CBC, Hct, bilirubin, LDH, alkaline phosphatase, Coombs' test monthly if patient is on long-term therapy
- Monitor electrolytes: potassium, sodium, chloride, magnesium monthly if patient is on long-term therapy
- Monitor for bleeding: ecchymosis, bleeding gums, hematuria, stool guaiac daily if on long-term therapy
- Assess for overgrowth of infection: perineal itching, fever, malaise, redness, pain, swelling, drainage, rash, diarrhea, change in cough, sputum
- Obtain weight before treatment; calculation of dosage is usually based on ideal body weight, but may be calculated on actual body weight
- Monitor I&O ratio; urinalysis daily for proteinuria, cells, casts; report sudden change in urine output
- Obtain serum peak 60 min after IM inj, trough level obtained just before next dose; blood level should be 2-4 × bacteriostatic level
- Monitor for deafness by audiometric testing, ringing, roaring in ears, vertigo; assess hearing before, during, after treatment
- Monitor for dehydration: high specific gravity, decrease in skin turgor, dry mucous membranes, dark urine

### Nursing diagnoses
- Diarrhea (adverse reactions)
- Infection, risk for (uses)
- Injury, risk for (adverse reactions)
- Knowledge, deficient (teaching)
- Noncompliance (teaching)

### Implementation
- Give deeply in large muscle mass
- Reconstitute with 4.2-4.5 ml of sterile water for inj or 0.9% NaCl/1 g (200 mg/ml), 3.2-3.5 ml/1 g (250 mg/ml), 17 ml/5 g (250 mg/ml); give at 500 mg/ml or less

*Syringe compatibilities:* Penicillin G sodium

*Syringe incompatibilities:* Heparin

*Y-site compatibilities:* Esmolol

*Additive compatibilities:* Bleomycin

### Patient/family education
- Teach patient to report sore throat, bruising, bleeding, joint pain, may indicate blood dyscrasias (rare); ringing, roaring in the ears
- Advise patient to contact prescriber if vaginal itching, loose foul-smelling stools, furry tongue occur; may indicate superinfection

### Evaluation
**Positive therapeutic outcome**
- Absence of signs/symptoms of infection
- Reported improvement in symptoms of infection

**Treatment of overdose:** Withdraw product, hemodialysis, monitor serum levels of product, may give ticarcillin or carbenicillin

---

### succimer (Rx)
(sux′i-mer)
Chemet
*Func. class:* Heavy metal antagonist
*Chem. class.:* Chelating agent
**Pregnancy category** C

**Action:** Binds with ions of lead to form a water-soluble complex that is excreted by kidneys

**Therapeutic outcome:** Removal of lead from the body

**Uses:** Lead poisoning in children with lead levels above 45 mcg/dl; may be beneficial in mercury, arsenic poisoning

### Dosage and routes
*Adult:* PO 10-30 mg/kg/day × 5 days

---

 Alert      Canada Only     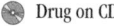 Drug on CD          * "Tall Man" lettering (See Preface)

*Child with lead level >45 mcg/dl:*
PO 10 mg/kg or 350 mg/m² q8hr × 5 days, then 10 mg/kg or 350 mg/m² q12hr × 2 wk; another course may be required depending on lead levels; allow 2 wk between courses

**Available forms:** Caps 100 mg

**Adverse effects**
*CNS:* Drowsiness, dizziness, paresthesia, sensorimotor neuropathy
*EENT:* Otitis media, watery eyes, film in eyes, plugged ears
*GI: Nausea, vomiting, diarrhea, metallic taste, anorexia*
*GU:* **Proteinuria,** decreased urination, voiding difficulties
*HEMA:* **Increased platelets, intermittent eosinophilia**
*INTEG:* Rash, urticaria, pruritus
*META:* Increased AST, ALT, alkaline phosphatase, cholesterol
*RESP:* Sore throat, rhinorrhea, nasal congestion, cough
*SYST:* Back, stomach, head, rib, flank pain; abdominal cramps; chills; fever; flulike symptoms; head cold; headache

**Contraindications:** Hypersensitivity

**Precautions:** Pregnancy **C,** breastfeeding, children <1 yr, renal/hepatic disease

| Pharmacokinetics | |
|---|---|
| Absorption | Rapidly absorbed |
| Distribution | Unknown |
| Metabolism | Liver—extensively |
| Excretion | Kidneys—unchanged |
| Half-life | 2 days |

| Pharmacodynamics | |
|---|---|
| Onset | Up to 2 hr |
| Peak | 2-4 hr |
| Duration | 8-12 hr |

**Interactions**
*Drug classifications*
Heavy metal antagonist, others: do not use together

**NURSING CONSIDERATIONS**
**Assessment**
• Assess VS, B/P, pulse, respirations, weigh daily
• Monitor I&O ratio, renal function tests, BUN, creatinine, CCr; watch for decreasing urine output
• Assess neurologic status: watch for paresthesias, beginning of seizures
• Monitor urine: pH, albumin, casts, blood, coproporphyrins, calcium
• Assess for febrile reactions that may occur 4-8 hr after product therapy
• Monitor for cardiac abnormalities: dysrhythmias, hypotension, tachycardia
• Assess for allergic reactions (rash, urticaria); if these occur, product should be discontinued

**Nursing diagnoses**
• Injury, risk for (uses, adverse reactions)
• Knowledge, deficient (teaching)
• Poisoning, risk for (uses)

**Implementation**
• Give whole or cap contents mixed with food or fluid

**Patient/family education**
• Explain reason for medication and expected results
• Provide a referral to health department to assess lead levels in home or workplace
• Teach patient to increase fluid intake

**Evaluation**
**Positive therapeutic outcome**
• Decreased symptoms of lead intoxication
• Decreased lead level <50 mcg/dl

! HIGH ALERT

**succinylcholine** (Rx)
(suk-sin-ill-koe′leen)
Anectine, Anectine Flo-Pack, Quelicin, succinylcholine chloride, Sucostrin, Suxamethonium
*Func. class.:* Neuromuscular blocker (depolarizing—ultra short)

**Pregnancy category C**

**Action:** Inhibits transmission of nerve impulses by binding with cholinergic receptor sites, antagonizing action of acetylcholine; causes release of histamine

**Therapeutic outcome:** Paralysis of skeletal muscles

**Uses:** Facilitation of endotracheal intubation, skeletal muscle relaxation during orthopedic manipulations

**Dosage and routes**
*Adult:* **IV** 1-1.5 mg/kg, max 150 mg, maintenance 0.04-0.07 mg/kg q5-10 min as needed; CONT **IV** INF dilute to concentration of 1-2 mg/ml in D₅W or NS 10-100 mcg/kg/min

Adverse effects: *italic* = common, **bold** = life-threatening

*Child:* **IV** Initially 1-2 mg/kg; CONT **IV** INF not recommended

**Available forms:** Inj 20, 50, 100 mg/ml; powder for inj 100, 500 mg/vial, 1 g/vial

### Adverse effects
*CV:* Bradycardia, tachycardia; increased, decreased B/P, **sinus arrest, dysrhythmias,** edema
*EENT:* Increased secretions, increased intraocular pressure
*HEMA:* **Myoglobulinemia**
*INTEG:* Rash, flushing, pruritus, urticaria
*MS:* Weakness, muscle pain, fasciculation, prolonged relaxation
*RESP:* **Prolonged apnea, bronchospasm, cyanosis, respiratory depression,** wheezing, dyspnea

**Contraindications:** Hypersensitivity, malignant hyperthermia, decreased plasma pseudocholinesterase, penetrating eye injuries, acute angle-closure glaucoma

**Precautions:** Pregnancy **C,** breastfeeding, children <2 yr, geriatric or debilitated patients, severe burns, fractures (fasciculation may increase damage), electrolyte imbalances, dehydration, neuromuscular disease, respiratory disease, collagen diseases, glaucoma, eye surgery, renal/hepatic/cardiac disease

### Pharmacokinetics
| | |
|---|---|
| Absorption | Well absorbed (IM) |
| Distribution | Widely distributed, crosses placenta |
| Metabolism | Plasma (90%) |
| Excretion | Hydrolyzed in blood, excreted in urine (active/inactive metabolites) |
| Half-life | Unknown |

### Pharmacodynamics
| | IM | IV |
|---|---|---|
| Onset | 2-3 min | 1 min |
| Peak | Unknown | 2-3 min |
| Duration | 10-30 min | 6-10 min |

### Interactions
*Individual products*
Clindamycin, enflurane, isoflurane, lincomycin, lithium, oxytocin, procainamide, quinidine: increased neuromuscular blockade
Theophylline: dysrhythmias
*Drug classifications*
Aminoglycosides, anesthetics (local), antibiotics (polymyxin), β-adrenergic blockers, cardiac glycosides, magnesium salts, opioids, thiazides: increased neuromuscular blockade

*Drug/herb*
Melatonin: blocks succinylcholine

### NURSING CONSIDERATIONS
**Assessment**
• Assess for electrolyte imbalances (potassium, magnesium); may lead to increased action of this product
• Monitor VS (B/P, pulse, respirations, airway) until fully recovered; rate, depth, pattern of respirations, strength of hand grip
• Monitor I&O ratio; check for urinary retention, frequency, hesitancy
• Assess for recovery: decreased paralysis of face, diaphragm, leg, arm, rest of body
• Assess for allergic reactions: rash, fever, respiratory distress, pruritus; product should be discontinued if these occur

**Nursing diagnoses**
• Breathing pattern, ineffective (uses)
• Communication, impaired verbal (adverse reactions)

**Implementation**
**IM route**
• Give inj deep IM, preferably high in deltoid muscle
• Store in refrigerator; store powder at room temperature; close container tightly
**IV route**
• Use nerve stimulator by anesthesiologist to determine neuromuscular blockade
• Give anticholinesterase to reverse neuromuscular blockade
• Give by **IV** inf; dilute 1-2 mg/ml in $D_5$, isotonic saline sol, give 0.5-10 mg/min, titrate to patient response; may be given directly over 1 min
*Syringe compatibilities:* Heparin
*Y-site compatibilities:* Etomidate, heparin, potassium chloride, propofol, vit B/C
*Additive compatibilities:* Amikacin, cephapirin, isoproterenol, meperidine, methyldopate, morphine, norepinephrine, scopolamine
*Additive incompatibilities:* Barbiturates, nafcillin, sodium bicarbonate

**Patient/family education**
• Explain reason for medication and expected results
• Provide reassurance if communication is difficult during recovery from neuromuscular blockade; postoperative stiffness is normal, soon subsides

### Evaluation
**Positive therapeutic outcome**
• Paralysis of jaw, eyelid, head, neck, rest of body

**Treatment of overdose:** Edrophonium or neostigmine, atropine, monitor VS; may require mechanical ventilation

---

## sucralfate (Rx)
(soo-kral′fate)
Carafate, Sulcrate ✤
*Func. class.:* Protectant; antiulcer
*Chem. class.:* Aluminum hydroxide/sulfated sucrose

**Pregnancy category B**

**Do not confuse:**
Carafate/Cafergot

**Action:** Forms a complex that adheres to ulcer site, adsorbs pepsin

**Therapeutic outcome:** Healing of ulcers

**Uses:** Duodenal ulcer, oral mucositis, stomatitis after radiation of head and neck

**Unlabeled uses:** Gastric ulcers, gastroesophageal reflux

### Dosage and routes
*Duodenal ulcers*
*Adult:* PO 1 g qid 1 hr before meals and at bedtime
*Child:* PO 40-80 mg/kg/day

**Available forms:** Tabs 1 g; oral susp 1 g/10 ml

### Adverse effects
*CNS:* Drowsiness, dizziness
*GI: Dry mouth, constipation,* nausea, gastric pain, vomiting
*INTEG:* Urticaria, rash, pruritus

**Contraindications:** Hypersensitivity

**Precautions:** Pregnancy **B,** breastfeeding, children, renal failure

#### Pharmacokinetics
| | |
|---|---|
| **Absorption** | Minimally absorbed |
| **Distribution** | Unknown |
| **Metabolism** | Not metabolized |
| **Excretion** | Feces (90%) |
| **Half-life** | 6-20 hr |

#### Pharmacodynamics
| | |
|---|---|
| **Onset** | ½ hr |
| **Peak** | Unknown |
| **Duration** | 6 hr |

### Interactions
*Individual drugs*
Cimetidine, digoxin, ketoconazole, phenytoin, ranitidine, tetracycline, theophylline: decreased action of each specific product
*Drug classifications*
Antacids: decreased absorption of sucralfate
Fat-soluble vitamins: decreased action of fat-soluble vitamins
Fluoroquinolones: decreased absorption

### NURSING CONSIDERATIONS
**Assessment**
• Monitor gastric pH (>5 should be maintained); blood in stools

**Nursing diagnoses**
• Constipation (adverse reactions)
• Knowledge, deficient (teaching)
• Pain, acute (uses)
• Pain, chronic (uses)

**Implementation**
• Do not break, crush, or chew tabs
• Give on empty stomach 1 hr before meals and at bedtime
• Avoid antacids ½ hr before or 1 hr after taking this product
• Store at room temperature

**Patient/family education**
• Instruct patient to take medication on empty stomach
• Caution patient to take full course of therapy, not to use over 8 wk, to avoid smoking
• Caution patient to avoid antacids within ½ hr of product or 1 hr after this product

**Evaluation**
**Positive therapeutic outcome**
• Absence of pain or GI complaints

S

---

Adverse effects: *italic* = common, **bold** = life-threatening

## sulfamethoxazole (Rx)

(sul-fa-meth-ox'a-zole)

Apo-Sulfamethoxazole , Gantanol, Urobak

*Func. class.:* Antiinfective

*Chem. class.:* Sulfonamide, intermediate-acting

**Pregnancy category C**

**Action:** Interferes with bacterial biosynthesis of proteins by competitive antagonism of *p*-aminobenzoic acid (PABA)

**Therapeutic outcome:** Bactericidal action against susceptible organisms: streptococci and staphylococci, *Clostridium perfringens, Clostridium tetani, Nocardia asteroides;* gram-negative pathogens, including *Enterobacter, Escherichia coli, Klebsiella, Proteus mirabilis, Proteus vulgaris, Salmonella, Shigella*

**Uses:** UTIs, chancroid, inclusion conjunctivitis, malaria, meningococcal meningitis, nocardiosis, acute otitis media, toxoplasmosis, trachoma

### Dosage and routes

*Adult:* PO 2 g, then 1 g bid or tid for 7-10 days

*Child >2 mo:* PO 50-60 mg/kg × 1 dose, then 25-30 mg/kg bid, max 75 mg/kg/day

### Renal dose

*Adult:* PO CCr <10-30 ml/min 50% of dose; CCr <10 ml/min give 25% of dose or extend interval

**Available forms:** Tabs 500 mg; oral susp 500 mg/5 ml

### Adverse effects

*CNS:* Headache, insomnia, hallucinations, depression, vertigo, fatigue, anxiety, seizures, product fever, chills, drowsiness

*CV:* **Allergic myocarditis**

*GI:* *Nausea, vomiting, abdominal pain,* stomatitis, **hepatitis**, glossitis, **pancreatitis**, diarrhea, **enterocolitis**, anorexia

*GU:* **Renal failure, toxic nephrosis,** increased BUN, creatinine, crystalluria, hematuria, proteinuria

*HEMA:* **Leukopenia, thrombocytopenia, agranulocytosis, hemolytic anemia, aplastic anemia**

*INTEG:* Rash, dermatitis, urticaria, erythema, photosensitivity, alopecia

*SYST:* **Anaphylaxis, Stevens-Johnson syndrome**

**Contraindications:** Pregnancy at term, breastfeeding, infants <2 mo (except congenital toxoplasmosis), hypersensitivity to sulfonamides, sulfonylureas, thiazide and loop diuretics, salicylates, sunscreen with PABA, porphyria, G6PD deficiency

**Precautions:** Pregnancy **C**, geriatric, impaired renal/hepatic function, severe allergy, bronchial asthma, UV exposure

### Pharmacokinetics

| | |
|---|---|
| **Absorption** | Well absorbed |
| **Distribution** | Widely distributed, crosses placenta |
| **Metabolism** | Liver, large amounts |
| **Excretion** | Unchanged kidneys (20%), enters breast milk |
| **Half-life** | 7-12 hr |

### Pharmacodynamics

| | |
|---|---|
| **Onset** | 1 hr |
| **Peak** | 3-4 hr |
| **Duration** | Unknown |

### Interactions

*Individual drugs*

CycloSPORINE: increased nephrotoxicity

Indomethacin, probenecid: increased product-free concentrations

Methenamine: increased crystalluria

Methotrexate: decreased renal excretion of methotrexate

Phenytoin: decreased hepatic clearance of phenytoin

Warfarin: increased anticoagulant effect

*Drug classifications*

Barbiturates, uricosuric agents: increased effects

Diuretics (thiazide): increased thrombocytopenia

Salicylates: increased product-free concentrations

Sulfonylurea agents: increased hypoglycemic response

*Drug/herb*

Acidophilus: do not use with antiinfectives; separate by several hours

*Drug/lab test*

False positive: urinary glucose test (Benedict's method)

### NURSING CONSIDERATIONS

**Assessment**

• Assess patient for previous sensitivity reaction

• Assess patient for signs and symptoms of infection including characteristics of wounds, sputum, urine, stool, WBC >10,000/mm³, elevated temp; obtain baseline information before and during treatment

• Complete C&S studies before beginning product therapy to identify if correct treatment has been initiated

• Assess for allergic reactions: rash, urticaria, pruritus, chills, fever, joint pain; angioedema may occur a few days after therapy begins; epINEPHrine, resuscitation equipment should be on unit for anaphylactic reaction; AIDS patients are more susceptible

• Monitor blood studies: CBC, Hct, bilirubin, alkaline phosphatase monthly if patient is on long-term therapy

• Monitor for bleeding: ecchymosis, bleeding gums, hematuria, stool guaiac daily if patient is on long-term therapy

• Assess for overgrowth of infection: perineal itching, fever, malaise, redness, pain, swelling, drainage, rash, diarrhea, change in cough, sputum

### Nursing diagnoses
• Diarrhea (adverse reactions)
• Infection, risk for (uses)
• Injury, risk for (adverse reactions)
• Knowledge, deficient (teaching)
• Noncompliance (teaching)

### Implementation
• Give around the clock to maintain proper blood levels; give on empty stomach to increase absorption of product; do not give within 3 hr of other agents, product actions may occur

### Patient/family education
• Teach patient to report sore throat, bruising, bleeding, joint pain; may indicate blood dyscrasias (rare)
• Instruct patient to take with 8 oz of water to prevent crystalluria
• Advise patient to contact prescriber if vaginal itching, loose foul-smelling stools, furry tongue occur; may indicate superinfection; report itching, rash, pruritus, urticaria
• Instruct patient to take all medication prescribed for the length of time ordered; product must be taken around the clock to maintain blood levels; do not give medication to others

### Evaluation
**Positive therapeutic outcome**
• Absence of signs/symptoms of infection (WBC <10,000/mm$^3$, temp WNL, absence of urinary pain, hematuria)
• Reported improvement in symptoms of infection
• Negative C&S

## sulfasalazine (Rx)
(sul-fa-sal'a-zeen)
Azulfidine, Azulfidine EN-tabs, PMS-Sulfasalazine ✦, S.A.S. ✦, Salazopyrin ✦, sulfasalazine
*Func. class.:* GI Antiinflammatory, antirheumatic (DMARD)
*Chem. class.:* GI Sulfonamide
**Pregnancy category B**

**Do not confuse:**
sulfasalazine/sulfiSOXAZOLE

**Action:** Proproduct to deliver sulfapyridine and 5-aminosalicylic acid to colon; antinflammatory in connective tissue

**Therapeutic outcome:** Treatment of ulcerative colitis, rheumatoid arthritis

**Uses:** Ulcerative colitis, rheumatoid arthritis (delayed rel tab) in patients who inadequately respond to or are intolerant of analgesics/NSAIDs, juvenile rheumatoid arthritis (Azulfidine EN-tabs)

**Unlabeled uses:** Crohn's disease

### Dosage and routes
*Bowel disease*
*Adult:* PO 3-4 g/day in divided doses; maintenance 2 g/day in divided doses q6hr
*Child ≥6 yr:* PO 40-60 mg/kg/day in 4-6 divided doses, then 30 mg/kg/day in 4 doses, max 2 g/day

*Rheumatoid arthritis*
*Adult:* PO 2 g/day in evenly divided doses, initiate treatment with a lower dose of enteric-coated tab

*Juvenile rheumatoid arthritis*
*Child ≥6 yr:* PO 30-50 mg/kg/24 hr, divided into 2 doses

*Renal dose*
*Adult:* PO CCr 10-30 ml/min bid; CCr <10 ml/min daily

**Available forms:** Tabs 500 mg; oral susp 250 mg/5 ml; delayed rel tabs 500 mg

### Adverse effects
*CNS:* Headache, confusion, insomnia, hallucinations, depression, vertigo, fatigue, anxiety, **seizures**, product fever, chills
*CV:* **Allergic myocarditis**
*GI:* *Nausea, vomiting, abdominal pain,* stomatitis, **hepatitis**, glossitis, **pancreatitis**, diarrhea
*GU:* **Renal failure, toxic nephrosis**, increased BUN, creatinine, crystalluria

S

***HEMA:*** **Leukopenia, neutropenia, thrombocytopenia, agranulocytosis, hemolytic anemia**
***INTEG:*** Rash, dermatitis, urticaria, **Stevens-Johnson syndrome**, erythema, photosensitivity
***SYST:*** **Anaphylaxis**

**Contraindications:** Pregnancy at term, children <2 yr, hypersensitivity to sulfonamides or salicylates, intestinal, urinary obstruction, porphyria

**Precautions:** Pregnancy **B**, breastfeeding, impaired renal/hepatic function, severe allergy, bronchial asthma, megaloblastic anemia

### Pharmacokinetics

| | |
|---|---|
| **Absorption** | Partially absorbed |
| **Distribution** | Crosses placenta |
| **Metabolism** | Liver |
| **Excretion** | Kidneys, breast milk |
| **Half-life** | 6 hr |

### Pharmacodynamics

| | |
|---|---|
| **Onset** | 1 hr |
| **Peak** | 1½-6 hr |
| **Duration** | 6-12 hr |

### Interactions
#### Individual drugs
Azathioprine, mercaptopurine: increased leucopenia risk
CycloSPORINE: decreased effect of cycloSPORINE
Digoxin: decreased digoxin effect
Folic acid: decreased folic acid effect
Methotrexate: decreased renal excretion
#### Drug classifications
Anticoagulants (oral): increased anticoagulant effect
Hypoglycemics (oral): increased hypoglycemic response
#### Drug/food
Iron, folic acid will be poorly absorbed
#### Drug/lab test
False positive: urinary glucose test

### NURSING CONSIDERATIONS
#### Assessment
• Monitor I&O ratio; note color, amount, character, pH of urine if product administered for UTIs; output should be 800 ml less than intake; if urine is highly acidic, alkalization may be needed
• Monitor kidney function tests: BUN, creatinine, urinalysis if on long-term therapy
• Monitor blood dyscrasias: skin rash, fever, sore throat, bruising, bleeding, fatigue, joint pain; monitor CBC before, during therapy (q3 mo)
• Assess for allergic reaction: rash, dermatitis, urticaria, pruritus, dyspnea, bronchospasm

#### Nursing diagnoses
• Injury, risk for (uses)
• Knowledge, deficient (teaching)

#### Implementation
• Give with full glass of water to maintain adequate hydration; increase fluids to 2 L/day to decrease crystallization in kidneys; contact lens, urine, skin may be yellow-orange
• Give total daily dose in evenly spaced doses and after meals to help minimize GI intolerance
• Give at bedtime
• Store in airtight, light-resistant container at room temperature

#### Patient/family education
• Advise patient to take each oral dose with full glass of water to prevent crystalluria
• Teach patient to avoid sunlight or to use sunscreen to prevent burns
• Teach patient to avoid OTC medication (aspirin, vit C) unless directed by prescriber
• Advise patient to notify prescriber if skin rash, sore throat, fever, mouth sores, unusual bruising, bleeding occur
• Advise patient to use rectal susp at bedtime and retain all night

#### Evaluation
**Positive therapeutic outcome**
• Absence of fever, mucus in stools or pain in joints

---

## sulfinpyrazone (Rx)
(sul-fin-peer'a-zone)
Anturan ✤, Anturane, sulfinpyrazone
*Func. class.:* Uricosuric
*Chem. class.:* Pyrazolone
**Pregnancy category C**

**Action:** Inhibits tubular reabsorption of urates, with increased excretion of uric acid; inhibits prostaglandin synthesis, which decreases platelet aggregation

**Therapeutic outcome:** Decreased uric acid levels, absence of platelet aggregation

**Uses:** Gout, gouty arthritis

### Dosage and routes
#### Gout/gouty arthritis
***Adult:*** PO 100-200 mg bid × 1 wk, then 200-400 mg bid, not to exceed 800 mg/day
***Child:*** PO 10 mg/kg/day in 3-4 divided doses

 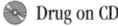

**Renal dose**
CCr <50 ml/min, avoid use

**Available forms:** Tabs 100 mg; caps 200 mg

**Adverse effects**
*CNS:* Dizziness, **seizures, coma**
*EENT:* Tinnitus
*GI: Gastric irritation, nausea, vomiting, anorexia,* **hepatic necrosis, GI bleeding**
*GU:* Renal calculi, hypoglycemia
*HEMA:* **Agranulocytosis** (rare)
*INTEG:* Rash, dermatitis, pruritus, fever, photosensitivity
*RESP:* **Apnea,** irregular respirations

**Contraindications:** Hypersensitivity to pyrazolone derivatives, salicylates, blood dyscrasias, CCr <50 ml/min, active peptic ulcer, GI inflammation, nephrolithiasis

**Precautions:** Pregnancy **C,** renal disease, NSAIDs hypersensitivity

| Pharmacokinetics | |
| --- | --- |
| **Absorption** | Well absorbed |
| **Distribution** | Unknown |
| **Metabolism** | Liver |
| **Excretion** | Feces (metabolites/active products) |
| **Half-life** | 4 hr |

| Pharmacodynamics | |
| --- | --- |
| **Onset** | Unknown |
| **Peak** | 1-2 hr |
| **Duration** | 4-6 hr |

**Interactions**
*Individual drugs*
Acetaminophen: increased toxicity
Niacin: decreased effects of sulfinpyrazone
Theophylline, verapamil: decreased effect of each specific product
TOLBUTamide, warfarin: increased effect of each specific product
*Drug classifications*
NSAIDs: increased bleeding risk
Salicylates: decreased effect of sulfinpyrazone
*Drug/lab test*
Increased: PSP, aminohippuric acid
False positive: Clinitest

**NURSING CONSIDERATIONS**
**Assessment**
• Monitor I&O ratio; observe for decrease in urinary output; increase fluids to 2-3 L/day
• Monitor CBC, platelets, reticulocytes before, during therapy (q3 mo)
• Assess mobility, joint pain, and swelling in the joints

**Nursing diagnoses**
• Knowledge, deficient (teaching)
• Mobility, impaired physical (uses)
• Pain, chronic (uses)

**Implementation**
• Give with food or antacid to decrease GI upset
• Reduce dose gradually if uric acid levels are normal after 6 mo

**Patient/family education**
• Advise patient to increase fluids to 3-4 L/day
• Caution patient to avoid alcohol, OTC preparations that contain alcohol; skin rashes may occur
• Advise patient to report any pain, redness, or hard area, usually in legs
• Instruct patient on importance of complying with medical regimen; bone marrow depression may occur

**Evaluation**
**Positive therapeutic outcome**
• Decreased pain in joints
• Normal serum uric acid levels
• Increased duration of antiinfectives

**\*sulfiSOXAZOLE** (Rx)
(sul-fi-sox′a-zole)
Gantrisin, Gantrisin Pediatric, Novo-Soxazole ✦, sulfiSOXAZOLE
*Func. class.:* Antiinfective
*Chem. class.:* Sulfonamide, short-acting
**Pregnancy category C**

**Do not confuse:**
sulfiSOXAZOLE/sulfasalazine/sulfADIAZINE

**Action:** Inhibits folic acid synthesis

**Therapeutic outcome:** Bactericidal action against susceptible organisms: gram-positive pathogens, including streptococci and staphylococci, *Clostridium perfringens, Clostridium tetani, Nocardia asteroides;* gram-negative pathogens, including *Enterobacter, Escherichia coli, Klebsiella, Proteus mirabilis, Proteus vulgaris, Salmonella, Shigella*

**Uses:** UTIs; chancroid, trachoma, toxoplasmosis, acute otitis media, malaria, *Haemophilus influenzae* meningitis, meningococcal meningitis, nocardiosis

### Dosage and routes
*UTIs, other systemic infections*
**Adult:** PO 2-4 g loading dose, then 1-2 g qid × 7-10 days, max 12 g/day
**Child >2 mo:** PO 75 mg/kg or 2 g/m² loading dose, then 120-150 mg/kg/day or 4 g/m²/day in divided doses q6hr, max 6 g/day

*Chlamydia trachomatis*
**Adult:** PO 500 mg-1 g qid × 3 wk

*Renal dose*
**Adult:** PO CCr 10-50 ml/min q8-12hr; CCr <10 ml/min q12-24hr

**Available forms:** Tabs 500 mg; sulfiSOX-AZOLE acetyl: liquid 500 mg/5 ml

### Adverse effects
***CNS:*** Headache, insomnia, hallucinations, depression, vertigo, fatigue, anxiety, **seizures,** product fever, chills, drowsiness
***CV:*** **Allergic myocarditis, tachycardia**
***GI:*** *Nausea, vomiting, abdominal pain,* stomatitis, **hepatitis,** glossitis, pancreatitis, diarrhea, **enterocolitis,** anorexia, **pseudomembranous colitis**
***GU:*** **Renal failure, toxic nephrosis,** increased BUN, creatinine, crystalluria, hematuria, proteinuria, urinary retention
***HEMA:*** **Leukopenia, thrombocytopenia, agranulocytosis, hemolytic anemia, aplastic anemia**
***INTEG:*** Rash, dermatitis, urticaria, erythema, photosensitivity, alopecia
***SYST:*** **Anaphylaxis, Stevens-Johnson syndrome**

**Contraindications:** Pregnancy at term, breastfeeding, infants <2 mo (except congenital toxoplasmosis), hypersensitivity to sulfonamides and sulfonylureas, thiazide and loop diuretics, salicylates; sunscreen with PABA, porphyria, G6PD deficiency

**Precautions:** Pregnancy **C,** breastfeeding, geriatric, impaired renal/hepatic function, severe allergy, bronchial asthma, UV exposure

| Pharmacokinetics | |
|---|---|
| **Absorption** | Well absorbed |
| **Distribution** | Widely distributed, crosses placenta |
| **Metabolism** | Liver, mostly |
| **Excretion** | Breast milk |
| **Half-life** | 4-7 hr |

| Pharmacodynamics | |
|---|---|
| **Onset** | Unknown |
| **Peak** | 2-4 hr |
| **Duration** | Unknown |

### Interactions
*Individual products*
CycloSPORINE: increased nephrotoxicity
Indomethacin, probenecid: increased product-free concentrations
Methenamine: increased crystalluria risk
Methotrexate: decreased renal excretion of methotrexate
Phenytoin: decreased hepatic clearance of phenytoin
TOLBUTamide: increased effects of TOLBUTamide
Warfarin: increased anticoagulant effect
*Drug classifications*
Barbiturates, uricosuric agents: increased effects of each specific product
Diuretics (thiazide): increased thrombocytopenia
Salicylates: increased product-free concentrations
Sulfonylurea agents: increased hypoglycemic response
*Drug/herb*
Acidophilus: do not use with antiinfectives; separate by several hours
*Drug/lab test*
False positive: urinary glucose test

### NURSING CONSIDERATIONS
**Assessment**
• Assess patient for previous sensitivity reaction
• Assess patient for signs and symptoms of infection including characteristics of wounds, sputum, urine, stool, WBC >10,000/mm³, temp; obtain baseline information before and during treatment
• Complete C&S testing before beginning product therapy to identify if correct treatment has been initiated
• Assess for allergic reactions: rash, urticaria, pruritus, chills, fever, joint pain; angioedema may occur a few days after therapy begins; epINEPHrine, resuscitation equipment should be available for anaphylactic reaction
• Monitor blood tests: CBC, Hct, bilirubin, alkaline phosphatase monthly if patient is on long-term therapy
• Monitor for bleeding: ecchymosis, bleeding gums, hematuria, stool guaiac daily if on long-term therapy
• Assess for overgrowth of infection: perineal itching, fever, malaise, redness, pain, swelling, drainage, rash, diarrhea, change in cough, sputum

**Nursing diagnoses**
• Diarrhea (adverse reactions)
• Infection, risk for (uses)

- Injury, risk for (adverse reactions)
- Knowledge, deficient (teaching)
- Noncompliance (teaching)

## Implementation

- Give around the clock to maintain proper blood levels; give on an empty stomach to increase absorption of product; do not give within 3 hr of other agents; product interactions may occur
- Give with 8 oz of water

## Patient/family education

- Teach patient to report sore throat, bruising, bleeding, joint pain; may indicate blood dyscrasias (rare)
- Advise patient to contact prescriber if vaginal itching; loose foul-smelling stools; or furry tongue occur; may indicate superinfection; report itching, rash, pruritus, urticaria
- Instruct patient to take all medication prescribed for the length of time ordered; product must be taken around the clock to maintain blood levels; medication should not be shared with others

## Evaluation

**Positive therapeutic outcome**

- Absence of signs/symptoms of infection (WBC <10,000/mm$^3$, temp WNL, absence of urinary pain, hematuria)
- Reported improvement in symptoms of infection
- Negative C&S

---

## sulindac (Rx)

(sul-in'dak)

Apo-Sulin ✦, Clinoril, Novosundac ✦, sulindac

*Func. class.:* Nonsteroidal antiinflammatory, antirheumatic

*Chem. class.:* Indeneacetic acid derivative

**Pregnancy category C**

## Do not confuse:

Clinoril/Clozaril/Oruvail

**Action:** Inhibits prostaglandin synthesis by decreasing an enzyme needed for biosynthesis; analgesic, antiinflammatory, antipyretic

**Therapeutic outcome:** Decreased pain, inflammation

**Uses:** Mild to moderate pain, osteoarthritis, rheumatoid, gouty arthritis, ankylosing spondylitis, bursitis, juvenile arthritis

## Dosage and routes

*Arthritis*

*Adult:* PO 150 mg bid, may increase to 200 mg bid, max 400 mg/day

*Child:* PO 2-4 mg/kg/day in divided doses, max 6 mg/kg/day or 200 mg bid, whichever is less (safe/effective dose not established)

*Bursitis/acute arthritis*

*Adult:* PO 200 mg bid × 1-2 wk, then reduce dose

**Available forms:** Tabs 150, 200 mg

## Adverse effects

*CNS:* Dizziness, drowsiness, fatigue, tremors, confusion, insomnia, anxiety, depression, *headache*

*CV:* Tachycardia, peripheral edema, palpitations, dysrhythmias, **MI, stroke**

*EENT:* Tinnitus, hearing loss, blurred vision

*GI: Nausea, anorexia, vomiting, diarrhea,* jaundice, **cholestatic hepatitis,** constipation, flatulence, cramps, dry mouth, peptic ulcer, **bleeding, ulceration, perforation**

*GU:* **Nephrotoxicity: dysuria, hematuria, oliguria, azotemia**

*HEMA:* **Blood dyscrasias with prolonged use**

*INTEG:* Purpura, *rash, pruritus,* sweating, photosensitivity

**Contraindications:** Hypersensitivity, asthma, severe renal/hepatic disease, active ulcers, perioperative pain

**Precautions:** Pregnancy C (1st trimester), breastfeeding, children, bleeding disorders, GI/cardiac/renal disorders, hypersensitivity to other antiinflammatory agents

### Pharmacokinetics

| | |
|---|---|
| **Absorption** | Well absorbed |
| **Distribution** | Not known |
| **Metabolism** | Converted to active product—liver |
| **Excretion** | Minimal unchanged kidneys, breast milk |
| **Half-life** | 7.8 hr; 16.4 hr active metabolite |

### Pharmacodynamics

| | |
|---|---|
| **Onset** | Unknown |
| **Peak** | 2 hr |
| **Duration** | Unknown |

## Interactions

*Individual drugs*

Aspirin: increased GI reactions

Clopidogrel, eptifibatide, plicamycin, ticlopidine, tirofiban, valproic acid: increased bleeding risk

CycloSPORINE: increased nephrotoxicity
Diflunisal: decreased sulindac effect
Methotrexate, probenecid: increased toxicity

**Drug classifications**
Antacids: decreased sulindac effect
Anticoagulants, cephalosporins (some), thrombolytics: increased bleeding risk
Glucocorticoids, NSAIDs: increased GI reactions
Sulfonamides, sulfonylurea: increased toxicity

**Drug/herb**
Arginine, gossypol: increased gastric irritation
Bearberry, bilberry: increased NSAIDs effect
Bogbean, chondroitin: increased bleeding risk

**NURSING CONSIDERATIONS**
**Assessment**
• Monitor blood counts during therapy; watch for decreasing platelets; if low, therapy may need to be discontinued, restarted after hematologic recovery; and for blood dyscrasia (thrombocytopenia): bruising, fatigue, bleeding, poor healing
• Assess pain: frequency, intensity, characteristics, relief 1-2 hr after medication
• Assess for asthma, aspirin hypersensitivity, nasal polyps; hypersensitivity may develop, watch for rash

**Nursing diagnoses**
• Injury, risk for (adverse reactions)
• Knowledge, deficient (teaching)
• Mobility, impaired physical (uses)
• Pain, chronic (uses)

**Implementation**
• Do not break, crush, or chew tabs
• Give with full glass of water to enhance absorption
• Administer with food or milk to decrease gastric symptoms; food slows absorption slightly, does not decrease absorption

**Patient/family education**
• Advise patient that product must be continued for prescribed time to be effective; to avoid aspirin, alcoholic beverages
• Caution patient to report bleeding, bruising, fatigue, malaise because blood dyscrasias do occur
• Instruct patient to use caution when driving; drowsiness, dizziness may occur
• Teach patient to take with a full glass of water to enhance absorption

**Evaluation**
**Positive therapeutic outcome**
• Decreased pain
• Decreased inflammation
• Increased mobility

---

**sumatriptan** (Rx)
(soo-ma-trip'tan)
Imitrex
*Func. class.:* Antimigraine agent
*Chem. class.:* 5-HT₁ receptor agonist

**Pregnancy category C**

**Action:** Binds selectively to the vascular 5-HT₁ receptor subtype and exerts antimigraine effect; causes vasoconstriction in cranial arteries

**Therapeutic outcome:** Absence of migraines

**Uses:** Acute treatment of migraine with or without aura and cluster headache

**Dosage and routes**
*Adult:* SUBCUT 6 mg or less; may repeat in 1 hr; not to exceed 12 mg/24 hr; PO 25 mg with fluids if no relief in 2 hr, give another dose, max 200 mg/day; NASAL 1 dose of 5, 10, or 20 mg in one nostril, may repeat in 2 hr, max 40 mg/24 hr

**Hepatic dose**
*Adult:* PO 25 mg, if no response after 2 hr, give up to 50 mg

**Available forms:** Inj 6 mg (12 mg/ml); tabs 25, 50, 100 mg; nasal spray 5 mg/100 mcl-units dose spray device 20 mg/100 mcl-units

**Adverse effects**
*CNS: Tingling, hot sensation, burning, feeling of pressure, tightness, numbness, dizziness, sedation,* headache, anxiety, fatigue, cold sensation
*CV: Flushing,* **MI**
*EENT:* Throat, mouth, nasal discomfort, vision changes
*GI:* Abdominal discomfort
*INTEG: Inj site reaction,* sweating
*MS: Weakness, neck stiffness,* myalgia
*RESP:* Chest tightness, pressure

**Contraindications:** Angina pectoris, history of MI, documented silent ischemia, Prinzmetal's angina, ischemic heart disease, **IV** use, concurrent ergotamine-containing preparations, uncontrolled hypertension, hypersensitivity, basilar or hemiplegic migraine

**Precautions:** Pregnancy **C**, breastfeeding, children <18 yr, postmenopausal women, men >40 yr, geriatric, risk factors for CAD, hypercholesterolemia, obesity, diabetes, impaired renal/hepatic function

---

## Pharmacokinetics

| | |
|---|---|
| **Absorption** | Well absorbed (SUBCUT) |
| **Distribution** | 10%-20% plasma protein binding |
| **Metabolism** | Liver (metabolite) |
| **Excretion** | Urine, feces |
| **Half-life** | 2 hr |

## Pharmacodynamics

| | SUBCUT |
|---|---|
| **Onset** | 10-20 min |
| **Peak** | 10 min-2 hr |
| **Duration** | Up to 24 hr (pain relief) |

## Interactions
### Individual drugs
Ergotamine: increased risk of vasospastic reaction
### Drug classifications
Ergot derivatives: extended vasospastic effects
MAOIs, selective serotonin reuptake inhibitors: increased sumatriptan levels
### Drug/herb
Butterbur, feverfew: increased effect
SAM-e, St. John's wort: serotonin syndrome

## NURSING CONSIDERATIONS
### Assessment
• Assess for tingling, hot sensation, burning, feeling of pressure, numbness, flushing, inj site reaction
• Assess B/P; signs/symptoms of coronary vasospasm
• Monitor stress level, activity, reaction, coping mechanisms of patient
• Assess neurologic status: LOC, blurring vision, nausea, vomiting, tingling in extremities preceding headache
• Assess for ingestion of tyramine-containing foods (pickled products, beer, wine, aged cheese), food additives, preservatives, colorings, artificial sweeteners, chocolate, caffeine, which may precipitate these types of headaches

### Nursing diagnoses
• Knowledge, deficient (teaching)
• Pain, chronic (uses)

### Implementation
#### PO route
• Swallow tab whole; do not break, crush, or chew
• Take with fluids as soon as symptoms appear; may take a second dose >4 hr, max 200 mg/24 hr
#### SUBCUT route
• Give by SUBCUT route only, avoid IM or **IV** administration, use only for actual migraine attack

### Nasal route
• Spray once in 1 nostril, may repeat if headache returns, do not repeat if pain continues after 1st dose

### Patient/family education
• Caution patient not to take more than 2 doses/day or 12 mg/day; allow at least 1 hr between doses
• Caution patient to avoid driving or hazardous activities if dizziness or drowsiness occurs
• Teach patient to report chest tightness, heat, flushing, drowsiness, dizziness, fatigue, sudden severe abdominal pain or any allergic reactions that occur to prescriber immediately
• Inform patient to report any side effects to prescriber
• Caution patient to use contraception when taking product, to notify prescriber if pregnancy is suspected or planned

### Evaluation
#### Positive therapeutic outcome
• Decrease in frequency, severity of headache

## sunitinib (Rx)
(soo-nit′-in-ib)
Sutent
*Func. class.:* Antineoplastic—miscellaneous
*Chem. class.:* Protein-tyrosine kinase inhibitor
### Pregnancy category D

**Action:** Inhibits multiple receptor tyrosine kinases (RTKs), some are responsible for tumor growth

**Therapeutic outcome:** Decrease in size of tumor

**Uses:** Gastrointestinal stromal tumors (GIST) after disease progression or intolerance to imatinib; advanced renal carcinoma

### Dosage and routes
*Adult:* PO 50 mg/day × 4 wk, then 2 wk off; may increase or decrease dose by 12.5 mg; if administered with CYP3A4 inducers, give 87.5 mg/day; if given with CYP3A4 inhibitors give 37.5 mg/day

**Available forms:** Caps 12.5, 25, 50 mg

### Adverse effects
*CNS:* **CNS hemorrhage,** headache, dizziness, insomnia, **seizures,** fatigue
*CV:* Hypertension, **left ventricular dysfunction**
*GI:* *Nausea,* **hepatotoxicity, vomiting, dyspepsia,** *anorexia, abdominal pain,*

S

altered taste, constipation, stomatitis, mucositis, **pancreatitis**
**HEMA:** **Neutropenia, thrombocytopenia**
**INTEG:** *Rash,* skin discoloration, depigmentation of hair or skin, alopecia
**MS:** Pain, arthralgia, myalgia
**RESP:** Cough, dyspnea
**SYST:** **Bleeding,** electrolyte abnormalities

**Contraindications:** Pregnancy **D**, breast-feeding, hypersensitivity

**Precautions:** Children, geriatric, active infections

### Pharmacokinetics

| | |
|---|---|
| **Absorption** | Unknown |
| **Distribution** | Protein binding 95% |
| **Metabolism** | By CYP3A4 |
| **Excretion** | Feces, small amount in urine |
| **Half-life** | Terminal 40-60 hr (sunitinib); active metabolite 80-110 hr |

### Pharmacodynamics

| | |
|---|---|
| **Onset** | Unknown |
| **Peak** | 6-12 hr |
| **Duration** | Unknown |

### Interactions
*Individual drugs*
Acetaminophen: increased hepatotoxicity
Clarithromycin, erythromycin, itraconazole, ketoconazole: increased sunitinib concentrations
Dexamethasone, carbamazepine, phenobarbital, phenytoin, rifampin: decreased sunitinib concentrations
Simvastatin: increased plasma concentrations
Warfarin: increased plasma concentration; avoid use with warfarin, use low-molecular-weight anticoagulants instead
*Drug classifications*
Calcium channel blockers: increased plasma concentrations
*Drug/herb*
St. John's wort: decreased sunitinib concentration
*Drug/food*
Grapefruit juice: increased plasma concentrations

### NURSING CONSIDERATIONS
Assessment
• Monitor ANC and platelets; if ANC <1 × $10^9$/L and/or platelets <50 × $10^9$/L, stop until ANC >1.5 × $10^9$/L and platelets >75 × $10^9$/L ; if ANC <0.5 × $10^9$/L and/or platelets <10 × $10^9$/L, reduce dose by 200 mg, if cytopenia

continues, reduce dose by another 100 mg; if cytopenia continues for 4 wk, stop product until ANC ≥1 × $10^9$/L
• Assess CV status: hypertension, QT prolongation can occur; monitor left ventricular ejection fraction (LVEF) baseline periodically
• Assess for renal toxicity: if bilirubin >3 × IULN, withhold sunitinib until bilirubin levels return to <1.5 × IULN
• Monitor for hepatic toxicity: liver function tests, before treatment and qmo; if liver transaminases >5 × IULN, withhold sunitinib until transaminase levels return to <2.5 × IULN
• Monitor CBC, differential, platelet count weekly; withhold product if WBC is <3500/mm³, or platelet count <100,000/mm³; notify prescriber of these results; product should be discontinued
• Assess for CHF: adrenal insufficiency in those experiencing trauma
• Assess for bleeding: epistaxis rectal, gingival, upper GI, genital and wound bleeding; tumor-related hemorrhage may occur rapidly

### Nursing diagnoses
• Injury, risk for (uses, adverse reactions)
• Knowledge, deficient (teaching)

### Implementation
• Give with meal and large glass of water, to decrease GI symptoms
• Give nutritious diet with iron, vitamin supplement, low fiber, few dairy products
• Store at 25°C (77°F)

### Patient/family education
• Advise patient to report adverse reactions immediately: shortness of breath, bleeding
• Teach patient reason for treatment, expected result
• Teach patient that many adverse reactions may occur: high B/P, bleeding, mouth swelling, taste change, skin discoloration, depigmentation of hair/skin
• Teach patient to avoid persons with known upper respiratory infections; immunosuppression is common

### Evaluation
**Positive therapeutic outcome**
• Decrease in size of tumor

### suprofen ophthalmic
*See Appendix D*

## tacrine (Rx)

(tack'rin)

Cognex

*Func. class.:* Anti-Alzheimer agent
*Chem. class.:* Reversible cholinesterase inhibitor

### Pregnancy category C

### Do not confuse:

Cognex/Corgard

**Action:** Elevates acetylcholine concentrations (cerebral cortex) by slowing degrading of acetylcholine released in cholinergic neurons; does not alter underlying dementia

**Therapeutic outcome:** Improvement in symptoms of dementia in Alzheimer's disease

**Uses:** Treatment of mild to moderate dementia in Alzheimer's disease

### Dosage and routes

*Adult:* PO 10 mg qid × 4 wk, then 20 mg qid × 4 wk, increase at 4-wk intervals if patient tolerates product well and if transaminase is within normal limits, then titrate to higher doses (30-40 mg qid) at 4-wk intervals

**Available forms:** Caps 10, 20, 30, 40 mg

### Adverse effects

*CNS: Dizziness, confusion, insomnia,* tremor, *ataxia, somnolence, anxiety, agitation, depression, hallucinations, hostility, abnormal thinking,* chills, fever, headache, **seizures**

*CV:* Hypotension or hypertension, **bradycardia, heart block**

*GI: Nausea, vomiting, anorexia, abdominal pain, constipation,* dyspepsia, flatulence, **hepatotoxicity, GI bleeding,** diarrhea

*GU: Frequency, UTI, incontinence*

*INTEG: Rash,* flushing

*OTHER:* Myalgia

*RESP: Rhinitis, upper respiratory tract infection, cough,* pharyngitis

**Contraindications:** Hypersensitivity to this product or acridine derivatives, patients treated with this product who developed jaundice with a total bilirubin of >3 mg/dl

**Precautions:** Pregnancy **C,** breastfeeding, children, sick sinus syndrome, history of ulcers, GI bleeding, hepatic disease, bladder obstruction, asthma, seizure disorder, history of bradyarrhythmias

### Pharmacokinetics

| | |
|---|---|
| **Absorption** | Rapidly absorbed, low |
| **Distribution** | 55% plasma protein bound |
| **Metabolism** | Liver, extensively by CYP450 enzyme system |
| **Excretion** | Unknown |
| **Half-life** | 2-4 hr |

### Pharmacodynamics

Unknown

### Interactions

*Individual drugs*

Cimetidine, ciprofloxacin, fluvoxamine, ritonavir: increased tacrine level

Succinylcholine: synergistic effect

Theophylline: increased elimination half-life of theophylline

Smoking: may decrease product level

*Drug classifications*

Anticholinergics: decreased activity of anticholinergics

Cholinergic agonists, cholinesterase inhibitors: synergistic effect

NSAIDs: increased bleeding risk

*Drug/food*

May delay absorption; give 1 hr before meals

### NURSING CONSIDERATIONS

**Assessment**

• Monitor ALT qowk × 4-16 wk, then q3 mo; weekly ALT × 6 wk if dose is increased

• Monitor B/P for hypo/hypertension, heart rate

• Assess mental status: affect, mood, behavioral changes, depression, hallucinations, confusion; conduct suicide assessment

• Assess GI status: nausea, vomiting, anorexia, constipation, abdominal pain; add bulk and increase fluids for constipation

• Assess GU status: urinary frequency, incontinence

• Jaundice confirmed by significant increase in bilirubin (>3 mg/dl) and/or those with hypersensitivity (rash/fever) with increased ALT; should be immediately, permanently discontinued

**Nursing diagnoses**

• Injury, risk for (uses)

• Knowledge, deficient (teaching)

• Thought processes, disturbed (uses)

**Implementation**

• Give dosage adjusted to patient's response no more than q4 wk

• Provide assistance with ambulation if needed during beginning therapy; dizziness, ataxia may occur

T

Adverse effects: *italic* = common, **bold** = life-threatening

• Give between meals; if GI symptoms occur, may be given with meals

## Patient/family education

• Advise patient to report side effects: severe nausea, vomiting, sweating, salivation, bradycardia, hypotension, collapse, seizures, dizziness; may indicate overdose
• Instruct patient to use product exactly as prescribed at regular intervals, preferably between meals; may be taken with meals for GI upset; product is not a cure
• Advise patient to notify prescriber of nausea, vomiting, diarrhea (dose increased or beginning treatment) or rash, very dark or very light stools, jaundice (delayed onset)
• Caution patient not to increase or abruptly decrease dose; serious consequences may result

## Evaluation
**Positive therapeutic outcome**
• Decrease in confusion, improved mood

**Treatment of overdose:** Withdraw product, administer tertiary anticholinergics, provide supportive care

---

## tacrolimus (Rx)
(tak-roe'li-mus)
Prograf
## tacrolimus topical (Rx)
Protopic
*Func. class.:* Immunosuppressant
*Chem. clas.:* Macrolide

**Pregnancy category** C

**Action:** Produces immunosuppression by inhibiting lymphocytes (T)

**Therapeutic outcome:** Prevention of rejection in organ transplant

**Uses:** Organ transplants, to prevent rejection; topical: atopic dermatitis

**Unlabeled uses:** Autoimmune diseases, severe recalcitrant psoriasis

## Dosage and routes
*Adult and child:* IV 0.03-0.05 mg/kg/day × 3 days then PO 0.15 mg/kg bid; adjust dose in renal impairment
*Adult and child ≥2 yr:* Apply ointment bid × 7 days

**Available forms:** Inj **IV** 5 mg/ml; caps 0.5, 1, 5 mg; ointment 0.03%, 0.1%

## Adverse effects
*CNS: Tremors, headache,* insomnia, paresthesia, chills, fever, **seizures**
*CV:* Hypertension, myocardial hypertrophy

*EENT:* Blurred vision, photophobia
*GI:* Nausea, vomiting, diarrhea, constipation, GI bleeding
*GU:* Urinary tract infections, **albuminuria, hematuria, proteinuria, renal failure**
*HEMA:* Anemia, **leukocytosis, thrombocytopenia, purpura**
*INTEG:* Rash, flushing, itching, alopecia
*META:* Hirsutism, hyperglycemia, hyperuricemia, hypo/hyperkalemia, hypomagnesemia
*MS:* Back pain, muscle spasms
*RESP:* **Pleural effusion, atelectasis,** dyspnea
*SYST:* **Anaphylaxis**

**Contraindications:** Hypersensitivity to this product or to some kinds of castor oil, long-term use (topical), child <2 yr (topical)

**Precautions:** Pregnancy C, breastfeeding, children <12 yr, severe renal/hepatic disease, diabetes mellitus, hyperkalemia, hyperuricemia, lymphomas, hypertension

### Pharmacokinetics

| | |
|---|---|
| **Absorption** | Erractically absorbed (PO), completely absorbed (**IV**) |
| **Distribution** | Crosses placenta, 75% protein binding |
| **Metabolism** | Liver to metabolite |
| **Excretion** | Kidney—minimal, breast milk, bile |
| **Half-life** | 10 hr |

### Pharmacodynamics

| | PO | IV |
|---|---|---|
| **Onset** | Unknown | Unknown |
| **Peak** | 1-4 hr | Unknown |
| **Duration** | 12 hr | 12 hr |

## Interactions
### Individual drugs
Carbamazepine, phenobarbital, phenytoin, rifamycin: decreased blood levels
Cimetidine, danazol, erythromycin, mycophenolate, mofetil: increased blood levels
Cisplatin, cycloSPORINE: increased toxicity
Ibuprofen: increased oliguria
### Drug classifications
Aminoglycosides: increased toxicity
Antifungals, calcium channel blockers: increased blood levels
Vaccines: decreased effect
### Drug/herb
Astragalus, echinacea, melatonin: decreased immunosuppression
Ginseng, maitake, mistletoe: decreased effect

---

## NURSING CONSIDERATIONS
### Assessment
• Monitor blood studies: Hgb, WBC, platelets during treatment monthly; if WBC is <3000/mm$^3$, or platelet count <100,000/mm$^3$, product should be discontinued or reduced; decreased Hgb level may indicate bone marrow suppression
• Monitor liver function tests: alkaline phosphatase, AST, ALT, amylase, bilirubin, and for hepatotoxicity: dark urine, jaundice, itching, light-colored stools; product should be discontinued
◆ Assess for anaphylaxis: rash, pruritus, wheezing, laryngeal edema; stop infusion, initiate emergency procedures

### Nursing diagnoses
• Infection, risk for (uses)
• Knowledge, deficient (teaching)

### Implementation
**PO route**
• Give all medications PO if possible; avoid IM inj because bleeding may occur
• Give with meals to reduce GI upset; nausea is common
• Give for several days before transplant surgery; patients should be placed in protective isolation
**IV route**
• Give after diluting in 0.9% NaCl or D$_5$W to a concentration of 0.004-0.02 mg/ml as a cont inf
*Y-site compatibilities:* Acyclovir, aminophylline, amphotericin B, ampicillin, ampicillin/sulbactam, benztropine, calcium gluconate, cefazolin, cefotetan, ceftazidime, ceftriaxone, cefuroxime, chloramphenicol, cimetidine, ciprofloxacin, clindamycin, dexamethasone, digoxin, diphenhydrAMINE, DOBUTamine, DOPamine, doxycycline, erythromycin, esmolol, fluconazole, furosemide, ganciclovir, gentamicin, haloperidol, heparin, hydrocortisone, imipenem/cilastatin, insulin (regular), isoproterenol, leucovorin, lorazepam, methylPREDNISolone, metoclopramide, metronidazole, mezlocillin, multivitamins, nitroglycerin, nitroprusside, oxacillin, penicillin G potassium, perphenazine, phenytoin, piperacillin, potassium chloride, propranolol, ranitidine, sodium bicarbonate, trimethoprim/sulfamethoxazole, vancomycin

### Patient/family education
• Instruct patient to report fever, rash, severe diarrhea, chills, sore throat, fatigue because serious infections may occur; clay-colored stools, cramping may indicate hepatotoxicity

• Caution patient to avoid crowds or persons with known infections to reduce risk of infection

### Evaluation
**Positive therapeutic outcome**
• Absence of graft rejection
• Immunosuppression in autoimmune disorders

---

## tadalafil (Rx)
(tah-dal′a-fil)
Cialis
*Func. class.:* Impotence agent
*Chem. class.:* Phosphodiesterase type 5 inhibitor

**Action:** Inhibits phosphodiesterase type 5 (PDE5); enhances erectile function by increasing the amount of cGMP, which causes smooth muscle relaxation and increased blood flow into the corpus cavernosum; improves erectile function for up to 36 hr

**Therapeutic outcome:** Erection

**Uses:** Treatment of erectile dysfunction

### Dosage and routes
*Adult:* PO 10 mg, taken prior to sexual activity, dose may be reduced to 5 mg or increased to a max of 20 mg; usual max dosing frequency is once per day

*Renal dose*
*Adult:* PO CCr 31-50 ml/min 5 mg/day, max 10 mg q48hr; CCr <30 ml/min, max 5 mg

*Hepatic dose*
*Adult:* PO Child-Pugh class A, B, max 10 mg/day; Child-Pugh class C, not recommended

*Concomitant medications*
Ketoconazole, ritonavir, max 10 mg q72hr

**Available forms:** Tabs 5, 10, 20 mg

### Adverse effects
*CNS: Headache, flushing, dizziness*
*CV:* **MI, sudden death, CV collapse,** hypo/hypertension, tachycardia
*MISC:* Back pain/myalgia, *dyspepsia, nasal congestion, UTI,* blurred vision, changes in color vision, *diarrhea,* pruritus, priapism, **nonarteritic ischemic optic neuropathy (NAION),** hearing loss

**Contraindications:** Newborns, women, children, hypersensitivity, patients taking organic nitrates regularly or intermittently, patients taking any α-adrenergic antagonist other than 0.4 mg once-daily tamsulosin

T

**Precautions:** Anatomic penile deformities, sickle cell anemia, leukemia, multiple myeloma, CV/renal/hepatic disease, bleeding disorders, active peptic ulcer, prolonged erection

| Pharmacokinetics | |
|---|---|
| Absorption | Rapid; rate and extent of absorption of tadalafil are not influenced by food |
| Distribution | 94% protein bound |
| Metabolism | Liver |
| Excretion | Excreted primarily as metabolites, feces, urine; plasma concentration 61% in feces, 36% in urine |
| Half-life | 17.5 hr |

| Pharmacodynamics | |
|---|---|
| Onset | Rapid |
| Peak | 6 hr |
| Duration | Unknown |

### Interactions
#### Individual drugs
Alcohol, amlodipine, enalapril: decreased B/P
Bosentan: decreased effects of tadalafil
Itraconazole, ketoconazole, ritonavir: increased levels (although not studied, may also include other HIV protease inhibitors)
#### Drug classifications
◆Do not use with nitrates because of unsafe drop in B/P that could result in heart attack or stroke
α-blockers, angiotensin II receptor blockers: decreased B/P
Antacids: decreased effects of tadalafil

### NURSING CONSIDERATIONS
#### Assessment
• Assess for organic nitrates that should not be used with this product
#### Nursing diagnoses
• Knowledge, deficient (teaching)
• Sexual dysfunction (uses)
#### Implementation
• Before sexual activity; do not use more than once a day
#### Patient/family education
• Advise that product does not protect against STDs, including HIV
• Instruct to tell physician if patient has a bleeding problem
• Advise that product should not be used with nitrates in any form
• Advise that product has no effect in the absence of sexual stimulation

• Instruct to seek medical help if an erection lasts more than 4 hr
• Advise to tell physician of all medicines, vitamins, and herbs patient is taking, especially α-blockers, erythromycin, indinavir, itraconazole, ketoconazole, nitrates, ritonavir
• Advise that tadalafil is contraindicated for use with α-blockers except 0.4 mg/daily tamsulosin
### Evaluation
#### Positive therapeutic outcome
• Sustainable erection

### tamoxifen (Rx)
(ta-mox'i-fen)
Alpha-Tamoxifen ✦, Med Tamoxifen ✦, Nolvadex, Nolvadex-D ✦, Novo-Tamoxifen ✦, Tamofen ✦, Tamone ✦, Tamoplex ✦
*Func. class.:* Antineoplastic
*Chem. class.:* Antiestrogen hormone
**Pregnancy category D**

**Action:** Inhibits cell division by binding to cytoplasmic estrogen receptors; resembles normal cell complex but inhibits DNA synthesis and estrogen response of target tissue

**Therapeutic outcome:** Prevention of rapidly growing malignant cells

**Uses:** Advanced breast carcinoma that has not responded to other therapy in estrogen receptor-positive patients (usually postmenopausal), prevention of breast cancer, after breast surgery/radiation in ductal carcinoma in situ

**Unlabeled uses:** Mastalgia, pain/size of gynecomastia, ovulation stimulation, malignant carcinoid tumor, carcinoid syndrome, metaplastic melanoma, desmoid tumors, McCune-Albright syndrome (female pediatric patients)

### Dosage and routes
#### Breast cancer
*Adult:* PO 20-40 mg/day, doses >20 mg/day divide AM/PM
#### High risk for breast cancer
*Adult:* PO 20 mg/day × 5 yr
#### Ductal carcinoma in situ
*Adult:* PO 20 mg/day × 5 yr
#### McCune-Albright syndrome (unlabeled)
*Child 2-10 yr (girls):* PO 20 mg/day for up to 1 yr

**Available forms:** Tabs 10, 20 mg; oral sol 10 mg/5 ml

**Adverse effects**

*CNS: Hot flashes, headache, light-headedness,* depression, mood changes

*CV:* Chest pain, stroke, fluid retention, flushing

*EENT:* Ocular lesions, retinopathy, corneal opacity, blurred vision (high doses)

*GI: Nausea, vomiting,* altered taste (anorexia)

*GU:* Vaginal bleeding, pruritus vulvae, uterine malignancies, altered menses

**HEMA: Thrombocytopenia, leukopenia,** deep vein thrombosis

*INTEG: Rash,* alopecia

*META:* Hypercalcemia

**RESP: Pulmonary embolism**

**Contraindications:** Pregnancy **D**, breast-feeding, hypersensitivity

**Precautions:** Leukopenia, thrombocytopenia, cataracts, women of childbearing age

| Pharmacokinetics | |
|---|---|
| **Absorption** | Adequately absorbed |
| **Distribution** | Unknown |
| **Metabolism** | Liver—extensively |
| **Excretion** | Feces—slowly, small amounts (kidneys) |
| **Half-life** | 1 wk |

| Pharmacodynamics | |
|---|---|
| **Onset** | Unknown |
| **Peak** | 4-7 hr |
| **Duration** | Unknown |

**Interactions**

*Individual drugs*

Aminoglutethimide, medroxyprogesterone, rifamycin: decreased tamoxifen levels

Bromocriptine: increased tamoxifen level

Letrozole: decreased levels of letrozole

Radiation: increased myelosuppression

*Drug classifications*

Anticoagulants: increased risk of bleeding

Cytotoxics: increased thromboembolic action

CYP3A4 inducers (barbiturates, bosentan, carbamazepine, efavirenz, phenytoin, nevirapine, rifabutin, rifampin): decreased tamoxifen effect

CYP3A4 inhibitors (aprepitant, antiretroviral protease inhibitors, clarithromycin, danazol, delavirdine, diltiazem, erythromycin, fluconazole, fluoxetine, fluvoxamine, imatinib, ketoconazole, mibefradil, nefazodone, telithromycin, voriconazole): increased toxicity

*Drug/herb*

St. John's wort, dong quai, black cohosh: avoid use

*Drug/lab test*

Increased: serum calcium, $T_4$, AST, ALT, cholesterol, triglycerides

**NURSING CONSIDERATIONS**

**Assessment**

• Monitor CBC, differential, platelet count weekly; withhold product if WBC is <4000/$mm^3$ or platelet count is <75,000/$mm^3$; notify prescriber of results; monitor calcium levels (hypercalcemia is common)

◆ Assess for tumor flare: increase in bone, tumor pain during beginning treatment; give analgesics as ordered to decrease pain

• Assess for bleeding: hematuria, guaiac, bruising or petechiae, mucosa or orifices q8hr, no rectal temp

◆ Assess for uterine malignancies: Symptoms of stroke, PE that may occur in women with ductal carcinoma in situ (DCIS) and women at high risk for breast cancer

**Nursing diagnoses**

• Injury, risk for (adverse reactions)

• Knowledge, deficient (teaching)

**Implementation**

• Do not break, crush, or chew tabs

• Give with food or fluids for GI upset; repeat dose may be needed if vomiting occurs

• Store in light-resistant container at room temperature

**Patient/family education**

• Instruct patient to report any complaints, side effects to prescriber; if dose is missed, do not double next dose

• Advise patient that vaginal bleeding, pruritus, hot flashes can occur and are reversible after discontinuing treatment

• Instruct patient to report immediately decreased visual acuity, which may be irreversible; stress need for routine eye exams

• Inform patient about who should be told about tamoxifen therapy

• Advise patient to report vaginal bleeding immediately; that tumor flare (increase in size or tumor, increased bone pain) may occur and will subside rapidly; may take analgesics for pain; that premenopausal women must use mechanical birth control method because ovulation may be induced (teratogenic product)

• Caution patient to use sunscreen and protective clothing to prevent burns because photosensitivity is common

T

Adverse effects: *italic* = common, **bold** = life-threatening

• Teach patient that hair loss may occur during treatment; a wig or hairpiece may make patient feel better; new hair may be different in color, texture
• Inform patient rash or lesions are temporary and may become large during beginning therapy
• Advise patient to increase fluids to 2 L/day unless contraindicated

### Evaluation
**Positive therapeutic outcome**
• Decreased spread of malignant cells in breast cancer

---

## tamsulosin (Rx)
(tam-sue-lo'sen)
Flomax
*Func. class.:* Selective α-adrenergic blocker
*Chem. class.:* Sulfamoyl phenethylamine derivative

### Pregnancy category B

**Do not confuse:**
Flomax/Fosamax/Volmax

**Action:** Binds preferentially to α IA-adrenoceptor subtype located mainly in the prostate

**Therapeutic outcome:** Decreased symptoms of benign prostatic hyperplasia (BPH)

**Uses:** Symptoms of BPH

### Dosage and routes
*Adult:* PO 0.4 mg/day, increasing to 0.8 mg/day if required

**Available forms:** Caps 0.4 mg

### Adverse effects
*CNS: Dizziness, headache,* asthenia, insomnia
*CV:* Chest pain
*EENT:* Amblyopia, floppy iris syndrome
*GI:* Nausea, diarrhea, dysgeusia
*GU:* Decreased libido, abnormal ejaculation
*MS:* Back pain
*RESP:* Rhinitis, pharyngitis, cough

**Contraindications:** Hypersensitivity

**Precautions:** Pregnancy **B,** breastfeeding, children, hepatic disease, CAD, severe renal disease

### Pharmacokinetics

| | |
|---|---|
| **Absorption** | Well absorbed |
| **Distribution** | Not known; 98% plasma protein bound |
| **Metabolism** | Liver, extensively |
| **Excretion** | Kidneys |
| **Half-life** | 9-15 hr |

### Pharmacodynamics
Unknown

### Interactions
*Individual drugs*
Cimetidine: increased toxicity
Doxazosin, prazosin, terazosin, vardenafil: do not use together
*Drug classifications*
β-Adrenergic blockers: do not use together
*Drug/food*
Decreased: absorption with food

### NURSING CONSIDERATIONS
### Assessment
• Monitor CBC with differential and liver function tests; B/P and heart rate
• Monitor urodynamic studies/urinary flow rates, residual volume
• Assess for BPH: change in urinary patterns, baseline and throughout treatment
• Monitor I&O ratios, weight daily, edema, report weight gain or edema

### Nursing diagnoses
• Cardiac output, decreased (uses)
• Injury, risk for (side effects)
• Knowledge, deficient (teaching)
• Noncompliance (teaching)

### Implementation
• Swallow caps whole; do not break, crush, or chew
• Store in airtight container at 86° F (30° C) or less
• May be given with food to prevent GI symptoms; ½ hr after same meal each day

### Patient/family education
• Teach patient not to discontinue product abruptly; emphasize the importance of complying with dosage schedule, even if feeling better; if dose is missed take as soon as remembered; take at same time each day
• Teach patient not to use OTC products (cough, cold, allergy) unless directed by prescriber; also to avoid large amounts of caffeine
• Caution patient that product may cause dizziness, may occur during 1st few days of therapy; to avoid hazardous activities

---

## Evaluation
**Positive therapeutic outcome**
- Decreased symptoms of BPH

## tazobactam
*See piperacillin/tazobactam*

## tegaserod (Rx)
(teg-as'er-odd)
Zelnorm
*Func. class.:* 5-HT$_4$ receptor partial agonist,
GI agent—miscellaneous

**Pregnancy category** B

**Action:** A 5-HT$_4$ receptor partial agonist that
binds 5-HT$_4$ receptors, stimulating peristalsis
and intestinal secretion

**Therapeutic outcome:** Decreased
constipation in irritable bowel syndrome (IBS)

**Uses:** IBS where primary bowel symptom is
constipation

## Dosage and routes
*Adult (females):* **PO** 6 mg bid before
meals × 4-6 wk

**Available forms:** Tabs 2, 6 mg

## Adverse effects
*CNS: Headache, dizziness, depression,
vertigo, fatigue,* suicide attempt, poor concentration
*CV:* Hypotension, angina, **dysrhythmias,
bundle branch block, supraventricular
tachycardia**
*GI: Nausea, abdominal pain, increased
appetite, eructation, increased AST, in
creased ALT, diarrhea, irritable colon,
tenesmus, flatulence*
*GU:* Polyuria, renal pain, ovarian cyst, miscar-
riage, albuminuria
*MISC:* Pain, facial edema, increased CPK,
asthma, breast carcinoma
*MS:* Back pain, arthralgia
*SYST:* Anaphylaxis

**Contraindications:** Hypersensitivity,
severe renal disease, moderate to severe
hepatic disease, history of bowel obstruction,
gallbladder disease, abdominal adhesions,
sphincter of Oddi dysfunction, hypotension

**Precautions:** Pregnancy **B**, breastfeeding,
children, diarrhea

### Pharmacokinetics
| | |
|---|---|
| **Absorption** | Unknown |
| **Distribution** | 98% protein binding |
| **Metabolism** | Unknown |
| **Excretion** | ⅔ unchanged in feces, remainder in urine as metabolites |
| **Half-life** | 11 hr |

### Pharmacodynamics
| | |
|---|---|
| **Onset** | Unknown |
| **Peak** | 1 hr |
| **Duration** | Unknown |

## Interactions
*Individual drug*
Digoxin: decreased effect of digoxin
*Drug classification*
Antimuscarinics: decreased tegaserod effect
*Drug/food*
Food: decreased absorption, but is minimized
when taken ½ hr before a meal

## NURSING CONSIDERATIONS
### Assessment
- This product is only available to women ≤55
yrs old who meet specific guidelines; it is off
the market to the general public
- Assess GI symptoms: nausea, abdominal pain
- Assess CV status: B/P, pulse, chest pain

### Nursing diagnoses
- Constipation, (uses)
- Knowledge, deficient (teaching)

### Implementation
- Give before meals, bid
- Store at room temperature

### Patient/family education
- Advise to notify prescriber of GI symptoms,
hypersensitivity reactions

### Evaluation
**Positive therapeutic outcome**
- Decreased constipation in IBS

## telbivudine (Rx)
(tel-bi'vyoo-deen)
Tyzeka
*Func. class.:* Antiretroviral
*Chem. class.:* Nucleoside reverse transcrip-
tase inhibitor (NRTI)

**Pregnancy category** B

**Action:** Inhibits replication of HBV DNA
polymerase, which inhibits HBV replication

**Therapeutic outcome:** Decreased
hepatitis B serology

**Uses:** Hepatitis B

T

Adverse effects: *italic* = common, **bold** = life-threatening

**Dosage and routes**
*Adult and adolescent >16 yr:* PO 600 mg/day; max 600 mg/day

**Available forms:** Tabs 600 mg

**Adverse effects**
*CNS:* Fever, headache, malaise, weakness, dizziness, insomnia
*EENT:* Taste change, hearing loss, photophobia
*GI:* Nausea, vomiting, diarrhea, anorexia, abdominal pain, hepatomegaly
*INTEG:* Rash
*MISC:* Lactic acidosis
*MS:* Myalgia, arthralgia, muscle cramps
*RESP:* Cough

**Contraindications:** Hypersensitivity, breastfeeding

**Precautions:** Pregnancy **B,** children, severe renal disease, impaired hepatic function, anemia, organ transplant, dialysis, HIV, lactic acidosis, obesity, alcoholism

| Pharmacokinetics | |
|---|---|
| **Absorption** | Unknown |
| **Distribution** | Steady state 5-7 days, protein binding 3.3% |
| **Metabolism** | Unknown |
| **Excretion** | Kidneys, unchanged |
| **Half-life** | Terminal 40-49 hr |

| Pharmacodynamics |
|---|
| Unknown |

**Interactions**
*Individual drugs*
CycloSPORINE, erythromycin, hydrochloro-quine, niacin, penicillamine, zidovudine, ZDV: increased myopathy risk
*Drug classifications*
Any agent altering renal function: altered telbivudine levels
Azole antifungals, corticosteroids, fibric acid derivatives, HMG-CoA reductase inhibitors: increased myopathy risk

**NURSING CONSIDERATIONS**
**Assessment**
• Monitor liver function tests, hepatitis B serology, creatine kinase, periodically

**Nursing diagnoses**
• Infection, risk for (uses)
• Knowledge, deficient (teaching)

**Implementation**
• Give with or without food with a full glass of water
• Store at room temperature

**Patient/family education**
• Advise patient that GI complaints and insomnia may resolve after 3-4 wk of treatment
• Teach patient that product does not cure hepatitis B and does not stop the spread to others
• Teach patient that follow-up visits must be continued
• Teach patient that serious product interactions may occur if OTC products are ingested; check with prescriber before taking
• Advise patient that product may cause dizziness; avoid hazardous activities until response is known
• Teach patient to report symptoms of cough, difficulty sleeping or excessive headache

**Evaluation**
**Positive therapeutic outcome**
• Decreased hepatitis B serology

**telithromycin** (Rx)
(teh-lih-throw-my'sin)
Ketek
*Func. class.:* Antiinfective
*Chem. class.:* Ketolides
**Pregnancy category  C**

**Action:** Binds to 50S ribosomal subunits of susceptible bacteria and suppresses protein synthesis

**Therapeutic outcome:** Bacterial action against *Streptococcus pneumoniae, Haemophilus influenzae, Moraxella catarrhalis, Staphylococcus aureus*

**Uses:** Acute bacterial exacerbation of chronic bronchitis caused by *Streptococcus pneumoniae, Haemophilus influenzae, Moraxella catarrhalis*; acute bacterial sinusitis caused by *S. pnuemoniae, H. influenzae, M. catarrhalis, Staphylococcus aureus*, community-acquired pneumonia

**Unlabeled uses:** Acute tonsillitis/pharyngitis

**Dosage and routes**
*Acute bacterial exacerbation of bronchitis*
*Adult:* PO 800 mg/day × 5 days

*Acute bacterial sinusitis*
*Adult:* PO 800 mg/day × 5 days

*Community-acquired pneumonia*
*Adult:* PO 800 mg/day × 7-10 days

**Available forms:** Tabs 300, 400 mg

## Adverse effects
**CNS:** Dizziness, headache, insomnia, increased sweating
**EENT:** Blurred vision, diplopia, difficulty focusing
**GI:** *Nausea, vomiting, diarrhea,* hepatitis, abdominal pain/distension, stomatitis, anorexia, **pseudomembranous colitis, pancreatitis**
**GU:** *Vaginitis, moniliasis*
**INTEG:** Rash, urticaria
**MISC:** **Atrial dysrhythmias, QT prolongation**
**MS:** Muscle cramps
**SYST:** **Anaphylaxis,** superinfection

**Contraindications:** Hypersensitivity to this product or macrolide antibiotics, myasthenia gravis

**Precautions:** Pregnancy **C**, breastfeeding, children, geriatric, ongoing prodysrhythmias, hepatic/GI disease, QT prolongation

| Pharmacokinetics | |
|---|---|
| **Absorption** | Unknown |
| **Distribution** | Protein binding 60%-70% |
| **Metabolism** | Liver |
| **Excretion** | Bile, feces |
| **Half-life** | Unknown |

| Pharmacodynamics | |
|---|---|
| **Onset** | Unknown |
| **Peak** | 1 hr |
| **Duration** | Unknown |

## Interactions
### Individual drugs
Atorvastatin, carbamazepine, cycloSPORINE, digoxin, ergots, lovastatin, metoprolol, midazolam, phenobarbital, phenytoin, simvastatin, sirolimus, tacrolimus, theophylline: increased action
Carbamazepine, phenobarbital, phenytoin, rifampin: decreased action of telithromycin
Itraconazole, ketoconazole: increased telithromycin
Pimozide: serious dysrhythmias; do not use together
Sotalol: decreased action
Verapamil: increased cardiotoxicity
### Drug classifications
Antidysrhythmics (amiodarone, bretylium, disopyramide, dofetilide, procainamide, quinidine, sotalol): serious dysrhythmias; do not use together
Antidysrhythmics (class IA, III): increased QT interval; do not use together

### Drug/herb
Acidophilus: do not use with antiinfectives; separate by several hours
### Drug/lab test
Increased: AST/ALT

## NURSING CONSIDERATIONS
### Assessment
• Assess for infection: temp, sputum, WBCs, baseline and periodically
• Assess for oliguria in renal disease
• Monitor liver function tests: AST, ALT, if patient is on long-term therapy
• Monitor C&S before product therapy; product may be given as soon as culture is taken; C&S may be repeated after treatment
• Monitor bowel pattern before, during treatment
• Assess for skin eruptions, itching

### Nursing diagnoses
• Infection, risk for (uses)

### Implementation
• May take without regard to food
• Store at room temperature
• Provide adequate intake of fluids (2 L) during diarrhea episodes

### Patient/family education
• Teach patient to report sore throat, fever, fatigue (could indicate superinfection)
• Teach patient to notify nurse of diarrhea stools, dark urine, pale stools, jaundice of eyes or skin, and severe abdominal pain
• Teach patient to report blurred vision, if interfering with daily activities
• Advise patient to avoid driving, hazardous activities if blurred vision occurs
• Instruct patient to take as prescribed, do not double or skip doses
• Instruct patient not to use this product if using Class 1A or III antidysrhythmics
• Advise patient to avoid simvastatin, lovastatin or atorvastatin
• Inform patient that medication may be taken without regard to meals

### Evaluation
**Positive therapeutic outcome**
• Decreased symptoms of infection

### Treatment of hypersensitivity:
Withdraw product; maintain airway; administer epINEPHrine, aminophylline, $O_2$, **IV** corticosteroids

T

---

Adverse effects: *italic* = common, **bold** = life-threatening

## telmisartan (Rx)
(tel-mih-sar'tan)
Micardis
*Func. class.:* Antihypertensive
*Chem. class.:* Angiotensin II receptor (type $AT_1$)

**Pregnancy category**
C (1st trimester),
D (2nd/3rd trimesters)

**Action:** Blocks the vasoconstrictor and aldosterone-secreting effects of angiotensin II; selectively blocks the binding of angiotensin II to the $AT_1$ receptor found in tissues

**Therapeutic outcome:** Decreased B/P

**Uses:** Hypertension, alone or in combination

**Unlabeled uses:** Heart failure

**Dosage and routes**
*Adult:* PO 40 mg/day; range 20-80 mg/day

**Available forms:** Tabs 20, 40, 80 mg

**Adverse effects**
*CNS:* Dizziness, insomnia, *anxiety,* headache, fatigue
*GI: Diarrhea,* dyspepsia, *anorexia, vomiting*
*MS: Myalgia, pain*
*RESP:* Cough, *upper respiratory tract infection,* sinusitis, pharyngitis

**Contraindications:** Pregnancy **D** (2nd/3rd trimesters), hypersensitivity

**Precautions:** Pregnancy **C** (1st trimester), breastfeeding, children, geriatric, hypersensitivity to angiotensin-converting enzyme (ACE) inhibitors, renal/hepatic disease, renal artery stenosis, dialysis, CHF

### Pharmacokinetics

| | |
|---|---|
| **Absorption** | Unknown |
| **Distribution** | Highly protein bound |
| **Metabolism** | Liver (extensively) |
| **Excretion** | Urine/feces |
| **Half-life** | Terminal 24 hr |

### Pharmacodynamics
Unknown

### Interactions
Digoxin: increased digoxin peak, trough concentrations
*Drug classifications*
Antihypertensives, diuretics: increased antihypertensive action
NSAIDs, salicylates: decreased antihypertensive effect

Potassium-sparing diuretics, potassium salt substitutes: increased hyperkalemia
*Drug/herb*
Aconite: increased toxicity, death
Astragalus, cola tree: increased or decreased antihypertensive effect
Barberry, betony, black catechu, black cohosh, bloodroot, broom, burdock, cat's claw, dandelion, goldenseal, Irish moss, Jamaican dogwood, kelp, khella, mistletoe, parsley: increased antihypertensive effect
Coltsfoot, guarana, khat, licorice, yohimbe: decreased antihypertensive effect

### NURSING CONSIDERATIONS
**Assessment**
• Monitor B/P, pulse q4hr; note rate, rhythm, quality
• Monitor electrolytes: potassium, sodium, chloride
• Monitor baselines in renal, liver function tests before therapy begins
• Assess edema in feet, legs daily
• Assess skin turgor, dryness of mucous membranes for hydration status

**Nursing diagnoses**
• Knowledge, deficient (teaching)
• Noncompliance (teaching)
• Tissue perfusion, ineffective (uses)

**Implementation**
• Give without regard to meals
• Give increased dose to African-American patients, B/P response may be reduced

**Patient/family education**
• Instruct patient to comply with dosage schedule, even if feeling better
• Advise patient to notify prescriber of mouth sores, fever, swelling of hands or feet, irregular heartbeat, chest pain
• Teach patient that excessive perspiration, dehydration, vomiting, diarrhea may lead to fall in blood pressure; consult prescriber if these occur
• Teach patient that product may cause dizziness, fainting; light-headedness may occur
• Advise patient to use contraception while taking this product
• Teach patient to notify prescriber of all prescriptions, OTC preparations, and supplements taken

**Evaluation**
**Positive therapeutic outcome**
• Decreased B/P

 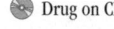

## temazepam (Rx)

(tem-az'a-pam)
Razepam, Restoril, Temazepam
*Func. class.:* Sedative/hypnotic
*Chem. class.:* Benzodiazepine, short-acting

**Pregnancy category X**

**Controlled substance
schedule IV (USA),
schedule F (Canada)**

**Action:** Produces CNS depression at limbic,
thalamic, hypothalamic levels of the CNS; may
be mediated by neurotransmitter
γ-aminobutyric acid (GABA); results are
sedation, hypnosis, skeletal muscle relaxation,
anticonvulsant activity, anxiolytic action

**Therapeutic outcome:** Decreased
insomnia

**Uses:** Insomnia (short-term)

**Dosage and routes**
*Adult:* PO 7.5-30 mg at bedtime
*Geriatric:* PO 7.5 mg at bedtime

**Available forms:** Caps 7.5, 15, 22.5,
30 mg

**Adverse effects**
*CNS: Lethargy, drowsiness, daytime seda-
tion,* dizziness, confusion, light-headedness,
headache, anxiety, irritability, complex sleep-
related reactions (sleep driving, sleep eating),
fatigue
*CV:* Chest pain, pulse changes, hypotension
*EENT:* Blurred vision
*GI:* Nausea, vomiting, diarrhea, heartburn,
abdominal pain, constipation, anorexia
*HEMA:* **Leukopenia, granulocytopenia**
(rare)
*SYST:* **Severe allergic reactions**

**Contraindications:** Pregnancy **X**, breastfeeding, hypersensitivity to benzodiazepines,
intermittent porphyria

**Precautions:** Children <15 yr, geriatric,
anemia, pulmonary/renal/hepatic disease,
suicidal individuals, product abuse, psychosis,
acute angle-closure glaucoma, seizure disorders, angioedema, sleep-related behaviors
(sleep walking)

### Pharmacokinetics

| Absorption | Well absorbed |
| --- | --- |
| Distribution | Widely distributed, crosses placenta, crosses blood-brain barrier |
| Metabolism | Liver |
| Excretion | Kidneys, breast milk |
| Half-life | 10-20 hr |

### Pharmacodynamics

| Onset | ½ hr |
| --- | --- |
| Peak | 2-3 hr |
| Duration | 6-8 hr |

**Interactions**
*Individual drugs*
Alcohol: increased actions of both products
Cimetidine, disulfiram: increased effect of each
  specific product
Rifampin: decreased action of rifampin
Theophylline: decreased effects of theophylline
*Drug classifications*
Antacids: decreased effect of antacids
Contraceptives (oral): increased effect
CNS depressants: increased action of both
  products
*Drug/herb*
Black cohosh: increased hypotension
Catnip, chamomile, clary, cowslip, hops, kava,
  lavender, mistletoe, nettle, pokeweed, poppy,
  Queen Anne's lace, senega, skullcap,
  valerian: increased CNS depression
*Drug/lab test*
Increased: AST/ALT, serum bilirubin
Decreased: radioactive iodine uptake
False increase: 17-OHCS

**NURSING CONSIDERATIONS**
**Assessment**
• Assess mental status: mood, sensorium,
anxiety, affect, sleeping pattern, drowsiness,
dizziness, especially geriatric; physical dependency, withdrawal symptoms: anxiety, panic
attacks, agitation, seizures, headache, nausea,
vomiting, muscle pain, weakness; suicidal
tendencies; for indications of increasing
tolerance and abuse
• Monitor B/P (lying, standing), pulse; if
systolic B/P drops 20 mm Hg, hold product,
notify prescriber
• Monitor blood studies: CBC during long-
term therapy; blood dyscrasias have occurred
rarely; decreased hematocrit, neutropenia may
occur
• Monitor hepatic studies: AST, ALT, bilirubin,
creatinine LDH, alkaline phosphatase
• Monitor I&O ratio; indicate renal dysfunction

**Nursing diagnoses**
• Anxiety (uses)
• Injury, risk for (adverse reactions)
• Knowledge, deficient (teaching)

**Implementation**
• Give with food or milk to decrease GI
symptoms; if patient is unable to swallow

T

medication whole, tab may be crushed and mixed with foods or fluids

• Give sugarless gum, hard candy, frequent sips of water for dry mouth

### Patient/family education

• Inform patient that product may be taken with food, and that fluids and tab may be crushed or swallowed whole

• Advise patient not to use for everyday stress or longer than 3 mo unless directed by prescriber; not to take more than prescribed amount; may be habit forming; not to double or skip doses

• Caution patient to avoid OTC preparations unless approved by prescriber; alcohol and CNS depressants will increase CNS depression

• Advise patient to avoid driving, activities that require alertness, because drowsiness may occur; to avoid alcohol ingestion or other psychotropic medications; to rise slowly or fainting may occur, especially in geriatric; that drowsiness may worsen at beginning of treatment

• Caution patient not to discontinue medication abruptly after long-term use; withdrawal symptoms include vomiting, cramping, tremors, seizures

• Advise patient to use contraception while taking this product

• Advise patient that complex sleep-related behaviors may occur (sleep driving/eating)

### Evaluation
**Positive therapeutic outcome**

• Decreased anxiety, restlessness, sleeplessness (short-term treatment only)

**Treatment of overdose:** Lavage, VS, supportive care

---

### temozolomide (Rx)
(tem-oo-zole'oo-mide)
Temodar
*Func. class.:* Antineoplastic alkylating agents
*Chem. class.:* Imidazotetrazine derivative

**Pregnancy category D**

**Action:** A proproduct that undergoes conversion to 5-(3-methyl-1-triazeno) imidazole-4-carboxamide (MTIC); MTIC action prevents DNA transcription

**Therapeutic outcome:** Prevention of rapidly growing malignant cells

**Uses:** Anaplastic astrocytoma with relapse, glioblastoma multiforme

**Unlabeled uses:** Metastatic melanoma

### Dosage and routes
*Anaplastic astrocytoma*
*Adult:* PO Adjust dose based on nadir neutrophil and platelet counts 150 mg/m$^2$/day × 5 days during 28-day cycle

*Glioblastoma multiforme*
*Adult:* PO 75 mg/m$^2$/day × 42 days with focal radiotherapy, then maintenance of 6 cycles

**Available forms:** Caps 5, 20, 100, 140, 180, 250 mg

### Adverse effects
*CNS: Seizures, hemiparesis, dizziness, poor coordination, amnesia, insomnia, paresthesia, somnolence, paresis, ataxia, anxiety, dysphagia, depression, confusion*
*GI: Nausea, anorexia, vomiting, abdominal pain, constipation*
*GU: Urinary incontinence, UTI, frequency*
*HEMA: Thrombocytopenia, leukopenia, anemia, myelosuppression, neutropenia*
*INTEG: Rash, pruritus*
*MISC: Headache, fatigue, asthenia, fever, edema, back pain, weight increase, diplopia*
*RESP: Upper respiratory tract infection, pharyngitis, sinusitis, coughing*
*SYST: Anaphylaxis, secondary malignancy*

**Contraindications:** Pregnancy **D**, breastfeeding, hypersensitivity to this product or carbazine

**Precautions:** Radiation therapy, renal/hepatic disease, bone marrow suppression, geriatric, myelosuppression

| Pharmacokinetics | |
|---|---|
| **Absorption** | Rapid, complete |
| **Distribution** | Crosses blood-brain barrier |
| **Metabolism** | To MTIC and metabolite |
| **Excretion** | Urine, feces |
| **Half-life** | 1.8 hr |

| Pharmacodynamics | |
|---|---|
| **Onset** | Unknown |
| **Peak** | 1 hr |
| **Duration** | Unknown |

### Interactions
*Individual drugs*
Digoxin: decreased action of digoxin
Filgrastim, G-CSF, pegfilgrastim, sargramostim: do not use within 24 hr of these products
Radiation: increased toxicity, bone marrow suppression

---

 Alert    Canada Only    Drug on CD       * "Tall Man" lettering (See Preface)

### Drug classifications
Anticoagulants, NSAIDs, platelet inhibitors, thrombolytics: increased bleeding risk
Antineoplastics, bone marrow–suppressing products: increased bone marrow suppression
Live virus vaccines, toxoids: increased adverse reactions, decreased antibody reaction

## NURSING CONSIDERATIONS
### Assessment
• Assess symptoms indicating severe allergic reaction: rash, pruritus, urticaria, purpuric skin lesions, itching, flushing; product should be discontinued
• Assess tumor response during treatment
• Obtain CBC on day 22 (21 days after 1st dose), CBC weekly until recovery if ANC is $<1.5 \times 10^9$/L and platelets $<100 \times 10^9$/L, do not administer to patients that do not tolerate 100 mg/m$^2$; myelosuppression usually occurs late in the treatment cycle
• Assess for seizures, mental status throughout treatment
• Monitor renal function studies: BUN, creatinine, urine CCr before and during therapy; I&O ratio; report fall in urine output to <30 ml/hr
• Monitor temp q4hr (may indicate beginning of infection)
• Monitor liver function tests before and during therapy (bilirubin, AST, ALT, LDH) as needed or monthly; note jaundice of skin or sclera, dark urine, clay-colored stools, itchy skin, abdominal pain, fever, diarrhea; hepatotoxicity can be serious and fatal
• Assess for bleeding: hematuria, stool guaiac, bruising or petechiae, mucosa or orifices; check for inflammation of mucosa, breaks in skin

### Nursing diagnoses
• Body image, disturbed (adverse reactions)
• Infection, risk for (adverse reactions)
• Injury, risk for (adverse reactions)
• Knowledge, deficient (teaching)

### Implementation
• Give fluids **IV** or PO before chemotherapy to hydrate patient
• Give antiemetic 30-60 min before giving product to prevent vomiting, and prn; antibiotics for prophylaxis of infection
• Provide liquid diet: carbonated beverages; gelatin may be added if patient is not nauseated or vomiting
• Capsules should not be opened; if accidentally damaged, do not allow contact with skin, or inhale; take caps one at a time with 8 oz of water at the same time of day; use cytotic handling procedure
• Give on empty stomach at bedtime to prevent nausea/vomiting

### Patient/family education
• Teach patient to avoid use of products containing aspirin or NSAIDs, razors, commercial mouthwash, since bleeding may occur; to report symptoms of bleeding (hematuria, tarry stools)
• Instruct patient to report signs of anemia (fatigue, headache, irritability, faintness, shortness of breath)
• Caution patient not to have any vaccinations without the advice of prescriber; serious reactions can occur
• Advise patient contraception is needed during treatment and for several months after completion of therapy; product has teratogenic properties

### Evaluation
**Positive therapeutic outcome**
• Prevention of rapid division of malignant cells

### temsirolimus (Rx)
(tem-sir-oh′li-mus)
Torisel
*Func. class.:* Biologic response modifier
*Chem. class.:* mTOR antagonist
**Pregnancy category D**

**Action:** Inhibits mammalian target of rapamycin (mTOR), a protein kinase

**Therapeutic outcome:** Decreased time of progression of renal cell carcinoma

**Uses:** Renal cell carcinoma

### Dosage and routes
*Adult:* **IV** 25 mg over 30-60 min qwk; treat until disease progression or severe toxicity occurs

**Available forms:** 25 mg/ml solution for inj kit

### Adverse effects
*CNS: Headache,* **seizures**
*CV:* Hypertension, **thrombophlebitis**
*ENDO:* Hypertriglyceridemia, hyperlipidemia, hyperglycemia
*GI:* Nausea, vomiting, diarrhea, constipation, **bowel perforation**
*GU:* UTIs, **albuminuria, hematuria, proteinuria, renal failure**

*HEMA:* **Anemia, leukopenia, thrombocy-topenia**
*INTEG:* *Rash,* pruritus
*META:* Metabolic acidosis
*RESP:* **Interstitial lung disease**
*SYST:* **Lymphoma**

**Contraindications:** Pregnancy **D**, breast-feeding, hypersensitivity to this product or to sirolimus, polysorbate 80

**Precautions:** Children <13 yr, females, severe pulmonary/renal/hepatic disease, diabetes mellitus, hyperkalemia, hyperurice-mia, hypertension, bone marrow suppression, hypertriglyceridemia/hyperlipidemia, surgery, brain tumors

### Pharmacokinetics

| | |
|---|---|
| **Absorption** | Rapidly |
| **Distribution** | Unknown |
| **Metabolism** | Extensively via liver by P450 3A4 |
| **Excretion** | Eliminated via feces |
| **Half-life** | Unknown |

### Pharmacodynamics

| | |
|---|---|
| **Onset** | Unknown |
| **Peak** | 0.5-2 hr |
| **Duration** | Unknown |

### Interactions
*Individual drugs*
Bromocriptine, cimetidine, cycloSPORINE, danazol, erythromycin, metoclopramide: increased blood levels
Carbamazepine, phenobarbital, phenytoin, rifamycin, rifapentine: decreased blood levels
*Drug classifications*
Antifungals, benzodiazepines, calcium channel blockers, CYP3A4 inhibitors, HIV-protease inhibitors, HMG-CoA reductase inhibitors: increased blood levels
CYP3A4 inducers: decreased blood levels
Vaccines: decreased effect of vaccines
*Drug/herb*
Astragalus, echinacea, melatonin: decreased immunosuppression
Ginseng, maitake, mistletoe: increased effect
St. John's wort: may decrease the effect of sirolimus
*Drug/food*
Alters bioavailability; use consistently with or without food; do not use with grapefruit juice

### NURSING CONSIDERATIONS
**Assessment**
• Assess for hypersensitive reactions: anaphy-laxis

• Monitor lipid profile: cholesterol, triglycer-ides, a lipid-lowering agent may be needed
 Assess for infection and development of lymphoma
 Monitor blood tests: Hgb, WBC, platelets during treatment qmo
• Monitor renal function tests: BUN, creati-nine, phosphate potassium; proteinuria, hematuria, albuminemia may indicate renal failure

**Nursing diagnoses**
• Injury, risk for (uses, adverse reactions)
• Knowledge, deficient (teaching)

**Implementation**
• Use in-line filter ≤5 microns and infusion pump
• Infuse over 30-60 min
• Complete infusion within 6 hr
• Dilute product with 1.8 ml of provided diluent, the result is 3 ml (10 mg/ml); invert to mix well; withdraw the required amount and inject rapidly into 250 ml of NS; do not use PVC infusion bags/sets
• Protect from light during preparation

**Patient/family education**
• Advise patient to report fever, rash, severe diarrhea, chills, sore throat, fatigue; serious infections may occur; clay-colored stools, cramping (hepatotoxicity)
• Advise patient to avoid crowds, persons with known infections to reduce risk of infection
• Teach patient to use contraception before, during, and 12 wk after product has been discontinued; avoid breastfeeding; men should also use reliable contraception during and 12 wk after cessation of product

**Evaluation**
**Positive therapeutic outcome**
• Decreased time of progression of renal cell carcinoma

### ! HIGH ALERT

## tenecteplase (Rx)
(ten-ek'ta-place)
TNKase
*Func. class.:* Thrombolytic enzyme
*Chem. class.:* Tissue plasminogen activator

### Pregnancy category C

**Action:** Activates conversion of plasminogen to plasmin (fibrinolysin): plasmin breaks down clots (fibrin), fibrinogen, factors V, VII; occlusion of venous access lines

**Therapeutic outcome:** Resolution of MI

**Uses:** Acute MI

**Dosage and routes**
*Adult <60 kg:* **IV** BOL 30 mg, give over 5 sec
*Adult ≥60-<70 kg:* **IV** BOL 35 mg, give over 5 sec
*Adult ≥70-<80 kg:* **IV** BOL 40 mg, give over 5 sec
*Adult ≥80-<90 kg:* **IV** BOL 45 mg, give over 5 sec
*Adult ≥90 kg:* **IV** BOL 50 mg, give over 5 sec

**Available forms:** Powder for inj, lyophilized 50 mg

**Adverse effects**
*CV:* Dysrhythmias, hypotension, pulmonary edema, **PE, cardiogenic shock, cardiac arrest, heart failure, myocardial reinfarction, myocardial rupture, tamponade, pericarditis, pericardial effusion, thrombosis**
*HEMA:* Decreased Hct, **bleeding**
*INTEG:* Rash, urticaria, phlebitis at **IV** inf site, itching, flushing
*SYST:* **GI, GU, intracranial, retroperitoneal bleeding, surface bleeding, anaphylaxis**

**Contraindications:** Hypersensitivity, arteriovenous malformation, aneurysm, active bleeding, intracranial, intraspinal surgery, CNS neoplasms, severe hypertension, severe renal disease, hepatic disease, history of CVA

**Precautions:** Pregnancy **C**, breastfeeding, children, geriatric, arterial emboli from left side of heart, ulcerative colitis, enteritis, hypocoagulation, COPD, subacute bacterial endocarditis, rheumatic valvular disease, cerebral embolism/thrombosis/hemorrhage, intraarterial diagnostic procedure or surgery (10 days), recent major surgery

| Pharmacokinetics | |
|---|---|
| **Absorption** | Unknown |
| **Distribution** | Unknown |
| **Metabolism** | Liver |
| **Excretion** | Unknown |
| **Half-life** | 20-24 min |

| Pharmacodynamics | |
|---|---|
| **Onset** | Immediate |
| **Peak** | Unknown |
| **Duration** | Unknown |

**Interactions**
*Individual drugs*
Aspirin; dipyridamole; glycoprotein IIb, IIIa inhibitors; indomethacin; phenylbutazone: increased bleeding potential
*Drug classifications*
Anticoagulants, antithrombolytics: increased bleeding potential
*Drug/herb*
Agrimony, alfalfa, angelica, anise, basil, bay, bilberry, black haw, bogbean, bromelain, buchu, chondroitin, cinchona bark, dong quai, fenugreek, feverfew, garlic, ginger, ginkgo, ginseng, horse chestnut, Irish moss, kelp, kelpware, khella, lovage, lungwort, meadowsweet, motherwort, mugwort, nettle, papaya, parsley (large amounts), pau d'arco, pineapple, poplar, prickly ash, safflower, saw palmetto, tonka bean, turmeric, wintergreen, yarrow: increased risk of bleeding
Chamomile, coenzyme Q10, flax, glucomannan, goldenseal, guar gum: decreased anticoagulant effect
*Drug/lab test*
Increased: pro-time, APTT, TT
Decreased: plasminogen, fibrinogen

**NURSING CONSIDERATIONS**
**Assessment**
• Assess for allergy: fever, rash, itching, chills; mild reaction may be treated with antihistamines
◆Assess for bleeding during 1st hr of treatment; hematuria, hematemesis, bleeding from mucous membranes, epistaxis, ecchymosis; may require transfusion (rare), continue to assess for bleeding for 24 hr
• Monitor blood tests (Hct, platelets, PTT, pro-time, TT, APTT) before starting therapy; protime or APTT must be less than 2 × control before starting therapy; PTT or pro-time q3-4hr during treatment
• Assess for hypersensitive reactions: fever, rash, dyspnea; product should be discontinued
• Monitor VS, B/P, pulse, respirations, neurologic signs, temp at least q4hr; temp >104° F (40° C) indicates internal bleeding; systolic pressure increase >25 mm Hg should be reported to prescriber
◆ Assess for neurologic changes that may indicate intracranial bleeding
◆ Assess for retroperitoneal bleeding: back pain, leg weakness, diminished pulses

**Nursing diagnoses**
• Cardiac output, decreased (uses)
• Knowledge, deficient (teaching)

**T**

Adverse effects: *italic* = common, **bold** = life-threatening

## Implementation
### IV route
• Give as soon as thrombi identified; not useful for thrombi >1 wk old
• Administer cryoprecipitate or fresh frozen plasma if bleeding occurs
• Give heparin after fibrinogen level >100 mg/dl; heparin infusion to increase PTT to 1.5-2 × baseline for 3-7 days; **IV** heparin with loading dose is recommended
• Aseptically withdraw 10 ml of sterile $H_2O$ for inj from diluent vial, use red cannula syringe-filling device, inject all contents of syringe into product vial, direct into powder, swirl, withdraw correct dose, discard any unused solution; stand the shield with dose vertically on flat surface and passively recap the red cannula, remove entire shield assembly by twisting counterclockwise, give by **IV** bol
• **IV** therapy: use upper extremity vessel that is accessible to manual compression
• Provide bed rest during entire course of treatment
• Avoid venous or arterial puncture, inj, rectal temp; any invasive treatment
• Treat fever with acetaminophen or aspirin
• Apply pressure for 30 sec to minor bleeding sites; inform prescriber if this does not attain hemostasis; apply pressure dressing

## Evaluation
### Positive therapeutic outcome
• Resolution of myocardial infarction

---

## tenofovir (Rx)
(ten-oh-foh'veer)
Viread
*Func. class.:* Antiretroviral
*Chem. class.:* Nucleoside analog reverse transcriptase inhibitor

**Pregnancy category** B

**Action:** Inhibits replication of HIV-1 virus by competing with the natural substrate and then incorporating into cellular DNA by viral reverse transcriptase, thereby terminating cellular DNA chain

**Therapeutic outcome:** Improved symptoms of HIV-1 infection

**Uses:** HIV-1 infection with other antiretrovirals

## Dosage and routes
*Adult:* PO 300 mg with meal; if used with didanosine, give tenofovir 2 hr before or 1 hr after didanosine

## Renal dose
CCr 30-49 ml/min 300 mg q48hr
CCr 10-29 ml/min 300 mg 2 ×/wk
CCr <10 ml/min not recommended

**Available forms:** Tabs 300 mg (300 mg of fumarate salt equivalent to 245 mg tenofovir disoproxil)

## Adverse effects
*CNS: Headache*
*GI: Nausea, vomiting, diarrhea,* anorexia, *flatulence, abdominal pain*
*GU:* Renal dysfunction
*SYST:* Change in body fat distribution

**Contraindications:** Hypersensitivity, lactic acidosis

**Precautions:** Pregnancy **B**, breastfeeding, children, geriatric, renal disease, hepatic insufficiency, CCr <60 ml/min, osteoporosis

### Pharmacokinetics
| | |
|---|---|
| **Absorption** | Rapidly absorbed |
| **Distribution** | Extravascular space; bound to serum plasma <0.7%, to serum proteins <7.2% |
| **Metabolism** | Unknown |
| **Excretion** | Urine, unchanged (70%-80%) |
| **Half-life** | Terminal 17 hr |

### Pharmacodynamics
| | |
|---|---|
| **Onset** | Unknown |
| **Peak** | 0.6-1.4 hr |
| **Duration** | Unknown |

## Interactions
### Individual drugs
Acyclovir, cidofovir, ganciclovir, valacyclovir, valganciclovir: increased level of tenofovir
Didanosine: increased level of didanosine when coadministered with tenofovir
### Drug classifications
Increased: levels of tenofovir with any product that decreased renal function

## NURSING CONSIDERATIONS
### Assessment
• Assess liver function tests: AST, ALT, bilirubin; amylase, lipase, triglycerides periodically during treatment
• Assess for bone, renal toxicity: if bone abnormalities are suspected, obtain tests: serum phosphorus, creatinine
• Assess for lactic acidosis, severe hepatomegaly with steatosis

---

 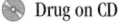

## Nursing diagnoses
- Infection, risk for (uses)
- Injury, risk for (adverse reactions)
- Knowledge, deficient (teaching)

## Implementation
- Administer PO daily with meal
- Store at 25° C (77° F)
- Give product 2 hr before or 1 hr after taking didanosine (if used)

## Patient/family education
- Instruct patient to take this product 2 hr before or 1 hr after taking didanosine (if used)
- Instruct patient to take product with meal
- Advise patients that GI complaints resolve after 3-4 wk of treatment
- Caution patient not to breastfeed while taking this product
- Inform patient that product must be taken daily even if patient feels better
- Advise patient to continue follow-up visits since serious toxicity may occur; blood counts must be done q2 wk
- Inform patient that product will control symptoms but is not a cure for HIV; patient is still infectious, may pass HIV virus on to others
- Advise patient that other products may be necessary to prevent other infections
- Advise patient that changes in body fat distribution may occur

## Evaluation
**Positive therapeutic outcome**
- Decrease in signs/symptoms of HIV

---

## terazosin (Rx)
(ter-ay'zoe-sin)
Hytrin
*Func. class.:* Antihypertensive
*Chem. class.:* α-Adrenergic blocker (peripherally acting)

### Pregnancy category C

**Action:** Peripheral blood vessels are dilated, peripheral resistance lowered; reduction in blood pressure results from α-adrenergic receptors being blocked

**Therapeutic outcome:** Decreased B/P in hypertension, decreased symptoms of benign prostatic hyperplasia (BPH)

**Uses:** Hypertension, as a single agent or in combination with diuretics or β-blockers, BPH

## Dosage and routes
### Hypertension
*Adult:* PO 1 mg at bedtime, may increase doses slowly to desired response; max 20 mg/day

### Benign prostatic hyperplasia
*Adult:* PO 1 mg at bedtime, gradually increase up to 5-10 mg, max 20 mg

**Available forms:** Tabs 1, 2, 5, 10 mg

### Adverse effects
*CNS: Dizziness, headache, drowsiness,* anxiety, depression, vertigo, weakness, fatigue
*CV:* Palpitations, orthostatic hypo/hypertension, tachycardia, edema, rebound hypertension
*EENT:* Blurred vision, epistaxis, tinnitus, dry mouth, red sclera, nasal congestion, sinusitis
*GI: Nausea,* vomiting, diarrhea, constipation, abdominal pain
*GU:* Urinary frequency, incontinence, impotence, priapism
*RESP:* Dyspnea, cough, pharyngitis

**Contraindications:** Hypersensitivity

**Precautions:** Pregnancy **C,** breastfeeding, children, prostate cancer

| Pharmacokinetics | |
|---|---|
| **Absorption** | Well absorbed |
| **Distribution** | Not known |
| **Metabolism** | Liver—50% |
| **Excretion** | Kidneys unchanged—10%, feces unchanged—20% |
| **Half-life** | 9-12 hr |

| Pharmacodynamics | |
|---|---|
| **Onset** | 15 min |
| **Peak** | 1 hr |
| **Duration** | 24 hr |

## Interactions
### Individual drugs
Alcohol, nitroglycerin, verapamil: increased hypotensive effects
### Drug classifications
Antihypertensives (other): increased hypotension
β-Blockers: increased hypotensive effects
Estrogens, NSAIDs, salicylates, sympathomimetics: decreased antihypertensive effect

## NURSING CONSIDERATIONS
### Assessment
- Monitor B/P, orthostatic hypotension, syncope; check for edema in feet, legs daily; I&O ratio; weight daily; notify prescriber of changes

T

Adverse effects: *italic* = common, **bold** = life-threatening

- Assess for allergic reactions: rash, fever, pruritus, urticaria; product should be discontinued if antihistamines fail to help

### Nursing diagnoses

- Cardiac output, decreased (uses)
- Injury, risk for (adverse reactions)
- Knowledge, deficient (teaching)
- Noncompliance (teaching)

### Implementation

- May be used in combination with other antihypertensives
- Give at same time each day
- May be given with food to prevent GI symptoms
- Store in airtight container at 86° F (30° C) or less

### Patient/family education

- Caution patient not to discontinue product abruptly; the importance of complying with dosage schedule, even if feeling better; if dose is missed take as soon as remembered; take medication at same time each day
- Teach patient not to use OTC products (cough, cold, allergy) unless directed by prescriber; also to avoid large amounts of caffeine
- Emphasize the need to rise slowly to sitting or standing position to minimize orthostatic hypotension
- Teach patient to notify prescriber of mouth sores, sore throat, fever, swelling of hands or feet, irregular heartbeat, chest pain
- Caution patient to report excessive perspiration, dehydration, vomiting, diarrhea; may lead to fall in B/P
- Caution patient that product may cause dizziness, fainting, light-headedness; may occur during 1st few days of therapy; to avoid hazardous activities
- Teach patient how to take B/P, and normal readings for age-group; to take B/P q7 days

### Evaluation

**Positive therapeutic outcome**

- Decreased B/P in hypertension
- Decreased symptoms of BPH

**Treatment of overdose:** Administer volume expanders or vasopressors; discontinue product; place patient in supine position

---

**terbinafine** (Rx)
(ter-bin′a-feen)
Lamisil
*Func. class.:* Antifungal, systemic
*Chem. class.:* Synthetic allylamine derivative

**Pregnancy category B**

**Do not confuse:**
Lamisil/lamotrigine

**Action:** Interferes with cell membrane permeability in fungi such as *Trichophyton rubrum, Trichophyton mentagrophytes, Trichophyton tonsurans, Epidermophyton floccosum, Microsporum canis, Microsporum audouinii, Microsporum gypseum, Candida,* broad-spectrum antifungal

**Therapeutic outcome:** Resolution of fungal infection

**Uses:** Onychomycosis of the toenail or fingernail due to dermatophytes

**Unlabeled uses:** Cutaneous candidiasis, tinea versicolor

**Dosage and routes**
*Fingernail:* PO 250 mg/day × 6 wk
*Toenail:* PO 250 mg/day × 12 wk

**Available forms:** Tabs 250 mg

**Adverse effects**
*GI:* Diarrhea, dyspepsia, abdominal pain, nausea, hepatitis
***HEMA:*** **Neutropenia**
*INTEG:* Rash, pruritus, urticaria, **Stevens-Johnson syndrome**
***MISC:*** Headache, hepatic enzyme changes, taste, visual disturbance

**Contraindications:** Hypersensitivity, chronic/active renal/hepatic disease GFR ≤50 mg/min

**Precautions:** Pregnancy **B**, breastfeeding, children, renal disease

#### Pharmacokinetics

| | |
|---|---|
| **Absorption** | 80% |
| **Distribution** | Extensive, most to hair, scalp, nails; excreted in breast milk; protein binding 99% |
| **Metabolism** | Liver, extensively |
| **Excretion** | Unknown |
| **Half-life** | 22 days or longer |

#### Pharmacodynamics

| | |
|---|---|
| **Onset** | Up to 1 wk |
| **Peak** | Several days-weeks |
| **Duration** | Several weeks |

---

### Interactions
*Individual drugs*
Cimetidine: increased effect
CycloSPORINE: increased cycloSPORINE clearance
Dextromethorphan: increased levels
Rifampin: increased terbinafine clearance
*Drug/herb*
Cola nut, guarana, yerba maté, tea (black, green), coffee: side effects

### NURSING CONSIDERATIONS
**Assessment**
• Assess hepatic studies (ALT, AST) prior to beginning treatment; do not use in presence of hepatic disease
• Monitor CBC in treatment >6 wk
• Assess for continuing infection

**Nursing diagnoses**
• Infection, risk for (uses)
• Knowledge, deficient (teaching)
• Noncompliance (teaching)

**Patient/family education**
• Teach patient to notify prescriber of nausea, vomiting, fatigue, jaundice, dark urine, clay-colored stool, RUQ pain, that may indicate hepatic dysfunction
• Teach patient to avoid using OTC medication unless approved by prescriber

**Evaluation**
**Positive therapeutic outcome**
• Decrease in size, number of lesions

---

### terbinafine topical
*See Appendix D*

---

### terbutaline (Rx)
(ter-byoo'te-leen)
Brethine, Bricanyl
*Func. class.:* Selective $\beta_2$-agonist; broncho-dilator
*Chem. class.:* Catecholamine
**Pregnancy category B**

**Action:** Relaxes bronchial smooth muscle by direct action on $\beta_2$-adrenergic receptors through accumulation of cAMP at β-adrenergic receptor sites; results are bronchodilation, diuresis, and CNS and cardiac stimulation; relaxes uterine smooth muscle

**Therapeutic outcome:** Bronchodilation with ease of breathing

**Uses:** Bronchospasm, hyperkalemia

**Unlabeled uses:** Premature labor

### Dosage and routes
*Bronchospasm*
**Adult and child >12 yr:** PO 2.5-5 mg q8hr; SUBCUT 0.25 mg q15-30 min, max 0.5 mg in 4 hr

*Bronchodilation*
**Adult and child >15 yr:** PO 2.5-5 mg q6hr during day, max 15 mg/24 hr
**Child 12-15 yr:** PO 2.5 mg tid

*Renal dose*
**Adult:** PO GFR 10-50 ml/min 50% of dose

*Severe renal failure*
**Adult:** PO avoid if GFR <10 ml/min

*Tocolytic (preterm labor) (unlabeled)*
**Adult:** PO 2.5 mg q4-6hr until delivery

**Available forms:** Tabs 2.5, 5 mg; inj 1 mg/ml

### Adverse effects
*CNS:* Tremors, anxiety, insomnia, headache, dizziness, stimulation
*CV:* Palpitations, tachycardia, hypertension, dysrhythmias, **cardiac arrest**
*GI:* Nausea, vomiting

**Contraindications:** Hypersensitivity to sympathomimetics; angle-closure glaucoma, tachydysrhythmias

**Precautions:** Pregnancy **B**, breastfeeding, geriatric, cardiac disorders, hyperthyroidism, diabetes mellitus, prostatic hypertension, hypertension, seizure disorder

| Pharmacokinetics | |
|---|---|
| **Absorption** | Well absorbed (SUBCUT), partially absorbed (PO) |
| **Distribution** | Unknown |
| **Metabolism** | Liver—partially |
| **Excretion** | Unknown |
| **Half-life** | Unknown |

| Pharmacodynamics | | | | |
|---|---|---|---|---|
| | PO | INH | SUBCUT | IV |
| **Onset** | ½ hr | 5-15 min | 10-15 min | Rapid |
| **Peak** | 1-2 hr | 1-2 hr | ½-1 hr | Unknown |
| **Duration** | 4-8 hr | 4-6 hr | 1½-4 hr | Unknown |

### Interactions
*Individual drugs*
Bleomycin: products are incompatible
*Drug classifications*
β-Adrenergic blockers: block therapeutic effect
MAOIs: increased chance of hypertensive crisis

---

Adverse effects: *italic* = common, **bold** = life-threatening

Sympathomimetics: increased effects of both products
*Drug/herb*
Green tea (large amounts), guarana: increased effect

## NURSING CONSIDERATIONS
### Assessment
• Monitor respiratory function: vital capacity, FEV, ABGs, lung sounds, heart rate, rhythm (baseline)
• Determine that patient has not received theophylline therapy before giving dose; assess client's ability to self-medicate
• Monitor for evidence of allergic reactions; withhold dose and notify prescriber
• Assess for paradoxical bronchospasm: dyspnea, wheezing, keep emergency resuscitative equipment nearby
• Assess for labor: maternal heart rate, B/P, contractions, fetal heart rate

### Nursing diagnoses
• Airway clearance, ineffective (uses)
• Gas exchange, impaired (uses)
• Knowledge, deficient (teaching)
• Noncompliance (teaching)

### Implementation
• Use this medication before other medications and allow 5 min between each to prevent overstimulation
**PO route**
• Give PO with meals to decrease gastric irritation; tab may be crushed and mixed with foods and fluids
**SUBCUT route**
• May give by SUBCUT route; do not give by IM route
**Aerosol route**
• Give after shaking; ask patient to exhale, place mouthpiece in mouth, then inhale slowly; hold breath, remove, exhale slowly; allow at least 1 min between inhalations
• Store in light-resistant container, do not expose to temperatures over 86° F (30° C)
**IV route**
• Give at 5 mcg q10 min until contractions are stopped, use infusion pump for correct dose; after ½-1 hr with no contraction decrease dose by 5 mcg; switch to PO dose when possible

*Syringe compatibilities:* Doxapram
*Y-site compatibilities:* Regular insulin
*Additive compatibilities:* Aminophylline
*Additive incompatibilities:* Bleomycin

### Patient/family education
• Advise patient not to use OTC medications; extra stimulation may occur; to use this medication before other medications and allow at least 5 min between each to prevent overstimulation
• Teach patient how to use inhaler; to avoid getting aerosol in eyes because blurring may result; to wash inhaler in warm water daily and dry; to avoid smoking, smoke-filled rooms, persons with respiratory infections; review package insert with patient
• Teach patient that paradoxical bronchospasm may occur; to stop product immediately and notify prescriber; to limit caffeine products such as chocolate, coffee, tea, and colas
• Instruct patient on administration of dose, not to use more than prescribed; serious side effects may occur; if taking PO regularly and dose is missed, take when remembered; space other doses on new time schedule

### Evaluation
**Positive therapeutic outcome**
• Absence of dyspnea, wheezing after 1 hr
• Improved airway exchange
• Improved ABGs

**Treatment of overdose:** Administer a $\beta_2$-adrenergic blocker

## terconazole vaginal antifungal
*See Appendix D*

## teriparatide (Rx)
(tah-ree-par'ah-tide)
Forteo
*Func. class.:* Parathyroid hormone (rDNA)

**Pregnancy category** C

**Action:** Contains human recombinant parathyroid hormone, which stimulates new bone growth

**Therapeutic outcome:** Calcium levels at 9-10 mg/dl, decreased symptoms of hypocalcemia, hypoparathyroidism

**Uses:** Postmenopausal women with osteoporosis, men with primary or hypogonadal osteoporosis who are at high risk for fracture

### Dosage and routes
*Adult:* SUBCUT 20 mcg/day × 29 mo

**Available forms:** Prefilled pen delivery device (delivers 20 mcg/day)

## Adverse effects

*CNS:* Dizziness, headache, insomnia, depression, vertigo
*CV:* Hypertension, angina, syncope
*GI:* Nausea, diarrhea, dyspepsia, vomiting, constipation
*INTEG:* Rash, sweating
*MISC:* Pain, asthenia
*MS:* Arthralgia, leg cramps
*RESP:* Rhinitis, cough, pharyngitis, pneumonia, dyspnea

**Contraindications:** Hypersensitivity, increased baseline risk of osteosarcoma (Paget's disease, open epiphyses, previous bone radiation), bone metastases, history of skeletal malignancies, other metabolic bone diseases, preexisting hypercalcemia

**Precautions:** Pregnancy **C**, breastfeeding, urolithiasis, hypotension, use >2 yr

### Pharmacokinetics

| | |
|---|---|
| **Absorption** | Extensively, rapidly |
| **Distribution** | Unknown |
| **Metabolism** | Liver |
| **Excretion** | Kidneys |
| **Half-life** | Unknown |

### Pharmacodynamics

Unknown

## Interactions

*Individual drug*
Digoxin: increased digoxin toxicity
*Drug/lab test*
Calcium: increased levels

## NURSING CONSIDERATIONS
### Assessment

• Uric acid, chloride, magnesium, electrolytes, urine pH, vit D, phosphate for normal serum levels. Serum calcium may be transiently increased after dosing (max at 4-6 hr post-dose)
• For bone pain, headache, fatigue, changes in LOC, leg cramps
• For signs of persistent hypercalcemia: nausea, vomiting, constipation, lethargy, muscle weakness
• Nutritional status: diet for sources of vit D (milk, some seafood), calcium (dairy products, dark green vegetables), phosphates (dairy products)

### Nursing diagnoses

• Injury, risk for (uses)
• Knowledge, deficient (teaching)
• Mobility, impaired physical (uses)

## Implementation

• Store refrigerated, do not freeze
**SUBCUT route**
• Give by SUBCUT only, rotate inj sites

### Patient/family education

• Advise patient of the symptoms of hypercalcemia
• Teach about foods rich in calcium
• Teach how to use delivery device, dispose of needles, not to share pen with others
• To sit or lie down if dizziness or fast heartbeat occurs after the first few doses

### Evaluation

**Positive therapeutic outcome**
• Increased bone mineral density

---

## testosterone 🔄 (Rx)
(tess-toss´te-rone)
## testosterone, long acting (Rx)
## testosterone enanthate (Rx)
Andro LA, Andropository, Andryl, Delatest, Delatestryl, Everone, Malog-x ✦, Testone LA, Testrin-PA
## testosterone cypionate (Rx)
Andro-Cyp, Andronate, depAndro, Depotest, Depo-Testosterone, Dura-test, T-Cypionate, Testa-C, Testred, Testoject-LA, Virilon IM
## testosterone pellets (Rx)
Testopel
## testosterone transdermal (Rx)
Androderm, Androplex ✦, Testoderm, Testoderm TTS, Testoderm with Adhesive
## testosterone gel (Rx)
AndroGel 1%, Testim
## testosterone buccal (Rx)
Striant
*Func. class.:* Androgenic anabolic steroid
*Chem. class.:* Halogenated testosterone derivative

**Pregnancy category X**
**Controlled substance schedule III**

T

---

**Action:** Increases weight by building body tissue; increases potassium, phosphorus, chloride, nitrogen levels; increases bone development; responsible for maintenance of secondary sex characteristics (male)

**Therapeutic outcome:** Increased hormone levels in eunuchoidism, decreased tumor growth in female breast cancer, onset of male puberty

**Uses:** Female breast cancer, eunuchoidism, male climacteric, oligospermia, impotence, osteoporosis, weight loss in AIDS patients, vulvar dystrophies, low testosterone levels, delayed male puberty (Inj)

## Dosage and routes
### Replacement
*Adult:* **IM** 25-50 mg 2-3 ×/wk (base or propionate) or 50-400 mg q2-4 wk (enanthate or cypionate); TRANSDERMAL (Testoderm) 4-6 mg applied q24hr; (Androderm, Andro-Gel) 5 mg applied q24hr; once daily (gel); BUCCAL 1 buccal system (30 mg) to the gum region q12hr before meals/PM

### Breast cancer
*Adult:* IM 50-100 mg 3 ×/wk (propionate) or 200-400 mg q2-4 wk (cypionate or enanthate)

### Delayed male puberty
*Child >12 yr:* IM up to 100 mg/mo for up to 6 mo

**Available forms:** Enanthate: inj 200 mg/ml; cypionate: inj 100, 200 mg/ml; pellets 75 mg; transdermal 2.5, 4, 5, 6 mg/24 hr; gel 1% buccal system 30 mg

## Adverse effects
***CNS:*** Dizziness, headache, fatigue, tremors, paresthesias, flushing, sweating, anxiety, lability, insomnia, carpal tunnel syndrome
***CV:*** Increased B/P
***EENT:*** Conjunctival edema, nasal congestion
***ENDO:*** Abnormal GTT
***GI:*** Nausea, vomiting, constipation, weight gain, **cholestatic jaundice**
***GU:*** Hematuria, amenorrhea, vaginitis, decreased libido, decreased breast size, clitoral hypertrophy, testicular atrophy
***INTEG:*** Rash, acneiform lesions, oily hair and skin, flushing, sweating, acne vulgaris, alopecia, hirsutism
***MS:*** Cramps, spasms

**Contraindications:** Pregnancy **X**, breastfeeding, severe renal/cardiac/hepatic disease, hypersensitivity, genital bleeding (rare)

**Precautions:** Diabetes mellitus, CV disease, MI, urinary tract disorders, prostate cancer, breast cancer (male)

| Pharmacokinetics | |
|---|---|
| **Absorption** | Well but slowly absorbed |
| **Distribution** | Crosses placenta |
| **Metabolism** | Liver |
| **Excretion** | Kidneys, breast milk |
| **Half-life** | 8 days (cypionate) |
| | 10-100 min (base) |

| Pharmacodynamics | | | | |
|---|---|---|---|---|
| | **IM (base)** | **IM (cypionate)** | **IM (enanthate)** | **IM (propionate)** |
| **Onset** | Unknown | Unknown | Unknown | Unknown |
| **Peak** | Unknown | Unknown | Unknown | Unknown |
| **Duration** | 1-3 days | 2-4 wk | 2-4 wk | 1-3 days |

## Interactions
### Individual drugs
ACTH, buPROPion: increased edema
Insulin: decreased glucose levels may alter need for insulin
Oxyphenbutazone: increased effects of oxyphenbutazone
### Drug classifications
Adrenal steroids: increased edema
Anticoagulants: increased pro-time
Antidiabetics, oral: decreased need for oral antidiabetics
### Drug/lab test
Increased: serum cholesterol, blood glucose, urine glucose
Decreased: serum Ca, serum K, $T_4$, $T_3$, thyroid [131]I uptake test, urine 17-OHCS, 17-KS, PBI

## NURSING CONSIDERATIONS
### Assessment
• Monitor patient's weight daily; notify prescriber if weekly weight gain is >5 lb; assess I&O ratio; be alert for decreasing urinary output, increasing edema
• Monitor B/P q4hr
• Assess growth rate in adolescent because growth rate may be uneven (linear/bone growth) if used for extended periods
• Monitor electrolytes: potassium, sodium, chloride, calcium; cholesterol
• Monitor liver function tests: ALT, AST, bilirubin
• Assess edema, hypertension, cardiac symptoms, jaundice
• Assess mental status: affect, mood, behavioral changes, aggression
• Assess signs of masculinization in female: increased libido, deepening of voice, decreased breast tissue, enlarged clitoris, menstrual irregularities; male: gynecomastia, impotence, testicular atrophy
• Assess hypercalcemia: lethargy, polyuria, polydipsia, nausea, vomiting, constipation; product may have to be decreased
• Assess hypoglycemia in diabetics because oral antidiabetic action is increased

**Nursing diagnoses**
- Infection, risk for (adverse reactions)
- Injury, risk for (adverse reactions)
- Knowledge, deficient (teaching)

**Implementation**
- Administer diet with increased calories, protein; decreased sodium if edema occurs
- Administer supportive product if anemia occurs
- Give titrated dose; use lowest effective dose
- Give IM inj deep into upper outer quadrant of gluteal muscle; route can be painful

**Transdermal route**
- Apply Testoderm to skin of scrotum, Androderm to skin of back, upper arms, thighs, abdomen; area must be clean and dry, free of hair

**Patient/family education**
- Inform patient that product needs to be combined with complete health plan: diet, rest, exercise
- Caution patient to notify prescriber if therapeutic response decreases; not to discontinue this medication abruptly
- Inform women patients to report menstrual irregularities; about changes in sex characteristics
- Discuss that 1-3 mo course is necessary for response in breast cancer
- Inform patient about application of transdermal patches: Testoderm to skin of scrotum, Androderm to skin of back, upper arms, thighs, abdomen; area must be dry and free of hair; may be reapplied after bathing, swimming

**Evaluation**
**Positive therapeutic outcome**
- Decrease size of tumor in breast cancer
- Increased androgen levels

---

**tetracaine ophthalmic**
*See Appendix D*

---

**tetracaine topical**
*See Appendix D*

---

**tetracycline** (Rx)
(tet-ra-sye′kleen)
Achromycin V, Actisite (dental product), Apo-Tetra ✦, Novotetra ✦, Nu-Tetra ✦, Panmycin, Robitet, Sumycin, Teline, Tetracap, tetracycline HCl, Tetracyn, Tetralan, Tetram
*Func. class.:* Antiinfective—broad-spectrum
*Chem. class.:* Tetracycline

**Pregnancy category D**

**Action:** Inhibits protein synthesis and phosphorylation in microorganisms; bacteriostatic

**Therapeutic outcome:** Bactericidal action against susceptible organisms: gram-positive pathogens *Bacillus anthracis, Clostridium perfringens, Clostridium tetani, Listeria monocytogenes, Nocardia, Propionibacterium acnes, Actinomyces israelii;* gram-negative pathogens *Haemophilus influenzae, Legionella pneumophila, Yersinia entercolitica, Yersinia pestis, Neisseria gonorrhoeae, Neisseria meningitidis*

**Uses:** Syphilis, *Chlamydia trachomatis,* gonorrhea, lymphogranuloma venereum, uncommon gram-positive, gram-negative organisms, rickettsial infections

**Dosage and routes**
*Susceptible gram-positive/gram-negative infections*
*Adult:* PO 250-500 mg q6hr
*Child >8 yr:* PO 25-50 mg/kg/day in divided doses q6hr

*Chlamydia trachomatis*
*Adult:* PO 500 mg qid × 7 days

*Syphilis*
*Adult and adolescent:* PO 500 mg qid × 2 wk; if syphilis duration >1 yr, must treat 30 days

*Brucellosis*
*Adult:* PO 500 mg qid × 3 wk with 1 g of streptomycin IM 2 ×/day × 1 wk, and 1 ×/day the 2nd wk

*Urethral, endocervical, rectal infections (C. trachomatis)*
*Adult:* PO 500 mg qid × 7 days

*Acne*
*Adult and adolescent:* PO 250 mg q6hr, then 125-500 mg/day or every other day

**Available forms:** Oral susp 125 mg/5 ml, caps 250, 500 mg

T

---

Adverse effects: *italic* = common, **bold** = life-threatening

## Adverse effects

***CNS:*** Fever, headache, paresthesia

***CV:*** Pericarditis

***EENT:*** Dysphagia, glossitis, decreased calcification (permanent discoloration) of deciduous teeth, oral candidiasis, oral ulcers

***GI:*** *Nausea,* abdominal pain, *vomiting, diarrhea,* anorexia, enterocolitis, **hepatotoxicity,** flatulence, abdominal cramps, epigastric burning, stomatitis, hepatitis

***GU:*** *Increased BUN*

***HEMA:*** **Eosinophilia, neutropenia, thrombocytopenia, leukocytosis, hemolytic anemia**

***INTEG:*** *Rash, urticaria, photosensitivity, increased pigmentation,* **exfoliative dermatitis,** pruritus, **angioedema, Stevens-Johnson syndrome**

**Contraindications:** Pregnancy **D,** breastfeeding, children <8 yr, hypersensitivity to tetracyclines

**Precautions:** Renal/hepatic disease, UV exposure

### Pharmacokinetics

| | |
|---|---|
| **Absorption** | 60%-80% (PO), lower (IM) |
| **Distribution** | Widely distributed, some in CSF; crosses placenta |
| **Metabolism** | Not metabolized |
| **Excretion** | Unchanged—kidneys |
| **Half-life** | 6-10 hr |

### Pharmacodynamics

| | |
|---|---|
| **Onset** | 1-2 hr |
| **Peak** | 2-3 hr |
| **Duration** | Unknown |

## Interactions
### Individual drugs

Cimetidine, NaHCO₃: decreased tetracycline effect

Digoxin: increased digoxin effect

Iron: forms chelates, decreased absorption

Methoxyflurane: nephrotoxicity

Warfarin: increased warfarin effect

### Drug classifications

Alkali products, antacids: decreased tetracycline effect

Contraceptives (oral): decreased oral contraceptive effect

Penicillins: decreased penicillin effect

### Drug/herb

Acidophilus: Do not use with antiinfectives; separate by several hours

Dong quai: increased photosensitivity

### Drug/food

Decreased: absorption with dairy products; forms insoluble chelate

### Drug/lab test

False increase: urinary catecholamines

## NURSING CONSIDERATIONS
### Assessment

• Assess patient for previous sensitivity reaction

• Assess patient for signs and symptoms of infection including characteristics of wounds, sputum, urine, stool, WBC >10,000/mm³, temp; obtain baseline information before and during treatment

• Complete C&S testing before beginning product therapy to identify if correct treatment has been initiated

• Assess for allergic reactions: rash, urticaria, pruritus, chills, fever, joint pain; angioedema may occur a few days after therapy begins; epINEPHrine, resuscitation equipment should be available for anaphylactic reaction

• Identify urine output; if decreasing, notify prescriber (may indicate nephrotoxicity); also, increased BUN, creatinine

• Monitor blood studies: AST, ALT, CBC, Hct, bilirubin, LDH, alkaline phosphatase, monthly if patient is on long-term therapy

• Assess bowel pattern daily; if severe diarrhea occurs, product should be discontinued

• Monitor for bleeding: ecchymosis, bleeding gums, hematuria, stool guaiac daily if on long-term therapy; blood dyscrasias may occur

• Assess for overgrowth of infection: perineal itching, fever, malaise, redness, pain, swelling, drainage, rash, diarrhea, change in cough, sputum

### Nursing diagnoses

• Diarrhea (adverse reactions)
• Infection, risk for (uses)
• Injury, risk for (adverse reactions)
• Knowledge, deficient (teaching)
• Noncompliance (teaching)

### Implementation
#### PO route

• Give around the clock to maintain proper blood levels; give with food to increase absorption of product; do not give within 3 hr of other agents; product actions may occur; take on an empty stomach

• Give with 8 oz of water

• Shake liquid preparation well before giving; use calibrated device for proper dosing

---

 Alert      Canada Only      Drug on CD     * "Tall Man" lettering (See Preface)

## Patient/family education
- Teach patient to report sore throat, bruising, bleeding, joint pain; may indicate blood dyscrasias (rare)
- Advise patient to use sunscreen when outdoors to decrease photosensitivity reaction
- Advise patient to contact prescriber if vaginal itching; loose foul-smelling stools, furry tongue occur; may indicate superinfection; report itching, rash, pruritus, urticaria
- Instruct patient to take all medication prescribed for the length of time ordered; product must be taken around the clock to maintain blood levels; do not give medication to others

## Evaluation
**Positive therapeutic outcome**
- Absence of signs/symptoms of infection (WBC <10,000/mm$^3$, temp WNL, absence of red, draining wounds)
- Reported improvement in symptoms of infection

---

**tetrahydrozoline nasal agent**
*See Appendix D*

---

**tetrahydrozoline ophthalmic**
*See Appendix D*

---

**theophylline** 😊 (Rx)
(thee-off'i-lin)
Accurbron, Aquaphyllin, Asmalix, Bronkodyl, Elixomin, Elixophyllin, Lanophyllin, Quibron-T Dividose, Quibron-T/SR Dividose, Respbid, Slo-bid Gyrocaps, Slo-Phyllin, Sustaire, Theo-24, Theobid Duracaps, Theochron, Theoclear-80, Theoclear L.A., Theo-Dur, Theolair-SR,Theo-Sav, Theospan-SR, Theostat 80, Theovent, Theo-X, T-Phyl, Uni-Dur, Uniphyl
*Func. class.:* Spasmolytic, bronchodilator
*Chem. class.:* Xanthine, ethylenediamine

**Pregnancy category** C

**Action:** Relaxes smooth muscle of respiratory system by blocking phosphodiesterase, which increases cAMP, which increases bronchodilatation, diuresis, circulation, CNS stimulation

**Therapeutic outcome:** Ability to breathe without difficulty

**Uses:** Bronchial asthma, bronchospasm of COPD, chronic bronchitis, emphysema

## Dosage and routes
*Hepatic dose*
*Adult:* PO 6 mg/kg loading dose, then 2 mg/kg q8hr ×2 doses, then 1-2 mg/kg q12hr
*Adult:* IV 4.7 mg/kg then 0.39 mg/kg/hr for 12 hr, then 0.08-0.16 mg/kg/hr maintenance

*Bronchospasm, bronchial asthma*
*Adult:* PO 100-200 mg q6hr; dosage must be individualized; max 800 mg/day
*Child:* PO 50-100 mg q6hr, max 12 mg/kg/24 hr

*COPD, chronic bronchitis*
*Adult:* PO 330-800 q6-8hr after meals
*Child 1-9 yr:* PO 5 mg/kg loading dose, then 4 mg/kg q6hr
*Child 9-16 yr:* PO 5 mg/kg loading dose, then 4 mg/kg q6hr

*Apnea of prematurity*
*Neonate:* 2-10 mg/kg/day divided q8-12hr (usual loading dose is 4 mg/kg PO)

**Available forms:** Caps 50, 100, 200, 250 mg; tabs 100, 125, 200, 225, 250, 300 mg; time rel tabs 100, 200, 250, 300, 400, 500 mg; time rel caps 50, 65, 100, 125, 130, 200, 250, 260, 300, 400, 500 mg; elixir 80, 11.25 mg/15 mg; sol 80 mg/15 ml; liquid 80, 150, 160 mg/15 ml; susp 300 mg/15 ml

## Adverse effects
*CNS: Anxiety, restlessness, insomnia, dizziness, seizures,* headache, light-headedness, muscle twitching, tremors
*CV: Palpitations, sinus tachycardia,* hypotension, **dysrhythmias,** fluid retention with tachycardia
*ENDO:* Hyperglycemia
*GI: Nausea, vomiting, anorexia,* diarrhea, bitter taste, dyspepsia, gastric distress
*INTEG:* Flushing, urticaria
*MISC:* SIADH, urinary frequency
*RESP:* Increased rate, tachypnea

**Contraindications:** Hypersensitivity to xanthines, tachydysrhythmias

**Precautions:** Pregnancy **C**, children, geriatric, CHF, cor pulmonale, hepatic disease, active peptic ulcer disease, diabetes mellitus, hyperthyroidism, hypertension, seizure disorder

T

## Pharmacokinetics

| | |
|---|---|
| **Absorption** | Well absorbed (PO), slowly absorbed (ext rel) |
| **Distribution** | Crosses placenta, widely distributed |
| **Metabolism** | Liver |
| **Excretion** | Kidneys, breast milk |
| **Half-life** | 6.5-10.5 hr; increased in liver disease, CHF, geriatric |

## Pharmacodynamics

| | PO | PO–TIME REL | IV |
|---|---|---|---|
| **Onset** | Rapid | Slow | Immediate |
| **Peak** | 1 hr | 4-8 hr | Inf end |
| **Duration** | 6 hr | 12-24 hr | 6-8 hr |

## Interactions
### Individual drugs
Carbamazepine: decreased theophylline level
Cimetidine, disulfiram, erythromycin, fluvoxamine, influenza vaccine, mexiletine, propranolol: increased theophylline action
Lithium: decreased effect of lithium
Phenobarbital, phenytoin, rifampin: decreased theophylline
### Drug classifications
Anticoagulants: increased anticoagulant level
β-Adrenergic blockers: cardiotoxicity
Contraceptives (oral), corticosteroids, fluoroquinolones, interferons: increased theophylline action
Smoking: decreased theophylline level
### Drug/herb
Coffee, cola nut, guarana, tea (black, green), yerba maté: increased toxicity
St. John's wort: decreased theophylline level
Ma huang (ephedra): increased toxicity

## NURSING CONSIDERATIONS
### Assessment
• Monitor theophylline blood levels (therapeutic level is 5-15 mcg/ml); toxicity may occur with small increase above 15 mcg/ml
• Monitor I&O; diuresis occurs; dehydration may result in children or geriatric
• Assess for signs of toxicity: irritability, insomnia, restlessness, tremors, nausea, vomiting
• Monitor respiratory rate, rhythm, depth; auscultate lung fields bilaterally; notify prescriber of abnormalities
• Assess for allergic reactions: rash, urticaria; if these occur, product should be discontinued

### Nursing diagnoses
• Airway clearance, ineffective (uses)
• Knowledge, deficient (teaching)

## Implementation
### PO route
• Do not crush or chew time release products
• Contents of bead-filled cap may be sprinkled over food for children's use
• Give PO with 8 oz water; to decrease GI symptoms; avoid food, absorption may be affected
### IV route
• Give loading dose over 20-30 min, max 20-25 mg/min, do not give by rapid **IV**, use only by cont inf
*Y-site compatibilities:* Acyclovir, ampicillin, aztreonam, cefazolin, cefotetan, ceftazidime, ceftriaxone, cimetidine, clindamycin, dexamethasone, diltiazem, DOBUTamine, DOPamine, doxycycline, erythromycin, famotidine, fluconazole, gentamicin, haloperidol, heparin, hydrocortisone, lidocaine, methyldopate, methylPREDNISolone, metronidazole, midazolam, nafcillin, nitroglycerin, nitroprusside, penicillin G potassium, piperacillin, potassium chloride, ranitidine, ticarcillin, ticarcillin/clavulanate, tobramycin, vancomycin
*Additive compatibilities:* Cefepime, chlorproMAZINE, fluconazole, methylPREDNISolone, verapamil

### Patient/family education
• Advise patient to check OTC medications, current prescription medications for epHEDrine, which will increase stimulation, and to avoid alcohol, caffeine
• Caution patient to avoid hazardous activities; dizziness may occur
• Inform patient that if GI upset occurs, to take product with 8 oz of water; avoid food; absorption may be decreased
• Advise patient to notify prescriber of toxicity: nausea, vomiting, anxiety, insomnia, seizures
• Advise patient to notify prescriber of change in smoking habit; dosage may have to be changed

### Evaluation
**Positive therapeutic outcome**
• Ability to breathe more easily

 Alert      Canada Only     ◉ Drug on CD     * "Tall Man" lettering (See Preface)

# thiamine (vitamin B₁) (PO, OTC; **IV**, IM, Rx)

Betaxin ✤, Betalin S, Biamine, Revitonus, Thiamilate, thiamine HCl
*Func. class.:* Vitamin B₁
*Chem. class.:* Water soluble

**Pregnancy category A**

**Do not confuse:**
thiamine/Tenormin

**Action:** Needed for pyruvate metabolism, carbohydrate metabolism

**Therapeutic outcome:** Prevention and treatment of thiamine deficiency

**Uses:** Vit B₁ deficiency or polyneuritis, cheilosis adjunct with thiamine beriberi, Wernicke-Korsakoff syndrome, pellagra, metabolic disorders, alcoholism

**Dosage and routes**
*RDA*
*Adult:* PO (Male) 1.2-1.5 mg; (females) 1.1 mg; (pregnancy) 1.5 mg; (breastfeeding) 1.6 mg
*Child 7-10 yr:* PO 1.3 mg
*Child 4-6 yr:* PO 0.9 mg
*Child 1-3 yr:* PO 0.7 mg
*Infant 6 mo-1 yr:* PO 0.4 mg
*Neonate and infant to 6 mo:* PO 0.3 mg

*Beriberi*
*Adult:* IM 10-20 mg tid × 2 wk, then 5-10 mg/day × 1 mo

*Beriberi with cardiac failure*
*Adult and child:* **IV** 10-30 mg tid

**Available forms:** Tabs 50, 100, 250, 500 mg; inj 100 mg/ml; enteric-coated tabs 20 mg

**Adverse effects**
*CNS:* Weakness, restlessness
*CV:* **Collapse, pulmonary edema,** hypotension
*EENT:* Tightness of throat
*GI:* Hemorrhage, *nausea, diarrhea*
*INTEG:* **Angioneurotic edema,** cyanosis, sweating, warmth
*SYST:* **Anaphylaxis**

**Contraindications:** Hypersensitivity

**Precautions:** Pregnancy **A**

## Pharmacokinetics

| | |
|---|---|
| **Absorption** | Well absorbed (PO, IM), completely absorbed (**IV**) |
| **Distribution** | Widely distributed |
| **Metabolism** | Liver |
| **Excretion** | Kidneys (unchanged—excess amounts) |
| **Half-life** | Unknown |

## Pharmacodynamics
Unknown

## NURSING CONSIDERATIONS
**Assessment**
• Assess nutritional status: yeast, beef, liver, whole or enriched grains, legumes

**Nursing diagnoses**
• Knowledge, deficient (teaching)
• Nutrition: less than body requirements, imbalanced (uses)

**Implementation**
**IM route**
• Give by IM inj; rotate sites if pain and inflammation occur; do not mix with alkaline sol; Z-track to minimize pain
• Application of cold compress may decrease pain
• Store in airtight, light-resistant container
**IV route**
• **IV** undiluted given over 5 min or diluted with **IV** sol and given as an INF at a rate of 100 mg or less/5 min or more
*Syringe compatibilities:* Doxapram
*Y-site compatibilities:* Famotidine
*Additive incompatibilities:*
Barbiturates; sol with neutral or alkaline pH, such as carbonates, bicarbonates, citrates and acetates; erythromycin, kanamycin, or streptomycin

**Patient/family education**
• Teach patient necessary foods to be included in diet: yeast, beef, liver, legumes, whole grains

**Evaluation**
**Positive therapeutic outcome**
• Absence of nausea, vomiting, anorexia, insomnia, tachycardia, paresthesias, depression, muscle weakness

T

Adverse effects: *italic* = common, **bold** = life-threatening

## thiethylperazine (Rx)
(thye-eth-il-per'a-zeen)

Norzine, Torecan

*Func. class.:* Antiemetic

*Chem. class.:* Phenothiazine, piperazine derivative

**Pregnancy category X**

**Do not confuse:**
Torecan/Toradol

**Action:** Acts centrally by blocking chemoreceptor trigger zone, which in turn acts on vomiting center; dopamine blocker

**Therapeutic outcome:** Control of nausea, vomiting

**Uses:** Nausea, vomiting

**Dosage and routes**
*Adult:* PO/IM 10 mg/day-tid

**Available forms:** Tabs 10 mg; inj 5 mg/ml

**Adverse effects**

*CNS: Euphoria, depression,* restlessness, tremor, EPS, **seizures,** drowsiness, confusion, **neuroleptic malignant syndrome**

*CV:* **Circulatory failure, tachycardia,** postural hypotension, ECG changes

*GI:* Nausea, vomiting, anorexia, dry mouth, diarrhea, constipation, weight loss, metallic taste, cramps

*GU:* Urinary retention, dark urine

*HEMA:* **Agranulocytosis, leukopenia**

*RESP:* **Respiratory depression**

**Contraindications:** Pregnancy **X,** hypersensitivity to phenothiazines, coma, seizure, encephalopathy, bone marrow depression

**Precautions:** Breastfeeding, children <2 yr, geriatric, Parkinson's disease

### Pharmacokinetics

| Absorption | Readily absorbed |
|---|---|
| **Distribution** | Crosses placenta |
| **Metabolism** | Liver |
| **Excretion** | Kidneys, breast milk |
| **Half-life** | Unknown |

### Pharmacodynamics

|  | PO | IM |
|---|---|---|
| **Onset** | 45-60 min | Unknown |
| **Peak** | Unknown | Unknown |
| **Duration** | 4 hr | Unknown |

**Interactions**
*Individual drugs*
Ethanol: increased sedation

*Drug classifications*
Anesthetics (general), anxiolytics, sedatives/hypnotics, benzodiazepines, opiate agonists: increased sedation

Antacids: decreased effect of thiethylperazine

Anticholinergics, antiparkinson products, antidepressants (tricylics): increased anticholinergic action

Barbiturates: decreased effect of thiethylperazine, increased sedation

Phenothiazines: avoid use, seizures may occur

## NURSING CONSIDERATIONS
**Assessment**

• Monitor I&O ratio, palpate bladder if low urinary output occurs, especially in geriatric; urinalysis recommended before, during prolonged therapy

• Monitor bilirubin, CBC, liver function tests monthly

• Assess affect, orientation, LOC, reflexes, gait, coordination, sleep pattern disturbances

• Monitor B/P with patient in sitting, standing, and lying positions; take pulse and respirations q4hr during initial treatment; establish baseline before starting treatment; report drops of 30 mm Hg

• Check for dizziness, faintness, palpitations, tachycardia on rising; severe orthostatic hypotension is common

 Identify for neuroleptic malignant syndrome: hyperpyrexia, muscle rigidity, increased CPK, altered mental status, seizures, fatigue, loss of urinary control, tachycardia; product should be discontinued; have emergency equipment nearby

• Assess for EPS including akathisia (inability to sit still, no pattern to movements), tardive dyskinesia (bizarre movements of the jaw, mouth, tongue, extremities), pseudoparkinsonism (tremors, pill rolling, shuffling gait); antiparkinsonian product should be prescribed

• Assess for constipation, urinary retention daily; if these occur, increase bulk, water in diet

**Nursing diagnoses**
• Coping, ineffective (uses)
• Knowledge, deficient (teaching)
• Noncompliance (teaching)
• Thought processes, disturbed (uses)

**Implementation**
**IM route**
• Give IM inj in large muscle mass; aspirate to avoid **IV** administration; give slowly; have patient remain supine for at least 30 min after administration

---

*Syringe compatibilities:* Butorphanol, hydromorphone, midazolam, ranitidine
*Y-site compatibilities:* Aldesleukin

## Patient/family education

• Teach patient to use good oral hygiene; frequent rinsing of mouth, sugarless gum for dry mouth
• Caution patient to avoid hazardous activities until product response is determined; dizziness, blurred vision may occur
• Inform patient that orthostatic hypotension often occurs and to rise gradually from sitting or lying position; avoid hot tubs, hot showers, and tub baths since hypotension may occur
• Instruct patient to remain lying down after IM inj for at least 30 min
• Inform patient that heat stroke may occur in hot weather, and to take extra precautions to stay cool
• Teach patient to avoid OTC preparations (cough, hay fever, cold) unless approved by prescriber because serious product interactions may occur; avoid use with alcohol, CNS depressants because increased drowsiness may occur
• Inform patient to use sunglasses and sunscreen to prevent burns
• Teach patient about EPS
• Instruct patient to report sore throat, malaise, fever, bleeding, mouth sores; if these occur, CBC should be performed and product discontinued

## Evaluation

**Positive therapeutic outcome**
• Absence of nausea, vomiting

---

## thioridazine (Rx)
(thye-or-rid′a-zeen)
Apo-Thioridazine ✦, Mellaril, Mellaril Concentrate, Mellaril-5, Novo-Ridazine ✦, PMS-Thioridazine ✦, thioridazine HCl
*Func. class.:* Antipsychotic/neuroleptic
*Chem. class.:* Phenothiazine, piperidine
**Pregnancy category C**

## Do not confuse:
Mellaril/Elavil

**Action:** Depresses cerebral cortex, hypothalamus, limbic system, which control activity, aggression; blocks neurotransmission produced by dopamine at synapse; exhibits strong α-adrenergic, anticholinergic blocking action; mechanism for antipsychotic effects is unclear

**Therapeutic outcome:** Decreased signs and symptoms of psychosis

**Uses:** Psychotic disorders, schizophrenia, behavioral problems in children, anxiety, major depressive disorders, organic brain syndrome

## Dosage and routes
*Psychosis*
**Adult:** PO 25-100 mg tid, max dose 800 mg/day; dose is gradually increased to desired response, then reduced to minimum maintenance

*Depression/behavioral problems/ organic brain syndrome*
**Adult:** PO 25 tid, range from 10 mg bid-qid to 50 mg tid-qid; max 800 mg/day
**Geriatric:** PO 10-25 mg daily-bid, increase 4-7 days by 10-25 mg to desired dose, max 800 mg/day
**Child 2-12 yr:** PO 0.5-3 mg/kg/day in divided doses, max 3 mg/kg/day

**Available forms:** Tabs 10, 15, 25, 50, 100, 150, 200 mg; conc 30, 100 mg/ml; susp 25, 100 mg/5 ml; syr 10 mg/15 ml

## Adverse effects
*CNS: EPS (rare) (pseudoparkinsonism, akathisia, dystonia, tardive dyskinesia),* seizures, *headache,* confusion, **neuroleptic malignant syndrome, dizziness**
*CV:* Orthostatic hypotension, **cardiac arrest,** ECG changes, **tachycardia**
*EENT:* Blurred vision, glaucoma, dry eyes
*GI: Dry mouth, nausea, vomiting, anorexia, constipation,* diarrhea, jaundice, weight gain
*GU:* Urinary retention, urinary frequency, enuresis, impotence, amenorrhea, gynecomastia
*HEMA:* Anemia, **leukopenia, leukocytosis, agranulocytosis**
*INTEG: Rash,* photosensitivity, dermatitis
*RESP:* **Laryngospasm,** dyspnea, **respiratory depression**

**Contraindications:** Children <2 yr, hypersensitivity, blood dyscrasias, coma, brain damage, bone marrow depression

**Precautions:** Pregnancy **C**, breastfeeding, seizure disorders, hypertension, cardiac/hepatic disease, renal failure, BPH, glaucoma

| Pharmacokinetics | |
|---|---|
| Absorption | Variably absorbed (tab) |
| Distribution | Widely distributed, high concentrations in CNS, crosses placenta, protein binding 91%-99% |
| Metabolism | Liver, extensively; GI mucosa |
| Excretion | Kidneys, breast milk |
| Half-life | 26-36 hr |

Adverse effects: *italic* = common, **bold** = life-threatening

| Pharmacodynamics | |
|---|---|
| **Onset** | Erratic |
| **Peak** | 2-4 hr |
| **Duration** | 8-12 hr |

## Interactions
### Individual drugs
Alcohol: oversedation

Aluminum hydroxide, magnesium hydroxide: decreased absorption

Lithium: decreased thioridazine levels

### Drug classifications
Anesthetics (barbiturate), CNS depressants: oversedation

Antacids: decreased absorption

Anticholinergics: increased anticholinergic effects

Antiparkinson agents: decreased effect of these agents

Barbiturates: decreased thioridazine effect

Centrally acting antihypertensives: decreased antihypertensive effect

CYP2D6 inducers: decreased thioridazine levels

CYP2D6 inhibitors: increased thioridazine levels

### Drug/herb
Betel palm, kava: increased EPS

Cola tree, hops, nettle, nutmeg: increased effect

Kava: increased CNS depression

### Drug/lab test
Increased: liver function tests, cardiac enzymes, cholesterol, blood glucose, prolactin, bilirubin, cholinesterase, $^{131}$I

Decreased: hormones (blood and urine)

False positive: pregnancy tests, PKU

False negative: urinary steroids, pregnancy test

## NURSING CONSIDERATIONS
### Assessment
• Assess mental status: orientation, mood, behavior, presence of hallucinations, and type before initial administration and monthly; this product should significantly reduce psychotic behavior

• Check for swallowing of PO medication; check for hoarding or giving of medication to other patients

• Monitor I&O ratio, palpate bladder if low urinary output occurs, especially in geriatric; urinalysis recommended before, during prolonged therapy

• Monitor bilirubin, CBC, liver function tests monthly

• Assess affect, orientation, LOC, reflexes, gait, coordination, sleep pattern disturbances

• Monitor B/P sitting, standing, and lying, take pulse and respirations q4hr during initial treatment; establish baseline before starting treatment; report drops of 30 mm Hg; obtain baseline ECG, monitor Q- and T-wave changes

• Check for dizziness, faintness, palpitations, tachycardia on rising; severe orthostatic hypotension is common

 Identify for neuroleptic malignant syndrome: hyperpyrexia, muscle rigidity, increased CPK, altered mental status, dyspnea, fatigue; product should be discontinued

• Assess for EPS including akathisia (inability to sit still, no pattern to movements), tardive dyskinesia (bizarre movements of the jaw, mouth, tongue, extremities), pseudoparkinsonism (ragged tremors, pill rolling, shuffling gate); an antiparkinsonian product should be prescribed

• Assess for constipation, urinary retention daily; if these occur, increase bulk, water in diet

### Nursing diagnoses
• Coping, ineffective (uses)
• Knowledge, deficient (teaching)
• Noncompliance (teaching)
• Thought processes, disturbed (uses)

### Implementation
• Administer product in liquid form mixed in glass of juice if hoarding is suspected; do not mix in caffeine drinks, tannics, pectins, antacids separated by ≥2 hr

• Decrease dose in geriatric because metabolism is slowed

• Administer PO with full glass of water, milk; or give with food to decrease GI upset

• Give antacids 2 hr before or after this product

• Store in airtight, light-resistant container, oral sol in amber bottle

### Patient/family education
• Teach patient to use good oral hygiene; frequent rinsing of mouth, sugarless gum for dry mouth

• Advise patient to avoid hazardous activities until product response is determined; dizziness, blurred vision are common

• Inform patient that orthostatic hypotension occurs often and to rise from sitting or lying position gradually; to avoid hot tubs, hot showers, tub baths because hypotension may occur

• Instruct patient that in hot weather, heat stroke may occur; take extra precautions to stay cool

- Caution patient to avoid abrupt withdrawal of this product, or EPS may result; product should be withdrawn slowly
- Teach patient to avoid OTC preparations (cough, hay fever, cold) unless approved by prescriber; serious product interactions may occur; avoid use with alcohol, CNS depressants; increased drowsiness may occur
- Advise patient to use sunglasses and sunscreen to prevent burns
- Teach patient about EPS and necessity for meticulous oral hygiene because oral candidiasis may occur
- Advise patient to take antacids 2 hr before or after this product
- Instruct patient to report sore throat, malaise, fever, bleeding, mouth sores; if these occur, CBC should be performed and product discontinued; may cause vision impairment, report to prescriber
- Advise patient that urine may be discolored

### Evaluation
**Positive therapeutic outcome**
- Decrease in emotional excitement, hallucinations, delusions, paranoia
- Reorganization of patterns of thought, speech

**Treatment of overdose:** Lavage if orally ingested; provide airway; *do not induce vomiting or use epINEPHrine,* CV monitoring, continuous ECG

---

## thyroid USP (desiccated) (Rx)
(thye'roid)
Armour Thyroid, Thyrar, Thyroid Strong, Westhroid
*Func. class.:* Thyroid hormone
*Chem. class.:* Active thyroid hormone in natural state and ratio
**Pregnancy category A**

**Do not confuse:**
Thyrar/Thyrolar

**Action:** Increases metabolic rates; controls protein synthesis; increases cardiac output, renal blood flow, $O_2$ consumption, body temp, blood volume, growth, development at cellular level

**Therapeutic outcome:** Correction of lack of thyroid hormone

**Uses:** Hypothyroidism, cretinism (juvenile hypothyroidism), myxedema

## Dosage and routes
### Hypothyroidism
**Adult:** PO 65 mg/day, increased by 65 mg q30 days until desired response; maintenance dose 65-195 mg/day
**Geriatric:** PO 7.5-15 mg/day, double dose q6-8 wk until desired response

### Cretinism/juvenile hypothyroidism
**Child >1 yr:** PO Up to 180 mg/day titrated to response
**Child 4-12 mo:** PO 30-60 mg/day
**Child 1-4 mo:** PO 15-30 mg/day; may increase q2 wk; titrated to response; maintenance dose 30-45 mg/day

### Myxedema
**Adult:** PO 16 mg/day, double dose q2 wk, maintenance 65-195 mg/day

**Available forms:** Tabs 16, 32, 65, 98, 130, 195, 260, 325 mg; enteric-coated tabs 32, 65, 130 mg; sugar-coated tabs 32, 65, 130, 195 mg; caps 65, 130, 195, 325 mg

## Adverse effects
***CNS:*** *Insomnia, tremors,* headache, thyroid storm
***CV:*** *Tachycardia, palpitations, angina,* **dysrhythmias,** hypertension, **cardiac arrest**
***GI:*** Nausea, diarrhea, increased or decreased appetite, cramps
***MISC:*** Menstrual irregularities, weight loss, sweating, heat intolerance, fever

**Contraindications:** Adrenal insufficiency, MI, thyrotoxicosis

**Precautions:** Pregnancy **A,** breastfeeding, geriatric, angina pectoris, hypertension, ischemia, cardiac disease

| Pharmacokinetics | |
|---|---|
| Absorption | Well absorbed |
| Distribution | Widely distributed, does not cross placenta |
| Metabolism | Liver, tissues |
| Excretion | Feces via bile, breast milk |
| Half-life | $T_3$—2 days; $T_4$—1 wk |

T

| Pharmacodynamics | |
|---|---|
| Onset | 1 hr |
| Peak | 12-48 hr |
| Duration | Unknown |

## Interactions
### Individual drugs
Digoxin: decreased effect of digoxin
Insulin: increased requirement for insulin

---

Adverse effects: *italic* = common, **bold** = life-threatening

*Drug classifications*

Anticoagulants, oral: increased effects of anticoagulants

Antidepressants (tricyclic): increased antidepressants (tricylics) effect

Bile acid sequestrants: decreased thyroid absorption

Catecholamines: increased effects of catecholamines

Estrogens: decreased thyroid hormone effect

Hypoglycemics: decreased effect of hypoglycemics

Sympathomimetics: increased effects of sympathomimetics

*Drug/herb*

Agar, bugleweed, carnitine, kelpware, soy, spirulina: decreased thyroid effect

*Drug/lab test*

Increased: CPK, LDH, AST, PBI, blood glucose

Decreased: thyroid function tests

## NURSING CONSIDERATIONS
### Assessment

• Identify if the patient is taking anticoagulants, antidiabetic agents; document on chart

• Take B/P, pulse before each dose; monitor I&O ratio and weight every day in same clothing, using same scale, at same time of day

• Monitor height, weight, psychomotor development, and growth rate if given to a child

• Monitor $T_3$, $T_4$, FTIs, which are decreased; radioimmunoassay of TSH, which is increased; radioactive iodine uptake (RAIU), which is increased if patient's dose of medication is too low

• Monitor pro-time; patient may require decreased dosage of anticoagulant; check for bleeding, bruising

• Assess for increased nervousness, excitability, irritability, which may indicate that dose of medication is too high, usually after 1-3 wk of treatment

• Assess cardiac status: angina, palpitation, chest pain, change in VS; the geriatric patient may have undetected cardiac problems and baseline ECG should be completed before treatment

### Nursing diagnoses

• Knowledge, deficient (teaching)
• Noncompliance (teaching)

### Implementation

• Give in AM if possible as a single dose to decrease sleeplessness; at same time each day to maintain product level

• Do not give with food as absorption will be decreased

• Give only for hormone imbalances; not to be used for obesity, male infertility, menstrual conditions, lethargy; give lowest dose that relieves symptoms; lower dose to the geriatric and in cardiac diseases

• Store in airtight, light-resistant container

• Wean patient off medication 4 wk before RAIU test

### Patient/family education

• Teach patient that product is not a cure but controls symptoms and that treatment is long-term

• Instruct patient to report excitability, irritability, anxiety, sweating, heat intolerance, chest pain, palpitations, which indicate overdose

• Advise patient not to switch brands unless approved by prescriber; bioavailability may differ; do not take with food; absorption will be decreased

• Teach patient that product may be discontinued after giving birth; thyroid panel will be evaluated after 1-2 mo

• Teach patient that hyperthyroid child will show almost immediate behavior/personality change; that hair loss will occur in child and is temporary

• Caution patient that product is not to be taken to reduce weight

• Caution patient to avoid OTC preparations containing iodine; read labels; other medications should not be used unless approved by prescriber

• Teach patient to avoid iodine-containing food: iodized salt, soybeans, tofu, turnips, certain kinds of seafood and bread

### Evaluation
**Positive therapeutic outcome**

• Absence of depression
• Weight loss, increased diuresis, pulse, appetite
• Absence of constipation, peripheral edema, cold intolerance, pale, cool dry skin, brittle nails, alopecia, coarse hair, menorrhagia, night blindness, paresthesias, syncope, stupor, coma, rosy cheeks
• Improved levels of $T_3$, $T_4$ by laboratory tests
• Child: Age-appropriate weight, height, and psychomotor development

**Treatment of overdose:** Withhold dose for up to 1 wk, acute overdose—gastric lavage or induce emesis, then activated charcoal; provide supportive treatment to control symptoms

## tiagabine (Rx)
(tie-ah-ga'been)
Gabitril
*Func. class.:* Anticonvulsant

**Pregnancy category C**

**Action:** Inhibits reuptake and metabolism of GABA; may increase seizure threshold, structurally similar to GABA; tiagabine binding sites in neocortex, hippocampus

**Uses:** Adjunct treatment of partial seizures

### Dosage and routes
*Adult:* PO 4 mg/day in divided doses, may increase by 4-8 mg qwk until desired response, max 56 mg/day
*Child 12-18 yr:* PO 4 mg/day, may increase by 4 mg at beginning of wk 2, may increase by 4-8 mg qwk until desired response, max 32 mg/day

**Available forms:** Tabs 2, 4, 12, 16 mg

### Adverse effects
*CNS: Dizziness, anxiety,* somnolence, ataxia, confusion, *asthenia,* unsteady gait, depression
*CV:* Vasodilatation
*GI:* Nausea, diarrhea, vomiting, increased appetite
*INTEG:* Pruritus, rash
*RESP:* Pharyngitis, coughing

**Contraindications:** Hypersensitivity to this product

**Precautions:** Pregnancy C, breastfeeding, child <12 yr, geriatric, renal/hepatic disease

| Pharmacokinetics | |
|---|---|
| Absorption | >95% |
| Distribution | Protein binding 96% |
| Metabolism | Liver |
| Excretion | Kidneys |
| Half-life | 7-9 hr |

| Pharmacodynamics | |
|---|---|
| Onset | Unknown |
| Peak | 45 min |
| Duration | Unknown |

### Interactions
*Individual drugs*
Carbamazepine, phenobarbital, phenytoin, primidone: decreased effect of these products
Sevelamer: decreased tiagabine effect
Valproate: lower dose of tiagabine may be required

*Drug classifications*
CNS depressants: increased CNS depression
*Drug/food*
High-fat meal: decreased rate of absorption

### NURSING CONSIDERATIONS
**Assessment**
• Monitor renal function tests: urinalysis, BUN, urine creatinine q3 mo
• Monitor liver function tests: ALT, AST, bilirubin
• Assess description of seizures: location, duration, presence of aura
• Assess mental status: mood, sensorium, affect, behavioral changes; if mental status changes, notify prescriber

**Nursing diagnoses**
• Injury, risk for (uses, adverse reactions)
• Knowledge, deficient (teaching)
• Noncompliance (teaching)

**Implementation**
• Store at room temperature away from heat and light
• Provide assistance with ambulation during early part of treatment; dizziness occurs
• Provide seizure precautions: padded side rails; move objects that may harm patient

**Patient/family education**
• Advise patient to carry/wear emergency ID stating patient's name, products taken, condition, prescriber's name and phone number
• Advise patient to avoid driving, other activities that require alertness
• Teach patient not to discontinue medication quickly after long-term use

**Evaluation**
**Positive therapeutic outcome**
• Decreased seizure activity; document on patient's chart

**Treatment of overdose:** Lavage, VS

## ticarcillin (Rx)
(tye-kar-sill'in)
Ticar
*Func. class.:* Broad-spectrum antiinfective
*Chem. class.:* Extended-spectrum penicillin

**Pregnancy category B**

**Action:** Interferes with cell wall replication of susceptible organisms; osmotically unstable cell wall swells, bursts from osmotic pressure

**Therapeutic outcome:** Decreased symptoms of infection

**Uses:** Respiratory, soft tissue, urinary tract infections, bacterial septicemia; effective for gram-positive cocci *(Staphylococcus aureus, Streptococcus faecalis, Streptococcus pneumoniae)*, gram-negative cocci *(Neisseria gonorrhoeae)*, gram-positive bacilli *(Clostridium perfringens, Clostridium tetani)*, gram-negative bacilli *(Bacteroides, Fusobacterium nucleatum, Escherichia coli, Proteus mirabilis, Salmonella, Morganella morganii, Proteus rettgeri, Enterobacter, Pseudomonas aeruginosa, Serratia; and Peptococcus, Peptostreptococcus, Eubacterium)*

## Dosage and routes
### Bacterial septicemia, respiratory, skin, soft tissue, intraabdominal, reproductive infections
*Adult:* **IV** INF 200-300 mg/kg/day in divided doses q4-6hr
*Child <40 kg:* **IV** INF 33.3-50 mg/kg/q4hr or 50-75 mg/kg q6hr

### Urinary tract complicated infections
*Adult and child:* **IV** INF 150-200 mg/kg/day in divided doses q4-6hr

### Uncomplicated urinary infections
*Adult:* **IM/IV** DIRECT 1 g q6hr
*Child <40 kg:* **IM/IV** DIRECT 50-100 mg/kg/day q6-8hr

### Severe infections (Pseudomonas, Proteus, E. coli)
*Neonate <2 kg:* **IM/IV** 75 mg/kg q8-12hr
*Neonate >2 kg:* **IM/IV** 75-100 mg/kg q8hr

### Renal/hepatic dose
*Adult:* CCr >60 ml/min 3 g q4hr; CCr 30-60 ml/min 2 g q4hr; CCr 10-30 ml/min 2 g q8hr; CCr <10 ml/min 2 g q12hr or 1 g q6hr; CCr <10 ml/min and hepatic dysfunction 2 g q24hr or 1 g q12hr

**Available forms:** Inj 1, 3, 6, 20, 30 g

### Adverse effects
*CNS:* Lethargy, hallucinations, anxiety, depression, twitching, **coma, seizures**
*GI:* Nausea, vomiting, diarrhea; increased AST, ALT, abdominal pain, glossitis, colitis, **pseudomembranous colitis**
*GU:* Oliguria, proteinuria, hematuria, *vaginitis, moniliasis,* **glomerulonephritis**
*HEMA:* Anemia, increased bleeding time, **bone marrow depression, granulocytopenia**
*INTEG:* Rash, **Stevens-Johnson syndrome**
*META:* Hypokalemia
*SYST:* **Anaphylaxis**

**Contraindications:** Hypersensitivity to penicillins

**Precautions:** Pregnancy **B,** breastfeeding, hypersensitivity to cephalosporins, renal/GI disease, diabetes, electrolyte imbalances

### Pharmacokinetics

| | |
|---|---|
| **Absorption** | Unknown |
| **Distribution** | Widely, breast milk |
| **Metabolism** | Liver, small amount |
| **Excretion** | Kidneys |
| **Half-life** | 70 min |

### Pharmacodynamics

| | IM | IV |
|---|---|---|
| **Onset** | Unknown | Unknown |
| **Peak** | 1 hr | 30-45 min |
| **Duration** | 4-6 hr | 4 hr |

## Interactions
### Individual drugs
Aspirin, probenecid: increased ticarcillin concentration
Erythromycin: decreased effect of erthromycin
Heparin: increased effect of heparin
Methotrexate: increased effect of methotrexate
### Drug classifications
Aminoglycosides (**IV**), tetracyclines: decreased effect of ticarcillin
Anticoagulants: increased effect of anticoagulants
Contraceptives (oral): decreased effect of oral contraceptives
Neuromuscular blockers: increased effect of neuromuscular blockers
### Drug/lab test
False positive: urine glucose, urine protein

## NURSING CONSIDERATIONS
### Assessment
• Monitor I&O ratio; report hematuria, oliguria, since penicillin in high doses is nephrotoxic
 Monitor any patient with compromised renal system, since product is excreted slowly in poor renal system function; toxicity may occur rapidly
• Monitor liver function tests: AST, ALT
• Monitor blood tests: WBC, RBC, Hgb, Hct, bleeding time
• Monitor renal function tests: urinalysis, protein, blood, BUN, creatinine
• Monitor C&S before product therapy; product may be given as soon as culture is performed
• Assess bowel pattern before, during treatment
• Check for skin eruptions after administra-

 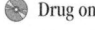

tion of penicillin to 1 wk after discontinuing product

◆ Assess for anaphylaxis: wheezing, rash, pruritus, laryngeal edema, keep emergency equipment nearby

• Assess allergies before initiation of treatment, reaction of each medication

## Nursing diagnoses

• Infection, risk for (uses)
• Knowledge, deficient (teaching)

## Implementation

• Give product after C&S has been completed
• Have adrenalin, suction, tracheostomy set, endotracheal intubation equipment
• Provide adequate fluid intake (2 L) during diarrhea episodes
• Provide scratch test to assess allergy on order from prescriber; usually done when penicillin is only product of choice
• Store at room temperature, reconstituted sol 72 hr at room temperature

**IM route**

• Inject into well-developed muscle
• Reconstitute ticarcillin 1 g/2 ml sterile water for inj, NaCl inj, 1% lidocaine HCl without epINEPHrine (385 mg/ml)

**IV route**

• Give **IV** after diluting 1 g or less/4 ml of sterile H₂O for inj; dilute further with 10-20 ml or more D₅W, 0.9% NaCl, or sterile H₂O for inj sol; give 1 g or less/5 min or more or by intermittent inf over ½-2 hr or by continuous inf at prescribed rate

*Y-site compatibilities:* Acyclovir, allopurinol, amifostine, aztreonam, cyclophosphamide, diltiazem, famotidine, filgrastim, fludarabine, granisetron, hydromorphone, heparin, IL-2, insulin (regular), magnesium sulfate, melphalan, meperidine, morphine, ondansetron, perphenazine, propofol, sargramostim, teniposide, theophylline, thiotepa, verapamil, vinorelbine

*Additive compatibilities:* Ranitidine, verapamil

## Patient/family education

• Advise patient that culture may be done after completed course of medication
• Teach patient to report sore throat, fever, fatigue (may indicate superinfection)
• Teach patient to carry/wear emergency ID if allergic to penicillins
• Advise patient to notify nurse of diarrhea

## Evaluation

**Positive therapeutic outcome**

• Absence of fever, purulent drainage, redness, inflammation

**Treatment of overdose:** Withdraw product, maintain airway, administer epINEPHrine, aminophylline, O₂, **IV** corticosteroids for anaphylaxis

---

### ticarcillin/clavulanate (Rx)
(tye-kar-sill′in)
Timentin
*Func. class.:* Extended-spectrum penicillin
*Chem. class:* Antiinfective—broad-spectrum
**Pregnancy category B**

---

**Action:** Interferes with cell wall replication of susceptible organisms; osmotically unstable cell wall swells, bursts from osmotic pressure; clavulanate inhibits β-lactamase and protects against enzymatic degradation of ticarcillin

**Therapeutic outcome:** Resolution of infection

**Uses:** Respiratory, soft tissue, urinary tract infections; bacterial septicemia; effective for gram-positive cocci *(Staphylococcus aureus, Streptococcus faecalis, Streptococcus pneumoniae),* gram-negative cocci *(Neisseria gonorrhoeae),* gram-positive bacilli *(Clostridium perfringens, Clostridium tetani),* gram-negative bacilli *(Bacteroides, Fusobacterium nucleatum, Escherichia coli, Proteus mirabilis, Salmonella, Morganella morganii, Proteus rettgeri, Enterobacter, Pseudomonas aeruginosa, Serratia, Peptococcus, Peptostreptococcus, Eubacterium)*

## Dosage and routes
*Renal dose*
*Adult:* **IV** INF Loading dose 3.1 g; CCr 60 ml/min 3.1 g q4hr; CCr 30-60 ml/min 2 g q4hr; CCr 10-30 ml/min 2g q8hr; CCr <10 ml/min 2 g q12hr; CCr <10 ml/min with hepatic dysfunction 2 g q24hr

*Systemic/urinary tract infections, serious infections*
*Adult ≥60 kg:* **IV** INF 3.1 g q4-6hr
*Adult <60 kg:* **IV** INF 200-300 mg/kg/day q4-6hr
*Child >60 kg:* **IV** INF 3.1 g q4hr
*Child <60 kg:* **IV** INF 300 mg/kg/day q4hr

*Mild/moderate infections*
*Child ≥60 kg:* **IV** INF 3.1 g q6hr
*Child <60 kg:* **IV** INF 200 mg/kg/day q6hr

**Available forms:** Inj IM, **IV** 3 g ticarcillin and 0.1 g clavulanate; **IV** inf 3 g ticarcillin and 0.1 g clavulanate; powder for inj 3 g ticarcillin, 0.1 g clavulanate

T

---

Adverse effects: *italic* = common, **bold** = life-threatening

## Adverse effects

*CNS:* Lethargy, hallucinations, anxiety, depression, twitching, **coma, seizures**

*GI: Nausea, vomiting, diarrhea,* increased AST, ALT, abdominal pain, glossitis, colitis, **pseudomembranous colitis**

*GU:* Oliguria, proteinuria, hematuria, *vaginitis, moniliasis,* **glomerulonephritis**

*HEMA:* Anemia, increased bleeding time, **bone marrow depression, granulocytopenia**

*META:* Hypokalemia, hyperkalemia, alkalosis, hypernatremia

*SYST:* **Anaphylaxis, Stevens-Johnson syndrome**

**Contraindications:** Hypersensitivity to penicillins; neonates

**Precautions:** Pregnancy **B**, hypersensitivity to cephalosporins, renal disease

### Pharmacokinetics

| | |
|---|---|
| **Absorption** | Completely absorbed (**IV**) |
| **Distribution** | Widely distributed, crosses blood-brain barrier |
| **Metabolism** | Liver |
| **Excretion** | Kidneys |
| **Half-life** | 64-68 min |

### Pharmacodynamics

| | IV |
|---|---|
| **Onset** | Unknown |
| **Peak** | 30-45 min |
| **Duration** | 4 hr |

## Interactions

### Individual drugs
Heparin: increased effect of heparin
Methotrexate: increased methotrexate level
Probenecid: increased ticarcillin concentration

### Drug classifications
Aminoglycosides (**IV**): decreased antimicrobial effect of ticarcillin
Anticoagulants: increased bleeding
Contraceptives (oral): decreased effect of oral contraceptives
Erythromycins: decreased absorption
Macrolides, sulfonamides, tetracyclines: decreased ticarcillin effect

### Drug/herb
Acidophilus: do not use with antiinfectives; separate by several hours

### Drug/lab test
False positive: urine glucose, urine protein, Coombs' test

## NURSING CONSIDERATIONS

### Assessment
• Monitor I&O ratio; report hematuria, oliguria because penicillin in high doses is nephrotoxic
• Monitor any patient with compromised renal system because product is excreted slowly in poor renal system function; toxicity may occur rapidly
• Monitor liver function tests: AST, ALT
• Monitor blood tests: WBC, RBC, Hgb, Hct, bleeding time
• Monitor renal function tests: urinalysis, protein, blood
• Obtain C&S test results before initiating product therapy; product may be given as soon as culture is performed
• Assess bowel pattern before, during treatment
• Assess skin eruptions after administration of penicillin to 1 wk after discontinuing product
 Assess for anaphylaxis: wheezing, rash, laryngeal edema; have emergency equipment nearby
• Assess allergies before initiation of treatment, reaction of each medication

### Nursing diagnoses
• Infection, risk for (uses)
• Knowledge, deficient (teaching)

### Implementation
• Give product after C&S has been completed
• Have adrenalin, suction, tracheostomy set, endotracheal intubation equipment available
• Give adequate fluid intake (2 L) during diarrhea episodes
• Obtain scratch test results to assess allergy after securing order from prescriber; usually done when penicillin is only product of choice
• Store at room temperature, reconstituted sol for 12-24 hr or 3-7 days refrigerated

**IV route**
• Give **IV** after diluting 3.1 g or less/13 ml of sterile $H_2O$ or NaCl (200 mg/ml), shake; may further dilute in 50-100 ml or more 0.9% NaCl, $D_5W$, or LR sol and run over ½ hr

**Y-site compatibilities:** Allopurinol, aztreonam, cefepime, cyclophosphamide, diltiazem, famotidine, filgrastim, fluconazole, fludarabine, foscarnet, heparin, insulin (regular), melphalan, meperidine, morphine, ondansetron, perphenazine, sargramostim, teniposide, theophylline, vinorelbine

### Patient/family education
• Advise patient that C&S may be performed after completed course of medication
• Instruct patient to report sore throat, fever, fatigue (may indicate superinfection)

- Advise patient to carry/wear emergency ID if allergic to penicillins
- Advise patient to use alternative birth control methods

### Evaluation
**Positive therapeutic outcome**
- Absence of fever, purulent drainage, redness, inflammation

**Treatment of overdose:** Withdraw product, maintain airway, administer epINEPHrine, aminophylline, O$_2$, **IV** corticosteroids for anaphylaxis

---

### ticlopidine (Rx)
(tye-cloe′pi-deen)
Ticlid
*Func. class.:* Platelet aggregation inhibitor
*Chem. class.:* Thienopyridine compound

**Pregnancy category B**

**Action:** Irreversible inhibition of platelet aggregation through antagonism of ADP

**Therapeutic outcome:** Decreased stroke by decreasing platelet aggregation

**Uses:** Reducing the risk of stroke in high-risk patients

**Unlabeled uses:** Intermittent claudication, chronic arterial occlusion, subarachnoid hemorrhage, uremic patients with AV shunts/fistulas, open heart surgery, coronary artery bypass grafts, primary glomerulonephritis, diabetic neuropathy

**Dosage and routes**
*Adult:* PO 250 mg bid with food

**Available forms:** Tabs 250 mg

**Adverse effects**
*CNS:* Dizziness
*GI:* Nausea, vomiting, diarrhea, GI discomfort, **cholestatic jaundice, hepatitis,** increased cholesterol LDL, VLDL, TG
*HEMA:* **Bleeding (epistaxis, hematuria, conjunctival hemorrhage, GI bleeding), agranulocytosis, neutropenia, thrombocytopenia, thrombotic thrombocytopenic purpura**
*INTEG:* Rash, pruritus

**Contraindications:** Hypersensitivity, severe liver disease, blood dyscrasias, active bleeding, coagulopathy

**Precautions:** Pregnancy **B,** breastfeeding, children, geriatric, past liver disease, renal disease, increased bleeding risk, anemia, peptic ulcer disease, surgery

### Pharmacokinetics
| | |
|---|---|
| **Absorption** | Well absorbed |
| **Distribution** | Unknown |
| **Metabolism** | Liver—extensively, 98% protein binding |
| **Excretion** | Kidneys—unchanged product |
| **Half-life** | Increased with repeat dosing; 4-5 days (multiple doses) |

### Pharmacodynamics
| | |
|---|---|
| **Onset** | Unknown |
| **Peak** | 1-3 hr |
| **Duration** | Unknown |

### Interactions
*Individual drugs*
Cimetidine: increased effects of ticlopidine
Digoxin: decreased plasma levels of digoxin
Fosphenytoin, phenytoin: increased levels of phenytoin
Theophylline: increased effects of theophylline
*Drug classifications*
Antacids: decreased plasma levels of ticlopidine
Anticoagulants, NSAIDs, salicylates, thrombolytics: increased bleeding risk
*Drug/herb*
Ginger, gingko, garlic, feverfew, horse chestnut, green tea: increased bleeding risk

### NURSING CONSIDERATIONS
**Assessment**
- Monitor liver function tests: AST, ALT, bilirubin, creatinine if patient is on long-term therapy (4 mo or more)
- Monitor blood tests: CBC, Hct, Hgb, protime if patient is on long-term therapy; CBC q2 wk × 3 mo therapy; thrombocytopenia, neutropenia may occur
- Monitor bleeding time baseline and throughout therapy, levels may be 2-5 × normal limit

**Nursing diagnoses**
- Injury, risk for (uses)
- Knowledge, deficient (teaching)

**Implementation**
- Give with food or after eating to decrease GI effects

**Patient/family education**
- Advise patient that blood studies will be necessary during treatment
- Advise patient to report any unusual bleeding to prescriber
- Instruct patient to take with food or just after eating to minimize GI discomfort, not to double missed dose

T

Adverse effects: *italic* = common, **bold** = life-threatening

• Caution patient to report side effects such as diarrhea, skin rashes, subcutaneous bleeding, signs of cholestasis (yellow skin and sclera, dark urine, light-colored stools)

• Advise patient that product should be discontinued 10-14 days prior to surgery

### Evaluation
**Positive therapeutic outcome**
• Absence of stroke

---

### tigecycline (Rx)
(tye-ge-sye′kleen)
Tygacil
*Func. class.:* Broad-spectrum antiinfective
*Chem. class.:* Glycylcyclines

**Pregnancy category D**

**Action:** Inhibits protein synthesis and phosphorylation in microorganisms; bacteriostatic, structurally similar to the tetracyclines

**Therapeutic outcome:** Resolution of infection

**Uses:** Complicated skin/skin structure infections (*Escherichia coli, Enterococcus faecalis* (vancomycin-susceptible only) *Staphylococcus aureus, Streptococcus agalactiae, S. anginosus* group, *S. pyogenes, Bacteroides fragilis*; complicated intraabdominal infections *(Citrobacter freundii)*, *Enterobacter cloacae, E. coli, Klebsiella oxytoca, K. pneumoniae, E. faecalis* (vancomycin-susceptible only), *S. aureus* (methicillin-susceptible only), *S. anginosus* group, *B. fragilis, Bacteroides thetaiotaomicron, B. uniformis, B. vulgatus, Clostridium perfringens, Peptostreptococcus micros*

### Dosage and routes
*Adult:* **IV** 100 mg, then 50 mg q12hr, **IV** INF is given over 30 min to 60 min q12 hr; given for 5-14 days depending on infection

*Hepatic dose (Child-Pugh C)*
*Adult:* **IV** 100 mg, then 25 mg q12hr

**Available forms:** Powder for inj, lyophilized 50 mg

### Adverse effects
*CNS:* Headache, dizziness, insomnia
*CV:* Hypo/hypertension, phlebitis
*GI: Nausea, vomiting, diarrhea,* anorexia, constipation, dyspepsia
*HEMA:* **Anemia, leukocytosis, thrombocytopenia**
*INTEG: Rash,* pruritus, sweating, photosensitivity

*META:* Increased ALT, AST, BUN, lactic acid, alkaline phosphatase, amylase, hyperglycemia, hypokalemia, hypoproteinemia, bilirubinemia
*MISC:* Back pain, fever, abnormal healing, abdominal pain, abscess, asthenia, infection, pain, peripheral edema, local reactions
*RESP:* Cough, dyspnea

**Contraindications:** Pregnancy **D**, breast-feeding, children <18 yr, hypersensitivity to tigecycline

**Precautions:** Renal/hepatic disease, hypersensitivity to tetracyclines

### Pharmacokinetics

| | |
|---|---|
| **Absorption** | Unknown |
| **Distribution** | Unknown |
| **Metabolism** | Not extensively |
| **Excretion** | 22% unchanged, urine; primarily biliarily excreted |
| **Half-life** | Terminal 42 hr |

### Pharmacodynamics
Unknown

### Interactions
*Individual drugs*
Warfarin: increased effect of tigecycline
*Drug classifications*
Oral contraceptives: decreased effect of tigecycline

### NURSING CONSIDERATIONS
**Assessment**
🔷 Assess for pseudomembranous colitis
• Assess for signs of anemia: Hct, Hgb, fatigue
• Monitor blood tests: PT, CBC, AST, ALT, BUN creatinine
• Assess for allergic reactions: rash, itching, pruritus, angioedema
• Assess for nausea, vomiting, diarrhea; administer antiemetic, antacids as ordered
• Assess for overgrowth of infection: fever, malaise, redness, pain, swelling, drainage, perineal itching, diarrhea, changes in cough or sputum

### Nursing diagnoses
• Infection, risk for (use)
• Knowledge, deficient (teaching)

### Implementation
• Give after C&S obtained
**IV route**
• Reconstitute each vial with 5.3 ml of 0.9% NaCl, or $D_5$ (10 mg/ml); swirl to dissolve; immediately withdraw 5 ml of the reconstituted sol and add to a 100-ml **IV** bag for inf (1 mg/ml); may be yellow or orange, if not, sol

---

should be discarded; do not give if particulate matter is present
• Store in tight, light-resistant container at room temperature

### Patient/family education
• Teach patient to avoid sun exposure; sunscreen does not seem to decrease photosensitivity
• Teach patient to avoid pregnancy while taking this product; fetal harm may occur

### Evaluation
**Positive therapeutic outcome**
• Decreased temp, absence of lesions, negative C&S

---

### tiludronate (Rx)
(till-oo'droe-nate)
Skelid
*Func. class.:* Bone resorption inhibitor
*Chem. class.:* Bisphosphonate

### Pregnancy category C

**Action:** Decreases bone reabsorption and new bone development, inhibits osteoclasts

**Therapeutic outcome:** Decreased bone reabsorption and reduced calcium levels WNL

**Uses:** Paget's disease in those with alkaline phosphatase at 2 × upper limit, patients at risk of future complications of Paget's disease

### Dosage and routes
*Adult:* PO 400 mg/day, with 8 oz of water × 3 mo

*Renal dose*
*Adult:* PO CCr <30 ml/min do not use

**Available forms:** Tabs 240 mg (equivalent to 200 mg tiludronic acid)

### Adverse effects
*CNS:* Headache, somnolence, dizziness, anxiety, vertigo, nervousness, involuntary movements
*CV:* Chest pain, edema, hypertension, peripheral edema, **atrial fibrillation**
*EENT:* Cataracts, ocular hypertension/inflammation/pain, sinusitis
*ENDO:* Hyperparathyroidism
*GI:* *Nausea, diarrhea,* dry mouth, gastritis, vomiting, flatulence, gastric ulcers, dyspepsia
*GU:* **Nephrotoxicity,** UTI
*INTEG:* Rash, epidermal necrosis, pruritus, sweating
*MS:* *Bone pain,* decreased mineralization of nonaffected bones, pathologic fractures, osteonecrosis of the jaw

*RESP:* Bronchitis, rhinitis, crackles, sinusitis, upper respiratory tract infection
*SYST:* **Stevens-Johnson syndrome**

**Contraindications:** Hypersensitivity to bisphosphonates, severe renal disease with creatinine >5 mg/dl, breastfeeding, CCr <30 ml/min

**Precautions:** Pregnancy **C**, GI/renal disease, restricted vit D/Ca, asthma, anemia coagulopathy, dental disease, GERD, hiatal hernia, hypocalcemia, infection

| Pharmacokinetics | |
|---|---|
| **Absorption** | Rapid |
| **Distribution** | Unknown, steady state 10 days |
| **Metabolism** | Protein binding 90% |
| **Excretion** | Feces (unabsorbed), kidney (unchanged) |
| **Half-life** | 150 hr |

| Pharmacodynamics | |
|---|---|
| **Onset** | Up to 4 wk |
| **Peak** | Unknown |
| **Duration** | Unknown |

### Interactions
*Individual drugs*
Aspirin: decreased tiludronate absorption
Indomethacin: increased effect of tiludronate
*Drug classifications*
Aminoglycosides, NSAIDs: increased tiludronate level
Antacids, mineral supplements with magnesium, calcium, or aluminum: decreased absorption of tiludronate, separate by ≥2 hr

### NURSING CONSIDERATIONS
**Assessment**
• Assess for GI symptoms, polyuria, flushing, head swelling, tingling, headache; may indicate hypercalcemia; nervousness, irritability, twitching, seizures, spasm, paresthesia indicates hypocalcemia at start of treatment
• Identify nutritional status; evaluate diet for sources of vit D (milk, some seafood), calcium (dairy products, dark green vegetables), phosphates; dental health
• Monitor BUN, creatinine, uric acid, chloride, electrolytes, urine pH, urinary calcium, magnesium, phosphate, urinalysis (calcium should be kept at 9-10 mg/dl), albumin, alkaline phosphatase baseline and q3-6 mo; check urine sediment for casts throughout treatment
• Assess for increased product level; toxic reactions occur rapidly; have calcium chloride

T

Adverse effects: *italic* = common, **bold** = life-threatening

or gluconate on hand if calcium level drops too low; check for tetany

### Nursing diagnoses
• Injury, risk for (adverse reactions)
• Knowledge, deficient (teaching)
• Pain, chronic (uses)

### Implementation
• Administer on empty stomach to improve absorption (2 hr before meals), with 6-8 oz of water; do not use with mineral water, juice, or coffee; take calcium or mineral supplements 2 hr before or 2 hr after tiludronate; take aluminum or magnesium antacids ≥2 hr after tiludronate; do not take indomethacin within 2 hr
• Remove tabs from foil strip immediately before use

### Patient/family education
• Caution patient to notify prescriber of hypercalcemic relapse: renal calculi, nausea, vomiting, thirst, lethargy, deep bone or flank pain
• Teach patient to follow a low-calcium diet as prescribed (Paget's disease, hypercalcemia)
• Advise patient to notify prescriber of diarrhea, nausea; dose may be divided to lessen these symptoms

### Evaluation
**Positive therapeutic outcome**
• Calcium levels 9-10 mg/dl
• Decreasing symptoms of Paget's disease including pain

---

### timolol (Rx)
(tye'moe-lole)
Apo-Timol ♦, Blocadren, Novo-Timol ♦, timolol maleate, Timoptic
*Func. class.:* Antihypertensive; antiglaucoma
*Chem. class.:* Nonselective β-blocker

**Pregnancy category C**

**Do not confuse:**
Timoptic/Viroptic

**Action:** Competitively blocks stimulation of β-adrenergic receptor within vascular smooth muscle (decreases rate of SA node discharge, increases recovery time), slows conduction of AV node, decreases heart rate, which decreases $O_2$ consumption in myocardium; also decreases renin-aldosterone-angiotensin system; at high doses inhibits $β_2$ receptors in bronchial system

**Therapeutic outcome:** Decreased B/P, decreased arrhythmias, absence of death from MI, decreased aqueous humor in the eye, absence of migraine headaches

**Uses:** Mild to moderate hypertension, migraine prophylaxis

**Unlabeled uses:** Tremors, angina pectoris

### Dosage and routes
*Hypertension*
*Adult:* PO 10 mg bid, or 20 mg/day, may increase by 10 mg q7 days, not to exceed 60 mg/day

*Myocardial infarction*
*Adult:* 10 mg bid beginning 1-4 wk after MI

*Glaucoma*
*Adult:* Ophth 1 gtt daily or bid
*Child:* Ophth 1 gtt daily or bid (0.25% sol only)

*Migraine headache prevention*
*Adult:* PO 10 mg bid, or 20 mg/day; may increase to 30 mg/day, 20 mg in AM, 10 mg in PM; discontinue if not effective after 8 wk

**Available forms:** Tabs 5, 10, 20 mg

### Adverse effects
*CNS: Insomnia, dizziness,* hallucinations, anxiety, fatigue, depression, headache
*CV:* Hypotension, bradycardia, **CHF,** edema, chest pain, bradycardia, claudication, angina, AV block, ventricular dysrhythmias
*EENT: Visual changes,* sore throat, *double vision,* dry burning eyes
*GI: Nausea,* vomiting, **ischemic colitis,** diarrhea, *abdominal pain,* **mesenteric arterial thrombosis,** flatulence, constipation
*GU:* Impotence, urinary frequency
*HEMA:* **Agranulocytosis, thrombocytopenia, purpura**
*INTEG:* Rash, alopecia, pruritus, fever
*META:* Hypoglycemia
*MUSC: Joint pain, muscle pain*
*RESP:* **Bronchospasm,** dyspnea, cough, crackles, nasal stuffiness

**Contraindications:** Hypersensitivity to β-blockers, cardiogenic shock, heart block (2nd or 3rd degree), sinus bradycardia, CHF, cardiac failure, severe COPD, asthma

**Precautions:** Pregnancy **C,** breastfeeding, major surgery, diabetes mellitus, thyroid/renal/hepatic disease, COPD, well-compensated heart failure, CAD, nonallergic bronchospasm, peripheral vascular disease

## Pharmacokinetics

| | |
|---|---|
| **Absorption** | Well absorbed (PO), minimal (ophth) |
| **Distribution** | Protein binding <10% |
| **Metabolism** | Liver—extensively |
| **Excretion** | Breast milk |
| **Half-life** | 3 hr |

## Pharmacodynamics

| | PO |
|---|---|
| **Onset** | Unknown |
| **Peak** | 2-4 hr |
| **Duration** | 12-24 hr |

## Interactions
### Individual drugs
Alcohol: increased hypotension, bradycardia (large amounts)

HydrALAZINE, methyldopa, prazosin: increased hypotension, bradycardia

Insulin: decreased hypoglycemia

Thyroid hormones: decreased antihypertensive effect

### Drug classifications
Anticholinergics, nitrates: increased hypotension, increased bradycardia

$\beta_2$-Adrenergic agonists: increased $\beta$-blocking effect

Calcium channel blockers: increased effects of calcium channel blockers

NSAIDs, salicylates, sympathomimetics: decreased antihypertensive effect

Sulfonylureas: decreased hypoglycemic effect

Theophyllines: decreased bronchodilatation

### Drug/herb
Aconite: increased toxicity, death

Astragalus, cola tree: increased or decreased antihypertensive effect

Barberry, betony, black catechu, black cohosh, bloodroot, broom, burdock, cat's claw, dandelion, goldenseal, Irish moss, Jamaican dogwood, kelp, khella, mistletoe, parsley: increased antihypertensive effect

Coltsfoot, guarana, khat, licorice, yohimbe: decreased antihypertensive effect

### Drug/lab test
Increased: renal, liver function tests, potassium, uric acid

Decreased: Hct, Hgb, HDL

Interference: glucose, insulin tolerance test

## NURSING CONSIDERATIONS
### Assessment
• Assess for headaches: location, severity, duration, frequency baseline and throughout treatment

• Monitor B/P during beginning treatment, periodically thereafter; pulse q4hr; note rate, rhythm, quality: apical/radial pulse before administration; notify prescriber of any significant changes (pulse <50 bpm)

• Check for baselines in renal, liver function tests before therapy begins

• Assess for edema in feet, legs daily, monitor I&O ratio, daily weight; check for jugular vein distention, crackles, bilaterally, dyspnea (CHF)

• Monitor skin turgor, dryness of mucous membranes for hydration status, especially geriatric

### Nursing diagnoses
• Cardiac output, decreased (uses)
• Injury, risk for (side effects)
• Knowledge, deficient (teaching)
• Noncompliance (teaching)

### Implementation
• Given before meals, at bedtime; tab may be crushed or swallowed whole; give with food to prevent GI upset; reduced dosage in renal dysfunction

• Store protected from light, moisture; place in cool environment

### Patient/family education
• Teach patient not to discontinue product abruptly; taper over 2 wk; may cause precipitate angina if stopped abruptly

• Advise patient not to use OTC products containing $\alpha$-adrenergic stimulants (such as nasal decongestants, cold preparations); to avoid alcohol, smoking and to limit sodium intake as prescribed

• Teach patient how to take pulse and B/P at home; advise patient when to notify prescriber

• Instruct patient to comply with weight control, dietary adjustments, modified exercise program

• Advise patient to carry/wear emergency ID to identify product being taken, any allergies; tell patient product controls symptoms but does not cure

• Caution patient to avoid hazardous activities if dizziness, drowsiness is present

• Teach patient to report symptoms of CHF; difficult breathing, especially on exertion or when lying down; night cough; swelling of extremities or bradycardia; dizziness; confusion; depression; fever

• Teach patient to take product as prescribed, not to double dose, skip doses; take any missed doses as soon as remembered if at least 4 hr until next dose

### Evaluation
**Positive therapeutic outcome**
• Decreased B/P in hypertension (after 1-2 wk)
• Absence of dysrhythmias

**Treatment of overdose:** Lavage, **IV** atropine for bradycardia, **IV** theophylline for bronchospasm, digoxin, O₂, diuretic for cardiac failure, hemodialysis, **IV** glucose for hyperglycemia, **IV** diazepam (or phenytoin) for seizures

## timolol ophthalmic
*See Appendix D*

## tinidazole (Rx)
(tye-ni'da-zole)
Tindamax
*Func. class.:* Antiprotozoal
*Chem. class.:* Nitroimidazole derivative

**Pregnancy category C**

**Action:** Interferes with DNA/RNA synthesis in protozoa

**Therapeutic outcome:** Decrease in infection

**Uses:** Amebiasis, giardiasis, trichomoniasis

### Dosage and routes
*Amebiasis*
*Adult:* PO 2 g/day × 3-5 days
*Child >3 yr:* PO 50 mg/kg/day × 3-5 days, max 2 g

*Giardiasis*
*Adult:* PO 2 g as a single dose
*Child >3 yr:* PO 50 mg/kg as a single dose, max 2 g

*Trichomoniasis*
*Adult:* PO 2 g as a single dose

*Bacterial vaginosis*
*Adult (nonpregnant woman):* PO 2 g/day × 2 days with food or 1 g/day × 5 days with food

**Available forms:** Tabs 250, 500 mg

### Adverse effects
*CNS: Dizziness, headache,* **seizures,** *peripheral neuropathy,* malaise, fatigue
*GI: Nausea, vomiting,* anorexia, increased AST and ALT, constipation, abdominal pain, indigestion, altered sense of taste
*HEMA:* **Leukopenia,** neutropenia
*INTEG:* Pruritus, urticaria, *rash,* oral monilia
*SYST:* **Angioedema,** cramping

**Contraindications:** Hypersensitivity to this product or nitroimidazole derivative, pregnancy 1st trimester

**Precautions:** Pregnancy **C**, breastfeeding, children, geriatric, hepatic disease, CNS depression, blood dyscrasias, candidiasis

### Pharmacokinetics
| | |
|---|---|
| **Absorption** | Unknown |
| **Distribution** | Crosses blood/brain barrier |
| **Metabolism** | Extensively in the liver |
| **Excretion** | Unchanged (20-25%) in urine, (12%) feces |
| **Half-life** | 12-14 hr |

### Pharmacodynamics
Unknown

### Interactions
*Individual drugs*
Do not use within 2 wk of taking disulfiram
Cholestyramine, oxytetracycline: decreased action of tinidazole
CycloSPORINE, tacrolimus, fluorouracil, lithium: increased action
*Drug classifications*
Anticoagulants, hydantoins: increased action
CYP 3A4 inducers (phenobarbital, rifampin, phenytoin): decreased action of tinidazole
CYP 3A4 inhibitors (cimetidine, ketoconazole): increased action of tinidazole

### NURSING CONSIDERATIONS
**Assessment**
• Assess for amebic liver absess: CBC, ESR, amebic gel diffusion test, ultrasound, total and differential leukocyte count
• Assess for signs of infection, anemia
• Assess bowel pattern before, during treatment

**Nursing diagnoses**
• Infection, risk for (uses)
• Knowledge, deficient (teaching)

**Implementation**
• Administer to those over 3 yr old
• Give with food; tabs can be crushed and mixed with artificial cherry syrup

**Patient/family education**
• Instruct patient to take with food to increase plasma concentrations, minimize epigastric distress and other GI effects; not to use alcoholic beverages during or for 3 days afterward
• Advise patient that in cases of trichomoniasis, both partners should be treated at the same time

**Evaluation**
**Positive therapeutic outcome**
• Decrease in infection as evidenced by negative culture

peptic ulcer disease, thrombocytopenic
purpura, heparin-induced thrombocytopenia

## ! HIGH ALERT

### tinzaparin (Rx)
(tin-zay-par'in)
Innohep
*Func. class.:* Anticoagulant
*Chem. class.:* Unfractionated porcine
heparin

#### Pregnancy category C

**Action:** Prevents conversion of fibrinogen to
fibrin and prothrombin to thrombin by enhancing inhibitory effects of antithrombin III;
produces higher ratio of antifactor Xa to
antifactor IIa

**Therapeutic outcome:** Resolution of
DVT

**Uses:** Treatment of DVT, pulmonary emboli
after abdominal, knee, hip surgery or knee,
hip replacement

**Unlabeled uses:** DVT prophylaxis

**Dosage and routes**
*Treatment of deep vein
thrombosis*
*Adult:* SUBCUT 175 anti-Xa international
units/kg daily ≥6 days and until adequate
anticoagulation with warfarin (INR ≥2 for 2
consecutive days)

*Prophylaxis of deep vein
thrombosis (unlabeled)*
*Adult:* 3500 anti-Xa units (50 anti-Xa units/
kg) daily beginning 1-2 hr prior to surgery and
continued for 5-10 days

*Prophylaxis of deep vein
thrombosis in orthopedic
procedures (unlabeled)*
*Adult:* 75 anti-Xa units/kg/day started 12-24
hr after surgery

**Available forms:** Inj 40,000 international
units/1 ml

**Adverse effects**
*CNS:* Fever, confusion, dizziness, insomnia
*CV:* Angina, dysrhythmias, peripheral edema,
tachycardia, hypo/hypertension
*GI:* Nausea, constipation, flatulence, dyspepsia,
**hepatitis**
*GU:* UTI, hematuria, urinary retention, dysuria
*HEMA:* Hemorrhage, **anemia, thrombocyto-
penia,** bleeding
*INTEG:* Ecchymosis, inj site reaction
*MISC:* Headache, chest pain, hypersensitivity

**Contraindications:** Hypersensitivity to
this product, heparin, pork or benzyl alcohol,
sulfites; hemophilia, leukemia with bleeding,
peptic ulcer disease, thrombocytopenic
purpura, heparin-induced thrombocytopenia

**Precautions:** Pregnancy **C,** breastfeeding,
children, geriatric, alcoholism, severe renal/
hepatic disease, blood dyscrasias, severe
uncontrolled hypertension, subacute bacterial
endocarditis, acute nephritis

### Pharmacokinetics

| | |
|---|---|
| **Absorption** | Unknown |
| **Distribution** | Unknown |
| **Metabolism** | Unknown |
| **Excretion** | Unknown |
| **Half-life** | 4.5 hr |

### Pharmacodynamics

| | |
|---|---|
| **Onset** | Unknown |
| **Peak** | 3-5 hr (max antithrombin activity) |
| **Duration** | Unknown |

### Interactions
*Individual drug*
Ticlopidine: increased tinzaparin action
*Drug classifications*
Anticoagulants (oral), NSAIDs, platelet inhibitors, salicylates, thrombolytics: increased
tinzaparin action
*Drug/herb*
Agrimony, alfalfa, angelica, anise, basil, bay,
bilberry, black haw, bogbean, bromelain,
buchu, chondroitin, cinchona bark, dong
quai, fenugreek, feverfew, garlic, ginger,
ginkgo, ginseng, horse chestnut, Irish moss,
kelp, kelpware, khella, lovage, lungwort,
meadowsweet, motherwort, mugwort, nettle,
papaya, parsley (large amounts), pau
d'arco, pineapple, poplar, prickly ash,
safflower, saw palmetto, tonka bean, turmeric, wintergreen, yarrow: increased risk
of bleeding
Chamomile, coenzyme Q10, flax, glucomannan, goldenseal, guar gum: decreased
anticoagulant effect

### NURSING CONSIDERATIONS
**Assessment**
• Monitor blood tests (Hct, platelets, occult
blood in stools), anti-Xa; thrombocytopenia
may occur
• Assess for bleeding gums, petechiae, ecchymosis, black tarry stools, hematuria

**Nursing diagnoses**
• Cardiac output, decreased (uses)
• Knowledge, deficient (teaching)

T

Adverse effects: *italic* = common, **bold** = life-threatening

## Implementation
- Give only after screening patient for bleeding disorders
- Give SUBCUT only; do not give IM
- Give SUBCUT to recumbent patient; rotate inj sites (left/right anterolateral, left/right posterolateral abdominal wall)
- Insert whole length of needle into skin fold held with thumb and forefinger
◆ Use only this product when ordered; not interchangeable with heparin or LMWHs
- Give at same time each day to maintain steady blood levels
- Do not massage area or aspirate when giving SUBCUT inj
- Avoid all IM inj that may cause bleeding
- Do not mix with other products or infusion fluids
- Store at 77° F (25° C); do not freeze

## Patient/family education
- Advise patient to use soft-bristle toothbrush to avoid bleeding gums, to use electric razor
- Instruct patient to report any signs of bleeding: gums, under skin, urine, stools

## Evaluation
**Positive therapeutic outcome**
- Resolution of deep vein thrombosis

**Treatment of overdose:** Protamine 1 mg/100 anti-Xa international units of tinzaparin

---

## tioconazole vaginal antifungal
*See Appendix D*

---

## tiotropium (Rx)
(ty-oh′tro-pee-um)
Spiriva
*Func. class.:* Anticholinergic, bronchodilator
*Chem. class.:* Synthetic quaternary ammonium compound

**Pregnancy category C**

**Action:** Inhibits interaction of acetylcholine at receptor sites on the bronchial smooth muscle, resulting in decreased cGMP and bronchodilation

**Therapeutic outcome:** Improved breathing

**Uses:** COPD, for long-term treatment, once daily maintenance of bronchospasm, associated with COPD including chronic bronchitis and emphysema

## Dosage and routes
*Adult:* INH content of 1 cap/day using HandiHaler inhalation device

**Available forms:** Powder for inhalation 18 mcg in blister packs containing 6 caps with inhaler; 30 caps with inhaler

## Adverse effects
*CNS:* Depression, paresthesia
*CV:* Chest pain, increased heart rate
*EENT:* Dry mouth, blurred vision, glaucoma
*GI: Vomiting,* abdominal pain, constipation, dyspepsia
*INTEG:* Rash
*MISC:* Urinary difficulty, urinary retention
*RESP: Cough, worsening of symptoms,* sinusitis, URI, epistaxis, pharyngitis

**Contraindications:** Hypersensitivity to this product, atropine or its derivatives

**Precautions:** Pregnancy **C**, breastfeeding, children, geriatric, angle-closure glaucoma, prostatic hypertrophy, bladder neck obstruction, renal disease

### Pharmacokinetics

| | |
|---|---|
| **Absorption** | Unknown |
| **Distribution** | Does not cross blood-brain barrier |
| **Metabolism** | Very little metabolized in the liver |
| **Excretion** | Excreted in urine |
| **Half-life** | 5-6 days in animals |

### Pharmacodynamics
Unknown

## Interactions
*Drug classifications*
Anticholinergics: avoid use with other anticholinergics
*Drug/herb*
Black catechu: increased constipation
Butterbur, jimsonweed: increased anticholinergic effect
Green tea (large amts), guarana: increased bronchodilator effect
Jaborandi tree, pill-bearing spurge: decreased anticholinergic effect

## NURSING CONSIDERATIONS
## Assessment
- For tolerance over long-term therapy; dose may have to be increased or changed

## Nursing diagnoses
- Breathing pattern, ineffective (uses)
- Knowledge, deficient (teaching)

---

 Alert   ♣ Canada Only    Drug on CD   * "Tall Man" lettering (See Preface)

## Implementation
- Caps are for INH only; do not swallow
- Immediately prior to administration, peel back foil until cap is visible; until "stop" line, open dust cap of HandiHaler by pulling upward, then open mouthpiece
- Place cap in center chamber; firmly close mouthpiece until it clicks, leaving dust cap open
- Hold HandiHaler with mouthpiece upward; press button in once, completely, and release; this allows for medication to be released
- Breathe out completely; do not breathe into mouthpiece at any time
- Raise device to mouth and close lips tightly around mouthpiece
- With head upright, breathe in slowly/deeply, but allowing the cap to vibrate; breathe until lungs fill; hold breath and remove mouthpiece; resume normal breathing
- Repeat
- Remove used capsule and dispose; close the mouthpiece and dust cap; store

## Patient/family education
- Teach patient how to use Handihaler
- Teach patient signs of angle-closure glaucoma
- Advise patient that product is used for long-term maintenance, not for immediate relief of breathing problems
- Caution patient to avoid getting the powder in the eyes; may cause blurred vision and pupil dilation

## Evaluation
**Positive therapeutic outcome**
- Ability to breathe easier

## tipranavir (Rx)
(ti-pran'a-veer)
Aptivus
*Func. class.:* Antiretroviral
*Chem. class.:* Protease inhibitor
**Pregnancy category** C

**Action:** Inhibits human immunodeficiency virus (HIV) protease; this prevents the maturation of virus

**Therapeutic outcome:** Prevent worsening of HIV

**Uses:** HIV in combination with other antiretrovirals

## Dosage and routes
Reduce dose in mild or moderate hepatic impairment and ketoconazole coadministration

*Adult:* PO 500 mg coadministered with ritonavir 200 mg bid with food

**Available forms:** Caps 250 mg

## Adverse effects
*CNS: Headache, insomnia,* dizziness, somnolence, fatigue
*GI: Diarrhea, abdominal pain, nausea, vomiting,* anorexia, dry mouth, **hepatitis B or C, fatalities when given with ritonavir**
*GU:* Nephrolithiasis
*INTEG:* Rash, urticaria, lipodystrophy
*MS:* Pain
*OTHER:* Asthenia, **insulin-resistant hyperglycemia,** hyperlipidemia, **ketoacidosis**

**Contraindications:** Hypersensitivity, hepatic disease (Child-Pugh B to C)

**Precautions:** Pregnancy **C**, breastfeeding, children, renal disease, history of renal stones, sulfa allergy, hemophilia, diabetes mellitus, pancreatitis

### Pharmacokinetics
| | |
|---|---|
| **Absorption** | Unknown |
| **Distribution** | Protein binding, 99.9%, steady state 7-10 days |
| **Metabolism** | CYP3A4 |
| **Excretion** | 80% feces |
| **Half-life** | Terminal 6 hr |

### Pharmacodynamics
Unknown

## Interactions
*Individual drugs*
Clarithromycin, zidovudine: increased levels of both products
Delavirdine, itraconazole, ketoconazole: increased tipranavir levels
Efavirenz, fluconazole, nevirapine: decreased tipranavir levels
Lovastatin, simvastatin: increased myopathy
◆Midazolam, rifampin, triazolam: life-threatening dysrhythmias
*Drug classifications*
◆ Ergots: life-threatening dysrhythmias
Oral contraceptives: increased levels of tipranavir
Rifamycins: decreased tipranavir levels
*Drug/herb*
St. John's wort: decreased tipranavir levels; avoid concurrent use
*Drug/food*
Grapefruit juice, high-fat, high-protein foods: decreased tipranavir absorption
*Drug/lab test*
Increased: AST, ALT

Adverse effects: *italic* = common, **bold** = life-threatening

## NURSING CONSIDERATIONS
### Assessment
• Monitor for complaints of lower back, flank pain; indicates kidney stones
• Assess for signs of infection, anemia, the presence of other STDs
• Assess for hepatic studies: ALT, AST; total bilirubin, amylase, all may be elevated
• Monitor viral load, CD4 during treatment
• Monitor bowel pattern before, during treatment; if severe abdominal pain with bleeding occurs, product should be discontinued; monitor hydration
• Monitor skin eruptions; rash, urticaria, itching
• Assess for allergies before treatment, reaction of each medication; place allergies on chart

### Nursing Diagnoses
• Infection, risk for (use, adverse reactions)
• Knowledge, deficient (teaching)

### Implementation
• Swallow cap whole; do not break, crush, or chew
• Give after meals
• Give in equal intervals around the clock to maintain blood levels

### Patient/family education
• Teach patient to take as prescribed; if dose is missed, take as soon as remembered up to 1 hr before next dose; do not double dose
• Teach patient that product must be taken in equal intervals around the clock to maintain blood levels for duration of therapy
◆ That hyperglycemia may occur; watch for increased thirst, weight loss, hunger, dry, itchy skin; notify prescriber
• Teach patient to increase fluids to prevent kidney stones, if stone formation occurs, treatment may need to be interrupted
• Advise patient that product does not cure AIDS, only controls symptoms; not to donate blood

### Evaluation
**Positive therapeutic outcome**
• Prevention of viral replication

---

**❗ HIGH ALERT**

# tirofiban (Rx)
(tie-roh-fee′ban)
Aggrastat
*Func. class.:* Antiplatelet
*Chem. class.:* Glycoprotein IIb/IIIa inhibitor

**Pregnancy category B**

**Action:** Antagonist of platelet glycoprotein (GP) IIb/IIIa receptor that leads to binding of fibrinogen and von Willebrand's factor, which inhibits platelet aggregation

**Therapeutic outcome:** Decreased platelet count

**Uses:** Acute coronary syndrome in combination with heparin

### Dosage and routes
*Adult:* IV 0.4 mcg/kg/min × 30 min, then 0.1 mcg/kg/min for 12-24 hr after angioplasty or atherectomy

*Renal dose*
*Adult:* IV CCr <30 ml/min 0.2 mcg/kg/min × 30 min, then 0.05 mcg/kg/min, during angiography and for up to 24 hr after angioplasty

**Available forms:** Inj for sol 250 mcg/ml, inj 50 mcg/ml

### Adverse effects
*CNS:* Dizziness, headache
*CV:* Bradycardia, hypotension
*GI:* Nausea, vomiting
*HEMA:* Bleeding, **thrombocytopenia**
*INTEG:* Rash
*MISC:* Dissection, coronary artery edema, pain in legs/pelvis, sweating

**Contraindications:** Hypersensitivity, active internal bleeding, stroke, major surgery, severe trauma, intracranial neoplasm, aneurysm, hemorrhage, acute pericarditis, platelets <100,000/mm$^3$, history of thrombocytopenia, coagulopathy

**Precautions:** Pregnancy **B**, breastfeeding, children, geriatric, renal disease, bleeding tendencies, hypertension

| Pharmacokinetics | |
|---|---|
| **Absorption** | Unknown |
| **Distribution** | Plasma clearance 20%-25% |
| **Metabolism** | Liver |
| **Excretion** | Urine/feces |
| **Half-life** | 2 hr |

| Pharmacodynamics | |
|---|---|
| Unknown | |

---

## Interactions
### Individual drugs
Abciximab, aspirin, cefamandole, cefoperazone, cefotetan, clopidogrel, dipyridamole, eptifibatide, heparin, ticlopidine, valproic acid: increased bleeding risk
### Drug classifications
NSAIDs: increased bleeding risk
### Drug/herb
Agrimony, alfalfa, angelica, anise, basil, bay, bilberry, black haw, bogbean, bromelain, buchu, chondroitin, cinchona bark, dong quai, fenugreek, feverfew, garlic, ginger, ginkgo, ginseng, green tea, horse chestnut, Irish moss, kelp, kelpware, khella, lovage, lungwort, meadowsweet, motherwort, mugwort, nettle, papaya, parsley (large amounts), pau d'arco, pineapple, poplar, prickly ash, safflower, saw palmetto, tonka bean, turmeric, wintergreen, yarrow: increased risk of bleeding
Chamomile, coenzyme Q10, flax, glucomannan, goldenseal, guar gum: decreased anticoagulant effect

## NURSING CONSIDERATIONS
### Assessment
- Monitor platelet counts, Hct, Hgb, before treatment, within 6 hr of loading dose and at least daily thereafter; watch for bleeding from puncture sites, catheters or in stools, urine

### Nursing diagnoses
- Tissue perfusion, ineffective (uses)

### Implementation
- Dilute inj: withdraw and discard 100 ml from a 500-ml bag of sterile 0.9% NaCl or $D_5$ and replace this vol with 100 ml of tirofiban inj from two vials
- Tirofiban inj for sol is premixed in containers of 500 ml 0.9% NaCl (50 mg/ml)
- Minimize other arterial/venous punctures IM inj, catheter use, intubation, to reduce bleeding risks
### Y-site compatibility: Heparin

### Patient/family education
- Advise patient that it is necessary to quit smoking to prevent excessive vasoconstriction

### Evaluation
**Positive therapeutic outcome**
- Treatment of acute coronary syndrome

---

## tizanidine (Rx)
(tye-za'na-deen)
Zanaflex
*Func. class.:* Skeletal muscle relaxant, central acting
*Chem. class.:* Imidazole
**Pregnancy category C**

**Action:** Unknown; possesses central $\alpha_2$-adrenergic agonist properties; reduces excitation of spinal cord interneurons; also acts on the basal ganglia, producing muscle relaxation

**Therapeutic outcome:** Decreased spasticity of muscles

**Uses:** Spinal cord injury, spasticity in multiple sclerosis, tension headache, symptoms of multiple sclerosis

### Dosage and routes
*Adult:* PO 4-8 mg q6-8hr increase gradually by 2-4 mg increments, may repeat q6-8hr up to 3 doses/24 hr, max 36 mg/day

**Available forms:** Tabs 2, 4 mg; caps 2, 4, 6 mg

### Adverse effects
*CNS: Dizziness,* somnolence, speech disorder, dyskinesia, nervousness, hallucination, psychosis
*CV:* Hypotension, bradycardia
*GI: Constipation, vomiting, dry mouth,* increased ALT, abnormal liver function tests
*GU:* Urinary frequency
*OTHER:* Blurred vision, pharyngitis, rhinitis, tremor, rash, muscle weakness

**Contraindications:** Hypersensitivity

**Precautions:** Pregnancy **C**, breastfeeding, children, geriatric, renal/hepatic disease, hypotension

| Pharmacokinetics | |
|---|---|
| **Absorption** | Complete |
| **Distribution** | Widely |
| **Metabolism** | Liver, extensively |
| **Excretion** | Kidneys, feces |
| **Half-life** | 2½ hr |

| Pharmacodynamics | |
|---|---|
| **Onset** | Unknown |
| **Peak** | 1-2 hr |
| **Duration** | 3-6 hr |

## Interactions
### Individual drugs
Alcohol: CNS depression
Amiodarone, ciprofloxacin, famotidine,

T

---

Adverse effects: *italic* = common, **bold** = life-threatening

fluvoxamine: increased tizanidine levels; do not use together

### Drug classifications

CNS depressants: increased CNS depression

Contraceptives (oral): decreased clearance of tizanidine

### Drug/lab test

Increased: AST, alkaline phosphatase, ALT, serum glucose

## NURSING CONSIDERATIONS

### Assessment

• Assess for muscle spasticity baseline and throughout treatment

• Monitor B/P, heart rate

• Perform neurologic exam in spasticity: deep tendon reflexes, muscle tone, clonus, sensory function

• Monitor renal/liver function tests, electrolytes, CBC with differential during long-term treatment

• Assess for allergic reactions: rash, fever, respiratory distress; severe weakness, numbness in extremities

• Assess CNS depression: dizziness, drowsiness, psychiatric symptoms

• Check dosage, as individual titration is required

### Nursing diagnoses

• Injury, risk for (adverse reactions)

• Knowledge, deficient (teaching)

• Mobility, impaired physical (uses)

### Implementation

• Give with meals for GI symptoms

• Store in airtight container at room temperature

• Give consistently either with or without food; food may affect absorption

• Titrate dose carefully

### Patient/family education

• Advise patient not to discontinue medication quickly; spasticity will occur; product should be tapered off over 1-2 wk

• Advise patient not to take with alcohol, other CNS depressants, take as directed, if dose is missed, take as soon as remembered, unless it is almost time for next dose

• Caution patient to avoid altering activities while taking this product; to avoid hazardous activities if drowsiness or dizziness occurs; to rise from sitting or lying slowly to prevent fainting

• Teach patient to use gum, frequent sips of water for dry mouth

• Advise patient to avoid using OTC medications (cough preparations, antihistamines) unless directed by prescriber

• Notify prescriber if fainting, hallucinations, dark urine, stomach pain, yellowing of skin/eyes occurs

### Evaluation

**Positive therapeutic outcome**

• Decreased pain, spasticity

---

### tobramycin (Rx)

(toe-bra-mye'sin)

Nebcin, tobramycin sulfate, TOBI

*Func. class.:* Antiinfective

*Chem. class.:* Aminoglycoside

### Pregnancy category  D

**Action:** Interferes with protein synthesis in bacterial cell by binding to ribosomal subunit, causing inaccurate peptide sequence to form in protein chain, causing bacterial death

**Therapeutic outcome:** Bactericidal effects for the following organisms: *Pseudomonas aeruginosa, Enterobacter, Escherichia coli, Providencia, Citrobacter, Staphylococcus, Proteus, Klebsiella, Serratia*

**Uses:** Severe systemic infections of CNS, respiratory, GI, urinary tract, bone, skin, soft tissues, eye, cystic fibrosis (nebulizer) for *P. aeruginosa*

### Dosage and routes

*Adult:* IM/**IV** 3 mg/kg/day in divided doses q8hr; may give up to 5 mg/kg/day in divided doses q6-8hr; once-daily dosing is an option

*Child:* IM/**IV** 6-7.5 mg/kg/day in 3-4 equal divided doses

*Child ≥6 yr:* NEB 300 mg bid in repeating cycles of 28 days on/28 days off; give inh over 10-15 min using a hand-held PARI LC PLUS reusable nebulizer with a DeVilbiss Pulmo-Aid compressor

*Neonate <1 wk:* IM up to 4 mg/kg/day in divided doses q12hr; **IV** up to 4 mg/kg/day in divided doses q12hr diluted in 50-100 mg NS or D₅W; give over 30-60 min

### Renal dose

*Adult:* IM/**IV** 1 mg/kg, then dose determined by blood levels

**Available forms:** Inj 10, 40 mg/ml; powder for inj 1.2 g; neb sol 300 mg/5 ml

### Adverse effects

*CNS:* Confusion, depression, numbness, tremors, **seizures,** muscle twitching, **neurotoxicity,** dizziness, vertigo

*CV:* Hypo/hypertension, palpitations

*EENT: Ototoxicity,* deafness, visual disturbances, tinnitus

---

*GI: Nausea, vomiting, anorexia,* increased ALT, AST, bilirubin, hepatomegaly, **hepatic necrosis,** splenomegaly
*GU:* **Oliguria, hematuria, renal damage, azotemia, renal failure, nephrotoxicity**
*HEMA:* **Agranulocytosis, thrombocytopenia, leukopenia, eosinophilia,** anemia
*INTEG: Rash,* burning, urticaria, dermatitis, alopecia

**Contraindications:** Pregnancy **D**, severe renal disease, hypersensitivity to aminoglycosides

**Precautions:** Breastfeeding, geriatric, neonates, mild renal disease, myasthenia gravis, hearing deficits, Parkinson's disease

### Pharmacokinetics

| | |
|---|---|
| **Absorption** | Well absorbed (IM), completely absorbed (**IV**) |
| **Distribution** | Widely distributed in extracellular fluids |
| **Metabolism** | Minimal—liver |
| **Excretion** | Mostly unchanged (>90%) kidneys |
| **Half-life** | 2-3 hr, increased in renal disease, neonates |

### Pharmacodynamics

| | IM | IV | OPHTH |
|---|---|---|---|
| **Onset** | Rapid | Rapid | Rapid |
| **Peak** | 1 hr | Inf end | Unknown |
| **Duration** | Unknown | Unknown | Unknown |

### Interactions
#### Individual drugs
Acyclovir, amphotericin B, bacitracin, cidofovir, cisplatin, ethacrynic acid, furosemide, mannitol, methoxyflurane, polymyxin, vancomycin: increased ototoxicity, neurotoxicity, nephrotoxicity
#### Drug classifications
Aminoglycosides, cephalosporins, penicillins: increased otoxicity, neurotoxicity, nephrotoxicity
#### Drug/herb
Acidophilus: do not use with antiinfectives; separate by several hours
Lysine (large amounts): increased toxicity

### NURSING CONSIDERATIONS
#### Assessment
• Assess patient for previous sensitivity reaction
#### Systemic route
• Assess patient for signs and symptoms of infection including characteristics of wounds, sputum, urine, stool WBC >10,000/mm$^3$, temp; baseline and during treatment
• Complete C&S testing before beginning product therapy to identify if correct treatment has been initiated
• Assess for allergic reactions: rash, urticaria, pruritus, chills, fever, joint pain
• Identify urine output; if decreasing, notify prescriber (may indicate nephrotoxicity); also, obtain BUN, creatinine, urine CCr (<80 ml/min) values; urinalysis daily for proteinuria, cells, casts; report sudden change in urine output
• Monitor blood studies: AST, ALT, CBC, Hct, bilirubin, LDH, alkaline phosphatase, Coombs' test monthly if patient is on long-term therapy
• Monitor electrolytes: potassium, sodium, chloride, magnesium monthly if patient is on long-term therapy
• Monitor for bleeding: ecchymosis, bleeding gums, hematuria, stool guaiac daily if patient is on long-term therapy
• Assess for overgrowth of infection: perineal itching, fever, malaise, redness, pain, swelling, drainage, rash, diarrhea, change in cough, sputum
• Obtain weight before treatment; calculation of dosage is usually based on ideal body weight, but may be calculated on actual body weight
• Monitor VS during infusion, watch for hypotension, change in pulse
• Assess **IV** site for thrombophlebitis including pain, redness, swelling q30 min, change site if needed; apply warm compresses to discontinued site
• Obtain serum peak, drawn at 30-60 min after **IV** inf or 60 min after IM inj, trough level drawn just before next dose; peak 4-12 mcg/ml, trough 1-2 mcg/ml
• Monitor for deafness by audiometric testing, ringing, roaring in ears, vertigo; assess hearing before, during, after treatment
• Monitor for dehydration: high specific gravity, decrease in skin turgor, dry mucous membranes, dark urine
• Monitor for overgrowth of infection including increased temp, malaise, redness, pain, swelling, perineal itching, diarrhea, stomatitis, change in cough, sputum

#### Nursing diagnoses
• Diarrhea (adverse reactions)
• Infection, risk for (uses)
• Injury, risk for (adverse reactions)
• Knowledge, deficient (teaching)
• Noncompliance (teaching)

T

## Implementation
**IM route**
- Give inj deeply in large muscle mass

**Nebulizer route**
- Give as close to q12hr apart as possible; do not use <6 hr apart
- Do not mix with dornase alfa in the nebulizer
- Inhale sitting or standing, breathe normally through the mouthpiece, may use nose clips

**IV route**
- Give **IV** diluted in 50-100 ml of 0.9% NaCl, $D_{10}W$, $D_5$/0.9% NaCl, 0.9% NaCl, Ringer's, LR, $D_5W$ (adult), infuse over 20-60 min
- Flush after inf with $D_5W$, 0.9% NaCl
- Separate aminoglycosides and penicillins by ≥1 hr

*Syringe compatibilities:* Doxapram
*Syringe incompatibilities:* Cefamandole, clindamycin, heparin, sargramostim
*Y-site compatibilities:* Acyclovir, amifostine, amiodarone, amsacrine, aztreonam, ciprofloxacin, cyclophosphamide, diltiazem, enalaprilat, esmolol, filgrastim, fluconazole, fludarabine, foscarnet, furosemide, granisetron, hydromorphone, IL-2, insulin (regular), labetalol, magnesium sulfate, melphalan, meperidine, midazolam, morphine, perphenazine, tacrolimus, teniposide, theophylline, thiotepa, tolazoline, vinorelbine, zidovudine
*Additive compatibilities:* Aztreonam, bleomycin, calcium gluconate, cefoxitin, ciprofloxacin, clindamycin, furosemide, metronidazole, ofloxacin, ranitidine, verapamil
*Additive incompatibilities:* Cefamandole, floxacillin

## Patient/family education
- Advise patient to use multiple therapies first, then tobramycin
- Teach patient to report sore throat, bruising, bleeding, joint pain; may indicate blood dyscrasias (rare)
- Advise patient to contact prescriber if vaginal itching, loose foul-smelling stools, furry tongue occur; may indicate superinfection
- Advise patient to notify prescriber of diarrhea with blood or pus; may indicate pseudomembranous colitis

## Evaluation
**Positive therapeutic outcome**
- Absence of signs/symptoms of infection (WBC <10,000/mm³, temp WNL, absence of red, draining wounds)
- Reported improvement in symptoms of infection

**Treatment of overdose:** Withdraw product, hemodialysis, exchange transfusion in the newborn, monitor serum levels of product, may give ticarcillin or carbenicillin

## tobramycin ophthalmic
*See Appendix D*

## tocainide (Rx)
(toe-kay'nide)
Tonocard
*Func. class.:* Antidysrhythmic (class IB)
*Chem. class.:* Lidocaine analog
**Pregnancy category C**

**Action:** Produces dose-dependent decreases in sodium and potassium conduction, thereby decreasing the excitability of myocardial cells; does not affect heart rate or B/P

**Therapeutic outcome:** Decreased ventricular dysrhythmia

**Uses:** Life-threatening ventricular dysrhythmias (multifocal/unifocal premature ventricular contractions [PVCs]), ventricular tachycardia

## Dosage and routes
*Adult:* PO 400 mg q8hr, may increase to 1.2-1.8 g/day in divided doses q8-12hr

**Available forms:** Tabs 400, 600 mg

## Adverse effects
***CNS:*** *Headache, dizziness,* involuntary movement, confusion, psychosis, restlessness, irritability, paresthesias, tremors, **seizures**
***CV:*** *Hypotension, bradycardia,* angina, PVCs, **heart block, CV collapse, sinus arrest, CHF,** chest pain, tachycardia, prodysrhythmias
***EENT:*** Tinnitus, blurred vision, hearing loss
***GI:*** Nausea, vomiting, anorexia, diarrhea, hepatitis
***HEMA:*** **Blood dyscrasias: leukopenia, agranulocytosis, hypoplastic anemia, thrombocytopenia,** bone marrow depression
***INTEG:*** Rash, urticaria, lupus, alopecia, sweating
***RESP:*** Dyspnea, **respiratory depression, pulmonary fibrosis,** pulmonary edema, interstitial pneumonitis pneumonia

**Contraindications:** Hypersensitivity to amides, severe heart block

**Precautions:** Pregnancy **C**, breastfeeding, children, geriatric, pulmonary/renal/hepatic disease, CHF, myasthenia gravis, blood dyscrasias, hypokalemia, atrial flutter/fibrillation

### Pharmacokinetics

| | |
|---|---|
| **Absorption** | Well absorbed |
| **Distribution** | Widely distributed, crossed blood-brain barrier |
| **Metabolism** | Liver |
| **Excretion** | Kidney (up to 40% unchanged) |
| **Half-life** | 10-17 hr |

### Pharmacodynamics

| | |
|---|---|
| **Onset** | 1 hr |
| **Peak** | ½-2 hr |
| **Duration** | 8-12 hr |

### Interactions
*Individual drugs*
Cimetidine, rifampin: decreased effects of tocainide
Metropolol: increased tocainide effects
*Drug/herb*
Aconite: increased toxicity, death
Aloe, broom, buckthorn (chronic use), cascara sagrada (chronic use), Chinese rhubarb, figwort, fumitory, goldenseal, kudzu, licorice: increased effect
Coltsfoot: decreased effect
Horehound: increased serotonin effect
*Drug/lab test*
Increased: CPK
False positive: ANA titer

### NURSING CONSIDERATIONS
**Assessment**
• Assess for oxygenation or perfusion deficit: decreased B/P, chest pain, dizziness, loss of consciousness
• Assess respiratory status: auscultate lung fields for bibasilar crackles in patients with advanced CHF
• Assess for urinary retention: check for pain, abdominal absorption, palpate bladder; check males with benign prostatic hypertrophy; anticholinergic reaction may cause retention
• Monitor I&O ratio; electrolytes (potassium, sodium, chloride); watch for decreasing urinary output, possible retention
• Monitor liver function tests: AST, ALT, bilirubin, alkaline phosphatase
• Monitor ECG to determine product effectiveness; measure PR, QRS, QT intervals; check for PVCs, other dysrhythmias; monitor B/P for hypotension, hypertension; for rebound hypertension after 1-2 hr
• Monitor patient for CNS symptoms: confusion, psychosis, numbness, depression,

involuntary movements; if these occur, product should be discontinued
• Assess pulmonary toxicity: dyspnea, fatigue, cough, fever, chest pain; product should be discontinued if these occur
• Assess cardiac rate, respiration (rate, rhythm, character), chest pain, ventricular tachycardia, supraventricular tachycardia or fibrillation

**Nursing diagnoses**
• Cardiac output, decreased (uses)
• Gas exchange, impaired (adverse reactions)
• Knowledge, deficient (teaching)

**Implementation**
• Give with meals to decrease GI upset

**Patient/family education**
• Inform patient or family of reason for medication and expected results
• Teach patient method for taking pulse at home and what to report to prescriber
• Advise patient to avoid hazardous activities until product response is known; dizziness, confusion, sedation may occur
• Advise patient to carry/wear emergency ID indicating medications taken, condition, and prescriber's name and phone number
• Instruct patient to report bleeding, bruising, respiratory symptoms, chills, fever, sore throat to prescriber

**Evaluation**
**Positive therapeutic outcome**
• Decreased dysrhythmias

**Treatment of overdose:** Defibrillation, vasopressor for hypotension

---

## tolcapone (Rx)
(toll'cah-pone)
Tasmar
*Func. class.:* Antiparkinson agent
*Chem. class.:* Catecholamine inhibitor (COMT)
**Pregnancy category C**

**Action:** Selective, reversible inhibitor of catecholamine; used as adjunct to levodopa/carbidopa therapy

**Therapeutic outcome:** Increased ability to move and speak

**Uses:** Parkinsonism

**Dosage and routes**
*Adult:* PO 100-200 mg tid, with levodopa/carbidopa therapy; max 600 mg/day; discontinue if no benefit in 3 wk

T

### Renal dose
*Adult:* PO 100 mg tid or less

**Available forms:** Tabs 100, 200 mg

### Adverse effects
*CNS:* Dystonia, dyskinesia, dreaming, *fatigue, headache, confusion,* psychosis, hallucination, dizziness

*CV: Orthostatic hypotension,* chest pain, hypotension

*EENT:* Cataract, eye inflammation

*GI: Nausea, vomiting, abdominal distress,* diarrhea, constipation, **fatal liver failure,** elevated liver function tests

*GU:* UTI, urine discoloration, uterine tumor, micturition disorder, hematuria

*HEMA:* **Hemolytic anemia, leukopenia, agranulocytosis**

*INTEG:* Sweating, alopecia

**Contraindications:** Hypersensitivity

**Precautions:** Pregnancy **C,** breastfeeding, cardiac/renal/hepatic disease, hypertension, asthma

| Pharmacokinetics | |
|---|---|
| **Absorption** | Rapidly |
| **Distribution** | Protein binding 99% |
| **Metabolism** | Liver (extensively) |
| **Excretion** | Urine (60%), feces (40%) |
| **Half-life** | 2-3 hr |

| Pharmacodynamics | |
|---|---|
| **Onset** | Unknown |
| **Peak** | 2 hr |
| **Duration** | Unknown |

### Interactions
*Individual drugs*
Apomorphine, DOBUTamine, isoproterenol, α-methyldopa: may influence pharmacokinetics

*Drug classifications*
MAOIs: decreased normal catecholamine metabolism; MAO-B inhibitor may be used

*Drug/herb*
Kava: decreased effect

### NURSING CONSIDERATIONS
**Assessment**
• Monitor liver function tests: AST, ALT, alkaline phosphatase, LDH, bilirubin, CBC
• Assess involuntary movements in parkinsonism: akinesia, tremors, staggering gait, muscle rigidity, drooling
• Monitor B/P, respiration during initial treatment; hypo/hypertension should be reported

• Monitor mental status: affect, mood, behavioral changes

### Nursing diagnoses
• Injury, risk for (uses)
• Knowledge, deficient (teaching)
• Mobility, impaired physical (uses)

### Implementation
• Administer tid with levodopa/carbidopa therapy
• Food taken within 1 hr before or 2 hr after meals increases action of product by 20%
• Provide assistance with ambulation during beginning therapy

### Patient/family education
• Advise patient to change positions slowly to prevent orthostatic hypotension
• Advise patient that urine, sweat may change color
• Teach patient to report nausea, vomiting, anorexia

### Evaluation
**Positive therapeutic outcome**
• Decrease in akathisia, increased mood

---

## tolnaftate topical
*See Appendix D*

---

## tolterodine (Rx)
(tol-tehr'oh-deen)
Detrol, Detrol LA
*Func. class.:* Overactive bladder product
*Chem. class.:* Muscarinic receptor antagonist

**Pregnancy category** C

**Action:** Relaxes smooth muscles in urinary tract by inhibiting acetylcholine at postganglionic sites

**Therapeutic outcome:** Decreased symptoms of overactive bladder

**Uses:** Overactive bladder (frequency, urgency)

### Dosage and routes
*Adult:* PO 2 mg bid, hepatic disease 1 mg bid; EXT REL 4 mg/day, may decrease to 2 mg if needed, max 4 mg/day

### Renal dose
*Adult:* PO CCr ≤30 ml/min reduce by 50%

**Available forms:** Tabs 1, 2 mg; ext rel caps 2, 4 mg

---

## Adverse effects

**CNS:** *Anxiety,* paresthesia, fatigue, *dizziness,* headache, increasing dementia, memory impairment
**CV:** Chest pain, hypertension
**EENT:** Vision abnormalities, xerophthalmia
**GI:** *Nausea, vomiting, anorexia,* abdominal pain, constipation, dry mouth, dyspepsia
**GU:** Dysuria, retention, frequency, UTI
**INTEG:** Rash, pruritus
**RESP:** Bronchitis, cough, pharyngitis, upper respiratory tract infection
**SYST: Angioedema**

**Contraindications:** Hypersensitivity, uncontrolled angle-closure glaucoma, urinary retention, gastric retention

**Precautions:** Pregnancy C, breastfeeding, children, renal/hepatic disease, controlled angle-closure glaucoma, bladder obstruction, QT prolongation

### Pharmacokinetics

| | |
|---|---|
| **Absorption** | Rapidly |
| **Distribution** | Highly protein bound |
| **Metabolism** | Liver (extensively) |
| **Excretion** | Urine/feces |
| **Half-life** | Unknown |

### Pharmacodynamics
Unknown

## Interactions
### Drug classifications
Antibiotics (macrolide), antifungal agents, antiretroviral protease inhibitors: increased action of tolterodine
Antimuscarinics: increased anticholinergic effect
Diuretics: increased urinary frequency
### Drug/food
Increased: bioavailability of tolterodine

## NURSING CONSIDERATIONS
### Assessment
• Assess urinary patterns: distension, nocturia, frequency, urgency, incontinence
• Assess allergic reactions: rash; if this occurs, product should be discontinued

### Nursing diagnoses
• Activity intolerance (uses)
• Incontinence, functional urinary (uses)
• Knowledge, deficient (teaching)
• Urinary elimination, impaired (uses)

### Implementation
• Swallow whole; give with liquids

## Patient/family education
• Advise patient to avoid hazardous activities; dizziness may occur
• Advise patient not to drink liquids before bedtime
• Teach patient importance of bladder maintenance
• Teach patient to take with liquids; swallow whole

## Evaluation
### Positive therapeutic outcome
• Decreased urinary frequency, urgency

---

## topiramate (Rx)
(to-pi-ra′mate)
Topamax
*Func. class.:* Anticonvulsant—miscellaneous
*Chem. class.:* Monosaccharide derivative

### Pregnancy category  C

**Action:** Increase GABA activity; may prevent seizure spread as opposed to an elevation of seizure threshold

**Therapeutic outcome:** Absence of seizures

**Uses:** Partial seizures in adults and children 2-16 yr old; tonic-clonic seizures; seizures in Lennox-Gastaut syndrome

**Unlabeled uses:** Infantile spasms

### Dosage and routes
#### Adjunctive therapy
**Adult:** PO 25-50 mg/day initially, titrate by 25-50 mg/wk, up to 400 mg/day in 2 divided doses

#### Renal dose
**Adult:** PO CCr <70 ml/min ½ dose

**Available forms:** Tabs 25, 100, 200 mg; sprinkle caps 15, 25 mg

### Adverse effects
**CNS:** Dizziness, fatigue, cognitive disorder, *insomnia,* anxiety, depression, paresthesia, motor retardation
**EENT:** Diplopia, vision abnormality
**GI:** *Diarrhea, anorexia,* nausea, dyspepsia, abdominal pain, constipation, dry mouth, **pancreatitis**
**GU:** Breast pain, dysmenorrhea, menstrual disorder
**INTEG:** Rash
**MISC:** Weight loss, leukopenia, metabolic acidosis, increased body temperature

T

---

Adverse effects: *italic* = common, **bold** = life-threatening

*RESP:* Upper respiratory tract infection, pharyngitis

**Contraindications:** Hypersensitivity, metabolic acidosis

**Precautions:** Pregnancy **C,** breastfeeding, children, renal/hepatic disease, acute myopia, secondary angle-closure glaucoma, behavioral disorders

### Pharmacokinetics

| | |
|---|---|
| **Absorption** | Well absorbed |
| **Distribution** | Crosses placenta, plasma protein binding (9%-17%), steady state 4 days |
| **Metabolism** | Unknown |
| **Excretion** | Kidneys unchanged 55%-97% |
| **Half-life** | 19-25 hr |

### Pharmacodynamics

| | |
|---|---|
| **Onset** | Unknown |
| **Peak** | 2-4 hr |
| **Duration** | Unknown |

### Interactions
*Individual drugs*
Alcohol: increased CNS depression
Carbamazepine, phenytoin, probenecid: decreased levels of topiramate
Digoxin: decreased levels of digoxin
Metformin: increased topiramate levels
Valproic acid: decreased levels of both products
*Drug classifications*
Carbonic anhydrase inhibitors: increased kidney stone formation
Contraceptives, oral: decreased level of oral contraceptives
CNS depressants: increased CNS depression
*Drug/herb*
Ginkgo: increased effect
Ginseng, santonica: decreased effect

### NURSING CONSIDERATIONS
Assessment
• Assess mental status: mood, sensorium, affect, memory (long, short), especially in geriatric
• Assess for blood dyscrasias: fever, sore throat, bruising, rash, jaundice, epistaxis (long-term treatment only)
• Assess seizure activity including type, location, duration, and character; provide seizure precaution
• Monitor CBC during long-term therapy
• Assess body weight and evidence of cognitive disorder

### Nursing diagnoses
• Injury, risk for (side effects)
• Knowledge, deficient (teaching)
### Implementation
• Do not break, crush, or chew tabs; very bitter
• May take without regard to meals
• Sprinkle cap can be given whole or opened and sprinkled on soft food; do not chew
### Patient/family education
• Teach patient to carry/wear emergency ID stating name, products taken, condition, prescriber's name and phone number
• Advise patient to avoid driving, other activities that require alertness
• Teach patient not to discontinue medication abruptly after long-term use
### Evaluation
**Positive therapeutic outcome**
• Decreased seizure activity
**Treatment of overdose:** Lavage, VS

---

### ! HIGH ALERT

## topotecan (Rx)
(to-poe'ti-kan)
Hycamtin
*Func. class:* Antineoplastic natural
*Chem. class:* Camptothecin analog
**Pregnancy category D**

**Action:** Antitumor product with topo-isomerase I–inhibitory activity; topoisomerase I relieves torsional strain in DNA by causing single-strand breaks; causes double-strand DNA damage

**Therapeutic outcome:** Decreased tumor size

**Uses:** Metastatic ovarian cancer after failure of traditional chemotherapy, relapsed small cell lung cancer, cervical cancer

### Dosage and routes
*Adult:* **IV** INF 1.5 mg/m² over 30 min/day × 5 days starting on day 1 of a 21-day course × 4 courses; may be reduced to 0.25 mg/m² for subsequent courses if severe neutropenia occurs; PO 2.3 mg/m²/day on days 1-5 of a 21-day course (relapsed small cell lung cancer in those with prior response)

*Renal dose*
*Adult:* **IV** CCr 20-39 ml/min 0.75 mg/m²/day × 5 days on day 1 of a 21-day course

**Available forms:** lyophilized powder for inj 4 mg; cap 0.25, 1 mg

---

 Alert      Canada Only      Drug on CD          * "Tall Man" lettering (See Preface)

## Adverse effects

*CNS:* Arthralgia, asthenia, headache, myalgia, pain, weakness
*GI:* Abdominal pain, constipation, diarrhea, obstruction, nausea, stomatitis, vomiting, increased ALT, AST, anorexia
**HEMA: Neutropenia, leukopenia, thrombocytopenia, anemia, sepsis**
*INTEG:* Total alopecia
*RESP:* Dyspnea, cough

**Contraindications:** Pregnancy **D**, breastfeeding, hypersensitivity, severe bone marrow depression

**Precautions:** Children, renal disease

### Pharmacokinetics

| | |
|---|---|
| **Absorption** | Rapidly/completely |
| **Distribution** | 7%-35% protein binding |
| **Metabolism** | Liver |
| **Excretion** | Urine, feces to metabolites |
| **Half-life** | 2.8 hr |

### Pharmacodynamics
Unknown

## Interactions
### Individual drugs
Cisplatin: increased myelosuppression
Granulocyte colony-stimulating factor: increased duration of neutropenia

### Drug classifications
Anticoagulants, NSAIDs, platelet inhibitors, thrombolytics: increased bleeding risk
P-glycoprotein, breast cancer resistance protein inhibitors (amiodarone, clarithromycin, diltiazem, erythromycin, indinavir, itraconazole, mefloquine, niCARdipine, quinidine, RU-486, tamoxifen, testosterone, verapamil: avoid using together

## NURSING CONSIDERATIONS
### Assessment
• Monitor liver function tests: AST, ALT, alkaline phosphatase, which may be elevated
• Monitor CBC, differential, platelet count weekly; withhold product if WBC is <3500/mm³ or platelet count is <100,000/mm³; notify prescriber of these results; product should be discontinued
• Assess buccal cavity for dryness, sores or ulceration, white patches, oral pain, bleeding, dysphagia
• Assess GI symptoms: frequency of stools, cramping

• Assess signs of dehydration: rapid respiration, poor skin turgor, decreased urine output, dry skin, restlessness, weakness

### Nursing diagnoses
• Infection, risk for (adverse reactions)
• Knowledge, deficient (teaching)

### Implementation
• Provide increased fluid intake to 2-3 L/day to prevent dehydration, unless contraindicated
• Change **IV** site q48hr

### Patient/family education
• Advise patient to avoid foods with citric acid or hot or rough texture if stomatitis is present; to drink adequate fluids
• Provide patient with nutritious diet of iron, vit K supplements, low fiber, few dairy products
• Advise patient that total alopecia may occur; hair grows back but may be different in color and texture
• Advise patient to report stomatitis; any bleeding, white spots, ulcerations in mouth; tell patient to examine mouth daily; report symptoms
• Assess patient to report signs of anemia; fatigue, headache, faintness, shortness of breath, irritability
• Teach patient to rinse mouth tid-qid with water, club soda; brush teeth bid-tid with soft brush or cotton-tipped applicator for stomatitis; use unwaxed dental floss
• Teach patient to use effective contraception during treatment, avoid breastfeeding
• Advise patient to avoid OTC products without approval of prescriber

### Evaluation
**Positive therapeutic outcome**
• Decreased tumor size, spread of malignancy

## toremifene (Rx)
(tore′me-feen)
Fareston
*Func. class.:* Antineoplastic
*Chem. class.:* Antiestrogen hormone
**Pregnancy category D**

**Action:** Inhibits cell division by binding to cytoplasmic estrogen receptors; resembles normal cell complex but inhibits DNA synthesis and estrogen response of target tissue

**Therapeutic outcome:** Prevention of rapidly growing malignant cells

**Uses:** Advanced breast carcinoma that has not responded to other therapy in estrogen-receptor-positive patients (usually postmenopausal)

## Dosage and routes
*Adult:* PO 60 mg/day

## Available forms: Tabs 60 mg

## Adverse effects
*CNS:* Hot flashes, headache, lightheadedness, depression
*CV:* Chest pain, **CHF**, **MI**, **PE**, chest pain, angina
*EENT:* Ocular lesions, retinopathy, corneal opacity, blurred vision (high doses)
*GI:* Nausea, vomiting, altered taste (anorexia)
*GU:* Vaginal bleeding, pruritus vulvae
*HEMA:* **Thrombocytopenia, leukopenia**
*INTEG:* Rash, alopecia
*META:* Hypercalcemia

**Contraindications:** Pregnancy **D**, hypersensitivity, history of thromboembolism

**Precautions:** Breastfeeding, children, leukopenia, thrombocytopenia, cataracts, hypercalcemia, leukopenia, hepatic disease, thrombocytopenia

### Pharmacokinetics

| | |
|---|---|
| **Absorption** | Adequately absorbed |
| **Distribution** | 99% protein binding |
| **Metabolism** | Liver, extensively |
| **Excretion** | Feces, slowly, small amounts (kidneys) |
| **Half-life** | Terminal 5-6 days |

### Pharmacodynamics

| | |
|---|---|
| **Onset** | Unknown |
| **Peak** | 3 hr |
| **Duration** | Unknown |

## Interactions
### Individual drugs
Warfarin: increased warfarin effect
### Drug classifications
CYP3A4 inducers (barbiturates, bosentan, carbamazepine, efavirenz, phenytoins, nevirapine, rifabutin, rifampin): decreased toremifene effect
CYP3A4 inhibitors (aprepitant, antiretroviral protease inhibitors, clarithromycin, danazol, delivirdine, diltiazem, erythromycin, fluconazole, fluoxetine, fluvoxamine, imatinib, ketoconazole, mibefradil, nefazodone, telithromycin, voriconazole): increased toxicity
### Drug/herb
St. John's wort: avoid use

### Drug/lab test
Increased: serum Ca

## NURSING CONSIDERATIONS
### Assessment
• Monitor CBC, differential, platelet count weekly; withhold product if WBC is <4000/mm$^3$ or platelet count is <75,000/mm$^3$; notify prescriber of results; monitor calcium levels (hypercalcemia is common)
• Assess for tumor flare: increase in bone, tumor pain during beginning treatment; give analgesics as ordered to decrease pain
• Assess for bleeding: hematuria, guaiac, bruising or petechiae, mucosa or orifices q8hr, no rectal temp

### Nursing diagnoses
• Injury, risk for (adverse reactions)
• Knowledge, deficient (teaching)

### Implementation
• Do not break, crush, or chew tabs
• Give with food or fluids to decrease GI upset; repeat dose may be needed if vomiting occurs
• Store in light-resistant container at room temperature

### Patient/family education
• Instruct patient to report any complaints, side effects to prescriber; if dose is missed, do not double next dose
• Advise patient that vaginal bleeding, pruritus, hot flashes can occur and are reversible after discontinuing treatment
• Instruct patient to report immediately decreased visual acuity, which may be irreversible; stress need for routine eye exams
• Inform patient about who should be told about toremifene therapy
• Advise patient to report vaginal bleeding immediately; that tumor flare (increase in size of tumor, increased bone pain) may occur and will subside rapidly; may take analgesics for pain; that premenopausal women must use mechanical birth control method because ovulation may be induced (teratogenic product)
• Caution patient to use sunscreen and protective clothing to prevent burns because photosensitivity is common
• Teach patient that hair loss may occur during treatment; a wig or hairpiece may make patient feel better; new hair may be different in color, texture
• Inform patient rash or lesions are temporary and may become large during beginning therapy

 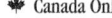

## Evaluation
**Positive therapeutic outcome**
• Decreased spread of malignant cells in breast cancer

---

## trace elements (chromium, copper, iodide, manganese, selenium, zinc) (Rx)
Concentrated Multiple Trace Elements, ConTE-PAK-4, M.T.E.-4, M.T.E.-4 Concentrated, M.T.E.-5, M.T.E.-5 Concentrated, M.T.E.-6, M.T.E.-6 Concentrated, M.T.E.-7, MulTE-PAK-4, MulTE-PAK-5, Multiple Trace Element, Multiple Trace Element Neonatal, Multiple Trace Element Pediatric, Neotrace 4, Ped TE-PAK-4, Pedtrice-4, P.T.E.-4, P.T.E.-5
*Func. class.:* Mineral supplement

### Pregnancy category C

**Action:** Needed for adequate absorption and synthesis of amino acids

**Therapeutic outcome:** Replacement for mineral deficiencies

**Uses:** Prevention of trace element deficiency, a component of TPN

### Dosage and routes
Usual dosage may be given in TPN sol

*Chromium*
*Adult:* **IV** 10-15 mcg/day
*Child:* **IV** 0.14-0.20 mcg/ kg/day

*Copper*
*Adult:* **IV** 0.5-1.5 mg/day
*Child:* **IV** 0.05-0.2 mg/kg/day

*Iodide*
*Adult:* **IV** 1 mcg/kg/day

*Manganese*
*Adult:* **IV** 0.15-0.8 mg/day

*Selenium*
*Adult:* **IV** 20-40 mcg/day
*Child:* **IV** 3 mcg/kg/day

*Zinc*
*Adult:* **IV** 2-4 mg/day
*Child:* **IV** 0.05 mg/kg/day

**Available forms:** Many forms available; see particular elements

### Adverse effects
*CHROMIUM:* **Seizures, coma,** nausea, vomiting, ulcers, **renal/hepatic toxicity**
*COPPER:* Personality changes, diarrhea, weakness, photophobia, muscle weakness

*IODINE:* Headache, edema of eyelids, acne, metallic taste, sore mouth, runny nose
*MANGANESE:* Incoordination, headache, irritability, lability, slurred speech, impotence
*SELENIUM:* Alopecia, depression, vomiting, GI cramping, nervousness, garlic smell
*ZINC:* Vomiting, oliguria, **hypothermia,** vision changes, **tachycardia,** jaundice, **coma**

**Precautions:** Pregnancy **C,** breastfeeding, liver, biliary disease, vomiting or diarrhea

### Pharmacokinetics
| | |
|---|---|
| **Absorption** | Completely absorbed |
| **Distribution** | Widely distributed |
| **Metabolism** | Unknown |
| **Excretion** | Depends on element |
| **Half-life** | Unknown |

### Pharmacodynamics
Unknown

## NURSING CONSIDERATIONS
### Assessment
• Assess trace element levels; notify prescriber if low copper 0.07-0.15 mg/ml, zinc 0.05-0.15 mg/100 ml, manganese 4-20 mcg/100 ml, selenium 0.1-0.19 mcg/ml
• Assess trace element deficiency if patient is receiving TPN for extended period
• Obtain calorie count to identify nutritional deficiencies
• Assess for toxicity to individual element (see Adverse effects)

### Nursing diagnoses
• Knowledge, deficient (teaching)
• Nutrition: less than body requirements, imbalanced (uses)

### Implementation
• Give by **IV** inf, often mixed with TPN sol
• Discard unused portions
• Give by continuous inf diluted in 1 L or more **IV** sol; give at prescribed rate

### Patient/family education
• Explain to patient reason for and expected results of medication

### Evaluation
**Positive therapeutic outcome**
• Absence of element deficiency

T

---

Adverse effects: *italic* = common, **bold** = life-threatening

## tramadol (Rx)
(trah'mah-dol)

Raliva ER, Raliva Flashdose, Ultram, Ultram ER, Ultram ODT

*Func. class.:* Analgesic, miscellaneous

**Pregnancy category C**

### Do not confuse:
tramadol/Toradol

**Action:** Not completely understood, binds to opioid receptors and inhibits reuptake of norepinephrine, serotonin; does not cause histamine release or affect heart rate

**Therapeutic outcome:** Relief of pain

**Uses:** Management of moderate to severe pain

### Dosage and routes
*Mild to moderate pain*
**Adult:** PO 50-100 mg prn q4-6hr, max 400 mg/day
**Geriatric >75 yr:** PO <300 mg/day in divided dose

*Hepatic dose*
**Adult:** PO 50 mg q12hr

*Renal dose*
**Adult:** PO CCr <30 ml/min q12hr, max 200 mg/day

*Moderate to severe pain*
**Adult:** PO-ER 100 mg, titrate upward q5 days by 100 mg, max 300 mg/day

**Available forms:** Tabs 50 mg; ext rel tab 100, 200, 300 mg; orally disintegrating tab 50 mg

### Adverse effects
***CNS:*** Dizziness, CNS stimulation, somnolence, headache, anxiety, confusion, euphoria, **seizures,** hallucinations, flushing, sedation
***CV:*** Vasodilatation, orthostatic hypotension, tachycardia, hypertension, abnormal ECG
***EENT:*** Visual disturbances
***GI:*** Nausea, constipation, vomiting, dry mouth, diarrhea, abdominal pain, anorexia, flatulence, GI bleeding
***GU:*** Urinary retention/frequency, menopausal symptoms, dysuria, menstrual disorder
***INTEG:*** Pruritus, rash, urticaria, vesicles
***SYST:*** **Anaphylaxis, Stevens-Johnson syndrome, toxic epidermal necrolysis, serotonin syndrome**

**Contraindications:** Hypersensitivity, acute intoxication with any CNS depressant

**Precautions:** Pregnancy **C,** breastfeeding, children, geriatric, seizure disorder, renal/ hepatic disease, respiratory depression, head trauma, increased ICP, acute abdominal condition, product abuse

### Pharmacokinetics
| | |
|---|---|
| **Absorption** | Rapidly, almost completely absorbed |
| **Distribution** | Steady state 2 days |
| **Metabolism** | Extensively in liver, may cross blood-brain barrier |
| **Excretion** | Unchanged product 30% in urine |
| **Half-life** | Unknown |

### Pharmacodynamics
Unknown

### Interactions
*Individual drugs*
Alcohol: increased CNS depression
Carbamazepine: decreased tramadol level
*Drug classifications*
CYP3A4 inducers (barbiturates, bosentan, carbamazepine, efavirenz, nevirapine, phenytoin, rifabutin, rifampin): decreased tramadol effect
CYP3A4 inhibitors (aprepitant, antiretroviral protease inhibitors, clarithromycin, danazol, delavirdine, diltiazem, erythromycin, fluconazole, fluoxetine, fluvoxamine, imatinib, ketoconazole, mibefradil, nefazodone, telithromycin, voriconazole): increased tramadol levels
MAOIs: inhibition of norepinephrine and serotonin reuptake; use together with caution
Opiates, sedative/hypnotics: increased CNS depression
Selective serotonin reuptake inhibitors: increased serotonin syndrome
*Drug/herb*
Chamomile, hops, kava, skullcap, valerian: increased CNS depression
St. John's wort: avoid use
*Drug/lab test*
Increased: creatinine, liver enzymes
Decreased: Hgb

### NURSING CONSIDERATIONS
**Assessment**
• Assess pain: location, type, character; give before pain becomes extreme
• Assess for increased side effects in renal/ hepatic disease
• Monitor I&O ratio: check for decreasing output; may indicate urinary retention
• Assess need for product

 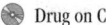

- Assess for constipation and bowel pattern; increase fluids, bulk in diet
- Monitor CNS changes: dizziness, drowsiness, hallucinations, euphoria, LOC, pupil reaction
- Determine allergic reactions: rash, urticaria

## Nursing diagnoses
- Injury, risk for (adverse reactions)
- Knowledge, deficient (teaching)
- Pain, acute (uses)
- Pain, chronic (uses)
- Sensory perception, disturbed: visual, auditory (adverse reactions)

## Implementation
- Do not break, crush, or chew ER product
- Give with antiemetic for nausea, vomiting
- Administer when pain is beginning to return; determine dosage interval by patient response
- Store in cool environment, protect from sunlight

## Patient/family education
- Teach patient to report any symptoms of CNS changes, allergic reactions
- Teach patient that drowsiness, dizziness, and confusion may occur; to call for assistance
- Instruct patient to make position changes slowly; orthostatic hypotension may occur
- Tell patient to avoid OTC medication and alcohol unless approved by prescriber

## Evaluation
**Positive therapeutic outcome**
- Decreased pain

## trandolapril (Rx)
(tran-doe'la-prill)
Mavik
*Func. class.:* Antihypertensive
*Chem. class.:* Angiotensin-converting enzyme (ACE) inhibitor

### Pregnancy category D

**Action:** Selectively suppresses renin-angiotensin-aldosterone system; inhibits ACE; prevents conversion of angiotensin I to angiotensin II, resulting in dilatation of arterial and venous vessels and lowered B/P

**Therapeutic outcome:** Decreased B/P in hypertension

**Uses:** Hypertension alone or in combination, heart failure, after MI/left ventricular dysfunction after MI

## Dosage and routes
### Hypertension
*Adult:* PO 1 mg/day, 2 mg/day in African Americans, make dosage adjustment ≥wk; up to 8 mg/day

### Heart failure (after MI/left ventricular dysfunction)
*Adult:* PO 1 mg/day, titrate upward to 4 mg/day if tolerated

### Renal dose/hepatic dose
*Adult:* PO CCr <30 ml/min 0.5 mg/day, may increase gradually up to 4 mg/day

**Available forms:** Tabs 1, 2, 4 mg

## Adverse effects
*CNS: Dizziness,* paresthesias, headache, *syncope,* fatigue, drowsiness, depression, sleep disturbances, anxiety
*CV: Hypotension,* **MI,** palpitations, angina, TIAs, **stroke,** bradycardia, dysrhythmias
*GI:* Nausea, vomiting, cramps, diarrhea, constipation, pancreatitis, *dyspepsia*
*GU:* **Proteinuria, renal failure**
*HEMA:* **Agranulocytosis, neutropenia, leukopenia,** anemia
*INTEG:* Rash, purpura, pruritus
*MISC:* Hyperkalemia, hyponatremia, impotence, *myalgia,* **angioedema,** muscle cramps, asthenia, hypocalcemia, gout
*RESP:* Dyspnea, cough

**Contraindications:** Pregnancy **D**, hypersensitivity, history of angioedema

**Precautions:** Geriatric, hyperkalemia, hepatic disease, bilateral renal stenosis, post kidney transplant, aortal/mitral valve stenosis, cirrhosis, severe renal disease, untreated CHF, autoimmune diseases, cough

### Pharmacokinetics
| | |
|---|---|
| Absorption | 40-60% |
| Distribution | Unknown |
| Metabolism | Liver |
| Excretion | Kidneys, feces |
| Half-life | 0.6-1.1 hr, 16-24 hr |

### Pharmacodynamics
| | |
|---|---|
| Onset | ½ hr |
| Peak | 4-10 hr |
| Duration | >8 days |

## Interactions
### Individual drugs
Levodopa, reserpine: increased effect of each specific product

*Drug classifications*
Antacids, NSAIDs, salicylates: decreased effect of trandolapril
Antihypertensives, diuretics: increased severe hypotension
Barbiturates, ergots, hypoglycemics, neuromuscular blocking agents: increased effects of each specific product
Diuretics (potassium-sparing): increased potassium levels
Phenothiazines: increased antihypertensive effects
Potassium supplements: increased potassium levels
Salt substitutes: increased potassium levels

*Drug/herb*
Aconite: increased toxicity, death
Astragalus, cola tree: increased or decreased antihypertensive effect
Barberry, betony, black catechu, black cohosh, bloodroot, broom, burdock, cat's claw, dandelion, goldenseal, Irish moss, Jamaican dogwood, kelp, khella, mistletoe, parsley: increased antihypertensive effect
Coltsfoot, guarana, khat, licorice, yohimbe: decreased antihypertensive effect

**NURSING CONSIDERATIONS**
**Assessment**
• Monitor blood tests: neutrophils, decreased platelets
• Monitor B/P, orthostatic hypotension, syncope; if changes occur dosage change may be required
• Monitor renal studies: protein, BUN, creatinine; increased levels may indicate nephrotic syndrome and renal failure
• Monitor renal symptoms: polyuria, oliguria, frequency, dysuria
• Establish baselines in renal, liver function tests before therapy begins
• Check potassium levels throughout treatment, although hyperkalemia rarely occurs
• Check for edema in feet, legs daily
• Assess for allergic reactions: rash, fever, pruritus, urticaria; product should be discontinued if antihistamines fail to help

**Nursing diagnoses**
• Cardiac output, decreased (uses)
• Injury, risk for (adverse reactions)
• Knowledge, deficient (teaching)
• Noncompliance (teaching)

**Implementation**
• Store in airtight container at ≤77° F (≤25° C) or less

**Patient/family education**
• Advise patient not to discontinue product abruptly; advise patient to tell all persons associated with health care
• Teach patient not to use OTC products (cough, cold, allergy medications) unless directed by physician; serious side effects can occur; xanthines, such as coffee, tea, chocolate, cola, can prevent action of product
• Instruct patient on the importance of complying with dosage schedule, even if feeling better; to continue with medical regimen to decrease B/P: exercise, cessation of smoking, decreasing stress, diet modifications
• Emphasize the need to rise slowly to sitting or standing position to minimize orthostatic hypotension; not to exercise in hot weather, which can cause increased hypotension
• Advise patient to notify prescriber of mouth sores, sore throat, fever, swelling of hands or feet, irregular heartbeat, chest pain, coughing, shortness of breath
• Caution patient to report excessive perspiration, dehydration, vomiting, diarrhea; may lead to fall in B/P
• Caution patient that product may cause dizziness, fainting, light-headedness; may occur during 1st few days of therapy; to avoid activities that may be hazardous
• Teach patient how to take B/P, and normal readings for age-group

**Evaluation**
**Positive therapeutic outcome**
• Decreased B/P in hypertension

**Treatment of overdose:** Lavage, **IV** atropine for bradycardia, **IV** theophylline for bronchospasm, digoxin, $O_2$, diuretic for cardiac failure, hemodialysis

---

**❗HIGH ALERT**

**trastuzumab** (Rx)
(tras-tuz'uh-mab)
Herceptin
*Func. class.:* Antineoplastic—miscellaneous
*Chem. class.:* Humanized monoclonal antibody

**Pregnancy category B**

**Action:** DNA-derived monoclonal antibody selectively binds to extracellular portion of human epidermal growth factor receptor 2 (HER2); it inhibits proliferation of cancer cells

**Therapeutic outcome:** Decreasing symptoms of breast cancer

**Uses:** Breast cancer; metastatic with overexpression of HER2, early breast cancer (adjuvant)

## Dosage and routes
*Adult:* **IV** 4 mg/kg given over 90 min, then maintenance 2 mg/kg given over 30 min; do not give as **IV** PUSH or BOL

## Available forms: Lyophilized powder 440 mg

## Adverse effects
*CNS: Dizziness, numbness, paresthesias,* depression, insomnia, neuropathy, peripheral neuritis
*CV:* **Tachycardia, CHF**
*GI:* Nausea, vomiting, anorexia, diarrhea
*HEMA:* Anemia, **leukopenia**
*INTEG: Rash,* acne, herpes simplex
*META:* Edema, peripheral edema
*MISC: Flulike symptoms; fever, headache, chills*
*MS:* Arthralgia, bone pain
*RESP:* Cough, dyspnea, pharyngitis, rhinitis, sinusitis
*SYST:* **Anaphylaxis, angioedema**

**Contraindications:** Hypersensitivity to this product, Chinese hamster ovary cell protein

**Precautions:** Pregnancy **B,** breastfeeding, children, geriatric, cardiac/pulmonary disease, anemia, leukopenia

### Pharmacokinetics
| | |
|---|---|
| **Absorption** | Unknown |
| **Distribution** | Unknown |
| **Metabolism** | Unknown |
| **Excretion** | Unknown |
| **Half-life** | 1-32 days |

### Pharmacodynamics
Unknown

## Interactions
*Individual drugs*
Cyclophosphamide: increased cardiomyopathy risk; avoid use
*Drug classifications*
Anthracyclines: increased cardiomyopathy risk
Vaccines/toxoids: decreased immune response

## NURSING CONSIDERATIONS
### Assessment
• Assess for symptoms of infection; may be masked by product
• Assess CNS reaction: LOC, mental status, dizziness, confusion

• Assess for CHF and other cardiac symptoms: dyspnea, coughing, gallop; obtain a full cardiac workup including ECG, echocardiogram, multigated angiogram
• Assess for hypersensitivity reactions, anaphylaxis
• Monitor for potentially fatal infusion reactions: fever, chills, nausea, vomiting, pain, headache, dizziness, hypotension; discontinue product

### Nursing diagnoses
• Infection, risk for (side effects)
• Knowledge, deficient (teaching)
• Nutrition: less than body requirements, imbalanced (side effects)

### Implementation
• Give acetaminophen as ordered to alleviate fever and headache
• Increase fluid intake to 2-3 L/day
**IV route**
• Administer after reconstituting vial with 20 ml of bacteriostatic water for inj, 1.1% benzyl alcohol preserved (supplied) to yield 21 mg/ml, mark date on vial 28 days from reconstitution date, if patient is allergic to benzyl alcohol, reconstitute with sterile water for inj; use immediately
• Do not mix or dilute with other products or dextrose sol

### Patient/family education
• Advise patient to take acetaminophen for fever
• Teach patient to avoid hazardous tasks, since confusion, dizziness may occur
• Teach patient to report signs of infection: sore throat, fever, diarrhea, vomiting
• Inform patient that emotional lability is common; instruct patient to notify prescriber if severe or incapacitating

### Evaluation
**Positive therapeutic outcome**
• Decrease in size of tumors

## travoprost ophthalmic
*See Appendix D*

## trazodone (Rx)
(tray′zoe-done)
Desyrel, Desyrel Dividose, trazodone HCl
*Func. class.:* Antidepressant—
miscellaneous
*Chem. class.:* Triazolopyridine
**Pregnancy category C**

**Action:** Selectively inhibits serotonin, norepinephrine uptake by brain, potentiates behavioral changes

**Therapeutic outcome:** Decreased symptoms of depression after 2-3 wk

**Uses:** Depression

**Unlabeled uses:** Chronic pain syndromes, aggressive behavior, cocaine withdrawal

**Dosage and routes:**
*Adult:* PO 150 mg/day in divided doses; may increase by 50 mg/day q3-4 days, not to exceed 600 mg/day
*Geriatric:* PO 25-50 at bedtime, increase by 25-50 mg q3-7 days to desired dose, usual 75-150 mg/day
*Child 6-18 yr:* PO 1.5-2 mg/kg/day in divided doses, may increase q3-4 days up to 6 mg/kg/day or 400 mg/day in divided doses, whichever is less

**Available forms:** Tabs 50, 100, 150, 300 mg

**Adverse effects**
*CNS: Dizziness, drowsiness,* confusion, headache, anxiety, tremors, stimulation, weakness, insomnia, nightmares, EPS (geriatric), increase in psychiatric symptoms, **suicide in children/adolescents**
*CV: Orthostatic hypotension, ECG changes, tachycardia,* **hypertension,** palpitations
*EENT: Blurred vision,* tinnitus, mydriasis
*GI: Diarrhea, dry mouth,* nausea, vomiting, **paralytic ileus,** increased appetite, cramps, epigastric distress, jaundice, **hepatitis,** stomatitis, constipation
*GU: Retention,* **acute renal failure, priapism**
*HEMA: Agranulocytosis, thrombocytopenia, eosinophilia, leukopenia*
*INTEG:* Rash, urticaria, sweating, pruritus, photosensitivity

**Contraindications:** Hypersensitivity to tricyclics, recovery phase of MI, seizure disorders, prostatic hypertrophy

**Precautions:** Pregnancy **C**, suicidal patients, severe depression, increased intraocular pressure, angle-closure glaucoma, urinary retention, cardiac/hepatic disease, hyperthyroidism, electroshock therapy, elective surgery, suicidal ideation in children/adolescents

### Pharmacokinetics
| | |
|---|---|
| **Absorption** | Well absorbed |
| **Distribution** | Widely distributed |
| **Metabolism** | Liver, extensively |
| **Excretion** | Kidneys—unchanged minimally |
| **Half-life** | 4½-7½ hr |

### Pharmacodynamics
| | |
|---|---|
| **Onset** | Unknown |
| **Peak** | 1 hr without food, 2 hr with food |
| **Duration** | Unknown |

### Interactions
*Individual drugs*
Alcohol, carbamazepine, digoxin, phenytoin: increased effect of each product
Clonidine, guanethidine: decreased effects
Fluoxetine, nefazodone: increased levels, increased toxicity, serotonin syndrome
Warfarin: increased or decreased effects of warfarin
*Drug classifications*
Barbiturates, benzodiazepines, CNS depressants: increased effects
CYP3A4, 2D6 inhibitors (phenothiazenes, protease inhibitors, azole antifungals): increased effects of trazodone
MAOIs: increased hyperpyretic crisis, seizures, hypertensive episode
Selective serotonin reuptake inhibitors: increased toxicity, serotonin syndrome
Sympathomimetics (direct-acting): increased sympathomimetic effects
Sympathomimetics (indirect-acting): decreased effects
*Drug/herb*
Chamomile, hops, kava, lavender, skullcap, valerian: increased CNS depression
Corkwood, jimsonweed: increased anticholinergic effect
SAM-e, St. John's wort: increased serotonin syndrome
*Drug/lab test*
Increased: serum bilirubin, blood glucose, alkaline phosphatase
Decreased: VMA, 5-HIAA
False increase: urinary catecholamines

## NURSING CONSIDERATIONS
### Assessment
- Assess for pain: location, duration, intensity before and 1-2 hr after medication
- Monitor B/P (lying, standing), pulse q4hr; if systolic B/P drops 20 mm Hg hold product, notify prescriber; take vital signs q4hr in patients with CV disease
- Monitor blood tests: CBC, leukocytes, differential, cardiac enzymes if patient is receiving long-term therapy
- Monitor liver function tests: AST, ALT, bilirubin
- Check weight qwk; appetite may increase with product
- Assess ECG for flattening of T wave, bundle branch block, AV block, dysrhythmias in cardiac patients
- Assess for EPS primarily in geriatric: rigidity, dystonia, akathisia
- Assess mental status: mood, sensorium, affect, suicidal tendencies; increase in psychiatric symptoms: depression, panic
- Monitor urinary retention, constipation; constipation is more likely to occur in children or geriatric
- Assess for withdrawal symptoms: headache, nausea, vomiting, muscle pain, weakness; do not usually occur unless product was discontinued abruptly
- Identify alcohol consumption; if alcohol is consumed, hold dose until AM

### Nursing diagnoses
- Coping, ineffective (uses)
- Injury, risk for (adverse reactions)
- Knowledge, deficient (teaching)
- Noncompliance (teaching)

### Implementation
- Give with food or milk for GI symptoms; crush if patient is unable to swallow medication whole
- Give dosage at bedtime if oversedation occurs during day; may take entire dose at bedtime; geriatric may not tolerate once/day dosing
- Store at room temperature; do not freeze

### Patient/family education
- Teach patient that therapeutic effects may take 2-3 wk
- Teach patient to use caution in driving or other activities requiring alertness because of drowsiness, dizziness, blurred vision; to avoid rising quickly from sitting to standing, especially geriatric
- Caution patient to avoid alcohol ingestion, other CNS depressants

- Teach patient not to discontinue medication quickly after long-term use: may cause nausea, headache, malaise
- Advise patient to wear sunscreen or large hat because photosensitivity occurs
- Teach patient to increase fluids, bulk in diet if constipation, urinary retention occur, especially geriatric
- Advise patient to take gum, hard sugarless candy, or frequent sips of water for dry mouth
- Teach family to watch for suicidal ideation or tendencies usually in children/adolescents

### Evaluation
#### Positive therapeutic outcome
- Decrease in depression
- Absence of suicidal thoughts

**Treatment of overdose:** ECG monitoring, induce emesis, lavage, activated charcoal, administer anticonvulsant

---

## treprostinil (Rx)
(treh-prah'stin-ill)
Remodulin
*Func. class.:* Antiplatelet agent
*Chem. class.:* Tricyclic benzidine prostacyclin analog

### Pregnancy category B

**Action:** Direct vasodilatation of pulmonary, systemic arterial vascular beds, inhibition of platelet aggregation

**Therapeutic outcome:** Decreased pulmonary arterial hypertension (PAH)

**Uses:** Pulmonary arterial hypertension (PAH) NYHA class II through IV

### Dosage and routes
*Adult:* SUBCUT inf 1.25 ng/kg/min by cont inf, may reduce to 0.625 ng if not tolerated; may increase by 1.25 ng/kg/min qwk for first 4 wk, then 2.5 ng/kg/min/wk for remainder of infusion

#### Hepatic dose
*Adult:* SUBCUT INF 0.625 ng/kg ideal body weight/min and increase cautiously

**Available forms:** Inj 1, 2.5, 5, 10 ng/ml

### Adverse effects
*CNS:* Dizziness, headache
*CV:* Vasodilatation, hypotension, edema
*GI:* Nausea, *diarrhea*
*INTEG:* Rash, pruritus
*OTHER:* Jaw pain
*SYST:* Infusion site reactions, infusion site pain, increased risk of infection

T

Adverse effects: *italic* = common, **bold** = life-threatening

**Contraindications:** Hypersensitivity

**Precautions:** Pregnancy **B**, breastfeeding, children, geriatric, past hepatic disease, renal/thromboembolic disease

### Pharmacokinetics

| | |
|---|---|
| **Absorption** | Unknown |
| **Distribution** | Unknown |
| **Metabolism** | Liver, 90% protein binding |
| **Excretion** | Urine, feces |
| **Half-life** | 2-4 hr, terminal |

### Pharmacodynamics
Unknown

### Interactions
*Individual drug*
Aspirin: increased risk of bleeding
*Drug classifications*
Anticoagulants, NSAIDs: increased risk of bleeding
Antihypertensives, diuretics, MAOIs, vasodilators: increased hypotension

### NURSING CONSIDERATIONS
**Assessment**
• Monitor liver function tests: AST, ALT, bilirubin, creatinine (long-term therapy)
◆ Monitor blood tests: CBC; CBC q2 wk × 3 mo, Hct, Hgb, pro-time (long-term therapy)
◆ Monitor bleed time baseline and throughout; levels may be 2-5 × normal limit

**Nursing diagnoses**
• Knowledge, deficient (teaching)
• Tissue perfusion, ineffective (uses)

**Implementation**
• Give by continuous SUBCUT infusion or surgically placed indwelling central venous catheter via infusion pump
• Sudden decreased doses or abrupt withdrawal may worsen pulmonary atrial hypertension symptoms

**Patient/family education**
• Teach patient that blood work will be necessary during treatment
• Teach patient to report side effects such as diarrhea, skin rashes
• Teach patient that therapy will be needed for prolonged periods of time, sometimes years
• Advise patient that aseptic technique must be used in preparing and administration to prevent infection

**Evaluation**
**Positive therapeutic outcome**
• Decreased pulmonary arterial hypertension

---

## tretinoin (vitamin A acid, retinoic acid) (Rx)
(tret'i-noyn)
Avita, Renova, Retin-A, Retin-A Micro, Stievaa ♣
*Func. class.:* Vitamin A acid/acne product, antineoplastic—miscellaneous
*Chem. class.:* Tretinoin derivative

**Pregnancy category**
C (TOPICAL),
D (PO)

**Action:** (Topical) Decreases cohesiveness of follicular epithelium, decreases microcomedone formation; (PO) induces maturation of acute promyelocytic leukemia, exact action is unknown

**Therapeutic outcome:** Decreased signs/symptoms of leukemia

**Uses:** (Topical) Acne vulgaris (grades 1-3); (PO) acute promyelocytic leukemia, facial wrinkles, photoaging

**Unlabeled uses:** Acne rosacea, actinic keratosis, ichthyosis, Kaposi's sarcoma, keloids, keratosis follicularis, melasma

**Dosage and routes**
*Adult and child:* TOP Cleanse area, apply 0.025%-0.1% cream or 0.05% liquid at bedtime; cover lightly

*Promyelocytic leukemia*
*Adult:* PO 45 mg/m²/day given as 2 evenly divided doses until remission; discontinue treatment 30 days after remission or after 90 days of treatment, whichever is first

**Available forms:** Topical cream 0.01%, 0.02%, 0.025%, 0.05%, 0.01%; topical gel 0.025%, 0.01%, 0.04%, 0.1%; topical liquid 0.05%; caps 10 mg

**Adverse effects**
*PO route*
*CNS:* Headache, fever, sweating, fatigue
*CV:* Cardiac dysrhythmias, pericardial effusion
*GI:* Nausea, vomiting, **hemorrhage,** abdominal pain, diarrhea, constipation, dyspepsia, distention, **hepatitis**
*META:* Hypercholesterolemia, hypertriglyceridemia
*RESP:* Pneumonia, upper respiratory tract disease
*Topical route*
*INTEG:* Rash, stinging, warmth, redness, erythema, blistering, crusting, peeling, contact dermatitis, hypo/hyperpigmentation, dry skin, pruritus, scaly skin

---

**Contraindications:** Pregnancy **D** (PO), hypersensitivity to retinoids or sensitive to parabens

**Precautions:** Pregnancy **C** (topical), breastfeeding, eczema, sunburn, sun exposure, rapid-evolving leukocytosis, respiratory compromise

### Pharmacokinetics

| | |
|---|---|
| **Absorption** | Small amounts |
| **Distribution** | Unknown |
| **Metabolism** | Unknown |
| **Excretion** | Kidneys |
| **Half-life** | Unknown |

### Pharmacodynamics

Unknown

### Interactions
*Individual drugs*
Aminocaproic acid, aprotinin, tranexamic acid: increased thrombotic complications
Benzoyl peroxide, resorcinol, salicylic acid (topical), sulfur: increased peeling
Ketoconazole: increased plasma concentrations of tretinoin (oral)
*Drug classifications*
Medicated, abrasive soaps, alcohol, astringents, cleansers with drying effect: use with caution (topical)
Diuretics (thiazide), phenothiazines, quinolones, retinoids, sulfonamides, sulfonylureas: increased photosensitivity
Tetracyclines: increased ICP, risk of pseudotumor cerebri; do not use together
*Drug/lab test*
Increased: AST, ALT

### NURSING CONSIDERATIONS
#### Assessment
**Topical route**
• Assess part of body involved, including time involved, what helps or aggravates condition, cysts, dryness, itching; lesions may become worse at beginning of treatment

#### Nursing diagnoses
• Body image, disturbed (uses)
• Knowledge, deficient (teaching)
• Skin integrity, impaired (uses)

#### Implementation
**Topical route**
• Apply using gloves or cotton, once daily before bedtime; cover area lightly using gauze
• Store at room temperature
• Wash hands after application
• Apply only to affected areas

#### Patient/family education
**Topical route**
• Instruct patient to avoid application on normal skin, and to avoid getting cream in eyes, nose, other mucous membranes
• Advise patient to avoid sunlight, sunlamps or to use protective clothing or sunscreen to prevent burns
• Advise patient that treatment may cause warmth, stinging; dryness; peeling will occur
• Inform patient that cosmetics may be used over product; not to use shaving lotions
• Inform patient that rash may occur during first 1-3 wk of therapy
• Caution patient that product does not cure condition; only relieves symptoms; that therapeutic results may be seen in 2-3 wk but may not be optimal until after 6 wk

#### Evaluation
**Positive therapeutic outcome**
• Decrease in size and number of lesions

---

### tretinoin topical
*See Appendix D*

---

### triamcinolone (Rx)
(trye-am-sin'oh-lone)
Amcort, Aristocort, Aristocort Forte, Aristocort Intralesional, Aristospan Intra-Articular, Aristospan Intralesional, Articulose L.A., Atolone, Azmacort, Cenocort A-40, Cenocort Forte, Kenacort, Kenaject-40, Kenalog, Kenalog-10, Kenalog-40, Tac-3, Tac-40, Triam-A, triamcinolone, triamcinolone acetonide, Triam Forte, Triamolone 40, Triamonide 40, Tri-Kort, Trilog, Trilone, Trisoject
*Func. class.:* Corticosteroid, synthetic; antiinflammatory
*Chem. class.:* Glucocorticoid, intermediate-acting

#### Pregnancy category C

T

**Action:** Decreases inflammation by suppression of migration of polymorphonuclear leukocytes, fibroblasts, reversal of increased capillary permeability and lysosomal stabilization

**Therapeutic outcome:** Decreased inflammation, normal immune response

**Uses:** Severe inflammation, immunosuppression, neoplasms, asthma (steroid dependent), collagen, respiratory, dermatologic disorders, rheumatic disorders

Adverse effects: *italic* = common, **bold** = life-threatening

## Dosage and routes
***Adult:*** PO 4-12 mg/day in divided doses daily-qid; IM 40 mg q wk (acetonide, diacetate), 5-48 mg into neoplasms (diacetate, acetonide), 2-40 mg into joint or soft tissue (diacetate, acetonide), 0.5 mg/sq in of affected intralesional skin (hexacetonide), 2-20 mg into joint or soft tissue (hexacetonide)
***Child:*** PO 117 mcg/kg/day in divided doses

### Asthma
***Adult:*** INH 2 tid-qid, max 16 inh/day
***Child 6-12 yr:*** INH 1-2 tid-qid, max 12 inh/day

**Available forms:** Tabs 1, 2, 4, 8 mg; syr 2, 4.85 mg/5 ml; inj 25, 40 mg/ml diacetate; inj 3, 10, 40 mg/ml acetonide; inj 5, 20 mg/ml hexacetonide; inh 100 mcg/spray

## Adverse effects
***CNS:*** *Depression, flushing, sweating,* headache, mood changes
***CV:*** *Hypertension,* **circulatory collapse, thrombophlebitis, embolism,** tachycardia, edema
***EENT:*** Fungal infections, increased intraocular pressure, blurred vision
***GI:*** *Diarrhea, nausea, abdominal distention,* **GI hemorrhage,** *increased appetite,* **pancreatitis**
***HEMA:*** **Thrombocytopenia**
***INTEG:*** Acne, poor wound healing, ecchymosis, petechiae
***MS:*** Fractures, osteoporosis, weakness

**Contraindications:** Children <2 yr, psychosis, hypersensitivity, idiopathic thrombocytopenia, acute glomerulonephritis, amebiasis, fungal infections, nonasthmatic bronchial disease, AIDS, TB, adrenal insufficiency

**Precautions:** Pregnancy **C,** breastfeeding, diabetes mellitus, glaucoma, osteoporosis, seizure disorders, ulcerative colitis, CHF, myasthenia gravis, renal disease, esophagitis, peptic ulcer, acne, cataracts, coagulopathy

## Interactions
### Individual drugs
Alcohol, amphotericin B, cycloSPORINE, digoxin, indomethacin: increased side effects
Ambenonium, isoniazid, neostigmine, somatrem: decreased effects of each specific product

Cholestyramine, colestipol, ephEDrine, phenytoin, rifampin, theophylline: decreased action of triamcinolone
Indomethacin, ketoconazole: increased action of triamcinolone

### Drug classifications
Anticholinesterases, anticoagulants, anticonvulsants, antidiabetics, salicylates: decreased effects of each specific product
Antidiabetic agents: increased need for antidiabetic agents
Antiinfectives (macrolide), contraceptives (oral), estrogens, salicylates: increased action of triamcinolone
Barbiturates: decreased action of triamcinolone
Diuretics, salicylates: increased side effects
Toxoids, vaccines: decreased effects of toxoids, vaccines

### Drug/herb
Aloe, buckthorn, cascara sagrada, Chinese rhubarb, senna: increased hypokalemia

### Drug/lab test
Increased: cholesterol, sodium, blood glucose, uric acid, calcium, urine glucose
Decreased: calcium, potassium, $T_4$, $T_3$, thyroid $^{131}I$ uptake test, urine 17-OHCS, 17-KS
False negative: skin allergy tests

### Pharmacokinetics
| | |
|---|---|
| **Absorption** | Well absorbed (PO, IM) |
| **Distribution** | Crosses placenta, widely distributed |
| **Metabolism** | Liver—extensively |
| **Excretion** | Kidney, breast milk |
| **Half-life** | 2-5 hr, adrenal suppression 3-4 days |

## NURSING CONSIDERATIONS
### Assessment
- Monitor potassium, blood glucose, urine glucose while on long-term therapy; hypokalemia and hyperglycemia
- Monitor weight daily; notify prescriber of weekly gain >5 lb; I&O ratio; be alert for decreasing urinary output and increasing edema
- Monitor B/P q4hr, pulse; notify prescriber if chest pain occurs

### Pharmacodynamics
| | PO | IM | TOPICAL | INH | INTRANASAL |
|---|---|---|---|---|---|
| **Onset** | Unknown | Unknown | Min to hr | 1-2 wk | Unknown |
| **Peak** | 1-2 hr | 1-2 hr | Hr to days | Unknown | 2-3 wk |
| **Duration** | 3 days | Unknown | Hr to days | Unknown | Unknown |

• Monitor plasma cortisol levels during long-term therapy (normal level; 138-635 nmol/L [SI units] when measured at 8 AM); adrenal function periodically for hypothalamic-pituitary-adrenal axis suppression

• Assess for infection: increased temp, WBC even after withdrawal of medication; product masks infection symptoms

• Assess for potassium depletion: paresthesias, fatigue, nausea, vomiting, depression, polyuria, dysrhythmias, weakness

• Assess mental status: affect, mood, behavioral changes, aggression

• Assess nasal passages during long-term treatment for changes in mucus (nasal)

• Monitor temp; if fever develops, product should be discontinued

• Assess for systemic absorption: increased temp, inflammation, irritation (topical)

## Nursing diagnoses

• Infection, risk for (adverse reactions)
• Knowledge, deficient (teaching)
• Noncompliance (teaching)

## Implementation

### PO route

• Give with food or milk to decrease GI symptoms, tablet may be crushed

### IM route

• Give IM inj deeply in large muscle mass, rotate sites, avoid deltoid, use 21G needle

• Give in one dose in AM to prevent adrenal suppression; avoid SUBCUT administration; may damage tissue

### Inhalation route

• Use spacer device for geriatric

• Give inh with water to decrease possibility of fungal infections; titrated dose, use lowest effective dose

• Give after cleaning aerosol top daily with warm water, dry thoroughly

• Store in cool environment; do not puncture or incinerate container

### Topical route

• Apply only to affected areas; do not get in eyes

• Apply medication, then cover with occlusive dressing (only if prescribed), seal to normal skin, change q12hr; systemic absorption may occur

• Apply only to dermatoses; do not use on weeping, denuded, or infected areas

• Cleanse skin before applying product

• Continue treatment for a few days after area has cleared

• Store at room temperature

### Nasal route

• Have patient clear nasal passages before administration; use decongestant if needed; shake inhaler, invert, tilt head backward, insert nozzle into nostril, away from septum; hold other nostril closed and depress activator, inhale through nose, exhale through mouth

## Patient/family education

• Advise patient that emergency ID as steroid user should be carried/worn

• Instruct patient to notify prescriber if therapeutic response decreases; dosage adjustment may be needed; not to discontinue abruptly; adrenal crisis can result

• Caution patient to avoid OTC products: salicylates, alcohol in cough products, cold preparations unless directed by prescriber

• Advise patient on all aspects of product usage including cushingoid symptoms

• Teach patient symptoms of adrenal insufficiency: nausea, anorexia, fatigue, dizziness, dyspnea, weakness, joint pain

• Teach patient that long-term therapy may be needed to clear infection (1-2 mo depending on type of infection)

### Inhalation route

• Teach patient proper administration technique; to wash inhaler with warm water and dry after each use

• Teach patient all aspects of product usage including cushingoid symptoms

### Topical route

• Instruct patient to avoid sunlight on affected area; burns may occur

### Nasal route

• Instruct patient to clear nasal passages if sneezing attack occurs, repeat dose

• Advise patient to continue using product even if mild nasal bleeding occurs; is usually transient

• Teach patient method of instillation after providing written instruction from manufacturer

## Evaluation

### Positive therapeutic outcome

• Decrease in runny nose (nasal)
• Decreased dyspnea, wheezing, dry crackles on auscultation (inh)
• Ease of respirations, decreased inflammation
• Absence of severe itching, patches on skin, flaking (topical)

T

### triamcinolone nasal agent
*See Appendix D*

Adverse effects: *italic* = common, **bold** = life-threatening

## triamcinolone ophthalmic
*See Appendix D*

## triamcinolone topical
*See Appendix D*

## triamterene (Rx)
(try-am'ter-een)
Dyrenium
*Func. class.:* Potassium-sparing diuretic
*Chem. class.:* Pteridine derivative

**Pregnancy category B**

**Action:** Acts primarily on distal tubule to inhibit reabsorption of sodium, chloride; increase potassium retention and conserve hydrogen ions

**Therapeutic outcome:** Diuretic and antihypertensive effect while retaining potassium

**Uses:** Edema, hypertension, diuretic-induced hypokalemia

**Dosage and routes**
*Adult:* PO 100 mg bid after meals, max 300 mg/day
*Geriatric:* PO 50 mg/day, max 100 mg/day

**Renal dose**
CCr <10 ml/min, do not use

**Available forms:** Caps 50, 100 mg

**Adverse effects**
*CNS:* Weakness, headache, dizziness, fatigue
*ELECT:* Hyperkalemia, hyponatremia, hypochloremia
*GI:* Nausea, diarrhea, vomiting, dry mouth, jaundice, constipation
*GU:* **Azotemia, interstitial nephritis,** increased BUN, creatinine, renal stones, bluish discoloration of urine, **nephrotoxicity**
*HEMA:* **Thrombocytopenia, megaloblastic anemia, agranulocytosis**
*INTEG:* Photosensitivity, rash
*RESP:* Dyspnea

**Contraindications:** Breastfeeding, hypersensitivity, anuria, severe renal/hepatic disease; hyperkalemia

**Precautions:** Pregnancy **B**, dehydration, renal/hepatic disease, CHF, cirrhosis, renal stenosis, hyperuricemia, electrolyte abnormalities

### Pharmacokinetics

| | |
|---|---|
| **Absorption** | GI tract; well absorbed |
| **Distribution** | Crosses placenta |
| **Metabolism** | Liver |
| **Excretion** | Renal; breast milk |
| **Half-life** | 3 hr |

### Pharmacodynamics

| | |
|---|---|
| **Onset** | 2 hr |
| **Peak** | 6-8 hr |
| **Duration** | 12-16 hr |

### Interactions
*Drug classifications*
Angiotensin-converting enzyme inhibitors, diuretics (potassium-sparing), potassium products, salt substitutes: increased hyperkalemia
Antihypertensives: increased action
*Drug/herb*
Arginine: fatal hypokalemia
Bearberry, gossypol: increased hypokalemia
Cucumber, dandelion, horsetail, licorice, nettle, pumpkin, Queen Anne's lace: increased diuretic effect
St. John's wort: severe photosensitivity
*Drug/lab test*
Interference: quinidine serum levels, LDH

### NURSING CONSIDERATIONS
**Assessment**
• Monitor for manifestations of hyperkalemia: *RENAL:* acidic urine, reduced urine osmolality, nocturia, polyuria, polydipsia; *CV:* hypotension, broad T wave, U wave, ectopy, tachycardia, weak pulse; *NEURO:* muscle weakness, altered LOC, drowsiness, apathy, lethargy, confusion, depression, anorexia, nausea, cramps, constipation, distention, paralytic ileus, hypoventilation, respiratory muscle weakness
• Monitor for manifestations of hyponatremia: *CV:* increased B/P, cold, clammy skin, hypo/hypervolemia; *GI:* anorexia, nausea, vomiting, diarrhea, abdominal cramps; *NEURO:* lethargy, increased ICP, confusion, headache, seizures, coma, fatigue, tremors, hyperreflexia
• Monitor for manifestations of hyperchloremia: *NEURO:* weakness, lethargy, coma; *RESP:* deep rapid breathing
• Assess fluid volume status: I&O ratios and record, weight, distended red veins, crackles in lung, color, quality, and specific gravity of urine, skin turgor, adequacy of pulses, moist mucous membranes, bilateral lung sounds, peripheral pitting edema; dehydration symptoms of decreasing output, thirst, hypotension,

dry mouth and mucous membranes should be reported
• Monitor electrolytes: potassium, sodium, calcium, magnesium; also include BUN, ABGs, uric acid, CBC, blood glucose

Nursing diagnoses
• Fluid volume, deficient (adverse reactions)
• Fluid volume, excess (uses)
• Knowledge, deficient (teaching)
• Urinary elimination, impaired (adverse reactions)

Implementation
• Give in AM to avoid interference with sleep
• Give after meals if nausea occurs

Patient/family education
• Teach patient to take medication early in the day to prevent nocturia
• Instruct the patient to take with meals if GI symptoms of nausea and anorexia occur
• Teach patient to maintain a record of weight on a weekly basis and notify prescriber of weight loss of 5 lb
• Caution the patient that this product causes an increase in potassium levels, that foods high in potassium should be avoided; refer to dietitian for assistance planning
• Caution the patient not to exercise in hot weather, stand for prolonged periods of time because orthostatic hypotension will be enhanced
• Advise patient to wear protective clothing and sunscreen in the sun to prevent photosensitivity
• Teach patient not to use alcohol or any OTC medications without prescriber's approval because serious product reactions may occur
• Emphasize the need to contact prescriber immediately if muscle cramps, weakness, nausea, dizziness, or numbness occur
• Teach patient to take own B/P and pulse and record
• Advise patient that dizziness and confusion may occur; avoid driving or other hazardous activities if alertness is decreased
• Teach patient to continue taking medication even if feeling better; this product controls symptoms but does not cure the condition
• Advise the patient with hypertension to continue other medical treatment (exercise, weight loss, relaxation techniques, cessation of smoking)

Evaluation
Positive therapeutic outcome
• Prevention of hypokalemia (diuretic use)
• Decreased edema
• Decreased B/P
• Increased diuresis

Treatment of overdose: Lavage if taken orally; monitor electrolytes; administer sodium bicarbonate for potassium 6.5 mEq/L; monitor hydration, CV, renal status

## triazolam (Rx)
(trye-az'oh-lam)
Apo-Triazo ✦, Gen-Triazolam ✦, Halcion, Novotriolam ✦, Nu-Triazol ✦
*Func. class.:* Sedative-hypnotic, antianxiety
*Chem. class.:* Benzodiazepine, short-intermediate acting

**Pregnancy category** X

**Controlled substance schedule IV (USA), targeted (CDSA IV) (Canada)**

Action: Produces CNS depression at limbic, thalamic, hypothalamic levels of CNS; may be mediated by neurotransmitter; γ-aminobutyric acid (GABA); results are sedation, hypnosis, skeletal muscle relaxation, anticonvulsant activity, anxiolytic action

Therapeutic outcome: Decreased anxiety, insomnia

Uses: Insomnia (short-term), sedative/hypnotic

Dosage and routes
*Adult:* PO 0.125-0.5 mg at bedtime, max 0.5 mg
*Geriatric:* PO 0.0625-0.125 mg at bedtime

Available forms: Tabs 0.125, 0.25 mg

Adverse effects
*CNS: Headache, lethargy, drowsiness, daytime sedation,* dizziness, confusion, lightheadedness, anxiety, irritability, amnesia, poor coordination, complex sleep-related reactions (sleep driving, sleep eating)
*CV:* Chest pain, pulse changes
*GI:* Nausea, vomiting, diarrhea, heartburn, abdominal pain, constipation, **hepatic injury**
*HEMA:* **Leukopenia, granulocytopenia (rare)**
*SYST:* **Severe allergic reactions**

Contraindications: Pregnancy X, breastfeeding, hypersensitivity to benzodiazepines, intermittent porphyria

Precautions: Children <15 yr, geriatric, anemia, renal/hepatic disease, suicidal individuals, product abuse, psychosis, acute angle-closure glaucoma, seizure disorders, angioedema, respiratory disease, depression, sleep-related behaviors (sleep walking)

T

Adverse effects: *italic* = common, **bold** = life-threatening

| Pharmacokinetics | |
|---|---|
| **Absorption** | Well absorbed |
| **Distribution** | Widely distributed, crosses placenta, crosses blood-brain barrier |
| **Metabolism** | Liver |
| **Excretion** | Kidneys, breast milk |
| **Half-life** | 2-3 hr |

| Pharmacodynamics | |
|---|---|
| **Onset** | ½ hr |
| **Peak** | Unknown |
| **Duration** | 6-8 hr |

## Interactions
### Individual drugs
Alcohol: increased action of both products
Cimetidine, disulfiram, isoniazid: increased action, do not use concurrently
Erythromycin, probenecid: increased effects, do not use concurrently
Rifampin: decreased action of rifampin
Theophylline: decreased effects of theophylline
### Drug classifications
Antacids: decreased effects of antacids
Antiinfectives (macrolide): increased effects
CNS depressants: increased effects of both products
Contraceptives (oral): increased effects; do not use concurrently
CYP3A4 inhibitors: increased triazolam levels
Smoking: decreased hypnotic effects
### Drug/herb
Black cohosh: increased hypotension
Catnip, clary, chamomile, cowslip, hops, kava, lavender, mistletoe, nettle, pokeweed, poppy, Queen Anne's lace, senega, skullcap, valerian: increased CNS depression
### Drug/lab test
Increased: AST, ALT, serum bilirubin
Decreased: radioactive iodine uptake
False increase: 17-OHCS

## NURSING CONSIDERATIONS
### Assessment
• Assess patient's mental status: mood, sensorium, anxiety, affect, sleeping pattern, drowsiness, dizziness, especially geriatric; physical dependency, withdrawal symptoms: anxiety, panic attacks, agitation, seizures, headache, nausea, vomiting, muscle pain, weakness; suicidal tendencies; for indications of increasing tolerance and abuse
• Monitor patient's B/P (lying, standing), pulse; if systolic B/P drops 20 mm Hg, hold product, notify prescriber
• Monitor blood tests: CBC during long-term therapy; blood dyscrasias have occurred rarely; decreased hematocrit, neutropenia may occur
• Monitor liver function tests: AST, ALT, bilirubin, creatinine LDH, alkaline phosphatase
• Monitor I&O ratio; indicate renal dysfunction

### Nursing diagnoses
• Anxiety (uses)
• Injury, risk for (adverse reactions)
• Knowledge, deficient (teaching)

### Implementation
• Give with food or milk to decrease GI symptoms; if patient is unable to swallow medication whole, tab may be crushed and mixed with foods or fluids
• Give sugarless gum, hard candy, frequent sips of water for dry mouth

### Patient/family education
• Advise patient that product may be taken with food or fluids, and tab may be crushed or swallowed whole
• Caution patient not to use for everyday stress or longer than 3 mo unless directed by prescriber; not to take more than prescribed amount; may be habit forming; not to double doses or skip doses
• Instruct patient to avoid OTC preparations unless approved by prescriber; alcohol and CNS depressants will increase CNS depression
• Caution patient to avoid driving, activities that require alertness because drowsiness may occur; to avoid alcohol ingestion or other psychotropic medications; to rise slowly or fainting may occur, especially geriatric; that drowsiness may worsen at beginning of treatment
• Teach patient to use reliable contraception
• Teach patient that complex sleep-related behaviors (sleep eating/driving) may occur
• Advise patient not to discontinue medication abruptly after long-term use; withdrawal symptoms include vomiting, cramping, tremors, seizures; decrease dose by 50% q2 nights until 0.125 mg for 2 nights, then stop

### Evaluation
**Positive therapeutic outcome**
• Decreased anxiety, restlessness, sleeplessness (short-term treatment only)

### Treatment of overdose: Lavage, VS, supportive care

## trifluoperazine (Rx)
(trye-floo-oh-per′a-zeen)
Apo-Trifluoperazine ✦, Novofluurazine ✦,
Solazine ✦, Stelazine, Suprazine,
Terfluzine, trifluoperazine HCl, Triflurin
*Func. class.:* Antipsychotic/neuroleptic
*Chem. class.:* Phenothiazine, piperazine
**Pregnancy category C**

### Do not confuse:
trifluoperazine/trihexyphenidyl

**Action:** Depresses cerebral cortex, hypothalamus, limbic system, which control activity, aggression; blocks neurotransmission produced by DOPamine at synapse; exhibits strong α-adrenergic, anticholinergic blocking action; mechanism for antipsychotic effects is unclear

**Therapeutic outcome:** Decreased signs and symptoms of psychosis

**Uses:** Psychotic disorders, nonpsychotic anxiety, schizophrenia

### Dosage and routes
#### Psychotic disorders
**Adult:** PO 2-5 mg bid, usual range 15-20 mg/day, may require 40 mg/day or more; IM 1-2 mg q4-6hr, max 100 mg/day
**Geriatric:** PO 0.5-1 mg daily-bid, increase q4-7 days by 0.5-1 mg/day to desired dose, max 100 mg/day
**Child >6 yr:** PO 1 mg/day or bid; IM *not recommended for children,* but 1 mg may be given daily or bid

#### Nonpsychotic anxiety
**Adult:** PO 1-2 mg bid, not to exceed 6 mg/day; do not give longer than 12 wk

**Available forms:** Tabs 1, 2, 5, 10 mg; conc 10 mg/ml; inj 2 mg/ml

### Adverse effects
*CNS: EPS (pseudoparkinsonism, akathisia, dystonia, tardive dyskinesia),* **seizures,** *headache,* **neuroleptic malignant syndrome,** dizziness
*CV: Orthostatic hypotension,* hypertension, **cardiac arrest,** ECG changes, **tachycardia**
*EENT:* Blurred vision, glaucoma, dry eyes
*GI: Dry mouth, nausea, vomiting, anorexia, constipation,* diarrhea, jaundice, weight gain
*GU:* Urinary retention, urinary frequency, enuresis, impotence, amenorrhea, gynecomastia
*HEMA:* Anemia, **leukopenia, leukocytosis, agranulocytosis**
*INTEG: Rash,* photosensitivity, dermatitis
*RESP:* **Laryngospasm,** dyspnea, **respiratory depression**

**Contraindications:** Children <6 yr, hypersensitivity, CV disease, coma, blood dyscrasias, severe hepatic disease, angle-closure glaucoma

**Precautions:** Pregnancy C, breastfeeding, geriatric, breast cancer, seizure disorders, diabetes mellitus, respiratory conditions, prostatic hypertrophy, Parkinson's disease, renal failure

### Pharmacokinetics
| | |
|---|---|
| **Absorption** | Variably absorbed (PO), well absorbed (IM) |
| **Distribution** | Widely distributed, high concentrations in CNS, crosses placenta, 91%-99% protein binding |
| **Metabolism** | Liver—extensively |
| **Excretion** | Kidneys, breast milk |
| **Half-life** | Unknown |

### Pharmacodynamics
| | PO | IM |
|---|---|---|
| **Onset** | Rapid | Immediate |
| **Peak** | 2-3 hr | 1 hr |
| **Duration** | 12 hr | 12 hr |

### Interactions
#### Individual drugs
Alcohol: increased effects of both products, oversedation
Aluminum hydroxide, magnesium hydroxide: decreased absorption
Levodopa: decreased antiparkinson activity
Lithium: decreased effects of lithium
#### Drug classifications
Anesthetics (barbiturate), CNS depressants: oversedation
Anesthetics (general), opiates, sedative/hypnotics: increased CNS depression
Antacids: decreased absorption
Anticholinergics: increased anticholinergic effects
Anticonvulsants: decreased effects of anticonvulsants
β-Adrenergic blockers: increased effects of both products
CYP2D6 inducers: decreased level of trifluoperazine
CYP2D6 inhibitors: increased level of trifluoperazine
#### Drug/herb
Chamomile, hops, kava, skullcap, valerian: increased CNS depression
Betel palm, kava: increased EPS
Cola tree, hops, nettle, nutmeg: increased action

Adverse effects: *italic* = common, **bold** = life-threatening

*Drug/lab test*

Increased: LFTs, cardiac enzymes, cholesterol, blood glucose, prolactin, bilirubin, cholinesterase, $^{131}$I

Decreased: hormones (blood and urine)

False positive: pregnancy tests, PKU

False negative: urinary steroids, 17-OHCS, pregnancy tests

## NURSING CONSIDERATIONS
### Assessment

• Assess mental status: orientation, mood, behavior, presence of hallucinations and type before initial administration and monthly; product should significantly reduce psychotic behavior

• Check for swallowing of PO medication; check for hoarding or giving of medication to other patients

• Monitor I&O ratio, palpate bladder if low urinary output occurs, especially in geriatric; urinalysis recommended before, during prolonged therapy

• Monitor bilirubin, CBC, liver function tests monthly

• Assess affect, orientation, LOC, reflexes, gait, coordination, sleep pattern disturbances

• Monitor B/P sitting, standing, and lying, take pulse and respirations q4hr during initial treatment; establish baseline before starting treatment; report drops of 30 mm Hg; obtain baseline ECG, monitor Q- and T-wave changes

• Check for dizziness, faintness, palpitations, tachycardia on rising; severe orthostatic hypotension is common

◆ Identify for neuroleptic malignant syndrome: hyperpyrexia, muscle rigidity, increased CPK, altered mental status; product should be discontinued

• Assess for EPS including akathisia (inability to sit still, no pattern to movements), tardive dyskinesia (bizarre movements of the jaw, mouth, tongue, extremities), pseudoparkinsonism (ragged tremors, pill rolling, shuffling gait); an antiparkinson product should be prescribed

• Assess for constipation, urinary retention daily; if these occur, increase bulk, water in diet

• Assess for hypo/hyperglycemia; appetite patterns

### Nursing diagnoses

• Coping, ineffective (uses)
• Knowledge, deficient (teaching)
• Noncompliance (teaching)
• Thought processes, disturbed (uses)

## Implementation
### PO route

• Give product in liquid form mixed in glass of juice if hoarding is suspected; do not mix in caffeine drinks, tannics, pectins

• Give decreased dose in geriatric; metabolism is slowed in the geriatric

• Give PO with full glass of water, milk; or give with food to decrease GI upset

• Give antacids 2 hr before or after this product

• Store in airtight, light-resistant container, oral sol in amber bottle

### IM route

• Inj in deep muscle mass, do not give SUBCUT; do not administer sol with a precipitate

• Patient should lie down for 30 min after IM inj

### IV route

• Give **IV** after diluting 10 mg/9 ml of 0.9% NaCl; give 1 mg or less/2 min

*Syringe compatibilities:* Glycopyrrolate
*Additive compatibilities:* Meperidine, netilmicin

### Patient/family education

• Teach patient to use good oral hygiene; frequent rinsing of mouth, sugarless gum for dry mouth; oral candidasis may occur

• Caution patient to avoid hazardous activities until product response is determined; dizziness, blurred vision is common

• Inform patient that orthostatic hypotension occurs often; to rise from sitting or lying position gradually; avoid tubs, hot showers, and tub baths because hypotension may occur

• Advise patient to remain lying down after IM inj for at least 30 min

• Instruct patient that heat stroke may occur in hot weather, so take extra precautions to stay cool

• Advise patient to avoid abrupt withdrawal of this product, or EPS may result; product should be withdrawn slowly

• Teach patient to avoid OTC preparations (cough, hay fever, cold) unless approved by prescriber because serious product interactions may occur; avoid use with alcohol, CNS depressants because increased drowsiness may occur

• Advise patient to use sunglasses and sunscreen to prevent burns

• Instruct patient to report sore throat, malaise, fever, bleeding, mouth sores; if these occur, CBC should be performed and product discontinued

### Evaluation
**Positive therapeutic outcome**
- Decrease in emotional excitement, hallucinations, delusions, paranoia
- Reorganization of patterns of thought, speech

**Treatment of overdose:** Lavage if orally ingested; provide airway; *do not induce vomiting or use epINEPHrine*

### trifluridine ophthalmic
*See Appendix D*

### trihexyphenidyl (Rx)
(trye-hex-ee-fen'i-dill)
Apo-Trihex ✦, Artane, Artane Sequels, Novohexidyl ✦, PMS-Trihexyphenidyl ✦, Trihexy-2, Trihexy-5, trihexyphenidyl HCl, Trihexane
*Func. class.:* Cholinergic blocker; antiparkinson
*Chem. class.:* Synthetic tertiary amine
**Pregnancy category C**

**Do not confuse:**
trihexyphenidyl/trifluoperazine, Artane/Altace

**Action:** Blocks central muscarinic receptors, which decreases involuntary movements, sweating, salivation

**Therapeutic outcome:** Decreased involuntary movements

**Uses:** Parkinsonian symptoms, product-induced EPS

**Unlabeled uses:** Hypersalivation

### Dosage and routes
*Parkinsonian symptoms*
*Adult:* PO 1 mg, increased by 2 mg q3-5 days to a total of 5-15 mg/day, given in 3-4 divided doses

*Drug-induced EPS*
*Adult:* PO 1 mg/day; usual dose 5-15 mg/day, given in 3-4 divided doses

**Available forms:** Tabs 2, 5 mg; elixir 2 mg/5 ml

### Adverse effects
*CNS:* Confusion, anxiety, restlessness, irritability, delusions, hallucinations, headache, sedation, depression, incoherence, dizziness, flushing, weakness
*CV:* Palpitations, tachycardia, postural hypotension

*EENT:* Blurred vision, photophobia, dilated pupils, difficulty swallowing, dry eyes, increased intraocular tension, angle-closure glaucoma
*GI: Dryness of mouth, constipation,* nausea, vomiting, abdominal distress, **paralytic ileus**
*GU:* Urinary hesitancy, urinary retention, dysuria
*INTEG:* Urticaria, rash, dry skin, photosensitivity
*MISC:* Suppression of lactation, nasal congestion, decreased sweating, hyperthermia, heat stroke, numbness of fingers
*MS:* Weakness, cramping

**Contraindications:** Hypersensitivity, tardive dyskinesia, angle-closure glaucoma, myasthenia gravis, GI/ GU obstruction

**Precautions:** Pregnancy **C,** breastfeeding, tachycardia, abdominal obstruction, infection, gastric ulcer, myocardial ischemia, unstable CV disease, prostatic hypertrophy

### Pharmacokinetics
| | |
|---|---|
| **Absorption** | Well absorbed |
| **Distribution** | Unknown |
| **Metabolism** | Unknown |
| **Excretion** | Unknown |
| **Half-life** | 5-10 hr |

### Pharmacodynamics
| | PO |
|---|---|
| **Onset** | 1 hr |
| **Peak** | 2-3 hr |
| **Duration** | 6-12 hr |

### Interactions
*Individual drugs*
Alcohol: increased CNS depression
Amantadine: increased cholinergic effects
Digoxin: increased levels of digoxin
Donepezil, galantamine, rivastigmine: decreased anticholinergic effect
Haloperidol: decreased action of haloperidol
Levodopa: decreased action of levodopa
*Drug classifications*
Analgesics, antihistamines, opioids, sedative/hypnotics: increased CNS depression
Antidepressants (tricyclics), antihistamines, phenothiazines: increased anticholinergic effects
*Drug/herb*
Henbane, jimsonweed, scopolia: increased trihexyphenidyl

T

## NURSING CONSIDERATIONS
### Assessment
- Monitor I&O ratio; retention commonly causes decreased urinary output, distention, frequency, incontinence
- Assess for parkinsonism, EPS: shuffling gait, muscle rigidity, involuntary movements, pill rolling, muscle spasms, drooling before and during treatment
- Monitor for urinary hesitancy, retention; palpate bladder if retention occurs
- Monitor for constipation, cramping, pain in abdomen, abdominal distention; increase fluids, bulk, exercise if this occurs
- Assess for tolerance over long-term therapy; dose may have to be increased or changed
- Assess for mental status: affect, mood, CNS depression, worsening of mental symptoms during early therapy

### Nursing diagnoses
- Knowledge, deficient (teaching)
- Mobility, impaired physical (uses)

### Implementation
- Give with or after meals to prevent GI upset; may give with fluids other than water
- Give at bedtime to avoid daytime drowsiness in patient with parkinsonism
- Store at room temperature

### Patient/family education
- Teach patient to use caution in hot weather; product may increase susceptibility to stroke because perspiration is decreased; patient should remain indoors
- Teach patient not to discontinue this product abruptly; to taper off over 1 wk to prevent withdrawal symptoms (insomnia, involuntary movements, anxiety, tachycardias)
- Caution patient to avoid driving or other hazardous activities; drowsiness, dizziness may occur
- Advise patient to avoid OTC medications (cough, cold preparations with alcohol, antihistamines) unless directed by prescriber; increased CNS depression may occur
- Instruct patient to rise from sitting or recumbent position slowly to minimize orthostatic hypotension
- Advise patient to use gum, hard candy, frequent sips of water to decrease dry mouth; if dry mouth continues, saliva substitutes may be prescribed
- Instruct patient that doses should not be doubled, but missed dose may be taken up to 2 hr before next dose

### Evaluation
**Positive therapeutic outcome**
- Absence of involuntary movements (pill rolling, tremors, muscle spasms)

---

### trimethobenzamide (Rx)
(trye-meth-oh-ben'za-mide)
Arrestin, Benzacot, Brogan, Stemetic, Ticon, Tigan, Tijet-20, Triban, trimethobenzamide, trimethobenzamide HCl
*Func. class.:* Antiemetic, anticholinergic
*Chem. class.:* Ethanolamine derivative

**Pregnancy category C**

**Action:** Acts centrally by blocking chemoreceptor trigger zone, which in turn acts on vomiting center

**Therapeutic outcome:** Absence of nausea and vomiting

**Uses:** Nausea, vomiting, prevention of postoperative vomiting

### Dosage and routes
*Postoperative vomiting*
*Adult:* IM/RECT 200 mg followed by a second dose 1 hr later

*Nausea/vomiting*
*Adult:* PO 300 mg tid-qid; IM/RECT 200 mg tid-qid

**Available forms:** Caps 300 mg; inj 100 mg/ml

### Adverse effects
*CNS: Drowsiness,* restlessness, headache, dizziness, confusion, *vertigo,* EPS, disorientation, **coma, seizures,** depression
*CV:* Hyper/hypotension, palpitations, **cardiac dysrhythmias**
*EENT:* Dry mouth, blurred vision, photosensitivity
*GI:* Nausea, diarrhea, vomiting, difficulty swallowing
*INTEG:* Rash, urticaria, fever, chills, flushing, hyperpyrexia

**Contraindications:** Children (parenterally), hypersensitivity to opioids, shock

**Precautions:** Pregnancy **C**, children, geriatric, cardiac dysrhythmias, acute febrile illness, encephalitis, gastroenteritis, dehydration, electrolyte imbalances, Reye's syndrome

---

 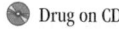

## Pharmacokinetics

| | |
|---|---|
| **Absorption** | Unknown |
| **Distribution** | Unknown |
| **Metabolism** | Liver, extensively |
| **Excretion** | Kidneys |
| **Half-life** | Unknown |

## Pharmacodynamics

| | PO | IM | RECT |
|---|---|---|---|
| **Onset** | 20-40 min | 15 min | 10-40 min |
| **Peak** | Unknown | Unknown | Unknown |
| **Duration** | 3-4 hr | 2-3 hr | 3-4 hr |

## Interactions
### Individual drugs
Alcohol: increased effect
### Drug classifications
CNS depressants: increased effect

## NURSING CONSIDERATIONS
### Assessment
• Monitor VS, B/P; check patients with cardiac disease more often
• Assess for signs of toxicity of other products or masking of symptoms of disease: brain tumor, intestinal obstructions
• Observe for drowsiness, dizziness
• Assess for nausea, vomiting before and after treatment

### Nursing diagnoses
• Knowledge, deficient (teaching)

### Implementation
#### PO route
• Cap may be swallowed whole or opened and mixed with food or fluids
#### IM route
• Administer IM inj in large muscle mass; aspirate to avoid **IV** administration
• Patient should remain lying down for 30 min after IM inj
**Syringe compatibilities:** Glycopyrrolate, hydromorphone, midazolam, nalbuphine
**Y-site compatibilities:** Heparin, hydrocortisone, potassium chloride, vit B/C

### Patient/family education
• Teach patient to use good oral hygiene; frequent rinsing of mouth, sugarless gum for dry mouth
• Caution patient to avoid hazardous activities until product response is determined, drowsiness may occur
• Inform patient that orthostatic hypotension occurs often and to rise from sitting or lying position gradually; avoid hot tubs, hot showers, and tub baths because hypotension may occur
• Advise patient to remain lying down after IM inj for at least 30 min
• Inform patient that in hot weather, heat stroke may occur; take extra precautions to stay cool
• Teach patient to avoid OTC preparations (cough, hayfever, cold) unless approved by prescriber because serious product interactions may occur; avoid use with alcohol, CNS depressants because increased drowsiness may occur
• Teach patient about EPS
• Instruct patient to report sore throat, malaise, fever, bleeding, mouth sores; if these occur, CBC should be performed and product discontinued

### Evaluation
**Positive therapeutic outcome**
• Decreased nausea, vomiting

## trimethoprim/ sulfamethoxazole (cotrimoxazole) (Rx)
(trye-meth'oh-prim/sul-fa-meth-ox'a-zole [ko-trye-mox'a-zole])
Apo-Sulfatrim*, Apo-Sulfatrim DS ✳, Bactrim, Bactrim IV, Bethaprim, Cotrim, Novo-Trimel ✳, Novo-Trimel DS ✳, Nu-Cotrimox ✳, Nu-Cotrimox DS ✳, Roubac ✳, Septra, Septra DS, SMZ/TMP, Sulfatrim
*Func. class.:* Antiinfective
*Chem. class.:* Sulfonamide—miscellaneous

### Pregnancy category C

**Action:** Sulfamethoxazole (SMZ) interferes with bacterial biosynthesis of proteins by competitive antagonism of PABA when adequate levels are maintained; trimethoprim (TMP) blocks synthesis of tetrahydrofolic acid; combination blocks two consecutive steps in bacterial synthesis of essential nucleic acids, protein

**Therapeutic outcome:** Absence of infection, based on C&S

**Uses:** UTI, otitis media, acute and chronic prostatitis, shigellosis, *Pneumocystis jiroveci* pneumonitis, chronic bronchitis, chancroid, traveler's diarrhea

T

## Dosage and routes
Based on TMP content

### UTI
*Adult:* PO 160 mg TMP q12hr × 10-14 days
*Child:* PO 8 mg/kg TMP daily in 2 divided doses q12hr

### Otitis media
*Child:* PO 8 mg/kg TMP daily in 2 divided doses q12hr × 10 days

### Chronic bronchitis
*Adult:* PO 160 mg TMP q12hr × 14 days

### Pneumocystis jiroveci pneumonitis
*Adult and child:* PO 20 mg/kg TMP daily in 4 divided doses q6hr × 14 days; **IV** 15-20 mg/kg/day (based on TMP) in 3-4 divided doses for up to 14 days

### Renal dose
Dosage reduction necessary in moderate to severe renal impairment (CCr <30 ml/min)

**Available forms:** Tabs 80 mg trimethoprim (TMP)/400 mg sulfamethoxazole (SMZ), 160 mg TMP/800 mg SMZ; susp 40 mg/200 mg/5 ml; **IV** 16 mg/80 mg/ml

## Adverse effects
*CNS:* Headache, insomnia, hallucinations, depression, vertigo, fatigue, anxiety, seizures, product fever, chills, **aseptic meningitis**
*CV:* **Allergic myocarditis**
*GI:* *Nausea, vomiting, abdominal pain,* stomatitis, **hepatitis**, glossitis, pancreatitis, diarrhea, **enterocolitis**, anorexia, **pseudomembranous colitis**
*GU:* **Renal failure, toxic nephrosis;** increased BUN, creatinine; crystalluria
*HEMA:* **Leukopenia, neutropenia, thrombocytopenia, agranulocytosis, hemolytic anemia, hypoprothrombinemia, Henoch-Schönlein purpura, methemoglobinemia, eosinophilia I**
*INTEG:* Rash, dermatitis, urticaria, erythema, photosensitivity, pain, inflammation at injection site, **toxic epidermal necrolysis, erythema multiforme**
*RESP:* Cough, shortness of breath
*SYST:* **Anaphylaxis, systemic lupus erythematosus, Stevens-Johnson syndrome**

**Contraindications:** Pregnancy at term, breastfeeding, infants <2 mo, hypersensitivity to trimethoprim or sulfonamides, megaloblastic anemia, CCr <15 ml/min, porphyria, hyperkalemia

**Precautions:** Pregnancy **C,** infants, geriatric, renal disease, glucose-6-phosphate dehydrogenase deficiency, impaired renal/hepatic function, possible folate deficiency, severe allergy, bronchial asthma, UV exposure

### Pharmacokinetics
| | |
|---|---|
| **Absorption** | Rapid |
| **Distribution** | Breast milk, crosses placenta, 68% protein bound |
| **Metabolism** | Liver |
| **Excretion** | Kidneys |
| **Half-life** | 8-13 hr |

### Pharmacodynamics
| | |
|---|---|
| **Onset** | Unknown |
| **Peak** | 1-4 hr |
| **Duration** | Unknown |

## Interactions
### Individual drugs
CycloSPORINE: decreased response
Dofetilide: increased levels of dofetilide
Methenamine: increased crystalluria
Methotrexate: increased bone marrow depression
Phenytoin: decreased hepatic clearance of phenytoin

### Drug classifications
Anticoagulants (oral): increased anticoagulant effect
Diuretics (potassium-sparing), potassium supplements: increased potassium levels
Diuretics (thiazide): increased thrombocytopenia
Sulfonylureas: increased hypoglycemic response

### Drug/herb
Acidophilus: do not use with antiinfectives; separate by several hours

### Drug/lab test
Increased: alkaline phosphatase, creatinine, bilirubin, AST, ALT

## NURSING CONSIDERATIONS
### Assessment
• Assess allergic reactions: rash, fever (AIDS patients more susceptible)
• Monitor I&O ratio; note color, character, pH of urine if product administered for UTI; output should be 800 ml less than intake; if urine is highly acidic, alkalization may be needed
• Monitor renal function tests: BUN, creatinine, urinalysis (long-term therapy)
• Assess type of infection; obtain C&S before starting therapy
• Assess blood dyscrasias, skin rash, fever, sore throat, bruising, bleeding, fatigue, joint pain

- Assess allergic reaction: rash, dermatitis, urticaria, pruritus, dyspnea, bronchospasm

## Nursing diagnoses
- Infection, risk for (uses)
- Knowledge, deficient (teaching)
- Noncompliance (teaching)

## Implementation
- Give with full glass of water to maintain adequate hydration; increase fluids to 2 L/day to decrease crystallization in kidneys
- Give medication after C&S; repeat C&S after full course of medication
- Store in airtight, light-resistant container at room temp

**IV route**
- Dilute 5 ml ampule/100-125 ml of $D_5W$, stable for 6 hr, give over 1½ hr, do not refrigerate

*Syringe compatibilities:* Heparin
*Y-site compatibilities:* Acyclovir, aldesleukin, allopurinol, amifostine, atracurium, aztreonam, cefepime, cyclophosphamide, diltiazem, enalaprilat, esmolol, filgrastim, fludarabine, gallium, granisetron, hydromorphone, labetalol, lorazepam, magnesium sulfate, melphalan, meperidine, morphine, pancuronium, perphenazine, piperacillin/tazobactam, sargramostim, tacrolimus, teniposide, thiotepa, vecuronium, zidovudine

## Patient family education
- Teach patient to take each oral dose with full glass of water to prevent crystalluria; drink 8-10 glasses of water/day
- Teach patient to complete full course of treatment to prevent superinfection
- Teach patient to avoid sunlight or use sunscreen to prevent burns
- Teach patient to avoid OTC medications (aspirin, vit C) unless directed by prescriber
- If diabetic, teach patient to use Clinistix or Tes-Tape
- Teach patient to use alternative contraceptive measures; decreased effectiveness of oral contraceptives may result
- Teach patient to notify prescriber if skin rash, sore throat, fever, mouth sores, unusual bruising, bleeding occur

## Evaluation
**Positive therapeutic outcome**
Absence of pain, fever, C&S negative

**triptorelin** (Rx)
(trip-toe'rel-in)
Trelstar Depot, Trelstar LA
*Func. class.:* Gonadotropin-releasing hormone antagonist
*Chem. class.:* Synthetic decapeptide analog of LHRH

**Pregnancy category** X

**Action:** Inhibitor of pituitary gonadotropin secretion; initially increases LH and FSH, with increases in testosterone, reduction in sex steroid levels

**Therapeutic outcome:** Decreased signs/symptoms of advanced prostate cancer

**Uses:** Advanced prostate cancer

**Dosage and routes**
*Adult:* IM 3.75 mg qmo; 11.75 mg q84 days

**Available forms:** Microgranules, depot inj 3.75 mg, 11.75 mg

**Adverse effects**
*CNS:* Headache, insomnia, dizziness, lability, fatigue
*CV: Hypertension,* peripheral edema
*ENDO:* Gynecomastia, breast tenderness, hot flashes
*GI:* Nausea, vomiting, diarrhea
*GU:* Impotence, urinary retention, UTI
*INTEG:* Rash, pain on injection, pruritus, hypersensitivity
*MISC:* **Anaphylaxis, angioedema**
*MS:* Osteoneuralgia

**Contraindications:** Pregnancy X, breastfeeding, hypersensitivity to this product or other LHRH agonists or LHRH

**Precautions:** Metastatic vertebral lesions, urinary tract obstruction, spinal cord compression, renal disease

| Pharmacokinetics | |
|---|---|
| Absorption | Unknown |
| Distribution | Unknown |
| Metabolism | CYP/450 |
| Excretion | Liver, kidneys |
| Half-life | 3 hr |

| Pharmacodynamics |
|---|
| Unknown |

**Interactions**
*Drug/lab test*
Increased: alkaline phosphatase, estradiol, FSH, LH, testosterone levels
Decreased: testosterone levels, progesterone

Adverse effects: *italic* = common, **bold** = life-threatening

## NURSING CONSIDERATIONS
### Assessment
- Assess for severe hypersensitivity: discontinue product and give antihistamines, have emergency equipment nearby
- Monitor I&O ratios; palpate bladder for distintion in urinary obstruction
- Monitor for relief of bone pain (back pain)
- Assess levels of testosterone and PSA

### Nursing diagnoses
- Diarrhea (adverse reactions)
- Knowledge, deficient (teaching)

### Implementation
- Give IM using implant, inserted by qualified person
- Use syringe with 20-G needle, withdraw 2 ml of sterile water for inj, inject into vial, shake well, withdraw vial contents, inject immediately

### Patient/family education
- Teach patient that gynecomastia may occur but will decrease after treatment is discontinued
- Advise patient to report allergic reaction immediately
- Teach patient that disease flare may occur at beginning of therapy

### Evaluation
**Positive therapeutic outcome**
- More normal levels of PSA, acid phosphatase, alkaline phosphatase, testosterone level of <25 ng/dl, tumor response

---

## tropicamide ophthalmic
*See Appendix D*

---

## trospium (Rx)
(trose′pee-um)
Sanctura
*Func. class.:* Anticholinergic, overactive bladder product
*Chem. class.:* Muscarinic receptor antagonist

**Pregnancy category C**

**Action:** Relaxes smooth muscles in bladder by inhibiting acetylcholine effect on muscarinic receptors

**Therapeutic outcome:** Absence of urinary distention, nocturia, frequency, urgency, incontinence

**Uses:** Overactive bladder (urinary frequency, urgency)

## Dosage and routes
*Adult:* PO 20 mg bid, give 5 ml ≥1 hr prior to meals or on empty stomach

*Renal dose*
*Adult:* PO CCr < 30 ml/min 20 mg/day at bedtime
*Geriatric ≥75 yr:* PO titrate down to 20 mg/day based on response and tolerance

**Available forms:** Tabs 20 mg

**Adverse effects**
*CNS:* Fatigue, dizziness, headache
*CV:* Tachycardia
*EENT:* Dry eyes, vision abnormalities
*GI:* Flatulence, abdominal pain, *constipation, dry mouth,* dyspepsia
*GU:* Urinary retention
*INTEG:* Dry skin

**Contraindications:** Hypersensitivity, uncontrolled angle-closure glaucoma, urinary retention, gastric retention, myasthenia gravis

**Precautions:** Pregnancy **C,** breastfeeding, children, renal/hepatic disease, controlled angle-closure glaucoma, ulcerative colitis, intestinal atony, bladder outflow obstruction

### Pharmacokinetics

| | |
|---|---|
| **Absorption** | Rapidly absorbed (10%) |
| **Distribution** | Protein bound (50–85%) |
| **Metabolism** | Not fully understood in humans; extensively metabolized |
| **Excretion** | Urine (6%), feces (85%); excreted in urine by active tubular secretion |
| **Half-life** | Unknown |

### Pharmacodynamics
Unknown

### Interactions
*Individual drugs*
Alcohol: increased drowsiness
Metformin, procainamide, quinidine, ranitidine, tenofovir, triamterene, vancomycin: increased or decreased action of trospium
*Drug classifications*
Products excreted by active renal secretion (amiloride, digoxin, morphine): increased or decreased action of trospium
*Drug/food*
High-fat meal: decreased absorption

## NURSING CONSIDERATIONS
### Assessment
- Assess urinary patterns: distention, nocturia, frequency, urgency, incontinence

---

 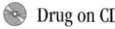

### Nursing diagnoses
• Knowledge, deficient (teaching)
• Urinary elimination, impaired (uses)

### Implementation
• Take 1 hr prior to meals or on empty stomach

### Patient/family education
• Advise patient to avoid hazardous activities; dizziness may occur
• Caution patient that alcohol may increase drowsiness
• Inform patient about anticholinergic effects that may occur

### Evaluation
**Positive therapeutic outcome**
• Correction of urinary status: absence of dysuria, frequency, nocturia, incontinence

---

### ⚠ HIGH ALERT

## tubocurarine 🔄 (Rx)
(too-boh-cure′a-reen)
Tubarine ✸, Tubocurarine
*Func. class.:* Neuromuscular blocker non-depolarizing
*Chem. class.:* Synthetic curariform

**Pregnancy category C**

**Action:** Inhibits transmission of nerve impulses by binding with cholinergic receptor sites, antagonizing action of acetylcholine; no analgesic response

**Therapeutic outcome:** Skeletal muscle paralysis during anesthesia

**Uses:** Facilitation of endotracheal intubation; skeletal muscle relaxation during mechanical ventilation, surgery, or general anesthesia; ECT contraction management

### Dosage and routes
*Electroconvulsive therapy*
*Adult:* **IV** 0.1-0.2 mg/kg slow **IV** after induction of anesthesia; 5 min prior to shock therapy
*Induction of neuromuscular blockade*
*Adult:* **IV** Mech vent 0.25-0.5 mg/kg q2-3hr
*Neonate ≤1 mo:* **IV** 0.25-0.5 mg/kg then ⅕-¼ of initial dose
*Child and infant:* **IV** 0.5 mg/kg
*Surgical procedure*
*Adult:* **IV** 6-9 mg or 0.165 mg/kg, give 3-4.5 mg 3 to 5 min later if needed
*Myasthenia gravis diagnosis*
*Adult:* **IV** 0.004-0.033 mg/kg

*Seizure*
*Adult:* **IV** 0.165 mg/kg over 30-90 sec
*Burn patients >40% total body surface area*
Increase dose 2.5-5 fold; if used with halothane or cyclopropane, reduce dose by 20%; if used with enflurane, isoflurane, methoxyflurane reduce dose by ⅓ to ½

**Available forms:** Inj 3 mg/ml (20 units/ml)

### Adverse effects
*CV:* Bradycardia, tachycardia, increased, decreased B/P
*EENT:* Increased secretions
*INTEG:* Rash, flushing, pruritus, urticaria
*RESP:* **Prolonged apnea, bronchospasm, cyanosis, respiratory depression,** wheezing, dyspnea

**Contraindications:** Hypersensitivity

**Precautions:** Pregnancy **C,** breastfeeding, children <2 yr, cardiac disease, electrolyte imbalances, dehydration, neuromuscular disease, respiratory disease, renal/hepatic disease

#### Pharmacokinetics
| | |
|---|---|
| **Absorption** | Complete bioavailability |
| **Distribution** | Extensive, crosses placenta |
| **Metabolism** | Liver, small amount |
| **Excretion** | Kidneys—unchanged (30%-75%), bile (11%) |
| **Half-life** | 1-3 hr |

#### Pharmacodynamics
| | IM | IV |
|---|---|---|
| **Onset** | 15-30 min | 3-5 min, dose dependent |
| **Peak** | Unknown | 2-3 min |
| **Duration** | Unknown | ½-1½ hr |

### Interactions
*Individual drugs*
Amphotericin B, clindamycin, enflurane, isoflurane, lidocaine, lincomycin, lithium, magnesium salts, trimethaphan, quinidine, verapamil: increased neuromuscular blockade
Theophylline: dysrhythmias
*Drug classifications*
Aminoglycosides, analgesics (opioid), anesthetics (local), antiinfectives (polymyxin), loop diuretics, thiazides: increased neuromuscular blockade

**T**

Adverse effects: *italic* = common, **bold** = life-threatening

## NURSING CONSIDERATIONS
### Assessment
• Monitor for electrolyte imbalances (potassium, magnesium) before product is used; electrolyte imbalances may lead to increased action of this product
• Monitor VS (B/P, pulse, respirations, airway) until fully recovered; rate, depth, pattern of respirations, strength of hand grip; patient should be intubated before use
• Monitor recovery: decreased paralysis of face, diaphragm, leg, arm, rest of body; residual weakness and respiratory problems may occur during recovery period
• Monitor allergic reactions: rash, fever, respiratory distress, pruritus; product should be discontinued

### Nursing diagnoses
• Breathing pattern, ineffective (uses)
• Communication, verbal, impaired (adverse reactions)
• Fear (adverse reactions)
• Knowledge, deficient (teaching)

### Implementation
• Use peripheral nerve stimulator by anesthesiologist to determine neuromuscular blockade; deep tendon reflexes should be monitored during extended periods
• Give **IV** undiluted by direct **IV** over 1-1½ min (only by qualified person, usually an anesthesiologist)
*Syringe compatibilities:* Pentobarbital, thiopental
*Additive incompatibilities:* Barbiturates, sodium bicarbonate
*Solution compatibilities:* $D_5$, $D_{10}W$, 0.9% NaCl, 0.45% NaCl, Ringer's, LR, dextrose/Ringer's or dextrose/LR combinations

### Patient/family education
• Provide patient reassurance if communication is difficult during recovery from neuromuscular blockade
• Provide explanation to patient regarding all procedures or treatments; patient will remain conscious if anesthesia is not given also

### Evaluation
**Positive therapeutic outcome**
• Paralysis of jaw, eyelid, head, neck, rest of body as evaluated by peripheral nerve stimulator

**Treatment of overdose:** Edrophonium or neostigmine, atropine, monitor VS; patient may require mechanical ventilation

---

## undecylenic acid topical
*See Appendix D*

---

## unoprostone ophthalmic
*See Appendix D*

---

### ! HIGH ALERT

## urokinase (Rx)
(yoor-oh-kin'ase)
Abbokinase, Abbokinase Open-Cath
*Func. class.:* Thrombolytic enzyme
*Chem. class.:* β-Hemolytic *Streptococcus* filtrate (purified)

**Pregnancy category** B

**Action:** Promotes thrombolysis by directly converting plasminogen to plasmin

**Therapeutic outcome:** Lysis of emboli, or thrombosis in various parts of the body

**Uses:** Venous thrombosis, PE, arterial thrombosis, arterial embolism, arteriovenous cannula occlusion, lysis of coronary artery thrombi after MI

### Dosage and routes
*Lysis of pulmonary emboli*
*Adult and child:* **IV** 4400 international units/kg/hr over 10 min (90 ml/hr); CONT **IV** INF 4400 international units/kg/hr × 12 hr (15 ml/hr); flush line at end of INF

*Coronary artery thrombosis*
*Adult:* Instill 6000 international units/min into occluded artery for 1-2 hr after giving **IV** BOL of heparin 2500-10,000 units; may also give as **IV** INF of 2-3 million units over 45-90 min

*Venous catheter occlusion*
*Adult and child:* Instill 5000 international units into line, wait 5 min, then aspirate; repeat aspiration attempts q5 min × ½ hr; if occlusion has not been removed, then cap line and wait ½-1 hr, then aspirate; may need 2nd dose if still occluded

**Available forms:** Powder for inj, lyophilized: 250,000 international units/vial; powder for catheter clearance

### Adverse effects
*CNS: Headache,* fever
*CV:* Hypotension, dysrhythmias
*GI: Nausea,* vomiting
*HEMA: Decreased Hct,* **bleeding**
*INTEG: Rash, urticaria,* phlebitis at **IV** inf site, itching, flushing

---

 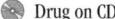

**MS:** Low back pain
**RESP:** Altered respirations, cyanosis, shortness of breath, **bronchospasm**
**SYST:** GI, GU, intracranial, retroperitoneal bleeding; surface bleeding; anaphylaxis (rare)

**Contraindications:** Hypersensitivity, internal active bleeding, intraspinal surgery, neoplasms of CNS, ulcerative colitis/enteritis, severe uncontrolled hypertension, renal/hepatic disease, hypocoagulation, COPD, subacute bacterial endocarditis, rheumatic valvular disease, cerebral embolism/thrombosis/hemorrhage, intraarterial diagnostic procedure or surgery (10 days), recent major surgery/trauma, aneurysm, AV malformation

**Precautions:** Pregnancy **B**, arterial emboli from left side of heart, hepatic disease

| Pharmacokinetics | |
|---|---|
| **Absorption** | Completely |
| **Distribution** | Unknown |
| **Metabolism** | Liver |
| **Excretion** | Kidneys |
| **Half-life** | 10-20 min |

| Pharmacodynamics | |
|---|---|
| **Onset** | Rapid |
| **Peak** | Rapid |
| **Duration** | 12 hr |

## Interactions
### Individual drugs
Abciximab, aspirin, clopidogrel, dipyridamole, eptifibatide, heparin, indomethacin, phenylbutazone, plicamycin, ticlopidine, tirofiban, valproic acid: increased bleeding potential
### Drug classifications
Anticoagulants (oral), cephalosporins (some), NSAIDs: increased bleeding potential
Glycoprotein IIb, IIIa inhibitors: increased bleeding risk
### Drug/lab test
Increased: pro-time, APTT, TT

## NURSING CONSIDERATIONS
### Assessment
• Monitor VS, B/P, pulse, respirations (including peripheral), neurologic signs, temp at least q4hr; temp >104° F (40° C) indicates internal bleeding; monitor rhythm closely; ventricular dysrhythmias may occur with hyperfusion; monitor heart, breath sounds, neurologic status, peripheral pulses
• Assess for bleeding during 1st hr of treatment: hematuria, hematemesis, bleeding from mucous membranes, epistaxis, ecchymosis; guaiac, all body fluids, stools; blood studies (Hct, platelets, PTT, pro-time, TT, APTT) before starting therapy (pro-time or APTT must be less than 2 × control); TT or pro-time q3-4hr during treatment
• Assess hypersensitivity: fever, rash, itching, chills, facial swelling, dyspnea; mild reaction may be treated with antihistamines; notify prescriber of severe reactions, stop product, keep resuscitative equipment nearby
• Monitor ECG on monitor, watch for segment changes, changes in rhythm; sinus bradycardia, ventricular tachycardia, accelerated idioventricular rhythm may occur because of reperfusion

### Nursing diagnoses
• Gas exchange, impaired (uses)
• Injury, risk for (adverse reactions)
• Tissue perfusion, ineffective (uses)

### Implementation
**Intermittent IV route**
• Give **IV** loading dose over 30 min to avoid hypotension
• **IV** after dilution with 4-5 g/250 ml of 0.9% NaCl, D₅W, LR, give over 1 hr; may give by continuous inf after loading dose(s) of 1 g/hr diluted in 50-100 ml of compatible sol; use infusion pump; do not give by direct **IV**
• Give heparin therapy after thrombolytic therapy is discontinued, TT, ACT, or APTT less than 2 × control (about 3-4 hr)
• Avoid invasive procedures, inj, rectal temp
• Apply pressure for 30 sec to minor bleeding sites, 30 min to sites of atrial puncture, followed by pressure dressing; inform prescriber if this does not attain hemostasis
• Store powder at room temperature or refrigerate; protect from excessive light
**Additive incompatibilities:** Do not mix with other medications

### Patient/family education
• Teach patient reason for medication, signs and symptoms of bleeding, allergic reactions, when to notify health care prescriber

### Evaluation
**Positive therapeutic outcome**
• Lysis of thrombi or emboli

U

Adverse effects: *italic* = common, **bold** = life-threatening

## valacyclovir (Rx)

(val-a-sye'kloh-vir)

Valtrex

*Func. class.:* Antiviral

*Chem. class.:* Acyclic purine nucleoside analog

### Pregnancy category B

**Do not confuse:**

valacyclovir/valganciclovir, Valtrex/Valcyte

**Action:** Interferes with DNA synthesis by conversion to acyclovir, causing decreased viral replication, time of lesional healing

**Therapeutic outcome:** Absence of itching, painful lesions; crusting and healing of lesions

**Uses:** Treatment or suppression of herpes zoster (shingles), recurrent genital herpes, herpes labialis (cold sores)

**Unlabeled uses:** Prevention of CMV infection, in advanced HIV posttransplant patients

### Dosage and routes
*Genital herpes (suppressive initial)*
*Adult:* PO 1 g bid × 10 days initially

*Genital herpes (recurrent episodes)*
*Adult:* PO 500 mg bid × 3 days

*Genital herpes (suppressive therapy)*
*Adult:* PO 1 g/day with normal immune function; 500 mg/day for those with ≤9 recurrences/yr; 500 mg bid in HIV-infected patients with CD4 ≥100

*Reduction of transmission*
*Adult:* PO 500 mg/day for source partner

*Herpes zoster*
*Adult:* PO 1 g tid × 1 wk

*Herpes labialis*
*Adult:* PO 2 g bid × 1 day

*Renal dose*
*Adult:* PO CCr 30-49 ml/min 1g q12hr (herpes zoster); 1 g q12hr × 1 day (herpes labalis); CCr 10-29 ml/min 1 g q24hr (genital herpes/herpes zoster); 500 mg q24hr (recurrent genital herpes); CCr <10 ml/min 500 mg q24hr (genital herpes/herpes zoster), 500 mg q24hr (recurrent genital herpes)

**Available forms:** Tabs 500, 1000 mg

### Adverse effects
*CNS:* Tremors, lethargy, *dizziness, headache, weakness,* depression
***ENDO:*** *Dysmennorhea*

*GI:* *Nausea, vomiting, diarrhea, abdominal pain, constipation,* increased AST
***HEMA:*** **Thrombocytopenic purpura, hemolytic uremic syndrome**
***INTEG:*** *Rash*

**Contraindications:** Hypersensitivity to this product, acyclovir, penciclovir, famciclovir, ganciclovir, valganciclovir

**Precautions:** Pregnancy **B**, breastfeeding, geriatric, renal/hepatic disease, electrolyte imbalance, dehydration, thrombotic thrombocytopenic purpura/hemolytic uremic syndrome (TTP/HUS), AIDS

### Pharmacokinetics

| | |
|---|---|
| **Absorption** | Unknown |
| **Distribution** | Crosses placenta, enters breast milk, protein binding 13.5%-17.9% |
| **Metabolism** | Converts to acyclovir |
| **Excretion** | Urine, as acyclovir |
| **Half-life** | 2½-3½ hr |

### Pharmacodynamics
Unknown

### Interactions
*Individual drugs*
Cimetidine, probenecid: increased blood levels of valacyclovir (only if renal disease is significant)

### NURSING CONSIDERATIONS
**Assessment**
• Assess for signs of infection; characteristics of lesions; therapy should be started at first sign of herpes and is most effective within 72 hr of outbreak
• Assess C&S before product therapy; product may be performed as soon as culture is performed; repeat C&S after treatment; determine the presence of other STDs
• Assess bowel pattern before, during treatment
• Assess for skin eruptions: rash
• Assess allergies before treatment, reaction of each medication
◆ Assess for thrombocytopenic purpura, hemolytic uremic syndrome, may be fatal

**Nursing diagnoses**
• Infection, risk for (uses)

**Implementation**
• Give within 72 hr of outbreak (herpes zoster); as soon as possible (herpes labialis, genital herpes)
• Give orally before infection occurs

  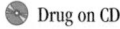

## Patient/family education
• Advise patient to take as prescribed; if dose is missed, take as soon as remembered up to 2 hr before next dose; do not double dose
• Instruct patient to take product orally before infection occurs; product should be taken when itching or pain occurs, usually before eruptions
• Inform patient that partners need to be told that patient has herpes; they can become infected; condoms must be worn to prevent reinfections
• Tell patient that product does not cure infection, just controls symptoms and does not prevent infection to others

## Evaluation
**Positive therapeutic outcome**
• Absence of itching, painful lesions; crusting and healed lesions

---

## valganciclovir (Rx)
(val-gan-sy'kloh-veer)
Valcyte
*Func. class:* Antiviral
*Chem. class:* Synthetic nucleoside analog

**Pregnancy category C**

**Do not confuse:**
valganciclovir/valacyclovir, Valcyte/Valtrex

**Action:** Valganciclovir is metabolized to ganciclovir; inhibits replication of human CMV in vivo and in vitro by selectively inhibiting viral DNA synthesis

**Therapeutic outcome:** Decreased proliferation of virus responsible for CMV retinitis

**Uses:** Cytomegalovirus (CMV) retinitis in immunocompromised persons, including those with AIDS, after indirect ophthalmoscopy confirms diagnosis; prevention of CMV in transplantation; prevention of CMV in transplant patients

## Dosage and routes
*Treatment of CMV*
**Adult:** PO Induction 900 mg bid × 21 days with food; maintenance 900 mg/day with food

*Transplant*
**Adult:** PO 900 mg/day with food starting within 10 days prior to transplantation until 100 days post transplantation

*Renal dose*
CCr ≥60 ml/min same dosage as above; CCr 40-59 ml/min 450 mg bid × 21 days, then 450 mg/day; CCr 25-39 ml/min 450 mg/day × 21 days, then 450 mg q2 days; CCr 10-24 ml/min 450 mg q2 days, then 450 mg 2×/week

**Available forms:** Tabs 450 mg

## Adverse effects
*CNS: Fever,* chills, **coma,** *confusion,* abnormal thoughts, dizziness, bizarre dreams, *headache,* psychosis, tremors, somnolence, *paresthesia, weakness,* **seizures,** insomnia
*EENT:* Retinal detachment in CMV retinitis
*GI: Abnormal liver function tests, nausea, vomiting, anorexia, diarrhea, abdominal pain,* **hemorrhage**
*GU:* **Hematuria,** increased creatinine, BUN
*HEMA:* **Granulocytopenia, thrombocytopenia, irreversible neutropenia, anemia, eosinophilia**
*INTEG: Rash,* alopecia, *pruritus,* urticaria, pain at inj site, phlebitis, **Stevens-Johnson syndrome**
*MISC:* Local and systemic infections and **sepsis**

**Contraindications:** Breastfeeding; hypersensitivity to acyclovir, ganciclovir, penciclovir, famciclovir, or valacyclovir; absolute neutrophil count <500/mm$^3$; platelet count <25,000/mm$^3$; hemodialysis; liver transplant

**Precautions:** Pregnancy **C,** children, geriatric, preexisting cytopenias, renal function impairment

### Pharmacokinetics

| | |
|---|---|
| **Absorption** | Well absorbed from GI tract |
| **Distribution** | Plasma protein binding unknown; crosses blood-brain barrier, CSF |
| **Metabolism** | Rapidly metabolized in intestinal wall and liver to ganciclovir |
| **Excretion** | Kidneys (ganciclovir) |
| **Half-life** | 3-4½ hr |

### Pharmacodynamics

| | |
|---|---|
| **Onset** | Unknown |
| **Peak** | 1-3 hr |
| **Duration** | Unknown |

## Interactions
*Individual drugs*
Adriamycin, amphotericin B, cycloSPORINE, dapsone, DOXOrubicin, flucytosine, pentamidine, trimethoprim/sulfamethoxazole, vinBLAStine, vinCRIStine: increased toxicity
Didanosine: decreased effect
Imipenem/cilastatin: increased seizures
Probenecid: decreased renal clearance of valganciclovir

V

Radiation, zidovudine: severe granulocytopenia; do not coadminister

*Drug classifications*

Antineoplastics: severe granulocytopenia; do not coadminister

Nucleoside analogs, other: increased toxicity

*Drug/food*

Absorption: increased

## NURSING CONSIDERATIONS
### Assessment

- Assess for leukopenia/neutropenia/thrombocytopenia: WBCs, platelets q2 days during 2×/day dosing and then qwk
- Assess for leukopenia daily with WBC count in patients with prior leukopenia using other nucleoside analogs or for whom leukopenia counts are <1000 cells/mm$^3$ at start of treatment
- Assess serum creatinine or CCr ≥q2 wk
- Assess for CMV retinitis by ophthalmoscopy before beginning treatment and q2wk
- Obtain culture for CMV
- Assess for infection: sore throat, cough, fever, chills, back pain; notify prescriber

### Nursing diagnoses

- Infection, risk for (uses)
- Injury, risk for (uses, adverse reactions)
- Knowledge, deficient (teaching)

### Implementation

- Give with food for better absorption

### Patient/family education

- Inform patient that product does not cure condition, that regular ophthalmologic and blood tests are necessary
- Caution patient that major toxicities may necessitate discontinuing product
- Caution patient to use contraception during treatment and that infertility may occur; men should use barrier contraception for 90 days after treatment
- Instruct patient to take with food
- ◑ Instruct patient to report infection: fever, chills, sore throat; blood dyscrasias: bruising, bleeding, petechiae
- Advise patient to avoid crowds, persons with respiratory infections
- Caution patient to use sunscreen to prevent burns

### Evaluation
**Positive therapeutic outcome**

- Decreased symptoms of CMV

**Treatment of overdose:** Maintain adequate hydration; dialysis may help reduce serum concentrations; consider use of hematopoietic growth factors

---

**valproate** (Rx)
(val-proh′ate)
Depacon
**valproic acid** (Rx)
Depakene
**divalproex sodium** (Rx)
Depakote, Depakote ER, Epival
*Func. class.:* Anticonvulsant, vascular headache suppressant
*Chem. class.:* Carboxylic acid derivative

**Pregnancy category  D**

**Action:** Increases levels of γ-aminobutyric acid (GABA) in brain, which decreases seizure activity

**Therapeutic outcome:** Decreased symptoms of epilepsy, bipolar disorder

**Uses:** Simple (petit mal), complex (petit mal), absence, mixed seizures, manic episode associated with bipolar disorder, prophylaxis of migraine, adjunct in schizophrenia, tardive dyskinesia, aggression in children with ADHD, organic brain syndrome, tonic-clonic (grand mal)/myoclonic seizures

**Unlabeled uses:** Rectal for seizures (valproic acid)

### Dosage and routes
*Epilepsy*
*Adult and child:* PO 10-15 mg/kg/day divided in 2-3 doses, may increase by 5-10 mg/kg/day qwk, max 60 mg/kg/day in 2-3 divided doses; **IV** ≤20 mg/min over 1 hr

*Mania (divalproex sodium)*
*Adult:* PO 750 mg/day in divided doses, max 60 mg/kg/day or 3000 mg/day

*Migraine (divalproex sodium)*
*Adult:* PO 250 mg bid, may increase to 1000 mg/day; or 500 mg (Depakote ER) daily × 7 days, then 1000 mg/day

**Available forms:** Valproic acid: caps 250 mg; syr 250 mg/5 ml; divalproex: delayed rel tabs 125, 250, 500 mg; ext rel tabs 250, 500 mg; sprinkle caps 125 mg; valproate: inj 100 mg/ml

### Adverse effects
*CNS: Sedation, drowsiness,* dizziness, headache, incoordination, depression, hallucinations, behavioral changes, tremors, aggression, weakness, **coma**
*EENT:* Visual disturbances, taste perversion
*GI: Nausea, vomiting, constipation, diarrhea, dyspepsia,* anorexia, cramps, **hepatic failure, pancreatitis, toxic hepatitis,** stomatitis, weight gain

---

*GU:* Enuresis, irregular menses
*HEMA:* **Thrombocytopenia, leukopenia, lymphocytosis,** increased pro-time, bruising, epistaxis
*INTEG:* *Rash,* alopecia, photosensitivity, dry skin

**Contraindications:** Pregnancy **D,** hypersensitivity, renal/hepatic disease, urea cycle disorders, pancreatitis

**Precautions:** Breastfeeding, children <2 yr, geriatric

### Pharmacokinetics

| | |
|---|---|
| **Absorption** | Unknown |
| **Distribution** | Breast milk, crosses placenta, widely distributed, protein binding 90% |
| **Metabolism** | Liver |
| **Excretion** | Kidneys |
| **Half-life** | 6-16 hr |

### Pharmacodynamics

| | |
|---|---|
| **Onset** | 15-30 min |
| **Peak** | 1-4 hr |
| **Duration** | 4-6 hr |

### Interactions
*Individual drugs*
Abciximab, cefoperazone, cefotetan, eptifibatide, heparin, tirofiban: increased bleeding risk
Alcohol: increased CNS depression
Carbamazepine, ethosuximide, lamotrigine, zidovudine: increased action and toxicity of these products
Carbamazepine, lamotrigine, rifampin: decreased valproic acid level
Cimetidine: decreased metabolism of valproic acid
Chlorpromazine, erythromycin, felbamate: increased valproic acid level
Phenytoin: increased action of phenytoin
*Drug classifications*
Antidepressants (tricyclics), barbiturates: increased action
Antihistamines, barbiturates, MAOIs, opioids, sedative/hypnotics: increased CNS depression
Antiplatelets, NSAIDs, thrombolytics: increased bleeding risk
Salicylates: increased toxicity of valproic acid
*Drug/lab test*
False positive: ketones
Interference: thyroid function tests

## NURSING CONSIDERATIONS
### Assessment
• Monitor blood tests: Hct, Hgb, RBC, serum folate, platelets, pro-time, vit D if on long-term therapy
• Monitor liver function tests: AST, ALT, bilirubin, creatinine, failure
• Monitor blood levels: therapeutic level 50-100 mcg/ml
• Assess seizure disorder: location, aura, activity, duration; seizure precautions should be in place
• Assess bipolar disorder: mood, activity, sleeping, eating, behavior
• Assess migraines: frequency, intensity
• Assess respiratory dysfunction: respiratory depression, character, rate, rhythm; hold product if respirations are <12/min or if pupils are dilated

### Nursing diagnoses
• Injury, risk for (uses, adverse reactions)
• Knowledge, deficient

### Implementation
• Swallow tabs and caps whole; do not break, crush, or chew; use sprinkle cap contents on food
• Give elixir alone; do not dilute with carbonated beverage; do not give syrup to patients on sodium restriction
• Give with food or milk to decrease GI symptoms

### Patient/family education
• Teach patient that physical dependency may result from extended use
• Instruct patient to avoid driving, other activities that require alertness
• Advise patient not to discontinue medication quickly after long-term use; seizures may result
• Advise patient to report visual disturbances, rash, diarrhea, light-colored stools, jaundice, protracted vomiting to prescriber

### Evaluation
**Positive therapeutic outcome**
• Decreased seizures

**V**

## valsartan (Rx)

(val-zar'tan)

Diovan

*Func. class.:* Antihypertensive

*Chem. class.:* Angiotensin II receptor antagonist (type $AT_1$)

**Pregnancy category** D

**Action:** Blocks the vasoconstrictor and aldosterone-secreting effects of angiotensin II; selectively blocks the binding of angiotensin II to the $AT_1$ receptor found in tissues

**Therapeutic outcome:** Decreased B/P

**Uses:** Hypertension, alone or in combination, CHF

### Dosage and routes

*Adult:* PO 80-160 mg/day alone or in combination with other antihypertensives, may increase to 320 mg CHF

### CHF

*Adult:* PO 40 mg bid, up to 60 mg bid

**Available forms:** Tabs 80, 160, 320 mg

### Adverse effects

*CNS: Dizziness, insomnia,* drowsiness, vertigo, headache, fatigue

*CV:* Angina pectoris, 2nd-degree AV block, **cerebrovascular accident,** hypotension, **MI, dysrhythmias**

*EENT:* Conjunctivitis

*GI:* Diarrhea, abdominal pain, nausea, **hepatotoxicity**

*GU:* Impotence, **nephrotoxicity**

*HEMA: Anemia,* neutropenia

*META:* Hyperkalemia

*MS:* Cramps, myalgia, pain, stiffness

*RESP: Cough*

**Contraindications:** Pregnancy **D** (2nd/3rd trimester), hypersensitivity, severe hepatic disease, bilateral renal artery stenosis

**Precautions:** Breastfeeding, children, geriatric, CHF, hypertrophic cardiomyopathy, aortic/mitral valve stenosis, CAD, angioedema, renal/hepatic disease, hypersensitivity to ACE inhibitors

### Pharmacokinetics

| | |
|---|---|
| **Absorption** | Well absorbed |
| **Distribution** | Bound to plasma proteins |
| **Metabolism** | Extensive |
| **Excretion** | Feces, urine, breast milk |
| **Half-life** | 9 hr |

### Pharmacodynamics

| | |
|---|---|
| **Onset** | Up to 2 hr |
| **Peak** | 4-6 hr |
| **Duration** | 24 hr |

### Interactions

*Individual drugs*

Lithium: increased effects of lithium

*Drug classifications*

Diuretics (potassium-sparing, potassium supplements, ACE inhibitors): increased hyperkalemia

NSAIDs, salicylates: decreased antihypertensive effects

*Drug/herb*

Aconite: increased toxicity, death

Astragalus, cola tree: increased or decreased antihypertensive effect

Barberry, betony, black catechu, black cohosh, bloodroot, broom, burdock, cat's claw, dandelion, goldenseal, Irish moss, Jamaican dogwood, kelp, khella, mistletoe, parsley: increased antihypertensive effect

Coltsfoot, guarana, khat, licorice, yohimbe: decreased antihypertensive effect

### NURSING CONSIDERATIONS

**Assessment**

• Assess B/P (lying, sitting, standing), pulse q4hr; note rate, rhythm, quality periodically

• Monitor electrolytes: potassium, sodium, chloride; total $CO_2$

• Assess for angioedema: facial swelling, shortness of breath

• Obtain baselines in renal, liver function tests before therapy begins

• Assess blood tests: BUN, creatinine, before treatment

• Monitor for edema in feet, legs daily

• Assess for skin turgor, dryness of mucous membranes for hydration status; correct volume depletion before initiating therapy

**Nursing diagnoses**

• Fluid volume, deficient (side effects)

• Knowledge, deficient (teaching)

• Noncompliance (teaching)

**Implementation**

• Administer without regard to meals

**Patient/family education**

• Teach patient not to take this product if breastfeeding or pregnant, or have had an allergic reaction to this product

• If a dose is missed, instruct patient to take as soon as possible, unless it is within an hour before next dose

• Advise patient to comply with dosage schedule, even if feeling better

- Teach patient to notify prescriber of fever, swelling of hands or feet, irregular heartbeat, chest pain
- Advise patient excessive perspiration, dehydration, diarrhea may lead to fall in blood pressure; consult prescriber if these occur
- Inform patient that product may cause dizziness, fainting; light-headedness may occur
- Caution patient to rise slowly to sitting or standing position to minimize orthostatic hypotension; how to take B/P

## Evaluation
**Positive therapeutic outcome**
- Decreased B/P

---

## vancomycin
(van-koe-mye′sin)
Vancocin, Vancoled, vancomycin HCl
*Func. clas.:* Antiinfective—miscellaneous
*Chem. class.:* Tricyclic glycopeptide
**Pregnancy category B**

---

**Action:** Inhibits bacterial cell wall synthesis

**Therapeutic outcome:** Bactericidal for the following organisms: staphylococci, streptococci, *Corynebacterium*, *Clostridium*

**Uses:** Resistant staphylococcal infections, pseudomembranous colitis, staphylococcal enterocolitis, group A β-hemolytic streptococci, endocarditis prophylaxis for dental procedures, diphtheroid endocarditis

### Dosage and routes
**Serious staphylococcal infections**
*Adult:* **IV** 500 mg (7.5 mg/kg) q6-8hr or 1 g (15 mg/kg) q12hr
*Child:* **IV** 40 mg/kg/day divided q6-8hr
*Neonate:* **IV** 15 mg/kg initially followed by 10 mg/kg q8-24hr

**Pseudomembranous/
staphylococcal enterocolitis**
*Adult:* PO 500 mg in divided doses for 7-10 days
*Child:* PO 40 mg/kg/day divided q6hr, max 2 g/day

**Endocarditis prophylaxis for dental procedure**
*Adult:* **IV** 1 g over 1 hr; 1 hr before dental procedure
*Child:* **IV** 20 mg/kg over 1 hr; 1 hr before procedure

**Renal dose**
*Adult:* **IV** Loading dose 750 mg-1 g but not <15 mg/kg; CCr 50-80 ml/min 1 g q1-3 days;

CCr 10-50 ml/min 1 g q3-7 days; CCr <10 ml/min 1 g q7-14 days

**Available forms:** Pulvules 125, 250 mg; powder for oral sol 250 mg/5 ml, 500 mg/6 ml; powder for inj **IV** 500 mg; vials 1, 5, 10 g

### Adverse effects
*CV:* **Cardiac arrest, vascular collapse (rare),** hypotension
*EENT: Ototoxicity, permanent deafness,* tinnitus, nystagmus
*GI:* **Nausea, pseudomembranous colitis**
*GU:* **Nephrotoxicity: increased BUN, creatinine, albumin, fatal uremia**
*HEMA:* **Leukopenia, eosinophilia, neutropenia**
*INTEG:* Chills, fever, rash, thrombophlebitis at inj site, urticaria, pruritus, necrosis (Red Man product syndrome)
*RESP:* Wheezing, dyspnea
*SYST:* **Anaphylaxis,** superinfection

**Contraindications:** Hypersensitivity, previous hearing loss

**Precautions:** Pregnancy **B**, breastfeeding, neonates, geriatric, renal disease

### Pharmacokinetics
| | |
|---|---|
| **Absorption** | Poorly absorbed (PO), completely absorbed (**IV**) |
| **Distribution** | Widely distributed, crosses placenta |
| **Metabolism** | Liver |
| **Excretion** | PO—feces, **IV**—kidneys |
| **Half-life** | 4-8 hr |

### Pharmacodynamics
| | IV |
|---|---|
| **Onset** | Immediate |
| **Peak** | Inf end |
| **Duration** | Unknown |

### Interactions
*Individual drugs*
Amphotericin B, bacitracin, cidofovir, cisplatin, colistin, polymyxin B: increased ototoxicity or nephrotoxicity
*Drug classifications*
Aminoglycosides, cephalosporins, nondepolarizing muscle relaxants: increased ototoxicity or nephrotoxicity

### NURSING CONSIDERATIONS
**Assessment**
- Assess for infection: WBC, urine, stools, sputum, wound characteristics, throughout treatment
- Monitor I&O ratio; report hematuria, oliguria because nephrotoxicity may occur

V

Adverse effects: *italic* = common, **bold** = life-threatening

- Monitor any patient with compromised renal system (BUN, creatinine); product is excreted slowly in poor renal function; toxicity may occur rapidly
- Monitor blood tests: WBC; serum levels; peak 1 hr after 1-hr inf 25-40 mg/ml; trough before next dose 5-10 mg/ml
- Obtain C&S before product therapy; product may be given as soon as culture is performed
- Assess auditory function during, after treatment; hearing loss, ringing, roaring in ears; product should be discontinued
- Monitor B/P during administration; sudden drop may indicate Red Man syndrome
- Assess for signs of infection
- Assess respiratory status: rate, character, wheezing, tightness in chest
- Identify allergies before treatment, reaction of each medication

### Nursing diagnoses
- Infection, risk for (uses)
- Knowledge, deficient (teaching)

### Implementation
- Give antihistamine if Red Man syndrome occurs: decreased B/P, flushing of neck, face
- Give dose based on serum concentration
- Give in equal intervals around the clock to maintain blood levels
- Store at room temperature for up to 2 wk after reconstitution
- Have adrenaline, suction, tracheostomy set, endotracheal intubation equipment on unit; anaphylaxis may occur
- Provide adequate intake of fluids (2 L) to prevent nephrotoxicity

**IT route**
- Use preservative-free 0.9% NaCl (2-5 mg/ml final conc)

**Intermittent IV route**
- Give after reconstitution with 10 ml of sterile water for inj (500 mg/10 ml); further dilution is needed for **IV**, 500 mg/100 ml of 0.9% NaCl, $D_5W$ given as intermittent inf over 1 hr; decrease rate of infusion if Red Man syndrome occurs

**Continuous IV INF route**
- Reconstitute, then may infuse 1-2 g in volume to give over 24 hr, if intermittent **IV** route cannot be used

***Y-site compatibilities:*** Acyclovir, allopurinol, amiodarone, amsacrine, atracurium, cyclophosphamide, diltiazem, enalaprilat, esmolol, filgrastim, fluconazole, fludarabine, gallium, granisetron, hydromorphone, insulin (regular), labetalol, lorazepam, magnesium sulfate, melphalan, meperidine, meropenem, midazolam, morphine, on-

dansetron, paclitaxel, pancuronium, perphenazine, propofol, sodium bicarbonate, tacrolimus, teniposide, theophylline, thiotepa, tolazoline, vecuronium, vinorelbine, warfarin, zidovudine

***Additive compatibilities:*** Amikacin, atracurium, calcium gluconate, cefepime, cimetidine, corticotropin, dimenhyDRINATE, hydrocortisone, meropenem, ofloxacin, potassium chloride, ranitidine, verapamil, vit B/C

### Patient/family education
- Teach patient aspects of product therapy: need to complete entire course of medication to ensure organism death (7-10 days); culture may be performed after completed course of medication
- Advise patient to report sore throat, fever, fatigue; could indicate superinfection
- Instruct patient that product must be taken in equal intervals around clock to maintain blood levels

### Evaluation
**Positive therapeutic outcome**
- Absence of fever, sore throat
- Negative culture after treatment

---

## vardenafil (Rx)
(var-den′a-fil)
Levitra
*Func. class.:* Impotence agent
*Chem. class.:* Phosphodiesterase type 5 inhibitor

**Pregnancy category** B

**Action:** Inhibits phosphodiesterase type 5 (PDE5); enhances erectile function by increasing the amount of cGMP, which causes smooth muscle relaxation and increased blood flow into the corpus cavernosum

**Therapeutic outcome:** Erection

**Uses:** Treatment of erectile dysfunction

### Dosage and routes
*Adult:* PO 10 mg, taken 1 hr before sexual activity, dose may be reduced to 5 mg or increased to a max of 20 mg; max dosing frequency is once/day
*Geriatric >65 yr:* PO 5 mg initially, titrate as needed

**Hepatic dose (Child-Pugh B)**
*Adult:* PO 5 mg, max 10 mg

### Concomitant medications
Ritonavir, max 2.5 mg q72 hr; for indinavir, ketoconazole 400 mg/day and itraconazole

---

400 mg/day, max 2.5 mg/day; for ketoconazole 200 mg/day, itraconazole 200 mg/day and erythromycin max 5 mg/day

**Available forms:** Tabs 2.5, 5, 10, 20 mg

**Adverse effects**

*CNS:* Headache, flushing, dizziness, insomnia

*CV:* Hypertension, **MI, CV collapse,** chest pain

*EENT:* Conjunctivitis, tinnitus, photophobia, diminished vision, glaucoma, hearing loss

*GU:* Abnormal ejaculation, priapism

*MISC:* Rash, GERD, GGTP increased, **NAION (nonarteritic ischemic optic neuropathy)**

*MS:* Myalgia, arthralgia, neck pain

*RESP:* Rhinitis, sinusitis, dyspnea, pharyngitis, epistaxis

**Contraindications:** Hypersensitivity, coadministration of α-blockers or nitrates, renal failure, congenital or acquired QT prolongation

**Precautions:** Pregnancy **B;** not indicated for women, children, or newborns; hepatic impairment; retinitis pigmentosa; cardiovascular disease; anatomic penile deformities; sickle cell anemia; leukemia; multiple myeloma; bleeding disorders; active peptic ulceration; renal disease

| Pharmacokinetics | |
|---|---|
| **Absorption** | Rapid; reduced absorption with high-fat meal |
| **Distribution** | Bioavailability 15%; protein binding 95% |
| **Metabolism** | Liver |
| **Excretion** | Primarily in feces (91%-95%) |
| **Half-life** | 4-5 hr |

| Pharmacodynamics | |
|---|---|
| **Onset** | 20 min |
| **Peak** | ½-1½ hr |
| **Duration** | <5 hr |

**Interactions**

*Individual drugs*

Alcohol, amlodipine, metoprolol, NIFEdipine: increased hypotension, do not use concurrently

Cimetidine, erythromycin, itraconazole, ketoconazole: increased levels

NIFEdipine: decreased B/P

*Drug classifications*

◆Do not use with nitrates because of unsafe decrease in B/P that could result in heart attack or stroke

α-Blockers, protease inhibitors: do not use concurrently

Angiotensin II receptor blockers: increased hypotension

Antidysrhythmics class Ia, III, quinolones: serious dysrhythmias; do not use together

Antiretroviral protease inhibitors: increased vardenafil levels

**NURSING CONSIDERATIONS**

**Assessment**

• Assess for use of organic nitrates that should not be used with this product

• Assess for severe loss of vision while taking this or any similar products; these products should not be used if vision loss has occurred

**Nursing diagnoses**

• Knowledge, deficient (teaching)

• Sexual dysfunction (uses)

**Implementation**

• Give approximately 1 hr before sexual activity, do not use more than once a day

**Patient/family education**

• Advise that product does not protect against STDs, including HIV

• Teach that product absorption is reduced with a high-fat meal

• Instruct that product should not be used with nitrates in any form

• Inform that product has no effect in the absence of sexual stimulation

• Teach that patient should seek immediate medical attention if erection lasts for more than 4 hr

• Advise to inform physician of all medications being taken

• Teach patient to notify prescriber immediately and stop taking product if vision loss occurs

**Evaluation**

**Positive therapeutic outcome**

• Sustainable erection

**varenicline (Rx)**

(var-e-ni′kleen)

Chantix

*Func. class.:* Smoking cessation agent

**Pregnancy category** C

**V**

**Action:** Partial agonist for nicotine receptors; partially activates receptors to help curb cravings; occupies receptors to prevent nicotine binding

**Therapeutic outcome:** Smoking cessation

Adverse effects: *italic* = common, **bold** = life-threatening

**Uses:** Smoking deterrent

### Dosage and routes
*Adult:* PO Therapy should begin 1 week prior to smoking stop date (i.e., take product plus tobacco for 7 days); titrate for 1 wk, days 1 through 3, 0.5 mg/day; days 4 through 7, 0.5 mg bid; day 8 through end of treatment 1 mg bid; treatment is 12 wk and may repeat for another 12 wk

### Available forms: Tabs 0.5, 1 mg

### Adverse effects
*CNS:* Headache, agitation, dizziness, insomnia, abnormal dreams, fatigue, malaise
*CV:* **Dysrhythmias,** hypertension, palpitations, **tachycardia,** angina, hypotension, **MI**
*EENT:* *Blurred vision,* tinnitus
*GI:* *Nausea, vomiting,* anorexia, *dry mouth,* increased/decreased appetite, *constipation,* flatulence, GERD
*GU:* Erectile dysfunction, urinary frequency, menstrual irregularities
*INTEG:* Rash, pruritus
*MISC:* Weight loss or gain
*RESP:* Dyspnea, rhinorrhea

**Contraindications:** Hypersensitivity, eating disorders

**Precautions:** Pregnancy **C,** breastfeeding, children <18 yr, geriatric, renal disease, recent MI

| Pharmacokinetics | |
|---|---|
| Absorption | Unknown |
| Distribution | Steady state 4 days |
| Metabolism | Minimal |
| Excretion | Urine 92%, unchanged |
| Half-life | Elimination 24 hr |

| Pharmacodynamics |
|---|
| Unknown |

### NURSING CONSIDERATIONS
#### Assessment
• Assess for renal function in geriatric
• Assess for smoking cessation after 12 wk; if progress has not been made, product may be used for an additional 12 wk
• Assess mental status: mood, sensorium, affect

#### Nursing diagnoses
• Coping, ineffective (uses)
• Knowledge, deficient (teaching)

#### Implementation
• Do not break, crush, or chew tabs

• Give increased fluids, bulk in diet if constipation occurs
• Give after eating with a full glass of water
• Give sugarless gum, hard candy, or frequent sips of water for dry mouth

### Patient/family education
• Teach patient that treatment for smoking cessation lasts 12 wk and another 12 wk may be required
• Teach patient to use caution in driving, other activities requiring alertness; blurred vision may occur
• Advise patient to set a date to quit smoking and initiate treatment 1 wk prior to that date
• Teach patient how to titrate product
• Advise patient not to use with nicotine patches unless directed by prescriber; may increase B/P
• Advise patient to notify prescriber if pregnancy is suspected or planned
• Teach patient common side effects to be expected

### Evaluation
#### Positive therapeutic outcome
• Smoking cessation

---

### vasopressin  (Rx)
(vay-soe-press'in)
Pitressin, Pressyn ✦
*Func. class.:* Pituitary hormone
*Chem. class.:* Lysine vasopressin
**Pregnancy category C**

**Action:** Promotes reabsorption of water by action on renal tubular epithelium, causes vasoconstriction on muscles in the GI system

**Therapeutic outcome:** Increased osmolality, decreased urine output in diabetes insipidus

**Uses:** Diabetes insipidus (nonnephrogenic/nonpsychogenic), abdominal distention postoperatively, bleeding esophageal varices

### Dosage and routes
*Diabetes insipidus*
*Adult:* IM/SUBCUT 5-10 units bid-qid prn; IM/SUBCUT 2.5-5 units q2-3 days (Pitressin Tannate) for chronic therapy; CONT **IV** INF 0.0005 units/kg/hr, (0.05 milliunit/kg/hr), double dose q30 min as needed
*Child:* IM/SUBCUT 2.5-10 units bid-qid prn; IM/SUBCUT 1.25-2.5 units q2-3 days (Pitressin Tannate) for chronic therapy

### Abdominal distention
**Adult:** IM 5 units, then q3-4 hr, increasing to 10 units if needed (aqueous)

**Available forms:** Inj 20, 5 units/ml (tannate), spray, cotton pledgets

### Adverse effects
*CNS:* Drowsiness, headache, lethargy, flushing, vertigo
*CV:* Increased B/P, dysrhythmias
*EENT:* Nasal irritation, congestion, rhinitis
*GI:* Nausea, heartburn, cramps, vomiting, flatus
*GU:* Vulval pain, uterine cramping
*MISC:* Tremor, sweating, vertigo, urticaria, bronchial constriction

**Contraindications:** Hypersensitivity, chronic nephritis

**Precautions:** Pregnancy **C**, breastfeeding, CAD, asthma, renal/vascular disease, migraines, seizures

#### Pharmacokinetics
| | |
|---|---|
| **Absorption** | Erratically absorbed (IM) |
| **Distribution** | Widely distributed extracellular fluid |
| **Metabolism** | Liver—rapidly |
| **Excretion** | Kidneys—unchanged |
| **Half-life** | 10-20 min |

#### Pharmacodynamics
| | IM | IV |
|---|---|---|
| **Onset** | 1 hr | Unknown |
| **Peak** | Unknown | Unknown |
| **Duration** | 3-8 hr | 3-8 hr |

### NURSING CONSIDERATIONS
#### Assessment
• Monitor nasal mucosa for irritation if given by intranasal spray
• Assess intranasal use: nausea, congestion, cramps, headache; usually decreased with decreased dose
• Monitor pulse, B/P when giving product **IV** or SUBCUT
• Monitor I&O ratio, weight daily, fluid/electrolyte balance; check for edema in extremities; if water retention is severe, diuretic may be prescribed; check for water intoxication: lethargy, behavioral changes, disorientation, neuromuscular excitability

#### Nursing diagnoses
• Fluid volume, deficit (uses)
• Fluid volume, excess (side effects)
• Knowledge, deficient (teaching)

### Implementation
#### IM/SUBCUT route
• May be given IM/SUBCUT for diagnosis of diabetes insipidus
• Give patient 16 oz water at administration to prevent nausea, vomiting, cramping

#### Patient/family education
• Teach patient technique for nasal instillation: to insert tube into nasal cavity to instill product
• Caution patient to avoid OTC products for cough, hay fever because these preparations may contain epINEPHrine, decrease product response; do not use with alcohol
• Advise patient to carry/wear emergency ID specifying therapy, disease process (diabetes insipidus)
• Teach patient to measure/record I&O
• Teach patient to avoid alcohol, all OTC medications unless approved by prescription

### Evaluation
#### Positive therapeutic outcome
• Absence of severe thirst
• Decreased urine output, osmolality

---

**❗ HIGH ALERT**

## vecuronium (Rx)
(ve-kure-oh'nee-yum)
Norcuron
*Func. class.:* Neuromuscular blocker—nondepolarizing
*Chem. class.:* Synthetic curariform

**Pregnancy category C**

**Do not confuse:**
Nocuron/Narcan

**Action:** Inhibits transmission of nerve impulses by binding with cholinergic receptor sites, antagonizing action of acetylcholine; no analgesic response

**Therapeutic outcome:** Skeletal muscle paralysis during anesthesia

**Uses:** Facilitation of endotracheal intubation; skeletal muscle relaxation during mechanical ventilation, surgery, or general anesthesia

### Dosage and routes
**Adult and child >1 yr: IV** Initially 0.08-0.1 mg/kg or 0.04-0.06 mg/kg if given with succinylcholine, maintenance 0.01-0.015 mg/kg 25-40 min after initial dose, then 0.01-0.015 mg/kg q12-15 min
**Infant 1 yr->7 wk: IV** 0.08-0.1 mg/kg, maintenance 0.05-0.1 mg/kg q60 min as needed

**V**

*Neonate:* **IV** 0.1 mg/kg/dose, maintenance 0.03-0.15 mg/kg/dose q1-2 hr as needed

**Available forms:** 10 mg/5 ml vial

**Adverse effects**
*CNS:* Skeletal muscle weakness or paralysis (rarely), flushing
*INTEG:* Urticaria
*MISC:* Myopathy, hypotension
*RESP:* **Prolonged apnea, possible respiratory paralysis,** bronchospasm, tachycardia, flushing, wheezing, dyspnea
*SYST:* **Anaphylaxis**

**Contraindications:** Hypersensitivity

**Precautions:** Pregnancy **C**, breastfeeding, children <2 yr, electrolyte imbalances, dehydration, neuromuscular/respiratory/cardiac/hepatic disease

### Pharmacokinetics

| | |
|---|---|
| **Absorption** | Completely absorbed |
| **Distribution** | Rapid—to extracellular fluids |
| **Metabolism** | Liver (20%) |
| **Excretion** | Kidneys—unchanged (35%) |
| **Half-life** | 1½ hr, increased in hepatic disease |

### Pharmacodynamics

| | |
|---|---|
| **Onset** | 1 min |
| **Peak** | 3-5 min |
| **Duration** | 15-25 min (recovery index) |

### Interactions
*Individual products*
Amphotericin B, clindamycin, lithium, phenytoin, piperacillin, polymyxin B, quinidine, succinylcholine, verapamil: increased paralysis, length and intensity
Enflurane, isoflurane, lincomycin: increased neuromuscular blockade
Theophylline: dysrhythmias

*Drug classifications*
Aminoglycosides: increased paralysis, length and intensity
Analgesics (opioid), local anesthetics, thiazides: increased neuromuscular blockade

### NURSING CONSIDERATIONS
**Assessment**
• Monitor for electrolyte imbalances (potassium, magnesium) before product is used; electrolyte imbalances may lead to increased action of this product
• Monitor patient's vital signs (B/P, pulse, respirations, airway) until fully recovered; rate, depth, pattern of respirations, strength of hand grip; patient should be intubated before use
• Monitor patient's recovery: decreased paralysis of face, diaphragm, leg, arm, rest of body; residual weakness and respiratory problems may occur during recovery period
• Monitor allergic reactions: rash, fever, respiratory distress, pruritus; product should be discontinued

**Nursing diagnoses**
• Breathing pattern, ineffective (uses)
• Communication, impaired verbal (adverse reactions)
• Fear (adverse reactions)
• Knowledge, deficient (teaching)

**Implementation**
• Use peripheral nerve stimulator by anesthesiologist to determine neuromuscular blockade; deep tendon reflexes should be monitored during extended periods
• Give by direct **IV** after reconstituting with bacteriostatic water, over 5 min, D₅W, 0.9% NaCl or LR
• Give by direct **IV** after reconstituting dose in 5-10 ml of provided diluent; give by titrating to patient response
• Give by continuous inf after diluting to 10-20 mg/100 ml and by titrating to patient response (only by qualified person, usually an anesthesiologist); do not administer IM
• Store in light-resistant area

*Syringe incompatibilities:* Barbiturates

*Y-site compatibilities:* Aminophylline, cefazolin, cefuroxime, cimetidine, diltiazem, DOBUTamine, DOPamine, epINEPHrine, esmolol, fentanyl, fluconazole, gentamicin, heparin, hydrocortisone, hydromorphone, isoproterenol, labetalol, lorazepam, midazolam, milrinone, morphine, niCARdipine, nitroglycerin, nitroprusside, norepinephrine, propofol, ranitidine, trimethoprim/sulfamethoxazole, vancomycin

*Y-site incompatibilities:* Barbiturates

**Patient/family education**
• Provide patient reassurance if communication is difficult during recovery from neuromuscular blockade
• Provide explanation to patients regarding all procedures or treatments; patient will remain conscious if anesthesia is not given also

**Evaluation**
**Positive therapeutic outcome**
• Paralysis of jaw, eyelid, head, neck, rest of body as evaluated by peripheral nerve stimulator

**Treatment of overdose:** Edrophonium or neostigmine, atropine, monitor VS; may require mechanical ventilation

---

**venlafaxine** (Rx)
(ven-la-fax'een)
Effexor, Effexor XR
*Func. class.:* Second-generation antidepressant—miscellaneous

**Pregnancy category** C

**Action:** Potent inhibitor of neuronal serotonin and norepinephrine uptake, weak inhibitor of dopamine; no muscarinic, histaminergic, or α-adrenergic receptors in vitro

**Therapeutic outcome:** Relief of depression

**Uses:** Prevention/treatment of major depression, to treat depression at end of life; long-term treatment of generalized anxiety disorder, social anxiety disorder (Effexor XR only)

**Unlabeled uses:** Hot flashes, obsessive-compulsive disorder (OCD), premenstrual dysphoric disorder (PMDD), posttraumatic stress disorder (PTSD)

**Dosage and routes**
*Depression*
*Adult:* PO 75 mg/day in 2 or 3 divided doses; taken with food, may be increased to 150 mg/day; if needed may be further increased to 225 mg/day; increments of 75 mg/day should be made at intervals of no less than 4 days; some hospitalized patients may require up to 375 mg/day in 3 divided doses; EXT REL 37.5-75 mg PO daily, max 225 mg/day; give Effexor XR daily

*Hepatic dose*
*Adult:* PO Moderate impairment 50% of dose

*Renal dose*
*Adult:* PO Mild to moderate impairment 75% of dose

*Hot flashes (unlabeled)*
*Adult:* PO 12.5 mg bid × 4 wk or ext rel cap 37.5 mg × 4 wk

**Available forms:** Tabs scored (Effexor) 25, 37.5, 50, 75, 100 mg; ext rel caps (Effexor XR) 37.5, 75, 150 mg

**Adverse effects**
*CNS: Emotional lability, vertigo,* apathy, ataxia, CNS stimulation, euphoria, hallucinations, hostility, increased libido, hypertonia, hypotonia, psychosis, insomnia, anxiety, suicidal ideation in children/adolescents, seizures
*CV: Migraine,* angina pectoris, extrasystoles, postural hypotension, syncope, thrombophlebitis, hypertension
*EENT: Abnormal vision,* taste, *ear pain,* cataract, conjunctivitis, corneal lesions, dry eyes, otitis media, photophobia
*GI: Dysphagia, eructation,* colitis, gastritis, gingivitis, **rectal hemorrhage,** stomatitis, stomach and mouth ulceration, nausea, anorexia, dry mouth
*GU: Anorgasmia,* abnormal ejaculation, *dysuria, hematuria, metrorrhagia, vaginitis, impaired urination,* albuminuria, amenorrhea, kidney calculus, cystitis, nocturia, breast and bladder pain, polyuria, **uterine hemorrhage, vaginal hemorrhage,** moniliasis
*HEMA: **Agranulocytosis, aplastic anemia, neutropenia, pancytopenia***
*INTEG:* Ecchymosis, acne, alopecia, brittle nails, dry skin, photosensitivity, sweating
*META: Peripheral edema, weight loss or gain,* diabetes mellitus, edema, glycosuria, hyperlipemia, hypokalemia
*MS:* Arthritis, bone pain, bursitis, myasthenia, tenosynovitis, arthralgia
*RESP: Bronchitis, dyspnea,* asthma, chest congestion, epistaxis, hyperventilation, laryngitis
*SYST: Malaise, neck pain,* enlarged abdomen, cyst, facial edema, hangover effect, hernia

**Contraindications:** Hypersensitivity, bipolar disorder, interstitial lung disease

**Precautions:** Pregnancy C, breastfeeding, children, geriatric, mania, recent MI, cardiac/renal/hepatic disease, seizure disorder, hypertension, eosinophilic pneumonia, suicidal ideation

**Pharmacokinetics**

| | |
|---|---|
| **Absorption** | Well absorbed |
| **Distribution** | Widely distributed, 27% protein binding |
| **Metabolism** | Liver—extensively |
| **Excretion** | Kidneys, 87% |
| **Half-life** | 5-7 hr, 11-13 hr (active metabolite) |

**Pharmacodynamics**
Unknown

V

**Interactions**
*Individual drugs*
Alcohol: increased CNS depression
Cimetidine: increased venlafaxine effect
Clozapine, desipramine, haloperidol, warfarin: increased levels of these products

*Adverse effects: italic = common, **bold** = life-threatening*

Cyproheptadine: decreased venlafaxine effect

Indinavir: decreased effect of indinavir

Sibutramine, sumatriptan, trazodone: increased serotonin syndrome

### Drug classifications

Antihistamines, opioids, sedative/hypnotics: increased CNS depression

MAOIs: hyperthermia, rigidity, rapid fluctuations of vital signs, mental status changes, neuroleptic malignant syndrome

### Drug/herb

Chamomile, hops, kava, lavender, skullcap, valerian: increased CNS depression

Corkwood, jimsonweed: increased anticholinergic effect

SAM-e, St. John's wort: serotonin syndrome

Yohimbe: increased hypertension

### Drug/lab test

Increased: alkaline phosphatase, bilirubin, AST, ALT, BUN, creatinine, serum cholesterol, CPK, LDH

## NURSING CONSIDERATIONS

### Assessment

• Monitor B/P (lying, standing), pulse q4hr; if systolic B/P drops 20 mm Hg hold product, notify prescriber; take vital signs q4hr in patients with CV disease

• Monitor blood tests: CBC, leukocytes, differential, cardiac enzymes if patient is receiving long-term therapy

• Monitor liver function tests: AST, ALT, bilirubin

• Check weight qwk; weight loss or gain; appetite may increase, peripheral edema may occur

• Assess mental status: mood, sensorium, affect; increase in psychiatric symptoms: depression, panic; for suicidal ideation in children/adolescents

• Monitor urinary retention, constipation; constipation is more likely to occur in children or geriatric

• Assess for withdrawal symptoms: headache, nausea, vomiting, muscle pain, weakness; do not usually occur unless product was discontinued abruptly

• Identify alcohol consumption; if alcohol is consumed, hold dose

### Nursing diagnoses

• Coping, ineffective (uses)
• Injury, risk for (side effects)
• Knowledge, deficient (teaching)
• Noncompliance (teaching)

### Implementation

• Give with food or milk for GI symptoms

• Crush if patient is unable to swallow medication whole

• Store at room temperature; do not freeze

### Patient/family education

• Advise patient to notify prescriber of rash, hives, or allergic reactions

• Teach patient that therapeutic effects may take 2-3 wk

• Teach patient to use caution in driving or other activities requiring alertness because of drowsiness, dizziness, blurred vision; to avoid rising quickly from sitting to standing, especially geriatric

• Teach patient to avoid alcohol ingestion, other CNS depressants

• Advise patient to avoid pregnancy, breastfeeding while taking this product

• Teach patient that worsening of symptoms, suicidal thoughts/behavior may occur in children, young adults

### Evaluation

#### Positive therapeutic outcome

• Decreased depression, anxiety; sense of well-being

• Absence of suicidal thoughts

**Treatment of overdose:** ECG monitoring, induce emesis, lavage, activated charcoal, administer anticonvulsant

---

**verapamil** 🔘 (Rx)

(ver-ap'a-mil)

Apo-Verap, Calan, Calan SR, Covera-HS, Isoptin, Isoptin SR, Novo-Verapamil ✦, Nu-Verap ✦, verapamil HCl, verapamil HCl SR, Verelan PM

*Func. class.:* Calcium-channel blocker; antihypertensive; antianginal, antidysrhythmic (Class IV)

*Chem. class.:* Diphenylalkylamine

### Pregnancy category C

---

**Action:** Inhibits calcium ion influx across cell membrane during cardiac depolarization; produces relaxation of coronary vascular smooth muscle; peripheral vascular smooth muscle; dilates coronary vascular arteries; increases myocardial oxygen delivery in patients with vasospastic angina

**Therapeutic outcome:** Decreased angina pectoris, dysrhythmias, B/P

**Uses:** Chronic stable vasospastic, unstable angina; dysrhythmias, hypertension, supraventricular tachycardia, atrial flutter or fibrillation

**Unlabeled uses:** Prevention of migraine headaches, claudication, mania

## Dosage and routes
### Angina
*Adult:* PO 80-120 mg tid, increase qwk

### Dysrhythmias
*Adult:* PO 240-320 mg/day in 3-4 divided doses in digitalized patients
*Adult:* **IV** BOL 5-10 mg (0.075-0.15 mg/kg) over 2 min, may repeat 10 mg (0.15 mg/kg) ½ hr after first dose
*Child 1-15 yr:* **IV** BOL 0.1-0.3 mg/kg over >2 min, repeat in 30 min, not to exceed 5 mg in a single dose
*Child 0-1 yr:* **IV** BOL 0.1-0.2 mg/kg over ≥2 min, may repeat after 30 min

### Hypertension
*Adult:* PO 80 mg tid, may titrate upward; EXT REL 120-240 mg/day as a single dose, may increase to 240-480 mg/day

### Hepatic dose/geriatric/compromised ventricular function
*Adult:* PO 40 mg tid initially, increased as tolerated

**Available forms:** Tabs 40, 80, 120 mg; ext rel tabs 120, 180, 240 mg; inj 2.5 mg/ml in ampules, syringes, vials; ext rel caps 100, 120, 180, 200, 240, 300 mg

## Adverse effects
*CNS: Headache, drowsiness,* dizziness, anxiety, depression, weakness, asthenia, fatigue, insomnia, confusion, light-headedness
*CV: Edema,* **CHF,** bradycardia, hypotension, palpitations, AV block, **dysrhythmias**
*GI: Nausea,* diarrhea, gastric upset, *constipation,* elevated liver function tests
*GU:* Impotence, nocturia, polyuria, gynecomastia
*HEMA:* Bruising, petechiae, bleeding
*INTEG:* Rash, bruising
*MISC:* Gingival hyperplasia
*SYST:* **Stevens-Johnson syndrome**

**Contraindications:** Sick sinus syndrome, 2nd- or 3rd-degree heart block, hypotension <90 mm Hg systolic, cardiogenic shock, severe CHF

**Precautions:** Pregnancy **C,** breastfeeding, children, geriatric, CHF, hypotension, hepatic injury, renal disease, concomitant β-blocker therapy

### Pharmacokinetics
| | |
|---|---|
| **Absorption** | Well absorbed (PO) |
| **Distribution** | Not known |
| **Metabolism** | Liver—extensively |
| **Excretion** | Kidneys (70%) |
| **Half-life** | Biphasic 4 min, 3-7 hr |

### Pharmacodynamics
| | PO | PO-EXT REL | IV |
|---|---|---|---|
| **Onset** | 1-2 hr | Unknown | 1-5 min |
| **Peak** | ½-1½ hr | 5-7 hr | 3-5 min |
| **Duration** | 3-7 hr | 24 hr | 2 hr |

## Interactions
### Individual drugs
Carbamazepine, cycloSPORINE, digoxin, theophylline: increased levels of each specific product
Cimetidine, telithromycin: increased effect of verapamil
Fentanyl, prazosin, quinidine: increased hypotension
Lithium: decreased lithium levels
### Drug classifications
Antihypertensive, nitrates, β-adrenergic blockers: increased effects of verapamil
Nondepolarizing muscle relaxants: increased effect
NSAIDs: decreased antihypertensive effect
### Drug/herb
Barberry, betel palm, burdock, goldenseal, khat, lily of the valley, plantain: increased effect
Yohimbe: decreased effect
### Drug/food
Grapefruit juice: increased hypotension
### Drug/lab test
Increased: alkaline phosphatase, AST, ALT, BUN, creatinine, serum cholesterol

## NURSING CONSIDERATIONS
### Assessment
• Assess fluid volume status: I&O ratio and record; weight; distended red veins; crackles in lung; color; quality, specific gravity of urine; skin turgor; adequacy of pulses; moist mucous membranes; bilateral lung sounds; peripheral pitting edema; dehydration symptoms of decreasing output, thirst, hypotension, dry mouth, and mucous membranes should be reported
• Monitor B/P and pulse, pulmonary capillary wedge pressure (PCWP), central venous pressure, index, often during inf; notify prescriber if <50 bpm, systolic B/P <90 mm Hg
• Monitor ALT, AST, bilirubin daily; if these are elevated, hepatotoxicity is suspected

- Monitor if platelets are <150,000/mm³, if so, product is usually discontinued and another product started
- Assess for extravasation; change site q48hr
- Monitor cardiac status: B/P, pulse, respiration, ECG
- Monitor renal/hepatic function tests during long-term treatment, serum potassium, periodically

**Nursing diagnoses**
- Cardiac output, decreased (uses)
- Knowledge, deficient (teaching)

**Implementation**
**PO route**
- Do not crush or chew ext rel products
- Cap may be opened and contents sprinkled on food; do not dissolve chew cap
- Give once a day before meals at bedtime; sus rel give with food to decrease GI symptoms

**IV route**
- Give by direct **IV** undiluted (Y-site, 3-way stopcock) over at least 2 min, or 3 min geriatric; discard unused solution; to prevent serious hypotension, patient should be recumbent for 1 hr or more

*Syringe compatibilities:* Inamrinone, heparin, milrinone

*Y-site compatibilities:* Aprofloxacin, dobutamine, DOPamine, famotidine, hydrALAZINE, inamrinone, meperidine, methicillin, milrinone, penicillin G potassium, piperacillin, propofol, ticarcillin

*Y-site incompatibilities:* Albumin, ampicillin, mezlocillin, nafcillin, oxacillin, sodium bicarbonate

*Additive compatibilities:* Amikacin, amiodarone, ascorbic acid, atropine, bretylium, calcium chloride, calcium gluconate, cefamandole, cefazolin, cefotaxime, cefoxitin, cephapirin, chloramphenicol, cimetidine, clindamycin, dexamethasone, diazepam, digoxin, DOPamine, epINEPHrine, erythromycin, gentamicin, heparin, hydrocortisone, hydromorphone, hydrocortisone sodium phosphate, insulin (regular), isoproterenol, lidocaine, magnesium sulfate, mannitol, meperidine, metaraminol, methicillin, methyldopate, methylPREDNISolone, metoclopramide, mezlocillin, morphine, moxalactam, multivitamins, naloxone, nitroglycerin, norepinephrine, oxytocin, pancuronium, penicillin G potassium, penicillin G sodium, pentobarbital, phenobarbital, phentolamine, phenytoin, piperacillin, potassium chloride, potassium phosphates, procainamide, propranolol, protamine, quinidine, sodium bicarbonate, sodium nitroprusside, theophylline, ticarcillin,

tobramycin, tolazoline, vancomycin, vasopressin, vit B/C

**Patient/family education**
- Advise patient to increase fluids/fiber to counteract constipation
- Caution patient to avoid hazardous activities until stabilized on product and dizziness is no longer a problem
- Teach patient how to take pulse, B/P before taking product; to keep record or graph
- Instruct patient to limit caffeine consumption; to avoid alcohol, grapefruit, and OTC products unless directed by prescriber
- Advise patient to comply with medical regimen: diet, exercise, stress reduction, product therapy; to notify prescriber of irregular heartbeat, shortness of breath, swelling of feet and hands, pronounced dizziness, constipation, nausea, hypotension, **IV** calcium
- Teach patient to use as directed even if feeling better; may be taken with other CV products (nitrates, β-blockers)
- Caution patient not to discontinue abruptly; chest pain may occur

**Evaluation**
**Positive therapeutic outcome**
- Decreased anginal pain
- Decreased dysrhythmias
- Decreased B/P

**Treatment of overdose:** Defibrillation, atropine for AV block, vasopressor for hypotension, **IV** calcium

---

**vidarabine ophthalmic**
*See Appendix D*

---

**⚠ HIGH ALERT**

***vinBLAStine (VLB)** (Rx)
(vin-blast'een)
Velban, Velbe ✦, vinBLAStine sulfate
*Func. class.:* Antineoplastic
*Chem. class.:* Vinca rosea alkaloid

**Pregnancy category** D

**Do not confuse:**
vinBLAStine/vinCRIStine

**Action:** Inhibits mitotic activity, arrests cell cycle at metaphase; inhibits RNA synthesis, blocks cellular use of glutamic acid needed for purine synthesis; a vesicant

**Therapeutic outcome:** Prevention of rapid growth of malignant cells, immunosuppressive

---

**Uses:** Breast, testicular cancer; lymphomas; neuroblastoma; Hodgkin's, non-Hodgkin's lymphomas; mycosis fungoides; histiocytosis; Kaposi's sarcoma

### Dosage and routes
*Adult:* **IV** 0.1 mg/kg or 3-6 mg/m² qwk or q2 wk, max 0.5 mg/kg or 18.5 mg/m² qwk
*Child:* **IV** 2.5 mg/m² then dose of 3.75, 5.0, 6.25, and 7.5 at 7-day intervals

**Available forms:** Inj powder 10 mg for 10 ml **IV** inj

### Adverse effects
*CNS:* Paresthesias, peripheral neuropathy, depression, headache, **seizures**
*CV:* Tachycardia, orthostatic hypotension, hypertension
*GI: Nausea, vomiting,* ileus, *anorexia, stomatitis,* constipation, abdominal pain, GI and rectal bleeding, **hepatotoxicity,** pharyngitis
*GU:* Urinary retention, **renal failure**
*HEMA:* **Thrombocytopenia, leukopenia, myelosuppression,** agranulocytosis, granulocytosis, aplastic anemia, neutropenia, pancytopenia
*INTEG: Rash,* alopecia, photosensitivity, **extravasation, tissue necrosis**
*META:* SIADH
*SYST:* **Tumor lysis syndrome (TLS)**
*RESP:* **Fibrosis, pulmonary infiltrate, bronchospasm**

**Contraindications:** Pregnancy **D**, breastfeeding, infants, hypersensitivity, leukopenia, granulocytopenia

**Precautions:** Renal/hepatic disease

#### Pharmacokinetics
| | |
|---|---|
| Absorption | Complete bioavailability |
| Distribution | Crosses blood-brain barrier slightly |
| Metabolism | Liver—active antineoplastic |
| Excretion | Biliary, kidneys |
| Half-life | Triphasic—<5 min, 50-155 min, 23-85 hr |

#### Pharmacodynamics
Unknown

### Interactions
#### Individual drugs
Bleomycin: increased synergism
Methotrexate: increased methotrexate action
Mitomycin: increased bronchospasm
Phenytoin: decreased phenytoin level
Radiation: increased toxicity, bone marrow suppression; do not use together

### Drug classifications
Anticoagulants, NSAIDs: increased bleeding risk
Antineoplastics: increased toxicity, bone marrow suppression
CYP3A4 inducers (barbiturates, bosentan, carbamazepine, efavirenz, phenytoin, nevirapine, rifabutin, rifampin): decreased vinBLAStine effect
CYP3A4 inhibitors (aprepitant, antiretroviral protease inhibitors, clarithromycin, danazol, delavirdine, diltiazem, erythromycin, fluconazole, fluoxetine, fluvoxamine, imatinib, ketoconazole, mebefradil, nefazodone, telithromycin, voriconazole): increased toxicity
Live virus vaccines: increased adverse reactions

#### Drug/herb
St. John's wort: avoid use

### NURSING CONSIDERATIONS
#### Assessment
• Monitor B/P (baseline and q15 min) during administration
• Monitor CBC, differential, platelet count weekly; withhold product if WBC is <2000/mm³ or platelet count is <75,000/mm³; notify prescriber of results, recovery will take 3 wk; RBC, Hct, Hgb may be decreased
• Assess for dyspnea, crackles, unproductive cough, chest pain, tachypnea
• Monitor renal function tests: BUN, serum uric acid, urine CCr before, during therapy; I&O ratio; report fall in urine output of 30 ml/hr; for decreased hyperuricemia
• Monitor for cold, fever, sore throat (may indicate beginning of infection); notify prescriber if these occur
• Assess for bleeding: hematuria, guaiac, bruising or petechiae, mucosa or orifices q8hr, no rectal temp; avoid IM inj; use pressure to venipuncture sites
• Identify nutritional status: an antiemetic may need to be prescribed
• Assess for gout, joint pain, swelling, increased uric acid; allopurinol or other treatment may be used
• Assess for symptoms indicating severe allergic reactions: rash, pruritus, urticaria, itching, flushing, bronchospasm, hypotension; epINEPHrine and resuscitative equipment should be nearby

#### Nursing diagnoses
• Body image, disturbed (adverse reactions)
• Infection, risk for (adverse reactions)
• Injury, risk for (adverse reactions)
• Knowledge, deficient (teaching)

**V**

Adverse effects: *italic* = common, **bold** = life-threatening

## Implementation

- Give by intermittent infusion
- Sol should be prepared by qualified personnel only under controlled conditions
- Use Luer-Lok tubing to prevent leakage; do not let sol come in contact with skin; if contact occurs, wash well with soap and water
- Administer **IV** after diluting 10 mg/10 ml NaCl; give through Y-tube or 3-way stopcock or directly over 1 min
- Give hyaluronidase 150 units/ml in 1 ml of NaCl, warm compress for extravasation for vesicant activity treatment

*Syringe compatibilities:* Bleomycin, cisplatin, cyclophosphamide, droperidol, fluorouracil, leucovorin, methotrexate, metoclopramide, mitomycin, vinCRIStine

*Y-site compatibilities:* Allopurinol, amifostine, aztreonam, bleomycin, cisplatin, cyclophosphamide, DOXOrubicin, droperidol, filgrastim, fludarabine, fluorouracil, granisetron, heparin, leucovorin, melphalan, methotrexate, metoclopramide, mitomycin, ondansetron, paclitaxel, piperacillin/tazobactam, sargramostim, teniposide, thiotepa, vinCRIStine, vinorelbine

*Y-site incompatibilities:* Furosemide
*Additive compatibilities:* Bleomycin

## Patient/family education

- Teach patient to avoid use of products containing aspirin or NSAIDs, razors, commercial mouthwash because bleeding may occur; to report symptoms of bleeding (hematuria, tarry stools)
- Instruct patient to report signs of anemia, (fatigue, headache, irritability, faintness, shortness of breath)
- Caution patient to report any changes in breathing or coughing even several mo after treatment
- Advise patient that contraception will be necessary during treatment; teratogenesis may occur
- Advise patient to use sunscreen, wear protective clothing, and sunglasses
- Inform patient that hair may be lost during treatment; a wig or hairpiece may make patient feel better; new hair will be different in color, texture
- Advise patient to avoid vaccinations during treatment; serious reactions may occur
- Teach patient to report signs/symptoms of infection: fever, chills, sore throat; patient should avoid crowds and persons with known infections

## Evaluation

**Positive therapeutic outcome**

- Decreased spread of malignant cells

---

**⚠ HIGH ALERT**

## *vinCRIStine (VCR) 🌀 (Rx)
(vin-kris′teen)
Oncovin, Vincasar PFS, vinCRIStine sulfate
*Func. class.:* Antineoplastic—miscellaneous
*Chem. class.:* Vinca alkaloid

**Pregnancy category D**

**Do not confuse:**
vinCRIStine/vinBLAStine

**Action:** Inhibits mitotic activity, arrests cell cycle at metaphase; inhibits RNA synthesis, blocks cellular use of glutamic acid needed for purine synthesis; a vesicant

**Therapeutic outcome:** Prevention of rapid growth of malignant cells, immunosuppression

**Uses:** Lymphomas, neuroblastomas, Hodgkin's disease, acute lymphoblastic and other leukemias, rhabdomyosarcoma, Wilms' tumor

## Dosage and routes
*Adult:* **IV** 1-2 mg/m$^2$/wk, max 2 mg
*Child:* **IV** 1.5-2 mg/m$^2$/wk, max 2 mg

**Available forms:** Inj 1 mg/ml; powder for inj 5 mg/vial

## Adverse effects
*CNS: Decreased reflexes, numbness, weakness, motor difficulties,* CNS depression, cranial nerve paralysis, **seizures,** peripheral neuropathy
*CV:* Orthostatic hypotension
*GI: Nausea, vomiting, anorexia, stomatitis, constipation,* **paralytic ileus, abdominal pain, hepatotoxicity**
*GU:* **Renal tubular obstruction**
*HEMA:* **Thrombocytopenia, leukopenia, myelosuppression, anemia**
*INTEG: Alopecia,* extravasation
*SYST:* **Tumor lysis syndrome (TLS)**

**Contraindications:** Pregnancy **D,** breastfeeding, infants, hypersensitivity, radiation therapy

**Precautions:** Renal/hepatic disease, hypertension, neuromuscular disease

---

## Pharmacokinetics

| | |
|---|---|
| **Absorption** | Complete bioavailability |
| **Distribution** | Rapidly, widely distributed; blood-brain barrier |
| **Metabolism** | Liver |
| **Excretion** | Biliary, in feces, crosses placenta |
| **Half-life** | Triphasic <5 min, 50-155 min, 23-85 hr |

## Pharmacodynamics

| | |
|---|---|
| **Onset** | Unknown |
| **Peak** | Unknown |
| **Duration** | 1 wk |

## Interactions
### Individual drugs
Digoxin: decreased digoxin level

Methotrexate: increased action of methotrexate

Mitomycin-C: increased acute pulmonary reactions

Radiation: increased toxicity, bone marrow suppression; do not use together

### Drug classifications
CYP3A4 inducers (barbiturates, bosentan, carbamazepine, efavirenz, phenytoins, nevirapine, rifabutin, rifampin): decreased vinCRIStine effect

CYP3A4 inhibitors (aprepitant, antiretroviral protease inhibitors, clarithromycin, danazol, delavirdine, diltiazem, erythromycin, fluconazole, fluoxetine, fluvoxamine, imatinib, ketoconazole, mibefradil, nefazodone, telithromycin, voriconazole): increased toxicity

Peripheral nervous system products: neurotoxicity

Vaccines/toxoids: decreased immune response

### Drug/herb
St. John's wort: avoid use

## NURSING CONSIDERATIONS
### Assessment
• Monitor CBC, differential, platelet count weekly; withhold product if WBC is <4000/mm³ or platelet count is <75,000/mm³; notify prescriber of results; platelets may increase or decrease

• Assess neurologic status: paresthesia, weakness, cranial nerve palsies, orthostatic hypotension, lethargy, agitation, psychosis; notify prescriber

• Monitor renal function tests: BUN, serum uric acid, urine CCr before, during therapy; I&O ratio; report fall in urine output of 30 ml/hr; for decreased hyperuricemia, hyponatremia, and increased fluid retention (SIADH)

• Monitor for cold, fever, sore throat (may indicate beginning of infection)

• Identify for increased uric acid levels, joint pain in extremities; increase fluid intake to 2-3 L/day unless contraindicated

### Nursing diagnoses
• Body image, disturbed (adverse reactions)
• Infection, risk for (adverse reactions)
• Injury, risk for (adverse reactions)
• Knowledge, deficient (teaching)

### Implementation
• Administer **IV** after diluting with diluent provided or 1 mg/10 ml of sterile water or 0.9% NaCl; give through Y-tube or 3-way stopcock or directly over 1 min

• Hyaluronidase 150 units/ml in 1 ml of NaCl; apply warm compress for extravasation

**Syringe compatibilities:** Bleomycin, cisplatin, cyclophosphamide, doxapram, DOXOrubicin, droperidol, fluorouracil, heparin, leucovorin, methotrexate, metoclopramide, mitomycin, ondansetron, vinCRIStine

**Syringe incompatibilities:** Furosemide

**Y-site compatibilities:** Allopurinol, amifostine, aztreonam, bleomycin, cisplatin, cladribine, cyclophosphamide, DOXOrubicin, droperidol, filgrastim, fludarabine, fluorouracil, granisetron, heparin, leucovorin, methotrexate, metoclopramide, mitomycin, ondansetron, paclitaxel, sargramostim, teniposide, thiotepa, vinCRIStine, vinorelbine

**Y-site incompatibilities:** Furosemide

### Patient/family education
• Teach patient to avoid use of products containing aspirin or NSAIDs, razors, commercial mouthwash because bleeding may occur; to report symptoms of bleeding (hematuria, tarry stools)

• Instruct patient to report signs of anemia (fatigue, headache, irritability, faintness, shortness of breath)

• Caution patient to report any changes in breathing or coughing, even several mo after treatment

• Advise patient that contraception will be necessary during treatment; teratogenesis may occur

• Inform patient that hair may be lost during treatment; a wig or hairpiece may make patient feel better; new hair will be different in color, texture

• Advise patient to avoid vaccinations during treatment; serious reactions may occur

• Teach patient to report signs/symptoms of infection: fever, chills, sore throat; patient should avoid crowds or persons with known infections

V

Adverse effects: *italic* = common, **bold** = life-threatening

- Advise patient to increase fluids, bulk in diet, exercise to prevent constipation

## Evaluation
**Positive therapeutic outcome**
- Decreased spread of malignancies

---

**⚠ HIGH ALERT**

# vinorelbine (Rx)
(vi-nor'el-bine)
Navelbine
*Func. class.:* Antineoplastic—miscellaneous
*Chem. class.:* Semisynthetic vinca alkaloid

**Pregnancy category D**

**Action:** Inhibits mitotic spindle activity, arrests cell cycle at metaphase; inhibits RNA synthesis, blocks cellular use of glutamic acid needed for purine synthesis; a vesicant

**Therapeutic outcome:** Decreased spread of malignancy

**Uses:** Unresectable, advanced non–small-cell lung cancer (NSCLC) stage IV; may be used alone or in combination with cisplatin for stage III or IV NSCLC

## Dosage and routes
*Adult:* IV 30 mg/m² qwk
*ANC:* 1000-1499, give 50% dose; <1000 hold dose; <1000 × 3 wk, discontinue

## Hepatic dose
*Adult:* IV Total bilirubin 2.1-3 mg/dl 15 mg/m² qwk; total bilirubin ≥3 mg/dl 7.5 mg/m²/day

**Available forms:** Inj 10 mg/ml

## Adverse effects
*CNS:* Paresthesias, peripheral neuropathy, depression, headache, **seizures**, weakness, jaw pain
*CV:* Chest pain
*GI:* *Nausea, vomiting,* ileus, *anorexia, stomatitis,* constipation, abdominal pain, diarrhea, **hepatotoxicity**
*HEMA:* **Neutropenia, anemia, thrombocytopenia, granulocytopenia**
*INTEG:* *Rash,* alopecia, photosensitivity
*META:* Syndrome of inappropriate diuretic hormone
*MS:* Myalgia
*RESP:* Shortness of breath

**Contraindications:** Pregnancy **D**, breastfeeding, hypersensitivity, infants, granulocyte count <1000 cells/mm³ pretreatment, severe neutropenia

**Precautions:** Children, geriatric, hepatic/pulmonary/neurologic/renal disease

## Pharmacokinetics
| | |
|---|---|
| **Absorption** | Poor bioavailability (<50%) |
| **Distribution** | Highly bound to platelets, lymphocytes |
| **Metabolism** | Liver—to metabolite |
| **Excretion** | Bile |
| **Half-life** | 43 hr |

## Pharmacodynamics
| | |
|---|---|
| **Onset** | Unknown |
| **Peak** | 1-2 hr |
| **Duration** | Unknown |

## Interactions
*Individual products*
Fluorouracil: increased toxicity a possibility

## NURSING CONSIDERATIONS
### Assessment
- Monitor B/P (baseline and q15 min) during administration
- Monitor CBC, differential, platelet count weekly; withhold product if WBC is <4000/mm³ or platelet count is <75,000/mm³; notify prescriber of results, recovery will take 3 wk; liver function tests: AST, ALT, bilirubin, LDH
- Assess for dyspnea, crackles, unproductive cough, chest pain, tachypnea
- Monitor renal function tests: BUN, serum uric acid, urine CCr before, during therapy, I&O ratio; report fall in urine output of 30 ml/hr; for decreased hyperuricemia
- Monitor for cold, fever, sore throat (may indicate beginning infection); notify health care prescriber if these occur; effects of alopecia on body image
- Assess for bleeding: hematuria, guaiac, bruising or petechiae, mucosa or orifices q8hr: no rectal temp; avoid IM inj; use pressure on venipuncture sites
- Identify nutritional status: an antiemetic may need to be prescribed
- Assess for symptoms indicating severe allergic reactions: rash, pruritus, urticaria, itching, flushing, mucosa or bronchospasm, hypotension; epINEPHrine and resuscitative equipment should be nearby
- Assess neurologic status: numbness, pain, tingling, loss of Achilles reflex, weakness, palsies
- Assess for gout: pain, swelling, increased uric acid levels

---

**Nursing diagnoses**
- Body image, disturbed (adverse reactions)
- Infection, risk for (adverse reactions)
- Injury, risk for (adverse reactions)
- Knowledge, deficient (teaching)

**Implementation**
- Hyaluronidase 150 units/ml in 1 ml of NaCl, warm compress for extravasation for vesicant activity treatment
- Antacid before oral agent; give product after evening meal before bedtime
- Antiemetic 30-60 min before giving product and prn to prevent vomiting

**Intermittent IV INF route**
- Dilute to 0.5-2 mg/ml with 0.9% NaCl, 0.45% NaCl, $D_5W$, $D_5$/0.45% NaCl, LR, Ringer's; give over 6-10 min into Y-site or central line; flush line

**Continuous infusion**
- Give 40 mg/m$^2$ q3 wk after **IV** bol of 8 mg/m$^2$; may be given in combination with DOXOrubicin, fluorouracil, cisplatin

**Y-site compatibilities:**
Amikacin, aztreonam, bleomycin, buprenorphine, butorphanol, calcium gluconate, carboplatin, cefotaxime, cisplatin, cimetidine, clindamycin, dexamethasone, enalaprilat, etoposide, famotidine, filgrastim, fluconazole, fludarabine, gentamicin, hydrocortisone, lorazepam, meperidine, morphine, netilmicin, ondansetron, plicamycin, streptozocin, teniposide, ticarcillin, tobramycin, vancomycin, vinBLAStine, vinCRIStine, zidovudine

**Patient/family education**
- Teach patient to use liquid diet: cola, Jell-O; dry toast or crackers may be added if patient is not nauseated or vomiting
- Advise patient to rinse mouth 3-4 ×/day with water and brush teeth 2-3 ×/day with soft brush or cotton-tipped applicators for stomatitis; use unwaxed dental floss
- Inform patient that a nutritious diet with iron, vitamin supplements is necessary; avoid herbals, OTC products
- Advise patient to avoid crowds, people with infections, vaccinations
- Advise patient to use effective contraception during and for ≥2 mo after product is discontinued; avoid breastfeeding
- Teach patient hair may be lost but will grow back; new hair may be different texture, color

**Evaluation**
**Positive therapeutic outcome**
- Decreased spread of malignant cells

**vitamin A** (PO, OTC; IM, Rx)
Aquasol A, Del-Vi-A, Vitamin A
*Func. class.:* Vitamin, fat-soluble
*Chem. class.:* Retinol
**Pregnancy category C**

**Action:** Needed for normal bone and tooth development, visual dark adaptation, skin disease, mucosa tissue repair, assists in production of adrenal steroids, cholesterol, RNA

**Therapeutic outcome:** Prevention, absence of vit A deficiency

**Uses:** Vit A deficiency

**Dosage and routes**
*Adult and child >8 yr:* PO 100,000-500,000 international units/day × 3 days, then 50,000/day × 2 wk; dose based on severity of deficiency; maintenance 10,000-20,000 international units for 2 mo
*Child 1-8 yr:* IM 5000-15,000 international units/day × 10 days
*Infant <1 yr:* IM 5000-15,000 international units × 10 days

*Maintenance*
*Child 4-8 yr:* IM 15,000 international units/day × 2 mo
*Child <4 yr:* IM 10,000 international units/day × 2 mo

**Available forms:** Caps 10,000, 25,000, 50,000 international units; drops 5000 international units; inj 50,000 international units/ml; tabs 10,000, 25,000, 50,000 international units

**Adverse effects**
*CNS:* Headache, **increased ICP, intracranial hypertension,** lethargy, malaise
*EENT:* Gingivitis, papilledema, exophthalmos, inflammation of tongue and lips
*GI:* Nausea, vomiting, anorexia, abdominal pain, *jaundice*
*INTEG:* Drying of skin, pruritus, increased pigmentation, night sweats, alopecia
*META:* Hypomenorrhea, hypercalcemia
*MS:* Arthralgia, retarded growth, hard areas on bone

**Contraindications:** Hypersensitivity to vit A, malabsorption syndrome (PO)

**Precautions:** Pregnancy **C**, breastfeeding, impaired renal function

V

| Pharmacokinetics | |
|---|---|
| Absorption | Rapidly absorbed |
| Distribution | Stored in liver, kidneys, lungs |
| Metabolism | Liver |
| Excretion | Breast milk |
| Half-life | Unknown |

| Pharmacodynamics | |
|---|---|
| Unknown | |

## Interactions
### Individual drugs
Cholestyramine, colestipol, mineral oil: decreased absorption of vit A
### Drug classifications
Contraceptives (oral), corticosteroids: increased levels of vit A
### Drug/lab test
False increase: bilirubin, serum cholesterol

## NURSING CONSIDERATIONS
### Assessment
• Assess nutritional status: increase intake of yellow and dark green vegetables, yellow/orange fruits, vit A–fortified foods, liver, egg yolks
• Assess vit A deficiency: decreased growth; night blindness; dry, brittle nails; hair loss; urinary stones; increased infection; hyperkeratosis of skin; drying of cornea
• Identify vit A deficiency by plasma vit A, carotene level
• Assess for chronic vit A toxicity: increased calcium, BUN, glucose, cholesterol, triglyceride level

### Nursing diagnoses
• Knowledge, deficient (teaching)
• Nutrition: less than body requirements, imbalances (uses)

### Implementation
#### PO route
• Give with food (PO) for better absorption; do not give **IV** because anaphylaxis may occur, IM only
• Oral preparations are not indicated for vit A deficiency in those with malabsorption syndrome
• Store in airtight, light-resistant container
#### IM route
• Give deep in large muscle mass; do not use deltoid muscle for administration of >1 ml

### Patient/family education
• Instruct patient that if dose is missed, it should be omitted
• Inform patient that ophth exams may be required periodically throughout therapy
• Instruct patient not to use mineral oil while taking this product because absorption will be decreased
• Advise patient to notify prescriber of nausea, vomiting, lip cracking, loss of hair, headache
• Caution patient not to take more than the prescribed amount

### Evaluation
#### Positive therapeutic outcome
• Increase in growth rate, weight
• Absence of dry skin and mucous membranes, night blindness

**Treatment of overdose:** Discontinue product

## vitamin A acid
*See tretinoin*

## vitamin B₁
*See thiamine*

## (vitamin B₁₂) cyanocobalamin (PO, OTC; IM/SUBCUT, Rx)
(sye-an-oh-koe-bal'a-min)
Alphamin, Anacobin ♣, Bedoz ♣, Cobex, Cobolin-M Crystamine, Crysti-1000, Cyanabin ♣ Cyanoject, Cyomin, Ener-B, Hydrobexan, Hydro Cobex, Hydro-Crysti-12
*Func. class.:* Vitamin B₁₂, water-soluble vitamin

## (vitamin B₁₂a) hydroxocobalamin (vit B₁₂) (Rx)
(hye-drox'-o-ko-bal'-a-min)
Hydroxycobal, LA-12, Nascobal, Neuroforter, Rubesol-1000, Rubramin PC, Shovite, Vibral LA, Vibral, Vitamin B₁₂

**Pregnancy category** A

**Action:** Needed for adequate nerve functioning, protein and carbohydrate metabolism, normal growth, RBC development and cell reproduction

**Therapeutic outcome:** Prevention, correction of vit B₁₂ deficiency

**Uses:** Vit B₁₂ deficiency; pernicious anemia; vit B₁₂ malabsorption syndrome; Schilling test; increased requirements with pregnancy, thyrotoxicosis, hemolytic anemia, hemorrhage, renal and hepatic disease

## Dosage and routes
### Cyanocobalamin
*Adult:* PO Up to 1000 mcg/day SUBCUT/IM 30-100 mcg/day × 1 wk, then 100-200 mcg/mo

### Shilling test
*Adult and child:* IM 1000 mcg in 1 dose
*Child:* PO Up to 1000 mcg/day SUBCUT/IM 30-50 mcg/day × 2 wk, then 100 mcg/mo; NASAL 500 mcg qwk

### Hydroxocobalamin
*Adult:* SUBCUT/IM 30-50 mcg/day × 5-10 days, then 100-200 mcg/mo
*Child:* SUBCUT/IM 30-50 mcg/day × 5-10 days, then 30-50 mcg/mo

**Available forms:** Cyanocobalamin: tabs 25, 50, 100, 250, 500, 1000, 5000 mcg; ext rel tabs 100, 200, 500, 1000 mcg; lozenges: 100, 250, 500 mcg; nasal gel 500 mcg/spray; inj 100, 1000 mcg/ml; hydroxocobalamin: inj 1000 mcg/ml

## Adverse effects
*CNS:* Flushing, optic nerve atrophy
*CV:* **CHF,** peripheral vascular thrombosis, **pulmonary edema**
*GI:* *Diarrhea*
*INTEG:* Itching, rash, pain at inj site
*META:* Hypokalemia
*SYST:* **Anaphylactic shock**

**Contraindications:** Hypersensitivity, optic nerve atrophy

**Precautions:** Pregnancy **A,** breastfeeding, children

### Pharmacokinetics
| | |
|---|---|
| **Absorption** | Well absorbed (IM, SUBCUT) |
| **Distribution** | Crosses placenta |
| **Metabolism** | Stored in liver, kidney, stomach |
| **Excretion** | 50%-90% (urine), breast milk |
| **Half-life** | Unknown |

### Pharmacodynamics
Unknown

## Interactions
### Individual drugs
Aminosalicylic acid, chloramphenicol, cimetidine, colchicine: decreased absorption
Prednisone: increased absorption
### Drug classifications
Aminoglycosides, anticonvulsants, potassium products: decreased absorption
### Drug/herb
Goldenseal: decreased vit B$_{12}$ absorption
### Drug/lab test
False positive: intrinsic factor

## NURSING CONSIDERATIONS
### Assessment
• Assess for deficiency: anorexia, dyspepsia on exertion, palpitations, paresthesias, psychosis, visual disturbances, pallor, red inflamed tongue, neuropathy, edema of legs
• Monitor potassium levels during beginning treatment in patients with megaloblastic anemia
• Monitor CBC for increase in reticulocyte count during 1st wk of therapy, then increase in RBC and hemoglobin; folic acid levels, vit B$_{12}$ levels
• Assess nutritional status: egg yolks, fish, organ meats, dairy products, clams, oysters, which are good sources of vit B$_{12}$
• Monitor for pulmonary edema or worsening of CHF in cardiac patients

### Nursing diagnoses
• Knowledge, deficient (teaching)
• Noncompliance (teaching) (overuse)
• Nutrition: less than body requirements, imbalanced (uses)

### Implementation
#### PO route
• Give with fruit juice to disguise taste; administer immediately after mixing
• Give with meals if possible for better absorption; large doses should not be used because most is excreted
#### IM route
• Give by IM inj for pernicious anemia for life unless contraindicated
#### IV route
• May be mixed with TPN sol, but **IV** route is not recommended
*Y-site compatibilities:* Heparin, hydrocortisone sodium succinate, potassium chloride
*Solution compatibilities:* Dextrose/Ringer's or LR's combinations, dextrose/saline combinations, D$_5$W, D$_{10}$W, 0.45% NaCl, Ringer's or LR's sol, ascorbic acid

### Patient/family education
• Instruct patient that treatment must continue for life if diagnosed as having pernicious anemia
• Advise patient to eat well-balanced diet from the food pyramid and comply with dietary recommendation
• Caution patient not to exceed the RDA of vit B$_{12}$ because adverse reactions may occur

### Evaluation
#### Positive therapeutic outcome
• Decreased anorexia, dyspnea on exertion, palpitations, paresthesias, psychosis, visual disturbances, edema of legs

V

Adverse effects: *italic* = common, **bold** = life-threatening

• Prevention or correction of vit $B_{12}$ deficiency

**Treatment of overdose:** Discontinue products

---

## vitamin D (cholecalciferol, vitamin D₃ or ergocalciferol, vitamin D₂) (Rx, OTC)

Calciferol, Delta-D, Drisdol, Radiostol ♣, Radiostol Forte ♣, vitamin D, vitamin D₃

*Func. class.:* Vitamin D
*Chem. class:* Fat-soluble vitamin

### Pregnancy category C

**Do not confuse:**
Calciferol/calcitriol

**Action:** Needed for regulation of calcium, phosphate levels; normal bone development; parathyroid activity; neuromuscular functioning

**Therapeutic outcome:** Prevention of rickets, osteomalacia, normal calcium/phosphate levels

**Uses:** Vit D deficiency, rickets, renal osteodystrophy, hypoparathyroidism, hypophosphatemia, psoriasis, rheumatoid arthritis

### Dosage and routes
*Deficiency*
*Adult:* PO/IM 12,000 international units/day, then increased to 500,000 international units/day
*Child:* PO/IM 1500-5000 international units/day × 2-4 wk, may repeat after 2 wk or 600,000 international units as single dose

*Hypoparathyroidism*
*Adult and child:* PO/IM 200,000 international units given with 4 g calcium tab

**Available forms:** Tabs 400, 1000, 50,000 international units; caps 25,000, 50,000; oral sol 8000 international units/ml; inj 500,000 international units/ml, 500,000 international units/5 ml

### Adverse effects
*CNS:* Fatigue, weakness, drowsiness, **seizures,** headache, psychosis
*CV:* Hypertension, dysrhythmias
*GI:* Nausea, vomiting, anorexia, cramps, diarrhea, constipation, metallic taste, dry mouth
*GU:* Polyuria, nocturia, **hematuria, albuminuria, renal failure,** decreased libido

*INTEG:* Pruritus, photophobia
*MS:* Decreased bone growth, early joint pain, early muscle pain

**Contraindications:** Hypersensitivity, hypercalcemia, renal dysfunction, hyperphosphatemia

**Precautions:** Pregnancy **C,** CV disease, renal calculi

### Pharmacokinetics

| | |
|---|---|
| **Absorption** | Well absorbed |
| **Distribution** | Stored in liver |
| **Metabolism** | Liver, sun |
| **Excretion** | Bile, kidney |
| **Half-life** | 12-22 hr |

### Pharmacodynamics

| | PO | IM |
|---|---|---|
| **Onset** | Unknown | Unknown |
| **Peak** | 4 hr | Unknown |
| **Duration** | 15-20 days | Unknown |

### Interactions
*Individual drugs*
Cholestyramine, colestipol, phenobarbital, phenytoin: decreased effects of vit D
Verapamil: increased toxicity
*Drug classifications*
Antacids, diuretics (thiazide): increased toxicity

### NURSING CONSIDERATIONS
*Assessment*
• Monitor BUN, urinary calcium, AST, ALT, cholesterol, creatinine, uric acid, chloride, magnesium, electrolytes, urine pH, phosphate—may increase; calcium should be kept at 9-10 mg/dl; vit D at 50-135 international units/dl, phosphate at 70 mg/dl; alkaline phosphatase may be decreased
• Monitor for increased blood level; toxic reactions may occur rapidly
• Assess for dry mouth, metallic taste, polyuria, bone pain, muscle weakness, headache, fatigue, tinnitus, change in LOC, irregular pulse, dysrhythmias, increased respirations, anorexia, nausea, vomiting, cramps, diarrhea, constipation; may indicate hypercalcemia
• Assess renal status: decreased urinary output (oliguria, anuria), edema in extremities, weight gain 5 lb, periorbital edema
• Assess nutritional status, diet for sources of vit D (milk, cod, halibut, salmon, sardines, egg yolk) calcium (dairy products, dark green vegetables), phosphates (dairy products)

---

 Alert     Canada Only    🌐 Drug on CD    * "Tall Man" lettering (See Preface)

## Nursing diagnoses
- Knowledge, deficient (teaching)
- Nutrition, less than body requirements, imbalanced (uses)

## Implementation
**PO route**
- PO may be increased q4 wk depending on blood level
- Store in airtight, light-resistant container at room temperature

**IM route**
- Give inj deeply in large muscle mass, administer slowly, aspirate to avoid **IV** administration, rotate inj site

## Patient/family education
- Advise patient to omit dose if missed; to avoid vitamin supplements unless directed by prescriber
- Inform patient of necessary foods to be included in diet
- Advise patient to keep appointments for evaluation because therapeutic and toxic levels are narrow
- Instruct patient to report weakness, lethargy, headache, anorexia, loss of weight; to report nausea, vomiting, abdominal cramps, diarrhea, constipation, excessive thirst, polyuria, muscle and bone pain
- Caution patient to decrease intake of antacids and laxatives containing magnesium

## Evaluation
**Positive therapeutic outcome**
- Calcium levels 9-10 ml/dl
- Decreasing symptoms of bone disease

---

## vitamin E (OTC)
Amino-Opti-E, Aquasol E, Daltose ✤, E-Complex-600, E-Ferol, E-Vitamin Succinate, E-200 I.U. Softgels, Gordo-Vite E, Tocopherol, vitamin E, Vita-Plus E Softgels, Vitec
*Func. class.:* Vitamin E
*Chem. class.:* Fat-soluble vitamin

**Pregnancy category  A**

**Action:** Needed for digestion and metabolism of polyunsaturated fats, decreases platelet aggregation, decreases blood clot formation, promotes normal growth and development of muscle tissue, prostaglandin synthesis

**Therapeutic outcome:** Prevention and treatment of vit E deficiency

**Uses:** Vit E deficiency, impaired fat absorption, hemolytic anemia in premature neonates, prevention of retrolental fibroplasia, sickle cell anemia, supplement in malabsorption syndrome

## Dosage and routes
*Deficiency*
*Adult:* PO 60-75 international units/day
*Child:* PO 1 international unit/kg (malabsorption)

*Prevention of deficiency*
*Adult:* PO 30 international units/day
*Infant:* PO 5 international units/day

*Topical route*
*Adult and child:* TOP Apply to affected areas as needed

**Available forms:** Caps 100, 200, 400, 500, 600, 1000 international units; tabs 100, 200, 400 international units; drops 50 mg/ml; chew tabs 400 units; ointment, cream, lotion, oil

## Adverse effects
*CNS:* Headache, fatigue
*CV:* Increased risk of thrombophlebitis
*EENT:* Blurred vision
*GI:* Nausea, cramps, diarrhea
*GU:* Gonadal dysfunction
*INTEG:* Sterile abscess, contact dermatitis
*META:* Altered metabolism of hormones (thyroid, pituitary, adrenal), altered immunity
*MS:* Weakness

**Contraindications:** **IV** use in infants

**Precautions:** Pregnancy **A**

| Pharmacokinetics | |
|---|---|
| Absorption | 20%-80% (PO) |
| Distribution | Widely distributed, stored in fat |
| Metabolism | Liver |
| Excretion | Bile |
| Half-life | Unknown |

| Pharmacodynamics |
|---|
| Unknown |

## Interactions
*Individual drugs*
Cholestyramine, colestipol, mineral oil, sucralfate: decreased absorption
*Drug classification*
Anticoagulants (oral): increased action of anticoagulants

V

Adverse effects: *italic* = common, **bold** = life-threatening

## NURSING CONSIDERATIONS
### Assessment
- Assess nutritional status: intake of wheat germ, dark green leafy vegetables, nuts, eggs, liver, vegetable oils, dairy products, cereals
- Assess for vit E deficiency (usually in neonates): irritability, restlessness, hemolytic anemia

### Nursing diagnoses
- Knowledge, deficient (teaching)
- Nutrition: less than body requirements, imbalanced (uses)

### Implementation
**PO route**
- Chew chewable tabs well
- Sol: may be dropped in mouth or mixed with food
- Store in airtight, light-resistant container
**Topical route**
- Apply topical to moisturize dry skin

### Patient/family education
- Inform patient necessary foods to be included in diet high in vit E
- Instruct patient to omit if dose missed
- Instruct patient to avoid vit supplements unless directed by prescriber because overdose may occur

### Evaluation
**Positive therapeutic outcome**
- Absence of hemolytic anemia
- Adequate vit E levels
- Improvement in skin lesions
- Decrease in edema

---

## voriconazole (Rx)
(vohr-i-kahn'a-zol)
Vfend
*Func. class:* Antifungal
**Pregnancy category D**

**Action:** Inhibits fungal CYP450-mediation demethylation, needed for biosynthesis

**Therapeutic outcome:** Decreasing signs, symptoms of infection

**Uses:** Invasive aspergillosis, serious fungal infections (*Scedosporium apiospermum, Fusarium* sp.), *Monosportum, Apiospermum*

### Dosage and routes
*Adult:* PO Give 1 hr before or after meals; ≥40 kg, 200 mg q12hr; <40 kg, 100 mg q12hr
*Adult:* IV Loading dose 6 mg/kg q12hr × 2 dose, then 4 mg/kg q12hr; may switch to oral dosing

*Renal dose*
*Adult:* PO CCr <50 ml/min, use only orally

*Hepatic dose*
*Adult:* PO 6 mg/kg q12hr × 2 doses, then 2 mg/kg q12hr or 100 mg q12hr if >40 kg; 50 mg q12hr if <40 kg

**Available forms:** Tabs 50, 200 mg; powder for inj, lyophilized 200 mg voriconazole, powder for oral susp 45 g (40 mg/ml after reconstitution)

### Adverse effects
*CNS: Headache,* paresthesias, peripheral neuropathy, hallucinations, psychosis, EPS, depression, Guillain-Barré syndrome, insomnia, suicidal ideation, dizziness
*CV:* **Tachycardia,** hyper/hypotension, vasodilatation, **atrial dysrhythmias, atrial fibrillation, AV block, bradycardia, CHF, MI**
*EENT:* Blurred vision, eye hemorrhage
*INTEG: Burning, irritation,* pain, necrosis at inj site with extravasation, dermatitis, rash, photosensitivity
*GI: Nausea, vomiting, anorexia,* diarrhea, cramps, **hemorrhagic gastroenteritis, acute liver failure, hepatitis, intestinal perforation, pancreatitis**
*GU: Hypokalemia,* azotemia, **renal tubular necrosis, permanent renal impairment, anuria, oliguria**
*HEMA:* Anemia, **eosinophilia,** hypomagnesemia, **thrombocytopenia, leukopenia, pancytopenia**
*MISC:* Respiratory disorder
*SYST:* **Stevens-Johnson syndrome, toxic epidermal necrolysis, sepsis**

**Contraindications:** Pregnancy **D**, breastfeeding, children, hypersensitivity, severe bone marrow depression, severe hepatic disease

**Precautions:** Renal disease (**IV**)

### Pharmacokinetics
| | |
|---|---|
| **Absorption** | Unknown |
| **Distribution** | Protein binding 58% |
| **Metabolism** | By CYP45 enzyme |
| **Excretion** | Via hepatic metabolism |
| **Half-life** | Unknown |

### Pharmacodynamics
| | |
|---|---|
| **Onset** | Unknown |
| **Peak** | 1-2 hr |
| **Duration** | Unknown |

### Interactions
*Individual drugs*
Cisplatin, cycloSPORINE, polymyxin B, vancomycin: increased nephrotoxicity

---

CycloSPORINE, phenytoin, pimozide, prednisolone, quinidine, rifabutin, sirolimus, tacrolimus, warfarin: increased effects of each
specific product
Digoxin: increased hypokalemia
*Drug classifications*
Aminoglycosides: increased nephrotoxicity
Benzodiazepines, calcium channel blockers,
ergots, HMG-CoA reductase inhibitors,
non-nucleoside reverse transcriptase inhibitors, protease inhibitors, proton pump
inhibitors, sulfonylureas, vinca alkaloids:
increased effects of each specific product
Corticosteroids, diuretics (thiazide), skeletal
muscle relaxants: increased hypokalemia
*Drug/herb*
Gossypol: increased nephrotoxicity
*Drug/food*
High-fat foods: avoid use with high-fat meals

## NURSING CONSIDERATIONS
### Assessment
• Monitor VS q15-30 min during first
infusion; note changes in pulse, B/P
• Monitor I&O ratio; watch for decreasing
urinary output, change in specific gravity;
discontinue product to prevent permanent
damage to renal tubules
• Monitor blood tests: CBC, K, Na, Ca, Mg q2
wk; BUN, creatinine weekly
• Monitor weight weekly; if weight increases
over 2 lb/wk, edema is present; renal damage
should be considered
◆ Assess for renal toxicity: increasing BUN,
serum creatinine; if BUN is >40 mg/dl or if
serum creatinine >3 mg/dl, product may be
discontinued or dosage reduced
◆ Assess for hepatotoxicity: increasing AST,
ALT, alkaline phosphatase, bilirubin
• Assess for allergic reaction: dermatitis, rash;
product should be discontinued, antihistamines (mild reaction) or epINEPHrine (severe
reaction) administered
• Assess for hypokalemia: anorexia, drowsiness, weakness, decreased reflexes, dizziness,
increased urinary output, increased thirst,
paresthesias
• Assess for ototoxicity: tinnitus (ringing,
roaring in ears), vertigo, loss of hearing (rare)
### Nursing diagnoses
• Infection, risk for (uses)
• Injury, risk for (uses, adverse reactions)
• Knowledge, deficient (teaching)
### Implementation
• Give 1 hr before or after meals
• Store at room temperature (powder, tabs)

### IV route
• Give product only after C&S confirms
organism, product needed to treat condition;
make sure product is used in life-threatening
infections
• Reconstitute powder with 19 ml water for
inj to 10 mg/ml, shake until dissolved; infuse
over 1-2 hr at a conc of 5 mg/ml or less; do
not admix with other products, 4.2% sodium
bicarbonate inf

### Patient/family education
• Teach that long-term therapy may be needed
to clear infection (2 wk-3 mo depending on
type of infection)
• Advise patient to notify prescriber of bleed-
ing, bruising, or soft tissue swelling
• Teach to take 1 hr before or after meal
• Advise patient not to drive at night because
of vision changes
• Advise to avoid strong, direct sunlight
• Advise that women of childbearing age
should use effective contraceptive
### Evaluation
**Positive therapeutic outcome**
• Decreased fever, malaise, rash, negative C&S
for infecting organism

---

### ⚠ HIGH ALERT

**warfarin** 🔄 (Rx)
(war′far-in)
Coumadin, Jantoven, warfarin sodium,
Warfilone ✦
*Func. class.:* Anticoagulant
**Pregnancy category X**

**Do not confuse:**
Coumadin/Cardura/Compazine

**Action:** Interferes with blood clotting by
indirect means; depresses hepatic synthesis of
vit K–dependent coagulation factors (II, VII,
IX, X)

**Therapeutic outcome:** Prevention of
clotting

**Uses:** Deep vein thrombosis, prevention or
treatment of venous thrombosis, pulmonary
embolism, thromboembolic complications
associated with atrial fibrillation or cardiac
valve replacement, after MI to reduce risk of
death

**Dosage and routes**
*Adult:* PO/**IV** 2.5-10 mg/day × 3 days, then
titrated to INR
*Geriatric:* PO/**IV** 2-10 mg/day
*Child:* PO/**IV** 0.1 mg/kg/day titrated to INR

W

Adverse effects: *italic* = common, **bold** = life-threatening

**Available forms:** Tabs 1, 2, 2.5, 3, 4, 5, 6, 7.5, 10 mg; 5.4 mg powder for inj

**Adverse effects**

*CNS: Fever*

*CV:* Angina, chest pain

*GI: Diarrhea,* nausea, vomiting, anorexia, stomatitis, cramps, **hepatitis**

*GU:* **Hematuria**

*HEMA:* **Hemorrhage, agranulocytosis, leukopenia, eosinophilia,** ecchymosis, anemia, petechiae

*INTEG: Rash,* dermatitis, urticaria, alopecia, pruritus

*MISC:* Epistaxis, hemoptysis

*MS:* Bone fractures

*SYST:* **Anaphylaxis,** coma, cholesterol, microembolisms, **exfoliative dermatitis, purple toe syndrome**

**Contraindications:** Pregnancy **X,** breast-feeding, hypersensitivity, hemophilia, leukemia with bleeding, peptic ulcer disease, thrombocytopenic purpura, hepatic disease (severe), malignant hypertension, subacute bacterial endocarditis, acute nephritis, blood dyscrasias, preeclampsia, eclampsia, hemorrhagic tendencies; surgery of CNS, eye; traumatic surgery with large open surface, bleeding tendencies of GI/GU/respiratory, stroke, aneurysms, pericardial effusion, spinal puncture, major regional/lumbar block anesthesia

**Precautions:** Alcoholism, geriatric, CHF, debilitated patients, trauma, indwelling catheters, severe hypertension, active infections, protein C deficiency, polycythemia vera, vasculitis, severe diabetes

## Pharmacokinetics

| | |
|---|---|
| **Absorption** | Well absorbed (PO), completely absorbed |
| **Distribution** | Crosses placenta, 99% plasma protein binding |
| **Metabolism** | Liver |
| **Excretion** | Kidney, feces (active, inactive metabolites) |
| **Half-life** | Effective ½-2½ days |

## Pharmacodynamics

| | PO |
|---|---|
| **Onset** | 12-24 hr |
| **Peak** | ½-4 days |
| **Duration** | 3-5 days |

## Interactions
### Individual drugs

Allopurinol, amiodarone, chloral hydrate, chloramphenicol, cimetidine, clofibrate, clotrimoxazole, dextrothyroxine, diflunisal, disulfiram, erythromycin, furosemide, glucagon, heparin, indomethacin, isoniazid, mefenamic acid, metronidazole, mifepristone, phenylbutazone, quinidine, RU-486, sulfinpyrazone, sulindac, thyroid: increased warfarin action

Aprepitant, azothioprine, bosentan, carbamazepine, dicloxicillin, ethchlorvynol, factor IX/VIIa, griseofulvin, nafcillin, phenytoin, rifampin, sucralfate, sulfasalazine, thyroid, vitamin K: decreased warfarin action

Phenytoin: increased toxicity

Digoxin: increased hypokalemia increased toxicity

### Drug classifications

Antidepressants (tricyclic), ethacrynic acids, HMG-CoA reductase inhibitors, NSAIDs, oxyphenbutazones, COX-2 selective inhibitors, penicillins, quinolones, salicylates, selective serotonin reuptake inhibitors, steroids, sulfonamides, thrombolytics: increased warfarin action

Barbiturates, bile acid sequestrants, contraceptives (oral), estrogens: decreased warfarin action

Sulfonylureas (oral): increased toxicity

### Drug/herb

Agrimony, angelica, anise, basil, bay, bilberry, black currant, black haw, bogbean, bromelain, buchu, cat's claw, chamomile, chondroitin, cinchona bark, cranberry, danshen, devil's claw, dong quai, evening primrose, fenugreek, feverfew, garlic, ginger, ginkgo, ginseng, horse chestnut, Irish moss, kava, kelp, kelpware, khella, licorice, lovage, lungwort, meadowsweet, melatonin, motherwort, mugwort, nettle, papaya, parsley (large amounts), pau d'arco, pineapple, poplar, prickly ash, red clover, red yeast rice, safflower, saw palmetto, skullcap, tonka bean, turmeric, wintergreen, yarrow: increased risk of bleeding

Alfalfa, coenzyme Q10, flax, glucomannan, goldenseal, guar gum, St. John's wort: decreased anticoagulant effect

### Drug/food

Vit K foods: decreased warfarin action

### Drug/lab test

Increased: $T_3$ uptake, liver function tests

Decreased: uric acid

## NURSING CONSIDERATIONS
### Assessment

• Monitor blood studies (Hct, occult blood in stools) q3 mo; partial pro-time, which should be 1½-2 × control, PTT; often done daily, APTT, ACT; platelet count q2-3 days; thrombocytopenia may occur

- Monitor B/P, watch for increasing signs of hypertension
◆ Assess for bleeding: bleeding gums, petechiae, ecchymosis, black tarry stools, hematuria, epistaxis; decreased B/P may indicate bleeding and possible hemorrhage; fatal hemorrhage can occur
- Assess for fever, skin rash, urticaria
- Assess for needed dosage change q1-2 wk
◆ Assess patients carefully for symptoms of Churg-Strauss syndrome (rare): eosinophilia, vasculitis, rash, worsening pulmonary symptoms, cardiac complications, neuropathy

### Nursing diagnoses
- Injury, risk for (uses, adverse reactions)
- Knowledge, deficient (teaching)
- Tissue perfusion, ineffective (uses)

### Implementation
**PO route**
- Warfarin is usually given with **IV** heparin for 3 or more days, warfarin blood level may take several days
**IV route**
- Reconstitute with 2.7 ml of sterile water for inj; do not use solution that is discolored or has particulates
- Give over 1-2 min into peripheral vein
*Y-site compatibilities:* Cefazolin, ceftriaxone, DOPamine, heparin, lidocaine, morphine, nitroglycerin, potassium chloride, ranitidine

### Patient/family education
- Caution patient to avoid OTC preparations unless directed by prescriber; may cause serious product interactions
- Advise patient that product may be withheld during active bleeding (menstruation), depending on condition
- Advise patient to use soft-bristle toothbrush to avoid bleeding gums, avoid contact sports, use electric razor, avoid IM inj
- Instruct patient to carry/wear emergency ID identifying product taken
- Advise patient to report any signs of bleeding: gums, under skin, urine, stools
- Teach patient to read food labels; limited intake of vit K foods (green leafy vegetables) is necessary to maintain consistent prothrombin levels

### Evaluation
**Positive therapeutic outcome**
- Decrease of deep vein thrombosis
- Pro-time (1.3-2.0 × control)

## xylometazoline nasal agent
*See Appendix D*

## zafirlukast (Rx)
(za-feer'loo-cast)
Accolate
*Func. class.:* Bronchodilator
*Chem. class:* Leukotriene receptor antagonist

**Pregnancy category B**

**Action:** Antagonizes the contractile action of leukotrienes ($LTC_4$, $LTD_4$, $LTE_4$) in airway smooth muscle; inhibits bronchoconstriction caused by antigens

**Therapeutic outcome:** Ability to breathe more easily

**Uses:** Prophylaxis and chronic treatment of asthma in adults/children >5 yr

**Unlabeled uses:** Chronic urticaria

**Dosage and routes**
*Adult and child ≥12 yr:* PO 20 mg bid, take 1 hr before or 2 hr after meals
*Child 5-11 yr:* PO 10 mg bid

**Available forms:** Tabs 10, 20 mg

**Adverse effects**
*CNS:* Headache, dizziness
*GI:* Nausea, diarrhea, abdominal pain, vomiting, dyspepsia
*MISC:* Infections, pain, asthenia, myalgia, fever, increased ALT, urticaria, rash, **angioedema**

**Contraindications:** Hypersensitivity

**Precautions:** Pregnancy **B**, breastfeeding, children, geriatric, hepatic disease

| Pharmacokinetics | |
| --- | --- |
| Absorption | Rapidly |
| Distribution | Unknown |
| Metabolism | Extensively by CYP450 2C9, 3A4 enzyme systems, protein binding (99%) |
| Excretion | Feces |
| Half-life | 10 hr |

| Pharmacodynamics | |
| --- | --- |
| Onset | Unknown |
| Peak | 3 hr |
| Duration | Unknown |

## Interactions
### Individual drugs
Aspirin: increased plasma levels of zafirlukast
Erythromycin, theophylline: decreased plasma levels of zafirlukast
Warfarin: increased pro-time
### Drug/herb
Green tea (large amounts), guarana: increased effect
### Drug/food
Decreased: bioavailability of zafirlukast

## NURSING CONSIDERATIONS
### Assessment
• Assess respiratory rate, rhythm, depth; auscultate lung fields bilaterally; notify prescriber of abnormalities

### Nursing diagnoses
• Breathing pattern, ineffective (uses)
• Knowledge, deficient (teaching)
• Noncompliance (teaching)

### Implementation
• Give PO 1 hr before or 2 hr after meals; absorption may be decreased if given with food
• Give with 8 oz of water if GI upset occurs

### Patient/family education
• Advise patient to check OTC medications, current prescription medications, which will increase stimulation
• Advise patient to avoid hazardous activities; dizziness may occur
• Advise patient that if GI upset occurs, to take product with 8 oz of water; avoid food if possible, absorption may be decreased
• Advise to take even if symptom free
• Advise patient to notify prescriber of nausea, vomiting, diarrhea, abdominal pain, fatigue, jaundice, anorexia, flulike symptoms (hepatic dysfunction)
• Advise patient not to use for acute asthma episodes, or to use while breastfeeding

### Evaluation
**Positive therapeutic outcome**
• Ability to breathe more easily

## zaleplon (Rx)
(zale'plon)
Sonata
*Func. class.:* Sedative-hypnotic, antianxiety, non-barbiturate
*Chem. class.:* Pyrazolopyrimidine

**Pregnancy category C**

**Controlled substance schedule IV**

**Action:** Binds selectively to ω-1 receptor of the γ-aminobutyric acid type A ($GABA_A$) receptor complex; results are sedation, hypnosis, skeletal muscle relaxation, anticonvulsant activity, anxiolytic action

**Therapeutic outcome:** Ability to sleep

**Uses:** Insomnia

### Dosage and routes
*Adult:* PO 10 mg at bedtime; may increase dose to 20 mg at bedtime if needed; 5 mg may be used in low-weight persons
*Geriatric:* PO 5 mg at bedtime; may increase if needed

**Available forms:** Caps 5, 10 mg

### Adverse effects
*CNS: Drowsiness,* amnesia, depersonalization, hallucinations, hypesthesia, paresthesia, somnolence, tremor, vertigo, dizziness, anxiety, *lethargy, daytime sedation,* confusion, complex sleep-related reactions (sleep driving, sleep eating)
*EENT:* Vision changes, ear/eye pain, hyperacusis, parosmia
*GI:* Nausea, anorexia, colitis, dyspepsia, dry mouth, constipation, abdominal pain
*MISC:* Asthenia, fever, headache, myalgia, dysmenorrhea
*SYST:* **Severe allergic reactions**

**Contraindications:** Hypersensitivity, severe hepatic disease

**Precautions:** Pregnancy **C**, breastfeeding, children <15 yr, geriatric, renal/hepatic disease, psychosis, angioedema, respiratory disease, depression, sleep-related behaviors (sleep walking)

### Pharmacokinetics

| | |
|---|---|
| **Absorption** | Rapidly absorbed |
| **Distribution** | Extravascular tissues, crosses blood-brain barrier; crosses placenta |
| **Metabolism** | Extensively, liver to inactive metabolites |
| **Excretion** | Kidneys |
| **Half-life** | 1 hr |

## Pharmacodynamics

| | |
|---|---|
| **Onset** | Rapid |
| **Peak** | 1 hr |
| **Duration** | Unknown |

## Interactions
### Individual drugs
Cimetidine: increased action of zaleplon
Rifampin: decreased zaleplon levels
### Drug classifications
CYP3A4 inhibitors/inducers: increased or decreased
### Drug/herb
Black cohosh: increased hypotension
Catnip, chamomile, clary, cowslip, hops, kava, lavender, mistletoe, nettle, pokeweed, poppy, Queen Anne's lace, senega, skullcap, valerian: increased CNS depression
### Drug/food
High-fat/heavy meal: prolonged absorption, sleep onset reduced

## NURSING CONSIDERATIONS
### Assessment
• Assess for previous product dependence or tolerance; if product dependent or tolerant, amount of medication should be restricted
• Monitor patient's mental status: mood, sensorium, affect, sleeping patterns, drowsiness, dizziness, suicidal tendencies, excessive sedation, impaired coordination

### Nursing diagnoses
• Knowledge, deficient (teaching)
• Noncompliance (teaching)
• Sleep deprivation (uses)

### Implementation
• Give ½-1 hr before bedtime for sleeplessness; give on empty stomach

### Patient/family education
• Inform patient that product is for short-term use only
• Teach patient to take immediately before going to bed
• Advise patient that product may cause memory problems, dependence (if used for longer periods of time), changes in behavior/thinking, complex sleep-related behaviors (sleep eating/driving)
• Advise patient not to ingest a high-fat/heavy meal before taking
• Advise patient to avoid OTC preparations unless approved by a physician, to avoid alcohol ingestion or other psychotropic medications unless prescribed by a health care provider, that 1-2 wk of therapy may be required before therapeutic effects occur
• Caution patient to avoid driving, activities requiring alertness; drowsiness may occur; until medication response is known, tell patient that drowsiness may worsen at beginning of treatment
• Instruct patient not to discontinue medication abruptly after long-term use

### Evaluation
**Positive therapeutic outcome**
• Decreased sleeplessness

## zanamivir (Rx)
(zan-a-mee'veer)
Relenza
*Func. class.:* Antiviral
*Chem class.:* Nevramidase inhibitor

**Pregnancy category C**

**Action:** Inhibits neuramidase enzyme needed for influenza virus replication

**Therapeutic outcome:** Decreased symptoms of influenza types A and B for those who have been symptomatic for no more than 2 days

**Uses:** Treatment of influenza types A and B

**Unlabeled uses:** Prophylaxis against influenza A and B infections; avian flu (H5N1)

### Dosage and routes
**Adult and child >7 yr:** INH 2 inh (two 5-mg blisters) q12hr × 5 days, on the 1st day 2 doses should be taken with at least 2 hr between doses

**Available forms:** Blisters of powder for inhalation 5 mg

### Adverse effects
*CNS: Headache, dizziness,* fatigue
*EENT:* Ear, nose, throat infections
*GI: Nausea, vomiting, diarrhea*
*RESP:* Nasal symptoms, cough, sinusitis, bronchitis

**Contraindications:** Hypersensitivity

**Precautions:** Pregnancy **C**, breastfeeding, children <7 yr, geriatric, respiratory disease

## Pharmacokinetics

| | |
|---|---|
| **Absorption** | 4%-17% absorbed |
| **Distribution** | <10% protein binding |
| **Metabolism** | Not metabolized |
| **Excretion** | Kidneys unchanged |
| **Half-life** | 2½-5 hr |

## Pharmacodynamics
Unknown

---

Adverse effects: *italic* = common, **bold** = life-threatening     **Z**

## Interactions
### Individual drugs
Intranasal influenza vaccine: decreased effect; separate by ≥48 hr

## NURSING CONSIDERATIONS
### Assessment
- Assess for symptoms of influenza A: increased temp, malaise, aches and pains
- Assess for skin eruptions, photosensitivity after administration of product
- Monitor respiratory status: rate, character, wheezing, tightness in chest
- Assess for allergies before initiation of treatment, reaction of each medication

### Nursing diagnoses
- Infection, risk for (uses)
- Knowledge, deficient (teaching)

### Implementation
- Give before exposure to influenza; continue for 5 days after contact
- Store in airtight, dry container

### Patient/family education
- Give patient "Patient's instructions for use" and review all points before using delivery system
- Teach patient to avoid hazardous activities if dizziness occurs
- Teach patient to take product exactly as prescribed; to use for the entire 5 days
- Inform patient that this product does not reduce transmission risk of influenza to others
- Advise patients with asthma or COPD to carry a fast-acting inhaled bronchodilator since bronchospasm may occur; to use scheduled inhaled bronchodilators before using this product

### Evaluation
**Positive therapeutic outcome**
- Absence of fever, malaise, cough, dyspnea in influenza A

---

**zidovudine**  (Rx)
(zye-doe'vue-deen)
Apo-Zidovudine ✦, Azidothymidine, AZT, Novo-AZT ✦, Retrovir
*Func. class.:* Antiretroviral
*Chem. class.:* (NRTI) Nucleoside reverse transcriptase inhibitor

**Pregnancy category** C

**Action:** Inhibits replication of HIV-1 by incorporating into cellular DNA by viral reverse transcriptase, thereby terminating the cellular DNA chain

**Therapeutic outcome:** Decreased symptoms of HIV-1 infection

**Uses:** Used in combination with other antiretrovirals for HIV-1 infection

### Dosage and routes
*Adult:* PO 600 mg/day in divided doses, either 200 mg tid or 300 mg bid in combination with other antiretrovirals; **IV** 1-2 mg/kg q4hr, initiate PO as soon as possible, up to 1000 mg
*Child 6 wk-12 yr:* PO 160 mg/m² q8hr (480 mg/m²/day, max 200 mg q8hr) in combination with other antiretrovirals; **IV** same as adult
*Neonate:* PO 2-3 mg/kg/dose q6hr; **IV** 1.5 mg/kg infused over 30 min q6hr

*Perinatal transmission prophylaxis*
*Full-term neonate:* PO 2 mg/kg or **IV** 1.5 mg/kg q6hr starting 12 hr after birth; continue up to 6 wk of age
*Preterm neonate:* PO 2 mg/kg or **IV** 1.5 mg/kg q12hr; if >30 wk gestation at birth, advance to q8hr at 2 wk of age; if <30 wk gestation at birth, advance to q8hr at 4 wk of age

*Prevention of maternal-fetal HIV transmission*
*Neonatal:* PO 2 mg/kg/dose q6hr × 6 wk beginning 8-12 hr after birth; **IV** 1.5 mg/kg/dose over 30 min q6hr until able to take PO
*Maternal (>14 wk gestation):* PO 100 mg 5 ×/day until start of labor, then during labor/delivery **IV** 2 mg/kg over 1 hr followed by **IV** INF 1 mg/kg/hr until umbilical cord clamped

*Symptomatic HIV infection*
*Child 3 mo-12 yr:* PO 90-180 mg/m² q6hr, max 200 mg q6hr; **IV** 1-2 mg/kg over 1 hr q4hr
*Adult:* PO 100 mg q4hr; **IV** 1-2 mg/kg over 1 hr q4hr

*Prevention of HIV after needlestick*
*Adult:* PO 200 mg tid plus lamivudine 150 mg bid, plus a protease inhibitor for high-risk exposure; begin within 2 hr of exposure

**Available forms:** Caps 100 mg; tabs 300 mg; inj 200 mg/20 ml; oral syr 50 mg/5 ml

### Adverse effects
*CNS: Fever, headache, malaise,* diaphoresis, *dizziness, insomnia,* paresthesia, somnolence, chills, tremor, twitching, anxiety, confusion, depression, lability, vertigo, loss of mental acuity, **seizures**

---

 Alert    ✦ Canada Only     Drug on CD      * "Tall Man" lettering (See Preface)

*EENT:* Taste change, hearing loss, photophobia

*GI: Nausea, vomiting, diarrhea,* anorexia, cramps, *dyspepsia,* constipation, dysphagia, *flatulence,* rectal bleeding, mouth ulcer, abdominal pain

*GU:* Dysuria, polyuria, frequency, hesitancy

*HEMA:* **Granulocytopenia, anemia**

*INTEG: Rash,* acne, pruritus, urticaria

*MS:* Myalgia, arthralgia, muscle spasm

*RESP:* Dyspnea

**Contraindications:** Hypersensitivity

**Precautions:** Pregnancy **C**, breastfeeding, children, granulocyte count <1000/mm$^3$ or Hgb <9.5 g/dl, severe renal disease, impaired hepatic function, anemia

### Pharmacokinetics

| | |
|---|---|
| **Absorption** | Well absorbed (PO), completely absorbed (**IV**) |
| **Distribution** | Widely distributed—crosses placenta, CSF, protein binding 38% |
| **Metabolism** | Liver—mostly |
| **Excretion** | Kidneys |
| **Half-life** | Terminal ½-3 hr |

### Pharmacodynamics

| | PO | IV |
|---|---|---|
| **Onset** | Unknown | Rapid |
| **Peak** | ½-1½ hr | Inf end |
| **Duration** | Unknown | Unknown |

### Interactions
*Individual drugs*

Fluconazole, probenecid: increased toxicity

Ganciclovir, radiation, valganciclovir, SMX/ TMP: increased bone marrow suppression

Methadone: increased zidovudine level

*Drug classifications*

Antineoplastics: increased bone marrow suppression

### NURSING CONSIDERATIONS
### Assessment

• Assess for peripheral neuropathy: tingling or pain in hands and feet, distal numbness; if these occur, product may be decreased or discontinued

• Assess for pancreatitis: abdominal pain, nausea, vomiting, elevated liver enzymes; product should be discontinued because condition can be fatal

• Assess children by dilated retinal examination q6 mo to rule out retinal depigmentation

• Monitor CBC, differential, platelet count qmo; withhold product if WBC is <4000/mm$^3$ or platelet count is <75,000/mm$^3$; notify prescriber of results; monitor viral load, CD4 counts baseline and throughout treatment

• Monitor renal function tests: BUN, serum uric acid, urine CCr before, during therapy; these may be elevated throughout treatment

• Monitor temp q4hr, may indicate beginning of infection

• Monitor liver function tests before, during therapy (bilirubin, AST, ALT amylase, alkaline phosphatase) prn or qmo

### Nursing diagnoses
• Infection, risk for (uses)
• Injury, risk for (adverse reactions)
• Knowledge, deficient (teaching)

### Implementation
**PO route**
• Give on empty stomach, bid or tid
• Do not take dapsone at same time as didanosine

**IV route**
• Give by intermittent inf after diluting with D$_5$W; give over 1 hr (<4 mg/ml), do not give by direct **IV**

*Y-site compatibilities:* Acyclovir, allopurinol, amikacin, amphotericin B, aztreonam, ceftazidime, ceftriaxone, cimetidine, clindamycin, dexamethasone, DOBUTamine, DOPamine, erythromycin, fluconazole, fludarabine, gentamicin, heparin, imipenem/ cilastatin, lorazepam, metoclopramide, morphine, nafcillin, ondansetron, oxacillin, pentamidine, phenylephrine, piperacillin, potassium chloride, ranitidine, sargramostim, tobramycin, trimethoprim/sulfamethoxazole, vancomycin

*Additive incompatibilities:* Blood products or protein solutions

### Patient/family education
• Caution patient to take on empty stomach; to use exactly as prescribed

• Advise patient to report signs of infection: increased temp, sore throat, flulike symptoms; to avoid crowds and those with known infections

• Instruct patient to report signs of anemia: fatigue, headache, faintness, shortness of breath, irritability

• Advise patient to report bleeding; avoid use of razors or commercial mouthwash

• Inform patient that hair may be lost during therapy (rare); a wig or hairpiece may make patient feel better

• Caution patient to avoid OTC products or other medications without approval of prescriber

• Caution patient not to have any sexual contact without use of a condom; needles

Adverse effects: *italic* = common, **bold** = life-threatening  Z should not be shared; blood from infected individual should not come in contact with another's mucous membranes

### Evaluation
**Positive therapeutic outcome**
• Decreased infection; symptoms of HIV infection

---

## zinc
### (PO, OTC; **IV**, Rx)
(zink sul'fate)
Orazinc, PMS Egozine ✤, Verazinc, Zinca-Pak, Zincate, Zinc 15, Zinc-220, zinc sulfate
*Func. class.:* Trace element; nutritional supplement

### Pregnancy category  A

**Action:** Needed for adequate healing, bone and joint development, taste and smell (23% zinc)

**Therapeutic outcome:** Replacement of zinc

**Uses:** Prevention of zinc deficiency, adjunct to vit A therapy

**Unlabeled uses:** Wound healing

### Dosage and routes
*Dietary supplement*
*Adult:* PO 25-50 mg/day

*Nutritional supplement* (**IV**)
*Adult:* **IV** 2.5-4 mg/day, may increase by 2 mg/day if needed
*Child to 5 yr:* **IV** 100 mcg/kg/day
*Infant <1500 g-3 kg:* **IV** 300 mcg/kg/day

*Wound healing*
*Adult:* PO 50 mg/day × 1-2 mo

**Available forms:** Tabs 66, 110 mg; caps 220 mg; inj 1, 5 mg/ml

### Adverse effects
*GI:* Nausea, vomiting, cramps, heartburn, ulcer formation
*OVERDOSE:* Diarrhea, rash, dehydration, restlessness

**Precautions:** Pregnancy **A**

### Pharmacokinetics
| | |
|---|---|
| **Absorption** | Poorly absorbed (PO), completely absorbed (**IV**) |
| **Distribution** | Widely distributed |
| **Metabolism** | Liver |
| **Excretion** | 90%—feces, 10%—kidneys |
| **Half-life** | Unknown |

### Pharmacodynamics
Unknown

### Interactions
*Drug classifications*
Fluoroquinolones, tetracyclines: decreased absorption

### NURSING CONSIDERATIONS
### Assessment
• Monitor zinc levels during treatment

### Nursing diagnoses
• Knowledge, deficient (teaching)
• Nutrition: less than body requirements, imbalanced (uses)

### Implementation
**PO route**
• Give with meals to decrease gastric upset; restrict dairy products, caffeine, which decrease absorption
**IV route**
• Part of TPN

### Patient/family education
• Inform patient that element must be taken for 3 mo to be effective
• Advise patient to report immediately nausea, diarrhea, rash, severe vomiting, restlessness, abdominal pain, tarry stools

### Evaluation
**Positive therapeutic outcome**
• Absence of zinc deficiency
• Improved wound healing

---

## ziprasidone (Rx)
(zi-praz'ih-dohn)
Geodon
*Func. class.:* Antipsychotic/neuroleptic
*Chem. class.:* Benzisoxazole derivative

### Pregnancy category  C

**Action:** Unknown; may be mediated through both dopamine type 2 ($D_2$) and serotonin type 2 (5-$HT_2$) antagonism

**Therapeutic outcome:** Decreased signs/symptoms of psychosis

**Uses:** Schizophrenia, acute agitation

### Dosage and routes
*Adult:* PO 20 mg bid with food, adjust dosage every 2 days upward to max of 80 mg bid; IM 10-20 mg; may give 10 mg q2hr, doses of 20 mg may be given q4hr, max 40 mg/day

**Available forms:** Tabs 20, 40, 60, 80 mg; inj 20 mg/ml

---

### Adverse effects
*CNS:* *EPS (pseudoparkinsonism, akathisia, dystonia, tardive dyskinesia), drowsiness, insomnia, agitation, anxiety, headache,* **seizures, neuroleptic malignant syndrome,** dizziness, tremor, facial droop
*CV:* Orthostatic hypotension, **tachycardia, prolonged QT/QTc, sudden death, heart failure (geriatric), torsade de pointes**
*EENT:* Blurred vision, swollen tongue
*GI:* *Nausea,* vomiting, *anorexia, constipation,* jaundice, weight gain, diarrhea, dry mouth, abdominal pain
*GU:* Enuresis, urinary incontinence
*RESP:* Rhinitis, dyspnea

### Contraindications: Hypersensitivity, breastfeeding, seizure disorders

### Precautions: Pregnancy **C**, children, geriatric, renal/cardiac/hepatic disease, breast cancer, diabetes

#### Pharmacokinetics
| | |
|---|---|
| **Absorption** | Unknown |
| **Distribution** | Protein binding 90% |
| **Metabolism** | Liver—extensively to metabolite |
| **Excretion** | Unknown |
| **Half-life** | Terminal 7 hr |

#### Pharmacodynamics
| | |
|---|---|
| **Onset** | Unknown |
| **Peak** | 6-8 hr |
| **Duration** | Unknown |

### Interactions
*Individual drugs*
Alcohol: increased sedation
Carbamazepine: increased excretion of ziprasidone
Ketoconazole: increased ziprasidone level
Lithium: increased EPS
*Drug classifications*
Antihypertensives: increased hypotension
Antipsychotics: increased EPS
CNS depressants: increased sedation
*Drug/herb*
Betel palm, kava: increased EPS
Chamomile, hops, kava, skullcap, valerian: increased CNS depression
Cola tree, hops, nettle, nutmeg: increased action

### NURSING CONSIDERATIONS
#### Assessment
• Assess mental status before initial administration
• Check swallowing of PO medication; check

for hoarding or giving of medication to other patients
• Monitor I&O ratio; palpate bladder if urinary output is low
• Monitor bilirubin, CBC, liver function tests, fasting blood glucose qmo
• Monitor urinalysis before, during prolonged therapy
• Assess affect, orientation, LOC, reflexes, gait, coordination, sleep pattern disturbances
• Monitor B/P standing and lying; also pulse, respirations; take these q4hr during initial treatment; establish baseline before starting treatment; report drops of 30 mm Hg; watch for ECG changes
• Assess dizziness, faintness, palpitations, tachycardia on rising
• Assess EPS, including akathisia (inability to sit still, no pattern to movements), tardive dyskinesia (bizarre movements of the jaw, mouth, tongue, extremities), pseudoparkinsonism (rigidity, tremors, pill rolling, shuffling gait)
◆ Assess for neuroleptic malignant syndrome: hyperthermia, increased CPK, altered mental status, muscle rigidity
• Assess skin turgor daily
• Assess constipation, urinary retention daily; if these occur, increase bulk and water in diet

#### Nursing diagnoses
• Coping, ineffective (uses)
• Knowledge, deficient (teaching)
• Noncompliance (teaching)
• Thought processes, disturbed (uses)

#### Implementation
• Give reduced dose in geriatric
• Give antiparkinsonian agent on order from prescriber, to be used for EPS
• Provide decreased stimulus by dimming lights, avoiding loud noises
• Provide supervised ambulation until patient is stabilized on medication; do not involve in strenuous exercise program because fainting is possible; patient should not stand still for a long time
**PO route**
• Food increases absorption
• Store in airtight, light-resistant container
**IM route**
• Add 1.2 ml sterile water for inj to vial, shake vigorously until product is dissolved, do not admix

#### Patient/family education
• Advise patient that orthostatic hypotension may occur and to rise from sitting or lying position gradually; avoid hot tubs, hot showers, tub baths because hypotension may occur

- Advise patient to avoid abrupt withdrawal of this product; EPS may result; product should be withdrawn slowly
- Advise patient to avoid OTC preparations (cough, hay fever, cold) unless approved by prescriber, since serious product interactions may occur; avoid use with alcohol, CNS depressants; increased drowsiness may occur
- Teach patient to avoid hazardous activities if drowsy or dizzy
- Advise patient to increase fluids to prevent constipation
- Teach patient to use sips of water, candy, gum for dry mouth
- Teach patient compliance with product regimen
- Teach patient to report impaired vision, tremors, muscle twitching
- Teach patient that in hot weather, heat stroke may occur; take extra precautions to stay cool

### Evaluation
**Positive therapeutic outcome**
- Decrease in emotional excitement, hallucinations, delusions, paranoia; reorganization of patterns of thought, speech

**Treatment of overdose:** Lavage if orally ingested; provide airway; *do not induce vomiting*

---

## zoledronic acid (Rx)
(zoh'leh-drah'nick ass'id))
Reclast, Zometa
*Func. class.:* Bone-resorption inhibitor
*Chem. class.:* Bisphosphonate
**Pregnancy category D**

**Action:** Inhibits normal and abnormal bone resorption; potent inhibitor of osteoclastic bone resorption; inhibits osteoclastic activity, reduces bone resorption and inhibits skeletal calcium release caused by stimulating factors released by tumors; reduction of abnormal bone resorption is responsible for therapeutic effect in hypercalcemia; may directly block dissolution of hydroxyapatite bone crystals

**Therapeutic outcome:** Serum calcium at normal level

**Uses:** Moderate to severe hypercalcemia associated with malignancy; multiple myeloma; bone metastases from solid tumors (used with antineoplastics)

**Unlabeled uses:** Osteoporosis prophylaxis (yearly), osteoporosis

## Dosage and routes
### Hypercalemia of malignancy
**Adult:** **IV** INF 4 mg, given as a single INF over ≥15 min, may re-treat with 4 mg if serum calcium does not return to normal within 1 wk

### Multiple myeloma/metastatic bone lesions
**Adult:** **IV** INF 4 mg, given over 15 min q3-4 wk; may continue treatment for 9-15 mo, depending on condition

### Osteoporosis prophylaxis (yearly)/ osteoporosis
**Adult:** **IV** 5 mg over 15 min or more q12mo

**Available forms:** Powder for inj 4 mg; inj 5 mg/100 ml (Reclast)

## Adverse effects
*CNS:* Dizziness, headache, anxiety, confusion, insomnia, agitation
*CV:* Hypotension, leg edema
*GI:* Abdominal pain, anorexia, constipation, nausea, diarrhea, vomiting, mucositis
*GU:* UTI, possible reduced renal function
*META:* Anemia, hypokalemia, hypomagnesemia, hypophosphatemia, hypocalcemia, increased serum creatinine
*MISC: Fever, chills, flulike symptoms*
*MS:* Bone pain, *arthralgias, myalgias,* osteonecrosis of the jaw

**Contraindications:** Pregnancy **D**, breast-feeding, hypocalcemia, hypersensitivity to this product or bisphosphonates

**Precautions:** Children, geriatric, renal dysfunction, aspirin-sensitive asthma, asthmatic patients, asthma, acute bronchospasm, anemia, chemotherapy, coagulopathy, dehydration, dental disease, diabetes mellitus, renal disease, electrolyte imbalance, hypertension, infection, multiple myeloma

| Pharmacokinetics | |
|---|---|
| Absorption | Rapidly cleared from circulation |
| Distribution | Taken up mainly by bones; plasma protein binding ~22% |
| Metabolism | Not metabolized |
| Excretion | Kidneys (~50% eliminated in urine within 24 hr) |
| Half-life | 146 hr |

| Pharmacodynamics | |
|---|---|
| Onset | Unknown |
| Peak | 15 min |
| Duration | Max effect 7 days |

## Interactions
### Individual drugs
Calcium, vitamin D: decreased zoledronic acid effect

Digoxin: hypomagnesemia, hypokalemia

Infusion solutions (calcium-containing): do not mix with calcium-containing infusion sol such as lactated Ringer's sol

### Drug classifications
Aminoglycosides, NSAIDs, radiopaque contrast agents: increased neurotoxicity

Aminoglycosides, loop diuretics: decreased serum calcium

## NURSING CONSIDERATIONS
### Assessment
• Assess renal function tests and Ca, P, Mg, K, creatinine, if creatinine is elevated hold treatment
• Assess for hypercalcemia: paresthesia, twitching, laryngospasm; Chvostek's, Trousseau's signs

### Nursing diagnoses
• Fluid, volume excess (side effects)
• Injury, risk for (uses, adverse reactions)
• Knowledge, deficient (teaching)

### Implementation
• Saline hydration must be performed before administration; urine output should be 2 L/day during treatment, do not overhydrate
• Sol reconstituted with sterile water may be stored under refrigeration for up to 24 hr **IV**
• Administer in separate **IV** line from all other products
• Administer after reconstituting by adding 5 ml of sterile water for inj to each vial, then add up to ≥100 ml of sterile 0.9% NaCl, D₅W, run over ≥15 min

### Patient/family education
• Instruct patient to report hypercalcemic relapse: nausea, vomiting, bone pain, thirst
• Advise patient to continue with dietary recommendations including calcium and vit D; take a multiple vitamin daily, 500 mg of calcium, 400 international units vit D in multiple myeloma
• Teach patient if nausea/vomiting occur, eat small meals, use lozenges, or chewing gum
• Advise patient if bone pain occurs, notify prescriber to obtain analgesic
• Advise patient to avoid pregnancy

### Evaluation
**Positive therapeutic outcome**
• Calcium levels decreased to normal

**Treatment of overdose:** Correct clinically relevant reductions in serum calcium by administering **IV** calcium gluconate; in serum phosphorus, with potassium or sodium phosphate; in serum magnesium, with magnesium sulfate

## zolmitriptan (Rx)
(zole-mih-trip'tan)
Zomig, Zomig-ZMT
*Func. class.:* Migraine agent
*Chem. class.:* 5-HT₁ receptor agonist
**Pregnancy category C**

**Action:** Binds selectively to the vascular serotonin type 1 (5-HT₁) receptor subtype, exerts antimigraine effect; causes vasoconstriction in cranial arteries

**Therapeutic outcome:** Decreased severity, frequency of headache

**Uses:** Acute treatment of migraine with or without aura

**Dosage and routes:**
*Adult:* PO Start at 2.5 mg or lower (tab may be broken), may repeat after 2 hr, max 10 mg/24 hr; NASAL 1 spray in each nostril at onset of migraine, repeat in 2 hr if no relief

**Available forms:** Tabs 2.5, 5 mg; orally disintegrating tabs 2.5, 5 mg; nasal spray 5 mg

**Adverse effects**
*CNS: Tingling, hot sensation, burning, feeling of pressure, tightness, numbness, dizziness, sedation*
*CV:* Palpitations, chest pain
*GI:* Abdominal discomfort, nausea, dry mouth, dyspepsia, dysphagia
*MISC:* Odd taste (spray)
*MS: Weakness, neck stiffness, myalgia*
*RESP: Chest tightness, pressure*

**Contraindications:** Angina pectoris, history of MI, documented silent ischemia, ischemic heart disease, concurrent ergotamine-containing preparations, uncontrolled hypertension, hypersensitivity, basilar or hemiplegic migraine, risk of CV events

**Precautions:** Pregnancy **C**, breastfeeding, children, postmenopausal women, men >40 yr, geriatric, risk factors for CAD, hypercholesterolemia, obesity, diabetes, impaired renal/hepatic function

---

Adverse effects: *italic* = common, **bold** = life-threatening    Z

## Pharmacokinetics

| | |
|---|---|
| **Absorption** | Unknown |
| **Distribution** | 25% plasma protein binding |
| **Metabolism** | Liver |
| **Excretion** | Urine, feces |
| **Half-life** | 3-3½ hr |

## Pharmacodynamics

| | |
|---|---|
| **Onset** | Unknown |
| **Peak** | Unknown |
| **Duration** | 2-3½ hr |

## Interactions
### Individual drugs
Cimetidine: increased half-life of zolmitriptan
Ergot: increased vasospastic effects
Fluoxetine, fluvoxamine, paroxetine, sertraline: increased weakness, hyperreflexia, incoordination
Sibutramine: increased zolmitriptan levels
### Drug classifications
Contraceptives (oral): increased half-life of zolmitriptan
Ergot derivatives: increased vasospastic effects
MAOIs: do not use within 2 wk
Selective serotonin reuptake inhibitors (selective serotonin reuptake inhibitors): increased weakness, hyperreflexia, incoordination
### Drug/herb
Butterbur, feverfew: increased effect
SAM-e, St. John's wort: serotonin syndrome

## NURSING CONSIDERATIONS
### Assessment
• Assess tingling, hot sensation, burning, feeling of pressure, numbness, flushing
• Assess for stress level, activity, recreation, coping mechanisms
• Assess neurologic status: LOC, blurring vision, nausea, vomiting, tingling in extremities preceding headache
• Monitor ingestion of tyramine foods (pickled products, beer, wine, aged cheese), food additives, preservatives, colorings, artifical sweeteners, chocolate, caffeine, which may precipitate these types of headaches
• Assess for serotonin syndrome, if also taking a selective serotonin reuptake inhibitor

### Nursing diagnoses
• Knowledge, deficient (teaching)
• Noncompliance (teaching)
• Pain, acute (uses)

### Implementation
• Give with fluids as soon as symptoms of migraine occur

• Provide quiet, calm environment with decreased stimulation for noise, bright light, excessive talking

### Patient/family education
• Teach patient to report any side effects to prescriber
• Advise patient to use contraception while taking product

### Evaluation
**Positive therapeutic outcome**
• Decrease in frequency, severity of headache

## zolpidem (Rx)
(zole-pi'dem)
Ambien, Ambien CR, Tovalt ODT
*Func. class.:* Sedative-hypnotic
*Chem. class.:* Nonbenzodiazepine of imidazopyridine class

**Pregnancy category** C
**Controlled substance schedule** IV

**Action:** Produces CNS depression at limbic, thalamic, hypothalamic levels of CNS; may be mediated by neurotransmitter γ-aminobutyric acid (GABA); results are sedation, hypnosis, skeletal muscle relaxation, anticonvulsant activity, anxiolytic action

**Therapeutic outcome:** Ability to sleep, sedation

**Uses:** Insomnia, short-term treatment; insomnia with difficulty of sleep onset/maintenance (ext rel)

### Dosage and routes
*Adult:* PO 10 mg at bedtime × 7-10 days only; total dose should not exceed 10 mg; orally disintegrating tabs use immediately before retiring; EXT REL 12.5 mg immediately before bedtime
*Geriatric:* PO 5 mg at bedtime

**Available forms:** Tabs 5, 10 mg; ext rel tabs 6.25, 12.5 mg; orally disintegrating tabs 5, 10 mg

### Adverse effects
*CNS:* Headache, lethargy, drowsiness, daytime sedation, dizziness, confusion, lightheadedness, anxiety, irritability, amnesia, poor coordination, complex sleep-related reactions (sleep driving, sleep eating), depression, somnolence, suicidal ideation
*CV:* Chest pain, palpitation
*GI:* Nausea, vomiting, diarrhea, heartburn, abdominal pain, constipation

*HEMA:* **Leukopenia, granulocytopenia** (rare)
*MISC:* Myalgia
*SYST:* **Severe allergic reactions**

**Contraindications:** Hypersensitivity to benzodiazepines

**Precautions:** Pregnancy **C**, breastfeeding, children <18 yr, geriatric, anemia, renal/hepatic disease, suicidal individuals, product abuse, psychosis, seizure disorders, angioedema, depression, respiratory disease, sleep apnea, sleep-related behavior (sleep walking)

### Pharmacokinetics

| | |
|---|---|
| **Absorption** | Rapidly absorbed |
| **Distribution** | Unknown |
| **Metabolism** | Liver—inactive metabolite |
| **Excretion** | Kidneys, breast milk |
| **Half-life** | 2½ hr, increased in geriatric |

### Pharmacodynamics

Unknown

### Interactions
*Individual drugs*
Alcohol: increased action of both products
*Drug classifications*
CNS depressants: increased action of both products
*Drug/herb*
Chamomile, hops, kava, skullcap, valerian: increased CNS depression
*Drug/lab test*
Increased: ALT, AST, serum bilirubin
Decreased: radioactive iodine uptake
False increase: urinary 17-OHCS

### NURSING CONSIDERATIONS
**Assessment**
• Assess mental status: mood, sensorium, anxiety, affect, sleeping pattern, drowsiness, dizziness, especially geriatric; physical dependency, withdrawal symptoms: anxiety, panic attacks, agitation, seizures, headache, nausea, vomiting, muscle pain, weakness; suicidal tendencies; for indications of increasing tolerance and abuse
• Monitor B/P (lying, standing), pulse; if systolic B/P drops 20 mm Hg, hold product, notify prescriber
• Monitor I&O ratio for renal dysfunction

**Nursing diagnoses**
• Anxiety (uses)
• Injury, risk for (adverse reactions)
• Knowledge, deficient (teaching)

### Implementation
• Do not break, crush, or chew ext rel product or orally disintegrating tab
• Give ½-1 hr before bedtime for sleeplessness; give several hr before patient is to rise (to avoid hangover)
• Give with food or fluids; tab may be crushed or swallowed whole
• Store in airtight container in cool environment

### Patient/family education
• Advise patient that complex sleep-related behaviors may occur (sleep driving/eating)
• Instruct patient that product may be taken with food or fluids
• Caution patient not to use for everyday stress or longer than 3 mo unless directed by prescriber; not to take more than prescribed amount; may be habit forming; not to double or skip doses
• Caution patient to avoid OTC preparations unless approved by prescriber; alcohol and CNS depressants will increase CNS depression
• Advise patient to avoid driving, activities that require alertness, because drowsiness may occur; to avoid alcohol ingestion or other psychotropic medications; to rise slowly or fainting may occur, especially geriatric; that drowsiness may worsen at beginning of treatment
• Instruct patient not to discontinue medication abruptly after long-term use; withdrawal symptoms include vomiting, cramping, tremors, seizures
• Teach patient use of orally disintegrating tabs: place on tongue, allow to dissolve before swallowing

### Evaluation
**Positive therapeutic outcome**
• Ability to sleep at night
• Decreased amount of early-morning awakening if taking product for insomnia

**Treatment of overdose:** Lavage, VS, supportive care

---

### zonisamide (Rx)
(zone-is′a-mide)
Zonegran
*Func. class.:* Anticonvulsant
*Chem. class.:* Sulfonamides
**Pregnancy category** C

---

**Action:** May act through sodium and calcium channels, but exact action is unknown; serotonergic action

Adverse effects: *italic* = common, **bold** = life-threatening    **Z**

**Therapeutic outcome:** Decreased seizures

**Uses:** Epilepsy, adjunctive therapy of partial seizures

### Dosage and routes
*Adults and child >16 yr:* PO 100 mg/day, may increase after 2 wk to 200 mg/day, may increase q2 wk, max dose 600 mg/day

**Available forms:** Caps 25, 50, 100 mg

### Adverse effects
*CNS:* Dizziness, insomnia, paresthesias, depression, fatigue, headache, confusion, somnolence, agitation, irritability, speech disturbance
*EENT:* Diplopia, verbal difficulty, speech abnormalities, taste perversion
*GI:* Nausea, constipation, anorexia, weight loss, diarrhea, dyspepsia
*HEMA:* **Aplastic anemia, granulocytopenia** (rare)
*INTEG:* Rash
*SYST:* **Stevens-Johnson syndrome**

**Contraindications:** Hypersensitivity to this product or sulfonamides, psychiatric condition, hepatic failure

**Precautions:** Pregnancy **C,** breastfeeding, children <16 yr, geriatric, allergies, renal/hepatic disease

#### Pharmacokinetics
| | |
|---|---|
| Absorption | Unknown |
| Distribution | Protein binding 40% |
| Metabolism | Liver |
| Excretion | Kidneys |
| Half-life | 63 hr |

#### Pharmacodynamics
| | |
|---|---|
| Onset | Unknown |
| Peak | 2-6 hr |
| Duration | Unknown |

### Interactions
*Drug classifications*
Products inducing CYP450 enzyme (carbamazepine, phenytoin, phenobarbital): decreased half-life of zonisamide
*Drug/herb*
St. John's wort: increased effect of zonisamide
*Drug/food*
Grapefruit: do not use together

### NURSING CONSIDERATIONS
**Assessment**
- Assess for seizures: duration, type, intensity, precipitating factors
- Renal function: albumin conc
- Assess mental status: mood, sensorium, affect, memory (long, short)
- Assess for rash, hypersensitivity reaction

**Nursing diagnoses**
- Injury, risk for (uses, adverse reactions)
- Knowledge, deficient (teaching)
- Noncompliance (teaching)

**Patient/family education**
- Advise patient not to discontinue product abruptly; seizures may occur
- Advise patient to avoid hazardous activities until stabilized on product
- Advise patient to carry/wear emergency ID stating product use
- Teach patient to take adequate fluids; not to use grapefruit juice

**Evaluation**
**Positive therapeutic outcome**
- Decrease in severity of seizures

## ALPHA-ADRENERGIC BLOCKERS

**Action:** α-Adrenergic blockers bind to α-adrenergic receptors, causing dilatation of peripheral blood vessels; lower peripheral resistance resulting in decreased blood pressure.

**Uses:** α-Adrenergic blockers are used for pheochromocytoma, prevention of tissue necrosis, and sloughing associated with extravasation of IV vasopressors.

**Adverse effects:** The most common side effects are hypotension, tachycardia, nasal stuffiness, nausea, vomiting, and diarrhea.

**Contraindications:** Hypersensitive reactions may occur, and allergies should be identified before these products are given. Patients with myocardial infarction, coronary insufficiency, angina, or other evidence of coronary artery disease should not use these products.

**Pharmacokinetics:** Onset, peak, and duration vary among products.

**Interactions:** Vasoconstrictive and hypertensive effects of epinephrine are antagonized by α-adrenergic blockers.

### NURSING CONSIDERATIONS
#### Assessment
• Monitor electrolytes: potassium, sodium chloride, carbon dioxide
• Monitor weight daily, I&O
• Monitor B/P with patient lying, standing before starting treatment, q4hr thereafter
• Assess for nausea, vomiting, diarrhea
• Assess for skin turgor, dryness of mucous membranes for hydration status

#### Nursing diagnoses
• Injury, risk for (adverse reactions)
• Sleep deprivation (adverse reactions)
• Tissue perfusion, ineffective (uses)

#### Implementation
**PO route**
• Start with low dose, gradually increasing to prevent side effects
• Give with food or milk for GI symptoms

#### Patient/family education
• Caution patient to avoid alcoholic beverages
• Advise patient to report dizziness, palpitations, fainting
• Instruct patient to change position slowly or fainting may occur
• Teach patient to take product exactly as prescribed; to avoid all OTC products (cough, cold, allergy) unless directed by prescriber

#### Evaluation
**Positive therapeutic outcome**
• Decreased B/P
• Increased peripheral pulses

### Generic Names
phentolamine

## ANESTHETICS—GENERAL/LOCAL

**Action:** Anesthetics (general) act on the CNS to produce tranquilization and sleep before invasive procedures. Anesthetics (local) inhibit conduction of nerve impulses from sensory nerves.

**Uses:** General anesthetics are used to premedicate for surgery, and for induction and maintenance in general anesthesia. For local anesthetics, refer to individual product listing for indications.

**Adverse effects:** The most common side effects are dystonia, akathisia, flexion of arms, fine tremors, drowsiness, restlessness, and hypotension. Also common are chills, respiratory depression, and laryngospasm.

**Contraindications:** Persons with CVA, increased ICP, severe hypertension, and cardiac decompensation should not use these products since severe adverse reactions can occur.

**Precautions:** Anesthetics (general) should be used with caution in the geriatric, children <2 yr, and those with cardiovascular disease (hypotension, bradydysrhythmias), renal/hepatic disease, and Parkinson's disease. The precaution for anesthetics (local) is pregnancy.

**Pharmacokinetics:** Onset, peak, and duration vary widely among products. Most products are metabolized in the liver and excreted in urine.

**Interactions:** MAOIs, tricyclics, and phenothiazines may cause severe hypo/hypertension when used with local anesthetics. CNS depressants will potentiate general and local anesthetics.

### NURSING CONSIDERATIONS
#### Assessment
• Monitor VS q10 min during **IV** administration, q30 min after IM dose

#### Nursing diagnoses
**General**
• Injury, risk for (adverse reactions)
• Knowledge, deficient (teaching)

---

Adverse effects: *italic* = common, **bold** = life-threatening

1024    Antacids

**Local**
- Pain, acute (uses)
- Knowledge, deficient (teaching)

## Implementation
- Give anticholinergic preoperatively to decrease secretions
- Administer only with resuscitative equipment nearby
- Provide quiet environment for recovery to decrease psychotic symptoms

### Evaluation
**Positive therapeutic outcome**
- Maintenance of anesthesia
- Decreased pain

---

## Generic Names

*General anesthetics:*
**droperidol** (high alert)
etomidate
**fentanyl** (high alert)
fentanyl transdermal
midazolam
**propofol** (high alert)

*Local anesthetics:*
 **lidocaine, parenteral** (high alert)
ropivacaine
tetracaine

---

## ANTACIDS

**Action:** Antacids are basic compounds that neutralize gastric acidity and decrease the rate of gastric emptying. Products are divided into those containing aluminum, magnesium, calcium, or a combination of these.

**Uses:** Antacids decrease hyperacidity in conditions such as peptic ulcer disease, reflux esophagitis, gastritis, or hiatal hernia.

**Adverse effects:** The most common side effect caused by aluminum-containing antacids is constipation, which may lead to fecal impaction and bowel obstruction. Diarrhea occurs often when magnesium products are given. Alkalosis may occur when systemic products are used. Constipation occurs more frequently than laxation with calcium carbonate. The release of $CO_2$ from carbonate-containing antacids causes belching, abdominal distention, and flatulence. Sodium bicarbonate may act as a systemic antacid and produce systemic electrolyte disturbances and alkalosis. Calcium carbonate and sodium bicarbonate may cause rebound hyperacidity and milk-alkali syndrome. Alkaluria may occur when products are

used on a long-term basis, particularly in persons with abnormal renal function.

**Contraindications:** Sensitivity to aluminum or magnesium products may cause hypersensitive reactions. Aluminum products should not be used by persons sensitive to aluminum. Magnesium products should not be used by persons sensitive to magnesium. Check for sensitivity before administering.

**Precautions:** Magnesium products should be given cautiously to patients with renal insufficiency, and during pregnancy and breastfeeding. Sodium content of antacids may be significant. Use with caution for patients with hypertension, CHF or those on a low-sodium diet.

**Pharmacokinetics:** Duration is 20-40 min. If ingested 1 hr after meals, acidity is reduced for at least 3 hr.

**Interactions:** Products whose effects may be increased by some antacids include quinidine, amphetamines, pseudoephedrine, levodopa, valproic acid, and dicumarol. Products whose effects may be decreased by some antacids include cimetidine, corticosteroids, ranitidine, iron salts, phenothiazines, phenytoin, digoxin, tetracyclines, ketoconazole, salicylates, and isoniazid.

## NURSING CONSIDERATIONS
### Assessment
- Assess for aggravating and alleviating factors of epigastric pain or hyperacidity; identify the location, duration, and characteristics of epigastric pain
- Assess GI symptoms, including constipation, diarrhea, abdominal pain; if severe abdominal pain with fever occurs, these products should not be given
- Assess renal symptoms, including increasing urinary pH, electrolytes

### Nursing diagnoses
- Constipation (adverse reactions)
- Diarrhea (adverse reactions)
- Pain, chronic (uses)

### Implementation
- Advise patient not to take other products within 1-2 hr of antacid administration, since antacids may impair absorption of other products
- Give all products with an 8-oz glass of water to ensure absorption in the stomach
- Give another antacid if constipation occurs with aluminum products

 Alert     Canada Only     Drug on CD          * "Tall Man" lettering (See Preface)

## Evaluation
**Positive therapeutic outcome**
- Absence of epigastric pain
- Decreased acidity

---

## Generic Names

aluminum hydroxide
bismuth subsalicylate
calcium carbonate
magaldrate
magnesium oxide
sodium bicarbonate

### ANTI-ALZHEIMER AGENTS

**Action:** Anti-Alzheimer agents improve cognitive functioning by increasing acetylcholine and inhibiting cholinesterase in the CNS. Does not cure condition, but improves symptoms.

**Uses:** Anti-Alzheimer agents are used for the treatment of Alzheimer's symptoms.

**Adverse effects:** The most common side effects are *nausea, vomiting, diarrhea, dry mouth, insomnia, dizziness,* as well as *urinary frequency, incontinence,* and *rash.* The most serious side effects are **seizures** and **dysrhythmias.**

**Contraindications:** Persons with hypersensitivity reactions should not use these products.

**Precautions:** Anti-Alzheimer agents should be used cautiously in pregnancy **(C),** breastfeeding, sick sinus syndrome, GI bleeding, bladder obstruction, and seizures.

**Pharmacokinetics:** Onset, peak, and duration vary widely among products. Most products are metabolized in the liver and excreted by the kidneys.

**Interactions:** Increased synergistic reactions may occur with succinylcholine, cholinesterase inhibitors, and cholingeric agonists. There may be a decrease in the action of anticholinergics, and there may be additive effects when used with cholinergic agents.

## NURSING CONSIDERATIONS
### Assessment
- B/P, hypo/hypertension
- Mental status: affect, mood, behavioral changes, depression, confusion
- GI status: nausea, vomiting, anorexia, diarrhea
- GU status: urinary frequency, incontinence

### Nursing diagnoses
- Knowledge, deficient (teaching)
- Noncompliance (teaching)
- Thought processes, disturbed (uses)

### Implementation
- Give lowest possible dose for therapeutic result; adjust dose to response
- Provide assistance with ambulation during beginning therapy if dizziness, ataxia occur

### Patient/family education
- Instruct patient to report side effects, adverse reactions to health care provider
- Advise patient to use exactly as prescribed, at regular intervals
- Caution patient not to increase or abruptly decrease dose; serious consequences may result
- Inform patient that product is not a cure, but relieves symptoms

### Evaluation
**Positive therapeutic outcome**
- Decrease in confusion
- Improved mood

---

## Generic Names

donepezil
galanthamine
memantine
rivastigmine
tacrine

### ANTIANGINALS

**Action:** Antianginals are divided into the nitrates, calcium channel blockers, and β-adrenergic blockers. The nitrates dilate coronary arteries, causing decreased preload, and dilate systemic arteries, causing decreased afterload. Calcium channel blockers dilate coronary arteries and decrease SA/AV node conduction. β-Adrenergic blockers decrease heart rate so that myocardial $O_2$ use is decreased. Dipyridamole selectively dilates coronary arteries to increase coronary blood flow.

**Uses:** Antianginals are used in chronic stable angina pectoris, unstable angina and vasospastic angina. Some (i.e., calcium channel blockers and β-blockers) may be used as dysrhythmias and in hypertension.

**Adverse effects:** The most common side effects are *postural hypotension, headache, flushing, dizziness, nausea, edema,* and *drowsiness.* Also common are *rash,* **dysrhythmias,** and *fatigue.*

Adverse effects: *italic* = common, **bold** = life-threatening

**Contraindications:** Persons with known hypersensitivity, increased ICP, or cerebral hemorrhage should not use some of these products.

**Precautions:** Antianginals should be used with caution in pregnancy, breastfeeding, children, postural hypotension, renal disease, and hepatic injury.

**Pharmacokinetics:** Onset, peak, and duration vary widely among coronary products. Most products are metabolized in the liver and excreted in urine.

**Interactions:** Interactions vary widely among products. Check individual monographs for specific information.

## NURSING CONSIDERATIONS
### Assessment
• Monitor orthostatic B/P, pulse
• Assess for pain: duration, time started, activity being performed, character
• Assess for tolerance if taken over long period
• Assess for headache, light-headedness, decreased B/P; may indicate a need for decreased dosage

### Nursing diagnoses
• Cardiac output, decreased (adverse reactions)
• Injury, risk for (uses)
• Knowledge, deficient (teaching)
• Pain, acute (uses)
• Tissue perfusion, ineffective (uses)

### Implementation
• Store protected from light, moisture; place in cool environment

### Patient/family education
• Instruct patient to keep tabs in original container
• Instruct patient not to use OTC products unless directed by prescriber
• Advise patient to report bradycardia, dizziness, confusion, depression, fever
• Teach patient to take pulse at home; advise when to notify prescriber
• Advise patient to avoid alcohol, smoking, sodium intake
• Advise patient to comply with weight control, dietary adjustments, modified exercise program
• Teach patient to carry/wear emergency ID to identify product being taken, allergies
• Caution patient to make position changes slowly to prevent fainting

### Evaluation
**Positive therapeutic outcome**
• Decrease, prevention of anginal pain

## Generic Names

*Nitrates:*
amyl nitrite
isosorbide
🔘 nitroglycerin

*β-Adrenergic blockers:*
atenolol
dipyridamole
metoprolol
nadolol
propranolol

*Calcium channel blockers:*
amlodipine
bepridil
**diltiazem** (high alert)
niCARdipine
NIFEdipine
🔘 verapamil

*Miscellaneous:*
ranolazine

## ANTIANXIETY AGENTS

**Action:** Benzodiazepines potentiate the action of GABA, including any other inhibitory transmitters in the CNS, resulting in decreased anxiety. Most agents cause a decrease in CNS excitability.

**Uses:** Anxiety is relieved in conditions such as generalized anxiety disorder and phobic disorders. Benzodiazepines are also used for acute alcohol withdrawal to prevent delirium tremens, and some products are used for relaxation before surgery.

**Adverse effects:** The most common side effects are dizziness, drowsiness, blurred vision, and orthostatic hypotension. Most adverse reactions are mediated through the CNS. There is potential for abuse and physical dependence with some products.

**Contraindications:** These products are contraindicated in hypersensitivity, acute angle-closure glaucoma, breastfeeding (diazepam), children <6 mo, and hepatic disease (clonazepam).

**Precautions:** Antianxiety agents should be used cautiously in geriatric or debilitated patients. Usually smaller doses are needed since metabolism is slowed. Persons with renal/hepatic disease may show delayed excretion. Clonazepam may increase the incidence of seizures.

**Pharmacokinetics:** Most of these agents are metabolized by the liver and excreted via the kidneys.

**Interactions:** Increased CNS depression may occur when given with other CNS depressants. These products should be used together cautiously. Alcohol should not be used, as fatal reactions have occurred. The serum concentration and toxicity may be increased when used with benzodiazepines.

## NURSING CONSIDERATIONS
### Assessment
• Assess B/P (lying and standing), pulse; if systolic B/P drops 20 mm Hg, hold product and notify prescriber; orthostatic hypotension can be severe
• Monitor renal/hepatic function tests: AST, ALT, bilirubin, creatinine, LDH, alkaline phosphatase
• Monitor physical dependency and withdrawal with some products, including headache, nausea, vomiting, muscle pain, and weakness after long-term use

### Nursing diagnoses
• Anxiety (uses)
• Injury, risk for, physical (adverse reactions)
• Knowledge, deficient (teaching)

### Implementation
• Give with food or milk for GI symptoms; may give crushed if patient is unable to swallow whole (tabs only, no controlled or sustained-release products)

### Patient/family education
• Inform patient that product should not be used for everyday stress or long-term use; not to take more than prescribed amount since product is habit forming
• Caution patient to avoid driving and activities that require alertness since drowsiness and dizziness may occur
• Instruct patient to abstain from alcohol, other psychotropic medications unless directed by prescriber
• Caution patient not to discontinue abruptly; after extended periods, withdrawal symptoms may occur

### Evaluation
**Positive therapeutic outcome**
• Decreased anxiety
• Increased relaxation

---

### Generic Names
*Benzodiazepines:*
alprazolam
chlordiazepoxide
clonazepam
diazepam
lorazepam
midazolam
oxazepine
temazepine
triazolam

*Miscellaneous:*
busPIRone
doxepin
hydrOXYzine
meprobamate
paroxetine
venlafaxine

## ANTIASTHMATICS

**Action:** Bronchodilators are divided into anticholinergics, α/β-adrenergic agonists, β-adrenergic agonists, and phosphodiesterase inhibitors. Also included in antiasthmatic agents are corticosteroids, leukotriene antagonists, mast cell stabilizers, and monoclonal antibodies. Anticholinergics act by inhibiting interaction of acetylcholine at receptor sites on bronchial smooth muscle. α/β-Adrenergic agonists act by relaxing bronchial smooth muscle and increasing diameter of nasal passages. β-Adrenergic agonists act by action on $\beta_2$-receptors, which relaxes bronchial smooth muscle. Phosphodiesterase inhibitors act by blocking phosphodiesterase and increasing cAMP, which mediates smooth muscle relaxation in the respiratory system. Corticosteroids act by decreasing inflammation in the bronchial system. Leukotriene receptor antagonists decrease leukotrienes and mast cell stabilizers decrease histamine; both act to decrease bronchospasm.

**Uses:** Antiasthmatics are used for bronchial asthma; bronchospasm associated with bronchitis, emphysema, or other obstructive pulmonary diseases; Cheyne-Stokes respirations and prevention of exercise-induced asthma. Some products are used for rhinitis and other allergic reactions.

**Adverse effects:** The most common side effects are tremors, anxiety, nausea, vomiting and irritation in the throat. The most serious adverse reactions are bronchospasm and dyspnea.

**Contraindications:** Persons with hypersensitivity, angle-closure glaucoma, tachydysrhythmias, and severe cardiac disease should not use some of these products.

---

Adverse effects: *italic* = common, **bold** = life-threatening

**Precautions:** Antiasthmatics should be used with caution in pregnancy, breastfeeding, hyperthyroidism, hypertension, prostatic hypertrophy, and seizure disorders.

**Pharmacokinetics:** Onset, peak, and duration vary widely among products. Most products are metabolized by the liver and excreted in urine.

**Interactions:** Interactions vary widely among products. Check individual monographs for specific information.

### NURSING CONSIDERATIONS
#### Assessment
• Monitor respiratory function: vital capacity, forced expiratory volume, ABGs, lung sounds, heart rate and rhythm, aggravating and alleviating factors

#### Nursing diagnoses
• Activity intolerance (uses)
• Airway clearance, ineffective (uses)
• Injury, risk for, physical (adverse reactions)
• Knowledge, deficient (teaching)
• Noncompliance (teaching)

#### Implementation
• Give inhaled product after shaking; exhale, place mouthpiece in mouth, inhale slowly, hold breath, remove, exhale slowly
• Give PO product with meals to decrease gastric irritation
• Store inhaled product in light-resistant container; do not expose to temperatures >86° F (30° C)
• Give gum, small sips of water for dry mouth

#### Patient/family education
• Caution patient to avoid hazardous activities; drowsiness or dizziness may occur with some products
• Instruct patient to obtain bloodwork as required; some products require blood levels to be drawn
• Advise patient to avoid all OTC medications unless approved by provider
• Instruct patient to report side effects, including insomnia, heart palpitations, lightheadedness; these side effects may occur with some products

#### Evaluation
**Positive therapeutic outcome**
• Decrease severity and number of asthma attacks
• Absence of dyspnea, wheezing

### Generic Names

*Bronchodilators:*
albuterol
arformoterol
**atropine** (high alert)
bitolterol
dyphylline
formoterol
ipratropium
isoproterenol
levalbuterol
metaproterenol
pirbuterol
terbutaline
theophylline
tiotropium

*Adrenergics:*
**epINEPHrine** (high alert)

*Corticosteroids:*
beclomethasone
betamethasone
budesonide
cortisone
dexamethasone
flunisolide
fluticasone
hydrocortisone
methylPREDNISolone
predniSONE
trimicinolone

*Leukotriene antagonists:*
zafirlukast

*Mast cell stabilizers:*
cromolyn
nedocromil

*Monoclonal antibodies:*
omalizumab

### ANTICHOLINERGICS

**Action:** Anticholinergics inhibit the muscarinic actions of acetylcholine at receptor sites in the autonomic nervous system. Anticholinergics are also known as antimuscarinic products.

**Uses:** Anticholinergics are used for a variety of conditions: decreasing involuntary movements in parkinsonism (benztropine, trihexyphenidyl); bradydysrhythmias (atropine); nausea and vomiting (scopolamine); and as cycloplegic mydriatics (atropine, hematropine, scopalamine, cyclopentolate, tropicamide). Gastrointestinal anticholinergics are used to decrease motility (smooth muscle tone) in the GI, biliary, and urinary tracts and for their ability to decrease gastric secretions (propantheline, glycopyrrolate).

**Adverse effects:** The most common side effects are dry mouth, constipation, urinary retention, urinary hesitancy, headache, and dizziness. Also common is paralytic ileus.

**Contraindications:** Persons with angle-closure glaucoma, myasthenia gravis, or GI/GU obstruction should not use some of these products.

**Precautions:** Anticholinergics should be used with caution in pregnant, breastfeeding, or geriatric patients, or in those with prostatic hypertrophy, CHF, or hypertension. Use with caution in the presence of high environmental temperature.

**Pharmacokinetics:** Onset, peak, and duration vary widely among products. Most products are metabolized in the liver and excreted in urine.

**Interactions:** Increased anticholinergic effects may occur when used with MAOIs, tricyclics, and amantadine. Anticholinergics may cause a decreased effect of phenothiazines and levodopa.

### NURSING CONSIDERATIONS
#### Assessment
- Assess I&O ratio; retention commonly causes decreased urinary output
- Assess for urinary hesitancy, retention; palpate bladder if retention occurs
- Assess for constipation; increase fluids, bulk, exercise if this occurs
- Identify tolerance over long-term therapy; dosage may need to be increased or changed
- Assess mental status: affect, mood, CNS depression, worsening of mental symptoms during early therapy

#### Nursing diagnoses
- Cardiac output, decreased (uses)
- Constipation (adverse reactions)
- Knowledge, deficient (teaching)

#### Implementation
**PO route**
- Give with or after meals to prevent GI upset; may give with fluids other than water
- Store at room temperature
- Give hard candy, frequent drinks, sugarless gum to relieve dry mouth

**IM/IV route**
- Give parenteral dose with patient recumbent to prevent postural hypotension
- Give parenteral dose slowly; keep in bed for at least 1 hr after dose; monitor VS

- Give after checking dose carefully; even slight overdose could lead to toxicity

#### Patient/family education
- Caution patient to avoid driving and other hazardous activities; drowsiness may occur
- Advise patient to avoid OTC medication: cough, cold preparations with alcohol, antihistamines unless directed by prescriber

#### Evaluation
**Positive therapeutic outcome**
- Decreased secretions
- Absence of nausea and vomiting

### Generic Names

 atropine (high alert)
benztropine
biperiden
glycopyrrolate
hyoscyamine
propantheline
scopolamine (transdermal)
solifenacin
trihexyphenidyl

## ANTICOAGULANTS

**Action:** Anticoagulants interfere with blood clotting by preventing clot formation.

**Uses:** Anticoagulants are used for DVT, pulmonary emboli, myocardial infarction, open heart surgery, disseminated intravascular clotting syndrome, atrial fibrillation with embolization, and in transfusion and dialysis.

**Adverse effects:** The most serious adverse reactions are hemorrhage, agranulocytosis, leukopenia, eosinophilia, and thrombocytopenia, depending on the specific product. The most common side effects are diarrhea, rash, and fever.

**Contraindications:** Persons with hemophilia, leukemia with bleeding, peptic ulcer disease, thrombocytopenic purpura, blood dyscrasias, acute nephritis, and subacute bacterial endocarditis should not use these products.

**Precautions:** Anticoagulants should be used with caution in pregnancy, geriatric, and alcoholism.

**Pharmacokinetics:** Onset, peak, and duration vary widely among products. Most products are metabolized in the liver and excreted in urine.

**Interactions:** Salicylates, steroids, and nonsteroidal antiinflammatories will potentiate the action of anticoagulants. Anticoagulants may cause serious effects. Check individual monographs for specific information.

## NURSING CONSIDERATIONS
### Assessment
- Monitor blood tests (Hct, platelets, occult blood in stools) q3 mo
- Monitor PTT, which should be 1½-2 × control, PPT; often daily, APTT, ACT, INR
- Monitor B/P; watch for increasing signs of hypertension
- Monitor for bleeding gums, petechiae, ecchymosis, black tarry stools, hematuria
- Monitor for fever, skin rash, urticaria
- Monitor for needed dosage change q1-2 wk

### Nursing diagnoses
- Injury, risk for (side effects)
- Knowledge, deficient (teaching)
- Tissue perfusion, ineffective (uses)

### Implementation
- Store in tight container (PO dose)

**SUBCUT route**
- Give at same time each day to maintain steady blood levels
- Do not massage area or aspirate when giving SUBCUT inj; give in abdomen between pelvic bones; rotate sites; do not pull back on plunger, leave in for 10 sec; apply gentle pressure for 1 min
- Do not change needles
- Avoid all IM inj that may cause bleeding

### Patient/family education
- Advise patient to avoid OTC preparations that may cause serious product interactions unless directed by prescriber
- Inform patient that product may be held during active bleeding (menstruation), depending on condition
- Caution patient to use soft-bristle toothbrush to avoid bleeding gums; avoid contact sports; use electric razor
- Instruct patient to carry/wear emergency ID identifying product taken
- Instruct patient to report any signs of bleeding: gums, under skin, urine, stools

### Evaluation
**Positive therapeutic outcome**
- Decrease of DVT

---

### Generic Names
argatroban
**dalteparin** (high alert)
desirudin
**enoxaparin** (high alert)
fondaparinux
**heparin** (high alert)
**lepirudin** (high alert)
**tinzaparin** (high alert)
**warfarin** (high alert)

---

## ANTICONVULSANTS

**Action:** Anticonvulsants are divided into the barbiturates, benzodiazepines, hydantoins, succinimides, and miscellaneous products. Barbiturates and benzodiazepines are discussed in separate sections. Hydantoins act by inhibiting the spread of seizure activity in the motor cortex. Succinimides act by inhibiting spike and wave formation; they also decrease amplitude, frequency, duration, and spread of discharge in seizures.

**Uses:** Hydantoins are used in generalized tonic-clonic seizures, status epilepticus, and psychomotor seizures. Succinimides are used for absence (or petit mal) seizures. Barbiturates are used in generalized tonic-clonic and cortical focal seizures.

**Adverse effects:** Bone marrow depression is the most life-threatening adverse reaction associated with hydantoins or succinimides. The most common side effects are GI symptoms. Other common side effects for hydantoins are gingival hyperplasia and CNS effects such as nystagmus, ataxia, slurred speech, and confusion.

**Contraindications:** Hypersensitive reactions may occur, and allergies should be identified before these products are given.

**Precautions:** Persons with renal/hepatic disease should be watched closely.

**Pharmacokinetics:** Onset, peak, and duration vary widely among products. Most products are metabolized in the liver and excreted in urine, bile, and feces.

**Interactions:** Decreased effects of estrogens, oral contraceptives (hydantoins).

## NURSING CONSIDERATIONS
### Assessment
- Monitor renal function tests, including BUN, creatinine, serum uric acid, urine CCr before and during therapy
- Monitor blood tests: RBC, Hct, Hgb, reticulocyte counts weekly for 4 wk then monthly
- Monitor hepatic function tests: AST, ALT, bilirubin, creatinine

---

- Assess mental status, including mood, sensorium, affect, behavioral changes; if mental status changes, notify prescriber
- Assess for eye problems, including need for ophth examinations before, during, and after treatment (slit lamp, fundoscopy, tonometry)
- Assess for allergic reaction, including red, raised rash; if this occurs, product should be discontinued
- Assess for blood dyscrasias, including fever, sore throat, bruising, rash, jaundice
- Monitor toxicity, including bone marrow depression, nausea, vomiting, ataxia, diplopia, cardiovascular collapse, Stevens-Johnson syndrome

### Nursing diagnoses
- Injury, risk for (uses)
- Noncompliance (teaching)
- Sleep deprivation (adverse reactions)

### Implementation
**PO route**
- Give with food, milk to decrease GI symptoms
- Provide good oral hygiene as it is important for patients taking hydantoins

### Patient/family education
- Advise patient to carry/wear emergency ID stating products taken, condition, prescriber's name, phone number
- Advise patient to avoid driving, other activities that require alertness

### Evaluation
**Positive therapeutic outcome**
- Decreased seizure activity; document on patient's chart

---

### Generic Names

*Hydantoins:*
fosphenytoin
🔵 phenytoin

*Miscellaneous:*
acetazolamide
carbamazepine
clonazepam
🔵 diazepam
felbamate
gabapentin
lamotrigine
**magnesium sulfate** (high alert)
tiagabine
topiramate
valproate/valproic acid/divalproex sodium
zonisamide

*Barbiturates:*
🔵 **phenobarbital** (high alert)
primidone
**thiopental** (high alert)

---

### ANTIDEPRESSANTS

**Action:** Antidepressants are divided into the tricyclics, MAOIs, and miscellaneous antidepressants. The tricyclics work by blocking reuptake of norepinephrine and serotonin into nerve endings and increasing action of norepinephrine and serotonin in nerve cells. MAOIs act by increasing concentrations of endogenous epINEPHrine, norepinephrine, serotonin, dopamine in storage sites in CNS by inhibition of MAO; increased concentration reduces depression.

**Uses:** Antidepressants are used for depression, and in some cases, enuresis in children.

**Adverse effects:** The most serious adverse reactions are paralytic ileus, acute renal failure, hypertension, and hypertensive crisis, depending on the specific product. Common side effects are dizziness, drowsiness, diarrhea, dry mouth, urinary retention, and orthostatic hypotension.

**Contraindications:** The contraindications for antidepressants are seizure disorders, prostatic hypertrophy, severe renal/hepatic/cardiac disease depending on the type of medication.

**Precautions:** Antidepressants should be used cautiously in pregnant, geriatric, and suicidal patients; severe depression; schizophrenia; hyperactivity; and diabetes mellitus.

**Pharmacokinetics:** Onset, peak, and duration vary widely among products. Most products are metabolized in the liver and excreted in urine.

**Interactions:** Interactions vary widely among products. Check individual monographs for specific information.

### NURSING CONSIDERATIONS
**Assessment**
- Monitor B/P (lying, standing), pulse q4hr; if systolic B/P drops 20 mm Hg, hold product, notify prescriber; take VS q4hr in patients with CV disease
- Monitor blood tests: CBC, leukocytes, differential, cardiac enzymes if patient is receiving long-term therapy

Adverse effects: *italic* = common, **bold** = life-threatening

- Monitor hepatic function tests: AST, ALT, bilirubin, creatinine
- Monitor weight weekly; appetite may increase with product
- Monitor for EPS primarily in geriatric: rigidity, dystonia, akathisia
- Assess mental status: mood, sensorium, affect, suicidal tendencies, increase in psychiatric symptoms (depression, panic)
- Check for urinary retention, constipation; constipation is more likely to occur in children, geriatric patients
- Assess for withdrawal symptoms: headache, nausea, vomiting, muscle pain, weakness; do not usually occur unless product was discontinued abruptly
- Identify alcohol consumption; if alcohol is consumed, hold dose until AM

### Nursing diagnoses
- Coping, ineffective (uses)
- Injury, risk for (uses/adverse reactions)
- Knowledge, deficient (teaching)

### Implementation
**PO route**
- Give increased fluids, bulk in diet if constipation, urinary retention occur
- Give with food or milk for GI symptoms
- Give gum, hard candy, or frequent sips of water for dry mouth
- Store in airtight container at room temperature; do not refreeze
- Provide assistance with ambulation during beginning therapy since drowsiness/dizziness occurs

### Patient/family education
- Teach patient that therapeutic effects may take 2-3 wk
- Advise patient to use caution in driving or other activities requiring alertness because of drowsiness, dizziness, blurred vision
- Caution patient to avoid alcohol ingestion, other CNS depressants
- Instruct patient not to discontinue medication quickly after long-term use; may cause nausea, headache, malaise
- Instruct patient to wear sunscreen or large hat, since photosensitivity may occur

### Evaluation
**Positive therapeutic outcome**
- Decreased depression

### Generic Names
*Tetracyclics:*
mirtazapine

*Tricyclics:*
amitriptyline
amoxapine
clomiPRAMINE
desipramine
doxepin
 imipramine
nortriptyline
trimipramine

*Miscellaneous:*
buPROPion
duloxetine
trazodone
venlafaxine

*MAOIs:*
phenelzine
tranylcypromine

*SSRIs:*
citalopram
escitalopram
fluoxetine
paroxetine
sertraline

## ANTIDIABETICS

**Action:** Antidiabetics are divided into the insulins that decrease blood glucose, phosphate, and potassium and increase blood pyruvate and lactate; and oral antidiabetics that cause functioning β-cells in the pancreas to release insulin, improves the effect of endogenous and exogenous insulin.

**Uses:** Insulins are used for ketoacidosis and diabetes mellitus types 1 and 2; oral antidiabetics are used for diabetes mellitus type 2.

**Adverse effects:** The most common side effect of insulin and oral antidiabetics is hypoglycemia. Other adverse reactions for oral antidiabetics include blood dyscrasias, hepatotoxicity, and, rarely, cholestatic jaundice. Adverse reactions for insulin products include allergic responses and, more rarely, anaphylaxis.

**Contraindications:** Hypersensitive reactions may occur, and allergies should be identified before these products are given. Oral antidiabetics should not be used in juvenile or brittle diabetes, diabetic ketoacidosis, or severe renal/hepatic disease.

**Precautions:** Oral antidiabetics should be used with caution in pregnancy, breastfeeding, geriatric, cardiac disease, and in the presence of alcohol.

**Pharmacokinetics:** Onset, peak, and duration vary widely among products. Oral antidiabetics are metabolized in the liver, with metabolites excreted in urine, bile, and feces.

**Interactions:** Interactions vary widely among products. Check individual monographs for specific information.

## NURSING CONSIDERATIONS
### Assessment
• Monitor blood, urine glucose levels during treatment to determine diabetes control (oral products)
• Monitor fasting blood glucose, 2 hr PP (60-100 mg/dl normal fasting level) (70-130 mg/dl—normal 2-hr level)
• Assess for hypoglycemic reaction that can occur during peak time

### Nursing diagnoses
• Nutrition: more than body requirements, imbalanced (uses)

### Implementation
**PO route**
• Give oral antidiabetic 30 min before meals
**SUBCUT route**
• Give insulin after warming to room temperature by rotating in palms to prevent lipodystrophy from injecting cold insulin
• Give human insulin to those allergic to beef or pork
• Rotate inj sites when giving insulin; use abdomen, upper back, thighs, upper arm, buttocks; keep a record of sites

### Patient/family education
• Advise patient to avoid alcohol and salicylates except on advice of prescriber
• Teach patient symptoms of ketoacidosis: nausea, thirst, polyuria, dry mouth, decreased B/P, dry, flushed skin, acetone breath, drowsiness, Kussmaul respirations
• Teach patient symptoms of hypoglycemia: headache, tremors, fatigue, weakness; that candy or sugar should be carried to treat hypoglycemia
• Advise patient to test urine for glucose/ketones tid if this product is replacing insulin
• Advise patient to continue weight control, dietary restrictions, exercise, hygiene

### Evaluation
**Positive therapeutic outcome**
• Decrease in polyuria, polydipsia, polyphagia
• Clear sensorium
• Absence of dizziness
• Stable gait

### Generic Names
chlorproPAMIDE
glipiZIDE
glyBURIDE
**insulin aspart** (high alert)
**insulin detemir** (high alert)
**insulin glargine** (high alert)
**insulin glulisine** (high alert)
**insulin isophane suspension (NPH)** (high alert)
**insulin lispro** (high alert)
**insulin regular** (high alert)
**insulin regular concentrated** (high alert)
**insulin zinc suspension (Lente)** (high alert)
metformin
miglitol
pioglitazone
repaglinide
rosiglitazone
sitagliptin

## ANTIDIARRHEALS

**Action:** Antidiarrheals work by various actions including direct action on intestinal muscles to decrease GI peristalsis; or by inhibiting prostaglandin synthesis responsible for GI hypermotility; acting on mucosal receptors responsible for peristalsis; or decreasing water content of stools.

**Uses:** Antidiarrheals are used for diarrhea of undetermined causes.

**Adverse effects:** The most serious adverse reactions of some products are paralytic ileus, toxic megacolon, and angioneurotic edema. The most common side effects are constipation, nausea, dry mouth, and abdominal pain.

**Contraindications:** Persons with severe ulcerative colitis, pseudomembranous colitis with some products.

**Precautions:** Antidiarrheals should be used with caution in pregnancy, breastfeeding, children, geriatric patients, dehydration.

**Pharmacokinetics:** Onset, peak, and duration vary widely among products. Most products are metabolized in the liver and excreted in urine.

**Interactions:** Interactions vary widely among products. Check individual monographs for specific information.

## NURSING CONSIDERATIONS
### Assessment
- Monitor electrolytes (potassium, sodium, chloride) if on long-term therapy
- Monitor bowel pattern before; for rebound constipation after termination of medication
- Assess response after 48 hr; if no response, product should be discontinued
- Identify dehydration in children

### Nursing diagnoses
- Constipation (adverse reactions)
- Diarrhea (uses)
- Fluid volume, risk for deficient (adverse reactions)
- Knowledge, deficient (teaching)

### Implementation
**PO route**
- Give for 48 hr only

### Patient/family education
- Advise patient to avoid OTC products
- Caution patient not to exceed recommended dose

### Evaluation
**Positive therapeutic outcome**
- Decreased diarrhea

---

## Generic Names

bismuth subsalicylate
kaolin/pectin
loperamide

---

## ANTIDYSRHYTHMICS

**Action:** Antidysrhythmics are divided into four classes and miscellaneous antidysrhythmics:
- Class I increases the duration of action potential and the effective refractory period and reduces disparity in the refractory period between a normal and infarcted myocardium; further subclasses include Ia, Ib, Ic
- Class II decreases the rate of SA node discharge, increases recovery time, slows conduction through the AV node, and decreases heart rate, which decreases $O_2$ consumption in the myocardium
- Class III increases the duration of action potential and the effective refractory period
- Class IV inhibits calcium ion influx across the cell membrane during cardiac depolarization; decreases SA node discharge, decreases conduction velocity through the AV node
- Miscellaneous antidysrhythmics include those such as adenosine, which slows conduction through the AV node, and digoxin, which decreases conduction velocity and prolongs the effective refractory period in the AV node

**Uses:** Antidysrhythmics are used for PVCs, tachycardia, hypertension, atrial fibrillation, and angina pectoris.

**Adverse effects:** Side effects and adverse reactions vary widely among products.

**Contraindications:** Contraindications vary widely among products.

**Precautions:** Precautions vary widely among products.

**Pharmacokinetics:** Onset, peak, and duration vary widely among products.

**Interactions:** Interactions vary widely among products. Check individual monographs for specific information.

## NURSING CONSIDERATIONS
### Assessment
- Monitor ECG continuously to determine product effectiveness, PVCs, or other dysrhythmias
- Assess for dehydration or hypovolemia
- Monitor B/P continuously for hypo/hypertension
- Monitor I&O ratio
- Monitor serum potassium
- Assess for edema in feet and legs daily

### Nursing diagnoses
- Cardiac output, decreased (uses)
- Diarrhea (adverse reactions)
- Gas exchange, impaired (adverse reactions)
- Tissue perfusion, ineffective (uses)

### Patient/family education
- Advise patient to comply with dosage schedule, even if patient is feeling better
- Instruct patient to report bradycardia, dizziness, confusion, depression, fever

### Evaluation
**Positive therapeutic outcome**
- Decrease in B/P in hypertension
- Decreased B/P, edema, moist crackles in CHF

---

## Generic Names

*Class I:*
moricizine

*Class Ia:*
disopyramide
 procainamide
quinidine

---

*Class Ib:*
**lidocaine, parenteral** (high alert)
mexiletine
phenytoin
tocainide

*Class Ic:*
flecainide
propafenone

*Class II:*
acebutolol
esmolol
propranolol
sotalol

*Class III:*
**amiodarone** (high alert)
**ibutilide** (high alert)

*Class IV:*
verapamil

*Miscellaneous:*
**adenosine** (high alert)
**atropine** (high alert)
**digoxin** (high alert)

---

## ANTIEMETICS

**Action:** The antiemetics are divided into the 5-HT3 receptor antagonists, the phenothiazines and the miscellaneous products. The 5-HT3 receptor antagonists work by blocking serotonin peripherally, centrally, and in the small intestine. The phenothiazines act by blocking the chemoreceptor trigger zone in the brain. The miscellaneous products work by either decreasing motion sickness or delaying gastric emptying.

**Uses:** Antiemetics are used to prevent nausea and vomiting due to cancer chemotherapy, radiotherapy, and surgery (5-HT3 receptor antagonists); some of the miscellaneous products (antihistamines) work by decreasing motion sickness. Most other products are used for many types of nausea and vomiting.

**Adverse effects:** The most common side effects are headache, dizziness, fatigue, and diarrhea.

**Contraindications:** Persons developing hypersensitive reactions should not use these products.

**Precautions:** Antiemetics should be used cautiously in pregnancy, breastfeeding, hepatic disease, and some GI disorders.

**Pharmacokinetics:** Onset, peak, and duration vary widely among products. Most products are metabolized by the liver and excreted by the kidneys.

**Interactions:** Interactions vary widely among products. Check individual monographs for specific information. Other CNS depressants increase CNS depression.

### NURSING CONSIDERATIONS
**Assessment**
• Assess reason for nausea, vomiting; absence of nausea and vomiting after giving product
• Monitor hypersensitivity reactions: rash, bronchospasm with some products

**Nursing diagnoses**
• Fluid volume, risk for deficient (uses)
• Injury, risk for, physical (uses, adverse reactions)
• Knowledge, deficient (teaching)
• Nutrition: less than body requirements, imbalanced (uses)

**Implementation**
• Give prophylactically, before nausea and vomiting occur, in cancer chemotherapy
• Store at room temperature vial/ampules, oral products

**Patient/family education**
• Caution patient to avoid hazardous activities if dizziness occurs; ask for assistance if hospitalized
• Instruct patient to rise slowly to prevent orthostatic hypotension
• Teach patient all aspects of product usage
• Teach patient conservative methods to control nausea and vomiting such as sips of water or other fluids and dry crackers

**Evaluation**
**Positive therapeutic outcome**
• Absence or decreasing nausea and vomiting after use

---

### Generic Names

*5-HT3 antagonists:*
dolasetron
granisetron
ondansetron
palonosetron

*Phenothiazines:*
chlorproMAZINE
prochlorperazine
promethazine
thiethylperazine

*Miscellaneous:*
aprepitant
dimenhyDRINATE

---

Adverse effects: *italic* = common, **bold** = life-threatening

meclizine
metoclopramide
scopolamine
trimethobenzamide

## ANTIFUNGALS (SYSTEMIC)

**Action:** Antifungals act by increasing cell membrane permeability in susceptible organisms by binding sterols and decreasing potassium, sodium, and nutrients in the cell.

**Uses:** Antifungals are used for infections of histoplasmosis, blastomycosis, coccidioidomycosis, cryptococcosis, aspergillosis, phycomycosis, candidiasis, sporotrichosis causing severe meningitis, septicemia, and skin infections.

**Adverse effects:** The most serious adverse reactions include renal tubular acidosis, permanent renal impairment, anuria, oliguria, hemorrhagic gastroenteritis, acute liver failure, and blood dyscrasias. Some common side effects include hypokalemia, nausea, vomiting, anorexia, headache, fever, and chills.

**Contraindications:** Persons with severe bone depression or hypersensitivity should not use these products.

**Precautions:** Antifungals should be used with caution in renal/hepatic disease and pregnancy.

**Pharmacokinetics:** Onset, peak, and duration vary widely among products. Most products are metabolized in the liver and excreted in urine.

**Interactions:** Interactions vary widely among products. Check individual monographs for specific information.

## NURSING CONSIDERATIONS
### Assessment
• Monitor VS q15-30 min during first infusion; note changes in pulse, B/P
• Monitor I&O ratio; watch for decreasing urinary output, change in specific gravity; discontinue product to prevent permanent damage to renal tubules
• Monitor blood tests; CBC, potassium, sodium, calcium, magnesium q2 wk
• Monitor weight weekly; if weight increases over 2 lb/wk, edema is present; renal damage should be considered
• Assess for renal toxicity: increasing BUN, is >40 mg/dl or if serum creatinine >3 mg/dl; product may be discontinued or dosage reduced
• Assess for hepatotoxicity: increasing AST, ALT, alkaline phosphatase, bilirubin

• Assess for allergic reaction: dermatitis, rash; product should be discontinued; antihistamines (mild reaction) or epINEPHrine (severe reaction) administered
• Assess for hypokalemia: anorexia, drowsiness, weakness, decreased reflexes, dizziness, increased urinary output, increased thirst, paresthesias
• Assess for ototoxicity: tinnitus (ringing, roaring in ears), vertigo, loss of hearing (rare)

### Nursing diagnoses
• Infection, risk for (uses)
• Injury, risk for (adverse reactions)
• Knowledge, deficient (teaching)

### Implementation
#### IV route
• Give by **IV** using in-line filter (mean pore diameter >1 µm) using distal veins; check for extravasation, necrosis q8hr
• Give product only after C&S confirms organism, make sure product is used in life-threatening infections
• Provide protection from light during infusion; cover with foil
• Give symptomatic treatment as ordered for adverse reactions: aspirin, antihistamines, antiemetics, antispasmodics
• Store protected from moisture and light; diluted sol is stable for 24 hr

### Patient/family education
• Teach patient that long-term therapy may be needed to clear infection (2 wk-3 mo depending on type of infection)

### Evaluation
#### Positive therapeutic outcome
• Decreased fever, malaise, rash
• Negative C&S for infecting organism

### Generic Names
amphotericin B
anidulafungin
fluconazole
griseofulvin
itraconazole
ketoconazole
nystatin
voriconazole

## ANTIHISTAMINES

**Action:** Antihistamines compete with histamines for $H_1$ receptor sites. They antagonize in varying degrees most of the pharmacologic effects of histamines.

**Uses:** Antihistamines are used to control the symptoms of allergies, rhinitis, and pruritus.

**Adverse effects:** Most products cause drowsiness; however, two of the newer products, loratadine and fexofenadine, produce little, if any, drowsiness. Other common side effects are headache and thickening of bronchial secretions. Serious blood dyscrasias may occur, but are rare. Urinary retention, GI effects occur with many of these products.

**Contraindications:** Hypersensitivity to $H_1$-receptor antagonists occurs rarely. Patients with acute asthma and lower respiratory tract disease should not use these products since thick secretions may result. Other contraindications include angle-closure glaucoma, bladder neck obstruction, stenosing peptic ulcer, symptomatic prostatic hypertrophy, breastfeeding, newborn.

**Precautions:** Antihistamines must be used cautiously in conjunction with intraocular pressure since they increase intraocular pressure. Caution should also be used in pregnancy, breastfeeding, and geriatric patients; patients with renal/cardiac disease, hypertension, and seizure disorders.

**Pharmacokinetics:** Onset varies from 20-60 min, with duration lasting 4-12 hr. In general, pharmacokinetics vary widely among products.

**Interactions:** Barbiturates, opioids, hypnotics, tricyclics, and alcohol can increase CNS depression when taken with antihistamines.

## NURSING CONSIDERATIONS
### Assessment
• Check I&O ratio; be alert for urinary retention, frequency, dysuria; product should be discontinued if these occur
• Assess for blood dyscrasias: thrombocytopenia, agranulocytosis (rare)
• Assess for respiratory status, including rate, rhythm, increase in bronchial secretions, wheezing, chest tightness
• Assess for cardiac status, including palpitations, increased pulse, hypotension
• Assess CBC during long-term therapy, since hemolytic anemia, although rare, may occur
• Administer with food or milk to decrease GI symptoms; absorption may be decreased slightly
• Administer whole (sus rel tab)
• Provide hard candy, gum, frequent rinsing of mouth for dryness

### Nursing diagnoses
• Airway clearance, ineffective (uses)

### Patient/family education
• Advise patient to notify prescriber if confusion, sedation, hypotension occur
• Caution patient to avoid driving and other hazardous activity if drowsiness occurs
• Instruct patient to avoid concurrent use of alcohol and other CNS depressants
• Inform patient to discontinue a few days before skin testing

### Evaluation
**Positive therapeutic outcome**
• Absence of allergy symptoms, itching

---

## Generic Names
brompheniramine
budesonide
cetirizine
chlorpheniramine
cyproheptadine
desloratadine
diphenhydrAMINE
fexofenadine
levocetirizine
loratadine
promethazine

## ANTIHYPERTENSIVES

**Action:** Antihypertensives are divided into angiotensin converting enzyme (ACE) inhibitors, β-adrenergic blockers, calcium channel blockers, centrally acting adrenergics, diuretics, peripherally acting antiadrenergics, and vasodilators. β-Blockers, calcium channel blockers, and diuretics are discussed in separate sections. ACE inhibitors selectively suppress conversion of renin-angiotensin I to angiotensin II; dilatation of arterial and venous vessels occurs. Centrally acting adrenergics act by inhibiting the sympathetic vasomotor center in the CNS, which reduces impulses in the sympathetic nervous system; blood pressure, pulse rate, and cardiac output decrease. Peripherally acting antiadrenergics inhibit sympathetic vasoconstriction by inhibiting release of norepinephrine and/or depleting norepinephrine stores in adrenergic nerve endings. Vasodilators act on arteriolar smooth muscle by producing direct relaxation or vasodilatation; a reduction in blood pressure, with concomitant increases in heart rate and cardiac output, occurs.

**Uses:** Antihypertensives are used for hypertension and for heart failure not responsive to conventional therapy. Some products are used in hypertensive crisis, angina, and for some cardiac dysrhythmias.

Adverse effects: *italic* = common, **bold** = life-threatening

**Adverse effects:** The most common side effects are marked hypotension, bradycardia, tachycardia, headache, nausea, and vomiting. Side effects and adverse reactions may vary widely between classes and specific products.

**Contraindications:** Hypersensitive reactions may occur, and allergies should be identified before these products are given. Antihypertensives should not be used in children or in patients with heart block.

**Precautions:** Antihypertensives should be used with caution in geriatric and dialysis patients, and in the presence of hypovolemia, leukemia, and electrolyte imbalances.

**Pharmacokinetics:** Onset, peak, and duration vary widely among products. Most products are metabolized in the liver, with metabolites excreted in urine, bile, and feces.

**Interactions:** Interactions vary widely among products. Check individual monographs for specific information.

## NURSING CONSIDERATIONS
### Assessment
• Monitor blood tests: neutrophil; decreased platelets occur with many of the products
• Monitor renal function tests: protein, BUN, creatinine; watch for increased levels, which may indicate nephrotic syndrome; obtain baselines in renal/hepatic function tests before beginning treatment
• Assess for edema in feet and legs daily
• Identify allergic reaction, including rash, fever, pruritus, urticaria: product should be discontinued if antihistamines fail to help
• Identify symptoms of CHF: edema, dyspnea, wet crackles, B/P
• Assess for renal symptoms: polyuria, oliguria, frequency

### Nursing diagnoses
• Cardiac output, decreased (uses)
• Diarrhea (adverse reactions)
• Gas exchange, impaired (adverse reactions)
• Tissue perfusion, ineffective (uses)

### Implementation
• Place patient in supine or Trendelenburg position for severe hypotension

### Patient/family education
• Instruct patient to comply with dosage schedule, even if feeling better
• Advise patient to rise slowly to sitting or standing position to minimize orthostatic hypotension

### Evaluation
**Positive therapeutic outcome**
• Decrease in B/P in hypotension
• Decreased B/P, edema, moist crackles in CHF

## Generic Names
*Aldosterone receptor antagonist:*
eplerone

*Angiotensin-converting enzyme inhibitors:*
benazepril
enalapril
fosinopril
lisinopril
quinapril
ramipril
trandolapril

*Angiotensin II receptor blockers:*
candesartan
eprosartan
irbesartan
losartan
olmesartan
telmisartan
valsartan

*Centrally acting adrenergics:*
clonidine
guanfacine
methyldopa

*Peripherally acting antiadrenergics:*
doxazosin
prazosin
reserpine
terazosin

*Vasodilators:*
ambrisentan
diazoxide
fenoldopam
hydrALAZINE
minoxidil
**nitroprusside** (high alert)

*Antiadrenergic: Combined α/β-blocker:*
labetalol

*Direct renin inhibitors:*
aliskiren

## ANTIINFECTIVES

**Action:** Antiinfectives are divided into several groups, which include but are not limited to penicillins, cephalosporins, aminoglycosides, sulfonamides, tetracyclines, monobactam, erythromycins, and quinolones. These products inhibit the growth and replication of susceptible bacterial organisms.

**Uses:** Antiinfectives are used for infections of susceptible organisms. These products are effective against bacterial, rickettsial, and spirochete infections.

**Adverse effects:** The most common side effects are nausea, vomiting, and diarrhea. Adverse reactions include bone marrow depression and anaphylaxis.

**Contraindications:** Hypersensitive reactions may occur, and allergies should be identified before these products are given. Cross-sensitivity can occur between products of different classes (penicillins or cephalosporins). Often persons allergic to penicillins are also allergic to cephalosporins.

**Precautions:** Antiinfectives should be used with caution in persons with renal/hepatic disease.

**Pharmacokinetics:** Onset, peak, and duration vary widely among products. Most products are metabolized in the liver. Metabolites are excreted in urine, bile, and feces.

**Interactions:** Interactions vary widely among products. Check individual monographs for specific information.

## NURSING CONSIDERATIONS
### Assessment
- Assess for nephrotoxicity: increased BUN, creatinine
- Monitor blood tests: AST, ALT, CBC, Hct, bilirubin; test monthly if patient is on long-term therapy
- Monitor bowel pattern daily; if severe diarrhea occurs, product should be discontinued
- Monitor urine output; if decreasing, notify prescriber; may indicate nephrotoxicity
- Assess for allergic reaction: rash, fever, pruritus, urticaria; product should be discontinued
- Assess for bleeding: ecchymosis, bleeding gums, hematuria, stool guaiac daily
- Assess for overgrowth of infection: perineal itching, fever, malaise, redness, pain, swelling, drainage, rash, diarrhea, change in cough, sputum

### Nursing diagnoses
- Diarrhea (adverse reactions)
- Infection, risk for (uses)

### Implementation
- Give for 10-14 days to ensure organism death, prevention of superinfection
- Give after C&S completed; product may be taken as soon as culture is obtained

### Patient/family education
- Teach patient to comply with dosage schedule, even if feeling better
- Advise patient to report sore throat, bruising, bleeding, joint pain; may indicate blood dyscrasias (rare)

### Evaluation
**Positive therapeutic outcome**
- Absence of fever, fatigue, malaise, draining wounds

---

## Generic Names

*Aminoglycosides:*
amikacin
azithromycin
clarithromycin
gentamicin
kanamycin
neomycin
streptomycin
tobramycin

*Cephalosporins:*
cefaclor
cefadroxil
cefazolin
cefdinir
cefditoren
cefepime
cefonicid
cefoperazone
cefotaxime
cefprozil
ceftibuten
cefuroxime
cephalexin
cephapirin
cephradine

*Fluoroquinolones:*
alatrofloxacin/trovafloxacin
ciprofloxacin
enoxacin
gemifloxacin
levofloxacin
lomefloxacin
norfloxacin
ofloxacin
sparfloxacin

*Ketolides:*
telithromycin

*Miscellaneous:*
adefovir dipivoxil
daptomycin
doripenem

Adverse effects: *italic* = common, **bold** = life-threatening

ertapenem
meropenem
peginterferon alfa-2a

*Penicillins:*
amoxicillin/clavulanate
ampicillin/sulbactam
cloxacillin
dicloxacillin
imipenem/cilastatin
mezlocillin
nafcillin
oxacillin
penicillin G benzathine
penicillin G
penicillin G procaine
penicillin V
piperacillin
ticarcillin
ticarcillin/clavulanate

*Sulfonamides:*
sulfasalazine
sulfiSOXAZOLE

*Tetracyclines:*
doxycycline
minocycline
tetracycline

## ANTILIPIDEMICS

**Action:** Antilipidemics are divided into three categories or subclassifications; HMG-CoA reductase inhibitors (statins), bile acid sequestrants, and miscellaneous products. The HMG-CoA reductase inhibitors work by reduction of an enzyme that is responsible for the beginning step in cholesterol production. Bile acid sequestrants work by binding cholesterol in the GI system. The miscellaneous products work by various actions.

**Uses:** Primary hypercholesterolemia in individuals as an adjunct with other lifestyle changes.

**Adverse effects:** The most common side effects are headache, dizziness, fatigue, insomnia, peripheral edema, dysrhythmias, sinusitis, pharyngitis, abdominal pain, diarrhea, constipation, flatulence, and back pain.

**Contraindications:** Persons breastfeeding (some products) or those with hypersensitivity to any product or severe hepatic disease should not take these products. Antilipidemics are identified as pregnancy category **X** on some products.

**Precautions:** Some products are identified as pregnancy category **C.**

**Pharmacokinetics:** Pharmacokinetics and pharmacodynamics vary with each product.

**Interactions:** Interactions vary widely among products. Check individual monographs for specific information.

### NURSING CONSIDERATIONS
#### Assessment
• Obtain a diet and lifestyle history, including exercise, smoking, alcohol, and stress-related activities

#### Nursing diagnoses
• Constipation (adverse reactions)
• Diarrhea (adverse reactions)
• Knowledge, deficient (teaching)
• Noncompliance (teaching)

#### Implementation
• Give as directed by health care provider; times will vary with medication used
• Provide protection from sunlight and heat

#### Patient/family education
• Teach patient all aspects of medication use
• Instruct patient to combine medication with lifestyle changes, including low-cholesterol diet, decreasing LDL in diet; avoid smoking, alcohol, and sedentary daily routine

#### Evaluation
**Positive therapeutic outcome**
• Decrease in triglycerides and LDL cholesterol levels

### Generic Names
*HMG-CoA reductase inhibitors:*
atorvastatin
fluvastatin
lovastatin
pravastatin
rosovastatin
simvastatin

*Bile acid sequestrants:*
cholestyramine
colesevelam
colestipol

*Miscellaneous:*
ezetimibe
fenofibrate
gemfibrozil
niacin
niacinamide

 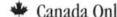

## ANTINEOPLASTICS

**Action:** Antineoplastics are divided into alkylating agents, antimetabolites, antibiotic agents, hormonal agents, and miscellaneous agents. Alkylating agents act by cross-linking strands of DNA. Antimetabolites act by inhibiting DNA synthesis. Antibiotic agents act by inhibiting RNA synthesis and by delaying or inhibiting mitosis. Hormones alter the effect of androgens, luteinizing hormone, follicle-stimulating hormone, or estrogen by changing the hormonal environment.

**Uses:** Antineoplastics vary widely among products and classes of products. They are used to treat leukemia, Hodgkin's disease, lymphomas, and other tumors throughout the body.

**Adverse effects:** Most products cause thrombocytopenia, leukopenia, and anemia. If these reactions occur, the product may need to be stopped until the problem is corrected. Other side effects include nausea, vomiting, glossitis, and hair loss. Some products also cause hepatotoxicity, nephrotoxicity, and cardiotoxicity.

**Contraindications:** Hypersensitive reactions may occur, and allergies should be identified before these products are given. Also, persons with severe renal/hepatic disease should not use these products unless the benefits outweigh the risks.

**Precautions:** Persons with bleeding, severe bone marrow depression, or renal/hepatic disease should be watched closely.

**Pharmacokinetics:** Onset, peak, and duration vary widely among products. Most products cross the placenta and are excreted in breast milk and in urine.

**Interactions:** Toxicity may occur when used with other antineoplastics or radiation.

## NURSING CONSIDERATIONS
### Assessment

• Monitor CBC, differential, platelet count weekly; withhold product if WBC is <4000 or platelet count is <75,000; notify prescriber of results
• Monitor renal function tests: BUN, creatinine, serum uric acid, and urine creatinine clearance before and during therapy
• Monitor I&O ratio; report fall in urine output of 30 ml/hr
• Monitor temp q4hr (may indicate beginning infection)

• Monitor hepatic function tests before and during therapy (bilirubin, AST, ALT, LDH) monthly or as needed
• Assess for bleeding, including hematuria, guaiac, bruising or petechiae, mucosa, or orifices q8hr; obtain prescription for viscous lidocaine (Xylocaine)
• Identify jaundice of skin, sclera, dark urine, clay-colored stools, itchy skin, abdominal pain, fever, diarrhea
• Assess for edema in feet, joint pain, stomach pain, shaking
• Assess for inflammation of mucosa, breaks in skin

### Nursing diagnoses
• Infection, risk for (adverse reactions)
• Nutrition: less than body requirements, imbalanced (adverse reactions)
• Oral mucous membrane, impaired (adverse reactions)

### Implementation
• Check **IV** site for irritation; phlebitis
• Have epINEPHrine available for hypersensitivity reaction
• Give antibiotics for prophylaxis of infection
• Provide strict medical asepsis, protective isolation if WBC levels are low
• Provide comprehensive oral hygiene, using careful technique and soft-bristle brush

### Patient/family education
• Advise patient to report signs of infection, including increased temp, sore throat, malaise
• Instruct patient to report signs of anemia, including fatigue, headache, faintness, shortness of breath, irritability
• Instruct patient to report bleeding and to avoid use of razors and commercial mouthwash

### Evaluation
**Positive therapeutic outcome**
• Decreased tumor size

### Generic Names

*Alkylating agents:*
**busulfan** (high alert)
**carboplatin** (high alert)
**carmustine** (high alert)
chlorambucil
**cisplatin** (high alert)
**cyclophosphamide** (high alert)
**dacarbazine** (high alert)
lomustine
mechlorethamine
**melphalan** (high alert)
oxaliplatin
thiotepa

Adverse effects: *italic* = common, **bold** = life-threatening

*Antimetabolites:*
capecitabine
**cytarabine** (high alert)
decitabine
**etoposide** (high alert)
fludarabine
**fluorouracil** (high alert)
mercaptopurine
pemetrexed
thioguanine (6-TG)

*Antibiotic agents:*
**bleomycin** (high alert)
**dactinomycin** (high alert)
**DAUNOrubicin** (high alert)
**DOXOrubicin** (high alert)
**epirubicin** (high alert)
**methotrexate** (high alert)
**mitomycin** (high alert)
**mitoxantrone** (high alert)

*Hormonal agents:*
flutamide
fulvestrant
goserelin
**irinotecan** (high alert)
**leuprolide** (high alert)
megestrol
mitotane
nilutamide
tamoxifen
testolactone
**topotecan** (high alert)

*Miscellaneous agents:*
alemtuzumab
altretamine
anastrozole
arsenic trioxide
**asparaginase** (high alert)
azacitidine
bortezomib
cetuximab
cladribine
dasatinib
erlotinib
gefitinib
gemcitabine
ibritumomab
imatinib
interferon alfa-2a
interferon alfa-2b
ixabepilone
lapatinib
nilotinib
panitumumab
**pentostatin** (high alert)
porfimer
procarbazine
ranibizumab

rituximab
sunitinib
**vinBLAStine** (high alert)
**vinCRIStine** (high alert)
**vinorelbine** (high alert)

## ANTIPARKINSONIAN AGENTS

**Action:** Antiparkinsonian agents are divided into cholinergics, dopamine agonists, and monoamine oxidase type B. Cholinergics work by blocking or competing at central acetylcholine receptors. Dopamine agonists work by decarboxylation to dopamine or by activation of dopamine receptors. Monoamine oxidase type B inhibitors increase dopamine activity by inhibiting MAO type B activity.

**Uses:** Antiparkinson agents are used alone or in combination for patients with Parkinson's disease.

**Adverse effects:** Side effects and adverse reactions vary widely among products. The most common side effects include involuntary movements, headache, numbness, insomnia, nightmares, nausea, vomiting, dry mouth, and orthostatic hypotension.

**Contraindications:** Persons with hypersensitivity, angle-closure glaucoma, and undiagnosed skin lesions should not use these products.

**Precautions:** Antiparkinsonian agents should be used with caution in pregnancy, breastfeeding, children, renal/cardiac/hepatic disease, and affective disorder.

**Pharmacokinetics:** Onset, peak, and duration vary widely among products. Most products are metabolized in the liver and excreted in urine.

**Interactions:** Interactions vary widely among products. Check individual monographs for specific information.

### NURSING CONSIDERATIONS
#### Assessment
- Monitor B/P, respiration
- Assess mental status: affect, behavioral changes, depression, complete suicide assessment

#### Nursing diagnoses
- Injury, risk for (uses)
- Knowledge, deficient (teaching)
- Mobility, impaired physical (uses)

#### Implementation
- Give product up until NPO before surgery
- Adjust dosage depending on patient response

- Give with meals; limit protein taken with product
- Give only after MAOIs have been discontinued for 2 wk
- Assist with ambulation, during beginning therapy if needed
- Test for diabetes mellitus and acromegaly if on long-term therapy

### Patient/family education
- Advise patient to change positions slowly to prevent orthostatic hypotension
- Instruct patient to report side effects: twitching, eye spasm; indicate overdose
- Advise patient to use product exactly as prescribed; if product is discontinued abruptly, parkinsonian crisis may occur

### Evaluation
**Positive therapeutic outcome**
- Decrease in akathisia
- Improvement in mood

---

### Generic Names
amantadine
apomorphine
benztropine
biperiden
bromocriptine
cabergoline
carbidopa-levodopa
levodopa
pramipexole
rasagiline
rotigotine
selegiline
tolcapone
trihexyphenidyl

---

## ANTIPLATELETS

**Action:** The antiplatelets are divided into the platelet aggregation inhibitors, platelet adhesion inhibitors, and the glycoprotein IIb, IIIa inhibitors. The platelet aggregation inhibitors work by action on thrombin; the platelet adhesion inhibitors work by inhibition of phosphodiesterase; and the glycoprotein IIb, IIIa inhibitors work by preventing fibrin from binding to glycoprotein IIb, IIIa receptors.

**Uses:** Antiplatelets are used to prevent myocardial infarction and stroke; other products are used for coronary syndromes.

**Adverse effects:** The most common side effects are headache, dizziness, bleeding, and diarrhea.

**Contraindications:** Persons developing hypersensitive reactions should not use these products.

**Precautions:** Antiplatelets should be used cautiously in pregnancy, breastfeeding, and bleeding disorders.

**Pharmacokinetics:** Onset, peak, and duration vary widely among products. Most products are metabolized by the liver and excreted by the kidneys.

**Interactions:** Interactions vary widely among products. Check individual monographs for specific information.

### NURSING CONSIDERATIONS
#### Assessment
- Assess reason for use of these products
- Monitor hypersensitivity reactions with some products
- Monitor bleeding from orifices, stool urine
- Monitor blood tests: platelets, Hgb, Hct, PT/APTT, and INR

#### Nursing diagnoses
- Injury, risk for, physical (uses, adverse reactions)
- Knowledge, deficient (teaching)

#### Implementation
- Give with heparin or other aspirin (some products)
- Store at room temperature vial/ampules, oral products

#### Patient/family education
- Caution patient to avoid hazardous activities if drowsiness, dizziness occurs; ask for assistance if hospitalized
- Teach patient all aspects of product usage

#### Evaluation
**Positive therapeutic outcome**
- Absence of MI, stroke, or other coronary syndromes

---

### Generic Names
*Platelet aggregation inhibitors:*
cilostazol
clopidogrel
ticlopidine

*Platelet adhesion inhibitors:*
dipyridamole

*Glycoprotein IIb, IIIa inhibitors:*
**eptifibatide** (high alert)
**tirofiban** (high alert)

## ANTIPSYCHOTICS

**Action:** Antipsychotics/neuroleptics are divided into several subgroups: phenothiazines, thioxanthenes, butyrophenones, dibenzoxazepines, dibenzodiazepines, and indolones and other heterocyclic compounds. Although chemically different, these subgroups share many pharmacologic and clinical properties. All antipsychotics work to block postsynaptic dopamine receptors in the brain that are responsible for psychotic behavior, including hallucinations, delusions, and paranoia.

**Uses:** Antipsychotic behavior is decreased in conditions such as schizophrenia, paranoia, and mania. These agents are also effective for severe anxiety, intractable hiccups, nausea, vomiting, behavioral problems in children, and for relaxation before surgery.

**Adverse effects:** The most common side effects include EPS such as pseudoparkinsonism, akathisia, dystonia, and tardive dyskinesia, which may be controlled by use of antiparkinsonian agents. Serious adverse reactions such as hypotension, agranulocytosis, cardiac arrest, and laryngospasm have occurred. Other common side effects include dry mouth and photosensitivity.

**Contraindications:** Persons with liver damage, severe hypertension or coronary disease, cerebral arteriosclerosis, blood dyscrasias, bone marrow depression, parkinsonism, severe depression, or angle-closure glaucoma, children <12 yr, or persons withdrawing from alcohol or barbiturates should not use antipsychotics until these conditions are corrected.

**Precautions:** Caution must be used when antipsychotics are given to geriatric patients, since metabolism is slowed and adverse reactions can occur rapidly. Renal/hepatic disease may cause poor metabolism and excretion of the product. Seizure threshold is decreased with these products; increases in the dose of anticonvulsants may be required. Persons with diabetes mellitus, prostatic hypertrophy, chronic respiratory disease, and peptic ulcer disease should be monitored closely.

**Pharmacokinetics:** Onset, peak, and duration vary widely with different products and routes. Products are metabolized by the liver, excreted in urine as metabolites, are highly bound to plasma proteins, cross the placenta, and enter breast milk. Half-life can be extended over 3 days.

**Interactions:** Because other CNS depressants can cause oversedation, these combinations should be used carefully. Anticholinergics may decrease the therapeutic actions of phenothiazines and also cause increased anticholinergic effects.

## NURSING CONSIDERATIONS
### Assessment
• Monitor bilirubin, CBC, hepatic function tests monthly, since these products are metabolized in the liver and excreted in urine
• Monitor I&O ratio: palpate bladder if low urinary output occurs, since urinary retention occurs with many of these products
• Assess affect, orientation, LOC, reflexes, gait, coordination, sleep pattern disturbances
• Assess dizziness, faintness, palpitations, tachycardia on rising
• Check B/P with patient lying and standing; wide fluctuations between lying and standing B/P may require dosage or product change, since orthostatic hypotension is occurring
• Assess for EPS, including akathisia, tardive dyskinesia, pseudoparkinsonism

### Nursing diagnoses
• Sensory perception, disturbed (uses)
• Thought processes, disturbed (uses)

### Implementation
• Give antiparkinsonian agent if EPS occur
• Administer liquid conc mixed in glass of juice or cola since taste is unpleasant; avoid contact with skin when preparing liquid conc or parenteral medications
• Supervise ambulation until stabilized on medication; do not involve in strenuous exercise program, since fainting is possible; patient should not stand still for long periods
• Increase fluids to prevent constipation
• Give sips of water, candy, gum for dry mouth
• Patient should remain lying down for at least 30 min after IM inj

### Patient/family education
• Advise patient to rise from sitting or lying position gradually, since fainting may occur
• Caution patient to avoid hot tubs, hot showers, or tub baths, since hypotension may occur
• Advise patient to wear sunscreen or protective clothing to prevent burns
• Advise patient to take extra precautions during hot weather to stay cool; heat stroke can occur
• Caution patient to avoid driving and other activities requiring alertness until response to medication is known

• Inform patient that drowsiness or impaired mental/motor activity is evident the first 2 wk, but tends to decrease over time

### Evaluation
**Positive therapeutic outcome**
• Decrease in excitement, hallucinations, delusions, paranoia
• Reorganization of thought patterns, speech

---

### Generic Names

*Phenothiazines:*
 chlorproMAZINE
fluphenazine
perphenazine
prochlorperazine
thioridazine
thiothixene
trifluoperazine

*Butyrophenone:*
haloperidol

*Miscellaneous:*
aripiprazole
loxapine
olanzapine
paliperidone
quetiapine
risperidone
ziprasidone

---

### NURSING CONSIDERATIONS
### Assessment
• Monitor temp frequently
• Assess reason for use and expected outcome
• Monitor hypersensitivity reactions: rash, bronchospasm with some products

### Nursing diagnoses
• Injury, risk for, physical (uses, adverse reactions)
• Knowledge, deficient (teaching)

### Implementation
• Give around the clock to keep fever reduced
• Store at room temperature

### Patient/family education
• Teach patient all aspects of product usage

### Evaluation
**Positive therapeutic outcome**
• Absence or decreasing fever after use

---

### Generic Names

acetaminophen
aspirin
choline/magnesium salicylates
choline salicylate
ibuprofen
ketoprofen
magnesium salicylate
naproxen
salsalate

---

## ANTIPYRETICS

**Action:** The antipyretics act on the CNS to control fever and also inhibit prostaglandin production.

**Uses:** Antipyretics are used to decrease fever.

**Adverse effects:** The most common side effects are nausea, vomiting, and rash.

**Contraindications:** Persons developing hypersensitive reactions should not use these products.

**Precautions:** Antipyretics should be used cautiously in pregnancy, breastfeeding, geriatric patients, hepatic disease, and those with certain GI disorders.

**Pharmacokinetics:** Onset, peak, and duration vary widely among products. Most products are metabolized by the liver and excreted by the kidneys.

**Interactions:** Interactions vary widely among products. Check individual monographs for specific information.

## ANTIRETROVIRALS

**Action:** Antiretrovirals act by blocking DNA synthesis.

**Uses:** Antiretrovirals are used in HIV infections to slow the progression of the disease.

**Adverse effects:** The most common side effects are nausea, vomiting, anorexia, headache, and diarrhea. The most serious adverse reactions are nephrotoxicity and blood dyscrasias.

**Contraindications:** Persons with hypersensitivity should not use these products.

**Precautions:** Antiretrovirals should be used cautiously in pregnancy, breastfeeding, and renal/hepatic disease. Protease inhibitors should be used cautiously in diabetes.

**Pharmacokinetics:** Onset, peak, and duration vary widely among products. Most products are metabolized by the liver and excreted by the kidneys.

---

**Interactions:** Interactions vary widely among products. Check individual monographs for specific information.

## NURSING CONSIDERATIONS
### Assessment
• Monitor for signs of HIV infection: increased CD4 counts, decreased viral load
• Monitor patients with compromised renal system; since product is excreted slowly in poor renal system function, toxicity may occur rapidly

### Nursing diagnoses
• Infection, risk for (uses)
• Injury, risk for (adverse reactions)
• Knowledge, deficient (teaching)
• Noncompliance (teaching)

### Implementation
• Give in equal intervals around the clock
• Store at room temperature

### Patient/family education
• Instruct patient to report sore throat, fever, fatigue; may indicate superinfection
• Caution patient that product does not cure condition or prevent infecting others, but controls symptoms
• Instruct patient that product must be taken around the clock, in equal intervals to maintain blood levels for duration of therapy
• Instruct patient to notify prescriber of side effects such as bruising, bleeding, fatigue, malaise; may indicate blood dyscrasias

### Evaluation
**Positive therapeutic outcome**
• Decreased viral load
• Increased CD4 count
• Improvement in the symptoms of HIV/AIDS

---

### Generic Names

*Nonnucleoside reverse transcriptase inhibitors:*
delavirdine
efavirenz
nevirapine

*Nucleoside reverse transcriptase inhibitors:*
abacavir
didanosine
emtricitabine
lamivudine
stavudine
tenofovir
zalcitabine
zidovudine

*Protease inhibitors:*
amprenavir

atazanavir
fosamprenavir
indinavir
nelfinavir
ritonavir
saquinavir
tipranavir

*Fusion inhibitors:*
enfuvirtide

*Miscellaneous:*
raltegravir

## ANTITUBERCULARS

**Action:** Antituberculars act by inhibiting RNA or DNA, or interfering with lipid and protein synthesis, thereby decreasing tubercle bacilli replication.

**Uses:** Antituberculars are used for pulmonary tuberculosis.

**Adverse effects:** They vary widely among products. Most products can cause nausea, vomiting, anorexia, and rash. Serious adverse reactions include renal failure, nephrotoxicity, ototoxicity, and hepatic necrosis.

**Contraindications:** Persons with severe renal disease or hypersensitivity should not use these products.

**Precautions:** Antituberculars should be used with caution in pregnancy, breastfeeding, and hepatic disease.

**Pharmacokinetics:** Onset, peak, and duration vary widely among products. Most products are metabolized in the liver and excreted in urine.

**Interactions:** Interactions vary widely among products. Check individual monographs for specific information.

## NURSING CONSIDERATIONS
### Assessment
• Assess for signs of anemia: Hct, Hgb, fatigue
• Monitor hepatic function tests weekly: ALT, AST, bilirubin
• Monitor renal status before treatment and monthly thereafter: BUN, creatinine, output, specific gravity, urinalysis
• Monitor hepatic status: decreased appetite, jaundice, dark urine, fatigue

### Nursing diagnoses
• Infection, risk for (uses)
• Injury, risk for (adverse reactions)
• Knowledge, deficient (teaching)
• Noncompliance (teaching)

## Implementation
- Give some of these agents on empty stomach, 1 hr before meals (only for isoniazid and rifampin) or 2 hr after meals
- Give antiemetic if vomiting occurs
- Give after C&S is completed; monthly to detect resistance

## Patient/family education
- Teach patient that compliance with dosage schedule, duration is necessary
- Teach patient that scheduled appointments must be kept; relapse may occur
- Advise patient to avoid alcohol while taking product
- Advise patient to report flulike symptoms: excessive fatigue, anorexia, vomiting, sore throat; unusual bleeding, yellowish discoloration of skin/eyes

## Evaluation
**Positive therapeutic outcome**
- Decreased symptoms of TB
- Culture negative

---

## Generic Names
ethambutol
isoniazid
pyrazinamide
rifabutin
rifampin
streptomycin

### ANTITUSSIVES/EXPECTORANTS

**Action:** Antitussives suppress the cough reflex by direct action on the cough center in the medulla. Expectorants act by liquefying and reducing the viscosity of thick, tenacious secretions.

**Uses:** Antitussives/expectorants are used to treat cough occurring in pneumonia, bronchitis, TB, cystic fibrosis, and emphysema; as an adjunct in atelectasis (expectorants); and for nonproductive cough (antitussives).

**Adverse effects:** The most common side effects are drowsiness, dizziness, and nausea.

**Contraindications:** Some products are contraindicated in pregnancy, breastfeeding, hypothyroidism, and iodine sensitivity.

**Precautions:** Some products should be used cautiously in asthma, and geriatric and debilitated patients.

**Pharmacokinetics:** Onset, peak, and duration vary widely among products. Some

products are metabolized in the liver and excreted in urine.

**Interactions:** Interactions vary widely among products. Check individual monographs for specific information.

## NURSING CONSIDERATIONS
### Assessment
- Assess cough: type, frequency, character including sputum

### Nursing diagnoses
- Airway clearance, ineffective (uses)
- Breathing pattern, ineffective (uses)
- Knowledge, deficient (teaching)

### Implementation
- Give decreased dosage to geriatric patients; their metabolism may be slowed
- Increase fluids to liquefy secretions
- Humidify patient's room

### Patient/family education
- Advise patient to avoid driving and other hazardous activities until stabilized on this medication
- Caution patient to avoid smoking, smoke-filled rooms, perfumes, dust, environmental pollutants, cleaners that increase cough

### Evaluation
**Positive therapeutic outcome**
- Absence of cough

---

## Generic Names
 acetylcysteine
benzonatate
 codeine
dextromethorphan
diphenhydrAMINE
guaifenesin
hydrocodone

### ANTIVIRALS

**Action:** Antivirals act by interfering with DNA synthesis that is needed for viral replication.

**Uses:** Antivirals are used for mucocutaneous herpes simplex virus, herpes genitalis (HSV-1, HSV-2), varicella infections, herpes zoster, and herpes simplex encephalitis.

**Adverse effects:** The most common side effects are nausea, vomiting, anorexia, headache, and diarrhea. The most serious adverse reactions are nephrotoxicity and blood dyscrasias.

**Contraindications:** Persons with hypersensitivity or immunosuppressed individuals should not use these products.

**Precautions:** Antivirals should be used cautiously in pregnancy, breastfeeding, and renal/hepatic disease.

**Pharmacokinetics:** Onset, peak, and duration vary widely among products. Most products are metabolized by the liver and excreted by the kidneys.

**Interactions:** Interactions vary widely among products. Check individual monographs for specific information.

## NURSING CONSIDERATIONS
### Assessment
• Monitor for signs of infection, anemia
• Monitor patients with a compromised renal system; since product is excreted slowly in poor renal system function, toxicity may occur rapidly
• Monitor renal function tests: urinalysis, BUN, serum creatinine or decreased CCr may indicate nephrotoxicity; I&O ratio; report hematuria, oliguria, fatigue, weakness; check for protein in the urine during treatment
• Assess C&S before treatment, agent may be taken as soon as culture is taken; repeat C&S after treatment
• Monitor bowel pattern before, during treatment; if severe abdominal pain with bleeding occurs, agent should be discontinued
• Monitor skin reactions: rash, urticaria, itching
• Monitor hepatic function tests: AST, ALT
• Monitor blood tests: WBC, RBC, Hct, Hgb, bleeding time; blood dyscrasias

### Nursing diagnoses
• Infection, risk for (uses)
• Injury, risk for (adverse reactions)
• Knowledge, deficient (teaching)

### Implementation
• Give increased fluids to 3 L/day to decrease crystalluria when given **IV**
• Store at room temperature for up to 12 hr after reconstitution

### Patient/family education
• Instruct patient to report sore throat, fever, fatigue; may indicate superinfection
• Caution patient that product does not prevent infecting others or cure condition but controls symptoms
• Instruct patient that product must be taken around the clock in equal intervals to maintain blood levels for duration of therapy
• Instruct patient to notify prescriber of side effects such as bruising, bleeding, fatigue, malaise; may indicate blood dyscrasias

### Evaluation
**Positive therapeutic outcome**
• Absence or control of infection

---

## Generic Names

 acyclovir
amantadine
cidofovir
docosanol
entecavir
famciclovir
foscarnet
ganciclovir
lamivudine
maraviroc
oseltamivir
penciclovir
ribavirin
valacyclovir
valganciclovir
zanamivir

---

### β-ADRENERGIC BLOCKERS

**Action:** β-Blockers are divided into selective and nonselective blockers. Selective β-blockers competitively block stimulation of $\beta_1$-receptors in cardiac smooth muscle; these products produce chronotropic and inotropic effects. Nonselective blockers produce a fall in blood pressure without reflex tachycardia or reduction in heart rate through a mixture of β-blocking effects; elevated plasma renins are reduced.

**Uses:** β-Blockers are used for hypertension, ventricular dysrhythmias, and prophylaxis of angina pectoris.

**Adverse effects:** The most common side effects are orthostatic hypotension, bradycardia, diarrhea, nausea, and vomiting. Serious adverse reactions include blood dyscrasias, bronchospasm, and CHF.

**Contraindications:** Hypersensitive reactions may occur, and allergies should be identified before these products are given. β-Adrenergic blockers should not be used in heart block, CHF, or cardiogenic shock.

**Precautions:** β-Blockers should be used with caution in pregnant and geriatric patients or in renal/thyroid disease, COPD, CAD, diabetes mellitus, and asthma.

**Pharmacokinetics:** Onset, peak, and duration vary widely among products. Most products are metabolized in the liver, with metabolites excreted in urine, bile, and feces.

**Interactions:** Interactions vary widely among products. Check individual monographs for specific information.

## NURSING CONSIDERATIONS
### Assessment
• Monitor renal function tests: protein, BUN, creatinine; watch for increased levels that may indicate nephrotic syndrome; obtain baselines in renal/hepatic function tests before beginning treatment
• Monitor I&O ratio, weight daily
• Monitor B/P during beginning treatment and periodically thereafter, pulse q4hr; note rate, rhythm, quality
• Monitor apical/radial pulse before administration; notify prescriber of significant changes
• Check for edema in feet and legs daily

### Nursing diagnoses
• Cardiac output, decreased (uses)
• Diarrhea (adverse reactions)
• Gas exchange, impaired (adverse reactions)
• Tissue perfusion, ineffective (uses)

### Implementation
• Give PO before meals and at bedtime; tab may be crushed or swallowed whole
• Give reduced dosage in renal dysfunction

### Patient/family education
• Instruct patient to comply with dosage schedule, even if feeling better
• Caution patient to rise slowly to sitting or standing position to minimize orthostatic hypotension
• Advise patient to report bradycardia, dizziness, confusion, depression, fever
• Teach patient to take pulse at home; advise when to notify prescriber
• Instruct patient to comply with weight control, dietary adjustment, modified exercise program
• Advise patient to wear support hose to minimize effects of orthostatic hypotension
• Advise patient not to discontinue product abruptly; taper over 2 wk; may precipitate angina

### Evaluation
**Positive therapeutic outcome**
• Decrease in B/P in hypertension
• Decreased B/P, edema, moist crackles in CHF

## Generic Names
*Selective β$_1$-receptor blockers:*
acebutolol
atenolol
esmolol
metoprolol
nebivolol

*Nonselective β$_1$ and β$_2$-blockers:*
carteolol
nadolol
pindolol
propranolol
timolol

*Combined α$_1$, β$_1$, and β$_2$-receptor blocker:*
labetalol

## BONE RESORPTION INHIBITORS

**Action:** Bone resorption inhibitors are divided into the biphosphonates and the selective estrogen receptor modulators. The biphosphonates act by absorbing calcium phosphate crystals in bone and may directly block dissolution of hydroxyapatite crystals of bone, inhibiting normal and abnormal bone resorption and mineralization. Selective estrogen receptor modulators act by reducing resorption of bone and decreasing bone turnover; medicated through estrogen receptor binding.

**Uses:** Bone resorption inhibitors are used for prevention and treatment of osteoporosis in postmenopausal women, treatment of Paget's disease, and treatment of osteoporosis in men.

**Adverse effects:** The most common side effects are nausea, vomiting, headache, bone pain, and rash.

**Contraindications:** Persons developing hypersensitive reactions or those with hypocalcemia should not use these products.

**Precautions:** Bone resorption inhibitors should be used cautiously in pregnancy, breastfeeding, the geriatric patient, renal/hepatic disease, and some GI disorders.

**Pharmacokinetics:** Onset, peak, and duration vary widely among products. Most products are taken up by the bones and excreted by the kidneys.

**Interactions:** Interactions vary widely among products. Check individual monographs for specific information.

## NURSING CONSIDERATIONS
### Assessment
- Assess reason for use and expected outcome
- Monitor bone density test; hormonal status (women) before starting treatment and thereafter
- Monitor hypercalcemia: paresthesia, twitching, laryngospasm; Chvostek's, Trousseau's signs

### Nursing diagnoses
- Injury, risk for, physical (uses, adverse reactions)
- Knowledge, deficient (teaching)

### Implementation
- Give for 6 months or more in Paget's disease
- Store at room temperature

### Patient/family education
- Instruct patient to remain upright for at least 30 min after taking to prevent esophageal irritation
- Teach patient all aspects of product usage
- Inform patient to use weight-bearing exercise to increase bone density

### Evaluation
**Positive therapeutic outcome**
- Increase in bone mass
- Absence of fractures

---

## Generic Names
*Bisphosphonates:*
alendronate
etidronate
ibandronate
pamidronate
risedronate

*Selective estrogen receptor modulators:*
raloxifene

---

## CALCIUM CHANNEL BLOCKERS

**Action:** Calcium channel blockers inhibit calcium ion influx across the cell membrane in cardiac and vascular smooth muscle. This action produces relaxation of coronary vascular smooth muscle, dilates coronary arteries, slows SA/AV node conduction, and dilates peripheral arteries.

**Uses:** Calcium channel blockers are used for chronic stable angina pectoris, vasospastic angina, dysrhythmias, hypertension, and unstable angina.

**Adverse effects:** The most common side effects are dysrhythmias and edema. Also common are headache, fatigue, drowsiness, and flushing.

**Contraindications:** Persons with 2nd- or 3rd-degree heart block, sick sinus syndrome, hypotension of <90 mm Hg systolic, Wolff-Parkinson-White syndrome, or cardiogenic shock should not use these products, since worsening of those conditions may occur.

**Precautions:** CHF may worsen since edema may be increased. Hypotension may worsen, since B/P is decreased. Patients with renal/hepatic disease should use these products cautiously since they are metabolized in the liver and excreted by the kidneys.

**Pharmacokinetics:** Onset, peak, and duration vary widely with route of administration. Products are metabolized by the liver and excreted in the urine primarily as metabolites.

**Interactions:** Increased levels of digoxin and theophylline may occur when used with these products. Increased effects of β-blockers and antihypertensives may occur with calcium channel blockers.

## NURSING CONSIDERATIONS
### Assessment
- Monitor cardiac system: B/P, pulse, respirations, ECG intervals (PR, QRS, QT)

### Nursing diagnoses
- Cardiac output, decreased (adverse reactions)
- Tissue perfusion, ineffective (uses)

### Implementation
- Give PO before meals and at bedtime

### Patient/family education
- Teach patient how to take pulse before taking product; patient should record or graph pulses to identify changes
- Advise patient to avoid hazardous activities until stabilized on this product since dizziness occurs frequently
- Inform patient of the need for compliance to all areas of medical regimen, including diet, exercise, stress reduction, and product therapy

### Evaluation
**Positive therapeutic outcome**
- Decreased anginal pain
- Decreased B/P, dysrhythmias

---

## Generic Names
amlodipine
**diltiazem** (high alert)
felodipine
isradipine

niCARdipine
NIFEdipine
 verapamil

## CARDIAC GLYCOSIDES

**Action:** Cardiac glycosides act by inhibiting sodium and potassium ATPase and then making more calcium available to activate contracted proteins. Cardiac contractility and cardiac output are increased.

**Uses:** Cardiac glycosides are used for CHF, atrial fibrillation, atrial flutter, atrial tachycardia, and rapid digitalization in these disorders.

**Adverse effects:** The most common side effects are cardiac disturbances, headache, hypotension, and GI symptoms. Also common are blurred vision and yellow-green halos.

**Contraindications:** Hypersensitive reactions may occur, and allergies should be identified before these products are given. Also, persons with ventricular tachycardia, ventricular fibrillation, and carotid sinus syndrome should not use these products.

**Precautions:** Persons with acute MI and those who have or may develop serum potassium, calcium, or magnesium imbalances should use these products cautiously. Also, geriatric patients and those with AV block, severe respiratory disease, hypothyroidism, renal/hepatic disease should exercise caution when these products are prescribed.

**Pharmacokinetics:** Onset, peak, and duration vary widely with the route of administration. Digitoxin is inactivated by the liver, and inactive metabolites are excreted in urine. Digoxin is excreted in urine mainly as the parent product and metabolites.

**Interactions:** Toxicity may occur when used with diuretics, succinylcholine, quinidine, and thioamines. Increased blood levels may occur with propantheline bromide, spironolactone, quinidine, verapamil, aminoglycosides (PO), amiodarone, anticholinergics, and quinine. Diuretics may increase toxicity.

### NURSING CONSIDERATIONS
#### Assessment
• Montior cardiac system: B/P, pulse, respirations, and increased urine output
• Monitor apical pulse for 1 min before giving product; if pulse <60, take again in 1 hr; if <60 notify prescriber
• Monitor electrolytes: potassium, sodium, chloride, calcium, magnesium; renal function

tests, including BUN and creatinine; and blood tests, including AST, ALT, bilirubin
• Monitor I&O ratio, daily weights
• Monitor therapeutic product levels

#### Nursing diagnoses
• Cardiac output, decreased (adverse reactions)
• Tissue perfusion, ineffective (uses)

#### Implementation
• Give potassium supplements if ordered for potassium levels <3

#### Patient/family education
• Teach patient how to take pulse before taking product; patient should record or graph pulse to identify changes
• Advise patient to avoid hazardous activities until stabilized on this product since dizziness occurs frequently
• Inform patient of the need for compliance to all areas of medical regimen, including diet, exercise, stress reduction, product therapy

#### Evaluation
**Positive therapeutic outcome**
• Decreased weight, edema, pulse, respiration
• Increased urine output

---

### Generic Names

 **digoxin** (high alert)

## CHOLINERGICS

**Action:** Cholinergics act by preventing destruction of acetylcholine, which increases concentration at sites where acetylcholine is released. This exaggerates the effects of acetylcholine and facilitates transmission of impulses across myoneural junction. Cholinergics may also act by stimulating receptors for acetylcholine.

**Uses:** Cholinergics are used for myasthenia gravis, as antagonists of nondepolarizing neuromuscular blockade, postoperative bladder distention and urinary distention, postoperative ileus.

**Adverse effects:** The most serious adverse reactions are respiratory depression, bronchospasm, constriction, laryngospasm, respiratory arrest, convulsions, and paralysis. The most common side effects are nausea, diarrhea, and vomiting.

**Contraindications:** Persons with obstruction of the intestine or renal system should not use these products.

**Precautions:** Caution should be used in patients with bradycardia, hypotension, seizure disorders, bronchial asthma, coronary occlusion, and hyperthyroidism, and in breastfeeding and children.

**Pharmacokinetics:** Onset, peak, and duration vary widely among products. Most products are metabolized in the liver and excreted in urine.

**Interactions:** Interactions vary widely among products. Check individual monographs for specific information.

## NURSING CONSIDERATIONS
### Assessment
• Monitor VS, respiration q8hr
• Monitor I&O ratio; check for urinary retention or incontinence
• Assess for bradycardia, hypotension, bronchospasm, headache, dizziness, seizures, respiratory depression; product should be discontinued if toxicity occurs

### Nursing diagnoses
• Breathing pattern, ineffective (uses)
• Knowledge, deficient (teaching)
• Noncompliance (teaching)
• Urinary elimination, impaired (uses)

### Implementation
• Give only with atropine sulfate available for cholinergic crisis
• Give only after all other cholinergics have been discontinued
• Give increased dosages if tolerance occurs
• Give larger doses after exercise or fatigue
• Give on empty stomach for better absorption
• Store at room temperature

### Patient/family education
• Inform patient that product is not a cure; it only relieves symptoms (myasthenia gravis)
• Advise patient to carry/wear emergency ID specifying myasthenia gravis, products taken

### Evaluation
**Positive therapeutic outcome**
• Increased muscle strength, hand grasp
• Improved muscle gait
• Absence of labored breathing (if severe)

---

### Generic Names
 bethanechol
edrophonium
neostigmine
physostigmine
pyridostigmine

## CHOLINERGIC BLOCKERS

**Action:** Cholinergic blockers inhibit or block acetylcholine at receptor sites in the autonomic nervous system.

**Uses:** Many cholinergic blockers are used to decrease secretions before surgery, to reverse neuromuscular blockade, and to decrease motility of GI, biliary, urinary tracts. Other products are used for parkinsonian symptoms, including dystonia associated with neuroleptic products.

**Adverse effects:** The most common side effects are dryness of the mouth and constipation, which can be prevented by frequent rinsing of the mouth and increasing water and bulk in the diet.

**Contraindications:** Hypersensitivity can occur, and allergies should be identified before administering these products. Persons with GI and GU obstruction should not use these products, since constipation and urinary retention may occur. They are also contraindicated in angle-closure glaucoma and myasthenia gravis.

**Precautions:** Caution must be used when these products are given to the geriatric patient, since metabolism is slowed. Also, persons with tachycardia or prostatic hypertrophy should use these products with caution.

**Pharmacokinetics:** Onset, peak, and duration vary with route.

**Interactions:** Increase in anticholinergic effect occurs when used with opioids, barbiturates, antihistamines, MAOIs, phenothiazines, amantadine.

## NURSING CONSIDERATIONS
### Assessment
• Assess I&O ratio; be alert for urinary retention, frequency, dysuria; product should be discontinued if these occur
• Assess urinary hesitancy, retention; palpate bladder if retention occurs
• Assess constipation; increase fluids, bulk, exercise
• Assess for tolerance over long-term therapy; dosage may need to be changed
• Assess mental status: affect, mood, CNS depression, worsening of mental symptoms during early therapy

### Nursing diagnoses
• Mobility, impaired physical (uses)
• Pain, chronic (uses)

---

## Implementation
• Give with food or milk to decrease GI symptoms
• Give parenteral dose with patient recumbent to prevent postural hypotension; give dose slowly, monitoring VS
• Give hard candy, gum, frequent rinsing of mouth for dryness

## Patient/family education
• Caution patient to avoid driving and other hazardous activities if drowsiness occurs
• Advise patient to avoid concurrent use of cough, cold preparations with alcohol, antihistamines unless directed by prescriber
• Caution patient to use with caution in hot weather, since medication may increase susceptibility to heat stroke

## Evaluation
**Positive therapeutic outcome**
• Absence of cramps
• Absence of EPS

## Generic Names

**atropine** (high alert)
benztropine
biperiden
glycopyrrolate
scopolamine
trihexyphenidyl

---

## CORTICOSTEROIDS

**Action:** Corticosteroids are divided into glucocorticoids and mineralocorticoids. Glucocorticoids decrease inflammation by the suppression of migration of polymorphonuclear leukocytes, fibroblasts, increased capillary permeability, and lysosomal stabilization. They also have varied metabolic effects and modify the body's immune responses to many different stimuli. Mineralocorticoids act by increasing resorption of sodium by increasing hydrogen and potassium excretion in the distal tubule.

**Uses:** Glucocorticoids are used to decrease inflammation and for immunosuppression. In addition, some products may be given for allergy, adrenal insufficiency, or cerebral edema. Mineralocorticoids are given for adrenal insufficiency or adrenogenital syndrome.

**Adverse effects:** The most common side effects include change in behavior, including insomnia and euphoria; GI irritation, including peptic ulcer; metabolic reactions, including hypokalemia, hyperglycemia, and carbohydrate intolerance; and sodium and fluid retention. Most adverse reactions are dose dependent.

**Contraindications:** Hypersensitivity may occur and should be identified before administering. Since these products mask infection, they should not be used in systemic fungal infections or amebiasis. Mothers taking pharmacologic doses of corticosteroids should not breastfeed.

**Precautions:** Caution must be used when these products are prescribed for diabetic patients since hyperglycemia may occur. Also, patients with glaucoma, seizure disorders, peptic ulcer, impaired renal function, CHF, hypertension, ulcerative colitis, or myasthenia gravis should be monitored closely if corticosteroids are given. Use with caution during pregnancy, in children, and in the geriatric patient.

**Pharmacokinetics:** For oral preparations the onset of action occurs between 1-2 hr, and duration can be up to 2 days, with a half-life of 2-4 days. Pharmacokinetics vary widely among products. These products cross the placenta and appear in breast milk.

**Interactions:** Decreased corticosteroid effect may occur with barbiturates, rifampin, and phenytoin; corticosteroid dosage may need to be increased. There is a possibility of GI bleeding when used with salicylates and indomethacin. Steroids may reduce salicylate levels. When using with digoxin glycosides, potassium-depleting diuretics, and amphotericin, serum potassium levels should be monitored.

## NURSING CONSIDERATIONS
### Assessment
• Monitor potassium, blood glucose, urine glucose while on long-term therapy; hypokalemia and hyperglycemia are common
• Monitor weight daily; notify prescriber if weekly gain of >5 lb since these products alter fluid and electrolyte balance
• Assess for potassium depletion: paresthesias, fatigue, nausea, vomiting, depression, polyuria, dysrhythmias, weakness
• Assess for mental status: affect, mood, behavioral changes, aggression; if severe personality changes occur, including depression, product may need to be tapered and then discontinued
• Monitor I&O ratio; be alert for decreasing urinary output and increasing edema
• Monitor plasma cortisol levels during long-term therapy (normal level is 138-635 nmol/L when drawn at 8 AM)

• Assess for infection: increased temp, WBC, even after withdrawal of medication; product masks symptoms of infection
• Assess for adrenal insufficiency: nausea, anorexia, fatigue, dizziness, dyspnea, weakness, joint pain

### Nursing diagnoses
• Body image, disturbed (adverse reactions)
• Infection, risk for (adverse reactions)
• Suicide, risk for (adverse reactions)

### Implementation
• Give with food or milk to decrease GI symptoms
• Give single daily or alternate-day doses in the morning before 9 AM (for replacement therapy)

### Patient/family education
• Advise patient that emergency ID as steroid user should be carried/worn
• Advise patient not to discontinue this medication abruptly; adrenal crisis can result
• Teach patient all aspects of product use, including cushingoid symptoms
• Instruct patient to take with meals or a snack
• Teach patient to avoid exposure to chickenpox or measles if taking immunosuppressives

### Evaluation
**Positive therapeutic outcome**
• Decreased inflammation

---

### Generic Names

*Glucocorticoids:*
beclomethasone
betamethasone
 cortisone
dexamethasone
hydrocortisone
methylPREDNISolone
predniSOLONE
predniSONE
triamcinolone

*Mineralocorticoid:*
fludrocortisone

---

### DIURETICS

**Action:** Diuretics are divided into subgroups: thiazides and thiazide-like diuretics, loop diuretics, carbonic anhydrase inhibitors, osmotic diuretics, and potassium-sparing diuretics. Each one of these subgroups differs in its mechanism of action. Thiazides and thiazide-like diuretics increase excretion of water and sodium by inhibiting resorption in the early distal tubule. Loop diuretics inhibit resorption of sodium and chloride in the thick ascending limb of the loop of Henle. Carbonic anhydrase inhibitors increase sodium excretion by decreasing sodium-hydrogen ion exchange throughout the renal tubule. Carbonic anhydrase inhibitors also decrease secretion of aqueous humor in the eye and thus decrease intraocular pressure. Osmotic diuretics increase the osmotic pressure of glomerular filtrate, thus decreasing net absorption of sodium. The potassium-sparing diuretics interfere with sodium resorption at the distal tubule, thus decreasing potassium excretion.

**Uses:** Blood pressure is reduced in hypertension; edema is reduced in CHF; intraocular pressure is decreased in glaucoma.

**Adverse effects:** Hypokalemia, hyperuricemia, and hyperglycemia occur most frequently with thiazide diuretics. Aplastic anemia, blood dyscrasias, volume depletion, and dehydration may occur when thiazide-like diuretics, loop diuretics, or carbonic anhydrase inhibitors are given. Side effects and adverse reactions vary widely for the miscellaneous products.

**Contraindications:** Persons with electrolyte imbalances (sodium, chloride, potassium), dehydration, or anuria should not be given these products until the problem is corrected.

**Precautions:** Caution must be used when diuretics are given to the geriatric patient, since electrolyte disturbances and dehydration can occur rapidly. Renal/hepatic disorders may cause poor metabolism and excretion of the product.

**Pharmacokinetics:** Onset, peak, and duration vary widely among the different subgroups of these products.

**Interactions:** Cholestyramine and colestipol decrease the absorption of thiazide diuretics. Concurrent use of thiazides with diazoxide may increase hyperuricemia, hyperglycemia, and antihypertensive effects of thiazides. Ototoxicity may occur when loop diuretics are used with aminoglycosides. Thiazide and loop diuretics may increase therapeutic and toxic effects of lithium.

### NURSING CONSIDERATIONS
### Assessment
• Monitor weight, I&O ratio daily to determine fluid loss; check skin turgor for dehydration
• Monitor electrolytes: potassium, sodium, chloride: include BUN, blood glucose, CBC, serum creatinine, blood pH, ABGs, uric acid, calcium; electrolyte imbalances may occur quickly

- Monitor B/P with patient lying, standing; postural hypotension may occur since fluid loss occurs from intravascular spaces first
- Assess for signs of metabolic alkalosis, including drowsiness and restlessness
- Assess for signs of hypokalemia with some products: postural hypotension, malaise, fatigue, tachycardia, leg cramps, weakness

### Nursing diagnoses
- Cardiac output, decreased (adverse reactions)
- Fluid volume, excess (uses)

### Implementation
- Give in AM to avoid interference with sleep if using product as a diuretic
- Give potassium replacement if potassium is less than 3 mg/dl

### Patient/family education
- Teach patient to take product early in the day (diuretic) to prevent nocturia

### Evaluation
**Positive therapeutic outcome**
- Improvement in edema of feet, legs, sacral area daily if medication is being used in CHF
- Improvement in B/P if medication is being used as a diuretic
- Improvement in intraocular pressure if medication is being used to decrease aqueous humor in the eye

### Generic Names

*Thiazides:*
chlorothiazide
hydrochlorothiazide

*Thiazide-like:*
chlorthalidone
indapamide
metolazone

*Loop:*
bumetanide
furosemide
torsemide

*Carbonic anhydrase inhibitors:*
acetaZOLAMIDE

*Potassium-sparing:*
amiloride
spironolactone
triamterene

*Osmotic:*
mannitol

**Action:** Histamine H₂ antagonists act by inhibiting histamine at H₂ receptor site in parietal cells, which inhibits gastric acid secretion.

**Uses:** Histamine H₂ antagonists are used for short-term treatment of duodenal and gastric ulcers and maintenance therapy for duodenal ulcer; and for gastroesophageal reflux disease.

**Adverse effects:** The most serious adverse reactions are agranulocytosis, thrombocytopenia, neutropenia, aplastic anemia, and exfoliative dermatitis. The most common side effects are confusion (not with rantidine), headache and diarrhea.

**Contraindications:** Persons with hypersensitivity should not use these products.

**Precautions:** Caution should be used in pregnancy, breastfeeding, children <16 yr, organic brain syndrome, renal/hepatic disease.

**Pharmacokinetics:** Onset, peak, and duration vary widely among products. Most products are metabolized in the liver and excreted in urine.

**Interactions:** Antacids interfere with absorption of histamine H₂ antagonists. Check individual monographs for specific information.

### NURSING CONSIDERATIONS
**Assessment**
- Monitor gastric pH (>5 should be maintained)
- Monitor I&O ratio, BUN, creatinine

### Nursing diagnoses
- Injury, risk for (bleeding)
- Knowledge, deficient (teaching)
- Pain, chronic (uses)

### Implementation
- Give with meals for prolonged product effect
- Give antacids 1 hr before or 1 hr after cimetidine
- Give **IV** slowly; bradycardia may occur; give over 30 min
- Store diluted sol at room temperature for up to 48 hr

### Patient/family education
- Advise patient that gynecomastia, impotence may occur but is reversible
- Caution patient to avoid driving and other hazardous activities until patient is stabilized on this medication
- Caution patient to avoid black pepper, caffeine, alcohol, harsh spices, extremes in temperature of food

Adverse effects: *italic* = common, **bold** = life-threatening

- Caution patient to avoid OTC preparations: aspirin, cough, cold preparations
- Inform patient that product must be continued for prescribed time to be effective
- Advise patient to report bruising, fatigue, malaise; blood dyscrasias may occur

### Evaluation
**Positive therapeutic outcome**
- Decreased pain in abdomen

---

### Generic Names
cimetidine
famotidine
ranitidine

## IMMUNOSUPPRESSANTS

**Action:** Immunosuppressants produce immunosuppression by inhibiting T lymphocytes.

**Uses:** Most immunosuppressants are used for organ transplants to prevent rejection.

**Adverse effects:** The most serious adverse reactions are albuminuria, hematuria, proteinuria, renal failure, and hepatotoxicity. The most common side effects are oral *Candida* infection, gum hyperplasia, tremors, and headache. The most serious adverse reactions for azathioprine are hematologic (leukopenia and thrombocytopenia) and GI (nausea and vomiting). There is a risk of secondary infection.

**Contraindications:** Products are contraindicated in hypersensitivity.

**Precautions:** Caution should be used in pregnancy and severe renal/hepatic disease

**Pharmacokinetics:** Onset, peak, and duration vary widely among products. Most products are metabolized in the liver and excreted in urine.

**Interactions:** Interactions vary widely among products. Check individual monographs for specific information.

### NURSING CONSIDERATIONS
**Assessment**
- Monitor renal function tests: BUN, creatinine at least monthly during treatment, 3 mo after treatment
- Monitor hepatic function tests: alkaline phosphatase, AST, ALT, bilirubin
- Monitor product blood levels during treatment

- Assess for hepatotoxicity: dark urine, jaundice, itching, light-colored stools; product should be discontinued

### Nursing diagnoses
- Infection, risk for (adverse reactions)
- Injury, risk for (uses)
- Knowledge, deficient (teaching)

### Implementation
- Give for several days before transplant surgery
- Give with meals for GI upset or place product in chocolate milk
- Give with oral antifungal for *Candida* infections

### Patient/family education
- Advise patient to report fever, chills, sore throat, fatigue since serious infections may occur
- Caution patient to use contraceptive measures during treatment and for 12 wk after ending therapy

### Evaluation
**Positive therapeutic outcome**
- Absence of rejection

---

### Generic Names
azathioprine
**basiliximab** (high alert)
cycloSPORINE
muromonab-CD3
sirolimus
tacrolimus

## LAXATIVES

**Action:** Laxatives are divided into bulk products, lubricants, osmotics, saline laxative stimulants, and stool softeners. Bulks work by absorbing water and expanding to increase moisture content and bulk in the stool. Lubricants increase water retention in the stool causing reabsorption of water in the bowel. Saline draws water into the intestinal lumen. Osmotics increase distention and promote peristalsis. Stimulants act by increasing peristalsis by direct effect on the intestine. Stool softeners reduce surface tension of liq in the bowel.

**Uses:** Laxatives are used as a preparation for bowel, rectal examination, constipation, or as stool softeners.

**Adverse effects:** The most common side effects are nausea, abdominal cramps, and diarrhea.

---

**Contraindications:** Persons with GI obstruction, perforation, gastric retention, toxic colitis, megacolon, abdominal pain, nausea, vomiting, and fecal impaction should not use these products.

**Precautions:** Caution should be used in rectal bleeding, large hemorrhoids, and anal excoriation.

**Pharmacokinetics:** Onset, peak, and duration vary among products.

**Interactions:** Interactions vary widely among products. Check individual monographs for specific information.

## NURSING CONSIDERATIONS
### Assessment
* Monitor blood, urine electrolytes if product is used often by patient
* Monitor I&O ratio to identify fluid loss
* Determine cause of constipation; identify whether fluids, bulk, or exercise is missing from lifestyle
* Assess for cramping, rectal bleeding, nausea, vomiting; if these symptoms occur, product should be discontinued

### Nursing diagnoses
* Constipation (uses)
* Diarrhea (adverse reactions)
* Knowledge, deficient (teaching)

### Implementation
* Give alone only with water for better absorption; do not take within 1 hr of antacids, milk, or cimetidine
* Swallow tab whole; do not break, crush, or chew

### Patient/family education
* Caution patient not to use laxatives for long-term therapy; bowel tone will be lost; that normal bowel movements do not always occur daily
* Caution patient not to use in presence of abdominal pain, nausea, vomiting
* Advise patient to notify prescriber of abdominal pain, nausea, vomiting
* Advise patient to notify prescriber if constipation is unrelieved or if symptoms of electrolyte imbalance occur: muscle cramps, pain, weakness, dizziness

### Evaluation
**Positive therapeutic outcome**
* Decrease in constipation

## Generic Names

*Bulk laxatives:*
calcium polycarbophil
psyllium

*Osmotic agents:*
glycerin
lactulose

*Saline laxatives:*
magnesium salts
sodium biphosphate/phosphate

*Stimulants:*
bisacodyl
cascara sagrada
senna

*Stool softeners:*
docusate

## NEUROMUSCULAR BLOCKING AGENTS

**Action:** Neuromuscular blocking agents are divided into depolarizing and nondepolarizing blockers. They act by inhibiting transmission of nerve impulses by binding with cholinergic receptor sites.

**Uses:** Neuromuscular blocking agents are used to facilitate endotracheal intubation and skeletal muscle relaxation during mechanical ventilation, surgery, or general anesthesia.

**Adverse effects:** The most serious adverse reactions are prolonged apnea, bronchospasm, cyanosis, respiratory depression, and malignant hyperthermia. The most common side effects are bradycardia and decreased motility.

**Contraindications:** Persons who are hypersensitive should not be given this product.

**Precautions:** Caution should be used in pregnancy, breastfeeding, children <2 yr, thyroid disease, collagen disease, cardiac disease, electrolyte imbalances, dehydration, neuromuscular disease (myasthenia gravis), and respiratory disease.

**Pharmacokinetics:** Onset, peak, and duration vary widely among products. Most products are metabolized in the liver and excreted in urine.

**Interactions:** Aminoglycosides potentiate neuromuscular blockade. Check individual monographs for specific information.

Adverse effects: *italic* = common, **bold** = life-threatening

## NURSING CONSIDERATIONS
### Assessment
- Monitor for electrolyte imbalances (potassium, magnesium); may lead to increased action of this product
- Monitor VS (B/P, pulse, respirations, airway) q15 min until fully recovered; rate, depth, pattern of respirations, strength of hand grip
- Monitor I&O ratio; check for urinary retention, frequency, hesitancy
- Assess for recovery: decreased paralysis of face, diaphragm, leg, arm, rest of body
- Assess for allergic reactions: rash, fever, respiratory distress, pruritus; product should be discontinued

### Nursing diagnoses
- Breathing pattern, ineffective (uses)
- Injury, risk for (adverse reactions)
- Knowledge, deficient (teaching)

### Implementation
- Administer using nerve stimulator by anesthesiologist to determine neuromuscular blockade
- Administer anticholinesterase to reverse neuromuscular blockade
- Give **IV** undiluted over 1-2 min (only by qualified person, usually an anesthesiologist)
- Store in light-resistant, cool area
- Reassure if communication is difficult during recovery from neuromuscular blockade

### Evaluation
**Positive therapeutic outcome**
- Paralysis of jaw, eyelid, head, neck, rest of body

---

### Generic Names
atracurium
doxacurium
gallamine
**pancuronium** (high alert)
**succinylcholine** (high alert)
**tubocurarine** (high alert)
**vecuronium** (high alert)

---

## NONSTEROIDAL ANTIINFLAMMATORIES

**Action:** Nonsteroidal antiinflammatories decrease prostaglandin synthesis by inhibiting an enzyme needed for biosynthesis.

**Uses:** Nonsteroidal antiinflammatories are used to treat mild to moderate pain, osteoarthritis, rheumatoid arthritis, and dysmenorrhea.

**Adverse effects:** The most serious adverse reactions are nephrotoxicity (dysuria, hematuria, oliguria, azotemia), blood dyscrasias, and cholestatic hepatitis. The most common side effects are nausea, abdominal pain, anorexia, dizziness, and drowsiness.

**Contraindications:** Persons with hypersensitivity, asthma, severe renal/hepatic disease should not use these products.

**Precautions:** Caution should be used in pregnancy, breastfeeding, children, geriatric patients, bleeding/GI/cardiac disorders, and hypersensitivity to other antiinflammatory agents.

**Pharmacokinetics:** Onset, peak, and duration vary widely among products. Most products are metabolized in the liver and excreted in urine.

**Interactions:** Interactions vary widely among products. Check individual monographs for specific information.

## NURSING CONSIDERATIONS
### Assessment
- Monitor renal, hepatic, blood tests: BUN, creatinine, AST, ALT, Hgb, before treatment, periodically thereafter
- Monitor audiometric, ophth examination before, during, and after treatment.
- Check for eye, ear problems: blurred vision, tinnitus, may indicate toxicity

### Nursing diagnoses
- Knowledge, deficient (teaching)
- Mobility, impaired physical (uses)
- Noncompliance (teaching)
- Pain, chronic (uses)

### Implementation
- Give with food to decrease GI symptoms; however, best to take on empty stomach to facilitate absorption
- Store at room temperature

### Patient/family education
- Advise patient to report blurred vision, ringing, roaring in ears; may indicate toxicity
- Caution patient to avoid driving, other hazardous activities if dizziness, drowsiness occurs, especially in geriatric patients
- Advise patient to report change in urine pattern, increased weight, edema, increased pain in joints, fever, blood in urine; indicate nephrotoxicity
- Inform patient that therapeutic effects may take up to 1 mo

---

## Evaluation
### Positive therapeutic outcome
- Decreased pain, stiffness in joints
- Decreased swelling in joints
- Ability to move more easily

## Generic Names

celecoxib
diclofenac
etodolac
fenoprofen
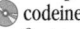 ibuprofen
indomethacin
ketoprofen
ketorolac
nabumetone
naproxen
piroxicam
sulindac

## OPIOID ANALGESICS

**Action:** These agents depress pain impulse transmission at the spinal cord level by interacting with opioid receptors. Products are divided into opiates and nonopiates.

**Uses:** Most opioid analgesics are used to control moderate to severe pain and are used before and after surgery.

**Adverse effects:** GI symptoms, including nausea, vomiting, anorexia, constipation, and cramps are the most common side effects. Other common side effects include light-headedness, dizziness, and sedation. Serious adverse reactions such as respiratory depression, respiratory arrest, circulatory depression, and increased ICP may result, but are less common and usually dose dependent.

**Contraindications:** Hypersensitive reactions occur frequently. Check for sensitivity before administering. These products should not be used if opioid addiction is suspected, and they are also contraindicated in acute bronchial asthma and upper airway obstruction.

**Precautions:** Caution must be used when these products are given to persons with an addictive personality, since the possibility of addiction is so great. Also, persons with increased ICP may experience an even greater increase in ICP. Persons with severe heart disease, renal/hepatic disease, respiratory conditions, and seizure disorders should be monitored closely for worsening condition.

**Pharmacokinetics:** Onset of action is immediate by **IV** route and rapid by IM and PO routes. Peak occurs from 1-2 hr, depending on route, with a duration of 2-8 hr. These agents cross the placenta and appear in breast milk.

**Interactions:** Barbiturates, other opioids, hypnotics, antipsychotics, or alcohol can increase CNS depression when taken with opioids.

## NURSING CONSIDERATIONS
### Assessment
- Monitor I&O ratio; be alert for urinary retention, frequency, dysuria; product should be discontinued if these occur
- Assess for respiratory dysfunction: respiratory depression, rate, rhythm, character; notify prescriber if respirations are <12/min
- Assess for CNS changes: dizziness, drowsiness, hallucinations, euphoria, LOC, pupil reaction
- Assess for allergic reactions: rash, urticaria
- Assess for need for pain medication, use pain scoring

### Nursing diagnoses
- Gas exchange, impaired (adverse reactions)
- Pain, acute (uses)

### Implementation
- Give with antiemetic if nausea or vomiting occurs
- Give when pain is beginning to return; determine dosage interval by patient response
- Provide assistance with ambulation; patient should not be ambulating during product peak

### Patient/family education
- Advise patient to report any symptoms of CNS changes, allergic reactions, or shortness of breath
- Caution patient that physical dependency may result when used for extended periods
- Teach patient that withdrawal symptoms may occur, including nausea, vomiting, cramps, fever, faintness, anorexia
- Advise patient to avoid alcohol and other CNS depressants

### Evaluation
#### Positive therapeutic outcome
- Decrease in pain

## Generic Names

alfentanil
buprenorphine
butorphanol
codeine
**fentanyl** (high alert)

Adverse effects: *italic* = common, **bold** = life-threatening

fentanyl transdermal
**hydromorphone** (high alert)
 **meperidine** (high alert)
**methadone** (high alert)
 **morphine** (high alert)
nalbuphine
**oxycodone** (high alert)
**oxymorphone** (high alert)
**pentazocine** (high alert)
**propoxyphene** (high alert)
**remifentanil** (high alert)

## SALICYLATES

**Action:** Salicylates have analgesic, antipyretic, and antiinflammatory effects. The analgesic and antiinflammatory activities may be mediated through the inhibition of prostaglandin synthesis. Antipyretic action results from inhibition of the hypothalamic heat-regulating center.

**Uses:** The primary uses of salicylates are relief of mild to moderate pain and fever and in inflammatory conditions such as arthritis, thromboembolic disorders, and rheumatic fever.

**Adverse effects:** The most common side effects are GI symptoms and rash. Serious blood dyscrasias and hepatotoxicity may result when used for long periods at high doses. Tinnitus or impaired hearing may indicate that blood salicylate levels are reaching or exceeding the upper limit of the therapeutic range.

**Contraindications:** Hypersensitivity to salicylates is common. Check for sensitivity before administering. Persons with bleeding disorders, GI bleeding, and vit K deficiency should not use these products since salicylates increase pro-time. Children should not use these products since salicylates have been associated with Reye's syndrome.

**Precautions:** Caution is needed when salicylates are given to patients with anemia, renal/hepatic disease, and Hodgkin's disease. Caution should also be exercised in pregnancy and breastfeeding.

**Pharmacokinetics:** Onset of action occurs in 15-30 min, with a peak of 1-2 hr and a duration up to 6 hr. These products are metabolized by the liver and excreted by the kidneys.

**Interactions:** Increased effects of anticoagulants, insulin, methotrexate, heparin, valproic acid, and oral sulfonylureas may occur when used with salicylates. Aspirin may decrease serum concentrations of nonsteroidal antiinflammatory agents.

## NURSING CONSIDERATIONS
### Assessment
• Monitor renal/hepatic function tests: AST, ALT, bilirubin, creatinine, LDH, alkaline phosphatase, BUN if patient is on long-term therapy since these products are metabolized and excreted by the liver and kidney
• Monitor blood tests: CBC, Hct, Hgb, and pro-time if patient is on long-term therapy, since these products increase the possibility of bleeding and blood dyscrasias
• Assess for hepatotoxicity: dark urine, clay-colored stools, jaundiced skin and sclera, itching, abdominal pain, fever, diarrhea, which may occur with long-term use
• Assess for ototoxicity: tinnitus, ringing, roaring in ears; audiometric testing is needed before and after long-term therapy

### Nursing diagnoses
• Activity intolerance (uses)
• Mobility, impaired physical (uses)
• Pain, acute (uses)
• Pain, chronic (uses)
• Sensory perception, disturbed (adverse reactions)
• Thermoregulation, ineffective (uses)

### Implementation
• Give with food or milk to decrease gastric irritation; give 30 min before or 1 hr after meals with a full glass of water

### Patient/family education
• Advise patient that blood sugar levels should be monitored closely, if patient is diabetic
• Caution patient not to exceed recommended dosage; acute poisoning may result
• Inform patient that therapeutic response takes 2 wk in arthritis
• Caution patient to avoid use of alcohol since GI bleeding may result
• Advise patient to notify prescriber if ringing in the ears or persistent GI pain occurs
• Advise patient to take with full glass of water to reduce risk of lodging in esophagus

### Evaluation
**Positive therapeutic outcome**
• Decreased pain, fever

---

### Generic Names
 aspirin
choline salicylate
magnesium salicylate
salsalate

## SEDATIVES/HYPNOTICS

**Action:** The sedatives/hypnotics depress the CNS; some products at the cerebral cortex, others inhibit transmitters in the CNS.

**Uses:** Sedatives/hypnotics are used for the treatment of sleep disorders, seizures, muscle spasms, and alcohol withdrawal.

**Adverse effects:** The most common side effects are nausea and drowsiness. The most serious side effects are Stevens-Johnson syndrome, blood dyscrasias, and risk of dependency.

**Contraindications:** Persons with hypersensitivity reactions should not use these products.

**Precautions:** Sedatives/hypnotics should be used cautiously in pregnancy **(C)** and breastfeeding.

**Pharmacokinetics:** Onset, peak, and duration vary widely among products. Most products are metabolized in the liver and excreted by the kidneys.

**Interactions:** Increased CNS depression may occur with other CNS depressants such as alcohol, opiates, antipsychotics, and antidepressants.

### NURSING CONSIDERATIONS
**Assessment**
- Monitor mental status: affect, mood, behavioral changes, depression, confusion; seizure activity

**Nursing diagnoses**
- Knowledge, deficient (teaching)
- Noncompliance (teaching)
- Sleep deprivation (uses)

**Implementation**
- Give lowest possible dose for therapeutic result; adjust dose to response
- Provide assistance with ambulation during beginning therapy if dizziness, ataxia occur

**Patient/family education**
- Inform patient that these products should only be used for short-term insomnia
- Caution patient not to drive or engage in other hazardous activities while taking these products
- Instruct patient to avoid breastfeeding while taking these products
- Instruct patient to avoid alcohol or other CNS depressants as drowsiness will increase
- Teach patient that some of the products take two nights to be effective

- Advise patient to report side effects, adverse reactions to health care provider
- Instruct patient to use exactly as prescribed, at regular intervals

**Evaluation**
**Positive therapeutic outcome**
- Ability to sleep throughout the night
- Absence or decreasing seizure activity

### Generic Names
*Barbiturates:*
**phenobarbital** (high alert)

*Benzodiazepines:*
chlordiazepoxide
clorazepate
diazepam
flurazepam
lorazepam
midazolam
oxazepam
temazepam
triazolam

*Miscellaneous products:*
chloral hydrate
dexmedetomidine
**droperidol** (high alert)
eszopiclone
hydrOXYzine
promethazine
ramelteon
zaleplon
zolpidem

## SKELETAL MUSCLE RELAXANTS

**Action:** Most skeletal muscle relaxants inhibit synaptic responses in the CNS by stimulating receptors and decreasing neurotransmission, decreasing pain and spasticity.

**Uses:** Skeletal muscle relaxants are used for musculoskeletal disorders with pain or spasticity related to spinal cord injuries.

**Adverse effects:** The most common side effects are dizziness, weakness, fatigue, drowsiness, and headache. Some products can cause seizures, cardiovascular collapse and severe CNS depression.

**Contraindications:** Persons with hypersensitivity should not use these products.

**Precautions:** Skeletal muscle relaxants should be used cautiously in pregnancy **(C)**, breastfeeding, the geriatric patient, peptic ulcer,

Adverse effects: *italic* = common, **bold** = life-threatening

renal/hepatic disease, stroke, seizure disorder, and diabetes.

**Pharmacokinetics:** Pharmacokinetics vary widely among products. Check individual monographs for specific information.

**Interactions:** CNS depressants used with skeletal muscle relaxants may lead to increased CNS depression.

## NURSING CONSIDERATIONS
### Assessment
• Monitor pain: character, location, duration, alleviating/aggravating factors

### Nursing diagnoses
• Injury, risk for (adverse reactions)
• Knowledge, deficient (teaching)
• Mobility, impaired physical (uses)
• Pain, acute (uses)
• Pain, chronic (uses)

### Implementation
• Give when pain is beginning to return, not after pain is severe
• Store in dry area, away from heat and sunlight

### Patient/family education
• Advise patient not to use with other CNS depressant unless prescriber approved
• Inform patient that many products require 1-2 mo of treatment for full effect
• Caution patient to avoid hazardous activities until response to medication is known
• Caution patient that most products should not be discontinued quickly, but tapered over 1-2 wk

### Evaluation
**Positive therapeutic outcome**
• Decrease in pain or spasticity

## Generic Names

*Centrally acting:*
baclofen
carisoprodol
chlorzoxazone
cyclobenzaprine
diazepam
metaxalone
methocarbamol
orphenadrine

*Direct-acting:*
dantrolene

## THROMBOLYTICS

**Action:** Thrombolytics activate conversion of plasminogen to plasmin (fibrinolysin). Plasmin is able to break down clots (fibrin).

**Uses:** Thrombolytics are used to treat DVT, PE, arterial thrombosis, arterial embolism, arteriovenous cannula occlusion, lysis of coronary artery thrombi after MI, acute evolving transmural MI.

**Adverse effects:** Serious adverse reactions include GI, GU, intracranial, and retroperitoneal bleeding, and anaphylaxis. The most common side effects are decreased Hct, urticaria, headache, and nausea.

**Contraindications:** Persons with hypersensitivity, active bleeding, intraspinal surgery, neoplasms of the CNS, ulcerative colitis/enteritis, severe hypertension, renal/hepatic disease, hypocoagulation, COPD, subacute bacterial endocarditis, rheumatic valvular disease, cerebral embolism/thrombosis/hemorrhage, intraarterial diagnostic procedure or surgery (10 days), and recent major surgery should not use these products.

**Precautions:** Caution should be used in arterial emboli from left side of heart and pregnancy.

**Pharmacokinetics:** Onset, peak, and duration vary widely among products. Most products are metabolized in the liver and excreted in urine.

**Interactions:** Interactions vary widely among products. Check individual monographs for specific information.

## NURSING CONSIDERATIONS
### Assessment
• Monitor VS, B/P, pulse, respirations, neurologic signs, temp at least q4hr, temp is an indicator of internal bleeding, cardiac rhythm following intracoronary administration; systolic pressure increase of >25 mm Hg should be reported to prescriber
• Assess for neurologic changes that may indicate intracranial bleeding
• Assess retroperitoneal bleeding: back pain, leg weakness, diminished pulses
• Assess for allergy: fever, rash, itching, chills; mild reaction may be treated with antihistamines
• Assess for bleeding during 1st hr of treatment: hematuria, hematemesis, bleeding from mucous membranes, epistaxis, ecchymosis
• Monitor blood tests (Hct, platelets, PTT, PT, TT, APTT) before starting therapy; PT or APTT

must be less than 2 times control before starting therapy TT or PT q3-4hr during treatment

## Nursing diagnoses
• Injury, risk for (uses)

## Implementation
• Administer as soon as thrombi identified; not useful for thrombi over 1 wk old
• Administer cryoprecipitate or fresh, frozen plasma if bleeding occurs
• Give loading dose at beginning of therapy; may require increased loading doses
• Give heparin after fibrinogen level is over 100 mg/dl; heparin inf to increase PTT to 1.5-2 times baseline for 3-7 days
• About 10% of patients have high streptococcal antibody titers requiring increased loading doses
• Give **IV** therapy using 0.8-μm filter
• Store reconstituted sol in refrigerator; discard after 24 hr
• Provide bed rest during entire course of treatment

## Patient/family education
• Teach patient to avoid venous or arterial puncture, injection, rectal temp
• Teach patient to treat fever with acetaminophen or aspirin
• Teach patient to apply pressure for 30 sec to minor bleeding sites; inform prescriber if this does not attain hemostasis; apply pressure dressing

## Evaluation
**Positive therapeutic outcome**
• Resolution of thrombosis, embolism

## Generic Names
alteplase (high alert)
anistreplase (high alert)
drotrecogin alfa
streptokinase (high alert)
tenecteplase (high alert)
urokinase (high alert)

## THYROID HORMONES

**Action:** Thyroid hormones increase metabolic rates resulting in increased cardiac output, $O_2$ consumption, body temp, blood volume, growth, development at cellular level, respiratory rate, and enzyme system activity

**Uses:** Thyroid hormones are used for thyroid replacement.

**Adverse effects:** The most common side effects include insomnia, tremors, tachycardia, palpitations, angina, dysrhythmias, weight loss, and changes in appetite. Serious adverse reactions include thyroid storm.

**Contraindications:** Persons with adrenal insufficiency, myocardial infarction, or thyrotoxicosis should not use these products.

**Precautions:** Caution should be used in pregnancy and breastfeeding. Geriatric patients and those with angina pectoris, hypertension, ischemia, cardiac disease, or diabetes mellitus or insipidus should be watched closely when using these products.

**Pharmacokinetics:** Pharmacokinetics vary widely among products. Check individual monographs for specific information.

## Interactions
• Impaired absorption of thyroid products may occur when administered with cholestyramine (separate by 4-5 hr)
• Increased effects of anticoagulants, sympathomimetics, tricyclics, catecholamines may occur
• Decreased effects of digoxin, glycosides, insulin, hypoglycemics may occur
• Decreased effects of thyroid products may occur with estrogens

## NURSING CONSIDERATIONS
### Assessment
• Monitor B/P, pulse before each dose
• Monitor I&O ratio
• Monitor weight daily in same clothing, using same scale, at same time of day
• Monitor height, growth rate if given to a child
• Monitor $T_3$, $T_4$, which are decreased; radioimmunoassay of TSH, which is increased; ratio uptake, which is decreased if patient is on too low a dosage of medication
• Assess for increased nervousness, excitability, irritability; may indicate too high a dosage of medication usually after 1-3 wk of treatment
• Assess for cardiac status: angina, palpitation, chest pain, change in VS

## Nursing diagnoses
• Body image, disturbed (adverse reactions)
• Knowledge, deficient (teaching)
• Noncompliance (teaching)

## Implementation
• Give at same time each day to maintain product level
• Give only for hormone imbalances; not to be used for obesity, male infertility, menstrual conditions, lethargy
• Remove medication 4 wk before RAIU test

Adverse effects: *italic* = common, **bold** = life-threatening

## Patient/family education

• Advise patient that hair loss will occur in children and is temporary
• Advise patient to report excitability, irritability, anxiety; indicates overdose
• Caution patient not to switch brands unless directed by prescriber
• Caution patient that hypothyroid children will show almost immediate behavior/personality change
• Advise patient that treatment product is not to be taken to reduce weight
• Advise patient to avoid OTC preparations with iodine; read labels; to avoid iodine-containing foods: iodized salt, soybeans, tofu, turnips, some seafood, some bread

## Evaluation

**Positive therapeutic outcome**

• Absence of depression
• Increased weight loss, diuresis, pulse, appetite
• Absence of constipation, peripheral edema, cold intolerance, pale, cool, dry skin, brittle nails, alopecia, coarse hair, menorrhagia, night blindness, paresthesias, syncope, stupor, coma, rosy cheeks

## Generic Names

 levothyroxine (T$_4$)
liothyronine (T$_3$)
liotrix
thyroid USP

## VASODILATORS

**Action:** Vasodilators act in various ways. Check individual monographs for specific action.

**Uses:** Vasodilators are used to treat intermittent claudication, arteriosclerosis obliterans, vasospasm and muscular ischemia, ischemic cerebral vascular disease, hypertension, and angina.

**Adverse effects:** The most common side effects are headache, nausea, hypotension, hypertension, and ECG changes.

**Contraindications:** Some products are contraindicated in acute MI, paroxysmal tachycardia, and thyrotoxicosis.

**Precautions:** Caution should be used in uncompensated heart disease or peptic ulcer disease.

**Pharmacokinetics:** Onset, peak, and duration vary widely among products. Most products are metabolized in the liver and excreted in urine.

**Interactions:** Interactions vary widely among products. Check individual monographs for specific information.

## NURSING CONSIDERATIONS
### Assessment

• Assess bleeding time in individuals with bleeding disorders
• Assess cardiac status: B/P, pulse, rate, rhythm, character; watch for increasing pulse

### Nursing diagnoses

• Cardiac output, decreased (uses)
• Knowledge, deficient (teaching)
• Tissue perfusion, ineffective (uses)

### Implementation

• Give with meals to reduce GI symptoms
• Store in tight container at room temperature

### Patient/family education

• Inform patient that medication is not cure, may need to be taken continuously
• Advise patient that it is necessary to quit smoking to prevent excessive vasoconstriction
• Advise patient that improvement may be sudden, but usually occurs gradually over several weeks
• Instruct patient to report headache, weakness, increased pulse, since product may need to be decreased or discontinued
• Instruct patient to avoid hazardous activities until stabilized on medication; dizziness may occur

### Evaluation

**Positive therapeutic outcome**

• Ability to walk without pain
• Increased temp in extremities
• Increased pulse volume

## Generic Names

amyl nitrite
bosentan
dipyridamole
hydrALAZINE
midodrine
minoxidil
nesiritide
papaverine

## VITAMINS

**Action:** The action of vitamins varies widely among products and classes. Check individual monographs for specific action.

**Uses:** Vitamins are used to correct and prevent vitamin deficiencies.

**Adverse effects:** There is an absence of side effects or adverse reactions with the water-soluble vitamins (C, B). However, fat-soluble vitamins (A, D, E, K) may accumulate in the body and cause adverse reactions (refer to individual monographs).

**Contraindications:** Hypersensitive reactions may occur, and allergies should be identified before these products are given.

**Pharmacokinetics:** Onset, peak, and duration vary widely among products. Check individual monographs for specific information.

### NURSING CONSIDERATIONS
**Nursing diagnoses**
• Nutrition: less than body requirements, imbalanced (uses)

### Implementation
• Give PO with food for better absorption
• Store in tight, light-resistant container

### Patient/family education
• Advise patient not to take more than prescribed amount

### Evaluation
**Positive therapeutic outcome**
• Absence of vitamin deficiency

### Generic Names

*Fat-soluble:*
phytonadione (vitamin $K_1$)
vitamin A
vitamin D
vitamin E

*Water-soluble:*
ascorbic acid (C)
pyridoxine ($B_6$)
riboflavin ($B_2$)
thiamine ($B_1$)

*Miscellaneous:*
multivitamins

## Appendix A

### Selected New Drugs

---

### aliskiren (Rx)
(a-lis'kir-en)
Tekturna
*Func. class.:* Antihypertensive
*Chem. class.:* Direct renin inhibitor

**Pregnancy category**
C (1st trimester)
D (2nd/3rd trimesters)

**Action:** Renin inhibitor that acts on the renin-angiotensin system (RAS)

**Therapeutic outcome:** Decrease in B/P

**Uses:** Hypertension, alone or in combination with other antihypertensives

**Dosage and routes**
*Adult:* PO 150 mg/day, may increase to 300 mg/day if needed, max 300 mg/day

**Available forms:** Tabs 150, 300 mg

**Adverse effects**
*CNS:* Headache, dizziness
*CV:* Orthostatic hypotension, hypotension
*GI:* Diarrhea
*GU:* Renal stones, increased uric acid
*INTEG:* Rash
*META:* Hyperkalemia
*MISC:* Angioedema

**Contraindications:** Pregnancy **D** (2nd/3rd trimester), hypersensitivity

**Precautions:** Pregnancy **C** (1st trimester), breastfeeding, children, geriatric, angioedema, aortic/renal artery stenosis, cirrhosis, CAD, dialysis, hyper/hypokalemia, hyponatremia, hypotension, hypovolemia, renal/hepatic disease, surgery

| Pharmacokinetics | |
|---|---|
| **Absorption** | Poorly, bioavailability 2.3% |
| **Distribution** | Steady state 7-8 days |
| **Metabolism** | Unknown |
| **Excretion** | 91% unchanged in the feces |
| **Half-life** | Unknown |

| Pharmacodynamics | |
|---|---|
| **Onset** | Unknown |
| **Peak** | 1-3 hr |
| **Duration** | Unknown |

**Interactions**
*Individual drugs*
Atorvastatin, ketoconazole: increased aliskiren levels
Warfarin: decreased levels of warfarin
*Drug classifications*
ACE inhibitors, angiotensin receptor antagonists: increased potassium levels
Diuretics, other antihypertensives: increased hypotension
*Drug/food*
High-fat meal: decreased absorption
*Drug/lab test*
Increased: uric acid, CPK, BUN, serum creatinine
Decreased: Hct, Hgb

**NURSING CONSIDERATIONS**
**Assessment**
• Monitor blood tests: CBC with differential; Hct, Hgb may be decreased; uric acid, serum creatinine, BUN may be increased; potassium, hyperkalemia may occur
• Assess for allergic reactions: angioedema may occur
• Monitor daily dependent edema in feet, legs; weight, B/P, orthostatic hypotension

**Nursing diagnoses**
• Cardiac output, decreased (uses)
• Knowledge, deficient (teaching)
• Noncompliance (teaching)

**Implementation**
• PO; do not use with a high-fat meal
• Give daily with a full glass of water
• Do not discontinue abruptly
• Store in tight container at room temperature

**Patient/family education**
• Teach patient the importance of complying with dosage schedule even if feeling better
• Instruct patient to notify if pregnancy is planned or suspected; if pregnant, product will need to be discontinued
• Teach patient how to take B/P and normal reading for age-group
• Advise patient that if dose is missed, take as soon as possible; if it is almost time for the next dose, take only that dose; do not double dose

---

 Alert     Canada Only     Drug on CD    * "Tall Man" lettering (See Preface)

- Instruct patient not to use OTC products, including herbs, supplements unless approved by prescriber
- Advise patient to report to prescriber immediately: dizziness, faintness, chest pain, palpitations, uneven or rapid heart beat, headache, severe diarrhea, swelling of tongue or lips, trouble breathing, difficulty swallowing, tightening of the throat
- Caution patient not to operate machinery or perform hazardous tasks if dizziness occurs
- Advise patient to avoid faintness; do not get up or stand up rapidly

## Evaluation
**Positive therapeutic outcome**
- Decrease in B/P

---

## ambrisentan (Rx)
(am-bri-sen'tan)
Letairis
*Func. class.:* Antihypertensive
*Chem class.:* Vasodilator/endothelin receptor antagonist

**Pregnancy category X**

**Action:** Endothelin-1 receptor antagonist; endothelin-1 is vasoconstrictor

**Therapeutic outcome:** Decreased shortness of breath, dizziness

**Uses:** Pulmonary arterial hypertension, alone or in combination with other antihypertensives

**Dosage and routes**
*Adult:* PO 5 mg/day; may increase to 10 mg if needed

**Available forms:** Tabs 5, 10 mg

**Adverse effects**
*CNS:* Headache, fever, flushing
*CV:* Orthostatic hypotension, hypotension, peripheral edema
*EENT:* Sinusitis, rhinitis
*GI:* Abdominal pain, constipation
*HEMA:* Anemia
*INTEG:* Rash
*RESP:* Pharyngitis, dyspnea

**Contraindications:** Pregnancy **X**, breast-feeding, hypersensitivity

**Precautions:** Children, women, geriatric, hepatitis, hepatic disease, anemia, heart failure, jaundice, peripheral edema

### Pharmacokinetics
| | |
|---|---|
| **Absorption** | Rapidly |
| **Distribution** | Protein binding 99% |
| **Metabolism** | By CYP3A4, CYP2C19 |
| **Excretion** | Unknown |
| **Half-life** | Terminal 15 hr |

### Pharmacodynamics
| | |
|---|---|
| **Onset** | Unknown |
| **Peak** | 2 hr |
| **Duration** | Unknown |

## Interactions
### Individual drugs
Cimetidine, clopidogrel, efavirenz, felbamate, fluoxetine, modafinil, omeprazole, oxcarbazepine, ticlopidine: possibly increased ambrisentan
CycloSPORINE: avoid concurrent use
Fosphenytoin, griseofulvin, nevirapine, phenytoin, rifabutin, rifampin, rifapentine: need for ambrisentan dosage change
Mefloquine, nicardipine, propafenone, quinidine, ranolazine, tacrolimus, testosterone: decreased ambrisentan absorption
### Drug classifications
Antihypertensives (other), diuretics, MAOIs: increased hypotension
Barbiturates: need for ambrisentan dosage change
CYP3A4 inhibitors (amprenavir, aprepitant, atazanavir, clarithromycin, conivaptan, dalfopristin, danazol, darunavir, erythromycin, estradiol, imatinib, itraconazole, ketoconazole, nefazodone, nelfinavir, propoxyphene, quinupristin, ritonavir, RU-486, saquinavir, tamoxifen, telithromycin, troleandomycin, zafirlukast), CYP2C19/CYP3A4 (chloramphenicol, delavirdine, fluconazole, fluvoxamine, isoniazid, voriconazole): increased ambrisentan
### Drug/herb
St. John's wort: need for ambrisentan dosage change
### Drug/food
Grapefruit products: avoid use
### Drug/lab test
Decreased: Hct, Hgb

## NURSING CONSIDERATIONS
### Assessment
- Monitor blood tests: CBC with differential; Hct, Hgb may be decreased
- Monitor daily edema in feet, legs; weight, B/P, orthostatic hypotension

---

Adverse effects: *italic* = common, **bold** = life-threatening

• Monitor hepatic function tests: AST, ALT, bilirubin
• Assess pregnancy status before giving this product; pregnancy category **X**

## Nursing diagnoses
• Activity intolerance (uses)
• Breathing pattern, ineffective (uses)
• Knowledge, deficient (teaching)

## Implementation
• Do not break, crush, or chew tabs
• Give daily with a full glass of water without regard to food
• Do not discontinue abruptly
• Only those facilities enrolled in the LEAP program may administer this product
• Store in tight container at room temperature

## Patient/family education
• Teach patient the importance of complying with dosage schedule even if feeling better
• Instruct patient to notify if pregnancy is planned or suspected; if pregnant, product will need to be discontinued
• Advise patient that if a dose is missed, take as soon as possible; if it is almost time for the next dose, take only that dose; do not double dose
• Instruct patient not to use OTC products, including herbs, supplements unless approved by prescriber
• Advise patient to report to prescriber immediately: dizziness, faintness, chest pain, palpitations, uneven or rapid heart rate, headache
• Caution patient not to operate machinery or perform hazardous tasks if dizziness occurs
• Advise patient to avoid faintness; do not get up or stand up rapidly

## Evaluation
### Positive therapeutic outcome
• Decrease in B/P
• Decreased shortness of breath

---

### RARELY USED

## armodafinil (Rx)
(ar-moe-daf'in-il)
Nuvigil

### Controlled substance schedule IV

**Dosage and routes**
*Narcolepsy, obstructive sleep apnea/hypoapnea syndrome*
*Adult and adolescent ≥17 yr:* PO 150-250 mg in AM

*Circadian rhythm disruption (shift work sleep problems)*
*Adult and adolescent ≥17 yr:* PO 150 mg at start of shift

**Uses:** Narcolepsy, obstructive sleep apnea/hypoapnea syndrome, circadian rhythm disruption (shift work sleep problems)

**Contraindications:** Hypersensitivity to this product or modafinil

---

## doripenem (Rx)
(dore-i-pen'em)
Doribax
*Func. class.:* Antiinfective—miscellaneous
*Chem. class.:* Carbapenem

### Pregnancy category B

**Action:** Bactericidal, interferes with cell wall replication of susceptible organisms; osmotically unstable cell wall swells, bursts from osmotic pressure

**Therapeutic outcome:** Negative C&S; decreasing symptoms and signs of infection

**Uses:** Serious infections caused by *Acinetobacter baumannii, Bacteroides caccae, Bacteroides fragilis, Bacteroides thetaiotaomicron, Bacteroides uniformis, Bacteroides vulgatus, Escherichia coli, Klebsiella pneumoniae, Peptostreptococcus micros, Proteus mirabilis, Pseudomonas aeruginosa, Streptococcus contellatus, Streptococcus intermedius;* complicated urinary tract infections, pyelonephritis, complicated intraabdominal infections

**Dosage and routes**
*Adult:* **IV** 500 mg every 8 hr × 5-14 days; if improvement occurs after 3 days, switch to an appropriate oral product

**Available forms:** Powder for inj 500 mg

---

**Adverse effects**

*CNS:* **Seizures,** headache

*GI:* Diarrhea, nausea, vomiting, **pseudomembranous colitis, hepatitis**

*INTEG: Rash,* urticaria, phlebitis, erythema at inj site, **Stevens-Johnson syndrome, toxic epidermal necrolysis,** pruritus

*SYST:* Anaphylaxis

**Contraindications:** Hypersensitivity to meropenem, doripenem, imipenem, penicillin, β-lactam; viral infection

**Precautions:** Pregnancy **B,** breastfeeding, geriatric, renal disease, seizure disorder

| Pharmacokinetics | |
|---|---|
| **Absorption** | Unknown |
| **Distribution** | To most body fluids/tissue |
| **Metabolism** | Unknown |
| **Excretion** | Mainly unchanged in urine, 70% recovered in 48 hr |
| **Half-life** | 1 hr, extended in renal disease |

| Pharmacodynamics |
|---|
| Unknown |

**Interactions**

*Individual drugs*

Probenecid: increased doripenem plasma levels

Divalproex sodium, valproic acid: decreased effects

*Drug/herb*

Acidophilus: do not use with antiinfectives; separate by several hours

*Drug/lab test*

Increased: AST, ALT, LDH, BUN, alkaline phosphatase, bilirubin, creatinine

False positive: direct Coombs' test

**NURSING CONSIDERATIONS**

**Assessment**

• Assess sensitivity to carbapenem antibiotics, penicillins

• Monitor renal disease: lower dose may be required

• Monitor bowel pattern daily; if severe diarrhea occurs, product should be discontinued; may indicate pseudomembranous colitis

• Monitor for infection: temp, sputum, characteristics of wound, before, during, and after treatment

◆ Monitor for allergic reactions, anaphylaxis: rash, urticaria, pruritus; may occur few days after therapy begins

• Monitor overgrowth of infection: perineal itching, fever, malaise, redness, pain, swelling,

drainage, rash, diarrhea, change in cough, sputum

**Nursing diagnoses**

• Infection, risk for (uses)

• Knowledge, deficient (teaching)

**Implementation**

• Give after C&S is taken

• When giving 500-mg dose: constitute vial with 10 ml of sterile water for inj or NaCl 0.9%; gently shake; (50 mg/ml); the solution must be further diluted using a 21-G needle; withdraw susp and add to 100-ml infusion bag of D₅W; gently shake until clear

• When giving 250-mg dose: constitute vial with 10 ml of sterile water for inj or NaCl 0.9%; gently shake; (50 mg/ml); the solution must be further diluted using a 21-G needle; withdraw susp and add to 100-ml infusion bag of D₅W; gently shake; remove 55 ml of solution; discard; the remaining solution contains 250 mg doripenem (4.5 mg/ml)

*Solution compatibilities:* D₅W, 0.9% NaCl, sterile water for inj

**Patient/family education**

• Instruct patient to report severe diarrhea; may indicate pseudomembranous colitis

• Instruct patient to report sore throat, bruising, bleeding, joint pain; may indicate blood dyscrasias (rare)

• Instruct patient to report overgrowth of infection: black, furry tongue; vaginal itching; foul-smelling stools

• Advise patient to avoid breastfeeding; product is excreted in breast milk

**Evaluation**

**Positive therapeutic outcome**

• Negative C&S

• Absence of symptoms and signs of infection

**Treatment of overdose:** EpINEPHrine, antihistamines; resuscitate if needed (anaphylaxis)

**RARELY USED**

**eculizumab** (Rx)

(ek-yoo-lye′zyoo-mab)

Soliris

*Func. class.:* Monoclonal antibody

**Dosage and routes**

*Adult:* **IV** INF 600 mg q7 days × 4 wk, then a single dose of 900 mg q7 days by **IV** INF after the 4th dose, then 900 mg q14 days by **IV** INF

Adverse effects: *italic* = common, **bold** = life-threatening

**Uses:** Proximal nocturnal hemoglobinuria (PNH) a rare, genetic form of hemolytic anemia

**Contraindications:** Hypersensitivity, discontinuing product rapidly (serious hemolysis)

## ixabepilone
Ixempra
*See p. 526*

### RARELY USED
## lanreotide (Rx)
(lan-ree'oh-tide)
Somatuline Depot

**Dosage and routes**
*Adult:* SUBCUT 90 mg injected deep q4 wk × 3 mo; after 3 mo if growth hormone is >1 ng/ml and ≤2.5 ng/ml, continue same dosage; if growth hormone is >2.5 ng/ml or insulin growth factor-1 (IGF-1) is elevated, increase dose to 120 mg q4 wk × 3 mo; if symptoms are controlled and growth hormone is <1 ng/ml, reduce dose to 60 mg q4 wk × 3 mo; thereafter adjust to patient response

**Uses:** Acromegaly in patients having an inadequate response to other treatments

**Contraindications:** Hypersensitivity to this product, latex allergy

## lapatinib
Tykerb
*See p. 539*

## lenalidomide
Revlimid
*See p. 541*

## levocetirizine
Xyzal
*See p. 551*

## lisdexamfetamine
Vyvanse
*See p. 564*

## maraviroc
Selzentry
*See p. 585*

## nebivolol (Rx)
(ne-biv'oh-lol)
Bystolic
*Func. class.:* Antihypertensive
*Chem. class.:* $\beta_1$-Blocker

**Pregnancy category C**

**Action:** Competitively blocks stimulation of β-adrenergic receptors within vascular smooth muscle; decreases rate of SA node discharge, increases recovery time, slows conduction of AV node resulting in decreased heart rate (negative chronotropic effect), which decreases $O_2$ consumption in myocardium due to $\beta_1$-receptor antagonism; also decreases renin-aldosterone-angiotensin system at high doses, inhibits $\beta_2$-receptors in bronchial system (high doses)

**Therapeutic outcome:** Decreased B/P after 1-2 wk

**Uses:** Hypertension alone or in combination

**Unlabeled uses:** Heart failure

**Dosage and routes**
*Hypertension*
*Adult:* PO 5 mg/day, may be increased to desired response q2 wk; max 40 mg/day
*Geriatric:* PO Not to exceed 40 mg/day

*Renal dose*
*Adult:* PO CCr <30 ml/min, 2.5 mg/day; may increase cautiously

*Heart failure (unlabeled)*
*Adult:* PO 1.25 mg titrated to max 10 mg/day

**Available forms:** Tabs 2.5, 5, 10 mg

**Adverse effects**
*CNS: Insomnia, fatigue, dizziness, mental changes,* drowsiness, headache
*CV:* **Bradycardia, MI,** AV heart block, edema
*GI: Nausea, diarrhea,* vomiting, abdominal pain
*GU: Impotence*
*HEMA:* **Thrombocytopenia**
*INTEG:* Rash, pruritus, vasculitis, urticaria, psoriasis, **angioedema**
*MISC:* **Renal failure, pulmonary edema,** hyperuricemia, hypercholesterolemia
*RESP:* **Bronchospasm,** dyspnea

**Contraindications:** Cardiogenic shock, sick sinus syndrome, abrupt discontinuation, acute bronchospasm, AV heart block, hypersensitivity to this agent or β-blockers

**Precautions:** Pregnancy **C**, breastfeeding, children, major surgery, peripheral vascular disease, diabetes mellitus, thyrotoxicosis disease, COPD, asthma, well-compensated heart failure, renal/hepatic disease

### Pharmacokinetics

| | |
|---|---|
| **Absorption** | Unknown |
| **Distribution** | Unknown |
| **Metabolism** | In liver by CYP2D6 |
| **Excretion** | 38% excreted in urine, 44% in feces |
| **Half-life** | 12 hr |

### Pharmacodynamics

| | |
|---|---|
| **Onset** | Unknown |
| **Peak** | 1.5-4 hr |
| **Duration** | Unknown |

### Interactions
#### Individual drugs
Cimetidine: increased nebivolol action
Mefloquine, sotalol: do not give
Sildenafil: decreased nebivolol action
#### Drug classifications
CYP2D6 inducers (rifampin): decreased nebivolol action
CYP2D6 inhibitors (amiodarone, buPROPion, chloroquine, chlorpheniramine, chlorproMAZINE, cinacalcet, diphenhydrAMINE, duloxetine, fluoxetine, haloperidol, imatinib, paroxetine, promethazine, propoxyphene, quinidine, quinine, ritonavir, terbinafine, thioridazine): increased nebivolol action
#### Drug/herb
Hawthorn: may increase nebivolol effect
#### Drug/lab test
Increased: serum lipoprotein levels, BUN, potassium, triglyceride, uric acid, LDH, AST, ALT, blood glucose, alkaline phosphatase
Positive: ANA titer

### NURSING CONSIDERATIONS
#### Assessment
• Monitor B/P during beginning treatment, periodically thereafter; pulse q4hr; note rate, rhythm, quality
• Assess apical/radial pulse before administration; notify prescriber of any significant changes (pulse <50 bpm); signs of CHF (dyspnea, crackles, weight gain, jugular vein distention)
• Assess baselines in renal/hepatic studies before therapy begins and periodically
• Monitor I&O, edema in feet, legs daily
• Monitor skin turgor, dryness of mucous membranes for hydration status, especially geriatric patients

### Nursing diagnoses
• Cardiac output, decreased (uses)
• Knowledge, deficient (teaching)
• Noncompliance (teaching)

### Implementation
#### PO route
• Give without regard for meals; tab may be crushed or swallowed whole; give with food to prevent GI upset
• Store protected from light, moisture; place in cool environment

### Patient/family education
◆ Caution patient not to discontinue product abruptly, severe cardiac reactions may occur, taper over 2 wk; do not double dose; if a dose is missed, take as soon as remembered up to 4 hr before next dose
• Inform patient product may mask signs of hypoglycemia or alter blood glucose levels
• Advise patient not to use OTC products containing α-adrenergic stimulants (such as nasal decongestants, OTC cold preparations) unless directed by prescriber
• Instruct patient to report low pulse, dizziness, confusion, depression, fever
• Teach patient to take pulse, B/P at home; advise when to notify prescriber
• Advise patient to comply with weight control, dietary adjustments, modified exercise program
• Instruct patient to carry emergency ID to identify product, allergies
• Caution patient to avoid hazardous activities if dizziness, drowsiness is present
• Instruct patient to report symptoms of CHF: difficulty breathing, especially on exertion or when lying down, night cough, swelling of extremities
• Teach patient to continue with required lifestyle changes (exercise, diet, weight loss, stress reduction)

### Evaluation
#### Positive therapeutic outcome
• Decreased B/P after 1-2 wk
• Decreased dysrhythmias

### Treatment of overdose: Lavage, **IV** atropine for bradycardia, **IV** theophylline for bronchospasm, digoxin, $O_2$, diuretic for cardiac failure, **IV** glucose for hypoglycemia, **IV** diazepam (or phenytoin) for seizures

---

Adverse effects: *italic* = common, **bold** = life-threatening

# nilotinib (Rx)
(nye-loe'ti-nib)
Tasigna
*Func. class.:* Antineoplastic—miscellaneous
*Chem. class.:* Protein-tyrosine kinase
inhibitor
## Pregnancy category D

**Action:** Inhibits BCR-ABL tyrosine kinase
created in chronic myeloid leukemia (CML)

**Therapeutic outcome:** Decrease in
progression of disease

**Uses:** Chronic phase/accelerated phase
Philadelphia chromosome positive chronic
myelogenous leukemia that is resistant/
intolerant to imatinib

## Dosage and routes
*Adult:* PO 400 mg bid, continue until disease
progression or unacceptable toxicity

### Escalation regimen for those
taking a strong CYP3A4 inducer
*Adult:* PO Increase dose as required

### Adjustment following
discontinuation of a strong
CYP3A4 inducer
*Adult:* PO Reduce to 400 mg/bid

### For those taking a strong CYP3A4
inhibitor
*Adult:* PO Reduce dose to 400 mg/day

### QT prolongation
*QTc >480 msec:* Withhold dose

### Myelosuppression
*ANC 1 x 10^9/L or platelets <50 x
10^9/L:* Withhold dose

**Available forms:** Caps 200 mg

## Adverse effects
*CNS:* Headache, dizziness, fatigue, fever,
flushing, paresthesia
*CV:* **QT prolongation**, palpitations, **torsade
de pointes**
*GI:* *Nausea*, **hepatotoxicity, vomiting,
dyspepsia,** *anorexia, abdominal pain,*
constipation, **pancreatitis,** diarrhea
*HEMA:* **Neutropenia, thrombocytopenia,
anemia, pancytopenia**
*INTEG:* *Rash,* alopecia, erythema
*META:* Hyperamylasemia, hyperbilirubinemia,
hyperglycemia, hyperkalemia, hypocalcemia,
hyponatremia, hypomagnesemia
*MISC:* Diaphoresis
*MS:* Arthralgia, myalgia, back/bone pain,
muscle cramps
*RESP:* Cough, dyspnea
*SYST:* **Bleeding**

**Contraindications:** Pregnancy **D**, breastfeeding, hypersensitivity, hypokalemia, hypomagnesemia, QT prolongation

**Precautions:** Children, women, geriatric
patients, active infections, anemia, cardiac/
hepatic disease, bone marrow suppression,
cholestasis, diabetes, gelatin hypersensitivity,
infertility, galactose-free diet, lactase deficiency, neutropenia, pancreatitis, thrombocytopenia

| Pharmacokinetics | |
|---|---|
| **Absorption** | Unknown |
| **Distribution** | Protein binding 98%, plasma levels 3 hr |
| **Metabolism** | By CYP3A4 |
| **Excretion** | Unknown |
| **Half-life** | Elimination 17 hr |

| Pharmacodynamics |
|---|
| Unknown |

## Interactions
### Individual drugs
• Product interactions are numerous
Acetaminophen: increased hepatotoxicity
Carbamazepine, dexamethasone, phenobarbi-
tal, phenytoin, rifampin: decreased concen-
trations
Clarithromycin, erythromycin, itraconazole,
ketoconazole: increased concentrations
Simvastatin: increased plasma concentrations
Warfarin: increased plasma concentration;
avoid use with warfarin, use low-molecular-
weight anticoagulants instead
### Drug classifications
Calcium channel blockers: increased plasma
concentrations
### Drug/herb
St. John's wort: decreased concentration
### Drug/food
Grapefruit juice: increased plasma concentrations

## NURSING CONSIDERATIONS
### Assessment
• Assess ANC and platelets; if ANC <1 × 10^9/L
and/or platelets <50 × 10^9/L, stop until ANC
>1.5 × 10^9/L and platelets >75 × 10^9/L
• Monitor CV status: hypertension, QT prolon-
gation can occur; monitor left ventricular
ejection fraction (LVEF) baseline periodically
• Assess for renal toxicity: if bilirubin >3 ×
IULN, withhold until bilirubin levels return to
<1.5 × IULN
• Assess for hepatotoxicity: monitor hepatic
function tests, before treatment and qmo; if

liver transaminases >5 × IULN, withhold until transaminase levels return to <2.5 × IULN
• Monitor CBC, differential, platelet count weekly; withhold product if WBC is <3500/mm³ or platelet count <100,000/mm³; notify prescriber of these results; product should be discontinued
• Monitor for bleeding: epistaxis, rectal, gingival, upper GI, genital, and wound bleeding; tumor-related hemorrhage may occur rapidly
• Monitor electrolytes: calcium, potassium, sodium; lipase, phosphate

**Nursing diagnoses**
• Knowledge, deficient (teaching)

**Implementation**
• Do not break, crush, or chew caps
• Give on an empty stomach; separate doses by 12 hr; a make-up dose should not be taken if a dose is missed
• Store at 15°–30° C (59°–86° F)

**Patient/family education**
• Instruct patient to report adverse reactions immediately: SOB, bleeding
• Inform patient reason for treatment, expected result
• Advise patient that many adverse reactions may occur
• Teach patient to avoid persons with known upper respiratory infections; immunosuppression is common

**Evaluation**
**Positive therapeutic outcome**
• Decrease in progression of disease

---

**RARELY USED**

**nitisinone** (Rx)
(ni-tiz'i-none)
Orfadin
*Func. class.:* Orphan drug

**Dosage and routes**
*Adult/adolescent/child/infant:* PO 1 mg/kg/day divided in AM and PM

**Uses:** Hereditary tyrosinemia type I

**Contraindications:** Hypersensitivity, tyrosine/phenylalanine intake

---

**paliperidone**
Invega
*See p. 725*

---

**raltegravir**
Isentress
*See p. 824*

---

**rotigotine**
Neupro
*See p. 858*

---

**temsirolimus**
Torisel
*See p. 915*

---

Adverse effects: *italic* = common, **bold** = life-threatening

## Appendix B

### Controlled Substance Chart

| DRUGS | UNITED STATES* |
|---|---|
| Heroin, LSD, peyote, marijuana, mescaline | Schedule I<br>• High abuse potential<br>• No currently accepted medical use |
| Opium (morphine), meperidine, amphetamines, cocaine, short-acting barbiturates (secobarbital) | Schedule II<br>• High abuse potential; potentially severe psychologic or physical dependence<br>• Currently accepted medical use but may be severely restricted<br>• Telephone orders only in emergencies if written Rx follows promptly<br>• No refills |
| Glutethimide, paregoric, phendimetrazine | Schedule III<br>• Abuse potential less than the drugs/substances in Schedules I and II; potentially moderate or low physical dependence or high psychologic dependence<br>• Currently accepted medical use<br>• Telephone orders permitted<br>• Prescriber may authorize limited refills |
| Chloral hydrate, chlordiazepoxide, diazepam, mazindol, meprobamate, phenobarbital | Schedule IV<br>• Low abuse potential relative to drugs/substances in Schedule III; potentially limited physical or psychologic dependence<br>• Currently accepted medical use<br>• Telephone orders permitted<br>• Prescriber may authorize limited refills |
| Antidiarrheals with opium, antitussives | Schedule V<br>• Lowest abuse potential; potentially very limited physical or psychologic dependence<br>• Currently accepted medical use<br>• Prescriber determines refills<br>• Some products containing limited amounts of Schedule V substances (e.g., cough suppressants) available OTC to patients >18 yr |

*For Canadian controlled substance chart, go to http://evolve.elsevier.com/nursingdrugupdates/Skidmore/NDG

## Appendix C

### Rarely Used Drugs

**abciximab** (Rx)
*Func. class.:* Platelet aggregation inhibitor

Dosage and routes
*Percutaneous coronary intervention (PCI)*
*Adult:* **IV** BOL 250 mcg (0.25 mg)/kg 10-60 min before PCI, followed by 0.125 mcg/kg/min CONT INF for 12 hr

*MI*
*Adult:* **IV** BOL 0.25 mg/kg over 5 min, then 0.125 mcg/kg/min, max 10 mcg/min; **IV** INF for 12 hr unless complications

Uses: Used with heparin and aspirin to prevent acute cardiac ischemia following PTCA in patients at high risk for reclosure of affected arteries

Unlabeled uses: Acute MI, Kawasaki disease (child)

Contraindications: Hypersensitivity to this product or murine protein; GI, GU bleeding; CVA within 2 yr, bleeding disorders, intracranial neoplasm, intracranial arteriovenous malformations, intracranial aneurysm, platelet count <100,000 cells/mm³, recent surgery, aneurysm, uncontrolled severe hypertension, vasculitis coagulopathy

**alefacept** (Rx)
*Func. class.:* Immunosuppressive

Dosage and routes
*Adult:* **IV** BOL 7.5 mg qwk or IM 15 mg qwk, for 12 wk

Uses: Adults with moderate to severe plaque psoriasis

Contraindications: Hypersensitivity

**alfentanil** (Rx)
*Func. class.:* Opioid analgesic
Controlled substance schedule **II**

Dosage and routes
*Anesthesia <30 min*
*Combination*
*Adult:* **IV** 8-50 mcg/kg, may increase by 3-15 mcg/kg

*Anesthetic induction*
*Adult:* **IV** 3-5 mcg/kg, then 0.5-1.5 mcg/kg/min; total dose is 8-40 mcg/kg

*Anesthesia 30-60 min*
*Induction*
*Adult:* **IV** 20-50 mcg/kg

*Maintenance*
*Adult:* **IV** 5-15 mcg/kg; may give up to 75 mcg/kg total dose

*Continuous anesthesia >45 min*
*Induction*
*Adult:* **IV** 50-75 mcg/kg

*Maintenance*
*Adult:* **IV** 0.5-3.0 mcg/kg/min; rate should be decreased by 30%-50% after 1 hr maintenance INF; may be increased to 4 mcg/kg/min or BOL doses of 7 mcg/kg

*Induction of anesthesia >45 min*
*Adult:* **IV** 130-245 mcg/kg, then 0.5-1.5 mcg/kg/min

*MAC*
*Induction*
*Adult:* **IV** Duration ≤½ hr 3-8 mcg/kg

*Maintenance*
*Adult:* 3-5 mcg/kg q5-20min to 1 mcg/kg/min, total dose 3-40 mcg/kg

Uses: In combination with other products in general anesthesia, as a primary anesthetic in general surgery, monitored anesthesia care (MAC)

Contraindications: Children <12 yr, hypersensitivity

Adverse effects: *italic* = common, **bold** = life-threatening

## alprostadil (Rx)
*Func. class.:* Hormone

### Dosage and routes
*Patent ductus arteriosus*
***Infant:*** **IV** INF 0.1 mcg/kg/min, until desired response, then reduce to lowest effective amount, 0.4 mcg/kg/min not likely to produce greater beneficial effects

*Erectile dysfunction of vasculogenic or mixed etiology, psychogenic*
***Men:*** INTRACAVERNOSAL 2.5 mcg may increase by 2.5 mcg; may then increase by 5-10 mcg until adequate response occurs; INTRAURETHRAL administer as needed to achieve erection

**Uses:** To maintain patent ductus arteriosus (temporary treatment), erectile dysfunction

**Contraindications:** Hypersensitivity, respiratory distress syndrome (RDS)

## altretamine (Rx)
*Func. class.:* Antineoplastic—miscellaneous

### Dosage and routes
***Adult:*** PO 260 mg/m$^2$ day for 14 or 21 days in a 28-day cycle; give in 4 divided doses after meals and at bedtime

**Uses:** Palliative treatment of recurrent, persistent ovarian cancer following first-line treatment with cisplatin or alkylating agent–based combination

**Unlabeled uses:** Lymphoma, lung cancer

**Contraindications:** Pregnancy **D**, hypersensitivity, severe bone marrow depression, severe neurologic toxicity

## amantadine (Rx)
*Func. class.:* Antiviral, antiparkinsonian agent

### Do not confuse:
amantadine/ranitidine/rimantidine, Symmetrel/ Synthroid

### Dosage and routes
*Influenza type A*
***Adult and child >12 yr:*** PO 200 mg/day in single dose or divided bid, max 400 mg/day
***Child 9-12 yr:*** PO 100 mg bid
***Child 1-9 yr:*** PO 5 mg/kg/day divided bid-tid, not to exceed 150 mg/day
***Geriatric:*** PO no more than 100 mg/day

*Extrapyramidal reaction/ parkinsonism*
***Adult:*** PO 100 mg bid, up to 400 mg/day in EPS; give for 1 wk, then 100 mg as needed up to 400 mg in parkinsonism

*Renal dose*
***Adult:*** PO CCr 40-50 ml/min 100 mg/day; CCr 30 ml/min 200 mg 2×/wk; CCr 20 ml/min 100 mg 3×/wk; CCr <10 ml/min 100 mg alternating with 200 mg q7 days

**Uses:** Prophylaxis or treatment of influenza type A, EPS, parkinsonism, Parkinson's disease

**Contraindications:** Breastfeeding, children <1 yr, hypersensitivity, eczematic rash

## aminocaproic acid (Rx)
*Func. class.:* Hemostatic

### Dosage and routes
***Adult:*** PO/**IV** 4-5 g loading dose, then 1-1.25 g q1hr

**Uses:** Severe hemorrhage from hyperfibrinolysis; adjunctive therapy in hemophilia

**Contraindications:** Hypersensitivity, abnormal bleeding, postpartum bleeding, DIC, upper urinary tract bleeding, new burns

## aminolevulinic acid (Rx)
*Func. class.:* Photochemotherapy

### Dosage and routes
***Adult:*** TOP 1 application of solution and 1 dose of illumination/treatment site × 8 wk

**Uses:** Face/scalp nonhyperkeratotic actinic keratoses

**Contraindications:** Hypersensitivity to porphyrins

## amyl nitrite (Rx)
*Func. class.:* Coronary vasodilator

### Dosage and routes
*Angina*
***Adult:*** INH 0.18-0.3 ml as needed, 1-6 puffs from 1 cap; may repeat in 3-5 min

*Cyanide poisoning*
***Adult:*** INH 0.3 ml ampule inhaled 15 sec until preparation of sodium nitrite inf is ready

**Uses:** Acute angina pectoris, cyanide poisoning

 Alert     Canada Only    🐱 Drug on CD    * "Tall Man" lettering (See Preface)

**Unlabeled uses:** Cardiac murmur diagnosis

**Contraindications:** Pregnancy **X,** hypersensitivity to nitrites, severe anemia, ICP, hypertension

---

! HIGH ALERT

## asparaginase (Rx)
*Func. class.:* Antineoplastic

### Dosage and routes
*In combination*
*Adult and child:* **IV** 1000 international units/kg/day × 10 days given over 30 min; IM 6000 international units/m²/day

*Sole induction*
*Adult and child:* **IV** 200 international units/kg/day × 28 days

*Desensitization*
*Adult and child:* Test dose adult and child ID 2 international units, then double dose q10 min, until total dose is administered or reaction occurs

**Uses:** Acute lymphocytic leukemia in combination with other antineoplastics

**Contraindications:** Breastfeeding, infants, hypersensitivity, pancreatitis

---

## atracurium (Rx)
*Func. class.:* Neuromuscular blocker (nondepolarizing)

### Dosage and routes
*Adult and child >2 yr:* **IV** BOL 0.4-0.5 mg/kg, then 0.08-0.10 mg/kg 20-45 min after first dose if needed for prolonged procedures
*Child 1 mo-2 yr:* **IV** BOL 0.3-0.4 mg/kg

**Uses:** Facilitation of endotracheal intubation, skeletal muscle relaxation during mechanical ventilation, surgery, or general anesthesia

**Contraindications:** Hypersensitivity

---

## auranofin (Rx)
*Func. class.:* Antiinflammatory

### Do not confuse:
Ridaura/Cardura

### Dosage and routes
*Adult:* PO 6 mg/day or 3 mg bid; may increase to 9 mg/day after 3 mo

**Uses:** Rheumatoid arthritis; not for first-line therapy

**Unlabeled uses:** SLE, psoriatic arthritis, pemphigus

**Contraindications:** Breastfeeding, child <6 yr, hypersensitivity to gold, necrotizing enterocolitis, bone marrow aplasia, pulmonary fibrosis, exfoliative dermatitis, blood dyscrasias, recent radiation therapy, renal/hepatic disease, marked hypertension, uncontrolled CHF

---

## aztreonam (Rx)
*Func. class.:* Antiinfective—miscellaneous

### Dosage and routes
*Urinary tract infections*
*Adult:* IM/**IV** 500 mg-1 g q8-12hr

*Systemic infections*
*Adult:* IM/**IV** 1-2 g q8-12hr
*Child:* IM/**IV** 90-120 mg/kg/day divided q6-8hr; max 8 g/day **IV**

*Severe systemic infections*
*Adult:* IM/**IV** 2 g q6-8hr; do not exceed 8 g/day
Continue treatment for 48 hr after negative culture or until patient is asymptomatic

**Uses:** Urinary tract infection; septicemia; skin, muscle, bone, lower respiratory tract, intraabdominal infections, and other infections caused by gram-negative organisms

**Contraindications:** Hypersensitivity to this product, penicillins, cephalosporins, severe renal disease

---

## bacitracin (Rx)
*Func. class.:* Antiinfective—miscellaneous

### Dosage and routes
*Child:* IM 800-1200 units/kg/day in divided doses q8-12hr; max 12 days of therapy
*Infant >2.5 kg:* IM 1000 units/kg/day in divided doses q8-12hr
*Infant ≤2.5 kg:* IM 900 units/kg/day in divided doses q8-12hr; max 12 days of therapy

*Renal dose*
*Adult:* CCr 10-30 ml/min, decrease dose by 50% q6-12hr after 0.5-2 g **IV** loading dose; CCr <10 ml/min, decrease dose by 75% q6-12hr after 0.5-2 g **IV** loading dose

---

Adverse effects: *italic* = common, **bold** = life-threatening

Uses: Staphylococcal pneumonia, empyema

**Contraindications:** Hypersensitivity, severe renal disease (IM use)

---

## benzonatate (Rx)
*Func. class.:* Antitussive, nonopioid

**Dosage and routes**
*Adult and child:* PO 100 mg up to q4hr, not to exceed 600 mg/day

**Uses:** Nonproductive cough

**Contraindications:** Hypersensitivity

---

## benzoyl peroxide (OTC)
*Func. class.:* Antiacne medication

**Dosage and routes**
*Adult and child:* TOP Apply to affected area daily or bid

**Uses:** Mild to moderate acne

**Contraindications:** Hypersensitivity to benzoic acid derivatives

---

## beractant (Rx)
*Func. class.:* Natural lung surfactant

**Dosage and routes**
*Newborn:* INTRATRACHEAL INSTILL 4 doses can be administered in the 1st 48 hr of life; give doses no more frequently than q6hr; each dose is 100 mg of phospholipids/kg birth weight (4 ml/kg)

**Uses:** Prevention and treatment (rescue) of respiratory distress syndrome in premature infants

---

## biperiden (Rx)
*Func. class.:* Antiparkinsonian agent, anti-cholinergic

**Dosage and routes**
*Extrapyramidal symptoms*
*Adult:* PO 2 mg daily-tid; IM/**IV** 2 mg q30 min, if needed, not to exceed 8 mg/24 hr
*Child:* IM 40 mcg/kg or 1.2 mg/m$^2$, may repeat q½hr

*Parkinsonian symptoms*
*Adult:* PO 2 mg tid-qid; max 16 mg/24 hr

**Uses:** Parkinsonian symptoms, EPS secondary to neuroleptic product therapy

**Contraindications:** Hypersensitivity, angle-closure glaucoma, myasthenia gravis, GI/GU obstruction, megacolon, stenosing peptic ulcers, prostatic hypertrophy

---

## calfactant (Rx)
*Func. class.:* Natural lung surfactant extract

**Dosage and routes**
*Newborn:* INTRATRACHEAL INSTILL 3 ml/kg of birth wt, given as 2 doses of 1.5 ml/kg, repeat doses of 3 ml/kg of birth wt until up to 3 doses 12 hr apart have been given

**Uses:** Prevention and treatment (rescue) of respiratory distress syndrome in premature infants

---

## *chlorproPAMIDE (Rx)
*Func. class.:* Antidiabetic

**Dosage and routes**
*Adult:* PO 100-250 mg/day initially, then 100-500 mg maintenance according to response; not to exceed 750 mg/day

**Uses:** Type 2 diabetes mellitus

**Contraindications:** Hypersensitivity to sulfonylureas, type 1 diabetes, severe liver disease, breastfeeding, renal failure

---

## cladribine (CdA) (Rx)
*Func. class.:* Antineoplastic antiinfective

**Dosage and routes**
*Adult:* **IV** 0.09 mg/kg diluted with 0.9% NaCl qs to 100 ml; pass through 0.22 μm microfilter, given for cont inf × 5-7 days

**Uses:** Treatment of active hairy cell leukemia; may be useful in chronic lymphocytic leukemia, non-Hodgkin's lymphomas, acute/chronic myeloid leukemia, autoimmune hemolytic anemia

**Contraindications:** Pregnancy **D**, breastfeeding, hypersensitivity

---

## clemastine (Rx)
*Func. class.:* Antihistamine

**Dosage and routes**
*Adult and child >12 yr:* PO 1.34-2.68 mg bid-tid, not to exceed 8.04 mg/day

**Uses:** Allergy symptoms, rhinitis, allergic dermatoses, nasal allergies, hypersensitive reactions including blood transfusion reactions, anaphylaxis

**Contraindications:** Hypersensitivity to $H_1$-receptor antagonists, acute asthma attack, lower respiratory tract disease

## corticotropin (ACTH) (Rx)
*Func. class.:* Pituitary hormone

**Dosage and routes**
*Acute exacerbations of multiple sclerosis*
*Adult:* IM 80-120 units/day × 14-21 days

*Infantile spasms*
*Infant:* IM Gel 20 units/day × 2 wk, increase if needed

**Uses:** Testing adrenocortical function, treatment of adrenal insufficiency caused by administration of corticosteroids (long term), multiple sclerosis, infantile spasms

**Contraindications:** Hypersensitivity, scleroderma, osteoporosis, CHF, peptic ulcer disease, hypertension, systemic fungal infections, smallpox vaccination, recent surgery, ocular herpes simplex, primary adrenocortical insufficiency/hyperfunction

## cosyntropin (Rx)
*Func. class.:* Pituitary hormone

**Dosage and routes**
*Adult and child >2 yr:* IM/ **IV** 0.25-1 mg between blood sampling
*Child <2 yr:* IM/**IV** 0.125 mg

**Uses:** Testing adrenocortical function

**Contraindications:** Hypersensitivity

## crotamiton (Rx)
*Func. class.:* Scabicide

**Dosage and routes**
*Scabies*
*Adult and child:* CREAM Wash area with soap, water; remove visible crusts; apply cream; apply another coat in 24 hr; remove with soap, water in 48 hr

*Pruritus:* CREAM Massage into affected area, repeat as necessary

**Uses:** Scabies, pruritus

**Contraindications:** Hypersensitivity, skin inflammation, abrasions, breaks in skin, mucous membranes

## deferasirox (Rx)
*Func. class.:* Heavy metal chelating agent

**Dosage and routes**
*Adult:* PO 20-30 mg/kg/day; oral dispersion tablet is dissolved in water <1 g in 3.5 oz; >1 g in 7 oz or more; give on empty stomach at least 30 min before meals

**Uses:** Chronic iron overload

**Contraindications:** Breastfeeding, children, hypersensitivity, severe renal/hepatic disease

## deferoxamine (Rx)
*Func. class.:* Heavy metal antagonist

**Do not confuse:**
deferoxamine/cefuroxime

**Dosage and routes**
*Acute iron toxicity*
*Adult and child:* IM/**IV** 1 g; then 500 mg q4hr × 2 doses; then 500 mg q4-12hr × 2 doses, not to exceed 15 mg/kg/hr or 6 g/24 hr

*Chronic iron toxicity*
*Adult and child:* IM 500 mg-1 g/day plus **IV** INF 2 g given by separate line with each blood transfusion, not to exceed 15 mg/kg/hr or 6 g/24 hr; SUBCUT 1-2 g over 8-24 hr by SUBCUT infusion pump

*Iron overload due to transfusion-dependent anemias*
*Adult:* IM 1 g/day plus **IV** 2 g/unit of blood, max 1 g/day with no blood; 6 g/day with 3 or more units of blood or packed RBC

**Uses:** Acute, chronic iron intoxication, hemochromatosis, hemosiderosis

**Contraindications:** Children <3 yr, hypersensitivity, anuria, severe renal disease

## demeclocycline (Rx)
*Func. class.:* Antiinfective

### Dosage and routes
*Adult:* PO 150 mg q6hr or 300 mg q12hr
*Child >8 yr:* PO 6-12 mg/kg/day in divided doses q6-12hr

*Gonorrhea*
*Adult:* PO 600 mg, then 300 mg q12hr × 4 days, total 3 g

**Uses:** Uncommon gram-positive/gram-negative bacteria, protozoa, *Rickettsia, Mycoplasma, Haemophilus ducreyi, Yersinia pestis, Campylobacter fetus, Chlamydia trachomatis,* psittacosis, granuloma inguinale

**Contraindications:** Pregnancy **D**, children <8 yr, hypersensitivity to tetracyclines

## desipramine
*Func. class.:* Antidepressant, tricyclic

### Dosage and routes
*Adult:* PO 100-200 mg/day in a single dose or in divided doses; max 300 mg/day
*Geriatric:* PO 25-50 mg/day, may increase to 150 mg/day
*Child >12 yr:* PO 25-50 mg/day in divided doses; max 100 mg/day
*Child 6-12 yr:* PO 10-30 mg/day or 1-5 mg/kg/day in divided doses; give >3 mg/kg/day with close medical monitoring

**Uses:** Depression

**Contraindications:** Hypersensitivity to tricyclics, angle-closure glaucoma

## desonide (Rx)
Desonate, Verdeso
*Func. class.:* Topical antiinflammatory

### Dosage and routes
*Adult:* TOP Apply to affected area; do not use more than 4 consecutive weeks

**Uses:** Atopic dermatitis

**Contraindications:** Open wounds, burns

## dicyclomine (Rx)
*Func. class.:* Gastrointestinal anticholinergic

### Dosage and routes
*Adult:* PO 10-20 mg tid-qid; IM 20 mg q4-6hr; max 160 mg/day

*Child >2 yr:* PO 10 mg tid-qid
*Child 6 mo-2 yr:* PO 5 mg tid-qid

**Uses:** Treatment of peptic ulcer disease in combination with other products; infant colic, urinary incontinence, IBS

**Contraindications:** Hypersensitivity to anticholinergics, angle-closure glaucoma, GI obstruction, myasthenia gravis, paralytic ileus, GI atony, toxic megacolon

## diflunisal (Rx)
*Func. class.:* Nonsteroidal anti-inflammatory/analgesic (nonopioid)

### Dosage and routes
*Adult:* PO Loading dose 1 g; then 500-1000 mg/day in 2 divided doses, q12hr, not to exceed 1500 mg/day

*Geriatric:* PO ½ adult dose

**Uses:** Mild to moderate pain or fever including arthritis; 3-4 × more potent than aspirin

**Contraindications:** Pregnancy (3rd trimester), children <12 yr, hypersensitivity to salicylates, GI bleeding, bleeding disorders, vit K deficiency, Reye's syndrome, perioperative pain of CABG

## disulfiram (Rx)
*Func. class.:* Alcohol deterrent

### Dosage and routes
*Adult:* PO 250-500 mg/day × 1-2 wk, then 125-500 mg/day until fully socially recovered

**Uses:** Chronic alcoholism (as adjunct)

**Contraindications:** Pregnancy **X,** breast-feeding, hypersensitivity, alcohol intoxication, psychoses, CV disease, ADD

## dornase alfa (Rx)
*Func. class.:* Cystic fibrosis agent (orphan product)

### Dosage and routes
*Adult and child >5 yr:* INH 2.5 mg/day by nebulizer

**Uses:** Management of cystic fibrosis

**Contraindications:** Hypersensitivity to this product or Chinese hamster ovary cell products

## edetate calcium disodium (Rx)
*Func. class.:* Heavy metal antagonist (antidote)

### Dosage and routes
**Lead mobilization test**
*Adult:* **IV** 25-30 mg/kg (up to 2 g) in 250-1000 ml $D_5W$ over 1-6 hr

**Acute lead encephalopathy (blood levels 20-70 mcg/dl)**
*Adult:* IM 1 g/m²/day divided q8-12hr ×5 days; skip 2-4 days; repeat course

**Acute lead poisoning (blood levels 20-70 mcg/dl)**
*Adult:* **IV** INF 1 g/m²/day over 8-12 hr ×5 days; skip 2-4 days and repeat as needed; max 75 mg/kg/day

**Chronic lead poisoning (blood levels 20-70 mcg/dl)**
*Adult:* **IV** INF 1 g/m²/day over 8-12 hr ×5 days; skip 2-4 days; repeat as needed

**Uses:** Lead poisoning, acute lead encephalopathy

**Contraindications:** Children <3 yr, hypersensitivity, anuria, poisoning of other metals, severe renal disease, hepatitis

## edetate disodium (Rx)
*Func. class.:* Heavy metal antagonist (chelator)

### Dosage and routes
**Digitalis glucoside toxicity/ ventricular dysrhythmias/ hypercalcemia crisis**
*Adult:* **IV** 50 mg/kg/day given over 3 hr or more, daily ×5 days; skip 2 days; repeat as needed up to 15 doses; max 3 g/day

**Uses:** Hypercalcemic crisis, control of ventricular dysrhythmias associated with digoxin toxicity

**Contraindications:** Child <3 yr, hypersensitivity, anuria, hepatic insufficiency, poisoning of other metals, severe renal disease, seizure disorders, active/inactive TB

## efalizumab (Rx)
*Func. class.:* Immunosuppressive

### Dosage and routes
*Adult:* SUBCUT 0.7 mg/kg as a conditioning dose, then SUBCUT 1 mg/kg qwk, max single dose 200 mg

**Uses:** Adults 18 years of age and older with moderate to severe plaque psoriasis

**Contraindications:** Hypersensitivity

## estramustine
*Func. class.:* Antineoplastic

### Dosage and routes
*Adult:* PO 10-16 mg/kg in 3-4 divided doses/day; treatment may continue for ≥3 mo or 600 mg/m²/day in 3 divided doses

**Uses:** Metastatic prostate cancer

**Contraindications:** Pregnancy **D**, hypersensitivity to estradiol, thromboembolic disorders

## etomidate (Rx)
*Func. class.:* General anesthetic

### Dosage and routes
**Adult and child >10 yr:** **IV** 0.2-0.6 mg/kg over ½-1 min

**Uses:** Induction of general anesthesia

**Contraindications:** Labor/delivery, hypersensitivity

## felbamate (Rx)
*Func. class.:* Anticonvulsant

### Dosage and routes
**Adjunctive therapy**
**Adult and child >14 yr:** PO Add 1.2 g/day in 3-4 divided doses; reduce other anticonvulsants (valproic acid, phenytoin, carbamazepine and derivatives) by 20% to control plasma concentrations; may increase felbamate in 1.2 g/day increments qwk, up to 3.6 g/day

**Monotherapy**
*Adult:* PO 1.2 g/day in 3-4 divided doses; titrate with close supervision; increase dose by 600 mg increments q2 wk to 3.6 g/day if needed

Adverse effects: *italic* = common, **bold** = life-threatening

*Lennox-Gastaut syndrome adjunctive therapy*
*Child 2-14 yr:* PO Add 15 mg/kg/day in 3-4 divided doses; reduce other anticonvulsants (valproic acid, phenytoin, carbamazepine and derivatives) by 20% to control plasma concentrations; may increase felbamate 15 mg/kg/day q wk up to 45 mg/kg/day; max 3600 mg/day

**Uses:** Partial seizures, with or without generalization in adults; partial and generalized seizures in children with Lennox-Gastaut syndrome

**Contraindications:** Hypersensitivity to this product, other carbamates, history of blood dyscrasia, aplastic anemia, hepatic disease

## fenoprofen (Rx)
*Func. class.:* Nonsteroidal antiinflammatory/nonopioid analgesic

**Dosage and routes**
*Pain*
*Adult:* PO 200 mg q4-6hr prn
*Arthritis*
*Adult:* PO 300-600 mg qid, not to exceed 3.2 g/day

**Uses:** Mild to moderate pain, osteoarthritis, rheumatoid arthritis, acute gout, arthritis, inflammation

**Contraindications:** Hypersensitivity, asthma, severe renal/hepatic disease

## flavoxate (Rx)
*Func. class.:* Spasmolytic

**Dosage and routes**
*Adult and child >12 yr:* PO 100-200 mg tid-qid

**Uses:** Relief of nocturia, incontinence, suprapubic pain, dysuria, frequency associated with urologic conditions (symptomatic only)

**Contraindications:** Hypersensitivity, GI obstruction, GI hemorrhage, GU obstruction

## floxuridine (Rx)
*Func. class.:* Antineoplastic, antimetabolite

**Dosage and routes**
*Adult:* INTRAARTERIAL by cont inf 0.1-0.6 mg/kg/day × 1-6 wk; HEPATIC ARTERY INJ 0.4-0.6 mg/kg/day × 1-6 wk

**Uses:** GI adenocarcinoma metastatic to liver; cancer of breast, head, neck, liver, brain, gallbladder, bile duct

**Contraindications:** Pregnancy **D**, breastfeeding, hypersensitivity, myelosuppression, poor nutritional status, serious infections

## fludarabine (Rx)
*Func. class.:* Antineoplastic, antimetabolite

**Dosage and routes**
*Adult:* IV 25 mg/m$^2$ over 30 min/day × 5 days, may repeat q28 days; reconstitute with 2 ml of sterile water for inj; dissolution should occur in <15 sec

**Uses:** Chronic lymphocytic leukemia, non-Hodgkin's lymphoma

**Contraindications:** Pregnancy **D**, breastfeeding, hypersensitivity

## galsulfase (Rx)
*Func. class.:* Miscellaneous drug

**Dosage and routes**
*Adult and child ≥5 yr:* IV 1 mg/kg infused over ≥4hr once per week

**Uses:** Mucopolysaccharidosis VI (MPS VI); Maroteaux-Lamy syndrome

**Contraindications:** Hypersensitivity, hamster allergy

## glycerin (OTC)
*Func. class.:* Laxative, hyperosmotic

**Dosage and routes**
*Laxative*
*Adult and child >6 yr:* RECT SUPP 3 g; enema 5-15 ml
*Child <6 yr:* RECT SUPP 1-1.5 g; enema 2-5 ml

*Intraocular pressure reduction*
*Adult:* PO 1-1.5 g/kg once, then may be given 500 mg/kg q6hr
*Child:* PO 1-1.5 g/kg once, then 500 mg/kg 4-8 hr after first dose

---

 Alert    Canada Only    Drug on CD      * "Tall Man" lettering (See Preface)

Uses: Constipation, intraocular pressure reduction

Contraindications: Hypersensitivity

## guanfacine (Rx)
*Func. class.:* Antihypertensive

**Dosage and routes**
*Adult:* PO 1 mg/day at bedtime; may increase dose in 3-4 wk to 2 mg/day, max 4 mg/day

Uses: Hypertension in individual using a thiazide diuretic or other antihypertensives

Unlabeled uses: Heroin withdrawal, ADHD

Contraindications: Hypersensitivity

## hydroxychloroquine (Rx)
*Func. class.:* Antimalarial, antirheumatic (DMARDs)

**Dosage and routes**
*Malaria*
*Adult:* PO Suppression or prevention 200 mg qwk, begin 1-2 wk before travel, continue 4 wk after returning; treatment 400 mg, then 200 mg at 6, 24, 48 hr after 1st dose
*Child:* PO Suppression or prevention 5 mg/kg qwk, begin 1-2 wk before travel, continue 4 wk after returning; treatment 10 mg/kg, then 5 mg/kg at 6, 18, 24 hr after 1st dose

*Lupus erythematosus*
*Adult:* PO 400 mg daily-bid; length depends on patient response; maintenance 200-400 mg/day

*Rheumatoid arthritis*
*Adult:* PO 400-600 mg/day for 4-12 wk, then 200-300 mg/day after good response
*Child:* PO 3-5 mg/kg/day; max 400 mg/day

Uses: Malaria caused by *Plasmodium vivax, P. malariae, P. ovale, P. falciparum* (some strains); SLE, rheumatoid arthritis

Contraindications: Children (long term), hypersensitivity, retinal field changes

## idursulfase (Rx)
Elaprase
*Func. class.:* Enzyme replacement

**Dosage and routes**
*Adult:* IV INF 0.5 mg/kg/wk; dilute calculated volume of concentrated drug in 100 ml of 0.9% NaCl; use a 0.2 micron filter
*Child >5 yr:* IV INF 0.5 mg/kg/wk given over 1-3 hr

Uses: Mucopolysaccharidosis II (Hunter's syndrome) (MPS-11)

Contraindications: Hypersensitivity, IM/intrathecal administration

## isotretinoin (Rx)
*Func. class.:* Antiacne agent, retinoid

**Dosage and routes**
*Adult:* PO 0.5-2 mg/kg/day in 2 divided doses × 15-20 wk; if relapse occurs, repeat after 2 mo off product

Uses: Severe recalcitrant cystic acne

Contraindications: Pregnancy **X,** hypersensitivity, inflamed skin

## kanamycin (Rx)
*Func. class.:* Antiinfective

**Dosage and routes**
*Severe systemic infections*
*Adult and child:* IV INF 15 mg/kg/day in divided doses q8-12hr; diluted 500 mg/200 ml of NS or D5W given over 30-60 min, not to exceed 1.5 g/day; IM 15 mg/kg/day in divided doses q8-12hr, not to exceed 1.5 g/day; irrigation not to exceed 1.5 g/day; NEB/INH 250 mg qid

*Preoperative bowel sterilization*
*Adult:* PO 1 g qhr × 4 doses, then q6hr × 36-72 hr

*Renal dose*
*Adult:* IM/IV 7.5 mg/kg, may increase or decrease dose based on renal status

Uses: Severe systemic infections of CNS; respiratory, GI, urinary tract; bone, skin, soft tissues caused by *Escherichia coli, Acinetobacter, Proteus, Klebsiella pneumoniae, Pseudomonas aeruginosa, Serratia marcescens;* also used as an adjunct in hepatic coma, peritonitis, preoperatively to sterilize bowel; decreases ammonia-producing bacteria in bowel and IP after fecal spill during surgery

**Contraindications:** Pregnancy **D,** bowel obstruction, severe renal disease, hypersensitivity

## kunecatechins (Rx)
Veregen
*Func. class.:* Topical keratolytic

**Dosage and routes**
*Adult:* TOP Apply ointment using a 0.5-cm strand applied to warts tid; continue treatment until complete clearance has occurred, max 16 wk

**Uses:** External genital/perianal warts

**Contraindications:** Hypersensitivity

## lanthanum (Rx)
*Func. class.:* Electrolyte/renal agent

**Dosage and routes**
*Adult:* PO 750-1500 mg/day in divided doses with meals; titrate dose q2-3 wk until an acceptable phosphate level is reached; tabs should be chewed completely before swallowing; intact tabs should not be swallowed

**Uses:** End-stage renal disease

**Contraindications:** Hypophosphatemia, hypersensitivity

## laronidase (Rx)
*Func. class.:* Metabolic agent/enzymes

**Dosage and routes**
*Adult:* IV INF 0.58 mg/kg qwk infused over 3-4 hr; pretreat with antipyretic and/or antihistamines 1 hr prior to **IV** INF; max rate 200 mcg/kg/hr

**Uses:** Mucopolysaccharidosis I (MPSI), patients with Hurler and Hurler-Scheie forms of MPSI

**Contraindications:** Hypersensitivity

## magnesium salicylate (Rx, OTC)
*Func. class.:* Nonopioid analgesic, nonsteroidal antiinflammatory

**Dosage and routes**
*Arthritis*
*Adult:* PO not to exceed 4.8 g/day in divided doses

*Pain/fever*
*Adult:* PO 600 mg qid or 1160 mg tid

**Uses:** Mild to moderate pain or fever including arthritis, juvenile rheumatoid arthritis

**Contraindications:** Pregnancy **D** (1st trimester), children <12 yr, hypersensitivity to salicylates, GI bleeding, bleeding disorders, vit K deficiency

## miglustat (Rx)
*Func. class.:* Miscellaneous agent

**Dosage and routes**
*Adult:* PO 100 mg tid, without regard to food

**Uses:** Adults with mild to moderate type 1 Gaucher disease

**Contraindications:** Pregnancy **X,** hypersensitivity

## mitotane (Rx)
*Func. class.:* Antineoplastic

**Do not confuse:**
mitotane/mitomycin/mithramycin/mitoxantrone

**Dosage and routes**
*Adult:* PO 9-10 g/day in divided doses tid or qid; may have to decrease dosage if severe reactions occur; start with reduced dose and gradually increase

**Uses:** Adrenocortical carcinoma

**Contraindications:** Hypersensitivity

## neomycin (Rx)
*Func. class.:* Antiinfective

**Dosage and routes**
*Hepatic encephalopathy*
*Adult:* PO 4-12 g/day in divided doses × 5-6 days
*Child:* PO 50-100 mg/kg/day in divided doses q6hr × 5-6 days

*Preoperative intestinal antisepsis*
*Adult:* PO 1 g qhr × 4 hr, then 1 g q4hr for remaining 24 hr

**Uses:** Severe systemic infections of CNS, respiratory tract, GI tract, urinary tract, eye, bone, skin, soft tissues caused by *Pseudomonas aeruginosa, Escherichia coli, Enterobacter, Klebsiella pneumoniae, Proteus vulgaris;* also used for hepatic coma, preoperatively to sterilize bowel, infectious diarrhea caused by enteropathogenic *E. coli*

**Contraindications:** Infants, children, bowel obstruction (PO use), severe renal disease, hypersensitivity, GI disease

---

**papaverine** (Rx)
*Func. class.:* Peripheral vasodilator

**Dosage and routes**
*Adult:* SUS REL cap 150-300 mg q8-12hr; IM/**IV** 30-120 mg

**Uses:** Arterial spasm resulting in cerebral and peripheral ischemia, myocardial ischemia associated with vascular spasm or dysrhythmias, angina pectoris, peripheral pulmonary embolism, visceral spasm as in ureteral, biliary, GI colic, peripheral vascular disease

**Contraindications:** Hypersensitivity, complete AV heart block

---

**paromomycin** (Rx)
*Func. class.:* Amebicide

**Dosage and routes**
*Intestinal amebiasis*
*Adult and child:* PO 25-35 mg/kg/day in 3 divided doses × 5-10 day after meals

*Hepatic coma*
*Adult:* PO 4 g/day in divided doses × 5-6 day

**Uses:** Intestinal amebiasis, adjunct in hepatic coma

**Contraindications:** Hypersensitivity, renal disease, GI obstruction

---

**pegvisomant** (Rx)
*Func. class.:* Agent—miscellaneous

**Dosage and routes**
*Adult:* SUBCUT Loading dose of 40 mg, under supervision of prescriber, then SUBCUT 10 mg/day; measure IGF-I levels q4-6 wk

**Uses:** Acromegaly, in those patients who have an inadequate response to other treatment

**Contraindications:** Hypersensitivity, latex allergy

---

**permethrin** (OTC, Rx)
*Func. class.:* Pediculicide

**Dosage and routes**
*Lice (head)*
*Adult and child:* Wash hair, towel dry; apply liberally to hair, leave on 10 min, rinse with water; repeat in 7-10 days

*Scabies*
*Adult and child:* TOP 5% cream applied and massaged into all skin surfaces; leave cream on 8-14 hr, then wash; repeat in 7-10 days

**Uses:** Lice, nits, ticks, flea nits

**Contraindications:** Hypersensitivity

---

**phenelzine** (Rx)
*Func. class.:* Antidepressant, MAOI

**Dosage and routes**
*Adult:* PO 45 mg/day in divided doses; may increase to 60 mg/day; dose should be reduced to 15 mg/day, not to exceed 90 mg/day
*Geriatric:* PO 7.5 mg/day, increase by 7.5-15 mg q3-4 days; usual dose 15-60 mg/day in divided doses

**Uses:** Depression, when uncontrolled by other means

**Contraindications:** Hypersensitivity to MAOIs, hypertension, CHF, severe renal/hepatic/cardiac disease, pheochromocytoma, active alcoholism

---

**physostigmine** (Rx)
*Func. class.:* Antidote, reversible anticholinesterase

**Dosage and routes**
*Overdose of anticholinergics*
*Adult:* IM/**IV**/SUBCUT 0.5-2 mg; give no more than 1 mg/min; may repeat q20 min until response or adverse reactions; repeat 1-4 mg q30-60 min as life-threatening signs reoccur
*Child:* IM/**IV** inj 0.02 mg/kg, not more than 0.5 mg/min; may repeat at 5-10 min intervals until max dose of 2 mg is reached or adverse reaction occurs

---

Adverse effects: *italic* = common, **bold** = life-threatening

**Uses:** To reverse CNS effects of anticholinergic

**Contraindications:** Hypotension, obstruction of intestine or renal system, asthma, gangrene, CV disease, choline esters, depolarizing neuromuscular blocking agents, diabetes

---

## ! HIGH ALERT

### poractant alfa (Rx)
*Func. class.:* Lung surfactant extract

**Dosage and routes**
*Premature infant:* INTRATRACHEAL INSTILL 2.5 ml/kg birth weight, up to 2 subsequent doses of 1.25 ml/kg birth weight can be administered at 12-hr intervals, max 5 ml/kg

**Uses:** Treatment (rescue) of respiratory distress syndrome (RDS) in premature infants

**Contraindications:** Full-term infant, hypersensitivity

---

### pralidoxime (Rx)
*Func. class.:* Cholinesterase reactivator, nerve gas antidote

**Dosage and routes**
*Anticholinesterase overdose*
*Adult:* **IV** 1-2 g, then 250 mg q5 min until desired response

*Organophosphate poisoning*
*Adult:* **IV** INF 1-2 g/100 ml 0.9% NaCl over 15-30 min; may repeat in 1 hr; PO 1-3 g q5hr
*Child:* **IV** INF 20-40 mg/kg/dose diluted in 100 ml 0.9% NaCl over 15-30 min

**Uses:** Cholinergic crisis in myasthenia gravis, organophosphate poisoning antidote (early), relief of paralysis of respiratory muscles; used as an adjunct to systemic atropine administration

**Contraindications:** Hypersensitivity, carbamate insecticide poisoning

---

### reserpine (Rx)
*Func. class.:* Antihypertensive, antiadrenergic agent, peripherally acting

**Do not confuse:**
reserpine/Risperdal

**Dosage and routes**
*Adult:* PO 0.05-0.1 mg/day × 1-2 wk, then 0.1-0.25 mg/day for maintenance

*Geriatric:* PO 0.05 mg/day, increase by 0.05 weekly to desired dose

**Uses:** Hypertension

**Contraindications:** Pregnancy **D**, hypersensitivity, depression, suicidal patients, active peptic ulcer disease, ulcerative colitis, Parkinson's disease, renal failure

---

## ! HIGH ALERT

### secobarbital (Rx)
*Func. class.:* Sedative/hypnotic-barbiturate

**Controlled substance schedule II (USA), schedule G (CDSA IV) (Canada)**

**Dosage and routes**
*Insomnia*
*Adult:* PO/IM 100-200 mg at bedtime
*Child:* IM 3-5 mg/kg, max 100 mg, do not inject >5 ml in one site

*Sedation/preoperatively*
*Adult:* PO 200-300 mg 1-2 hr preoperatively
*Child:* PO 2-6 mg/kg 1-2 hr prior to surgery, max 100 mg; IM 4-5 mg/kg, max 100 mg

*Status epilepticus*
*Adult and child:* IM/**IV** 250-350 mg

*Acute psychotic agitation*
*Adult and child:* IM/**IV** 5.5 mg/kg q3-4hr

**Uses:** Insomnia, sedation, preoperative medication, acute tetanus seizures

**Unlabeled uses:** Status epilepticus

**Contraindications:** Pregnancy **D**, hypersensitivity to barbiturates, respiratory depression, addiction to barbiturates, severe liver impairment, porphyria, uncontrolled severe pain

---

### sevelamer (Rx)
*Func. class.:* Polymeric phosphate binder

**Dosage and routes**
Reduction of serum phosphorus in adults not taking phosphate binders
*Adult:* PO Initially 800-1600 mg tid with meals based on serum phosphorus level (see below); adjust dose gradually at 2-wk intervals until serum phosphorus 6 mg/dl

*Adult, serum phosphorus ≥9 mg/dl:* 1600 mg tid with meals

---

 Alert    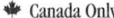 Canada Only    🕲 Drug on CD          * "Tall Man" lettering (See Preface)

*Adult, serum phosphorus ≥7.5 and <9 mg/dl:* 1200-1600 mg tid with meals

*Adult, serum phosphorus >6 and <7.5 mg/dl:* 800 mg tid with meals

**Uses:** End-stage renal disease (ESRD)

**Contraindications:** Hypophosphatemia, bowel obstruction, hypersensitivity

---

### sibutramine (Rx)
*Func. class.:* Appetite suppressant

**Controlled substance schedule IV**

**Dosage and routes**
*Adult:* PO 10 mg/day; may be increased to 15 mg/day after 4 wk, or lowered to 5 mg/day depending on response

**Uses:** Obesity in conjunction with other treatments

**Contraindications:** Breastfeeding, hypersensitivity, hypothyroidism, anorexia nervosa, severe renal/hepatic disease, uncontrolled hypertension, history of CAD, CHF, dysrhythmias, CVA

---

### teniposide (Rx)
*Func. class.:* Antineoplastic

**Dosage and routes**
*Child:* IV INF Combo teniposide 165 mg/m$^2$ and cytarabine 300 mg/m$^2$ 2×/wk × 8-9 doses or combo teniposide 250 mg/m$^2$ and vinCRIStine 1.5 mg/m$^2$ qwk × 4-8 wk and predniSONE 40 mg/m$^2$ PO × 28 days

**Uses:** Childhood acute lymphoblastic leukemia (ALL), refractory childhood acute lymphocytic leukemia

**Contraindications:** Pregnancy **D**, hypersensitivity, bone marrow depression, severe renal/hepatic disease, bacterial infection, polyoxethylated castor oil hypersensitivity

---

### testolactone (Rx)
*Func. class.:* Antineoplastic

**Controlled substance schedule III**

**Dosage and routes**
*Adult:* PO 250 mg qid

**Uses:** Advanced breast carcinoma in postmenopausal women

**Contraindications:** Breastfeeding, premenopausal women, hypersensitivity, carcinoma of male breast

---

### thioguanine (6-TG) (Rx)
*Func. class.:* Antineoplastic-antimetabolite

**Dosage and routes**
*Adult and child:* PO 2-2.5 mg/kg/day, then increase slowly to 3 mg/kg/day after 4 wk

**Uses:** Acute leukemias, chronic granulocytic leukemia, lymphomas, multiple myeloma, solid tumors

**Contraindications:** Pregnancy **D**, prior product resistance, leukopenia (WBC <2500/mm$^3$), thrombocytopenia (platelets <100,000/mm$^3$), anemia

---

### ⚠ HIGH ALERT

### thiopental (Rx)
*Func. class.:* General anesthetic

**Controlled substance schedule III**

**Dosage and routes**
*Induction and anesthesia*
*Adult:* IV 25-75 mg test dose, observe for 60 min; initial dose 50-100 mg given at 20-40 sec interval; additional 25-50 mg as needed
*Child 1-12 yr:* IV 5-6 mg/kg over 10-60 min, maintenance 1 mg/kg as needed
*Infant:* IV 5-8 mg/kg over 10-60 min
*Neonate:* IV 3-4 mg over 10-60 min

*Rapid induction*
*Adult:* IV 210-280 mg or 3-5 mg/kg in 2-4 divided doses
*Child:* IV 3-5 mg/kg over 20-30 sec, then 1 mg/kg as needed

*Narcoanalysis*
*Adult:* IV 100 mg/min, not to exceed 50 ml/min

*Sedation or narcosis*
*Adult:* RECT 30 mg/kg

**Uses:** Short, general anesthesia; narcoanalysis, induction anesthesia before other anesthetics, status epilepticus, increased ICP

**Contraindications:** Hypersensitivity, status asthmaticus, porphyrias

---

Adverse effects: *italic* = common, **bold** = life-threatening

## thiotepa (Rx)
*Func. class.:* Antineoplastic

**Dosage and routes**
*Adult:* **IV** 0.2 mg/kg q4 days, q2-4 wk
*Neoplastic effusions*
*Adult:* INTRACAVITY 0.6-0.8 mg/kg

*Bladder cancer*
*Adult:* INSTILL 60 mg/30-60 ml water for inj instilled in bladder for 2 hr once/wk × 4 wk

**Uses:** Hodgkin's disease, lymphomas; breast, ovarian, lung, bladder cancer; neoplastic effusions

**Contraindications:** Pregnancy **D**, hypersensitivity

## thiothixene (Rx)
*Func. class.:* Antipsychotic/neuroleptic

**Dosage and routes**
*Adult:* PO 2-5 mg bid-qid depending on severity of condition; dose gradually increased to 15-30 mg if needed; IM 4 mg bid-qid; max dose 30 mg/day; administer PO dose as soon as possible
*Geriatric:* PO 1-2 mg daily-bid, increase by 1-2 mg q4-7 days to desired dose

**Uses:** Psychotic disorders, schizophrenia, acute agitation

**Contraindications:** Child <12 yr, hypersensitivity, blood dyscrasias, bone marrow depression, circulatory collapse, CNS depression, coma, alcoholism, CV/hepatic disease, Reye's syndrome, angle-closure glaucoma

## tranylcypromine (Rx)
*Func. class.:* Antidepressant—MAOI

**Dosage and routes**
*Adult:* PO 10 mg bid; may increase to 30 mg/day after 2 wk; up to 60 mg/day

**Uses:** Depression, when uncontrolled by other means

**Unlabeled uses:** Bulimia, cocaine addiction, migraines, seasonal affective disorder, panic disorder

**Contraindications:** Geriatric, hypersensitivity to MAOIs, uncontrolled hypertension, CHF, severe renal/hepatic/cardiac disease, pheochromocytoma, suicidal patients

## trimipramine (Rx)
*Func. class.:* Antidepressant—tricyclic

**Dosage and routes**
*Adult:* PO 50-150 mg/day in divided doses, may be increased to 200 mg/day
*Geriatric:* PO 25 mg at bedtime, increase by 25 mg q3-7 days, max 100 mg/day
*Child >6 yr:* 25 mg at bedtime, may increase to 50 mg in children <12 yr or 75 mg in children >12 yr

**Uses:** Depression, enuresis in children

**Contraindications:** Hypersensitivity to tricyclics, recovery phase of MI, seizure disorders, prostatic hypertrophy

## Appendix D

### Ophthalmic, Nasal, Topical, and Otic Products

#### OPHTHALMIC PRODUCTS

**α-ADRENERGIC BLOCKER**
**dapiprazole (Rx)**
(da-pip'ra-zole)
Rev-Eyes

**ANESTHETICS**
**proparacaine (Rx)**
(proe-par'a-kane)
Alcaine, Diocaine ✤, Ophthaine,
Ophthetic
**tetracaine (Rx)**
(tet'ra-kane)
Minims Tetracaine ✤, Pontocaine,
Tetracaine

**ANTIHISTAMINES**
**azelastine (Rx)**
(ay-zell'ah-steen)
Optivar
**emedastine (Rx)**
(ee-med'-a-steen)
Emadine
**epinastine (Rx)**
(ep-een-as'teen)
Elestat
**ketotifen (Rx, OTC)**
(kee-toh-tif'en)
Zaditor
**levocabastine (Rx)**
(lee-voh-cab'ah-steen)
Livostin
**olopatadine (Rx)**
(oh-loh-pat'ah-deen)
Patanol

**ANTIINFECTIVES**
**azithromycin (Rx)**
(ay-zi-thro-my'sin)
AzaSite
**chloramphenicol (Rx)**
(klor-am-fen'i-kole)
AK-Chlor, Chloramphenicol, Chloromycetin
Ophthalmic, Chloroptic, Chloroptic S.O.P.,
Fenicol ✤, Isopto Fenical ✤,
Pentamycin ✤

**ciprofloxacin (Rx)**
(sip-ro-floks'a-sin)
Ciloxan
**erythromycin (Rx)**
(er-ith-roe-mye'sin)
Erythromycin, Ilotycin
**ganciclovir (Rx)**
(gan-sye'kloe-vir)
Virgan
**gatifloxacin (Rx)**
(gat-ih-floks'ah-sin)
Zymar
**gentamicin (Rx)**
(jen-ta-mye'sin)
Garamycin Ophthalmic, Genoptic
Ophthalmic, Genoptic S.O.P., Gentacidin,
Gentamicin Ophthalmic, Gentak
**levofloxacin (Rx)**
(lee-voh-flock'sah-sin)
Quixin
**moxifloxacin (Rx)**
(mox-i-flox'a-sin)
Vigamox
**natamycin (Rx)**
(nat-a-mye'sin)
Natacyn
**norfloxacin (Rx)**
(nor-floks'a-sin)
Chibroxin
**ofloxacin (Rx)**
(oh-floks'a-sin)
Ocuflox
**silver nitrate 1% (Rx)**
**silver nitrate**
**sulfacetamide sodium (Rx)**
(sul-fa-seet'a-mide)
AK-Sulf, Bleph-10, Bleph-10 S.O.P.,
Cetamide, Isopto Cetamide, Ocusulf-10,
Sodium Sulamyd, Sodium Sulfacetamide,
Storzsulf, Sulf-10, Sulster

Adverse effects: *italic* = common, **bold** = life-threatening

**tobramycin** (Rx)
(toe-bra-mye'sin)
AKTob, Defy, Tobrex
**trifluridine** (Rx)
(trye-floor'i-deen)
Viroptic
**vidarabine** (Rx)
(vye-dare'a-been)
Vira-A

**β-ADRENERGIC BLOCKERS**
**betaxolol** (Rx)
(beh-tax'oh-lole)
Betoptic, Betoptic S
**carteolol** (Rx)
(kar-tee'oh-lole)
Carteolol HCl, Ocupress
**levobetaxolol** (Rx)
(lee-voh-beh-tax'oh-lohl)
Betaxon
**levobunolol** (Rx)
(lee-voe-byoo'no-lole)
AK Beta, Betagen
**metipranolol** (Rx)
(met-ee-pran'oh-lole)
OptiPranolol
**timolol** (Rx)
(tym'-moe-lole)
Apo-Timop ✦, Betimol, Timoptic,
Timoptic-XE

**CARBONIC ANHYDRASE
INHIBITORS**
**brinzolamide** (Rx)
(brin-zoh'la-mide)
Azopt
**dorzolamide** (Rx)
(dor-zol'a-mide)
Trusopt

**CHOLINERGICS
(Direct-acting)**
**acetylcholine** (Rx)
(ah-see-til-koe'leen)
Miochol-E
**carbachol** (Rx)
(kar'ba-kole)
Carbastat, Carboptic, Isopto Carbachol,
Miostat

**pilocarpine** (Rx)
(pye-loe-kar'peen)
Adsorbocarpine, Akarpine, Isopto Carpine,
Ocu-Carpine, Ocusert Pilo-20, Ocusert Pilo-
40, Pilagan, Pilocar, pilocarpine, Pilopine
HS, Piloptic-½, Piloptic-1, Piloptic-2,
Piloptic-3, Piloptic-4, Piloptic-6, Pilostat,
Pilopto-Carpine

**CHOLINESTERASE INHIBITORS**
**demecarium** (Rx)
(dem-e-kare'ee-um)
Humorsol
**ecothiophate** (Rx)
(ek-oh-thye'oh-fate)
Phospholine Iodide
**isoflurophate** (Rx)
(i-se'flur-e'fate)
Floropryl
**physostigmine** (Rx)
(fi-zoe-stig'meen)
Eserine Salicylate, Isopto Eserine

**CORTICOSTEROIDS**
**dexamethasone** (Rx)
(dex-a-meth'a-sone)
AK-Dex, Decadron Phosphate,
Dexamethasone Ophthalmic Suspension,
Maxidex
**fluorometholone** (Rx)
(flure-oh-meth'oh-lone)
Flarex, Fluor-Op, FML, FML Forte, FML
S.O.P.
**loteprednol** (Rx)
(loe-tee-pred-nole)
Alrex, Lotemax
**medrysone** (Rx)
(me'dri-sone)
HMS
*****prednisoLONE** (Rx)
(pred-niss'oh-lone)
Econopred, Econopred Plus, AK-Pred,
Inflamase Forte, Inflamase Mild, Pred-Forte
**rimexolone** (Rx)
(ri-mex'a-lone)
Vexol
**triamcinolone** (Rx)
(trye-am-sin'oh-lone)
Triesence

**MYDRIATICS**
**atropine** (Rx)
(a′troe-peen)
Atropine-1, Atropine Care, Atropine Sulfate
Ophthalmic, Atropisol, Isopto Atropine
**cyclopentolate** (Rx)
(sye-kloe-pen′toe-late)
AK-Pentolate, Cyclogyl, Cyclopentolate HCl
**homatropine** (Rx)
(home-a′troe-peen)
Homatropine ✦, Homatropine HBr, Isopto
Homatropine, Minims
**phenylephrine** (OTC)
(fen-ill-ef′rin)
AK-Dilate, AK-Nefrin, Isopto Frin, Neo-
Synephrine 2.5%, Neo-Synephrine 10%,
phenylephrine HCl, 2.5% Mydfrin,
Phenoptic Relief, Prefrin
**scopolamine** (Rx)
(skoe-pol′a-meen)
Isopto Hyoscine
**tropicamide** (Rx)
(troe-pik′a-mide)
Mydriacyl, Opticyl, Tropicacyl, Tropicamide

**NONSTEROIDAL**
**ANTIINFLAMMATORIES**
**bromfenac** (Rx)
(brome′fen-ak)
Xibrom
**diclofenac** (Rx)
(dye-kloe′fen-ak)
Voltaran
**flurbiprofen** (Rx)
(flure-bi′-pro-fen)
Ocufen
**ketorolac** (Rx)
(kee-toe′role-ak)
Acular
**nepafenac** (Rx)
(ne-pa-fen′ak)
Nevanac
**suprofen** (Rx)
(soo-proe′fen)
Profenal

**SYMPATHOMIMETICS**
**apraclonidine** (Rx)
(a-pra-klon′i-deen)
Iopidine

**brimonidine** (Rx)
(brem-on′-i-dine)
Alphagan, Alphagan P
**dipivefrin** (Rx)
(dye-pi′vef-rin)
Propine, AKPro
*****epINEPHrine/epinephryl**
**borate** (Rx)
(ep-i-nef′rin)
Epifrin, Glaucon/Epinal, Eppy ✦

**OPHTHALMIC DECONGESTANTS/**
**VASOCONSTRICTORS**
**Iodoxamide**
(loe-dox′ah-mide)
Alomide
**naphazoline** (Rx, OTC)
(naf-az′oh-leen)
20/20 Eye Drops, AK-Con, Allergy Drops,
Albalon, Allerest Eye Drops, Clear Eyes,
Clear Eyes ACR, Comfort Eye Drops, Degest
2, Maximum Strength Allergy Drops,
Nafazair, naphazoline HCl, Naphcon,
Naphcon Forte, Opcon, Vasoclear, Vasocon
Regular
**oxymetazoline** (Rx)
(ox-i-met-ah-zoh′leen)
OcuClear, Visine L.R.
**tetrahydrozoline** (OTC)
(tet-ra-hye-dro′zoe-leen)
Collyrium Fresh, Eyesine, Geneye, Geneye
Extra, Mallazine Eye Drops, Murine Plus,
Optigene 3, tetrahydrozoline HCl,
Tetrasine, Tetrasine Extra, Visine
Moisturizing

**MISCELLANEOUS OPHTHALMICS**
**bimatoprost** (Rx)
(bih-mat′o-prost)
Lumigan
**latanoprost** (Rx)
(la-tan′oh-prost)
Xalatan
**travoprost** (Rx)
(tra′voe-prost)
Travatan
**unoprostone** (Rx)
(yoo-noe-pros′tone)
Rescula

**β-Adrenergic blockers**
**Action:** Reduces production of aqueous
humor by unknown mechanism

---

Adverse effects: *italic* = common, **bold** = life-threatening

**Uses:** Ocular hypertension, chronic open-angle glaucoma

### Anesthetics

**Action:** Decreases ion permeability by stabilizing neuronal membrane

**Uses:** Cataract extraction, tonometry, gonioscopy, removal of foreign objects, corneal suture removal, glaucoma surgery (ophthalmic); pruritus, sunburn, toothache, sore throat, cold sores, oral pain, rectal pain and irritation, control of gagging (topical)

### Antiinfectives

**Action:** Inhibits folic acid synthesis by preventing PABA use, which is necessary for bacterial growth

**Uses:** Conjunctivitis, superficial eye infections, corneal ulcers, prophylaxis against infection after removal of foreign matter from the eye

### Antiinflammatories

**Action:** Decreases inflammation, resulting in decreased pain, photophobia, hyperemia, cellular infiltration

**Uses:** Inflammation of eye, eyelids, conjunctiva, cornea; uveitis, iridocyclitis, allergic conditions, burns, foreign bodies, postoperatively in cataract

### Carbonic anhydrase inhibitor

**Action:** Converted to epINEPHrine, which decreases aqueous production and increases outflow

**Uses:** Open-angle glaucoma, ocular hypertension

### Direct-acting miotic

**Action:** Acts directly on cholinergic receptor sites; induces miosis, spasm of accommodation, fall in intraocular pressure, caused by stimulation of ciliary, pupillary sphincter muscles, which leads to pulling away of iris from filtration angle, resulting in increased outflow of aqueous humor

**Uses:** Primary glaucoma, early stages of wide-angle glaucoma (less useful in advanced stages), chronic open-angle glaucoma, acute angle-closure glaucoma before emergency surgery; also neutralizes mydriatics used during eye exam; may be used alternately with mydriatics to break adhesions between iris and lens

### Adverse effects

***CNS:*** Headache
***CV:*** Hypertension, tachycardia, dysrhythmias
***EENT:*** Burning, stinging
***GI:*** Bitter taste

**Contraindications:** Hypersensitivity

**Precautions:** Pregnancy, breastfeeding, children, aphakia, hypersensitivity to carbonic anhydrase inhibitors, sulfonamides, thiazide diuretics, ocular inhibitors, renal/hepatic insufficiency

### NURSING CONSIDERATIONS
### Assessment

* Monitor ophthalmic exams and intraocular pressure readings
* Monitor blood counts; renal/hepatic function tests and serum electrolytes during long-term treatment

### Nursing diagnoses

* Knowledge, deficient (teaching)
* Sensory perception, disturbed: visual (uses)

### Implementation

* Storage at room temperature away from light

### Patient/family education

* Teach how to instill drops
* Advise patient that product may cause burning, itching, blurring, dryness of eye area

### Evaluation

**Positive therapeutic outcome**
* Absence of increased intraocular pressure

## NASAL AGENTS

**NASAL DECONGESTANTS**
**azelastine** (Rx)
(ay-zell'ah-steen)
Astelin
**desoxyephedrine** (OTC)
(des-oxy-e-fed'rin)
Vicks Vapor Inhaler
***epHEDrine** (OTC)
(e-fed'rin)
Pretz-D
***epINEPHrine** (OTC)
(ep-i-neff'rin)
Adrenalin
**naphazoline** (OTC)
(naff-a-zoe'leen)
Privine

**oxymetazoline** (OTC)
(ox-i-met-az'oh-leen)

12 Hour Nasal, Afrin 12 Hour Original, Afrin 12-Hour Original Pump Mist, Afrin Severe Congestion With Menthol, Afrin Sinus With Vapornase, Afrin No-Drip 12-Hour, Afrin No-Drip 12-Hour Extra Moisturizing, Dristan, Duramist Plus, Duration, Genasal, Nafrine ✦, Neo-Synephrine 12 Hour, Nostrilla, oxymetazoline HCl, Nasal Relief, Nasal Decongestant Maximum Strength, Vicks Sinex 12 Hour Long-Acting, Vicks Sinex 12-Hour Ultra Fine Mist for Sinus Relief

**phenylephrine** (OTC)
(fen-ill-eff'rin)

Alconefrin 12, Children's Nostril, Neo-Synephrine, Sinex

**propylhexadrine** (OTC)
(proe-pil-hex'a-dreen)

Benzedrex Inhaler

**pseudoephedrine** (Rx, OTC)
(soo-doe-e-fed'rin)

Cenafed, Decofed, Dimetapp, Genaphed, Sudafed, Triaminic

**tetrahydrozoline** (OTC)
(tet-ra-hye-dro'zoe-leen)

Tyzine, Tyzine Pediatric

**xylometazoline** (OTC)
(zye-loh-meh-tazz'oh-leen)

Natru-vent, Otrivin, Otrivin Pediatric Nasal

**NASAL STEROIDS**
**beclomethasone** (Rx)
(be-kloe-meth'a-sone)

Beconase AQ Nasal, Beconase Inhalation, Vancenase AQ Nasal, Vancenase Pocket Inhaler

**budesonide** (Rx)
(byoo-des'oh-nide)

Rhinocort, Rhinocort Aqua

**flunisolide** (Rx)
(floo-niss'oh-lide)

Nasalide, Nasarel

**fluticasone** (Rx)
(floo-tic'a-son)

Flonase, Veramyst

**triamcinolone** (Rx)
(trye-am-sin'oh-lone)

Nasacort AQ

**Action:** Produces vasoconstriction (rapid, long acting) of arterioles, thereby decreasing fluid exudation, mucosal engorgement by stimulation of α-adrenergic receptors in vascular smooth muscle

**Therapeutic outcome:** Absence of nasal congestion

**Uses:** Nasal congestion

**Dosage and routes**
*Desoxyephedrine*
***Adult and child >6 yr:*** 1-2 INH in each nostril q2hr or less

*EpHEDrine*
***Adult:*** Fill dropper to the level marked, then use in each nostril q4hr or less

*EpINEPHrine*
***Adult and child >6 yr:*** Apply with swab, drops, spray prn

*Naphazoline*
***Adult and child >6 yr:*** 1-2 drops/spray q6hr or less

*Oxymetazoline*
***Adult and child >6 yr:*** INSTILL 2-3 gtt or sprays to each nostril bid
***Child 2-6 yr:*** INSTILL 2-3 gtt or sprays 0.025 sol bid, not to exceed 3 days

*Phenylephrine*
***Adult and child >12 yr:*** 2-3 drops/spray (0.25-0.5) in each nostril: q3-4hr or less; or 2-3 drops/spray (1%) in each nostril q4hr or less
***Child 6-12 yr:*** 2-3 drops/spray (0.25%) in each nostril q3-4hr
***Infant >6 mo:*** 1-2 drops (0.16%) in each nostril q3hr

*Propylhexadrine*
***Adult and child >6 yr:*** 1-2 INH in each nostril q2hr or less

*Tetrahydrozoline*
***Adult and child >6 yr:*** 2-4 drops (0.1%) q3-4hr prn or 3-4 sprays in each nostril q4hr prn
***Child 2-6 yr:*** 2-3 drops (0.05%) in each nostril q4-6hr prn

*Xylometazoline*
***Adult and child >12 yr:*** 2-3 drops/spray (0.1%) in each nostril q8-10hr
***Child 2-12 yr:*** 2-3 drops (0.05%) in each nostril q8-10hr

**Available forms:** Nasal sol 0.025%, 0.05%
**Adverse effects**
*CNS:* Anxiety, restlessness, tremors, weakness, insomnia, dizziness, fever, headache
*EENT:* Irritation, burning, sneezing, stinging, dryness, rebound congestion
*GI:* Nausea, vomiting, anorexia
*INTEG:* Contact dermatitis

Adverse effects: *italic* = common, **bold** = life-threatening

**Contraindications:** Hypersensitivity to sympathomimetic amines

**Precautions:** Pregnancy **C**, children <6 yr, geriatric, diabetes, CV disease, hypertension, hyperthyroidism, increased ICP, prostatic hypertrophy, glaucoma

## NURSING CONSIDERATIONS
### Assessment
• Assess for redness, swelling, pain in nasal passages before and during treatment
• Assess for systemic absorption; hypertension, tachycardia; notify prescriber; systemic absorption occurs at high doses or after prolonged use

### Nursing diagnoses
• Airway clearance, ineffective (uses)
• Knowledge, deficient (teaching)
• Noncompliance (teaching)

### Implementation
• Have patient tilt head back, squeeze bulb to create a vacuum, and draw correct amount of sol into dropper; insert 2 gtt of sol into nostril; repeat in other nostril
• Store in light-resistant container; do not expose to high temperature or let sol come into contact with aluminum
• Give for <4 consecutive days
• Provide environmental humidification to decrease nasal congestion, dryness

### Patient/family education
• Advise patient that stinging may occur for several applications; drying of mucosa may be decreased by environmental humidification
• Caution patient to notify prescriber if irregular pulse, insomnia, dizziness, or tremors occur
• Teach patient proper administration to avoid systemic absorption
• Advise patient to rinse dropper with very hot water to prevent contamination

### Evaluation
**Positive therapeutic outcome**
• Decreased nasal congestion

## TOPICAL GLUCOCORTICOIDS

**betamethasone** (Rx)
(bay-ta-meth'a-sone)
Alphatrex, Beben ♣, Betacort ♣, Betatrex, Beta-Val, Betnovate ♣, Celestoderm ♣, Diprosone, Ectosonel ♣, Luxiq, Maxivate, Metaderm ♣, Psorion, Valisone

**betamethasone (augmented)** (Rx)
(bay-ta-meth'a-sone)
Diprolene, Diprolene AF

**clobetasol** (Rx)
(kloe-bay'ta-sol)
Clobex, Cormax, Dermovate ♣, Embeline E 0.05%, Temovate

**desonide** (Rx)
(dess'oh-nide)
Verdeso Foam

**desoximetasone** (Rx)
(dess-ox-i-met'a-sone)
Topicort, Topicort LP

**dexamethasone** (Rx)
(dex-a-meth'a-sone)
Aeroseb-Dex, Decaspray

**fluocinolone** (Rx)
(floo-oh-sin'oh-lone)
Fluocin, Licon, Lidemol ♣, Lidex, Lyderm ♣, Topsyn ♣, Vasoderm

**flurandrenolide** (Rx)
(flure-an-dren'oh-lide)
Cordran, Cordran SP, Drenison 1/4 ♣, Drenison Tape ♣

**fluticasone** (Rx)
(floo-tik'a-sone)
Cutivate

**halcinonide** (Rx)
(hal-sin'oh-nide)
Halog, Halog-E

## hydrocortisone (Rx)
(hye-droe-kor'ti-sone)

Actiocort, Aeroseb-HC, Ala-Cort, Allercort, Alphaderm, Anusol HC, Bactine, Barriere-HC ♦, CaldeCORT Anti-Itch, Carmol HC, Cetacort, Cortacet ♦, Cortaid, Cortate ♦, Cort-Dome, Cortef ♦, Corticaine, Corticreme ♦, Cortifair, Cortizone, Cortoderm ♦, Cortril, Delcort, Dermacort, DemiCort, Dermtex HC, Emo-Cort, Epifoam, FoilleCort, Gly-Cort, Gynecort, Hi-Cor, Hycort, Hyderm ♦, Hydro-Tex, Hytone, Lacti-Care-HC, Lanacort, Lemoderm, Locoid, Locoid Lotion, My Cort, Novoehydrocort ♦, Nutracort Pharm, Pharmacort, Pentacort, Rederm, Rhulicort S-T Cort, Synacort, Sarna HC ♦, Texa-Cort, Unicort ♦, Westcort

## triamcinolone (Rx)
(trye-am-sin'oh-lone)

Aristocort, Delta-Tritex, Flutex, Kenac, Kenalog, Kenonel, Triaderm, Trianide ♦, Triderm, Trymex

**Action:** Antipruritic, antiinflammatory

**Therapeutic outcome:** Decreased itching, inflammation

**Uses:** Psoriasis, eczema, contact dermatitis, pruritus; usually reserved for severe dermatoses that have not responded to less potent formulation

### Dosage and routes
*Adult and child:* Apply to affected area

### Adverse effects
*INTEG: Acne, atrophy, epidermal thinning, purpura, striae*

**Contraindications:** Hypersensitivity, viral infections, fungal infections

**Precautions:** Pregnancy **C**

### NURSING CONSIDERATIONS
### Assessment
• Monitor temp; if fever develops, product should be discontinued
• Monitor for systemic absorption, increased temp, inflammation, irritation

### Nursing diagnoses
• Knowledge, deficient (teaching)
• Pain, chronic (uses)
• Skin integrity, impaired (uses)

### Implementation
• Apply only to affected areas; do not get in eyes
• Apply and leave site uncovered or lightly covered; occlusive dressing is not recommended—systemic absorption may occur
• Use only on dermatoses; do not use on weeping, denuded, or infected area
• Cleanse area before application of product
• Continue treatment for a few days after area has cleared
• Store at room temperature

### Patient/family education
• Teach patient to avoid sunlight on affected area, burns may occur
• Teach patient to limit treatment to 14 days

### Evaluation
**Positive therapeutic outcome**
• Absence of severe itching, patches on skin, flaking

## TOPICAL ANTIFUNGALS

## clotrimazole (OTC)
(kloe-trye'ma-zole)

Canestew ♦, Clotrimaderm ♦, Clotrimazole, Cruex, Desenex, Lotrimin AF, Myclo ♦, Neozol ♦

## econazole (OTC)
(ee-kon'a-zole)

Spectazole

## ketoconazole (OTC)
(kee-toe-kon'a-zole)

Nizoral, Xolegel

## miconazole (OTC)
(mye-kon'a-zole)

Absorbine Antifungal Foot Powder, Breeze Mist Antifungal, Fungoid Tincture, Lotrimin AF, Maximum Strength Desenex Antifungal, Micatin, Monistat-Derm, Ony-Clear, Tetterine, ZeaSob-AF

## nystatin (OTC)
(nye-stat'in)

Mycostatin, Nodostine ♦, Nilstat, Nyoderm ♦, Nystex

## selenium (OTC)
(see-leen'ee-um)

Exsel, Head and Shoulders Intensive Treatment, Selenium Sulfide, Selsun, Selsun Blue

## terbinafine (OTC)
(ter-bin'a-feen)

Lamisil

Adverse effects: *italic* = common, **bold** = life-threatening

## tolnaftate (OTC)
(tole-naf'tate)

Absorbine Athlete's Foot Cream, Aftate for Athlete's Foot, Aftate for Jock Itch, Genaspor, Quinsana Plus, Tinactin, Ting, tolnaftate

## undecylenic acid (OTC)
(un-deh-sih-len'ik)

Blis-To-Sol, Breeze Mist, Caldesene, Cruex, Decylenes, Desenex, Desenex Maximum Strength, Pedi-Pro, Phicon F, Protectol

**Action:** Interferes with fungal cell membrane permeability

**Therapeutic outcome:** Absence of itching and white patches of the skin

**Uses:** Tinea cruris, tinea pedis, diaper rash, minor skin irritations; amphotericin B is used for *Candida* infections

### Dosage and routes
Massage into affected area, surrounding area daily or bid, continue for 7-14 days, not to exceed 4 wk

### Adverse effects
***INTEG:*** Burning, stinging, dryness, itching, local irritation

**Contraindications:** Hypersensitivity

**Precautions:** Pregnancy **B,** breastfeeding, children

### NURSING CONSIDERATIONS
### Assessment
• Assess skin for fungal infections; peeling, dryness, itching before and throughout treatment
• Assess for continuing infection; increased size, number of lesions

### Nursing diagnoses
• Infection, risk for (uses)
• Knowledge, deficient (teaching)
• Skin integrity, impaired (uses)

### Implementation
• Apply to affected area, surrounding area; do not cover with occlusive dressings
• Store below 30° C (86° F)

### Teach patient/family
• Instruct to apply with glove to prevent further infection; not to cover with occlusive dressings
• Teach patient that long-term therapy may be needed to clear infection (2 wk-6 mo depending on organism); compliance is needed even after feeling better
• Teach patient proper hygiene; hand-washing technique, nail care, use of concomitant top agents if prescribed
• Caution patient to avoid use of OTC creams, ointments, lotions unless directed by prescriber
• Instruct patient to use medical asepsis (hand washing) before, after each application; to change socks and shoes once a day during treatment of tinea pedis
• Advise patient to report to health care prescriber if infection persists or recurs; if blisters, burning, oozing, swelling occur
• Caution patient to avoid alcohol because nausea, vomiting, hypertension may occur
• Caution patient to use sunscreen or avoid direct sunlight to prevent photosensitivity
• Advise patient to notify prescriber of sore throat, fever, skin rash, which may indicate overgrowth of organisms

### Evaluation
### Positive therapeutic outcome
• Decrease in size, number of lesions

## TOPICAL ANTIINFECTIVES

## azelaic acid (Rx)
(a-zuh-lay'ic)

Azelex, Finacea

## bacitracin (OTC)
(bass-i-tray'sin)

Bacitin ✦, Bacitracin

## clindamycin (Rx)
(klin-da-my'sin)

Cleocin T, Clindets, Clindagel, ClindaMax

## erythromycin (Rx, OTC)
(er-ith-roe-mye'sin)

A/T/S, Akne-Mycin, Eryderm, Erygel, Erythromycin, Staticin, T-Stat

## gentamicin (Rx)
(jen-ta-mye'sin)

Gentamicin

## mafenide (Rx)
(ma'fe-nide)

Sulfamylon

## metronidazole (Rx)
(met-roh-nye'da-zole)

MetroGel, MetroCream, MetroLotion, Noritate

## mupirocin (Rx)
(myoo-peer'oh-sin)

Bactroban

## neomycin (OTC)
(nee-oh-mye'sin)

Neomycin Sulfate

**nitrofurazone** (Rx)
(nye-troe-fyoor′a-zone)
Furacin, Nitrofurazone
**retapamulin** (Rx)
(re-tap′a-mue′lin)
Altabax
**salicylic acid** (Rx)
(sal′i-sil′ik)
Salitop
*__silver sulfADIAZINE__ (Rx)
(sul-fa-dye′a-zeen)
Flamazine ♣, Silvadene, SSD, SSD AF,
Thermazene
**tretinoin** (Rx)
(treh′tih-noyn)
Atralin

**Action:** Interferes with bacterial protein
synthesis

**Therapeutic outcome:** Resolution of
infection

**Uses:** Skin infections, minor burns, wounds,
skin grafts, primary pyodermas, otitis externa

**Adverse effects**
*INTEG:* Rash, urticaria, scaling, redness

**Contraindications:** Hypersensitivity, large
areas, burns, ulcerations

**Precautions:** Pregnancy **C**, breastfeeding,
impaired renal function, external ear or
perforated eardrum

**NURSING CONSIDERATIONS**
**Assessment**
• Assess for allergic reaction: burning, sting-
ing, swelling, redness
• Assess for signs of nephrotoxicity or ototox-
icity

**Nursing diagnoses**
• Infection, risk for (uses)
• Knowledge, deficient (teaching)
• Skin integrity, impaired (uses)

**Implementation**
• Apply enough medication to cover lesions
completely
• Apply after cleansing with soap, water
before each application; dry well
• Apply to less than 20% of body surface area
when patient has impaired renal function
• Store at room temperature in dry place

**Evaluation**
**Positive therapeutic outcome**
• Decrease in size, number of lesions

**TOPICAL ANTIVIRALS**

**acyclovir** (Rx)
(ay-sye′kloe-ver)
Zovirax
**penciclovir** (Rx)
(pen-sye′kloe-ver)
Denavir

**Action:** Interferes with viral DNA replication

**Therapeutic outcome:** Resolution of
infection

**Uses:** Simple mucocutaneous herpes simplex, in immunocompromised clients with
initial herpes genitalis

**Adverse effects**
*INTEG:* Rash, urticaria, stinging, burning,
pruritus, vulvitis

**Contraindications:** Hypersensitivity

**Precautions:** Pregnancy **C**, breastfeeding

**NURSING CONSIDERATIONS**
**Assessment**
• Assess for allergic reaction: burning, sting-
ing, swelling, redness, rash, vulvitis, pruritus
• Assess for signs of nephrotoxicity or ototox-
icity

**Nursing diagnoses**
• Infection, risk for (uses)
• Knowledge, deficient (teaching)
• Skin integrity, impaired (uses)

**Implementation**
• Apply with finger cot or rubber glove to
prevent further infection
• Apply enough medication to cover lesions
completely
• Apply after cleansing with soap, water
before each application; dry well
• Store at room temperature in dry place

**Patient/family education**
• Teach patient not to use in eyes or when
there is no evidence of infection
• Advise patient to apply with glove to prevent
further infection
• Advise patient to avoid use of OTC creams,
ointments, lotions unless directed by prescriber
• Advise patient to use medical asepsis (hand
washing) before, after each application and
avoid contact with eyes
• Advise patient to adhere strictly to prescribed regimen to maximize successful
treatment outcome
• Advise patient to begin taking product when
symptoms arise

Adverse effects: *italic* = common, **bold** = life-threatening

Evaluation
**Positive therapeutic outcome**
• Decrease in size, number of lesions

## TOPICAL ANESTHETICS

**benzocaine** (OTC)
(ben'zoe-kane)
Americaine Anesthetic, Anbesol Maximum Strength, Baby Anbesol, Biozene, Boil-Ease, Children's Chloraseptic, Dermoplast, Foille, Foille Plus, Hurricaine, Lanacane, Medamint, Orabase, Oracin, Ora-Jel
**dibucaine** (OTC)
(dye'byoo-kane)
Dibucaine, Nupercainal
**lidocaine** (Rx, OTC)
(lye'doe-kane)
Anestacon, Burn-O-Jel, Dentipatch, Derma Flex, ELA-Max, Lidocaine HCl Topical, Lidocaine Viscous, Numby Staff, Solarcaine Aloe Extra Burn Relief, Xylocaine, Xylocaine 10% Oral, Xylocaine Viscous, Zilactin-L
**pramoxine** (OTC)
(pra-mox'een)
Itch-X, PrameGel, Prax, Tronothane
**tetracaine** (OTC, Rx)
(tet'ra-cane)
Pontocaine, Viractin

**Action:** Inhibits conduction of nerve impulses from sensory nerves

**Therapeutic outcome:** Decreasing inflammation, itching, pain

**Uses:** Oral irritation, sore throat, toothache, cold sore, canker sore, sunburn, minor cuts, insect bites, pain, itching

**Dosage and routes**
*Adult and child:* TOP apply qid as needed; RECT insert tid and after each BM
**Adverse effects**
*INTEG:* Rash, irritation, sensitization

**Contraindications:** Hypersensitivity, infants <1 yr, application to large areas

**Precautions:** Pregnancy **C,** children <6 yr, sepsis, denuded skin

**NURSING CONSIDERATIONS**
**Assessment**
• Assess pain: location, duration, characteristics before and after administration
• Assess for infection: redness, drainage, inflammation; this product should not be used until infection is treated

**Nursing diagnoses**
• Knowledge, deficient (teaching)
• Pain, acute (uses)

**Implementation**
• Store in tight, light-resistant container; do not freeze, puncture, or incinerate aerosol container

**Patient/family education**
• Teach patient to avoid contact with eyes
• Teach patient not to use for prolonged periods: use for <1 wk; if condition remains, prescriber should be contacted

**Evaluation**
**Positive therapeutic outcome**
• Decreased redness, swelling, pain

## TOPICAL MISCELLANEOUS

**docosanol** (OTC)
(doh-koh'sah-nohl)
Abreva
**pimecrolimus** (Rx)
(pim-eh-kroh-ly'mus)
Elidel

**Action:** Docosanol unknown; pimecrolimus may bind with macrophilin and inhibit calcium-dependent phosphatase

**Therapeutic outcome:** Decreased redness, swelling, pain

**Uses:** Docosanol applied to fever blisters to promote more rapid healing; pimecrolimus used to treat mild to moderate atopic dermatitis in nonimmunocompromised patients ≥2 yr who are unresponsive to other treatment

**Dosage and routes**
*Docosanol*
*Adult:* TOP Rub into blisters 5×/day until healing occurs

*Pimecrolimus*
*Adult and child ≥2 yr:* TOP Apply thin layer 2×/day and rub in, use as long as needed

**Adverse effects**
*Docosanol*
None known

*Pimecrolimus*
*INTEG:* Burning

**Contraindications:** Hypersensitivity

**Precautions:** Pregnancy **C,** breastfeeding, dermal infections

## NURSING CONSIDERATIONS
### Assessment
• Assess skin condition (color, pain, inflammation) before and after administration
• Assess for signs and symptoms of skin infections (redness, draining lesions); if present, avoid use of product (pimecrolimus)

### Nursing diagnoses
• Skin integrity, impaired (uses)
• Infection, risk for (uses)
• Knowledge, deficient (teaching)

### Implementation
• Apply to skin, rub in gently

### Patient/family education
• Advise patient to avoid contact between medication and eyes
• Instruct patient to discontinue use of product when condition clears

### Evaluation
**Positive therapeutic outcome**
• Decreased inflammation, redness

## VAGINAL ANTIFUNGALS

**butoconazole** (OTC)
(byoo-toh-kone'ah-zole)
Femstat-3, Gynazol-1, Mycelex-3
**clotrimazole** (OTC)
(kloe-trye'ma-zole)
Canesten ✤, Clotriamazole, Gyne-Lotrimin 3, Gyne-Lotrimin 7, Mycelex 7, Myclo ✤
**miconazole** (OTC)
(mye-kon'a-zole)
Femizole-M, Monistat, Monistat 3, Monistat 7, Monistat Dual Pak, M-Zole 7 Dual Pack
**nystatin** (OTC)
(nye-stat'in)
Nystatin
**terconazole** (OTC)
(ter-kone'ah-zole)
Terazol 7, Tetrazol 3
**tioconazole** (OTC)
(tye-oh-kone'ah-zole)
Gyne-Trosyd ✤, Monistat 1, Vagistat-1

**Action:** Interferes with fungal DNA replication; binds sterols in fungal cell membranes, which increases permeability, leaking of nutrients

**Therapeutic outcome:** Fungistatic/fungicidal against susceptible organisms: *Candida* only

**Uses:** Vaginal, vulval, vulvovaginal candidiasis (moniliasis)

### Dosage and routes
*Butoconazole*
*Adult:* VAG 5 g (1 applicator) at bedtime × 3-6 days

*Clotrimazole*
*Adult:* 100 mg (1 vag tab, 100 mg) at bedtime × 1 wk, or 200 mg (2 vag tab, 100 mg) at bedtime × 3 nights, or 500 mg (1 vag tab, 500 mg); or 5 g (1 applicator) at bedtime × 1-2 wk

*Miconazole*
*Adult:* 200 mg supp at bedtime × 3 days or 100 mg supp × 1 wk

*Nystatin*
*Adult:* 100,000 units/day × 2 wk

*Terconazole*
*Adult:* VAG 5 g (1 applicator) at bedtime × 7 days

*Tioconazole*
*Adult:* 1 applicator at bedtime × 1 wk

### Adverse effects
*GU:* Vulvovaginal burning, itching, pelvic cramps
*INTEG:* Rash, urticaria, stinging, burning
*MISC:* **Headache**, body pain

**Contraindications:** Hypersensitivity

**Precautions:** Pregnancy, breastfeeding, children <2 yr

## NURSING CONSIDERATIONS
### Assessment
• Assess for allergic reaction: burning, stinging, itching, discharge, soreness

### Nursing diagnoses
• Infection, risk for (uses)
• Knowledge, deficient (teaching)
• Skin integrity, impaired (uses)

### Implementation
**Topical route**
• Administer one full applicator every night high into the vagina
• Store at room temperature in dry place

### Patient/family education
• Instruct patient in asepsis (hand washing) before, after each application
• Teach patient to apply with applicator only; to avoid use of any other vaginal product unless directed by prescriber; sanitary napkin may prevent soiling of undergarments
• Instruct patient to abstain from sexual intercourse until treatment is completed; reinfection and irritation may occur

Adverse effects: *italic* = common, **bold** = life-threatening

• Advise patient to notify prescriber if symptoms persist

Evaluation
**Positive therapeutic outcome**
• Decrease in itching or white discharge (vaginal)

## OTIC ANTIINFECTIVES

**boric acid** (OTC)
(bor'ik as'id)
Auro-Dri, Dri/Ear, Ear Dry
**chloramphenicol** (Rx)
(klor-am-fen'i-kole)
Chloromycetin Otic

**Action:** Inhibits protein synthesis in susceptible microorganisms

**Uses:** Ear infection (external), short-term use

Adverse effects
*EENT:* Itching, irritation in ear
*INTEG:* Rash, urticaria

**Contraindications:** Hypersensitivity, perforated eardrum

**Precautions:** Pregnancy **C**

NURSING CONSIDERATIONS
Assessment
• Assess for redness, swelling, fever, pain in ear, which indicates superinfection

Nursing diagnoses
• Infection, risk for uses
• Knowledge, deficient (teaching)

Implementation
• After removing impacted cerumen by irrigation
• After cleaning stopper with alcohol
• After restraining child if necessary
• After warming sol to body temp

Patient/family education
• The correct method of instillation using aseptic technique, including not touching dropper to ear
• That dizziness may occur after instillation

Evaluation
**Positive therapeutic outcome**
• Decreased ear pain

## Appendix E   Vaccines and Toxoids

| GENERIC NAME | TRADE NAME | USES | DOSAGES AND ROUTES | CONTRAINDICATIONS |
|---|---|---|---|---|
| anthrax vaccine | BioThrax | Pre/postexposure prophylaxis | **Preexposure**<br>Adult: SUBCUT 0.5 ml at 0, 2, 4, wk, then 0.5 ml at 6, 12, 18 mo<br>**Postexposure**<br>Adult: SUBCUT 0.5 ml 0, 2, 4 wk with antibiotics | Hypersensitivity |
| avian influenzae A (H5N1) virus vaccine | | Prophylaxis | Adult: IM 1 ml (90 mcg) 2 doses, 28 days apart | IV |
| BCG vaccine | TICE BCG | TB exposure | Adult/child >1 mo: 0.2-0.3 ml<br>Child <1 mo: Reduce dose by 50% using 2 ml of sterile water after reconstituting | Hypersensitivity, hypogamma-globulinemia, positive TB test, burns |
| cholera vaccine | No trade name | Immunization for cholera outside the U.S. | Adult/child >10 yr: IM/SUBCUT 2× of 0.5 ml, 7-30 days before traveling to areas with cholera<br>Booster is used q6 mo 0.5 ml prn | Hypersensitivity, acute febrile illness |
| diphtheria and tetanus toxoids, adsorbed | No trade name | Induces antitoxins to provide immunity to diphtheria, tetanus | Adult/child ≥7 yr: IM (adult strength) 0.5 ml q4-8 wk × 2 doses, then 3rd dose 6-12 mo after 2nd dose, booster IM 0.5 ml q10 yr<br>Child 1-6 yr: IM (pediatric strength) 0.5 ml q4 wk × 2 doses, booster 6-12 mo after 2nd dose<br>Infant 6 wk-1 yr: IM (pediatric strength) 0.5 ml q4 wk × 3 doses, booster 6-12 mo after 2nd dose | Hypersensitivity to mercury, thimerosal; immunocompromised patients; radiation; corticosteroids; acute illness |
| diphtheria and tetanus toxoids and whole-cell pertussis vaccine (DPT, DTP) | DTwP, Tr-Immunol | Prevention of diphtheria, tetanus, pertussis | Adult: Booster dose q10 yr<br>Child >6 wk-6 yr: IM 0.5 ml at 2, 4, 6 mo, 1½ yr; booster needed 0.5 ml at age 6 | Hypersensitivity, active infection, poliomyelitis outbreak, immunosuppression, febrile illness |
| diphtheria and tetanus toxoids and acellular pertussis vaccine | Acel-Imune, DTaP, Tripedia | | | |

*Continued*

*DPT,* Diphtheria-pertussis-tetanus (vaccine); *DTP,* diphtheria and tetanus toxoids and pertussis vaccine; *TB,* tuberculosis.

| GENERIC NAME | TRADE NAME | USES | DOSAGES AND ROUTES | CONTRAINDICATIONS |
|---|---|---|---|---|
| *Haemophilus* b conjugate vaccine, diphtheria CRM$_{197}$ protein conjugate (HbOC) *Haemophilus* b conjugate vaccine, meningococcal protein conjugate (PRP-OMP) | HibTITTER PedvaxHIB | Polysaccharide immunization of children 2-6 yr against *H. influenzae b*, conjugate immunization of child 2, 4, 6 mo | **HibTITTER (IM only)** Child: IM 0.5 ml Child 2-6 mo: 0.5 ml q2 mo × 3 inj Child 7-11 mo: Previously unvaccinated 0.5 ml q2 mo inj Child 12-14 mo: previously unvaccinated 0.5 ml × 1 inj **PEDVAXHIB (IM only)** Child 2-14 mo: 0.5 ml × 2 inj at 2, 4 mo of age (6 mo dose not needed), then booster at 12-18 mo against invasive disease Child ≥15 mo: Previously unvaccinated 0.5 ml inj | Hypersensitivity, febrile illness, active infection |
| hepatitis A vaccine, inactivated | Havrix, VAQTA | Active immunization against hepatitis A virus | Adults: IM 1, 440 EL units (Havrix) or 50 units (VAQTA) as a single dose, booster dose is the same given at 6, 12 mo Child 2-18 yr: IM 720 EL units (Havrix) or 25 units (VAQTA) as a single dose, booster dose is the same given at 6, 12 mo | Hypersensitivity |
| hepatitis B vaccine, recombinant | Engerix-B, Recombivax HB | Immunization against all subtypes of hepatitis B virus | Varies widely | Hypersensitivity to this vaccine or yeast |
| herpes zoster virus vaccine | Zostavax | Prevention of herpes zoster | Adult ≥60 yr: SUBCUT 0.65 ml | <60 yr, child, infant, AIDs, IM/IV, leukemia, lymphoma, pregnancy |
| human papillomavirus recombinant vaccine, quadrivalent | Gardasil | Prevention of HPV types 6, 11, 16, 18, cervical cancer, genital warts, precancerous dysplastic lesions | Adult and child >9 yr to 26 yr: IM Give as 3 separate doses; 1st dose as elected; 2nd dose 2 mo after 1st dose; 3rd dose 6 mo after 1st dose | Child <9 yr, pregnancy, breastfeeding, geriatric, active disease, hypersensitivity |

| Name | Uses | Trade names | Dosage | Cautions/Contraindications |
|---|---|---|---|---|
| influenza virus vaccine | Prevention of Russian, Chilean, Philippine influenza | Afluria, FluMist, Fluogen, FluShield, Fluviral ♣, Fluvirin, Fluzone, influenza virus vaccine, trivalent | Adult and child >12 yr: IM 0.5 ml in 1 dose; Child 3-12 yr: IM 0.5 ml, repeat in 1 mo (split) unless 1978-1985 vaccine was given; also given nasal; Child 6 mo to 3 yr: IM 0.25 ml, repeat in 1 mo (split) unless 1978-1985 vaccine was given; also given nasal | Hypersensitivity, active infection, chicken egg allergy, Guillain-Barré syndrome, active neurologic disorders |
| Japanese encephalitis virus vaccine, inactivated | Active immunity against Japanese encephalitis (JE) | JE-VAX | Adult and child ≥3 yr: SUBCUT 1 ml, days 0, 7, 30; booster SUBCUT 1 ml 2 yr after last dose; Child 1-3 yr: SUBCUT 0.5 ml, days 0, 7, 30; booster SUBCUT 0.5 ml 2 yr after last dose | Hypersensitivity to murine, thimerosal; allergic reactions to previous dose |
| Lyme disease vaccine (recombinant OspA) | Immunization against Lyme disease | LYMErix | Adult and adolescent 15-70 yr: IM 30 mcg in deltoid, repeat at 1, 12 mo after first dose | Hypersensitivity, antibiotic refractory Lyme arthritis |
| measles and rubella virus vaccine, live attenuated | Immunity to measles and rubella by antibody production | M-R-Vax II | Adult and child ≥15 mo: SUBCUT 0.5 ml (1000 units) | Hypersensitivity, immunocompromised patients, active untreated TB, cancer, blood dyscrasias, radiation, corticosteroids, pregnancy; allergic reactions to neomycin, eggs |
| measles, mumps, and rubella vaccine, live | Prevention of measles, mumps, rubella | M-M-R-II | Adult: SUBCUT 1 vial; 2 vials separated by 1 mo, in person born after 1957; Child >15 mo and adult: SUBCUT 0.5 ml | Hypersensitivity, blood dyscrasias, anemia, active infection, immunosuppression; egg, chicken allergy; pregnancy; febrile illness, neomycin allergy, neoplasms |

◆ Alert    ♣ Canada Only    ⊘ Drug on CD    * "Tall Man" lettering (See Preface)

Continued

| GENERIC NAME | TRADE NAME | USES | DOSAGES AND ROUTES | CONTRAINDICATIONS |
|---|---|---|---|---|
| measles virus vaccine, live attenuated | Attenuvax | Immunity to measles by antibody production | Adult and child ≥15 mo: SUBCUT 0.5 ml (1000 units), 1 dose 15 mo, 2nd dose age 4-6 or 11, or 12 | Hypersensitivity to eggs, neomycin; cancer, radiation, corticosteroids, pregnancy, immunocompromised patients, blood dyscrasias, active untreated TB |
| meningococcal polysaccharide vaccine | Menomune-A/C/Y/W-135, Menactra | Prophylaxis to meningococcal meningitis | Adult and child >2 yr: SUBCUT 0.5 ml | Hypersensitivity to thimerosal, pregnancy, acute illness |
| mumps virus vaccine, live | Mumpsvax | Active immunity to mumps | Adult and child ≥1 yr: SUBCUT 0.5 ml (20,000 units) | Hypersensitivity to eggs, neomycin; cancer, radiation, corticosteroids, pregnancy, immunocompromised patients, blood dyscrasias, active untreated TB |
| plague vaccine | No trade name | Active immunity to *Yersinia pestis* plague | Adult: IM 1 ml, then 0.2 ml in 4-12 wk, then 0.2 ml 5-6 mo after 2nd dose; booster 0.1-0.2 ml q6 mo when in area where plague is present | Hypersensitivity to phenol, sulfites, formaldehyde, beef, soy, casein; pregnancy; coagulation disorders |
| pneumococcal 7-valent conjugate vaccine | Prevnar | Immunity against *Streptococcus pneumoniae* | Child: IM 0.5 ml × 3 doses (7-11 mo); × 2 doses (12-23 mo); × 1 dose >2-9 yr | Hypersensitivity to diphtheria toxoid or this product |
| pneumococcal vaccine, polyvalent | Pneumovax 23, Pnu-Imune 23 | Pneumococcal immunization | Adult and child >2 yr: IM/SUBCUT 0.5 ml | Hypersensitivity, Hodgkin's disease, ARDS |
| poliovirus vaccine, live, oral, trivalent (TOPV) poliovirus vaccine (IPV) | Orimune, IPOL | Prevention of polio | Adult and child >2 yr: PO 0.5 ml, given q8 wk × 2 doses, then 0.5 ml ½-1 yr after dose 2<br>Infant: PO 0.5 at 2, 4, 18 mo; booster at 4-6 yr; may also be given IPV at 2, 4 mo, then TOPV at 12-18 mo, booster at 4-6 yr | Hypersensitivity, active infection, allergy to neomycin/streptomycin, immunosuppression, vomiting, diarrhea |

| | | | | |
|---|---|---|---|---|
| rabies vaccine, adsorbed | No trade name | Active immunity to rabies | **Preexposure** Adult and child: IM 1 ml day 0, 7, 21, or 28 days (total 3 doses); booster IM 1 ml prn q2-5 yr **Postexposure** Adult and child not vaccinated: IM 20 international units/kg of human rabies immune globulin (HRIG); 5 total doses of 1-ml inj of rabies vaccine on days 0, 3, 7, 14, 28 | Severe hypersensitivity to previous inj of vaccine, thimerosal |
| rabies vaccine, human diploid cell (HDCV) | IMOVax Rabies, IM-OVax Rabies I.D. | Active immunity to rabies | **Preexposure** Adult and child: IM 1 ml on days 0, 7, 21 or 28 (total 4 doses) **Postexposure** Adult and child: IM 1 ml on days 0, 3, 7, 14, 28 (total 5 doses) | No contraindications |
| rotovirus | RotaTeq | Prevents rotavirus | Infant: PO 3 doses given between 6 and 32 wk of age; 1st dose between 6-12 wk of age; 2nd and 3rd doses q4-10wk | Hypersensitivity, immunocompromised, blood products given within 6 wk, lymphatic disorders |
| rubella and mumps virus vaccine, live | Biavax II | Immunity to rubella and mumps by antibody production | Adult and child ≥1 yr: SUBCUT 0.5 ml | Hypersensitivity to eggs, neomycin; cancer, radiation, corticosteroids, pregnancy, immunocompromised patients, blood dyscrasias, active untreated TB |
| rubella virus vaccine, live attenuated (RA 27/3) | Meruvax II | Immunity to rubella by antibody production | Adult and child ≥1 yr: SUBCUT 0.5 ml (1000 units) | Hypersensitivity to eggs, neomycin; cancer, radiation, corticosteroids |
| smallpox vaccine | ACAM 2000, DryVax | Prevention of smallpox | See package insert | No contraindications |
| tetanus toxoid, adsorbed/tetanus toxoid | No trade name | Tetanus toxoid: used for prophylactic treatment of wounds | Adult and child: IM 0.5 ml q4-6 wk × 2 doses, then 0.5 ml 1 yr after dose 2 (adsorbed); SUBCUT/IM 0.5 ml q4-8 wk × 3 doses, then 0.5 ml ½-1 yr after dose 3, booster dose 0.5 ml q10 yr | Hypersensitivity, active infection, poliomyelitis outbreak, immunosuppression |

*ARDS*, Acute respiratory distress syndrome.

*Continued*

| GENERIC NAME | TRADE NAME | USES | DOSAGES AND ROUTES | CONTRAINDICATIONS |
|---|---|---|---|---|
| typhoid vaccine, parenteral | No trade name | Active immunity to typhoid fever | Adult: PO 1 cap 1 hr before meals × 4 doses, booster q5 yr | Parenteral: systemic or allergic reaction, acute respiratory or other acute infection, intensive physical exercise in high temperatures |
| typhoid vaccine, oral | Vivotif Berna Vaccine | | Adult and child >10 yr: SUBCUT 0.5 ml, repeat in 4 wk, booster q3 yr Child 6 mo-10 yr: SUBCUT 0.25 ml, repeat in 4 wk, booster q3 yr | Oral: hypersensitivity, acute febrile illness, suppressive or antibiotic products |
| typhoid Vi polysaccharide vaccine | Typhim Vi | Active immunity to typhoid fever | Adult and child ≥2 yr: IM 0.5 ml as a single dose, reimmunize q2 yr 0.5 ml IM, if needed | Hypersensitivity, chronic typhoid carriers |
| varicella virus vaccine | Varivax | Prevention of varicella-zoster (chickenpox) | Adult and child ≥13 yr: SUBCUT 0.5 ml, 2nd dose SUBCUT 0.5 ml 4-8 wk later | Hypersensitivity to neomycin; blood dyscrasias, immunosuppression, active untreated TB, acute illness, pregnancy, diseases of lymphatic system |
| yellow fever vaccine | YF-Vax | Active immunity to yellow fever | Adult and child ≥9 mo: SUBCUT 0.5 ml deeply, booster q10 yr Child 6-9 mo: same as above if exposed | Hypersensitivity to egg or chicken embryo protein, pregnancy, child <6 mo, immunodeficiency |
| zoster vaccine, live | Zostavax | Herpes zoster prevention | Reconstitute immediately after removing from freezer; give SUBCUT as a single dose; inject total amount of single-dose vial | Immunosuppression, children, TB, pregnancy C, neomycin/gelatin allergy |

# Appendix F

## Herbal Products

### acidophilus

**Uses:** Diarrhea, vaginal and other candida infections, urinary tract infections, atopic dermatitis (eczema), atopic disease, IBS, respiratory tract infections

### alfalfa

**Uses:**
• *External:* Boils and insect bites
• *Internal:* Constipation, arthritis, increase blood clotting, diuretic, relieve inflammation of the prostate, treat acute or chronic cystitis, nutrient source

### aloe

**Uses of aloe vera gel:** Minor burns, skin irritations, minor wounds, frostbite, radiation-caused injuries

### angelica

**Uses:** Poor blood flow to the extremities, headaches, backaches, osteoporosis, asthma, allergies, skin disorders, diuretic, antispasmodic, cholagogue, stomach cancer, mild antiseptic, expectorant, bronchitis, ease rheumatic pains, stomach cramps, muscle spasms

### anise

**Uses:**
• *External:* Treat catarrhs of respiratory system (asthma, bronchitis), cancer, cholera, colic, dysmenorrheal, epilepsy, indigestion, insomnia, lice, migraine, nausea, neuralgia, rash, scabies; given to children to reduce gas, colic, and respiratory symptoms
• *Internal:* Expectorant, bronchitis, emphysema, whooping cough, antibacterial, antispasmodic, abortifacient (large quantities), diaphoretic, diuretic, stimulant, tonic, flavoring in food

### astragalus

**Uses:** Bronchitis, COPD, colds, flu, gastrointestinal conditions, weakness, fatigue, chronic hepatitis, ulcers, hypertension and viral myocarditis, immune stimulant, aphrodisiac, and improve sperm motility

### bilberry

**Uses:** Improve night vision, prevent cataracts, macular degeneration, glaucoma, varicose veins, hemorrhoids, diabetic retinopathy, myopia, mild diarrhea, dyspepsia in adults or children, controlling insulin levels, diuretic, urinary antiseptic

### black cohosh

**Uses:** Smooth-muscle relaxant, antispasmodic, antitussive, astringent, diuretic, antidiarrheal, antiarthritic, hormone balancer in perimenopausal women, decrease uterine spasms in first trimester of pregnancy, antiabortion agent, dysmenorrheal

### buckthorn

**Uses:** Powerful laxative

Adapted from Skidmore-Roth L: *Mosby's Handbook of Herbs & Natural Supplements,* ed 3, St. Louis, 2006, Elsevier.

Adverse effects: *italic* = common, **bold** = life-threatening

## capsicum peppers

**Uses:**
- *External:* Diabetic neuropathy, psoriasis, postmastectomy pain, Raynaud's disease, herpes zoster, arthritis, muscular pain, poor peripheral circulation
- *Internal:* Cardiovascular health, CAD, reduce cholesterol and blood clotting, peptic ulcer disease, cold, flu

## cascara

**Uses:** Laxative

## chamomile

**Uses:**
- *External:* As an antiseptic and soothing agent for inflamed skin and minor wounds
- *Internal:* As an antispasmodic, antianxiety, gas-relieving, and antiinflammatory agent for the treatment of digestive problems; light sleep aid and sedative

## chondroitin

**Uses:** Alone or in combination with glucosamine for joint conditions, as an antithrombotic, extravasation therapy agent, for ischemic heart disease, hyperlipidemia

## chromium

**Uses:** Essential trace mineral required for proper metabolic functioning, decreases glucose tolerance, arteriosclerosis, elevated cholesterol, glaucoma, hypoglycemia, diabetes, obesity

## coenzyme Q10

**Uses:** Ischemic heart disease, CHF, angina pectoris, hypertension, arrhythmias, diabetes mellitus, deafness, Bell's palsy, decreased immunity, mitral valve prolapse, periodontal disease, infertility

## dong quai

**Uses:** Menopausal symptoms, menstrual irregularities, headache, neuralgia, herpes infections, malaria, vitiligo, anemia

## echinacea

**Uses:**
- *External:* Wound healing, bruises, burns, scratches, leg ulcers
- *Internal:* Immune stimulant, prophylaxis for colds, influenzae, other infections

## eyebright

**Uses:** Internally and externally to relieve eye fatigue, redness, sty and eye infections, nasal catarrh in sinusitis and hay fever

## feverfew

**Uses:** Menstrual irregularities, threatened spontaneous abortion, arthritis, fever

## flax

**Uses:**
- *External*: Inflammatory
- *Internal*: Laxative anticholesteremic

## garlic

**Uses:** Antilipidemic, antimicrobial, antiasthmatic, antiinflammatory, possible antihypertensive, treatment for some heavy metal poisonings

## ginger

**Uses:** Antioxidant, nausea, motion sickness, vomiting, sore throat, migraine headaches

 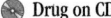

## ginkgo

Uses: Poor circulation, age-related decline in cognition, memory; vascular disease, antioxidant, depressive mood disorders, sexual dysfunction, asthma, glaucoma, menopausal symptoms, multiple sclerosis, headaches, tinnitus, dizziness, arthritis, altitude sickness, intermittent claudication

## ginseng

Uses: Physical and mental exhaustion, stress, sluggishness, fatigue, weak immunity, as a tonic

## goldenseal

Uses: Gastritis, gastrointestinal ulceration, peptic ulcer disease, mouth ulcer, bladder infection, sore throat, postpartum hemorrhage, skin disorders, cancer, tuberculosis, wound healing, antiinflammatory, in combination with echinacea for cold and flu

## green tea

Uses: Antioxidant, anticancer agent, diuretic, stimulant, antibacterial, antilipidemic, antiatherosclerotic

## hops

Uses: Analgesic, hyperactivity, anthelmintic, mild sedative, insomnia, menopausal symptoms

## kava

Uses: Anxiolytic, antiepileptic, antidepressant, antipsychotic, nervous anxiety, hyperactivity, restlessness, sleep disturbances, headache, muscle relaxant, wound healing

## khat

Uses: Fatigue, obesity, gastric ulcers, depression

## lemon balm

Uses:
• *External:* Cold sores
• *Internal:* Insomnia, anxiety, gastric conditions, psychiatric conditions, Graves' disease, attention deficit disorder (ADD)

## licorice

Uses: Allergies, arthritis, asthma, constipation, esophagitis, gastritis, hepatitis, inflammatory conditions, peptic ulcers, poor adrenal function, poor appetite

## lysine

Uses: Cold sores, herpes infections, Bell's palsy, rheumatoid arthritis, detoxify opiates

## maitake

Uses: Diabetes, hypertension, high cholesterol, obesity, cancer

## melatonin

Uses: Insomnia, inhibit cataract formation, increase longevity, epilepsy, hypertension, various cancers, jet lag, cancer protection, oral contraceptive

## panax ginseng

Uses: Physical and mental exhaustion, stress, sluggishness, fatigue, weak immunity, as a tonic

Adverse effects: *italic* = common, **bold** = life-threatening

## papaya

Uses:
• *External:* Debridement of wounds
• *Internal:* Intestinal worms, gastrointestinal disorders, injection in a herniated lumbar intervertebral disk

## raspberry

Uses:
• *External:* Leaves promote diuresis, treat inflammation, cough, wounds
• *Internal:* UTIs, renal calculi, antimicrobial action, morning sickness and speed, ease labor in pregnancy

## red clover

Uses: Antispasmodic, expectorant, sedative, psoriasis, eczema, amenorrhea

## St. John's wort

Uses:
• *External:* Antiinflammatory, relieve hemorrhoids, treat vitiligo, burns
• *Internal:* Depression, anxiety

## SAM-e

Uses: Depression, Alzheimer's disease, migraine headache, hypersensitivity, chronic liver disease, fibromyalgia pain, inflammation in osteoarthritis

## saw palmetto

Uses: Benign prostatic hypertrophy, mild diuretic, chronic and subacute cystitis, increase breast size, sperm count, sexual potency

## senna

Uses: Laxative

## siberian ginseng

Uses: Increase immunity, energy and performance, decrease inflammation and insomnia

## turmeric

Uses: Menstrual disorders, colic, inflammation, bruising, dyspepsia, hematuria, flatulence

## valerian

Uses: Sedative

## wintergreen

Uses:
• *External:* Sore, inflamed muscles and joints
• *Internal:* Bladder inflammation, urinary tract diseases, diseases of prostate and kidney

## yohimbe

Uses: Aphrodisiac, hallucinogenic

# Appendix G

## Combination Products

**A-200 Lice Killing Shampoo:**
0.33% pyrethrins
4% piperonyl butoxide
*Uses:* Scabicide, pediculicide
**Accuretic 10/12.5:**
quinapril 10 mg
hydrochlorthiazide 12.5 mg
*Uses:* Antihypertensive
**Accuretic 20/12.5:**
quinapril 20 mg
hydrochlorthiazide 12.5 mg
*Uses:* Antihypertensive
**Accuretic 20/25:**
quinapril 20 mg
hydrochlorthiazide 25 mg
*Uses:* Antihypertensive
**Aceta-Gesic:**
acetaminophen 325 mg
phenyltoloxamine 30 mg
*Uses:* Pain
**Activella Tablets:**
estriol 1 mg
norethindrone 0.5 mg
*Uses:* Vasomotor symptoms (menopause)
**Actonel with Calcium:**
calcium carbonate 1250 mg
risedronate 35 mg
*Uses:* Osteoporosis
**Actoplus Met:**
pioglitazone 15 mg
metformin 500 mg
pioglitazone 15 mg
metformin 850 mg
*Uses:* Type 2 diabetes
**Adderall 5 mg:**
dextroamphetamine sulfate 1.25 mg
dextroamphetamine saccharate 1.25 mg
amphetamine sulfate 1.25 mg
amphetamine aspartate 1.25 mg
*Uses:* CNS stimulant
**Adderall 7.5 mg:**
dextroamphetamine sulfate 1.875 mg
dextroamphetamine saccharate 1.875 mg
dextroamphetamine aspartate 1.875 mg
amphetamine sulfate 1.875 mg
*Uses:* CNS stimulant
**Adderall 10 mg:**
dextroamphetamine sulfate 5 mg
dextroamphetamine saccharate 2.5 mg
amphetamine sulfate 2.5 mg
amphetamine aspartate 2.5 mg
*Uses:* CNS stimulant
**Adderall 12.5 mg:**
dextroamphetamine sulfate 3.125 mg
dextroamphetamine saccharate 3.125 mg
dextroamphetamine aspartate 3.125 mg

amphetamine sulfate 3.125 mg
*Uses:* CNS stimulant
**Adderall 15 mg:**
dextroamphetamine sulfate 3.75 mg
dextroamphetamine saccharate 3.75 mg
dextroamphetamine aspartate 3.75 mg
amphetamine sulfate 3.75 mg
*Uses:* CNS stimulant
**Adderall 20 mg:**
dextroamphetamine sulfate 5 mg
dextroamphetamine saccharate 5 mg
amphetamine sulfate 5 mg
amphetamine aspartate 5 mg
*Uses:* CNS stimulant
**Adderall 30 mg:**
dextroamphetamine sulfate 7.5 mg
dextroamphetamine saccharate 7.5 mg
amphetamine sulfate 7.5 mg
amphetamine aspartate 7.5 mg
*Uses:* CNS stimulant
**Adderall XR 5 mg:**
dextroamphetamine sulfate 1.25 mg
dextroamphetamine saccharate 1.25 mg
amphetamine sulfate 1.25 mg
amphetamine aspartate 1.25 mg
*Uses:* CNS stimulant
**Adderall XR 10 mg:**
dextroamphetamine sulfate 2.5 mg
dextroamphetamine saccharate 2.5 mg
amphetamine sulfate 2.5 mg
amphetamine aspartate 2.5 mg
*Uses:* CNS stimulant
**Adderall XR 15 mg:**
dextroamphetamine sulfate 3.75 mg
dextroamphetamine saccharate 3.75 mg
amphetamine sulfate 3.75 mg
amphetamine aspartate 3.75 mg
*Uses:* CNS stimulant
**Adderall XR 20 mg:**
dextroamphetamine sulfate 5 mg
dextroamphetamine saccharate 5 mg
amphetamine sulfate 5 mg
amphetamine aspartate 5 mg
*Uses:* CNS stimulant
**Adderall XR 25 mg:**
dextroamphetamine sulfate 6.25 mg
dextroamphetamine saccharate 6.25 mg
amphetamine sulfate 6.25 mg
*Uses:* CNS stimulant
**Adderall XR 30 mg:**
dextroamphetamine sulfate 7.5 mg
dextroamphetamine saccharate 7.5 mg
amphetamine sulfate 7.5 mg
amphetamine aspartate 7.5 mg
*Uses:* CNS stimulant

Adverse effects: *italic* = common, **bold** = life-threatening

**Advair Diskus 100:**
fluticasone 100 mcg
salmeterol 50 mcg
*Uses:* Corticosteroid, bronchodilator

**Advair Diskus 250:**
fluticasone 250 mcg
salmeterol 50 mcg
*Uses:* Corticosteroid, bronchodilator

**Advair Diskus 500:**
fluticasone 500 mcg
salmeterol 50 mcg
*Uses:* Corticosteroid, bronchodilator

**Advicor 500:**
niacin 500 mg
lovastatin 20 mg
*Uses:* Antilipidemic

**Advicor 750:**
niacin 750 mg
lovastatin 20 mg
*Uses:* Antilipidemic

**Advicor 1000:**
niacin 1000 mg
lovastatin 20 mg
niacin 1000 mg
lovastatin 40 mg
*Uses:* Antilipidemic

**Advil Cold and Sinus Caplets:**
pseudoephedrine 30 mg
ibuprofen 200 mg
*Uses:* Decongestant

**Advil PM:**
diphenhydrAMINE 38 mg
ibuprofen 25 mg
diphenhydrAMINE 200 mg
ibuprofen 200 mg
*Uses:* Insomnia, pain

**Aggrenox:**
200 mg ext rel dipyridamole
25 mg aspirin
*Uses:* Antiplatelet

**AK-Cide Ophthalmic Suspension/Ointment:**
10% sulfacetamide sodium
0.5% prednisoLONE acetate
*Uses:* Ophthalmic antiinfective, antiinflammatory

**Aldactazide 25/25:**
spironolactone 25 mg
hydrochlorothiazide 25 mg
*Uses*: Diuretic

**Aldactazide 50/50:**
spironolactone 50 mg
hydrochlorothiazide 50 mg
*Uses*: Diuretic

**Aldoril 15:**
methyldopa 250 mg
hydrochlorothiazide 15 mg
*Uses*: Antihypertensive

**Aldoril 25:**
methyldopa 250 mg
hydrochlorothiazide 25 mg
*Uses*: Antihypertensive

**Aldoril D30:**
methyldopa 500 mg
hydrochlorothiazide 30 mg
*Uses:* Antihypertensive

**Aldoril D50:**
methyldopa 500 mg
hydrochlorothiazide 50 mg
*Uses:* Antihypertensive

**Aleve Cold and Sinus:**
naproxen 200 mg
ER pseudoephedrine 120 mg
*Uses:* Analgesic, adrenergic

**Aleve Sinus and Headache:**
naproxen 220 mg
ER pseudoephedrine 120 mg
*Uses:* Analgesic, adrenergic

**Alka-Seltzer Original:**
sodium bicarbonate 1916 mg
citric acid 1000 mg
aspirin 325 mg
*Uses:* Antacid, adsorbent, antiflatulent

**Alka-Seltzer Plus Cold Effervescent Tablets:**
acetaminophen 250 mg
chlorpheniramine 2 mg
phenylephrine 5 mg
*Uses:* Decongestant, analgesic, antihistamine

**Alka-Seltzer Plus Night-Time Cold Liqui-Gels:**
doxylamine 6.25 mg
dextromethorphan 10 mg
pseudoephedrine 30 mg
acetaminophen 325 mg
*Uses:* Antitussive, decongestant, antihistamine, analgesic

**Alka-Seltzer Plus Ready Relief Tablets:**
chlorpheniramine 2 mg
pseudoephedrine 30 mg
*Uses:* Antihistamine, decongestant

**Alka-Seltzer PM Effervescent Tablets:**
aspirin 325 mg
diphenhydrAMINE 38 mg
*Uses*: Analgesic, antihistamine

**Allegra-D:**
fexofenadine 60 mg
pseudoephedrine 120 mg
*Uses:* Antihistamine, adrenergic

**Allercon Tablets:**
triprolidine 2.5 mg
pseudoephedrine 60 mg
*Uses:* Antihistamine, adrenergic

**Allerest Maximum Strength Tablets:**
pseudoephedrine 30 mg
chlorpheniramine 2 mg
*Uses:* Decongestant, antihistamine

**Allerest Allergy Sinus Relief Maximum Strength:**
pseudoephedrine 30 mg
acetaminophen 325 mg
*Uses:* Antihistamine, analgesic

**Allerfrim Syrup:**
Per 5 ml:
triprolidine 1.25 mg
pseudoephedrine 30 mg
*Uses:* Antihistamine, adrenergic

**Allerfrim Tablets:**
triprolidine 2.5 mg
pseudoephedrine 60 mg
*Uses:* Antihistamine, adrenergic

◆ Alert     ♣ Canada Only     😎 Drug on CD     * "Tall Man" lettering (See Preface)

**All-Nite Cold Liquid:**
Per 15 ml:
pseudoephedrine 30 mg
doxylamine 6.25 mg
dextromethorphan 15 mg
acetaminophen 500 mg
*Uses:* Decongestant, antihistamine, analgesic

**Alor 5/500:**
hydrocodone 5 mg
aspirin 500 mg
*Uses:* Analgesic

**Amaphen:**
acetaminophen 325 mg
butalbital 50 mg
caffeine 40 mg
*Uses:* analgesic, barbiturate

**Ambenyl Cough Syrup:**
Per 5 ml:
bromodiphenhydramine 12.5 mg
codeine 10 mg
5% alcohol
*Uses:* Antihistamine, opioid analgesic

**Anacin:**
aspirin 400 mg
caffeine 32 mg
*Uses:* Analgesic

**Anacin Maximum Strength:**
aspirin 500 mg
caffeine 32 mg
*Uses:* Analgesic

**Anacin PM (Aspirin Free):**
diphenhydrAMINE 25 mg
acetaminophen 500 mg
*Uses:* Analgesic

**Anaplex DM:**
Per 5 ml:
brompheniramine 4 mg
dextromethorphan 30 mg
pseudoephedrine 60 mg
*Uses:* Decongestant, antitussive, antihistamine

**Anaplex DMX:**
Per 5 ml:
brompheniramine 8 mg
dextromethorphan 60 mg
pseudoephedrine 90 mg
*Uses:* Decongestant, antitussive, antihistamine

**Anaplex HD Oral Solution:**
Per 5 ml:
hydrocodone 1.7 mg
brompheniramine 2 mg
pseudoephedrine 30 mg
*Uses:* Antihistamine, decongestant, analgesic

**Angeliq:**
drospirenone 0.5 mg
estradiol 1 mg
*Uses:* Vasomotor symptoms (menopause)

**Apresazide 25/25:**
hydrALAZINE 25 mg
hydrochlorothiazide 25 mg
*Uses:* Antihypertensive

**Apresazide 50/50:**
hydrALAZINE 50 mg
hydrochlorothiazide 50 mg
*Uses:* Antihypertensive

**Apri 28-Day:**
desorgestrel 0.15 mg
ethinyl estradiol 30 mcg
*Uses:* Estrogen, progestin

**Arthrotec:**
diclofenac 50 or 75 mg
misoprostol 200 mcg
*Uses:* NSAID, gastric protectant

**Ascriptin:**
aspirin 325 mg
magnesium hydroxide 50 mg
aluminum hydroxide 50 mg
calcium carbonate 50 mg
*Uses:* Nonopioid analgesic, antipyretic

**Ascriptin A/D:**
aspirin 325 mg
aluminum hydroxide 75 mg
magnesium hydroxide 75 mg
calcium carbonate 75 mg
*Uses:* Analgesic

**Aspirin-Free Bayer Select Allergy Sinus:**
pseudoephedrine 30 mg
chlorpheniramine 2 mg
acetaminophen 500 mg
*Uses:* Adrenergic, antihistamine, analgesic

**Aspirin Free Excedrin:**
acetaminophen 500 mg
caffeine 65 mg
*Uses:* Analgesic

**Aspirin Free Excedrin Dual:**
acetaminophen 500 mg
calcium carbonate 111 mg
magnesium carbonate 64 mg
magnesium oxide 30 mg
*Uses:* Analgesic, antacid

**Atacand HCT 16:**
candesartan 16 mg
hydrochlorthiazide 12.5 mg
*Uses:* Antihypertensive

**Atacand HCT 32:**
candesartan 32 mg
hydrochlorthiazide 12.5 mg
*Uses:* Antihypertensive

**Atripla:**
efavirenz 600 mg
emtricitabine 200 mg
tenofovir 300 mg
*Uses:* HIV

**Augmentin 250:**
amoxicillin 250 mg
clavulanic acid 125 mg
*Uses:* Antiinfective

**Augmentin 500:**
amoxicillin 500 mg
clavulanic acid 125 mg
*Uses:* Antiinfective

**Augmentin 875:**
amoxicillin 875 mg
clavulanic acid 125 mg
*Uses:* Antiinfective

**Augmentin 125 Chewable:**
amoxicillin 125 mg
clavulanic acid 31.25 mg
*Uses:* Antiinfective

Adverse effects: *italic* = common, **bold** = life-threatening

**Augmentin 200 Chewable:**
amoxicillin 200 mg
clavulanic acid 28.5 mg
*Uses:* Antiinfective
**Augmentin 250 Chewable:**
amoxicillin 250 mg
clavulanic acid 62.5 mg
*Uses:* Antiinfective
**Augmentin 125 mg/5 ml Suspension:**
Per 5 ml:
amoxicillin 125 mg
clavulanic acid 31.25 mg
*Uses:* Antiinfective
**Augmentin 200 mg/5 ml Suspension:**
Per 5 ml:
amoxicillin 200 mg
clavulanic acid 28.5 mg
*Uses:* Antiinfective
**Augmentin 250 mg/5 ml Suspension:**
Per 5 ml:
amoxicillin 250 mg
clavulanic acid 62.5 mg
*Uses:* Antiinfective
**Augmentin 400 mg/5 ml Suspension:**
Per 5 ml:
amoxicillin 400 mg
clavulanic acid 57 mg
*Uses:* Antiinfective
**Auralgan Otic Solution:**
5.4% antipyrine
1.4% benzocaine
*Uses:* Otic analgesic
**Avalide:**
hydrochlorthiazide 12.5 mg
irbesartan 150 mg
*Uses:* Antihypertensive
**Avalide 300:**
hydrochlorthiazide 12.5 mg
irbesartan 300 mg
*Uses:* Antihypertensive
**Avandamet:**
rosiglitazone/metformin
1 mg/500 mg
2 mg/500 mg
2 mg/1000 mg
4 mg/500 mg
4 mg/1000 mg
*Uses:* Diabetes mellitus
**Avandaryl 4/1:**
rosiglitazone 4 mg
glimepiride 1 mg
*Uses:* Antidiabetic
**Avandaryl 4/2:**
rosiglitazone 4 mg
glimepiride 2 mg
*Uses:* Antidiabetic
**Avandaryl 4/4:**
rosiglitazone 4 mg
glimepiride 4 mg
*Uses:* Antidiabetic
**Azor:**
amlodipine 5 mg
olmesartan 20 mg
amlodipine 10 mg
olmesartan 20 mg

amlodipine 5 mg
olmesartan 40 mg
amlodipine 10 mg
olmesartan 40 mg
*Uses:* Hypertension
**Bactrim:**
trimethoprim 80 mg
sulfamethoxazole 400 mg
*Uses:* Antiinfective
**Bactrim DS:**
trimethoprim 160 mg
sulfamethoxazole 800 mg
*Uses:* Antiinfective
**Bancap HC:**
acetaminophen 500 mg
hydrocodone 5 mg
*Uses:* Analgesic
**Bellatal:**
phenobarbital 16.2 mg
hyoscyamine sulfate 0.1037 mg
atropine sulfate 0.0194 mg
scopolamine hydrobromide 0.0065 mg
*Uses:* Barbiturate, anticholinergic
**Bellergal-S:**
ergotamine 0.6 mg
belladonna alkaloids 0.2 mg
phenobarbital 40 mg
*Uses:* α-Adrenergic blocker, anticholinergic,
   barbiturate
**Bel-Phen-Ergot-SR:**
phenobarbital 40 mg
ergotamine tartrate 0.6 mg
belladonna alkaloids 0.2 mg
*Uses:* α-Adrenergic blocker, anticholinergic,
   barbiturate
**Benadryl Allergy Decongestant Liquid:**
Per 5 ml:
diphenhydrAMINE 12.5 mg
pseudoephedrine 30 mg
*Uses:* Antihistamine, adrenergic
**Benadryl Allergy/Sinus Headache Caplets:**
diphenhydrAMINE 12.5 mg
pseudoephedrine 30 mg
acetaminophen 500 mg
*Uses:* Antihistamine, adrenergic, analgesic
**Benadryl Decongestant
   Allergy:**
pseudoephedrine 60 mg
diphenhydrAMINE 25 mg
*Uses:* Adrenergic, antihistamine
**Benylin Expectorant Liquid:**
Per 5 ml:
dextromethorphan 5 mg
guaifenesin 100 mg
5% alcohol
*Uses:* Expectorant, antitussive
**Benylin Multi-Symptom Liquid:**
Per 5 ml:
dextromethorphan 5 mg
pseudoephedrine 15 mg
guaifenesin 100 mg
*Uses:* Antitussive, adrenergic, expectorant
**BenzaClin:**
clindamycin 10%
benzoyl peroxide 5%

*Uses:* Antiinfective
**Benzamycin:**
benzoyl peroxide 5%
erythromycin 3%
*Uses:* Antiinfective
**Beta Tan Suspension:**
Per 5 ml:
carbetapentane 30 mg
brompheniramine 4 mg
phenylephrine 7.5 mg
*Uses:* Antitussive
**BiDil:**
isosorbide 20 mg
hydrALAZINE 37.5 mg
*Uses:* Vasodilator
**Blephamide Ophthalmic Suspension/
 Ointment:**
0.2% prednisoLONE
10% sodium sulfacetamide
*Uses:* Ophthalmic antiinfective,
 antiinflammatory
**Butibel:**
belladonna extract 15 mg
butabarbital 15 mg
*Uses:* Anticholinergic, barbiturate
**Cafatine PB:**
ergotamine 1 mg
caffeine 100 mg
belladonna alkaloids 0.125 mg
pentobarbital 30 mg
*Uses:* Migraine agent
**Cafergot:**
ergotamine 1 mg
caffeine 100 mg
*Uses:* Adrenergic blocker
**Cafergot Suppositories:**
ergotamine 2 mg
caffeine 100 mg
*Uses:* Adrenergic blocker
**Caladryl:**
8% calamine, camphor
2.2% alcohol
1% pramoxine
*Uses:* Topical antihistamine
**Calcet:**
calcium 152.8 mg
vitamin D 100 international units
*Uses:* Supplement
**Caltrate 600+D:**
vitamin D 200 international units
calcium 600 mg
*Uses:* Supplement
**Cama Arthritis Pain Reliever:**
aspirin 500 mg
magnesium oxide 150 mg
aluminum hydroxide 125 mg
*Uses:* Nonopioid analgesic,
 antacid
**Capital w/Codeine:**
Per 5 ml:
acetaminophen 120 mg
codeine 12 mg
*Uses:* Opioid analgesic
**Capozide 25/15:**
captopril 25 mg

hydrochlorothiazide 15 mg
*Uses:* Antihypertensive
**Capozide 25/25:**
captopril 25 mg
hydrochorothiazide 25 mg
*Uses:* Antihypertensive
**Capozide 50/15:**
captopril 50 mg
hydrochlorothiazide 15 mg
*Uses:* Antihypertensive
**Capozide 50/25:**
captopril 50 mg
hydrochlorothiazide 25 mg
*Uses:* Antihypertensive
**Cardec DM Syrup:**
Per 5 ml:
pseudoephedrine 60 mg
carbinoxamine 4 mg
dextromethorphan 15 mg
*Uses:* Adrenergic, antitussive
**Cenafed Plus Tablets:**
triprolidine 2.5 mg
pseudoephedrine 60 mg
*Uses:* Antihistamine, adrenergic
**Cetapred Ophthalmic Ointment:**
0.25% prednisoLONE
10% sodium sulfacetamide
*Uses:* Ophthalmic antiinfective,
 antiinflammatory
**Cheracol Cough Syrup:**
Per 5 ml:
codeine 10 mg
guaifenesin 100 mg
*Uses:* Analgesic, expectorant
**Cheracol Syrup:**
Per 5 ml:
codeine 10 mg
guaifenesin 100 mg
*Uses:* Analgesic, expectorant
**Children's Cepacol Liquid:**
Per 5 ml:
acetaminophen 160 mg
pseudoephedrine 15 mg
*Uses:* Analgesic, adrenergic
**Chlor-Trimeton Allergy-D 4 Hour Relief:**
pseudoephedrine 60 mg
chlorpheniramine 4 mg
*Uses:* Antihistamine, adrenergic
**Chlor-Trimeton Allergy 12 Hour Relief
 Tablets:**
pseudoephedrine 120 mg
chlorpheniramine 8 mg
*Uses:* Antihistamine, adrenergic
**Chromagen:**
ferrous fumarate 66 mg
vitamin $B_{12}$ 10 mcg
vitamin C 250 mg
intrinsic factor 100 mg
*Uses:* Supplement
**Cipro HC Otic:**
Per 1 ml:
ciprofloxacin 2 mg
hydrocortisone 10 mg
*Uses:* Antiinfective/antiinflammatory

Adverse effects: *italic* = common, **bold** = life-threatening

**Citracal+D:**
calcium 315 mg
cholecalciferol 200 international units
*Uses:* Osteoporosis
**Claritin-D 12 Hour:**
loratidine 5 mg
pseudoephedrine 120 mg
*Uses:* Antihistamine, adrenergic
**Claritin-D 24-Hour:**
loratidine 10 mg
pseudoephedrine 240 mg
*Uses:* Antihistamine, adrenergic
**Climara Pro (transdermal)**
estradiol 0.045 mg
levonorgestrel 0.015 mg
*Uses:* Vasomotor symptoms (menopause)
**Clindex:**
chlordiazepoxide 5 mg
clidinium 2.5 mg
*Uses:* Antianxiety, anticholinergic
**Clomycin Ointment:**
bacitracin 500 units
neomycin sulfate 3.5 g
polymyxin B sulfate 500 units
lidocaine 40 mg
*Uses:* Antiinfective, local anesthetic
**Co-Apap:**
pseudoephedrine 30 mg
chlorpheniramine 2 mg
dextromethorphan 15 mg
acetaminophen 325 mg
*Uses:* Adrenergic, antihistamine, antitussive,
   analgesic
**Co-Gesic:**
acetaminophen 500 mg
hydrocodone 5 mg
*Uses:* Analgesic
**Codeprex Extended Release Suspension:**
Per 5 ml:
codeine 20 mg
chlorpheniramine 4 mg
*Uses:* Cough, rhinitis
**Codiclear DH Syrup:**
Per 5 ml:
hydrocodone 5 mg
guaifenesin 100 mg
*Uses:* Analgesic, expectorant
**Codimal:**
pseudoephedrine 30 mg
chlorpheniramine 2 mg
acetaminophen 500 mg
*Uses:* Adrenergic, antihistamine, analgesic
**Codimal DH Syrup:**
Per 5 ml:
hydrocodone 1.66 mg
phenylephrine 5 mg
pyrilamine 8.33 mg
*Uses:* Analgesic, adrenergic
**Codimal DM Syrup:**
Per 5 ml:
phenylephrine 5 mg
pyrilamine 8.33 mg
dextromethorphan 10 mg
*Uses:* Adrenergic, antitussive

**ColBenemid:**
probenecid 500 mg
colchicine 0.5 mg
*Uses:* Antigout agent
**Coldrine:**
pseudoephedrine 30 mg
acetaminophen 500 mg
*Uses:* Decongestant, nonopioid analgesic
**Col-Probenecid:**
probenecid 500 mg
colchicine 0.5 mg
*Uses:* Antigout
**Coly-Mycin S Otic Suspension:**
1% hydrocortisone
neomycin base 3.3 mg/ml
colistin 3 mg/ml
0.05% thonzonium bromide
*Uses:* Otic antiinfective
**Combigan:**
brimonidine 0.2%
timolol 0.5%
*Uses:* Glaucoma
**CombiPatch 0.05/0.14:**
estradiol 0.05 mg/day
norethindrone 0.14 mg/day
*Uses:* Hypoestrogenism
**CombiPatch 0.05/0.25:**
estradiol 0.05 mg/day
norethindrone 0.25 mg/day
*Uses:* Hypoestrogenism
**Combivent:**
ipratropium bromide 18 mcg
albuterol 103 mcg/actuation
*Uses:* Bronchodilator
**Combivir:**
lamivudine 150 mg
zidovudine 300 mg
*Uses:* HIV
**Comtrex Nighttime Acute Head Cold:**
Per 30 ml:
acetaminophen 1000 mg
brompheniramine 4 mg
pseudoephedrine 60 mg
*Uses:* Antihistamine, analgesic, decongestant
**Comtrex Nighttime Cold and Cough Liquid:**
Per 30 ml:
chlorpheniramine 4 mg
acetaminophen 1000 mg
pseudoephedrine 60 mg
dextromethorphan 30 mg
*Uses:* Antihistamine, analgesic, decongestant,
   antitussive
**Comtrex Nighttime Flu Therapy:**
Per 30 ml:
chlorpheniramine 4 mg
acetaminophen 1000 mg
pseudoephedrine 60 mg
*Uses:* Antihistamine, analgesic, decongestant
**Comvax:**
Per 0.5 ml:
*Haemophilus* b conjugate 7.5 mcg
meningococcal protein 125 mcg
hepatitis B recombinant 5 mcg
*Uses:* Vaccine

**Congestac:**
guaifenesin 400 mg
pseudoephedrine 60 mg
*Uses:* Expectorant, decongestant
**Contac Severe Cold & Flu:**
chlorpheniramine 2 mg
acetaminophen 500 mg
pseudoephedrine 30 mg
dextromethorphan 15 mg
18.5% alcohol
*Uses:* Decongestant, antihistamine, antitussive,
analgesic
**Cortisporin Ophthalmic/Otic Suspension:**
0.35% neomycin polymyxin B 10,000 units/ml
1% hydrocortisone
*Uses:* Ophthalmic antiinfective,
antiinflammatory
**Cortisporin Topical Cream:**
0.5% neomycin sulfate
polymyxin B 10,000 units
0.5% hydrocortisone
*Uses:* Topical antiinfective
**Cortisporin Topical Ointment:**
0.5% neomycin sulfate
bacitracin 400 units
polymyxin B 5000 units
1% hydrocortisone
*Uses:* Topical antiinfective
**Corzide 40/5:**
nadolol 40 mg
bendroflumethiazide 5 mg
*Uses:* Antihypertensive
**Corzide 80/5:**
nadolol 80 mg
bendroflumethiazide 5 mg
*Uses:* Antihypertensive
**Cosopt:**
dorzolamide 2%
timolol 0.5%
*Uses:* Antihypertensive
**Cough-X:**
dextromethorphan 5 mg
benzocaine 2 mg
*Uses:* Antitussive, local anesthetic
**Creon:**
lipase 8000 units
amylase 30,000 units
protease 13,000 units
pancreatin 300 mg
*Uses:* Digestive enzyme
**Cyclomydril Ophthalmic Solution:**
0.2% cyclopentolate
1% phenylephrine
*Uses:* Mydriatic
**Dallergy Tablets:**
chlorpheniramine 4 mg
phenylephrine 10 mg
methscopolamine 1.25 mg
*Uses:* Antihistamine, adrenergic
**Damason-P:**
hydrocodone 5 mg
aspirin 500 mg
*Uses:* Analgesic
**Darvocet-N 100:**
propoxyphene-N 100 mg

acetaminophen 650 mg
*Uses:* Analgesic
**Darvon Compound-65:**
propoxyphene 65 mg
aspirin 389 mg
caffeine 32.4 mg
*Uses:* Analgesic
♣ **Darvon-N Compound:**
aspirin 375 mg
propoxyphene 100 mg
caffeine 30 mg
*Uses:* Analgesic
♣ **Darvon-N w/A.S.A.:**
aspirin 325 mg
propoxyphene 100 mg
*Uses:* Analgesic
**Decadron Phosphate with Xylocaine:**
Per ml:
dexamethasone 4 mg
lidocaine 10 mg
*Uses:* Local anesthetic
**Deconamine:**
pseudoephedrine 60 mg
chlorpheniramine 4 mg
*Uses:* Antihistamine, decongestant
**Deconamine SR:**
pseudoephedrine 120 mg
chlorpheniramine 8 mg
*Uses:* Antihistamine, decongestant
**Deconamine Syrup:**
Per 5 ml:
pseudoephedrine 30 mg
chlorpheniramine 2 mg
*Uses:* Antihistamine, decongestant
**Demi-Regroton:**
chlorthalidone 25 mg
reserpine 0.125 mg
*Uses:* Antihypertensive
**Demulen 1/35:**
ethinyl estradiol 35 mcg
ethynodiol diacetate 1 mg
*Uses:* Oral contraceptive
**Demulen 1/50:**
ethinyl estradiol 50 mcg
ethynodiol diacetate 1 mg
*Uses:* Oral contraceptive
**Desogen:**
ethinyl estradiol 30 mcg
desorgestrel 0.15 mg
*Uses:* Estrogen, progestin
**Dexacidin Ophthalmic Ointment/Suspension:**
Per ml:
0.1% dexamethasone
0.35% neomycin
polymyxin B 10,000 units/g
*Uses:* Ophthalmic, antiinfective/
antiinflammatory
**Dexasporin Ophthalmic Ointment:**
Per gram:
0.1% dexamethasone
0.35% neomycin
polymyxin B 10,000 units
*Uses:* Ophthalmic, antiinfective/
antiinflammatory

Adverse effects: *italic* = common, **bold** = life-threatening

**DHC Plus:**
dihydrocodeine 16 mg
acetaminophen 356.4 mg
caffeine 30 mg
*Uses:* Analgesic
**Di-Gel Liquid:**
Per 5 ml:
aluminum hydroxide 200 mg
magnesium hydroxide 200 mg
simethicone 20 mg
*Uses:* Antacid, adsorbent, antiflatulent
**Dihistine DH Liquid:**
Per 5 ml:
pseudoephedrine 30 mg
chlorpheniramine 2 mg
codeine 10 mg
*Uses:* Decongestant, antihistamine, analgesic
**Dilaudid Cough Syrup:**
Per 5 ml:
guaifenesin 100 mg
hydromorphone 1 mg
5% alcohol
*Uses:* Expectorant, analgesic
**Dimetapp DM Elixir:**
Per 5 ml:
pseudoephedrine 5 mg
brompheniramine 2 mg
dextromethorphan 10 mg
*Uses:* Antihistamine, adrenergic, expectorant
**Dimetapp Sinus:**
pseudoephedrine 30 mg
ibuprofen 200 mg
*Uses:* Decongestant, analgesic
**Diovan 80 HCT:**
valsartan 80 mg
hydrochlorthiazide 12.5 mg
*Uses:* Antihypertensive
**Diovan 160 HCT:**
valsartan 160 mg
hydrochlorthiazide 12.5 mg
*Uses:* Antihypertensive
**Diurigen w/Reserpine:**
chlorothiazide 250 mg
reserpine 0.125 mg
*Uses:* Antihypertensive
**Diutensen-R:**
methylclothiazide 2.5 mg
reserpine 0.1 mg
*Uses:* Antihypertensive
**Doan's PM Extra Strength:**
magnesium salicylate 500 mg
diphenhydrAMINE 25 mg
*Uses:* Analgesic, antihistamine
**Dolacet:**
hydrocodone 5 mg
acetaminophen 500 mg
*Uses:* Analgesic
**Donnatal:**
phenobarbital 16.2 mg
hyoscyamine 0.1037 mg
atropine 0.0194 mg
scopolamine 0.0065 mg
*Uses:* Anticholinergic, barbiturate

**Donnatal Elixir:**
Per 5 ml:
phenobarbital 16.2 mg
hyoscyamine 0.1037 mg
atropine 0.0194 mg
scopolamine 0.0065 mg
23% alcohol
*Uses:* Anticholinergic, barbiturate
**Donnatal Extentabs:**
phenobarbital 48.6 mg
hyoscyamine 0.3111 mg
atropine 0.0582 mg
scopolamine 0.0195 mg
*Uses:* Anticholinergic, barbiturate
**Donnazyme:**
pancreatin 500 mg
lipase 1000 units
protease 12,500 units
amylase 12,500 units
*Uses:* Pancreatic enzymes
**Dristan Cold:**
pseudoephedrine 30 mg
acetaminophen 500 mg
*Uses:* Decongestant, analgesic
**Dristan Cold Maximum Strength Caplets:**
pseudoephedrine 30 mg
brompheniramine 2 mg
acetaminophen 500 mg
*Uses:* Decongestant, antihistamine, analgesic
**Dristan Cold Multi-Symptom Formula:**
acetaminophen 325 mg
phenylephrine 5 mg
chlorpheniramine 2 mg
*Uses:* Analgesic, adrenergic, antihistamine
**Dristan Sinus:**
pseudoephedrine 30 mg
ibuprofen 200 mg
*Uses:* Decongestant, analgesic
**Drixoral Allergy Sinus:**
pseudoephedrine 60 mg
dexbrompheniramine 3 mg
acetaminophen 500 mg
*Uses:* Decongestant, antihistamine, analgesic
**Drixoral Cold & Allergy:**
pseudoephedrine 120 mg
dexbrompheniramine 6 mg
*Uses:* Decongestant, antihistamine
**Drixoral Cold & Flu:**
pseudoephedrine 60 mg
dexbrompheniramine 3 mg
acetaminophen 500 mg
*Uses:* Decongestant, antihistamine, analgesic
**DT:**
Per 5 ml:
diphtheria toxoid 2 LfU
tetanus toxoid 5 LfU
*Uses:* Vaccine
**DTP:**
Per 0.5 ml:
diphtheria toxoid 6.5 LfU
tetanus toxoid 5 LfU
pertussis 4 LfU
*Uses:* Vaccine
**Duetact:**
glimepiride 2 mg

pioglitazone 30 mg
glimepiride 4 mg
pioglitazone 30 mg
*Uses:* Antidiabetic
**DuoDote:**
atropine 21 mg
pralidoxime 0.7 ml
atropine 600 mg
pralidoxime 2 ml
*Uses:* Organophate toxicity
**DuoNeb:**
Per 3 ml:
albuterol 3 mg
ipratroprium 0.5 mg
*Uses:* Bronchodilator
**Dura-Vent/DA:**
phenylephrine 20 mg
chlorpheniramine 8 mg
methscopolamine 2.5 mg
*Uses:* Adrenergic, antihistamine
**Durabac Forte:**
acetaminophen 500 mg
caffeine 50 mg
magnesium salicylate 500 mg
phenyltoloxamine 20 mg
*Uses:* Analgesic, antihistamine
**Duratuss AC 12:**
Per 5 ml:
dextromethorphan 15 mg
diphenhydrAMINE 12.5 mg
phenylephrine 15 mg
*Uses:* Allergic rhinitis, common cold, flu
**Dyazide:**
hydrochlorothiazide 25 mg
triamterene 37.5 mg
*Uses:* Diuretic
**Dylline-GG Tablets:**
dyphylline 200 mg
guaifenesin 200 mg
*Uses:* Bronchodilator, expectorant
**Dynafed Asthma Relief:**
epHEDrine 25 mg
guaifenesin 200 mg
*Uses:* Adrenergic, expectorant
**Dynafed Plus Maximum Strength:**
pseudoephedrine 30 mg
acetaminophen 500 mg
*Uses:* Decongestant, analgesic
**Dynex 12:**
Per 5 ml:
carbetapentane 22.5 mg
phenylephrine 9 mg
*Uses:* Antitussive, nasal decongestant
**Dyphylline GG:**
dyphylline 200 mg
guaifenesin 200 mg
*Uses:* Bronchodilator, expectorant
**Elase Ointment:**
Per gram:
fibrinolysin 1 unit
desoxyribonuclease 666.6 units
*Uses:* Enzyme
**Elixophyllin GG Liquid:**
Per 5 ml:
theophylline 100 mg

guaifenesin 100 mg
*Uses:* Expectorant, bronchodilator
**EMLA Cream:**
lidocaine 2.5 mg
prilocaine 2.5 mg
*Uses:* Local anesthetic
**Empirin w/Codeine #3:**
aspirin 325 mg
codeine phosphate 30 mg
*Uses:* Analgesic
**Empirin w/Codeine #4:**
aspirin 325 mg
codeine phosphate 60 mg
*Uses:* Analgesic
♣ **Empracet-60:**
acetaminophen 300 mg
codeine 60 mg
*Uses:* Analgesic
**Endocet:**
acetaminophen 325 mg
oxycodone 5 mg
*Uses:* Analgesic
♣ **Endodan:**
aspirin 325 mg
oxycodone 5 mg
*Uses:* Analgesic
**Entex PSE:**
pseudoephedrine 120 mg
guaifenesin 600 mg
*Uses:* Adrenergic, expectorant
**Epifoam Aerosol Foam:**
1% hydrocortisone
1% pramoxine
*Uses:* Topical corticosteroid
**Epzicom:**
abacavir 600 mg
lamivudine 300 mg
*Uses:* HIV infection
**Eryzole:**
Per 5 ml:
erythromycin 200 mg
sulfisoxazole 600 mg
*Uses:* Macrolide antiinfective
**Esgic-Plus:**
butalbital 50 mg
acetaminophen 500 mg
caffeine 40 mg
*Uses:* Barbiturate, analgesic
**Esimil:**
guanethidine 10 mg
hydrochlorothiazide 25 mg
*Uses:* Antihypertensive
**Estratest:**
esterified estrogens 1.25 mg
methyltestosterone 2.5 mg
*Uses:* Vasomotor symptoms (menopause)
**Estratest HS:**
esterified estrogens 1.25 mg
methyltestosterone 2.5 mg
*Uses:* Vasomotor symptoms (menopause)
**Excedrin Extra Strength:**
acetaminophen 250 mg
aspirin 250 mg
caffeine 65 mg
*Uses:* Analgesic

Adverse effects: *italic* = common, **bold** = life-threatening

**Excedrin Migraine:**
aspirin 250 mg
acetaminophen 250 mg
caffeine 65 mg
*Uses:* Migraine agent
**Excedrin P.M.:**
acetaminophen 500 mg
diphenhydrAMINE citrate 38 mg
*Uses:* Analgesic, antihistamine
**Exforge:**
amlodipine 5 mg
valsartan 160 mg
amlodipine 5 mg
valsartan 320 mg
amlodipine 10 mg
valsartan 160 mg
amlodipine 10 mg
valsartan 320 mg
*Uses:* Hypertension
**Extra Strength Alka-Seltzer:**
aspirin 500 mg
citric acid 1000 mg
sodium bicarbonate 1985 mg
*Uses:* Analgesic
**Fansidar:**
sulfidoxine 500 mg
pyrimethamine 25 mg
*Uses:* Antimalarial
**Fem-1:**
acetaminophen 500 mg
pamabrom 25 mg
*Uses:* Nonopioid analgesic
**Femhrt 1/5:**
norethindrone 1 mg
ethinyl estradiol 5 mcg
norethindrone 1 mg
ethinyl estradiol 5 mcg
*Uses:* Vasomotor symptoms (menopause)
**Ferro-Sequels:**
docusate sodium 100 mg
ferrous fumarate 150 mg
*Uses:* Laxative, hematinic
**Fioricet:**
acetaminophen 325 mg
caffeine 40 mg
butalbital 50 mg
*Uses:* Analgesic, barbiturate
**Fioricet w/Codeine:**
acetaminophen 325 mg
caffeine 40 mg
butalbital 50 mg
codeine 30 mg
*Uses:* Analgesic, barbiturate
**Fiorinal:**
aspirin 325 mg
caffeine 40 mg
butalbital 50 mg
*Uses:* Analgesic, barbiturate
**Fiorinal w/Codeine:**
aspirin 325 mg
caffeine 40 mg
butalbital 50 mg
codeine 30 mg
*Uses:* Analgesic, barbiturate

**FML-S Ophthalmic Suspension:**
0.1% fluorometholone
10% sulfacetamide
*Uses:* Ophthalmic, antiinfective/
    antiinflammatory
**Gas-Ban:**
calcium carbonate 500 mg
simethicone 40 mg
*Uses:* Antiflatulent, antacid
**Gaviscon:**
magnesium trisilicate 20 mg
aluminum hydroxide 80 mg
*Uses:* Antacid, adsorbent, antiflatulent
**Gaviscon Liquid:**
Per 5 ml:
aluminum hydroxide 31.7 mg
magnesium carbonate 119.3 mg
*Uses:* Antacid, adsorbent, antiflatulent
**Gelusil:**
aluminum hydroxide 200 mg
magnesium hydroxide 200 mg
simethicone 25 mg
*Uses:* Antacid, adsorbent, antiflatulent
**Genac Tablets:**
triprolidine 2.5 mg
pseudoephedrine 60 mg
*Uses:* Antihistamine
**Genatuss DM Syrup:**
Per 5 ml:
guaifenesin 100 mg
dextromethorphan 10 mg
*Uses:* Expectorant, antitussive
**Glucovance 1.25:**
glyBURIDE: 1.25 mg
metformin: 250 mg
*Uses:* Antidiabetic
**Glucovance 2.50:**
glyBURIDE: 2.5 mg
metformin: 500 mg
*Uses:* Antidiabetic
**Glucovance 5:**
glyBURIDE: 5 mg
metformin: 500 mg
*Uses:* Antidiabetic
**Guaifenex PSE 60:**
pseudoephedrine 60 mg
guaifenesin 600 mg
*Uses:* Decongestant, expectorant
**Guaifenex PSE 120:**
pseudoephedrine 120 mg
guaifenesin 600 mg
*Uses:* Decongestant, expectorant
**Guiatuss AC:**
Per 5 ml:
codeine 10 mg
guafenesin 100 mg
*Uses:* Analgesic, expectorant
**Haley's M-O Liquid:**
Per 15 ml:
magnesium hydroxide 900 mg
mineral oil 3.75 ml
*Uses:* Laxative
**Halotussin-DM Sugar Free Liquid:**
Per 5 ml:
guaifenesin 100 mg

dextromethorphan 10 mg
*Uses:* Expectorant, antitussive
**Helidac:**
In a compliance package:
bismuth subsalicylate 262.4-mg tabs
metronidazole 250-mg tabs
tetracycline 500-mg caps
*Uses:* Antiinfective
**Humalog KwikPen Mix 50/50:**
Per 1 ml:
insulin lispro protamine 50 units
insulin lispro 50 units
*Uses:* Antidiabetic
**Humalog KwikPen Mix 75/25:**
Per 1 ml:
insulin lispro protamine 75 units
insulin lispro 25 units
*Uses:* Antidiabetic
**Humalog Mix 50/50:**
insulin lispro protamine 50 units
insulin lispro (rDNA) 50 units
*Uses:* Antidiabetic
**Humalog Mix 75/25:**
insulin lispro protamine 75 units
insulin lispro (rDNA) 25 units
*Uses:* Antidiabetic
**Humibid DM Pediatric:**
dextromethorphan 15 mg
guaifenesin 300 mg
*Uses:* Expectorant, antitussive
**Humibid DM Tablets:**
dextromethorphan 30 mg
guaifenesin 600 mg
*Uses:* Expectorant, antitussive
**HycoClear Tuss:**
Per 5 ml:
hydrocodone 5 mg
guaifenesin 100 mg
*Uses:* Analgesic, expectorant
**Hycodan:**
hydrocodone 5 mg
homatropine 1.5 mg
*Uses:* Analgesic, mydriatic
**Hycodan Syrup:**
Per 5 ml:
hydrocodone 5 mg
homatropine 1.5 mg
*Uses:* Analgesic, mydriatic
**Hycomine Compound:**
chlorpheniramine 2 mg
acetaminophen 250 mg
phenylephrine 10 mg
hydrocodone 5 mg
caffeine 30 mg
*Uses:* Antihistamine, analgesic, adrenergic
**Hycotuss Expectorant Syrup:**
Per 5 ml:
guaifenesin 100 mg
hydrocodone 5 mg
10% alcohol
*Uses:* Expectorant
**Hydrocet:**
hydrocodone 5 mg
acetaminophen 500 mg
*Uses:* Opioid analgesic

**Hydrogesic:**
hydrocodone 5 mg
acetaminophen 500 mg
*Uses:* Opioid analgesic
**Hydropres-50:**
hydrochlorothiazide 50 mg
reserpine 0.125 mg
*Uses:* Antihypertensive
**Hyzaar:**
losartan potassium 50 mg
hydrochlorothiazide 12.5 mg
potassium 4.24 mg
*Uses:* Antihypertensive
**Imodium Advanced:**
loperamide 2 mg
simethicone 125 mg
*Uses:* Antidiarrheal, antiflatulent
**Innovar:**
Per ml:
droperidol 2.5 mg
fentanyl 0.05 mg
*Uses:* Opioid analgesic, general anesthetic
**Iofed:**
brompheniramine 12 mg
pseudoephedrine 120 mg
*Uses:* Antihistamine, adrenergic
**Iofed PD:**
brompheniramine 6 mg
pseudoephedrine 60 mg
*Uses:* Antihistamine, adrenergic
**Janumet:**
metformin 500 mg
sitagliptan 50 mg
metformin 1000 mg
sitagliptan 50 mg
*Uses:* Antidiabetic
**Kaletra Capsules:**
lopinavir 133.3 mg
ritonavir 33.3 mg
*Uses:* HIV
**Kaletra Solution:**
Per 1 ml:
lopinavir 80 mg
ritonavir 20 mg
*Uses:* HIV
**Kaletra Tablets**
lopinavir 200 mg
ritonavir 50 mg
*Uses:* HIV
**Lactinex:**
Mixed culture of:
*Lactobacillus acidophilus* and
*Lactobacillus bulgaricus*
*Uses:* Supplement
**Levell 12.5 ml Suspension:**
carbetapentane 30 mg
phenylephrine 30 mg
*Uses:* Antitussive
**Levlite:**
levonorgestrel 0.100 mg
ethinyl estradiol 20 mcg
*Uses:* Estrogen, progestin
**Levsin PB Drops:**
Per ml:
hyoscyamine 0.125 mg

Adverse effects: *italic* = common, **bold** = life-threatening

phenobarbital 15 mg
5% alcohol
*Uses:* Anticholinergic, barbiturate
**Levsin w/Phenobarbital:**
hyoscyamine 0.125 mg
phenobarbital 15 mg
*Uses:* Anticholinergic, barbiturate
**Lexxel 1:**
enalapril 5 mg
felodipine 5 mg
*Uses:* Antihypertensive
**Lexxel 2:**
enalapril 5 mg
felodipine 2.5 mg
*Uses:* Antihypertensive
**Librax:**
chlordiazepoxide 5 mg
clidinium 2.5 mg
*Uses:* Antianxiety, anticholinergic
**Lida-Mantel-HC-Cream:**
0.5% hydrocortisone
3% lidocaine
*Uses:* Antiinflammatory, analgesic
**Limbitrol DS 10-25:**
chlordiazepoxide 10 mg
amitriptyline 25 mg
*Uses:* Antidepressant, antianxiety
**Lobac:**
salicylamide 200 mg
phenyltoloxamine 20 mg
acetaminophen 300 mg
*Uses:* Skeletal muscle relaxant, analgesic
**Loestrin Fe 1/20:**
norethindrone acetate 1 mg/tablet
ethinyl estradiol 20 mcg/tablet
  with 7 tablets of ferrous fumarate
  75 mg/container
*Uses:* Oral contraceptive
**Loestrin Fe 1.5/30:**
norethindrone acetate 1.5 mg
ethinyl estradiol 30 mcg
*Uses:* Oral contraceptive
**Lomotil:**
diphenoxylate 2.5 mg
atropine 0.025 mg
*Uses:* Antidiarrheal, anticholinergic
**Lomotil Liquid:**
Per 5 ml:
diphenoxylate 2.5 mg
atropine 0.025 mg
*Uses:* Antidiarrheal, anticholinergic
**Lo Ovral:**
ethinyl estradiol 30 mcg
norgestrel 0.3 mg
*Uses:* Oral contraceptive
**Lopressor HCT 50/25:**
metoprolol 50 mg
hydrochlorothiazide 25 mg
*Uses:* Antihypertensive
**Lopressor HCT 100/25:**
metoprolol 100 mg
hydrochlorothiazide 25 mg
*Uses:* Antihypertensive
**Lopressor HCT 100/50:**
metoprolol 100 mg

hydrochlorothiazide 50 mg
*Uses:* Antihypertensive
**Lorcet 10/650:**
acetaminophen 650 mg
hydrocodone 10 mg
*Uses:* Analgesic
**Lorcet-HD:**
hydrocodone 10 mg
acetaminophen 300 mg
*Uses:* Analgesic
**Lorcet Plus:**
acetaminophen 650 mg
hydrocodone 7.5 mg
*Uses:* Analgesic
**Lortab 2.5/500:**
hydrocodone 2.5 mg
acetaminophen 500 mg
*Uses:* Analgesic
**Lortab 5/500:**
hydrocodone 5 mg
acetaminophen 500 mg
*Uses:* Analgesic
**Lortab 7.5/500:**
hydrocodone 7.5 mg
acetaminophen 500 mg
*Uses:* Analgesic
**Lortab 10/500:**
hydrocodone 10 mg
acetaminophen 500 mg
*Uses:* Analgesic
**Lortab Oral Sol:**
Per 15 ml:
hydrocodone 7.5 mg
acetaminophen 500 mg
*Uses:* Analgesic
♣ **Losec 1-2-3A:**
omeprazole 20 mg
clarithromycin 500 mg
amoxicillin 1 g
*Uses:* Antiinfective
♣ **Losec 1-2-3M:**
omeprazole 20 mg
clarithromycin 250 mg
metronidazole 500 mg
*Uses:* Antiinfective
**Lotrel 10/20:**
amlopidine 10 mg
benazepril 20 mg
*Uses:* Antihypertensive
**Lotrel 10/40:**
amlopidine 10 mg
benazepril 40 mg
*Uses:* Antihypertensive
**Lotrisone Topical:**
0.05% betamethasone
1% clotrimazole
*Uses:* Local antiinfective, antiinflammatory
**Lufyllin-EPG Elixir:**
Per 5 ml:
dyphylline 150 mg
epHEDrine 24 mg
guaifenesin 300 mg
phenobarbital 24 mg
*Uses:* Bronchodilator, expectorant

**Lufyllin-GG:**
dyphylline 200 mg
guaifenesin 200 mg
*Uses:* Bronchodilator, expectorant
**Lunelle Monthly Contraceptive Injection:**
25 mg medroxyprogesterone
5 mg estradiol/0.5 ml
*Uses:* Contraceptive
**Lybrel:**
ethinyl estridiol 20 mcg
levonorgestrel 90 mcg
*Uses:* Continuous contraceptive
**M-M-R-II:**
measles
mumps
rubella
*Uses:* Vaccine, toxoid
**Maalox:**
aluminum hydroxide 200 mg
magnesium hydroxide 200 mg
*Uses:* Antacid, adsorbent, antiflatulent
**Maalox Extra Strength Suspension:**
Per 5 ml:
aluminum hydroxide 500 mg
magnesium hydroxide 450 mg
simethicone 40 mg
*Uses:* Antacid, adsorbent, antiflatulent
**Maalox Plus:**
aluminum hydroxide 200 mg
magnesium hydroxide 200 mg
simethicone 25 mg
*Uses:* Antacid, adsorbent, antiflatulent
**Maalox Suspension:**
Per 5 ml:
aluminum hydroxide 225 mg
magnesium hydroxide 200 mg
*Uses:* Antacid, adsorbent, antiflatulent
**Macrobid:**
nitrofurantoin macrocrystals 25 mg
nitrofurantoin monohydrate 75 mg
*Uses:* Antiinfective
**Malarone:**
250 mg atovaquone
100 mg proguanil
*Uses:* Malaria
**Malarone Pediatric:**
62.5 mg atovaquone
25 mg proguanil
*Uses:* Malaria
**Mapap Cold Formula:**
acetaminophen 325 mg
chlorpheniramine 2 mg
pseudoephedrine 30 mg
dextromethorphan 15 mg
*Uses:* Bronchodilator, expectorant
**Maxitrol Ophthalmic Suspension/Ointment:**
Per ml:
0.35% neomycin
0.1% dexamethasone
polymyxin B 10,000 units
*Uses:* Ophthalmic antiinfective,
antiinflammatory
**Maxzide:**
hydrochlorothiazide 50 mg
triamterene 75 mg

*Uses:* Antihypertensive, diuretic
**Maxzide-25 MG:**
hydrochlorothiazide 25 mg
triamterene 37.5 mg
*Uses:* Diuretic
**Medigesic:**
acetaminophen 325 mg
caffeine 40 mg
butalbital 50 mg
*Uses:* Nonopioid analgesic
**Mepergan Fortis:**
meperidine 50 mg
promethazine 25 mg
*Uses:* Analgesic, antihistamine
**Mepergan Injection:**
meperidine 25 mg
promethazine 25 mg
*Uses:* Analgesic
**Metaglip 2.5:**
glipiZIDE/metformin 2.5 mg/250 mg, 2.5 mg/
500 mg, 5 mg/500 mg
*Uses:* Diabetes mellitus
**Metimyd Ophthalmic Suspension/Ointment:**
0.5% prednisoLONE
10% sodium sulfacetamide
*Uses:* Ophthalmic antiinfective,
antiinflammatory
**Micardis HCT 40/12.5:**
telmesartan 40 mg
hydrochlorthiazide 12.5 mg
*Uses:* Antihypertensive
**Micardis HCT 80/12.5:**
telmesartan 80 mg
hydrochlorthiazide 12.5 mg
*Uses:* Antihypertensive
**Micardis HCT 80/25:**
telmesartan 80 mg
hydrochlorothiazide 25 mg
*Uses:* Antihypertensive
**Microgestin Fe 1/20:**
norethindrone 1 mg
ethinyl estradiol 20 mcg
ferrous fumarate 75 mg in container
*Uses:* Estrogen, progestin
**Microgestin Fe 1.5/30:**
norethindrone 1.5 mg
ethinyl estradiol 30 mcg
ferrous fumarate 75 mg in container
*Uses:* Estrogen, progestin
**Midol Maximum Strength Multi-Symptom Menstrual Gelcaps:**
acetaminophen 500 mg
pyrilamine 15 mg
caffeine 60 mg
*Uses:* Analgesic
**Midol PM:**
acetaminophen 500 mg
diphenhydrAMINE 25 mg
*Uses:* Analgesic, antihistamine
**Midol PMS Maximum Strength Caplets:**
acetaminophen 500 mg
pyrilamine 15 mg
pamabrom 25 mg
*Uses:* Analgesic

**Midol, Teen:**
acetaminophen 400 mg
pamabrom 25 mg
*Uses:* Analgesic

**Midrin:**
isometheptene 65 mg
acetaminophen 325 mg
dichloralphenazone 100 mg
*Uses:* Analgesic

**Moduretic:**
hydrochlorothiazide 50 mg
amiloride 5 mg
*Uses:* Diuretic

**Monopril-HCT 10:**
fosinopril 10 mg
hydrochlorthiazine 12.5 mg
*Uses:* Antihypertensive

**Monopril-HCT 20:**
fosinopril 20 mg
hydrochlorthiazine 12.5 mg
*Uses:* Antihypertensive

**Motrin Children's Cold Suspension:**
Per 5 ml:
ibuprofen 100 mg
pseudoephedrine 15 mg
*Uses:* Nonopioid analgesic, decongestant

**Motrin Sinus Headache:**
pseudoephedrine 30 mg
ibuprofen 200 mg
*Uses:* Adrenergic, analgesic

**Mucinex D:**
guaifenesin/pseudoephedrine 1200 mg/
    120 mg, 600 mg/60 mg
*Uses:* Expectorant, decongestant

**Mucinex DM:**
dextromethorphan 30 mg
guaifenesin 600 mg
*Uses:* Antitussive, expectorant

**Murocoll-2 Ophthalmic Drops:**
0.3% scopolamine
10% phenylephrine
*Uses:* Ophthalmic anticholinergic,
    mydriatic

**Mycolog II Topical:**
Per gram:
0.1% triamcinolone acetonide
nystatin 100,000 units
*Uses:* Local antiinfective, antiinflammatory

**Mylanta:**
aluminum hydroxide 200 mg
magnesium hydroxide 200 mg
simethicone 20 mg
*Uses:* Antacid, adsorbent, antiflatulent

**Mylanta Double Strength Liquid:**
Per 5 ml:
aluminum hydroxide 400 mg
magnesium hydroxide 400 mg
simethicone 40 mg
*Uses:* Antacid, adsorbent, antiflatulent

**Mylanta Gelcaps:**
calcium carbonate 311 mg
magnesium carbonate 232 mg
*Uses:* Antacid, adsorbent, antiflatulent

**Naphcon-A Ophthalmic
    Solution:**
0.25% naphazoline
0.3% pheniramine
*Uses:* Ophthalmic vasoconstrictor

**Nasatab LA:**
guaifenesin 500 mg
pseudoephedrine 120 mg
*Uses:* Expectorant, decongestant

**NeoDecadron Ophthalmic Ointment:**
0.35% neomycin
0.05% dexamethasone
*Uses:* Ophthalmic antiinfective,
    antiinflammatory

**NeoDecadron Ophthalmic Solution:**
0.35% neomycin
0.1% dexamethasone
*Uses:* Ophthalmic antiinfective,
    antiinflammatory

**Neosporin Cream:**
Per gram:
polymyxin B 10,000 units
neomycin 3.5 mg
*Uses:* Topical antiinfective

**Neosporin G.U. Irrigant:**
Per ml:
neomycin 40 mg
polymyxin B 200,000 units
*Uses:* Antiinfective

**Neosporin Ophthalmic Ointment:**
Per gram:
neomycin 3.5 mg
polymyxin B 10,000 units
bacitracin zinc 400 units
*Uses:* Ophthalmic antiinfective

**Neosporin Ophthalmic Solution:**
Per ml:
neomycin 1.75 mg
polymyxin B 10,000 units
gramicidin 0.025 mg
*Uses:* Ophthalmic antiinfective

**Neosporin Plus Cream:**
polymyxin B 10,000 units
neomycin 3.5 mg
lidocaine 40 mg
*Uses:* Topical antiinfective

**Neosporin Topical Ointment:**
Per gram:
polymyxin B 5000 units
bacitracin zinc 400 units
neomycin 3.5 mg
*Uses:* Topical antiinfective

**Niferex-150 Forte:**
ferrous sulfate 150 mg
vitamin $B_{12}$ 25 mcg
folic acid 1 mg
*Uses:* Supplement

**Norco:**
hydrocodone 10 mg
acetaminophen 325 mg
*Uses:* Analgesic, opioid, nonopioid

**Norco 5/325:**
hydrocodone 5 mg
acetaminophen 325 mg
*Uses:* Analgesic, opioid, nonopioid

**Norgesic:**
orphenadrine 25 mg
aspirin 385 mg
caffeine 30 mg
*Uses:* Skeletal muscle relaxant, analgesic
**Norgesic Forte:**
orphenadrine 50 mg
aspirin 770 mg
caffeine 60 mg
*Uses:* Skeletal muscle relaxant, analgesic
**Novacet Lotion:**
sodium sulfacetamine 10%
sulfur 5%
*Uses:* Acne agent
**Novafed A:**
pseudoephedrine 120 mg
chlorpheniramine 8 mg
*Uses:* Adrenergic, antihistamine
♣ **Novo-Gesic C8:**
acetaminophen 300 mg
codeine 8 mg
caffeine 15 mg
*Uses:* Analgesic
**NuLytely:**
PEG 3350/420 g
sodium bicarbonate 5.72 g
sodium chloride 11.2 g
potassium chloride 1.48 g
*Uses:* Laxative
**NuvaRing:**
ethinyl estradiol 0.015 mg/24 hr
etonogestrel 0.12 mg/24 hr
*Uses:* Contraceptive
**Octicair Otic Suspension:**
1% hydrocortisone
neomycin 5 mg/ml
polymyxin B 10,000 units/ml
*Uses:* Otic antiinflammatory,
   antiinfective
**Opcon-A Ophthalmic Solution:**
0.027% naphazoline
0.315% pheniramine
*Uses:* Ophthalmic vasoconstrictor
**Ornade Spansules:**
phenylpropanolamine 75 mg
chlorpheniramine 12 mg
*Uses:* Antihistamine, decongestant
**Ornex:**
pseudoephedrine 30 mg
acetaminophen 500 mg
*Uses:* Adrenergic, analgesic
**Ornex No Drowsiness Caplets:**
acetaminophen 325 mg
pseudoephedrine 30 mg
*Uses:* Adrenergic, analgesic
**Orphengesic:**
orphenadrine 25 mg
aspirin 385 mg
caffeine 30 mg
*Uses:* Analgesic
**Orphengesic Forte:**
orphenadrine 50 mg
aspirin 770 mg
caffeine 60 mg
*Uses:* Analgesic

**Ortho-cept:**
ethinyl estradiol 30 mcg
desogestrel 0.15 mg
*Uses:* Oral contraceptive
**Ortho-cyclen:**
ethinyl estradiol 35 mcg
norgestimate 0.25 mg
*Uses:* Oral contraceptive
**Ortho-Prefest:**
estradiol 1 mg (15)
norgestimate 0.09 mg (15)
*Uses:* Vasomotor symptoms (menopause)
**Ovcon-50:**
ethinyl estradiol 50 mcg
norethindrone 1 mg
*Uses:* Oral contraceptive
♣ **Oxycocet:**
acetaminophen 325 mg
oxycodone 5 mg
*Uses:* Analgesic
**P-A-C Analgesic:**
aspirin 400 mg
caffeine 32 mg
*Uses:* Nonopioid analgesic
**Pain-X Topical:**
0.05% capsaicin
5% menthol
4% camphor
*Uses:* Topical analgesic
**Pamprin Maximum Pain Relief:**
acetaminophen 250 mg
pamabrom 25 mg
magnesium salicylate 250 mg
*Uses:* Analgesic
**Pamprin Multi-Symptom:**
acetaminophen 500 mg
pamabrom 25 mg
pyrilamine 15 mg
*Uses:* Analgesic
**Panacet 5/500:**
hydrocodone 5 mg
acetaminophen 500 mg
*Uses:* Analgesic
**Panasal 5/500:**
hydrocodone 5 mg
aspirin 500 mg
*Uses:* Analgesic
**Pancrease Capsules:**
amylase 20,000 units
protease 25,000 units
lipase 4500 units (microspheres)
*Uses:* Digestive enzyme
**Pedia Care Cold-Allergy Chewable:**
pseudoephedrine 15 mg
chlorpheniramine 1 mg
*Uses:* Adrenergic, antihistamine
**Pedia Care Cough-Cold Liquid:**
Per 5 ml:
pseudoephedrine 15 mg
chlorpheniramine 1 mg
dextromethorphan 5 mg
*Uses:* Adrenergic, antihistamine, antitussive
**Pedia Care NightRest Cough-Cold Liquid:**
Per 5 ml:
pseudoephedrine 15 mg

Adverse effects: *italic* = common, **bold** = life-threatening

chlorpheniramine 1 mg
dextromethorphan 7.5 mg
*Uses:* Adrenergic, antihistamine, antitussive
**Pediazole Suspension:**
Per 5 ml:
erythromycin 200 mg
sulfiSOXAZOLE 600 mg
*Uses:* Antiinfective
**Pepcid Complete:**
calcium carbonate 800 mg
magnesium hydroxide 165 mg
famotidine 10 mg
*Uses:* Antiulcer agent
**Percocet 2.5/325:**
oxycodone 2.5 mg
acetaminophen 325 mg
*Uses:* Analgesic
**Percocet 5/325:**
oxycodone 5 mg
acetaminophen 325 mg
*Uses:* Analgesic
**Percocet 7.5/500:**
oxycodone 7.5 mg
acetaminophen 500 mg
*Uses:* Analgesic
**Percocet 10/650:**
oxycodone 10 mg
acetaminophen 650 mg
*Uses:* Analgesic
**Percodan:**
oxycodone 4.88 mg
aspirin 325 mg
*Uses:* Analgesic
**Percogesic:**
phenyltoloxamine 30 mg
acetaminophen 325 mg
*Uses:* Analgesic
**Perdiem Granules:**
Per teaspoon:
senna 0.74 g
psyllium 3.25 g
sodium 1.8 mg
potassium 35.5 mg
*Uses:* Laxative
**Peri-Colace:**
docusate sodium 100 mg
casanthranol 30 mg
*Uses:* Laxative
**Peri-Colace Syrup:**
Per 15 ml:
docusate sodium 60 mg
casanthranol 30 mg
*Uses:* Laxative
**Phenerbel-S:**
ergotamine tartrate 0.6 mg
belladonna alkaloids 0.2 mg
phenobarbital 40 mg
*Uses:* α-Adrenergic blocker, anticholinergic
**Phenergan VC Syrup:**
Per 5 ml:
phenylephrine 5 mg
promethazine 6.25 mg
*Uses:* Adrenergic, antihistamine

**Phenergan VC w/Codeine Syrup:**
Per 5 ml:
phenylephrine 5 mg
promethazine 6.25 mg
codeine 10 mg
*Uses:* Adrenergic, antihistamine, opioid analgesic
**Phenergan w/Codeine Syrup:**
Per 5 ml:
promethazine 6.25 mg
codeine 10 mg
*Uses:* Antihistamine, analgesic
**Phenflu G:**
acetaminophen 500 mg
dextromethorphan 30 mg
guaifenesin 600 mg
phenylephrine 15 mg
*Uses:* Analgesic, antitussive, expectorant, decongestant
**Polaramine Expectorant Liquid:**
Per 5 ml:
guaifenesin 100 mg
dexchlorpheniramine 2 mg
pseudoephedrine 20 mg
7.5% alcohol
*Uses:* Expectorant
**Polycitra Syrup:**
Per 5 ml:
potassium citrate 550 mg
sodium citrate 500 mg
citric acid 334 mg
*Uses:* Laxative
**Poly-Histine Elixir:**
Per 5 ml:
pheniramine 4 mg
pyrilamine 4 mg
phenyltoloxamine 4 mg
4% alcohol
*Uses:* Antihistamine
**Polysporin Ophthalmic Ointment:**
Per gram:
polymyxin B 10,000 units
bacitracin zinc 500 units
*Uses:* Ophthalmic antiinfective
**Polysporin Topical Ointment:**
Per gram:
polymyxin B 10,000 units
bacitracin zinc 500 units
*Uses:* Topical antiinfective
**Polytrim Ophthalmic Solution:**
Per ml:
trimethoprim 1 mg
polymyxin B 10,000 units
*Uses:* Ophthalmic antiinfective
**Pravigard PAC:**
aspirin 81 mg
pravastatin 20, 40, 80 mg
aspirin 325 mg
pravastatin 20, 40, 80 mg
*Uses:* Antihyperlipidemic, antithrombotic
**Prefest:**
estradiol 1 mg
norgestimate 0.09 mg
*Uses:* Vasomotor symptoms (menopause)

 Alert      Canada Only     🜨 Drug on CD     * "Tall Man" lettering (See Preface)

**Premphase:**
In a compliance package:
conjugated estrogens 0.625 mg
medroxyPROGESTERone 5 mg
*Uses:* Vasomotor symptoms (menopause)
**Prempro:**
In a compliance package:
conjugated estrogens 0.3 mg
medroxyPROGESTERone 1.5 mg
conjugated estrogens 0.45 mg
medroxyPROGESTERone 1.5 mg
conjugated estrogens 0.625 mg
medroxyPROGESTERone 2.5 mg
conjugated estrogens 0.625 mg
medroxyPROGESTERone 5 mg
*Uses:* Vasomotor symptoms (menopause)
**Premsyn PMS:**
acetaminophen 500 mg
pamabrom 25 mg
pyrilamine 15 mg
*Uses:* Analgesic
**Prevpac:**
In a compliance package:
amoxicillin 500-mg caps
clarithromycin 500-mg tabs
lansoprazole 30-mg caps
*Uses:* Antiinfective
**Primaxin 250 mg IV for Injection:**
imipenem 250 mg
cilastatin sodium 250 mg
*Uses:* Antiinfective
**Primaxin 500 mg IV for Injection:**
imipenem 500 mg
cilastatin sodium 500 mg
*Uses:* Antiinfective
**Prinzide 10-12.5:**
lisinopril 10 mg
hydrochlorothiazide 12.5 mg
*Uses:* Antihypertensive
**Prinzide 20-12.5:**
lisinopril 20 mg
hydrochlorothiazide 12.5 mg
*Uses:* Antihypertensive
**Prinzide 20-25:**
lisinopril 20 mg
hydrochlorothiazide 25 mg
*Uses:* Antihypertensive
**Proben-C:**
colchicine 0.5 mg
probenecid 500 mg
*Uses:* Antigout agent
**Proctofoam-HC Aerosol Foam:**
1% hydrocortisone
1% pramoxine
*Uses:* Topical corticosteroid
**Pronto Plus Lice Killing Shampoo:**
piperonyl butoxide 4%
pyrethrum extract 0.33%
*Uses:* Lice
**Propacet 100:**
propoxyphene-N 100 mg
acetaminophen 650 mg
*Uses:* Analgesic
**Pseudo-Chlor:**
pseudoephedrine 120 mg

chlorpheniramine 8 mg
*Uses:* Antihistamine
**Pseudo-Gest Plus:**
pseudoephedrine 60 mg
chlorpheniramine 4 mg
*Uses:* Antihistamine
**Pylera:**
bismuth subcitrate potassium 140 mg
metronidazole 125 mg
tetracycline 125 mg
*Uses: Helicobacter pylori*
**Quadrinal:**
epHEDrine 24 mg
theophylline 65 mg
potassium iodide 320 mg
phenobarbital 24 mg
*Uses:* Adrenergic, bronchodilator, barbiturate
**Quibron-300:**
theophylline 300 mg
guaifenesin 180 mg
*Uses:* Bronchodilator, expectorant
**Rebetron:**
interferon alfa-2b 3 million units/0.5 ml
ribavirin, PO 200 mg
*Uses:* Biologic response modifier, antiviral
**Regulace:**
docusate sodium 100 mg
casanthranol 30 mg
*Uses:* Laxative
**Renese-R:**
polythiazide 2 mg
reserpine 0.25 mg
*Uses:* Diuretic, antihypertensive
**Respahist:**
pseudoephedrine 60 mg
brompheniramine 6 mg
*Uses:* Adrenergic, antihistamine
**Respaire-60:**
guaifenesin 200 mg
pseudoephedrine 60 mg
*Uses:* Expectorant, adrenergic
**Respi-TANN:**
Per 5 ml:
carbetapentane 20 mg
pseudoephedrine 30 mg
*Uses:* Cough suppressant, decongestant
**Respi-TANN Pd:**
Per 5 ml:
carbetapentane 7.5 mg
pseudoephedrine 30 mg
*Uses:* Cough suppressant, decongestant
**Rifamate:**
isoniazid 150 mg
rifampin 300 mg
*Uses:* Antitubercular, antileprotic
**Rifater:**
rifampin 120 mg
isoniazid 50 mg
pyrazinamide 300 mg
*Uses:* Antitubercular
**Riopan Plus Suspension:**
Per 5 ml:
magaldrate 540 mg
simethicone 40 mg
*Uses:* Antacid, adsorbent, antiflatulent

Adverse effects: *italic* = common, **bold** = life-threatening

**Robaxisal:**
methocarbamol 400 mg
aspirin 325 mg
*Uses:* Skeletal muscle relaxant, analgesic

**Robitussin A/C Syrup:**
codeine 10 mg
guaifenesin 100 mg
35% alcohol
*Uses:* Antitussive, opioid analgesic

**Robitussin Cold & Cough Liquigels:**
pseudoephedrine 30 mg
guaifenesin 200 mg
dextromethorphan 10 mg
*Uses:* Antitussive, expectorant, decongestant

**Robitussin-DM Liquid:**
Per 5 ml:
guaifenesin 100 mg
dextromethorphan 10 mg
*Uses:* Expectorant, antitussive

**Robitussin Honey Flu Multi-Symptom Liquid:**
dextromethorphan 6.6 mg
pseudoephedrine 20 mg
acetaminophen 166.7
*Uses:* Antitussive, decongestant, analgesic

**Robitussin Maximum Strength Cough and Cold Syrup:**
dextromethorphan 15 mg
pseudoephedrine 30 mg
*Uses:* Antitussive, adrenergic

**Robitussin Night Relief Liquid:**
dextromethorphan 5 mg
pyrilamine 8.3 mg
pseudoephedrine 10 mg
acetaminophen 108.3 mg
*Uses:* Antitussive, adrenergic

**Robitussin Pediatric Cough & Cold Liquid:**
Per 5 ml:
pseudoephedrine 15 mg
dextromethorphan 7.5 mg
*Uses:* Antitussive, adrenergic

**Rolaids Calcium Rich:**
magnesium hydroxide 80 mg
calcium carbonate 412 mg
*Uses:* Antacid, adsorbent, antiflatulent

**Rondec:**
pseudoephedrine 60 mg
carbinoxamine 4 mg
*Uses:* Adrenergic

**Rondec DM Drops:**
Per ml:
pseudoephedrine 25 mg
carbinoxamine 2 mg
dextromethorphan 4 mg
*Uses:* Adrenergic, antitussive

**Rondec DM Syrup:**
Per 5 ml:
pseudoephedrine 60 mg
carbinoxamine 4 mg
dextromethorphan 15 mg
*Uses:* Adrenergic, antitussive

**Rondec Oral Drops:**
Per 5 ml:
pseudoephedrine 25 mg
carbinoxamine 2 mg
*Uses:* Adrenergic

**Roxicet 5/325:**
acetaminophen 325 mg
oxycodone 5 mg
*Uses:* Opioid analgesic

**Roxicet 5/500:**
oxycodone 5 mg
acetaminophen 500 mg
*Uses:* Opioid analgesic

**Roxicet Oral Solution:**
Per 5 ml:
acetaminophen 325 mg
oxycodone 5 mg
*Uses:* Analgesic

**Roxiprin:**
aspirin 325 mg
oxycodone HCl 4.5 mg
oxycodone terephthalate 0.38 mg
*Uses:* Analgesic

**Salutensin Demi:**
hydroflumethiazide 25 mg
reserpine 0.125 mg
*Uses:* Antihypertensive

**Scot-Tussin DM Liquid:**
Per 5 ml:
chlorpheniramine 2 mg
dextromethorphan 15 mg
*Uses:* Antihistamine, antitussive

**Scot-Tussin Original 5-Action Liquid:**
phenylephrine 4.2 mg
pheniramine 13.3 mg
sodium citrate 83.3 mg
sodium salicylate 83.3 mg
caffeine citrate 25 mg
*Uses:* Adrenergic, analgesic

**Sedapap-10:**
acetaminophen 650 mg
butalbital 50 mg
*Uses:* Analgesic, barbiturate

**Semprex-D:**
acrivastine 8 mg
pseudoephedrine 60 mg
*Uses:* Adrenergic, bronchodilator

**Senokot-S:**
docusate 50 mg
senna concentrate 187 mg
*Uses:* Laxative

**Septra:**
sulfamethoxazole 400 mg
trimethroprim 80 mg
*Uses:* Antiinfective

**Septra DS:**
sulfamethoxazole 800 mg
trimethroprim 160 mg
*Uses:* Antiinfective

**Ser-Ap-Es:**
hydrochlorothiazide 15 mg
reserpine 0.1 mg
hydrALAZINE 25 mg
*Uses:* Diuretic, antihypertensive

**Silafed Syrup:**
Per 5 ml:
pseudoephedrine 30 mg
triprolidine 1.25 mg

 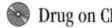

*Uses:* Adrenergic, antihistamine
**Silaminic Cold Syrup:**
Per 5 ml:
phenylpropanolamine 12.5 mg
chlorpheniramine 2 mg
*Uses:* Antihistamine, decongestant
**Sinemet 10/100:**
carbidopa 10 mg
levodopa 100 mg
*Uses:* Antiparkinsonian
**Sinemet 25/100:**
carbidopa 25 mg
levodopa 100 mg
*Uses:* Antiparkinsonian
**Sinemet 25/250:**
carbidopa 25 mg
levodopa 250 mg
*Uses:* Antiparkinsonian
**Sinemet CR 25-100:**
carbidopa 25 mg
levodopa 100 mg
*Uses:* Antiparkinsonian
**Sinemet CR 50-200:**
carbidopa 50 mg
levodopa 200 mg
*Uses:* Antiparkinsonian
**Sinus-Relief:**
acetaminophen 325 mg
pseudoephedrine 30 mg
*Uses:* Nonopioid analgesic
**Slo-Phyllin GG Syrup:**
theophylline 150 mg
guaifenesin 90 mg
*Uses:* Bronchodilator, expectorant
**Slow-Salt-K:**
sodium chloride 410 mg
potassium chloride 15 mg
*Uses:* Potassium, sodium supplement
**Solage:**
mequinol 2%
tretinoin 0.01%
*Uses:* Antineoplastic
**Soma Compound:**
carisoprodol 200 mg
aspirin 325 mg
*Uses:* Skeletal muscle relaxant
**Spec-T Lozenge:**
dextromethorphan 10 mg
benzocaine 10 mg
*Uses:* Antitussive, topical anesthetic
**Stalevo 50:**
carbidopa 12.5 mg
levodopa 50 mg
entacapone 200 mg
*Uses:* Parkinsonism
**Stalevo 100:**
carbidopa 25 mg
levodopa 100 mg
entacapone 200 mg
*Uses:* Parkinsonism
**Stalevo 150:**
carbidopa 37.5 mg
levodopa 150 mg
entacapone 200 mg
*Uses:* Parkinsonism

**Sudafed Sinus & Cold:**
pseudoephedrine 30 mg
acetaminophen 325 mg
*Uses:* Adrenergic, analgesic
**Sudal 60/500:**
pseudoephedrine 60 mg
guaifenesin 500 mg
*Uses:* Adrenergic, expectorant
**Sudal 120/600:**
pseudoephedrine 120 mg
guaifenesin 600 mg
*Uses:* Adrenergic, expectorant
**Sultrin Triple Sulfa Vaginal Cream:**
3.42% sulfathiazole
2.86% sulfacetamine
3.7% sulfabenzamide
*Uses:* Antiinfective
**Sultrin Triple Sulfa Vaginal Tablets:**
sulfathiazole 172.5 mg
sulfacetamide 143.75 mg
sulfabenzamide 184 mg
*Uses:* Antiinfective
**Symbicort:**
budesonide 80 mcg
formoterol 4.5 mcg
budesonide 160 mcg
formoterol 4.5 mcg
*Uses:* Asthma
**Symbyax:**
olanzapine 6 mg
fluoxetine 25 mg
olanzapine 6 mg
fluoxetine 50 mg
olanzapine 12 mg
fluoxetine 25 mg
olanzapine 12 mg
fluoxetine 50 mg
*Uses:* Bipolar disorder
**Synalgos-DC:**
aspirin 356.4 mg
caffeine 30 mg
dihydrocodeine 16 mg
*Uses:* Analgesic
**Synercid:**
quinupristin 150 mg
dalfopristin 350 mg
*Uses:* Antiinfective
**Syntest H.S.:**
esterified estrogens 0.625 mg
methylTESTOSTERone 1.25 mg
*Uses:* Vasomotor symptoms (menopause)
**Taclonex:**
betamethasone 0.064%
calcipotriene 0.005%
*Uses:* Plaque psoriasis
**Talacen:**
acetaminophen 650 mg
pentazocine 25 mg
*Uses:* Analgesic
**Talwin Compound:**
aspirin 325 mg
pentazocine 12.5 mg
*Uses:* Analgesic
**Talwin NX:**
pentazocine 50 mg

Adverse effects: *italic* = common, **bold** = life-threatening

naloxone 0.5 mg
*Uses:* Analgesic, opioid antagonist
**Tarka 182:**
trandolapril 2 mg (immed rel)
verapamil 180 mg (sus rel)
*Uses:* Antihypertensive, calcium channel
    blocker
**Tarka 241:**
trandolapril 1 mg (immed rel)
verapamil 240 mg (sus rel)
*Uses:* Antihypertensive, calcium channel
    blocker
**Tarka 242:**
trandolapril 2 mg (immed rel)
verapamil 240 mg (sus rel)
*Uses:* Antihypertensive, calcium channel
    blocker
**Tarka 244:**
trandolapril 4 mg (immed rel)
verapamil 240 mg (sus rel)
*Uses:* Antihypertensive, calcium channel
    blocker
**Tavist Allergy/Sinus Headache:**
clemastine 0.335 mg
pseudoephedrine 30 mg
acetaminophen 500 mg
*Uses:* Antihistamine, adrenergic, analgesic
**Tavist Sinus:**
acetaminophen 500 mg
pseudoephedrine 30 mg
*Uses:* Analgesic, adrenergic
✤ **Tecnal:**
aspirin 330 mg
caffeine 40 mg
butalbital 50 mg
*Uses:* Nonopioid analgesic
**Teczem:**
enalapril 5 mg (extended release)
diltiazem 180 mg (extended release)
*Uses:* Antihypertensive, calcium channel
    blocker
**Tegrin-LT Shampoo:**
0.33% pyrethrins
3.15% piperonyl butoxide
*Uses:* Scabicide, pediculicide
**Tenoretic 50:**
atenolol 50 mg
chlorthalidone 25 mg
*Uses:* Antihypertensive
**Tenoretic 100:**
atenolol 100 mg
chlorthalidone 25 mg
*Uses:* Antihypertensive
**Terra-Cortril Ophthalmic Suspension:**
1.5% hydrocortisone acetate
0.5% oxytetracycline
*Uses:* Ophthalmic antiinflammatory,
    antiinfective
**Terramycin w/Polymycin B Sulfate Ophthal-
mic Ointment:**
Per gram:
polymyxin B 10,000 units
oxytetracycline 5 mg
*Uses:* Ophthalmic antiinfective

**T-Gesic:**
hydrocodone 5 mg
acetaminophen 500 mg
*Uses:* Analgesic
**Thera-Flu Cold & Cough Powder:**
Per packet:
pseudoephedrine 60 mg
chlorpheniramine 4 mg
dextromethorphan 20 mg
acetaminophen 650 mg
*Uses:* Adrenergic, antihistamine, antitussive,
    analgesic
**Timentin for Injection:**
Per 3.1-g vial:
ticarcillin 3 g
clavulanic acid 0.1 g
*Uses:* Antiinfective
**Timolide 10/25:**
timolol 10 mg
hydrochlorothiazide 25 mg
*Uses:* Antihypertensive
**Titralac Plus:**
calcium carbonate 420 mg
simethicone 21 mg
*Uses:* Antacid, adsorbent, antiflatulent
**Tobra Dex Ophthalmic
    Suspension/Ointment:**
tobramycin 0.3%
dexamethasone 0.1%
*Uses:* Ophthalmic antiinfective,
    antiinflammatory
**Triacin-C Cough Syrup:**
Per 5 ml:
codeine 10 mg
pseudoephedrine 30 mg
triprolidine 1.25 mg
*Uses:* Analgesic, adrenergic, antihistamine
**Tri-Hydroserpine:**
hydrALAZINE 25 mg
hydrochlorothiazide 15 mg
reserpine 0.1 mg
*Uses:* Antihypertensive
**Trinalin Repetabs:**
azatadine maleate 1 mg
pseudoephedrine 120 mg
*Uses:* Antihistamine
**Triple Antibiotic Ophthalmic Ointment:**
Per gram:
polymyxin B 10,000 units
neomycin 3.5 mg
bacitracin 400 units
*Uses:* Antiinfective
**Triprolidine/Pseudoephedrine Syrup
    (generic):**
Per 5 ml
triprolidine 1.25 mg
pseudoephedrine 50 mg
*Uses:* Antihistamine, decongestant
**Triprolidine/Pseudoephedrine Tablets
    (generic):**
triprolidine 2.5 mg
pseudoephedrine 60 mg
*Uses:* Antihistamine, decongestant
**Trizivir:**
300 mg abacavir

150 mg lamivudine
300 mg zidovudine
*Uses:* HIV
**Tusibron-DM Syrup:**
Per 5 ml:
guaifenesin 100 mg
dextromethorphan 15 mg
*Uses:* Expectorant, antitussive
**Tylenol Allergy Sinus, DayTime Caplet:**
acetaminophen 500 mg
chlorpheniramine 2 mg
pseudoephedrine 30 mg
*Uses:* Antihistamine, adrenergic, analgesic
**Tylenol Children's Cold:**
acetaminophen 80 mg
chlorpheniramine 0.5 mg
pseudoephedrine 7.5 mg
*Uses:* Antihistamine, adrenergic, analgesic
**Tylenol Children's Cold Multi- Symptom
　Plus Cough Liquid:**
Per 5 ml:
acetaminophen 160 mg
dextromethorphan 5 mg
chlorpheniramine 1 mg
pseudoephedrine 15 mg
*Uses:* Antihistamine, adrenergic, analgesic
**Tylenol Children's Cold Plus Cough
　Chewable:**
acetaminophen 80 mg
pseudoephedrine 7.5 mg
dextromethorphan 2.5 mg
chlorpheniramine 0.5 mg
*Uses:* Antihistamine, adrenergic, analgesic
**Tylenol Cold & Flu Severe DayTime Liquid:**
dextromethorphan 5 mg
pseudoephedrine 10 mg
acetaminophen 166.7 mg
*Uses:* Antitussive, decongestant, analgesic
**Tylenol Cold Multi-Symptom Tablets:**
acetaminophen 325 mg
chlorpheniramine 2 mg
pseudoephedrine 30 mg
dextromethorphan 15 mg
*Uses:* Antihistamine, adrenergic, analgesic
**Tylenol Cold Severe Congestion Tablets:**
dextromethorphan 15 mg
guaifenesin 200 mg
pseudoephedrine 32 mg
acetaminophen 325 mg
*Uses:* Antitussive, expectorant, decongestant,
　analgesic
**Tylenol Cough & Sore Throat DayTime
　Liquid:**
dextromethorphan 5 mg
acetaminophen 166.7 mg
*Uses:* Antitussive, analgesic
**Tylenol Flu Day Non-Drowsy Gelcaps:**
diphenhydrAMINE 25 mg
pseudoephedrine 30 mg
acetaminophen 500 mg
*Uses:* Analgesic, adrenergic, antitussive
**Tylenol Flu NightTime Gelcaps:**
diphenhydrAMINE 25 mg
doxylamine 2.1 mg
pseudoephedrine 30 mg

acetaminophen 500 mg
*Uses:* Antihistamine, decongestant, analgesic
**Tylenol PM, Extra Strength:**
acetaminophen 500 mg
diphenhydrAMINE 25 mg
*Uses:* Analgesic, antihistamine
**Tylenol Severe Allergy:**
diphenhydrAMINE 12.5 mg
acetaminophen 500 mg
*Uses:* Analgesic, antihistamine
**Tylenol w/Codeine Elixir:**
Per 5 ml:
acetaminophen 120 mg
codeine 12 mg
*Uses:* Analgesic
**Tylenol w/Codeine No. 1:**
acetaminophen 300 mg
codeine 7.5 mg
*Uses:* Analgesic
**Tylenol w/Codeine No. 2:**
acetaminophen 300 mg
codeine 15 mg
**Tylenol w/Codeine No. 3:**
acetaminophen 300 mg
codeine 30 mg
*Uses:* Analgesic
**Tylenol w/Codeine No. 4:**
acetaminophen 300 mg
codeine 60 mg
*Uses:* Analgesic
**Tylox:**
oxycodone 5 mg
acetaminophen 500 mg
*Uses:* Analgesic
**Ultracet:**
tramadol 37.5 mg
acetaminophen 325 mg
*Uses:* Analgesic
**Unasyn for Injection 3 g:**
ampicillin 2 g
sulbactam 1 g
*Uses:* Antiinfective
**Uniretic:**
moexipril 7.5 mg
hydrochlorothiazide 12.5 mg
moexipril 15 mg
hydrochlorothiazide 25 mg
*Uses:* Antihypertensive, diuretic
**Urised:**
methenamine 40.8 mg
phenylsalicylate 18.1 mg
atropine 0.03 mg
hyoscyamine 0.03 mg
benzoic acid 4.5 mg
methylene blue 5.4 mg
*Uses:* Antiinfective
**Vanquish:**
aspirin 227 mg
acetaminophen 194 mg
caffeine 33 mg
aluminum hydroxide 25 mg
magnesium hydroxide 50 mg
*Uses:* Nonopioid analgesic
**Vaseretic 5-12.5:**
enalapril 5 mg

Adverse effects: *italic* = common, **bold** = life-threatening

hydrochlorthiazide 12.5 mg
*Uses:* Antihypertensive diuretic
**Vaseretic 10-25:**
enalapril 10 mg
hydrochlorothiazide 25 mg
*Uses:* Antihypertensive, diuretic
**Vasocidin Ophthalmic Ointment:**
sulfacetamide 10%
prednisoLONE 0.5%
*Uses:* Ophthalmic antiinfective,
  antiinflammatory
**Vasocidin Ophthalmic Solution:**
sulfacetamide 10%
prednisoLONE 0.25%
*Uses:* Ophthalmic antiinfective,
  antiinflammatory
**Vasocon-A Ophthalmic Solution:**
naphazoline 0.05%
antazoline 0.5%
*Uses:* Ophthalmic vasoconstrictor
**Vicks 44D Cough & Head Congestion
  Liquid:**
Per 5 ml:
dextromethorphan 10 mg
pseudoephedrine 20 mg
*Uses:* Antitussive, adrenergic
**Vicks 44E Liquid:**
Per 5 ml:
dextromethorphan 6.7 mg
guaifenesin 66.7 mg
*Uses:* Antitussive, expectorant
**Vicks 44M Cold, Flu, & Cough LiquiCaps:**
dextromethorphan 10 mg
pseudoephedrine 30 mg
chlorpheniramine 2 mg
acetaminophen 250 mg
*Uses:* Antitussive, adrenergic, antihistamine,
  analgesic
**Vicks 44M Pediatric Liquid:**
Per 5 ml:
pseudoephedrine 15 mg
chlorpheniramine 1 mg
*Uses:* Adrenergic, antihistamine, antitussive
**Vicks 44 Non-Drowsy Cold & Cough
  LiquiCaps:**
dextromethorphan 30 mg
pseudoephedrine 60 mg
*Uses:* Antitussive, adrenergic
**Vicks Children's NyQuil Nighttime Cough/
  Cold Liquid:**
Per 5 ml:
pseudoephedrine 10 mg
chlorpheniramine 0.67 mg
dextromethorphan 5 mg
*Uses:* Adrenergic, antihistamine,
  antitussive
**Vicks DayQuil Liquid:**
dextromethorphan 3.3 mg
pseudoephedrine 10 mg
acetaminophen 108.3 mg
guaifenesin 33.3 mg
*Uses:* Antitussive, adrenergic, analgesic, expectorant

**Vicks DayQuil Multi-Symptom Cold/Flu Re-
  lief Liquid:**
dextromethorphan 33 mg
pseudoephedrine 10 mg
acetaminophen 108.3 mg
*Uses:* Antitussive, decongestant, analgesic
**Vicks DayQuil Pressure & Pain Caplet:**
pseudoephedrine 30 mg
ibuprofen 200 mg
*Uses:* Adrenergic, analgesic
**Vicks NyQuil LiquiCaps:**
pseudoephedrine 30 mg
doxylamine 6.25 mg
dextromethorphan 10 mg
acetaminophen 250 mg
*Uses:* Adrenergic, antihistamine, antitussive,
  analgesic
**Vicks NyQuil Multi-Symptom Cold Flu Re-
  lief Liquid:**
pseudoephedrine 10 mg
doxylamine 2.1 mg
dextromethorphan 5 mg
acetaminophen 167 mg
*Uses:* Adrenergic, antihistamine, antitussive,
  analgesic
**Vicodin:**
acetaminophen 500 mg
hydrocodone 5 mg
*Uses:* Analgesic
**Vicodin ES:**
acetaminophen 750 mg
hydrocodone 7.5 mg
*Uses:* Analgesic
**Vicodin HP:**
acetaminophen 660 mg
hydrocodone 10 mg
*Uses:* Analgesic
**Vicodin Tuss:**
Per 5 ml:
hydrocodone 5 mg
guaifenesin 100 mg
*Uses:* Analgesic, expectorant
**Vicoprofen:**
hydrocodone 7.5 mg
ibuprofen 200 mg
*Uses:* Analgesic
**Vytorin:**
ezetimibe: 10, 10, 10, 10 mg
simvastatin: 10, 20, 40, 80 mg
*Uses:* Antihyperlipidemic
**Yasmin 28:**
ethinyl estadiol 30 mcg
dropirenone 3 mg
*Uses:* Oral contraceptive
**YAZ:**
prospirenone 3 mg
ethinyl estradiol 0.02 mg
*Uses:* Vasomotor symptoms (menopause)
**Zegerid Capsules:**
omeprazole 20 mg
sodium bicarbonate 1100 mg
omeprazole 40 mg
sodium bicarbonate 1100 mg
*Uses:* Gastric ulcer, GERD

**Zegerid Powder (Oral Solution):**
omeprazole 20 mg
sodium bicarbonate 1680 mg
omeprazole 40 mg
sodium bicarbonate 1680 mg
*Uses:* Gastric ulcer, GERD
**Zestoretic 10/12.5:**
lisinopril 10 mg
hydrochlorothiazide 12.5 mg
*Uses:* Antihypertensive
**Zestoretic 20/12.5:**
lisinopril 20 mg
hydrochlorothiazide 12.5 mg
*Uses:* Antihypertensive
**Zestoretic 20/25:**
lisinopril 20 mg
hydrochlorothiazide 25 mg
*Uses:* Antihypertensive
**Ziac 2.5:**
bisoprolol 2.5 mg
hydrochlorothiazide 6.25 mg

*Uses:* Antihypertensive
**Ziac 5:**
bisoprolol 5 mg
hydrochlorothiazide 6.25 mg
*Uses:* Antihypertensive
**Ziac 10:**
bisoprolol 10 mg
hydrochlorothiazide 6.25 mg
*Uses:* Antihypertensive
**Ziana:**
clindamycin 1.2%
tretinoin 0.025%
*Uses:* Acne vulgaris
**Zydone:**
hydrocodone 5 mg
acetaminophen 500 mg
*Uses:* Analgesic
**Zyrtec-D**
cetirizine 5 mg
pseudoephedrine 120 mg
*Uses:* Antihistamine, decongestant

## Appendix H

### High-Alert Drugs

The Institute for Safe Medication Practices (ISMP) compiled a list of the medications with the greatest potential for patient harm if they are used in error. These high-alert medications include drugs in the 19 classes listed below. To help nurses identify these drugs, we have listed the individual high-alert medications found in this book. Although care should be taken in giving any medication, nurses are advised to exercise extra precautions when administering these high-risk drugs.

### Class/Category of Medications

adrenergic agonists, **IV** (e.g., epINEPHrine, phenylephrine, norepinephrine)
adrenergic antagonists, **IV** (e.g., propranolol, metoprolol, labetalol)
anesthetic agents, general, inhaled, and **IV** (e.g., propofol, ketamine)
antiarrhythmics, **IV** (e.g., lidocaine, amiodarone)
antithrombic agents (anticoagulants), including warfarin, low-molecular-weight heparin, **IV** unfractionated heparin, factor Xa inhibitors (fondaparinux), direct thrombin inhibitors (e.g., argatroban, lepirudin, bivalirudin), thrombolytics (e.g., alteplase, reteplase, tenecteplase), and glycoprotein IIb/IIIa inhibitors (e.g., eptifibatide)
cardioplegic solutions
chemotherapeutic agents, parenteral and oral
dextrose, hypertonic, 20% or greater
dialysis solutions, peritoneal and hemodialysis
epidural or intrathecal medications
hypoglycemics, oral
inotropic medications, **IV** (e.g., digoxin, milrinone)
liposomal forms of drugs (e.g., liposomal amphotericin B)
moderate sedation agents, **IV** (e.g., midazolam)
moderate sedation agents, oral, for children (e.g., chloral hydrate)
narcotics/opiates, **IV**, transdermal, and oral (including liquid concentrates, immediate- and sustained-release formulations)
neuromuscular blocking agents (e.g., succinylcholine, rocuronium, vecuronium)
radiocontrast agents, **IV**
total parenteral nutrition solutions

### Individual Medications

abciximab
adenosine
aldesleukin, IL-2
alteplase
amiodarone
anistreplase
antihemophilic factor VIII (AHF)
argatroban
asparaginase
atropine
azacitidine
basiliximab
bevacizumab
bivalirudin
bleomycin
busulfan
carboplatin
carmustine
celecoxib
cisplatin
cyclophosphamide
cytarabine
dacarbazine
daclizumab
dactinomycin
dalteparin
DAUNOrubicin
DAUNOrubicin citrate liposome
digoxin
diltiazem
DOPamine
DOXOrubicin
droperidol

enoxaparin
epHEDrine
epINEPHrine
epirubicin
eptifibatide
etoposide
factor VIIa, recombinant
factor IX complex (human)
fentanyl
fluorouracil
gemtuzumab
heparin
hydromorphone
ibutilide
idarubicin
ifosfamide
inamrinone
insulins
irinotecan
lepirudin
leuprolide
lidocaine, parenteral
magnesium sulfate
melphalan
meperidine
methadone
methotrexate (amethopterin, MTX)
milrinone
mitomycin
mitoxantrone
morphine
nalbuphine

nesiritide
nitroprusside
oxycodone
oxymorphone
oxytocin
pancuronium
pegaspargase
pemetrexed
pentazocine
pentobarbital
pentostatin
phenobarbital
poractant alfa
propofol
propoxyphene
remifentanil
secobarbital
streptokinase
succinylcholine
tenecteplase
thiopental
tinzaparin
tirofiban
topotecan
trastuzumab
tubocurarine
urokinase
vecuronium
vinBLAStine
vinCRIStine
vinorelbine
warfarin

ISMP's List of High-Alert Medications, accessed on 3/19/08 at http://www.ismp.org/Tools/highalertmedications.pdf.

## Appendix I

### Abbreviations and Pregnancy Categories

| | | | |
|---|---|---|---|
| **abd** | abdomen | **CPK** | creatinine phosphokinase |
| **ABG** | arterial blood gas | **CPR** | cardiopulmonary resuscitation |
| **ac** | before meals | **CCr** | creatinine clearance |
| **ACE** | angiotensin-converting enzyme | **C&S** | culture and sensitivity |
| **ACT** | activated clotting time | **C sect** | cesarean section |
| **ADA** | American Diabetes Association | **CSF** | cerebrospinal fluid |
| **ADH** | antidiuretic hormone | **CTCL** | cutaneous T-cell lymphoma |
| **ALT** | alanine aminotransferase | **CV** | cardiovascular |
| **ANA** | antinuclear antibody | **CVA** | cerebrovascular accident |
| **AP** | anteroposterior | **CVP** | central venous pressure |
| **APLA** | antiphospholipid antibody syndrome | **D&C** | dilatation and curettage |
| **APTT** | activated partial thromboplastin time | **dir inf** | direct infusion |
| **ASA** | acetylsalicylic acid, aspirin | **dr** | dram |
| **ASHD** | arteriosclerotic heart disease | **$D_5W$** | 5% glucose in distilled water |
| **AST** | aspartate aminotransferase (SGOT) | **DVT** | deep vein thrombosis |
| **AV** | atrioventricular | **ECG** | electrocardiogram (EKG) |
| **bid** | twice a day | **EDTA** | ethylenediamine tetraacetic acid |
| **BM** | bowel movement | **EEG** | electroencephalogram |
| **BMR** | basal metabolic rate | **EENT** | ear, eye, nose, and throat |
| **B/P** | blood pressure | **EPS** | extrapyramidal symptoms |
| **BPH** | benign prostatic hypertrophy | **ESR** | erythrocyte sedimentation rate |
| **BPM** | beats per minute | **ext rel** | extended release |
| **BS** | blood sugar | **FBS** | fasting blood sugar |
| **BUN** | blood urea nitrogen | **FHT** | fetal heart tones |
| **C** | Celsius (centigrade) | **FSH** | follicle-stimulating hormone |
| **CAD** | coronary artery disease | **g** | gram |
| **cap** | capsule | **GABA** | γ-aminobutyric acid |
| **Cath** | catheterization or catheterize | **GI** | gastrointestinal |
| **CBC** | complete blood cell count | **GPC** | giant papillary conjunctivitis |
| **CHF** | congestive heart failure | **gr** | grain |
| **CHo** | carbohydrates | **GTT** | glucose tolerance test |
| **cm** | centimeter | **gtt** | drops |
| **CNS** | central nervous system | **GU** | genitourinary |
| **$CO_2$** | carbon dioxide | **GVHD** | graft-versus-host disease |
| **cont** | continuous | **$H_2$** | histamine$_2$ |
| **COPD** | chronic obstructive pulmonary disease | **hCG** | human chorionic gonadotropin |
| **CPAP** | continuous positive airway pressure | **Hct** | hematocrit |
| | | **HDCV** | human diploid cell rabies vaccine |

| | | | |
|---|---|---|---|
| **Hgb** | hemoglobin | **NHL** | non-Hodgkin's lymphoma |
| **H&H** | hematocrit and hemoglobin | **NPO** | nothing by mouth (Lat. *nulla per os*) |
| **5-HIAA** | 5-hydroxyindoleacetic acid | **NS** | normal saline |
| **HIV** | human immunodeficiency virus (AIDS) | **O$_2$** | oxygen |
| **H$_2$O** | water | **OBS** | organic brain syndrome |
| **HOB** | head of bed | **OD** | right eye |
| **HR** | heart rate | **OR** | operating room |
| **hr** | hour | **OS** | left eye |
| **IBD** | inflammatory bowel disease | **OTC** | over-the-counter |
| **IC** | intracardiac | **OU** | each eye |
| **ICP** | intracranial pressure | **oz** | ounce |
| **ID** | intradermal | **p̄** | after |
| **IgG** | immunoglobulin G | **P56** | Plasma-Lyte 56 |
| **IM** | intramuscular | **PaCO$_2$** | arterial carbon dioxide tension (pressure) |
| **inf** | infusion | **PaO$_2$** | arterial oxygen tension (pressure) |
| **INH** | inhalation | | |
| **inj** | injection | **PAT** | paroxysmal atrial tachycardia |
| **I&O** | intake and output | **PBI** | protein-bound iodine |
| **IPPB** | intermittent positive-pressure breathing | **pc** | after meals |
| **IT** | intrathecal | **PCI** | percutaneous coronary intervention |
| **ITP** | idiopathic thrombocyto-penic purpura | **PCWP** | pulmonary capillary wedge pressure |
| **IUD** | intrauterine device | **PEEP** | positive end-expiratory pressure |
| **IV** | intravenous | | |
| **IVP** | intravenous pyelogram | **PERRLA** | pupils equal, round, react to light and accommodation |
| **K** | potassium | | |
| **kg** | kilogram | **pH** | hydrogen ion concentration |
| **L** | liter | **PO** | by mouth |
| **lb** | pound | **postop** | postoperative |
| **LDH** | lactic dehydrogenase | **PP** | postprandial |
| **LE** | lupus erythematosus | **PPHN** | persistent pulmonary hyper-tension of the newborn |
| **LH** | luteinizing hormone | | |
| **LLQ** | left lower quadrant | **preop** | preoperative |
| **LMP** | last menstrual period | **prn** | as required |
| **LOC** | level of consciousness | **PT** | prothrombin time |
| **LR** | lactated Ringer's solution | **PTT** | partial thromboplastin time |
| **LUQ** | left upper quadrant | **PVC** | premature ventricular contraction |
| **M** | meter | | |
| **m** | minim | **q** | every |
| **m$^2$** | square meter | **qAM** | every morning |
| **MAOI** | monoamine oxidase inhibitor | **qhr** | every hour |
| | | **q2hr** | every 2 hours |
| **mcg** | microgram | **q3hr** | every 3 hours |
| **mEq** | milliequivalent | **q4hr** | every 4 hours |
| **mg** | milligram | **q6hr** | every 6 hours |
| **MI** | myocardial infarction | **q12hr** | every 12 hours |
| **min** | minute | **qid** | four times daily |
| **ml** | milliliter | **qmo** | every month |
| **mm** | millimeter | **qPM** | every night |
| **mo** | month | **qs** | sufficient quantity |
| **Na** | sodium | **qt** | quart |
| **neg** | negative | **qwk** | every week |
| **NGU** | nongonococcal urethritis | | |

| | | | |
|---|---|---|---|
| **R** | right | **temp** | temperature |
| **RAIU** | radioactive iodine uptake | **tid** | three times daily |
| **RBC** | red blood count or cell | **tinc** | tincture |
| **RLQ** | right lower quadrant | **TPN** | total parenteral nutrition |
| **ROM** | range of motion | **TOP** | topical |
| **RUQ** | right upper quadrant | **TSH** | thyroid-stimulating |
| **Rx** | prescription | | hormone |
| **SARS** | severe acute respiratory | **tsp** | teaspoon |
| | syndrome | **TT** | thrombin time |
| **SCr** | serum creatinine | **UA** | urinalysis |
| **SIMV** | synchronous intermittent | **UTI** | urinary tract infection |
| | mandatory ventilation | **UV** | ultraviolet |
| **SL** | sublingual | **vag** | vaginal |
| **SLE** | systemic lupus | **VMA** | vanillylmandelic acid |
| | erythematosus | **vol** | volume |
| **SOB** | shortness of breath | **VS** | vital sign |
| **sol** | solution | **WBC** | white blood cell count |
| **sp gr** | specific gravity | **wk** | week |
| **ss** | one half | **wt** | weight |
| **STD** | sexually transmitted disease | **yr** | year |
| **SUBCUT** | subcutaneous | **>** | greater than |
| **supp** | suppository | **<** | less than |
| **sus rel** | sustained release | **=** | equal |
| **syr** | syrup | **°** | degree |
| **T&A** | tonsillectomy and adenoid- | **%** | percent |
| | ectomy | **α** | alpha |
| **tab** | tablet | **γ** | gamma |
| **tbsp** | tablespoon | **β** | beta |
| **TD** | transdermal | | |

• For a list of the Institute for Safe Medicine Practices (ISMP) error-prone abbreviations, symbols, and dose designations, please see http://www.ismp.org/tools/errorproneabbreviations.pdf.
• For frequently asked questions regarding the 2008 National Patient Safety Goals, please visit The Joint Commission website at http://www.jointcommission.org/PatientSafety/NationalPatientSafetyGoals.

## FDA Pregnancy Categories

**A**    No risk demonstrated to the fetus in any trimester
**B**    No adverse effects in animals, no human studies available
**C**    Only given after risks to the fetus are considered; animal studies have shown adverse reactions, no human studies available
**D**    Definite fetal risks, may be given in spite of risks if needed in life-threatening conditions
**X**    Absolute fetal abnormalities; not to be used any time during pregnancy

*Note:* **UK** = Unknown fetal risk (used in this text but not an official FDA pregnancy category).

# Index

---

Entries can be identified as follows: generic name, Trade Name, DRUG CATEGORY, *Combination Product.*

---

Entries can be identified as follows: generic name, Trade Name, DRUG CATEGORY, *Combination Product.*

---

Entries can be identified as follows: generic name, Trade Name, DRUG CATEGORY, *Combination Product.*

Entries can be identified as follows: generic name, Trade Name, DRUG CATEGORY, *Combination Product.*

Entries can be identified as follows: generic name, Trade Name, DRUG CATEGORY, *Combination Product.*

Entries can be identified as follows: generic name, Trade Name, DRUG CATEGORY, *Combination Product.*

---

Entries can be identified as follows: generic name, Trade Name, DRUG CATEGORY, *Combination Product.*

Entries can be identified as follows: generic name, Trade Name, DRUG CATEGORY, *Combination Product.*

Major Acid Reducer, 224-226
*Malarone,* 1123
*Malarone Pediatric,* 1123
Mallamint, 163-164
Mallazine Eye Drops, 1091-1092
Malog-x, 923-925
manganese, 959
mannitol, 583-585, 1055
Maox, 581-583
Mapap, 38-40
*Mapap Cold Formula,* 1123
Maranox, 38-40
maraviroc, 585-586, 1048
marijuana, 1074
Marthritic, 860-861
Matulane, 793-794
Mavik, 961-962
Maxair, 772-773
Maxalt, 852-853
Maxalt-MLT, 852-853
Maxeran, 620-622
Maxidex, 1090, 1091-1092
Maximum Strength Allergy Drops, 1091-1092
Maximum Strength Desenex Antifungal, 1095-1096
Maximum Strength Gas Relief, 871
Maximum Strength Mylanta Gas Relief, 871
Maximum Strength Pepcid, 395-396
Maximum Strength Phazyme, 871
Maxipime, 191-198
*Maxitrol Ophthalmic Suspension/Ointment,* 1123
Maxivate, 1094, 1095
*Maxzide,* 1123
*Maxzide-25 MG,* 1123
mazindol, 1074
measles, mumps, and rubella vaccine, live, 1103
measles and rubella virus vaccine, live attenuated, 1103
measles virus vaccine, live attenuated, 1104
mebendazole, 586-587
mecasermin, 587-588
mechlorethamine, 588-589, 1041
meclizine, 589-590, 1036
meclizine HCl, 589-590

Meda, 38-40
Medamint, 1098
*Medigesic,* 1123
Medihaler, 358-359
Medipren, 487-488
Medralone, 618-620
Medrol, 618-620
medroxyprogesterone, 255-257, 590-591
medrysone, 1090, 1091-1092
Med Tamoxifen, 906-908
Mefoxin, 186-191
Mega-C/A Plus, 107-109
Megace, 592-593
Megace ES, 592-593
Megacillin, 741-744
megestrol, 592-593, 1042
melatonin, 1109
Mellaril, 931-933
Mellaril-5, 931-933
Mellaril Concentrate, 931-933
meloxicam, 593-594
melphalan, 594-596, 1041, 1135
memantine, 596, 1025
Menactra, 1104
Menadol, 487-488
Menaval, 378-380
Meni-D, 589-590
meningococcal polysaccharide vaccine, 1104
Menomune-A/C/Y/ W-135, 1104
Menopur, 596-597
menotropins, 596-597
*Mepergan Fortis,* 1123
*Mepergan Injection,* 1123
meperidine, 597-599, 1060, 1074, 1135
meperidine HCl, 597-599
Mephyton, 764-765
meprobamate, 1027, 1074
Mepron, 116-117
mercaptopurine, 599-601, 1042
meropenem, 601-602, 1040
Merrem IV, 601-602
Merumax II, 1105
mesalamine (5-ASA), 602-603
mescaline, 1074
Mestinon, 813-814
Mestinon SR, 813-814
Mestinon Timespan, 813-814
mestranol/norethindrone, 255-257
Metadate CD, 616-617

Metaderm, 1094, 1095
*Metaglip 2.5,* 1123
Metamucil, 811-812
Metamucil Lemon Lime, 811-812
Metamucil Orange Flavor, 811-812
Metamucil Sugar Free, 811-812
Metamucil Sugar Free Orange Flavor, 811-812
metaproterenol, 603-604, 1028
metaxalone, 1062
metformin, 605-606, 1033
methadone, 606-607, 1060, 1135
Methadose, 606-607
Methergine, 615-616
Methidate, 616-617
methimazole, 607-609
methocarbamol, 609-610, 1062
methotrexate (amethopterin, MTX), 610-613, 1135
Methotrexate, 610-613, 1042
methyldopa/ methyldopate, 613-615, 1038
methylergonovine, 615-616
Methylin, 616-617
Methylin ER, 616-617
methylphenidate, 616-617
methylprednisolone, 618-620, 1028, 1054
Meticorten, 786-787
*Metimyd Ophthalmic Suspension/Ointment,* 1123
metipranolol, 1090, 1091-1092
metoclopramide, 620-622, 1036
metolazone, 622-623, 1055
metoprolol, 624-625, 1026, 1049
MetroCream, 1096, 1097
MetroGel, 1096, 1097
MetroLotion, 1096, 1097
metronidazole, 626-627
Metronidazole, 626-627
metronidazole (topical), 1096, 1097
Mevacor, 575-577
mexiletine, 628-629, 1035
Mexitil, 628-629
mezlocillin, 1040

Entries can be identified as follows: generic name, Trade Name, DRUG CATEGORY, *Combination Product.*

Entries can be identified as follows: generic name, Trade Name, DRUG CATEGORY, *Combination Product.*

Entries can be identified as follows: generic name, Trade Name, DRUG CATEGORY, *Combination Product.*

Entries can be identified as follows: generic name, Trade Name, DRUG CATEGORY, *Combination Product.*

Entries can be identified as follows: generic name, Trade Name, DRUG CATEGORY, *Combination Product.*

Entries can be identified as follows: generic name, Trade Name, DRUG CATEGORY, *Combination Product.*

---

Entries can be identified as follows: generic name, Trade Name, DRUG CATEGORY, *Combination Product.*

Entries can be identified as follows: generic name, Trade Name, DRUG CATEGORY, *Combination Product.*

# 2010 Update to Mosby's Drug Guide for Nurses
## Eighth Edition

Following are the monographs for 21 drugs that have received FDA approval since the publication of *Mosby's Drug Guide for Nurses,* 8th edition. These monographs follow the same format as those in the book. They are arranged in alphabetical order by generic name, and trade names are given for all medications in common use. Each monograph contains the same subsections as those listed and described on pages x through xii of the preface to this book.

## Drug Monographs in this Update

| GENERIC | TRADE |
|---|---|
| alvimopan | Entereg |
| bendamustine | Treanda |
| c1 inhibitor, human | Cinryze |
| certolizumab | Cimzia |
| clevidipine | Cleviprex |
| etravirine | Intelence |
| fesoterodine | Toviaz |
| fluoxymesterone | Androxy |
| fosaprepitant | Emend |
| hydroxyethyl starch | Voluven |
| lacosamide | Vimpat |
| levoleucovorin | Isovorin, Fusilev |
| methoxy polyethylene glycol-epoetin beta | Mircera |
| methylnaltrexone | Relistor |
| pegademase bovine | Adagen |
| regadenoson | Lexiscan |
| romiplostim | Nplate |
| rufinamide | Banzel |
| sapropterin | Kuvan |
| silodosin | Rapaflo |
| tetrabenazine | Xenazine |

## alvimopan (Rx)
(al-vi′moe-pan)

Entereg
*Func. class.:* Functional GI disorder agent
*Chem. class.:* Peripheral μ-opioid receptor antagonist

**Pregnancy category** B

**Action:** Acts within the GI tract, antagonizes opioid induced GI dysfunction

**Therapeutic outcome:** Resolution of ileus

**Uses:** Ileus, post-operative

**Dosage and routes**
*Ileus, post-operative*
*Adult:* PO 12 mg given ½-5 hrs before surgery, then 12 mg bid the day after surgery, max 7 days (15 doses)

**Available forms:** Caps 12 mg

**Adverse effects**
*CV:* **MI**
*GI:* Dyspepsia, flatulence, constipation
*GU:* Urinary retention
*MISC:* **Anemia,** hypokalemia
*MS:* Back pain

**Contraindications:** Hypersensitivity

**Precautions:** Pregnancy **B,** breastfeeding, renal/hepatic disease, children, GI obstruction, MI, complete GI obstruction surgery

| Pharmacokinetics | |
|---|---|
| **Absorption** | High fat meal decreases absorption |
| **Distribution** | Protein binding 80%-94% |
| **Metabolism** | Unknown |
| **Excretion** | Kidneys (35%) |
| **Half-life** | Terminal 10-18 hr |

Pharmacodynamics
Unknown

## INTERACTIONS
*Individual drugs*
Amiodarone, bepridil, cycloSPORINE, diltiazem, itraconazole, quinidine, quinine, spironolactone, verapamil: increased alvimopan effect
Methylnaltrexone: duplicate therapy
*Drug classifications*
Opiate agonists: increased GI adverse reactions; do not give if opiate agonists were taken for ≥7 days
Opiate antagonists: duplicate therapy

## NURSING CONSIDERATIONS
**Assessment**
• Monitor Hgb/Hct, serum potassium

**Nursing diagnoses**
• Knowledge, deficient (teaching)

**Implementation**
• Use in hospital only; therapeutic doses of opiates should not be used for >7 consecutive days
• Give without regard to food
• Store at room temperature

**Patient/family education**
• Instruct the patient in the reason for the product

**Evaluation**
**Positive therapeutic outcome**
• Resolution of ileus

⚠ **HIGH ALERT**

## bendamustine (Rx)
(ben-da-muss′teen)

Treanda
*Func. class.:* Antineoplastic alkylating agent
*Chem. class.:* Nitrogen mustard

**Pregnancy category** Unknown

**Action:** Cross-linking DNA which causes single strand and double strand breaks, inhibits several mitotic checkpoints, combines alkylating and antimetabolite properties

**Therapeutic outcome:** Improvement in blood counts and morphology

**Uses:** Chronic lymphocytic leukemia, non-Hodgkin's lymphoma

**Dosage and routes**
*Chronic lymphocytic leukemia*
*Adult:* **IV** INF 100 mg/m² over 30 min on days 1, 2 q 28 days up to 6 cycles

*Non-Hodgkin's lymphoma*
*Adult:* **IV** INF 120 mg/m² over 60 min on days 1, 2 q 21 days up to 8 cycles

**Available forms:** Powder for inj 100 mg

**Adverse effects**
*CNS:* Asthenia, fatigue, fever, headache
*CV:* Hypertension, **hypertensive crisis**
*GI:* Nausea, *vomiting,* diarrhea, hyperbilirubinemia, constipation, stomatitis, anorexia
*GU:* **Renal failure**
*HEMA:* **Thrombocytopenia, leukopenia, anemia, lymphocytopenia, neutropenia, secondary malignancy, toxic epidermal necrolysis, tumor lysis syndrome**
*INTEG:* Bulbous rash, pruritus

**META:** Hyperuricemia
**SYST:** **Anaphylaxis,** infection, dehydration

**Contraindications:** Pregnancy category unknown, hypersensitivity to this product or mannitol, children, hepatic disease, renal impairment, breastfeeding

**Precautions:** Hyperuricemia, infusion-related reactions, myelosuppression, infection, skin-reactions

### Pharmacokinetics

| | |
|---|---|
| **Absorption** | Unknown |
| **Distribution** | Protein binding 95% |
| **Metabolism** | Hydrolysis via cytochrome P450 1A2; two metabolites are produced |
| **Excretion** | 90% unchanged (feces) |
| **Half-life** | 40 min |

### Pharmacodynamics

Unknown

## INTERACTIONS
### Individual drugs
Cimetidine: increased toxicity
Clozapine: do not use due to risk of agranulocytosis
### Drug classifications
Anticoagulants, aspirin, NSAIDs, platelet inhibitors, thrombolytics: increased risk of bleeding
Antineoplastics (other), radiation: increased toxicity
CYP1A2 inducers (barbiturates, carbamazepine, rifampin): decreased bendamustine
CYP1A2 inhibitors (atazanavir, cimetidine, ciprofloxacin, enoxacin, ethyl estradiol, fluvoxamine, mexiletine, norfloxacin, tacrine, thiabendazole, zileuton): increased bendamustine
Myelosuppressive agents: increased myelosuppression
Vaccines (live): increased adverse reactions, decreased antibody reaction
### Drug/lab test
Increased: LFTs

## NURSING CONSIDERATIONS
### Assessment
• Assess CBC, differential, platelet count weekly; withhold product if WBC is <1000 or platelet count is <75,000; notify prescriber of results
• Monitor hepatic studies: AST, ALT, bilirubin
• Monitor renal studies: BUN, serum uric acid, urine CCr before, during therapy; I&O ratio; report fall in urine output of 30 ml/hr; electrolytes
• Assess for cold, cough, fever (may indicate beginning infection)
• Assess bleeding: hematuria, guaiac, bruising, petechiae, mucosa, orifices q8hr
• Assess for tumor-lysis syndrome

### Nursing diagnoses
• Infection, risk for (adverse reactions)
• Injury, risk for (adverse reactions)
• Knowledge, deficient (teaching)
• Nutrition, less than body requirements, imbalanced (adverse reactions)

### Implementation
• Give blood transfusions or RBC colony-stimulating factors to counter anemia
• Give antiemetic 30-60 min before giving product to prevent vomiting
• Give all medications PO, if possible avoid IM inj if platelets are <100,000/mm$^3$
• Store reconstituted sol in refrigerator for 24 hr, or room temperature for 3 hr; protect from light; store vials at room temperature
**Intermittent IV INF route**
• Prepare in biologic cabinet wearing gown, gloves, mask; avoid contact with skin; can cause burning and staining the skin brown; use cytotoxic handling procedures
• After diluting 100 mg product/20 ml sterile water for inj (5 mg/ml), sol should be clear, colorless to pale yellow, completely dissolve in 5 min; if particulate is present, do not use
• Give within 30 min of reconstitution, withdraw the volume needed and further dilute in 500 ml NS or D$_{2.5/0.45}$% NS to a final conc 0.2-0.6 mg/ml; doses ≤100 mg/m$^2$, give over 30 min; doses >100 mg/m$^2$, give over 60 min

### Patient/family education
• Advise patient to avoid use of aspirin, ibuprofen, razors, commercial mouthwash
• Instruct patient to report signs of anemia (fatigue, irritability, shortness of breath, faintness)
• Instruct patient to report signs of infection

### Evaluation
**Positive therapeutic outcome**
• Improvement in blood counts and morphology

Adverse effects: *italic* = common, **bold** = life-threatening

## RARELY USED

### c1 inhibitor, human (Rx)
Cinryze
*Func. class.:* Hemostatic

### Dosage and routes
*Adult and adolescent:* **IV** 1000 units (10 ml) given over at least 10 min every 3-4 days

Uses: Angioedema prophylaxis

Contraindications: Hypersensitivity

---

### certolizumab (Rx)
(ser'tue-liz'oo-mab)
Cimzia
*Func. class.:* Biologic response modifier
*Chem. class.:* Anti-TNF (tissue necrosis factor) agent

**Pregnancy category B**

Action: Monoclonal antibody that neutralizes the activity of tumor necrosis factor alpha (TNF α) found in Crohn's disease; decreased infiltration of inflammatory cells

Therapeutic outcome: Absence of fever, mucus in stools

Uses: Crohn's disease (moderate-severe)

### Dosage and routes
*Crohn's disease (moderate-severe)*
*Adult:* SUBCUT 400 mg given as 2 inj at wks 0, 2, 4; if clinical response occurs, give 400 mg q 4 wks

*Rheumatoid arthritis*
*Adult:* SUBCUT 400 mg q 2 wks × 3 doses, then 200 mg q 2 wks; given with methotrexate

Available forms: Powder for inj 400 mg kit

### Adverse effects
*CNS: Dizziness,* syncope, peripheral neuropathy, fever, **seizures, demyelinating disease of CNS**
*CV:* Hypotension, **heart failure, MI, cardiac dysrhythmia**
*EENT:* Optic neuritis, retinal hemorrhage, uveitis
*GI:* Increased LFTs, **hepatitis, bowel obstruction**
*GU:* UTI, renal disease
*HEMA:* **Anemia, aplastic anemia, pancytopenia, thrombocytopenia**
*INTEG:* Rash, urticaria, **angioedema**
*RESP:* Dyspnea, URI

*SYST:* **Anaphylaxis, malignancies, serum sickness,** bleeding, antibody formation, infection, lupus-like symptoms, lymphadenopathy, arthralgia, **suicidal ideation**

Contraindications: Infection, influenzae, **IV** administration, sepsis, hypersensitivity

Precautions: Pregnancy **B**, breastfeeding, children, geriatric patients, AIDS, coagulopathy, diabetes, fungal infection, heart failure, hepatitis, human anti-chimeric antibody, immunosuppression, leukopenia, MS, cancer, neurologic disease, surgery, thrombocytopenia, TB, vaccinations, renal disease

### Pharmacokinetics
| | |
|---|---|
| **Absorption** | Unknown |
| **Distribution** | Unknown |
| **Metabolism** | Unknown |
| **Excretion** | Unknown |
| **Half-life** | Terminal 14 days |

### Pharmacodynamics
| | |
|---|---|
| **Onset** | Unknown |
| **Peak** | 54-171 hr |
| **Duration** | Unknown |

### Interactions
*Individual drugs*
Abatacept, adalimumab, anakinra, etanercept, infliximab, rilonacept: increased possible infections
Adalimumab, etanercept, infliximab: increased possible malignancies
*Drug classifications*
Immunosuppressive agents: increased possible infections
Live vaccines, toxoids: do not administer concurrently

### NURSING CONSIDERATIONS
**Assessment**
• Monitor antibody test (ANA), hepatitis B serology, CBC
• Assess for rheumatoid arthritis, ROM, pain
• Assess GI symptoms: nausea, vomiting, abdominal pain, hepatitis, increased LFTs
• Monitor periodic blood counts (CBC)
• Assess CV status: B/P, pulse, chest pain
⊕ Assess for allergic reaction, anaphylaxis: rash, dermatitis, urticaria, dyspnea, hypotension, fever, chills; discontinue if severe, administer epINEPHrine, corticosteroids, antihistamines; assess for allergies to murine proteins before starting therapy
• Assess infections: discontinue if infection occurs; do not administer to patients with active infections

- Identify TB, risk for HBV before beginning treatment; a TB test should be obtained, if present; TB should be treated prior to receiving infliximab

## Nursing diagnoses
- Diarrhea (uses)
- Knowledge, deficient (teaching)
- Mobility, impaired physical (uses)

## Implementation
- Store in refrigerator; do not freeze

**SUBCUT route**
- Give by SUBCUT only
- Allow reconstitution to warm to room temp; add 1 ml sterile water for inj to each vial; two vials will be needed for Crohn's disease
- Gently swirl; do not shake; full reconstitution may take up to 30 min; reconstituted product may remain at room temp for up to 2hr or refrigerated up to 24hr
- Warm to room temperature if reconstituted product has been refrigerated
- Use 2 syringes and 2-20 G needles
- Withdraw reconstituted sol from each vial into separate syringes; each will contain 200 mg; switch 20 G to 23 G needle; inject into 2 separate sites in abdomen or thigh

## Patient/family education
- Instruct patient not to breastfeed while taking this product
- Advise patient to notify prescriber of GI symptoms, hypersensitivity reactions
- Caution patient not to operate machinery, drive if dizziness, vertigo occur

## Evaluation
**Positive therapeutic outcome**
- Absence of fever, mucus in stools

---

## clevidipine (Rx)
(klev-id'i-peen)
Cleviprex
*Func. class.:* Calcium channel blocker (L-type)
*Chem. class.:* Dihydropyridine

**Pregnancy category** C

**Action:** L-type calcium channel mediate the influx of calcium during depolarization in arterial smooth muscle, reduces mean arterial B/P by decreasing systemic vascular resistance

**Therapeutic outcome:** Decreased B/P

**Uses:** Treatment of hypertension when oral therapy is not feasible

## Dosage and routes
*Adult:* CONT **IV** 1-2 mg/hr; dose may be doubled q 90 sec initially; as B/P reaches goal, adjust dose less frequently (5-10 min) with smaller increases in dose; most patients require 4-6 mg/hr, max 32 mg/hr; no more than 1000 ml should be infused per 24 hr period due to lipid load restrictions

**Available forms:** Single dose vial 50, 100 ml (0.5 mg/ml), intravenous emulsion

## Adverse effects
*CNS:* Headache
*CV:* Hypotension, **MI, sinus tachycardia,** syncope, **reflex tachycardia, atrial fibrillation**
*GI:* Nausea, vomiting
*GU:* Renal failure

**Contraindications:** Hypersensitivity to this product, eggs or soya lecithin; defective lipid metabolism; severe aortic stenosis

**Precautions:** Pregnancy **C**, breastfeeding, children <18 yr, geriatric patients, heart failure, hyperlipidemia, hypertension, labor, pancreatitis, phenochromocytoma

| Pharmacokinetics | |
|---|---|
| **Absorption** | Unknown |
| **Distribution** | Protein binding >99% |
| **Metabolism** | By esterases in blood, extravascular tissues |
| **Excretion** | Urine 63%-74%, feces 7%-22% |
| **Half-life** | Initially 1 min; terminal 15 min; increased in hepatic disease |

| Pharmacodynamics | |
|---|---|
| **Onset** | 2-4 min |
| **Peak** | 6-12 hr |
| **Duration** | Unknown |

## NURSING CONSIDERATIONS
### Assessment
- Assess cardiac status: B/P, pulse, respiration, ECG; some patients have developed severe angina, acute MI after calcium channel blockers if obstructive CAD is severe; if not transitioned to other antihypertensive therapies following clevidipine infusion, patients should be monitored ≥8 hr for rebound hypertension; monitor for rebound hypertension following drug stoppage
- Monitor I&O ratio, weight daily; peripheral edema, dyspnea, jugular vein distention, crackles

Adverse effects: *italic* = common, **bold** = life-threatening

### Nursing diagnoses
- Knowledge, deficient (teaching)
- Noncompliance (teaching)

### Implementation
- Do not give through same line as other medications
- Gently invert several times before use; do not use if discolored or particulate matter is present
- Give through central or peripheral line
- Use infusion device
- Store vials in refrigerator, do not freeze; leave vials in carton until use; product is photosensitive, however protection from light during administration is not required

### Patient/family education
- Instruct patient to notify prescriber immediately if neurological symptoms, visual changes or symptoms of CHF occur
- Instruct patient to continue follow up for hypertension

### Evaluation
**Positive therapeutic outcome**
- Decreased B/P

---

### etravirine (Rx)
(e-tra′veer-een)
Intelence
*Func. class.:* Antiretroviral
*Chem. class.:* Non-nucleoside reverse transcriptase inhibitor (NNRII)

### Pregnancy category B

**Action:** Binds directly to reverse transcriptase blocking the RNA and DNA dependent DNA polymerase action causing a disruption of the enzyme's catalytic site

**Therapeutic outcome:** Increased CD4 count, decrease viral load

**Uses:** In combination with other antiretroviral agents for HIV infection in treatment-experienced patients with evidence of HIV replication despite ongoing antiretroviral therapy

### Dosages and routes
*Adult:* PO 200 mg bid after a meal, max 400 mg/day; not established in naïve patients

**Available forms:** Tabs 100 mg

### Adverse effects
*CNS: Headache, insomnia,* amnesia, anxiety, confusion, fatigue, nightmares, peripheral neuropathy, **seizures, stroke,** tremor
*CV:* **Atrial fibrillation,** hypertension, MI

*EENT:* Blurred vision
*GI: Nausea, vomiting, diarrhea, anorexia,* abdominal pain, increased AST/ALT, constipation, flatulence, gastritis, GERD, **hematemesis, hepatitis,** hepatomegaly, **pancreatitis**
*GU:* Renal failure
*HEMA:* **Hemolytic anemia, neutropenia, thrombocytopenia, anemia**
*INTEG: Rash,* erythema multiforme, **angioedema, Stevens-Johnson syndrome**
*OTHER:* Diabetes mellitus, gynecomastia, hyperamylasemia, hypercholesterolemia, hyperglycemia, hyperlipidemia
*RESP:* Dyspnea, **bronchospasm**

**Contraindications:** Hypersensitivity, breastfeeding

**Precautions:** Pregnancy **B,** impaired hepatic function, children, antimicrobial resistance, geriatric patients, hepatitis, hypercholesterolemia, hypertriglycerides, immune reconstitution syndrome

### Pharmacokinetics

| | |
|---|---|
| **Absorption** | Unknown |
| **Distribution** | Plasma protein binding 99.9% |
| **Metabolism** | By CYP3A4, 2C9, 2C19 |
| **Excretion** | Feces |
| **Half-life** | 21-61 hr |

### Pharmacodynamics
Unknown

### Interactions
*Individual drugs*
Amiodarone, atazanavir, clarithromycin, flecainide, fosamprenavir, lidocaine, mexiletine, propafenone, quinidine, sildenafil, tadalafil, vardenafil: decreased levels
Atazanavir, carbamazepine, delavirdine, fosamprenavir, fosphenytoin, phenytoin, phenobarbital, rifapentine, rifampin, tipranavir: do not use concurrently
Bepridil, darunavir, dexamethasone, disopyramide, efavirenz, nevirapine, ritonavir, saquinavir, tipranavir: decreased etravirine levels
CycloSPORINE, sirolimus, tacrolimus: altered effect
Diazepam, rifampin, voriconazole, warfarin: increased levels
Fluconazole, itraconazole, ketoconazole, lopinavir, posaconazole, ritonavir, voriconazole: increased etravirine levels
Methadone: increased withdrawal symptoms

---

### Drug classifications
HMG-CoA reductase inhibitors: increased myopathy, rhabdomyolysis
### Drug/herb
St. John's wort: decreased etravirine

## NURSING CONSIDERATIONS
### Assessment
• Assess symptoms of HIV and for possible infections; increased temp

🔷 Monitor for fatal hypersensitivity reactions: fever, rash, nausea, vomiting, fatigue, cough, dyspnea, diarrhea, abdominal discomfort; treatment should be discontinued and not restarted

• Assess blood dyscrasias (anemia, granulocytopenia): bruising, fatigue, bleeding, poor healing
• Monitor renal studies: BUN, serum uric acid, CCr before, during therapy; these may be elevated throughout treatment
• Monitor hepatic studies before and during therapy: bilirubin, AST, ALT, amylase, alk phos, creatine phosphokinase, creatinine, qmo
• Monitor blood counts q2wk; monitor viral load and CD4 counts during treatment; watch for decreasing granulocytes, Hgb; if low, therapy may have to be discontinued and restarted after hematologic recovery; blood transfusions may be required
• Monitor cholesterol/lipid profile during treatment

### Nursing diagnoses
• Infection, risk for (uses)
• Knowledge, deficient (teaching)

### Implementation
• Give in combination with other antiretrovirals with food
• Store in cool environment; protect from light

### Patient/family education
• Inform patient that product is not a cure but will control symptoms; patient is still infective, may pass AIDS virus on to others
• Instruct patient to notify prescriber of sore throat, swollen lymph nodes, malaise, fever; other infections may occur; to stop product and notify prescriber immediately if skin rash, fever, cough, shortness of breath, GI symptoms; advise all health care providers that allergic reaction has occurred with etravirine
• Advise patient that follow-up visits must be continued since serious toxicity may occur; blood counts must be done
• Instruct patient to use contraception during treatment; still able to transmit disease

• Give patient Medication Guide and Warning Card, discuss points on guide
• Inform patient that other products may be necessary to prevent other infections
• Advise patient to take medication following a meal

### Evaluation
**Positive therapeutic outcome**
• Increased CD4 count, decrease viral load

---

## fesoterodine (Rx)
(fess'oh-ter-oh-deen)
Toviaz
*Func. class.:* Overactive bladder product
*Chem. class.:* Muscarinic receptor antagonist
### Pregnancy category C

**Action:** Relaxes smooth muscles in urinary tract by inhibiting acetylcholine at postganglionic sites

**Therapeutic outcome:** Absence of urinary frequency, urgency, incontinence

**Uses:** Overactive bladder (urinary frequency, urgency), urinary incontinence

### Dosage and routes
*Adult and geriatric:* PO EXT REL 4 mg/day, may increase to 8 mg/day based on response, max 4 mg/day in those taking potent CYP3A4 inhibitors

### Renal dose
*Adult:* PO EXT REL Max 4 mg/day in severe renal impairment

**Available forms:** Ext rel tabs 4, 8 mg
### Adverse effects
*CV:* Chest pain, angina, QT prolongation
*EENT:* Xerophthalmia
*GI: Nausea, vomiting,* abdominal pain, constipation, dry mouth
*GU:* Dysuria, urinary retention
*INTEG:* Rash
*MISC:* Peripheral edema
*MS:* Back pain
*RESP:* Cough
*SYST:* Infection

**Contraindications:** GI obstruction, ileus, pyloric stenosis, urinary retention, gastric retention, hypersensitivity

**Precautions:** Pregnancy C, breastfeeding, children, renal/hepatic disease, closed angle glaucoma, urinary tract obstruction, ambient temperature increase, autonomic neuropathy, constipation, contact lenses, hazardous activity,

Adverse effects: *italic* = common, **bold** = life-threatening

GERD, gastroparesis, myasthenia gravis, prostatic hypertrophy, toxic megacolon, ulcerative colitis

### Pharmacokinetics
| | |
|---|---|
| **Absorption** | Rapidly |
| **Distribution** | Protein binding 50% |
| **Metabolism** | Unknown |
| **Excretion** | Urine/feces |
| **Half-life** | 7 hr |

### Pharmacodynamics
Unknown

## Interactions
### Drug classifications
Anticholinergics, antimuscarinics: increased anticholinergic effect

Antiretroviral protease inhibitors, azole antifungals, macrolide antiinfectives: increased action of fesoterodine

Diuretics: increased urinary frequency

### Drug/herb
Caffeine, green tea, guarana: decreased fesoterodine

### Drug/food
Grapefruit juice: increased fesoterodine level

Cola, coffee, tea: decreased fesoterodine level

### Drug/lab test
Increased: LFTs

## NURSING CONSIDERATIONS
### Assessment
• Assess urinary patterns: distention, nocturia, frequency, urgency, incontinence
• Assess for allergic reactions: rash; if this occurs, product should be discontinued

### Nursing diagnoses
• Knowledge, deficient (teaching)
• Incontinence, urge urinary (uses)
• Urinary elimination, impaired (uses)

### Implementation
• Do not break, crush, or chew ext rel product
• Give without regard to meals
• Store at room temperature; protect from moisture

### Patient/family education
• Advise patient not to drink liquids before bedtime
• Instruct the patient on the importance of bladder maintenance

### Evaluation
**Positive therapeutic outcome**
• Absence of urinary frequency, urgency, incontinence

---

## fluoxymesterone (Rx)
(floo-oks-i-mes′te-rone)
Androxy
*Func. class.:* Hormone-androgen
*Chem. class.:* Alkylated derivative of testosterone

**Pregnancy category X**

**Controlled substance schedule C-III**

**Action:** Androgens are responsible for sexual maturation, suppression of gonadotropin-releasing hormones, LH, FSH, by a negative feedback mechanism

**Therapeutic outcome:** Decreased advance of inoperable female breast cancer, male puberty

**Uses:** Inoperable female breast cancer, male hypogonadism, delayed male puberty

### Dosage and routes
**Androgen replacement in male hypogonadism**
*Adult:* PO 5 mg 1-4 ×/day, may increase dose, max 40 mg/day

**Delayed male puberty**
*Adult and adolescent:* PO 2.5-10 mg/day × 4-6 mo, max 20 mg/day

**Inoperable female breast cancer**
*Adult:* PO 10-40 mg/day in divided doses, continue for ≥2-3 mo

**Available forms:** Tabs 10 mg

### Adverse effects
*CV:* **Heart failure**
*GI:* **Hepatitis**
*GU:* Amenorrhea, feminization, virilization, prostatic hypertrophy, priapism, oligospermia, oligomenorrhea, gynecomastia
*HEMA:* Coagulation disorders (clotting factors II, V, VII, X)
*INTEG:* Alopecia, acne, hirsutism, seborrhea
*MISC:* Edema, hypercalcemia

**Contraindications:** Pregnancy **X,** breastfeeding, prostate cancer, male breast cancer

**Precautions:** Diabetes mellitus, CV/hepatic/renal disease

### Pharmacokinetics
| | |
|---|---|
| **Absorption** | Unknown |
| **Distribution** | Unknown, crosses placenta |
| **Metabolism** | Liver |
| **Excretion** | Urine, breast milk |
| **Half-life** | 9.2 hr |

---

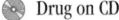

◆ Alert      ♣ Canada Only      ◉ Drug on CD      * "Tall Man" lettering (See Preface)

## Pharmacodynamics
Unknown

## Interactions
### Individual drugs
CycloSPORINE: increased nephrotoxicity

Darbepoetin, epoetin: increased erythropoiesis; avoid concurrent administration

Insulin: decreased glucose levels may alter need for insulin

Warfarin: increased PT

### Drug classifications
5-alpha reductase inhibitors (dutasteride, finasteride): decreased androgen effect

Antidiabetics (oral): decreased glucose levels may alter need for oral antidiabetics

Corticosteroids: edema

Hepatotoxic agents (other): increased hepatotoxicity

### Drug/herb
Saw palmetto: decreased fluoxymesterone effect

### Drug/food
Soy: decreased fluoxymesterone effect

## NURSING CONSIDERATIONS
### Assessment
- Monitor weight daily; notify prescriber if weekly weight gain is >5lb
- Monitor I&O ratio; be alert for decreasing urinary output, increasing edema
- Assess growth rate in children; growth rate may be uneven (linear/bone growth) with extended use
- Monitor electrolytes: K, Na, Cl, Ca; cholesterol
- Monitor hepatic studies: ALT, AST, bilirubin
- Assess edema, hypertension, cardiac symptoms
- Assess signs of masculinization in female: increased libido, deepening of voice, decreased breast tissue, enlarged clitoris, menstrual irregularities; male: gynecomastia, impotence, testicular atrophy
- Assess hypercalcemia: lethargy, polyuria, polydipsia, nausea, vomiting, constipation; product may have to be decreased
- Assess hypoglycemia in diabetics; oral antidiabetic action is increased

### Nursing diagnoses
- Injury, risk for (adverse reactions)
- Knowledge, deficient (teaching)

### Implementation
- Give as a single dose or up to 4×/day
- Store at controlled room temperature (68°-77° F)

## Patient/family education
- Instruct patient to notify prescriber if therapeutic response decreases; if edema occurs
- Teach patient about changes in sex characteristics
- Instruct women to report menstrual irregularities, voice changes, acne, facial hair growth
- Advise patient to notify prescriber if pregnancy is planned or suspected; use contraception while taking product
- Inform patient that 2-3-mo course is necessary to determine objective treatment in breast cancer
- Advise patient to report signs/symptoms of hepatic disorder

## Evaluation
### Positive therapeutic outcome
- Decreased advance of inoperable female breast cancer, male puberty

## fosaprepitant (Rx)
(phos-a-prep'ih-tant)
Emend
*Func. class.:* Antiemetic
*Chem. class.:* Miscellaneous
### Pregnancy category B

**Action:** A selective antagonist of human substance P/neurokinin 1 (NK$_1$) receptors decreasing emetic reflex, prodrug of aprepitant

**Therapeutic outcome:** Absence of nausea, vomiting during cancer chemotherapy

**Uses:** Prevention of nausea/vomiting associated with cancer chemotherapy (highly emetogenic/moderately emetogenic) including high-dose cisplatin, used in combination with other antiemetics; postoperative nausea/vomiting

### Dosage and routes
*Adult:* IV INF 115 mg over 15 min, 30 min prior to chemotherapy as an alternate to the 1st dose of aprepitant on day 1 of the aprepitant-CINV regimen

**Available forms:** Powder for inj 115 mg

### Adverse effects
*CNS: Headache, dizziness,* insomnia, anxiety, depression, confusion, peripheral neuropathy
*CV:* Bradycardia, tachycardia, DVT, hypo/hypertension
*GI: Diarrhea, constipation,* abdominal pain, anorexia, gastritis, increased AST/ALT, *nausea,* vomiting, heartburn

Adverse effects: *italic* = common, **bold** = life-threatening

*GU:* Increased BUN, serum creatine, protein-uria, dysuria
*HEMA:* Anemia, **thrombocytopenia, neutropenia**
*MISC:* Asthenia, fatigue, dehydration, fever, hiccups, tinnitus, Stevens-Johnson syndrome

**Contraindications:** Hypersensitivity

**Precautions:** Pregnancy **B**, breastfeeding, children, hepatic disease, geriatric patients, continuous use for nausea and vomiting not recommended

### Pharmacokinetics

| | |
|---|---|
| **Absorption** | Unknown |
| **Distribution** | Protein binding 95% |
| **Metabolism** | In liver by CYP3A4 enzymes to an active metabolite; rapidly converted to aprepitant (within 30 mins) |
| **Excretion** | Unknown |
| **Half-life** | 13 hr |

### Pharmacodynamics

Unknown

### Interactions
*Individual drugs*
Paroxetine: increased action of both products
*Drug classifications*
CYP2C9 substrates (warfarin, tolbutamide, phenytoin), oral contraceptives: decreased action
CYP3A4 inducers (rifampin, carbamazepine, phenytoin): decreased aprepitant action
CYP3A4 inhibitors (ketoconazole, itraconazole, nefazodone, troleandomycin, clarithromycin, ritonavir, nelfinavir, diltiazem): increased aprepitant action
CYP3A4 substrates (pimozide, cisapride, dexamethasone, terfenadine, astemizole, methylPREDNISolone, midazolam, alprazolam, triazolam, docetaxel, paclitaxel, etoposide, irinotecan, imatinib, ifosfamide, vinorelbine, vinBLAStine, vinCRIStine): increased action
*Drug/food*
Grapefruit juice: decreased effect

### NURSING CONSIDERATIONS
**Assessment**
• Assess CV status: hyper/hypotension, bradycardia, tachycardia, DVT
• Assess for absence of nausea, vomiting during chemotherapy
• Monitor LFTs

### Nursing diagnoses
• Knowledge, deficient (teaching)
• Nausea (uses)

### Implementation
**IV INF route**
• Give **IV** route
• Approved only as a substitute for the 1st dose of aprepitant in 3-day regimen
• Use aseptic technique for reconstitution; inject 5 ml of 0.9% NaCl into the vial directing stream to wall of vial to prevent foam; swirl; do not shake
• Prepare infusion bag with 110 ml of NS; do not dilute or reconstitute with any divalent cations such as calcium, magnesium, including LR, Hartmann's sol
• Withdraw the entire volume from vial and transfer to infusion bag; total volume 115 ml (1mg/1ml)
• Gently invert bag 2-3 times; reconstituted sol is stable for 24 hr at lower room temp or <25° C
• Visually inspect for particulates and discoloration
• Infuse over 15 min

### Patient/family education
• Instruct patient to report diarrhea, constipation
• Instruct patient to report all medications and herbals to prescriber prior to taking this medication
• Advise patient to use nonhormonal form of contraception while taking this agent; oral contraceptive effect may be decreased
• Advise patient on warfarin to have clotting monitored closely during 2-wk period following administration of aprepitant
• Instruct patient to avoid breastfeeding

### Evaluation
**Positive therapeutic outcome**
• Absence of nausea, vomiting during cancer chemotherapy

### RARELY USED

### hydroxyethyl starch (Rx)
Voluven
*Func. class.:* Hematolgic agent
*Chem. class.:* Plasma volume expander

### Dosage and routes
*Adult and child >12 yr:* **IV** INF 50 ml/kg/day; infuse the first 10-20 ml slowly; monitor for anaphylaxis

**Uses:** Treatment, prevention of hypovolemia

**Contraindications:** Hypervolemic, renal failure with oliguria, anuria not related to hypovolemia, dialysis, severe hypernatremia/hypercholeremia, intracranial bleeding, hypersensitivity to this agent

## lacosamide (Rx)
(la-koe′sa-mide)
Vimpat
*Func. class.:* Anticonvulsant
*Chem. class.:* Functionalized amino acid

**Pregnancy category** C

**Action:** May act through action at sodium channels; exact action is unknown

**Therapeutic outcome:** Decrease in severity of seizures

**Uses:** Adjunctive therapy of partial seizures

**Dosage and routes**
*Adult and child >17 yr:* PO 50 mg bid, may increase q wk by 50 mg bid to 200-400 mg/day; **IV** 50 mg 2×/day, infuse over 30-60 min, may be increased 100 mg/day weekly, up to 200-400 mg/day maintenance

**Available forms:** Film coated tabs 50, 100, 150, 200 mg; **IV** 20 ml single use vials (200 mg/20 ml)

**Adverse effects**
*CNS:* Dizziness, syncope, tremor, vertigo, ataxia, drowsiness, fever, hypoesthesia, paresthesias, depression, fatigue, headache, confusion, irritability, psychological dependence, **suicidal ideation**
*CV:* **Atrial fibrillation/flutter**, AV block, bradycardia, myocarditis, orthostatic hypotension, palpitations, **QT prolongation**
*EENT:* Diplopia, blurred vision, nystagmus, tinnitus
*GI:* Nausea, constipation, vomiting, **hepatitis**, diarrhea, dyspepsia
*HEMA:* **Anemia, neutropenia**
*INTEG:* Rash, erythemia, inj site reaction, pruritus, xerostomia
*MS:* Asthenia, dysarthria

**Contraindications:** Hypersensitivity

**Precautions:** Pregnancy C, breastfeeding, allergies, renal/hepatic disease, geriatric patients, child <17 yr, acute MI, atrial fibrillation/flutter, AV block, bradycardia, cardiac disease, congenital heart disease, dehydration, depression, dialysis, hazardous activity, electrolyte imbalance, heart failure, labor, QT prolongation, sick sinus syndrome, substance abuse, suicidal ideation, syncope, torsade de pointes

### Pharmacokinetics
| | |
|---|---|
| **Absorption** | Unknown |
| **Distribution** | Protein binding <15% |
| **Metabolism** | Liver |
| **Excretion** | Kidneys (95% unchanged) |
| **Half-life** | 13 hr (PO) |

### Pharmacodynamics
| | |
|---|---|
| **Onset** | Unknown |
| **Peak** | 1-4 hr (PO) |
| **Duration** | Unknown |

**Interactions**
*Individual drugs*
◆Bepridil, chloroquine, clarithromycin, droperidol, erythromycin, grepafloxacin, halofantrine, haloperidol, methadone, pentamidine, probucol, sparfloxacin: increased QT prolongation
*Drug classifications*
◆Anesthetics (local), β-agonists, class 1A/III antidysrhythmics, some phenothiazines, tricyclic antidepressants: increased QT prolongation
*Drug/lab test*
Increased: LFTs

**NURSING CONSIDERATIONS**
**Assessment**
• Assess for seizures: duration, type, intensity precipitating factors
• Monitor for albumin concentration
• Assess CV status: orthostatic hypotension, QT prolongation; monitor cardiac status throughout treatment
• Assess mental status: mood, sensorium, affect, memory (long, short), depression, suicidal ideation, psychological dependence
• Assess for rash, hypersensitivity reactions

**Nursing diagnoses**
• Injury, risk for (uses)
• Knowledge, deficient (teaching)

**Implementation**
**PO route**
• Give without regard to meals
**IV route**
• May give undiluted or mixed in 0.9% NaCl, D₅, or LR
• Infuse over 30-60 min
• Do not use if discolored or particulates are present; discard unused portions
• Store PO products/**IV** vials at room temperature; solution is stable for 24 hrs when

Adverse effects: *italic* = common, **bold** = life-threatening

mixed with compatible diluents in glass or PVC bags at room temperature

### Patient/family education
- Caution patient not to discontinue product abruptly; seizures may occur
- Advise patient to avoid hazardous activities until stabilized on product
- Instruct patient to carry emergency ID stating product use
- Advise patient to notify prescriber of suicidal thoughts or actions, syncope, cardiac changes
- Instruct patient to notify prescriber if pregnancy is planned or suspected
- Teach patient that interactions with other medications may occur
- Give patient MediGuide for proper use and risks

### Evaluation
**Positive therapeutic outcome**
- Decrease in severity of seizures

---

### levoleucovorin (Rx)
(lee-voe-loo-koe-voe′rin)
Isovorin, Fusilev
*Func. class.:* Chemotherapy protectant
*Chem. class.:* Tetrahydrofolic acid derivative

**Pregnancy category** C

**Action:** Acts as a replacement to rescue cells from the effects of folate antagonists

**Therapeutic outcome:** Prevention of methotrexate toxicity

**Uses:** For methotrexate toxicity prophylaxis

### Dosage and routes
*For levoleucovorin rescue following high-dose methotrexate treatment for osteosarcoma*
*Adult and child >6 yr:* **IV** 7.5 mg (approximately 5 mg/m$^2$) q6hr × 10 doses starting 24hr after the beginning of methotrexate infusion; do not give >16 ml (160 mg) of the reconstituted sol/min

*For inadvertent overdose of methotrexate*
*Adult and child >6 yr:* **IV** 7.5 mg q6hr until serum methotrexate conc <0.01 micromolar; do not give >16 ml (160 mg) of the reconstituted sol/min

**Available forms:** Powder for inj 50 mg

### Adverse effects
*CNS:* Seizures, syncope
*GI:* Nausea, vomiting, stomatitis
*GU:* Abnormal renal function
*INTEG:* Rash, pruritus, anaphylaxis, *urticaria*
*RESP:* Dyspnea

**Contraindications:** Hypersensitivity to this agent or folic acid, mannitol; intrathecal administration

**Precautions:** Pregnancy **C**, breastfeeding, children <6yr, megaloblastic/pernicious anemia, seizure disorder, vitamin B$_{12}$ deficiency

### Interactions
*Individual drugs*
Fluorouracil: increased toxicity
Methotrexate, pyrimethamine, trimethoprim, trimetrexate: decreased effect of these products
*Drug classifications*
Barbiturates, hydantoins: increased metabolism

### NURSING CONSIDERATIONS
### Assessment
- Monitor CCr, creatinine before levoleucovorin rescue and daily to detect methotrexate level
- Monitor CBC with differential
- Assess other products taken: hydantoins, trimethoprim may cause increased folic acid use by body
- Assess neurologic status (rescue): weakness, fatigue

### Nursing diagnoses
- Injury, risk for (uses)
- Knowledge, deficient (teaching)

### Implementation
- Give within 1 hr of folic acid antagonist
- Do not give concurrently with systemic methotrexate
- Increase fluid intake if used to treat folic acid inhibitor overdose
- Protect from light and heat
**IV route**
- For **IV** reconstitute 50 mg vial/5.3 ml of normal saline (10 mg/ml)
**IV, direct route**
- Give 160 mg/min or less (16 ml of 10 mg/ml sol/min)
**Intermittent IV route**
- Further dilute to a final concentration of 0.5 mg/ml – 5 mg/ml

### Patient/family education
- Teach patient to eat folic acid rich foods for folic acid deficiency: bran, yeast, dried beans, nuts, fresh, green leafy vegetables

---

 Alert      Canada Only     🌐 Drug on CD     * "Tall Man" lettering (See Preface)

- Advise patient to notify prescriber of side effects
- Instruct patient to report signs of hyposensitivity reaction immediately
- Inform patient to avoid breastfeeding

## Evaluation
**Positive therapeutic outcome**
- Prevention of methotrexate toxicity

---

## methoxy polyethylene glycol-epoetin beta (Rx)
(meth-ox'ee pol'ee-eth'i-leen glye'kol-e-poe'e-tin bay'ta)
Mircera
*Func. class.:* Antianemic, biologic modifier, hormone
*Chem. class.:* Amino acid polypeptide

**Pregnancy category C**

---

**Action:** Erythropoietin is one factor controlling rate of red cell production; product is developed by recombinant DNA technology

**Therapeutic outcome:** Increase in reticulocyte count in 2-6 wk, Hgb/Hct; increased appetite, enhanced sense of wellbeing

**Uses:** Anemia caused by reduced endogenous erythropoietin production, primarily end-stage renal disease; to correct hemostatic defect in uremia on all dosages

## Dosage and routes
*For all dosages*
*Adult and geriatric:* Reduce by 25% if Hgb >1 g/dl in any 2 wk period or if Hgb is close to 12 g/dl; if Hgb continues to rise after decrease, hold until Hgb starts to decrease

*Treatment of anemia in chronic renal failure (dialysis dependant/independent) — not currently using ESA*
*Adult and geriatric:* **IV**/SUBCUT 0.6 mcg q 2wk

*Using >80 mcg/wk darbepoetin or >16000 units/wk epoetin*
*Adult and geriatric:* **IV**/SUBCUT 180 mcg q 2 wk or 360 mcg q 4 wk

*Using 40-80 mcg/wk darbepoetin or 8000-16000 units/wk epoetin*
*Adult and geriatric:* **IV**/SUBCUT 100 mcg q 2 wk

*Using <40 mcg/wk darbepoetin or <8000 units/wk epoetin*
*Adult and geriatric:* **IV**/SUBCUT 60 mcg q 2 wk or 120 mcg g 4 wk

## Adverse effects
*CNS:* **Seizures, encephalopathy,** headache
*CV: Hypertension,* edema, **heart failure,** hypotension, **sinus tachycardia, stroke, myocardial infarction**
*GI:* Diarrhea
*HEMA:* **Anemia, red cell aplasia, thrombocytopenia, thromboembolism, thrombosis**
*INTEG:* Pruritus, rash, erythema, inj site reaction
*MS:* Muscle spasms, back pain
*SYST:* Antibody formation

**Contraindications:** Red cell aplasia, neoplastic disease, Hgb >12 g/dl, hypersensitivity to mannitol

**Precautions:** Pregnancy **C**, seizure disorder, porphyria, children <1 mo, breastfeeding, multidose preserved formulation contains benzyl alcohol and should not be used in premature infants, CV disease, hemodialysis, latex allergy, surgery, hypertension, history of CABG

### Pharmacokinetics
| | |
|---|---|
| **Absorption** | Unknown |
| **Distribution** | Unknown |
| **Metabolism** | Unknown |
| **Excretion** | Unknown |
| **Half-life** | Half-life 139 +/- 67 hr rise in reticulocytes on day 7, rise in Hgb in 7-14 days (SUBCUT); Half-life 134 +/- 65 hr (IV) |

### Pharmacodynamics
Unknown

## Interactions
*Drug classifications*
Androgens: increased action of methoxy polyethylene gycol-epoetin
Other erythropoiesis stimulating agents (ESA) (epoetin, darbepoetin): adverse reactions; do not give concurrently

## NURSING CONSIDERATIONS
### Assessment
- Monitor renal studies: urinalysis, protein, blood, BUN, creatinine; I&O, report drop in output <50 ml/hr
- ◆ Assess CBC, blood studies: ferritin, transferrin monthly; transferrin ≥20%, ferritin ≥100 ng/ml; Hct 2×/wk until stabilized in target range (30%-36%) then at regular intervals; those with endogenous erythropoietin levels of <500 units/L respond to this agent; monitor Hct 2×/wk in chronic renal failure; patients

---

Adverse effects: *italic* = common, **bold** = life-threatening

treated with zidovudine or cancer patients should be monitored weekly, then periodically after stabilization; death may occur in Hgb >12 g/dl

• Monitor B/P; check for rising B/P as Hct rises, antihypertensives may be needed; hypertension may occur rapidly leading to hypertensive encephalopathy

• Assess CNS symptoms: for seizures if Hct is increased within 2 wk by 4 pts

• Assess for hypersensitivity reactions: skin rashes, urticaria (rare), antibody development

◆ For pure cell aplasia (PRCA) in absence of other causes, evaluate by testing sera for recombinant erythropoetin antibodies; any loss of response to epoetin should be evaluated

• Assess dialysis patients: thrill, bruit of shunts, monitor for circulation impairment

### Nursing diagnoses
• Injury, risk for (uses)
• Knowledge, deficient (teaching)
• Urinary elimination, impaired (uses)

### Implementation
• Do not shake vial
• Give iron supplements as needed; adequate iron stores are needed for this agent to work properly

**SUBCUT route**
• Inject into outer aspect of upper arms, abdomen (except for 2 inches around navel) or front aspect of middle thigh; do not inject in areas that have stretch marks, or are scarred or bruised
• Rotate inj sites

**IV route**
• Giveadditional heparin to lower chance of clots
• Give by direct inj or bolus into venous line at end of dialysis

**Solution compatibilities:** Do not dilute or administer with other solutions

### Patient/family education
• Caution patient to avoid driving or hazardous activities during beginning of treatment
• Instruct patient to monitor B/P
• Instruct patient to take iron supplements, vitamin $B_{12}$, folic acid as directed

### Evaluation
**Positive therapeutic outcome**
• Increase in reticulocyte count in 2-6 wk, Hgb/Hct; increased appetite, enhanced sense of wellbeing

---

## methylnaltrexone (Rx)
(meth-il-nal-trex'one)
Relistor
*Func. class.:* Opioid antagonist

**Pregnancy category B**

**Action:** Peripheral mu-opioid receptor antagonist that reduces constipation associated with opiate agonists

**Therapeutic outcome:** Decreased constipation

**Uses:** Treatment of opioid-induced constipation in patients with advanced illness who are receiving palliative care when response to laxative therapy has been insufficient.

### Dosage and routes
*Opiate-agonist induced constipation*
*Adult >114 kg:* SUBCUT 0.15 mg/kg every other day prn
*Adult 62-114 kg:* SUBCUT 12 mg every other day prn
*Adult 38-<62 kg:* SUBCUT 8 mg every other day prn
*Adult <38 kg:* SUBCUT 0.15 mg/kg every other day prn

*Renal dose*
*Adult:* SUBCUT CCr <30 ml/min, reduce normal adult dose by 50%

**Available forms:** Solution for inj 12 mg/0.6 ml

### Adverse effects
*CNS:* Dizziness
*GI:* Nausea, vomiting, diarrhea, flatulence, abdominal pain

**Contraindications:** Hypersensitivity, GI obstruction, **IV** route

**Precautions:** Pregnancy **B**, breastfeeding, renal disease, children, diarrhea, driving, operating machinery, geriatric patients

| Pharmacokinetics | |
|---|---|
| Absorption | Unknown |
| Distribution | Protein binding 11%-15.3% |
| Metabolism | Unknown |
| Excretion | Unknown |
| Half-life | Terminal 8 hr |

| Pharmacodynamics | |
|---|---|
| Onset | Unknown |
| Peak | 30 min (SUBCUT) |
| Duration | Unknown |

---

## NURSING CONSIDERATIONS
### Assessment
- Monitor serum creatinine
- Assess for stool characteristics

### Nursing diagnoses
- Constipation (uses)
- Knowledge, deficient (teaching)

### Implementation
- Give SUBCUT only; oral dose is investigational and not currently available
- Do not give **IV**; **IV** dosing for urinary retention is investigational
- Store at 15°-30° C (59°-86° F); do not freeze
- Store away from light

**SUBCUT route**
- Inspect the solution before use; it should be a clear, colorless to pale yellow aqueous solution; do not use if particulate matter or discoloration are present
- Withdraw the needed amount of solution into a sterile syringe; if immediate administration is impossible, the syringe may be kept at room temperature for up to 24 hrs; the syringe does not need to be kept away from light during the 24-hr period; immediately discard any unused portion in the vile; no preservatives are present
- Administer into the upper arm, abdomen, or thigh no more than 1×/24 hr; rotate inj sites; do not inject into the same spot each time; do not inject into areas where skin is tender, bruised, red, or hard; avoid areas with scars or stretch marks
- If using with retractable needle, slowly push down on the plunger past the resistance point until the syringe is empty and a click is heard.

### Patient/family education
- Caution patient not to drive or operate machinery until effect is known

### Evaluation
**Positive therapeutic outcome**
- Decreasing constipation

---

**RARELY USED**

### pegademase bovine (Rx)
Adagen
*Func. class.:* Metabolic enzyme

### Dosage and routes
*Neonate/infant/child:* IM 10 units/kg (first dose), then 15 units/kg (second dose), then 20 units/kg (third dose and maintenance) given q 7 days; dose determined by laboratory monitoring

**Uses:** Severe combined immunodeficiency disease due to adenosine deaminase deficiency

**Contraindications:** Thrombocytopenia

---

**RARELY USED**

### regadenoson (Rx)
Lexiscan
*Func. class.:* Cardiovascular agent, diagnostic

### Dosage and routes
*Adult and geriatric:* **IV** 0.4 mg as a single dose

**Uses:** Coronary artery disease diagnosis

**Contraindications:** Hypersensitivity

---

### romiplostim (Rx)
(roe-mi-ploe'stim)
Nplate
*Func. class.:* Thrombopoietin receptor agonist
**Pregnancy category** C

**Action:** A thrombopoietin-like fusion protein produced by DNA recombinant technology

**Therapeutic outcome:** Increase in platelet counts, absence of bleeding

**Uses:** Chronic idiopathic thrombocytopenic purpura in patients who have had an insufficient response to corticosteroids, immunoglobulins, or splenectomy

### Dosage and routes
*Adult:* SUBCUT 1 mcg/kg q wk, increase q wk by 1 mcg/kg until platelets ≥50,000/mm$^3$, max 10 mcg/kg/wk

**Available forms:** Inj vials 250, 500 mcg

### Adverse effects
*CNS: Dizziness, insomnia, headache,* fatigue
*GI:* Abdominal pain, dyspepsia, diarrhea
*HEMA:* **Thromboembolism, thrombosis,** bleeding, myelofibrosis
*MS:* Myalgia
*SYST:* **Secondary malignancy,** antibody formation

**Contraindications:** Hypersensitivity to this product or mannitol

**Precautions:** Pregnancy C, breastfeeding, malignancies, bleeding, bone marrow suppression, children

---

Adverse effects: *italic* = common, **bold** = life-threatening

| Pharmacokinetics | |
|---|---|
| Absorption | Unknown |
| Distribution | Unknown |
| Metabolism | Unknown |
| Excretion | Unknown |
| Half-life | Terminal 1-34 days |

| Pharmacodynamics | |
|---|---|
| Onset | Unknown |
| Peak | 7-50 hr |
| Duration | Unknown |

## Interactions
### Drug classifications
Anticoagulants, NSAIDs, platelet inhibitors, thrombolytics, salicylates: possible risk of bleeding

## NURSING CONSIDERATIONS
### Assessment
• Assess blood studies: CBC during treatment weekly and for 2 wks after discontinuing

### Nursing diagnoses
• Injury, risk for (uses)
• Knowledge, deficient (teaching)

### Implementation
• Romiplostim is only available through Nplate NEXUS Program; call 1-877-675-2831 to enroll
• Store vials in refrigerator, do not freeze; protect from light; diluted sol is stable refrigerated or at room temperature for 24 hrs
**SUBCUT route**
• Use 0.01 ml graduations syringe
• Discard any unused portion in vial; do not pool unused portions from vials
• Dilute 250 mcg/0.72 preservative-free sterile water for inj; 500 mcg/1.2 preservative-free sterile water for inj; final concentration 500 mcg/ml
• Gently swirl until dissolved; do not shake
• Do not use if discolored or if particulate matter is present
• Inject into outer aspect of upper arm or abdomen except for 2 inches around navel or front aspect of middle thigh; do not use areas that are bruised, scratched or scarred
• Rotate injection sites

### Patient/family education
• Instruct patient to report bleeding
• Inform the patient the reason for product and expected results
• Advise patient to report a missed dose to prescriber due to increased risk of bleeding

## Evaluation
**Positive therapeutic outcome**
• Increase in platelet counts, absence of bleeding

## rufinamide (Rx)
(roo-fin'a-mide)
Banzel
*Func. class.:* Anticonvulsant
*Chem. class.:* Triazole derivative
**Pregnancy category C**

**Action:** May act through action at sodium channels; exact action is unknown

**Therapeutic outcome:** Decrease in severity of seizures

**Uses:** Lennox-Gastaut syndrome

### Dosage and routes
*Adult:* PO 400-800 mg/day divided bid, increase by 400-800 mg/day q 2 days to 3200 mg/day
*Child ≥4 yr:* PO 10 mg/kg/day divided equally bid; increase by 10 mg/kg/day every other day to 45 mg/kg/day or 3200 mg/day, whichever is less

**Available forms:** Tabs 200, 400 mg

### Adverse effects
*CNS:* Dizziness, ataxia, drowsiness, fever, seizures, tremor, fatigue, headache, gait disturbance
*EENT:* Diplopia, blurred vision, nystagmus
*GI:* Nausea, hepatitis, vomiting
*HEMA:* **Anemia, leukopenia, neutropenia, thrombocytopenia,** lymphadenopathy
*INTEG:* Rash, urticaria
*MISC:* Edema, hematuria, influenzae, nephrolithiasis

**Contraindications:** Hypersensitivity

**Precautions:** Pregnancy **C**, breastfeeding, renal/hepatic disease, geriatric patients, child <16 yr, depression, dialysis, hazardous activities, suicidal ideation

| Pharmacokinetics | |
|---|---|
| Absorption | Unknown |
| Distribution | Unknown |
| Metabolism | Liver |
| Excretion | Kidneys |
| Half-life | Terminal 6-10 hr |

## Pharmacodynamics

| | |
|---|---|
| **Onset** | Unknown |
| **Peak** | 4-6 hr |
| **Duration** | Unknown |

### Interactions
*Individual drugs*
Carbamazepine, phenobarbital, phenytoin, primidone: decreased effect of rufinamide
Valproate: increased rufinamide effect
*Drug classifications*
Hormonal contraceptives: decreased effect
*Drug/lab test*
Increased: LFTs

### NURSING CONSIDERATIONS
Assessment
• Assess for seizures: duration, type, intensity precipitating factors
◆ Assess mental status: mood, sensorium, affect, memory (long, short), increased suicidal thoughts/actions

### Nursing diagnoses
• Injury, risk for (uses)
• Knowledge, deficient (teaching)

### Patient/family education
• Caution patient not to discontinue product abruptly; seizures may occur
• Advise patient to avoid hazardous activities until stabilized on product
• Instruct patient to carry emergency ID stating product use
• Instruct patient to notify prescriber if pregnancy is planned or suspected
• Teach patient to use alternate form of contraception; hormonal contraceptives may be decreased
• Inform patient to take adequate fluids

### Evaluation
**Positive therapeutic outcome**
• Decrease in severity of seizures

### RARELY USED

## sapropterin (Rx)
Kuvan
*Func. class.:* Metablolic enzyme

### Dosage and routes
*Adult and child ≥4 yr:* PO 10 mg/kg/day; check blood phenylalanine (Phe) levels at baseline and after 1 wk

**Uses:** Treatment of hyperphenylalaninemia (HPA)

**Contraindications:** Hypersensitivity to this agent or mannitol

## silodosin (Rx)
(si-lo'do-seen)
Rapaflo
*Func. class.:* Selective $\alpha_1$ adrenergic blocker
*Chem. class.:* Sulfamoylphenethylamine derivative

### Pregnancy category B

**Action:** Binds preferentially to $\alpha_{1A}$-adrenoceptor subtype located mainly in the prostate

**Therapeutic outcome:** Decreased symptoms of benign prostatic hyperplasia

**Uses:** Symptoms of benign prostatic hyperplasia (BPH)

### Dosage and routes
*Adult:* PO 8 mg/day with a meal; max 8 mg/day

**Available forms:** Tabs 8 mg

### Adverse effects
*CNS: Dizziness, headache,* asthenia, insomnia, syncope
*CV:* Orthostatic hypotension
*EENT:* Nasal congestion, rhinorrhea, sinusitis
*GI:* Diarrhea, abdominal pain, jaundice
*GU:* Abnormal ejaculation, priapism, urinary incontinence
*HEMA:* Purpura

**Contraindications:** Hypersensitivity, renal failure

**Precautions:** Pregnancy **B**, breastfeeding, children, renal/hepatic disease, females, hypotension, ocular surgery, orthostatic hypotension, prostate cancer, syncope, geriatric patients

## Pharmacokinetics

| | |
|---|---|
| **Absorption** | Decreased with high fat/high calorie meal |
| **Distribution** | Extensive protein binding 97% |
| **Metabolism** | Liver |
| **Excretion** | Urine |
| **Half-life** | 24 hr (metabolite) |

## Pharmacodynamics
Unknown

Adverse effects: *italic* = common, **bold** = life-threatening

## Interactions
### Drug classifications
CYP3A4 inhibitors (clarithromycin, itraconazole, ritonavir, anti-retroviral protease inhibitors, aprepitant, chloramphenicol, conivaptan, dalfopristin, danazol, delavirdine, efavirenz, fosaprepitant, fluconazole, fluvoxamine, imatinib, isoniazid, mifepristone, nefazodone, tamoxifen, telithromycin, troleandomycin, voriconazole, zileuton, zafirlukast): increased silodosin effect
### Drug/food
Grapefruit juice: increased silodosin effect
### Drug/lab test
Increased: LFTs

## NURSING CONSIDERATIONS
### Assessment
• Assess prostatic hyperplasia: change in urinary patterns, baseline and throughout treatment
• Monitor CBC with diff and LFTs; B/P and heart rate
• Monitor BUN, uric acid, urodynamic studies (urinary flow rates, residual volume)
• Assess I&O ratios, weight daily, edema, report weight gain or edema

### Nursing diagnoses
• Urinary elimination, impaired (uses)
• Knowledge deficient (teaching)

## Implementation
• Give with meal at same time of day
• Store at room temperature; protect from light and moisture

### Patient/family education
• Caution patient not to drive or operate machinery until effect is known
• Advise patient not to use with grapefruit juice

### Evaluation
**Positive therapeutic outcome**
• Decreased symptoms of benign prostatic hyperplasia

### RARELY USED

### tetrabenazine (Rx)
Xenazine
*Func. class.:* Monoamine depleter

## Dosage and routes
*Adult:* PO 12.5 mg every morning; after 1 week increase to 12.5 mg bid; may increase by 12.5 mg after each week

**Uses:** Huntington's disease

**Contraindications:** Hypersensitivity, hepatic disease, torsade de pointes, MAOIs

# Notes

# Notes

# Notes

- Does the patient have any allergies?
- Is the patient NPO?
- Is the patient taking any other medication and/or herbal supplements that may interact with this drug?
- Are there any vital signs that I need to check before administering the drug?
- Are there any vital signs that I need to monitor after administering the drug?
- Do I need to check any lab values (i.e., glucose)?
- Are there any other assessments that I need to make before giving this drug?

## The 5 rights of medication administration

Always adhere to the 5 rights of medication administration when transcribing, preparing, administering, and documenting medications:

1. **Right patient:** Compare the patient's armband with the medication administration record. Compare the patient's name on the medication administration record (MAR) with that on the medication drawer or computerized equipment.
2. **Right drug:** Verify the correct medication by comparing the name on the label on the drug container with that written on the MAR.
3. **Right route:** Check the ordered route by reading the medication order, and verify the appropriateness of the route based on knowledge of the patient's condition.
4. **Right dose:** Always independently double-check dosages of medications with the pharmacy's calculations or with a second nurse. The nurse must also be aware of therapeutic dosages for each medication and question an order that is not within that range.
5. **Right time:** All medications should be administered within 30 minutes of the scheduled time. The medications must also be prepared to correlate appropriately with meal times and to avoid drug interactions.

Following appropriate drug administration, assess the patient for the expected therapeutic outcome and/or potential side effects.

## Nomogram for Calculation of Body Surface Area

Place a straight edge from the patient's height in the left column to his or her weight in the right column. The point of intersection on the body surface area column indicates the body surface area (BSA). (Reproduced in Behrman RE, Kliegman RM, Jenson HB: *Nelson Textbook of Pediatrics,* ed 18, Philadelphia, 2007, WB Saunders; nomogram modified from data of E. Boyd by CD West.)

Alternative (Mosteller's formula):

$$\text{Surface area (m}^2) = \sqrt{\frac{\text{Height (cm)} \times \text{Weight (kg)}}{3600}}$$

Surface area rule:

$$\text{Child dose} = \frac{\text{Surface area (m}^2)}{1.73 \text{ m}^2} \times \text{Adult dose}$$

BMI formula:

$$\text{BMI} = \frac{\text{Weight (kg)}}{\text{Height (m}^2)}$$

## Formulas for Drug Calculations

**Surface area rule:**

$$\text{Child dose} = \frac{\text{Surface area (m}^2\text{)}}{1.73 \text{ m}^2} \times \text{Adult dose}$$

**Calculating strength of a solution:**

*Solution Strength:*   *Desired Solution:*

$$\frac{x}{100} = \frac{\text{Amount of drug desired}}{\text{Amount of finished solution}}$$

**Calculating flow rate for IV:**

$$\text{Rate of flow} = \frac{\text{Amount of fluid} \times \text{Administration set calibration}}{\text{Running time}}$$

$$\frac{x}{1} = \frac{\text{(ml) (gtt/min)}}{\text{min}}$$

**Calculating medication dosages:**

**Formula method:**

$$\frac{\text{Amount ordered}}{\text{Amount on hand}} \times \text{Vehicle} = \text{Number of tablets, capsules, or amount of liquid}$$

Vehicle is the drug form or amount of liquid containing the dosage. Amounts used in calculation by formula must be in same system.

**Ratio–proportion method:**

1 tablet:tablet in mg on hand::$x$ tablet order in mg

Know or have::Want to know or order

Multiply means and extremes, divide both sides by known amount to get $x$. Amounts used in equation must be in same system.

**Dimensional analysis method:**

$$\text{Order in mg} \times \frac{1 \text{ tablet or capsule}}{\text{What 1 tablet or capsule is in mg}} = \text{Tablets or capsules to be given}$$

*If amounts are in different systems:*

$$\text{Order in mg} \times \frac{1 \text{ tablet or capsule}}{\text{What 1 tablet or capsule is in g}} \times \frac{1}{1000 \text{ mg}}$$

$$= \text{Tablets or capsules to be given}$$

# IV Drug/Solution Compatibility Chart

| | D$_5$ | D$_{10}$ | D$_5$ ½S | D$_5$ S | NS | R | LR | OTHER |
|---|---|---|---|---|---|---|---|---|
| AcetaZOLAMIDE | C | C | C | C | C | C | C | |
| Acyclovir | C | | | | | | | |
| Alpha$_1$-proteinase inhibitor | | | | | | | | Sterile water for inj |
| Alprostadil | C | C | | | C | | | |
| Alteplase | | | | | | | | Sterile water for inj |
| Amikacin | C | | | | C | | | |
| Aminocaproic acid | | | C | C | C | C | | D in distilled water |
| Ammonium Cl | | | | | C | | | May add KCl to solution |
| Amphotericin B | C | | | | | | | |
| Ampicillin | C | | | | C | | | |
| Antithrombin III | C | | | | C | | | Sterile water for inj |
| Ascorbic acid | C | | | | C | C | C | Sodium lactate |
| Atenolol | C | | | | C | | | 0.45% saline |
| Azlocillin | C | | C | | C | | | |
| Aztreonam | C | C | | | C | C | C | Normosol-R |
| Cefazolin | C | | | | C | | | |
| Cefotetan | C | | | | C | | | |
| Cefoxitin | C | C | | | C | C | C | Aminosol |
| Ceftrazidime | C | | C | C | C | C | C | M/G sodium lactate |
| Ceftriaxone | C | | | | C | | | |
| Cefuroxime | C | | C | C | | C | | M/G sodium lactate |

This chart is not inclusive and is based on manufacturers' recommendations.

**Key**

C   = Compatible
D$_5$  = Dextrose 5%
D$_{10}$ = Dextrose 10%
D$_5$½S = Dextrose 5% in saline 0.45%

D$_5$S = Dextrose 5% in saline 0.9%
NS  = Sodium chloride 0.9% (normal saline)
R   = Ringer's solution
LR  = Lactated Ringer's solution

| | $D_5$ | $D_{10}$ | $D_5$ | | NS | R | LR | OTHER |
| --- | --- | --- | --- | --- | --- | --- | --- | --- |
| | | | ½S | S | | | | |
| Ciprofloxacin | C | | | | C | | | |
| CycloSPORINE | C | | | | C | | | Use only glass containers |
| DOBUTamine | | | | | C | | | Sodium lactate |
| DOPamine | C | | C | C | C | | C | M/G sodium lactate |
| Doxycycline | C | | | | C | | | Invert sugar 10% |
| Edetate Na | C | C | | | | | | Isotonic saline |
| Ganciclovir | C | | | | C | C | C | |
| Gentamicin | C | | | | C | | | Normosol-R |
| Heparin Na | C | C | | | C | C | | |
| Ifosfamide | C | | | | C | | C | Sterile water for inj |
| Inamrinone lactate | | | | | C | | | 0.45% saline |
| Isoproterenol | C | | | C | C | C | | Invert sugar 5% & 10% |
| Kanamycin | C | | | | C | | | |
| Metaraminol | C | | | C | C | C | C | Normosol-R |
| Methicillin | C | | | C | | | | |
| Metoclopramide | C | | | C | | C | C | |
| Mezlocillin | C | C | C | C | C | C | C | Fructose 5% |
| Nitroglycerin | C | C | | | C | | | |
| Norepinephrine | C | C | | C | | | C | |
| Piperacillin | C | | | C | C | | C | |
| Ritodrine | C | | | | | | | |
| Ticarcillin | C | | | | C | | C | |
| Tobramycin | C | | | | C | | | |
| Vidarabine | C | C | | | C | | | |

# Syringe Compatibility

| | Atropine | Buprenorphine | Butorphanol | ChlorproMAZINE | Codeine | Diazepam | DimenhyDRINATE | DiphenhydrAMINE | Droperidol | Fentanyl | Glycopyrrolate | Heparin |
|---|---|---|---|---|---|---|---|---|---|---|---|---|
| Atropine | ■ | | C | C | | I | C | C | C | C | C | |
| Buprenorphine | | ■ | | | | | | | | | | |
| Butorphanol | C | | ■ | C | | I | I | C | C | C | | |
| ChlorproMAZINE | C | | C | ■ | | I | I | C | C | C | C | |
| Codeine | | | | | ■ | I | | | | | | |
| Diazepam | I | | I | I | I | ■ | I | I | I | I | I | |
| DimenhyDRINATE | C | | I | I | | I | ■ | C | C | C | I | |
| DiphenhydrAMINE | C | | C | C | | I | C | ■ | C | C | C | |
| Droperidol | C | | C | C | | I | C | C | ■ | C | C | I |
| Fentanyl | C | | C | C | | I | C | C | C | ■ | C | |
| Glycopyrrolate | C | | | C | | I | I | C | C | C | ■ | |
| Heparin | | | I | C | | I | | | I | | | ■ |
| HydrOXYzine | C | | C | C | | I | I | C | C | C | C | |
| Meperidine | C | | C | C | | I | C | C | C | C | C | I |
| Metoclopramide | C | | C | C | | I | C | C | C | C | | |
| Midazolam | C | | C | C | | I | C | C | C | C | | |
| Morphine | C | | C | C | | I | C | C | C | C | C | I |
| Nalbuphine | C | | | | | I | | | C | | | |
| Pentazocine | C | | C | C | | I | C | C | C | C | I | I |
| Pentobarbital | C | | I | I | I | I | I | I | I | I | I | |
| Perphenazine | C | | C | C | | I | C | C | C | C | | |
| Prochlorperazine | C | | C | C | | I | I | C | C | C | C | |
| Promazine | C | | | C | | I | I | C | C | C | C | |
| Promethazine | C | | C | C | | I | I | C | C | C | C | |
| Ranitidine | C | | | C | | | C | C | | C | C | |
| Scopolamine Hbr | C | | C | C | | I | C | C | C | C | C | |
| Secobarbital | I | | I | I | I | I | I | I | I | I | I | |
| Thiethylperazine | | | C | | | I | | | | | | |

Developed by Providence Memorial Hospital, El Paso, Texas.
NOTE: Give within 15 minutes of mixing.
C = compatible; I = incompatible; □ = no documented information.
* = compatibility depends on manufacturer, Wyeth and DuPont forms are incompatible.